17. **PHARMACOKINETICS** Important parameters described in the FDA-approved labeling, the majority of which are an average or the approximate values provided in the FDA-approved labeling. Only select parameters are included. Refer to the full FDA-approved labeling for more detailed pharmacokinetics information.

18. **ABSORPTION** The process by which the drug enters the bloodstream and becomes bioavailable; may include time to peak plasma concentration (T_{max}), area under the curve (AUC), peak plasma concentration (C_{max}), and absolute bioavailability.

19. **DISTRIBUTION** Parameters related to the dispersion and dissemination of the drug through bodily fluids and tissues; may include plasma protein binding and volume of distribution (V_d).

20. **METABOLISM** Summary of the biotransformation or detoxification of the parent compound into metabolites. Associated enzymes and active metabolites are included if applicable.

21. **ELIMINATION** Parameters associated with the removal of the drug from the body; may include elimination/terminal half-life ($T_{1/2}$) and percentage eliminated through urine or feces.

NURSING CONSIDERATIONS

22. **ASSESSMENT** Specific parameters and laboratory tests that the patient must be assessed for or undergo prior to starting treatment with the drug.

23. **MONITORING** Information used for monitoring patients currently treated with the drug; may include specific lab tests and drug-related or condition-specific information.

24. **PATIENT COUNSELING** Important treatment information to discuss with the patient.

25. **ADMINISTRATION** Guidelines for preparing the drug for administration, rate of administration, proper administration technique, and/or compatibility. For more details on the step-by-step administration process, refer to the full FDA-approved labeling.

26. **STORAGE** Instructions for safe storage and disposal of the drug.

1 Drug monographs contain concise information. Not all fields described here are included in every monograph. For more detailed information, please see the full, FDA-approved labeling information.

2 Abbreviations used within monographs are defined in the *Abbreviations, Acronyms, and Symbols* table on page A1 of the appendix.

---

18 20 19

MECHANISM OF ACTION ... omimetic agent that modulates gastric emptying, prevents postprandial rise in plasma glucagon, and produces satiety, which leads to a decreased caloric intake.

17 → **PHARMACOKINETICS: Absorption:** Absolute bioavailability (30-40%); SQ administration of variable doses resulted in different parameters. **Distribution:** Not extensively bound to blood cells or albumin (40% unbound). **Metabolism:** Kidneys (primarily). Des-lys pramlintide (primary active

21 → metabolite). **Elimination:** $T_{1/2}$=48 min.

NURSING CONSIDERATIONS

22 → **Assessment:** Assess whether patient does or does not have confirmed diagnosis of gastroparesis or hypoglycemia unawareness. Evaluate patient's HbA1c, recent blood glucose monitoring data, history of insulin-induced hypoglycemia, current insulin regimen, and body weight. Assess if patient has failed to achieve proper glycemic control despite individualized insulin management. Assess use in patients with visual or dexterity impairment. Assess for possible drug interactions and pregnancy/nursing status.

23 → **Monitoring:** Monitor for signs/symptoms of hypoglycemia (eg, hunger, headache, sweating, tremor) when using in combination with insulin. Monitor proper glucose control through serum blood glucose levels and HbA1c test.

24 → **Patient Counseling:** Instruct to never mix with insulin and not to transfer from pen injector to syringe. If dose missed, wait until next scheduled dose and administer usual amount. Administer immediately prior to each major meal (≥250 calories or ≥30g of carbohydrates). Insulin dose adjustments should be made only by healthcare professional. Patients should have fast-acting sugar (eg, hard candy, glucose tablet, juice) at all times. Self-glucose monitoring should be done on a daily basis. Counsel about signs/symptoms of hypoglycemia (eg, hunger, headache, sweating, tremor, irritability). Instruct regarding the critical importance of maintaining proper glucose control, especially when operating heavy machinery (eg, motor vehicles).

25 → **Administration:** SQ injection to abdomen or thigh; administration to the arm is not recommended because of variable absorption. Rotate injection sites; injection site should be distinct from site for any concomitant insulin injection. Allow to come to room temperature before injecting.

26 → **Storage:** Pen injectors and vials not in use: 2-8°C (36-40°F). Do not freeze. Do not use if frozen. Pen injectors and vials in use: After 1st use, refrigerate or keep at a temperature <30°C (86°F). Use within 30 days.

PDR® 2015 EDITION
NURSE'S
DRUG HANDBOOK

THE INFORMATION STANDARD FOR PRESCRIPTION DRUGS AND NURSING CONSIDERATIONS

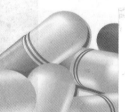
FOREWORD BY
Ivy M. Alexander, PhD, APRN, ANP-BC, FAAN
Clinical Professor, Director of Advanced Practice Programs
University of Connecticut School of Nursing

DATE DUE

NOV 0 8 2018	

BRODART, CO.   Cat. No. 23-221

PDR® NURSE'S DRUG HANDBOOK

2015 EDITION

Associate Vice President of Operations: Jeffrey D. Schaefer
Associate Director, Clinical Operations: Christine Sunwoo, PharmD
Associate Manager, Clinical Content Development: Anila Patel, PharmD
Associate Manager, Clinical Operations: Pauline Lee, PharmD
Senior Drug Information Specialists: Demyana Farag, PharmD; Kristine Mecca, PharmD
Drug Information Specialists: Vanessa De Almeida, PharmD; Autri Sajedeen, PharmD
Managing Clinical Editor: Julia Tonelli, MD
Medical Editor: Christa Mary Kronick, MA
Lead Project Manager: Gary Lew
Manager, Art Department: Livio Udina
Director, Manufacturing and Distribution: Thomas Westburgh

PDR NETWORK, LLC

Executive Chairman: Edward Fotsch, MD
President and Chief Executive Officer: Richard C. Altus
Chief Medical Officer: Salvatore Volpe, MD, FAAP, FACP, CHCQM
Executive Vice President and Chief Financial Officer: Gary Lubin
Chief Technology Officer: David Cheng
Senior Vice President, Corporate Development, and General Counsel: Andrew Gelman
Associate Vice President, Sales: Dennis McCormack
Senior Vice President, Marketing and Business Line Management: Barbara Senich, BSN, MBA, MPH

ISBN: 978-1-56363-828-2

Printed in Canada

DISCARD

CONTENTS

FOREWORD

The role of nursing professionals in safe medication administration and patient education has never been more crucial—especially as our national healthcare system responds to the expanded coverage provided by the Affordable Care Act.[1] The 2011 Institute of Medicine Report on the future of nursing[2] notes that nurses are being called on to practice at the fullest extent of their practice scope. Nurses are central to the goal of ensuring the highest quality healthcare while reducing costs. To accomplish this in the arena of pharmacotherapy and medication administration, nurses must decipher constantly changing information regarding medications, new therapies, and interactions, and rapidly assess patient responses to multiple variables that are important to medication administration. As such, it is vital for each nurse to have a reference that provides accurate and easily accessible drug information. The 2015 *PDR® Nurse's Drug Handbook* is this reference.

Physicians' Desk Reference® is a well-known and trusted resource for medication information—and the 2015 *PDR Nurse's Drug Handbook* follows this tradition. This important reference is specifically designed for nurses, with each entry providing the following, when applicable: therapeutic class, brand and generic names, indications, dosage, how the medication is supplied, contraindications, relevant warnings and precautions, key adverse reactions, interactions, pregnancy category, mechanism of action, pharmacokinetics, and nursing considerations—a special section that features content specific to assessing, monitoring, and counseling patients, as well as administering medications.

The 2015 *PDR Nurse's Drug Handbook* is organized to foster quick identification of key drug information; medications are identified by generic and brand names, as well as therapeutic class. Special sections provide important considerations to use when caring for children, older adults, and pregnant or breastfeeding patients. Other unique resources include: a multitude of tables on topics like medications for specific chronic problems such as hypertension, cholesterol, migraine, HIV, and diabetes; immunizations; poison antidotes; sugar-free products; drugs that should not be used in pregnancy; and a full-color visual identification guide. In the 2015 edition, there are multiple new tables covering important topics such as comparisons of antiviral treatments; indication-based approach for use of oral and systemic antibiotics; treatment options for angina, heart failure, pulmonary arterial hypertension, and mental health; and listings of easily confused drug names, and error-prone abbreviations, symbols, and dose designations (from ISMP). The 2015 edition also boasts tables providing detailed information about the most commonly used herbal products, cough-cold-allergy agents, obesity guidelines specific to adults and children, a listing of FDA newly approved drug products for 2013–2014, products for which the FDA has approved Risk Evaluation and Management Strategies (REMS), and treatment recommendations and algorithm for tuberculosis.

The 2015 *PDR Nurse's Drug Handbook* is an essential reference for enhancing full-scope nursing practice and patient education efforts. Its convenient size and clear layout provide fast access to concise, authoritative drug information, making this book a trusted resource among nurses.

Ivy M. Alexander, PhD, APRN, ANP-BC, FAAN
Clinical Professor
Director of Advanced Practice Programs
University of Connecticut School of Nursing

1. Affordable Care Act, available at: http://www.healthcare.gov/law/full/index.html.

2. Committee on the Robert Wood Johnson Foundation Initiative on the Future of Nursing, at the Institute of Medicine. (2011). The Future of Nursing: Leading Change, Advancing Health. The National Academies Press; Washington, DC. Available at: http://www.nap.edu/catalog.php?record_id=12956.

Concise Drug Monographs

ABELCET
amphotericin B lipid complex (Sigma-Tau)

RX

THERAPEUTIC CLASS: Polyene antifungal

INDICATIONS: Treatment of invasive fungal infections in patients refractory to or intolerant of conventional amphotericin B therapy.

DOSAGE: *Adults:* 5mg/kg given as a single IV infusion at 2.5mg/kg/hr.
Pediatrics: 5mg/kg given as a single IV infusion at 2.5mg/kg/hr.

HOW SUPPLIED: Inj: 5mg/mL

WARNINGS/PRECAUTIONS: Anaphylaxis reported; d/c infusion and do not give further infusions if severe respiratory distress occurs. Administer initial dose under close clinical observation. Acute reactions, including fever and chills, may occur 1-2 hrs after starting IV. Frequently monitor SrCr during therapy. Regularly monitor LFTs, serum electrolytes (particularly Mg^{2+} and K^+) and CBC.

ADVERSE REACTIONS: Chills, fever, increased SrCr, multiple organ failure, N/V, hypotension, respiratory failure, dyspnea, sepsis, diarrhea, headache, heart arrest, HTN, hypokalemia.

INTERACTIONS: Caution with antineoplastic agents; may enhance potential for renal toxicity, bronchospasm, and hypotension. Corticosteroids and corticotropin may potentiate hypokalemia. Initiation with cyclosporine A within several days of bone marrow ablation may be associated with increased nephrotoxicity. May induce hypokalemia and potentiate digitalis toxicity with digitalis glycosides. May increase flucytosine toxicity; use with caution. Antagonism with imidazole derivatives (eg, miconazole, ketoconazole) reported. Acute pulmonary toxicity reported with leukocyte transfusions; avoid concurrent use. Caution with nephrotoxic agents (eg, aminoglycosides, pentamidine); may enhance the potential for drug-induced renal toxicity. Amphotericin B-induced hypokalemia may enhance curariform effect of skeletal muscle relaxants (eg, tubocurarine) due to hypokalemia. Monitor renal and hematologic function with zidovudine.

PREGNANCY: Category B, not for use in nursing.

MECHANISM OF ACTION: Polyene antifungal; binds to sterols in the cell membrane of susceptible fungi, with a resultant change in membrane permeability.

PHARMACOKINETICS: Absorption: C_{max} =1.7µg/mL; AUC=14µg•hr/mL. **Distribution:** V_d=131L/kg. **Elimination:** Urine (0.9%); $T_{1/2}$=173.4 hrs.

NURSING CONSIDERATIONS

Assessment: Assess for previous hypersensitivity to the drug, pregnancy/nursing status, and possible drug interactions.

Monitoring: Monitor clinical condition, and cardiac/renal function. Monitor for anaphylaxis, severe respiratory distress, and acute reactions. Frequently monitor SrCr. Regularly monitor LFTs, serum electrolytes (particularly Mg^{2+} and K^+), and CBC.

Patient Counseling: Inform of risks and benefits of therapy. Advise to seek medical attention if any adverse reactions occur.

Administration: IV route. Shake the infusion bag q2h if the infusion time exceeds 2 hrs. Refer to PI for preparation of admixture for infusion. Do not dilute with saline sol or mix with other drugs or electrolytes. Do not use an in-line filter. **Storage:** 2-8°C (36-46°F). Protect from light. Do not freeze. Diluted Ready-For-Use Admixture: Stable for up to 48 hrs at 2-8°C (36-46°F) and an additional 6 hrs at room temperature. Do not freeze.

ABILIFY
aripiprazole (Bristol-Myers Squibb/Otsuka America)

RX

> Elderly patients with dementia-related psychosis treated with antipsychotic drugs are at an increased risk of death; most deaths appeared to be either cardiovascular (CV) (eg, heart failure [HF], sudden death) or infectious (eg, pneumonia) in nature. Not approved for treatment of patients with dementia-related psychosis. Antidepressants increased risk of suicidal thinking and behavior (suicidality) in children, adolescents, and young adults in short-term studies of major depressive disorder (MDD) and other psychiatric disorders. Monitor and observe closely for clinical worsening, suicidality, or unusual changes in behavior in patients who are started on antidepressant therapy. Not approved for use in pediatric patients with depression.

OTHER BRAND NAMES: Abilify Discmelt (Bristol-Myers Squibb/Otsuka America)

THERAPEUTIC CLASS: Partial $D_2/5HT_{1A}$ agonist/$5HT_{2A}$ antagonist

INDICATIONS: (PO) Treatment of schizophrenia in adults and adolescents (13-17 yrs of age). Acute treatment of manic and mixed episodes associated with bipolar I disorder, as monotherapy in adults and pediatric patients (10-17 yrs of age) and as an adjunct to lithium or valproate in adults. Maintenance treatment of bipolar I disorder, both as monotherapy and adjunct to either

1

lithium or valproate, in adults. Adjunctive therapy to antidepressants for treatment of MDD in adults. Treatment of irritability associated with autistic disorder in pediatric patients (6-17 yrs of age). (Inj) Acute treatment of agitation associated with schizophrenia or bipolar disorder, manic or mixed, in adults.

DOSAGE: *Adults;* Schizophrenia: Initial/Target: 10mg or 15mg qd. Titrate: Should not increase dose before 2 weeks. Usual: 10-30mg/day. Bipolar I Disorder: Initial: (Monotherapy) 15mg qd. (Adjunct) 10-15mg qd. Target: 15mg qd. Titrate: May increase to 30mg/day based on clinical response. Max: 30mg/day. MDD Adjunct: Initial: 2-5mg/day. Titrate: Dose adjustments of up to 5mg/day should occur gradually at intervals of no <1 week. Usual: 2-15mg/day. Reassess periodically to determine the need for maintenance treatment in all indications. Oral sol can be substituted for tabs on a mg-per-mg basis up to 25mg. Patients receiving 30mg tabs should receive 25mg of oral sol. (Inj) Agitation Associated with Schizophrenia or Bipolar Mania: 9.75mg IM. Usual: 5.25-15mg. A lower dose of 5.25mg may be considered when clinical factors warrant. If agitation warranting a 2nd dose persists following the initial dose, cumulative doses of up to a total of 30mg/day may be given. Max: 30mg/day. Not more frequent than q2h. If clinically indicated, may replace with PO at 10-30mg/day. Refer to PI for dose adjustments when used concomitantly with CYP3A4 inhibitors, CYP2D6 inhibitors, CYP3A4 inducers, and in CYP2D6 poor metabolizers.
Pediatrics: Schizophrenia (13-17 Yrs)/Bipolar I Disorder (Monotherapy or Adjunct) (10-17 Yrs): Initial: 2mg/day. Titrate: May increase to 5mg/day after 2 days and to the target dose of 10mg/day after 2 additional days. Subsequent dose increases, if needed, should be administered in 5mg increments. Max: 30mg/day. Irritability Associated with Autistic Disorder (6-17 Yrs): Individualize dose. Initial: 2mg/day. Titrate: Increase to 5mg/day. May increase to 10mg or 15mg/day if needed. Dose adjustments of up to 5mg/day should occur gradually at intervals of no <1 week. Usual: 5-15mg/day. Reassess periodically to determine the need for maintenance treatment in all indications. Oral sol can be substituted for tabs on a mg-per-mg basis up to the 25mg dose level. Patients receiving 30mg tabs should receive 25mg of the sol. Refer to PI for dose adjustments when used concomitantly with CYP3A4 inhibitors, CYP2D6 inhibitors, CYP3A4 inducers, and in CYP2D6 poor metabolizers.

HOW SUPPLIED: Inj: 7.5mg/mL [1.3mL]; Sol: 1mg/mL [150mL]; Tab: 2mg, 5mg, 10mg, 15mg, 20mg, 30mg; Tab, Disintegrating: (Discmelt) 10mg, 15mg

WARNINGS/PRECAUTIONS: Initiate in pediatric patients only after a thorough diagnostic evaluation has been conducted and careful consideration given to the risks associated with therapy. Neuroleptic malignant syndrome (NMS) reported; d/c immediately, institute symptomatic treatment and monitor. May cause tardive dyskinesia (TD), especially in the elderly; d/c if this occurs. Hyperglycemia, in some cases extreme and associated with ketoacidosis or hyperosmolar coma or death, reported; monitor glucose control regularly in patients with diabetes mellitus (DM) and FPG in patients at risk for DM. Dyslipidemia and weight gain reported. May cause orthostatic hypotension; caution with known CV disease (history of myocardial infarction or ischemic heart disease, HF or conduction abnormalities), cerebrovascular disease, or conditions that would predispose patients to hypotension. Leukopenia, neutropenia, and agranulocytosis reported; monitor CBC frequently during 1st few months in patients with history of clinically significant low WBC counts or drug-induced leukopenia/neutropenia. D/C at 1st sign of a clinically significant decline in WBC counts in the absence of other causative factors. D/C therapy and follow WBC counts until recovery in patients with severe neutropenia (absolute neutrophil counts <1000/mm³). Seizures reported; caution with history of seizures or with conditions that lower seizure threshold (eg, Alzheimer's dementia). May impair physical/mental abilities. May disrupt body's ability to reduce core body temperature; caution when exposed to conditions that may contribute to an elevation in core body temperature (eg, exercising strenuously, exposure to extreme heat, receiving concomitant medication with anticholinergic activity, or being subject to dehydration). May cause esophageal dysmotility and aspiration; caution in patients at risk for aspiration pneumonia.

ADVERSE REACTIONS: Headache, fatigue, tremor, anxiety, insomnia, increased appetite, N/V, somnolence, constipation, akathisia, extrapyramidal disorder, nasopharyngitis, dizziness, restlessness, weight increase.

INTERACTIONS: Caution with other centrally acting drugs. Avoid with alcohol. May potentiate the effect of certain antihypertensive agents. CYP3A4 inducers (eg, carbamazepine) may increase clearance and lower blood levels. CYP3A4 inhibitors (eg, ketoconazole, itraconazole) or CYP2D6 inhibitors (eg, quinidine, fluoxetine, paroxetine) may inhibit elimination and increase blood levels. (Inj) Greater intensity of sedation and greater orthostatic hypotension with lorazepam inj; monitor for excessive sedation and for orthostatic hypotension with parenteral benzodiazepines.

PREGNANCY: Category C, not for use in nursing.

MECHANISM OF ACTION: Partial D_2/$5HT_{1A}$ agonist/$5HT_{2A}$ antagonist; not established.

PHARMACOKINETICS: Absorption: Well-absorbed. Absolute bioavailability (87%, tab), (100%, IM); T_{max}=3-5 hrs (Tab), 1-3 hrs (IM, median). **Distribution:** V_d=404L (IV); plasma protein binding (>99%, albumin); found in breast milk. **Metabolism:** Hepatic via dehydrogenation, hydroxylation (CYP2D6 and CYP3A4), and N-dealkylation (CYP3A4). Dehydro-aripiprazole (active metabolite).

Elimination: (PO) Urine (25%, <1% unchanged), feces (55%, 18% unchanged); T$_{1/2}$=75 hrs (extensive metabolizers), 146 hrs (poor metabolizers).

NURSING CONSIDERATIONS

Assessment: Assess for dementia-related psychosis, drug hypersensitivity, psychiatric disorders or any other conditions where treatment is cautioned, pregnancy/nursing status, and possible drug interactions. Obtain baseline FPG in patients with DM or at risk for DM. Obtain baseline CBC if at risk for leukopenia/neutropenia.

Monitoring: Monitor for clinical worsening of depression, suicidality, unusual changes in behavior, NMS, TD, hyperglycemia, orthostatic hypotension, seizures/convulsions, esophageal dysmotility, aspiration, and other adverse effects. Monitor CBC frequently in patients with preexisting low WBC counts or drug-induced leukopenia/neutropenia. Monitor for fever or other signs/symptoms of infection in patients with neutropenia. Monitor weight regularly and FPG in patients with DM or at risk for DM periodically during therapy. Periodically reassess to determine the continued need for maintenance treatment.

Patient Counseling: Inform about the risks and benefits of treatment. Instruct patients, families, and caregivers to be alert to the emergence of anxiety, agitation, panic attacks, insomnia, irritability, hostility, aggressiveness, impulsivity, akathisia, hypomania, mania, other unusual changes in behavior, worsening of depression, and suicidal ideation; advise to contact physician if these symptoms occur. Instruct to use caution when operating hazardous machinery and to avoid alcohol use while on therapy. Counsel to avoid overheating and dehydration. Advise to notify physician if patient becomes pregnant or intends to become pregnant during therapy, and if patient is taking or plans to take any prescription or OTC drugs. Instruct to not breastfeed during therapy. (Discmelt) Inform phenylketonurics that product contains phenylalanine. Instruct to not open blister until ready to administer. Instruct that drug is to be taken without liquid. However, if needed, drug can be taken with liquid. Advise not to split the tab. (Sol) Inform that sol contains sucrose and fructose.

Administration: Oral/IM route. (Inj) Refer to PI for administration instructions. (PO) Administer without regard to meals. **Storage:** 25°C (77°F); excursions permitted to 15-30°C (59-86°F). Oral Sol: May be used for ≤6 months after opening. Inj: Store in original container; protect from light.

ABILIFY MAINTENA   RX
aripiprazole (Otsuka America)

> Elderly patients with dementia-related psychosis treated with antipsychotic drugs are at an increased risk of death. Not approved for the treatment of patients with dementia-related psychosis.

THERAPEUTIC CLASS: Partial D$_2$/5HT$_{1A}$ agonist/5HT$_{2A}$ antagonist

INDICATIONS: Treatment of schizophrenia.

DOSAGE: *Adults:* Establish tolerability with PO aripiprazole prior to initiating treatment in naive patients. Initial/Maint: 400mg monthly (no sooner than 26 days after the previous inj). After the 1st inj, continue treatment with PO aripiprazole (10-20mg) or other oral antipsychotic for 14 consecutive days. If adverse reactions occur with the 400mg dose, consider reducing dose to 300mg once monthly. Refer to PI for dosage adjustments, missed doses, patients who are CYP2D6 poor metabolizers, and with concomitant use of CYP2D6 inhibitors, CYP3A4 inhibitors, or CYP3A4 inducers.

HOW SUPPLIED: Inj, Extended-Release: 300mg, 400mg

WARNINGS/PRECAUTIONS: Do not substitute with other aripiprazole inj. Neuroleptic malignant syndrome (NMS) reported; d/c immediately and institute symptomatic treatment. May cause tardive dyskinesia (TD), especially in the elderly; d/c if this occurs. Hyperglycemia, in some cases extreme and associated with ketoacidosis or hyperosmolar coma or death, reported; monitor glucose control regularly in patients with diabetes mellitus (DM) and FPG in patients at risk for DM. Dyslipidemia and weight gain reported. May cause orthostatic hypotension. Leukopenia, neutropenia, and agranulocytosis reported; monitor CBC frequently during 1st few months in patients with history of clinically significant low WBC counts or drug-induced leukopenia/neutropenia, and d/c at 1st sign of decline in WBC counts without causative factors. D/C therapy and follow WBC counts until recovery in patients with severe neutropenia (absolute neutrophil counts <1000/mm^3). Caution with history of seizures or with conditions that lower seizure threshold. May impair mental/physical abilities. May disrupt body's ability to reduce core body temperature. May cause esophageal dysmotility and aspiration; caution in patients at risk for aspiration pneumonia.

ADVERSE REACTIONS: Inj-site reactions (eg, pain, swelling, redness, induration), akathisia, headache, agitation, insomnia, anxiety, N/V, constipation, dizziness, fatigue, extrapyramidal disorder, tremor, somnolence, restlessness.

ABRAXANE

INTERACTIONS: Avoid use with carbamazepine or other CYP3A4 inducers for >14 days. Concomitant use with ketoconazole, other strong CYP3A4 inhibitors (eg, itraconazole), quinidine, or other strong CYP2D6 inhibitors (eg, fluoxetine, paroxetine) for more than 14 days may increase levels; reduce dose. Caution with other centrally acting drugs or alcohol. May enhance effect of certain antihypertensives. Caution with anticholinergics.

PREGNANCY: Category C, not for use in nursing.

MECHANISM OF ACTION: Partial D_2/$5HT_{1A}$ agonist/$5HT_{2A}$ antagonist; not established.

PHARMACOKINETICS: Absorption: Slow and prolonged. T_{max}=5-7 days. **Distribution:** Found in breast milk. **Metabolism:** Hepatic via CYP2D6 and CYP3A4; dehydro-aripiprazole (major metabolite). **Elimination:** $T_{1/2}$=29.9 days (300mg), 46.5 days (400mg).

NURSING CONSIDERATIONS

Assessment: Assess for history of dementia-related psychosis, DM, drug hypersensitivity, any other conditions where treatment is cautioned, pregnancy/nursing status, and possible drug interactions. Obtain baseline FPG in patients with DM or at risk for DM. Obtain baseline CBC if at risk for leukopenia/neutropenia.

Monitoring: Monitor for NMS, TD, hyperglycemia, orthostatic hypotension, seizures, weight gain, dyslipidemia, esophageal dysmotility, aspiration, and other adverse effects. Monitor CBC frequently in patients with preexisting low WBC counts or history of drug-induced leukopenia/neutropenia. Monitor for fever or other symptoms/signs of infection in patients with neutropenia. Monitor FPG in patients with DM or at risk for DM.

Patient Counseling: Inform of the risks/benefits of therapy. Counsel about signs/symptoms of NMS (eg, hyperpyrexia, muscle rigidity, altered mental status, evidence of autonomic instability), hyperglycemia, and DM. Instruct to notify physician if any movements that cannot be controlled in the face, tongue, or other body part develop. Advise to use caution when operating hazardous machinery. Inform to avoid alcohol use while on therapy. Counsel to avoid overheating and dehydration. Instruct to notify physician if pregnant/intending to become pregnant or breastfeeding, and if taking/planning to take any prescription or OTC drugs.

Administration: IM route. Administer by deep IM inj into the gluteal muscle; do not administer by any other route. Inject immediately after reconstitution. Rotate inj sites between the two gluteal muscles. Refer to PI for preparation, reconstitution, and administration instructions. **Storage:** 25°C (77°F); excursions permitted to 15-30°C (59-86°F).

ABRAXANE   RX
paclitaxel protein-bound (Abraxis)

Do not administer to patients who have baseline neutrophil counts of <1500 cells/mm³. Perform frequent peripheral blood cell counts to monitor occurrence of bone marrow suppression, primarily neutropenia. Do not substitute for or with other paclitaxel formulations.

THERAPEUTIC CLASS: Antimicrotubule agent

INDICATIONS: Treatment of breast cancer after failure of combination chemotherapy for metastatic disease or relapse within 6 months of adjuvant chemotherapy. Prior therapy should have included an anthracycline unless clinically contraindicated. First-line treatment of locally advanced or metastatic non-small cell lung cancer (NSCLC), in combination with carboplatin, in patients who are not candidates for curative surgery or radiation therapy. First-line treatment of metastatic adenocarcinoma of the pancreas, in combination with gemcitabine.

DOSAGE: *Adults:* Metastatic Breast Cancer (MBC): 260mg/m² IV over 30 min every 3 weeks. Moderate Hepatic Impairment (AST <10X ULN and Bilirubin 1.26-2X ULN): Initial: 200mg/m² for the 1st course of therapy. Titrate: May adjust dose in subsequent courses based on tolerance. Severe Hepatic Impairment (AST <10X ULN and Bilirubin 2.01-5X ULN): Initial: 130mg/m² for the 1st course of therapy. Titrate: May increase up to 200mg/m² in subsequent courses based on tolerance. Withhold if AST >10X ULN or bilirubin >5X ULN. NSCLC: 100mg/m² IV infusion over 30 min on Days 1, 8, and 15 of each 21-day cycle. Give carboplatin on Day 1 of each 21-day cycle immediately after paclitaxel. Moderate Hepatic Impairment (AST <10X ULN and Bilirubin 1.26-2X ULN): Initial: 75mg/m² for the 1st course of therapy. Titrate: May adjust dose in subsequent courses based on tolerance. Severe Hepatic Impairment (AST <10X ULN and Bilirubin 2.01-5X ULN): Initial: 50mg/m² for the 1st course of therapy. Titrate: May increase to 75mg/m² in subsequent courses, as tolerated. Withhold if AST >10X ULN or bilirubin >5X ULN. Adenocarcinoma of the Pancreas: 125mg/m² IV infusion over 30-40 min on Days 1, 8, and 15 of each 28-day cycle. Give gemcitabine immediately after paclitaxel on Days 1, 8, and 15 of each 28-day cycle. Moderate Hepatic Impairment (AST <10X ULN and Bilirubin 1.26-2X ULN)/Severe Hepatic Impairment (AST <10X ULN and Bilirubin 2.01-5X ULN)/AST >10X ULN or Bilirubin >5X ULN: Not recommended. Refer to PI for dose reduction/discontinuation recommendations.

HOW SUPPLIED: Inj: 100mg

CONTRAINDICATIONS: Patients with baseline neutrophil counts of <1500 cells/mm³.

WARNINGS/PRECAUTIONS: Bone marrow suppression (primarily neutropenia) is dose-dependent and a dose-limiting toxicity. Frequently monitor CBC (including neutrophil counts); perform prior to dosing on Day 1 (for MBC) and Days 1, 8, and 15 (for NSCLC and pancreatic cancer). Resume treatment with every-3-week cycles after absolute neutrophil count (ANC) recovers to >1500 cells/mm³ and platelets recover to >100,000 cells/mm³ in MBC patients. Sensory neuropathy is dose- and schedule-dependent. Sepsis reported; initiate treatment with broad-spectrum antibiotics if patient becomes febrile (regardless of ANC). Pneumonitis reported; interrupt treatment and gemcitabine during evaluation of suspected pneumonitis. After ruling out infectious etiology and upon making a diagnosis of pneumonitis, permanently d/c combination therapy. Severe and sometimes fatal hypersensitivity reactions, including anaphylactic reactions, reported. Caution with hepatic impairment. Contains human albumin; may carry a remote risk for transmission of viral diseases. May cause fetal harm. Men should be advised not to father a child while receiving treatment.

ADVERSE REACTIONS: Alopecia, neutropenia, thrombocytopenia, sensory/peripheral neuropathy, abnormal ECG, fatigue/asthenia, myalgia/arthralgia, AST elevation, alkaline phosphatase elevation, anemia, nausea, infections, diarrhea.

INTERACTIONS: Caution with medicines known to inhibit (eg, ketoconazole and other imidazole antifungals, erythromycin, fluoxetine, gemfibrozil, cimetidine, ritonavir, saquinavir, indinavir, nelfinavir) or induce (eg, rifampicin, carbamazepine, phenytoin, efavirenz, nevirapine) either CYP2C8 or CYP3A4.

PREGNANCY: Category D, not for use in nursing.

MECHANISM OF ACTION: Antimicrotubule agent; promotes assembly of microtubules from tubulin dimers and stabilizes microtubules by preventing depolymerization. This stability results in inhibition of the normal dynamic reorganization of the microtubule network that is essential for vital interphase and mitotic cellular functions.

PHARMACOKINETICS: Absorption: C_{max}=18,741ng/mL. **Distribution:** V_d=632L/m²; plasma protein binding (89-98%). **Metabolism:** Liver via CYP2C8 to 6α-hydroxypaclitaxel (major metabolite), and CYP3A4. **Elimination:** Urine (4% unchanged, <1% metabolites), feces (20%); $T_{1/2}$=27 hrs.

NURSING CONSIDERATIONS

Assessment: Assess for previous hypersensitivity reactions to drug, pregnancy/nursing status, and possible drug interactions. Obtain baseline CBC, including neutrophil counts, and LFTs.

Monitoring: Monitor for bone marrow suppression, neutropenia, sensory neuropathy, sepsis, pneumonitis, hypersensitivity reactions, and other adverse reactions. Frequently monitor CBC (including neutrophil counts); perform prior to dosing on Day 1 (for MBC) and Days 1, 8, and 15 (for NSCLC and pancreatic cancer).

Patient Counseling: Inform that drug may cause fetal harm; advise women of childbearing potential to avoid becoming pregnant. Advise men not to father a child while on therapy. Inform of the risk of low blood cell counts and severe and life-threatening infections; instruct to contact physician immediately for fever or evidence of infection. Advise to contact physician for persistent vomiting, diarrhea, or signs of dehydration. Inform that sensory neuropathy occurs frequently and to report to physician any numbness, tingling, pain, or weakness involving the extremities. Inform that alopecia, fatigue/asthenia, and myalgia/arthralgia occur frequently with therapy. Instruct to contact physician for signs of an allergic reaction and for sudden onset of dry persistent cough, or SOB.

Administration: IV route. Refer to PI for preparation and administration precautions and instructions. **Storage:** 20-25°C (68-77°F). Retain in original packaging to protect from bright light. Reconstituted Sus in Vial: Use immediately or refrigerate at 2-8°C (36-46°F) for a max of 8 hrs if necessary and store in original carton to protect from bright light. Reconstituted Sus in Infusion Bag: Use immediately or store at ambient temperature (approximately 25°C [77°F]) and lighting conditions for up to 4 hrs.

ABSORICA RX
isotretinoin (Ranbaxy)

Not for use by females who are or may become pregnant. Severe birth defects (eg, internal/external abnormalities) may result if pregnancy occurs while on therapy. Some cases of death reported with certain abnormalities. Increased risk of spontaneous abortion and premature births reported; IQ scores <85 with or without other abnormalities reported. D/C immediately and refer to an Obstetrician-Gynecologist if pregnancy occurs during treatment. Available only through a restricted program under Risk Evaluation and Mitigation Strategy (REMS) called iPLEDGE. Prescribers, patients, pharmacies, and distributors must enroll and register in the program.

THERAPEUTIC CLASS: Retinoid

INDICATIONS: Treatment of severe recalcitrant nodular acne in patients ≥12 yrs and female patients who are not pregnant. Reserve for patients with multiple severe nodular acne who are unresponsive to conventional therapy, including systemic antibiotics.

DOSAGE: *Adults:* Usual: 0.5-1mg/kg/day given in 2 divided doses for 15-20 weeks. Refer to PI for dosing by body weight. Titrate: May adjust dose according to response of disease and/or appearance of clinical side effects. Very Severe Disease With Scarring or Primarily Manifested on Trunk: May adjust dose up to 2mg/kg/day, as tolerated. D/C if total nodule count has been reduced by >70% prior to completing 15-20 weeks. Initiate 2nd course of treatment with persistent or recurring severe nodular acne after a period of 2 months or more without therapy.
Pediatrics: ≥12 yrs: Usual: 0.5-1mg/kg/day given in 2 divided doses for 15-20 weeks. Refer to PI for dosing by body weight. Titrate: May adjust dose according to response of disease and/or appearance of clinical side effects. Very Severe Disease With Scarring or Primarily Manifested on Trunk: May adjust dose up to 2mg/kg/day, as tolerated. D/C if total nodule count has been reduced by >70% prior to completing 15-20 weeks. Initiate 2nd course of treatment with persistent or recurring severe nodular acne after a period of 2 months or more without therapy.

HOW SUPPLIED: Cap: 10mg, 20mg, 30mg, 40mg

CONTRAINDICATIONS: Pregnancy, vitamin A hypersensitivity.

WARNINGS/PRECAUTIONS: Avoid long-term use. Blood donation during therapy and for 1 month following d/c should be avoided. Micro-dosed progesterone preparations are an inadequate method of contraception during therapy. Do not initiate 2nd course of therapy until at least 8 weeks after completion of 1st course. Optimal interval before retreatment has not been defined in patients who have not completed skeletal growth. Acute pancreatitis, impaired hearing, inflammatory bowel disease, elevated TG and LFTs, decreased HDL, hepatotoxicity, premature epiphyseal closure, and hyperostosis reported. May cause depression, psychosis, aggressive and/or violent behaviors, suicidal ideation/attempts, and suicide. May cause dry eye, decreased night vision, and corneal opacities; may experience decreased tolerance to contact lenses during and after therapy. Associated with pseudotumor cerebri. Check lipid levels before therapy, and then at intervals until response is established (within 4 weeks). D/C if hearing or visual impairment, abdominal pain, rectal bleeding, or severe diarrhea occurs. May develop musculoskeletal symptoms. Caution with history of childhood osteoporosis, osteomalacia, other bone metabolism disorders or anorexia nervosa. Spontaneous osteoporosis, osteopenia, bone fractures, and delayed fracture healing reported; caution in sports with repetitive impact. Skeletal hyperostosis, calcification of ligaments and tendons, premature epiphyseal closure, and bone age changes reported. Erythema mutiforme, anaphylactic reactions, and other allergic reactions reported; d/c and institute appropriate therapy if severe allergic reactions occur. Rhabdomyolysis and elevated CPK reported. New cases of diabetes reported.

ADVERSE REACTIONS: Allergic reactions, vascular thrombotic disease, stroke, decreased appetite, weight fluctuation, lip dry, nausea, anemia, thrombocytopenia, infections, infestations.

INTERACTIONS: Avoid use with tetracyclines or vitamin supplements containing Vitamin A. Caution with phenytoin and systemic corticosteroids.

PREGNANCY: Category X, not for use in nursing.

MECHANISM OF ACTION: Retinoid; not established. Suspected to inhibit sebaceous gland function and keratinization.

PHARMACOKINETICS: Absorption: AUC=6095ng•hr/mL (fed), 4055ng•hr/mL (fasted); C_{max}= 395ng/mL (fed), 314ng/mL (fasted); T_{max}=6.4 hr (fed), 2.9 hr (fasted). **Distribution:** Plasma protein binding (>99%). **Metabolism:** Liver via CYP2C8, 2C9, 3A4, and 2B6; 4-oxo-isotretinoin, retinoic acid, and 4-oxo-retinoic acid (active metabolites). **Elimination:** Feces and urine (65%-83%); $T_{1/2}$=18 hrs (isotretinoin), 38 hrs (4-oxo-isotretinoin).

NURSING CONSIDERATIONS

Assessment: Assess that females have had 2 negative pregnancy tests separated by at least 19 days, and are on 2 forms of effective contraception: a primary form (eg, tubal sterilization, partner's vasectomy, intrauterine device, or hormonal) and a secondary form (barrier, vaginal sponge) for at least 1 month prior to administration. Assess for vitamin A or drug hypersensitivity, history of psychiatric disorder, depression, risk of hyperlipidemia (eg, diabetes mellitus, obesity, increased alcohol intake, history of or known lipid metabolism disorder), nursing/pregnancy status, and possible drug interactions. Obtain lipid profile and LFTs.

Monitoring: Monitor for signs/symptoms of psychiatric disorders, pseudotumor cerebri, lipid abnormalities, acute pancreatitis, hearing impairment, hepatotoxicity, inflammatory bowel disease (regional ileitis), decreased bone mineral density, hyperostosis, premature epiphyseal closure, musculoskeletal symptoms, hypersensitivity reactions, visual impairments, corneal opacities, and decreased night vision. Monitor lipid levels and LFTs (weekly or biweekly), glucose levels, and CPK levels until response is established. Monitor that females remain on 2 forms of contraception during and for 1 month following d/c of therapy.

Patient Counseling: Instruct to read the Medication Guide/iPledge and sign the Patient Information/Informed Consent form. Inform male and female patients, not of childbearing potential, the risks and benefits of the drug. Inform females of childbearing potential that 2 forms of contraception are required starting 1 month prior to initiation, during treatment, and for 1 month following d/c. Inform that monthly pregnancy tests are required before new prescription is issued. Counsel not to share drug with anyone and not to donate blood during therapy and 1 month following d/c. Instruct to swallow cap with full glass of liquid. Inform that transient flare of acne may occur. Notify physician if depression, mood disturbances, psychosis, or aggression occurs. Instruct to avoid wax epilation and skin resurfacing procedures during and for at least 6 months thereafter. Instruct to avoid prolonged UV rays or sunlight exposure. Inform that decreased tolerance to contact lenses during and after therapy may occur. Inform that musculoskeletal symptoms, transient chest pain, back pain in pediatrics, arthralgias, neutropenia, agranulocytosis, severe skin reactions, inflammatory bowel disease, and rhabdomyolysis may occur. Instruct to d/c the drug and notify physician if abdominal pain, rectal bleeding, or severe diarrhea occurs. Inform that increased risk of spondylolisthesis or hip growth plate injuries, fractures, and/or delayed healing may occur.

Administration: Oral route. **Storage:** 20-25°C (68-77°F); excursions permitted to 15-30°C (59-86°F). Protect from light.

ABSTRAL

CII

fentanyl (Galena Biopharma)

Fatal respiratory depression may occur. Contraindicated in the management of acute or postoperative pain (eg, headache/migraine) and in opioid-nontolerant patients. Keep out of reach of children. Concomitant use with CYP3A4 inhibitors may increase plasma levels, and may cause fatal respiratory depression. Do not convert patients on a mcg-per-mcg basis from any other fentanyl products to Abstral or substitute for any fentanyl products; may result in fatal overdose. Contains fentanyl with abuse liability similar to other opioid analgesics. Available only through a restricted program called TIRF REMS Access program (Transmucosal Immediate Release Fentanyl Risk Evaluation Mitigation Strategy) due to risk of misuse, abuse, addiction, and overdose. Outpatients, healthcare professionals who prescribe to outpatients, pharmacies, and distributors must enroll in this program.

THERAPEUTIC CLASS: Opioid analgesic

INDICATIONS: Management of breakthrough pain in cancer patients ≥18 yrs of age who are already receiving and are tolerant to around-the-clock opioid therapy for underlying persistent cancer pain.

DOSAGE: *Adults:* ≥18 Yrs: Initial: 100mcg. If adequate analgesia is obtained within 30 min of first 100mcg, continue to treat subsequent episodes of breakthrough pain with this dose. If adequate analgesia not obtained after initiation, use 2nd dose (after 30 min) ud. No more than 2 doses may be used to treat an episode of breakthrough pain and must wait at least 2 hrs before treating another episode. Titrate: If adequate analgesia is not obtained with the first 100mcg dose, continue dose escalation in a stepwise manner over consecutive breakthrough episodes until adequate analgesia with tolerable side effects is achieved. Increase dose by 100mcg multiples up to 400mcg PRN. If adequate analgesia is not obtained with 400mcg dose, titrate to 600mcg. If adequate analgesia is not obtained with a 600mcg dose, titrate to 800mcg. During titration, use multiples of 100mcg tabs and/or 200mcg tabs for any single dose. Do not use >4 tabs at one time. May repeat the same dose if adequate analgesia is not obtained 30 min after use. May use rescue medication ud if adequate analgesia not achieved. Refer to PI for information on dose readjustments, maintenance, and discontinuation of therapy.

HOW SUPPLIED: Tab, SL: 100mcg, 200mcg, 300mcg, 400mcg, 600mcg, 800mcg

CONTRAINDICATIONS: Opioid-nontolerant patients, management of acute or postoperative pain (eg, headache/migraine, dental pain, or use in emergency room).

WARNINGS/PRECAUTIONS: May cause anaphylaxis and hypersensitivity reactions. Increased risk of respiratory depression in patients with underlying respiratory disorders and in elderly/debilitated. May impair mental/physical abilities. Caution with chronic obstructive pulmonary disease or preexisting medical conditions predisposing to hypoventilation; may further decrease respiratory drive to the point of respiratory failure. Extreme caution in patients who may be susceptible to intracranial effects of CO_2 retention (eg, with evidence of increased intracranial pressure or impaired consciousness). May obscure clinical course of head injuries. Caution with bradyarrhythmias. Caution with hepatic/renal impairment.

ADVERSE REACTIONS: Respiratory depression, nausea, somnolence, dizziness, headache, constipation, stomatitis, dry mouth, dysgeusia, fatigue, dyspnea, hyperhidrosis, bradycardia, asthenia, anxiety.

INTERACTIONS: See Boxed Warning. May produce increased depressant effects with other CNS depressants (eg, other opioids, sedatives or hypnotics, general anesthetics, phenothiazines, tranquilizers, skeletal muscle relaxants, sedating antihistamines, and alcoholic beverages); adjust dose if warranted. May decrease levels and efficacy with CYP3A4 inducers (eg, barbiturates, carbamazepine, efavirenz, glucocorticoids, modafinil, nevirapine, oxcarbazepine, phenobarbital, phenytoin, pioglitazone, rifabutin, rifampin, St. John's wort, troglitazone). Not recommended with MAOIs or within 14 days of discontinuation of MAOIs. Respiratory depression may occur; more likely when given with other drugs that depress respiration.

PREGNANCY: Category C, not for use in nursing.

MECHANISM OF ACTION: Opioid analgesic; μ-opioid receptor agonist. Exact mechanism not established. Specific CNS opioid receptors for endogenous compounds with opioid-like activity have been identified throughout the brain and spinal cord and play a role in analgesic effects.

PHARMACOKINETICS: Absorption: Bioavailability (54%). Administration of various doses led to different parameters. **Distribution:** V_d=4L/kg; plasma protein binding (80-85%); crosses placenta; found in breast milk. **Metabolism:** Liver and intestinal mucosa via CYP3A4; norfentanyl (metabolite). **Elimination:** Urine (<7% unchanged), feces (1% unchanged); $T_{1/2}$=5.02 hrs (100mcg), 6.67 hrs (200mcg), 13.5 hrs (400mcg), 10.1 hrs (800mcg).

NURSING CONSIDERATIONS

Assessment: Assess for degree of opioid tolerance, previous opioid dose, level of pain intensity, type of pain, patient's general condition and medical status, and for any other conditions where treatment is contraindicated or cautioned. Assess for hypersensitivity to the drug, renal/hepatic function, pregnancy/nursing status, and possible drug interactions.

Monitoring: Monitor for signs/symptoms of respiratory depression, bradycardia, impairment of mental/physical abilities, drug abuse/addiction, hypersensitivity reactions, and other adverse reactions.

Patient Counseling: Inform outpatients to enroll in the TIRF REMS Access program. Counsel that therapy may be fatal in children, in individuals for whom it is not prescribed, and who are not opioid tolerant. Counsel on proper administration and disposal. Advise to take drug as prescribed and avoid sharing it with anyone else. Instruct not to take medication for acute or postoperative pain, pain from injuries, headache, migraine, or any other short-term pain. Instruct to notify physician if breakthrough pain is not alleviated or worsens after taking the drug. Inform that drug may impair mental/physical abilities; caution against performing activities that require high level of attention (eg, driving/using heavy machinery). Advise not to combine with alcohol, sleep aids, or tranquilizers except if ordered by the physician. Instruct to notify physician if pregnant or planning to become pregnant.

Administration: SL route. Do not chew, suck, or swallow tabs. Do not eat or drink until tab is completely dissolved. Refer to PI for complete administration instructions. **Storage:** 20-25°C (68-77°F); excursions permitted between 15-30°C (59-86°F). Protect from moisture.

ACANYA   RX
clindamycin phosphate - benzoyl peroxide (Coria Laboratories)

THERAPEUTIC CLASS: Antibacterial/keratolytic

INDICATIONS: Topical treatment of acne vulgaris in patients ≥12 yrs of age.

DOSAGE: *Adults:* Apply pea-sized amount to face qd.
Pediatrics: ≥12 Yrs: Apply pea-sized amount to face qd.

HOW SUPPLIED: Gel: (Clindamycin-Benzoyl Peroxide) 1.2%-2.5% [50g]

CONTRAINDICATIONS: History of regional enteritis, ulcerative colitis, or antibiotic-associated colitis.

WARNINGS/PRECAUTIONS: Diarrhea, bloody diarrhea, and colitis (including pseudomembranous colitis) reported; d/c if significant diarrhea occurs. Minimize sun exposure following application. Not for oral, ophthalmic, or intravaginal use. Use for >12 weeks has not been evaluated.

ADVERSE REACTIONS: Erythema, scaling, itching, burning, stinging.

INTERACTIONS: Avoid with topical or oral erythromycin-containing products. Caution with topical acne therapy (eg, peeling, desquamating, or abrasive agents) due to potential cumulative irritancy effects. Caution with other neuromuscular blocking agents. Antiperistaltic agents (eg, opiates, diphenoxylate with atropine) may prolong and/or worsen severe colitis.

PREGNANCY: Category C, not for use in nursing.

MECHANISM OF ACTION: Clindamycin phosphate: Antibacterial; binds to 50S ribosomal subunits of susceptible bacteria and prevents elongation of peptide chains, thereby suppressing bacterial protein synthesis. Benzoyl peroxide: Oxidizing agent; bacteriocidal and keratolytic effects.

NURSING CONSIDERATIONS

Assessment: Assess for history of regional enteritis, ulcerative colitis, or antibiotic-associated colitis, diarrhea, pregnancy/nursing status, and possible drug interactions.

Monitoring: Monitor for erythema, scaling, itching, burning, stinging, allergic reactions, diarrhea, bloody diarrhea, and colitis.

Patient Counseling: Instruct to apply medication ud and avoid other topical acne products unless directed by physician. Avoid washing of face >2-3X a day and direct contact with mouth, eyes, inside the nose, and all mucous membranes, cuts, or open wounds. Instruct to wash hands with soap and water after application. Advise to notify physician if any signs/symptoms of local skin irritation develop. Counsel to minimize exposure to natural sunlight and avoid artificial sunlight. Inform that medication may bleach hair or colored fabric. Advise to d/c and notify physician if severe diarrhea, GI discomfort, or allergic reaction occurs.

Administration: Topical route. Wash affected areas gently with mild soap and pat dry prior to application. Refer to PI for administration instructions. **Storage:** Prior to Dispensing: 2-8°C (36-46°F). After Dispensing: 25°C (77°F). Do not freeze. Keep container tightly closed.

ACCOLATE   RX
zafirlukast (AstraZeneca)

THERAPEUTIC CLASS: Leukotriene receptor antagonist

INDICATIONS: Prophylaxis and chronic treatment of asthma in adults and children ≥5 yrs of age.

DOSAGE: *Adults:* 20mg bid. Take at least 1 hr ac or 2 hrs pc.
Pediatrics: ≥12 Yrs: 20mg bid. 5-11 Yrs: 10mg bid. Take at least 1 hr ac or 2 hrs pc.

HOW SUPPLIED: Tab: 10mg, 20mg

CONTRAINDICATIONS: Hepatic impairment, including hepatic cirrhosis.

WARNINGS/PRECAUTIONS: Cases of life-threatening hepatic failure and cases of liver injury reported. D/C if liver dysfunction is suspected based upon clinical signs/symptoms; measure LFTs (particularly serum ALT) immediately and manage patient accordingly. Not for use in the reversal of bronchospasm in acute asthma attacks, including status asthmaticus. May continue therapy during acute exacerbations of asthma. Rarely, systemic eosinophilia, eosinophilic pneumonia, or clinical features of vasculitis consistent with Churg-Strauss syndrome may occur. Neuropsychiatric events (eg, insomnia, depression) reported; carefully evaluate risks and benefits of continuing treatment if such events occur.

ADVERSE REACTIONS: Headache, infection, nausea.

INTERACTIONS: Coadministration with warfarin results in a clinically significant increase in PT; when given with oral warfarin, monitor PT closely and adjust anticoagulant dose accordingly. Caution with drugs metabolized by CYP2C9 (eg, tolbutamide, phenytoin, carbamazepine). Decreased levels with erythromycin and liquid theophylline. May increase theophylline levels. Increased levels with aspirin and fluconazole (a moderate CYP2C9 inhibitor). Moderate and strong CYP2C9 inhibitors may increase exposure. Monitor when coadministered with drugs metabolized by CYP3A4 (eg, dihydropyridine calcium channel blockers, cyclosporine, cisapride).

PREGNANCY: Category B, not for use in nursing.

MECHANISM OF ACTION: Leukotriene receptor antagonist; selective and competitive receptor antagonist of leukotriene D_4 and E_4, components of slow-reacting substance of anaphylaxis. Inhibits bronchoconstriction caused by several kinds of inhalational challenges.

PHARMACOKINETICS: Absorption: Rapid. (Adults) C_{max}=326ng/mL; T_{max}=2 hrs (median); AUC=1137ng•h/mL. (7-11 Yrs of Age) C_{max}=601ng/mL; T_{max}=2.5 hrs; AUC=2027ng•h/mL. (5-6 Yrs of Age) C_{max}=756ng/mL; T_{max}=2.1 hrs; AUC=2458ng•h/mL. **Distribution:** V_d=70L; plasma protein binding (>99%); found in breast milk. **Metabolism:** Liver (extensive), hydroxylation via CYP2C9. **Elimination:** Urine (10%), feces. (Adults) $T_{1/2}$=13.3 hrs.

NURSING CONSIDERATIONS

Assessment: Assess for hepatic impairment, hepatic cirrhosis, drug hypersensitivity, asthma status, pregnancy/nursing status, and possible drug interactions.

Monitoring: Monitor for signs/symptoms of liver dysfunction, eosinophilia, vasculitic rash, worsening pulmonary symptoms, cardiac complications, neuropathy, neuropsychiatric events, and other adverse reactions. Monitor LFTs periodically. Closely monitor PT when given with oral warfarin.

Patient Counseling: Inform that hepatic dysfunction may occur; instruct to contact physician immediately if symptoms of hepatic dysfunction (eg, right upper quadrant abdominal pain, nausea, fatigue, lethargy, pruritus, jaundice, flu-like symptoms, anorexia) occur. Advise to take regularly as prescribed, even during symptom-free periods. Inform that it is not a bronchodilator and should not be used to treat acute episodes of asthma. Instruct not to decrease dose or stop taking any other antiasthma medications unless instructed by a physician. Instruct to notify physician if neuropsychiatric events occur. Instruct not to take the medication if breastfeeding.

Administration: Oral route. Take at least 1 hr ac or 2 hrs pc. **Storage:** 20-25°C (68-77°F). Protect from light and moisture.

ACCUPRIL   RX
quinapril HCl (Parke-Davis)

> D/C if pregnancy is detected. Drugs that act directly on the renin-angiotensin system (RAS) can cause injury/death to the developing fetus.

THERAPEUTIC CLASS: ACE inhibitor

INDICATIONS: Treatment of HTN, alone or in combination with thiazide diuretics. Management of heart failure (HF) as adjunctive therapy when added to conventional therapy, including diuretics and/or digitalis.

DOSAGE: *Adults:* HTN: If possible, d/c diuretic 2-3 days prior to therapy. Initial: 10mg or 20mg qd; 5mg qd if with concomitant diuretic, with careful monitoring until BP is stabilized. Titrate: May adjust dosage based on BP response at intervals of at least 2 weeks. Usual: 20mg, 40mg, or 80mg/day, given as single dose or in 2 equally divided doses. Max Initial for HTN with Renal Impairment: CrCl >60mL/min: 10mg/day. CrCl 30-60mL/min: 5mg/day. CrCl 10-30mL/min: 2.5mg/day. Elderly: Initial: 10mg qd. Titrate: Adjust to the optimal response. HF: Initial: 5mg bid. Titrate: Adjust weekly until effective dose achieved or hypotension/orthostasis/azotemia prohibits further adjustment. Usual: 20-40mg/day given in 2 equally divided doses. Initial for HF with Renal Impairment: CrCl >30mL/min: 5mg/day. CrCl 10-30mL/min: 2.5mg/day. Give bid in succeeding days if well tolerated. Titrate: Increase dose at weekly intervals based on clinical and hemodynamic response if without excessive hypotension or significant renal deterioration. Elderly: Start at lower end of dosing range.

HOW SUPPLIED: Tab: 5mg*, 10mg, 20mg, 40mg *scored

CONTRAINDICATIONS: History of ACE inhibitor-associated angioedema. Coadministration with aliskiren in patients with diabetes.

WARNINGS/PRECAUTIONS: Less effect on BP and more reports of angioedema in blacks than nonblacks. Angioedema of the face, extremities, lips, tongue, glottis, and larynx reported; d/c and administer appropriate therapy if laryngeal stridor or angioedema of the face, tongue, or glottis occurs. Intestinal angioedema reported; monitor for abdominal pain. Patients with history of angioedema unrelated to ACE inhibitor therapy may be at increased risk of angioedema during therapy. Anaphylactoid reactions reported during desensitization with hymenoptera venom, dialysis with high-flux membranes, and LDL apheresis with dextran sulfate absorption. Associated with syndrome that starts with cholestatic jaundice and progresses to fulminant hepatic necrosis, and sometimes death; d/c if jaundice or marked hepatic enzyme elevation occurs. Excessive hypotension sometimes associated with oliguria, azotemia, and (rarely) acute renal failure and/or death may occur. Risk factors for excessive hypotension include HF, hyponatremia, high-dose diuretic therapy, recent intensive diuresis, dialysis, or severe volume and/or salt depletion; eliminate or reduce the diuretic or cautiously increase salt intake (except with HF) prior to therapy and monitor closely. May cause agranulocytosis and bone marrow depression. May cause renal function changes. May increase BUN and SrCr levels with renal artery stenosis or without renal vascular disease. Risk of hyperkalemia with diabetes mellitus (DM) and renal dysfunction. Persistent nonproductive cough reported. Hypotension may occur with surgery or during anesthesia. Caution in elderly.

ADVERSE REACTIONS: Headache, dizziness, cough.

INTERACTIONS: See Contraindications. Dual blockade of the RAS is associated with increased risks of hypotension, hyperkalemia, and changes in renal function (including acute renal failure); closely monitor BP, renal function, and electrolytes with concomitant agents that also affect the RAS. Avoid concomitant use of aliskiren in patients with renal impairment (GFR <60mL/min). Hypotension risk and increased BUN and SrCr with diuretics. Coadministration with NSAIDs, including selective COX-2 inhibitors, may attenuate antihypertensive effect of ACE inhibitors, and may further deteriorate renal function. Decreases tetracycline absorption (possibly due to Mg^{2+} content in quinapril); consider interaction with drugs that interact with Mg^{2+}. Increased risk of hyperkalemia with K^+-sparing diuretics (eg, spironolactone, amiloride, triamterene), K^+ supplements, or K^+-containing salt substitutes; use caution and monitor serum K^+. May increase lithium levels and risk of toxicity; use caution and monitor serum lithium levels. Nitritoid reactions reported rarely with injectable gold (eg, sodium aurothiomalate). Increased risk for angioedema with mammalian target of rapamycin inhibitor (eg, temsirolimus) therapy.

PREGNANCY: Category D, caution in nursing.

MECHANISM OF ACTION: ACE inhibitor; decreases plasma angiotensin II, which leads to decreased vasopressor activity and decreased aldosterone secretion.

PHARMACOKINETICS: Absorption: T_{max}=1 hr, 2 hrs (quinaprilat). **Distribution:** Plasma protein binding (97%); crosses placenta; found in breast milk. **Metabolism:** Deesterification. Quinaprilat (active metabolite). **Elimination:** (IV) Renal (≤96% quinaprilat); $T_{1/2}$=2 hrs (quinaprilat).

NURSING CONSIDERATIONS

Assessment: Assess for history of angioedema, hypersensitivity to drug, volume/salt depletion, collagen vascular disease, DM, renal artery stenosis, ischemic heart disease, cerebrovascular disease, renal function, pregnancy/nursing status, and possible drug interactions.

Monitoring: Monitor for signs/symptoms of hypotension, anaphylactoid or hypersensitivity reactions, head/neck/intestinal angioedema, agranulocytosis, neutropenia, bone marrow depression, cholestatic jaundice, fulminant hepatic necrosis, and hyperkalemia. Monitor BP and renal function. Monitor WBC count periodically in patients with collagen vascular disease and/or renal disease.

Patient Counseling: Inform of pregnancy risks and instruct to notify physician as soon as possible if pregnant/planning to become pregnant. Instruct to d/c therapy and immediately report signs/symptoms of angioedema (eg, swelling of face, extremities, eyes, lips, or tongue; difficulty swallowing/breathing). Caution about lightheadedness, especially during the 1st few days of therapy and advise to report to physician. Instruct to d/c and consult physician if syncope occurs. Caution that inadequate fluid intake or excessive perspiration, diarrhea, or vomiting may lead to an excessive fall in BP, resulting in lightheadedness or syncope. Instruct to inform physician about therapy if planning to undergo surgery/anesthesia. Instruct to avoid K⁺ supplements or salt substitutes containing K⁺ without consulting physician. Advise to report any symptoms of infection (eg, sore throat, fever).

Administration: Oral route. **Storage:** 15-30°C (59-86°F). Protect from light.

ACCURETIC   RX
quinapril HCl - hydrochlorothiazide (Parke-Davis)

> D/C if pregnancy is detected. Drugs that act directly on the renin-angiotensin system (RAS) can cause injury/death to the developing fetus.

THERAPEUTIC CLASS: ACE inhibitor/thiazide diuretic

INDICATIONS: Treatment of HTN.

DOSAGE: *Adults:* Use only after failure to achieve desired effect with monotherapy. Not Controlled with Quinapril Monotherapy: Initial: 10mg-12.5mg or 20mg-12.5mg qd. Titrate: May increase dose based on clinical response. May increase HCTZ after 2-3 weeks. Controlled with HCTZ 25mg/day with Hypokalemia: 10mg-12.5mg or 20mg-12.5mg qd. Replacement Therapy: Patients adequately treated with 20mg quinapril and 25mg HCTZ without significant electrolyte disturbances may switch to 20mg-25mg qd. Elderly: Start at lower end of dosing range.

HOW SUPPLIED: Tab: (Quinapril-HCTZ) 10mg-12.5mg*, 20mg-12.5mg*, 20mg-25mg *scored

CONTRAINDICATIONS: Anuria, hypersensitivity to other sulfonamide-derived drugs, history of ACE inhibitor-associated angioedema. Coadministration with aliskiren in patients with diabetes.

WARNINGS/PRECAUTIONS: Not for initial therapy. Caution in elderly and with severe renal disease. Avoid if CrCl ≤30mL/min. Caution with liver dysfunction or progressive liver disease; may precipitate hepatic coma. Quinapril: Less effect on BP and more reports of angioedema in blacks than nonblacks. Angioedema of the face, extremities, lips, tongue, glottis, and larynx reported; d/c and administer appropriate therapy if laryngeal stridor or angioedema of the face, tongue, or glottis occurs. Intestinal angioedema reported; monitor for abdominal pain. Patients with history of angioedema unrelated to ACE inhibitor therapy may be at increased risk of angioedema during therapy. Anaphylactoid reactions reported during desensitization with hymenoptera venom, dialysis with high-flux membranes, and LDL apheresis with dextran sulfate absorption. Associated with syndrome that starts with cholestatic jaundice and progresses to fulminant hepatic necrosis, and sometimes death; d/c if jaundice or marked hepatic enzyme elevation occurs. Symptomatic hypotension sometimes associated with oliguria, azotemia, and, rarely, acute renal failure and/or death may occur. Risk factors for symptomatic hypotension include heart failure (HF), hyponatremia, high dose diuretic therapy, recent intensive diuresis, dialysis, or severe volume and/or salt depletion; correct volume/salt depletion prior to therapy and monitor closely. May cause renal function changes. May increase BUN and SrCr levels with renal artery stenosis or without renal vascular disease. May cause agranulocytosis and bone marrow depression. Hyperkalemia and persistent nonproductive cough reported. Hypotension may occur with surgery or during anesthesia. HCTZ: May precipitate azotemia with renal disease. May exacerbate/activate systemic lupus erythematosus (SLE). May cause idiosyncratic reaction, resulting in acute transient myopia and acute angle-closure glaucoma; d/c rapidly. May increase cholesterol, TG levels, and uric acid levels, and decrease glucose tolerance. Fluid/electrolyte imbalance (hyponatremia, hypokalemia, hypochloremic alkalosis, hypomagnesemia) may occur. Hypokalemia may sensitize or exaggerate the response of the heart to toxic effects of digitalis. Dilutional hyponatremia may occur in edematous patients during hot weather; water restriction rather than salt administration should be instituted, except for life-threatening hyponatremia. Pathological changes in parathyroid glands, with hypercalcemia and hypophosphatemia, observed with prolonged

11

therapy. Enhanced effects in postsympathectomy patients. May decrease protein-bound iodine levels without signs of thyroid disturbance. Interrupt treatment for a few days prior to carrying out parathyroid function tests.

ADVERSE REACTIONS: Headache, dizziness, cough, increases in SrCr and BUN levels.

INTERACTIONS: See Contraindications. Dual blockade of the RAS is associated with increased risk of hypotension, hyperkalemia, and changes in renal function (including acute renal failure); closely monitor BP, renal function, and electrolytes with concomitant agents that also affect the RAS. Increased risk for angioedema with mammalian target of rapamycin inhibitor (eg, temsirolimus) therapy. Quinapril: Decreases tetracycline absorption (possibly due to Mg^{2+} content in quinapril); consider interaction with drugs that interact with Mg^{2+}. Increased risk of hyperkalemia with K^+-sparing diuretics (eg, spironolactone, amiloride, triamterene), K^+ supplements, or K^+-containing salt substitutes; use caution and monitor serum K^+. May increase lithium levels and risk of toxicity; use caution and monitor lithium levels. Nitritoid reactions reported rarely with injectable gold (eg, sodium aurothiomalate). NSAIDs, including selective COX-2 inhibitors, may result in deterioration of renal function, including possible acute renal failure, and may attenuate antihypertensive effect. Avoid with aliskiren in patients with renal impairment (GFR <60mL/min). HCTZ: May potentiate orthostatic hypotension with alcohol, barbiturates, and narcotics. May need to adjust dose of antidiabetic drugs. Impaired absorption with cholestyramine and colestipol. Corticosteroids and adrenocorticotropic hormone intensify electrolyte depletion. May decrease response to pressor amines. May increase responsiveness to nondepolarizing skeletal muscle relaxants (eg, tubocurarine). NSAIDs may reduce diuretic, natriuretic, and antihypertensive effects of thiazide diuretics. May potentiate action of other antihypertensives, especially ganglionic or peripheral adrenergic-blocking drugs.

PREGNANCY: Category D, not for use in nursing.

MECHANISM OF ACTION: Quinapril: ACE inhibitor; decreases plasma angiotensin II, which leads to decreased vasopressor activity and decreased aldosterone secretion. HCTZ: Thiazide diuretic; affects renal tubular mechanism of electrolyte reabsorption, directly increasing excretion of Na^+ and Cl^-, and indirectly reducing plasma volume.

PHARMACOKINETICS: Absorption: Quinapril: T_{max}=1 hr, 2 hrs (quinaprilat). **Distribution:** Crosses placenta; found in breast milk. Quinapril: Plasma protein binding (97%). HCTZ: V_d=3.6-7.8L/kg; plasma protein binding (67.9%). **Metabolism:** Quinapril: Deesterification. Quinaprilat (metabolite). **Elimination:** Quinapril: (IV) Renal (≤96% quinaprilat); $T_{1/2}$=2 hrs. HCTZ: Kidney (at least 61% unchanged); $T_{1/2}$=4-15 hrs.

NURSING CONSIDERATIONS

Assessment: Assess for anuria, history of angioedema, volume/salt depletion, HF, SLE, and any other conditions where treatment is contraindicated or cautioned. Assess for hypersensitivity to drug or sulfonamides, pregnancy/nursing status, and possible drug interactions. Assess renal/hepatic function and electrolyte levels.

Monitoring: Monitor for angioedema, agranulocytosis, hyperkalemia, anaphylactoid reactions, hypotension, jaundice, hypersensitivity/idiosyncratic reactions, SLE, gout, myopia, and angle-closure glaucoma. Periodically monitor WBC counts in patients with collagen vascular disease and/or renal disease. Monitor serum electrolytes, BP, LFTs, BUN, SrCr, uric acid levels, and cholesterol/TG levels.

Patient Counseling: Inform females of childbearing age of the consequences of exposure during pregnancy and of the treatment options for women planning to become pregnant. Instruct to report pregnancy to the physician as soon as possible. Instruct to d/c therapy and immediately report signs/symptoms of angioedema (eg, swelling of face, eyes, lips, tongue, difficulty breathing). Caution about lightheadedness, especially during the 1st days of therapy and advise to report to physician. Instruct to d/c and consult physician if syncope occurs. Caution that inadequate fluid intake or excessive perspiration, diarrhea, or vomiting may lead to an excessive fall in BP, resulting in lightheadedness or syncope. Instruct to inform physician about therapy if planning to undergo surgery/anesthesia. Instruct to avoid K^+ supplements or salt substitutes containing K^+ without consulting physician. Instruct to report any symptoms of infection (eg, sore throat, fever).

Administration: Oral route. **Storage:** 20-25°C (68-77°F).

ACEON

perindopril erbumine (XOMA)   RX

D/C if pregnancy is detected. Drugs that act directly on the renin-angiotensin system (RAS) can cause injury/death to the developing fetus.

THERAPEUTIC CLASS: ACE inhibitor

INDICATIONS: Treatment of essential HTN alone or with other antihypertensives (eg, thiazide diuretics). Treatment of stable coronary artery disease (CAD) to reduce risk of cardiovascular mortality or nonfatal myocardial infarction (MI); may be used with conventional treatment for CAD (eg, antiplatelet, antihypertensive, or lipid-lowering therapy).

DOSAGE: *Adults:* HTN: Initial: 4mg qd. May be titrated PRN to max of 16mg/day. Maint: 4-8mg/day given in 1 or 2 divided doses. Elderly: Initial: 4mg/day given in 1 or 2 divided doses. Monitor BP and titrate carefully with doses >8mg. Use with Diuretics: Consider reducing diuretic dose prior to start of treatment. Stable CAD: Initial: 4mg qd for 2 weeks. Maint: 8mg qd if tolerated. Elderly (>70 Yrs): Initial: 2mg qd in the 1st week, followed by 4mg qd in the 2nd week. Maint: 8mg qd if tolerated. Renal Impairment: CrCl ≥30mL/min: Initial: 2mg/day. Max: 8mg/day.

HOW SUPPLIED: Tab: 2mg*, 4mg*, 8mg* *scored

CONTRAINDICATIONS: Hereditary or idiopathic angioedema. Coadministration with aliskiren in patients with diabetes.

WARNINGS/PRECAUTIONS: Not recommended with CrCl <30mL/min. Higher incidence of angioedema in blacks than nonblacks. Angioedema of the face, extremities, lips, tongue, glottis, or larynx reported; d/c and administer appropriate therapy. Intestinal angioedema reported; monitor for abdominal pain. Symptomatic hypotension may occur and is most likely in patients with volume/salt depletion. Closely monitor patients at risk for excessive hypotension, especially during the first 2 weeks of treatment and whenever dose is increased. May cause agranulocytosis and bone marrow depression, most frequently in renal impairment patients, especially with collagen vascular disease (eg, systemic lupus erythematosus [SLE] or scleroderma). May cause changes in renal function. Oliguria, progressive azotemia, and (rarely) acute renal failure and death may occur in patients with severe congestive heart failure (CHF). May increase BUN and SrCr in patients with renal artery stenosis. May cause hyperkalemia; risk factors include renal insufficiency and diabetes mellitus (DM). Persistent nonproductive cough reported. Rarely, associated with syndrome that starts with cholestatic jaundice and progresses to fulminant necrosis and sometimes death; d/c if jaundice or marked elevations of hepatic enzymes develop. Hypotension may occur with major surgery or during anesthesia.

ADVERSE REACTIONS: Cough, headache, asthenia, dizziness, back pain.

INTERACTIONS: See Contraindications. Dual blockade of the RAS is associated with increased risks of hypotension, hyperkalemia, and changes in renal function (including acute renal failure); closely monitor BP, renal function, and electrolytes with concomitant agents that affect the RAS. Avoid with aliskiren in patients with renal impairment (GFR <60mL/min). Hypotension risk, increased BUN and SrCr, and reduced perindoprilat bioavailability with diuretics. Increased risk of hyperkalemia with K^+-sparing diuretics (eg, spironolactone, amiloride, triamterene), drugs that increase serum K^+ (eg, indomethacin, heparin, cyclosporine), K^+ supplements and/or K^+-containing salt substitutes. May increase lithium levels and risk of toxicity; monitor lithium levels. Nitritoid reactions reported with injectable gold (sodium aurothiomalate). Caution with digoxin. Coadministration with NSAIDs, including selective COX-2 inhibitors, may attenuate antihypertensive effect of ACE inhibitors and may further deteriorate renal function.

PREGNANCY: Category D, caution in nursing.

MECHANISM OF ACTION: ACE inhibitor; inhibits ACE activity, resulting in decreased plasma angiotensin II, leading to decreased vasoconstriction, increased plasma renin activity, and decreased aldosterone secretion.

PHARMACOKINETICS: Absorption: Absolute bioavailability (75%, 25% perindoprilat); T_{max}=1 hr, 3-7 hrs (perindoprilat). **Distribution:** Plasma protein binding (60%, 10-20% perindoprilat); crosses placenta. **Metabolism:** Hepatic (extensive); hydrolysis, glucuronidation, cyclization via dehydration; perindoprilat (active metabolite). **Elimination:** Urine (4-12%, unchanged); $T_{1/2}$=0.8-1 hr, 3-10 hrs (perindoprilat).

NURSING CONSIDERATIONS

Assessment: Assess for hereditary or idiopathic angioedema, volume and/or salt depletion, CHF, renal artery stenosis, ischemic heart disease, cerebrovascular disease, hepatic/renal impairment, DM, collagen vascular disease (eg, SLE), previous hypersensitivity to the drug, pregnancy/nursing status, and possible drug interactions.

Monitoring: Monitor for signs/symptoms of anaphylactoid reactions, head/neck/intestinal angioedema, hypotension, agranulocytosis, bone marrow depression, cholestatic jaundice, fulminant hepatic necrosis, hepatic failure, hyperkalemia, persistent nonproductive cough, hypersensitivity reactions, and neutropenia. Monitor hepatic/renal function, BP, and K^+ levels.

Patient Counseling: Inform of pregnancy risks and discuss treatment options with women planning to become pregnant; advise to report pregnancy to physician as soon as possible. Instruct to d/c and immediately report to physician if any signs/symptoms of angioedema develop. Counsel to report any signs of infection (eg, sore throat, fever).

Administration: Oral route. **Storage:** 20-25°C (68-77°F). Protect from moisture.

ACETAMINOPHEN AND CODEINE TABLETS `CIII`

codeine phosphate - acetaminophen (Various)

Associated with cases of acute liver failure, at times resulting in liver transplant and death. Most cases of liver injury are associated with acetaminophen (APAP) use at doses >4000mg/day, and often involve >1 APAP-containing product. Respiratory depression and death reported in children who received codeine following tonsillectomy and/or adenoidectomy and had evidence of being ultra-rapid metabolizers of codeine due to a CYP2D6 polymorphism.

OTHER BRAND NAMES: Tylenol with Codeine (Janssen)

THERAPEUTIC CLASS: Opioid analgesic

INDICATIONS: Relief of mild to moderately severe pain.

DOSAGE: *Adults:* Adjust dose according to severity of pain and response. Usual Range (Single Dose): 15mg-60mg codeine; 300mg-1000mg APAP. May repeat doses up to q4h. Max: 360mg/24 hrs codeine; 4000mg/24 hrs APAP.

HOW SUPPLIED: Tab: (APAP-Codeine) 300mg-15mg; (Tylenol with Codeine) 300mg-30mg, 300mg-60mg

CONTRAINDICATIONS: Postoperative pain management in children who have undergone tonsillectomy and/or adenoidectomy.

WARNINGS/PRECAUTIONS: Increased risk of acute liver failure in patients with underlying liver disease. May cause serious skin reactions (eg, acute generalized exanthematous pustulosis, Stevens-Johnson syndrome, toxic epidermal necrolysis), which can be fatal; d/c at the 1st appearance of skin rash or any other sign of hypersensitivity. Deaths reported in nursing infants exposed to high levels of morphine because their mothers were ultra-rapid metabolizers of codeine. Ultra-rapid metabolizers, due to specific CYP2D6 genotype (gene duplications denoted as *1/*1xN or *1/*2xN), may have life-threatening or fatal respiratory depression or experience signs of overdose (eg, extreme sleepiness, confusion, shallow breathing). Choose lowest effective dose for the shortest period of time. Hypersensitivity and anaphylaxis reported; d/c if signs/symptoms occur. Respiratory-depressant effects and capacity for elevating CSF pressure may be markedly enhanced in the presence of head injury or other intracranial lesions. May obscure diagnosis or clinical course of head injuries and acute abdominal conditions. Habit-forming and potentially abusable; extended use is not recommended. Caution with severe renal/hepatic impairment, head injuries, elevated intracranial pressure, acute abdominal conditions, hypothyroidism, urethral stricture, Addison's disease, prostatic hypertrophy, and in the elderly or debilitated. May increase serum amylase levels. Lab test interactions may occur. Avoid during labor if delivery of a premature infant is anticipated. (Tylenol with Codeine) Contains sodium metabisulfite; may cause allergic-type reactions, including anaphylactic symptoms and life-threatening or less severe asthmatic episodes in certain susceptible people.

ADVERSE REACTIONS: Acute liver failure, drowsiness, lightheadedness, dizziness, sedation, SOB, N/V.

INTERACTIONS: Increased risk of acute liver failure with alcohol ingestion. May enhance effects of other narcotic analgesics, alcohol, general anesthetics, tranquilizers (eg, chlordiazepoxide), sedative-hypnotics, or other CNS depressants; may increase CNS depression.

PREGNANCY: Category C, not for use in nursing.

MECHANISM OF ACTION: Codeine: Narcotic analgesic; centrally acting analgesic. APAP: Nonopiate, nonsalicylate analgesic; peripherally acting analgesic.

PHARMACOKINETICS: Absorption: Rapid. **Distribution:** Found in breast milk. Codeine: Crosses placenta. **Metabolism:** Codeine: CYP2D6; morphine (active metabolite). APAP: Liver (conjugation). **Elimination:** Codeine: Urine (90%), feces; $T_{1/2}$=2.9 hrs. APAP: Urine (85%); $T_{1/2}$=1.25-3 hrs.

NURSING CONSIDERATIONS

Assessment: Assess for hypersensitivity to drug, hepatic/renal impairment, head injury, intracranial lesions, acute abdominal conditions, any other conditions where treatment is contraindicated or cautioned, pregnancy/nursing status, and possible drug interactions.

Monitoring: Monitor for signs/symptoms of hepatotoxicity, respiratory depression, skin reactions, hypersensitivity, anaphylaxis, elevation in CSF pressure, drug abuse, tolerance, dependence, and other adverse reactions. Monitor effects of therapy with serial LFTs and/or renal function tests in patients with severe hepatic/renal disease. Closely monitor newborn infants for signs of respiratory depression if the mother received the drug during labor.

Patient Counseling: Instruct to d/c therapy and contact physician immediately if signs of allergy (eg, rash, difficulty breathing) develop. Instruct to look for APAP on package labels and not to use >1 APAP-containing product. Instruct to seek medical attention immediately upon ingestion of >4000mg/day APAP, even if patient is feeling well. Advise that drug may impair mental/physical abilities. Instruct to avoid performing potentially hazardous tasks (eg, driving, operating machinery), drinking alcohol, or taking other CNS depressants while on therapy. Inform that drug may be habit-forming; instruct to take ud.

Administration: Oral route. **Storage:** 20-25°C (68-77°F).

ACIPHEX RX
rabeprazole sodium (Eisai)

OTHER BRAND NAMES: Aciphex Sprinkle (Eisai)

THERAPEUTIC CLASS: Proton pump inhibitor

INDICATIONS: Short-term treatment (4-8 weeks) in the healing and symptomatic relief of erosive or ulcerative gastroesophageal reflux disease (GERD). Maintenance of healing and reduction in relapse rates of heartburn symptoms with erosive or ulcerative GERD. Treatment of daytime and nighttime heartburn and other symptoms associated with GERD. Short-term treatment (up to 4 weeks) in the healing and symptomatic relief of duodenal ulcers (DU). In combination with amoxicillin and clarithromycin as a 3-drug regimen for the treatment of *Helicobacter pylori* infection and DU disease (active or history within the past 5 yrs); for *H. pylori* eradication to reduce the risk of DU recurrence. Long-term treatment of pathological hypersecretory conditions, including Zollinger-Ellison syndrome. Treatment of symptomatic GERD in adolescents ≥12 yrs of age for up to 8 weeks. Treatment of GERD in children 1-11 yrs of age for up to 12 weeks.

DOSAGE: *Adults:* (Tab) Erosive/Ulcerative GERD: Healing: 20mg qd for 4-8 weeks. Consider an additional 8 weeks if not healed after 8 weeks of treatment. Maint of Healing: 20mg qd; controlled studies do not extend beyond 12 months. Symptomatic GERD: 20mg qd for 4 weeks. Consider an additional course if symptoms do not resolve completely after 4 weeks. Healing of DU: 20mg qd after am meal for up to 4 weeks; may need additional therapy to achieve healing. *H. pylori* Eradication: 20mg + clarithromycin 500mg + amoxicillin 1000mg, all bid with am and pm meals for 7 days. Pathological Hypersecretory Conditions: Individualize dose. Initial: 60mg qd or in divided doses. Titrate: Adjust to individual needs and continue for as long as clinically indicated. Doses up to 100mg qd and 60mg bid have been administered. Some have been treated for up to 1 yr.
Pediatrics: ≥12 Yrs: (Tab) Symptomatic GERD: 20mg qd for up to 8 weeks. (Cap) Take 30 min ac. 1-11 Yrs: GERD: Usual: ≥15kg: 10mg qd for up to 12 weeks. <15kg: 5mg qd for up to 12 weeks with the option to increase to 10mg if inadequate response.

HOW SUPPLIED: Cap, Delayed-Release (Sprinkle): 5mg, 10mg; Tab, Delayed-Release: 20mg

WARNINGS/PRECAUTIONS: Symptomatic response does not preclude the presence of gastric malignancy. May increase risk of *Clostridium difficile* associated diarrhea (CDAD), especially in hospitalized patients. May increase risk of osteoporosis-related fractures of the hip, wrist, or spine, especially with high-dose and long-term therapy. Use lowest dose and shortest duration appropriate to the condition being treated. Hypomagnesemia reported and may require Mg²⁺ replacement and discontinuation of therapy; consider monitoring of Mg²⁺ levels prior to therapy and periodically with prolonged treatment. Caution with severe hepatic impairment.

ADVERSE REACTIONS: Headache, flatulence, pain, pharyngitis, diarrhea, N/V, abdominal pain.

INTERACTIONS: May substantially decrease atazanavir levels; avoid concurrent use. May interfere with the absorption of drugs dependent on gastric pH for absorption (eg, ketoconazole, digoxin). May inhibit cyclosporine metabolism. Monitor for increases in INR and PT with warfarin. Combination with amoxicillin and clarithromycin may increase levels of rabeprazole and 14-hydroxyclarithromycin. May elevate and prolong levels of methotrexate (MTX) and/or its metabolite, possibly leading to toxicities; consider temporary withdrawal of therapy with high-dose MTX. Caution with digoxin or with drugs that may cause hypomagnesemia (eg, diuretics).

PREGNANCY: Category B, caution in nursing.

MECHANISM OF ACTION: Proton pump inhibitor; suppresses gastric acid secretion by inhibiting the gastric H⁺/K⁺-ATPase at the secretory surface of the gastric parietal cell. Blocks the final step of gastric acid secretion.

PHARMACOKINETICS: Absorption: (Tab) T_{max}=2-5 hrs; absolute bioavailability (52%). (Cap) T_{max}=2.5 hrs (median). **Distribution:** Plasma protein binding (96.3%). **Metabolism:** Extensive; CYP3A, CYP2C19; thioether and sulphone (primary metabolites). **Elimination:** Urine (90% metabolites), feces; $T_{1/2}$=1-2 hrs.

NURSING CONSIDERATIONS

Assessment: Assess for drug hypersensitivity, hepatic impairment, risk for osteoporosis-related fractures, pregnancy/nursing status, and possible drug interactions. Obtain baseline Mg²⁺ levels.

Monitoring: Monitor for signs/symptoms of CDAD, bone fractures, hypersensitivity reactions, and other adverse reactions. Monitor Mg²⁺ levels periodically. Monitor INR and PT when given with warfarin.

Patient Counseling: Instruct to take ud. Advise to immediately report and seek care for diarrhea that does not improve.

Administration: Oral route. (Tab) May be taken with or without food. Swallow whole; do not chew, crush, or split. (Cap) Take 30 min ac. Do not chew or crush granules. Open cap and sprinkle entire contents on a small amount of soft food (eg, applesauce, fruit/vegetable-based baby food, yogurt), or empty contents into a small amount of liquid (eg, infant formula, apple juice, pediatric electrolyte sol). Take whole dose within 15 min of preparation; do not store mixture for future use. **Storage:** 25°C (77°F); excursions permitted to 15-30°C (59-86°F). Protect from moisture.

ACTEMRA   RX
tocilizumab (Genentech)

> Increased risk for developing serious infections (eg, active tuberculosis [TB], invasive fungal infections, bacterial/viral infections due to opportunistic pathogens) that may lead to hospitalization or death. Most patients who developed these infections were taking concomitant immunosuppressants (eg, methotrexate [MTX], corticosteroids). If serious infection develops, interrupt treatment until infection is controlled. Test for latent TB prior to and during therapy; initiate latent TB treatment prior to therapy. Consider risks and benefits prior to initiating therapy in patients with chronic or recurrent infection. Monitor for development of signs and symptoms of infection during and after treatment.

THERAPEUTIC CLASS: Interleukin-6 receptor antagonist

INDICATIONS: Treatment of moderate to severe active rheumatoid arthritis (RA) in adults who have had an inadequate response to one or more disease-modifying anti-rheumatic drugs (DMARDs). Treatment of active polyarticular juvenile idiopathic arthritis (PJIA) and active systemic juvenile idiopathic arthritis (SJIA) in patients ≥2 yrs of age.

DOSAGE: *Adults:* RA: Monotherapy/With MTX or Other Nonbiologic DMARDs: (IV) Usual: 4mg/kg every 4 weeks as 60-min single IV drip infusion. Titrate: Increase to 8mg/kg every 4 weeks based on clinical response. Max: 800mg/infusion. (SQ) ≥100kg: 162mg every week. <100kg: 162mg every other week. Titrate: Increase dose every week based on clinical response. Transition from IV to SQ: Administer 1st SQ dose instead of the next scheduled IV dose. Refer to PI for dose modifications based on liver enzyme abnormalities, absolute neutrophil count (ANC), and platelet count.
Pediatrics: ≥2 Yrs: Administer as a 60-min single IV drip infusion. (IV) PJIA: Monotherapy/With MTX: ≥30kg: 8mg/kg once every 4 weeks. <30kg: 10mg/kg once every 4 weeks. SJIA: Monotherapy/With MTX: ≥30kg: 8mg/kg once every 2 weeks. <30kg: 12mg/kg once every 2 weeks. Change in dose should not be made solely on a single visit body weight measurement. May interrupt dose for management of dose-related lab abnormalities (eg, elevated liver enzymes, neutropenia, thrombocytopenia); refer to PI.

HOW SUPPLIED: Inj: 20mg/mL [4mL, 10mL, 20mL vials]; 162mg/0.9mL [prefilled syringe]

WARNINGS/PRECAUTIONS: Avoid with active infection, including localized infections. Caution in patients with chronic/recurrent infections, who have been exposed to TB, with history of serious/opportunistic infection, who resided or traveled in areas of endemic TB/mycoses, or with underlying conditions that may predispose them to infection. Viral reactivation and herpes zoster exacerbation observed. GI perforation reported; caution in patients at risk for GI perforation. Neutropenia, thrombocytopenia, elevation of liver enzymes, and increase in lipid parameters reported; do not initiate treatment if ANC <2000/mm³, platelets <100,000/mm³, or ALT/AST >1.5X ULN. D/C treatment with ANC <500/mm³, platelets <50,000/mm³, or ALT/AST >5X ULN. May increase risk of malignancies. Hypersensitivity reactions, including anaphylaxis and death, reported; d/c immediately and permanently if anaphylaxis or other hypersensitivity reaction occurs. Should only be infused IV by a healthcare professional with appropriate medical support to manage anaphylaxis. Multiple sclerosis and chronic inflammatory demyelinating polyneuropathy reported rarely in RA studies; caution with preexisting or recent onset demyelinating disorders. Not recommended in patients with active hepatic disease or hepatic impairment. Caution in elderly.

ADVERSE REACTIONS: Upper respiratory tract infections, nasopharyngitis, headache, HTN, increased ALT/AST, dizziness, bronchitis, infusion reaction, neutropenia, diarrhea, inj-site reaction, total cholesterol elevation, increased LDL.

INTERACTIONS: See Boxed Warning. Avoid with live vaccines. May increase metabolism of CYP450 substrates (eg, 1A2, 2B6, 2C9, 2C19, 2D6, 3A4). Upon initiation or discontinuation of tocilizumab, monitor therapeutic effect (eg, warfarin) or drug concentrations (eg, cyclosporine, theophylline) and adjust dose PRN. Caution with CYP3A4 substrates where decrease in effectiveness is undesirable (eg, oral contraceptives, lovastatin, atorvastatin). Avoid with biological DMARDs (eg, TNF antagonists, interleukin [IL]-1R antagonists, anti-CD20 monoclonal antibodies, selective costimulation modulators) due to increased immunosuppression. Increased frequency and magnitude of transaminase elevations with hepatotoxic drugs (eg, MTX). Decreased exposure of simvastatin and omeprazole.

PREGNANCY: Category C, not for use in nursing.

MECHANISM OF ACTION: IL-6 receptor antagonist monoclonal antibody; binds specifically to both soluble and membrane-bound IL-6 receptors (sIL-6R and mIL-6R) and inhibits IL-6-mediated signaling through these receptors.

PHARMACOKINETICS: Absorption: Administration of variable doses resulted in different pharmacokinetic parameters. **Distribution:** V_d=6.4L (RA), 4.08L (PJIA), 2.54L (SJIA). **Elimination:** (RA) (4mg/kg IV) $T_{1/2}$=≤11 days; (8mg/kg IV, 162mg every week SQ) $T_{1/2}$=≤13 days; (162mg every other week SQ) $T_{1/2}$=5 days. (SJIA) $T_{1/2}$=≤23 days, (PJIA) $T_{1/2}$=≤16 days.

NURSING CONSIDERATIONS

Assessment: Assess for infections (eg, bacteria, fungi, viruses), including latent TB. Assess for demyelinating disorders, risk of GI perforation, active hepatic disease or impairment, hypersensitivity to drug, pregnancy/nursing status, and possible drug interactions. Obtain baseline lipid levels and platelet, liver transaminases, and neutrophil counts.

Monitoring: Monitor for signs/symptoms of TB and other infections. Monitor for hypersensitivity reactions, GI perforation, malignancies, and demyelinating disorders. Monitor neutrophil counts, platelet counts, and LFTs, after 4-8 weeks and every 3 months thereafter in RA patients, or at the time of 2nd infusion and every 4-8 weeks thereafter in PJIA patients, or every 2-4 weeks thereafter in SJIA patients. Monitor lipid levels 4-8 weeks after initiation then at approximately 24-week intervals.

Patient Counseling: Advise of the potential risks/benefits of therapy. Inform that therapy may lower resistance to infections and may cause serious GI side effects; instruct to contact physician if symptoms of infection or severe, persistent abdominal pain appear. Advise to inform physician of travel history, especially to places that are endemic for TB/mycoses. Inform that some patients have developed serious allergic reactions, including anaphylaxis. Advise to seek immediate medical attention if any symptoms of serious allergic reactions develop. Inform of inj techniques and procedures. Advise not to reuse needles/syringes and instruct on proper disposal procedures.

Administration: IV/SQ route. Do not administer as an IV bolus or push. Refer to PI for preparation and administration instructions. **Storage:** 2-8°C (36-46°F). Do not freeze. Protect from light; store in original package until time of use. Keep syringes dry. Diluted Sol for Infusion: 2-8°C (36-46°F) or room temperature for up to 24 hrs. Protect from light. Discard unused portion.

ACTIQ
fentanyl citrate (Cephalon)

CII

> Fatal respiratory depression may occur. Contraindicated in the management of acute or postoperative pain (eg, headache/migraine) and in opioid-nontolerant patients. Death reported upon accidental ingestion in children; must keep out of reach of children. Concomitant use with CYP3A4 inhibitors may increase plasma levels, and may cause fatal respiratory depression. Do not convert patients on a mcg-per-mcg basis from any other fentanyl products to Actiq. Do not substitute for any other fentanyl products; may result in fatal overdose. Contains fentanyl with abuse liability similar to other opioid analgesics. Available only through a restricted program called Transmucosal Immediate Release Fentanyl (TIRF) Risk Evaluation Mitigation Strategy (REMS) Access program due to risk of misuse, abuse, addiction, and overdose. Outpatients, healthcare professionals who prescribe to outpatients, pharmacies, and distributors must enroll in the program.

THERAPEUTIC CLASS: Opioid analgesic

INDICATIONS: Management of breakthrough pain in cancer patients ≥16 yrs of age who are already receiving and are tolerant to around-the-clock opioid therapy for their underlying persistent cancer pain.

DOSAGE: *Adults:* ≥16 Yrs: Initial: 200mcg (consume over 15 min). Titrate: May take only 1 additional dose of the same strength if breakthrough pain episode is not relieved 15 min after completion of previous dose. Max: 2 doses/breakthrough pain episode; must wait at least 4 hrs before treating another episode of breakthrough pain. Prescribe an initial titration supply of six 200mcg units. Maint: Once titrated to an effective dose, use only 1 unit of the appropriate strength per breakthrough pain episode; limit consumption to 4 or fewer units/day. If >4 breakthrough pain episodes/day are experienced, reevaluate maint dose (around-the-clock) used for persistent pain. Upon discontinuation, gradually titrate dose downward.

HOW SUPPLIED: Loz: 200mcg, 400mcg, 600mcg, 800mcg, 1200mcg, 1600mcg

CONTRAINDICATIONS: Opioid-nontolerant patients, management of acute or postoperative pain, including headache/migraine and dental pain.

WARNINGS/PRECAUTIONS: Increased risk of respiratory depression in patients with underlying respiratory disorders and in elderly/debilitated. May impair mental/physical abilities. Caution with chronic obstructive pulmonary disease or preexisting medical conditions predisposing to respiratory depression; may further decrease respiratory drive to the point of respiratory failure. Extreme caution in patients who may be susceptible to the intracranial effects of CO_2 retention (eg, with evidence of increased intracranial pressure or impaired consciousness). May obscure clinical course of head injuries. Caution with bradyarrhythmias. Anaphylaxis and hypersensitivity reported. Avoid use during labor and delivery. Caution with renal/hepatic impairment.

ADVERSE REACTIONS: Respiratory depression, circulatory depression, hypotension, shock, N/V, headache, constipation, dizziness, dyspnea, anxiety, somnolence, asthenia, confusion, depression.

INTERACTIONS: See Boxed Warning. Respiratory depression is more likely to occur when given with other drugs that depress respiration. Increased depressant effects with other CNS depressants (eg, other opioids, sedatives, hypnotics, general anesthetics, phenothiazines, tranquilizers, skeletal muscle relaxants, sedating antihistamines, alcoholic beverages); adjust dose if warranted. Avoid with grapefruit and grapefruit juice. CYP3A4 inducers may decrease levels. Not recommended with MAOIs or within 14 days of discontinuation of MAOIs.

PREGNANCY: Category C, not for use in nursing.

MECHANISM OF ACTION: Opioid analgesic; has not been established. Known to be μ-opioid receptor agonist; specific CNS opioid receptors for endogenous compounds with opioid-like activity have been identified throughout the brain and spinal cord and play a role in analgesic effects.

PHARMACOKINETICS: Absorption: Rapidly absorbed from buccal mucosa; more prolonged absorption of swallowed fentanyl from GI tract. Absolute bioavailability (50%). Administration of variable doses resulted in different pharmacokinetic parameters. **Distribution:** V_d=4L/kg; plasma protein binding (80-85%); crosses the placenta; found in breast milk. **Metabolism:** Liver and intestinal mucosa via CYP3A4; norfentanyl (metabolite). **Elimination:** Urine (<7%, unchanged), feces (1%, unchanged); $T_{1/2}$=7 hrs.

NURSING CONSIDERATIONS

Assessment: Assess for degree of opioid tolerance, previous opioid dose, level of pain intensity, type of pain, patient's general condition and medical status, and any other conditions where treatment is contraindicated or cautioned. Assess for hypersensitivity to the drug, renal/hepatic function, pregnancy/nursing status, and possible drug interactions.

Monitoring: Monitor for signs/symptoms of respiratory depression, impairment of mental/physical abilities, bradycardia, anaphylaxis/hypersensitivity, abuse/addiction, and other adverse reactions.

Patient Counseling: Advise to enroll in TIRF REMS Access program. Instruct to keep drug out of reach of children. Advise to take drug as prescribed and avoid sharing it with anyone else. Instruct to notify physician if breakthrough pain is not alleviated or worsens after taking the drug. Inform that drug may impair mental/physical abilities; caution against performing activities that require high level of attention (eg, driving/using heavy machinery). Advise not to combine with alcohol, sleep aids, or tranquilizers, except if ordered by the physician. Instruct to notify physician if pregnant or planning to become pregnant. Inform that frequent consumption may increase risk of dental decay; advise to consult dentist to ensure appropriate oral hygiene. Inform diabetics that drug contains approximately 2g sugar/U. Inform of proper storage, administration, and disposal.

Administration: Oral route. Should be sucked, not chewed, and consumed over 15 min. Refer to PI for proper administration. **Storage:** 20-25°C (68-77°F); excursions permitted between 15-30°C (59-86°F). Protect from freezing and moisture.

ACTIVASE   RX
alteplase (Genentech)

THERAPEUTIC CLASS: Thrombolytic agent

INDICATIONS: Management of acute myocardial infarction (AMI) in adults for the improvement of ventricular function following AMI, the reduction of incidence of congestive heart failure, and the reduction of mortality associated with AMI. Management of acute ischemic stroke (AIS) for improving neurological recovery and reducing the incidence of disability. Management of acute massive pulmonary embolism (PE) in adults for the lysis of acute pulmonary emboli, and for the lysis of pulmonary emboli accompanied by unstable hemodynamics.

DOSAGE: *Adults:* AMI: Administer as soon as possible after the onset of symptoms. Accelerated Infusion: Max Total Dose: 100mg. >67kg: Usual: 15mg IV bolus, then 50mg over next 30 min, and then 35mg over next 60 min. ≤67kg: Usual: 15mg IV bolus, then 0.75mg/kg (max 50mg) over next 30 min, then 0.50mg/kg (max 35mg) over the next 60 min. 3-hr Infusion: ≥65kg: Usual: 60mg in 1st hr (give 6-10mg as IV bolus), then 20mg over 2nd hr, and 20mg over 3rd hr. <65kg: 1.25mg/kg over 3 hrs. Refer to PI for further administration instructions. AIS: Usual: 0.9mg/kg IV over 1 hr with 10% of total dose as initial IV bolus over 1 min. Max Total Dose: 90mg. PE: Usual: 100mg IV infusion over 2 hrs. Institute or reinstitute heparin at end or immediately after infusion when PTT or thrombin time returns to ≤2X normal.

HOW SUPPLIED: Inj: 50mg, 100mg

CONTRAINDICATIONS: (AMI, PE) Active internal bleeding, history of cerebrovascular accident (CVA), recent intracranial/intraspinal surgery or trauma, intracranial neoplasm, arteriovenous (AV) malformation, or aneurysm, known bleeding diathesis, and severe uncontrolled HTN. (AIS) Evidence of intracranial hemorrhage on pretreatment evaluation; suspicion of subarachnoid hemorrhage on pretreatment evaluation; recent (within 3 months) intracranial or intraspinal surgery, serious head trauma or previous stroke; history of intracranial hemorrhage; uncontrolled HTN; seizure at the onset of stroke; active internal bleeding; intracranial neoplasm, AV malformation, or aneurysm; and known bleeding diathesis including current use of oral anticoagulants (eg, warfarin) or an INR >1.7 or a PT >15 sec, administration of heparin within 48 hrs preceding the onset of stroke and have an elevated activated PTT at presentation, and platelet count <100,000/mm^3.

WARNINGS/PRECAUTIONS: Internal bleeding and superficial/surface bleeding reported. Bleeding from recent puncture sites may occur as fibrin is lysed; careful attention to all potential bleeding sites (eg, catheter insertion sites, arterial/venous puncture sites, cutdown sites, needle puncture sites) is required. Avoid IM injection and nonessential handling of the patient; perform venipunctures carefully and only as required. Use an upper extremity vessel that is accessible to manual compression if an arterial puncture is necessary during infusion; apply pressure for at least 30 min, use a pressure dressing, and frequently check puncture site for evidence of bleeding. Immediately terminate infusion and any concomitant heparin if serious bleeding (not controllable by local pressure) occurs. Weigh benefits/risks of therapy with recent major surgery, cerebrovascular disease, recent GI or genitourinary bleeding, recent trauma, HTN (systolic BP ≥175mmHg and/or diastolic BP >110mmHg), left heart thrombus, acute pericarditis, subacute bacterial endocarditis, hemostatic defects (including those secondary to severe hepatic/renal disease), significant hepatic dysfunction, pregnancy, diabetic hemorrhagic retinopathy or other hemorrhagic ophthalmic conditions, septic thrombophlebitis or occluded AV cannula at a seriously infected site, advanced age (eg, >75 yrs old), and any other condition in which bleeding constitutes a significant hazard or would be particularly difficult to manage because of its location. Cholesterol embolism reported. Coronary thrombolysis may result in arrhythmias associated with reperfusion; antiarrhythmic therapy for bradycardia and/or ventricular irritability should be available when infusion is administered. Avoid noncompressible arterial puncture, and internal jugular and subclavian venous punctures. Minimize arterial and venous punctures. Orolingual angioedema reported in patients treated for AIS and AMI; monitor during and for several hrs after infusion for signs of orolingual angioedema. Promptly institute appropriate therapy and d/c infusion if angioedema is noted. Rare fatal cases of hemorrhage associated with traumatic intubation reported. D/C therapy if an anaphylactoid reaction occurs; caution with readministration. Lab test interaction may occur. (AIS) Initiate treatment within 3 hrs after the onset of stroke symptoms, and after exclusion of intracranial hemorrhage by a cranial computerized tomography (CT) scan or other diagnostic imaging method sensitive for the presence of hemorrhage. May initiate treatment prior to availability of coagulation study results in patients without recent use of PO anticoagulants or heparin. D/C infusion if pretreatment INR >1.7 or PT >15 sec or elevated active PTT is identified. Weigh benefits/risks of therapy with severe neurological deficit or major early infarct signs on a cranial CT scan. Treatment of patients with minor neurological deficit or with rapidly improving symptoms is not recommended. BP should be monitored frequently and controlled during and following administration. (AMI) Risk of stroke may offset the survival benefit of therapy in patients at a low risk for death from cardiac causes and who have high BP at the time of presentation. (PE) Treatment has not been shown to constitute adequate clinical treatment of underlying deep vein thrombosis (DVT). Consider possible risk of reembolization due to the lysis of underlying DVT.

ADVERSE REACTIONS: Bleeding, allergic-type reactions.

INTERACTIONS: See Contraindications. Increased risk of bleeding with heparin, vitamin K antagonists and drugs that alter platelets (eg, ASA, dipyridamole, abciximab) given before, during, or after alteplase therapy. Orolingual angioedema reported with concomitant ACE inhibitors.

PREGNANCY: Category C, caution in nursing.

MECHANISM OF ACTION: Tissue plasminogen activator; serine protease enzyme that has the property of fibrin-enhanced conversion of plasminogen to plasmin. Produces limited conversion of plasminogen in absence of fibrin. Binds to fibrin in thrombus and converts entrapped plasminogen to plasmin. Initiates local fibrinolysis with limited systemic proteolysis.

PHARMACOKINETICS: Metabolism: Liver. **Elimination:** $T_{1/2}$=<5 min (initial).

NURSING CONSIDERATIONS

Assessment: Assess for active internal bleeding, history of CVA; intracranial or intraspinal surgery or trauma; intracranial neoplasm, AV malformation, or aneurysm; known bleeding diathesis; presence or history of intracranial hemorrhage; recent (within 3 months) intracranial or intraspinal surgery, serious head trauma, or previous stroke; uncontrolled HTN; pregnancy/nursing status; and for any other conditions where treatment is contraindicated or cautioned. Assess for possible drug interactions. Confirm diagnosis of acute massive PE by objective means (eg, pulmonary angiography, noninvasive procedures). Assess INR, PT, activated PTT, and platelet count.

Monitoring: Monitor for signs/symptoms of bleeding, cholesterol embolism, allergic reactions, and other adverse reactions. Monitor for bleeding from recent puncture sites. Monitor during and for several hrs after infusion for signs of orolingual angioedema. In the management of AIS, monitor BP frequently and control during and following administration.

Patient Counseling: Inform about potential risks/benefits of therapy. Inform about risk of bleeding. Instruct to notify physician if any type of allergic reaction or any other adverse reaction develops during therapy.

Administration: IV route. Refer to PI for reconstitution and dilution instructions. **Storage:** Lyophilized: Controlled room temperature not to exceed 30°C (86°F), or under refrigeration 2-8°C (36-46°F). Protect from excessive exposure to light. Reconstituted: 2-30°C (36-86°F); use within 8 hrs following reconstitution.

ACTIVELLA   RX
norethindrone acetate - estradiol (Novo Nordisk)

> Should not be used for the prevention of cardiovascular (CV) disease or dementia. Increased risk of myocardial infarction (MI), stroke, invasive breast cancer, pulmonary embolism (PE), and deep vein thrombosis (DVT) in postmenopausal women (50-79 yrs of age) reported. Increased risk of developing probable dementia in postmenopausal women ≥65 yrs of age reported. Increased risk of endometrial cancer in women with a uterus who use unopposed estrogens. Perform adequate diagnostic measures, including endometrial sampling, to rule out malignancy in postmenopausal women with undiagnosed persistent or recurrent abnormal genital bleeding. Should be prescribed at the lowest effective dose and for the shortest duration consistent with treatment goals and risks.

THERAPEUTIC CLASS: Estrogen/progestogen combination

INDICATIONS: Treatment of moderate to severe vasomotor symptoms and/or vulvar/vaginal atrophy due to menopause and prevention of postmenopausal osteoporosis.

DOSAGE: *Adults:* Moderate to Severe Vasomotor Symptoms/Prevention of Postmenopausal Osteoporosis: 1 tab (1mg-0.5mg or 0.5mg-0.1mg) qd. Moderate to Severe Vulvar and Vaginal Atrophy: 1 tab (1mg-0.5mg) qd. Reevaluate treatment need periodically.

HOW SUPPLIED: Tab: (Estradiol-Norethindrone) 1mg-0.5mg, 0.5mg-0.1mg

CONTRAINDICATIONS: Undiagnosed abnormal genital bleeding, known/suspected/history of breast cancer, known/suspected estrogen-dependent neoplasia, active/history of DVT/PE, active/history of arterial thromboembolic disease (eg, stroke, MI), liver impairment or disease, known protein C/protein S/antithrombin deficiency or other known thrombophilic disorders, known/suspected pregnancy.

WARNINGS/PRECAUTIONS: D/C immediately if stroke, DVT, PE, or MI occurs or is suspected. Caution with risk factors for arterial vascular disease and/or venous thromboembolism. If feasible, d/c at least 4-6 weeks before surgery of the type associated with an increased risk of thromboembolism, or during periods of prolonged immobilization. May increase risk of ovarian cancer and gallbladder disease. May lead to severe hypercalcemia in patients with breast cancer and bone metastases; d/c and take appropriate measures if hypercalcemia occurs. Retinal vascular thrombosis reported; d/c pending exam if sudden partial/complete loss of vision, or sudden onset of proptosis, diplopia, or migraine occurs. D/C permanently if exam reveals papilledema or retinal vascular lesions. May elevate BP and thyroid-binding globulin levels. May elevate plasma TG levels leading to pancreatitis in women with preexisting hypertriglyceridemia; consider discontinuation if pancreatitis occurs. Caution with history of cholestatic jaundice associated with past estrogen use or with pregnancy; d/c in case of recurrence. May cause fluid retention; caution with conditions that might be influenced by this factor (eg, cardiac/renal impairment). Caution with hypoparathyroidism as estrogen-induced hypocalcemia may occur. May exacerbate endometriosis, asthma, diabetes mellitus, epilepsy, migraine, porphyria, systemic lupus erythematosus, and hepatic hemangiomas; use with caution. May exacerbate symptoms of angioedema in women with hereditary angioedema. May affect certain endocrine and blood components in lab tests.

ADVERSE REACTIONS: Back pain, headache, nasopharyngitis, sinusitis, insomnia, upper respiratory tract infection, breast pain, postmenopausal bleeding, vaginal hemorrhage, endometrial thickening, uterine fibroid, pain in extremities, nausea, diarrhea, viral infection.

INTERACTIONS: CYP3A4 inducers (eg, St. John's wort preparations, phenobarbital, carbamazepine) may decrease levels, which may decrease therapeutic effects and/or change uterine bleeding profile. CYP3A4 inhibitors (eg, erythromycin, ketoconazole, ritonavir) may increase levels, which may result in side effects. Patients concomitantly receiving thyroid hormone replacement therapy and estrogens may require increased doses of their thyroid replacement therapy; monitor thyroid function.

PREGNANCY: Contraindicated in pregnancy, not for use in nursing.

MECHANISM OF ACTION: Estradiol: Estrogen; binds to nuclear receptors in estrogen-responsive tissues. Reduces elevated levels of gonadotropins, luteinizing hormone, and follicle-stimulating hormone in postmenopausal women. Norethindrone: Progestin; enhances cellular differentiation and opposes actions of estrogens by decreasing estrogen receptor levels, increasing local metabolism of estrogens to less active metabolites, or inducing gene products that blunt cellular responses to estrogen.

PHARMACOKINETICS: Absorption: Administration of various doses resulted in different parameters. **Distribution:** Found in breast milk. Estradiol: Sex hormone-binding globulin (SHBG) (37%); albumin (61%). Norethindrone: SHBG (36%); albumin (61%). **Metabolism:** Estradiol: Liver to estrone (metabolite); estriol (major urinary metabolite); enterohepatic recirculation via sulfate and glucuronide conjugation; biliary secretion of conjugates into the intestine; hydrolysis in the intestine followed by reabsorption. Norethindrone: isomers of 5α-dihydro-norethindrone, tetrahydro-norethindrone (metabolites). **Elimination:** Estradiol: Urine (unchanged and metabolites); $T_{1/2}$=12-14 hrs. Norethindrone: $T_{1/2}$=8-11 hrs.

NURSING CONSIDERATIONS

Assessment: Assess for undiagnosed abnormal genital bleeding, presence/history of breast cancer, estrogen-dependent neoplasia, active/history of DVT/PE/arterial thromboembolic disease, liver impairment/disease, thrombophilic disorders, drug hypersensitivity, pregnancy/nursing status, any other conditions where treatment is contraindicated or cautioned, and for possible drug interactions.

Monitoring: Monitor for signs/symptoms of CV disease, malignant neoplasms, dementia, gallbladder disease, hypercalcemia, visual abnormalities, BP and plasma TG level elevations, pancreatitis, cholestatic jaundice, fluid retention, exacerbation of endometriosis and other conditions, and other adverse reactions. Perform annual breast exam; schedule mammography based on age, risk factors, and prior mammogram results. Perform adequate diagnostic measures (eg, endometrial sampling) to rule out malignancies in cases of undiagnosed, persistent, or recurring abnormal genital bleeding. Regularly monitor thyroid function if on thyroid hormone replacement therapy.

Patient Counseling: Inform of the importance of reporting vaginal bleeding to physician as soon as possible. Advise of possible serious adverse reactions of therapy (eg, CV disorders, malignant neoplasms, probable dementia) and of possible less serious, but common adverse reactions (eg, headache, breast pain and tenderness, N/V). Instruct to have yearly breast examinations by a healthcare provider and to perform monthly breast self-examinations.

Administration: Oral route. **Storage:** 20-25°C (68-77°F); excursions permitted to 15-30°C (59-86°F). Protect from light.

ACTONEL   RX
risedronate sodium (Warner Chilcott)

THERAPEUTIC CLASS: Bisphosphonate

INDICATIONS: Treatment and prevention of osteoporosis in postmenopausal women, and glucocorticoid-induced osteoporosis in men and women who are either initiating or continuing systemic glucocorticoid treatment (daily dosage of ≥7.5mg of prednisone or equivalent) for chronic diseases. Treatment to increase bone mass in men with osteoporosis, and of Paget's disease of bone in men and women.

DOSAGE: *Adults:* Treatment/Prevention of Postmenopausal Osteoporosis: 5mg qd, or 35mg once a week, or 150mg once a month. To Increase Bone Mass in Men with Osteoporosis: 35mg once a week. Treatment/Prevention of Glucocorticoid-Induced Osteoporosis: 5mg qd. Paget's Disease: 30mg qd for 2 months. May consider retreatment (following post-treatment observation of at least 2 months) if relapse occurs, or if treatment fails to normalize serum alkaline phosphatase. Periodically reevaluate the need for continued therapy. Refer to PI for instructions for missed doses.

HOW SUPPLIED: Tab: 5mg, 30mg, 35mg, 150mg

CONTRAINDICATIONS: Esophageal abnormalities that delay esophageal emptying (eg, stricture or achalasia), inability to stand or sit upright for at least 30 min, and hypocalcemia.

WARNINGS/PRECAUTIONS: Consider discontinuation after 3-5 yrs of use in patients at low-risk for fracture; periodically reevaluate risk for fracture in patients who d/c therapy. Contains same active ingredient as Atelvia; do not treat with Actonel if on concomitant therapy with Atelvia. May cause local irritation of the upper GI mucosa; caution with active upper GI problems (eg, Barrett's esophagus, dysphagia, esophageal diseases, gastritis, duodenitis, ulcers). Esophageal reactions (eg, esophagitis, esophageal ulcers/erosions) reported; d/c if dysphagia, odynophagia, retrosternal pain, or new/worsening heartburn develops. Use therapy under appropriate supervision in patients who cannot comply with dosing instructions due to mental disability. Gastric and duodenal ulcers reported. Hypocalcemia reported; treat hypocalcemia and other disturbances of bone and mineral metabolism before therapy, and ensure adequate Ca^{2+} and vitamin D intake. Osteonecrosis of the jaw (ONJ) reported; risk may increase with duration of exposure to drug.

ACTOPLUS MET XR

For patients requiring invasive dental procedures, discontinuation of treatment may reduce risk for ONJ. Consider discontinuation if ONJ develops. Severe and occasionally incapacitating bone, joint, and/or muscle pain reported; consider discontinuation if severe symptoms develop. Atypical, low-energy, or low-trauma fractures of the femoral shaft reported; evaluate any patient with a history of bisphosphonate exposure who presents with thigh/groin pain to rule out an incomplete femur fracture, and consider interruption of therapy. Not recommended with severe renal impairment (CrCl <30mL/min). Ascertain sex steroid hormonal status and consider appropriate replacement before initiating therapy for the treatment and prevention of glucocorticoid-induced osteoporosis. May interfere with the use of bone-imaging agents.

ADVERSE REACTIONS: Back pain, arthralgia, abdominal pain, dyspepsia, acute phase reaction, allergic reaction, arthritis, diarrhea, headache, infection, urinary tract infection, bronchitis, HTN, nausea, rash.

INTERACTIONS: Ca^{2+} supplements, antacids, or oral medications containing divalent cations will interfere with absorption; take such medications at a different time of the day.

PREGNANCY: Category C, not for use in nursing.

MECHANISM OF ACTION: Bisphosphonate; has an affinity for hydroxyapatite crystals in bone and acts as an antiresorptive agent. Inhibits osteoclast.

PHARMACOKINETICS: Absorption: Absolute bioavailability (0.63%) (30mg); T_{max}=1 hr. **Distribution:** V_d=13.8L/kg; plasma protein binding (24%). **Elimination:** Urine (1/2 of the absorbed dose), feces (unchanged [unabsorbed drug]); $T_{1/2}$=561 hrs (osteopenic postmenopausal women).

NURSING CONSIDERATIONS

Assessment: Assess for esophageal abnormalities, ability to stand or sit upright for at least 30 min, active upper GI problems, mental disability, hypocalcemia, disturbances of bone and mineral metabolism, risk for ONJ, renal impairment, drug hypersensitivity, any other conditions where treatment is contraindicated or cautioned, pregnancy/nursing status, and possible drug interactions. For glucocorticoid-induced osteoporosis treatment/prevention, assess sex steroid hormonal status.

Monitoring: Monitor for signs/symptoms of ONJ, atypical femoral fracture, esophageal reactions, hypocalcemia, musculoskeletal pain, and other adverse events. Periodically reevaluate the need for continued therapy.

Patient Counseling: Instruct to carefully follow dosing instructions and on what to do if doses are missed. Advise to consult physician before continuing treatment if symptoms of esophageal disease develop. Advise that drug should be taken at least 30 min before the 1st food or drink of the day other than water. Advise to take with a full glass of plain water (6-8 oz.) and to avoid the use of water with supplements (eg, mineral water). Advise to avoid lying down for 30 min after taking the drug. Instruct to take supplemental Ca^{2+} and vitamin D if dietary intake is inadequate. Counsel to consider weight-bearing exercise along with the modification of certain behavioral factors (eg, excessive cigarette smoking and/or alcohol consumption) if these factors exist. Advise to consult physician any time they have a medical problem they think may be from treatment.

Administration: Oral route. Take at least 30 min before the 1st food or drink of the day other than water, and before taking any oral medication or supplementation. Swallow tabs whole; do not chew or suck the tab. **Storage:** 20-25°C (68-77°F).

ACTOPLUS MET XR   RX

metformin HCl - pioglitazone (Takeda)

> Thiazolidinediones, including pioglitazone, cause or exacerbate congestive heart failure (CHF) in some patients. After initiation and dose increases, monitor carefully for signs and symptoms of heart failure (HF); manage accordingly and consider discontinuation or dose reduction if HF develops. Not recommended with symptomatic HF. Contraindicated with established NYHA Class III or IV HF. Lactic acidosis may occur due to metformin accumulation; risk increases with conditions such as sepsis, dehydration, excess alcohol intake, hepatic/renal impairment, and acute CHF. If acidosis is suspected, d/c therapy and hospitalize patient immediately.

OTHER BRAND NAMES: Actoplus Met (Takeda)

THERAPEUTIC CLASS: Biguanide/thiazolidinedione

INDICATIONS: Adjunct to diet and exercise to improve glycemic control in adults with type 2 diabetes mellitus (DM) when treatment with both pioglitazone and metformin is appropriate.

DOSAGE: *Adults:* Take with meals to reduce GI side effects of metformin. Initial: 15mg-500mg bid or 15mg-850mg qd (tab), or 15mg-1000mg or 30mg-1000mg qd (tab, Extended-Release [ER]). With NYHA Class I or II CHF: 15mg-500mg or 15mg-850mg qd (tab), or 15mg-1000mg or 30mg-1000mg qd (tab, ER). Inadequately Controlled on Metformin Monotherapy: 15mg-500mg bid or 15mg-850mg qd or bid (tab), or 15mg-1000mg bid or 30mg-1000mg qd (tab, ER), depending on the dose of metformin already being taken. Inadequately Controlled on

Pioglitazone Monotherapy: 15mg-500mg bid or 15mg-850mg qd (tab), or 15mg-1000mg bid or 30mg-1000mg qd (tab, ER). Titrate: Gradually adjust, PRN, after assessing adequacy of response and tolerability. Changing from Combination Therapy of Pioglitazone plus Metformin as Separate Tabs: Take at doses that are as close as possible to the dose of pioglitazone and metformin already being taken. Max: 45mg-2550mg/day (tab) or 45mg-2000mg/day (tab, ER). Metformin doses >2000mg may be better tolerated given tid. Concomitant Use with an Insulin Secretagogue (eg, Sulfonylurea): Reduce insulin secretagogue dose if hypoglycemia occurs. Concomitant Use with an Insulin: Decrease insulin dose by 10-25% if hypoglycemia occurs; further insulin dose adjustments should be individualized based on glycemic response. Concomitant Use with Strong CYP2C8 Inhibitors (eg, Gemfibrozil): Max: 15mg-850mg/day (tab) or 15mg-1000mg/day (tab, ER). Elderly: Do not titrate to max dose.

HOW SUPPLIED: (Pioglitazone-Metformin) Tab, ER (XR): 15mg-1000mg, 30mg-1000mg; (Actoplus Met) Tab: 15mg-500mg, 15mg-850mg

CONTRAINDICATIONS: NYHA Class III or IV HF, renal impairment (eg, SrCr ≥1.5mg/dL [males], ≥1.4mg/dL [females], or abnormal CrCl), metabolic acidosis, including diabetic ketoacidosis.

WARNINGS/PRECAUTIONS: Not for use in type 1 DM or for treatment of diabetic ketoacidosis. Dose-related edema reported; caution in patients with edema or at risk for CHF. Fatal and nonfatal hepatic failure reported; obtain LFTs prior to initiation; caution with abnormal LFTs. Measure LFTs promptly in patients who report symptoms that may indicate liver injury. D/C if ALT >3X ULN; do not restart if cause of abnormal LFTs not established or if ALT remains >3X ULN with total bilirubin >2X ULN without alternative etiologies. May use with caution in patients with lesser ALT elevations or bilirubin and with an alternate probable cause. Avoid with clinical or laboratory evidence of hepatic disease. Increased incidence of bone fracture reported in females. Not for use in patients with active bladder cancer; consider benefits versus risks in patients with a prior history of bladder cancer. Caution in patients susceptible to hypoglycemic effects, such as elderly, debilitated/malnourished patients, and those with adrenal/pituitary insufficiency, or alcohol intoxication. Macular edema reported; promptly refer to an ophthalmologist if visual symptoms occur. May result in ovulation in some premenopausal anovulatory women, which may increase risk for pregnancy; adequate contraception is recommended. Assess renal function before initiation of therapy and at least annually thereafter; d/c evidence of renal impairment. D/C at the time of or prior to radiologic studies involving the use of intravascular iodinated contrast materials, withhold for 48 hrs subsequent to the procedure, and reinstitute only if renal function is normal. D/C in hypoxic states (eg, acute CHF, shock, acute myocardial infarction). Temporarily suspend for any surgical procedure (except minor procedures not associated with restricted food and fluid intake); restart when oral intake is resumed and renal function is normal. May decrease serum vitamin B12 levels; monitor hematologic parameters annually. Caution in elderly.

ADVERSE REACTIONS: Lactic acidosis, CHF, diarrhea, headache, edema, upper respiratory tract infection, weight gain.

INTERACTIONS: See Dosage. Risk for hypoglycemia with insulin or other antidiabetic medications (particularly insulin secretagogues [eg, sulfonylureas]); may require a reduction in the dose of the concomitant antidiabetic medication. May be difficult to recognize hypoglycemia with β-adrenergic blocking drugs. Caution with drugs that may affect renal function or result in significant hemodynamic change or may interfere with the disposition of metformin (eg, cationic drugs eliminated by renal tubular secretion). Alcohol potentiates the effect of metformin on lactate metabolism; avoid excessive alcohol intake. Increased exposure and $T_{1/2}$ with strong CYP2C8 inhibitors (eg, gemfibrozil). CYP2C8 inducers (eg, rifampin) may decrease exposure; if a CYP2C8 inducer is started or stopped during treatment, changes in diabetes treatment may be needed based on clinical response. Topiramate or other carbonic anhydrase inhibitors (eg, zonisamide, acetazolamide, dichlorphenamide) may induce metabolic acidosis; use with caution. Cationic drugs that are eliminated by renal tubular secretion (eg, cimetidine, amiloride, digoxin, morphine, procainamide, quinidine, quinine, ranitidine, triamterene, trimethoprim, vancomycin) may potentially produce an interaction; monitor and adjust dose of therapy and/or the interfering drug. Observe for loss of blood glucose control with thiazides and other diuretics, corticosteroids, phenothiazines, thyroid products, estrogens, oral contraceptives, phenytoin, nicotinic acid, sympathomimetics, calcium channel blockers, and isoniazid; observe for hypoglycemia when such drugs are withdrawn during therapy. Pioglitazone: May cause dose-related fluid retention when used with other antidiabetic medications, most commonly with insulin.

PREGNANCY: Category C, not for use in nursing.

MECHANISM OF ACTION: Pioglitazone: Thiazolidinedione; insulin-sensitizing agent that acts primarily by enhancing peripheral glucose utilization. Decreases insulin resistance in the periphery and in the liver resulting in increased insulin-dependent glucose disposal and decreased hepatic glucose output. Metformin: Biguanide; decreases endogenous hepatic glucose production, decreases intestinal absorption of glucose, and improves insulin sensitivity by increasing peripheral glucose uptake and utilization.

PHARMACOKINETICS: Absorption: Pioglitazone: T_{max}=within 2 hrs, 3-4 hrs (with food). Metformin: Absolute bioavailability (50-60%) (fasted). **Distribution:** Pioglitazone: V_d=0.63L/kg; plasma protein binding (>99%). Metformin: V_d=654L (immediate-release). **Metabolism:**

Pioglitazone: Hydroxylation and oxidation (extensive), CYP2C8, CYP3A4; M-III [keto derivative] and M-IV [hydroxyl derivative] (major active metabolites). **Elimination:** Pioglitazone: Urine (15-30%), bile and feces; $T_{1/2}$=3-7 hrs, 16-24 hrs (metabolites). Metformin: Urine (90%); $T_{1/2}$=6.2 hrs (plasma), 17.6 hrs (blood).

NURSING CONSIDERATIONS

Assessment: Assess for HF or risk of HF, metabolic acidosis, risk factors for lactic acidosis, previous hypersensitivity to the drug, type of DM, diabetic ketoacidosis, edema, bone health, active/history of bladder cancer, inadequate vitamin B12 or Ca^{2+} intake/absorption, any other conditions where treatment is cautioned, pregnancy/nursing status, and possible drug interactions. Assess if patient is planning to undergo any surgical procedure or radiologic studies involving the use of intravascular iodinated contrast materials. Obtain baseline LFTs, renal function, FPG and HbA1c levels, and hematologic parameters.

Monitoring: Monitor for signs/symptoms of HF, liver injury, lactic acidosis, edema, fractures, visual symptoms, hypoxic states, and other adverse reactions. Monitor renal function, especially in elderly, at least annually. Monitor hematologic parameters annually. Perform routine serum vitamin B12 measurements at 2- to 3-yr intervals in patients predisposed to developing subnormal vitamin B12 levels. Monitor FPG, and HbA1c. Periodically monitor LFTs in patients with liver disease.

Patient Counseling: Advise on the importance of adherence to dietary instructions and regular testing of blood glucose, HbA1c, renal function, and hematologic parameters. Advise to seek medical advice promptly during periods of stress (eg, fever, trauma, infection, or surgery) as medication requirements may change. Instruct to promptly report any signs/symptoms of bladder cancer (eg, macroscopic hematuria, dysuria, urinary urgency), or HF (eg, unusually rapid increase in weight or edema, SOB). Inform of the risk of lactic acidosis; instruct to d/c therapy immediately and notify physician if unexplained hyperventilation, myalgia, GI symptoms, malaise, unusual somnolence, or other nonspecific symptoms occur. Counsel against excessive alcohol intake while on therapy. Instruct to d/c use and seek medical advice promptly if signs/symptoms of hepatotoxicity (eg, unexplained N/V, abdominal pain, fatigue, anorexia, or dark urine) occur. Counsel premenopausal women to use adequate contraception during treatment. Inform that hypoglycemia can occur; explain the risks, symptoms, and appropriate management. Instruct to take drug as prescribed and that any change in dosing should only be done if directed by physician. (Tab, ER) Inform that the inactive ingredients may occasionally be eliminated in the feces as a soft mass that may resemble the original tab.

Administration: Oral route. Take with meals. (Tab, ER) Swallow whole; do not chew, cut, or crush.
Storage: 25°C (77°F); excursions permitted to 15-30°C (59-86°F). Keep container tightly closed, and protect from moisture and humidity.

ACTOS   RX
pioglitazone (Takeda)

> Thiazolidinediones cause or exacerbate congestive heart failure (CHF) in some patients. After initiation and dose increases, monitor carefully for signs and symptoms of heart failure (HF) and manage accordingly; consider discontinuation or dose reduction. Not recommended in patients with symptomatic HF. Contraindicated with established NYHA Class III or IV HF.

THERAPEUTIC CLASS: Thiazolidinedione

INDICATIONS: Adjunct to diet and exercise to improve glycemic control in adults with type 2 diabetes mellitus (DM).

DOSAGE: *Adults:* Without CHF: Initial: 15mg or 30mg qd. With CHF (NYHA Class I or II): Initial: 15mg qd. Titrate: In increments of 15mg. Max: 45mg qd. With Insulin Secretagogue: Reduce dose of insulin secretagogue if hypoglycemia occurs. With Insulin: Decrease insulin dose by 10-25% if hypoglycemia occurs. Further insulin dose adjustment should be individualized based on glycemic response. With Gemfibrozil/Other Strong CYP2C8 Inhibitors: Max: 15mg qd.

HOW SUPPLIED: Tab: 15mg, 30mg, 45mg

CONTRAINDICATIONS: Established NYHA Class III or IV HF.

WARNINGS/PRECAUTIONS: Not for use in treatment of type 1 DM or diabetic ketoacidosis. Fatal and nonfatal hepatic failure reported. May use with caution in patients with lesser ALT elevations or bilirubin and with an alternate probable cause. Obtain LFTs prior to initiation; caution with liver disease/abnormal LFTs. D/C if ALT >3X ULN; do not restart if cause of abnormal LFTs not established or if ALT remains >3X ULN with total bilirubin >2X ULN without alternative etiologies. Not for use in patients with active bladder cancer; consider benefits versus risks in patients with a prior or history of bladder cancer. New onset or worsening of edema reported; caution in patients with edema and in patients at risk for CHF. Increased incidence of bone fractures reported in females.

Macular edema reported; refer to an ophthalmologist if visual symptoms develop. Ovulation in premenopausal anovulatory patients may occur; use adequate contraception.

ADVERSE REACTIONS: CHF, upper respiratory tract infection, hypoglycemia, edema, headache, cardiac failure, pain in extremity, sinusitis, back pain, myalgia, pharyngitis, chest pain.

INTERACTIONS: Increased exposure and $T_{1/2}$ with CYP2C8 inhibitors (eg, gemfibrozil). Decreased exposure with CYP2C8 inducers (eg, rifampin). Risk of fluid retention and hypoglycemia with insulin and other antidiabetic medications (eg, insulin secretagogues such as sulfonylureas).

PREGNANCY: Category C, not for use in nursing.

MECHANISM OF ACTION: Thiazolidinedione; decreases insulin resistance in the periphery and liver, resulting in increased insulin-dependent glucose disposal and decreased hepatic glucose output.

PHARMACOKINETICS: Absorption: T_{max}=Within 2 hrs, 3-4 hrs (with food). **Distribution:** V_d=0.63L/kg; plasma protein binding (>99%). **Metabolism:** Hydroxylation and oxidation (extensive), CYP2C8, CYP3A4; M-III [keto derivative] and M-IV [hydroxyl derivative] (active metabolites). **Elimination:** Urine (15-30%), bile and feces; $T_{1/2}$=3-7 hrs (pioglitazone), 16-24 hrs (metabolites).

NURSING CONSIDERATIONS

Assessment: Assess for previous hypersensitivity, HF, edema, risk factors for developing HF, liver disease, bone health, active/history of bladder cancer, pregnancy/nursing status, and possible drug interactions. Obtain baseline LFTs.

Monitoring: Monitor for signs and symptoms of HF, edema, weight gain, hematological changes (eg, decreases in Hgb, Hct), liver injury, macular edema, bone fractures, ovulation in premenopausal anovulatory women, and other adverse reactions. Perform periodic measurements of FPG and HbA1c. Periodically monitor LFTs in patients with liver disease. Perform periodic eye exams.

Patient Counseling: Advise to adhere to dietary instructions and have blood glucose and glycosylated Hgb levels tested regularly. Instruct to seek medical advice promptly during periods of stress (eg, fever, trauma, infection, or surgery) and report rapid increase in weight or edema, SOB, or other symptoms of HF to physician. Instruct to d/c and consult physician if unexplained N/V, abdominal pain, anorexia, fatigue, or dark urine occurs. Advise to report any signs of macroscopic hematuria or other symptoms such as dysuria or urinary urgency. Advise to take qd with or without meals. If dose is missed, advise to not double the dose the following day. Inform about the risk of hypoglycemia when using with insulin or other antidiabetic medications. Inform that therapy may result in ovulation in some premenopausal anovulatory women; recommend adequate contraception for all premenopausal women.

Administration: Oral route. Take without regard to meals. **Storage:** 25°C (77°F); excursions permitted to 15-30°C (59-86°F). Protect from light, moisture, and humidity.

ACULAR   RX
ketorolac tromethamine (Allergan)

THERAPEUTIC CLASS: NSAID

INDICATIONS: Temporary relief of ocular itching due to seasonal allergic conjunctivitis. Treatment of postoperative inflammation in patients who have undergone cataract extraction.

DOSAGE: *Adults:* Ocular Itching: 1 drop qid to the affected eye(s). Postoperative Inflammation: 1 drop to affected eye(s) qid beginning 24 hrs after cataract surgery and continuing through the first 2 weeks of the postoperative period. With Other Topical Eye Medications: Give at least 5 min apart.
Pediatrics: ≥2 Yrs: Ocular Itching: 1 drop qid to the affected eye(s). Postoperative Inflammation: 1 drop to affected eye(s) qid beginning 24 hrs after cataract surgery and continuing through the first 2 weeks of the postoperative period. With Other Topical Eye Medications: Give at least 5 min apart.

HOW SUPPLIED: Sol: 0.5% [5mL]

WARNINGS/PRECAUTIONS: May slow or delay healing, or result in keratitis. Potential for cross-sensitivity to acetylsalicylic acid (ASA), phenylacetic acid derivatives, and other NSAIDs; caution with previous sensitivities to these agents. Bronchospasm or exacerbation of asthma reported with known hypersensitivity to ASA/NSAIDs or past history of asthma. Increased bleeding of ocular tissues (eg, hyphemas) reported in conjunction with ocular surgery; caution with known bleeding tendencies. Continued use may result in sight-threatening epithelial breakdown, corneal thinning, erosion, ulceration, or perforation; d/c if corneal epithelial breakdown occurs and monitor for corneal health. Caution with complicated ocular surgeries, corneal denervation, corneal epithelial defects, diabetes mellitus (DM), ocular surface diseases (eg, dry eye syndrome), rheumatoid arthritis (RA), or repeat ocular surgeries within a short period of time. Use for >1 day prior to surgery or beyond 14 days postsurgery may increase risk for occurrence and severity of corneal adverse events. Do not administer while patient is wearing contact lenses. Avoid in late pregnancy.

ADVERSE REACTIONS: Stinging, burning, superficial keratitis, ocular infections, allergic reactions, ocular inflammation/irritation, corneal edema, iritis.

INTERACTIONS: Caution with medications that may prolong bleeding time. May increase potential for healing problems with topical steroids.

PREGNANCY: Category C, caution in nursing.

MECHANISM OF ACTION: NSAID; thought to inhibit prostaglandin biosynthesis.

NURSING CONSIDERATIONS

Assessment: Assess for previous hypersensitivity to the drug or cross-sensitivity to ASA, phenylacetic acid derivatives, and other NSAIDs, history of asthma, bleeding tendencies, complicated or repeated ocular surgeries, corneal denervation, corneal epithelial defects, DM, ocular surface diseases, RA, contact lens use, pregnancy/nursing status, and possible drug interactions.

Monitoring: Monitor for hypersensitivity reactions, healing problems, keratitis, increased bleeding of ocular tissues in conjunction with ocular surgery, and evidence of epithelial corneal breakdown.

Patient Counseling: Inform of the possibility that slow or delayed healing may occur. Instruct to avoid allowing the tip of the bottle to contact the eye or surrounding structures. Advise to use 1 bottle for ou following bilateral ocular surgery. Advise not to administer while wearing contact lenses and to seek physician's advice if an intercurrent ocular condition (eg, trauma or infection) develops, or in case of ocular surgery. Advise to administer at least 5 min apart if >1 ophthalmic medication is being used.

Administration: Ocular route. **Storage:** 15-25°C (59-77°F). Protect from light.

ACULAR LS   RX
ketorolac tromethamine (Allergan)

THERAPEUTIC CLASS: NSAID

INDICATIONS: Reduction of ocular pain and burning/stinging following corneal refractive surgery.

DOSAGE: *Adults:* 1 drop qid in the operated eye PRN for up to 4 days following surgery. *Pediatrics:* ≥3 Yrs: 1 drop qid in the operated eye PRN for up to 4 days following surgery.

HOW SUPPLIED: Sol: 0.4% [5mL]

WARNINGS/PRECAUTIONS: Potential cross-sensitivity to acetylsalicylic acid, phenylacetic acid derivatives, and other NSAIDs; caution with previous sensitivities to these drugs. May increase bleeding of ocular tissues (including hyphemas) in conjunction with ocular surgery; caution with known bleeding tendencies. May slow/delay healing or result in keratitis. Continued use may result in epithelial breakdown, corneal thinning, erosion, ulceration, or perforation; d/c if corneal epithelium breakdown occurs and closely monitor for corneal health. Caution with complicated ocular surgeries, corneal denervation, corneal epithelial defects, diabetes mellitus (DM), ocular surface diseases (eg, dry eye syndrome), rheumatoid arthritis (RA), or repeat ocular surgeries within a short period of time. Use for >24 hrs prior to surgery or beyond 14 days postsurgery may increase risk for occurrence and severity of corneal adverse events. Avoid in late pregnancy.

ADVERSE REACTIONS: Transient stinging/burning, allergic reactions, corneal edema, iritis, ocular inflammation/irritation/pain, superficial keratitis, superficial ocular infections.

INTERACTIONS: Concomitant use of topical NSAIDs and topical steroids may increase potential for healing problems. Caution with other medications that may prolong bleeding time.

PREGNANCY: Category C, caution in nursing.

MECHANISM OF ACTION: NSAID; inhibits prostaglandin biosynthesis.

PHARMACOKINETICS: Absorption: C_{max}=960ng/mL (10mg administered systemically).

NURSING CONSIDERATIONS

Assessment: Assess for drug hypersensitivity, cross-sensitivity reactions, bleeding tendencies, complicated ocular surgeries, corneal denervation, corneal epithelial defects, DM, ocular surface diseases, RA, and possible drug interactions.

Monitoring: Monitor for bleeding of ocular tissues, healing problems, keratitis, corneal epithelial breakdown, and corneal thinning/erosion/ulceration/perforation.

Patient Counseling: Advise not to use while wearing contact lenses.

Ocular route. Storage: 15-25°C (59-77°F).

ADALAT CC   RX
nifedipine (Bayer Healthcare)

OTHER BRAND NAMES: Nifediac CC (Teva) - Afeditab CR (Watson)

THERAPEUTIC CLASS: Calcium channel blocker (dihydropyridine)

INDICATIONS: Treatment of HTN alone or in combination with other antihypertensive agents.

DOSAGE: *Adults:* Individualize dose. Initial: 30mg qd on an empty stomach. Titrate: Increase dose over a 7-14 day period based on therapeutic efficacy and safety. Maint: Usual: 30-60mg qd. Max: 90mg qd. Elderly: Start at low end of dosing range.

HOW SUPPLIED: Tab, Extended-Release: (Adalat CC) 30mg, 60mg, 90mg, (Afeditab CR) 30mg, 60mg, (Nifediac CC) 30mg, 60mg, 90mg

CONTRAINDICATIONS: (Adalat CC) Cardiogenic shock and concomitant use with strong P450 inducers (eg, rifampin).

WARNINGS/PRECAUTIONS: May cause hypotension; monitor BP initially or with titration. May increase frequency, duration, and/or severity of angina or acute myocardial infarction (MI) upon starting or at time of dose increase, particularly with severe obstructive coronary artery disease (CAD). May develop congestive heart failure (CHF), especially with tight aortic stenosis or β-blockers. Peripheral edema may occur; rule out peripheral edema caused by left ventricular dysfunction if HTN is complicated by CHF. Transient elevations of enzymes (eg, alkaline phosphatase, CPK, LDH, SGOT, SGPT), cholestasis with/without jaundice, and allergic hepatitis reported rarely. May decrease platelet aggregation and increase bleeding time. Lab test interactions may occur. Reversible elevations in BUN and SrCr reported rarely in patients with chronic renal insufficiency. Caution with renal/hepatic impairment and in elderly. Adalat CC: Reduced clearance in cirrhosis; initiate lowest dose possible. Contains lactose; avoid with hereditary galactose intolerance problems, Lapp lactase deficiency, and glucose-galactose malabsorption. Nifediac CC: Contains tartrazine, which may cause allergic-type reactions in certain susceptible persons (eg, patients with aspirin hypersensitivity).

ADVERSE REACTIONS: Peripheral edema, headache, flushing, heat sensation, dizziness, fatigue, asthenia, nausea, constipation.

INTERACTIONS: See Contraindications. β-blockers may increase risk of CHF, severe hypotension, or angina exacerbation; avoid abrupt β-blocker withdrawal. Severe hypotension and/or increased fluid volume may occur with β-blockers and fentanyl or other narcotic analgesics. May increase plasma levels of digoxin; monitor digoxin levels when initiating, adjusting, and discontinuing therapy. May increase PT with coumarin anticoagulants. Monitor with other medications known to lower BP. Enhanced hypotensive effect with benazepril and timolol. Avoid with grapefruit juice; stop grapefruit juice intake at least 3 days prior to therapy. Increased exposure with CYP3A inhibitors (eg, ketoconazole, itraconazole, fluconazole, erythromycin, clarithromycin, nefazodone, fluoxetine, diltiazem, verapamil, cimetidine, quinupristin/dalfopristin, amprenavir, atazanavir, delavirdine, fosamprenavir, indinavir, nelfinavir, ritonavir, saquinavir), valproic acid, and doxazosin; monitor BP and consider dose reduction. Increased levels with quinidine; monitor HR and adjust dose if necessary. Monitor blood glucose levels and consider dose adjustment with acarbose. May increase plasma levels of metformin. May increase exposure of tacrolimus; monitor blood levels and consider dose reduction. May decrease doxazosin levels; monitor BP and reduce dose. May inhibit metabolism of CYP3A substrates. Afeditab CR/Nifediac CC: Decreased exposure with CYP3A4 inducers (eg, rifampin, rifapentine, phenytoin, phenobarbitone, carbamazepine, St. John's wort); monitor BP and consider dose adjustment. Adalat CC: May increase the BP-lowering effects of diuretics, PDE-5 inhibitors, and α-methyldopa. Magnesium sulfate IV in pregnant women may cause excessive fall in BP. Increased plasma concentrations with cisapride.

PREGNANCY: Category C, not for use in nursing.

MECHANISM OF ACTION: Calcium channel blocker (dihydropyridine); inhibits the transmembrane influx of Ca^{2+} ions into vascular smooth muscle and cardiac muscle. Involves peripheral arterial vasodilation and reduction in peripheral vascular resistance, resulting in reduced arterial BP.

PHARMACOKINETICS: Absorption: Complete; T_{max}=2.5-5 hrs; (90mg) C_{max}=115ng/mL. **Distribution:** Plasma protein binding (92-98%); found in breast milk. **Metabolism:** Liver via CYP3A4. **Elimination:** Urine (60-80%, metabolite; <0.1%, unchanged); feces (metabolite); $T_{1/2}$=7 hrs.

NURSING CONSIDERATIONS

Assessment: Assess for previous hypersensitivity to the drug, CHF, severe obstructive CAD, aortic stenosis, hepatic/renal impairment, pregnancy/nursing status, and possible drug interactions. (Adalat CC) Assess for cirrhosis, hereditary galactose intolerance problems, Lapp lactase deficiency, and glucose-galactose malabsorption. (Nifediac CC) Assess for susceptibility for tartrazine hypersensitivity (eg, aspirin hypersensitivity).

Monitoring: Monitor for excessive hypotension, increased frequency, duration and/or severity of angina and/or acute MI (especially during initiation and dose titration), CHF, peripheral edema, cholestasis with/without jaundice, and allergic hepatitis. Monitor BP, LFTs, BUN, SrCr, and increased bleeding time.

Patient Counseling: Inform about potential benefits/risks of therapy. Instruct to notify physician if pregnant/nursing or if any adverse reactions occur. (Afeditab CR) Advise patients that empty matrix "ghost" tab may pass via colostomy or in the stool and this should not be a concern.

Administration: Oral route. Swallow tab whole; do not chew, crush, or divide. **Storage:** Adalat CC/Afeditab CR: <30°C (86°F). Nifediac CC: 25°C (77°F); excursions permitted to 15-30°C (59-86°F). Protect from light and moisture.

ADCETRIS   RX
brentuximab vedotin (Seattle Genetics)

> JC virus infection resulting in progressive multifocal leukoencephalopathy (PML) and death may occur.

THERAPEUTIC CLASS: CD30-directed antibody-drug conjugate

INDICATIONS: Treatment of Hodgkin lymphoma after failure of autologous stem cell transplant (ASCT) or after failure of at least two prior multi-agent chemotherapy regimens in patients who are not ASCT candidates. Treatment of systemic anaplastic large cell lymphoma after failure of at least one prior multi-agent chemotherapy regimen.

DOSAGE: *Adults:* Usual: 1.8mg/kg as IV infusion over 30 min every 3 weeks. Continue treatment until max of 16 cycles, disease progression, or unacceptable toxicity. Patients ≥100kg: Calculate based on a weight of 100kg. Peripheral Neuropathy: Use a combination of dose delay and reduction to 1.2mg/kg. Grade 2 or 3 Neuropathy: Hold until neuropathy improves to Grade 1 or baseline, then restart at 1.2mg/kg. Grade 4 Neuropathy: D/C therapy. Neutropenia: Manage by dose delays and reductions. Grade 3 or 4 Neutropenia: Hold until resolution to baseline or Grade 2 or lower. Consider growth factor support for subsequent cycles. Recurrent Grade 4 Neutropenia Despite Growth Factor Support: D/C or reduce dose to 1.2mg/kg.

HOW SUPPLIED: Inj: 50mg

CONTRAINDICATIONS: Concomitant bleomycin due to pulmonary toxicity.

WARNINGS/PRECAUTIONS: Do not administer as IV push or bolus. Peripheral neuropathy (sensory and motor) reported; may require a delay, change in dose, or discontinuation. Infusion-related reactions, including anaphylaxis, reported; d/c and institute appropriate therapy if infusion reaction occurs. Premedicate if patient experienced a prior infusion-related reaction. Prolonged severe neutropenia may occur; monitor CBC prior to each dose, and monitor frequently with Grade 3 or 4 neutropenia. Tumor lysis syndrome may occur; monitor closely and take appropriate measures. Hold dosing for any suspected case of PML and d/c if diagnosis is confirmed. Stevens-Johnson syndrome (SJS) reported; d/c and administer appropriate therapy if SJS occurs. May cause fetal harm.

ADVERSE REACTIONS: Neutropenia, peripheral sensory neuropathy, anemia, fatigue, upper respiratory tract infection, N/V, pyrexia, diarrhea, rash, thrombocytopenia, pain, abdominal pain, cough.

INTERACTIONS: See Contraindications. Concomitant ketoconazole may increase exposure to monomethyl auristatin E (MMAE). Monitor closely for adverse reactions when given concomitantly with strong CYP3A4 inhibitors. Rifampin may decrease exposure to MMAE.

PREGNANCY: Category D, not for use in nursing.

MECHANISM OF ACTION: CD30-directed antibody-drug conjugate (ADC); binds ADC to CD30-expressing cells, followed by internalization of ADC-CD30 complex, and release of MMAE via proteolytic cleavage. Binding of MMAE to tubulin disrupts the microtubule network within the cell, subsequently inducing cell cycle arrest and apoptotic death of the cell.

PHARMACOKINETICS: Absorption: (MMAE) T_{max}=1-3 days. **Distribution:** (MMAE) Plasma protein binding (68-82%); (ADC) V_d=6-10L. **Metabolism:** (MMAE) Via oxidation by CYP3A4/5. **Elimination:** (MMAE) Urine, feces (24%); (ADC) $T_{1/2}$=4-6 days.

NURSING CONSIDERATIONS

Assessment: Assess for history of infusion-related reactions, pregnancy/nursing status, and for possible drug interactions. Assess if tumor is rapidly proliferating and if there is high tumor burden. Obtain CBC.

Monitoring: Monitor for peripheral neuropathy, infusion reactions, tumor lysis syndrome, SJS, and PML. Monitor CBC prior to each dose and perform more frequent monitoring with Grade 3 or 4 neutropenia.

Patient Counseling: Advise to contact physician if symptoms of peripheral neuropathy, an infection, or if an infusion reaction occurs. Instruct to immediately report changes in mood/usual behavior, confusion, thinking problems, loss of memory, changes in vision, speech, or walking, or if decreased strength or weakness on one side of the body occur. Advise to avoid pregnancy or nursing while receiving therapy and to contact physician immediately if pregnant.

Administration: IV route. Do not mix with, or administer as an infusion with, other medicinal products. Refer to PI for preparation and administration. Use diluted sol immediately. **Storage:** 2-8°C (36-46°F). Protect from light. Reconstituted Sol: Dilute immediately or use within 24 hrs. Do not freeze.

ADDERALL
amphetamine salt combo (Teva)

CII

> High potential for abuse; prolonged use may lead to drug dependence and must be avoided. Misuse of amphetamine may cause sudden death and serious cardiovascular (CV) adverse events.

THERAPEUTIC CLASS: Sympathomimetic amine

INDICATIONS: Treatment of attention-deficit hyperactivity disorder (ADHD) and narcolepsy.

DOSAGE: *Adults:* Individualize dose and administer at the lowest effective dose. Give 1st dose on awakening; additional doses (1 or 2) at intervals of 4-6 hrs. Narcolepsy: Initial: 10mg/day. Titrate: May increase in increments of 10mg at weekly intervals until optimal response is obtained. Usual: 5-60mg/day in divided doses. Reduce dose if bothersome adverse reactions appear (eg, insomnia or anorexia).
Pediatrics: Individualize dose and administer at the lowest effective dose. Give 1st dose on awakening; additional doses (1 or 2) at intervals of 4-6 hrs. ADHD: ≥6 Yrs: Initial: 5mg qd or bid. Titrate: May increase in increments of 5mg at weekly intervals until optimal response is obtained. Only in rare cases will it be necessary to exceed a total of 40mg/day. 3-5 Yrs: Initial: 2.5mg/day. Titrate: May increase in increments of 2.5mg at weekly intervals until optimal response is obtained. Narcolepsy: ≥12 Yrs: Initial: 10mg/day. Titrate: May increase in increments of 10mg at weekly intervals until optimal response is obtained. 6-12 Yrs: Initial: 5mg/day. Titrate: May increase in increments of 5mg at weekly intervals until optimal response is obtained. Usual: 5-60mg/day in divided doses. Reduce dose if bothersome adverse reactions appear (eg, insomnia or anorexia).

HOW SUPPLIED: Tab: 5mg*, 7.5mg*, 10mg*, 12.5mg*, 15mg*, 20mg*, 30mg* *scored

CONTRAINDICATIONS: Advanced arteriosclerosis, symptomatic CV disease, moderate to severe HTN, hyperthyroidism, glaucoma, agitated states, history of drug abuse, during or within 14 days of MAOI use.

WARNINGS/PRECAUTIONS: Sudden death reported in children and adolescents with structural cardiac abnormalities or other serious heart problems. Sudden death, stroke, and myocardial infarction (MI) reported in adults. Avoid use in patients with serious structural cardiac abnormalities, cardiomyopathy, serious heart rhythm abnormalities, coronary artery disease (CAD), or other serious cardiac problems. May cause modest increase in average BP and HR; caution with conditions that could be compromised by BP or HR elevation (eg, preexisting HTN, heart failure, recent MI, ventricular arrhythmia). Perform prompt cardiac evaluation when symptoms suggestive of cardiac disease develop. May exacerbate symptoms of behavior disturbance and thought disorder in patients with preexisting psychotic disorder. Caution in patients with comorbid bipolar disorder; may induce mixed/manic episodes. May cause treatment-emergent psychotic/manic symptoms (eg, hallucinations, delusional thinking, mania) in children and adolescents without prior history of psychotic illness or mania; consider discontinuation if such symptoms occur. Aggressive behavior or hostility reported in children and adolescents with ADHD; monitor for appearance of or worsening. May cause long-term suppression of growth in children; monitor growth, and may need to interrupt treatment if patients are not growing or gaining weight as expected. May lower convulsive threshold; d/c if seizures develop. Difficulties with accommodation and blurring of vision reported. May exacerbate motor and phonic tics, and Tourette's syndrome. May significantly elevate plasma corticosteroid levels or interfere with urinary steroid determinations.

ADVERSE REACTIONS: Palpitations, tachycardia, BP elevation, psychotic episodes, tremor, blurred vision, mydriasis, dryness of mouth, unpleasant taste, anorexia, urticaria, rash, impotence, libido changes, alopecia.

INTERACTIONS: See Contraindications. GI alkalinizing agents (eg, sodium bicarbonate, antacids) and urinary alkalinizing agents (eg, acetazolamide, some thiazides) may increase blood levels and potentiate effects; avoid with GI alkalinizing agents. GI acidifying agents (eg, guanethidine, reserpine, glutamic acid HCl, ascorbic acid, fruit juices) and urinary acidifying agents (eg, ammonium chloride, sodium acid phosphate) may lower blood levels and efficacy. May inhibit adrenergic blockers. May enhance activity of TCAs or sympathomimetic agents; caution with other sympathomimetic drugs. Increased d-amphetamine levels in the brain with desipramine or protriptyline and possibly other tricyclics. May counteract sedative effect of antihistamines. May antagonize the hypotensive effects of antihypertensives. Chlorpromazine and haloperidol may inhibit the central stimulant effects. Lithium carbonate may inhibit the anorectic and stimulatory effects. May delay intestinal absorption of ethosuximide, phenobarbital, and phenytoin; may produce a synergistic anticonvulsant action if coadministered with phenobarbital or phenytoin. May potentiate analgesic effect of meperidine. May enhance the adrenergic effect of norepinephrine. Use in cases of propoxyphene overdose may potentiate CNS stimulation and cause fatal convulsions. Monitor for changes in clinical effect when coadministered with proton pump inhibitors. May inhibit the hypotensive effect of veratrum alkaloids.

PREGNANCY: Category C, not for use in nursing.

MECHANISM OF ACTION: Sympathomimetic amine; has not been established. Thought to block the reuptake of norepinephrine and dopamine into the presynaptic neuron and increase the release of these monoamines into the extraneuronal space.

PHARMACOKINETICS: Absorption: T_{max}=3 hrs (fasted). **Distribution:** Found in breast milk. **Metabolism:** CYP2D6 (oxidation); 4-hydroxy-amphetamine and norephedrine (active metabolites). **Elimination:** Urine (normal pH) (30-40%, unchanged; 50%, α-hydroxy-amphetamine derivatives). $T_{1/2}$=9.77-11 hrs (d-amphetamine), 11.5-13.8 hrs (l-amphetamine).

NURSING CONSIDERATIONS

Assessment: Assess for advanced arteriosclerosis, symptomatic CV disease (structural/rhythm abnormalities, CAD, recent MI), moderate to severe HTN, hyperthyroidism, hypersensitivity or idiosyncrasy to sympathomimetic amines, glaucoma, agitation, history of drug abuse, psychiatric history, history of seizure, tics or Tourette's syndrome, pregnancy/nursing status, and possible drug interactions. Prior to treatment, adequately screen patients to determine risk for bipolar disorder.

Monitoring: Monitor for CV abnormalities, exacerbations of behavior disturbances and thought disorder, psychotic or manic symptoms, aggressive behavior, hostility, seizures, visual disturbances, exacerbation of motor and phonic tics and Tourette's syndrome, and other adverse reactions. Monitor BP and HR. Monitor growth and weight in children. Periodically reevaluate long-term usefulness of therapy.

Patient Counseling: Inform about benefits and risks of treatment, appropriate use, and about the potential for abuse/dependence. Advise to avoid breastfeeding and to notify physician if pregnant/planning to become pregnant. Instruct to use caution when engaging in potentially hazardous activities (eg, operating machinery or vehicles).

Administration: PO route. Give 1st dose on awakening; avoid late pm doses due to potential for insomnia. **Storage:** 20-25°C (68-77°F).

ADDERALL XR

CII

amphetamine salt combo (Shire)

> High potential for abuse; prolonged use may lead to drug dependence. Misuse may cause sudden death and serious cardiovascular (CV) adverse reactions.

THERAPEUTIC CLASS: Sympathomimetic amine

INDICATIONS: Treatment of attention-deficit hyperactivity disorder.

DOSAGE: *Adults:* Individualize dose. Amphetamine-Naive/Switching from Another Medication: 20mg qam. Switching from Amphetamine Immediate-Release (IR): Give the same total daily dose, qd. Titrate at weekly intervals as indicated.
Pediatrics: Individualize dose. Switching from Amphetamine IR: Give the same total daily dose, qd. Titrate at weekly intervals as indicated. Amphetamine-Naive/Switching from Another Medication: 13-17 Yrs: Initial: 10mg qam. Titrate: May increase to 20mg/day after 1 week if symptoms are not controlled. 6-12 Yrs: Initial: 10mg qam or 5mg qam when lower initial dose is appropriate. Titrate: Adjust daily dosage in increments of 5mg or 10mg at weekly intervals. Max: 30mg/day.

HOW SUPPLIED: Cap, Extended-Release: 5mg, 10mg, 15mg, 20mg, 25mg, 30mg

CONTRAINDICATIONS: Advanced arteriosclerosis, symptomatic CV disease, moderate to severe HTN, hyperthyroidism, glaucoma, agitated states, history of drug abuse, during or within 14 days following MAOI use.

WARNINGS/PRECAUTIONS: Sudden death, stroke, and myocardial infarction (MI) reported in adults. Sudden death reported in children and adolescents with structural cardiac abnormalities or other serious heart problems. Avoid use in patients with known serious structural cardiac and heart rhythm abnormalities, cardiomyopathy, coronary artery disease (CAD), or other serious cardiac problems. May cause modest increase in BP and HR. May exacerbate symptoms of behavior disturbance and thought disorder in patients with preexisting psychotic disorder. Caution in patients with comorbid bipolar disorder; may cause induction of mixed/manic episode. May cause treatment-emergent psychotic/manic symptoms (eg, hallucinations, delusional thinking, mania) in children and adolescents without a prior history of psychotic illness or mania; consider discontinuation if such symptoms occur. Aggressive behavior or hostility reported; monitor for appearance or worsening. May cause long-term suppression of growth in children; may need to d/c if patients are not growing or gaining weight as expected. May lower convulsive threshold; d/c if seizures develop. Associated with peripheral vasculopathy, including Raynaud's phenomenon. Difficulties with accommodation and blurring of vision reported. Exacerbation of motor and phonic tics and Tourette's syndrome reported. May significantly elevate plasma corticosteroid levels or interfere with urinary steroid determinations. Where possible, interrupt occasionally to determine the need for continued therapy.

ADVERSE REACTIONS: Dry mouth, loss of appetite, insomnia, headache, abdominal pain, weight loss, agitation, anxiety, N/V, dizziness, tachycardia, nervousness, asthenia, diarrhea, urinary tract infection.

INTERACTIONS: See Contraindications. Avoid with GI alkalinizing agents (eg, sodium bicarbonate, antacids). Urinary alkalinizing agents (eg, acetazolamide, some thiazides) may increase blood levels and potentiate effects. GI acidifying agents (eg, guanethidine, reserpine, ascorbic acid) and urinary acidifying agents (eg, ammonium chloride, sodium acid phosphate, methenamine salts) may lower blood levels and efficacy. May reduce CV effects of adrenergic blockers. May counteract sedative effects of antihistamines. May antagonize effects of antihypertensives. May inhibit hypotensive effect of veratrum alkaloids. May delay intestinal absorption of phenobarbital, phenytoin, and ethosuximide. May enhance activity of TCAs or sympathomimetic agents. Increased d-amphetamine levels in the brain with desipramine or protriptyline and possibly other tricyclics. May potentiate analgesic effect of meperidine. May enhance the adrenergic effect of norepinephrine. Chlorpromazine and haloperidol may inhibit central stimulant effects. Lithium carbonate may inhibit anorectic and stimulatory effects. Norepinephrine may enhance the adrenergic effect. Use in cases of propoxyphene overdose may potentiate CNS stimulation and cause fatal convulsions. Monitor for changes in clinical effect when coadministered with proton pump inhibitors.

PREGNANCY: Category C, not for use in nursing.

MECHANISM OF ACTION: Sympathomimetic amine; has not been established. Thought to block the reuptake of norepinephrine and dopamine into the presynaptic neuron and increase the release of these monoamines into the extraneuronal space.

PHARMACOKINETICS: Absorption: T_{max}=7 hrs. **Distribution:** Found in breast milk. **Metabolism:** CYP2D6 (oxidation); 4-hydroxy-amphetamine and norephedrine (active metabolites). **Elimination:** Urine (normal pH) (30-40%, unchanged; 50%, α-hydroxy-amphetamine derivatives). (20mg single dose) d-amphetamine: $T_{1/2}$=10 hrs (adults), 11 hrs (13-17 yrs of age), 9 hrs (6-12 yrs of age). l-amphetamine: $T_{1/2}$=13 hrs (adults), 13-14 hrs (13-17 yrs of age), 11 hrs (6-12 yrs of age).

NURSING CONSIDERATIONS

Assessment: Assess for advanced arteriosclerosis, symptomatic CV disease, moderate to severe HTN, hyperthyroidism, hypersensitivity or idiosyncrasy to sympathomimetic amines, glaucoma, agitation, history of drug abuse, psychiatric history, history of seizure, tics or Tourette's syndrome, hepatic/renal dysfunction, pregnancy/nursing status, and possible drug interactions.

Monitoring: Monitor for CV abnormalities, exacerbations of behavior disturbances and thought disorder, psychotic or manic symptoms, aggressive behavior, hostility, seizures, visual disturbances, exacerbation of motor and phonic tics and Tourette's syndrome, and other adverse reactions. Monitor BP and HR. Monitor height and weight in children. Observe carefully for signs and symptoms of peripheral vasculopathy; further clinical evaluation (eg, rheumatology referral) may be appropriate for certain patients.

Patient Counseling: Inform about benefits and risks of treatment, appropriate use, and about the potential for abuse/dependence. Advise about serious CV risks. Inform that treatment-emergent psychotic or manic symptoms may occur. Instruct to report signs/symptoms of peripheral vasculopathy, including Raynaud's phenomenon. Advise parents or guardians of pediatric patients to monitor growth and weight during treatment. Advise to notify physician if pregnant or planning to become pregnant. Advise to avoid breastfeeding. Advise to use caution when engaging in potentially hazardous activities.

Administration: Oral route. Give upon awakening; avoid pm doses due to potential for insomnia. Take with or without food. Take caps whole or sprinkle entire contents on applesauce. Consume sprinkled applesauce immediately without chewing the sprinkled beads. Do not divide the dose of a single cap or take anything <1 cap/day. **Storage:** 25°C (77°F); excursions permitted to 15-30°C (59-86°F).

ADEMPAS   RX
riociguat (Bayer Healthcare)

Do not administer to a pregnant female; may cause fetal harm. Exclude pregnancy before the start of treatment, monthly during treatment, and 1 month after stopping treatment. Prevent pregnancy during and for 1 month after stopping treatment; use acceptable methods of contraception. For all female patients, available only through a restricted program called the Adempas Risk Evaluation and Mitigation Strategy (REMS) Program.

THERAPEUTIC CLASS: Soluble guanylate cyclase (sGC) stimulator

INDICATIONS: Treatment of adults with persistent/recurrent chronic thromboembolic pulmonary HTN (CTEPH), (World Health Organization [WHO] Group 4) after surgical treatment, or inoperable CTEPH, to improve exercise capacity and WHO functional class. Treatment of adults with pulmonary arterial HTN, (WHO Group 1), to improve exercise capacity, WHO functional class, and to delay clinical worsening.

DOSAGE: *Adults:* Initial: 1mg tid; consider 0.5mg tid for patients who may not tolerate the hypotensive effect. Titrate: Increase by 0.5mg tid if systolic BP remains >95mmHg and patient has no signs/symptoms of hypotension. Dose increases should be no sooner than 2 weeks apart. Max: 2.5mg tid. If at any time, symptoms of hypotension occur, decrease dosage by 0.5mg tid. Dose Interruption: Retitrate if treatment is interrupted for ≥3 days. Patients Who Smoke: Consider titrating to dosages >2.5mg tid if tolerated. May require a dose decrease in patients who stop smoking. With Strong CYP and P-glycoprotein/Breast Cancer Resistant Protein (P-gp/BCRP) Inhibitors (eg, azole antimycotics, HIV protease inhibitors): Initial: 0.5mg tid.

HOW SUPPLIED: Tab: 0.5mg, 1mg, 1.5mg, 2mg, 2.5mg

CONTRAINDICATIONS: Pregnancy. Coadministration with nitrates or nitric oxide (NO) donors (eg, amyl nitrite) in any form, or PDE inhibitors, including specific PDE-5 inhibitors (eg, sildenafil, tadalafil, vardenafil) or nonspecific PDE inhibitors (eg, dipyridamole, theophylline).

WARNINGS/PRECAUTIONS: Reduces BP; consider the potential for symptomatic hypotension or ischemia in patients with hypovolemia, severe left ventricular outflow obstruction, resting hypotension, or autonomic dysfunction. Serious bleeding/hemoptysis/hemorrhagic events reported. May significantly worsen the cardiovascular status of patients with pulmonary veno-occlusive disease (PVOD); administration to such patients is not recommended. If signs of pulmonary edema occur, consider possibility of associated PVOD and, if confirmed, d/c treatment. Caution in the elderly. Safety and efficacy have not been demonstrated in patients with CrCl <15mL/min, in patients on dialysis, or in patients with severe hepatic impairment (Child-Pugh C).

ADVERSE REACTIONS: Headache, dyspepsia, gastritis, dizziness, N/V, diarrhea, hypotension, anemia, gastroesophageal reflux disease, constipation.

INTERACTIONS: See Contraindications. Consider the potential for symptomatic hypotension or ischemia with concomitant antihypertensives. Smoking may reduce concentrations; consider dose adjustment. Strong CYP inhibitors and P-gp/BCRP inhibitors (eg, azole antimycotics [eg, ketoconazole, itraconazole], HIV protease inhibitors [eg, ritonavir]) increase exposure and may result in hypotension; consider dose adjustment of riociguat. Strong CYP3A inducers (eg, rifampin, phenytoin, carbamazepine, phenobarbital, St. John's wort) may significantly reduce exposure. Antacids (eg, aluminum hydroxide, magnesium hydroxide) decrease absorption and should not be taken within 1 hr of taking riociguat.

PREGNANCY: Category X, not for use in nursing.

MECHANISM OF ACTION: sGC stimulator; sensitizes sGC to endogenous NO by stabilizing the NO-sGC binding. Also, directly stimulates sGC via a different binding site, independently of NO. Stimulates the NO-sGC-cGMP pathway and leads to increased generation of cGMP with subsequent vasodilation.

PHARMACOKINETICS: Absorption: Absolute bioavailability (94%); T_{max} =1.5 hrs. **Distribution:** V_d =30L; plasma protein binding (95%). **Metabolism:** CYP1A1, CYP3A, CYP2C8, CYP2J2; M1 (major active metabolite) (catalyzed by CYP1A1). **Elimination:** Urine (40%), feces (53%); $T_{1/2}$ =12 hrs.

NURSING CONSIDERATIONS

Assessment: Assess for hypovolemia, severe left ventricular outflow obstruction, resting hypotension, autonomic dysfunction, PVOD, renal/hepatic impairment, pregnancy/nursing status, and possible drug interactions.

Monitoring: Monitor for signs/symptoms of hypotension, bleeding, pulmonary edema, and other adverse reactions. Obtain pregnancy tests monthly during treatment and one month after discontinuation of treatment.

Patient Counseling: Counsel on the risk of fetal harm when used during pregnancy; instruct females of reproductive potential to use effective contraception during therapy and for one month after stopping treatment. Instruct to contact physician immediately if pregnancy is suspected. Inform female patients that they must enroll in the Adempas REMS Program. Inform of the contraindication of treatment with nitrates or NO donors or PDE-5 inhibitors. Advise about the potential risks/signs of hemoptysis and to report any potential signs of hemoptysis to physician. Instruct on the dosing, titration, and maintenance of therapy. Advise regarding activities that may impact the pharmacology of drug (strong multipathway CYP inhibitors and P-gp/BCRP inhibitors and smoking); instruct to report all current and new medications to physician. Advise that antacids should not be taken within 1 hr of taking the drug. Inform that drug can cause dizziness, which can affect the ability to drive and use machines.

Administration: Oral route. May take with or without food. **Storage:** 25°C (77°F); excursions permitted from 15-30°C (59-86°F).

ADENOCARD   RX
adenosine (Astellas)

THERAPEUTIC CLASS: Endogenous nucleoside

INDICATIONS: Conversion to sinus rhythm (SR) of paroxysmal supraventricular tachycardia (PSVT), including that associated with accessory bypass tracts (Wolff-Parkinson-White syndrome).

DOSAGE: *Adults:* Initial: 6mg rapid IV bolus over 1-2 sec. If not converted to SR within 1-2 min, give 12mg rapid IV bolus; may give second 12mg dose if needed. Max: 12mg/dose.
Pediatrics: ≥50kg: Initial: 6mg rapid IV bolus over 1-2 sec. If not converted to SR within 1-2 min, give 12mg rapid IV bolus; may give second 12mg dose if needed. Max: 12mg/dose. <50kg: Initial: 0.05-0.1mg/kg rapid IV bolus. If not converted to SR within 1-2 min, give additional bolus doses, incrementally increasing amount by 0.05-0.1mg/kg. Continue process until SR or a max single dose of 0.3mg/kg is used.

HOW SUPPLIED: Inj: 3mg/mL [2mL, 4mL]

CONTRAINDICATIONS: 2nd- or 3rd-degree atrioventricular (AV) block, and sinus node disease (eg, sinus syndrome or symptomatic bradycardia), except with functioning artificial pacemaker.

WARNINGS/PRECAUTIONS: May produce short-lasting 1st-, 2nd-, or 3rd-degree heart block; institute appropriate therapy PRN. Do not give additional doses if high-level block develops on 1st dose. Transient or prolonged asystole, respiratory alkalosis, ventricular fibrillation reported. New arrhythmias may appear on ECG at time of conversion. Caution with obstructive lung disease not associated with bronchoconstriction (eg, emphysema, bronchitis). Avoid with bronchoconstriction/bronchospasm (eg, asthma). D/C if severe respiratory difficulties develop. Caution in elderly. Does not convert atrial fibrillation/atrial flutter (A-fib/flutter), or ventricular tachycardia to normal SR. A transient modest slowing of ventricular response may occur immediately following administration in the presence of A-fib/flutter.

ADVERSE REACTIONS: Arrhythmias, facial flushing, dyspnea/SOB, chest pressure, nausea.

INTERACTIONS: Antagonized by methylxanthines (eg, theophylline, caffeine); may need larger dose. Potentiated by nucleoside transport inhibitors (eg, dipyridamole); use lower dose. Potential additive or synergistic depressant effects on the sinoatrial and AV nodes with other cardioactive drugs (eg, β-adrenergic blockers, quinidine, calcium channel blockers [CCBs]). Caution when used in combination with digoxin/verapamil; ventricular fibrillation reported with digoxin, verapamil, and digitalis. Possible higher degrees of heart block with carbamazepine.

PREGNANCY: Category C, safety in nursing not known.

MECHANISM OF ACTION: Endogenous nucleoside; slows conduction time through AV node, can interrupt reentry pathways through the AV node, and can restore normal SR in patients with PSVT, including PSVT associated with Wolff-Parkinson-White syndrome.

PHARMACOKINETICS: Metabolism: Rapid (intracellular); via phosphorylation or deamination. **Elimination:** $T_{1/2}$=<10 sec (extracellular).

NURSING CONSIDERATIONS

Assessment: Assess for A-fib/flutter, ventricular tachycardia, presence of functioning pacemaker, AV block, sinus node disease, arrhythmias, obstructive lung disease, bronchoconstriction/bronchospasm, hypersensitivity to drug, pregnancy status, and possible drug interactions. Obtain baseline ECG and vital signs.

Monitoring: Monitor for heart block, bradycardia, ventricular fibrillation, asystole, and arrhythmias, respiratory alkalosis/difficulties, or hypersensitivity reactions. Monitor ECG and vital signs.

Patient Counseling: Inform about benefits/risks of therapy. Advise to promptly report any adverse reactions to physician.

Administration: IV route. Administer by rapid IV bolus, either directly into a vein, or given as close to the patient as possible if via IV line. Follow each bolus with a rapid saline flush. **Storage:** 15-30°C (59-86°F). Do not refrigerate. Dissolve crystals by warming to room temperature if crystallization occurs. Discard unused portion. Do not break by hand, recap, or purposely bend needles.

ADRENACLICK   RX
epinephrine (Amedra)

THERAPEUTIC CLASS: Sympathomimetic catecholamine

INDICATIONS: Emergency treatment of severe allergic reactions (Type 1), including anaphylaxis to stinging insects (eg, order Hymenoptera, which includes bees, wasps, hornets, yellow jackets, and fire ants) and biting insects (eg, triatoma, mosquitoes), allergen immunotherapy, foods, drugs, diagnostic testing substances (eg, radiocontrast media), and other allergens, as well as anaphylaxis to unknown substances (idiopathic anaphylaxis) or exercise-induced anaphylaxis.

DOSAGE: *Adults:* Carefully assess each patient to determine the most appropriate dose. ≥30kg: Inject 0.3mg IM/SQ. 15-30kg: 0.15mg IM/SQ.
Pediatrics: Carefully assess each patient to determine the most appropriate dose. ≥30kg: Inject 0.3mg IM/SQ. 15-30kg: 0.15mg IM/SQ.

HOW SUPPLIED: Inj: 0.15mg/0.15mL, 0.3mg/0.3mL

WARNINGS/PRECAUTIONS: Intended for immediate administration in patients with a history of anaphylactic reactions. Designed as emergency supportive therapy only and is not a replacement or substitute for immediate medical care. May result in loss of blood flow to the affected area if accidentally injected into the hands or feet; avoid injecting into these areas. Do not inject into buttock. Do not inject IV. Large doses or accidental IV inj use may result in cerebral hemorrhage due to sharp rise in BP; rapidly acting vasodilators can counteract the marked pressor effect of epinephrine. Contains sodium bisulfite; may cause allergic-type reactions, including anaphylactic symptoms or life-threatening or less severe asthmatic episodes in certain susceptible persons. Caution in patients with cardiac arrhythmias, coronary artery or organic heart disease, or HTN. May precipitate/aggravate angina pectoris as well as produce ventricular arrhythmias in patients with coronary insufficiency or ischemic heart disease. More than two sequential doses should only be administered under direct medical supervision. Higher risk of developing adverse reactions with hyperthyroidism, cardiovascular disease, HTN, diabetes mellitus (DM), in elderly, and pregnant women.

ADVERSE REACTIONS: Anxiety, apprehensiveness, restlessness, tremor, weakness, dizziness, sweating, palpitations, pallor, N/V, headache, respiratory difficulties.

INTERACTIONS: May precipitate/aggravate angina pectoris as well as produce ventricular arrhythmias with drugs that may sensitize the heart to arrhythmias (eg, digitalis, diuretics, or antiarrhythmics); use with caution. Monitor for cardiac arrhythmias with cardiac glycosides or diuretics. Effects may be potentiated by TCAs, MAOIs, sodium levothyroxine, and certain antihistamines (eg, chlorpheniramine, tripelennamine, diphenhydramine). Cardiostimulating and bronchodilating effects antagonized by β-adrenergic blockers (eg, propranolol). Vasoconstricting and hypertensive effects antagonized by α-adrenergic blockers (eg, phentolamine). Ergot alkaloids and phenothiazines may reverse pressor effects.

PREGNANCY: Category C, safety not known in nursing.

MECHANISM OF ACTION: Sympathomimetic catecholamine; acts on α-adrenergic receptors and lessens the vasodilation and increased vascular permeability that occurs during anaphylactic reaction. Action on β-adrenergic receptors causes bronchial smooth muscle relaxation and helps alleviate bronchospasm, wheezing, and dyspnea that may occur during anaphylaxis. Also alleviates pruritus, urticaria, and angioedema and may relieve GI and genitourinary symptoms of anaphylaxis because of its relaxer effects on the smooth muscle of the stomach, intestine, uterus, and urinary bladder.

NURSING CONSIDERATIONS

Assessment: Assess for risk of anaphylaxis, heart disease, cardiac arrhythmias, HTN, DM, hyperthyroidism, pregnancy/nursing status, and for possible drug interactions.

Monitoring: Monitor for allergic-type reactions, angina pectoris, ventricular arrhythmias, cerebral hemorrhage, and for other adverse reactions. Monitor HR and BP.

Patient Counseling: Advise that therapy may produce signs and symptoms that include increased pulse rate, sensation of more forceful heartbeat, palpitations, a throbbing headache, pallor, feelings of overstimulation, anxiety, weakness, shakiness, dizziness, or nausea; advise that these signs and symptoms usually subside rapidly, especially with rest, quiet, and recumbency. Inform that more severe or persistent effects may develop if patient has HTN or hyperthyroidism. Inform that angina may be experienced if patient has coronary artery disease. Advise that patient may develop increased blood glucose levels following administration if patient has DM. Advise that a temporary worsening of symptoms may be noticed if patient has Parkinson's disease.

Administration: SQ/IM route. Inject into the anterolateral aspect of the thigh, through clothing if necessary. **Storage:** 20-25°C (68-77°F); excursions permitted to 15-30°C (59-86°F). Protect from light and freezing. Do not refrigerate. Discard if discolored, cloudy, or has particulate matter. The remaining volume left after the fixed dose should not be further administered and should be discarded.

ADRENALIN   RX
epinephrine (JHP)

THERAPEUTIC CLASS: Sympathomimetic catecholamine

INDICATIONS: Emergency treatment of allergic reactions (Type I), including anaphylaxis, which may result from allergic reactions to insect stings, biting insects, foods, drugs, sera, diagnostic testing substances and other allergens, as well as idiopathic anaphylaxis or exercise-induced anaphylaxis. Induction and maintenance of mydriasis during intraocular surgery.

DOSAGE: *Adults:* Anaphylaxis: ≥30kg: 0.3-0.5mg (0.3-0.5mL) of undiluted epinephrine IM or SQ into the anterolateral aspect of the thigh, repeated every 5-10 min PRN. Max: 0.5mg (0.5mL)/inj. Elderly: Start at a lower dose. Induction/Maint of Mydriasis: Use the irrigating sol PRN for the surgical procedure at a concentration of 1:100,000 to 1:1,000,000 (10mcg/mL to 1mcg/mL). May also be injected intracamerally as a bolus dose of 0.1mL at a dilution of 1:100,000 to 1:400,000 (10mcg/mL to 2.5mcg/mL).
Pediatrics: Anaphylaxis: ≥30kg: 0.3-0.5mg (0.3-0.5mL) of undiluted epinephrine IM or SQ into the anterolateral aspect of the thigh, repeated every 5-10 min PRN. Max: 0.5mg (0.5mL)/inj. <30kg: 0.01mg/kg (0.01mL/kg) of undiluted epinephrine IM or SQ into the anterolateral aspect of the thigh, repeated every 5-10 min PRN. Max: 0.3mg (0.3mL)/inj. Induction/Maint of Mydriasis: Use the irrigating sol PRN for the surgical procedure at a concentration of 1:100,000 to 1:1,000,000 (10mcg/mL to 1mcg/mL). May also be injected intracamerally as a bolus dose of 0.1mL at a dilution of 1:100,000 to 1:400,000 (10mcg/mL to 2.5mcg/mL).

HOW SUPPLIED: Inj: 1mg/mL [1mL]

WARNINGS/PRECAUTIONS: Must be diluted before intraocular use; epinephrine containing sodium bisulfite associated with corneal endothelial damage when used in the eye at undiluted concentrations. Not recommended for inj into or near smaller muscles (eg, deltoid) due to possible differences in absorption. Do not repeat inj at the same site; may cause tissue necrosis. Do not inject into buttock; may not provide effective treatment of anaphylaxis and gas gangrene may develop. May result in loss of blood flow to the affected areas if accidentally injected into digits, hands, or feet. Higher risk of adverse reactions in patients with heart disease (eg, cardiac arrhythmias, coronary artery or organic heart disease, cerebrovascular disease, HTN), hyperthyroidism, Parkinson's disease, diabetes mellitus (DM), pheochromocytoma, pregnant women, and in elderly; use with caution. Contains sodium bisulfite; may cause allergic reactions including anaphylaxis or asthmatic episodes in susceptible individuals.

ADVERSE REACTIONS: Anxiety, apprehensiveness, restlessness, tremor, weakness, dizziness, sweating, palpitations, pallor, N/V, headache, respiratory difficulties.

INTERACTIONS: Do not use to counteract circulatory collapse or hypotension caused by phenothiazines; may result in further lowering of BP. May cause additive effects with other sympathomimetics; coadminister with caution. Arrhythmias may occur with concomitant use with cardiac glycosides, digitalis, diuretics, quinidine, and other antiarrhythmics, or halogenated hydrocarbon general anesthetics (eg, halothane). Effects may be potentiated by TCAs (eg, imipramine), MAOIs, levothyroxine sodium, and certain antihistamines, notably diphenhydramine, tripelennamine, and dexchlorpheniramine. Cardiostimulating and bronchodilating effects antagonized by β-adrenergic blocking drugs (eg, propranolol). Vasoconstricting and hypertensive effects antagonized by α-adrenergic blocking drugs (eg, phentolamine). Ergot alkaloids may reverse pressor effects.

PREGNANCY: Category C, caution in nursing.

MECHANISM OF ACTION: Sympathomimetic catecholamine; acts on α- and β-adrenergic receptors.

NURSING CONSIDERATIONS

Assessment: Assess for sulfite sensitivity, heart disease, DM, hyperthyroidism, Parkinson's disease, pheochromocytoma, pregnancy/nursing status, and possible drug interactions.

Monitoring: Monitor for signs/symptoms of angina pectoris, ventricular arrhythmias, allergic reactions, and other adverse reactions. Monitor glucose levels in patients with DM. Monitor for worsening of symptoms in patients with Parkinson's disease. Monitor HR and BP. Monitor the patient clinically for the severity of the allergic reaction and potential cardiac effects of the drug, with repeat doses titrated to effect.

Patient Counseling: Inform about the common side effects of therapy and advise that these signs/symptoms usually subside rapidly, especially with rest, quiet, and recumbent positioning. Warn patients who have a good response to initial therapy about the possible recurrence of symptoms and instruct to obtain proper medical attention if symptoms return. Warn diabetic patients that increased blood sugar levels may develop following administration.

Administration: IM/SQ/Ocular route. Inject into the anterolateral aspect of the thigh; do not administer repeated inj at the same site. Refer to PI for dilution instructions for intraocular use.
Storage: 20-25°C (68-77°F). Protect from light and freezing.

ADVAIR DISKUS   RX
fluticasone propionate - salmeterol (GlaxoSmithKline)

> Long-acting β₂-adrenergic agonists (LABAs), such as salmeterol, increase the risk of asthma-related death. LABAs may increase the risk of asthma-related hospitalization in pediatrics and adolescents. Use only for patients not adequately controlled on a long-term asthma control medication (eg, inhaled corticosteroid) or whose disease severity clearly warrants initiation of treatment with both an inhaled corticosteroid and a LABA. Do not use if asthma is adequately controlled on low- or medium-dose inhaled corticosteroids.

THERAPEUTIC CLASS: Beta₂-agonist/corticosteroid

INDICATIONS: Treatment of asthma in patients ≥4 yrs of age. (250/50) Maintenance treatment of airflow obstruction in patients with chronic obstructive pulmonary disease (COPD), including chronic bronchitis and/or emphysema, and to reduce exacerbations of COPD in patients with history of exacerbations.

DOSAGE: *Adults:* Asthma: Initial: Based upon asthma severity. Usual: 1 inh bid (am/pm, q12h). Max: 500/50 bid. Increase to higher strength if response to initial dose is inadequate after 2 weeks. COPD: (250/50): 1 inh bid (am/pm, q12h). If asthma symptoms or SOB occurs between doses, use short-acting β₂-agonist for immediate relief.
Pediatrics: ≥12 Yrs: Asthma: Initial: Based upon asthma severity. Usual: 1 inh bid (am/pm, q12h). Max: 500/50 bid. Increase to higher strength if response to initial dose is inadequate after 2 weeks. If asthma symptoms arise between doses, use short-acting β₂-agonist for immediate relief. 4-11 Yrs: (100/50): Not Controlled on Inhaled Corticosteroid: 1 inh bid (am/pm, q12h).

HOW SUPPLIED: Disk: (Fluticasone Propionate-Salmeterol) (100/50) 100mcg-50mcg/inh, (250/50) 250mcg-50mcg/inh, (500/50) 500mcg-50mcg/inh [14, 60 blisters]

CONTRAINDICATIONS: Primary treatment of status asthmaticus or other acute episodes of asthma or COPD where intensive measures are required; severe hypersensitivity to milk proteins.

WARNINGS/PRECAUTIONS: Should not be initiated during rapidly deteriorating or potentially life-threatening episodes of asthma or COPD. Increased use of inhaled, short-acting β₂-agonists (SABAs) is a marker of deteriorating asthma; reevaluate and reassess treatment regimen. Should not be used for relief of acute symptoms; use SABA to relieve acute symptoms. Should not be used more often or at higher doses than recommended or in conjunction with other medications containing LABA; cardiovascular (CV) effects and fatalities reported with excessive use. *Candida albicans* infections of mouth and pharynx reported; treat and/or d/c if needed. Lower respiratory tract infections (eg, pneumonia) reported in patients with COPD. Increased susceptibility to infections (eg, chickenpox, measles); may lead to serious/fatal course; if exposed consider prophylaxis/treatment. Caution with tuberculosis (TB), untreated systemic fungal, bacterial, viral or parasitic infections, and ocular herpes simplex. Deaths due to adrenal insufficiency reported with transfer from systemic to inhaled corticosteroids (ICS); if oral corticosteroids required, wean slowly from systemic steroid use after transferring to ICS. Transfer from systemic to inhalation therapy may unmask allergic conditions (eg, rhinitis, conjunctivitis). May produce paradoxical bronchospasm; d/c immediately, treat, and institute alternative therapy. Upper airway symptoms reported. Decreases in bone mineral density (BMD) reported; caution with major risk factors for decreased bone mineral content, including chronic use of drugs that can reduce bone mass (eg, anticonvulsants, corticosteroids). May cause reduction in growth velocity in pediatrics. Glaucoma, increased intraocular pressure (IOP), cataracts, rare cases of systemic eosinophilic conditions and vasculitis consistent with Churg-Strauss syndrome reported. Observe for systemic corticosteroid effects; if hypercorticism and adrenal suppression appear, reduce dose slowly. Immediate hypersensitivity reactions, hypokalemia, and dose-related changes in blood glucose and/or serum K⁺ may occur. ECG changes (eg, flattening of T wave, QTc interval prolongation, and ST segment depression) reported. Caution with CV disorders, convulsive disorders, thyrotoxicosis, hepatic disease, diabetes mellitus (DM), those who are unusually responsive to sympathomimetic amines, and in elderly.

ADVERSE REACTIONS: Upper respiratory tract infection/inflammation, pharyngitis, dysphonia, oral candidiasis, bronchitis, cough, headache, N/V, pneumonia, throat irritation, viral respiratory infection, musculoskeletal pain.

INTERACTIONS: Avoid with strong CYP3A4 inhibitors (eg, ritonavir, atazanavir, clarithromycin, indinavir, itraconazole, nefazodone, nelfinavir, saquinavir, ketoconazole, telithromycin). Avoid use with other medications containing LABAs. Salmeterol: Extreme caution with TCAs or MAOIs, or within 2 weeks of discontinuing such products. Use with β-blockers may produce severe bronchospasm; if needed, consider cardioselective β-blocker with caution. ECG changes and/or hypokalemia that may result from non-K⁺-sparing diuretics (eg, loop/thiazide diuretics) can be acutely worsened; use with caution. May increase levels, increase HR, and prolong QTc interval with erythromycin. May increase exposure with ketoconazole; combination may be associated with QTc prolongation. Fluticasone: May increase exposure and reduce cortisol levels with ritonavir and ketoconazole.

PREGNANCY: Category C, not for use in nursing.

MECHANISM OF ACTION: Fluticasone: Corticosteroid with anti-inflammatory activity. Inhibits multiple cell types (eg, mast cells, eosinophils, basophils, lymphocytes, macrophages, neutrophils) and mediator production or secretion (eg, histamine, eicosanoids, leukotrienes, cytokines) involved in the asthmatic response. Salmeterol: Selective LABA; stimulates intracellular adenyl cyclase, which catalyzes conversion of ATP to cAMP, producing relaxation of bronchial smooth muscle and inhibits mediator release of immediate hypersensitivity from cells, especially from mast cells.

PHARMACOKINETICS: Absorption: Administration in healthy, asthmatic, and COPD patients resulted in different pharmacokinetic parameters. **Distribution:** Fluticasone: V_d=4.2L/kg; plasma protein binding (91%). Salmeterol: Plasma protein binding (96%). **Metabolism:** Fluticasone: Liver via CYP3A4; 17 β-carboxylic acid derivative (metabolite). Salmeterol: Liver, via CYP3A4 to α-hydroxysalmeterol (metabolite). **Elimination:** Fluticasone: (PO) Urine (<5%); (Inh) $T_{1/2}$=5.6 hrs. Salmeterol (PO): Urine (25%), feces (60%); $T_{1/2}$=5.5 hrs.

NURSING CONSIDERATIONS

Assessment: Assess for hypersensitivity to milk proteins, acute asthma/COPD episodes, status asthmaticus, rapidly deteriorating asthma or COPD, risk factors for decreased bone mineral content, CV disease, convulsive disorder, thyrotoxicosis, DM, history of IOP, glaucoma, cataracts, active or quiescent pulmonary TB, ocular herpes simplex, untreated systemic infections, hepatic disease, pregnancy/nursing status, and possible drug interactions. Obtain baseline serum K⁺, blood glucose levels, BMD, eye exam, and lung function prior to therapy.

Monitoring: Monitor for localized oral *C. albicans* infections, upper airway symptoms, worsening or acutely deteriorating asthma, development of glaucoma, increased IOP, CV, CNS effects, cataracts, hypercorticism, adrenal suppression, paradoxical bronchospasm, eosinophilic conditions, hypokalemia, hyperglycemia, and hypersensitivity reactions. Monitor ECG changes, BMD, and lung function periodically. Perform periodic eye exams. Monitor growth in pediatric patients. Monitor for lower respiratory tract infections in patients with COPD.

Patient Counseling: Inform about the risks and benefits of therapy. Advise that medication is not for the relief of acute asthma symptoms or exacerbations of COPD and extra doses should not be used for this purpose. Inform not to d/c unless directed by physician and counsel on administration instructions. Advise to rinse mouth after inhalation and to spit water out; instruct to not swallow water. Instruct to avoid exposure to chickenpox or measles; consult physician if exposed, if existing TB infections or ocular herpes simplex symptoms do not improve or worsen, or if hypersensitivity reactions occur.

Administration: Oral inhalation. Rinse mouth with water without swallowing after inhalation. Refer to PI for further administration instructions. **Storage:** 20-25°C (68-77°F). Keep in a dry place, away from direct heat or sunlight. Discard 1 month after removal from pouch or when indicator reads "0," whichever comes first.

ADVAIR HFA   RX
fluticasone propionate - salmeterol (GlaxoSmithKline)

> Long-acting β₂-adrenergic agonists (LABAs), such as salmeterol, increase the risk of asthma-related death. LABAs may increase the risk of asthma-related hospitalization in pediatrics and adolescents. Use only for patients not adequately controlled on a long-term asthma control medication (eg, inhaled corticosteroid) or whose disease severity clearly warrants initiation of treatment with both an inhaled corticosteroid and a LABA. Do not use if asthma is adequately controlled on low- or medium-dose inhaled corticosteroids.

THERAPEUTIC CLASS: Beta₂-agonist/corticosteroid

INDICATIONS: Treatment of asthma in patients ≥12 yrs of age.

DOSAGE: *Adults:* Initial: Based upon asthma severity. Usual: 2 inh bid (am and pm, q12h). May replace current strength with a higher strength if response to initial dose after 2 weeks is inadequate. Max: 2 inh of 230/21 bid. Elderly: Start at lower end of dosing range.
Pediatrics: ≥12 Yrs: Initial: Based upon asthma severity. Usual: 2 inh bid (am and pm, q12h). May replace current strength with a higher strength if response to initial dose after 2 weeks is inadequate. Max: 2 inh of 230/21 bid.

ADVAIR HFA

HOW SUPPLIED: MDI: (Fluticasone Propionate-Salmeterol) (45/21) 45mcg-21mcg/inh, (115/21) 115mcg-21mcg/inh, (230/21) 230mcg-21mcg/inh [60, 120 inhalations]

CONTRAINDICATIONS: Primary treatment of status asthmaticus or other acute episodes of asthma where intensive measures are required.

WARNINGS/PRECAUTIONS: Do not initiate during rapidly deteriorating or potentially life-threatening episodes of asthma; serious acute respiratory events, including fatalities, reported. Do not use for the relief of acute symptoms; use inhaled short-acting β_2-agonists (SABAs). D/C regular use of oral/inhaled SABAs when beginning treatment. Do not use more often or at higher doses than recommended; clinically significant cardiovascular (CV) effects and fatalities reported with excessive use. *Candida albicans* infections of mouth and pharynx reported; treat and if needed, interrupt therapy. Lower respiratory tract infections (eg, pneumonia) reported in patients with chronic obstructive pulmonary disease (COPD). Increased susceptibility to infections. May lead to serious/fatal course of chickenpox or measles; avoid exposure and if exposed, consider prophylaxis/treatment. Caution in patients with active/quiescent tuberculosis (TB), untreated systemic fungal, bacterial, viral, or parasitic infections, or ocular herpes simplex. Deaths due to adrenal insufficiency reported during and after transfer from systemic to inhaled corticosteroids. Resume oral corticosteroids during periods of stress or a severe asthma attack in patients previously withdrawn from systemic corticosteroids. Wean slowly from systemic corticosteroid use after transferring to therapy. Transferring from systemic to inhaled corticosteroid may unmask conditions previously suppressed by systemic therapy (eg, rhinitis, conjunctivitis, eczema, arthritis, eosinophilic conditions). Monitor for systemic corticosteroid effects. Reduce dose slowly if hypercorticism and adrenal suppression appear. May produce paradoxical bronchospasm; treat immediately, d/c therapy, and institute alternative therapy. Upper airway symptoms reported. Immediate hypersensitivity reactions may occur. CV and CNS effects may occur. Caution with CV disorders. Decreases in bone mineral density (BMD) reported with long-term use; caution with major risk factors for decreased bone mineral content, including chronic use of drugs that can reduce bone mass (eg, anticonvulsants, corticosteroids). May reduce growth velocity in pediatrics; monitor growth routinely. Glaucoma, increased intraocular pressure (IOP), and cataracts reported with long-term use. Systemic eosinophilic conditions (eg, Churg-Strauss syndrome) may occur. Caution with convulsive disorders or thyrotoxicosis, diabetes mellitus (DM), ketoacidosis, hepatic disease, in patients unusually responsive to sympathomimetic amines, and elderly. Clinically significant changes in blood glucose and/or serum K^+ reported.

ADVERSE REACTIONS: Upper respiratory tract infection, headache, throat irritation, musculoskeletal pain, N/V, dizziness, viral GI/respiratory infection, hoarseness/dysphonia, GI signs and symptoms, upper respiratory inflammation.

INTERACTIONS: Do not use with other medications containing a LABA. Not recommended with strong CYP3A4 inhibitors (eg, ritonavir, atazanavir, clarithromycin, indinavir, itraconazole, nefazodone, nelfinavir, saquinavir, ketoconazole, telithromycin); increased systemic corticosteroid and increased CV adverse effects may occur. Extreme caution with TCAs or MAOIs, or within 2 weeks of discontinuing of such agents; action on the vascular system may be potentiated by these agents. β-blockers may block pulmonary effects and produce severe bronchospasm in patients with reversible obstructive airways disease; if such therapy is needed, consider cardioselective β-blockers and use them with caution. ECG changes and/or hypokalemia that may result from non-K^+-sparing diuretics (eg, loop or thiazide diuretics) may be acutely worsened; use with caution.

PREGNANCY: Category C, caution in nursing.

MECHANISM OF ACTION: Fluticasone: Corticosteroid; shown to inhibit multiple cell types (eg, mast cells, eosinophils, basophils, lymphocytes, macrophages, neutrophils) and mediator production or secretion (eg, histamine, eicosanoids, leukotrienes, cytokines) involved in the asthmatic response. Salmeterol: LABA; attributable to stimulation of intracellular adenyl cyclase, the enzyme that catalyzes the conversion of ATP to cAMP. Increased cAMP levels cause relaxation of bronchial smooth muscle and inhibition of release of mediators of immediate hypersensitivity from cells, especially from mast cells.

PHARMACOKINETICS: Absorption: Fluticasone: Absolute bioavailability (5.3%); AUC=274pg•hr/mL; C_{max}=41pg/mL (45/21), 108pg/mL (115/21), 173pg/mL (230/21); T_{max}=0.33-1.5 hrs. Salmeterol: AUC=53pg•hr/mL; C_{max}=220-470pg/mL; T_{max}=5-10 min. **Distribution:** Fluticasone: (IV) V_d=4.2L/kg; plasma protein binding (99%). Salmeterol: Plasma protein binding (96%). **Metabolism:** Fluticasone: 17β-carboxylic acid via CYP3A4. Salmeterol: Extensive by hydroxylation; α-hydroxysalmeterol via CYP3A4. **Elimination:** Fluticasone: Urine (<5%, metabolites), feces; $T_{1/2}$=5.6 hrs. Salmeterol: Feces (60%), urine (25%); $T_{1/2}$=5.5 hrs.

NURSING CONSIDERATIONS

Assessment: Assess for status asthmaticus, acute asthma episodes, rapidly deteriorating asthma, COPD, active/quiescent TB, untreated systemic infections, ocular herpes simplex, CV disorders, risk factors for decreased bone mineral content, history of increased IOP, glaucoma, and/or cataracts, convulsive disorders, thyrotoxicosis, DM, ketoacidosis, hepatic disease, drug hypersensitivity, pregnancy/nursing status, and possible drug interactions. Assess use in patients unusually responsive to sympathomimetic amines.

Monitoring: Monitor for localized oral *C. albicans* infections, lower respiratory tract infections, deteriorating asthma, hypercorticism, adrenal suppression, paradoxical bronchospasm, upper airway symptoms, hypersensitivity reactions, CV/CNS effects, glaucoma, cataracts, IOP, eosinophilic conditions, and other adverse reactions. Monitor growth in pediatrics, BMD, blood glucose, and serum K+ levels.

Patient Counseling: Inform about increased risk of asthma-related hospitalization in pediatric/adolescent patients and asthma-related death. Advise not to use to relieve acute asthma symptoms, and, if symptoms arise in the period between doses, to use an inhaled SABA for immediate relief. Instruct to seek medical attention immediately if experiencing a decrease in effectiveness of inhaled SABA, a need for more inhalations than usual of inhaled SABA, or a significant decrease in lung function. Advise not to d/c therapy without physician's guidance and not to use additional LABA. Instruct to contact physician if oropharyngeal candidiasis or symptoms of pneumonia develop. Advise to avoid exposure to chickenpox or measles, and, if exposed, to consult physician without delay. Inform about risk of immunosuppression, hypercorticism and adrenal suppression, reduction in BMD, reduced growth velocity in pediatrics, ocular effects, and of adverse effects such as palpitations, chest pain, rapid HR, tremor, or nervousness.

Administration: Oral inhalation route. After inhalation, rinse mouth with water without swallowing. Shake well for 5 sec before using. Refer to PI for priming and administration instructions.
Storage: 25°C (77°F); excursions permitted to 15-30°C (59-86°F). Store with the mouthpiece down. Do not puncture, use/store near heat or open flame, or throw container into fire/incinerator. Discard when the counter reads "000."

ADVICOR   RX
niacin - lovastatin (AbbVie)

THERAPEUTIC CLASS: HMG-CoA reductase inhibitor/nicotinic acid

INDICATIONS: Niacin Extended-Release (ER): Adjunct to diet to reduce elevated total cholesterol (total-C), LDL, apolipoprotein B, and TG levels, and to increase HDL in primary hypercholesterolemia and mixed dyslipidemia. To reduce the risk of recurrent nonfatal myocardial infarction (MI) in patients with history of MI and hypercholesterolemia. Adjunctive therapy for treatment of adults with very high serum TG levels who present a risk of pancreatitis who do not respond adequately to diet. Lovastatin: Adjunct to diet to reduce elevated total-C and LDL in primary hypercholesterolemia. To reduce risk of MI, unstable angina, and coronary revascularization procedures in patients without symptomatic cardiovascular disease, average to moderately elevated total-C and LDL and below-average HDL. To slow progression of coronary atherosclerosis in patients with coronary heart disease by lowering total-C and LDL to target levels.

DOSAGE: *Adults:* Individualize dose. Take at hs with a low-fat snack. Not Currently on Niacin ER: Initial: 500mg-20mg qd. Titrate: Increase by no more than 500mg qd (based on niacin ER component) every 4 weeks. Max: 2000mg-40mg qd. Women may respond at lower niacin doses than men. Concomitant Danazol/Diltiazem/Verapamil: (Lovastatin Content): Initial: 10mg/day. Max: 20mg/day. Concomitant Amiodarone: (Lovastatin Content): Max: 40mg/day. Severe Renal Insufficiency (CrCl <30mL/min): Carefully consider lovastatin dose increases >20mg/day; give cautiously if deemed necessary. May take aspirin (ASA) (up to 325mg) 30 min prior to treatment to reduce flushing. Do not interchange two of 500mg-20mg and one of 1000mg-40mg tab. If therapy is discontinued for an extended period (>7 days), reinstitution should begin with lowest dose. Refer to PI for further dosing information.

HOW SUPPLIED: Tab: (Niacin ER-Lovastatin) 500mg-20mg, 750mg-20mg, 1000mg-20mg, 1000mg-40mg

CONTRAINDICATIONS: Active liver disease or unexplained persistent elevations in serum transaminases, active peptic ulcer disease (PUD), arterial bleeding, pregnancy, women of childbearing age who may become pregnant, and nursing mothers. Concomitant administration with strong CYP3A4 inhibitors (eg, itraconazole, ketoconazole, posaconazole, HIV protease inhibitors, boceprevir, telaprevir, erythromycin, clarithromycin, telithromycin, nefazodone).

WARNINGS/PRECAUTIONS: Do not substitute for equivalent doses of immediate-release (IR) (crystalline) niacin or other modified-release (sustained-release or time-release) niacin preparations other than Niaspan. Severe hepatic toxicity, including fulminant hepatic necrosis, reported when substituting sustained-release niacin for IR niacin at equivalent doses. If switching from IR niacin, initiate with low doses (500mg qhs) and titrate to desired therapeutic response. Caution with renal impairment, or with substantial alcohol consumption and/or history of liver disease. Associated with abnormal LFTs; obtain LFTs prior to initiation and repeat as clinically indicated. Fatal and nonfatal hepatic failure (rare) reported; promptly interrupt therapy if serious liver injury with clinical symptoms and/or hyperbilirubinemia or jaundice occurs and do not restart if no alternate etiology found. Myopathy and/or rhabdomyolysis reported when lovastatin is used with lipid-altering doses (≥1g/day) of niacin; d/c if markedly elevated CPK levels occur or myopathy is diagnosed/suspected, and temporarily withhold in any patient experiencing acute or serious condition predisposing to development of renal failure secondary to rhabdomyolysis. Immune-mediated necrotizing myopathy (IMNM) reported. Closely observe patients with history of jaundice, hepatobiliary disease, or peptic ulcer. Increases in HbA1c and FPG levels reported; closely monitor diabetic/potentially diabetic patients, and adjust diet and/or hypoglycemic therapy if necessary. May increase PT and reduce platelet counts; carefully evaluate patients undergoing surgery. Associated with dose-related reductions in phosphorus (P) levels; periodically monitor P levels in patients at risk for hypophosphatemia. Caution with unstable angina or in the acute phase of MI, particularly when such patients are also receiving vasoactive drugs (eg, nitrates, calcium channel blockers, adrenergic blocking agents). Elevated uric acid levels reported; caution in patients predisposed to gout. Evaluate patients who develop endocrine dysfunction. Lab test interactions may occur.

ADVERSE REACTIONS: Flushing, infection, headache, pain, N/V, pruritus, flu syndrome, diarrhea, back pain, asthenia, rash, hyperglycemia, abdominal pain, myalgia, dyspepsia.

INTERACTIONS: See Contraindications and Dosage. Lovastatin: Due to the risk of myopathy, avoid with gemfibrozil, cyclosporine, and large quantities of grapefruit juice (>1 quart/day); caution with fibrates, colchicine, danazol, diltiazem, verapamil, and amiodarone. Voriconazole may increase concentrations and may increase risk of myopathy/rhabdomyolysis; consider dose adjustment of lovastatin. Ranolazine may increase risk of myopathy/rhabdomyolysis; consider dose adjustment of lovastatin. Caution with drugs (eg, spironolactone, cimetidine) that may decrease the levels or activity of endogenous steroid hormones. Determine PT before initiation and frequently during therapy with coumarin anticoagulants. Niacin ER: Avoid ingestion of alcohol, hot drinks, or spicy foods around the time of administration; may increase flushing and pruritus. May potentiate the effects of ganglionic blocking agents and vasoactive drugs, resulting in postural hypotension. ASA may decrease the metabolic clearance. Separate dosing from bile acid-binding resins (eg, colestipol, cholestyramine) by at least 4-6 hrs. Vitamins or other nutritional supplements containing large doses of niacin or related compounds (eg, nicotinamide) may potentiate adverse effects.

PREGNANCY: Category X, not for use in nursing.

MECHANISM OF ACTION: Niacin ER: Nicotinic acid; has not been established. May partially inhibit release of free fatty acids from adipose tissue, and increase lipoprotein lipase activity (which may increase the rate of chylomicron TG removal from plasma). Decreases the rate of hepatic synthesis of VLDL and LDL. Lovastatin: HMG-CoA reductase inhibitor; may involve both reduction of VLDL concentration and induction of LDL receptor, leading to reduced production and/or increased catabolism of LDL.

PHARMACOKINETICS: Absorption: Niacin ER: C_{max}=18mcg/mL, T_{max}=5 hrs. Lovastatin: Incomplete. C_{max}=11ng/mL, T_{max}=2 hrs. **Distribution:** Niacin ER: Plasma protein binding (<20%); found in breast milk. Lovastatin: Plasma protein binding (>95%). **Metabolism:** Niacin ER: Liver (rapid and extensive 1st-pass); nicotinuric acid (via conjugation), nicotinamide adenine dinucleotide (metabolites). Lovastatin: Liver (extensive 1st-pass) via CYP3A4; β-hydroxyacid and 6'-hydroxy derivative (major active metabolites). **Elimination:** Niacin ER: Urine (≥60%); $T_{1/2}$=20-48 min. Lovastatin: (Mevacor) Urine (10%), feces (83%); $T_{1/2}$=4.5 hrs.

NURSING CONSIDERATIONS

Assessment: Assess for history of/active liver disease or PUD, unexplained persistent hepatic transaminase elevations, arterial bleeding, history of jaundice or hepatobiliary disease, renal impairment, diabetes, risk for hypophosphatemia, any other conditions where treatment is contraindicated or cautioned, drug hypersensitivity, pregnancy/nursing status, and possible drug interactions. Assess lipid profile and LFTs.

Monitoring: Monitor for signs/symptoms of myopathy (including IMNM), rhabdomyolysis, liver/renal/endocrine dysfunction, decreases in platelet counts, increases in PT and uric acid levels, and other adverse reactions. Monitor LFTs, blood glucose, and CPK levels. Perform lipid determinations at intervals of ≥4 weeks. Periodically monitor P levels in patients at risk for hypophosphatemia. Check PT with coumarin anticoagulants.

Patient Counseling: Instruct to report promptly any unexplained muscle pain, tenderness, or weakness, particularly if accompanied by malaise or fever or if muscle signs and symptoms persist after discontinuation. Instruct to report promptly any symptoms that may indicate liver injury (eg, fatigue, anorexia, right upper abdominal discomfort, dark urine, jaundice). Advise to carefully follow the prescribed dosing regimen. Inform that flushing may occur, but usually subsides after several weeks of consistent use of therapy. Instruct that if awakened by flushing, especially if taking antihypertensives, to rise slowly to minimize the potential for dizziness and/or syncope. Instruct to avoid ingestion of alcohol, hot beverages, or spicy foods around the time of administration to minimize flushing. Counsel to avoid administration with grapefruit juice. Instruct to contact physician prior to restarting therapy if therapy is discontinued for an extended length of time. Advise to notify physician if taking vitamins or other nutritional supplements containing niacin or related compounds, and if symptoms of dizziness occur. Instruct diabetic patients to notify physician of changes in blood glucose. Instruct to immediately d/c use and notify physician as soon as pregnancy is recognized.

Administration: Oral route. Take at hs with a low-fat snack. Take tab whole; do not break, crush, or chew. Avoid administration on an empty stomach to reduce flushing, pruritus, and GI distress.

Storage: 20-25°C (68-77°F).

AFINITOR RX
everolimus (Novartis)

OTHER BRAND NAMES: Afinitor Disperz (Novartis)

THERAPEUTIC CLASS: Kinase inhibitor

INDICATIONS: Indicated in pediatric and adult patients with tuberous sclerosis complex (TSC) for the treatment of subependymal giant cell astrocytoma (SEGA) that requires therapeutic intervention but cannot be curatively resected. (Tab) Treatment of postmenopausal women with advanced hormone receptor-positive, HER2-negative breast cancer (advanced HR+ BC) in combination with exemestane, after failure of treatment with letrozole or anastrozole. Treatment of adults with progressive neuroendocrine tumors of pancreatic origin (PNET) with unresectable, locally advanced, or metastatic disease. Treatment of adults with advanced renal cell carcinoma (RCC) after failure of treatment with sunitinib or sorafenib. Treatment of adults with renal angiomyolipoma and TSC, not requiring immediate surgery.

DOSAGE: *Adults:* (Tab) HR+ BC/RCC/PNET/Renal Angiomyolipoma with TSC: Usual: 10mg qd. (Sus/Tab) SEGA with TSC: Initial: 4.5mg/m^2 qd. Severe Hepatic Impairment (Child-Pugh Class C) or with Moderate CYP3A4/P-glycoprotein (P-gp) Inhibitors: Initial: 2.5mg/m^2 qd. Concomitant Strong CYP3A4 Inducers: Initial: 9mg/m^2 qd. Adjust dose based on therapeutic drug monitoring. Refer to PI for therapeutic drug monitoring and for dose modifications with hepatic impairment, adverse reactions, and concomitant moderate CYP3A4/P-gp inhibitors, and strong CYP3A4/P-gp inducers. Continue treatment until disease progression or unacceptable toxicity occurs. *Pediatrics:* ≥1 Yr: (Sus/Tab) SEGA with TSC: Initial: 4.5mg/m^2 qd. Severe Hepatic Impairment (Child-Pugh Class C) or with Moderate CYP3A4/P-gp Inhibitors: Initial: 2.5mg/m^2 qd. Concomitant Strong CYP3A4 Inducers: Initial: 9mg/m^2 qd. Adjust dose based on therapeutic drug monitoring. Refer to PI for therapeutic drug monitoring and for dose modifications with hepatic impairment, adverse reactions, and concomitant moderate CYP3A4/P-gp inhibitors, and strong CYP3A4/P-gp inducers. Continue treatment until disease progression or unacceptable toxicity occurs.

HOW SUPPLIED: Sus (Tab): (Disperz) 2mg, 3mg, 5mg; Tab: 2.5mg, 5mg, 7.5mg, 10mg

WARNINGS/PRECAUTIONS: Not indicated for the treatment of functional carcinoid tumors. Noninfectious pneumonitis reported; for moderate symptoms, consider interrupting therapy until symptoms resolve and consider corticosteroid use. Immunosuppressive properties may predispose patients to localized and systemic infections, including infections with opportunistic pathogens. Treat preexisting invasive fungal infections completely prior to therapy. Institute appropriate treatment if diagnosis of an infection is made and consider interruption or discontinuation of therapy. Mouth ulcers, stomatitis, and oral mucositis reported. May delay wound healing and may increase the occurrence of wound-related complications (eg, wound dehiscence, wound infection, incisional hernia, lymphocele, seroma). Caution use in the perisurgical period. Cases of renal failure observed; monitor renal function in patients with additional risk factors that may further impair renal function. Elevated SrCr, proteinuria, hyperglycemia, hyperlipidemia, hypertriglyceridemia, decreased Hgb, lymphocytes, neutrophils, and platelets reported; monitor parameters prior to initiating therapy and periodically thereafter as well as management with appropriate therapy. Exposure is increased in patients with hepatic impairment. Avoid close contact with those who have received live vaccines during treatment. Pediatric patients with SEGA that do not require immediate treatment should complete the recommended childhood series of live virus vaccinations prior to therapy; an accelerated vaccination schedule may be appropriate. May cause fetal harm. Caution in elderly.

ADVERSE REACTIONS: Stomatitis, infections, rash, diarrhea, fatigue, edema, abdominal pain, nausea, fever, headache, respiratory tract infection, asthenia, cough, decreased appetite.

INTERACTIONS: Reduce dose and use with caution in combination with moderate CYP3A4/P-gp inhibitors (eg, amprenavir, fosamprenavir, aprepitant, erythromycin, fluconazole, verapamil, diltiazem) and avoid use with strong inhibitors of CYP3A4/P-gp (eg, ketoconazole, itraconazole, clarithromycin, atazanavir, nefazodone, saquinavir, telithromycin, ritonavir, indinavir, nelfinavir, voriconazole); may increase levels. Strong CYP3A4/P-gp inducers (eg, phenytoin, carbamazepine, rifampin, rifabutin, rifapentine, phenobarbital) may decrease levels; avoid use, and if combination cannot be avoided, increase dose of everolimus. Avoid use with St. John's wort; may decrease levels. Avoid use with grapefruit, grapefruit juice, and other foods that are known to inhibit CYP450 and P-gp activity; may increase exposures. May increase midazolam levels and exposure. May increase octreotide levels. Avoid use of live vaccines while on therapy. May alter exemestane levels. More frequent monitoring is recommended when coadministered with other drugs that may induce hyperglycemia.

PREGNANCY: Category D, not for use in nursing.

MECHANISM OF ACTION: Kinase inhibitor; binds to an intracellular protein, FKBP-12, resulting in an inhibitory complex formation with mammalian target of rapamycin (mTOR) complex 1 and leading to inhibition of mTOR kinase activity. Inhibition of mTOR has been shown to reduce cell proliferation, angiogenesis, and glucose uptake. Also, inhibits the expression of hypoxia-inducible factor and reduces the expression of vascular endothelial growth factor.

PHARMACOKINETICS: Absorption: T_{max}=1-2 hrs. **Distribution:** Plasma protein binding (74%). **Metabolism:** CYP3A4 and P-gp. **Elimination:** Urine (5%), feces (80%); $T_{1/2}$=30 hrs.

NURSING CONSIDERATIONS

Assessment: Assess for hypersensitivity reactions, preexisting fungal infections, pregnancy/nursing status, and possible drug interactions. Assess renal/hepatic function. Obtain FPG, lipid profile, and CBC prior to start of therapy. Assess vaccination history in pediatric patients with SEGA.

Monitoring: Monitor for signs/symptoms of hypersensitivity reactions, noninfectious pneumonitis, infections, mouth ulcers, stomatitis, oral mucositis, and other adverse reactions. Monitor renal/hepatic function, FPG, lipid profile, and CBC periodically. Routine therapeutic drug monitoring is recommended.

Patient Counseling: Inform that noninfectious pneumonitis or infections may develop; advise to report new or worsening respiratory symptoms or any signs or symptoms of infection. Inform of the possibility of developing mouth ulcers, stomatitis, and oral mucositis; instruct to use topical treatments and mouthwashes (without alcohol, peroxide, iodine, or thyme) in such cases. Inform of the possibility of developing kidney failure and the need to monitor kidney function. Inform of the possibility of impaired wound healing or dehiscence during therapy. Inform of the need to monitor blood chemistry and hematology prior to therapy and periodically thereafter. Advise to notify physician of all concomitant medications, including OTC medications and dietary supplements. Advise of risk of fetal harm. Advise female patients of reproductive potential to avoid becoming pregnant and to use highly effective contraception while on treatment and for up to 8 weeks after ending treatment. Advise to avoid the use of live vaccines and close contact with those who have received live vaccines. Instruct to follow the dosing instructions ud and if a dose is missed, to take it up to 6 hrs after the time they would normally take it. Advise to read and carefully follow the FDA-approved "Instructions for Use" to minimize unintended exposure.

Administration: Oral route. Administer at the same time every day, either consistently with food or consistently without food. Do not combine the 2 dosage forms to achieve the desired total dose. (Tab) Swallow whole with a glass of water; do not break or crush. Do not take tabs that are crushed or broken. (Sus) Prepare only in water. Refer to PI for further administration and preparation instructions. **Storage:** 25°C (77°F); excursions permitted between 15-30°C (59-86°F). Store in the original container, protect from light and moisture.

AFLURIA RX
influenza virus vaccine (Merck)

THERAPEUTIC CLASS: Vaccine

INDICATIONS: Active immunization against influenza disease caused by influenza virus subtypes A and B in persons ≥5 yrs of age.

DOSAGE: *Adults:* 0.5mL IM, preferably in the deltoid muscle of the upper arm.
Pediatrics: ≥9 Yrs: 0.5mL IM. 5-8 Yrs: Not Previously Vaccinated/Vaccinated for the 1st Time Last Season with Only 1 Dose: 0.5mL IM on Day 1, then 0.5mL IM approximately 4 weeks later. Previously Vaccinated with 2 Doses Last Season/At Least 1 Dose ≥2 Yrs Ago: 0.5mL IM. Inject preferably in the deltoid muscle of the upper arm.

HOW SUPPLIED: Inj: 0.5mL [prefilled syringe], 5mL [multi-dose vial]

CONTRAINDICATIONS: Known severe allergic reactions to egg protein.

WARNINGS/PRECAUTIONS: Increased rates of fever and febrile seizures reported in children predominantly <5 yrs of age; febrile events were also reported in children 5 to <9 yrs of age. Caution if Guillain-Barre syndrome (GBS) occurred within 6 weeks of previous influenza vaccination. Appropriate medical treatment and supervision must be available to manage possible anaphylactic reactions. Immune response may be diminished in immunocompromised individuals. May not protect all recipients.

ADVERSE REACTIONS: Inj-site reactions (pain, redness, swelling, tenderness, erythema, induration), headache, myalgia, malaise, N/V, fever, cough, diarrhea.

INTERACTIONS: Corticosteroids or immunosuppressive therapies may diminish immunological response to vaccine.

PREGNANCY: Category B, caution in nursing.

MECHANISM OF ACTION: Vaccine; elicits the formation of antibodies that may protect against influenza virus subtypes A and B.

NURSING CONSIDERATIONS

Assessment: Review immunization history and for previous hypersensitivity to any component of the vaccine (eg, egg protein) or to a previous influenza vaccine, development of GBS following a prior dose of influenza vaccine, pregnancy/nursing status, and for possible drug interactions.

Monitoring: Monitor for signs/symptoms of GBS, allergic reactions, fever and febrile seizures, local inj-site reactions, immune response, and other adverse reactions.

Patient Counseling: Inform of the potential benefits/risks of immunization. Inform that vaccine cannot cause influenza but produces antibodies that protect against influenza and that the full effect of the vaccine is achieved approximately 3 weeks after vaccination. Instruct to report any severe or unusual adverse reactions to physician. Instruct that annual revaccination is recommended.

Administration: IM route. Shake thoroughly before use and administer dose immediately. Administer at different inj sites if to be given at the same time as another injectable vaccine(s). Do not mix with any other vaccine in the same syringe or vial. **Storage:** 2-8°C (36-46°F). Do not freeze. Protect from light. Discard vial within 28 days once stopper has been pierced.

AGGRASTAT RX
tirofiban HCl (Medicure)

THERAPEUTIC CLASS: Glycoprotein IIb/IIIa inhibitor

INDICATIONS: To reduce the rate of thrombotic cardiovascular events (combined endpoint of death, myocardial infarction, or refractory ischemia/repeat cardiac procedure) in patients with non-ST elevation acute coronary syndrome.

DOSAGE: *Adults:* 25mcg/kg IV over 3 min, then 0.15mcg/kg/min (or 0.075mcg/kg/min for patients with SrCr ≤60mL/min), for up to 18 hrs. Refer to PI for dosing by weight and CrCl.

HOW SUPPLIED: Inj: 50mcg/mL [100mL, 250mL]

CONTRAINDICATIONS: Active internal bleeding, history of bleeding diathesis, major surgical procedure or severe physical trauma within the previous month, history of thrombocytopenia following prior drug exposure.

WARNINGS/PRECAUTIONS: Most bleeding associated with therapy occurs at the arterial access site for cardiac catheterization. Minimize the use of traumatic or potentially traumatic procedures (eg, arterial and venous punctures, IM inj, nasotracheal intubation). Fatal bleeding events reported. Profound thrombocytopenia reported; monitor platelet counts beginning about 6 hrs after treatment initiation and daily thereafter. Monitor platelet counts to exclude pseudothrombocytopenia if platelet count decreases to <90,000/mm^3; d/c therapy and heparin if thrombocytopenia is confirmed. Previous exposure to a glycoprotein (GP) IIb/IIIa receptor antagonist may increase the risk of developing thrombocytopenia.

ADVERSE REACTIONS: Bleeding, pelvic pain, bradycardia, coronary artery dissection, leg pain, dizziness.

INTERACTIONS: Concomitant use of antiplatelet agents, thrombolytics, oral anticoagulants, heparin, and aspirin increases the risk of bleeding.

PREGNANCY: Category B, not for use in nursing.

MECHANISM OF ACTION: GP IIb/IIIa inhibitor; inhibits platelet function by inhibiting adenosine phosphate-induced platelet aggregation and prolongs bleeding time.

PHARMACOKINETICS: Distribution: Plasma protein binding (65%); V_d=22-42L. **Metabolism:** Limited. **Elimination:** Urine (65% unchanged), feces (25% unchanged); $T_{1/2}$=2 hrs.

NURSING CONSIDERATIONS

Assessment: Assess for drug hypersensitivity, active internal bleeding, history of bleeding diathesis, major surgical procedure or severe physical trauma within the previous month, history of thrombocytopenia following prior exposure to drug, pregnancy/nursing status, and possible drug interactions. Assess use of traumatic or potentially traumatic procedures. Obtain baseline platelet count.

Monitoring: Monitor for signs/symptoms of bleeding, hypersensitivity reaction (eg, anaphylaxis), thrombocytopenia, and other adverse reactions. Monitor platelet counts beginning about 6 hrs after treatment initiation and daily thereafter.

Patient Counseling: Advise to watch closely for any signs of bleeding or bruising and to report to physician if these occur. Advise to notify physician of use of any other medications, including OTC or herbal products prior to drug use.

Administration: IV route. Do not administer through the same IV line as diazepam; may administer in the same IV line as atropine sulfate, dobutamine, dopamine, epinephrine HCl, famotidine inj, furosemide, lidocaine, midazolam HCl, morphine sulfate, nitroglycerin, potassium chloride, and propranolol HCl. Refer to PI for further administration instructions. **Storage:** 25°C (77°F); excursions permitted between 15-30°C (59-86°F). Protect from light. Do not freeze.

Aggrenox   RX
aspirin - dipyridamole (Boehringer Ingelheim)

THERAPEUTIC CLASS: Platelet aggregation inhibitor

INDICATIONS: To reduce risk of stroke in patients who have had transient ischemia of the brain or completed ischemic stroke due to thrombosis.

DOSAGE: *Adults:* Usual: 1 cap bid (1 in am and 1 in pm). Intolerable Headaches During Initial Treatment: Switch to 1 cap at hs and low-dose aspirin (ASA) in am. Return to usual regimen as soon as possible, usually within 1 week.

HOW SUPPLIED: Cap: (ASA-Dipyridamole Extended-Release) 25mg-200mg

CONTRAINDICATIONS: NSAID allergy, syndrome of asthma, rhinitis, and nasal polyps, and children or teenagers with viral infections.

WARNINGS/PRECAUTIONS: May increase risk of bleeding. Intracranial hemorrhage reported. Risk of GI side effects (eg, stomach pain, heartburn, N/V, gross GI bleeding, dyspepsia); monitor for signs of ulceration and bleeding. May cause fetal harm; avoid in 3rd trimester of pregnancy. Not interchangeable with individual components of ASA and dipyridamole tabs. ASA: Avoid with history of active peptic ulcer disease (PUD) or with severe hepatic or severe renal (GFR <10mL/min) dysfunction. Bleeding risks reported with chronic, heavy alcohol use (≥3 alcoholic drinks/day). May not provide adequate treatment for cardiac indications for stroke/transient ischemic attack patients for whom ASA is indicated to prevent recurrent myocardial infarction or angina pectoris. Dipyridamole: Elevations of hepatic enzymes and hepatic failure reported. Has a vasodilatory effect; may precipitate/aggravate chest pain in patients with underlying coronary artery disease (CAD). May exacerbate preexisting hypotension.

ADVERSE REACTIONS: Headache, dyspepsia, abdominal pain, N/V, diarrhea, fatigue, arthralgia, pain, back pain, GI bleeding, hemorrhage.

INTERACTIONS: Increased risk of bleeding with other drugs that increase the risk of bleeding (eg, anticoagulants, antiplatelet agents, heparin, fibrinolytics, NSAIDs). Dipyridamole: May increase plasma levels and cardiovascular (CV) effects of adenosine. May counteract effect of cholinesterase inhibitors, potentially aggravating myasthenia gravis. ASA: May decrease effects of ACE inhibitors and β-blockers. Concurrent use with acetazolamide may lead to high serum concentrations of acetazolamide (and toxicity). May displace warfarin from protein binding sites, leading to prolongation of both PT and bleeding time. May decrease total concentration of phenytoin. May increase serum valproic acid levels. May decrease effects of diuretics in renal or CV disease. May inhibit renal clearance of methotrexate, leading to bone marrow toxicity (especially in elderly/renally impaired). Decreased renal function with NSAIDs. Moderate doses may increase effectiveness of PO hypoglycemics. May antagonize uricosuric agents (probenecid and sulfinpyrazone).

PREGNANCY: Category D, caution in nursing.

MECHANISM OF ACTION: Dipyridamole: Platelet aggregation inhibitor. Inhibits uptake of adenosine into platelets, endothelial cells, and erythrocytes. ASA: Platelet aggregation inhibitor. Irreversibly inhibits platelet cyclooxygenase and thus inhibits the generation of thromboxane A_2, a powerful inducer of platelet aggregation and vasoconstriction.

PHARMACOKINETICS: Absorption: Dipyridamole: C_{max}=1.98mcg/mL; T_{max}=2 hrs. ASA: C_{max}=319ng/mL; T_{max}=0.63 hrs. **Distribution:** Found in breast milk. Dipyridamole: V_d=92L; plasma protein binding (99%). ASA: V_d=10L; plasma protein binding (concentration-dependent). **Metabolism:** Dipyridamole: Liver (conjugation); monoglucuronide (primary metabolite). ASA: Plasma (hydrolysis) into salicylic acid (metabolite) then liver (conjugation). **Elimination:** Dipyridamole: Feces, urine; $T_{1/2}$=13.6 hrs. ASA: Urine (10% salicylic acid, 75% salicyluric acid); $T_{1/2}$=0.33 hrs, 1.71 hrs (salicylic acid).

NURSING CONSIDERATIONS

Assessment: Assess for NSAID allergy, syndrome of asthma, rhinitis and nasal polyps, renal/hepatic dysfunction, history of active PUD, alcohol use, CAD, hypotension, hypersensitivity, pregnancy/nursing status, and possible drug interactions.

Monitoring: Monitor for signs/symptoms of allergic reactions, GI effects, elevated hepatic enzymes, hepatic failure, and for bleeding.

Patient Counseling: Inform of risk and signs/symptoms of bleeding (eg, occult bleeding). Instruct to notify physician of all medications and supplements being taken, especially drugs that may increase risk of bleeding. Counsel patients who consume ≥3 alcoholic drinks daily about the bleeding risks. Inform that transient headache may occur; instruct to notify physician if an intolerable headache develops. Inform about signs and symptoms of GI side effects and what steps to take if they occur. Advise that if a dose is missed, take next dose on regular schedule and not to take a double dose. Inform of potential hazard to fetus if used during pregnancy; instruct to notify physician if patient is pregnant or becomes pregnant.

Administration: Oral route. Swallow whole; do not chew or crush. Take with or without food.
Storage: 25°C (77°F); excursions permitted to 15-30°C (59-86°F). Protect from excessive moisture.

ALACORT   RX
hydrocortisone (Crown Laboratories)

OTHER BRAND NAMES: U-cort (Taro)

THERAPEUTIC CLASS: Corticosteroid

INDICATIONS: Relief of the inflammatory and pruritic manifestations of corticosteroid-responsive dermatoses.

DOSAGE: *Adults:* Apply a thin film to affected area(s) bid-qid depending on the severity of the condition.
Pediatrics: Apply a thin film to affected area(s) bid-qid depending on the severity of the condition.

HOW SUPPLIED: Cre: 1% [28.4g, 85.2g]; (U-cort [acetate]) 1% [28.35g, 85g, 123g]

WARNINGS/PRECAUTIONS: Reversible hypothalamic-pituitary-adrenal (HPA) axis suppression, Cushing's syndrome, hyperglycemia and glucosuria reported with systemic absorption. Application of more potent steroids, use over large areas, and use with occlusive dressings augment systemic absorption. Monitor for HPA-axis suppression; d/c, reduce frequency, or substitute with less-potent steroid if occurs. Signs and symptoms of steroid withdrawal may occur infrequently; may require supplemental systemic corticosteroids. D/C if irritation develops. Use appropriate antifungal or antibacterial agent with dermatological infections. Pediatric patients may be more susceptible to systemic toxicity, Cushing's syndrome, intracranial HTN (eg, bulging fontanelles, headaches, bilateral papilledema), and adrenal suppression (eg, linear growth retardation, delayed weight gain, low plasma cortisol levels and absence of response to adrenocorticotropic hormone [ACTH] stimulation). Chronic corticosteroid therapy may interfere with growth and development of children. (Alacort) Not for ophthalmic use. (U-cort) Contains sodium bisulfite; may cause allergic-type reactions in susceptible people; caution with asthmatics. Atrophy of skin and SQ tissues may occur with prolonged use and even with short-term use when used on intertriginous or flexor areas, or on the face.

ADVERSE REACTIONS: HPA-axis suppression, Cushing's syndrome, burning/itching/irritation/dryness at application site, growth retardation, skin atrophy, allergic contact dermatitis, hypertrichosis, maceration of the skin, miliaria, striae, hypopigmentation, folliculitis.

PREGNANCY: Category C, caution in nursing.

MECHANISM OF ACTION: Corticosteroid; possesses anti-inflammatory, antipruritic, and vasoconstrictive properties. Mechanism of anti-inflammatory effects has not been established.

PHARMACOKINETICS: Absorption: Extent of percutaneous absorption depends on skin integrity, vehicle, and use of occlusive dressing. Inflammation and/or other disease processes in the skin increase absorption. **Metabolism:** Liver. **Elimination:** Urine, bile.

NURSING CONSIDERATIONS

Assessment: Assess for dermatological infections, hypersensitivity, pregnancy/nursing status, and possible drug interactions.

Monitoring: Monitor for signs/symptoms of glucocorticoid insufficiency, hyperglycemia, glucosuria, skin irritation, and skin infections (eg, fungal, bacterial). Monitor for HPA-axis suppression by using periodic ACTH stimulation and urinary free cortisol tests in patients applying medication to large surface areas or using occlusive dressings. Monitor for signs/symptoms of systemic toxicity in pediatrics.

Patient Counseling: Instruct patient to use medication ud by the physician and to avoid contact with the eyes. Advise not to use medication for any disorder other than for which it was prescribed. Instruct not to wrap, cover, or bandage treated skin unless directed by physician. Instruct patients to report adverse reactions. Advise not to use tight-fitting diapers or plastic pants on a child being treated in the diaper area.

Administration: Topical route. Occlusive dressings may be used for psoriasis or recalcitrant conditions; d/c if infection develops. **Storage:** (U-cort) 15-30°C (59-86°F). Protect from freezing. Dispense in tight container.

ALBUTEROL   RX
albuterol sulfate (Various)

THERAPEUTIC CLASS: Beta$_2$-agonist

INDICATIONS: (Sol) Relief of bronchospasm in patients ≥2 yrs of age with reversible obstructive airway disease and acute attacks of bronchospasm. (Syrup) Relief of bronchospasm in patients ≥2 yrs of age with reversible obstructive airway disease. (Tab) Relief of bronchospasm in patients ≥6 yrs of age with reversible obstructive airway disease.

DOSAGE: *Adults:* Individualize dose. (Sol) Usual: 2.5mg tid-qid by nebulizer. (Syrup/Tab) Initial: 2mg or 4mg tid or qid. Max: 8mg qid. Elderly/Patients Sensitive to β-Adrenergic Stimulators: (Syrup/Tab) Initial: 2mg tid or qid.
Pediatrics: Individualize dose. (Syrup) >14 Yrs: Initial: 2mg or 4mg tid or qid. Max: 8mg qid. 6-14 Yrs: Initial: 2mg tid or qid. Max: 24mg/day in divided doses. 2-5 Yrs: Initial: 0.1mg/kg tid; not to exceed 2mg tid. Titrate: May increase to 0.2mg/kg tid. Max: 4mg tid. (Tab) >12 Yrs: Initial: 2mg or 4mg tid or qid. Max: 8mg qid. 6-12 Yrs: Initial: 2mg tid or qid. Max: 24mg/day in divided doses. (Syrup/Tab) Patients Sensitive to β-Adrenergic Stimulators: Initial: 2mg tid or qid. 0.5% (Sol) >12 Yrs: Usual: 2.5mg tid-qid by nebulizer. 2-12 Yrs: Initial: 0.1-0.15mg/kg/dose. Max: 2.5mg tid-qid by nebulizer. Refer to PI for approximate dosing according to body weight. 0.083% (Sol) ≥2 Yrs: Usual: ≥15kg: 2.5mg (1 vial) tid-qid by nebulizer. <15kg: Use 0.5% sol if <2.5mg/dose is required.

HOW SUPPLIED: Sol, Inhalation: 0.083% [3mL], 0.5% [20mL]; Syrup: 2mg/5mL [16 fl. oz.]; Tab: 2mg*, 4mg* *scored

WARNINGS/PRECAUTIONS: D/C if paradoxical bronchospasm or cardiovascular (CV) effects occur. Caution with CV disorders (eg, coronary insufficiency, cardiac arrhythmias, HTN), convulsive disorders, hyperthyroidism, diabetes mellitus (DM), and in patients unusually responsive to sympathomimetic amines. Immediate hypersensitivity reactions may occur. Aggravation of pre-existing DM and ketoacidosis reported with large doses of IV albuterol. May produce significant hypokalemia. Reevaluate patient and treatment regimen if deterioration of asthma is observed. Consider adding anti-inflammatory agents (eg, corticosteroids) to adequately control asthma. (Sol) Fatalities reported with excessive use and with the home use of nebulizers. (Syrup/Tab) Rarely, erythema multiforme and Stevens-Johnson syndrome have been associated with oral administration in children.

ADVERSE REACTIONS: Tremors, nervousness, headache, tachycardia, dizziness, palpitations, bronchospasm. (Sol/Tab) Nausea. (Sol/Syrup) Cough. (Sol) Bronchitis. (Syrup) Shakiness, increased appetite, excitement, hyperkinesia. (Tab) Muscle cramps.

INTERACTIONS: Use extreme caution with MAOIs or TCAs, or within 2 weeks of discontinuation of such agents; action of albuterol may be potentiated. β-blockers and albuterol inhibit the effect of each other. (Sol) Do not use with other sympathomimetic aerosol bronchodilators or epinephrine; if additional adrenergic drugs are to be administered by any route, use with caution. (Syrup/Tab) Not recommended with other oral sympathomimetic agents; consider alternative therapy if regular coadministration with an aerosol bronchodilator of the adrenergic stimulant type is required. (0.5% Sol/Syrup/Tab) β-blockers may block pulmonary effects and produce severe bronchospasm in asthmatic patients; avoid concomitant use, but if needed, consider cardioselective β-blockers and use with caution. May acutely worsen ECG changes and/or hypokalemia caused by non-K$^+$-sparing diuretics (eg, loop or thiazide diuretics); use with caution. May decrease digoxin levels; monitor levels.

PREGNANCY: Category C, not for use in nursing.

MECHANISM OF ACTION: β$_2$-agonist; stimulates intracellular adenyl cyclase, the enzyme that catalyzes the conversion of ATP to cAMP. Increased cAMP levels are associated with relaxation of bronchial smooth muscle and inhibition of release of mediators of immediate hypersensitivity from cells, especially from mast cells.

PHARMACOKINETICS: Absorption: (Syrup/Tab) Rapid. C_{max}=18ng/mL, T_{max}=2 hrs. (Sol) C_{max}=2.1ng/mL, T_{max}=0.5 hr. **Elimination:** (Syrup/Tab) Urine (76%), feces (4%); $T_{1/2}$=5 hrs.

NURSING CONSIDERATIONS

Assessment: Assess for history of drug hypersensitivity, CV disorders, convulsive disorders, hyperthyroidism, DM, pregnancy/nursing status, and possible drug interactions. Assess use in patients unusually responsive to sympathomimetic amines.

Monitoring: Monitor for paradoxical bronchospasm, CV effects, deterioration of asthma, immediate hypersensitivity reactions, hypokalemia, and other adverse effects.

Patient Counseling: Instruct not to use more frequently than recommended; advise not to increase dose or frequency without consulting physician. Instruct to seek medical attention immediately if treatment becomes less effective for symptomatic relief, symptoms worsen, and/or there is a need to use the product more frequently than usual. Counsel to take other asthma medications and inhaled drugs only ud by the physician. Inform of the common adverse effects.

Instruct to inform physician if pregnant/nursing. Advise not to use the inh sol if it changes color or becomes cloudy. (0.5% Sol) Instruct to avoid microbial contamination by using proper aseptic techniques each time the bottle is opened.

Administration: Oral and inh route. (Sol) Refer to PI for preparation and administration instructions. **Storage:** (Sol) 2-25°C (36-77°F). (0.083% Sol) Protect from light. Store in pouch until time of use. (Syrup/Tab) 20-25°C (68-77°F).

ALCORTIN-A   RX
hydrocortisone - iodoquinol (Primus)

THERAPEUTIC CLASS: Anti-infective/corticosteroid

INDICATIONS: Possibly effective in contact or atopic dermatitis, impetiginized eczema, nummular eczema, endogenous chronic infectious dermatitis, stasis dermatitis, pyoderma, nuchal eczema and chronic eczematoid otitis externa, acne urticata, localized or disseminated neurodermatitis, lichen simplex chronicus, anogenital pruritus (vulvae, scroti, ani), folliculitis, bacterial dermatoses, mycotic dermatoses (eg, tinea [capitis, cruris, corporis, pedis]), moniliasis, intertrigo.

DOSAGE: *Adults:* Apply to affected area tid-qid or ud.
Pediatrics: ≥12 yrs: Apply to affected area tid-qid or ud.

HOW SUPPLIED: Gel: (Hydrocortisone-Iodoquinol) 2%-1% [2g]

WARNINGS/PRECAUTIONS: For external use only. Keep away from eyes. D/C and institute appropriate therapy if irritation develops. May stain skin, hair, or fabrics. Not for use on infants or under diapers or occlusive dressings. Risk of increased systemic absorption with treatment of extensive areas or use of occlusive dressings; take suitable precautions. Children may absorb larger amounts and be more susceptible to systemic toxicity. Prolonged use may result in overgrowth of nonsusceptible organisms requiring appropriate therapy. Burning, itching, irritation, and dryness reported infrequently. Iodoquinol: May be absorbed through the skin and interfere with thyroid function tests; wait at least 1 month after d/c of therapy to perform tests. Ferric chloride test for phenylketonuria may yield false (+) result if present in the diaper or urine.

ADVERSE REACTIONS: Burning, itching, irritation, dryness, folliculitis, hypertrichosis, acneiform eruptions, hypopigmentation, perioral dermatitis, allergic contact dermatitis, skin maceration, secondary infections, skin atrophy, striae, miliaria.

PREGNANCY: Category C, caution in nursing.

MECHANISM OF ACTION: Hydrocortisone: Corticosteroid; possesses anti-inflammatory, antipruritic, and vasoconstrictive properties. Anti-inflammatory action not established; however, there is a recognizable correlation between vasoconstrictor potency and therapeutic efficacy. Iodoquinol: Anti-infective; possesses both antifungal and antibacterial properties.

PHARMACOKINETICS: Absorption: Hydrocortisone: Percutaneous; inflammation, other disease processes in the skin, and occlusive dressings may increase absorption. **Metabolism:** Glucuronidation. Hydrocortisone: Tetrahydrocortisone and tetrahydrocortisol (metabolites). **Elimination:** Hydrocortisone: Urine. Iodoquinol: (PO) Urine (3-5% glucuronide).

NURSING CONSIDERATIONS

Assessment: Assess for known hypersensitivity to any components of the preparation and pregnancy/nursing status.

Monitoring: Monitor for irritation, development of systemic toxicity in children, and overgrowth of nonsusceptible organisms. If extensive areas are treated or if occlusive dressings are used, monitor for systemic absorption.

Patient Counseling: Instruct parents of pediatric patients not to use tight-fitting diapers or plastic pants on child being treated in diaper area. Counsel to keep medication away from eyes. Instruct to use the medication ud. If irritation develops, counsel to d/c medication and institute appropriate therapy. Inform that medication may cause staining of skin, hair, or fabrics and burning, itching, irritation, or dryness.

Administration: Topical route. **Storage:** 15-30°C (59-86°F). Keep tightly closed.

ALDACTAZIDE   RX
hydrochlorothiazide - spironolactone (G.D. Searle)

> Tumorigenic in chronic toxicity animal studies; avoid unnecessary use. Not for initial therapy of edema or HTN. Edema or HTN requires therapy titrated and treatment must be reevaluated as conditions in each patient warrant.

THERAPEUTIC CLASS: Aldosterone blocker/thiazide diuretic

INDICATIONS: Management of edematous conditions (for patients with congestive heart failure, cirrhosis of the liver accompanied by edema and/or ascites, nephrotic syndrome), essential HTN, and edema during pregnancy due to pathologic causes.

DOSAGE: *Adults:* Establish by individual titration of the components. Edema: Maint: 100mg of each component daily or in divided doses. Range: 25-200mg/day of each component depending on response to initial titration. HTN: Usual: 50-100mg of each component as single dose or in divided doses.

HOW SUPPLIED: Tab: (Spironolactone-HCTZ) 25mg-25mg, 50mg-50mg* *scored

CONTRAINDICATIONS: Anuria, acute renal insufficiency, significant impairment of renal excretory function, hypercalcemia, hyperkalemia, Addison's disease or other conditions associated with hyperkalemia, sulfonamide-derived drug hypersensitivity, acute or severe hepatic failure.

WARNINGS/PRECAUTIONS: Caution with hepatic dysfunction; alterations of fluid and electrolyte balance may precipitate hepatic coma. Somnolence and dizziness reported; may impair mental/physical abilities. HCTZ: Caution with severe renal disease; may precipitate azotemia. Sensitivity reactions with or without a history of allergy or bronchial asthma may occur. May exacerbate or activate systemic lupus erythematosus (SLE). Idiosyncratic reaction, resulting in acute transient myopia and acute angle-closure glaucoma may occur; d/c treatment as rapidly as possible and consider medical/surgical treatment if intraocular pressure remains uncontrolled. Hypokalemia, hyponatremia, and hypercalcemia may occur. May alter glucose tolerance and increase cholesterol and TG levels. May increase uric acid levels and cause or exacerbate hyperuricemia and precipitate gout in susceptible patients. Spironolactone: May increase risk of hyperkalemia in patients with renal insufficiency and diabetes mellitus (DM). Gynecomastia may occur. (Rare) Breast enlargement may persist when therapy is discontinued.

ADVERSE REACTIONS: Gastric bleeding, ulceration, gynecomastia, leukopenia, fever, urticaria, mental confusion, ataxia, renal dysfunction, electrolyte disturbances, weakness, irregular menses, toxic epidermal necrolysis, vertigo, muscle spasm.

INTERACTIONS: Avoid with K^+ supplements, K^+-sparing diuretics, or a diet rich in K^+; hyperkalemia may occur. Extreme caution with NSAIDs (eg, indomethacin), ACE inhibitors, angiotensin II receptor antagonists, aldosterone blockers, heparin, low molecular weight heparin, other drugs known to cause hyperkalemia, and salt substitutes containing K^+; severe hyperkalemia may occur. Alcohol, barbiturates, or narcotics may potentiate orthostatic hypotension. Dose adjustment of antidiabetic drugs (eg, oral agents, insulin) may be required. Intensified electrolyte depletion, particularly hypokalemia, may occur with corticosteroids and adrenocorticotropic hormone (ACTH). Reduced vascular responsiveness to norepinephrine. Caution with regional or general anesthesia. Increased responsiveness to nondepolarizing skeletal muscle relaxants (eg, tubocurarine). Increased risk of lithium toxicity; avoid with lithium. HCTZ: May add to or potentiate the action of other antihypertensive drugs. Electrolyte disturbances (eg, hypokalemia, hypomagnesia) may increase risk of digoxin toxicity. Spironolactone: May increase levels of digoxin; monitor digoxin levels and adjust dose accordingly. Hyperkalemic metabolic acidosis reported with cholestyramine.

PREGNANCY: Category C, not for use in nursing.

MECHANISM OF ACTION: Spironolactone: Aldosterone antagonist; acts primarily by competitive binding of receptors at the aldosterone-dependent Na^+-K^+ exchange site in the distal convoluted renal tubule. HCTZ: Thiazide diuretic and antihypertensive; promotes the excretion of Na^+ and water by inhibiting reabsorption in the cortical diluting segment of the distal renal tubule.

PHARMACOKINETICS: Absorption: Spironolactone: C_{max}=80ng/mL, 181ng/mL (canrenone); T_{max}=2.6 hrs, 4.3 hrs (canrenone); AUC_{0-24}=1.30ng•hr/mL, 1.41ng•hr/mL (canrenone). HCTZ: Rapid; T_{max}=1-2 hrs. **Distribution:** Spironolactone: Plasma protein binding (>90%). Canrenone: Found in breast milk. **Metabolism:** Spironolactone: Rapid and extensive; canrenone (active metabolite). **Elimination:** Spironolactone: Urine (major), bile (minor); $T_{1/2}$=1.4 hrs, 16.5 hrs (canrenone). HCTZ: Urine; $T_{1/2}$=4-5 hrs.

NURSING CONSIDERATIONS

Assessment: Assess for anuria, acute renal insufficiency, hypercalcemia, renal/hepatic impairment, risk factors for acute angle-closure glaucoma (eg, history of sulfonamide/penicillin allergy), hyperkalemia, SLE, DM, history of allergy or bronchial asthma, any other conditions where treatment is contraindicated or cautioned, pregnancy/nursing status, and possible drug interactions.

Monitoring: Monitor for signs/symptoms of serum electrolyte abnormalities, hyperkalemia, gynecomastia, exacerbation or activation of SLE, hyperuricemia or precipitation of gout, hypersensitivity reactions, idiosyncratic reactions, and other adverse reactions. Monitor serum electrolytes, TG, cholesterol, and Ca^{2+} levels, and renal/hepatic function.

Patient Counseling: Instruct to avoid K^+ supplements and foods containing high levels of K^+, including salt substitutes. Inform of pregnancy risks. Advise to seek medical attention if signs/symptoms of serum electrolyte abnormalities, hypersensitivity reactions, or other adverse events occur.

Administration: Oral route. **Storage:** <25°C (77°F).

ALDACTONE   RX
spironolactone (G.D. Searle)

Tumorigenic in chronic toxicity animal studies; avoid unnecessary use.

THERAPEUTIC CLASS: Aldosterone blocker

INDICATIONS: Management of primary hyperaldosteronism (diagnosis, short-term preoperative and long-term maintenance treatment for patients with discrete aldosterone-producing adrenal adenomas who are judged to be poor operative risks or who decline surgery, and for patients with bilateral micro- or macronodular adrenal hyperplasia [idiopathic hyperaldosteronism]), edematous conditions (for patients with congestive heart failure [CHF], hepatic cirrhosis with edema/ascites, nephrotic syndrome), essential HTN (usually in combination with other drugs), and edema during pregnancy due to pathologic causes. Treatment and prophylaxis of hypokalemia. To increase survival, and to reduce the need for hospitalization for severe heart failure (HF) (NYHA Class III-IV) in addition to standard therapy.

DOSAGE: *Adults:* Primary Hyperaldosteronism: (Diagnostic) Long Test: 400mg/day for 3-4 weeks. Short Test: 400mg/day for 4 days. Preoperative: 100-400mg/day. Unsuitable for Surgery: Maint: Lowest effective dose. Edema (CHF, Hepatic Cirrhosis, Nephrotic Syndrome): Initial: 100mg/day given in either single or divided doses for at least 5 days. Range: 25-200mg/day. Titrate: May adjust to optimal therapeutic or maintenance level in single or divided daily doses. May add 2nd diuretic that acts more proximally in the renal tubule if no adequate diuretic response after 5 days. Do not change spironolactone dose when other diuretic therapy is added. HTN: Initial: 50-100mg/day given in single or divided doses for at least 2 weeks. Titrate: Adjust dose according to response. Diuretic-Induced Hypokalemia: 25-100mg/day. Severe HF in Conjunction with Standard Therapy (Serum K⁺ ≤5.0mEq/L, SrCr ≤2.5mg/dL): Initial: 25mg qd. Titrate: If tolerated, may increase to 50mg qd as clinically indicated. May reduce to 25mg qod if not tolerated.

HOW SUPPLIED: Tab: 25mg, 50mg*, 100mg* *scored

CONTRAINDICATIONS: Anuria, acute renal insufficiency, significant impairment of renal excretory function, hyperkalemia, Addison's disease or other conditions associated with hyperkalemia. Concomitant use of eplerenone.

WARNINGS/PRECAUTIONS: Hyperkalemia may be fatal; monitor and manage serum K⁺ in patients with severe HF. If hyperkalemia is suspected, obtain an ECG, monitor serum K⁺, and d/c or interrupt treatment for serum K⁺ >5mEq/L or SrCr >4mg/dL. Caution with hepatic impairment; may precipitate hepatic coma. Monitor for fluid/electrolyte imbalance (eg, hypomagnesemia, hyponatremia, hypochloremic alkalosis, hyperkalemia). Reversible hyperchloremic metabolic acidosis reported in patients with decompensated hepatic cirrhosis. Dilutional hyponatremia may occur in edematous patients in hot weather. May cause transient BUN elevation, especially with preexisting renal impairment. Mild acidosis and dose-related gynecomastia may occur. Somnolence and dizziness reported; may impair mental/physical abilities.

ADVERSE REACTIONS: Gastric bleeding, ulceration, inability to achieve or maintain erection, leukopenia, fever, urticaria, hyperkalemia, mental confusion, ataxia, renal dysfunction, irregular menses, postmenopausal bleeding, N/V, diarrhea, breast pain.

INTERACTIONS: See Contraindications. Concomitant administration of K⁺ supplements, other K⁺-sparing diuretics, ACE inhibitors, angiotensin II antagonists, aldosterone blockers, NSAIDs (eg, indomethacin), heparin and low molecular weight heparin, other drugs known to cause hyperkalemia, diet rich in K⁺, or salt substitutes containing K⁺, may lead to severe hyperkalemia; avoid with other K⁺-sparing diuretics. Avoid using oral K⁺ supplements in patients with serum K⁺ >3.5mEq/L. Extreme caution with NSAIDs (eg, indomethacin) and ACE inhibitors. Alcohol, barbiturates, or narcotics may potentiate orthostatic hypotension. Corticosteroids and adrenocorticotropic hormone may intensify electrolyte depletion, particularly hypokalemia. Reduced vascular responsiveness to norepinephrine, a pressor amine; caution with regional/general anesthesia. May increase responsiveness to nondepolarizing skeletal muscle relaxants (eg, tubocurarine). May increase digoxin levels and subsequent digitalis toxicity; may need to reduce maintenance and digitalization doses and carefully monitor. Avoid with lithium; may reduce clearance of lithium and add a high risk of lithium toxicity. Dilutional hyponatremia may be caused or aggravated with other diuretics. Hyperkalemic metabolic acidosis reported with cholestyramine.

PREGNANCY: Category C, not for use in nursing.

MECHANISM OF ACTION: Aldosterone antagonist; competitively binds to receptors at aldosterone-dependent Na⁺-K⁺ exchange site in distal convoluted renal tubule, causing increased Na⁺ and water excretion, and K⁺ retention.

PHARMACOKINETICS: Absorption: (Healthy) C_{max}=80ng/mL, 181ng/mL (canrenone); T_{max}=2.6 hrs, 4.3 hrs (canrenone). **Distribution:** Plasma protein binding (>90%); found in breast milk (canrenone). **Metabolism:** Rapid and extensive; canrenone (active metabolite). **Elimination:** Urine (major), bile (minor); $T_{1/2}$=1.4 hrs, 16.5 hrs (canrenone).

NURSING CONSIDERATIONS

Assessment: Assess for renal/hepatic impairment, hyperkalemia, Addison's disease or other conditions associated with hyperkalemia, anuria, any other conditions where treatment is contraindicated or cautioned, pregnancy/nursing status, and for possible drug interactions.

Monitoring: Monitor for signs/symptoms of fluid/electrolyte imbalance, dilutional hyponatremia, BUN elevation, hyperchloremic metabolic acidosis, somnolence, dizziness, gynecomastia, and other adverse reactions. Monitor serum electrolytes periodically at appropriate intervals particularly in the elderly and with significant renal/hepatic impairment. Monitor serum K^+ and SrCr one week after initiation or dose increase, monthly for the first 3 months, then quarterly for a yr, and then every 6 months with severe HF.

Patient Counseling: Instruct to avoid K^+ supplements and foods containing high levels of K^+, including salt substitutes. Inform that somnolence and dizziness may occur; advise to use caution when driving or operating machinery until response to initial treatment has been determined.

Administration: Oral route. **Storage:** <25°C (77°F).

ALDARA   RX
imiquimod (Medicis)

THERAPEUTIC CLASS: Immune response modifier

INDICATIONS: Topical treatment of clinically typical, nonhyperkeratotic, nonhypertrophic actinic keratoses on face or scalp in immunocompetent adults. Topical treatment of biopsy-confirmed, primary superficial basal cell carcinoma (sBCC), with a max tumor diameter of 2cm, located on trunk (excluding anogenital skin), neck, or extremities (excluding hands and feet) in immunocompetent adults, only when surgical methods are medically less appropriate and follow-up can be assured. Treatment of external genital and perianal warts/condyloma acuminata in patients ≥12 yrs of age.

DOSAGE: *Adults:* Apply before hs and rub in until no longer visible. Actinic Keratosis: Usual: Apply 2X/week (eg, Monday, Thursday) for a full 16 weeks to defined treatment area (contiguous area 25cm² [eg, 5cm X 5cm]) on face (forehead or 1 cheek) or on scalp (but not both concurrently). Wash off after 8 hrs. Max: 36 pkts for 16 weeks. Use 1 pkt/application. External Genital and Perianal Warts/Condyloma Acuminata: Usual: Apply a thin layer 3X/week until warts are totally cleared. Wash off after 6-10 hrs. Max: 16 weeks. sBCC: Apply a sufficient amount to cover treatment area including 1 cm of skin surrounding tumor 5X/week for a full 6 weeks. Tumor Diameter: 1.5-2cm: 7mm cre droplet (40mg). 1-<1.5cm: 5mm cre droplet (25mg). 0.5-<1cm: 4mm cre droplet (10mg). Wash off after 8 hrs. Max: 36 pkts for 6 weeks. Do not occlude treatment area. *Pediatrics:* ≥12 Yrs: External Genital and Perianal Warts/Condyloma Acuminata: Usual: Apply a thin layer before hs and rub in until no longer visible 3X/week until warts are totally cleared. Wash off after 6-10 hrs. Max: 16 weeks. Do not occlude treatment area.

HOW SUPPLIED: Cre: 5% [250mg, 12ˢ]

WARNINGS/PRECAUTIONS: Caution in patients with preexisting autoimmune conditions. Not recommended for treatment of BCC subtypes other than sBCC. Not for oral, ophthalmic, or intravaginal use. Not recommended until completely healed from any previous drug/surgical treatment, or sunburn. Avoid contact with eyes, lips, and nostrils. Local skin reactions are common; a rest period of several days may be taken if required by patient's discomfort or severity of local skin reaction. Do not extend treatment beyond 16 weeks due to missed doses or rest periods. Non-occlusive dressings (eg, cotton gauze, cotton underwear) may be used in the management of skin reactions. Early clinical clearance cannot be adequately assessed until resolution of local skin reactions (eg, 12 weeks post-treatment). Consider biopsy or other alternative interventions if there is evidence of persistent tumor. Carefully reevaluate treatment and reconsider management with lesions that do not respond to treatment. Avoid or minimize exposure to sunlight (including sunlamps); sunburn susceptibility may be heightened. Caution in patients with considerable sun exposure (eg, due to occupation) and those with inherent sensitivity to sunlight. Intense local inflammatory reactions (eg, skin weeping or erosion, severe vulvar swelling that can lead to urinary retention) may occur and may be accompanied or preceded by flu-like signs/symptoms. May exacerbate inflammatory skin conditions, including chronic graft versus host disease. Interruption of dosing should be considered if systemic/local inflammatory reactions occur.

ADVERSE REACTIONS: Application-site reaction, local skin reactions, upper respiratory tract infection, sinusitis, headache, squamous cell carcinoma, diarrhea, back pain, rhinitis, lymphadenopathy, influenza-like symptoms.

PREGNANCY: Category C, caution in nursing.

MECHANISM OF ACTION: Immune response modifier; has not been established. In actinic keratosis, suspected to increase biomarker levels (CD3, CD4, CD8, CD11c, CD68). In sBCC, suspected to increase infiltration of lymphocytes, dendritic cells, and macrophages into the tumor lesion. In external genital warts, suspected to induce mRNA encoding cytokines, including interferon-α at the treatment site.

PHARMACOKINETICS: Absorption: C_{max}=0.1ng/mL (12.5mg face), 0.2ng/mL (25mg scalp), 3.5ng/mL (75mg hands/arms), 0.4ng/mL (4.6mg average dose). **Elimination:** Urine (4.6mg average dose) (0.11% [males], 2.41% [females]); (75mg dose) (0.08% [males], 0.15% [females]).

NURSING CONSIDERATIONS

Assessment: Assess for preexisting autoimmune conditions, immunosuppression, previous drug/surgical treatment, sunburn, inherent sensitivity to sunlight, and pregnancy/nursing status. For treatment of sBCC, perform biopsy to confirm diagnosis.

Monitoring: Monitor for local inflammatory reactions (eg, weeping or erosion, vulvar swelling), application-site reactions, systemic reactions (eg, flu-like symptoms), and other adverse reactions. For sBCC, monitor treatment site regularly; assess at 12 weeks post-treatment for clinical clearance.

Patient Counseling: Instruct on proper application technique and to use ud. Instruct to avoid contact with eyes, lips, and nostrils. Instruct not to bandage or occlude treatment area. Inform that local skin reactions may occur; instruct to contact physician promptly if experiencing any sign/symptom at application site that restricts/prohibits daily activities or makes continued application difficult. For patients being treated for actinic keratosis and sBCC, encourage using sunscreen and minimizing or avoiding exposure to natural or artificial sunlight (tanning beds, UVA/B treatment) while on therapy. Inform that subclinical lesions may appear in treatment area and may subsequently resolve. For patients being treated for external genital warts, instruct to avoid sexual (genital, anal, oral) contact while cream is on the skin. Advise female patients to avoid vaginal application and caution when applying cream at the vaginal opening. Instruct uncircumcised males treating warts under the foreskin to retract foreskin and clean area daily. Inform that new warts may develop during therapy, as drug is not a cure. Inform that drug may also weaken condoms and vaginal diaphragms and that concurrent use is not recommended.

Administration: Topical route. Prior to application, wash treatment area with mild soap and water and allow to dry thoroughly for at least 10 min. Wash hands before and after application. Wash off with mild soap and water. **Storage:** 4-25°C (39-77°F). Do not freeze. Discard unused and partially used pkts; do not reuse partially used pkts.

ALENDRONATE   RX
alendronate sodium (Various)

OTHER BRAND NAMES: Fosamax (Merck)

THERAPEUTIC CLASS: Bisphosphonate

INDICATIONS: Treatment of osteoporosis in postmenopausal women. Treatment to increase bone mass in men with osteoporosis. (Tab) Prevention of osteoporosis in postmenopausal women. Treatment of glucocorticoid-induced osteoporosis in men and women receiving glucocorticoids in a daily dosage equivalent to 7.5mg or greater of prednisone and who have low bone mineral density (BMD). Treatment of Paget's disease of bone in men and women.

DOSAGE: *Adults:* Postmenopausal Osteoporosis Treatment/Increase Bone Mass in Men with Osteoporosis: 70mg tab/sol once weekly or 10mg tab qd. (Tab) Postmenopausal Osteoporosis Prevention: 35mg once weekly or 5mg qd. Glucocorticoid-Induced Osteoporosis: 5mg qd; 10mg qd for postmenopausal women not on estrogen. Paget's Disease: 40mg qd for 6 months. May consider retreatment (following a 6-month post-treatment evaluation period) if relapse occurs (based on increases in serum alkaline phosphatase), or if treatment fails to normalize serum alkaline phosphatase. (Tab/Sol) Periodically reevaluate the need for continued therapy. Refer to PI for recommendations for Ca^{2+} and vitamin D supplementation.

HOW SUPPLIED: Sol: 70mg [75mL]; Tab: 5mg, 10mg, 35mg, 40mg; (Fosamax) 70mg

CONTRAINDICATIONS: Esophageal abnormalities that delay esophageal emptying (eg, stricture or achalasia), inability to stand or sit upright for at least 30 min, hypocalcemia. (Sol) Patients at increased risk of aspiration.

WARNINGS/PRECAUTIONS: Not recommended with CrCl <35mL/min. May cause local irritation of the upper GI mucosa; caution with active upper GI problems (eg, Barrett's esophagus, dysphagia, other esophageal diseases, gastritis, duodenitis, ulcers). Esophageal reactions (eg, esophagitis, esophageal ulcers/erosions) reported; d/c if dysphagia, odynophagia, retrosternal pain, or new/worsening heartburn develops. Use therapy under appropriate supervision in patients who cannot comply with dosing instructions due to mental disability. Gastric and duodenal ulcers reported. Treat hypocalcemia and other disorders affecting mineral metabolism (eg, vitamin D deficiency) prior to therapy; monitor serum Ca^{2+} and for symptoms of hypocalcemia during therapy. Asymptomatic decreases in serum Ca^{2+} and phosphate may occur; ensure adequate Ca^{2+} and vitamin D intake. Severe and occasionally incapacitating bone, joint, and/or muscle pain reported; d/c if severe symptoms develop. Osteonecrosis of the jaw (ONJ) reported; risk may increase with duration of exposure to drug. If invasive dental procedures are required, discontinuation of treatment may reduce risk for ONJ. Consider discontinuation if ONJ develops. Atypical, low-energy, or low-trauma fractures of the femoral shaft reported; evaluate any patient with a history of bisphosphonate exposure who presents with thigh/groin pain to rule out incomplete femur fracture, and consider interruption of therapy. (Tab) Consider discontinuation after 3-5 yrs of use in patients at low risk for fracture; periodically reevaluate risk for fracture in patients who d/c therapy. Ascertain gonadal hormonal status and consider replacement therapy before initiating therapy for glucocorticoid-induced osteoporosis; measure BMD at initiation and repeat after 6-12 months of combined alendronate and glucocorticoid treatment.

ADVERSE REACTIONS: Nausea, abdominal pain, musculoskeletal pain, acid regurgitation, flatulence, dyspepsia, constipation, diarrhea.

INTERACTIONS: Ca^{2+} supplements, antacids, or oral medications containing multivalent cations will interfere with absorption; wait at least 1/2 hr after taking alendronate before taking any other oral medications. Increased incidence of upper GI adverse events in patients receiving concomitant therapy with daily doses of alendronate >10mg and aspirin-containing products. NSAID use is associated with GI irritation; use with caution.

PREGNANCY: Category C, caution in nursing.

MECHANISM OF ACTION: Bisphosphonate; binds to hydroxyapatite found in bone, and specifically inhibits the osteoclast-mediated bone resorption.

PHARMACOKINETICS: Absorption: Absolute bioavailability (0.64% in women), (0.59% in men). **Distribution:** V_d= at least 28L; plasma protein binding (78%). **Elimination:** (IV) Urine (50%); $T_{1/2}$>10 yrs.

NURSING CONSIDERATIONS

Assessment: Assess for esophageal abnormalities, ability to stand or sit upright for at least 30 min, hypocalcemia, risk for ONJ, active upper GI problems, mental disability, renal impairment, drug hypersensitivity, any other conditions where treatment is contraindicated or cautioned, pregnancy/nursing status, and possible drug interactions. (Tab) For glucocorticoid-induced osteoporosis treatment, assess gonadal hormonal status and obtain BMD.

Monitoring: Monitor for signs/symptoms of ONJ, atypical fractures, esophageal reactions, musculoskeletal pain, hypocalcemia, and other adverse reactions. Monitor serum Ca^{2+} levels. Periodically reevaluate the need for continued therapy. (Tab) Monitor BMD after 6-12 months of combined alendronate and glucocorticoid treatment. For Paget's disease treatment, monitor serum alkaline phosphatase.

Patient Counseling: Inform about benefits/risks of therapy. Instruct to follow all dosing instructions and inform that failure to follow them may increase risk of esophageal problems. Instruct to take upon arising for the day and at least 1/2 hr before the 1st food, beverage, or medication of the day with plain water only; advise to swallow tab with 6-8 oz. of water and to follow oral sol by at least 2 oz. of water. Advise to avoid lying down for at least 30 min after taking the drug and until after 1st food of the day. Instruct to take supplemental Ca^{2+} and vitamin D if daily dietary intake is inadequate. Counsel to consider weight-bearing exercise along with the modification of certain behavioral factors (eg, cigarette smoking, excessive alcohol use), if these factors exist. Advise to d/c and consult physician if symptoms of esophageal disease develop. Instruct that if a once-weekly dose is missed, to take 1 dose on the am after they remember and to return to taking the dose, as originally scheduled on their chosen day; instruct not to take 2 doses on the same day.

Administration: Oral route. Take upon arising for the day. Take at least 1/2 hr before the 1st food, beverage, or medication of the day with plain water only. Do not chew or suck on the tab. **Storage:** Sol: 25°C (77°F); excursions permitted to 15-30°C (59-86°F). Do not freeze. Tab: 20-25°C (68-77°F); (Fosamax) 15-30°C (59-86°F).

ALIMTA   RX
pemetrexed (Lilly)

THERAPEUTIC CLASS: Antifolate

INDICATIONS: Initial treatment of locally advanced or metastatic nonsquamous non-small cell lung cancer (NSCLC) in combination with cisplatin. Maintenance treatment of patients with locally advanced or metastatic nonsquamous NSCLC whose disease has not progressed after 4 cycles of platinum-based first-line chemotherapy. Single-agent for the treatment of patients with locally advanced or metastatic nonsquamous NSCLC after prior chemotherapy. Treatment of patients with malignant pleural mesothelioma whose disease is unresectable or who are otherwise not candidates for curative surgery in combination with cisplatin.

DOSAGE: *Adults:* Premedication: Initiate folic acid (400-1000mcg) PO qd beginning 7 days before the 1st dose; continue during the full course of therapy and for 21 days after the last dose of therapy. Administer vitamin B12 1mg IM 1 week prior to the 1st dose and every 3 cycles thereafter. Subsequent vitamin B12 inj may be given the same day as treatment. Give dexamethasone 4mg PO bid the day before, the day of, and the day after administration of therapy. Combination with Cisplatin: Nonsquamous NSCLC/Mesothelioma: Usual: 500mg/m² IV infused over 10 min on Day 1 of each 21-day cycle. Give cisplatin 75mg/m² infused over 2 hrs beginning 30 min after the end of administration. Single Agent: Nonsquamous NSCLC: Usual: 500mg/m² IV infused over 10 min on Day 1 of each 21-day cycle. Refer to PI for dose adjustments for hematologic toxicities, nonhematologic toxicities, and neurotoxicities.

HOW SUPPLIED: Inj: 100mg, 500mg

WARNINGS/PRECAUTIONS: Not indicated for the treatment of patients with squamous cell NSCLC. Premedicate with folic acid and vitamin B12 to reduce hematologic/GI toxicity, and with dexamethasone. Do not substitute oral vitamin B12 for IM vitamin B12. Bone marrow suppression may occur; myelosuppression is usually the dose-limiting toxicity. Caution with renal/hepatic impairment and in elderly. Avoid in patients with CrCl <45mL/min. D/C if hematologic or nonhematologic Grade 3 or 4 toxicity after two dose reductions or immediately if Grade 3 or 4 neurotoxicity is observed. Do not start a cycle of treatment unless CrCl is ≥45mL/min, absolute neutrophil count is ≥1500 cells/mm³, and platelet count is ≥100,000 cells/mm³; obtain CBC and renal function tests at the beginning of each cycle and PRN. May cause fetal harm; use effective contraception to prevent pregnancy.

ADVERSE REACTIONS: Anemia, anorexia, fatigue, leukopenia, N/V, stomatitis, neutropenia, rash/desquamation, thrombocytopenia, constipation, pharyngitis, diarrhea.

INTERACTIONS: Reduced clearance with ibuprofen. In patients with mild to moderate renal insufficiency (CrCl 45-79mL/min), caution with NSAIDs; avoid NSAIDs with short $T_{1/2}$ (eg, diclofenac, indomethacin) for 2 days before, the day of, and 2 days following therapy. Interrupt dosing of NSAIDs with longer $T_{1/2}$ (eg, meloxicam, nabumetone) for at least 5 days before, the day of, and 2 days following therapy. If concomitant NSAIDs administration is necessary, monitor for toxicity. Delayed clearance with nephrotoxic or tubularly secreted drugs (eg, probenecid).

PREGNANCY: Category D, not for use in nursing.

MECHANISM OF ACTION: Antifolate; disrupts folate-dependent metabolic processes essential for cell replication. Inhibits thymidylate synthase, dihydrofolate reductase, and glycinamide ribonucleotide formyltransferase.

PHARMACOKINETICS: Distribution: V_d=16.1L; plasma protein binding (81%). **Elimination:** Urine (70-90% unchanged); $T_{1/2}$=3.5 hrs (normal renal function).

NURSING CONSIDERATIONS

Assessment: Assess for drug hypersensitivity, renal/hepatic impairment, pregnancy/nursing status, and possible drug interactions. Obtain CBC and renal function tests at the beginning of each cycle.

Monitoring: Monitor for signs and symptoms of hematologic/nonhematologic toxicities, bone marrow suppression (eg, neutropenia, thrombocytopenia, anemia), GI toxicity, neurotoxicity, and other adverse events. Monitor CBC with platelet counts and for nadir and recovery. Perform renal and hepatic function tests periodically.

Patient Counseling: Inform about benefits and risks of therapy. Instruct on the need for folic acid and vitamin B12 supplementation to reduce treatment-related hematological and GI toxicities, and of the need for corticosteroids to reduce treatment-related dermatologic toxicity. Inform about risks of low blood cell counts and instruct to contact physician immediately if signs of infection (eg, fever, bleeding or symptoms of anemia) occur. Instruct to contact physician if persistent vomiting, diarrhea, or signs of dehydration appear. Instruct to inform physician of all concomitant prescription or OTC medications (eg, NSAIDs). Inform female patients of the potential hazard to fetus; advise to avoid pregnancy and to use effective contraceptive measures to prevent pregnancy during treatment.

Administration: IV route. Refer to PI for preparation/administration precautions and preparation for IV infusion administration. **Storage:** Unreconstituted: 25°C (77°F); excursions permitted to 15-30°C (59-86°F). Reconstituted and Infusion Sol: Stable at 2-8°C (36-46°F) for up to 24 hrs.

ALOPRIM   RX
allopurinol sodium (Mylan)

THERAPEUTIC CLASS: Xanthine oxidase inhibitor

INDICATIONS: Management of patients with leukemia, lymphoma, and solid tumor malignancies who are receiving cancer therapy which causes elevations of serum and urinary uric acid levels and who cannot tolerate oral therapy.

DOSAGE: *Adults:* Individualize dose. Initiate 24-48 hrs before the start of chemotherapy. Usual: 200-400mg/m^2/day as single IV infusion or in equally divided infusions at 6-, 8-, or 12-hr intervals. Max: 600mg/day. Renal Impairment: CrCl 10-20mL/min: 200mg/day. CrCl 3-10mL/min: 100mg/day. CrCl <3mL/min: 100mg/day at extended intervals. Elderly: Start at lower end of dosing range.
Pediatrics: Individualize dose. Initiate 24-48 hrs before the start of chemotherapy. Initial: 200mg/m^2/day as single IV infusion or in equally divided infusions at 6-, 8-, or 12-hr intervals. Renal Impairment: CrCl 10-20mL/min: 200mg/day. CrCl 3-10mL/min: 100mg/day. CrCl <3mL/min: 100mg/day at extended intervals.

HOW SUPPLIED: Inj: 500mg

WARNINGS/PRECAUTIONS: D/C at 1st appearance of skin rash or other signs of an allergic reaction. Hepatotoxicity and elevated serum alkaline phosphatase/transaminase reported with PO allopurinol. Bone marrow suppression reported. Evaluate liver function if anorexia, weight loss, or pruritus develops. Periodically monitor LFTs during early stages of therapy in patients with preexisting liver disease. May impair mental/physical abilities. Maintain sufficient fluid intake to yield a daily urinary output in adults of at least 2L and maintain neutral or slightly alkaline urine. Caution with renal impairment or concurrent illnesses affecting renal function (eg, HTN, diabetes mellitus); periodically monitor renal function. Caution in elderly.

ADVERSE REACTIONS: Rash, eosinophilia, local inj-site reaction, diarrhea, nausea, decreased renal function, generalized seizure.

INTERACTIONS: Inhibits oxidation of mercaptopurine and azathioprine; reduce mercaptopurine or azathioprine dose to 1/3-1/4 of usual dose when given with 300-600mg of allopurinol. May prolong $T_{1/2}$ of dicumarol; monitor PT with concomitant use. Inhibition of xanthine oxidase by oxypurinol may be decreased and urinary excretion of uric acid may be increased with concomitant uricosuric agents. May increase toxicity and occurrence of hypersensitivity reactions with concomitant thiazide diuretics in patients with decreased renal function; monitor renal function. May increase frequency of skin rash when used with ampicillin or amoxicillin. Bone marrow suppression may be enhanced with cyclophosphamide and other cytotoxic agents among patients with neoplastic disease, except leukemia. May increase risk of hypoglycemia in the presence of renal insufficiency with concomitant chlorpropamide. May increase cyclosporine levels; monitor cyclosporine levels and consider possible adjustment of cyclosporine dose.

PREGNANCY: Category C, caution in nursing.

MECHANISM OF ACTION: Xanthine oxidase inhibitor; reduces production of uric acid by inhibiting the biochemical reactions immediately preceding its formation.

PHARMACOKINETICS: Absorption: Allopurinol: C_{max}=1.58mcg/mL (100mg), 5.12mcg/mL (300mg); T_{max}=0.5 hr; AUC=1.99 hr•mcg/mL (100mg), 7.1 hr•mcg/mL (300mg). Oxypurinol: C_{max}=2.2mcg/mL (100mg), 6.18mcg/mL (300mg); T_{max}=3.89 hrs (100mg), 4.16 hrs (300mg); AUC=80 hr•mcg/mL (100mg), 231 hr•mcg/mL (300mg). **Distribution:** Found in breast milk. Allopurinol: V_d=0.84L/kg (100mg), 0.87L/kg (300mg). **Metabolism:** Oxidation; oxypurinol (active metabolite). **Elimination:** Urine (12% unchanged, 76% oxypurinol). Allopurinol: $T_{1/2}$=1 hr (100mg), 1.21 hrs (300mg). Oxypurinol: $T_{1/2}$=24.1 hrs (100mg), 23.5 hrs (300mg).

NURSING CONSIDERATIONS

Assessment: Assess for renal/hepatic disease, concurrent illnesses affecting renal function, previous severe reaction to the drug, pregnancy/nursing status, and possible drug interactions. Obtain serum uric acid level to provide correct dosage and schedule.

Monitoring: Monitor for signs/symptoms of hypersensitivity/allergic reactions, drowsiness, bone marrow suppression, and other adverse reactions. Monitor fluid intake, LFTs, renal function (BUN, SrCr, CrCl), and serum uric acid level.

Patient Counseling: Inform of risks and benefits of therapy. Counsel that drug may impair mental/physical abilities. Advise to take sufficient fluid to yield urinary output of at least 2L/day in adults and inform of the need to maintain a neutral or, preferably, slightly alkaline urine. Instruct to report any adverse events to physician.

Administration: IV route. Refer to PI for preparation of sol and administration instructions. Begin administration within 10 hrs after reconstitution. **Storage:** 20-25°C (68-77°F). Do not refrigerate reconstituted/diluted sol.

ALOXI   RX
palonosetron HCl (Eisai)

THERAPEUTIC CLASS: 5-HT$_3$ receptor antagonist

INDICATIONS: Prevention of acute and delayed N/V associated with initial and repeat courses of moderately emetogenic cancer chemotherapy. Prevention of acute N/V associated with initial and repeat courses of highly emetogenic cancer chemotherapy. Prevention of postoperative N/V (PONV) for up to 24 hrs following surgery.

DOSAGE: *Adults:* Chemotherapy-Induced N/V: 0.25mg IV single dose administered over 30 sec; administer dose 30 min before the start of chemotherapy. PONV: 0.075mg IV single dose administered over 10 sec immediately before induction of anesthesia.

HOW SUPPLIED: Inj: 0.075mg/1.5mL, 0.25mg/5mL

WARNINGS/PRECAUTIONS: Hypersensitivity reactions, including anaphylaxis, reported with or without known hypersensitivity to other 5-HT$_3$ receptor antagonists. Routine prophylaxis is not recommended in patients who demonstrate low risk of PONV. Therapy is recommended in patients where N/V must be avoided during the postoperative period.

ADVERSE REACTIONS: Headache, constipation, QT prolongation, bradycardia.

PREGNANCY: Category B, not for use in nursing.

MECHANISM OF ACTION: 5-HT$_3$ receptor antagonist; antiemetic and antinauseant.

PHARMACOKINETICS: Absorption: (3mcg/kg single dose) C_{max}=5.6ng/mL, AUC=35.8ng•hr/mL. **Distribution:** V_d=8.3L/kg; plasma protein binding (62%). **Metabolism:** Via CYP2D6, CYP3A4, CYP1A2; N-oxide-palonosetron and 6-S-hydroxy-palonosetron (primary metabolites). **Elimination:** (10mcg/kg single dose) Urine (80%, 40% unchanged); $T_{1/2}$=40 hrs.

NURSING CONSIDERATIONS

Assessment: Assess for hypersensitivity to drug, risk/possibility of PONV, emetogenicity of cancer chemotherapy, and pregnancy/nursing status.

Monitoring: Monitor for hypersensitivity reactions including anaphylaxis, and other adverse reactions.

Patient Counseling: Inform of the benefits/risks of therapy. Advise to report to physician all medical conditions, any pain, redness, or swelling in and around infusion site.

Administration: IV route. Flush infusion line with normal saline before and after administration. Do not mix with other drugs. **Storage:** 20-25°C (68-77°F); excursions permitted to 15-30°C (59-86°F). Protect from light and freezing.

ALPHAGAN P   RX
brimonidine tartrate (Allergan)

THERAPEUTIC CLASS: Selective alpha$_2$ agonist

INDICATIONS: Reduction of elevated intraocular pressure in patients with open-angle glaucoma or ocular HTN.

DOSAGE: *Adults:* 1 drop in affected eye(s) tid (8 hrs apart). Space by at least 5 min if using >1 topical ophthalmic drug.
Pediatrics: ≥2 Yrs: 1 drop in affected eye(s) tid (8 hrs apart). Space by at least 5 min if using >1 topical ophthalmic drug.

HOW SUPPLIED: Sol: 0.1%, 0.15% [5mL, 10mL, 15mL]

CONTRAINDICATIONS: Neonates and infants <2 yrs of age.

WARNINGS/PRECAUTIONS: May potentiate syndromes associated with vascular insufficiency. Caution with severe cardiovascular disease (CVD), depression, cerebral or coronary insufficiency, Raynaud's phenomenon, orthostatic hypotension, or thromboangiitis obliterans. Bacterial keratitis reported with multidose containers.

ADVERSE REACTIONS: Allergic conjunctivitis, conjunctival hyperemia, eye pruritus, burning sensation, conjunctival folliculosis, HTN, oral dryness, ocular allergic reaction, visual disturbance, somnolence, decreased alertness.

INTERACTIONS: May potentiate effect with CNS depressants (alcohol, barbiturates, opiates, sedatives, anesthetics). Caution with antihypertensives, cardiac glycosides, and TCAs. May increase systemic side effects (eg, hypotension) with MAOIs; caution is advised.

PREGNANCY: Category B, not for use in nursing.

MECHANISM OF ACTION: Selective α$_2$ agonist; reduces aqueous humor production and increases uveoscleral outflow.

PHARMACOKINETICS: Absorption: T_{max}=0.5-2.5 hrs. **Metabolism:** Liver (extensive). **Elimination:** (Oral) Urine (74% unchanged and metabolites); $T_{1/2}$=2 hrs.

NURSING CONSIDERATIONS

Assessment: Assess for hypersensitivity, severe CVD, depression, cerebral or coronary insufficiency, Raynaud's phenomenon, orthostatic hypotension, thromboangiitis obliterans, pregnancy/nursing, and possible drug interactions.

Monitoring: Monitor vascular insufficiency, bacterial keratitis, and other adverse reactions.

Patient Counseling: Advise to avoid touching tip of applicator to eye or surrounding areas. Instruct patient to notify physician if they have ocular surgery or develop an intercurrent ocular condition (eg, trauma or infection). Inform patients that fatigue and/or drowsiness may occur; may impair physical or mental abilities. Instruct to space by at least 5 min if using >1 topical ophthalmic drug.

Administration: Ocular route. **Storage:** 15-25°C (59-77°F).

ALREX   RX
loteprednol etabonate (Bausch & Lomb)

THERAPEUTIC CLASS: Corticosteroid

INDICATIONS: Temporary relief of signs and symptoms of seasonal allergic conjunctivitis.

DOSAGE: *Adults:* 1 drop into the affected eye(s) qid.

HOW SUPPLIED: Sus: 0.2% [5mL, 10mL]

CONTRAINDICATIONS: Viral diseases of the cornea and conjunctiva, including epithelial herpes simplex keratitis (dendritic keratitis), vaccinia, and varicella. Mycobacterial infection of the eye and fungal diseases of the ocular structures.

WARNINGS/PRECAUTIONS: Prolonged use may result in glaucoma with optic nerve damage, visual acuity and visual field defects, and posterior subcapsular cataract formation. Caution with glaucoma. Prolonged use may increase the hazard of secondary ocular infections. Caution with diseases causing thinning of the cornea/sclera; perforations may occur. May mask/enhance existing infection in acute purulent conditions of the eye. May prolong the course or exacerbate severity of many viral infections of the eye. Caution with history of herpes simplex virus. Perform eye exam (eg, slit-lamp biomicroscopy, fluorescein staining) prior to therapy and renewal of medication order >14 days. Reevaluate if signs/symptoms failed to improve after 2 days. Monitor intraocular pressure (IOP) if used >10 days. Fungal infections of the cornea may develop with long-term use; consider fungal invasion in any persistent corneal ulceration.

ADVERSE REACTIONS: Elevated IOP, abnormal vision/blurring, burning on instillation, chemosis, discharge, dry eyes, epiphora, foreign body sensation, itching, photophobia, headache, rhinitis, pharyngitis.

PREGNANCY: Category C, caution in nursing.

MECHANISM OF ACTION: Corticosteroid; not established. Suspected to act by induction of phospholipase A_2 inhibitory proteins, collectively called lipocortins. Inhibits the inflammatory response to a variety of inciting agents and probably delays or slows healing. Inhibits edema, fibrin deposition, capillary dilation, leukocyte migration, fibroblast proliferation, deposition of collagen, and scar formation associated with inflammation.

PHARMACOKINETICS: Distribution: Found in breast milk (systemic use).

NURSING CONSIDERATIONS

Assessment: Assess for hypersensitivity to the drug, viral diseases of the cornea and conjunctiva, vaccinia varicella, mycobacterial eye infection, fungal diseases of the ocular structures, glaucoma, diseases causing thinning of the cornea/sclera, acute purulent conditions of the eye, and pregnancy/nursing status. Perform eye exam (eg, slit-lamp biomicroscopy, fluorescein staining) prior to therapy.

Monitoring: Monitor for signs and symptoms of glaucoma, optic nerve damage, visual acuity and visual field defects, posterior subcapsular cataracts, sclera/corneal perforations, masking or enhancement of existing infections in acute purulent conditions of the eye, and other adverse reactions. Monitor IOP and perform eye exams.

Patient Counseling: ≤Advise not to touch dropper tip to any surface to avoid contamination. Instruct to contact physician if redness or itching becomes aggravated. Instruct not wear contact lenses if eyes are red. Counsel not to use for contact lens-related irritation. Inform that the medication contains benzalkonium chloride that may be absorbed by soft contact lenses. Instruct to wait ≥10 min after administration before wearing soft contact lenses.

Administration: Ocular route. **Storage:** 15-25°C (59-77°F). Store upright. Do not freeze.

ALSUMA   RX
sumatriptan (Pfizer)

THERAPEUTIC CLASS: 5-HT$_{1B/1D}$ agonist

INDICATIONS: Acute treatment of migraine attacks, with or without aura, and cluster headache episodes.

DOSAGE: *Adults:* Max Single Dose: 6mg SQ. Max Dose/24 Hrs: Two 6mg inj separated by at least 1 hr.

HOW SUPPLIED: Inj: 6mg/0.5mL

CONTRAINDICATIONS: IV administration, ischemic heart disease (eg, angina pectoris, history of myocardial infarction [MI], or documented silent ischemia) or symptoms/findings consistent with ischemic heart disease, coronary artery vasospasm (eg, Prinzmetal's variant angina) or other significant underlying cardiovascular (CV) disease, cerebrovascular syndromes (eg, stroke, transient ischemic attacks), peripheral vascular disease (eg, ischemic bowel disease), uncontrolled HTN, hemiplegic or basilar migraine, use within 24 hrs of ergotamine-containing or ergot-type medications (eg, dihydroergotamine, methysergide) or of another 5-HT$_1$ agonist (eg, triptan).

WARNINGS/PRECAUTIONS: May cause coronary artery vasospasm; avoid in patients with potential unrecognized coronary artery disease (CAD) with unsatisfactory CV evaluation. Administer 1st dose under medical supervision; obtain ECG on the 1st occasion of therapy during the interval immediately following administration. Perform periodic CV evaluation in patients on long-term intermittent use with risk factors for CAD. Serious adverse cardiac events (eg, MI, life-threatening cardiac rhythm disturbances) and death reported. Cerebral/subarachnoid hemorrhage, stroke, other cerebrovascular events, and vasospastic reactions (eg, peripheral vascular ischemia and colonic ischemia with abdominal pain and bloody diarrhea) reported. Exclude other potentially serious neurologic conditions before therapy. May cause transient and permanent blindness and significant partial vision loss (very rare). Serotonin syndrome may occur. Significant elevation in BP, including hypertensive crisis reported rarely. Hypersensitivity reactions may occur. Sensations of tightness, pain, pressure, and heaviness in the precordium, throat, neck, and jaw may occur. Evaluate for atherosclerosis or predisposition to vasospasm if signs/symptoms suggestive of decreased arterial flow occur. Seizures reported; caution with history of epilepsy or conditions associated with a lowered seizure threshold. Reconsider the diagnosis of migraine or cluster headache before giving a 2nd dose if patient does not respond to the 1st dose of therapy. Overuse of acute migraine drugs may lead to exacerbation of headache; detoxification, including withdrawal of the overused drugs, and treatment of withdrawal symptoms may be necessary. Corneal opacities may occur. Not for prophylactic therapy of migraine. Should only be used where a clear diagnosis of migraine or cluster headache has been established. Avoid IM or intravascular delivery. Not recommended in elderly.

ADVERSE REACTIONS: Inj-site reactions (bruising, pain, hemorrhage), tingling, warm sensation, dizziness, burning sensation, feeling of heaviness, pressure sensation, flushing, feeling of tightness, numbness, chest tightness, weakness, neck pain.

INTERACTIONS: See Contraindications. Not recommended with MAO-A inhibitors; may increase sumatriptan exposure. If therapy is clinically warranted, dose reduction of sumatriptan (using a different sumatriptan product) and appropriate observation of patient are advised. Serotonin syndrome reported during combined use with SSRIs (eg, fluoxetine, paroxetine, sertraline, fluvoxamine, citalopram, escitalopram), or SNRIs (eg, venlafaxine, duloxetine); if concomitant therapy is clinically warranted, monitor patient during treatment initiation and dose increases.

PREGNANCY: Category C, caution in nursing.

MECHANISM OF ACTION: Selective 5-HT$_{1B/1D}$ agonist; binds to vascular 5-HT$_1$-type receptors in basilar artery and vasculature of isolated dura mater, resulting in vasoconstriction.

PHARMACOKINETICS: Absorption: (Healthy) Bioavailability (97%); (Deltoid) C_{max}=74ng/mL; T_{max}=12 min. (Thigh) C_{max}=61ng/mL (manual inj), 52ng/mL (auto-injector). **Distribution:** V_d=50L; plasma protein binding (14-21%), found in breast milk. **Metabolism:** Indole acetic acid (metabolite). **Elimination:** Urine (22% unchanged, 38% metabolite); $T_{1/2}$=115 min.

NURSING CONSIDERATIONS

Assessment: Confirm diagnosis of migraine or cluster headache and exclude other potentially serious neurologic conditions prior to therapy. Assess for CV disease, HTN, hemiplegic/basilar migraine, any conditions where treatment is cautioned or contraindicated, drug hypersensitivity, pregnancy/nursing status, and possible drug interactions.

Monitoring: Monitor for signs/symptoms of cardiac events (eg, coronary vasospasm, acute MI, arrhythmia, ECG changes), cerebrovascular events (eg, hemorrhage, stroke, transient ischemic attacks), peripheral vascular ischemia, colonic ischemia, serotonin syndrome, hypersensitivity reactions, HTN, ophthalmic changes, and other adverse reactions. Perform periodic CV evaluation in patients on long-term intermittent use with risk factors for CAD.

Patient Counseling: Inform that therapy may cause serious CV side effects; instruct to seek medical attention if chest pain, SOB, weakness, or slurring of speech occurs. Caution about the risk of serotonin syndrome, particularly with SSRIs or SNRIs. Inform that drug should not be used during pregnancy unless the potential benefit justifies the potential risk to fetus. Advise to notify physician if breastfeeding or planning to breastfeed. Instruct on proper use of product and to avoid IM or intravascular delivery. Instruct to use inj sites with adequate skin and SQ thickness (eg, lateral thigh, upper arms) to accommodate the length of the needle.

Administration: SQ route. **Storage:** 25°C (77°F); excursions permitted to 15-30°C (59-86°F). Protect from light. Do not refrigerate.

ALTABAX   RX
retapamulin (Stiefel)

THERAPEUTIC CLASS: Pleuromutilin antibacterial

INDICATIONS: Topical treatment of impetigo due to *Staphylococcus aureus* (methicillin-susceptible isolates only) or *Streptococcus pyogenes* in patients ≥9 months of age.

DOSAGE: *Adults:* Apply thin layer to the affected area (up to 100cm^2 in total area) bid for 5 days. May be covered with sterile bandage or gauze dressing if desired.
Pediatrics: ≥9 Months: Apply thin layer to the affected area (up to 2% total BSA) bid for 5 days. May be covered with sterile bandage or gauze dressing if desired.

HOW SUPPLIED: Oint: 1% [15g, 30g]

WARNINGS/PRECAUTIONS: In the event of sensitization or severe local irritation, d/c use, wipe off oint, and institute appropriate alternative therapy. Not intended for oral, intranasal, ophthalmic, or intravaginal use; epistaxis reported with use on nasal mucosa. May result in bacterial resistance with use in the absence of proven or suspected bacterial infection; take appropriate measures if superinfection occurs.

ADVERSE REACTIONS: Application-site irritation and pruritus, headache, diarrhea, nausea, nasopharyngitis, pruritus, pyrexia, eczema, increased CPK.

INTERACTIONS: Oral ketoconazole may increase levels. Not recommended with strong CYP3A4 inhibitors in patients <24 months of age.

PREGNANCY: Category B, caution in nursing.

MECHANISM OF ACTION: Semisynthetic pleuromutilin antibacterial; selectively inhibits bacterial protein synthesis by interacting at a site on the 50S subunit of the bacterial ribosome. The binding site involves ribosomal protein L3 and is in the region of the ribosomal P site and peptidyl transferase center. By virtue of binding to this site, peptidyl transfer is inhibited, P-site interactions are blocked, and the normal formation of active 50S ribosomal subunits is prevented.

PHARMACOKINETICS: Absorption: C$_{max}$=18.5ng/mL (2-17 yrs of age), 10.7ng/mL (adults). **Distribution:** Plasma protein binding (94%). **Metabolism:** Liver (extensive) by mono-oxygenation and N-demethylation via CYP3A4.

NURSING CONSIDERATIONS

Assessment: Assess pregnancy/nursing status, and for possible drug interactions.

Monitoring: Monitor for sensitization or severe local irritation, superinfection, and other adverse reactions.

Patient Counseling: Instruct to use medication externally ud and to wash hands after application (if hands are not the area for treatment). Instruct not to swallow drug or use in the eyes, on the mouth or lips, inside the nose, or inside the female genital area. Inform that treated area may be covered by sterile bandage or gauze dressing if desired. Instruct to use the medication for the full time recommended by physician, even though symptoms may improve. Advise to notify physician if symptoms do not improve within 3-4 days after starting treatment, and if area of application worsens in irritation, redness, itching, burning, swelling, blistering, or oozing.

Administration: Topical route. **Storage:** 25°C (77°F); excursions permitted to 15-30°C (59-86°F).

ALTACE   RX
ramipril (Pfizer)

> D/C when pregnancy is detected. Drugs that act directly on the renin-angiotensin system (RAS) can cause injury/death to the developing fetus.

THERAPEUTIC CLASS: ACE inhibitor

INDICATIONS: Treatment of HTN, alone or in combination with thiazide diuretics. To reduce risk of myocardial infarction (MI), stroke, or death from cardiovascular (CV) causes in patients ≥55 yrs of age at high risk of developing a major CV event due to history of coronary artery disease, stroke, peripheral vascular disease, or diabetes with at least 1 other CV risk factor. For use in stable patients who have demonstrated signs of congestive heart failure (CHF) within the 1st few days after sustaining acute MI.

DOSAGE: *Adults:* HTN: Not Receiving a Diuretic: Initial: 2.5mg qd. Titrate: Adjust dose according to BP response. Maint: 2.5-20mg/day as single dose or in 2 equally divided doses. May add diuretic if BP is not controlled. Renal Impairment (CrCl ≤40mL/min): Initial: 1.25mg qd. Titrate: May increase dosage until BP is controlled. Max: 5mg/day. Risk Reduction of MI, Stroke, CV Death: ≥55 Yrs: Initial: 2.5mg qd for 1 week. Titrate: Increase to 5mg qd for next 3 weeks, and then increase as tolerated. Maint: 10mg qd. May be given as a divided dose if hypertensive or recently post-MI. CHF Post-MI: Initial: 2.5mg bid (5mg/day), or may switch to 1.25mg bid if hypotensive at this dose. After initial dose, observe for at least 2 hrs and until BP has stabilized for at least an additional hr. Titrate: If tolerated, increase to target dose of 5mg bid at 3-week intervals after 1 week of initial dose. Renal Impairment (CrCl ≤40mL/min): Initial: 1.25mg qd. Titrate: May increase to 1.25mg bid, depending on clinical response and tolerability. Max: 2.5mg bid. With Renal Artery Stenosis/Volume Depletion (eg, Past and Current Diuretic Use): Initial: 1.25mg qd. Titrate: Adjust dosage according to BP response.

HOW SUPPLIED: Cap: 1.25mg, 2.5mg, 5mg, 10mg

CONTRAINDICATIONS: History of ACE inhibitor-associated angioedema. Coadministration with aliskiren in patients with diabetes.

WARNINGS/PRECAUTIONS: Increased risk of angioedema in patients with history of angioedema unrelated to ACE inhibitor therapy. Head/neck angioedema reported; d/c and institute appropriate therapy if laryngeal stridor or angioedema of the face, tongue, or glottis occurs. Higher rate of angioedema in blacks than nonblacks. Intestinal angioedema reported; monitor for abdominal pain. Anaphylactoid reactions reported during desensitization with hymenoptera venom, dialysis with high-flux membranes, and LDL apheresis with dextran sulfate absorption. Rarely, associated with a syndrome that starts with cholestatic jaundice and progresses to fulminant hepatic necrosis and sometimes death reported; d/c if jaundice or marked hepatic enzyme elevations develop. May cause changes in renal function. Excessive hypotension associated with oliguria or azotemia and, rarely, with acute renal failure and death may occur in patients with CHF; closely monitor during first 2 weeks of therapy and whenever the dose is increased. Increases in BUN and SrCr may occur in hypertensive patients with renal artery stenosis or without preexisting renal vascular disease; dosage reduction of therapy and/or discontinuation of diuretic may be required. Agranulocytosis, pancytopenia, bone marrow depression, and mild reductions in RBC count and Hgb content, blood cell, or platelet counts may occur; consider monitoring WBCs in patients with collagen vascular disease (eg, systemic lupus erythematosus, scleroderma), especially with renal impairment. Symptomatic hypotension may occur and is most likely in patients with volume and/or salt depletion; correct depletion prior to therapy. Hypotension may occur with surgery or during anesthesia. Hyperkalemia reported; risk factors include renal insufficiency and diabetes mellitus (DM). Persistent nonproductive cough reported.

ADVERSE REACTIONS: Hypotension, cough increased, dizziness, angina pectoris, headache, asthenia, fatigue.

INTERACTIONS: See Contraindications. Dual blockade of the RAS is associated with increased risks of hypotension, hyperkalemia, and changes in renal function (including acute renal failure); closely monitor BP, renal function, and electrolytes with concomitant agents that also affect the RAS. Avoid with aliskiren in patients with renal impairment (GFR <60mL/min). Hypotension risk, and increased BUN and SrCr with diuretics. Increased risk of hyperkalemia with K^+-sparing diuretics, K^+ supplements, and/or K^+-containing salt substitutes; use with caution and frequently monitor serum K^+. Not recommended with telmisartan; increased risk of renal dysfunction. Increased lithium levels and symptoms of lithium toxicity reported; frequently monitor serum lithium levels. Diuretics may further increase risk of lithium toxicity. Nitritoid reactions reported rarely with injectable gold (sodium aurothiomalate). Coadministration with NSAIDs, including selective COX-2 inhibitors, may deteriorate renal function and attenuate antihypertensive effect. Increased risk for angioedema with mammalian target of rapamycin inhibitor (eg, temsirolimus).

PREGNANCY: Category D, not for use in nursing.

MECHANISM OF ACTION: ACE inhibitor; decreases plasma angiotensin II, which leads to decreased vasopressor activity and aldosterone secretion.

PHARMACOKINETICS: Absorption: Absolute bioavailability (28%, 44% ramiprilat); T_{max}=1 hr, 2-4 hrs (ramiprilat). **Distribution:** Plasma protein binding (73%, 56% ramiprilat); crosses placenta; found in breast milk. **Metabolism:** Cleavage of ester group (primarily in the liver); ramiprilat (active metabolite). **Elimination:** Urine (60%, <2% unchanged), feces (40%); $T_{1/2}$>50 hrs (ramiprilat), 13-17 hrs (multiple daily doses, ramiprilat).

NURSING CONSIDERATIONS

Assessment: Assess for history of angioedema, CHF, renal artery stenosis, collagen vascular disease, volume/salt depletion, DM, hepatic impairment, hypersensitivity to drug, pregnancy/nursing status, and possible drug interactions. Obtain baseline renal function.

Monitoring: Monitor for signs/symptoms of angioedema, abdominal pain, anaphylactoid reactions, jaundice, hypotension, hyperkalemia, cough, and other adverse reactions. Consider monitoring WBCs in patients with collagen vascular disease, especially with renal impairment. Monitor BP and renal/hepatic function.

Patient Counseling: Instruct to d/c therapy and to immediately report any signs/symptoms of angioedema. Advise to promptly report any indication of infection (eg, sore throat, fever). Instruct to report lightheadedness, especially during 1st days of therapy; advise to d/c and consult with a physician if syncope occurs. Inform that inadequate fluid intake or excessive perspiration, diarrhea, or vomiting may lead to an excessive fall in BP, with the same consequences of lightheadedness and possible syncope. Inform females of childbearing age about the consequences of exposure during pregnancy and discuss treatment options in women planning to become pregnant; instruct to report pregnancy to physician as soon as possible. Advise not to use salt substitutes containing K⁺ without consulting physician.

Administration: Oral route. Swallow whole. May sprinkle contents on a small amount (about 4 oz.) of applesauce or mix in 4 oz. (120mL) of water or apple juice. Consume mixture in its entirety. May pre-prepare described mixtures. **Storage:** 15-30°C (59-86°F). Pre-prepared Mixtures: Up to 24 hrs at room temperature or up to 48 hrs under refrigeration.

ALTOPREV   RX
lovastatin (Shionogi)

THERAPEUTIC CLASS: HMG-CoA reductase inhibitor

INDICATIONS: Adjunct to diet to decrease total cholesterol, LDL, apolipoprotein B, and TG levels, and to increase HDL levels in primary hypercholesterolemia, mixed dyslipidemia, and for prevention of coronary heart disease.

DOSAGE: *Adults:* Individualize dose. Initial: 20, 40, or 60mg qhs. Usual: 20-60mg/day in single doses. May consider immediate-release lovastatin in patients requiring smaller reductions. Titrate: Adjust at ≥4-week intervals. Consider dose reduction if cholesterol levels fall significantly below the targeted range. Elderly/Complicated Medical Conditions (Renal Insufficiency, Diabetes): Initial: 20mg qhs. Concomitant Danazol/Diltiazem/Verapamil: Max: 20mg/day. Concomitant Amiodarone: Max: 40mg/day. Severe Renal Insufficiency (CrCl <30mL/min): Carefully consider dosage increases >20mg/day; give cautiously if deemed necessary.

HOW SUPPLIED: Tab, Extended-Release: 20mg, 40mg, 60mg

CONTRAINDICATIONS: Concomitant strong CYP3A4 inhibitors (eg, itraconazole, ketoconazole, posaconazole, HIV protease inhibitors, boceprevir, telaprevir, erythromycin, clarithromycin, telithromycin, nefazodone). Active liver disease or unexplained persistent elevations of serum transaminases, pregnancy, women of childbearing age who may become pregnant, and nursing mothers.

WARNINGS/PRECAUTIONS: Myopathy (including immune-mediated necrotizing myopathy [IMNM]) and rhabdomyolysis reported; d/c if markedly elevated CPK levels occur or myopathy is diagnosed/suspected. Temporarily withhold in any patient experiencing an acute or serious condition predisposing to development of renal failure secondary to rhabdomyolysis. Persistent increases in serum transaminases reported; obtain liver enzyme tests prior to initiation and repeat as clinically indicated. Fatal and nonfatal hepatic failure rarely reported; promptly interrupt therapy if serious liver injury with clinical symptoms and/or hyperbilirubinemia or jaundice occurs and do not restart if no alternate etiology found. Caution in patients who consume substantial quantities of alcohol and/or have history of liver disease. Increases in HbA1c and FPG levels reported. Evaluate patients who develop endocrine dysfunction. Caution in elderly.

ADVERSE REACTIONS: Nausea, abdominal pain, insomnia, dyspepsia, headache, asthenia, myalgia, infection, back pain, flu syndrome, arthralgia, sinusitis, diarrhea.

INTERACTIONS: See Contraindications and Dosage. Voriconazole, which may increase concentration, and ranolazine may increase risk of myopathy/rhabdomyolysis; consider dose adjustment. Due to the risk of myopathy, avoid with gemfibrozil, cyclosporine, and large quantities of grapefruit juice (>1 quart/day) and caution with other fibrates, lipid-lowering doses (≥1g/day) of niacin, colchicine, danazol, diltiazem, verapamil, or amiodarone. Determine PT before initiation and frequently during early therapy when used with coumarin anticoagulants. Caution with drugs that may decrease the levels or activity of endogenous steroid hormones (eg, spironolactone, cimetidine).

PREGNANCY: Category X, not for use in nursing.

MECHANISM OF ACTION: HMG-CoA reductase inhibitor; involves reduction of VLDL concentration and induction of LDL receptor, leading to reduced production and/or increased catabolism of LDL.

PHARMACOKINETICS: Absorption: Lovastatin: C_{max}=5.5ng/mL, T_{max}=14.2 hrs; AUC=77ng•hr/mL. Lovastatin Acid: C_{max}=5.8ng/mL, T_{max}=11.8 hrs; AUC=87ng•hr/mL. **Distribution:** Plasma protein binding (>95%). **Metabolism:** Liver (extensive), by hydrolysis via CYP3A4; β-hydroxyacid and 6'-hydroxy derivative (major active metabolites). **Elimination:** Bile.

NURSING CONSIDERATIONS

Assessment: Assess for active/history of liver disease or unexplained persistent elevations of serum transaminase, diabetes, alcohol use, hypersensitivity, pregnancy/nursing status, and possible drug interactions. Perform baseline LFTs, lipid profile, renal function, and check PT with coumarin anticoagulants.

Monitoring: Monitor for signs/symptoms of myopathy (including IMNM), rhabdomyolysis, liver/renal/endocrine dysfunction, and other adverse effects. Monitor cholesterol levels, creatine kinase, and LFTs. Check PT with coumarin anticoagulants.

Patient Counseling: Advise to promptly report unexplained muscle pain, tenderness, or weakness, particularly if accompanied by malaise or fever or if muscle signs and symptoms persist after discontinuation. Advise to promptly report any symptoms that may indicate liver injury (eg, fatigue, anorexia, right upper abdominal discomfort, dark urine, jaundice).

Administration: Oral route. Swallow whole; do not chew, crush, or cut. **Storage:** 20-25°C (68-77°F); excursions permitted to 15-30°C (59-86°F). Avoid excessive heat and humidity.

ALVESCO RX
ciclesonide (Sunovion)

THERAPEUTIC CLASS: Non-halogenated glucocorticoid

INDICATIONS: Maintenance treatment of asthma as prophylactic therapy in adults and adolescents ≥12 yrs of age.

DOSAGE: *Adults:* Previous Bronchodilators Alone: Initial: 80mcg bid. Max: 160mcg bid. Previous Inhaled Corticosteroids: Initial: 80mcg bid. Max: 320mcg bid. Previous Oral Corticosteroids: Initial/Max 320mcg bid. Titrate: Reduce to lowest effective dose once asthma stability is achieved. May increase to higher dose if response to initial dose is inadequate after 4 weeks. Elderly: Start at lower end of dosing range.
Pediatrics: ≥12 Yrs: Previous Bronchodilators Alone: Initial: 80mcg bid. Max: 160mcg bid. Previous Inhaled Corticosteroids: Initial: 80mcg bid. Max: 320mcg bid. Previous Oral Corticosteroids: Initial/Max 320mcg bid. Titrate: Reduce to lowest effective dose once asthma stability is achieved. May increase to higher dose if response to initial dose is inadequate after 4 weeks.

HOW SUPPLIED: MDI: 80mcg/actuation, 160mcg/actuation [60 actuations]

CONTRAINDICATIONS: Primary treatment of status asthmaticus or other acute episodes of asthma where intensive measures are required.

WARNINGS/PRECAUTIONS: Localized *Candida albicans* infections of mouth and pharynx reported; treat appropriately while remaining on treatment, or interrupt treatment if needed. Not indicated for rapid relief of bronchospasm or other acute episodes of asthma. Increased susceptibility to infections (eg, chickenpox, measles); may lead to serious/fatal course. Avoid exposure to chickenpox and measles; if exposed, consider prophylaxis/treatment. Caution with active/quiescent tuberculosis (TB), untreated systemic fungal, bacterial, viral, or parasitic infections, or ocular herpes simplex. Deaths due to adrenal insufficiency reported with transfer from systemic to inhaled corticosteroids; if oral corticosteroid is required, wean slowly from systemic corticosteroid use after transferring to therapy. Resume oral corticosteroids immediately during periods of stress or a severe asthma attack if previously withdrawn from systemic corticosteroids. Transferring from systemic to inhalation therapy may unmask allergic conditions previously suppressed (eg, rhinitis, conjunctivitis, eczema, arthritis, eosinophilic conditions). Systemic corticosteroid withdrawal effects may occur during withdrawal from oral steroids. Reduce dose slowly if hypercorticism and adrenal suppression occur. Decreases in bone mineral density (BMD) reported with long-term use; caution with major risk factors for decreased bone mineral content (eg, prolonged immobilization, family history of osteoporosis, chronic use of drugs that can reduce bone mass [eg, anticonvulsants, corticosteroids]). May reduce growth velocity in pediatric patients; monitor growth of pediatric patients routinely (eg, via stadiometry). Glaucoma, increased intraocular pressure (IOP), and cataracts reported. Bronchospasm may occur; d/c use, treat immediately, and institute alternative treatment. Caution in elderly.

ADVERSE REACTIONS: Headache, nasopharyngitis, sinusitis, pharyngolaryngeal pain, upper respiratory infection, arthralgia, nasal congestion, pain in extremity, back pain.

AMANTADINE

INTERACTIONS: Oral ketoconazole may increase the exposure of the active metabolite des-ciclesonide.

PREGNANCY: Category C, caution in nursing.

MECHANISM OF ACTION: Nonhalogenated glucocorticoid; not established. Has anti-inflammatory activity with affinity for glucocorticoid receptors. Shown to inhibit multiple cell types (eg, mast cells, eosinophils, basophils, lymphocytes, macrophages, neutrophils) and mediators (eg, histamine, eicosanoids, leukotrienes, cytokines) involved in the asthmatic response.

PHARMACOKINETICS: Absorption: Ciclesonide: Absolute bioavailability (22%). Des-ciclesonide: AUC=2.18ng•hr/mL; C_{max}=0.369ng/mL; T_{max}=1.04 hrs. **Distribution:** Plasma protein binding (≥99%). Ciclesonide: (IV) V_d=2.9L/kg. Des-ciclesonide: (IV) V_d=12.1L/kg. **Metabolism:** Hydrolyzed to des-ciclesonide (active metabolite); further metabolism in liver via CYP3A4 (major) and CYP2D6 (minor). **Elimination:** Ciclesonide: (IV) Feces (66%); $T_{1/2}$=0.71 hrs. Des-ciclesonide: (IV) Urine (≤20%); $T_{1/2}$=6-7 hrs.

NURSING CONSIDERATIONS

Assessment: Assess for status asthmaticus or other acute episodes of asthma, active/quiescent TB, untreated systemic infections, ocular herpes simplex, risk factors for decreased bone mineral content, previous hypersensitivity, pregnancy/nursing status, and possible drug interactions. Assess for history of increased IOP, glaucoma, and/or cataracts.

Monitoring: Monitor for infections, TB, chickenpox, measles, hypercorticism, adrenal suppression, decreased BMD, glaucoma, increased IOP, cataracts, bronchospasm, and other adverse events. Monitor growth routinely (eg, via stadiometry) in pediatric patients.

Patient Counseling: Advise that localized infections with *C. albicans* may occur in the mouth and pharynx; advise to rinse mouth after use and to notify physician if oropharyngeal candidiasis develops. Inform that drug is not a bronchodilator and is not for use as rescue medication for acute asthma exacerbations; instruct to contact physician immediately if deterioration of asthma occurs. Advise to avoid exposure to chickenpox or measles, and, if exposed, to consult physician immediately. Counsel on risks of immunosuppression, hypercorticism, adrenal suppression, and decreased BMD. Inform of risk of reduced growth velocity in pediatric patients. Advise to use medication at regular intervals, not to increase the prescribed dosage, not to stop use abruptly, and to contact physician if symptoms do not improve, condition worsens, or if use is discontinued. Inform to use only with the actuator supplied with the product.

Administration: Oral inhalation route. Prime inhaler before using for the 1st time or when inhaler has not been used for >10 days by actuating 3 times. Refer to PI for further administration instructions. **Storage:** 25°C (77°F); excursions permitted to 15-30°C (59-86°F). Do not puncture or use/store near heat or open flame. Exposure to temperatures >49°C (120°F) may cause bursting. Discard when dose indicator display window shows zero.

AMANTADINE   RX
amantadine HCl (Various)

THERAPEUTIC CLASS: Dopamine receptor agonist

INDICATIONS: Prophylaxis and treatment of uncomplicated influenza A infections. Treatment of parkinsonism and drug-induced extrapyramidal reactions.

DOSAGE: *Adults:* Influenza A Virus Prophylaxis/Treatment: 200mg/day as 2 caps/tabs or 4 tsp sol qd, or as 1 cap/tab or 2 tsp sol bid if CNS effects develop. Elderly/Intolerant to 200mg/day: 100mg/day. Refer to PI for commencement/duration of therapy and coadministration with inactivated influenza A vaccine. Parkinsonism: Usual: 100mg bid. Serious Associated Illness/Concomitant High-Dose Antiparkinson Agent: Initial: 100mg qd. Titrate: May increase to 100mg bid after 1 to several weeks. Max: 400mg/day in divided doses. Drug-Induced Extrapyramidal Reactions: Usual: 100mg bid. Max: 300mg/day in divided doses. CrCl 30-50mL/min: 200mg on Day 1, then 100mg qd. CrCl 15-29mL/min: 200mg on Day 1, then 100mg qod. CrCl <15mL/min or Hemodialysis: 200mg every 7 days.
Pediatrics: Influenza A Virus Prophylaxis/Treatment: 9-12 Yrs: 200mg/day as 1 cap/tab or 2 tsp sol bid. 1-9 Yrs: 4.4-8.8mg/kg/day. Max: 150mg/day.

HOW SUPPLIED: Cap: 100mg; Sol: 50mg/5mL; Tab: 100mg

WARNINGS/PRECAUTIONS: May need dose reduction with congestive heart failure (CHF), peripheral edema, orthostatic hypotension, or renal impairment. Deaths reported from overdose. Neuroleptic malignant syndrome (NMS) reported in association with dose reduction or withdrawal. Impulse control/compulsive behaviors reported; consider dose reduction or d/c if such behaviors develop. Suicide attempts reported. May exacerbate mental problems in patients with history of psychiatric disorder or substance abuse. May increase seizure activity. May impair mental/physical abilities. May cause mydriasis; avoid with untreated angle-closure glaucoma. Do not d/c abruptly in Parkinson's disease patients. Caution with liver disease, history of recurrent eczematoid rash, and uncontrolled psychosis or severe psychoneurosis. Monitor for melanomas frequently and regularly. Not shown to prevent complications secondary to influenza-like symptoms or concurrent bacterial infections.

ADVERSE REACTIONS: Nausea, dizziness, insomnia, depression, anxiety, hallucinations, confusion, anorexia, dry mouth, constipation, ataxia, livedo reticularis, peripheral edema, orthostatic hypotension, headache.

INTERACTIONS: Avoid live attenuated influenza vaccines within 2 weeks before or 48 hrs after therapy. Caution with neuroleptics and drugs having CNS effects. Triamterene/HCTZ may increase concentration. Quinine or quinidine may reduce renal clearance. Urine acidifying drugs may increase elimination. Anticholinergic agents may potentiate the anticholinergic-like side effects. May worsen tremor in elderly Parkinson's patients with thioridazine.

PREGNANCY: Category C, not for use in nursing.

MECHANISM OF ACTION: Dopamine receptor agonist; not established. Antiviral: Appears to prevent release of infectious viral nucleic acid into host cell by interfering with function of transmembrane domain of viral M2 protein. Also prevents virus assembly during replication. Parkinson's disease: May have direct/indirect effect on dopamine neurons and is a weak, noncompetitive *N*-methyl *D*-aspartate receptor antagonist.

PHARMACOKINETICS: Absorption: Well-absorbed. (Cap) C_{max}=0.22mcg/mL, T_{max}=3.3 hrs. (Sol) C_{max}=0.24mcg/mL (single dose), 0.47mcg/mL (multiple dose). (Tab) C_{max}=0.51mcg/mL, T_{max}=2-4 hrs. **Distribution:** V_d=3-8L/kg (IV); plasma protein binding (67%); found in breast milk. **Metabolism:** N-acetylation; acetylamantadine (metabolite). **Elimination:** Urine (unchanged); $T_{1/2}$=16 hrs.

NURSING CONSIDERATIONS

Assessment: Assess for CHF, peripheral edema, orthostatic hypotension, history of psychiatric disorders, substance abuse, epilepsy or other "seizures," and recurrent eczematoid rash, untreated angle-closure glaucoma, renal/hepatic impairment, hypersensitivity to the drug, pregnancy/nursing status, and possible drug interactions.

Monitoring: Monitor for signs/symptoms of suicide attempt, increased seizures, CNS and anticholinergic effects, NMS, impulse control/compulsive behaviors, melanoma, and renal/hepatic dysfunction.

Patient Counseling: Advise that blurry vision and/or impaired mental acuity may occur. Instruct to avoid excessive alcohol use, getting up suddenly from sitting or lying position, and taking more than prescribed. Instruct to notify physician if mood/mental changes, swelling of extremities, difficulty urinating, SOB, and intense urges occur, no improvement in a few days or drug appears less effective after a few weeks, or if suspicious that overdose has been taken. Advise to consult physician before discontinuing medication. Instruct Parkinson's disease patients to gradually increase physical activity as symptoms improve.

Administration: Oral route. **Storage:** 20-25°C (68-77°F). (Cap) Protect from moisture.

AMARYL RX
glimepiride (Sanofi-Aventis)

THERAPEUTIC CLASS: Sulfonylurea (2nd generation)

INDICATIONS: Adjunct to diet and exercise to improve glycemic control in adults with type 2 diabetes mellitus (DM).

DOSAGE: *Adults:* Administer with breakfast or the 1st main meal of the day. Initial: 1mg or 2mg qd. Titrate: After reaching 2mg/day, may further increase dose in increments of 1mg or 2mg based on glycemic response, not more frequently than every 1-2 weeks. Max: 8mg qd. Patients at Increased Risk for Hypoglycemia (eg, Elderly or with Renal Impairment): Initial: 1mg qd. Titrate: Adjust conservatively. Max: 8mg qd. Coadministration with Colesevelam: Administer at least 4 hrs prior to colesevelam.

HOW SUPPLIED: Tab: 1mg*, 2mg*, 4mg* *scored

WARNINGS/PRECAUTIONS: Not for the treatment of type 1 DM or diabetic ketoacidosis. Patients being transferred from longer $T_{1/2}$ sulfonylureas (eg, chlorpropamide) may have overlapping drug effect for 1-2 weeks; monitor for hypoglycemia. May cause severe hypoglycemia, which may impair mental/physical abilities; caution in patients predisposed to hypoglycemia. Early warning symptoms of hypoglycemia may be different/less pronounced in patients with autonomic neuropathy and in the elderly. Hypersensitivity reactions (eg, anaphylaxis, angioedema, Stevens-Johnson syndrome) reported; if suspected, promptly d/c therapy, assess for other potential causes for the reaction, and institute alternative treatment. May cause hemolytic anemia; caution with G6PD deficiency and consider the use of a non-sulfonylurea alternative. Increased risk of cardiovascular mortality.

ADVERSE REACTIONS: Dizziness, nausea, asthenia, headache, hypoglycemia, flu syndrome.

INTERACTIONS: See Dosage. Oral antidiabetic medications, pramlintide acetate, insulin, ACE inhibitors, H$_2$-receptor antagonists, fibrates, propoxyphene, pentoxifylline, somatostatin analogs, anabolic steroids and androgens, cyclophosphamide, phenyramidol, guanethidine, fluconazole, sulfinpyrazone, tetracyclines, clarithromycin, disopyramide, quinolones, and drugs that are highly protein-bound (eg, fluoxetine, NSAIDs, salicylates, sulfonamides, chloramphenicol, coumarins, probenecid, MAOIs) may increase glucose-lowering effect; monitor for hypoglycemia during coadministration and for worsening glycemic control during withdrawal of these drugs. Danazol, glucagon, somatropin, protease inhibitors, atypical antipsychotics (eg, olanzapine, clozapine), barbiturates, diazoxide, laxatives, rifampin, thiazides and other diuretics, corticosteroids, phenothiazines, thyroid hormones, estrogens, oral contraceptives, phenytoin, nicotinic acid, sympathomimetics (eg, epinephrine, albuterol, terbutaline), and isoniazid may reduce glucose-lowering effect; monitor for worsening glycemic control during coadministration and for hypoglycemia during withdrawal of these drugs. β-blockers, clonidine, reserpine, and acute/chronic alcohol intake may potentiate or weaken glucose-lowering effect. Signs of hypoglycemia may be reduced or absent with sympatholytic drugs (eg, β-blockers, clonidine, guanethidine, reserpine). Potential interaction leading to severe hypoglycemia reported with oral miconazole. May interact with inhibitors (eg, fluconazole) and inducers (eg, rifampin) of CYP2C9. Colesevelam may reduce levels.

PREGNANCY: Category C, not for use in nursing.

MECHANISM OF ACTION: Sulfonylurea (2nd generation); lowers blood glucose by stimulating insulin release from pancreatic β cells.

PHARMACOKINETICS: Absorption: T_{max}=2-3 hrs. **Distribution:** (IV) V_d=8.8L; plasma protein binding (>99.5%). **Metabolism:** Complete by oxidation; cyclohexyl hydroxy methyl derivative (M1) (via CYP2C9) and carboxyl derivative (M2) (major metabolites). **Elimination:** Urine (60%, 80-90% metabolites), feces (40%, 70% metabolites).

NURSING CONSIDERATIONS

Assessment: Assess for hypersensitivity to drug or sulfonamide derivatives, type of DM, diabetic ketoacidosis, predisposition to hypoglycemia, autonomic neuropathy, G6PD deficiency, pregnancy/nursing status, and possible drug interactions.

Monitoring: Monitor for hypoglycemia, hypersensitivity reactions, hemolytic anemia, and other adverse reactions.

Patient Counseling: Inform about importance of adherence to dietary instructions, a regular exercise program, and regular testing of blood glucose. Advise about potential side effects (eg, hypoglycemia, weight gain). Inform about the symptoms and treatment of hypoglycemia, and the conditions that predispose to it. Inform that ability to concentrate and react may be impaired as a result of hypoglycemia; caution when driving/operating machinery. Advise to inform physician if pregnant/breastfeeding or contemplating pregnancy/breastfeeding.

Administration: Oral route. Administer with breakfast or the 1st main meal of the day. **Storage:** 25°C (77°F); excursions permitted to 20-25°C (68-77°F).

AMBIEN
zolpidem tartrate (Sanofi-Aventis)

`CIV`

THERAPEUTIC CLASS: Imidazopyridine hypnotic

INDICATIONS: Short-term treatment of insomnia characterized by difficulties with sleep initiation.

DOSAGE: *Adults:* Use lowest effective dose. Initial: 5mg for women and either 5mg or 10mg for men, taken only once per night immediately before hs with at least 7-8 hrs remaining before the planned time of awakening. Titrate: May increase to 10mg if the 5mg dose is not effective. Max: 10mg qd immediately before hs. Elderly/Debilitated/Hepatic Insufficiency: 5mg qd immediately before hs. Use with CNS Depressants: May need to adjust dose.

HOW SUPPLIED: Tab: 5mg, 10mg

WARNINGS/PRECAUTIONS: Increased risk of next-day psychomotor impairment if taken with less than a full night of sleep remaining (7-8 hrs). May impair mental/physical abilities. Initiate only after careful evaluation; failure of insomnia to remit after 7-10 days of treatment may indicate presence of a primary psychiatric and/or medical illness. Cases of angioedema involving the tongue, glottis, or larynx reported; do not rechallenge if angioedema develops. Abnormal thinking, behavior changes, and visual and auditory hallucinations reported. Complex behaviors (eg, sleep-driving) reported; consider discontinuation if a sleep-driving episode occurs. Amnesia, anxiety, and other neuropsychiatric symptoms may occur. Worsening of depression and suicidal thoughts and actions (including completed suicides) reported primarily in depressed patients; prescribe the lowest feasible number of tabs at a time. Caution with compromised respiratory function; prior to prescribing, consider the risk of respiratory depression in patients with respiratory impairment (eg, sleep apnea, myasthenia gravis). Withdrawal signs and symptoms reported following rapid dose decrease or abrupt discontinuation; monitor for tolerance, abuse, and dependence.

ADVERSE REACTIONS: Drowsiness, dizziness, headache, diarrhea, drugged feeling, lethargy, dry mouth, back pain, pharyngitis, sinusitis, allergy.

INTERACTIONS: See Dosage. Increased risk of CNS depression and complex behaviors with other CNS depressants (eg, benzodiazepines, opioids, TCAs, alcohol). Use with other sedative-hypnotics (eg, other zolpidem products) at hs or the middle of the night is not recommended. Increased risk of next-day psychomotor impairment with other CNS depressants or drugs that increase zolpidem levels. May decrease peak levels of imipramine. Additive effect of decreased alertness with imipramine or chlorpromazine. Additive adverse effect on psychomotor performance with chlorpromazine or alcohol. Sertraline and CYP3A inhibitors may increase exposure. Fluoxetine may increase $T_{1/2}$. Rifampin (a CYP3A4 inducer) may reduce exposure, pharmacodynamic effects, and efficacy. Ketoconazole (a potent CYP3A4 inhibitor) may increase pharmacodynamic effects; consider lower dose of zolpidem.

PREGNANCY: Category C, caution in nursing.

MECHANISM OF ACTION: Imidazopyridine, nonbenzodiazepine hypnotic; interacts with a gamma-aminobutyric acid-BZ receptor complex. Binds the BZ_1 receptor preferentially with a high affinity ratio of the α_1/α_5 subunits.

PHARMACOKINETICS: Absorption: Rapid. (Healthy) C_{max}=59ng/mL (5mg), 121ng/mL (10mg); T_{max}=1.6 hrs (5mg, 10mg). **Distribution:** Plasma protein binding (92.5%); found in breast milk. **Elimination**: Renal; (Healthy) $T_{1/2}$=2.6 hrs (5mg), 2.5 hrs (10mg).

NURSING CONSIDERATIONS

Assessment: Assess for physical and/or psychiatric disorder, depression, compromised respiratory function, sleep apnea, myasthenia gravis, hepatic impairment, history of drug/alcohol addiction or abuse, hypersensitivity to the drug, pregnancy/nursing status, and possible drug interactions.

Monitoring: Monitor for angioedema, emergence of any new behavioral signs/symptoms of concern, respiratory depression, withdrawal signs/symptoms, tolerance, abuse, dependence, and other adverse reactions.

Patient Counseling: Inform about the benefits and risks of treatment. Instruct to take only as prescribed; advise to wait at least 8 hrs after dosing before driving or engaging in other activities requiring full mental alertness. Instruct to contact physician immediately if any adverse reactions (eg, severe anaphylactic/anaphylactoid reactions, sleep-driving, other complex behaviors, suicidal thoughts) develop. Advise not to use the drug if patient drank alcohol that pm or before bed.

Administration: Oral route. Take immediately before hs with at least 7-8 hrs remaining before the planned time of awakening. Do not administer with or immediately after a meal. **Storage:** 20-25°C (68-77°F).

AMBIEN CR
zolpidem tartrate (Sanofi-Aventis)

CIV

THERAPEUTIC CLASS: Imidazopyridine hypnotic

INDICATIONS: Treatment of insomnia characterized by difficulties with sleep onset and/or sleep maintenance.

DOSAGE: *Adults:* Use lowest effective dose. Initial: 6.25mg for women and either 6.25mg or 12.5mg for men, taken only once per night immediately before hs with at least 7-8 hrs remaining before the planned time of awakening. Titrate: May increase to 12.5mg if the 6.25mg dose is not effective. Max: 12.5mg qd immediately before hs. Elderly/Debilitated/Hepatic Insufficiency: 6.25mg qd immediately before hs. Use with CNS Depressants: May need to adjust dose.

HOW SUPPLIED: Tab, Extended-Release: 6.25mg, 12.5mg

WARNINGS/PRECAUTIONS: May impair daytime function; monitor for excess depressant effects. May impair mental/physical abilities. Increased risk of next-day psychomotor impairment if taken with less than a full night of sleep remaining (7-8 hrs). Initiate only after careful evaluation; failure of insomnia to remit after 7-10 days of treatment may indicate presence of a primary psychiatric and/or medical illness. Cases of angioedema involving the tongue, glottis, or larynx reported; do not rechallenge if angioedema develops. Abnormal thinking, behavior changes, and visual and auditory hallucinations reported. Complex behaviors (eg, sleep-driving) reported; consider discontinuation if a sleep-driving episode occurs. Amnesia, anxiety, and other neuropsychiatric symptoms may occur. Worsening of depression and suicidal thoughts and actions (including completed suicides) reported primarily in depressed patients; prescribe the lowest feasible number of tabs at a time. Caution with compromised respiratory function; consider the risk of respiratory depression prior to prescribing in patients with respiratory impairment (eg, sleep apnea, myasthenia gravis). Withdrawal signs and symptoms reported following rapid dose decrease or abrupt discontinuation; monitor for tolerance, abuse, and dependence.

ADVERSE REACTIONS: Headache, somnolence, dizziness, anxiety, nausea, influenza, hallucinations, back pain, myalgia, fatigue, disorientation, memory disorder, visual disturbance, nasopharyngitis.

INTERACTIONS: See Dosage. Additive effects with other CNS depressants (eg, benzodiazepines, opioids, TCAs, alcohol), including daytime use. Use with other sedative-hypnotics (eg, other zolpidem products) at hs or the middle of the night is not recommended. Increased risk of next-day psychomotor impairment with other CNS depressants or drugs that increase zolpidem levels. Increased risk of complex behaviors with alcohol and other CNS depressants. May decrease peak levels of imipramine. Additive effect of decreased alertness with imipramine or chlorpromazine. Additive adverse effect on psychomotor performance with chlorpromazine or alcohol. Sertraline and CYP3A inhibitors may increase exposure. Fluoxetine may increase $T_{1/2}$. Rifampin (a CYP3A4 inducer) may reduce exposure, pharmacodynamic effects, and efficacy. Ketoconazole (a potent CYP3A4 inhibitor) may increase pharmacodynamic effects; consider lower dose of zolpidem.

PREGNANCY: Category C, caution in nursing.

MECHANISM OF ACTION: Imidazopyridine, nonbenzodiazepine hypnotic; interacts with a gamma-aminobutyric acid-BZ receptor complex. Binds the BZ_1 receptor preferentially with a high affinity ratio of the α_1/α_5 subunits.

PHARMACOKINETICS: Absorption: Biphasic. (Healthy) C_{max}=134ng/mL; T_{max}=1.5 hrs (median); AUC=740ng•hr/mL. **Distribution:** Plasma protein binding (92.5%); found in breast milk. **Elimination:** Renal; (Healthy) $T_{1/2}$=2.8 hrs.

NURSING CONSIDERATIONS

Assessment: Assess for physical and/or psychiatric disorder, depression, compromised respiratory function, sleep apnea, myasthenia gravis, hepatic impairment, history of drug/alcohol addiction or abuse, hypersensitivity to the drug, pregnancy/nursing status, and possible drug interactions.

Monitoring: Monitor for angioedema, emergence of any new behavioral signs/symptoms of concern, respiratory depression, withdrawal signs/symptoms, tolerance, abuse, dependence, and other adverse reactions. Monitor for excess depressant effects.

Patient Counseling: Inform about the benefits and risks of treatment. Instruct to take only as prescribed. Caution against driving and other activities requiring complete mental alertness the day after use. Instruct to contact physician immediately if any adverse reactions (eg, severe anaphylactic/anaphylactoid reactions, sleep-driving, other complex behaviors, suicidal thoughts) develop. Advise not to use the drug if patient drank alcohol that pm or before bed.

Administration: Oral route. Swallow whole; do not divide, crush, or chew. Take immediately before hs with at least 7-8 hrs remaining before the planned time of awakening. Do not administer with or immediately after a meal. **Storage:** 15-25°C (59-77°F); limited excursions permissible up to 30°C (86°F).

AMBISOME   RX
amphotericin B liposome (Astellas)

THERAPEUTIC CLASS: Polyene antifungal

INDICATIONS: Empirical therapy for presumed fungal infection in febrile, neutropenic patients. Treatment of cryptococcal meningitis in HIV-infected patients. Treatment of *Aspergillus*, *Candida*, and/or *Cryptococcus* infections refractory to amphotericin B deoxycholate or where renal impairment or unacceptable toxicity precludes the use of amphotericin B deoxycholate. Treatment of visceral leishmaniasis.

DOSAGE: *Adults:* Individualize dose. Infuse over 120 min; may reduce to 60 min if well tolerated or increase duration if experiencing discomfort. Empirical Therapy: 3mg/kg/day IV. Systemic Infections (*Aspergillus*, *Candida*, *Cryptococcus*): 3-5mg/kg/day IV. Cryptococcal Meningitis in HIV: 6mg/kg/day IV. Visceral Leishmaniasis: Immunocompetent: 3mg/kg/day IV on Days 1-5, 14, 21. May repeat course PRN. Immunocompromised: 4mg/kg/day IV on Days 1-5, 10, 17, 24, 31, 38. *Pediatrics:* ≥1 Month: Individualize dose. Infuse over 120 min; may reduce to 60 min if well tolerated or increase duration if experiencing discomfort. Empirical Therapy: 3mg/kg/day IV. Systemic Infections (*Aspergillus*, *Candida*, *Cryptococcus*): 3-5mg/kg/day IV. Cryptococcal Meningitis in HIV: 6mg/kg/day IV. Visceral Leishmaniasis: Immunocompetent: 3mg/kg/day IV on Days 1-5, 14, 21. May repeat course PRN. Immunocompromised: 4mg/kg/day IV on Days 1-5, 10, 17, 24, 31, 38.

HOW SUPPLIED: Inj: 50mg

WARNINGS/PRECAUTIONS: Anaphylaxis reported; d/c immediately and do not give further infusions if severe anaphylactic reaction occurs. Should be administered by medically trained personnel; monitor closely during the initial dosing period. Significantly less toxic than amphotericin B deoxycholate. False elevations of serum phosphate seen with PHOSm assays.

ADVERSE REACTIONS: Hypokalemia, chills/rigors, SrCr elevation, anemia, N/V, diarrhea, hypomagnesemia, rash, dyspnea, bilirubinemia, BUN increased, headache, abdominal pain.

INTERACTIONS: Antineoplastic agents may enhance potential for renal toxicity, bronchospasm, and hypotension. Corticosteroids and adrenocorticotropic hormone may potentiate hypokalemia; closely monitor serum electrolytes and cardiac function. May induce hypokalemia and potentiate digitalis toxicity with digitalis glycosides; closely monitor serum K⁺ levels. May increase flucytosine toxicity. Imidazoles (eg, ketoconazole, miconazole, clotrimazole, fluconazole) may induce fungal resistance; use with caution, especially in immunocompromised patients. Acute pulmonary toxicity reported with simultaneous leukocyte transfusions. Nephrotoxic drugs may enhance drug-induced renal toxicity; intensive monitoring of renal function is recommended. Amphotericin B-induced hypokalemia may enhance curariform effect of skeletal muscle relaxants (eg, tubocurarine); closely monitor serum K⁺ levels.

PREGNANCY: Category B, not for use in nursing.

MECHANISM OF ACTION: Polyene antifungal; acts by binding to the sterol component, ergosterol, of the cell membrane in susceptible fungi, leading to alterations in cell permeability and cell death. Also binds to the cholesterol component of the mammalian cell, leading to cytotoxicity. Has been shown to penetrate the cell wall of both extracellular and intracellular forms of susceptible fungi.

PHARMACOKINETICS: Absorption: IV administration of variable doses resulted in different pharmacokinetic parameters. **Elimination:** $T_{1/2}$=7-10 hrs (24-hr dosing interval), 100-153 hrs (49 days after dosing).

NURSING CONSIDERATIONS

Assessment: Assess for hypersensitivity, health status, pregnancy/nursing status, and possible drug interactions.

Monitoring: Monitor for severe anaphylactic and other adverse reactions. Monitor renal, hepatic and hematopoietic function, and serum electrolytes (particularly Mg^{2+} and K⁺).

Patient Counseling: Inform of risks and benefits of therapy. Advise to seek medical attention if any adverse reactions occur.

Administration: IV route. An in-line membrane filter may be used provided the mean pore diameter of the filter is not <1.0 micron. Flush existing IV line with D5W prior to infusion; if not feasible, use a separate line. Refer to PI for directions for reconstitution, filtration, and dilution. **Storage:** Unopened Vials: ≤25°C (77°F). Reconstituted Concentrate: 2-8°C (36-46°F) for up to 24 hrs. Do not freeze. Diluted Product: Inj should commence within 6 hrs of dilution with D5W.

AMERGE   RX
naratriptan HCl (GlaxoSmithKline)

THERAPEUTIC CLASS: 5-HT₁ᵦ/₁ᴅ agonist

INDICATIONS: Acute treatment of migraine with or without aura in adults.

DOSAGE: *Adults:* Usual: 1mg or 2.5mg. May repeat dose once after 4 hrs if migraine returns or with partial response. Max: 5mg/24 hrs. Safety of treating an average of >4 migraine attacks in a 30-day period has not been established. Mild-Moderate Renal/Hepatic Impairment: Initial: 1mg. Max: 2.5mg/24 hrs. Elderly: Start at lower end of dosing range.

HOW SUPPLIED: Tab: 1mg, 2.5mg

CONTRAINDICATIONS: Ischemic coronary artery disease (CAD) (angina pectoris, history of myocardial infarction [MI], documented silent ischemia), or coronary artery vasospasm, including Prinzmetal's angina; Wolff-Parkinson-White syndrome or arrhythmias associated with other cardiac accessory conduction pathway disorders; history of stroke or transient ischemic attack or history of hemiplegic or basilar migraine; peripheral vascular disease; ischemic bowel disease; uncontrolled HTN, recent use (eg, within 24 hrs) of another 5-HT₁ agonist, ergotamine-containing medication, ergot-type medication (eg, dihydroergotamine, methysergide); severe renal/hepatic impairment.

WARNINGS/PRECAUTIONS: Rare reports of serious cardiac adverse reactions, including acute MI, occurring within a few hrs following administration. May cause coronary artery vasospasm (Prinzmetal's angina). Perform cardiovascular (CV) evaluation in triptan-naive patients who have multiple CV risk factors. If patient has a negative CV evaluation, consider administering 1st dose in a medically supervised setting, performing an ECG immediately following administration, and consider periodic CV evaluation with long-term intermittent use. Life-threatening disturbances of cardiac rhythm, including ventricular tachycardia and ventricular fibrillation leading to death, reported; d/c if these disturbances occur. Sensations of tightness, pain, and pressure in the chest, throat, neck, and jaw may occur after treatment and are usually noncardiac in origin; perform a cardiac evaluation if these patients are at high cardiac risk. Cerebral hemorrhage, subarachnoid hemorrhage, and stroke reported; d/c if a cerebrovascular event occurs. Exclude other potentially serious neurological conditions before treating headaches in patients not previously diagnosed as migraineurs and in migraineurs who present with symptoms atypical for migraine. May cause noncoronary vasospastic reactions (eg, peripheral vascular ischemia, GI vascular ischemia and infarction, splenic infarction, Raynaud's syndrome); rule out a vasospastic reaction, before receiving additional doses. Transient and permanent blindness and significant partial vision loss reported. Overuse of acute migraine drugs may lead to exacerbation of headache; detoxification, including withdrawal of overused drugs, and treatment of withdrawal symptoms may be necessary. Serotonin syndrome may occur; d/c if suspected. Significant BP elevation, including hypertensive crisis with acute impairment of organ systems reported; monitor BP. Anaphylaxis/anaphylactoid/hypersensitivity reactions, including angioedema reported. Caution in elderly.

ADVERSE REACTIONS: Paresthesias, nausea, dizziness, drowsiness, malaise/fatigue, throat and neck symptoms.

INTERACTIONS: See Contraindications. Serotonin syndrome reported during coadministration of triptans and SSRIs, SNRIs, TCAs, and MAOIs.

PREGNANCY: Category C, not for use in nursing.

MECHANISM OF ACTION: Selective 5-HT$_{1B/1D}$ receptor agonist; binds with high affinity to human cloned 5-HT$_{1B/1D}$ receptors. Therapeutic activity is thought to be due to the agonist effects at the 5-HT$_{1B/1D}$ receptors on intracranial blood vessels (including the arteriovenous anastomoses) and sensory nerves of the trigeminal system, which result in cranial vessel constriction and inhibition of pro-inflammatory neuropeptide release.

PHARMACOKINETICS: Absorption: Well-absorbed; oral bioavailability (70%); T$_{max}$=2-3 hrs (2.5mg), 3-4 hrs (during a migraine attack). **Distribution:** V$_d$=170L, plasma protein binding (28-31%). **Metabolism:** Via CYP450 isoenzymes. **Elimination:** Urine (50% unchanged, 30% metabolites); T$_{1/2}$=6 hrs.

NURSING CONSIDERATIONS

Assessment: Confirm diagnosis of migraine before therapy. Assess for CAD, uncontrolled HTN, history of hemiplegic/basilar migraine, ECG changes, renal/hepatic impairment, or any conditions where treatment is cautioned or contraindicated. Assess for pregnancy/nursing status and for possible drug interactions. Exclude other potentially serious neurological conditions before therapy. Perform a CV evaluation in triptan-naive patients who have multiple CV risk factors (eg, increased age, diabetes, HTN, smoking, obesity, strong family history of CAD).

Monitoring: Monitor for serious cardiac adverse reactions, arrhythmias, cerebrovascular events, noncoronary vasospastic reactions, exacerbation of headache, serotonin syndrome, increase in BP, anaphylactic/anaphylactoid reactions, and other adverse reactions. Perform ECG immediately after administration of 1st dose in patients with multiple CV risk factors. Consider periodic cardiac evaluation in patients who have multiple CV risk factors and are long-term intermittent users.

Patient Counseling: Inform that drug may cause serious CV effects (eg, MI, stroke); instruct to be alert for signs/symptoms of chest pain, SOB, irregular heartbeat, significant rise in BP, weakness, and slurring of speech, and ask for medical advice if any indicative sign/symptoms are observed. Inform that anaphylactic/anaphylactoid reactions may occur. Inform that use of drug within 24 hrs of another triptan or an ergot-type medication is contraindicated. Caution about the risk of serotonin syndrome, particularly during combined use with SSRIs, SNRIs, TCAs, and MAOIs. Inform that use of acute migraine drugs for ≥10 days/month may lead to an exacerbation of headache, and encourage to record headache frequency and drug use (eg, by keeping a headache diary). Inform that drug should not be used during pregnancy unless the potential benefit justifies the potential risk to the fetus. Advise to notify physician if breastfeeding or planning to breastfeed. Inform that treatment may cause somnolence and dizziness; instruct to evaluate the ability to perform complex tasks after drug administration.

Administration: Oral route. **Storage:** 20-25°C (68-77°F).

AMIKACIN

amikacin sulfate (Various)

> Potential for nephrotoxicity, neurotoxicity, and ototoxicity; adjust dose or d/c on evidence of ototoxicity/nephrotoxicity. Risk of nephrotoxicity is greater with impaired renal function and in those who receive high dose or prolonged therapy. Neurotoxicity (eg, vestibular and permanent bilateral auditory ototoxicity) can occur with preexisting renal damage and normal renal function treated at higher doses and/or longer treatment periods than recommended. Hearing loss may increase with the degree of exposure to either high peak or high trough serum concentrations. After the drug has been discontinued, total or partial irreversible bilateral deafness may occur. Neuromuscular blockade, respiratory paralysis reported following parenteral inj, topical instillation (as in orthopedic and abdominal irrigation or in local treatment of empyema), and oral use of therapy. Increased risk of neuromuscular blockade and respiratory paralysis with anesthetics, neuromuscular blockers or massive transfusions of citrate-anticoagulated blood. Closely monitor renal and 8th cranial nerve function. Examine urine for decreased specific gravity, increased protein excretion, and presence of cells/casts. Obtain serial audiograms in patients old enough to be tested. Avoid concurrent and/or sequential neurotoxic or nephrotoxic drugs and potent diuretics (eg, ethacrynic acid, furosemide). Advanced age and dehydration may increase risk of toxicity.

THERAPEUTIC CLASS: Aminoglycoside

INDICATIONS: Short-term treatment of serious infections due to susceptible strains of gram-negative bacteria. Shown to be effective in bacterial septicemia (including neonatal sepsis); serious infections of respiratory tract, bones and joints, CNS (including meningitis); skin and soft tissue; intra-abdominal infections (including peritonitis); burns and postoperative infections (including post-vascular surgery); serious complicated and recurrent urinary tract infections (UTIs) due to susceptible strains of microorganisms; infections caused by gentamicin- and/or tobramycin-resistant strains of gram-negative organisms, particularly *Proteus rettgeri*, *Providencia stuartii*, *Serratia marcescens*, and *Pseudomonas aeruginosa*; staphylococcal infections; and severe infections in combination with a penicillin-type drug.

DOSAGE: *Adults:* IM/IV: 15mg/kg/day divided into 2 or 3 equal doses given at equally divided intervals. Max: 15mg/kg/day. Heavier Weight Patients: Max: 1.5g/day. Uncomplicated UTI: 250mg bid. Usual Duration: 7-10 days. D/C therapy if no response after 3-5 days. Reevaluate if considering therapy beyond 10 days in difficult and complicated infections. Renal Impairment: Reduce dose or prolong intervals. Refer to PI for dosing guidelines.
Pediatrics: IM/IV: 15mg/kg/day divided into 2 or 3 equal doses given at equally divided intervals. Max: 15mg/kg/day. Newborns: LD: 10mg/kg. Maint: 7.5mg/kg q12h. Uncomplicated UTI: 250mg bid. Usual Duration: 7-10 days. D/C therapy if no response after 3-5 days. Reevaluate if considering therapy beyond 10 days in difficult and complicated infections. Renal Impairment: Reduce dose or prolong intervals. Refer to PI for dosing guidelines.

HOW SUPPLIED: Inj: 250mg/mL [2mL, 4mL]

WARNINGS/PRECAUTIONS: Avoid peak levels >35mcg/mL and trough levels >10mcg/mL. Not for uncomplicated initial episodes of UTI unless the causative organisms are are not susceptible to antibiotics having less potential for toxicity. May cause fetal harm. Contains sodium metabisulfite; allergic-type reactions may occur more frequently in asthmatics. *Clostridium difficile*-associated diarrhea (CDAD) reported; d/c if CDAD is suspected or confirmed. May result in overgrowth of nonsusceptible organisms with prolonged use; take appropriate measures if superinfection develops. Use in the absence of a proven or strongly suspected bacterial infection or prophylactic indication is unlikely to provide benefit and increases the risk of the development of drug-resistant bacteria. Signs of renal irritation may occur (casts, white/red cells/albumin); increase hydration. D/C therapy if azotemia increases or if a progressive decrease in urinary output occurs. May aggravate muscle weakness. Cross-allergenicity among aminoglycosides demonstrated. Caution in elderly, and premature and neonatal infants.

ADVERSE REACTIONS: Ototoxicity, neurotoxicity, nephrotoxicity, skin rash, drug fever, headache, paresthesia, tremor, N/V, eosinophilia, arthralgia, anemia, hypotension, hypomagnesemia.

INTERACTIONS: See Boxed Warning. Increased nephrotoxicity with parenteral administration of aminoglycosides, antibiotics, and cephalosporins. Significant mutual inactivation may occur with β-lactam antibiotics.

PREGNANCY: Category D, not for use in nursing.

MECHANISM OF ACTION: Semisynthetic aminoglycoside antibiotic.

PHARMACOKINETICS: Absorption: (IM) Rapid. (IV) C_{max}=38mcg/mL. **Distribution:** V_d=24L; plasma protein binding (0-11%); crosses placenta. **Elimination:** Urine (91.9-98.2% unchanged, IM), (84-94% IV); $T_{1/2}$=>2 hrs.

NURSING CONSIDERATIONS

Assessment: Assess for history of hypersensitivity to drug, other aminoglycosides, or to sulfites. Assess for muscular disorders, renal impairment, pregnancy/nursing status, and possible drug interactions. Obtain pretreatment body weight for calculation of correct dosage. Assess and document bacterial infection using culture and susceptibility techniques.

Monitoring: Monitor for signs/symptoms of nephrotoxicity, neurotoxicity, ototoxicity, neuromuscular blockade, respiratory paralysis, and other adverse reactions. Monitor 8th cranial nerve function, hydration status, and drug serum concentrations, and perform urinalysis.

Patient Counseling: Inform about potential risks/benefits of therapy. Inform that drug only treats bacterial, not viral, infections. Instruct to take exactly ud; explaining that skipping doses or not completing full course of therapy may decrease effectiveness and increase the likelihood of bacterial resistance. Inform that diarrhea may occur and will usually end if therapy is discontinued. Instruct to contact physician as soon as possible if watery/bloody stools (with/without stomach cramps, fever) develop even as late as 2 months after having taken the last dose of therapy.

Administration: IV/IM route. Do not physically premix with other drugs; administer separately. Infuse over a period of 30-60 min; infuse over 1-2 hrs in infants. Refer to PI for proper administration, compatibility, and stability information. **Storage:** 20-25°C (68-77°F).

AMITIZA   RX
lubiprostone (Sucampo/Takeda)

THERAPEUTIC CLASS: Chloride channel activator

INDICATIONS: Treatment of chronic idiopathic constipation in adults, opioid-induced constipation (OIC) in adults with chronic non-cancer pain, and irritable bowel syndrome with constipation (IBS-C) in women ≥18 yrs of age.

DOSAGE: *Adults:* Chronic Idiopathic Constipation/OIC: 24mcg bid with food and water. Hepatic Dysfunction: Moderate (Child-Pugh Class B): Initial: 16mcg bid. Severe (Child-Pugh Class C): Initial: 8mcg bid. If dose is tolerated but adequate response not obtained, may escalate to full dose with appropriate monitoring. IBS-C: 8mcg bid with food and water. Severe Hepatic Dysfunction (Child-Pugh Class C): Initial: 8mcg qd. If dose is tolerated but adequate response not obtained, may escalate to full dose with appropriate monitoring.

HOW SUPPLIED: Cap: 8mcg, 24mcg

CONTRAINDICATIONS: Known or suspected mechanical GI obstruction.

WARNINGS/PRECAUTIONS: Effectiveness not established in treatment of OIC in patients taking diphenylheptane opioids (eg, methadone). May cause nausea; give with food to reduce symptoms of nausea. Diarrhea may occur; avoid in patients with severe diarrhea and d/c therapy if severe diarrhea occurs. Dyspnea reported; resolves within a few hrs after dose but may recur with subsequent doses. Thoroughly evaluate patients with symptoms suggestive of mechanical GI obstruction prior to initiation of therapy.

ADVERSE REACTIONS: N/V, diarrhea, headache, abdominal pain/distention, flatulence, loose stools, dizziness, edema, dyspnea, abdominal discomfort.

INTERACTIONS: Diphenylheptane opioids (eg, methadone) may cause dose-dependent decrease in efficacy.

PREGNANCY: Category C, caution in nursing.

MECHANISM OF ACTION: Chloride channel activator; enhances chloride-rich intestinal fluid secretion, increasing motility in the intestine, thereby facilitating the passage of stool.

PHARMACOKINETICS: Absorption: (24mcg single dose) (M3) C_{max}=41.5pg/mL, T_{max}=1.1 hrs, AUC_{0-t}=57.1pg•hr/mL. **Distribution:** Plasma protein binding (94%). **Metabolism:** Rapid and extensive; reduction and oxidation by carbonyl reductase; M3 (active metabolite). **Elimination:** Urine (60%), feces (30%); (M3) $T_{1/2}$=0.9-1.4 hrs.

NURSING CONSIDERATIONS

Assessment: Assess for known or suspected mechanical GI obstruction, severe diarrhea, pregnancy/nursing status, and possible drug interactions.

Monitoring: Monitor for nausea, dyspnea, severe diarrhea, and other adverse reactions. Periodically assess the need for continued therapy.

Patient Counseling: Instruct to notify physician if experiencing severe nausea, diarrhea, or dyspnea during treatment. Inform that dyspnea may occur within an hr after 1st dose and resolves within 3 hrs, but may recur with repeat dosing. Advise lactating women to monitor their breastfed infants for diarrhea while on therapy.

Administration: Oral route. Take with food and water. Swallow caps whole; do not break or chew. **Storage:** 25°C (77°F); excursions permitted to 15-30°C (59-86°F). Protect from light and extreme temperatures.

AMNESTEEM
isotretinoin (Mylan)

Not for use by females who are or may become pregnant. Severe birth defects, including death, have been documented. Increased risk of spontaneous abortion and premature births reported. D/C immediately if pregnancy occurs during treatment and refer to an obstetrician-gynecologist experienced in reproductive toxicity for evaluation and counseling. Approved only under special restricted distribution program called iPLEDGE™. Prescribers, patients, pharmacies, and distributors must be registered and activated with the program.

OTHER BRAND NAMES: Claravis (Barr) - Sotret (Ranbaxy)

THERAPEUTIC CLASS: Retinoid

INDICATIONS: Severe recalcitrant nodular acne unresponsive to conventional therapy, including systemic antibiotics.

DOSAGE: *Adults:* Take with food. Usual: 0.5-1mg/kg/day given in 2 divided doses for 15-20 weeks. Refer to PI for dosing by body weight. Titrate: May adjust dose according to response and/or tolerability. Very Severe Disease with Scarring or Primarily Manifested on Trunk: May adjust dose up to 2mg/kg/day, as tolerated. D/C if total nodule count has been reduced by >70% prior to completing 15-20 weeks. May initiate 2nd course of treatment after a period of ≥2 months off therapy.
Pediatrics: Take with food. ≥12 Yrs: Usual: 0.5-1mg/kg/day given in 2 divided doses for 15-20 weeks. Refer to PI for dosing by body weight. Titrate: May adjust dose according to response and/or tolerability. Very Severe Disease with Scarring or Primarily Manifested on Trunk: May adjust dose up to 2mg/kg/day, as tolerated. D/C if total nodule count has been reduced by >70% prior to completing 15-20 weeks. May initiate 2nd course of treatment after a period of ≥2 months off therapy.

HOW SUPPLIED: Cap: 10mg, 20mg, 40mg, (Claravis, Sotret) 10mg, 20mg, 30mg, 40mg

CONTRAINDICATIONS: Pregnancy, paraben sensitivity (Sotret).

WARNINGS/PRECAUTIONS: Avoid long-term use. Blood donation during therapy and for 1 month following discontinuation should be avoided. Do not initiate 2nd course of therapy until at least 8 weeks after completion of 1st course. Hypersensitivity reactions reported; d/c therapy and institute appropriate management if severe allergic reactions occur. Acute pancreatitis, impaired hearing, inflammatory bowel disease, elevated TGs, decreased HDL, hepatotoxicity, premature epiphyseal closure, skeletal hyperostosis, corneal opacities, decreased night vision, and impaired glucose control reported. May cause depression, psychosis, suicidal ideation/attempts, suicide, and aggressive and/or violent behaviors. Associated with pseudotumor cerebri (benign intracranial HTN). D/C if significant decrease in WBC count, hearing or visual impairment, abdominal pain, rectal bleeding, severe diarrhea, or hepatitis occurs, or if liver enzyme levels do not normalize. Spontaneous osteoporosis, osteopenia, bone fractures, and delayed fracture healing reported; caution with genetic predisposition for osteoporosis, history of childhood osteoporosis conditions, osteomalacia, other bone metabolism disorders, anorexia nervosa, and in patients participating in sports with repetitive impact. Micro-dosed progesterone preparations may be an inadequate method of contraception during therapy. (Amnesteem/Claravis) Erythema multiforme and severe skin reactions (eg, Stevens-Johnson syndrome, toxic epidermal necrolysis) reported; closely monitor for severe skin reactions and consider discontinuation of therapy.

ADVERSE REACTIONS: Cheilitis, hypertriglyceridemia, allergic reactions, inflammatory bowel disease, skeletal hyperostosis, pseudotumor cerebri, suicidal ideation/attempt, abnormal menses, bronchospasms, hearing impairment, corneal opacities.

INTERACTIONS: Avoid use with tetracyclines or vitamin supplements containing vitamin A. Caution with drugs that cause drug-induced osteoporosis/osteomalacia and/or affect vitamin D metabolism (eg, systemic corticosteroids, any anticonvulsant).

PREGNANCY: Category X, not for use in nursing.

MECHANISM OF ACTION: Retinoid; not established. Suspected to inhibit sebaceous gland function and keratinization.

PHARMACOKINETICS: Absorption: Administration of various doses and age resulted in different parameters. **Distribution:** Plasma protein binding (>99.9%). **Metabolism:** Liver via CYP2C8, 2C9, 3A4, and 2B6; 4-*oxo*-isotretinoin, retinoic acid, and 4-*oxo*-retinoic acid (active metabolites). **Elimination:** Feces and urine (65%-83%); (Healthy) $T_{1/2}$=21 hrs (isotretinoin), 24 hrs (4-*oxo*-isotretinoin).

NURSING CONSIDERATIONS

Assessment: Assess that females have had 2 (-) urine or serum pregnancy tests separated by at least 19 days, and are on 2 forms of effective contraception. Assess for hypersensitivity to parabens, history of psychiatric disorder, depression, risk of hyperlipidemia, pregnancy/nursing status, and possible drug interactions. Obtain blood lipids and LFTs.

AMOXICILLIN

Monitoring: Monitor for signs/symptoms of psychiatric disorders, pseudotumor cerebri, lipid abnormalities, acute pancreatitis, hearing impairment, hepatotoxicity, inflammatory bowel disease (regional ileitis), decreased bone mineral density, hyperostosis, premature epiphyseal closure, and other adverse reactions. Monitor lipid levels and LFTs (weekly or biweekly), glucose levels, and CPK levels until response to drug is established. Monitor that females remain on 2 forms of contraception during and for 1 month following discontinuation of therapy.

Patient Counseling: Instruct to read the Medication Guide/iPLEDGE and sign the Patient Information/Informed Consent form. Inform females of childbearing potential that 2 forms of effective contraception are required starting 1 month prior to initiation, during treatment, and for 1 month following discontinuation. Inform that monthly pregnancy tests are required before new prescription is issued. Instruct patients to d/c therapy if signs/symptoms of pseudotumor cerebri (eg, papilledema, headache, N/V) occur. Counsel not to share drug with anyone and not to donate blood during therapy and for 1 month following discontinuation. Instruct to take with a meal and swallow cap with a full glass of liquid. Inform that transient exacerbation (flare) of acne may occur. Advice to notify physician if depression, mood disturbances, psychosis, or aggression occurs. Instruct to avoid wax epilation and skin resurfacing procedures during and for at least 6 months following therapy; instruct to avoid prolonged exposure to UV rays or sunlight. Inform that decreased tolerance to contact lenses during and after therapy may occur. Inform that musculoskeletal symptoms, transient pain in chest, back pain in pediatrics, arthralgias, neutropenia, agranulocytosis, anaphylactic reactions, allergic vasculitis, purpura of the extremities, and extraneous involvement may occur. (Amnesteem/Claravis) Advise that severe skin reactions may occur.

Administration: Oral route. Take with food. **Storage:** 20-25°C (68-77°F). Protect from light.

AMOXICILLIN
amoxicillin (Various)   RX

THERAPEUTIC CLASS: Semisynthetic ampicillin derivative

INDICATIONS: Treatment of infections of the ear, nose, throat, and genitourinary tract (GU); skin and skin structure infections (SSSIs); lower respiratory tract infections (LRTIs); and acute, uncomplicated gonorrhea (anogenital and urethral infections) due to susceptible (β-lactamase negative) strains of microorganisms. Combination therapy for *Helicobacter pylori* eradication to reduce the risk of duodenal ulcer recurrence.

DOSAGE: *Adults:* Ear/Nose/Throat/GU Infections/SSSIs: (Mild/Moderate) 500mg q12h or 250mg q8h. (Severe) 875mg q12h or 500mg q8h. LRTIs: 875mg q12h or 500mg q8h. Continue for a minimum of 48-72 hrs beyond the time that patient becomes asymptomatic or evidence of bacterial eradication has been obtained. *Streptococcus pyogenes* Infections: At least 10 days. Acute Gonorrhea/Uncomplicated Anogenital and Urethral Infections: 3g as single dose. *H. pylori*: (Dual Therapy) 1g + 30mg lansoprazole, both q8h for 14 days. (Triple Therapy) 1g + 30mg lansoprazole + 500mg clarithromycin, all q12h for 14 days. GFR 10-30mL/min: 250-500mg q12h. GFR <10mL/min: 250-500mg q24h. Hemodialysis: 250-500mg q24h; additional dose during and at end of dialysis.
Pediatrics: >3 Months: ≥40kg: Dose as adult. <40kg: Ear/Nose/Throat/GU Infections/SSSIs: (Mild/Moderate) 25mg/kg/day given in divided doses q12h or 20mg/kg/day given in divided doses q8h. (Severe) 45mg/kg/day given in divided doses q12h or 40mg/kg/day given in divided doses q8h. LRTIs: 45mg/kg/day given in divided doses q12h or 40mg/kg/day given in divided doses q8h. Continue for a minimum of 48-72 hrs beyond the time that patient becomes asymptomatic or evidence of bacterial eradication has been obtained. *S. pyogenes* Infections: At least 10 days. Acute Gonorrhea/Uncomplicated Anogenital and Urethral Infections: Prepubertal: 50mg/kg with 25mg/kg probenecid as single dose (not for <2 yrs of age). Neonates/Infants: ≤12 Weeks: Max: 30mg/kg/day divided q12h.

HOW SUPPLIED: Cap: 250mg, 500mg; Sus: 125mg/5mL [80mL, 100mL, 150mL], 200mg/5mL [50mL, 75mL, 100mL], 250mg/5mL [80mL, 100mL, 150mL], 400mg/5mL [50mL, 75mL, 100mL]; Tab: 500mg, 875mg*; Tab, Chewable: 125mg, 250mg *scored

WARNINGS/PRECAUTIONS: Serious and occasionally fatal, hypersensitivity (anaphylactic) reactions reported with penicillin (PCN) therapy. *Clostridium difficile*-associated diarrhea (CDAD) reported; d/c if CDAD is suspected or confirmed. Avoid use with mononucleosis; erythematous skin rash may develop in these patients. May result in bacterial resistance if used in the absence of a proven/suspected bacterial indication; d/c and institute appropriate therapy if superinfection develops. Lab test interactions may occur. Caution in elderly; monitor renal function.

ADVERSE REACTIONS: N/V, diarrhea, rash.

INTERACTIONS: Decreased renal tubular secretion and increased/prolonged levels with probenecid. May reduce efficacy of combined oral estrogen/progesterone contraceptives. Chloramphenicol, macrolides, sulfonamides, and tetracyclines may interfere with bactericidal effects of PCN. PT prolongation (increased INR) reported with oral anticoagulants;

dose adjustment of oral anticoagulant may be necessary. Increased incidence of rashes with allopurinol.

PREGNANCY: Category B, caution in nursing.

MECHANISM OF ACTION: Ampicillin analog; has broad-spectrum bactericidal activity against susceptible organisms during active multiplication; acts through inhibition of biosynthesis of cell wall.

PHARMACOKINETICS: Absorption: Rapid. Cap: (250mg) T_{max}=1-2 hrs, C_{max}=3.5-5mcg/mL; (500mg) T_{max}=1-2 hrs, C_{max}=5.5-7.5mcg/mL. Tab: (875mg) C_{max}=13.8mcg/mL, AUC=35.4mcg•hr/mL. Sus: (125mg/5mL) T_{max}=1-2 hrs, C_{max}=1.5-3mcg/mL; (250mg/5mL) T_{max}=1-2 hrs, C_{max}=3.5-5mcg/mL; (400mg/5mL) T_{max}=1 hr, C_{max}=5.92mcg/mL, AUC=17.1mcg•hr/mL. Tab, Chewable: (400mg) T_{max}=1 hr, C_{max}=5.18mcg/mL, AUC=17.9mcg•hr/mL. **Distribution:** Plasma protein binding (20%); found in breast milk. **Elimination:** Urine (60%, unchanged); $T_{1/2}$=61.3 min.

NURSING CONSIDERATIONS

Assessment: Assess for history of allergic reaction to PCNs, cephalosporins, or other allergens, mononucleosis, renal function, pregnancy/nursing status, and possible drug interactions.

Monitoring: Monitor for serious anaphylactic reactions, erythematous skin rash, development of drug-resistant bacteria or superinfection, and CDAD. Monitor renal function. Monitor PT and INR if coadministered with an oral anticoagulant.

Patient Counseling: Inform that drug treats only bacterial, not viral (eg, common colds), infections. Instruct to take exactly ud; inform that skipping doses or not completing full course of therapy may decrease effectiveness and increase resistance. Instruct to notify physician as soon as possible if watery and bloody stools (with/without stomach cramps and fever) develop, even as late as ≥2 months after having last dose. Advise patients that drug may cause allergic reactions.

Administration: Oral route. (Sus) Refer to PI for directions for mixing. Shake well before use. Can be added to formula, milk, fruit juice, water, ginger ale, or cold drinks; take immediately. **Storage:** 20-25°C (68-77°F). (Sus) Discard any unused portion after 14 days. Refrigeration preferable but not required.

AMOXICILLIN/CLAVULANATE 600/42.9   RX
clavulanate potassium - amoxicillin (Various)

THERAPEUTIC CLASS: Aminopenicillin/beta lactamase inhibitor

INDICATIONS: Treatment of pediatric patients with recurrent or persistent acute otitis media due to susceptible strains of microorganisms.

DOSAGE: *Pediatrics:* ≥3 Months <40kg: 90mg/kg/day divided q12h for 10 days based on amoxicillin component (600mg/5mL). Refer to PI for dosing based on weight.

HOW SUPPLIED: Sus: (Amoxicillin-Clavulanate) 600mg-42.9mg/5mL [75mL, 125mL, 200mL]

CONTRAINDICATIONS: History of penicillin (PCN) allergy or amoxicillin/clavulanate-associated cholestatic jaundice/hepatic dysfunction.

WARNINGS/PRECAUTIONS: Serious, occasionally fatal, hypersensitivity reactions reported with PCN therapy; d/c if allergic reaction occurs and institute appropriate therapy. Pseudomembranous colitis/*Clostridium difficile* colitis reported. Caution with hepatic dysfunction. Monitor renal, hepatic, and hematopoietic functions with prolonged use. May result in bacterial resistance with prolonged use or use in the absence of a proven/suspected bacterial infection or a prophylactic indication; take appropriate measures if superinfection develops. Avoid with mononucleosis. Each 5mL of 600mg/42.9mg sus contains 1.4mg of phenylalanine. Lab test interactions may occur. Do not substitute 200mg/28.5mg per 5mL and 400mg/57mg per 5mL amoxicillin/clavulanate potassium sus for 600mg/42.9mg per 5mL amoxicillin/clavulanate potassium PO sus.

ADVERSE REACTIONS: Contact dermatitis (diaper rash), diarrhea, vomiting, moniliasis, rash.

INTERACTIONS: Probenecid may increase levels; coadministration not recommended. Increased PT reported with anticoagulants; may require oral anticoagulant dose adjustment. Allopurinol may increase incidence of rashes. May reduce efficacy of oral contraceptives.

PREGNANCY: Category B, caution in nursing.

MECHANISM OF ACTION: Amoxicillin: Aminopenicillin; semisynthetic antibiotic with a broad spectrum of bactericidal activity against gram-positive and gram-negative organisms. Clavulanate: β-lactamase inhibitor; possesses ability to inactivate a wide range of β-lactamase enzymes commonly found in microorganisms resistant to PCN and cephalosporins.

PHARMACOKINETICS: Absorption: Amoxicillin: C_{max}=15.7mcg/mL, T_{max}=2 hrs; AUC=59.8mcg•hr/mL. Clavulanate: C_{max}=1.7mcg/mL, T_{max}=1.1 hrs; AUC=4mcg•hr/mL. **Distribution:** Plasma protein binding: Amoxicillin (18%), clavulanate (25%). Amoxicillin: Found in breast milk. **Elimination:**

Amoxicillin: Urine (50-70% unchanged); $T_{1/2}$=1.4 hrs. Clavulanate: Urine (25-40% unchanged); $T_{1/2}$=1.1 hrs.

NURSING CONSIDERATIONS

Assessment: Assess for history of allergic reactions to PCNs, cephalosporins or other allergens, cholestatic jaundice, and hepatic dysfunction. Assess for infectious mononucleosis, phenylketo-nuria, and possible drug interactions.

Monitoring: Periodically monitor renal, hepatic, and hematopoietic organ functions with pro-longed use. Monitor for anaphylactic reactions, development of superinfection, skin rash, and pseudomembranous/*C. difficile* colitis.

Patient Counseling: Instruct to take q12h with a meal or snack to reduce possibility of GI upset. Advise to consult physician if severe diarrhea or watery/bloody stools occur, even as late as ≥2 months after having taken the last dose. Instruct to take ud; skipping doses or not complet-ing the full course of therapy may decrease effectiveness of the drug and increase bacterial resistance. Instruct to use a dosing spoon or medicine dropper when dosing, and rinse them after each use. Instruct to discard any unused medicine. Instruct to shake sus bottle well before each use.

Administration: Oral route. Take at the start of a meal. Refer to PI for mixing directions. Shake well before use. **Storage:** 20-25°C (68-77°F). Refrigerate reconstituted sus; discard after 10 days.

AMPHOTEC   RX
amphotericin B lipid complex (InterMune)

THERAPEUTIC CLASS: Polyene antifungal

INDICATIONS: Treatment of invasive aspergillosis in patients where renal impairment or unac-ceptable toxicity precludes the use of amphotericin B deoxycholate in effective doses, and in patients with invasive aspergillosis where prior amphotericin B deoxycholate therapy has failed.

DOSAGE: *Adults:* Test Dose: Infuse small amount over 15-30 min. Treatment: 3-4mg/kg as re-quired, qd, at infusion rate of 1mg/kg/hr.
Pediatrics: Test Dose: Infuse small amount over 15-30 min. Treatment: 3-4mg/kg as required, qd, at infusion rate of 1mg/kg/hr.

HOW SUPPLIED: Inj: 50mg [20mL], 100mg [50mL]

WARNINGS/PRECAUTIONS: Anaphylaxis reported; administer epinephrine, oxygen, IV steroids, and airway management as indicated. D/C if severe respiratory distress occurs; do not give further infusions. Acute infusion-related reactions may occur 1-3 hrs after starting IV infusion; manage by pretreatment with antihistamines and corticosteroids and/or by reducing the rate of infusion and by prompt administration of antihistamines and corticosteroids. Avoid rapid IV infu-sion. Monitor renal and hepatic function, serum electrolytes, CBC, and PT as medically indicated.

ADVERSE REACTIONS: Chills, fever, tachycardia, N/V, increased creatinine, hypotension, HTN, headache, thrombocytopenia, hypokalemia, hypomagnesemia, hypoxia, abnormal LFTs, dyspnea.

INTERACTIONS: Caution with antineoplastic agents; may enhance potential for renal toxicity, bronchospasm, hypotension. Corticosteroids and corticotropin may potentiate hypokalemia; monitor serum electrolytes and cardiac function. Cyclosporine and tacrolimus may cause renal toxicity. Concurrent use with digitalis glycosides may induce hypokalemia and may potentiate digitalis toxicity of digitalis glycosides; closely monitor serum K^+ levels. May increase flucyto-sine toxicity; use with caution. Antagonism with imidazole derivatives (eg, miconazole, keto-conazole) reported. Nephrotoxic agents (eg, aminoglycosides, pentamidine) may enhance the potential for drug-induced renal toxicity; use with caution and intensively monitor renal function. Amphotericin B-induced hypokalemia may enhance curariform effect of skeletal muscle relax-ants (eg, tubocurarine) due to hypokalemia; closely monitor serum K^+ levels.

PREGNANCY: Category B, not for use in nursing.

MECHANISM OF ACTION: Polyene antifungal; binds to sterols (primarily ergosterol) in cell mem-branes of sensitive fungi, with subsequent leakage of intracellular contents and cell death due to changes in membrane permeability. Also binds to cholesterol in mammalian cell membranes, which may account for human toxicity.

PHARMACOKINETICS: Absorption: (3mg/kg/day) AUC=29mcg/mL•hr; C_{max}=2.6mcg/mL. (4mg/kg/day) AUC=36mcg/mL•hr; C_{max}=2.9mcg/mL. **Distribution:** V_d=3.8L/kg (3mg/kg/day), 4.1L/kg (4mg/kg/day). **Elimination:** $T_{1/2}$=27.5 hrs (3mg/kg/day), 28.2 hrs (4mg/kg/day).

NURSING CONSIDERATIONS

Assessment: Assess for previous hypersensitivity to the drug, pregnancy/nursing status, and for possible drug interactions. Assess renal function.

Monitoring: Monitor for anaphylaxis, respiratory distress, and acute infusion-related reactions. Monitor renal and hepatic function, serum electrolytes, CBC, and PT. Monitor patients for 30 min after administering the test dose.

Patient Counseling: Inform of risks and benefits of therapy. Advise to seek medical attention if any adverse reactions occur.

Administration: IV route. Refer to PI for further instructions on preparation and administration.

Storage: Unopened Vials: 15-30°C (59-86°F). Retain in carton until time of use. Reconstituted: 2-8°C (36-46°F). Use within 24 hrs. Do not freeze. Further Diluted with D5W for Inj: 2-8°C (36-46°F). Use within 24 hrs.

AMPICILLIN INJECTION   RX
ampicillin sodium (Various)

THERAPEUTIC CLASS: Semisynthetic penicillin derivative

INDICATIONS: Treatment of respiratory tract, urinary tract, and GI infections, bacterial meningitis, septicemia, and endocarditis caused by susceptible strains of microorganisms.

DOSAGE: *Adults:* IM/IV: Respiratory Tract/Soft Tissue Infections: ≥40kg: 250-500mg q6h. <40kg: 25-50mg/kg/day given in equally divided doses at 6- to 8-hr intervals. GI/Genitourinary Tract Infections (Including *Neisseria gonorrhoeae* Infections in Females): ≥40kg: 500mg q6h. <40kg: 50mg/kg/day given in equally divided doses at 6- to 8-hr intervals. Urethritis (Caused by *N. gonorrhoeae* in Males): 2 doses of 500mg at an interval of 8-12 hrs; may be repeated if necessary or extended if required. Bacterial Meningitis: 150-200mg/kg/day given in equally divided doses q3-4h. Septicemia: 150-200mg/kg/day IV for at least 3 days and continue with IM q3-4h. Treatment of all infections should be continued for a minimum of 48-72 hrs after becoming asymptomatic or evidence of bacterial eradication has been obtained. Treatment recommended for a minimum of 10 days for any infection caused by Group A β-hemolytic streptococci. *Pediatrics:* Bacterial Meningitis: 150-200mg/kg/day given in equally divided doses q3-4h. Septicemia: 150-200mg/kg/day IV for at least 3 days and continue with IM q3-4h. Treatment of all infections should be continued for a minimum of 48-72 hrs after becoming asymptomatic or evidence of bacterial eradication has been obtained. Treatment recommended for a minimum of 10 days for any infection caused by Group A β-hemolytic streptococci.

HOW SUPPLIED: Inj: 125mg, 250mg, 500mg, 1g, 2g. Also available as a Pharmacy Bulk Package. Refer to individual package insert for more information.

WARNINGS/PRECAUTIONS: Reserve this drug for moderately severe and severe infections and for patients unable to take the oral forms; change to oral form may be made as soon as appropriate. Serious and occasionally fatal hypersensitivity (anaphylactoid) reactions with penicillin (PCN) therapy reported. Prior to therapy, assess for previous hypersensitivity reactions to PCNs, cephalosporins, and other allergens. D/C and institute appropriate therapy if an allergic reaction occurs. *Clostridium difficile*-associated diarrhea (CDAD) reported; d/c therapy if CDAD is suspected/confirmed. Avoid in infectious mononucleosis; skin rash reported. Use in the absence of a proven or strongly suspected bacterial infection or a prophylactic indication is unlikely to provide benefit and increases the risk of development of drug-resistant bacteria; d/c and substitute appropriate treatment if superinfection occurs. Lab test interactions may occur. More rapid administration may result in convulsive seizures.

ADVERSE REACTIONS: Skin rashes, urticaria, glossitis, N/V, diarrhea, black hairy tongue, stomatitis, enterocolitis, anemia, thrombocytopenia, eosinophilia, leukopenia, agranulocytosis.

INTERACTIONS: Increased incidence of skin rash with allopurinol.

PREGNANCY: Category B, caution in nursing.

MECHANISM OF ACTION: PCN derivative; bactericidal against PCN-susceptible gram-positive organisms and many common gram-negative pathogens.

PHARMACOKINETICS: Distribution: Plasma protein binding (20%), found in breast milk. Penetrates to CSF and brain only when meninges are inflamed. **Elimination:** Urine (unchanged).

NURSING CONSIDERATIONS

Assessment: Assess for hypersensitivity to PCNs/cephalosporins or other allergens, infectious mononucleosis, pregnancy/nursing status, and possible drug interactions. Conduct culture and susceptibility testing prior to therapy. In gonorrhea with a suspected primary lesion of syphilis, perform a dark-field exam before therapy.

Monitoring: Monitor for signs/symptoms of hypersensitivity reactions, CDAD, superinfection, skin rashes, and other adverse reactions. Perform periodic monitoring of organ system function, including renal, hepatic, and hematopoietic function with prolonged therapy. Where concomitant syphilis is suspected, perform serological tests monthly for at least 4 months.

Patient Counseling: Inform that drug treats bacterial, not viral, infections. Instruct to take exactly ud; skipping dose or not completing full course of therapy may decrease effectiveness and increase the likelihood of bacterial resistance. Instruct to contact physician as soon as possible if watery and bloody stools (with/without stomach cramps, fever) develop even as late as 2 or more months after having taken the last dose of therapy.

Administration: IM/IV routes. Administer within 1 hr after preparation. Administer IV slowly over at least 10-15 min to avoid convulsive seizures. Refer to PI for information regarding dilution, storage, and administration instructions.

AMPICILLIN ORAL   RX
ampicillin (Various)

THERAPEUTIC CLASS: Semisynthetic penicillin derivative

INDICATIONS: Treatment of meningitis and infections of genitourinary (GU) tract (including gonorrhea), respiratory tract, and GI tract caused by susceptible strains of microorganisms.

DOSAGE: *Adults:* GI/GU Infections: 500mg qid in equally spaced doses. Gonorrhea: 3.5g single dose with 1g probenecid. Respiratory Tract Infections: 250mg qid in equally spaced doses. May need larger doses in chronic or severe infections. Treat hemolytic strains of streptococci for a minimum of 10 days. Except for single dose regimen of gonorrhea, continue therapy for a minimum of 48-72 hrs after patient becomes asymptomatic or evidence of bacterial eradication has been obtained.
Pediatrics: >20kg: GI/GU Infections: 500mg qid in equally spaced doses. Gonorrhea: 3.5g single dose with 1g probenecid. Respiratory Tract Infections: 250mg qid in equally spaced doses. ≤20kg: GI/GU: Usual: 100mg/kg/day total, qid in equally divided and spaced doses. Respiratory Tract Infections: Usual: 50mg/kg/day total tid-qid, in equally divided and spaced doses. Do not exceed adult doses. May need larger doses in chronic or severe infections. Treat hemolytic strains of streptococci for a minimum of 10 days. Except for single dose regimen of gonorrhea, continue therapy for a minimum of 48-72 hrs after patient becomes asymptomatic or evidence of bacterial eradication has been obtained.

HOW SUPPLIED: Cap: 250mg, 500mg; Sus: 125mg/5mL, 250mg/5mL [100mL, 200mL]

CONTRAINDICATIONS: Infections caused by penicillinase-producing organisms.

WARNINGS/PRECAUTIONS: Serious and fatal hypersensitivity reactions reported with penicillin (PCN) therapy; anaphylactoid reactions require immediate treatment with epinephrine, oxygen, IV steroids, and airway management. Possible cross-sensitivity with cephalosporins. Pseudomembranous colitis reported; initiate therapeutic measures if diagnosed and consider discontinuation of treatment. May result in bacterial resistance with prolonged use or use in the absence of a proven or suspected bacterial infection or a prophylactic indication; take appropriate measures if superinfection develops. Give additional parenteral PCN in patients with gonorrhea who also have syphilis. Treatment does not preclude the need for surgical procedures, particularly in staphylococcal infections. Lab test interactions may occur.

ADVERSE REACTIONS: Stomatitis, N/V, diarrhea, rash, SGOT elevation, agranulocytosis, anemia, eosinophilia, leukopenia, thrombocytopenia, thrombocytopenic purpura, hypersensitivity reactions.

INTERACTIONS: Increased risk of rash with allopurinol. Bacteriostatic antibiotics (eg, chloramphenicol, erythromycins, sulfonamides, tetracyclines) may interfere with bactericidal activity. May increase breakthrough bleeding with oral contraceptives and decrease oral contraceptive effectiveness. Increased blood levels and toxicity with probenecid.

PREGNANCY: Category B, not for use in nursing.

MECHANISM OF ACTION: PCN derivative; bactericidal against non-penicillinase-producing gram-positive and gram-negative organisms.

PHARMACOKINETICS: Absorption: Well-absorbed; (500mg Cap) C_{max}=3mcg/mL; (250mg Sus) C_{max}=2.3mcg/mL. **Distribution:** Plasma protein binding (20%); found in breast milk. **Elimination:** Urine (unchanged).

NURSING CONSIDERATIONS

Assessment: Assess for previous hypersensitivity reactions to PCNs, cephalosporins, or other allergens; history of allergy, asthma, hay fever, or urticaria; pregnancy/nursing status, syphilis, and possible drug interactions. Conduct susceptibility testing as guide to therapy.

Monitoring: Monitor for hypersensitivity reactions, pseudomembranous colitis, and overgrowth of nonsusceptible organisms. Evaluate renal/hepatic/hematopoietic systems periodically with prolonged therapy. Upon completion, obtain cultures to determine organism eradication. Monitor for masked syphilis; perform follow-up serologic test for each month for 4 months for syphilis in patients without suspected lesions of syphilis.

Patient Counseling: Instruct to notify physician of history of hypersensitivity to PCNs, cephalosporins, or other allergens. Inform diabetics to consult with physician prior to changing diet or dosage of diabetic medication. Inform to take exactly ud; skipping doses or not completing full course decreases effectiveness and increases bacterial resistance. Instruct to d/c and notify physician if side effects occur. Inform that therapy only treats bacterial, and not viral, infections. **Administration:** Oral route. Take at least 30 min before or 2 hrs pc with a full glass of water. Refer to PI for reconstitution directions. **Storage:** 20-25°C (68-77°F). (Sus) Store reconstituted sus in the refrigerator; discard unused portion after 14 days.

AMPYRA RX
dalfampridine (Acorda)

THERAPEUTIC CLASS: Potassium channel blocker

INDICATIONS: Treatment to improve walking in patients with multiple sclerosis (MS).

DOSAGE: *Adults:* Max: 10mg bid (approximately 12 hrs apart).

HOW SUPPLIED: Tab, Extended-Release: 10mg

CONTRAINDICATIONS: History of seizure, moderate or severe renal impairment (CrCl ≤50mL/min).

WARNINGS/PRECAUTIONS: May cause seizures; d/c and do not restart in patients who experience a seizure while on therapy. Caution with mild renal impairment (CrCl 51-80mL/min). Avoid with other forms of 4-aminopyridine; d/c use of any product containing 4-aminopyridine prior to initiating therapy. May cause anaphylaxis and severe allergic reactions; d/c if signs and symptoms occur. Urinary tract infections (UTIs) reported; evaluate and treat patients as clinically indicated.

ADVERSE REACTIONS: UTI, insomnia, dizziness, headache, nausea, asthenia, back pain, balance disorder, MS relapse, paresthesia, nasopharyngitis, constipation.

PREGNANCY: Category C, not for use in nursing.

MECHANISM OF ACTION: Broad-spectrum K+ channel blocker; has not been established. Has been shown to increase conduction of action potentials in demyelinated axons through inhibition of K+ channels.

PHARMACOKINETICS: Absorption: Rapid and complete. C_{max}=17.3-21.6ng/mL (fasted), T_{max}=3-4 hrs (fasted). **Distribution:** Plasma protein binding (1-3%); V_d=2.6L/kg. **Metabolism:** Hydroxylation; CYP2E1 (major). **Elimination:** Urine (95.9%, 90.3% parent drug), feces (0.5%); $T_{1/2}$=5.2-6.5 hrs.

NURSING CONSIDERATIONS

Assessment: Assess for hypersensitivity to the drug or 4-aminopyridine, history of seizures, and pregnancy/nursing status. Obtain baseline CrCl.

Monitoring: Monitor for seizures, anaphylaxis, severe allergic reactions, UTIs, and other adverse reactions. Monitor CrCl at least annually.

Patient Counseling: Inform that therapy may cause seizures and to d/c treatment if seizure is experienced. Instruct to take exactly ud and not take a double dose if a dose is missed. Instruct not to take more than 2 tabs in a 24-hr period and to make sure that there is an approximate 12-hr interval between doses. Inform of the signs/symptoms of anaphylaxis; instruct to d/c therapy and seek medical care if anaphylaxis develops.

Administration: Oral route. Take with or without food. Take tab whole; do not divide, crush, chew, or dissolve. **Storage:** 25°C (77°F); excursions permitted to 15-30°C (59-86°F).

AMRIX RX
cyclobenzaprine HCl (Cephalon)

THERAPEUTIC CLASS: Skeletal muscle relaxant (central-acting)

INDICATIONS: Adjunct to rest and physical therapy for relief of muscle spasm associated with acute, painful musculoskeletal conditions.

DOSAGE: *Adults:* Usual: 15mg qd; may require up to 30mg qd. Take at the same time each day.

HOW SUPPLIED: Cap, Extended-Release: 15mg, 30mg

CONTRAINDICATIONS: Concomitant use of MAOIs or within 14 days after their discontinuation. During the acute recovery phase of myocardial infarction (MI). Arrhythmias, heart block or conduction disturbances, congestive heart failure (CHF), hyperthyroidism.

WARNINGS/PRECAUTIONS: Use for periods longer than 2 or 3 weeks is not recommended. Not effective in the treatment of spasticity associated with cerebral or spinal cord disease or in children with cerebral palsy. May produce arrhythmias, sinus tachycardia, and conduction time prolongation leading to MI and stroke; consider discontinuation if clinically significant CNS symptoms develop. Not recommended with hepatic impairment and in elderly. Caution with history of urinary retention, angle-closure glaucoma, and increased intraocular pressure (IOP). Consider certain withdrawal symptoms; abrupt cessation after prolonged administration rarely may produce nausea, headache, and malaise.

ADVERSE REACTIONS: Dry mouth, dizziness, somnolence, fatigue, constipation, nausea, dyspepsia.

INTERACTIONS: See Contraindications. Serotonin syndrome reported when used with SSRIs, SNRIs, TCAs, tramadol, bupropion, meperidine, verapamil, or MAOIs; d/c immediately if this occurs. Observe carefully, particularly during treatment initiation or dose increases, if concomitant use with other serotonergic drugs is warranted. May enhance effects of alcohol, barbiturates, and other CNS depressants. Caution with anticholinergics. May block the antihypertensive action of guanethidine and similarly acting compounds. May enhance seizure risk with tramadol.

PREGNANCY: Category B, caution in nursing.

MECHANISM OF ACTION: Skeletal muscle relaxant (central-acting); relieves skeletal muscle spasm of local origin without interfering with muscle function. Reduces tonic somatic motor activity, influencing both gamma and α motor systems.

PHARMACOKINETICS: Absorption: T_{max} =7-8 hrs. **Metabolism:** Extensive; N-demethylation via CYP3A4, 1A2, and 2D6. **Elimination:** Kidney (glucuronides); $T_{1/2}$=32 hrs.

NURSING CONSIDERATIONS

Assessment: Assess for arrhythmias, heart block or conduction disturbances, CHF, hyperthyroidism, acute recovery phase of MI, history of urinary retention, angle-closure glaucoma, increased IOP, hepatic impairment, drug hypersensitivity, pregnancy/nursing status, and possible drug interactions.

Monitoring: Monitor for arrhythmias, sinus tachycardia, conduction time prolongation, CNS symptoms, withdrawal symptoms, and other adverse reactions.

Patient Counseling: Advise to d/c use and notify physician immediately if experiencing symptoms of an allergic reaction (eg, difficulty breathing, hives, swelling of face/tongue, itching), arrhythmias, or tachycardia. Caution about the risk of serotonin syndrome; instruct to seek medical care immediately if signs/symptoms occur. Inform that drug may enhance impairment effects of alcohol and other CNS depressants. Caution about operating an automobile or other hazardous machinery until accustomed to effects of medication.

Administration: Oral route. **Storage:** 25°C (77°F); excursions permitted to 15-30°C (59-86°F).

AMTURNIDE   RX
aliskiren - hydrochlorothiazide - amlodipine (Novartis)

> D/C when pregnancy is detected. Drugs that act directly on the renin-angiotensin system can cause injury/death to the developing fetus.

THERAPEUTIC CLASS: Calcium channel blocker (dihydropyridine)/renin inhibitor/thiazide diuretic

INDICATIONS: Treatment of HTN.

DOSAGE: *Adults:* Usual: Dose qd. Titrate: May increase after 2 weeks of therapy. Max: 300mg-10mg-25mg. Add-On/Switch Therapy: Use if not adequately controlled with any 2 of the following: aliskiren, dihydropyridine calcium channel blockers (CCBs), and thiazide diuretics. With dose-limiting adverse reactions to any component on dual therapy, switch to triple therapy at a lower dose of that component. Replacement Therapy: Substitute for individually titrated components. Hepatic/Renal Impairment: Consider lower doses. Elderly: Consider lower initial doses.

HOW SUPPLIED: Tab: (Aliskiren-Amlodipine-HCTZ) 150mg-5mg-12.5mg, 300mg-5mg-12.5mg, 300mg-5mg-25mg, 300mg-10mg-12.5mg, 300mg-10mg-25mg

CONTRAINDICATIONS: Anuria, sulfonamide-derived drug hypersensitivity. Concomitant use with ARBs or ACE inhibitors in patients with diabetes.

WARNINGS/PRECAUTIONS: Not indicated for initial therapy of HTN. Symptomatic hypotension may occur in patients with marked volume depletion or with salt depletion; correct volume/salt depletion prior to administration, or start treatment under close medical supervision. May cause changes in renal function, including acute renal failure; consider withholding or discontinuing therapy if significant decrease in renal function develops; caution with renal artery stenosis, severe heart failure [HF], post-myocardial infarction [MI], or volume depletion. May cause serum electrolyte abnormalities (eg, hyperkalemia, hypokalemia, hyponatremia, hypomagnesemia); correct hypokalemia and any coexisting hypomagnesemia prior to initiation of therapy. D/C if hypokalemia is accompanied by clinical signs (eg, muscular weakness, paresis, ECG alterations). Aliskiren: Hypersensitivity reactions and head/neck angioedema reported; d/c therapy immediately and do not readminister if anaphylactic reactions or angioedema develop. Amlodipine: May cause symptomatic hypotension, particularly in patients with severe aortic stenosis. May develop worsening of angina and acute MI after starting or increasing the dose, particularly with severe obstructive coronary artery disease (CAD). HCTZ: May cause hypersensitivity reactions and exacerbation or activation of systemic lupus erythematosus (SLE). Minor alterations of fluid and electrolyte balance may precipitate hepatic coma in patients with hepatic impairment or progressive liver disease. May cause idiosyncratic reaction, resulting in transient myopia and acute angle-closure glaucoma; d/c as rapidly as possible. May alter glucose tolerance, increase serum cholesterol/TG levels, and cause hypercalcemia. May cause or exacerbate hyperuricemia and precipitate gout in susceptible patients.

ADVERSE REACTIONS: Peripheral edema, dizziness, headache.

INTERACTIONS: See Contraindications. Avoid with ARBs or ACE inhibitors in patients with moderate renal impairment (GFR <60mL/min). Aliskiren: Cyclosporine or itraconazole may increase levels; avoid concomitant use with such drugs. NSAIDs, including selective COX-2 inhibitors, may deteriorate renal function and attenuate antihypertensive effect. Dual blockade of the renin-angiotensin-aldosterone system (RAAS) is associated with increased risks of hypotension, hyperkalemia, and changes in renal function (including acute renal failure); monitor BP, renal function, and electrolytes with concomitant agents that affect the RAAS. Oral coadministration with furosemide reduced exposure to furosemide; monitor diuretic effects when coadministered. May develop hyperkalemia with NSAIDs, K^+ supplements, or K^+-sparing diuretics. Amlodipine: May increase simvastatin exposure; limit simvastatin dose to 20mg/day. Increased systemic exposure with CYP3A inhibitors (moderate and strong) warranting dose reduction; monitor for symptoms of hypotension and edema with CYP3A4 inhibitors to determine the need for dose adjustment. Monitor BP when coadministered with CYP3A4 inducers. HCTZ: Dosage adjustment of antidiabetic drugs (insulin or oral hypoglycemic agents) may be required. Ion exchange resins (eg, cholestyramine, colestipol) may reduce exposure; space dosing at least 4 hrs before or 4-6 hrs after the administration of ion exchange resins. Increased risk of lithium toxicity; avoid concomitant use.

PREGNANCY: Category D, not for use in nursing.

MECHANISM OF ACTION: Aliskiren: Direct renin inhibitor; decreases plasma renin activity and inhibits conversion of angiotensinogen to angiotensin I. Amlodipine: Dihydropyridine CCB; inhibits the transmembrane influx of Ca^{2+} ions into vascular smooth muscle and cardiac muscle, causing a reduction in peripheral vascular resistance and BP. HCTZ: Thiazide diuretic; has not been established. Affects renal tubular mechanisms of electrolyte reabsorption, directly increasing excretion of Na^+ and Cl^- in approximately equivalent amounts.

PHARMACOKINETICS: Absorption: Aliskiren: Poor; T_{max}=1-2 hrs; bioavailability (2.5%). Amlodipine: Absolute bioavailability (64-90%); T_{max}=6-12 hrs. HCTZ: Absolute bioavailability (70%); T_{max}=1-4 hrs. **Distribution:** Amlodipine: Plasma protein binding (93%); V_d=21L/kg. HCTZ: Albumin binding (40-70%). Crosses the placenta; found in breast milk. **Metabolism:** Aliskiren: via CYP3A4. Amlodipine: Hepatic; extensive. **Elimination:** Aliskiren: Urine (25% parent drug). Amlodipine: Urine (10% parent compound, 60% metabolites), $T_{1/2}$=30-50 hrs. HCTZ: Urine (70% unchanged), $T_{1/2}$=10 hrs.

NURSING CONSIDERATIONS

Assessment: Assess for drug hypersensitivity, hepatic/renal impairment, anuria, CAD, renal artery stenosis, HF, post-MI status, sulfonamide or penicillin allergy, volume/salt depletion, SLE, severe aortic stenosis, pregnancy/nursing status, and possible drug interactions.

Monitoring: Monitor for hypersensitivity/anaphylactic reactions, head/neck angioedema, airway obstruction, worsening of angina and MI, exacerbation of SLE, idiosyncratic reaction, transient myopia, acute angle-closure glaucoma, and other adverse reactions. Monitor BP, hepatic/renal function, serum uric acid, serum electrolytes, and glucose/cholesterol/TG levels.

Patient Counseling: Counsel women of childbearing age about consequences of exposure during pregnancy and of the treatment options with women planning to become pregnant. Instruct to report pregnancy to physician as soon as possible. Caution that lightheadedness may occur, especially during the 1st days of therapy; instruct to contact physician if lightheadedness occurs. Advise to d/c treatment and to consult physician if syncope occurs. Caution that inadequate fluid intake, excessive perspiration, diarrhea, or vomiting can lead to excessive fall in BP. Advise to d/c and immediately report any signs/symptoms of severe allergic reaction or angioedema. Inform that angioedema, including laryngeal edema, may occur any time during treatment. Instruct not to use K^+ supplements or salt substitutes containing K^+ without consulting physician.

Administration: Oral route. Establish a routine pattern for taking the drug with or without a meal; high-fat meals decrease absorption substantially. **Storage:** 25°C (77°F); excursions permitted to 15-30°C (59-86°F). Protect from heat and moisture.

ANAGRELIDE   RX
anagrelide HCl (Various)

OTHER BRAND NAMES: Agrylin (Shire)

Ancobon

THERAPEUTIC CLASS: Platelet-reducing agent

INDICATIONS: Treatment of thrombocythemia, secondary to myeloproliferative disorders, to reduce elevated platelet counts and the risk of thrombosis and to ameliorate associated symptoms (eg, thrombohemorrhagic events).

DOSAGE: *Adults:* Initial: 0.5mg qid or 1mg bid for ≥1 week. Titrate: Increase by not more than 0.5mg/day in any 1 week. Max: 10mg/day or 2.5mg/dose. Adjust to lowest effective dose to reduce and maintain platelet count <600,000/μL, and ideally to the normal range. Moderate Hepatic Impairment: Initial: 0.5mg/day for ≥1 week. Titrate: Increase by not more than 0.5mg/day in any 1 week.
Pediatrics: Initial: 0.5mg qd. Initial Range: 0.5mg qd-0.5mg qid. Titrate: Increase by not more than 0.5mg/day in any 1 week. Max: 10mg/day or 2.5mg/dose. Adjust to lowest effective dose to reduce and maintain platelet count <600,000/μL, and ideally to the normal range.

HOW SUPPLIED: Cap: 0.5mg, 1mg, (Agrylin) 0.5mg

CONTRAINDICATIONS: Severe hepatic impairment.

WARNINGS/PRECAUTIONS: Initiate therapy under close medical supervision. Torsades de pointes and ventricular tachycardia reported; perform pretreatment cardiovascular (CV) exam (eg, ECG) and monitor during treatment. Caution with known/suspected heart disease; may cause vasodilation, tachycardia, palpitations, and congestive heart failure. Caution with mild and moderate hepatic impairment; reduce dose in moderate hepatic impairment and monitor for CV effects. Interstitial lung diseases (eg, allergic alveolitis, eosinophilic pneumonia, interstitial pneumonitis) reported. Monitor blood counts (Hgb, WBC) and renal function (SrCr, BUN). Cases of hepatotoxicity (eg, symptomatic ALT and AST elevations, elevation >3X ULN) reported; measure LFTs prior to and during therapy. Fall in standing BP accompanied by dizziness reported. Interruption of treatment may be followed by an increase in platelet count.

ADVERSE REACTIONS: Headache, palpitations, diarrhea, asthenia, edema, N/V, abdominal pain, dizziness, pain, dyspnea, flatulence, fever, peripheral edema, rash (including urticaria).

INTERACTIONS: Aspirin may increase major hemorrhagic events; assess potential risks and benefits for concomitant use, prior to coadministration, particularly in patients with a high-risk profile for hemorrhage. CYP1A2 inhibitors (eg, fluvoxamine) may adversely influence clearance. Potential interaction with CYP1A2 substrates (eg, theophylline). May exacerbate effects of cAMP phosphodiesterase III (PDE III) inhibitors (eg, inotropes milrinone, enoximone, amrinone, olprinone, cilostazol). Sucralfate may interfere with absorption.

PREGNANCY: Category C, not for use in nursing.

MECHANISM OF ACTION: Platelet-reducing agent; not established. Suspected to reduce platelet production through a decrease in megakaryocyte hypermaturation. Inhibits cAMP PDE III. PDE III inhibitors can also inhibit platelet aggregation.

PHARMACOKINETICS: Metabolism: RL603 and 3-hydroxy anagrelide (major metabolites). **Elimination:** Urine (>70%); $T_{1/2}$=1.3 hrs (0.5mg, fasted).

NURSING CONSIDERATIONS

Assessment: Assess for hepatic/renal impairment, known/suspected heart disease, pregnancy/nursing status, and possible drug interactions. Perform CV exam and LFTs. Assess potential risks and benefits of therapy before starting treatment in patients with mild or moderate hepatic impairment.

Monitoring: Monitor for signs/symptoms of torsades de pointes, ventricular tachycardia, CV effects, interstitial lung diseases, thrombocytopenia, and other adverse reactions. Monitor platelet counts every 2 days during the 1st week of treatment and at least weekly thereafter until the maintenance dosage is reached. Monitor blood counts, renal function, and LFTs.

Patient Counseling: Inform of risks/benefits of therapy. Instruct women of childbearing potential to avoid pregnancy and to use contraception during therapy.

Administration: Oral route. **Storage:** 20-25°C (68-77°F). (Agrylin) 25°C (77°F); excursions permitted to 15-30°C (59-86°F).

Ancobon   RX
flucytosine (Valeant)

> Extreme caution in patients with renal impairment. Monitor hematologic, renal, and hepatic status closely.

THERAPEUTIC CLASS: 5-fluorocytosine antifungal

INDICATIONS: Treatment of serious infections caused by susceptible strains of *Candida* (eg, septicemia, endocarditis, urinary system infections) and/or *Cryptococcus* (eg, meningitis, pulmonary infections) in combination with amphotericin B.

DOSAGE: *Adults:* Usual: 50-150mg/kg/day in divided doses at 6-hr intervals. Give a few caps at a time over a 15-min period to reduce or avoid N/V. Renal Impairment: Initial: Give at a lower level.

HOW SUPPLIED: Cap: 250mg, 500mg

WARNINGS/PRECAUTIONS: Extreme caution with bone marrow depression. Patients with hematologic disease, patients being treated with radiation or drugs that depress bone marrow, or patients who have a history of treatment with such drugs or radiation may be more prone to bone marrow depression. Bone marrow toxicity can be irreversible and may lead to death in immunosuppressed patients.

ADVERSE REACTIONS: Myocardial toxicity, chest pain, dyspnea, rash, pruritus, urticaria, nausea, jaundice, renal failure, azotemia, crystalluria, anemia, leukopenia, ataxia, confusion.

INTERACTIONS: Cytosine arabinoside reported to inactivate antifungal activity by competitive inhibition. Drugs that impair glomerular filtration may prolong the biological $T_{1/2}$.

PREGNANCY: Category C, not for use in nursing.

MECHANISM OF ACTION: 5-fluorocytosine antifungal; exerts antifungal activity through the subsequent conversion into several active metabolites, which inhibit protein synthesis by being falsely incorporated into fungal RNA or interfere with biosynthesis of fungal DNA through inhibition of enzyme thymidylate synthetase.

PHARMACOKINETICS: Absorption: Rapid and complete. Absolute bioavailability (78-89%); (2g, Healthy) C_{max}=30-40mcg/mL, T_{max}=2 hrs. **Distribution:** Plasma protein binding (2.9-4%). **Metabolism:** Deamination (by gut bacteria) to 5-fluorouracil; α-fluoro-β-ureido-propionic acid (metabolite). **Elimination:** Urine (>90% unchanged, 1% metabolite), feces; $T_{1/2}$=2.4-4.8 hrs (healthy), 85 hrs (nephrectomized/anuric).

NURSING CONSIDERATIONS

Assessment: Assess for hypersensitivity to the drug, renal impairment, bone marrow depression, immunosuppressed patients, pregnancy/nursing status, and possible drug interactions. Determine serum electrolytes and hematologic status prior to treatment.

Monitoring: Monitor for adverse reactions. Monitor renal function and blood concentrations. Monitor hematologic status (leukocyte and thrombocyte count) and hepatic function frequently.

Patient Counseling: Inform of the risks and benefits of therapy. Advise to take a few caps at a time over a 15-min period to reduce or avoid N/V.

Administration: Oral route. **Storage:** 25°C (77°F); excursions permitted to 15-30°C (59-86°F).

ANDRODERM
testosterone (Watson)

CIII

THERAPEUTIC CLASS: Androgen

INDICATIONS: Replacement therapy in adult males for conditions associated with a deficiency or absence of endogenous testosterone (eg, congenital/acquired primary hypogonadism or hypogonadotropic hypogonadism).

DOSAGE: *Adults:* ≥18 Yrs: Initial: One 4mg/day system applied nightly for 24 hrs to a clean dry area of the skin on the back, abdomen, upper arms, or thighs. Measure early am serum testosterone concentrations, approximately 2 weeks after starting. If outside the range of 400-930ng/dL, increase daily dose to 6mg (one 4mg/day and one 2mg/day system) or decrease to 2mg (one 2mg/day system), maintaining nightly application. Patients currently maintained on 2.5mg/day, 5mg/day, or 7.5mg/day systems may be switched to 2mg/day, 4mg/day, or 6mg/day (2mg/day and 4mg/day) systems respectively, at the next scheduled dose. Measure early am serum testosterone concentration approximately 2 weeks after switching to ensure proper dosing.

HOW SUPPLIED: Patch: 2mg/day [60^s], 4mg/day [30^s]

CONTRAINDICATIONS: Breast carcinoma or known/suspected prostate carcinoma in men, women who are or may become pregnant, and women who are breastfeeding.

WARNINGS/PRECAUTIONS: Monitor patients with BPH for worsening of signs/symptoms of BPH. May increase risk for prostate cancer; evaluate for prostate cancer prior to and during therapy. Increases in Hct/RBC mass may increase risk for thromboembolic events; lower dose or d/c therapy; may restart when Hct decreases to acceptable level. Suppression of spermatogenesis may occur at large doses. Risk of edema with or without congestive heart failure (CHF) with preexisting cardiac, renal, or hepatic disease. Gynecomastia may develop and persist. May potentiate sleep apnea. Changes in serum lipid profile may require dose adjustment or discontinuation of therapy. Caution in cancer patients at risk of hypercalcemia and associated hypercalciuria; monitor serum Ca^{2+} concentrations regularly. May decrease concentrations of thyroxine-binding globulin, resulting in decreased total T4 serum concentrations and increased resin uptake of T3 and T4. Skin burns reported at application site in patients wearing an aluminized transdermal system during a magnetic resonance imaging scan (MRI); remove the system before patient undergoes an MRI. Not indicated for use in women and children.

ADVERSE REACTIONS: Application-site reactions (pruritus, blistering, erythema, vesicles, burning, induration), back pain, prostatic abnormalities, headache, contact dermatitis, depression.

INTERACTIONS: Changes in insulin sensitivity or glycemic control may occur; may decrease blood glucose and therefore, decrease insulin requirements in diabetic patients. Changes in anticoagulant activity may occur; frequently monitor INR and PT in patients taking anticoagulants, especially at initiation and termination of androgen therapy. Adrenocorticotropic hormone or corticosteroids may increase fluid retention; caution in patients with cardiac, renal, or hepatic disease. Pretreatment with triamcinolone ointment formulation reduces testosterone absorption.

PREGNANCY: Category X, not for use in nursing.

MECHANISM OF ACTION: Androgen; responsible for normal growth and development of male sex organs and for maintenance of secondary sex characteristics.

PHARMACOKINETICS: Absorption: T_{max}=8 hrs (median). **Distribution:** Sex hormone-binding globulin binding (40%), albumin and plasma protein binding (58%). **Metabolism:** Estradiol and dihydrotestosterone (major active metabolites). **Elimination:** (IM) Urine (90% glucuronic and sulfuric acid conjugates), feces (6% unconjugated); $T_{1/2}$=10-100 min, $T_{1/2}$=70 min (upon removal).

NURSING CONSIDERATIONS

Assessment: Assess for breast carcinoma, prostate cancer, BPH, cardiac/renal/hepatic disease, obesity, chronic lung disease, cancer patients at risk for hypercalcemia, upcoming MRI exam, and possible drug interactions. Obtain Hct prior to therapy.

Monitoring: Monitor for signs/symptoms of edema with or without CHF, gynecomastia, sleep apnea, and worsening of BPH. Monitor Hgb, prostate-specific antigen, serum lipid profile, liver function, and serum testosterone levels periodically. In cancer patients at risk for hypercalcemia, regularly monitor serum Ca^{2+} levels. Reevaluate for prostate cancer 3-6 months after initiation, and then in accordance with prostate cancer screening practices. Reevaluate Hct 3-6 months after start of therapy, then annually. Monitor PT/INR more frequently with concomitant anticoagulants.

Patient Counseling: Inform that men with known or suspected prostate/breast cancer should not use androgen therapy. Inform about potential adverse reactions. Instruct to apply ud. Advise not to apply to the scrotum, over a bony prominence, or any part of the body that could be subject to prolonged pressure during sleep or sitting. Advise not to remove during sexual intercourse, nor while taking a shower or bath. Inform that strenuous exercise or excessive perspiration may loosen a patch or cause it to fall off; if patch falls off, advise not to tape to skin. Advise to avoid swimming or showering until 3 hrs following application. Instruct to use OTC topical hydrocortisone cre after system removal in order to ameliorate mild skin irritation. Advise to remove the patch before undergoing MRI. Advise not to cut the patches.

Administration: Transdermal route. Immediately apply adhesive side of the system to a clean, dry area of the skin on the back, abdomen, upper arms, or thighs. Rotate application site with an interval of 7 days between applications to the same site. Refer to PI for further application instructions. **Storage:** 20-25° (68-77°F). Do not store outside the pouch provided.

ANDROGEL
testosterone (AbbVie)

 CIII

> Virilization reported in children secondarily exposed to testosterone gel. Children should avoid contact with unwashed or unclothed application sites in men using testosterone gel. Advise patients to strictly adhere to recommended instructions for use.

THERAPEUTIC CLASS: Androgen

INDICATIONS: Replacement therapy in adult males for conditions associated with a deficiency or absence of endogenous testosterone (congenital/acquired primary hypogonadism or hypogonadotropic hypogonadism).

DOSAGE: *Adults:* (1%) Initial: Apply 50mg (4 pump actuations, two 25mg pkts, or one 50mg pkt) qd in am (preferably at the same time every day) to shoulders and upper arms and/or abdomen. Titrate: May increase to 75mg qd and then to 100mg qd as instructed by physician if serum testosterone is below normal range. May decrease daily dose if serum testosterone exceeds normal range. D/C therapy if serum testosterone consistently exceeds the normal range at a daily dose of 50mg. Assess serum testosterone concentrations periodically. Refer to PI for specific dosing guidelines using the multidose pump. (1.62%) Initial: Apply 40.5mg (2 pump actuations or a single 40.5mg pkt) qd in am to shoulders and upper arms. Titrate: May adjust dose between a minimum of 20.25mg (1 pump actuation or a single 20.25mg pkt) and a max of 81mg (4 pump actuations or two 40.5mg pkts). Titrate based on the pre-dose am serum testosterone concentration from a single blood draw at approximately 14 days and 28 days after starting treatment or following dose adjustment. Assess serum testosterone concentrations periodically. Refer to PI for dose adjustments required at each titration step.

HOW SUPPLIED: Gel: 1% [2.5g, 5g pkt; 75g pump], 1.62% [1.25g, 2.5g pkt; 88g pump]

CONTRAINDICATIONS: Breast carcinoma or known/suspected prostate carcinoma in men; women who are or may become pregnant, or are breastfeeding.

WARNINGS/PRECAUTIONS: Topical testosterone products may have different doses, strengths, or application instructions that may result in different systemic exposure. Application site and dose are not interchangeable with other topical testosterone products. Patients with BPH may be at increased risk for worsening of signs/symptoms of BPH. May increase risk for prostate cancer; evaluate for prostate cancer prior to and during therapy. Increases in Hct/RBC mass may increase risk for thromboembolic events; may require dose reduction or discontinuation of therapy. Not indicated for use in women. Suppression of spermatogenesis may occur with large doses. Risk of edema with or without congestive heart failure (CHF) with preexisting cardiac, renal, or hepatic disease. Gynecomastia may develop and persist. May potentiate sleep apnea. Changes in serum lipid profile may require dose adjustment or discontinuation of therapy. Caution in cancer patients at risk of hypercalcemia and associated hypercalciuria; monitor serum Ca^{2+} concentrations regularly. May decrease levels of thyroxin-binding globulins, resulting in decreased total T4 serum concentrations and increased resin uptake of T3 and T4. Flammable; avoid fire, flame, or smoking until the gel has dried.

ADVERSE REACTIONS: Prostate specific antigen (PSA) increase, acne, application-site reactions, prostatic/urinary/testicular disorders, abnormal lab tests, headache, emotional lability, gynecomastia, HTN, nervousness, asthenia, decreased libido.

INTERACTIONS: Changes in insulin sensitivity or glycemic control may occur; may decrease blood glucose and, therefore, may decrease insulin requirements in diabetic patients. Changes in anticoagulant activity may occur; frequently monitor INR and PT in patients taking anticoagulants, especially at initiation and termination of androgen therapy. Adrenocorticotropic hormone or corticosteroids may increase fluid retention; caution in patients with cardiac, renal, or hepatic disease.

PREGNANCY: Category X, not for use in nursing.

MECHANISM OF ACTION: Androgen; responsible for normal growth and development of male sex organs and for maintenance of secondary sex characteristics.

PHARMACOKINETICS: Distribution: Sex hormone-binding globulin binding (40%), albumin and other plasma protein binding (58%), unbound (2%). **Metabolism:** Estradiol and dihydrotestosterone (major active metabolites). **Elimination:** (IM) Urine (90% glucuronic and sulfuric acid conjugates), feces (6% unconjugated); $T_{1/2}$=10-100 min.

NURSING CONSIDERATIONS

Assessment: Assess for BPH, prostate cancer, cardiac/renal/hepatic disease, obesity, chronic lung disease, conditions where treatment is contraindicated or cautioned, and possible drug interactions. Obtain Hct prior to therapy.

Monitoring: Monitor for prostate cancer, edema with or without CHF, gynecomastia, sleep apnea, virilization, and worsening of signs/symptoms of BPH. Perform periodic monitoring of Hct, Hgb, PSA, serum lipid profile, LFTs, and serum testosterone concentrations. In cancer patients at risk for hypercalcemia, regularly monitor serum Ca^{2+} levels. Reevaluate Hct 3-6 months after start of therapy, then annually. Frequently monitor INR/PT during coadministration with anticoagulants.

Patient Counseling: Inform that men with known or suspected prostate/breast cancer should not use androgen therapy. Advise to report signs and symptoms of secondary exposure in children and women to the physician. Instruct to avoid contact with unwashed or unclothed application sites of men. Instruct to apply ud and to wash hands with soap and water after application, cover application site with clothing after gel dries, and wash application site with soap and water prior to direct skin-to-skin contact with others. Inform about possible adverse reactions. Advise to read Medication Guide before therapy and reread each time the prescription is renewed. Inform that drug is flammable; instruct to avoid fire, flame, or smoking until the gel has dried. Instruct to keep out of reach of children. Advise not to share the medication with anyone. Inform about importance of adhering to all the recommended monitoring, to report changes in their state of health, and to wait 5 hrs (1%) or 2 hrs (1.62%) before swimming or bathing.

Administration: Topical route. Apply to clean, dry, healthy, intact skin. (1%) Apply to right and left upper arms/shoulders and/or right and left abdomen; do not apply to genitals, chest, or back. (1.62%) Apply to upper arms and shoulders; do not apply to any other parts of the body (eg, abdomen, genitals). Refer to PI for administration instructions. **Storage:** (1%) 25°C (77°F); excursions permitted to 15-30°C (59-86°F). (1.62%) 20-25°C (68-77°F); excursions permitted to 15-30°C (59-86°F).

ANGELIQ

RX

drospirenone - estradiol (Bayer Healthcare)

> Estrogens increase the risk of endometrial cancer. Perform adequate diagnostic measures, including endometrial sampling, to rule out malignancy in postmenopausal women with undiagnosed persistent or recurring abnormal genital bleeding. Should not be used for the prevention of cardiovascular disease (CVD) or dementia. Increased risk of myocardial infarction (MI), stroke, invasive breast cancer, pulmonary embolism (PE), and deep vein thrombosis (DVT) in postmenopausal women (50-79 yrs of age) reported. Increased risk of developing probable dementia in postmenopausal women ≥65 yrs of age reported. Should be prescribed at the lowest effective dose and for the shortest duration consistent with treatment goals and risks.

THERAPEUTIC CLASS: Estrogen/progestogen combination

INDICATIONS: Treatment of moderate to severe vasomotor symptoms and/or vulvar and vaginal atrophy due to menopause in women who have a uterus.

DOSAGE: *Adults:* Moderate to Severe Vasomotor Symptoms: 1 tab (0.25mg-0.5mg or 0.5-1mg) qd. Moderate to Severe Vulvar and Vaginal Atrophy: 1 tab (0.5mg-1mg) qd. Reevaluate periodically.

HOW SUPPLIED: Tab: (Drospirenone [DSRP]-Estradiol [E2]) 0.25mg-0.5mg, 0.5mg-1mg

CONTRAINDICATIONS: Undiagnosed abnormal genital bleeding, known/suspected/history of breast cancer, known/suspected estrogen-dependent neoplasia, active or history of DVT/PE/ arterial thromboembolic disease (eg, stroke, MI), renal impairment, liver impairment/disease, adrenal insufficiency, protein C, protein S, antithrombin deficiency, or other known thrombophilic disorders; known/suspected pregnancy.

WARNINGS/PRECAUTIONS: D/C immediately if PE, DVT, stroke, or MI occur or are suspected. Caution in patients with risk factors for arterial vascular disease (eg, HTN, diabetes mellitus [DM], tobacco use, hypercholesterolemia, obesity) and/or venous thromboembolism (VTE) (eg, personal/family history of VTE, obesity, systemic lupus erythematosus [SLE]). If feasible, d/c therapy at least 4-6 weeks before surgery of the type associated with increased risk of thromboembolism, or during periods of prolonged immobilization. Potential for hyperkalemia development in high-risk patients; contraindicated with conditions that predispose to hyperkalemia. May increase risk of ovarian cancer and gallbladder disease. May lead to severe hypercalcemia in patients with breast cancer and bone metastases; d/c and take appropriate measures if hypercalcemia occurs. Retinal vascular thrombosis reported; d/c pending examination if sudden partial or complete loss of vision, sudden onset of proptosis, diplopia, or migraine occurs. D/C permanently if examination reveals papilledema or retinal vascular lesions. May elevate BP, thyroid-binding globulin levels, and plasma TG levels (with preexisting hypertriglyceridemia); d/c if pancreatitis occurs. Caution with history of cholestatic jaundice associated with past estrogen use or with pregnancy; d/c in case of recurrence. May cause fluid retention; caution with cardiac/renal dysfunction. Caution with hypoparathyroidism; hypocalcemia may occur. May increase possibility of hyponatremia in high-risk patients. May induce or exacerbate symptoms of angioedema in women with hereditary angioedema. May exacerbate endometriosis, asthma, DM, epilepsy, migraine, porphyria, SLE, otosclerosis, chorea minor, and hepatic hemangiomas; use with caution. May affect certain endocrine and blood components in lab tests.

ADVERSE REACTIONS: GI and abdominal pain, female genital tract bleeding, headache, breast pain, vulvovaginal fungal infections, nausea.

INTERACTIONS: CYP3A4 inducers (eg, St. John's wort, phenobarbital, carbamazepine, rifampin) may decrease levels, which may decrease therapeutic effects and/or change uterine bleeding profile. CYP3A4 inhibitors (eg, erythromycin, clarithromycin, ketoconazole, itraconazole, ritonavir, grapefruit juice) may increase levels that may result in side effects. May increase risk of hyperkalemia with regular intake of other medications that can increase K^+ (eg, NSAIDs, K^+-sparing diuretics, K^+ supplements, ACE inhibitors, ARBs, heparin, aldosterone antagonists). Patients concomitantly receiving thyroid hormone replacement therapy and estrogens may require increased doses of their thyroid replacement therapy. Acute alcohol ingestion may elevate circulating E2 concentrations.

PREGNANCY: Contraindicated in pregnancy, caution in nursing.

MECHANISM OF ACTION: Estrogen/progestogen combination. E2: Binds to nuclear receptors in estrogen-responsive tissues. Modulates pituitary secretion of gonadotropins, luteinizing hormone and follicle-stimulating hormone, through negative feedback mechanism. DRSP: Synthetic progestin and spironolactone analog with antimineralocorticoid activity. Possesses antiandrogenic activity. Counters estrogenic effects by decreasing number of nuclear estradiol receptors and suppressing epithelial DNA synthesis in endometrial tissue.

PHARMACOKINETICS: Absorption: DRSP: Absolute bioavailability (76-85%). Administration of variable doses resulted in different pharmacokinetic parameters. **Distribution:** Found in breast milk. DRSP: V_d=4.2L/kg, serum protein binding (97%). E2: Sex hormone-binding globulin (37%); albumin binding (61%). **Metabolism:** DRSP: Extensive; CYP3A4 (minor). E2: Liver to estrone (metabolite) and estriol (major urinary metabolite); enterohepatic recirculation via sulfate and glucuronide conjugation in the liver; biliary secretion of conjugates in the intestine; hydrolysis in the gut; reabsorption. **Elimination:** DRSP: Urine (38-47%, glucuronide and sulfate conjugates), feces (17-20%, glucuronide and sulfate conjugates); $T_{1/2}$=36-42 hrs. E2/Estrone: Urine.

NURSING CONSIDERATIONS

Assessment: Assess for undiagnosed abnormal genital bleeding, presence/history of breast cancer, estrogen-dependent neoplasia, arterial thromboembolic disease, pregnancy/nursing status, other conditions where treatment is cautioned/contraindicated, and possible drug interactions.

Monitoring: Monitor for signs/symptoms of CVD, malignant neoplasms, dementia, gallbladder disease, visual abnormalities, BP and plasma TG elevations, pancreatitis, cholestatic jaundice, hypothyroidism, fluid retention, hyperkalemia, hyponatremia, and exacerbation of endometriosis and other conditions. Perform annual breast examination; schedule mammography based on patient's age, risk factors, and prior mammogram results. Monitor thyroid function in patients on thyroid hormone replacement therapy. Monitor serum K⁺ levels during 1st month of dosing in patients at risk for hyperkalemia. Perform adequate diagnostic measures (eg, endometrial sampling) in patients with undiagnosed persistent or recurrent genital bleeding. Perform periodic evaluation to determine treatment need.

Patient Counseling: Inform postmenopausal women of the importance of reporting abnormal vaginal bleeding as soon as possible. Advise of possible adverse reactions. Instruct to have yearly breast exams by a healthcare provider and perform monthly breast self-examinations.

Administration: Oral route. Swallow whole with some liquid irrespective of food. Take at the same time qd. **Storage:** 25°C (77°F); excursions permitted to 15-30°C (59-86°F).

ANGIOMAX   RX
bivalirudin (The Medicines Company)

THERAPEUTIC CLASS: Direct thrombin inhibitor

INDICATIONS: As an anticoagulant in patients with unstable angina undergoing percutaneous transluminal coronary angioplasty (PTCA). As an anticoagulant in patients undergoing percutaneous coronary intervention (PCI) with provisional use of glycoprotein IIb/IIIa inhibitor (GPI). For patients with, or at risk of, heparin-induced thrombocytopenia (HIT) or heparin-induced thrombocytopenia and thrombosis syndrome (HITTS) undergoing PCI.

DOSAGE: *Adults:* Give with aspirin (300-325mg/day). Patients Without HIT/HITTS: 0.75mg/kg IV bolus, then 1.75mg/kg/hr infusion for the duration of the PCI/PTCA procedure. An activated clotting time should be performed 5 min after the bolus dose and an additional 0.3mg/kg should be given if needed. Consider GPI administration in the event that any condition listed in the REPLACE-2 clinical trial description is present; refer to PI. Patients With HIT/HITTS Undergoing PCI: 0.75mg/kg IV bolus, then 1.75mg/kg/hr infusion for the duration of the procedure. Ongoing Treatment Post-Procedure: Continuation of infusion following PCI/PTCA for up to 4 hrs postprocedure is optional. After 4 hrs, an additional infusion may be initiated at a rate of 0.2mg/kg/hr (low-rate infusion), for up to 20 hrs, if needed. Renal Impairment: Moderate (CrCl 30-59mL/min): 1.75mg/kg/hr infusion. Severe (CrCl <30mL/min): Consider reducing infusion to 1mg/kg/hr. Hemodialysis: 0.25mg/kg/hr infusion. Refer to PI for the dosing table based on weight.

HOW SUPPLIED: Inj: 250mg

CONTRAINDICATIONS: Active major bleeding.

WARNINGS/PRECAUTIONS: Hemorrhage may occur at any site; caution with disease states associated with increased risk of bleeding. D/C with unexplained fall in BP or Hct. Associated with increased risk of thrombus formation, including fatal outcomes in gamma brachytherapy; maintain meticulous catheter technique, with frequent aspiration and flushing, paying special attention to minimize stasis condition within the catheter/vessels. May need to reduce infusion dose and monitor anticoagulant status in patients with renal impairment.

ADVERSE REACTIONS: Bleeding, back pain, pain, N/V, headache, hypotension, HTN, bradycardia, dyspepsia, insomnia, pelvic pain, anxiety, abdominal pain, fever, inj-site pain.

INTERACTIONS: Increased risk of major bleeding events with heparin, warfarin, thrombolytics, or GPIs.

PREGNANCY: Category B, caution in nursing.

MECHANISM OF ACTION: Direct thrombin inhibitor; inhibits thrombin by specifically binding both to the catalytic site and to anion-binding exosite of circulating and clot-bound thrombin.

PHARMACOKINETICS: Metabolism: Proteolytic cleavage. **Elimination:** Renal. $T_{1/2}$=25 min (plasma).

NURSING CONSIDERATIONS

Assessment: Assess for drug hypersensitivity, active major bleeding, renal impairment, disease states associated with increased risk of bleeding, pregnancy/nursing status, and for possible drug interactions.

Monitoring: Monitor for signs/symptoms of hemorrhage, thrombus formation in gamma brachytherapy, and other adverse reactions. For patients with renal impairment, monitor anticoagulant status.

Patient Counseling: Advise to watch for any signs of bleeding/bruising and to report to physician if these occur. Advise to inform physician about the use of any other medications (eg, warfarin and heparin), including OTC medicines or herbal products, prior to therapy.

Administration: IV route. Refer to PI for administration instructions. **Storage:** 20-25°C (68-77°F); excursions permitted to 15-30°C (59-86°F). Reconstituted: 2-8°C (36-46°F) for up to 24 hrs. Diluted concentration of between 0.5mg/mL and 5mg/mL is stable at room temperature for up to 24 hrs. Do not freeze.

ANTARA   RX
fenofibrate (Lupin)

THERAPEUTIC CLASS: Fibric acid derivative

INDICATIONS: Adjunct to diet to reduce elevated LDL, total cholesterol, TG levels, and apolipoprotein B, and to increase HDL in adults with primary hypercholesterolemia or mixed dyslipidemia. Adjunct to diet for treatment of adults with severe hypertriglyceridemia.

DOSAGE: *Adults:* Primary Hypercholesterolemia/Mixed Dyslipidemia: Initial/Max: 90mg/day. Severe Hypertriglyceridemia: Initial: 30-90mg/day. Titrate: Adjust dose if necessary following repeat lipid determinations at 4- to 8- week intervals; individualize dose. Max: 90mg/day. Mild to Moderate Renal Impairment: Initial: 30mg/day. Titrate: Increase only after evaluation of effects on renal function and lipid levels. Elderly: Dose based on renal function. Consider dose reduction if lipid levels fall significantly below the targeted range. D/C if no adequate response after 2 months of therapy with max dose.

HOW SUPPLIED: Cap: 30mg, 90mg

CONTRAINDICATIONS: Severe renal impairment (including dialysis), active liver disease (including primary biliary cirrhosis and unexplained persistent liver function abnormalities), preexisting gallbladder disease, and nursing mothers.

WARNINGS/PRECAUTIONS: Not shown to reduce coronary heart disease morbidity and mortality in patients with type 2 diabetes mellitus (DM). Increased risk of myopathy and rhabdomyolysis; risk increased with diabetes, renal failure, hypothyroidism, and in elderly. D/C therapy if markedly elevated CPK levels occur or myopathy/myositis is suspected or diagnosed. Increases in serum transaminases, hepatocellular, chronic active and cholestatic hepatitis, and cirrhosis (extremely rare) reported; perform baseline and regular monitoring of LFTs, and d/c therapy if enzyme levels persist >3X the normal limit. Elevations in SrCr reported; monitor renal function in patients with renal impairment or at risk for renal insufficiency. May cause cholelithiasis; d/c if gallstones are found. Acute hypersensitivity reactions and pancreatitis reported. Mild to moderate decreases in Hgb, Hct, and WBCs, thrombocytopenia, and agranulocytosis reported; periodically monitor RBC and WBC counts during the first 12 months of therapy. May cause venothromboembolic disease (eg, pulmonary embolism [PE], deep vein thrombosis [DVT]). Severe decreases in HDL levels reported; check HDL levels within the 1st few months after initiation of therapy. If a severely depressed HDL level is detected, withdraw therapy, monitor HDL level until it has returned to baseline, and do not reinitiate therapy. Estrogen therapy, thiazide diuretics, and β-blockers may be associated with massive rises in plasma TG levels; discontinuation of the specific etiologic agent may obviate the need for specific drug therapy of hypertriglyceridemia.

ADVERSE REACTIONS: Abdominal pain, back pain, headache, abnormal LFTs, respiratory disorder, increased AST/ALT/CPK.

INTERACTIONS: May potentiate coumarin anticoagulant effects; use with caution, reduce anticoagulant dose, and monitor PT/INR frequently. Increased risk of rhabdomyolysis with HMG-CoA reductase inhibitors (statins); avoid combination unless benefits outweigh risks. Bile acid-binding resins may bind other drugs given concurrently; take at least 1 hr before or 4-6 hrs after the bile acid-binding resin. Immunosuppressants (eg, cyclosporine, tacrolimus) may produce nephrotoxicity; consider benefits and risks of use with immunosuppressants and other potentially nephrotoxic agents, and use lowest effective dose. Cases of myopathy, including rhabdomyolysis, reported when coadministered with colchicine; caution when prescribing with colchicine.

PREGNANCY: Category C, not for use in nursing.

MECHANISM OF ACTION: Fibric acid derivative; activates peroxisome proliferator activated receptor α. Increases lipolysis and elimination of TG-rich particles from plasma by activating lipoprotein lipase and reducing production of apoprotein C-III (lipoprotein lipase activity inhibitor). Also, induces an increase in the synthesis of apoproteins A-I, A-II and HDL.

PHARMACOKINETICS: Absorption: Well-absorbed. T_{max}=2-6 hrs (90mg dose). **Distribution:** Plasma protein binding (99%). **Metabolism:** Rapid via ester hydrolysis to fenofibric acid (active metabolite); conjugation with glucuronic acid. **Elimination:** Urine (60%, primarily fenofibric acid and glucuronate conjugate), feces (25%); $T_{1/2}$=23 hrs.

NURSING CONSIDERATIONS

Assessment: Assess for hypersensitivity to the drug, renal impairment, active liver disease, preexisting gallbladder disease, other medical conditions (eg, DM, hypothyroidism), pregnancy/ nursing status, and for possible drug interactions. Obtain baseline LFTs.

Monitoring: Monitor for cholelithiasis, pancreatitis, hypersensitivity reactions, PE, and DVT. Monitor renal function, LFTs, CBC, and lipid levels. Monitor for signs/symptoms of myositis, myopathy, or rhabdomyolysis; measure CPK levels in patients reporting such symptoms. Monitor PT/ INR frequently with coumarin anticoagulants.

Patient Counseling: Advise of potential risks and benefits of therapy and medications to avoid during treatment. Instruct to continue to follow appropriate lipid-modifying diet during therapy and to take drug ud. Instruct to inform physician of all medications, supplements, and herbal preparations being taken; any changes in medical condition; development of muscle pain, tenderness, or weakness; onset of abdominal pain; or any other new symptoms. Advise to return to the physician's office for routine monitoring.

Administration: Oral route. May be taken without regard to meals. Swallow cap whole; do not open, crush, dissolve, or chew. **Storage:** 25°C (77°F); excursions permitted to 15-30°C (59-86°F).

ANZEMET   RX
dolasetron mesylate (Sanofi-Aventis)

THERAPEUTIC CLASS: 5-HT$_3$ receptor antagonist

INDICATIONS: (Inj) Prevention and treatment of postoperative nausea and/or vomiting (PONV) in patients ≥2 yrs of age. (Tab) Prevention of N/V associated with moderately emetogenic cancer chemotherapy, including initial and repeat courses in patients ≥2 yrs of age.

DOSAGE: *Adults:* (Inj) Prevention/Treatment of PONV: 12.5mg IV as a single dose 15 min before cessation of anesthesia (prevention) or as soon as N/V presents (treatment). (Tab) Usual: 100mg within 1 hr before chemotherapy.
Pediatrics: 2-16 Yrs: (Inj) Prevention/Treatment of PONV: 0.35mg/kg IV as a single dose 15 min before cessation of anesthesia or as soon as N/V presents. Max: 12.5mg. May mix inj sol into apple or apple-grape juice for PO dosing of 1.2mg/kg up to a max 100mg dose, given within 2 hrs before surgery. (Tab) Usual: 1.8mg/kg within 1 hr before chemotherapy. Max: 100mg.

HOW SUPPLIED: Inj: 20mg/mL [0.625mL, 5mL, 25mL]; Tab: 50mg, 100mg

CONTRAINDICATIONS: (Inj) Prevention of N/V associated with initial and repeat courses of emetogenic cancer chemotherapy in adults and pediatric patients due to dose dependent QT prolongation.

WARNINGS/PRECAUTIONS: May prolong QT interval; avoid with congenital long QT syndrome. Correct hypokalemia and hypomagnesemia before administration and monitor these electrolytes after administration. Monitor ECG in patients with congestive heart failure (CHF), bradycardia, renal impairment, and in elderly. May cause PR and QRS interval prolongation, 2nd- or 3rd-degree atrioventricular block, cardiac arrest and serious ventricular arrhythmias; use with caution and with ECG monitoring in patients with underlying structural heart disease, preexisting conduction system abnormalities, sick sinus syndrome, atrial fibrillation with slow ventricular response, or myocardial ischemia. Avoid in patients with or at risk for complete heart block, unless implanted pacemaker is present. Caution in elderly. (Inj) When prophylaxis has failed, a repeat dose should not be initiated as rescue therapy.

ADVERSE REACTIONS: Headache, dizziness, pain, tachycardia, bradycardia, hypotension, dyspepsia. (Inj) Drowsiness, urinary retention. (Tab) Pruritus, fatigue, diarrhea, fever.

INTERACTIONS: Caution with QT, PR (eg, verapamil), and QRS (eg, flecainide, quinidine) interval prolonging drugs, diuretics with potential for inducing electrolyte abnormalities, antiarrhythmics, cumulative high-dose anthracycline therapy, and drugs that cause hypokalemia or hypomagnesemia. (Inj) Atenolol may decrease clearance. (PO) Cimetidine may increase levels. Rifampin may decrease levels.

PREGNANCY: Category B, caution in nursing.

MECHANISM OF ACTION: 5-HT$_3$ receptor antagonist; antiemetic and antinauseant.

PHARMACOKINETICS: Absorption: (Inj) T_{max}=0.6 hr (hydrodolasetron). (Tab) Well-absorbed. Absolute bioavailability (75%); T_{max}=1 hr (hydrodolasetron). **Distribution:** V_d=5.8L/kg (hydrodolasetron); plasma protein binding (69-77% hydrodolasetron). **Metabolism:** Complete. Reduction via carbonyl reductase to hydrodolasetron (active, major metabolite); CYP2D6 (hydroxylation of hydrodolasetron); CYP3A and flavin monooxygenase (N-oxidation of hydrodolasetron). **Elimination:** (Inj) Urine (53%, unchanged hydrodolasetron), feces; $T_{1/2}$=<10 min, 7.3 hrs (hydrodolasetron). (Tab) Urine (61%, unchanged hydrodolasetron), feces; $T_{1/2}$=8.1 hrs (hydrodolasetron). Refer to PI for hydrodolasetron pharmacokinetic values in special and targeted patient populations.

NURSING CONSIDERATIONS

Assessment: Assess for presence or possibility of cardiac conduction interval prolongation, renal impairment, pregnancy/nursing status, possible drug interactions and other conditions where treatment is cautioned or contraindicated.

Monitoring: Monitor ECG, especially in patients with CHF, bradycardia, renal impairment, or those at risk for cardiac conduction interval prolongation. Monitor serum electrolytes (K^+, Mg^{2+}).

Patient Counseling: Inform that drug may cause serious cardiac complications; instruct to contact physician immediately if perceiving change in HR, experiencing lightheadedness or a syncopal episode.

Administration: IV/Oral route. (Inj) Infuse as rapidly as 30 sec, or dilute in a compatible IV sol to 50mL and infuse over a period of up to 15 min. Do not mix with other drugs. Flush the infusion line before and after administration. **Storage:** (Inj) 20-25°C (68-77°F); excursions permitted to 15-30°C (59-86°F). Protect from light. Diluted IV Sol: Room temperature for 24 hrs or under refrigeration for 48 hrs. Diluted Sol with Apple or Apple-grape Juice: Room temperature for up to 2 hrs before use. (Tab) 20-25°C (68-77°F). Protect from light.

APIDRA   RX
insulin glulisine, rdna origin (Sanofi-Aventis)

OTHER BRAND NAMES: Apidra Solostar (Sanofi-Aventis)

THERAPEUTIC CLASS: Insulin

INDICATIONS: To improve glycemic control in adults and children with diabetes mellitus.

DOSAGE: *Adults:* Individualize dose. Total Daily Insulin Requirement: Usual: 0.5-1 U/kg/day. (SQ) Give within 15 min ac or within 20 min after starting a meal. Use with an intermediate or long-acting insulin. Continuous SQ Insulin Infusion (CSII) by External Pump: Based on the total daily insulin dose of the previous regimen. (IV) Use at concentrations from 0.05-1 U/mL in infusion systems using polyvinyl chloride bags. Hepatic/Renal Impairment: May require dose reduction. *Pediatrics:* ≥4 Yrs: Individualize dose. Total Daily Insulin Requirement: Usual: 0.5-1 U/kg/day. (SQ) Give within 15 min ac or within 20 min after starting a meal. Use with an intermediate or long-acting insulin. CSII by External Pump: Based on the total daily insulin dose of the previous regimen. Hepatic/Renal Impairment: May require dose reduction.

HOW SUPPLIED: Inj: 100 U/mL [3mL, SoloStar; 10mL, vial]

CONTRAINDICATIONS: During episodes of hypoglycemia.

WARNINGS/PRECAUTIONS: Any change in insulin regimen should be made cautiously and only under medical supervision. Changes in insulin strength, manufacturer, type, or method of administration may result in the need for a change in dosage or adjustment in concomitant oral antidiabetic treatment. Insulin requirements may be altered during stress, major illness, or with changes in exercise, meal patterns, or coadministered drugs. Hypoglycemia may occur and may impair ability to concentrate and react; caution in patients with hypoglycemia unawareness and in patients predisposed to hypoglycemia. Severe, life-threatening, generalized allergy, including anaphylaxis, may occur. Hypokalemia may occur; caution in patients who may be at risk. May be administered IV under medical supervision with close monitoring of blood glucose and serum K^+ to avoid potentially fatal hypoglycemia and hypokalemia. Frequent glucose monitoring and dose reduction may be required in patients with renal/hepatic impairment. Do not mix with insulin preparations other than NPH insulin for SQ inj, or with other insulins for IV administration or for use in a SQ continuous infusion pump. Malfunction of insulin pump or infusion set, handling errors, or insulin degradation can rapidly lead to hyperglycemia, ketosis, and diabetic ketoacidosis; prompt identification/correction of the cause is necessary and interim SQ inj may be required. Train patients using CSII pump therapy how to administer by inj and to have alternate insulin therapy available in case of pump failure. Caution in elderly patients.

ADVERSE REACTIONS: Allergic reactions, infusion-site reactions, hypoglycemia, influenza, nasopharyngitis, upper respiratory tract infection, arthralgia, HTN, headache, peripheral edema.

INTERACTIONS: Dose adjustment and close monitoring may be necessary with drugs that may increase blood-glucose-lowering effect and susceptibility to hypoglycemia (eg, oral antidiabetic products, pramlintide, ACE inhibitors, disopyramide, fibrates, fluoxetine, MAOIs, propoxyphene, pentoxifylline, salicylates, somatostatin analogs, sulfonamide antibiotics), drugs that may reduce blood-glucose-lowering effect (eg, corticosteroids, danazol, niacin, diuretics, sympathomimetics [eg, epinephrine, albuterol, terbutaline], glucagon, isoniazid, phenothiazine derivatives, somatropin, thyroid hormones, estrogens, progestogens [eg, in oral contraceptives], protease inhibitors, atypical antipsychotics), or drugs that may either increase or decrease blood-glucose-lowering effect (eg, β-blockers, clonidine, lithium salts, alcohol). Pentamidine may cause hypoglycemia, sometimes followed by hyperglycemia. Hypoglycemic signs may be reduced or absent with antiadrenergic drugs (eg, β-blockers, clonidine, guanethidine, reserpine). Caution with K⁺-lowering drugs and drugs sensitive to serum K⁺ levels.

PREGNANCY: Category C, caution in nursing.

MECHANISM OF ACTION: Insulin glulisine (rDNA origin); regulates glucose metabolism. Lowers blood glucose by stimulating peripheral glucose uptake by skeletal muscle and fat, and by inhibiting hepatic glucose production. Also inhibits lipolysis and proteolysis, and enhances protein synthesis.

PHARMACOKINETICS: Absorption: (SQ) Absolute bioavailability (70%); C_{max}=83μU/mL (0.15 U/kg), 84μU/mL (median) (0.2 U/kg); T_{max}=60 min (median) (0.15 U/kg), 100 min (median) (0.2 U/kg). **Distribution:** (IV) V_d=13L. **Elimination:** (SQ) $T_{1/2}$=42 min, (IV) $T_{1/2}$=13 min.

NURSING CONSIDERATIONS

Assessment: Assess for predisposition to hypoglycemia, risk of hypokalemia, hypersensitivity to drug or to any of its excipients, renal/hepatic impairment, pregnancy/nursing status, and possible drug interactions. Obtain baseline blood glucose and HbA1c levels.

Monitoring: Monitor for signs/symptoms of hypoglycemia, hypokalemia, allergic reactions, and other adverse reactions. Monitor blood glucose, HbA1c levels, and renal/hepatic function. Monitor glucose and K⁺ levels frequently during IV administration.

Patient Counseling: Counsel on self-management procedures including glucose monitoring, proper inj technique, and management of hypoglycemia and hyperglycemia. Instruct on handling of special situations, such as intercurrent conditions, inadequate or skipped dose, inadvertent administration of increased dose, inadequate food intake, and skipped meals. Advise to inform physician if pregnant or are contemplating pregnancy. Instruct to always check the label before each inj to avoid medication errors. Instruct on how to use an external infusion pump.

Administration: SQ/IV route. Inject SQ in the abdominal wall, thigh, or upper arm, or give by continuous SQ infusion in the abdominal wall by an external insulin pump; rotate inj sites within the same region. Do not mix with insulin preparations other than NPH insulin for SQ inj; if mixed with NPH insulin, draw Apidra into syringe 1st, and inject mixture immediately after mixing. Do not use diluted or mixed insulins in external insulin pumps. Do not administer insulin mixtures intravenously. Refer to PI for further instructions on preparation, handling, and administration. **Storage:** Unopened: 2-8°C (36-46°F). Do not freeze; discard if frozen. Protect from light. Must be used within 28 days if not stored in a refrigerator. Open (In-Use): <25°C (77°F). Discard after 28 days. Protect from direct heat and light. Do not refrigerate opened (in-use) SoloStar. Discard infusion sets and insulin in reservoir after 48 hrs of use or after exposure to temperatures >37°C (98.6°F). Prepared Infusion Bags: Room temperature for 48 hrs.

APLENZIN   RX
bupropion hydrobromide (Sanofi-Aventis)

> Antidepressants increased the risk of suicidal thinking and behavior (suicidality) in short-term studies in children, adolescents, and young adults with major depressive disorder (MDD) and other psychiatric disorders. Monitor and observe closely for clinical worsening, suicidality, or unusual changes in behavior. Advise families and caregivers of the need for close observation and communication with the prescriber. Not approved for smoking cessation; serious neuropsychiatric reactions have occurred in patients taking bupropion for smoking cessation. Instruct patient to contact a healthcare provider if such reactions occur.

THERAPEUTIC CLASS: Aminoketone

INDICATIONS: Treatment of MDD and prevention of seasonal major depressive episodes in patients with seasonal affective disorder (SAD).

DOSAGE: *Adults:* MDD: Initial: 174mg qam. Titrate: After 4 days of dosing, may increase to 348mg qam. Maint: Reassess periodically to determine the need for maintenance treatment and the appropriate dose. SAD: Initial: 174mg qam. Titrate: After 7 days of dosing, may increase to 348mg qam. Prevention of Seasonal MDD Episodes Associated with SAD: Initiate treatment in autumn prior to onset of depressive symptoms and continue through the winter season. Taper and d/c in early spring. Patients Treated with 348mg/day: Decrease dose to 150mg qd before discontinuation. Individualize timing of initiation and duration of treatment based on patient's historical pattern of seasonal MDD episodes. To D/C Treatment: From 348mg qd, decrease dose to 174mg qd prior to discontinuation. Severe Hepatic Impairment: Max: 174mg qod. Refer to PI for equivalent daily doses of bupropion HBr and bupropion HCl.

APLENZIN

HOW SUPPLIED: Tab, Extended-Release: 174mg, 348mg, 522mg

CONTRAINDICATIONS: Seizure disorder or conditions that increase the risk of seizure (eg, arteriovenous malformation, severe head injury, CNS tumor or CNS infection, severe stroke, anorexia nervosa or bulimia, or abrupt discontinuation of alcohol, benzodiazepines, barbiturates, and antiepileptic drugs), and concurrent use of MAOIs or within 14 days of use.

WARNINGS/PRECAUTIONS: Dose-related risk of seizures; do not exceed 522mg qd. D/C and do not restart treatment if seizure occurs. May precipitate manic, mixed, or hypomanic manic episode. Screen for bipolar disorder; not approved for use in treating bipolar depression. Neuropsychiatric signs and symptoms (eg, delusions, hallucinations, psychosis, concentration disturbance, paranoia, confusion) reported; d/c if these reactions occur. HTN reported; assess BP before initiating and monitor periodically during treatment. D/C treatment and consult healthcare provider if anaphylactoid/anaphylactic reactions occur (eg, skin rash, pruritus, hives, chest pain, edema, SOB). Arthralgia, myalgia, fever with rash, and other symptoms of serum sickness suggestive of delayed hypersensitivity reported. Caution with recent myocardial infarction, unstable heart disease, renal/hepatic impairment, and in elderly. False-positive urine immunoassay screening tests for amphetamines reported.

ADVERSE REACTIONS: Dry mouth, sweating, headache/migraine, insomnia, anxiety, agitation, weight loss, N/V, constipation, dizziness, pharyngitis, tinnitus, rash.

INTERACTIONS: See Contraindications. Primarily metabolized by CYP2B6. Dose adjustments may be necessary when coadministered with CYP2B6 inducers/inhibitors. Decreased levels with CYP2B6 inducers (eg, ritonavir, lopinavir, and efavirenz) and other CYP inducers (eg, carbamazepine, phenobarbital, phenytoin). Increased levels with CYP2B6 inhibitors (eg, ticlopidine, clopidogrel, prasugrel), paroxetine, sertraline, norfluoxetine, fluvoxamine, and nelfinavir. Inhibits CYP2D6; increases exposures of drugs that are metabolized by CYP2D6 (eg, certain antidepressants, antipsychotics, β-blockers, and type 1C antiarrhythmics). May reduce efficacy of drugs that require metabolic activation by CYP2D6 to be effective (eg, tamoxifen). Extreme caution with drugs that lower seizure threshold (eg, other bupropion products, antipsychotics, antidepressants, theophylline, or systemic corticosteroids); use low initial dose and increase gradually. CNS toxicity has been reported when coadministered with levodopa or amantadine; use with caution. Cimetidine may increase levels of some active metabolites. Increased citalopram levels. Increased seizure risk with sedatives/hypnotics or opiates; cocaine, or stimulant addiction; abuse or misuse of prescription drugs such as CNS stimulants, oral hypoglycemic drugs, or insulin. Altered PT and/or INR with warfarin.

PREGNANCY: Category C, caution in nursing.

MECHANISM OF ACTION: Aminoketone antidepressant; has not been established. Weak inhibitor of the neuronal uptake of norepinephrine and dopamine. Presumed that action is mediated by noradrenergic and/or dopaminergic mechanisms.

PHARMACOKINETICS: Absorption: (348mg) C_{max}=134.3ng/mL; AUC=1409ng•hr/mL; T_{max}=5 hrs, 6 hrs (hydroxybupropion). **Distribution:** Plasma protein binding (84%); found in breast milk. **Metabolism:** Extensive; via hydroxylation (CYP2B6) and reduction of carbonyl group; hydroxybupropion, threohydrobupropion, and erythrohydrobupropion (active metabolites). **Elimination:** Urine (87%), feces (10%), (0.5% unchanged). $T_{1/2}$= 21.3hrs, 24.3 hrs (hydroxybupropion), 31.1 hrs (erythrohydrobupropion), 50.8 hrs (threohydrobupropion).

NURSING CONSIDERATIONS

Assessment: Assess for seizure disorders or conditions that may increase risk of seizure, hypersensitivity, BP, bipolar disorder, hepatic/renal function, pregnancy/nursing status, possible drug interactions, or any other conditions where treatment is contraindicated or cautioned.

Monitoring: Monitor for clinical worsening, suicidality, or unusual changes in behavior, seizures, increased restlessness, agitation, anxiety, insomnia, neuropsychiatric signs/symptoms, changes in weight or appetite, anaphylactoid/anaphylactic reactions, delayed hypersensitivity reactions, HTN, and other adverse reactions.

Patient Counseling: Inform about benefits/risks of therapy. Advise patients and caregivers of need for close observation for clinical worsening and suicidal risks. Educate patients of the symptoms of hypersensitivity and to d/c if severe allergic reaction occurs. Instruct to d/c and not restart if seizure occurs while on therapy. Inform that excessive use or abrupt discontinuation of alcohol or sedatives may alter seizure threshold; advise to minimize or avoid alcohol use. Inform that therapy may impair mental/physical abilities; advise to use caution while operating hazardous machinery/driving. Instruct to notify physician if taking/planning to take any prescription or OTC medications. Advise to contact physician if pregnancy occurs or is planned during therapy. Inform that it is normal to notice something that looks like a tab in the stool.

Administration: Oral route. Swallow whole; do not chew, divide, or crush. Take with or without food. **Storage:** 25°C (77°F); excursions permitted to 15-30°C (59-86°F).

APOKYN
apomorphine HCl (Ipsen/Tercica)

RX

THERAPEUTIC CLASS: Non-ergoline dopamine agonist

INDICATIONS: Acute, intermittent treatment of hypomobility, "off" episodes ("end-of-dose wearing off" and unpredictable "on/off" episodes) associated with advanced Parkinson's disease.

DOSAGE: *Adults:* Start trimethobenzamide (300mg tid PO) 3 days prior to the initial dose and continue at least during the first 2 months of therapy. Test Dose: 0.2mL (2mg) SQ to patients in an "off" state. Closely monitor BP; do not treat if clinically significant orthostatic hypotension occurs. Initial: 0.2mL (2mg) PRN if test dose is tolerated. Titrate: Increase in increments of 0.1mL (1mg) every few days, if needed, on an outpatient basis. 0.2mL (2mg) Test Dose Tolerated But No Response: Test Dose: 0.4mL (4mg) given at next "off" period (no sooner than 2 hrs after the first test dose). Initial: 0.3mL (3mg) PRN if 0.4mL (4mg) test dose is tolerated. Titrate: Increase in increments of 0.1mL (1mg) every few days, if needed, on an outpatient basis. 0.4mL (4mg) Test Dose not Tolerated: Test Dose: 0.3mL (3mg) during a separate "off" period (no sooner than 2 hrs after the prior test dose). Initial: 0.2mL (2mg) PRN if 0.3mL test dose is tolerated. Titrate: Increase to 0.3mL (3mg) after a few days, if needed; assess efficacy/tolerability; do not increase to 0.4mL on an outpatient basis. Do not give second dose for an "off" period if the first was ineffective. Usual: 0.3-0.6mL (3-6mg) tid. Max: 0.6mL (6mg)/dose. If therapy is interrupted (>1 week), restart at 0.2mL (2mg) and gradually titrate. Renal Impairment: Test Dose/Initial: 0.1mL (1mg) SQ.

HOW SUPPLIED: Inj: 10mg/mL [3mL]

CONTRAINDICATIONS: Concomitant use with $5HT_3$ antagonists (eg, ondansetron, granisetron, dolasetron, palonosetron, alosetron).

WARNINGS/PRECAUTIONS: Avoid IV administration; serious adverse events reported. N/V, syncope, orthostatic hypotension, falling, and inj-site reactions reported. May prolong the QT interval and potential for proarrhythmic effects; caution with hypokalemia, hypomagnesemia, bradycardia, or genetic predisposition (eg, congenital prolongation of the QT interval). Hallucinations/psychotic-like behavior reported; avoid with major psychotic disorder. Falling asleep during activities of daily living may occur; d/c if daytime sleepiness or episodes of falling asleep develop. May impair mental/physical abilities. Coronary events (eg, angina, myocardial infarction [MI], cardiac arrest, sudden death) reported; caution with known cardiovascular (CV)/cerebrovascular disease. Contains sodium metabisulfite; caution with sulfite sensitivity. Potential for abuse. May cause or worsen dyskinesias. Monitor for withdrawal-emergent hyperpyrexia and confusion, fibrotic complications (eg, retroperitoneal fibrosis, pulmonary infiltrates, pleural effusion/thickening, cardiac valvulopathy) and melanoma. May cause priapism. Caution with hepatic/renal impairment.

ADVERSE REACTIONS: Yawning, dyskinesia, N/V, somnolence, dizziness, rhinorrhea, hallucinations, edema, chest pain, increased sweating, flushing, pallor, postural hypotension, angina.

INTERACTIONS: See Contraindications. Antihypertensives and vasodilators may increase risk of hypotension, MI, serious pneumonia, falls, bone and joint injuries. Dopamine antagonists, such as neuroleptics (eg, phenothiazines, butyrophenones, thioxanthenes) and metoclopramide, may diminish effectiveness. Caution with drugs that prolong QT/QTc interval. May increase drowsiness with sedating medications. Avoid with alcohol. May significantly reduce levodopa concentration threshold necessary for improved motor response.

PREGNANCY: Category C, not for use in nursing.

MECHANISM OF ACTION: Non-ergoline dopamine agonist; not established, suspected to stimulate postsynaptic dopamine D_2-type receptors within the caudate-putamen in the brain.

PHARMACOKINETICS: Absorption: Rapid; T_{max}=10-60 min. **Distribution:** V_d=218L. **Metabolism:** Sulfation, N-demethylation, glucuronidation, and oxidation. **Elimination:** $T_{1/2}$=40 min.

NURSING CONSIDERATIONS

Assessment: Assess for hypersensitivity to the drug, sulfite sensitivity, asthma, risk for QT prolongation, history of psychotic disorders, CV/cerebrovascular disease, dyskinesia, hepatic/renal dysfunction, pregnancy/nursing status, and possible drug interactions. Obtain baseline BP (supine and standing).

Monitoring: Monitor for N/V, syncope, QT/QTc interval prolongation and other proarrhythmic effects, hypotension, hallucinations/psychotic-like behavior, coronary/cerebral ischemia, dyskinesia (or exacerbation), hepatic/renal impairment, withdrawal-emergent hyperpyrexia and confusion, fibrotic complications, priapism, drug abuse, and other adverse reactions. Perform periodic skin exams to monitor for melanomas. Monitor BP closely.

Patient Counseling: Inform that medication is intended only for SQ and not IV use. Instruct to take as prescribed. Instruct to rotate the inj site and observe proper aseptic technique. Inform of the potential for hallucination, psychotic-like behavior, hypotension, sedating effects including somnolence, and the possibility of falling asleep. Caution against rising rapidly after sitting or lying down, especially if patient has been sitting or lying for prolonged periods, and during initiation of treatment. Advise not to drive a car or engage in any other potentially dangerous activities while on treatment. Instruct to notify physician if pregnancy occurs, or if intending to become pregnant and/or breastfeed. Advise to avoid alcohol. Advise to inform physician if new or increased gambling urges, increased sexual urges, or other intense urges develop while on treatment.

Administration: SQ route. **Storage:** 25°C (77°F); excursions permitted to 15-30°C (59-86°F).

APRISO

mesalamine (Salix)

RX

THERAPEUTIC CLASS: 5-aminosalicylic acid derivative

INDICATIONS: Maintenance of remission of ulcerative colitis in patients ≥18 yrs of age.

DOSAGE: *Adults:* 1.5g (4 caps) PO qam.

HOW SUPPLIED: Cap, Extended Release: 0.375g

WARNINGS/PRECAUTIONS: Renal impairment, including minimal change nephropathy, acute and chronic interstitial nephritis, and, rarely, renal failure reported; caution with renal dysfunction or history of renal disease. Evaluate renal function prior to therapy and periodically thereafter. May cause acute intolerance syndrome (eg, acute abdominal pain, cramping, bloody diarrhea); d/c if suspected. Hepatic failure reported in patients with preexisting liver disease; caution with liver disease. Caution with sulfasalazine hypersensitivity and in elderly.

ADVERSE REACTIONS: Headache, diarrhea, upper abdominal pain, nausea, nasopharyngitis, influenza/influenza-like illness, sinusitis.

INTERACTIONS: Avoid with antacids.

PREGNANCY: Category B, caution in nursing.

MECHANISM OF ACTION: 5-aminosalicylic acid derivative; has not been established. Suspected to diminish inflammation by blocking production of arachidonic acid metabolites.

PHARMACOKINETICS: Absorption: (Single dose) T_{max}=4 hrs, C_{max}=2.1mcg/mL, AUC_{0-24}=11mcg•h/mL, AUC_{0-inf}=14mcg•h/mL. Refer to PI for parameters using multiple doses and of major metabolite. **Distribution:** Plasma protein binding (43%); crosses placenta; found in breast milk. **Metabolism:** Liver and intestinal mucosa; N-acetyl-5-aminosalicylic acid (major metabolite). **Elimination:** Urine (2% unchanged; 30% N-acetyl-5-aminosalicylic acid); $T_{1/2}$=9-10 hrs.

NURSING CONSIDERATIONS

Assessment: Assess for previous hypersensitivity to sulfasalazine or salicylates, history of or known renal/hepatic dysfunction, phenylketonuria, pregnancy/nursing status, and possible drug interactions. Evaluate renal function prior to initiation of therapy.

Monitoring: Monitor for renal impairment, hepatic failure, acute intolerance syndrome, and hypersensitivity reactions. Perform periodic monitoring of renal function and blood cell counts (in elderly).

Patient Counseling: Inform patients with phenylketonuria that each cap contains aspartame. Instruct not to take with antacids. Instruct to contact a healthcare provider if symptoms of ulcerative colitis worsen.

Administration: Oral route. **Storage:** 20-25°C (68-77°F); excursions permitted between 15-30°C (59-86°F).

APTIOM

eslicarbazepine acetate (Sunovion)

RX

THERAPEUTIC CLASS: Dibenzazepine

INDICATIONS: Adjunctive treatment of partial-onset seizures.

DOSAGE: *Adults:* Initial: 400mg qd. Titrate: Increase to 800mg qd after 1 week. Maint: 800mg qd. Max Maint: 1200mg qd. Initiate max dose only after patient has tolerated 800mg/day for at least a week. May initiate at 800mg qd for some patients if the need for additional seizure reduction outweighs an increased risk of adverse reactions during initiation. Dose Modifications with Other Antiepileptic Drugs (AEDs): Concomitant Use with Carbamazepine: May need to adjust dose of both drugs based on efficacy and tolerability. Concomitant Use with Other Enzyme-Inducing AEDs (eg, phenobarbital, phenytoin, primidone): May need higher doses of eslicarbazepine. Moderate and Severe Renal Impairment (CrCl <50mL/min): Initial: 200mg qd. Titrate: Increase to 400mg qd after 2 weeks. Max Maint: 600mg qd. Discontinuation of Therapy: Reduce dose gradually and avoid abrupt discontinuation.

HOW SUPPLIED: Tab: 200mg*, 400mg, 600mg*, 800mg* *scored

WARNINGS/PRECAUTIONS: Increased risk of suicidal thoughts or behavior; monitor for emergence/worsening of depression, suicidal thoughts or behavior, and/or any unusual changes in mood or behavior. Serious dermatological reactions (eg, Stevens-Johnson syndrome) reported; d/c use if dermatologic reaction develops, unless the reaction is not drug-related. Drug reaction with eosinophilia and systemic symptoms (DRESS), also known as multiorgan hypersensitivity, reported; evaluate immediately if signs/symptoms of hypersensitivity (eg, fever, lymphadenopathy) are present and d/c if alternative etiology cannot be established. Anaphylaxis and angioedema reported; d/c if any of these reactions develop. Avoid in patients with prior DRESS reaction or anaphylactic-type reaction with either the drug or oxcarbazepine. Consider measuring serum Na$^+$ and Cl$^-$ levels during maintenance treatment; clinically significant hyponatremia with concurrent hypochloremia may develop requiring dose reduction/discontinuation. Associated with dose-related increases in adverse reactions related to dizziness and disturbance in gait and coordination, somnolence and fatigue, cognitive dysfunction, and visual changes. May impair mental/physical abilities. Withdraw gradually due to risk of increased seizure frequency and status epilepticus. Hepatic effects reported; d/c in patients with jaundice or other evidence of significant liver injury. Dose-dependent decreases in serum T3 and T4 (free and total) observed. Not recommended with severe hepatic impairment. Caution in elderly.

ADVERSE REACTIONS: Dizziness, somnolence, N/V, headache, diplopia, fatigue, vertigo, ataxia, blurred vision, tremor, diarrhea.

INTERACTIONS: See Dosage. Greater incidence of dizziness reported with the concomitant use of carbamazepine. Do not use as an adjunctive therapy with oxcarbazepine. Several AEDs (eg, carbamazepine, phenobarbital, phenytoin, primidone) can induce enzymes that metabolize eslicarbazepine and can cause decreased plasma concentrations. May increase levels of CYP2C19 substrates (eg, phenytoin, clobazam, omeprazole). Monitor plasma phenytoin concentration; in epilepsy, dose adjustment may be needed based on clinical response and serum levels of phenytoin. May decrease levels of CYP3A4 substrates (eg, simvastatin). Adjust dose of simvastatin or rosuvastatin if a clinically significant change in lipids is noted. May decrease levels of oral contraceptives (eg, ethinyl estradiol, levonorgestrel); use additional or alternative nonhormonal birth control. Monitor to maintain INR in patients on warfarin.

PREGNANCY: Category C, not for use in nursing.

MECHANISM OF ACTION: Dibenzazepine; has not been established. Thought to involve inhibition of voltage-gated Na$^+$ channels.

PHARMACOKINETICS: Absorption: T_{max}=1-4 hrs (post-dose). **Distribution:** Found in breast milk. V_d=61L; plasma protein binding (<40%). **Metabolism:** Rapid and extensive by hydrolytic 1st pass metabolism to eslicarbazepine (major active metabolite); (R)-licarbazepine and oxcarbazepine (minor active metabolites). **Elimination:** Urine (90% metabolites; 2/3 unchanged, 1/3 glucuronide conjugate, and 10% minor metabolites); $T_{1/2}$=13-20 hrs.

NURSING CONSIDERATIONS

Assessment: Assess for history of hypersensitivity to the drug or oxcarbazepine, renal/hepatic impairment, pregnancy/nursing status, and possible drug interactions.

Monitoring: Monitor for suicidal thoughts or behavior, any unusual changes in mood or behavior, dermatologic reactions, multiorgan hypersensitivity reaction, hyponatremia, anaphylaxis, angioedema, dizziness, disturbance in gait and coordination, somnolence, fatigue, cognitive dysfunction, visual changes, and other adverse reactions. Monitor Na$^+$ and Cl$^-$ levels. Monitor to maintain INR in patients on warfarin.

Patient Counseling: Inform of the availability of a Medication Guide and instruct to read the Medication Guide prior to treatment. Instruct to take ud. Advise of the need to be alert for the emergence/worsening of symptoms of depression, any unusual changes in mood/behavior, or the emergence of suicidal thoughts, behavior, or thoughts about self-harm; instruct to immediately report behaviors of concern to physician. Educate about signs/symptoms of a skin reaction; instruct to consult physician immediately if a skin reaction occurs. Inform that a fever associated with signs of other organ system involvement may be drug-related; instruct to contact physician immediately if such signs/symptoms occur. Instruct to d/c and contact physician immediately if signs/symptoms suggesting angioedema develop. Advise to report symptoms of low Na$^+$ to physician. Inform that drug may cause dizziness, gait disturbance, somnolence/fatigue, cognitive function, and visual changes; advise not to drive or operate machinery until effects have been determined. Instruct not to d/c use without consulting physician. Recommend female patients of childbearing age to use additional nonhormonal forms of contraception during treatment and after treatment has been discontinued for at least 1 menstrual cycle or until otherwise instructed by physician. Encourage to enroll in the North American Antiepileptic Drug Pregnancy Registry if patient becomes pregnant.

Administration: Oral route. Administer as whole or as crushed tabs. Take with or without food.
Storage: 20-25°C (68-77°F); excursions permitted to 15-30°C (59-86°F).

APTIVUS   RX
tipranavir (Boehringer Ingelheim)

> Both fatal and nonfatal intracranial hemorrhage reported. Clinical hepatitis and hepatic decompensation, including some fatalities, reported. Extra vigilance needed in patients with chronic hepatitis B or hepatitis C coinfection due to increased risk of hepatotoxicity.

THERAPEUTIC CLASS: Protease inhibitor

INDICATIONS: Coadministered with ritonavir for combination antiretroviral treatment of HIV-1 infected patients who are treatment-experienced and infected with HIV-1 strains resistant to >1 protease inhibitor.

DOSAGE: *Adults:* 500mg with 200mg ritonavir bid.
Pediatrics: 2-18 Yrs: 14mg/kg with 6mg/kg ritonavir (or 375mg/m^2 with ritonavir 150mg/m^2) bid. Max: 500mg with 200mg ritonavir bid. Intolerance/Toxicity: Decrease dose to 12mg/kg with 5mg/kg ritonavir (or 290mg/m^2 with ritonavir 115mg/m^2) bid. May switch to PO sol if unable to swallow caps.

HOW SUPPLIED: Cap: 250mg; Sol: 100mg/mL [95mL]

CONTRAINDICATIONS: Moderate or severe (Child-Pugh Class B or C) hepatic impairment. Coadministration with drugs that are highly dependent on CYP3A for clearance or are potent CYP3A inducers (eg, amiodarone, bepridil, flecainide, propafenone, quinidine, rifampin, dihydroergotamine, ergonovine, ergotamine, methylergonovine, cisapride, St. John's wort, lovastatin, simvastatin, pimozide, oral midazolam, triazolam, alfuzosin, and sildenafil [for treatment of pulmonary arterial HTN]). Refer to the individual monograph for ritonavir.

WARNINGS/PRECAUTIONS: Not recommended for treatment-naive patients. Caution with elevated transaminases, hepatitis B or C coinfection, with mild hepatic impairment (Child-Pugh Class A), with medications known to increase the risk of bleeding (eg, antiplatelet and anticoagulants) or with supplemental high doses of vitamin E, known sulfonamide allergy, patients at risk of increased bleeding from trauma, surgery, or other medical conditions, and in elderly. D/C if signs and symptoms of clinical hepatitis develop. D/C if asymptomatic elevations in AST or ALT >10X the ULN or if asymptomatic elevations in AST or ALT between 5-10X the ULN and increases in total bilirubin >2.5X the ULN occur. Monitor LFTs prior to and during therapy. New onset diabetes mellitus (DM), exacerbation of preexisting DM, hyperglycemia, and diabetic ketoacidosis reported. Increased bleeding in patients with hemophilia type A and B reported; additional factor VIII may be required. Rash (eg, urticarial/maculopapular, possible photosensitivity) accompanied by joint pain/stiffness, throat tightness, and generalized pruritus reported; d/c with severe skin rash. Increased total cholesterol and TG levels reported; assess lipid levels prior to and during therapy. Possible redistribution/accumulation of body fat. Immune reconstitution syndrome reported; autoimmune disorders (eg, Graves' disease, polymyositis, and Guillain-Barre syndrome) have also been reported in the setting of immune reconstitution. (Sol) Avoid supplemental vitamin E greater than a standard multivitamin as sol contains 116 IU/mL of vitamin E, which is higher than the Reference Daily Intake (adults 30 IU, pediatrics approximately 10 IU). Refer to individual monograph for ritonavir.

ADVERSE REACTIONS: Clinical hepatitis, hepatic decompensation, intracranial hemorrhage, diarrhea, N/V, abdominal pain, pyrexia, fatigue, headache, cough, rash, anemia, weight loss, hypertriglyceridemia, bleeding.

INTERACTIONS: See Contraindications. Not recommended with other protease inhibitors, salmeterol, and fluticasone. Avoid with colchicine in renally/hepatically impaired. Avoid with atorvastatin. May increase levels of SSRIs (eg, fluoxetine, paroxetine, sertraline), atorvastatin, rosuvastatin, trazodone, desipramine, colchicine, bosentan, itraconazole, ketoconazole, clarithromycin, rifabutin, parenteral midazolam, normeperidine, and PDE-5 inhibitors. May decrease levels of abacavir, atazanavir, didanosine, zidovudine, amprenavir, lopinavir, saquinavir, raltegravir, valproic acid, methadone, meperidine, and omeprazole. Increased levels with fluconazole, enfuvirtide, clarithromycin, atorvastatin, and atazanavir. Decreased levels with buprenorphine/naloxone, carbamazepine, phenobarbital, and phenytoin. May alter levels of voriconazole, calcium channel blockers, and immunosuppressants. May decrease levels of ethinyl estradiol by 50%; use alternative methods of nonhormonal contraception. Monitor glucose with hypoglycemic agents. Monitor INR with warfarin. (Cap) May produce disulfiram-like reactions with disulfiram or other drugs that produce the reaction (eg, metronidazole). See Prescribing Information for detailed information.

PREGNANCY: Category C, not for use in nursing.

MECHANISM OF ACTION: Protease inhibitor; inhibits virus-specific processing of viral Gag and Gag-Pol polyproteins in HIV-1 infected cells, thus preventing formation of mature virions.

PHARMACOKINETICS: Absorption: Tipranavir/Ritonavir: (Female) C_{max}=94.8µM, T_{max}=2.9 hrs, AUC_{0-12h}=851µM•h; (Male) C_{max}=77.6µM, T_{max}=3.0 hrs, AUC_{0-12h}=710µM•h. Refer to PI for pediatric parameters by age. **Distribution:** Plasma protein binding (>99.9%). **Metabolism:** Liver via

CYP3A4. **Elimination:** Tipranavir/Ritonavir: Feces (82.3%, 79.9% unchanged), urine (4.4%, 0.5% unchanged); $T_{1/2}$=5.5 hrs (females), 6 hrs (males).

NURSING CONSIDERATIONS

Assessment: Assess for hepatitis B or C infection, hepatic impairment, increased bleeding risk, hemophilia, sulfonamide allergy, DM, pregnancy/nursing status, and possible drug interactions. Assess LFTs and lipid levels. Assess the ability to swallow caps in pediatrics.

Monitoring: Monitor for signs and symptoms of clinical hepatitis, hepatic decompensation, severe skin reaction, DM, intracranial hemorrhage, bleeding, immune reconstitution syndrome, autoimmune disorders, and fat redistribution. Monitor for LFTs and lipid levels periodically during treatment.

Patient Counseling: Inform that therapy is not a cure for HIV-1 infection; may continue to experience illnesses associated with HIV-1 infections (eg, opportunistic infections). Advise to avoid doing things that can spread HIV-1 infection to others. Inform that redistribution/accumulation of body fat may occur. Instruct to notify physician if pregnant, planning to become pregnant, or if breastfeeding. Advise to seek medical attention for symptoms of hepatitis, bleeding, and severe skin reaction. Advise to inform physician about all medications, including prescription or nonprescription medications (eg, St. John's wort) before initiating therapy. Instruct to report any history of sulfonamide allergy. Instruct to avoid vitamin E supplements greater than a standard multivitamin when taking PO sol. Instruct to use additional or alternative contraceptive measures for patients taking estrogen-based hormonal contraceptives. Inform that drug must be taken with ritonavir.

Administration: Oral route. Take with meals with ritonavir tabs; take with/without meals with ritonavir caps/sol. **Storage:** Must be used within 60 days after 1st opening the bottle. (Cap) 2-8°C (36-46°F) prior to opening the bottle. After Opening the Bottle: 25°C (77°F); excursions permitted to 15-30°C (59-86°F). (Sol) 25°C (77°F); excursions permitted to 15-30°C (59-86°F). Do not refrigerate or freeze.

ARANESP   RX
darbepoetin alfa (Amgen)

> Increased risk of death, myocardial infarction (MI), stroke, venous thromboembolism (VTE), thrombosis of vascular access, and tumor progression or recurrence. Use the lowest dose sufficient to reduce/avoid the need for RBC transfusions. Chronic Kidney Disease (CKD): Greater risks for death, serious adverse cardiovascular (CV) reactions, and stroke when administered to target Hgb level of >11g/dL. Cancer: Shortened overall survival and/or increased risk of tumor progression or recurrence in patients with breast, non-small cell lung, head and neck, lymphoid, and cervical cancers. Must enroll in and comply with the ESA APPRISE Oncology Program to prescribe and/or dispense drug to patients. Use only for anemia from myelosuppressive chemotherapy. Not indicated for patients receiving myelosuppressive chemotherapy when anticipated outcome is cure. D/C following completion of chemotherapy course.

THERAPEUTIC CLASS: Erythropoiesis stimulator

INDICATIONS: Treatment of anemia due to CKD, including patients on and not on dialysis. Treatment of anemia in patients with nonmyeloid malignancies where anemia is due to the effect of concomitant myelosuppressive chemotherapy, and upon initiation, there is a minimum of 2 additional months of planned chemotherapy.

DOSAGE: *Adults:* Initiate when Hgb is <10g/dL (see PI for additional parameters). CKD on Dialysis: Initial: 0.45mcg/kg IV/SQ weekly or 0.75mcg/kg IV/SQ once every 2 weeks. IV route is recommended for hemodialysis patients. Titrate: Adjust dose based on Hgb levels; see PI. CKD Not on Dialysis: Initial: 0.45mcg/kg IV/SQ once every 4 weeks. Titrate: Adjust dose based on Hgb levels; see PI. Conversion from Epoetin Alfa with CKD on Dialysis: Administer less frequently than epoetin alfa, and estimate the starting weekly dose based on weekly epoetin alfa dose at the time of substitution; see PI. Maintain the route of administration. Patients on Chemotherapy: Initial: 2.25mcg/kg SQ weekly or 500mcg SQ every 3 weeks until completion of a chemotherapy course. Titrate: Adjust dose based on Hgb levels; see PI.
Pediatrics: >1 Yr: Conversion from Epoetin Alfa with CKD on Dialysis: Administer less frequently than epoetin alfa, and estimate the starting weekly dose based on weekly epoetin alfa dose at the time of substitution; see PI. Maintain the route of administration.

HOW SUPPLIED: Inj: 25mcg/mL, 40mcg/mL, 60mcg/mL, 100mcg/mL, 150mcg/0.75mL, 200mcg/mL, 300mcg/mL [single-dose vial]; 25mcg/0.42mL, 40mcg/0.4mL, 60mcg/0.3mL, 100mcg/0.5mL, 150mcg/0.3mL, 200mcg/0.4mL, 300mcg/0.6mL, 500mcg/mL [single-dose prefilled syringe]

CONTRAINDICATIONS: Uncontrolled HTN, pure red cell aplasia (PRCA) that begins after treatment with darbepoetin alfa or other erythropoietin protein drugs.

WARNINGS/PRECAUTIONS: Not indicated for use in patients with cancer receiving hormonal agents, biologic products, or radiotherapy, unless also receiving concomitant myelosuppressive chemotherapy, or as a substitute for RBC transfusions in patients requiring immediate correction of anemia. Evaluate transferrin saturation and serum ferritin prior to and during treatment; administer supplemental iron when serum ferritin is <100mcg/L or serum transferrin saturation is <20%. Correct/exclude other causes of anemia (eg, vitamin deficiency, metabolic/chronic inflammatory conditions, bleeding) before initiating therapy. Caution in patients with coexistent CV disease and stroke. Not approved for reduction of RBC transfusions in patients scheduled for surgical procedures. Hypertensive encephalopathy and seizures reported in patients with CKD. Appropriately control HTN prior to initiation of and during treatment; reduce/withhold therapy if BP becomes difficult to control. Cases of PRCA and severe anemia, with or without other cytopenias that arise following development of neutralizing antibodies to erythropoietin reported. Withhold and evaluate for neutralizing antibodies to erythropoietin if severe anemia and low reticulocyte count develop; d/c permanently if PRCA develops, and do not switch to other erythropoiesis-stimulating agents. Serious allergic reactions may occur; immediately and permanently d/c treatment and administer appropriate therapy if a serious allergic/anaphylactic reaction occurs. Patients may require adjustments in dialysis prescriptions after initiation of therapy, or require increased anticoagulation with heparin to prevent clotting of extracorporeal circuit during hemodialysis. Needle cover of the prefilled syringe contains dry natural rubber (a derivative of latex), which may cause allergic reactions.

ADVERSE REACTIONS: MI, stroke, VTE, thrombosis of vascular access, tumor progression/recurrence, HTN, dyspnea, peripheral edema, cough, procedural hypotension, angina pectoris, fluid overload, rash/erythema.

PREGNANCY: Category C, caution in nursing.

MECHANISM OF ACTION: Erythropoiesis-stimulating protein; stimulates erythropoiesis by the same mechanism as endogenous erythropoietin.

PHARMACOKINETICS: Absorption: Adults with CKD: (SQ) Slow. Bioavailability (37%) (on dialysis); T_{max}=48 hrs. Pediatric Patients with CKD: (SQ) Bioavailability (54%). Adults with Cancer: (SQ, 6.75mcg/kg) T_{max}=71 hrs. **Elimination:** Adults with CKD: (IV) $T_{1/2}$=21 hrs (on dialysis). (SQ) $T_{1/2}$=46 hrs (on dialysis), 70 hrs (not on dialysis). Adults with Cancer: (SQ, 6.75mcg/kg) $T_{1/2}$=74 hrs.

NURSING CONSIDERATIONS

Assessment: Assess for uncontrolled HTN, previous hypersensitivity to the drug, latex allergy, causes of anemia, pregnancy/nursing status, and other conditions where treatment is cautioned/contraindicated. Obtain baseline Hgb levels, transferrin saturation, and serum ferritin.

Monitoring: Monitor for signs/symptoms of an allergic reaction, CV/thromboembolic events, stroke, premonitory neurologic symptoms, PRCA, severe anemia, progression/recurrence of tumor, and other adverse reactions. Monitor BP, transferrin saturation, and serum ferritin. Following initiation of therapy and after each dose adjustment, monitor Hgb weekly until Hgb is stable and sufficient to minimize need for RBC transfusion, then monitor Hgb less frequently, provided Hgb levels remain stable.

Patient Counseling: Inform of the risks/benefits of therapy and of the increased risks of mortality, serious CV reactions, thromboembolic reactions, stroke, and tumor progression. Advise of the need to have regular lab tests for Hgb. Inform cancer patients that they must sign the patient-physician acknowledgment form prior to the start of each treatment course. Instruct to undergo regular BP monitoring, adhere to prescribed antihypertensive regimen, and follow recommended dietary restrictions. Advise to contact physician for new-onset neurologic symptoms or change in seizure frequency. Instruct regarding proper disposal and caution against reuse of needles, syringes, or unused portions of single-dose vials.

Administration: IV/SQ route. IV route is recommended for hemodialysis patients. Do not shake. Do not dilute and do not administer in conjunction with other drug sol. Refer to PI for further preparation and administration instructions. **Storage:** 2-8°C (36-46°F). Do not freeze; do not use if it has been frozen. Protect from light.

ARAVA   RX
leflunomide (Sanofi-Aventis)

> Pregnancy must be excluded before start of treatment. Avoid pregnancy during treatment or before completion of drug elimination procedure after treatment. Severe liver injury, including fatal liver failure, reported; not for use with pre-existing acute or chronic liver disease, or those with serum ALT >2X ULN before initiating treatment. Caution with other potentially hepatotoxic drugs. Monitor ALT levels at least monthly for 6 months after starting therapy, and thereafter every 6-8 weeks. Interrupt therapy if ALT elevation >3X ULN; if likely leflunomide-induced, start cholestyramine washout and monitor liver tests weekly until normalized. If leflunomide-induced liver injury is unlikely, may consider resuming therapy.

THERAPEUTIC CLASS: Pyrimidine synthesis inhibitor

INDICATIONS: Treatment of active rheumatoid arthritis (RA) in adults to reduce signs/symptoms, inhibit structural damage as evidenced by x-ray erosions and joint space narrowing, and to improve physical function.

DOSAGE: *Adults:* LD: 100mg qd for 3 days. Maint: 20mg qd. If not well tolerated, reduce to 10mg qd. Max: 20mg qd.

HOW SUPPLIED: Tab: 10mg, 20mg, 100mg

CONTRAINDICATIONS: Women who are or may become pregnant.

WARNINGS/PRECAUTIONS: Avoid with severe immunodeficiency, bone marrow dysplasia, or severe, uncontrolled infections. May cause immunosuppression, increased susceptibility to infections, especially *Pneumocystis jiroveci* pneumonia, tuberculosis (TB), and aspergillosis, or increase risk of malignancy. Rare cases of pancytopenia, agranulocytosis, and thrombocytopenia reported. D/C with evidence of bone marrow suppression. Monitor for hematologic toxicity if switching to another antirheumatic agent with a known potential for hematologic suppression. Serious toxicity (eg, hypersensitivity), peripheral neuropathy, and rare cases of Stevens-Johnson syndrome and toxic epidermal necrolysis reported; discontinuing therapy and drug elimination procedure are recommended if any of these occur. Interstitial lung disease reported. New onset or worsening of pulmonary symptoms (eg, cough, dyspnea), with or without associated fever, may be a reason for discontinuation; consider washout procedures if discontinuation is necessary. Screen for latent TB infection with a tuberculin skin test prior to initiating therapy. Caution in patients with renal impairment. Monitor BP before start of therapy and periodically thereafter. Has uricosuric effect and a separate effect of hypophosphaturia seen in some patients. Men wishing to father a child should consider discontinuing use and taking cholestyramine 8g tid for 11 days.

ADVERSE REACTIONS: Severe liver injury, diarrhea, respiratory infection, alopecia, headache, nausea, rash, HTN, joint disorder, dyspepsia, bronchitis, urinary tract infection, abdominal/back/ GI pain.

INTERACTIONS: See Boxed Warning. Avoid with live vaccines. Decreased plasma levels of M1 (metabolite) with cholestyramine or activated charcoal. Multiple doses of rifampin may increase levels; use with caution. May increase levels of diclofenac, ibuprofen, or tolbutamide. May increase risk of hepatotoxicity with methotrexate or peripheral neuropathy with neurotoxic medications. Increased INR with warfarin (rare). Concomitant immunosuppressant therapy may increase susceptibility to infections.

PREGNANCY: Category X, not for use in nursing.

MECHANISM OF ACTION: Pyrimidine synthesis inhibitor; isoxazole immunomodulatory agent. Inhibits dihydroorotate dehydrogenase and has antiproliferative activity. Has demonstrated an anti-inflammatory effect.

PHARMACOKINETICS: Absorption: T_{max}=6-12 hrs (M1). Oral administration of various doses led to different parameters. **Distribution:** M1: V_d=0.13L/kg; plasma protein binding (>99.3%). **Metabolism:** A77 1726 (M1) (primary active metabolite). **Elimination:** Urine (43%), feces (48%). (M1) $T_{1/2}$=2 weeks.

NURSING CONSIDERATIONS

Assessment: Assess for severe immunodeficiency, bone marrow dysplasia, severe uncontrolled infections, hepatic/renal impairment, comorbid illnesses, latent TB infection, drug hypersensitivity, pregnancy/nursing status, and possible drug interactions. Obtain baseline BP, platelet, WBC count, Hgb, Hct, and ALT levels.

Monitoring: Monitor for signs/symptoms of immunosuppression and opportunistic infections, sepsis, pancytopenia, agranulocytosis, thrombocytopenia, severe liver injury, skin reactions, interstitial lung disease, malignancy, hypersensitivity, and other adverse effects. Monitor BP periodically. Monitor platelets, WBC count, Hgb/Hct, and ALT levels monthly for 6 months and every 6-8 weeks thereafter. Monitor for hematologic toxicity when switching to another antirheumatic agent with known potential for hematologic suppression. Monitor for bone marrow suppression monthly if used concomitantly with immunosuppressants.

Patient Counseling: Advise women of increased risks of birth defects if used during pregnancy, or if the patient becomes pregnant while the drug has not been completely eliminated from the body. Instruct women of childbearing potential to use reliable form of contraception while on therapy. Advise to notify physician if patient develops any type of skin rash or mucous membrane lesions, hepatotoxicity, or interstitial lung disease. Inform of the need for monitoring liver enzymes while on therapy. Advise that lowering of blood counts may develop; instruct to have frequent monitoring and notify physician if symptoms of pancytopenia develop.

Administration: Oral route. **Storage:** 25°C (77°F); excursions permitted to 15-30°C (59-86°F). Protect from light.

ARCAPTA   RX
indacaterol (Novartis)

> Long-acting β₂-adrenergic agonists (LABAs) may increase the risk of asthma-related death. Not indicated for treatment of asthma.

THERAPEUTIC CLASS: Beta₂-agonist

INDICATIONS: Long-term, once-daily maintenance bronchodilator treatment of airflow obstruction in patients with chronic obstructive pulmonary disease (COPD), including chronic bronchitis and/or emphysema.

DOSAGE: *Adults:* 1 inhalation of the contents of 1 cap (75mcg) qd via Neohaler device.

HOW SUPPLIED: Cap, Inhalation: 75mcg

CONTRAINDICATIONS: Asthma without use of a long-term asthma control medication. Not indicated for treatment of asthma.

WARNINGS/PRECAUTIONS: Not for acutely deteriorating COPD, or relief of acute symptoms (eg, as rescue therapy for treatment of acute episodes of bronchospasm). Cardiovascular (CV) effects and fatalities reported with excessive use; do not use excessively or with other LABA. D/C if paradoxical bronchospasm or CV effects occur. ECG changes reported. Caution with CV disorders (eg, coronary insufficiency, cardiac arrhythmias, HTN), convulsive disorders, thyrotoxicosis, and in patients unusually responsive to sympathomimetic amines. Hypokalemia, hyperglycemia, and immediate hypersensitivity reactions may occur. D/C immediately and institute alternative therapy if signs suggesting allergic reactions occur.

ADVERSE REACTIONS: Cough, nasopharyngitis, headache, COPD exacerbation, pneumonia, angina pectoris, atrial fibrillation.

INTERACTIONS: Adrenergic drugs may potentiate effects; use with caution. Xanthine derivatives, steroids, or diuretics may potentiate any hypokalemic effect. ECG changes or hypokalemia that may result from non-K⁺-sparing diuretics (eg, loop/thiazide diuretics) can be acutely worsened; use with caution. MAOIs, TCAs, and drugs known to prolong QTc interval may potentiate effect on CV system; use with extreme caution. Drugs that are known to prolong the QTc interval may increase risk of ventricular arrhythmias. β-blockers may block effects and produce severe bronchospasm in COPD patients; if needed, consider cardioselective β-blocker with caution. May result in overdose if used in conjunction with other medications containing LABAs. Increased plasma levels with ketoconazole, verapamil, erythromycin, and ritonavir.

PREGNANCY: Category C, caution in nursing.

MECHANISM OF ACTION: LABA; stimulates intracellular adenyl cyclase, the enzyme that catalyzes the conversion of ATP to cAMP. Increases cAMP levels, causing relaxation of bronchial smooth muscles.

PHARMACOKINETICS: Absorption: Absolute bioavailability (43-45%); T_{max}=15 min. **Distribution:** (IV) V_d=2361-2557L; plasma protein binding (95.1-96.2%). **Metabolism:** Hydroxylation, glucuronidation, N-dealkylation; CYP3A4, UGT1A1; hydroxylated indacaterol (most prominent metabolite). **Elimination:** Urine (<2% unchanged), feces (54% unchanged, 23% metabolites); $T_{1/2}$=45.5-126 hrs.

NURSING CONSIDERATIONS

Assessment: Assess for previous hypersensitivity to the drug, acute COPD deteriorations, asthma and use of control medication, CV disorders, convulsive disorders, thyrotoxicosis, diabetes mellitus, pregnancy/nursing status, and possible drug interactions. Assess use in patients unusually responsive to sympathomimetic amines. Obtain baseline serum K⁺ and blood glucose levels.

Monitoring: Monitor lung function periodically. Monitor for signs of worsening asthma, CV effects, paradoxical bronchospasm, and immediate hypersensitivity reactions. Monitor pulse rate, BP, ECG changes, and serum K⁺ and glucose levels.

Patient Counseling: Inform of the risks and benefits of therapy. Instruct on proper administration of caps using the inhaler device and not to swallow caps. Caution that inhaler cannot be used more than once a day. Advise to d/c the regular use of short acting β₂-agonist (SABA) and use them only for the symptomatic relief of acute symptoms. Instruct to notify physician immediately if worsening of symptoms, decreasing effectiveness of inhaled SABA, need for more inhalations than usual of inhaled SABA, and significant decrease in lung function occur. Instruct not to stop therapy without physician's guidance. Inform patients not to use other inhaled medications containing LABAs. Inform about associated adverse effects, such as palpitations, chest pain, rapid HR, tremor, or nervousness.

Administration: Oral inhalation route. Use only with Neohaler device. Remove cap from blister only immediately before use. Refer to PI for proper administration and use. **Storage:** 25°C (77°F); excursions permitted to 15-30°C (59-86°F). Protect from light and moisture.

ARGATROBAN
argatroban (Various)

RX

THERAPEUTIC CLASS: Direct thrombin inhibitor

INDICATIONS: Prophylaxis or treatment of thrombosis in adult patients with heparin-induced thrombocytopenia (HIT). As an anticoagulant in adult patients with or at risk for HIT undergoing percutaneous coronary intervention (PCI).

DOSAGE: *Adults:* HIT/HIT and Thrombosis Syndrome (HITTS): Initial: 2mcg/kg/min as a continuous IV infusion. Check aPTT after 2 hrs. Titrate: Adjust dose as necessary until aPTT is 1.5-3X the initial baseline value (not to exceed 100 sec). Check aPTT after any dose change. Max: 10mcg/kg/min. PCI: Initial: 25mcg/kg/min IV infusion and a bolus of 350mcg/kg via a large-bore IV line over 3-5 min. Check activated clotting time (ACT) 5-10 min after bolus dose is completed. Proceed with PCI if ACT >300 sec. Titrate: If ACT <300 sec, give additional 150mcg/kg IV bolus and increase infusion to 30mcg/kg/min; check ACT after 5-10 min. If ACT >450 sec, decrease infusion to 15mcg/kg/min; check ACT after 5-10 min. Continue titration until a therapeutic ACT (between 300-450 sec) has been achieved; continue the same infusion rate for the duration of PCI procedure. May give additional 150mcg/kg bolus and increase infusion to 40mcg/kg/min in case of dissection, impending abrupt closure, thrombus formation, or inability to achieve/maintain ACT >300 sec. Check ACT after each additional bolus or change in rate of infusion. If anticoagulation is required after PCI, may continue at rate of 2mcg/kg/min; adjust PRN to maintain the aPTT in the desired range. Refer to PI for further dosing information, including dosing in patients with hepatic impairment, and for instructions for conversion to oral anticoagulant therapy. *Pediatrics:* HIT/HITTS: Normal Hepatic Function: Initial: 0.75mcg/kg/min continuous IV infusion. Check aPTT after 2 hrs. Titrate: May adjust in increments of 0.1-0.25mcg/kg/min until aPTT is 1.5-3X the baseline value (not to exceed 100 sec). Hepatic Impairment: Initial: 0.2mcg/kg/min continuous IV infusion. Check aPTT after 2 hrs. Titrate: May adjust in increments of ≤0.05mcg/kg/min until aPTT is 1.5-3X baseline value (not to exceed 100 sec).

HOW SUPPLIED: Inj: 100mg/mL [2.5mL]; 1mg/mL [50mL, 125mL]

CONTRAINDICATIONS: Major bleeding.

WARNINGS/PRECAUTIONS: Hemorrhage may occur at any site in the body; may increase risk of hemorrhage with severe HTN, immediately following lumbar puncture, spinal anesthesia, major surgery (especially involving the brain, spinal cord, or eye), hematologic conditions associated with increased bleeding tendencies, and GI lesions. Caution with hepatic impairment; full reversal of anticoagulation may require >4 hrs upon cessation of infusion. Avoid use of high doses in PCI patients with significant hepatic disease or AST/ALT ≥3X ULN.

ADVERSE REACTIONS: Hemorrhage, Hct/Hgb decrease, dyspnea, hypotension, fever, diarrhea, sepsis, cardiac arrest, N/V, ventricular tachycardia, chest pain, back pain, headache, bradycardia, abdominal pain.

INTERACTIONS: D/C all parenteral anticoagulants before administration. If therapy is to be initiated after cessation of heparin, allow sufficient time for heparin's effect on the aPTT to decrease prior to initiation of argatroban therapy. Prolonged PT and INR with warfarin. Antiplatelet agents, thrombolytics, and other anticoagulants may increase risk of bleeding.

PREGNANCY: Category B, not for use in nursing.

MECHANISM OF ACTION: Direct thrombin inhibitor; inhibits thrombin-catalyzed or thrombin-induced reactions, including fibrin formation; activation of coagulation factors V, VIII, XIII, and protein C; and platelet aggregation. Capable of inhibiting both free and clot-associated thrombin.

PHARMACOKINETICS: Distribution: V_d=174mL/kg; plasma protein binding (54%). **Metabolism:** Liver via hydroxylation and aromatization; CYP3A4/5; M1 (primary metabolite). **Elimination:** Feces (65%, ≥14% unchanged), urine (22%, 16% unchanged); $T_{1/2}$=39-51 min.

NURSING CONSIDERATIONS

Assessment: Assess for hypersensitivity to drug, hepatic impairment, major bleeding, conditions at risk for a hemorrhagic event, pregnancy/nursing status, and possible drug interactions. Obtain baseline aPTT and ACT.

Monitoring: Monitor for signs/symptoms of hemorrhagic events and other adverse reactions. In patients with HIT, monitor aPTT 2 hrs after initiation of therapy and after any dose changes. In patients undergoing a PCI, monitor ACT 5-10 min after bolus dosing, after changes in infusion rate, at the end of the PCI procedure, and every 20-30 min during a prolonged procedure. Monitor PT/INR when coadministered with warfarin.

Patient Counseling: Inform of the risks of therapy as well as the plan for regular monitoring during therapy. Instruct to tell physician if using any other products known to affect bleeding, if any medical history exists that may increase the risk for bleeding, if experiencing any bleeding signs/symptoms, or if any signs/symptoms of an allergic reaction develop.

Administration: IV route. (100mg/mL) Do not mix with other drugs prior to dilution. Refer to PI for further preparation and administration instructions. **Storage:** (1mg/mL) 20-25°C (68-77°F). Do not freeze. Protect from light. (100mg/mL) Undiluted Vial: 25°C (77°F); excursions permitted to 15-30°C (59-86°F). Do not freeze. Protect from light. Diluted Sol: 20-25°C (68-77°F) in ambient indoor light for 24 hrs; or stable for up to 96 hrs when protected from light at 20-25°C (68-77°F) or at 5°C (41°F). Do not expose to direct sunlight.

ARICEPT   RX
donepezil HCl (Eisai)

THERAPEUTIC CLASS: Acetylcholinesterase inhibitor

INDICATIONS: Treatment of dementia of the Alzheimer's type.

DOSAGE: *Adults:* Take qhs. Mild to Moderate: Initial: 5mg qd. Usual: 5-10mg qd. Titrate: May increase to 10mg qd after 4-6 weeks. Moderate to Severe: Initial: 5mg qd. Usual: 10-23mg qd. Titrate: May increase to 10mg qd after 4-6 weeks, then to 23mg qd after at least 3 months.

HOW SUPPLIED: Tab: 5mg, 10mg, 23mg; Tab, Disintegrating: (ODT) 5mg, 10mg

WARNINGS/PRECAUTIONS: May exaggerate succinylcholine-type muscle relaxation during anesthesia. May have vagotonic effects on sinoatrial (SA) and atrioventricular (AV) nodes, manifesting as bradycardia or heart block. Syncopal episodes reported. May produce diarrhea, N/V; observe closely at initiation of treatment and after dose increases. May increase gastric acid secretion; monitor for active or occult GI bleeding. Caution with increased risk for developing ulcers (eg, history of ulcer disease). May cause weight loss, generalized convulsions, and bladder outflow obstruction. Caution with history of asthma or obstructive pulmonary disease.

ADVERSE REACTIONS: N/V, diarrhea, insomnia, muscle cramps, fatigue, anorexia, headache, dizziness, weight decrease, infection, HTN, back pain, abnormal dreams, ecchymosis.

INTERACTIONS: Monitor closely for GI bleeding with concurrent NSAID use. Ketoconazole and quinidine, inhibitors of CYP3A4 and CYP2D6, respectively, inhibit metabolism in vitro. Increased concentrations with ketoconazole. Decreased clearance with a known CYP2D6 inhibitor. CYP2D6 and CYP3A4 inducers (eg, phenytoin, carbamazepine, dexamethasone, rifampin, phenobarbital) may increase elimination rate. May interfere with activity of anticholinergic medications. Synergistic effect with neuromuscular blocking agents (eg, succinylcholine) or cholinergic agonists (eg, bethanechol).

PREGNANCY: Category C, caution in nursing.

MECHANISM OF ACTION: Acetylcholinesterase inhibitor; may exert effect by increasing acetylcholine concentrations through reversible inhibition of its hydrolysis by acetylcholinesterase.

PHARMACOKINETICS: Absorption: T_{max}=3 hrs (10mg), 8 hrs (23mg). **Distribution:** V_d=12-16L/kg; plasma protein binding (96%). **Metabolism:** Hepatic via CYP2D6 and CYP3A4; glucuronidation. **Elimination:** Urine (57%, 17% unchanged), feces (15%); $T_{1/2}$=70 hrs.

NURSING CONSIDERATIONS

Assessment: Assess for hypersensitivity to the drug or piperidine derivatives, underlying cardiac conduction abnormalities, risks for developing ulcers, asthma, obstructive pulmonary disease, pregnancy/nursing status, and possible drug interactions.

Monitoring: Monitor for vagotonic effects on SA and AV nodes, syncopal episodes, diarrhea, N/V, active/occult GI bleeding, weight loss, bladder outflow obstruction, generalized convulsions, and other possible adverse reactions.

Patient Counseling: Instruct to take qhs without regard to meals, as prescribed. Instruct to swallow the 23mg tab whole; do not split, crush, or chew. For ODT, dissolve on tongue and follow with water. Caution with NSAID use. Advise that N/V, diarrhea, insomnia, muscle cramps, fatigue, and decreased appetite may occur.

Administration: Oral route. Take qhs. (23mg) Do not split, crush, or chew. (ODT) Allow to dissolve on the tongue and follow with water. **Storage:** 15-30°C (59-86°F).

ARIMIDEX   RX
anastrozole (AstraZeneca)

THERAPEUTIC CLASS: Nonsteroidal aromatase inhibitor

INDICATIONS: Adjuvant treatment of postmenopausal women with hormone receptor-positive early breast cancer. First-line treatment of postmenopausal women with hormone receptor-positive or hormone receptor-unknown locally advanced or metastatic breast cancer. Treatment of advanced breast cancer in postmenopausal women with disease progression following tamoxifen therapy.

DOSAGE: *Adults:* 1mg qd. Continue until tumor progression with advanced breast cancer.

HOW SUPPLIED: Tab: 1mg

CONTRAINDICATIONS: Women who are or may become pregnant, premenopausal women.

WARNINGS/PRECAUTIONS: Increased incidence of ischemic cardiovascular (CV) events in patients with preexisting ischemic heart disease reported; consider risks and benefits. May decrease bone mineral density (BMD); consider BMD monitoring. Elevated serum cholesterol reported.

ADVERSE REACTIONS: Hot flashes, asthenia, arthritis, pain, pharyngitis, HTN, depression, N/V, rash, osteoporosis, fractures, headache, bone pain, peripheral edema.

INTERACTIONS: Tamoxifen may decrease levels; avoid concomitant use. Avoid with estrogen-containing therapies.

PREGNANCY: Category X, not for use in nursing.

MECHANISM OF ACTION: Nonsteroidal aromatase inhibitor; lowers serum estradiol concentrations and has no detectable effect on formation of adrenal corticosteroids or aldosterone.

PHARMACOKINETICS: Absorption: (Fasted state) Rapid, T_{max}=2 hrs. **Distribution:** Plasma protein binding (40%). **Metabolism:** Liver via N-dealkylation, hydroxylation, and glucuronidation; triazole (major metabolite). **Elimination:** Hepatic (85%), renal (10%); $T_{1/2}$=50 hrs.

NURSING CONSIDERATIONS

Assessment: Assess for hypersensitivity to drug, preexisting ischemic cardiac disease, menopausal status, pregnancy/nursing status, and possible drug interactions. Obtain baseline BMD, and serum cholesterol levels.

Monitoring: Monitor BMD and cholesterol levels. Monitor for hypersensitivity reactions and other adverse reactions.

Patient Counseling: Inform that drug may cause fetal harm, and is not for use in premenopausal women. Instruct to notify physician if pregnant/nursing or intending to become pregnant. Instruct to report to physician if serious allergic reactions (angioedema) occur. Inform patients with preexisting ischemic heart disease that increased incidence of CV events has been observed. Advise to seek medical attention immediately if new or worsening chest pain or SOB occurs. Inform that drug may lower the level of estrogen that may lead to a loss of the mineral content of bones, and might decrease the bone strength, leading to increased risk of fractures. Inform that cholesterol levels may increase. Advise not to take drug with tamoxifen. Instruct to take the missed dose as soon as remembered; instruct that if it is almost time for the next dose, to skip the missed dose and take the next regularly scheduled dose. Advise not to take 2 doses at the same time.

Administration: Oral route. Take with or without food. **Storage:** 20-25°C (68-77°F).

ARIXTRA   RX
fondaparinux sodium (GlaxoSmithKline)

> Epidural or spinal hematomas may occur in patients who are anticoagulated with low molecular weight heparins (LMWHs), heparinoids, or fondaparinux sodium and who are receiving neuraxial anesthesia or undergoing spinal puncture; may result in long-term or permanent paralysis. Increased risk of developing epidural or spinal hematomas in patients using indwelling epidural catheters, concomitant use of other drugs that affect hemostasis (eg, NSAIDs, platelet inhibitors, other anticoagulants), history of traumatic or repeated epidural or spinal puncture, or a history of spinal deformity or spinal surgery. Monitor frequently for signs/symptoms of neurologic impairment; if neurologic compromise noted, urgent treatment is necessary. Consider benefit and risks before neuraxial intervention in patients anticoagulated or to be anticoagulated for thromboprophylaxis.

THERAPEUTIC CLASS: Selective factor Xa inhibitor

INDICATIONS: Prophylaxis of deep vein thrombosis (DVT), which may lead to pulmonary embolism (PE), in patients undergoing hip fracture surgery, including extended prophylaxis, hip replacement surgery, knee replacement surgery, and abdominal surgery who are at risk of thromboembolic complications. Treatment of acute DVT when administered in conjunction with warfarin sodium. Treatment of acute PE when administered in conjunction with warfarin sodium when initial therapy is administered in the hospital.

DOSAGE: *Adults:* DVT Prophylaxis: Usual: 2.5mg SQ qd after hemostasis has been established. Administer initial dose no earlier than 6-8 hrs after surgery. Usual Duration: 5-9 days. Hip Fracture Surgery Prophylaxis: Extended prophylaxis course of up to 24 additional days recommended. DVT/PE Treatment: Usual: >100kg: 10mg SQ qd. 50-100kg: 7.5mg SQ qd. <50kg: 5mg SQ qd. Initiate concomitant treatment with warfarin sodium as soon as possible, usually within 72 hrs. Continue for at least 5 days and until therapeutic oral anticoagulant effect is established (INR 2-3). Usual Duration: 5-9 days.

HOW SUPPLIED: Inj: 2.5mg/0.5mL, 5mg/0.4mL, 7.5mg/0.6mL, 10mg/0.8mL

CONTRAINDICATIONS: Severe renal impairment (CrCl <30mL/min), active major bleeding, bacterial endocarditis, thrombocytopenia associated with a positive in vitro test for antiplatelet antibody in the presence of fondaparinux sodium, body weight <50kg (venous thromboembolism prophylaxis only).

WARNINGS/PRECAUTIONS: Extreme caution in conditions with increased risk of hemorrhage (eg, congenital or acquired bleeding disorders, active ulcerative and angiodysplastic GI disease, hemorrhagic stroke, uncontrolled arterial HTN, diabetic retinopathy, or shortly after brain, spinal, or ophthalmological surgery). Elevated activated PTT temporally associated with bleeding events reported. Administration of initial dose earlier than 6 hrs after surgery increases risk of major bleeding. Increased risk of bleeding in patients with impaired renal function due to reduced clearance; monitor renal function periodically and d/c therapy immediately if severe renal impairment develops. Caution with CrCl 30-50mL/min. Increased risk of bleeding in patients who weigh <50kg; caution in treatment of PE and DVT. Thrombocytopenia reported; monitor closely. D/C if platelet count falls <100,000/mm^3. D/C if unexpected changes in coagulation parameters or major bleeding occur during therapy. Anti-factor Xa (FXa) activity can be measured by anti-Xa assay using appropriate calibrator (fondaparinux); activity is expressed in mg of fondaparinux and cannot be compared with the activities of heparin or LMWH. Needle guard of the prefilled syringe contains dry natural latex rubber that may cause allergic reactions in latex-sensitive individuals. Periodic CBC, including platelet count, SrCr level, and stool occult blood tests recommended. Caution with moderate hepatic impairment (Child-Pugh Category B) and in elderly.

ADVERSE REACTIONS: Bleeding complications, thrombocytopenia, local irritation (inj-site bleeding, rash, pruritus), anemia, insomnia, increased wound drainage, hypokalemia, dizziness, purpura, hypotension, confusion.

INTERACTIONS: See Boxed Warning. Agents that may enhance the risk of hemorrhage should be discontinued prior to initiation of therapy unless these agents are essential; if coadministration is necessary, monitor closely for hemorrhage.

PREGNANCY: Category B, caution in nursing.

MECHANISM OF ACTION: Specific FXa inhibitor; selectively binds to antithrombin III (ATIII) and potentiates the innate neutralization of FXa by ATIII, thereby interrupting the blood coagulation cascade and inhibiting thrombin formation and thrombus development.

PHARMACOKINETICS: Absorption: Rapid, complete. Absolute bioavailability (100%). (2.5mg qd) C_{max}=0.39-0.50mg/L, T_{max}=3 hrs. (5mg, 7.5mg, 10mg qd) C_{max}=1.2-1.26mg/L. **Distribution:** V_d=7-11L; plasma protein binding (≥94%, bound to ATIII). **Elimination:** Urine (≤77%, unchanged); $T_{1/2}$=17-21 hrs.

NURSING CONSIDERATIONS

Assessment: Assess for history of serious hypersensitivity reaction to the drug, conditions that increase the risk of hemorrhage, or any other conditions where treatment is cautioned or contraindicated, renal/hepatic impairment, latex sensitivity, pregnancy/nursing status, and for possible drug interactions.

Monitoring: Monitor for signs/symptoms of bleeding, thrombocytopenia, and other adverse reactions. In patients undergoing neuraxial anesthesia or spinal puncture, monitor for epidural or spinal hematomas and neurologic impairment. Perform periodic CBC (including platelet count), stool occult blood tests, and renal function (including SrCr level) tests.

Patient Counseling: Advise patients who have had neuraxial anesthesia or spinal puncture to watch for signs and symptoms of spinal/epidural hematoma (eg, tingling, numbness, muscular weakness), especially if concomitantly taking NSAIDs, platelet inhibitors, or other anticoagulants; instruct to contact physician immediately if symptoms occur. Advise patient that the use of aspirin and other NSAIDs may enhance the risk of hemorrhage. Instruct on proper administration technique. Counsel on signs and symptoms of possible bleeding. Inform patients that it may take longer than usual to stop bleeding and that they may bruise and/or bleed more easily while on therapy. Instruct to report any unusual bleeding, bruising, or signs of thrombocytopenia to the physician. Instruct to notify physician or dentist of all prescription and nonprescription medications currently being taken.

Administration: SQ route. Do not inject IM. Do not mix with other medications or sol. Do not expel air bubble from syringe before the inj. Administer in fatty tissue, alternating inj sites. Refer to PI for further instructions for use. **Storage:** 25°C (77°F); excursions permitted to 15-30°C (59-86°F).

ARMOUR THYROID   RX
thyroid (Forest)

Do not use for the treatment of obesity or weight loss; doses within range of daily hormonal requirements are ineffective for weight reduction in euthyroid patients. Serious or life-threatening manifestations of toxicity may occur when given in larger doses, particularly when given in association with sympathomimetic amines.

THERAPEUTIC CLASS: Thyroid replacement hormone

INDICATIONS: Replacement or supplemental therapy in hypothyroidism of any etiology, except transient hypothyroidism during the recovery phase of subacute thyroiditis. As a pituitary TSH suppressant in the treatment or prevention of various types of euthyroid goiters (eg, thyroid nodules, subacute or chronic lymphocytic thyroiditis [Hashimoto's], multinodular goiter). Management of thyroid cancer.

DOSAGE: *Adults:* Individualize dose. Hypothyroidism: Initial: 30mg/day; 15mg/day in patients with long-standing myxedema. Titrate: Increase by 15mg every 2-3 weeks. Readjust dose within the first 4 weeks. Maint: 60-120mg/day. Myxedema Coma: Resume to PO therapy when clinical situation has been stabilized after IV administration and patient is able to take PO medications. Thyroid Cancer: Give larger doses than those used for replacement therapy. Thyroid Suppression: 1.56mcg/kg/day T4 for 7-10 days.
Pediatrics: Individualize dose. Hypothyroidism: >12 Yrs: 1.2-1.8mg/kg/day. 6-12 Yrs: 2.4-3mg/kg/day. 1-5 Yrs: 3-3.6mg/kg/day. 6-12 months: 3.6-4.8mg/kg/day. 0-6 months: 4.8-6mg/kg/day.

HOW SUPPLIED: Tab: 15mg, 30mg, 60mg, 90mg, 120mg, 180mg*, 240mg, 300mg* *scored

CONTRAINDICATIONS: Uncorrected adrenal cortical insufficiency, untreated thyrotoxicosis.

WARNINGS/PRECAUTIONS: Use is unjustified for the treatment of male or female infertility unless accompanied by hypothyroidism. Caution with cardiovascular (CV) disorders (eg, angina pectoris) and elderly with risk of occult cardiac disease; initiate at low doses (eg, 15-30mg/day) and reduce dose if euthyroid state can only be reached at the expense of aggravation of CV disease. May aggravate diabetes mellitus (DM), diabetes insipidus (DI), and adrenal cortical insufficiency. Treatment of myxedema coma requires simultaneous administration of glucocorticoids. Excessive doses in infants may cause craniosynostosis. Caution with strong suspicion of thyroid gland autonomy. Androgens, corticosteroids, estrogens, iodine-containing preparations, and salicylates may interfere with lab tests.

INTERACTIONS: See Boxed Warning. Closely monitor PT in patients on oral anticoagulants; dose reduction of anticoagulant may be required. May increase insulin or oral hypoglycemic requirements. Impaired absorption with cholestyramine and colestipol; space dosing by 4-5 hrs. Estrogens may increase thyroxine-binding globulin and may decrease free T4; increase in thyroid dose may be needed.

PREGNANCY: Category A, caution in nursing.

MECHANISM OF ACTION: Thyroid hormone; not established. Enhances oxygen consumption by most body tissues, increases basal metabolic rate and metabolism of carbohydrates, lipids, and proteins.

PHARMACOKINETICS: Absorption: (T3) Almost total; (T4) partial. **Distribution:** Plasma protein binding (>99%), found in breast milk. **Metabolism:** (T4) Deiodination in liver, kidneys, other tissues.

NURSING CONSIDERATIONS

Assessment: Assess for adrenal cortical insufficiency, thyrotoxicosis, previous hypersensitivity to the drug, CV disorders (eg, coronary artery disease, angina pectoris), DM, DI, myxedema coma, nursing status, and possible drug interactions.

Monitoring: Monitor response to treatment, urinary glucose levels in patients with DM, PT in patients receiving anticoagulants, and aggravation of diabetes or CV disease. Monitor thyroid function periodically.

Patient Counseling: Inform that replacement therapy is to be taken essentially for life, except in transient hypothyroidism. Instruct to immediately report any signs/symptoms of thyroid hormone toxicity (eg, chest pain, increased pulse rate, palpitations, excessive sweating, heat intolerance, nervousness). Inform about the importance of frequent/close monitoring of PT and urinary glucose and the need for dose adjustment of antidiabetic and/or oral anticoagulant medication. Inform that partial hair loss may be seen in children in 1st few months of therapy. Inform that drug is not for treatment of obesity or weight loss.

Administration: Oral route. **Storage:** 15-30°C (59-86°F). Protect from light and moisture.

AROMASIN   RX
exemestane (Pharmacia & Upjohn)

THERAPEUTIC CLASS: Aromatase inactivator

INDICATIONS: Adjuvant treatment of postmenopausal women with estrogen-receptor positive early breast cancer who have received 2-3 yrs of tamoxifen and are switched to exemestane for completion of a total of 5 consecutive yrs of adjuvant hormonal therapy. Treatment of advanced breast cancer in postmenopausal women whose disease has progressed following tamoxifen therapy.

DOSAGE: *Adults:* Early/Advanced: Usual: 25mg qd after a meal. Concomitant Potent CYP3A4 Inducer (eg, Rifampicin, Phenytoin): 50mg qd after a meal.

HOW SUPPLIED: Tab: 25mg

CONTRAINDICATIONS: Women who are or may become pregnant, premenopausal women.

WARNINGS/PRECAUTIONS: Lymphocytopenia (common toxicity criteria [CTC] Grade 3 or 4) reported with advanced breast cancer; most had a preexisting lower grade lymphopenia. Elevations of serum levels of AST, ALT, alkaline phosphatase, and gamma-glutamyl transferase >5X ULN (eg, ≥CTC Grade 3) have been rarely reported with advanced breast cancer, but appear mostly attributable to the underlying presence of liver and/or bone metastases. Elevations in bilirubin, alkaline phosphatase, and creatinine reported with early breast cancer. Reductions in bone mineral density (BMD) over time reported. Assess BMD in women with osteoporosis or at risk of osteoporosis at the commencement of treatment; monitor patients carefully and initiate appropriate treatment for osteoporosis. Perform routine assessment of 25-hydroxy vitamin D levels prior to treatment; give vitamin D supplementation in women with vitamin D deficiency.

ADVERSE REACTIONS: Hot flashes/flushes, arthralgia, fatigue, N/V, increased sweating, HTN, alopecia, insomnia, headache, pain, depression, anxiety, dyspnea.

INTERACTIONS: Avoid coadministration with estrogen-containing agents. Potent CYP3A4 inducers (eg, rifampicin, phenytoin, carbamazepine, phenobarbital, St. John's wort) may significantly decrease exposure.

PREGNANCY: Category X, not for use in nursing.

MECHANISM OF ACTION: Aromatase inactivator; acts as false substrate for aromatase enzyme and is processed to an intermediate that binds irreversibly to the active site of the enzyme, causing inactivation.

PHARMACOKINETICS: Absorption: Rapid. (Breast cancer) T_{max}=1.2 hrs; AUC=75.4ng•hr/mL. **Distribution:** Plasma protein binding (90%). **Metabolism:** Oxidation and reduction; CYP3A4, aldoketoreductases. **Elimination:** (Healthy) Urine (42%, <1% unchanged), feces (42%); $T_{1/2}$=24 hrs.

NURSING CONSIDERATIONS

Assessment: Assess for hypersensitivity, preexisting lower grade lymphopenia, liver and/or bone metastases, osteoporosis/at risk of osteoporosis, pregnancy/nursing status, and for possible drug interactions. Perform routine assessment of 25-hydroxy vitamin D levels prior to treatment. Assess BMD in women with osteoporosis/at risk of osteoporosis.

Monitoring: Monitor for hematological abnormalities, reduction in BMD, osteoporosis, and other adverse reactions. Monitor for LFTs, creatinine, and bilirubin levels.

Patient Counseling: Advise that drug is not for use in premenopausal women. Inform not to take concomitant estrogen-containing agents. Counsel that drug lowers estrogen level in the body, which may lead to reduction in BMD over time, and that the lower the BMD, the greater the risk of osteoporosis and fracture.

Administration: Oral route. **Storage:** 25°C (77°F); excursions permitted to 15-30°C (59-86°F).

ARTHROTEC   RX
diclofenac sodium - misoprostol (G.D. Searle)

Misoprostol can cause abortion, premature birth or birth defects. Uterine rupture reported when used to induce labor or abortion beyond 8th week of pregnancy. Has an abortifacient property and must not be given to others. Should not be taken by pregnant women. Use only in women of childbearing potential if at high risk for gastric or duodenal ulcers or complications with NSAID therapy; must have had a negative serum pregnancy test within 2 weeks before therapy, must be capable of complying with effective contraceptive measures, and must have received both oral and written warnings of the hazards of misoprostol, risk of contraceptive failure, the danger to other women of childbearing potential should the drug be taken by mistake, and to begin therapy on 2nd or 3rd day of menstrual period. NSAIDs may increase risk of serious cardiovascular (CV) thrombotic events, myocardial infarction (MI), stroke, and serious GI adverse events including bleeding, ulceration, and perforation of the stomach or intestines. Increased risk of serious GI events in elderly. Contraindicated for the treatment of perioperative pain in the setting of coronary artery bypass graft (CABG) surgery.

THERAPEUTIC CLASS: NSAID/prostaglandin E_1 analogue

INDICATIONS: Treatment of the signs/symptoms of osteoarthritis (OA) or rheumatoid arthritis (RA) in patients at high risk of developing NSAID-induced gastric and duodenal ulcers and their complications.

DOSAGE: *Adults:* OA: 50mg-200mcg tid. RA: 50mg-200mcg tid or qid. OA/RA: If intolerable, may give 50mg-200mcg or 75mg-200mcg bid. May adjust dose and frequency according to individual needs after observing response to initial therapy. Refer to PI for special dosing considerations.

HOW SUPPLIED: Tab: (Diclofenac-Misoprostol) 50mg-200mcg, 75mg-200mcg

CONTRAINDICATIONS: Pregnant women, aspirin (ASA) or other NSAID allergy that precipitates asthma, urticaria, or allergic-type reactions. Treatment of perioperative pain in the setting of CABG.

WARNINGS/PRECAUTIONS: Use lowest effective dose for the shortest duration possible. Not a substitute for corticosteroids or treatment of corticosteroid insufficiency. May lead to onset of new HTN or worsening of preexisting HTN; monitor BP. Fluid retention and edema reported; caution with fluid retention or heart failure (HF). Extreme caution with a prior history of ulcer disease, and/or GI bleeding. May increase risk of GI bleeding with smoking, older age, debilitation, and poor general health status. D/C if a serious GI event occurs. Renal papillary necrosis and other renal injury reported after long-term use. Renal toxicity reported in patients in whom renal prostaglandins have a compensatory role in the maintenance of renal perfusion; caution with impaired renal function, HF, or liver dysfunction. Not recommended for use with advanced renal disease. May cause hepatotoxicity and elevation of transaminases; monitor transaminases periodically. D/C immediately if abnormal liver tests persist or worsen, if clinical signs and/or symptoms consistent with liver disease develop, or if systemic manifestations occur. Anaphylactic reactions may occur; avoid in patients with ASA-triad. May cause serious skin adverse events (eg, exfoliative dermatitis, Stevens-Johnson syndrome [SJS], toxic epidermal necrolysis); d/c if skin rash or hypersensitivity occurs. Anemia may occur; monitor Hgb/Hct if signs/symptoms of anemia develop. May inhibit platelet aggregation and prolong bleeding time; monitor with coagulation disorders. Caution with preexisting asthma. Aseptic meningitis with fever and coma reported. Avoid with hepatic porphyria. Caution in elderly and debilitated patients.

ADVERSE REACTIONS: Abdominal pain, diarrhea, dyspepsia, nausea, flatulence.

INTERACTIONS: Not recommended with Mg^{2+}-containing antacids. Diclofenac Sodium: Increased adverse effects with ASA; avoid with ASA. May diminish the antihypertensive effect of ACE inhibitors and increase the risk of renal toxicity. May increase the risk of renal toxicity with diuretics; may reduce the natriuretic effect of furosemide and thiazides. Increased serum potassium with K^+-sparing diuretics. Loop diuretics and thiazides may have impaired response when given concomitantly with NSAIDs. Synergistic GI bleeding effects when used concomitantly with warfarin. May increase risk of serious GI bleeding when used concomitantly with oral corticosteroids, anticoagulants, or alcohol. May alter response to insulin or oral hypoglycemics. Monitor for digoxin, methotrexate, cyclosporine, phenobarbital, and lithium toxicities. Caution with drugs that are known to be potentially hepatotoxic (eg, antibiotics, antiepileptics). Voriconazole may increase levels. May minimally interfere with protein binding of prednisolone. Antacids may delay absorption. Misoprostol: Antacids reduce the bioavailability. Mg^{2+}-containing antacids exacerbate misoprostol-associated diarrhea.

PREGNANCY: Category X, caution in nursing.

MECHANISM OF ACTION: Diclofenac: NSAID; not established. May be related to prostaglandin synthetase inhibition. Possesses anti-inflammatory, analgesic, and antipyretic properties. Misoprostol: Synthetic prostaglandin E_1 analogue; has both antisecretory and mucosal protective properties. Inhibits basal and nocturnal gastric acid secretion and acid secretion in response to stimuli (eg, meals, histamine, pentagastrin, coffee).

PHARMACOKINETICS: Absorption: Oral administration of a single dose or multiple doses is similar to pharmacokinetics of two individual components. Refer to PI for further information. **Distribution:** Found in breast milk. Diclofenac: V_d=550mL/kg; plasma protein binding (>99%). Misoprostol: Plasma protein binding (<90%). **Metabolism:** Diclofenac: Glucuronide and sulfate conjugation via CYP2C8, 2C9, 3A4; 4'-hydroxy diclofenac (major metabolite). Misoprostol: Rapid; misoprostol acid (active metabolite). **Elimination:** Diclofenac: Urine (65%), bile (35%); $T_{1/2}$=2 hrs. Misoprostol: Urine (70%); $T_{1/2}$=30 min.

NURSING CONSIDERATIONS

Assessment: Assess for history of hypersensitivity to ASA or other NSAIDs, presence of or risk factors for CV disease, HTN, HF, fluid retention, history of ulcer disease or GI bleeding, and any other conditions where treatment is contraindicated or cautioned. Assess renal/hepatic function, pregnancy/nursing status, and possible drug interactions. Assess use of effective contraceptive measures. Obtain baseline BP and perform pregnancy test 2 weeks prior to therapy.

Monitoring: Monitor for CV thrombotic events, new onset or worsening HTN, fluid retention, GI bleeding, perforation or ulceration, HF, allergic, anaphylactic or skin reactions, renal papillary necrosis or other renal injury/toxicity, hepatotoxicity, systemic manifestations, anemia, prolonged bleeding time, bronchospasm, aseptic meningitis, and porphyria. Monitor BP and renal function. Monitor Hgb/Hct if anemia is suspected. Monitor transaminases within 4-8 weeks after initiating therapy. Periodically monitor CBC and chemistry profile for long-term use. Monitor use of effective contraception.

Patient Counseling: Advise of pregnancy risks; inform women of childbearing potential that they must not be pregnant when therapy is initiated and must use an effective contraception during treatment. Inform that therapy should not be taken by nursing mothers. Instruct not to give medication to other individuals. Instruct to contact physician if signs/symptoms of CV effects (eg, chest pain, SOB, weakness, slurring of speech), GI effects (eg, epigastric pain, dyspepsia, melena, hematemesis), or unexplained weight gain and edema occur. Instruct to contact physician and d/c if signs of skin reactions (eg, rash, blisters, fever, itching) or hepatotoxicity (eg, nausea, fatigue, jaundice) occur. Instruct to seek immediate medical attention if an anaphylactic reaction occurs (eg, breathing difficulty, facial or throat swelling). Instruct to take with meals and avoid the use of Mg^{2+}-containing antacids. Instruct to swallow tab whole; do not chew, crush, or dissolve.

Administration: Oral route. **Storage:** ≤25°C (77°F), in a dry area.

ARZERRA   RX
ofatumumab (GlaxoSmithKline)

> Hepatitis B virus (HBV) reactivation may occur, in some cases resulting in fulminant hepatitis, hepatic failure, and death. Progressive multifocal leukoencephalopathy (PML) resulting in death may occur.

THERAPEUTIC CLASS: Monoclonal antibody/CD20-blocker

INDICATIONS: Treatment of patients with chronic lymphocytic leukemia refractory to fludarabine and alemtuzumab.

DOSAGE: *Adults:* 300mg initial dose (Dose 1), followed 1 week later by 2000mg weekly for 7 doses (Doses 2 through 8), followed 4 weeks later by 2000mg every 4 weeks for 4 doses (Doses 9 through 12). Premedicate 30 min to 2 hrs prior to each dose with oral acetaminophen 1000mg, oral/IV antihistamine (cetirizine 10mg or equivalent), and IV corticosteroid (prednisolone 100mg or equivalent). Refer to PI for instructions on infusion rates, dose modification, and premedication.

HOW SUPPLIED: Inj: 20mg/mL [5mL, 50mL]

WARNINGS/PRECAUTIONS: Administer in an environment where facilities to adequately monitor and treat infusion reactions are available. May cause serious infusion reactions; interrupt infusion for infusion reactions of any severity and institute medical management for severe reactions, including angina or other signs/symptoms of myocardial ischemia. Tumor lysis syndrome (TLS) reported; administer aggressive IV hydration and antihyperuricemic agents, correct electrolyte abnormalities, and monitor renal function. Prolonged (≥1 week) severe neutropenia and thrombocytopenia may occur; monitor CBC and platelet counts at regular intervals during therapy and at increased frequency in patients who develop grade 3 or 4 cytopenias. Screen for HBV infection by measuring hepatitis B surface antigen and hepatitis B core antibody before initiating treatment. Monitor patients with evidence of current or prior HBV infection for clinical and laboratory signs of hepatitis or HBV reactivation during and for several months following treatment. Immediately d/c therapy and any concomitant chemotherapy, and institute appropriate treatment if HBV reactivation develops. Fatal infection due to hepatitis B in patients who have not been previously infected reported; monitor for clinical and laboratory signs of hepatitis. Consider PML in any patient with new onset of or changes in preexisting neurological signs/symptoms; if PML is suspected, d/c therapy and initiate evaluation for PML. Obstruction of small intestine may occur; evaluate if symptoms (eg, abdominal pain, repeated vomiting) occur.

ADVERSE REACTIONS: HBV reactivation, fulminant hepatitis, hepatic failure, PML, neutropenia, pneumonia, pyrexia, cough, diarrhea, anemia, fatigue, dyspnea, rash, nausea, bronchitis, upper respiratory tract infections.

INTERACTIONS: Do not administer live viral vaccines to recently treated patients.

PREGNANCY: Category C, caution in nursing.

MECHANISM OF ACTION: CD20-directed cytolytic monoclonal antibody; binds specifically to both the small and large extracellular loops of CD20 molecule. The Fab domain of ofatumumab binds to the CD20 molecule and the Fc domain mediates immune effector functions to result in B-cell lysis in vitro. Possible mechanisms of cell lysis include complement-dependent cytotoxicity and antibody-dependent, cell-mediated cytotoxicity.

PHARMACOKINETICS: Distribution: V_d=1.7-5.1L. **Elimination:** $T_{1/2}$=14 days (between the 4th and 12th infusions).

NURSING CONSIDERATIONS

Assessment: Assess for electrolyte abnormalities, current/prior HBV infection, pregnancy/nursing status, and possible drug interactions.

Monitoring: Monitor for signs/symptoms of HBV reactivation, hepatitis, PML, infusion reactions (eg, angina, myocardial ischemia), TLS, intestinal obstruction, and other adverse reactions. Monitor renal function. Monitor CBC and platelet counts at regular intervals during therapy and at increased frequency in patients who develop grade 3 or 4 cytopenias.

Patient Counseling: Instruct to inform physician of signs/symptoms of infusion reactions; bleeding, easy bruising, petechiae, pallor, worsening weakness, or fatigue; signs of infections; symptoms of hepatitis (eg, worsening fatigue, yellow discoloration of skin/eyes); new neurological symptoms (eg, confusion, dizziness or loss of balance, difficulty talking/walking, vision problems); new/worsening abdominal pain or nausea or a significant increase in feeling unwell. Advise to notify physician if pregnant/nursing. Advise of the need for periodic monitoring of blood counts and for avoiding vaccination with live viral vaccines.

Administration: IV route. Do not administer as an IV push/bolus. Do not shake. Start infusion within 12 hrs of preparation. Refer to PI for preparation and administration instructions. **Storage:** 2-8°C (36-46°F). Do not freeze. Protect from light. Discard prepared solution after 24 hrs.

ASACOL HD   RX
mesalamine (Warner Chilcott)

THERAPEUTIC CLASS: 5-aminosalicylic acid derivative

INDICATIONS: Treatment of moderately active ulcerative colitis (UC) in adults.

DOSAGE: *Adults:* Usual: Two 800mg tabs tid for 6 weeks.

HOW SUPPLIED: Tab, Delayed-Release: 800mg

WARNINGS/PRECAUTIONS: Renal impairment, including minimal change nephropathy, acute and chronic interstitial nephritis, and, rarely, renal failure reported; evaluate renal function prior to therapy and periodically thereafter. Has been associated with an acute intolerance syndrome that may be difficult to distinguish from an exacerbation of UC. Exacerbation of symptoms of colitis reported; symptoms usually abate when therapy is discontinued. Patients with sulfasalazine hypersensitivity may have similar reaction to therapy. Mesalamine-induced cardiac hypersensitivity reactions (myocarditis and pericarditis) reported; caution with conditions that predispose to the development of myocarditis or pericarditis. Hepatic failure reported in patients with preexisting liver disease; caution with liver disease. Organic or functional obstruction in the upper GI tract may cause prolonged gastric retention of the drug, which could delay the release of mesalamine in the colon. Caution in elderly.

ADVERSE REACTIONS: Headache.

INTERACTIONS: Known nephrotoxic agents, including NSAIDs, may increase the risk of renal reactions. Azathioprine or 6-mercaptopurine may increase the risk for blood disorders.

PREGNANCY: Category C, caution in nursing.

MECHANISM OF ACTION: 5-aminosalicylic acid derivative; has not been established. Suspected to diminish inflammation by blocking cyclooxygenase and inhibiting prostaglandin production in the colon.

PHARMACOKINETICS: Absorption: T_{max}=10-16 hrs (median), C_{max}=5mcg/mL (mesalamine), 4.6mcg/mL (N-acetyl-5-aminosalicylic acid); AUC_{tau}=20mcg•hr/mL (mesalamine), 25mcg•hr/mL (N-acetyl-5-aminosalicylic acid). **Distribution:** Found in breast milk; crosses placenta. **Metabolism:** Gut mucosal wall and liver via rapid acetylation; N-acetyl-5-aminosalicylic acid (metabolite). **Elimination:** Urine (N-acetyl-5-aminosalicylic acid); $T_{1/2}$=12.6 hrs (mesalamine), 23.6 hrs (N-acetyl-5-aminosalicylic acid).

NURSING CONSIDERATIONS

Assessment: Assess for hypersensitivity to sulfasalazine, salicylates, or aminosalicylates; conditions that predispose to the development of myocarditis or pericarditis; organic or functional obstruction in the upper GI tract; hepatic impairment; pregnancy/nursing status; and possible drug interactions. Evaluate renal function prior to initiation of therapy.

Monitoring: Monitor for acute intolerance syndrome, exacerbation of symptoms of colitis, myocarditis, pericarditis, hepatic failure, hypersensitivity reactions, and other adverse reactions. Perform periodic monitoring of renal function. Monitor blood cell counts in elderly patients.

Patient Counseling: Instruct to swallow tabs whole and not to break, cut, or chew tabs. Advise to d/c previous oral mesalamine therapy and follow dosing instructions if switching therapy. Instruct to contact physician if intact, partially intact, and/or tab shells are seen in stool repeatedly. Advise pregnant and breastfeeding women, or women of childbearing potential that the medication contains dibutyl phthalate, which is excreted in breast milk and could possibly cause fetal malformations. Instruct to leave any desiccant pouches present in the bottle.

Administration: Oral route. Swallow tab whole; do not cut, break, or chew. Take with or without food. **Storage:** 20-25°C (68-77°F); excursions permitted 15-30°C (59-86°F). Protect from moisture.

ASMANEX   RX
mometasone furoate (Merck)

THERAPEUTIC CLASS: Corticosteroid

INDICATIONS: Maintenance treatment of asthma as prophylactic therapy in patients ≥4 yrs of age.

DOSAGE: *Adults:* Previous Therapy with Bronchodilators Alone or Inhaled Corticosteroids: Initial: 220mcg qpm. Max: 440mcg qpm or 220mcg bid. Previous Therapy with Oral Corticosteroids: Initial: 440mcg bid. Max: 880mcg/day. Titrate: May give higher dose if response is inadequate after 2 weeks. Adjust to lowest effective dose once asthma stability is achieved.
Pediatrics: ≥12 Yrs: Previous Therapy with Bronchodilators Alone or Inhaled Corticosteroids: Initial: 220mcg qpm. Max: 440mcg qpm or 220mcg bid. Previous Therapy with Oral Corticosteroids: Initial: 440mcg bid. Max: 880mcg/day. Titrate: May give higher dose if response is inadequate after 2 weeks. Adjust to lowest effective dose once asthma stability is achieved.
4-11 Yrs: Initial/Max: 110mcg qpm regardless of prior therapy.

HOW SUPPLIED: Powder, Inhalation: 110mcg/actuation, 220mcg/actuation

CONTRAINDICATIONS: Primary treatment of status asthmaticus or other acute episodes of asthma where intensive measures are required. Hypersensitivity to milk proteins.

WARNINGS/PRECAUTIONS: Not for the relief of acute bronchospasm. Localized *Candida albicans* infections of the mouth and pharynx reported; treat accordingly or interrupt therapy if needed. D/C if hypersensitivity reactions occur. Contains small amount of lactose that contains milk proteins; anaphylactic reactions with milk protein allergy reported. May increase susceptibility to infections; caution with active or quiescent tuberculosis (TB) infection, untreated systemic fungal, bacterial, viral, or parasitic infections, or ocular herpes simplex. Avoid exposure to chickenpox and measles. Deaths due to adrenal insufficiency have occurred with transfer from systemic to inhaled corticosteroids; wean slowly from systemic corticosteroid therapy. Resume oral corticosteroids immediately during periods of stress or severe asthma attack. Transferring from systemic corticosteroid may unmask allergic conditions (eg, rhinitis, conjunctivitis, eczema, arthritis, eosinophilic conditions). Monitor for systemic corticosteroid effects, such as hypercorticism and adrenal suppression; reduce dose slowly when the effects occur. Prolonged use may result in decrease of bone mineral density (BMD); caution in patients at risk (eg, prolonged immobilization, family history of osteoporosis, chronic use of drugs that reduce bone mass [eg, anticonvulsants, corticosteroids]). May cause reduction in growth velocity in pediatric patients; monitor growth routinely. Glaucoma, increased intraocular pressure (IOP), and cataracts reported. Bronchospasm may occur with an increase in wheezing after dosing; d/c treatment and institute alternative therapy.

ADVERSE REACTIONS: Headache, allergic rhinitis, pharyngitis, upper respiratory tract infection, sinusitis, oral candidiasis, dysmenorrhea, musculoskeletal pain, back pain, dyspepsia, myalgia, abdominal pain, nausea.

INTERACTIONS: Ketoconazole may increase plasma levels.

PREGNANCY: Category C, caution in nursing.

MECHANISM OF ACTION: Corticosteroid; not established. Shown to have inhibitory effects on multiple cell types (eg, mast cells, eosinophils, neutrophils, macrophages, and lymphocytes) and mediators (eg, histamine, eicosanoids, leukotrienes, and cytokines) involved in inflammatory and asthmatic response.

PHARMACOKINETICS: Absorption: Absolute bioavailability (<1%); C_{max}=94-114pcg/mL; T_{max}=1-2.5 hrs. **Distribution:** (IV) V_d=152L; plasma protein binding (98-99%). **Metabolism:** Liver via CYP3A4. **Elimination:** Feces (74%), urine (8%); (IV) $T_{1/2}$=5 hrs.

NURSING CONSIDERATIONS

Assessment: Assess for status asthmaticus, acute asthma episodes, known hypersensitivity to milk proteins or to any drug component, risk factors for decreased BMD, history of increased IOP/glaucoma/cataracts, active or quiescent pulmonary TB, ocular herpes simplex, untreated systemic infections, chickenpox, measles, pregnancy/nursing status, and possible drug interactions.

Monitoring: Monitor for localized infections of mouth and pharynx with *C. albicans*, decreased BMD, asthma instability, growth in pediatrics routinely, development of glaucoma, increased IOP, cataracts, change in vision, hypercorticism, signs and symptoms of adrenal insufficiency, paradoxical bronchospasm, hypersensitivity reactions, and immunosuppression. Monitor for lung function, β-agonist use, and asthma symptoms during withdrawal of oral corticosteroids

Patient Counseling: Advise that localized infection with *C. albicans* may occur in mouth and pharynx; instruct to rinse mouth after inhalation. Inform that therapy should not be used to treat status asthmaticus or to relieve acute asthma symptoms. Counsel to d/c if hypersensitivity reactions occur. Advise to avoid exposure to chickenpox or measles and to seek medical attention if exposed. Inform of potential worsening of existing TB, other infections, or ocular herpes simplex. Inform that drug may cause systemic corticosteroid effects of hypercorticism and adrenal suppression, may reduce BMD, and may cause reduction in growth rate (pediatrics). Advise to take ud, to use medication at regular intervals, and to contact physician if symptoms do not improve or if condition worsens. Instruct on proper administration procedures and on when to discard inhaler.

Administration: Oral inhalation. Inhale rapidly and deeply. Rinse mouth after inhalation. Refer to PI for further administration instructions. **Storage:** 25°C (77°F); excursions permitted to 15-30°C (59-86°F). Store in dry place. Discard inhaler 45 days after opening foil pouch or when dose counter reads "00," whichever comes 1st.

ASTELIN   RX
azelastine HCl (Meda)

THERAPEUTIC CLASS: Antihistamine

INDICATIONS: Treatment of the symptoms of seasonal allergic rhinitis (eg, rhinorrhea, sneezing, and nasal pruritus) in patients ≥5 yrs of age. Treatment of the symptoms of vasomotor rhinitis (eg, rhinorrhea, nasal congestion, and postnasal drip) in patients ≥12 yrs of age.

DOSAGE: *Adults:* Vasomotor Rhinitis: Usual: 2 sprays/nostril bid. Seasonal Allergic Rhinitis: Usual: 1-2 sprays/nostril bid. Elderly: Start at lower end of dosing range.
Pediatrics: Vasomotor Rhinitis: ≥12 Yrs: Usual: 2 sprays/nostril bid. Seasonal Allergic Rhinitis: Usual: ≥12 Yrs: 1-2 sprays/nostril bid. 5-11 Yrs: 1 spray/nostril bid.

HOW SUPPLIED: Spray: 137mcg/spray [30mL]

WARNINGS/PRECAUTIONS: Occurrence of somnolence reported. May impair physical/mental abilities. Caution in elderly.

ADVERSE REACTIONS: Bitter taste, headache, somnolence, dysesthesia, rhinitis, epistaxis, sinusitis, nasal burning, pharyngitis, paroxysmal sneezing.

INTERACTIONS: Avoid alcohol or other CNS depressants; additional reductions in alertness and CNS performance impairment may occur. Increased levels of PO azelastine with cimetidine.

PREGNANCY: Category C, caution in nursing.

MECHANISM OF ACTION: Phthalazinone derivative; exhibits histamine H_1-receptor antagonist activity in isolated tissues.

PHARMACOKINETICS: Absorption: T_{max}=2-3 hrs; bioavailability (40%). **Distribution:** V_d=14.5L/kg (PO/IV); plasma protein binding (88%, 97% metabolite). **Metabolism:** Oxidation via CYP450; desmethylazelastine (major metabolite). **Elimination:** (PO) Feces (75%, <10% unchanged); $T_{1/2}$=22 hrs (PO/IV), 54 hrs (PO, metabolite).

NURSING CONSIDERATIONS

Assessment: Assess for known hypersensitivity to the drug, pregnancy/nursing status, and possible drug interactions.

Monitoring: Monitor for somnolence and other adverse reactions.

Patient Counseling: Instruct to use only as prescribed. Instruct to prime the delivery system before initial use and after storage for ≥3 days. Instruct to store the bottle upright at room temperature with pump tightly closed and out of reach of children. Advise to seek professional assistance or contact poison control center in case of accidental ingestion by a young child. Advise to assess individual responses to the drug before engaging in any activity requiring mental alertness (eg, driving a car or operating machinery). Advise against concurrent use with other antihistamines without consulting a physician. Advise that concurrent use with alcohol or other CNS depressants may lead to additional reductions in alertness or CNS performance impairment and to avoid concurrent use. Instruct to consult physician if pregnant/nursing or planning to become pregnant.

Administration: Intranasal route. Avoid spraying in the eyes. Before initial use, the delivery system should be primed with 4 sprays or until a fine mist appears. When ≥3 days have elapsed since the last use, pump should be reprimed with 2 sprays or until a fine mist appears. **Storage:** 20-25°C (68-77°F). Protect from freezing.

ASTEPRO
azelastine HCl (Meda)

RX

THERAPEUTIC CLASS: H₁-antagonist

INDICATIONS: Relief of symptoms of seasonal and perennial allergic rhinitis in patients ≥6 yrs of age.

DOSAGE: *Adults:* Seasonal Allergic Rhinitis: 1 or 2 sprays/nostril bid or 2 sprays/nostril qd. Perennial Allergic Rhinitis: 2 sprays/nostril bid. Elderly: Start at lower end of dosing range. *Pediatrics:* Seasonal Allergic Rhinitis: ≥12 Yrs: 1 or 2 sprays/nostril bid or 2 sprays/nostril qd. 6-11 Yrs: 1 spray/nostril bid. Perennial Allergic Rhinitis: ≥12 Yrs: 2 sprays/nostril bid. 6-11 Yrs: 1 spray/nostril bid.

HOW SUPPLIED: Spray: 0.15% [30mL]

WARNINGS/PRECAUTIONS: Somnolence reported. May impair mental/physical abilities. Caution in elderly.

ADVERSE REACTIONS: Bitter taste, nasal discomfort, headache, sinusitis, epistaxis, dysgeusia, upper respiratory infection, sneezing.

INTERACTIONS: Avoid with alcohol or other CNS depressants; additional reductions in alertness and additional impairment of CNS performance may occur. Cimetidine increased levels of orally administered azelastine.

PREGNANCY: Category C, caution in nursing.

MECHANISM OF ACTION: H₁-receptor antagonist; phthalazinone derivative.

PHARMACOKINETICS: Absorption: Bioavailability (40%). C_{max}=409pg/mL; T_{max}=4 hrs (median); AUC=9312pg•hr/mL. Desmethylazelastine: C_{max}=38pg/mL; T_{max}=24 hrs (median); AUC=3824pg•hr/mL. **Distribution:** V_d=14.5L/kg (IV/PO); plasma protein binding (88%). Desmethylazelastine: Plasma protein binding (97%). **Metabolism:** Oxidation via CYP450; desmethylazelastine (major active metabolite). **Elimination:** $T_{1/2}$=25 hrs; (PO) feces (75%, <10% unchanged). Desmethylazelastine: $T_{1/2}$=57 hrs.

NURSING CONSIDERATIONS

Assessment: Assess pregnancy/nursing status and for possible drug interactions.

Monitoring: Monitor for somnolence and other adverse reactions.

Patient Counseling: Caution against engaging in hazardous occupations requiring complete mental alertness and motor coordination (eg, driving, operating machinery). Advise to avoid alcohol or other CNS depressants. Inform that treatment may lead to adverse reactions, most common of which include bitter taste, nasal discomfort, epistaxis, headache, sneezing, fatigue, somnolence, and respiratory infection. Advise to avoid spraying into eyes.

Administration: Intranasal route. Prime before initial use by releasing 6 sprays or until a fine mist appears. When not used for ≥3 days, reprime with 2 sprays or until a fine mist appears. **Storage:** 20-25°C (68-77°F). Protect from freezing. Discard after 200 sprays have been used.

ATACAND
candesartan cilexetil (AstraZeneca)

RX

> D/C when pregnancy is detected. Drugs that act directly on the renin-angiotensin system (RAS) can cause injury/death to the developing fetus.

THERAPEUTIC CLASS: Angiotensin II receptor antagonist

INDICATIONS: Treatment of HTN in adults and children 1-<17 yrs, alone or in combination with other antihypertensive agents. Treatment of heart failure (HF) (NYHA Class II-IV) in adults with left ventricular systolic dysfunction (ejection fraction ≤40%) to reduce cardiovascular death and HF hospitalizations; has an added effect when used with an ACE inhibitor.

DOSAGE: *Adults:* HTN: Individualize dose. Monotherapy Without Volume Depletion: Initial: 16mg qd. Usual: 8-32mg/day given qd or bid. May add diuretic if BP not controlled. Moderate Hepatic Impairment: Initial: 8mg. HF: Initial: 4mg qd. Titrate: Double the dose at 2-week intervals, as tolerated, to the target dose of 32mg qd. *Pediatrics:* HTN: May be administered qd or divided into 2 equal doses. Adjust dosage according to BP response. 6-<17 Yrs: >50kg: Initial: 8-16mg. Usual: 4-32mg/day. <50kg: Initial: 4-8mg. Usual: 2-16mg/day. 1-<6 Yrs: Initial: 0.20mg/kg (PO Sus). Usual: 0.05-0.4mg/kg/day. Intravascular Volume Depletion: Consider initiating at a lower dose.

HOW SUPPLIED: Tab: 4mg*, 8mg*, 16mg*, 32mg* *scored

WARNINGS/PRECAUTIONS: Symptomatic hypotension may occur in patients who have been volume- and/or salt-depleted (eg, prolonged diuretic therapy, dietary salt restriction, dialysis, diarrhea, vomiting); correct volume and/or salt depletion prior to therapy and temporary dose reduction of candesartan, diuretic, or both may be required. Monitor BP during dose escalation and periodically thereafter. Hypotension may occur during major surgery and anesthesia. Renal function changes may occur. Oliguria, progressive azotemia or acute renal failure may occur in patients whose renal function is dependent on the RAS (eg, severe HF, renal artery stenosis, volume depletion); consider withholding or discontinuing therapy if clinically significant decrease in renal function develops. May cause hyperkalemia; monitor serum K^+ periodically. Do not give in pediatric patients with GFR <30mL/min.

ADVERSE REACTIONS: Upper respiratory tract infection, dizziness, back pain.

INTERACTIONS: Dual blockade of the RAS is associated with increased risk of hypotension, hyperkalemia, and changes in renal function (including acute renal failure); closely monitor BP, renal function, and electrolytes with concomitant agents that also affect the RAS. Do not coadminister aliskiren in patients with diabetes, and in patients with renal impairment (GFR <60mL/min). NSAIDs, including selective COX-2 inhibitors, may deteriorate renal function and attenuate the antihypertensive effect; monitor renal function periodically. May increase lithium levels and risk of lithium toxicity; monitor serum lithium levels carefully.

PREGNANCY: Category D, not for use in nursing.

MECHANISM OF ACTION: Angiotensin II receptor antagonist; blocks vasoconstrictor and aldosterone-secreting effects of angiotensin II by selectively blocking the binding of angiotensin II to the AT_1 receptor in many tissues.

PHARMACOKINETICS: Absorption: Rapid and complete. Absolute bioavailability (15%); T_{max}=3-4 hrs. **Distribution:** V_d=0.13L/kg; plasma protein binding (>99%). **Metabolism:** Ester hydrolysis, liver via O-deethylation (minor). **Elimination:** Feces (67%), urine (33%, 26% unchanged); $T_{1/2}$=9 hrs.

NURSING CONSIDERATIONS

Assessment: Assess for hypersensitivity to drug, hepatic/renal impairment, volume/salt depletion, HF, renal artery stenosis, pregnancy/nursing status, and possible drug interactions.

Monitoring: Monitor for signs/symptoms of hypotension, renal function changes, and other adverse reactions. Monitor serum K^+ periodically and BP during dose escalation and periodically thereafter.

Patient Counseling: Inform of pregnancy risks; instruct to notify physician if pregnant as soon as possible.

Administration: Oral route. Take with or without food. For children who cannot swallow tabs, suspension may be substituted; refer to PI for preparation. **Storage:** 25°C (77°F); excursions permitted to 15-30°C (59-86°F). (Sus) <30°C (86°F). Shake well before each use. Use within 30 days after 1st opening. Do not freeze.

ATACAND HCT   RX
candesartan cilexetil - hydrochlorothiazide (AstraZeneca)

D/C when pregnancy is detected. Drugs that act directly on the renin-angiotensin system (RAS) can cause injury/death to developing fetus.

THERAPEUTIC CLASS: Angiotensin II receptor antagonist/thiazide diuretic

INDICATIONS: Treatment of HTN.

DOSAGE: *Adults:* BP Uncontrolled on 25mg HCTZ qd or Controlled on 25mg HCTZ qd with Hypokalemia: 16mg-12.5mg qd. BP Uncontrolled on 32mg Candesartan qd: 32mg-12.5mg qd, and then 32mg-25mg qd. Replacement Therapy: May be substituted for the titrated individual components.

HOW SUPPLIED: Tab: (Candesartan-HCTZ) 16mg-12.5mg*, 32mg-12.5mg*, 32mg-25mg* *scored

CONTRAINDICATIONS: Anuria, hypersensitivity to other sulfonamide-derived drugs. Coadministration with aliskiren in patients with diabetes.

WARNINGS/PRECAUTIONS: Not for initial therapy. Not recommended for initiation with moderate to severe hepatic impairment. Symptomatic hypotension may occur in patients who have been volume- and/or Na$^+$-depleted (eg, prolonged diuretic therapy, dietary salt restriction, dialysis, diarrhea, vomiting); correct volume and/or salt depletion prior to therapy and may require temporary dose reduction. May cause excessive hypotension leading to oliguria, azotemia, and (rarely) with acute renal failure and death in patients with heart failure (HF); monitor closely for the first 2 weeks of therapy and whenever dose is increased. Oliguria, progressive azotemia, or acute renal failure may occur in patients whose renal function is dependent on the RAS (eg, severe HF, renal artery stenosis, chronic kidney disease, volume depletion); consider withholding or discontinuing therapy if clinically significant decrease in renal function develops. Caution with severe renal disease; dosing recommendations in patients with CrCl <30mL/min cannot be provided. Caution with hepatic impairment or progressive liver disease; may precipitate hepatic coma. HCTZ: May cause hypokalemia and hyponatremia; monitor serum electrolytes periodically. May cause idiosyncratic reaction, resulting in acute transient myopia and acute angle-closure glaucoma; d/c as rapidly as possible. May cause hypersensitivity reactions (with or without history of allergy or bronchial asthma), alter glucose tolerance, raise serum levels of cholesterol/TG/uric acid, cause/exacerbate hyperuricemia and precipitate gout, and exacerbate/activate systemic lupus erythematosus (SLE). May decrease urinary Ca^{2+} excretion and cause mild elevation of serum Ca^{2+}; avoid with hypercalcemia.

ADVERSE REACTIONS: Upper respiratory tract infection, back pain.

INTERACTIONS: See Contraindications. NSAIDs, including selective COX-2 inhibitors, may deteriorate renal function and attenuate the antihypertensive effect; monitor renal function periodically. May increase lithium levels and risk of lithium toxicity; monitor serum lithium levels. Candesartan: Dual blockade of the RAS is associated with increased risk of hypotension, hyperkalemia, and changes in renal function (including acute renal failure); closely monitor BP, renal function, and electrolytes with concomitant agents that also affect the RAS. Avoid with aliskiren in patients with renal impairment (GFR <60mL/min). HCTZ: Alcohol, barbiturates, or narcotics may potentiate orthostatic hypotension. Dose adjustment of antidiabetic drugs (oral agents and insulin) may be required. Single doses of either cholestyramine or colestipol resins may impair absorption; administer therapy at least 4 hrs before or 4-6 hrs after administration of resins. May increase responsiveness to nondepolarizing skeletal muscle relaxants (eg, tubocurarine). Thiazide-induced hypokalemia or hypomagnesemia may predispose to digoxin toxicity.

PREGNANCY: Category D, not for use in nursing.

MECHANISM OF ACTION: Candesartan: Angiotensin II receptor antagonist; blocks vasoconstrictor and aldosterone-secreting effects of angiotensin II by selectively blocking the binding of angiotensin II to AT_1 receptor in many tissues. HCTZ: Thiazide diuretic; has not been established. Affects renal tubular mechanisms of electrolyte reabsorption, directly increasing excretion of Na^+ and Cl- and indirectly reducing plasma volume.

PHARMACOKINETICS: Absorption: Candesartan: Rapid and complete. Absolute bioavailability (15%); T_{max}=3-4 hrs. **Distribution:** Candesartan: Plasma protein binding (>99%); V_d=0.13L/kg. HCTZ: Crosses placenta; found in breast milk. **Metabolism:** Candesartan: Ester hydrolysis, liver via O-deethylation (minor). **Elimination:** Candesartan: Feces (67%), Urine (33%, 26% unchanged); $T_{1/2}$=9 hrs. HCTZ: Urine (61% unchanged); $T_{1/2}$=5.6-14.8 hrs.

NURSING CONSIDERATIONS

Assessment: Assess for hypersensitivity to the drugs and their components, anuria, sulfonamide-derived drug hypersensitivity, history of penicillin allergy, volume/salt depletion, SLE, diabetes, HF, hepatic/renal impairment, renal artery stenosis, pregnancy/nursing status, and possible drug interactions.

Monitoring: Monitor for signs/symptoms of fluid/electrolyte imbalance, exacerbation or activation of SLE, hypotension, hypersensitivity reactions, idiosyncratic reaction, renal function changes, and other adverse reactions. Monitor BP and serum electrolytes periodically.

Patient Counseling: Inform females of childbearing potential of the consequences of exposure during pregnancy and of the treatment options for women planning to become pregnant; instruct to notify physician as soon as possible if pregnant. Inform that lightheadedness may occur, especially during the 1st days of therapy; instruct to d/c therapy if syncope occurs and seek consult. Caution that adequate fluid intake, excessive perspiration, diarrhea, or vomiting may lead to an excessive fall in BP, with the same consequences of lightheadedness and possible syncope. Instruct not to use K^+ supplements or salt substitutes containing K^+ without consulting physician.

Administration: Oral route. Take with or without food. **Storage:** 25°C (77°F); excursions permitted to 15-30°C (59-86°F).

ATELVIA   RX
risedronate sodium (Warner Chilcott)

THERAPEUTIC CLASS: Bisphosphonate

INDICATIONS: Treatment of osteoporosis in postmenopausal women.

DOSAGE: *Adults:* 35mg once weekly. Take in the am immediately following breakfast. Swallow tab whole while in an upright position and with at least 4 oz. of plain water. Do not lie down for 30 min after dose.

HOW SUPPLIED: Tab, Delayed-Release: 35mg

CONTRAINDICATIONS: Esophageal abnormalities that delay esophageal emptying (eg, stricture or achalasia), inability to stand or sit upright for at least 30 min, hypocalcemia.

WARNINGS/PRECAUTIONS: Not recommended with severe renal impairment (CrCl <30mL/min). Should not be given in patients treated with Actonel; contains the same active ingredient.

May cause local irritation of the upper GI mucosa; caution with active upper GI problems (eg, Barrett's esophagus, dysphagia, other esophageal diseases, gastritis, duodenitis, ulcers). D/C if dysphagia, odynophagia, retrosternal pain, or new/worsening heartburn occurs. Gastric and duodenal ulcers reported. Treat hypocalcemia and other disturbances of bone and mineral metabolism before therapy; give supplemental Ca^{2+} and vitamin D. Osteonecrosis of the jaw (ONJ) reported; consider discontinuing in patients requiring invasive dental procedures or if ONJ develops. Severe and occasionally incapacitating bone, joint, and/or muscle pain reported; consider discontinuing use if severe symptoms develop. Atypical, low-energy, or low trauma fractures of the femoral shaft reported; consider interruption of therapy. Periodically reevaluate the need for continued therapy.

ADVERSE REACTIONS: Diarrhea, abdominal pain, constipation, N/V, dyspepsia, influenza, bronchitis, upper respiratory tract infection, arthralgia, back pain, pain in extremity.

INTERACTIONS: Ca^{2+} supplements, antacids, Mg^{2+}-based supplements or laxatives, and iron preparations interfere with absorption; take at a different time of the day. Drugs that raise stomach pH (eg, histamine 2 blockers, proton pump inhibitors) may cause faster drug release from the enteric coating; increased bioavailability reported with esomeprazole; avoid coadministration. Increased risk of upper GI adverse reactions with aspirin/NSAIDs. Risk for ONJ with concomitant corticosteroid/chemotherapy. May interfere with the use of bone-imaging agents.

PREGNANCY: Category C, not for use in nursing.

MECHANISM OF ACTION: Bisphosphonate; has an affinity for hydroxyapatite crystals in bone and acts as an antiresorptive agent. Inhibits osteoclasts.

PHARMACOKINETICS: Absorption: T_{max}=3 hrs. **Distribution:** V_d=13.8L/kg; plasma protein binding (24%). **Elimination:** (IV) Urine (50% in 24 hrs; 85% in 28 days), feces (unabsorbed dose); $T_{1/2}$=561 hrs.

NURSING CONSIDERATIONS

Assessment: Assess for previous drug hypersensitivity, esophageal abnormalities, ability to stand or sit upright for at least 30 min, hypocalcemia, active upper GI problems, disturbances of bone and mineral metabolism, risk for ONJ, renal function (CrCl), pregnancy/nursing status, and for possible drug interactions.

Monitoring: Monitor for signs/symptoms of upper GI disorders, ONJ, musculoskeletal pain, atypical femur fractures (eg, thigh or groin pain), hypocalcemia, disturbance of bone and mineral metabolism, and other adverse events.

Patient Counseling: Instruct to pay particular attention to the dosing instructions; advise that benefits may be compromised by failure to take drug accordingly. Advise to d/c and consult physician if symptoms of esophageal disease or severe bone, joint, or muscle pain develop. Instruct to take supplemental Ca^{2+} and vitamin D; inform to take Ca^{2+} supplements, antacids, Mg^{2+}-based supplements or laxatives, and iron preparations at a different time of the day. Counsel about possible adverse reactions. Counsel to consider weight-bearing exercise along with the modification of certain behavioral factors (eg, cigarette smoking, excessive alcohol consumption), if these factors exist. Instruct that if a dose is missed, to take 1 tab on am after they remember and to return to taking dose as originally scheduled on their chosen day; instruct not to take 2 tabs on the same day.

Administration: Oral route. Swallow tab whole; do not cut, crush or chew. **Storage:** 20-25°C (68-77°F).

ATIVAN INJECTION   CIV
lorazepam (Baxter)

THERAPEUTIC CLASS: Benzodiazepine

INDICATIONS: Treatment of status epilepticus and preanesthetic medication in adults.

DOSAGE: *Adults:* ≥18 Yrs: Status Epilepticus: 4mg IV (given slowly at 2mg/min); may repeat 1 dose after 10-15 min if seizures recur or fail to cease. Preanesthetic Sedation: Usual: (IM) 0.05mg/kg given at least 2 hrs prior to operation; (IV) 2mg or 0.044mg/kg IV (whichever is smaller) 15-20 min prior to procedure. Max: 4mg IM/IV. Elderly: Start at the low end of the dosing range.

HOW SUPPLIED: Inj: 2mg/mL, 4mg/mL [1mL, 10mL]

CONTRAINDICATIONS: Acute narrow-angle glaucoma, sleep apnea syndrome, severe respiratory insufficiency. Not for intra-arterial inj.

WARNINGS/PRECAUTIONS: May produce heavy sedation. Airway obstruction and respiratory depression may occur; ensure airway patency and monitor respiration. May impair mental/physical abilities. Avoid in patients with hepatic and/or renal failure; caution in patients with hepatic and/or renal impairment. May cause fetal damage during pregnancy. When used for peroral endoscopic procedures, adequate topical/regional anesthesia is recommended to minimize reflex activity. Extreme caution when administering injections to elderly, very ill, or to patients with limited pulmonary reserve; hypoventilation and/or hypoxic cardiac arrest may occur. Paradoxical reaction, propylene glycol toxicity (eg, lactic acidosis, hyperosmolality, hypotension) and polyethylene glycol toxicity (eg, acute tubular necrosis) reported; premature and low birth weight infants as well pediatric patients receiving high-doses may be at higher risk. Pediatric patients may exhibit sensitivity to benzyl alcohol; "gasping syndrome" associated with administration of IV sol containing benzyl alcohol in neonates. Repeated doses over a prolonged period of time may result in physical and psychological dependence and withdrawal symptoms following abrupt discontinuation.

ADVERSE REACTIONS: Respiratory depression/failure, hypotension, somnolence, headache, hypoventilation, inj-site reactions, paradoxical excitement.

INTERACTIONS: Additive CNS depression with other CNS depressants (eg, ethyl alcohol, phenothiazines, barbiturates, MAOIs, antidepressants). Increased sedation, hallucinations and irrational behavior with scopolamine. Reduce dose by 50% when given in combination with valproate or probenecid due to decreased clearance. Increased clearance with oral contraceptives. Severe adverse effects with clozapine, loxapine, and haloperidol reported. Prolonged and profound effect with concomitant sedatives, tranquilizers, narcotic analgesics.

PREGNANCY: Category D, not for use in nursing.

MECHANISM OF ACTION: Benzodiazepine; antianxiety, sedative, and anticonvulsant effects. Interacts with gamma-aminobutyric acid (GABA)-benzodiazepine receptor complex in human brain. Exhibits relatively high and specific affinity for its recognition site but does not displace GABA. Attachment to the specific binding site enhances the affinity of GABA for its receptor site on the same receptor complex.

PHARMACOKINETICS: Absorption: Complete, rapid; (IM) C_{max}=48ng/mL, T_{max}=within 3 hrs. **Distribution:** V_d=1.3L/kg, plasma protein binding (91%), crosses blood brain barrier. **Metabolism:** Liver. **Elimination:** Urine (88%), feces (7%), (0.3% unchanged); $T_{1/2}$=14 hrs.

NURSING CONSIDERATIONS

Assessment: Perform a comprehensive review of benefits/risks in status epilepticus. Assess for hypersensitivity to benzodiazepine or its vehicle, acute-angle glaucoma, preexisting respiratory impairment, hepatic/renal impairment, pregnancy/nursing status, and possible drug interactions.

Monitoring: Monitor for respiratory depression, airway obstruction, heavy sedation, drowsiness, excessive sleepiness, hypoglycemia and hyponatremia in status epilepticus, seizures, myoclonus, somnolence, inj-site reactions, and paradoxical reactions. Monitor for signs of toxicity to the vehicle's components (eg, lactic acidosis, hyperosmolarity, hypotension, acute tubular necrosis). Monitor for hypersensitivity reactions.

Patient Counseling: Inform of risks/benefits. Advise to use caution with hazardous tasks. Instruct to not get out of bed unassisted. Advise to avoid alcoholic beverages for at least 24-48 hrs after receiving drug. Advise about potential for physical/psychological dependence and withdrawal symptoms.

Administration: IM/IV route. IV must be diluted with an equal volume of compatible sol. **Storage:** Refrigerate; protect from light.

ATRIPLA   RX

tenofovir disoproxil fumarate - emtricitabine - efavirenz (Bristol-Myers Squibb/Gilead Sciences)

> Lactic acidosis and severe hepatomegaly with steatosis, including fatal cases, reported with the use of nucleoside analogues. Not approved for the treatment of chronic hepatitis B virus (HBV) infection. Severe acute exacerbations of hepatitis B reported in patients coinfected with HBV upon discontinuation of therapy; closely monitor hepatic function for at least several months. If appropriate, initiation of anti-hepatitis B therapy may be warranted.

THERAPEUTIC CLASS: Non-nucleoside reverse transcriptase inhibitor/nucleoside analogue combination

INDICATIONS: For use alone as a complete regimen or in combination with other antiretroviral agents for the treatment of HIV-1 infection in adults and pediatric patients ≥12 yrs of age.

DOSAGE: *Adults:* ≥40kg: 1 tab qd on an empty stomach; hs dosing may improve tolerability of nervous system symptoms. Concomitant Rifampin: ≥50kg: Additional 200mg/day of efavirenz is recommended.
Pediatrics: ≥12 Yrs: ≥40kg: 1 tab qd on an empty stomach; hs dosing may improve tolerability of nervous system symptoms. Concomitant Rifampin: ≥50kg: Additional 200mg/day of efavirenz is recommended.

HOW SUPPLIED: Tab: (Efavirenz-Emtricitabine-Tenofovir Disoproxil Fumarate [TDF]) 600mg-200mg-300mg

CONTRAINDICATIONS: Coadministration with CYP3A substrates for which elevated plasma concentrations are associated with serious and/or life-threatening reactions (eg, dihydroergotamine, ergonovine, ergotamine, methylergonovine, midazolam, triazolam, bepridil, cisapride, pimozide), voriconazole, or St. John's wort.

WARNINGS/PRECAUTIONS: Not for patients requiring dosage adjustment (eg, moderate or severe renal impairment [estimated CrCl <50mL/min]). Test for presence of chronic HBV prior to treatment. Monitor LFTs before and during treatment. Not recommended in moderate or severe hepatic impairment. Immune reconstitution syndrome, autoimmune disorders (eg, Graves' disease, polymyositis, Guillain-Barre syndrome) in the setting of immune reconstitution reported. Redistribution/accumulation of body fat has been observed. Caution in elderly. Efavirenz: Serious psychiatric adverse events and CNS symptoms reported. May impair mental/physical abilities. May cause fetal harm if administered during 1st trimester of pregnancy; avoid pregnancy during use. Use adequate contraceptive measures for 12 weeks after discontinuation. Skin rash reported; d/c if severe rash associated with blistering, desquamation, mucosal involvement, or fever develops. Consider alternative therapy in patients who have had a life-threatening cutaneous reaction (eg, Stevens-Johnson syndrome). Convulsions reported; caution with history of seizures. TDF: Obesity and prolonged nucleoside exposure may be risk factors for lactic acidosis and severe hepatomegaly with steatosis. Caution with known risk factors for liver disease. D/C if lactic acidosis or pronounced hepatotoxicity occurs. Renal impairment reported; assess estimated CrCl prior to and during therapy. Decreased bone mineral density (BMD), increased biochemical markers of bone metabolism, and osteomalacia reported; consider assessment of BMD in patients with history of pathologic bone fracture or other risk factors for osteoporosis or bone loss. Arthralgias and muscle pain/weakness reported in cases of proximal renal tubulopathy. Consider hypophosphatemia and osteomalacia secondary to proximal renal tubulopathy in patients at risk of renal dysfunction who present with persistent or worsening bone or muscle symptoms.

ADVERSE REACTIONS: Lactic acidosis, severe hepatomegaly with steatosis, diarrhea, nausea, fatigue, depression, dizziness, sinusitis, upper respiratory tract infection, rash, headache, insomnia, abnormal dreams, anxiety, nasopharyngitis.

INTERACTIONS: See Contraindications. Avoid with adefovir dipivoxil, atazanavir, drugs containing same component or lamivudine, other NNRTIs, boceprevir, posaconazole, or nephrotoxic agents (eg, high dose or multiple NSAIDs). Potential additive CNS effects with alcohol or psychoactive drugs. May increase levels of didanosine and ritonavir (RTV). May decrease levels of amprenavir, lopinavir, saquinavir, raltegravir, telaprevir, bupropion, sertraline, itraconazole, ketoconazole, clarithromycin, rifabutin, diltiazem and other calcium channel blockers, atorvastatin, pravastatin, simvastatin, indinavir, maraviroc, carbamazepine, anticonvulsants, norelgestromin, levonorgestrel, etonogestrel, immunosuppressants, and methadone. May alter levels of warfarin and substrates of CYP2C9, 2C19, 3A4, or 2B6. Efavirenz: RTV may increase levels. Telaprevir, carbamazepine, anticonvulsants, rifabutin, and rifamph may decrease levels. CYP3A substrates, inhibitors, or inducers may alter levels. TDF/Emtricitabine: Coadministration of drugs that reduce renal function or compete for active tubular secretion (eg, acyclovir, adefovir dipivoxil, cidofovir, ganciclovir, valacyclovir, valganciclovir, aminoglycosides [eg, gentamicin], and high-dose or multiple NSAIDs) may increase levels of emtricitabine, TDF, and/or other renally eliminated drugs. Darunavir with RTV and lopinavir/RTV may increase TDF levels. An increase in absorption may be observed when TDF is coadministered with an inhibitor of p-glycoprotein or breast cancer resistance protein. Refer to PI for further information on drug interactions.

PREGNANCY: Category D, not for use in nursing.

MECHANISM OF ACTION: Efavirenz: NNRTI; noncompetitive inhibition of HIV-1 reverse transcriptase (RT). Emtricitabine: Nucleoside analogue of cytidine; inhibits activity of HIV-1 RT by competing with natural substrate deoxycytidine 5'-triphosphate and incorporating into nascent viral DNA, resulting in chain termination. TDF: Acyclic nucleoside phosphonate diester analogue of adenosine monophosphate; inhibits activity of HIV-1 RT by competing with the natural substrate deoxyadenosine 5'-triphosphate and, after incorporation into the DNA, by DNA chain termination.

PHARMACOKINETICS: Absorption: Efavirenz: C_{max}=12.9μM, T_{max}=3-5 hrs, AUC=184μM•hr. Emtricitabine: Rapid; absolute bioavailability (93%), C_{max}=1.8mcg/mL, T_{max}=1-2 hrs, AUC=10mcg•hr/mL. TDF: bioavailability (25%), C_{max}=296ng/mL, T_{max}=1 hr, AUC=2287ng•hr/mL. **Distribution:** Efavirenz: Plasma protein binding (99.5-99.75%). Emtricitabine: Plasma protein binding (<4%); found in breast milk. TDF: Plasma protein binding (<0.7%); found in breast milk. **Metabolism:** Efavirenz: Via CYP3A and CYP2B6. Emtricitabine: 3'-sulfoxide diastereomers and glucuronic acid conjugate (metabolites). **Elimination:** Efavirenz: Urine (14-34% mostly metabolites, <1% unchanged), feces (16-61% mostly parent drug); $T_{1/2}$=52-76 hrs (single dose), 40-55 hrs (multiple doses). Emtricitabine: Urine (86%, 13% metabolites); $T_{1/2}$=10 hrs (single dose). TDF: (IV) Urine (70-80% unchanged); $T_{1/2}$=17 hrs (single dose).

NURSING CONSIDERATIONS

Assessment: Assess for obesity, prolonged nucleoside exposure, liver dysfunction or risk factors for liver disease, renal dysfunction, HBV infection, psychiatric history, history of injection drug use/seizures/cutaneous reaction, hypersensitivity, pregnancy/nursing status, and possible drug interactions. Assess BMD in patients with a history of pathological bone fracture or with other risk factors for osteoporosis or bone loss. Assess estimated CrCl, serum P, urine glucose and urine protein in patients at risk for renal dysfunction.

Monitoring: Monitor for signs/symptoms of lactic acidosis, severe hepatomegaly with steatosis, psychiatric/nervous system symptoms, new onset/worsening renal impairment, decreased BMD, increased biochemical markers for bone metabolism, osteomalacia, convulsions, immune reconstitution syndrome (eg, opportunistic infections), fat redistribution/accumulation, skin rash, and other adverse reactions. Monitor for acute exacerbations of hepatitis B in patients with coinfection upon discontinuation of therapy. Monitor LFTs. Monitor estimated CrCl, serum P, urine glucose, and urine protein periodically in patients at risk for renal dysfunction.

Patient Counseling: Inform that therapy is not a cure for HIV-1 infection and illnesses associated with HIV-1 infection may still be experienced. Advise to practice safe sex, use latex or polyurethane condoms, not to share personal items (eg, toothbrush, razor blades), needles, or other inj equipment, and not to breastfeed. Instruct to contact physician if N/V, unusual stomach discomfort, weakness, aggressive behavior, severe depression, suicide attempts, delusions, paranoia, psychosis-like symptoms, dizziness, insomnia, impaired concentration, drowsiness, abnormal dreams, or skin rash develops. Advise that fat redistribution/accumulation and decreases in BMD may occur. Counsel to avoid pregnancy while on therapy and use adequate contraceptive measures for 12 weeks after discontinuation; instruct that barrier contraception must always be used in combination with other methods of contraception. Advise to avoid potentially hazardous tasks if experiencing CNS/psychiatric symptoms or taking alcohol or psychoactive drugs. Advise that severe acute exacerbation of hepatitis B may occur if coinfected. Advise to report use of any prescription, nonprescription medication, or herbal products, particularly St. John's wort.

Administration: Oral route. Take on an empty stomach. **Storage:** 25°C (77°F); excursions permitted to 15-30°C (59-86°F).

ATROVENT **HFA** RX
ipratropium bromide (Boehringer Ingelheim)

THERAPEUTIC CLASS: Anticholinergic bronchodilator

INDICATIONS: Maintenance treatment of bronchospasm associated with chronic obstructive pulmonary disease (COPD), including chronic bronchitis and emphysema.

DOSAGE: *Adults:* Initial: 2 inh qid. May take additional inh PRN. Max: 12 inh/24 hrs.

HOW SUPPLIED: MDI: 17mcg/inh [12.9g]

CONTRAINDICATIONS: Hypersensitivity to atropine or any of its derivatives.

WARNINGS/PRECAUTIONS: Not for initial treatment of acute episodes of bronchospasm. Hypersensitivity reactions and/or paradoxical bronchospasm may occur; d/c at once and consider alternative treatment if any of these occur. May increase intraocular pressure (IOP), which may result in precipitation/worsening of narrow-angle glaucoma; caution with narrow-angle glaucoma. Avoid spraying into eyes; may cause eye pain/discomfort, temporary blurring of vision, mydriasis, visual halos, or colored images in association with red eyes from conjunctival or corneal congestion. May cause urinary retention; caution with prostatic hyperplasia or bladder neck obstruction.

ADVERSE REACTIONS: Bronchitis, COPD exacerbation, sinusitis, urinary tract infection, influenza-like symptoms, dyspnea, back pain, dyspepsia, headache, dizziness, nausea, dry mouth.

INTERACTIONS: Avoid with other anticholinergic-containing drugs; may lead to an increase in anticholinergic adverse effects.

PREGNANCY: Category B, caution in nursing.

MECHANISM OF ACTION: Anticholinergic bronchodilator; appears to inhibit vagally-mediated reflexes by antagonizing the action of acetylcholine. Prevents the increase in intracellular concentration of Ca^{2+} that is caused by interaction of acetylcholine with the muscarinic receptors on bronchial smooth muscle.

PHARMACOKINETICS: Absorption: Not readily absorbed. C_{max}=59pg/mL (4 inh, single dose), 82pg/mL (4 inh, qid). **Distribution:** Plasma protein binding (0-9%). **Metabolism:** Partial; ester hydrolysis. **Elimination:** Urine (1/2 of the IV dose, unchanged); $T_{1/2}$=2 hrs.

NURSING CONSIDERATIONS

Assessment: Assess for hypersensitivity to drug and/or hypersensitivity to atropine or any of its derivatives, narrow-angle glaucoma, prostatic hyperplasia, bladder neck obstruction, pregnancy/nursing status, and possible drug interactions.

Monitoring: Monitor for hypersensitivity reactions, paradoxical bronchospasm, increased IOP, urinary retention, and other adverse reactions.

Patient Counseling: Inform that drug is not for initial treatment of acute episodes of broncho-spasm. Instruct to d/c use if paradoxical bronchospasm occurs. Advise to consult physician if experiencing difficulty with urination. Instruct to avoid spraying aerosol into the eyes and to consult physician immediately if precipitation or worsening of narrow-angle glaucoma, mydriasis, increased IOP, eye pain/discomfort, blurring of vision, visual halos or colored images develop. Caution about engaging in activities requiring balance and visual acuity (eg, driving or operating appliances/machinery). Instruct to use drug consistently as prescribed throughout the course of therapy, not to increase the dose or frequency without consulting the physician, and to seek im-mediate medical attention if treatment becomes less effective for symptomatic relief, symptoms become worse, and/or use of product is more frequent than usual. Advise on the use of medica-tion in relation to other inhaled drugs.

Administration: Oral inhalation route. Prime medication before first use with 2 sprays. If not used for >3 days, reprime with 2 sprays. Refer to PI for further administration instructions. **Storage:** 25°C (77°F); excursions permitted to 15-30°C (59-86°F). Do not puncture or use/store near heat or open flame.

ATROVENT NASAL   RX
ipratropium bromide (Boehringer Ingelheim)

THERAPEUTIC CLASS: Anticholinergic

INDICATIONS: (0.03%) Symptomatic relief of rhinorrhea associated with allergic and nonallergic perennial rhinitis in adults and children ≥6 yrs of age. (0.06%) Symptomatic relief of rhinorrhea associated with the common cold or seasonal allergic rhinitis in adults and children ≥5 yrs of age.

DOSAGE: *Adults:* (0.03%) Rhinorrhea with Allergic/Nonallergic Perennial Rhinitis: 2 sprays/nostril bid-tid. (0.06%) Rhinorrhea Associated with Common Cold: 2 sprays/nostril tid-qid for ≤4 days. Rhinorrhea Associated with Seasonal Allergic Rhinitis: 2 sprays/nostril qid for ≤3 weeks. *Pediatrics:* (0.03%) ≥6 Yrs: Rhinorrhea with Allergic/Nonallergic Perennial Rhinitis: 2 sprays/nostril bid-tid. (0.06%) Rhinorrhea Associated with Common Cold: ≥12 Yrs: 2 sprays/nostril tid-qid for ≤4 days. 5-11 Yrs: 2 sprays/nostril tid for ≤4 days. Rhinorrhea Associated with Seasonal Allergic Rhinitis: ≥5 Yrs: 2 sprays/nostril qid for ≤3 weeks.

HOW SUPPLIED: Spray: (0.03%) 21mcg/spray [31.1g], (0.06%) 42mcg/spray [16.6g]

CONTRAINDICATIONS: Hypersensitivity to atropine or its derivatives.

WARNINGS/PRECAUTIONS: Immediate hypersensitivity reactions reported; d/c at once if reac-tion occurs and consider alternative treatment. Caution with narrow-angle glaucoma, prostatic hyperplasia, bladder neck obstruction, and hepatic or renal insufficiency.

ADVERSE REACTIONS: Epistaxis, pharyngitis, upper respiratory tract infection, nasal dryness, dry mouth/throat, headache, taste perversion.

INTERACTIONS: May produce additive effects with other anticholinergic agents.

PREGNANCY: Category B, caution in nursing.

MECHANISM OF ACTION: Anticholinergic; inhibits vagally mediated reflexes by antagonizing ac-tion of acetylcholine at the cholinergic receptor. Inhibits secretions from serous and seromucous glands lining the nasal mucosa.

PHARMACOKINETICS: Absorption: Bioavailability (<20%). **Distribution:** Plasma protein binding (0-9%). **Metabolism:** Partial; ester hydrolysis products, tropic acid, tropane. **Elimination:** Urine (half of administered dose, unchanged). (IV) $T_{1/2}$=1.6 hrs.

NURSING CONSIDERATIONS

Assessment: Assess for hypersensitivity to atropine or its derivatives, narrow-angle glaucoma, prostatic hyperplasia, bladder-neck obstruction, hepatic/renal insufficiency, pregnancy/nursing status, and possible drug interactions.

Monitoring: Monitor for signs and symptoms of hypersensitivity reactions (eg, urticaria, angioe-dema, rash, bronchospasm, anaphylaxis, oropharyngeal edema). Monitor visual changes and nasal symptoms.

Patient Counseling: Advise not to alter size of nasal spray opening. Instruct to avoid spraying medication into the eyes. Inform that temporary blurring of vision, precipitation or worsening of narrow-angle glaucoma, mydriasis, increased intraocular pressure, acute eye pain or discom-fort, visual halos, or colored images in association with red eyes from conjunctival and corneal congestion may occur if medication comes into direct contact with the eyes. Instruct to contact physician if eye pain, blurred vision, excessive nasal dryness, or episodes of nasal bleeding occur. Caution about engaging in activities requiring balance and visual acuity (eg, driving or operating machines).

Administration: Intranasal route. Prime the nasal spray pump and blow nose to clear nostrils before first use. Refer to PI for proper administration. **Storage:** 25°C (77°F); excursions permitted to 15-30°C (59-86°F). Avoid freezing.

AUBAGIO RX
teriflunomide (Genzyme)

> Severe liver injury, including fatal liver failure, reported in patients treated with leflunomide; similar risk would be expected because recommended doses of teriflunomide and leflunomide result in a similar range of plasma concentrations of teriflunomide. Concomitant use with other potentially hepatotoxic drugs may increase risk of severe liver injury. Obtain transaminase and bilirubin levels within 6 months before initiation of therapy. Monitor ALT levels at least monthly for 6 months after starting therapy. D/C therapy and start an accelerated elimination procedure with cholestyramine or charcoal if drug-induced liver injury is suspected. Contraindicated in patients with severe hepatic impairment. Increased risk of developing elevated serum transaminases in patients with preexisting liver disease. May cause major birth defects if used during pregnancy. Contraindicated in pregnant women or women of childbearing potential who are not using reliable contraception. Avoid pregnancy during treatment or before completion of an accelerated elimination procedure after treatment.

THERAPEUTIC CLASS: Pyrimidine synthesis inhibitor

INDICATIONS: Treatment of patients with relapsing forms of multiple sclerosis.

DOSAGE: *Adults:* Usual: 7mg or 14mg PO qd.

HOW SUPPLIED: Tab: 7mg, 14mg

CONTRAINDICATIONS: Severe hepatic impairment, women who are pregnant or of childbearing potential not using reliable contraception, concomitant use of leflunomide.

WARNINGS/PRECAUTIONS: Not for use with preexisting acute or chronic liver disease, or those with serum ALT >2X ULN before initiating therapy. Eliminated slowly from the plasma. An accelerated elimination procedure can be used at any time after discontinuation of therapy; refer to PI. Decrease in WBC count and platelet count reported; obtain CBC within 6 months before initiation of treatment, and base further monitoring on signs and symptoms of bone marrow suppression. Do not start treatment until the infection(s) is resolved with active acute or chronic infections. Consider suspending treatment and using an accelerated elimination procedure if serious infection develops. Avoid with severe immunodeficiency, bone marrow disease, or severe, uncontrolled infections. May cause immunosuppression and increased susceptibility to infections. Screen for latent tuberculosis (TB) infection prior to initiating therapy. May increase risk of malignancy. Peripheral neuropathy may occur; increased risk with age >60 yrs, concomitant neurotoxic medications, and diabetes. Consider discontinuing and performing an accelerated elimination procedure if peripheral neuropathy symptoms develop. Acute renal failure and hyperkalemia reported; check serum K⁺ level in patients with symptoms of hyperkalemia or with acute renal failure. Stevens-Johnson syndrome and toxic epidermal necrolysis may occur; d/c and perform an accelerated elimination procedure. HTN was reported; monitor BP before start of therapy and periodically thereafter. Interstitial lung disease (ILD) and worsening of preexisting ILD may occur. New onset or worsening of pulmonary symptoms, with or without associated fever, may be a reason for discontinuation; consider initiation of an accelerated elimination procedure. Monitor for hematologic toxicity if switching to another agent with a known potential for hematologic suppression.

ADVERSE REACTIONS: Severe liver injury, ALT increased, influenza, upper respiratory tract infection, headache, paresthesia, bronchitis, sinusitis, anxiety, HTN, diarrhea, nausea, abdominal pain upper, alopecia, neutropenia.

INTERACTIONS: See Boxed Warning and Contraindications. Vaccination with live vaccines not recommended. May increase levels of repaglinide; monitor patients with concomitant CYP2C8 substrates (eg, repaglinide, paclitaxel, pioglitazone, or rosiglitazone). May decrease the peak INR of warfarin; close INR follow-up and monitoring is recommended. May increase levels of ethinyl estradiol and levonorgestrel; consider the type or dose of oral contraceptives to be used. May decrease levels of caffeine; monitor patients with concomitant CYP1A2 substrates (eg, duloxetine, alosetron, theophylline, tizanidine). Breast cancer-resistant protein inhibitors (eg, cyclosporine, eltrombopag, gefitinib) may increase exposure.

PREGNANCY: Category X, not for use in nursing.

MECHANISM OF ACTION: Pyrimidine synthesis inhibitor; inhibits dihydroorotate dehydrogenase. May involve a reduction in the number of activated lymphocytes in CNS.

PHARMACOKINETICS: Absorption: T_{max}=1-4 hrs. **Distribution:** V_d=11L (IV); plasma protein binding (>99%). **Metabolism:** Hydrolysis (primary), oxidation (minor), N-acetylation, sulfate conjugation. **Elimination:** Urine (22.6%); feces (37.5%).

NURSING CONSIDERATIONS

Assessment: Assess for severe immunodeficiency, bone marrow disease, severe uncontrolled infections, ILD, hepatic/renal function, diabetes, pregnancy/nursing status, other conditions where treatment is cautioned or contraindicated, and for possible drug interactions. Obtain transaminase levels, bilirubin levels, and CBC within 6 months before initiation of therapy. Obtain BP. Screen for latent TB infection with a tuberculin skin test.

Monitoring: Monitor for signs/symptoms of immunosuppression and infections, bone marrow suppression (eg, pancytopenia, agranulocytosis, thrombocytopenia), severe liver injury, acute renal failure, skin reactions, ILD, new onset or worsening of pulmonary symptoms, malignancy, and other adverse reactions. Monitor ALT levels at least monthly for 6 months after starting therapy. Monitor BP periodically thereafter.

Patient Counseling: Inform of benefits and potential risks of treatment. Inform not to d/c treatment without first discussing with physician. Instruct to contact physician if unexplained N/V, abdominal pain, fatigue, anorexia, jaundice, dark urine, or symptoms of infection develop. Advise women of childbearing potential and men and their female partners to use effective contraception during and until completion of an accelerated elimination procedure. Advise that therapy may stay in the blood for up to 2 yrs after the last dose and that accelerated elimination procedure may be used if needed. Instruct to avoid some vaccines during treatment and for at least 6 months after discontinuation. Advise to contact physician if symptoms of peripheral neuropathy (eg, numbness or tingling of the hands or feet) develop. Inform that treatment may increase BP. Advise to either d/c breastfeeding or d/c therapy.

Administration: Oral route. May be taken with or without food. **Storage:** 20-25°C (68-77°F); excursions permitted between 15-30°C (59-86°F).

AUGMENTIN   RX
clavulanate potassium - amoxicillin (Dr. Reddy's)

THERAPEUTIC CLASS: Aminopenicillin/beta lactamase inhibitor

INDICATIONS: Treatment of skin and skin structure and urinary tract infections, lower respiratory tract infections (LRTIs), acute bacterial otitis media (OM), and sinusitis caused by susceptible strains of microorganisms.

DOSAGE: *Adults:* (Dose based on amoxicillin) Usual: One 500mg tab q12h or one 250mg tab q8h. Severe/Respiratory Tract Infections: One 875mg tab q12h or one 500mg tab q8h. May use 125mg/5mL or 250mg/5mL sus in place of 500mg tab and 200mg/5mL or 400mg/5mL sus in place of 875mg tab. Renal Impairment: Dose depending on severity of infection. GFR <30mL/min: Do not give 875mg dose. GFR 10-30mL/min: 500mg or 250mg q12h. GFR <10mL/min: 500mg or 250mg q24h. Hemodialysis: 500mg or 250mg q24h; give additional dose during and at end of dialysis. Take at the start of a meal.
Pediatrics: (Dose based on amoxicillin) ≥40kg: Use adult dose. ≥12 Weeks: Sinusitis/OM/LRTI/ Severe Infections: (Sus/Tab, Chewable) 45mg/kg/day q12h or 40mg/kg/day q8h. Treat acute OM for 10 days. Less Severe Infections: 25mg/kg/day q12h or 20mg/kg/day q8h. <12 Weeks: 30mg/kg/day divided q12h (use 125mg/5mL sus). Renal Impairment: Dose depending on severity of infection. GFR <30mL/min: Do not give 875mg dose. GFR 10-30mL/min: 500mg or 250mg q12h. GFR <10mL/min: 500mg or 250mg q24h. Hemodialysis: 500mg or 250mg q24h; give additional dose during and at end of dialysis. Take at the start of a meal.

HOW SUPPLIED: (Amoxicillin-Clavulanic Acid) Sus: 125mg-31.25mg/5mL, 250mg-62.5mg/5mL [75mL, 100mL, 150mL], 200mg-28.5mg/5mL, 400mg-57mg/5mL [50mL, 75mL, 100mL]; Tab: 250mg-125mg, 500mg-125mg, 875mg-125mg*; Tab, Chewable: 125mg-31.25mg, 200mg-28.5mg, 250mg-62.5mg, 400mg-57mg *scored

CONTRAINDICATIONS: History of amoxicillin/clavulanate-associated cholestatic jaundice/hepatic dysfunction.

WARNINGS/PRECAUTIONS: Serious and occasionally fatal hypersensitivity (anaphylactic) reactions reported; d/c if an allergic reaction occurs and institute appropriate therapy. Hepatic dysfunction, including hepatitis and cholestatic jaundice, may occur. *Clostridium difficile*-associated diarrhea (CDAD) reported; d/c if CDAD is suspected or confirmed. Avoid with mononucleosis. May result in bacterial resistance with prolonged use in the absence of a proven/ suspected bacterial infection; take appropriate measures if superinfection develops. The 200mg and 400mg chewable tabs and 200mg/5mL and 400mg/5mL sus contain phenylalanine; avoid with phenylketonurics. The 250mg tab and 250mg chewable tab are not interchangeable due to unequal clavulanic acid amounts; do not use 250mg tab in pediatric patients until child weighs at least 40kg. Do not substitute two 250mg tabs for one 500mg tab. May decrease estrogen levels in pregnant women. Lab test interactions may occur. Caution in elderly.

ADVERSE REACTIONS: Diarrhea/loose stools, nausea, skin rashes, urticaria

INTERACTIONS: Probenecid may increase/prolong levels of amoxicillin; coadministration not recommended. Abnormal prolongation of PT (increased INR) reported with oral anticoagulants; may require oral anticoagulant dose adjustment. Allopurinol may increase incidence of rashes. May reduce efficacy of combined oral estrogen/progesterone contraceptives.

PREGNANCY: Category B, caution in nursing.

MECHANISM OF ACTION: Amoxicillin: Aminopenicillin; semisynthetic antibiotic with broad spectrum of bactericidal activity against gram-positive and gram-negative organisms. Clavulanate: β-lactamase inhibitor; possesses ability to inactivate a wide range of β-lactamase enzymes commonly found in microorganisms resistant to penicillin (PCN) and cephalosporins.

PHARMACOKINETICS: Absorption: Refer to PI for absorption parameters. **Distribution:** Plasma protein binding: Amoxicillin (18%); clavulanic acid (25%). Amoxicillin: Found in breast milk. **Elimination:** Amoxicillin: Urine (50-70% unchanged); $T_{1/2}$=1.3 hrs. Clavulanic Acid: Urine (25-40% unchanged); $T_{1/2}$=1 hr.

NURSING CONSIDERATIONS

Assessment: Assess for history of serious hypersensitivity reactions to other β-lactam antibacterial drugs (eg, PCN, cephalosporins) or other allergens, history of amoxicillin/clavulanate-associated cholestatic jaundice/hepatic dysfunction, hepatic/renal impairment, mononucleosis, phenylketonuria, pregnancy/nursing status, and possible drug interactions.

Monitoring: Monitor for anaphylactic reactions, superinfection, skin rash, CDAD, and other adverse reactions. Periodically monitor renal (especially in elderly) and hepatic function. Monitor PT/INR with oral anticoagulants.

Patient Counseling: Instruct to take each dose with a meal or snack to reduce possibility of GI upset. Counsel that drug only treats bacterial, not viral (eg, common cold), infections. Instruct to take ud; inform that skipping doses or not completing the full course of therapy may decrease effectiveness of the drug and increase resistance of bacteria. Advise to consult physician if severe diarrhea or watery/bloody stools occur (even as late as ≥2 months after treatment). Instruct to use a dosing spoon or medicine dropper when dosing a child with sus, and rinse measuring device after each use. Instruct to discard any unused medicine.

Administration: Oral route. May be taken without regard to meal; take at start of a meal to reduce GI intolerance. (Sus) Shake well before use. Refer to PI for mixing directions. **Storage:** ≤25°C (77°F). Reconstituted Sus: Refrigerate; discard after 10 days.

AUGMENTIN XR   RX
clavulanate potassium - amoxicillin (Dr. Reddy's)

THERAPEUTIC CLASS: Aminopenicillin/beta lactamase inhibitor

INDICATIONS: Treatment of community-acquired pneumonia (CAP) or acute bacterial sinusitis due to confirmed or suspected β-lactamase-producing pathogens and *Streptococcus pneumoniae* with reduced susceptibility to penicillin (PCN).

DOSAGE: *Adults:* Sinusitis: 2 tabs q12h for 10 days. CAP: 2 tabs q12h for 7-10 days. Take at the start of a meal.
Pediatrics: ≥40kg (Able to Swallow Tab): Sinusitis: 2 tabs q12h for 10 days. CAP: 2 tabs q12h for 7-10 days. Take at the start of a meal.

HOW SUPPLIED: Tab, Extended-Release: (Amoxicillin-Clavulanic Acid) 1000mg-62.5mg* *scored

CONTRAINDICATIONS: Severe renal impairment (CrCl <30mL/min), hemodialysis, history of amoxicillin/clavulanate-associated cholestatic jaundice/hepatic dysfunction.

WARNINGS/PRECAUTIONS: Serious, occasionally fatal, hypersensitivity reactions reported with PCN therapy; d/c if allergic reaction occurs and institute appropriate therapy. *Clostridium difficile*-associated diarrhea (CDAD) reported; d/c if CDAD is suspected or confirmed. Caution with hepatic dysfunction. Avoid with mononucleosis. May result in bacterial resistance with prolonged use or use in the absence of a proven/suspected bacterial infection or a prophylactic indication; take appropriate measures if superinfection develops. May decrease estrogen levels in pregnant women. Lab test interactions may occur. Not recommended to be taken with a high-fat meal.

ADVERSE REACTIONS: Diarrhea, vaginal mycosis.

INTERACTIONS: Probenecid may increase/prolong levels; coadministration not recommended. Abnormal prolongation of PT (increased INR) reported with oral anticoagulants; may require anticoagulant dose adjustment. Allopurinol may increase incidence of rashes. May reduce efficacy of oral contraceptives.

PREGNANCY: Category B, caution in nursing.

MECHANISM OF ACTION: Amoxicillin: Aminopenicillin; semisynthetic antibiotic that binds to penicillin-binding proteins within the bacterial cell wall and inhibits its synthesis. Clavulanate:

β-lactamase inhibitor; possesses ability to inactivate a wide range of β-lactamase enzymes commonly found in microorganisms resistant to PCN and cephalosporins.

PHARMACOKINETICS: Absorption: Well-absorbed. Refer to PI for absorption parameters in adults and pediatric patients. **Distribution:** Plasma protein binding: Amoxicillin (18%), clavulanate (25%). Amoxicillin: Found in breast milk. **Elimination:** Amoxicillin: Urine (60-80% unchanged); $T_{1/2}$=1.3 hrs. Clavulanate: Urine (30-50% unchanged); $T_{1/2}$=1 hr.

NURSING CONSIDERATIONS

Assessment: Assess for history of serious hypersensitivity reactions to other β-lactam antibacterial drugs (eg, PCN, cephalosporins) or other allergens, history of amoxicillin/clavulanate-associated cholestatic jaundice/hepatic dysfunction, hepatic/renal impairment, mononucleosis, pregnancy/nursing status, and possible drug interactions.

Monitoring: Monitor for anaphylactic reactions, hepatic toxicity, superinfection, skin rash, diarrhea, CDAD, and other adverse reactions. Monitor PT/INR with oral anticoagulants. Monitor renal function in elderly. Monitor renal, hepatic, and hematopoietic functions with prolonged use.

Patient Counseling: Instruct to take q12h with a meal or snack to reduce possibility of GI upset. Advise to consult physician if severe diarrhea or watery/bloody stools occur (even as late as ≥2 months after treatment). Instruct to take ud; skipping doses or not completing the full course of therapy may decrease effectiveness of the drug and increase resistance of bacteria. Instruct to discard any unused medicine.

Administration: Oral route. Take at the start of a meal. **Storage:** ≤25°C (77°F).

AVALIDE   RX
hydrochlorothiazide - irbesartan (Sanofi-Aventis)

> D/C when pregnancy is detected. Drugs that act directly on the renin-angiotensin system (RAS) can cause injury and death to the developing fetus.

THERAPEUTIC CLASS: Angiotensin II receptor antagonist/thiazide diuretic

INDICATIONS: Treatment of HTN. May be used in patients whose BP is not adequately controlled on monotherapy. May also be used as initial therapy in patients likely to need multiple drugs to achieve BP goals.

DOSAGE: *Adults:* May be administered with other antihypertensive agents. Initial Therapy: 150mg-12.5mg qd. Titrate: May increase after 1-2 weeks of therapy. Max: 300mg-25mg qd. Add-On Therapy: Use if not controlled on monotherapy with irbesartan or HCTZ. Recommended doses in order of increasing mean effect are 150mg-12.5mg, 300mg-12.5mg, and 300mg-25mg. Replacement Therapy: May substitute for titrated components.

HOW SUPPLIED: Tab: (Irbesartan-HCTZ) 150mg-12.5mg, 300mg-12.5mg

CONTRAINDICATIONS: Anuria, sulfonamide-derived drug hypersensitivity. Coadministration with aliskiren in patients with diabetes.

WARNINGS/PRECAUTIONS: Not for initial therapy with intravascular volume depletion. Not recommended with severe renal impairment (CrCl ≤30mL/min). Symptomatic hypotension may occur in intravascular volume- or Na$^+$-depleted patients (eg, patients treated vigorously with diuretics or on dialysis); correct volume depletion before therapy. Hypokalemia and hyperkalemia reported; monitor serum electrolytes periodically. Irbesartan: May increase BUN and SrCr levels in patients with renal artery stenosis. Oliguria and/or progressive azotemia, and (rarely) acute renal failure and/or death may occur in patients whose renal function is dependent on the renin-angiotensin-aldosterone system activity (eg, severe congestive heart failure [CHF]). HCTZ: May cause hypersensitivity reactions, exacerbation or activation of systemic lupus erythematosus (SLE), hyponatremia, hypomagnesemia, and hyperuricemia or precipitation of frank gout. May alter glucose tolerance and increase cholesterol, TG, and Ca^{2+} levels. D/C before testing for parathyroid function. May cause idiosyncratic reaction, resulting in transient myopia and acute angle-closure glaucoma; d/c as rapidly as possible. May enhance effects in postsympathectomy patients. Caution with hepatic impairment or progressive liver disease; may precipitate hepatic coma. May precipitate azotemia in patients with renal disease.

ADVERSE REACTIONS: Dizziness, hypokalemia, fatigue, musculoskeletal pain, influenza, edema, N/V, headache.

INTERACTIONS: See Contraindications. NSAIDs, including selective COX-2 inhibitors, may decrease effects of diuretics and angiotensin II receptor antagonists and may deteriorate renal function. Irbesartan: Dual blockade of the RAS is associated with increased risks of hypotension, hyperkalemia, and changes in renal function (including acute renal failure); closely monitor BP, renal function, and electrolytes with concomitant agents that also affect the RAS. Avoid with aliskiren in patients with renal impairment (GFR <60mL/min). Concomitant use with K$^+$-sparing diuretics, K$^+$ supplements, or salt substitutes containing K$^+$ may increase serum K$^+$. HCTZ: Alcohol, barbiturates, and narcotics may potentiate orthostatic hypotension. Dosage adjustment of antidiabetic drugs may be required. Anionic exchange resins (eg, cholestyramine or colestipol) may impair absorption; take at least 1 hr before or 4 hrs after these medications. Additive effect or potentiation with other antihypertensive drugs. Corticosteroids and adrenocorticotropic hormone may intensify electrolyte depletion, particularly hypokalemia. May decrease response to pressor amines (eg, norepinephrine). May increase responsiveness to nondepolarizing skeletal muscle relaxants (eg, tubocurarine). Increased risk of lithium toxicity; avoid concurrent use. Risk of symptomatic hyponatremia with carbamazepine; monitor serum electrolytes.

PREGNANCY: Category D, not for use in nursing.

MECHANISM OF ACTION: Irbesartan: Angiotensin II receptor antagonist; blocks the vasoconstrictor and aldosterone-secreting effects of angiotensin II by selectively binding to the AT_1 angiotensin II receptor. HCTZ: Thiazide diuretic; not established. Affects renal tubular mechanisms of electrolyte reabsorption, directly increasing Na^+ and Cl^- excretion in approximately equivalent amounts, and indirectly reducing plasma volume.

PHARMACOKINETICS: Absorption: Irbesartan: Rapid and complete. Absolute bioavailability (60-80%); T_{max}=1.5-2 hrs. **Distribution:** Irbesartan: V_d=53-93L; plasma protein binding (90%). HCTZ: Crosses placenta; found in breast milk. **Metabolism:** Irbesartan: Oxidation by CYP2C9 and glucuronide conjugation. **Elimination:** Irbesartan: Urine (20%), feces; $T_{1/2}$=11-15 hrs. HCTZ: Kidney (at least 61%, unchanged); $T_{1/2}$=5.6-14.8 hrs.

NURSING CONSIDERATIONS

Assessment: Assess for hypersensitivity to drug and its components, anuria, sulfonamide-derived drug hypersensitivity, diabetes, history of penicillin allergy, volume/salt depletion, SLE, CHF, renal/hepatic function, postsympathectomy status, renal artery stenosis, pregnancy/nursing status, and possible drug interactions.

Monitoring: Monitor for hypersensitivity reactions, exacerbation/activation of SLE, precipitation of gout, idiosyncratic reaction, decreased visual acuity, ocular pain, and other adverse reactions. Monitor BP, serum electrolytes, cholesterol and TG levels, and hepatic/renal function.

Patient Counseling: Inform of potential risks if exposure occurs during pregnancy and of treatment options in women planning to become pregnant. Instruct to report pregnancies to physician as soon as possible. Inform that lightheadedness may occur, especially during 1st days of use; instruct to d/c use and contact physician if fainting occurs. Inform that dehydration, which may occur with excessive sweating, diarrhea, vomiting, and not drinking enough liquids, may lower BP too much and lead to lightheadedness and possibly fainting.

Administration: Oral route. Take with or without food. **Storage:** 25°C (77°F); excursions permitted to 15-30°C (59-86°F).

AVANDAMET   RX
metformin HCl - rosiglitazone maleate (GlaxoSmithKline)

> Thiazolidinediones cause or exacerbate congestive heart failure (CHF) in some patients. After initiation and dose increases, observe for signs and symptoms of heart failure (HF) and manage accordingly; consider discontinuation or dose reduction. Not recommended in patients with symptomatic HF. Contraindicated with established NYHA Class III or IV HF. Meta-analysis showed association with increased risk of myocardial infarction (MI). Lactic acidosis reported due to metformin accumulation (rare); d/c if suspected. Available only through a restricted distribution program called AVANDIA-Rosiglitazone Medicines Access Program.

THERAPEUTIC CLASS: Biguanide/thiazolidinedione

INDICATIONS: Adjunct to diet and exercise to improve glycemic control when treatment with both rosiglitazone and metformin is appropriate in adults with type 2 diabetes mellitus (DM) already taking rosiglitazone, or not taking rosiglitazone and unable to achieve glycemic control on other diabetes medication, and have decided not to take pioglitazone or pioglitazone-containing products upon consultation.

DOSAGE: *Adults:* Take in divided doses with meals. Initial: Take rosiglitazone component at lowest recommended dose. Switching From Prior Metformin Therapy of 1000mg/day: Initial: 2mg-500mg tab bid. Prior Metformin Therapy of 2000mg/day: Initial: 2mg-1000mg tab bid. Prior Rosiglitazone Therapy of 4mg/day: Initial: 2mg-500mg tab bid. Prior Rosiglitazone Therapy of 8mg/day: 4mg-500mg tab bid. Titrate: May increase by increments of 4mg rosiglitazone and/or 500mg metformin. After increasing metformin, titrate if inadequate after 1-2 weeks. After increasing rosiglitazone, titrate if inadequate after 8-12 weeks. Max: 8mg-2000mg/day. Elderly: Conservative dosing. Elderly/Debilitated/Malnourished: Do not titrate to max dose.

HOW SUPPLIED: Tab: (Rosiglitazone-Metformin) 2mg-500mg, 4mg-500mg, 2mg-1000mg, 4mg-1000mg

CONTRAINDICATIONS: Established NYHA Class III or IV HF, renal disease/dysfunction (SrCr ≥1.5mg/dL [males], ≥1.4mg/dL [females], or abnormal CrCl), acute or chronic metabolic acidosis (eg, diabetic ketoacidosis with or without coma). Temporarily d/c if undergoing radiologic studies involving IV administration of iodinated contrast materials.

WARNINGS/PRECAUTIONS: Not for use in type 1 DM. Initiation with patients experiencing acute coronary event is not recommended; consider discontinuing during the acute phase. Caution with edema and patients at risk for HF. Avoid with active liver disease or if ALT levels >2.5X ULN. May start or continue therapy with caution if ALT levels ≤2.5X ULN; monitor LFTs periodically. D/C if ALT levels remain >3X ULN or if jaundice occurs. Check LFTs if hepatic dysfunction symptoms occur. May lose glycemic control with stress; withhold therapy and temporarily administer insulin. Caution in elderly. Metformin: Avoid use in patients ≥80 yrs of age unless renal function is normal. Elderly, debilitated/malnourished, with adrenal/pituitary insufficiency, or alcohol intoxication may have increased susceptibility to hypoglycemia. Rosiglitazone: Increased risk of cardiovascular events with CHF NYHA Class I and II. Dose-related edema and weight gain reported. Macular edema reported; refer to an ophthalmologist if visual symptoms develop. Increased incidence of bone fracture; risk appears higher in females than males. May decrease Hgb and Hct. Decreased serum vitamin B12 levels reported. Ovulation in premenopausal anovulatory patients may occur, resulting in an increased risk of pregnancy; adequate contraception should be recommended. Review benefits of continued therapy if menstrual dysfunction occurs.

ADVERSE REACTIONS: CHF, lactic acidosis, upper respiratory tract infection, headache, back pain, fatigue, sinusitis, diarrhea, viral infection, arthralgia, anemia.

INTERACTIONS: See Contraindications. Avoid use with insulin. Metformin: Alcohol may potentiate effect on lactate metabolism. Caution with drugs that may affect renal function or result in significant hemodynamic change or may interfere with the disposition of metformin (eg, cationic drugs eliminated by renal tubular secretion). Hypoglycemia may occur with concomitant use of hypoglycemic agents or ethanol. May be difficult to recognize hypoglycemia with concomitant use of β-adrenergic blocking drugs. Increased levels with furosemide, nifedipine, cimetidine, and cationic drugs (eg, digoxin, amiloride, procainamide, quinidine, etc.). Observe for loss of glycemic control with thiazides and other diuretics, corticosteroids, phenothiazines, thyroid products, estrogens, oral contraceptives, phenytoin, nicotinic acid, sympathomimetics, calcium channel blockers, and isoniazid. May decrease furosemide levels. Rosiglitazone: Higher incidence of MI with ramipril. Dose-related weight gain and risk of hypoglycemia with other hypoglycemic agents. Increased levels with CYP2C8 inhibitors (eg, gemfibrozil). Decreased levels with CYP2C8 inducers (eg, rifampin).

PREGNANCY: Category C, not for use in nursing.

MECHANISM OF ACTION: Rosiglitazone: Thiazolidinedione; insulin-sensitizing agent that enhances peripheral glucose utilization. Metformin: Biguanide; decreases hepatic glucose production, decreases intestinal absorption of glucose, and increases peripheral glucose uptake and utilization.

PHARMACOKINETICS: Absorption: Rosiglitazone: Absolute bioavailability (99%). (4mg) AUC_{0-inf}=1442ng•h/mL; C_{max}=242ng/mL; T_{max}=0.95 hr. Metformin: (500mg) Absolute bioavailability (50-60%) (fasted); AUC_{0-inf}=7116ng•h/mL; C_{max}=1106ng/mL; T_{max}=2.97 hrs. **Distribution:** Rosiglitazone: V_d=17.6L; plasma protein binding (99.8%); crosses the placenta. Metformin: (850mg) V_d=654L. **Metabolism:** Extensive by N-demethylation and hydroxylation, then conjugation with sulfate and glucuronic acid; CYP2C8 (major), 2C9 (minor). **Elimination:** Rosiglitazone: Urine (64%), feces (23%); $T_{1/2}$=3-4 hrs. Metformin: Urine (90%); $T_{1/2}$=6.2 hrs (plasma), 17.6 hrs (blood).

NURSING CONSIDERATIONS

Assessment: Assess for renal/hepatic dysfunction, CHF, hypoxemia, dehydration, active liver disease, acute coronary event, edema, risk factors for HF, pregnancy/nursing status, and possible drug interactions. Obtain baseline FPG, HbA1c, renal function, LFTs, and hematological parameters.

Monitoring: Monitor for signs/symptoms of lactic acidosis, HF, MI, acute coronary event, edema, weight gain, hepatic function, macular edema, bone fractures, hematologic changes, hypoglycemia, menstrual function. Monitor renal function, especially in elderly, at least annually. Monitor vitamin B12 levels in patients predisposed to develop subnormal vitamin B12 levels. Periodically monitor LFTs, FPG, HbA1c, CBC, bone health, and hematologic parameters. Perform periodic eye exams in DM.

Patient Counseling: Inform about benefits/risks of therapy and that patient must be enrolled in the AVANDIA-Rosiglitazone Medicines Access Program. Inform on importance of adherence to dietary instructions and regular testing of blood glucose, HbA1c, renal function, and hematologic parameters. Advise to d/c and notify physician if unexplained hyperventilation, myalgia, malaise, unusual somnolence, or nonspecific symptoms occur. Instuct to immediately report rapid increase in weight or edema, or SOB and to avoid excessive alcohol intake. Inform that the drug is not recommended with symptomatic HF and patients taking insulin.

Administration: Oral route. **Storage:** 25°C (77°F); excursions permitted to 15-30°C (59-86°F).

AVANDARYL   RX
rosiglitazone maleate - glimepiride (GlaxoSmithKline)

> Thiazolidinediones cause or exacerbate congestive heart failure (CHF) in some patients. After initiation and dose increases, observe for signs and symptoms of heart failure (HF) and manage accordingly; consider discontinuation or dose reduction. Not recommended in patients with symptomatic HF. Contraindicated with established NYHA Class III or IV HF. Meta-analysis has shown to be associated with increased risk of myocardial infarction (MI). Available only through a restricted distribution program called AVANDIA-Rosiglitazone Medicines Access Program.

THERAPEUTIC CLASS: Sulfonylurea/thiazolidinedione

INDICATIONS: Adjunct to diet and exercise to improve glycemic control when treatment with both rosiglitazone and glimepiride is appropriate in adults with type 2 diabetes mellitus (DM) who are already taking rosiglitazone or not taking rosiglitazone and unable to achieve glycemic control on other diabetes medication, and have decided not to take pioglitazone or pioglitazone-containing products upon consultation.

DOSAGE: *Adults:* Initial: 4mg-1mg qd with 1st meal of day. Already Treated with Sulfonylurea or Rosiglitazone: Initial: 4mg-2mg qd. Switching from Prior Combination Therapy as Separate Tab: Start with dose of each component already being taken. Switching from Current Rosiglitazone Monotherapy: Increase glimepiride component in no >2mg increments if inadequately controlled after 1-2 weeks. After an increase in glimepiride component, titrate Avandaryl if inadequately controlled after 1-2 weeks. Switching from Current Sulfonylurea Monotherapy: Titrate rosiglitazone component if inadequately controlled after 8-12 weeks. After an increase in rosiglitazone component, titrate Avandaryl if inadequately controlled after 2-3 months. Max: 8mg-4mg/day. Elderly/Debilitated/Malnourished/Renal, Hepatic, or Adrenal Insufficiency: Initial: 4mg-1mg qd. Titrate carefully. Consider dose reduction of glimepiride component if hypoglycemia occurs during up-titration or maintenance.

HOW SUPPLIED: Tab: (Rosiglitazone-Glimepiride) 4mg-1mg, 4mg-2mg, 4mg-4mg, 8mg-2mg, 8mg-4mg

CONTRAINDICATIONS: Established NYHA Class III or IV HF.

WARNINGS/PRECAUTIONS: Not for use in type 1 DM or for treatment of diabetic ketoacidosis. Avoid with active liver disease or if ALT levels >2.5X ULN. Caution with mildly elevated liver enzymes (ALT levels ≤2.5X ULN). D/C if ALT levels remain >3X ULN on therapy or if jaundice occurs. Check LFTs if hepatic dysfunction symptoms occur. May lose glycemic control with stress; withhold therapy and temporarily administer insulin. Rosiglitazone: Increased risk of cardiovascular (CV) events with CHF NYHA Class I and II. Initiation with patients experiencing acute coronary event is not recommended; consider discontinuing during the acute phase. Caution with edema and patients at risk for HF. Edema and weight gain reported. Macular edema reported; refer to an ophthalmologist if visual symptoms develop. Increased incidence of bone fracture; risk appears higher in females than in males. May decrease Hgb and Hct. Ovulation in premenopausal anovulatory patients may occur, resulting in an increased risk of pregnancy; adequate contraception should be recommended. Review benefits of continued therapy if menstrual dysfunction occurs. Glimepiride: Increased risk of CV mortality. Hypoglycemia may be masked in elderly; risk in debilitated, malnourished, or with adrenal, pituitary, renal or hepatic insufficiency. May elevate liver enzyme levels in rare cases. Hemolytic anemia reported; caution with G6PD deficiency.

ADVERSE REACTIONS: Headache, hypoglycemia, anemia. (Rosiglitazone) CHF, upper respiratory tract infection, nasopharyngitis, HTN, back pain, arthralgia. (Glimepiride) Dizziness, asthenia, nausea.

INTERACTIONS: Severe hypoglycemia with oral miconazole. Avoid use with insulin. Glimepiride: Hypoglycemia may be masked with β-blockers and other sympatholytic agents. Increased hypoglycemia risk with alcohol or use of >1 glucose-lowering drug. Observe for loss of glycemic control with thiazides and other diuretics, corticosteroids, phenothiazines, thyroid products, estrogens, oral contraceptives, phenytoin, nicotinic acid, sympathomimetics, and isoniazid. Hypoglycemic action may be potentiated by certain drugs, including NSAIDs and other drugs that are highly protein bound (eg, salicylates, sulfonamides, chloramphenicol, coumarins, probenecid, MAOIs, β-blockers). Potential interactions with inhibitors (eg, fluconazole), inducers (eg, rifampicin), other drugs metabolized by CYP2C9 (eg, phenytoin, ibuprofen, mefenamic acid). Changes in levels with aspirin and propranolol. Decrease in the pharmacodynamic response to warfarin. Rosiglitazone: Dose-related weight gain with other hypoglycemic agents. Higher incidence of MI with ramipril. Increased levels with CYP2C8 inhibitors (eg, gemfibrozil). Decreased levels with CYP2C8 inducers (eg, rifampin).

PREGNANCY: Category C, not for use in nursing.

MECHANISM OF ACTION: Glimepiride: Sulfonylurea; stimulates insulin release from functional pancreatic β cells. Rosiglitazone: Thiazolidinedione; insulin-sensitizing agent that acts by enhancing peripheral glucose utilization.

PHARMACOKINETICS: Absorption: Glimepiride: Complete; T_{max}=2-3 hrs; (4mg) C_{max}=151ng/mL; $AUC_{(0-inf, 0-t)}$=1052ng•hr/mL, 944ng•hr/mL. Rosiglitazone: Absolute bioavailability (99%); T_{max}=1 hr; (4mg) C_{max}=257ng/mL; $AUC_{(0-inf, 0-t)}$=1259ng•hr/mL, 1231ng•hr/mL. **Distribution:** Glimepiride: Protein binding (>99.5%). Rosiglitazone: V_d=17.6L; plasma protein binding (99.8%); crosses the placenta. **Metabolism:** Glimepiride: Liver (complete) via oxidative biotransformation; cyclohexyl hydroxy methyl (M1) and carboxyl (M2) derivative (major metabolites); CYP2C9. Rosiglitazone: Liver (extensive) via N-demethylation and hydroxylation then conjugation with sulfate and glucuronic acid; CYP2C8 (major), 2C9 (minor). **Elimination:** Glimepiride: Urine (60%, 80-90% major metabolites), feces (40%, 70% major metabolites). Rosiglitazone: Urine (64%), feces (23%); $T_{1/2}$=3-4 hrs.

NURSING CONSIDERATIONS

Assessment: Assess for HF, active liver disease, acute coronary event, edema, G6PD deficiency, premenopausal anovulation, risk factors for HF, pregnancy/nursing status, and for possible drug interactions. Assess baseline renal function, LFTs, CBC, and bone health.

Monitoring: Monitor for adverse events related to fluid retention during dose increases. Periodically monitor LFTs, FPG, HbA1c, CBC, and bone health. Monitor for signs and symptoms of HF, MI, acute coronary event, edema, weight gain, hepatic function, macular edema, bone fractures, hematologic changes, hypoglycemia, hypersensitivity reactions, ovulation in premenopausal anovulatory women, and menstrual function. Perform periodic eye exams. Monitor renal function in elderly.

Patient Counseling: Inform about benefits/risks of therapy and that patient must be enrolled in the AVANDIA-Rosiglitazone Medicines Access Program. Inform about importance of caloric restrictions, weight loss, exercise, and regular testing of blood glucose levels. Advise to immediately report unexplained N/V, anorexia, abdominal pain, fatigue, dark urine, unusual rapid increase in weight or edema, SOB, or other symptoms of HF to physician. Instruct to take drug with 1st meal of the day. Explain to patients and their family members the risks, symptoms, treatment, and conditions that predispose to the development of hypoglycemia.

Administration: Oral route. **Storage:** 25°C (77°F); excursions permitted to 15-30°C (59-86°F).

AVANDIA   RX
rosiglitazone maleate (GlaxoSmithKline)

Thiazolidinediones, including rosiglitazone, cause or exacerbate congestive heart failure (CHF) in some patients. After initiation and dose increases, observe for signs and symptoms of heart failure (HF) and manage accordingly; consider discontinuation or dose reduction. Not recommended in patients with symptomatic HF. Contraindicated with established NYHA Class III or IV HF. Meta-analysis has shown to be associated with increased risk of myocardial infarction (MI). Available only through a restricted distribution program called AVANDIA-Rosiglitazone Medicines Access Program.

THERAPEUTIC CLASS: Thiazolidinedione

INDICATIONS: Adjunct to diet and exercise to improve glycemic control in adults with type 2 diabetes mellitus (DM) who either are already taking rosiglitazone or not already taking rosiglitazone and have inadequate glycemic control on other diabetes medications, and have decided not to take pioglitazone upon consultation.

DOSAGE: *Adults:* Initial: 4mg as qd dose or in 2 divided doses. Titrate: May increase to 8mg/day after 8-12 weeks if response to treatment is inadequate. Max: 8mg/day.

HOW SUPPLIED: Tab: 2mg, 4mg, 8mg

CONTRAINDICATIONS: Established NYHA Class III or IV HF.

WARNINGS/PRECAUTIONS: Avoid with type 1 DM or diabetic ketoacidosis. Increased risk of cardiovascular events with CHF NYHA Class I and II. Initiation not recommended if experiencing an acute coronary event; consider discontinuing therapy during the acute phase. Caution with edema and patients at risk for HF. Edema and weight gain reported. Monitor LFTs prior to initiation of and during therapy. Avoid with active liver disease or if ALT levels >2.5X ULN. Caution if liver enzymes are mildly elevated (ALT levels ≤2.5X ULN). D/C if ALT levels remain >3X ULN while on therapy or if jaundice occurs. Check LFTs if hepatic dysfunction symptoms occur. Macular edema reported; refer to an ophthalmologist if visual symptoms develop. Increased incidence of bone fracture; risk appears higher in females than in males. Decreases in Hgb and Hct reported. Perform periodic measurements of FPG and HbA1c to monitor therapeutic response. May cause ovulation in premenopausal anovulatory patients, resulting in an increased risk of pregnancy. Review benefits of continued therapy if menstrual dysfunction occurs.

ADVERSE REACTIONS: CHF, upper respiratory tract infection, headache, back pain, hyperglycemia, fatigue, sinusitis, edema.

INTERACTIONS: Risk of hypoglycemia when used with other hypoglycemic agents. May increase levels with CYP2C8 inhibitors (eg, gemfibrozil). May decrease levels with CYP2C8 inducers (eg, rifampin). Coadministration with insulin is not recommended; may increase risk of CHF and MI. Higher incidence of MI reported with ramipril.

PREGNANCY: Category C, not for use in nursing.

MECHANISM OF ACTION: Thiazolidinedione; improves insulin sensitivity.

PHARMACOKINETICS: Absorption: Administration of variable doses resulted in different parameters. Absolute bioavailability (99%); T_{max}=1 hr. **Distribution:** V_d=17.6L; plasma protein binding (99.8%); crosses the placenta. **Metabolism:** N-demethylation and hydroxylation followed by conjugation (extensive); CYP2C8 (major), 2C9 (minor); **Elimination:** Urine (64%), feces (23%); $T_{1/2}$=3-4 hrs.

NURSING CONSIDERATIONS

Assessment: Assess for CHF or risk factors for HF, symptomatic HF, type 1 DM, diabetic ketoacidosis, presence of an acute coronary event, hepatic dysfunction, edema, pregnancy/nursing status, and possible drug interactions. Assess baseline LFTs, CBC, and bone health.

Monitoring: Monitor for signs/symptoms of HF, MI, edema, weight gain, hepatic dysfunction, macular edema, bone fractures, hematologic changes, ovulation in premenopausal anovulatory women, and menstrual dysfunction. Perform periodic eye exams. Periodically monitor LFTs, fasting blood glucose, HbA1c, CBC, and bone health.

Patient Counseling: Advise of risks and benefits of therapy. Inform that drug may be taken with or without food. Inform about importance of caloric restriction, weight loss, exercise, and regular testing of blood glucose levels. Instruct to immediately report to physician any symptoms of HF or hepatic dysfunction. Inform about risk of hypoglycemia, its symptoms and treatment, and conditions that predispose to its development. Advise that ovulation may occur in some premenopausal anovulatory women and adequate contraception should be used.

Administration: Oral route. **Storage:** 25°C (77°F); excursions permitted to 15-30°C (59-86°F).

AVAPRO   RX
irbesartan (Sanofi-Aventis)

> D/C when pregnancy is detected. Drugs that act directly on the renin-angiotensin system (RAS) can cause injury/death to the developing fetus.

THERAPEUTIC CLASS: Angiotensin II receptor antagonist

INDICATIONS: Treatment of HTN alone or in combination with other antihypertensives. Treatment of diabetic nephropathy with an elevated SrCr and proteinuria (>300mg/day) in patients with type 2 diabetes and HTN.

DOSAGE: *Adults:* HTN: Initial: 150mg qd. Titrate: May increase to 300mg qd. A low dose diuretic may be added if BP is not controlled. Max: 300mg qd. Intravascular Volume/Salt Depletion: Initial: 75mg qd. Nephropathy: Maint: 300mg qd.

HOW SUPPLIED: Tab: 75mg, 150mg, 300mg

CONTRAINDICATIONS: Coadministration with aliskiren in patients with diabetes.

WARNINGS/PRECAUTIONS: Symptomatic hypotension may occur in volume- or salt-depleted patients (eg, patients treated vigorously with diuretics or on dialysis); correct volume depletion prior to therapy or use low starting dose. May cause changes in renal function. Oliguria and/or progressive azotemia and (rarely) acute renal failure and/or death may occur in patients whose renal function may depend on the renin-angiotensin-aldosterone system (eg, severe congestive heart failure [CHF]). Increased SrCr or BUN may occur in patients with renal artery stenosis.

ADVERSE REACTIONS: Hyperkalemia, dizziness, orthostatic dizziness, orthostatic hypotension, fatigue, diarrhea, dyspepsia, heartburn.

INTERACTIONS: See Contraindications. Dual blockade of the RAS is associated with increased risks of hypotension, hyperkalemia, and changes in renal function (including acute renal failure); closely monitor BP, renal function, and electrolytes with concomitant agents that also affect the RAS. Avoid with aliskiren in patients with renal impairment (GFR <60mL/min). CYP2C9 substrates/inhibitors sulphenazole, tolbutamide, and nifedipine significantly inhibited metabolism in vitro. Increased serum K+ with K+-sparing diuretics, K+ supplements, or salt substitutes containing K+. May deteriorate renal function and attenuate antihypertensive effect with NSAIDs, including selective COX-2 inhibitors; monitor renal function periodically.

PREGNANCY: Category D, not for use in nursing.

MECHANISM OF ACTION: Angiotensin II receptor antagonist; blocks the vasoconstrictor and aldosterone-secreting effects of angiotensin II by selectively binding to the AT_1 angiotensin II receptor.

PHARMACOKINETICS: Absorption: Rapid and complete. Absolute bioavailability (60-80%); T_{max}=1.5-2 hrs. **Distribution:** V_d=53-93L; plasma protein binding (90%). **Metabolism:** CYP2C9 (oxidation), glucuronide conjugation. **Elimination:** Urine (20%), feces; $T_{1/2}$=11-15 hrs.

NURSING CONSIDERATIONS

Assessment: Assess for intravascular volume/salt depletion, renal impairment, CHF, renal artery stenosis, diabetes, hypersensitivity, pregnancy/nursing status, and possible drug interactions.

Monitoring: Monitor for signs/symptoms of hypotension, hyperkalemia, and other adverse reactions. Monitor BP and renal function periodically.

Patient Counseling: Inform about the consequences of exposure during pregnancy in females of childbearing age. Discuss treatment options with women planning to become pregnant. Instruct to report pregnancies to physician as soon as possible.

Administration: Oral route. Take with or without food. **Storage:** 25°C (77°F); excursions permitted to 15-30°C (59-86°F).

AVASTIN   RX
bevacizumab (Genentech)

GI perforation reported; d/c with GI perforation. Increased incidence of wound-healing and surgical complications; d/c at least 28 days prior to elective surgery. Do not initiate for at least 28 days after surgery and until surgical wound is fully healed. D/C with wound dehiscence. Severe or fatal hemorrhage, including hemoptysis, GI bleeding, CNS hemorrhage, epistaxis, and vaginal bleeding have occurred; avoid with serious hemorrhage or recent hemoptysis.

THERAPEUTIC CLASS: Vascular endothelial growth factor (VEGF) inhibitor

INDICATIONS: 1st- or 2nd-line treatment of metastatic colorectal cancer (mCRC) in combination with IV 5-fluorouracil (5-FU)-based chemotherapy. Second-line treatment of patients with mCRC, in combination with fluoropyrimidine-irinotecan- or fluoropyrimidine-oxaliplatin-based chemotherapy, who have progressed on a 1st-line bevacizumab-containing regimen. First-line treatment of unresectable, locally advanced, recurrent, or metastatic nonsquamous non-small cell lung cancer (NSCLC) in combination with carboplatin and paclitaxel. Treatment of glioblastoma with progressive disease in adults following prior therapy as a single agent. Treatment of metastatic renal cell carcinoma (mRCC) in combination with interferon alfa.

DOSAGE: *Adults:* Administer as an IV infusion. Continue treatment until disease progression or unacceptable toxicity. mCRC: In Combination with Bolus-IFL: Usual: 5mg/kg every 2 weeks. In Combination with FOLFOX4: Usual: 10mg/kg every 2 weeks. In Combination with Fluoropyrimidine-Irinotecan or Fluoropyrimidine-Oxaliplatin-Based Chemotherapy: Usual: 5mg/kg every 2 weeks or 7.5mg/kg every 3 weeks. NSCLC: Usual: 15mg/kg every 3 weeks (with carboplatin and paclitaxel). Glioblastoma: Usual: 10mg/kg every 2 weeks. mRCC: Usual: 10mg/kg every 2 weeks (with interferon alfa).

HOW SUPPLIED: Inj: 100mg/4mL, 400mg/16mL

WARNINGS/PRECAUTIONS: Not indicated for adjuvant treatment of colon cancer. D/C in patients with wound-healing complications requiring medical intervention. Necrotizing fasciitis, usually secondary to wound-healing complications, GI perforation, or fistula formation reported; d/c therapy if necrotizing fasciitis develops. D/C if hemorrhage occurs. Serious and fatal non-GI fistula formation involving tracheoesophageal, bronchopleural, biliary, vaginal, renal, and bladder sites may occur; d/c with fistula formation involving an internal organ. Arterial thromboembolic events (ATEs) (eg, cerebral infarction, transient ischemic attacks, myocardial infarction, angina) reported; increased risk with history of arterial thromboembolism, diabetes, or age >65 yrs. D/C if severe ATE develops. Increased incidence of severe HTN; d/c if hypertensive crisis or hypertensive encephalopathy occurs and temporarily suspend for severe uncontrolled HTN. Reversible posterior leukoencephalopathy syndrome (RPLS) reported; d/c if RPLS develops. Monitor for the development or worsening of proteinuria with serial urinalyses by dipstick urine analysis. Suspend therapy for ≥2g proteinuria/24 hrs and resume when proteinuria is <2g/24 hrs. D/C in patients with nephrotic syndrome. Infusion reactions (eg, HTN, hypertensive crisis with neurologic signs/symptoms, wheezing, oxygen desaturation, Grade 3 hypersensitivity, chest pain, headaches, rigors, diaphoresis) reported; stop infusion if a severe infusion reaction occurs and administer appropriate medical therapy. Increases the risk of ovarian failure and may impair fertility.

ADVERSE REACTIONS: GI perforation, wound-healing and surgical complications, hemorrhage, epistaxis, headache, HTN, rhinitis, proteinuria, taste alteration, dry skin, rectal hemorrhage, lacrimation disorder, back pain, exfoliative dermatitis, diarrhea.

INTERACTIONS: May decrease paclitaxel exposure with paclitaxel/carboplatin.

PREGNANCY: Category C, not for use in nursing.

MECHANISM OF ACTION: VEGF inhibitor; binds VEGF and prevents the interaction of VEGF to its receptors (Flt-1, KDR) on the surface of endothelial cells. The interaction of VEGF with its receptors leads to endothelial cell proliferation and new blood vessel formation.

PHARMACOKINETICS: Elimination: $T_{1/2}$=20 days.

NURSING CONSIDERATIONS

Assessment: Assess for recent hemoptysis, serious hemorrhage, HTN, proteinuria, history of arterial thromboembolism, diabetes, pregnancy/nursing status, and possible drug interactions. Assess for prior surgical history and for any scheduled elective surgeries.

Monitoring: Monitor for GI perforation, fistula formation, wound-healing complications, hemorrhage, ATE, hypertensive crisis, hypertensive encephalopathy, RPLS, nephrotic syndrome, severe infusion reactions, and other adverse reactions. Monitor BP every 2-3 weeks, treat with appropriate anti-hypertensive therapy and monitor BP regularly; continue to monitor BP at regular intervals with drug-induced or -exacerbated HTN after drug discontinuation. Monitor for proteinuria by dipstick urine analysis for the development or worsening of proteinuria with serial urinalyses.

Patient Counseling: Advise to undergo routine BP monitoring and contact physician if BP is elevated. Instruct to immediately seek medical attention if unusual bleeding, high fever, rigors, sudden onset of worsening neurological function, persistent/severe abdominal pain, severe constipation, or vomiting occurs. Inform of pregnancy risks and the need to continue adequate contraception for at least 6 months after therapy. Inform of the increased risk for wound healing complications, ovarian failure, and ATE.

Administration: IV route. Do not administer as an IV push/bolus; administer only as an IV infusion. First Infusion: Give over 90 min. Subsequent Infusions: Give 2nd infusion over 60 min if 1st infusion is tolerated. Give all subsequent infusions over 30 min if infusion over 60 min is tolerated. Refer to PI for further preparation and administration instructions. **Storage:** 2-8°C (36-46°F). Protect from light. Do not freeze or shake. Diluted Sol: 2-8°C (36-46°F) for up to 8 hrs. Store in original carton until time of use.

AVELOX   RX
moxifloxacin HCl (Merck)

> Fluoroquinolones are associated with an increased risk of tendinitis and tendon rupture in all ages. Risk is further increased in patients >60 yrs of age, patients taking corticosteroids, and with kidney, heart, or lung transplants. May exacerbate muscle weakness with myasthenia gravis; avoid in patients with known history of myasthenia gravis.

THERAPEUTIC CLASS: Fluoroquinolone

INDICATIONS: Treatment of acute bacterial sinusitis, acute bacterial exacerbation of chronic bronchitis (ABECB), community-acquired pneumonia (CAP), uncomplicated and complicated skin and skin structure infections (SSSIs), and complicated intra-abdominal infections including polymicrobial infections (eg, abscess) caused by susceptible isolates of microorganisms, in adults ≥18 yrs of age.

DOSAGE: Adults: ≥18 Yrs: Sinusitis: 400mg PO/IV q24h for 10 days. ABECB: 400mg PO/IV q24h for 5 days. CAP: 400mg PO/IV q24h for 7-14 days. Uncomplicated SSSIs: 400mg PO/IV q24h for 7 days. Complicated SSSIs: 400mg PO/IV q24h for 7-21 days. Complicated Intra-Abdominal Infections: 400mg PO/IV q24h for 5-14 days. Infuse IV over 60 min.

HOW SUPPLIED: Inj: 400mg/250mL; Tab: 400mg

WARNINGS/PRECAUTIONS: D/C if pain, swelling, inflammation, or rupture of a tendon occurs. May prolong QT interval; avoid with QT interval prolongation or uncorrected hypokalemia. Caution with ongoing proarrhythmic conditions (eg, clinically significant bradycardia, acute myocardial ischemia) and liver cirrhosis. Serious anaphylactic reactions and other serious and sometimes fatal events reported; d/c immediately and institute supportive measures if skin rash, jaundice, or any other signs of hypersensitivity occur. Convulsions, increased intracranial pressure (including pseudotumor cerebri), and other CNS events reported; d/c and institute appropriate measures if CNS events (eg, dizziness, confusion, tremors, hallucinations, depression, and rarely, suicidal thoughts/acts) occur. Caution with CNS disorders (eg, severe cerebral arteriosclerosis, epilepsy) or risk factors that may predispose to seizures or lower seizure threshold. Clostridium difficile-associated diarrhea (CDAD) reported; d/c if CDAD is suspected or confirmed. Cases of sensory or sensorimotor axonal polyneuropathy, resulting in paresthesias, hypoesthesias, dysesthesias, and weakness reported; d/c if symptoms of peripheral neuropathy occur. May cause photosensitivity/phototoxicity reactions; d/c if phototoxicity occurs. Avoid excessive exposure to sun/UV light. May result in bacterial resistance if used in the absence of a proven/strongly suspected bacterial infection or a prophylactic indication. Caution in elderly and in patients with hepatic impairment.

ADVERSE REACTIONS: Tendinitis, tendon rupture, nausea, diarrhea, headache, dizziness.

INTERACTIONS: See Boxed Warning. May prolong QT interval; avoid Class IA (eg, quinidine, procainamide) or Class III (eg, amiodarone, sotalol) antiarrhythmics. Caution with other drugs that prolong the QT interval (eg, cisapride, erythromycin, antipsychotics, TCAs). NSAIDs may increase risk of CNS stimulation and convulsions. May enhance anticoagulant effects of warfarin or its derivatives; monitor PT and INR. (PO) Administration with antacids containing Mg^{2+} or aluminum, sucralfate, metal cations (eg, iron), multivitamins containing iron or zinc, or formulations containing divalent and trivalent cations such as Videx (didanosine) chewable/buffered tabs or the pediatric powder for oral sol, may substantially interfere with absorption and lower systemic concentrations; take at least 4 hrs before or 8 hrs after these agents.

PREGNANCY: Category C, not for use in nursing.

MECHANISM OF ACTION: Fluoroquinolone; inhibits topoisomerase II (DNA gyrase) and topoisomerase IV, which are required for bacterial DNA replication, transcription, repair, and recombination.

PHARMACOKINETICS: Absorption: Administration of variable doses resulted in different parameters. (PO) Well-absorbed; absolute bioavailability (90%). **Distribution:** V_d=1.7-2.7L/kg; plasma protein binding (30-50%). **Metabolism:** Glucuronide and sulfate conjugation. **Elimination:** 45% unchanged; urine (20%), feces (25%). Single dose: $T_{1/2}$=11.5-15.6 hrs (PO), 8.2-15.4 hrs (IV). Multiple doses: $T_{1/2}$=12.7 hrs (PO), 14.8 hrs (IV).

NURSING CONSIDERATIONS

Assessment: Assess for risk factors for developing tendinitis and tendon rupture, history of myasthenia gravis, drug hypersensitivity, QT interval prolongation, uncorrected hypokalemia, ongoing proarrhythmic conditions, liver cirrhosis, CNS disorders or risk factors that may predispose to seizures or lower seizure threshold, hepatic impairment, pregnancy/nursing status, and possible drug interactions. Obtain baseline culture and susceptibility tests.

Monitoring: Monitor for ECG changes (eg, QT interval prolongation), signs/symptoms of anaphylactic reactions, CNS events, drug resistance, CDAD, peripheral neuropathy, tendon rupture, tendinitis, photosensitivity/phototoxicity reactions, and other adverse reactions. Monitor for muscle weakness in patients with myasthenia gravis. Monitor PT and INR if administered with warfarin or its derivatives.

Patient Counseling: Inform that drug treats only bacterial, not viral (eg, common cold), infections. Instruct to take exactly ud; skipping doses or not completing full course may decrease effectiveness and increase bacterial resistance. Instruct to notify physician if pain, swelling, or inflammation of a tendon, or weakness or inability to move joints occurs; advise to rest and refrain from exercise and to d/c therapy. Instruct to notify physician if experiencing worsening muscle weakness or breathing problems, palpitations or fainting spells, sunburn-like reaction or skin eruption, or if watery and bloody stools (even ≥2 months after last dose) develop. Advise to notify physician of all medications and supplements currently being used. Instruct to inform physician of any personal or family history of QT prolongation, proarrhythmic conditions, convulsions, or psychiatric illness. Instruct to d/c and notify physician if an allergic reaction, skin rash, or symptoms of peripheral neuropathy develop. Inform that drug may cause dizziness, lightheadedness, and vision disorders; instruct to use caution with activities requiring mental alertness or coordination. Advise to minimize or avoid exposure to natural or artificial light (eg, tanning beds or UVA/B treatment).

Administration: Oral, IV routes. (Tab) May take with or without food; drink fluids liberally. Administer at least 4 hrs before or 8 hrs after multivitamins containing iron or zinc, antacids containing Mg^{2+} or aluminum, sucralfate, and Videx (didanosine) chewable/buffered tabs or the pediatric powder for oral sol. (Inj) Avoid rapid or bolus IV infusion. Do not add other IV substances, additives, or other medications to inj or infuse simultaneously through same IV line. Refer to PI for further preparation and administration instructions. **Storage:** 25°C (77°F); excursions permitted to 15-30°C (59-86°F). (Tab) Avoid high humidity. (Inj) Do not refrigerate.

AVIANE   RX
ethinyl estradiol - levonorgestrel (Barr)

Cigarette smoking increases the risk of serious cardiovascular (CV) side effects. This risk increases with age (>35 yrs) and with heavy smoking (≥15 cigarettes/day). Women who use oral contraceptives should be strongly advised not to smoke.

OTHER BRAND NAMES: Orsythia (Qualitest)

THERAPEUTIC CLASS: Estrogen/progestogen combination

INDICATIONS: Prevention of pregnancy.

DOSAGE: *Adults:* 1 tab qd for 28 days, then repeat. Start 1st Sunday after menses begins or on Day 1 of cycle.
Pediatrics: Postpubertal: 1 tab qd for 28 days, then repeat. Start 1st Sunday after menses begins or on Day 1 of cycle.

AVIANE

HOW SUPPLIED: Tab: (Ethinyl Estradiol-Levonorgestrel) 0.02mg-0.1mg

CONTRAINDICATIONS: Thrombophlebitis or history of deep vein thrombophlebitis, presence or history of thromboembolic disorders, presence or history of cerebrovascular or coronary artery disease, valvular heart disease with thrombogenic complications, thrombogenic rhythm disorders, hereditary or acquired thrombophilias, major surgery with prolonged immobilization, uncontrolled HTN, diabetes mellitus (DM) with vascular involvement, headaches with focal neurological symptoms, presence or history of breast cancer, carcinoma of the endometrium or other known or suspected estrogen-dependent neoplasia, undiagnosed abnormal genital bleeding, cholestatic jaundice of pregnancy or jaundice with prior pill use, hepatic adenomas/carcinomas or active liver disease, known/suspected pregnancy.

WARNINGS/PRECAUTIONS: Increased risk of myocardial infarction (MI), vascular disease, thromboembolism, stroke, hepatic neoplasia, and gallbladder disease. Increased risk of morbidity and mortality with certain inherited/acquired thrombophilias, HTN, hyperlipidemia, obesity, DM, and surgery or trauma with increased risk of thrombosis. D/C at least 4 weeks before and for 2 weeks after elective surgery with increased risk of thromboembolism, and during or following prolonged immobilization. Caution with CV disease risk factors. May develop visual changes with contact lens. Retinal thrombosis reported; d/c if unexplained partial/complete loss of vision or other ophthalmic irregularities develop. May cause glucose intolerance, elevated LDL or other lipid abnormalities, or exacerbate migraine headaches. Caution with history of depression; d/c if symptoms recur or worsen. May cause increased BP and fluid retention; d/c if significant BP elevations occur. Breakthrough bleeding and spotting reported; rule out malignancies or pregnancy. Diarrhea and/or vomiting may reduce hormone absorption, resulting in decreased serum concentrations. Not indicated for use before menarche. May affect certain endocrine, LFTs, and blood components in lab tests. Perform periodic history/physical exam; monitor patients with a strong family history of breast cancer.

ADVERSE REACTIONS: N/V, breakthrough bleeding, spotting, amenorrhea, migraine, depression, vaginal candidiasis, edema, weight changes, melasma, breast changes, changes in cervical erosion and secretion, allergic rash.

INTERACTIONS: Reduced effects result in pregnancy or breakthrough bleeding with antibiotics, anticonvulsants, and other drugs that increase the metabolism of contraceptive steroids (eg, rifampin, rifabutin, barbiturates, primidone, phenylbutazone, phenytoin, dexamethasone, carbamazepine, felbamate, oxcarbazepine, topiramate, griseofulvin, modafinil, ampicillin, other penicillins, tetracyclines, St. John's wort). Anti-HIV protease inhibitors may increase or decrease plasma levels. Atorvastatin, ascorbic acid, acetaminophen (APAP), CYP3A4 inhibitors (eg, indinavir, ketoconazole, troleandomycin) may increase plasma ethinyl estradiol levels. Increased risk of intrahepatic cholestasis with troleandomycin. Increased plasma levels of cyclosporine, prednisolone and other corticosteroids, and theophylline have been reported. Decreased plasma concentrations of APAP and increased clearance of temazepam, salicylic acid, morphine, and clofibric acid have also been reported.

PREGNANCY: Category X, not for use in nursing.

MECHANISM OF ACTION: Estrogen/progestogen oral contraceptive; acts by suppressing gonadotropins and inhibiting ovulation. Also causes changes in cervical mucus (increasing difficulty of sperm entry into uterus) and endometrium (reducing likelihood of implantation).

PHARMACOKINETICS: Absorption: Levonorgestrel: Rapid and complete. Bioavailability (100%); C_{max}=2.8ng/mL (single dose), 6.0ng/mL (multiple doses); T_{max}=1.6 hrs (single dose), 1.5 hrs (multiple doses). Ethinyl Estradiol: Rapid. Bioavailability (38-48%); C_{max}=62pg/mL (single dose), 77pg/mL (multiple doses); T_{max}=1.5 hrs (single dose), 1.3 hrs (multiple doses). **Distribution:** Levonorgestrel: Primarily bound to sex hormone-binding globulin. Ethinyl estradiol: Plasma protein binding (97%); found in breast milk. **Metabolism:** Levonorgestrel: Reduction, hydroxylation, and conjugation. Ethinyl Estradiol: Hepatic, via CYP3A4 (hydroxylation), methylation, and glucuronidation. **Elimination:** Levonorgestrel: Urine (40-68%), feces (16-48%); $T_{1/2}$=36 hrs. Ethinyl Estradiol: $T_{1/2}$=18 hrs.

NURSING CONSIDERATIONS

Assessment: Assess for current or history of thrombophlebitis or thromboembolic disorders, history of HTN, hyperlipidemia, DM, obesity, breast cancer, and any other conditions where treatment is contraindicated or cautioned. Assess use in patients >35 yrs of age and heavy smokers (≥15 cigarettes/day). Assess pregnancy/nursing status and for possible drug interactions.

Monitoring: Monitor for signs/symptoms of MI, thromboembolism, stroke, hepatic neoplasia, and other adverse effects. Monitor BP with history of HTN, serum glucose levels in DM or prediabetic patients, lipid levels with history of hyperlipidemia, and for signs of worsening depression if with history of the disorder. Monitor liver function and for signs of liver toxicity (eg, jaundice). Refer to an ophthalmologist if ocular changes develop.

Patient Counseling: Inform that the drug does not protect against HIV infection and other sexually transmitted diseases. Counsel about potential adverse effects. Advise to avoid smoking. Instruct to take exactly ud at intervals not exceeding 24 hrs. Advise about risks of pregnancy if dose is missed; counsel to have a back-up nonhormonal birth control method (eg, condoms, spermicide) at all times. Instruct that if one dose is missed, take as soon as possible and take next pill at regular scheduled time. Inform that spotting, light bleeding, or nausea may occur during the first 1-3 packs of pills; advise not to d/c medication and if symptoms persist, to notify physician. Instruct to d/c if pregnancy is confirmed/suspected.

Administration: Oral route. **Storage:** 20-25°C (68-77°F).

AVINZA
morphine sulfate (King)

> Contains pellets of morphine sulfate, an opioid agonist and Schedule II controlled substance with an abuse liability similar to other opioid agonists, legal or illicit; assess each patient's risk for opioid abuse or addiction prior to prescribing. Routinely monitor for signs of misuse, abuse, and addiction. Respiratory depression, including fatal cases, may occur even when used as recommended; proper dosing and titration are essential. Monitor for respiratory depression, especially during initiation or following a dose increase. Should only be prescribed by healthcare professionals who are knowledgeable in the use of potent opioids for the management of chronic pain. Swallow cap whole or sprinkle contents on applesauce; crushing, chewing, or dissolving the pellets within the cap can cause rapid release and absorption of a potentially fatal dose. Accidental ingestion, especially in children, can result in fatal overdose. Avoid alcohol and alcohol-containing medications while on therapy; may result in an increase of plasma levels and potentially fatal overdose of morphine.

THERAPEUTIC CLASS: Opioid analgesic

INDICATIONS: Management of moderate to severe pain when a continuous, around-the-clock opioid analgesic is needed for an extended period of time.

DOSAGE: *Adults:* Individualize dose. Refer to PI for the factors to consider when selecting an initial dose. First Opioid Analgesic: Initial: 30mg qd at 24-hr intervals. Titrate: Adjust dose in increments ≤30mg every 4 days. 90mg and 120mg caps are for opioid-tolerant patients only. Conversion from Other Oral Morphine Products: Give total daily dose as qd, not to be given more frequently than q24h. Conversion from Parenteral Morphine: 2-6mg may be required to provide analgesia equivalent to 1mg of parenteral. Give about 3X the previous daily parenteral requirement. Conversion from Other Parenteral or Oral Non-Morphine Opioids: Initial: Give 1/2 of estimated daily requirement q24h. Supplement with immediate-release (IR) morphine. May give first dose with the last dose of any IR opioid. Titrate and Maint: Individualize. Titrate to a dose that provides adequate analgesia and minimizes adverse reactions. Breakthrough Pain: May require dose adjustment or rescue medication with a small dose of IR medication. Max: 1600mg/day. If signs of excessive opioid-related adverse reactions are observed, reduce next dose; adjust dose to obtain appropriate balance between management of pain and opioid-related adverse reactions. Discontinuation: Gradual downward titration every 2 to 4 days; avoid abrupt discontinuation.

HOW SUPPLIED: Cap, Extended-Release: 30mg, 45mg, 60mg, 75mg, 90mg, 120mg

CONTRAINDICATIONS: Significant respiratory depression, acute or severe bronchial asthma in an unmonitored setting or in the absence of resuscitative equipment, and known or suspected paralytic ileus.

WARNINGS/PRECAUTIONS: Doses >1600mg/day contain a quantity of fumaric acid that may cause serious renal toxicity. Not for use as PRN analgesic, for acute or mild pain, pain not expected to persist for an extended period of time, and postoperative pain unless the patient is already receiving chronic opioid therapy prior to surgery, or postoperative pain is expected to be moderate to severe and persist for an extended period. Respiratory depression is more likely to occur in elderly, cachectic, or debilitated patients; monitor closely when initiating and titrating, and when given with drugs that depress respiration. Monitor for respiratory depression and consider alternative nonopioid analgesics in patients with significant chronic obstructive pulmonary disease (COPD) or cor pulmonale, patients having a substantially decreased respiratory reserve, hypoxia, hypercapnia, or preexisting respiratory depression. May cause severe hypotension, including orthostatic hypotension and syncope, in ambulatory patients; monitor for signs of hypotension after initiation or titration. Avoid with circulatory shock, impaired consciousness, or coma. Monitor for signs of sedation and respiratory depression in patients susceptible to the intracranial effects of carbon dioxide retention (eg, those with increased intracranial pressure [ICP] or brain tumors). May obscure clinical course in patients with head injury. Avoid with GI obstruction. May cause spasm of sphincter of Oddi and increases in serum amylase; monitor for worsening symptoms in patients with biliary tract disease (eg, acute pancreatitis). May aggravate convulsions in patients with convulsive disorders, and may induce or aggravate seizures in some clinical settings; monitor for worsened seizure control in patients with history of seizure disorders. May impair mental/physical abilities. Not for use in women during and immediately prior to labor, when use of shorter acting analgesics or other analgesic techniques are more appropriate.

ADVERSE REACTIONS: Constipation, N/V, somnolence, headache, peripheral edema, diarrhea, abdominal pain, infection, urinary tract infection, flu syndrome, back pain, rash, insomnia, depression.

INTERACTIONS: See Boxed Warning. Respiratory depression, hypotension, profound sedation or coma may occur with other CNS depressants (eg, antiemetics, phenothiazines, alcohol); when combination is contemplated, reduce the initial dose of one or both agents. Avoid use of mixed agonist/antagonists (eg, pentazocine, nalbuphine, butorphanol); may reduce analgesic effect or precipitate withdrawal symptoms. May enhance neuromuscular blocking action of skeletal muscle relaxants and increase respiratory depression. MAOIs may potentiate the effects of morphine anxiety, confusion, and significant respiratory depression or coma; avoid use with MAOIs or within 14 days of stopping such treatment. Confusion and severe respiratory depression in a patient undergoing hemodialysis reported with concurrent cimetidine. May reduce efficacy of diuretics. Anticholinergics may increase risk of urinary retention and/or severe constipation, which may lead to paralytic ileus. May increase absorption/exposure with p-glycoprotein (P-gp) inhibitors (eg, quinidine) by about two-fold.

PREGNANCY: Category C, not for use in nursing.

MECHANISM OF ACTION: Opioid analgesic; acts as a full agonist, binds with and activates opioid receptors at sites in the periaqueductal and periventricular grey matter, the ventromedial medulla and the spinal cord to produce analgesia.

PHARMACOKINETICS: Absorption: C_{max}=18.65ng/mL; AUC=273.25ng/mL•hr. **Distribution:** V_d=1-6L/kg, plasma protein binding (20-35%); crosses the placenta; found in breast milk. **Metabolism:** Liver via conjugation and sulfation; (metabolites) morphine-3-glucuronide (M3G, about 50%), morphine-6-glucuronide (M6G, about 5-15%), morphine-3-etheral sulfate. **Elimination:** Urine (M3G/M6G, 10% unchanged), bile (small amount), feces (7-10%); $T_{1/2}$=approximately 24 hrs.

NURSING CONSIDERATIONS

Assessment: Assess for risk factors for drug abuse or addiction, general condition and medical status, opioid experience/tolerance, pain type/severity, previous opioid daily dose, potency, and type of prior analgesics used, respiratory depression, COPD or other respiratory complications, GI obstruction, renal/hepatic impairment, pregnancy/nursing status, possible drug interactions, or any other condition where treatment is contraindicated or cautioned.

Monitoring: Monitor for respiratory depression, sedation, CNS depression, increase in ICP, orthostatic hypotension, syncope, symptoms of worsening biliary tract disease, aggravation/induction of seizure/convulsions, tolerance, physical dependence, mental/physical impairment, withdrawal syndrome, and other adverse reactions. Monitor BP and serum amylase levels. Monitor for relief of pain and need for IR morphine. Routinely monitor for signs of misuse, abuse, and addiction. Periodically reassess the continued need for therapy.

Patient Counseling: Inform that drug has potential for abuse; instruct not to share drug with others and to take steps to protect from theft or misuse. Discuss risks of respiratory depression. Inform that accidental exposure, especially in children, may result in serious harm or death; advise to store securely and dispose unused cap by flushing down the toilet. Inform that the concomitant use of alcohol can increase the risk of life-threatening respiratory depression. Instruct to not consume alcoholic beverages, or take prescription and OTC products that contain alcohol, during treatment. Inform that drug may cause orthostatic hypotension and syncope. Advise that drug may impair the ability to perform potentially hazardous activities and to avoid such tasks until they know how they will react to treatment. Advise of potential for severe constipation, including management instructions and when to seek medical attention. Advise how to recognize anaphylaxis and when to seek medical attention. Instruct to inform physician if pregnant or planning to become pregnant. Instruct to take exactly as prescribed and not to d/c without discussing the need for a tapering regimen with the prescriber.

Administration: Oral route. Swallow cap whole or sprinkle contents on applesauce and then swallow immediately without chewing. Do not crush, chew, or dissolve pellets in the cap. Do not administer pellets through a NG or gastric tube. **Storage:** 25°C (77°F); excursions permitted to 15-30°C (59-86°F). Protect from light and moisture.

AVODART   RX
dutasteride (GlaxoSmithKline)

THERAPEUTIC CLASS: Type I and II 5 alpha-reductase inhibitor (2nd generation)

INDICATIONS: Treatment of symptomatic BPH in men with an enlarged prostate, either as monotherapy or in combination with the α-adrenergic antagonist, tamsulosin.

DOSAGE: *Adults:* Monotherapy: 1 cap (0.5mg) qd. With Tamsulosin: 1 cap (0.5mg) qd and tamsulosin 0.4mg qd.

HOW SUPPLIED: Cap: 0.5mg

CONTRAINDICATIONS: Pregnancy, women of childbearing potential, pediatric patients.

WARNINGS/PRECAUTIONS: Not approved for the prevention of prostate cancer. May decrease serum prostate specific antigen (PSA) concentration during therapy or in the presence of prostate cancer; establish a new baseline PSA at least 3 months after starting treatment and monitor PSA periodically thereafter. Any confirmed increase from lowest PSA value during treatment may signal presence of prostate cancer. May increase risk of high-grade prostate cancer. Prior to treatment initiation, consider other urological conditions that may cause similar symptoms; BPH and prostate cancer may coexist. Risk to male fetus; cap should not be handled by pregnant women or women who could become pregnant. Avoid donating blood until at least 6 months after last dose. Reduced total sperm count, semen volume, and sperm motility reported.

ADVERSE REACTIONS: Impotence, decreased libido, breast disorders, ejaculation disorders.

INTERACTIONS: Caution with potent, chronic CYP3A4 inhibitors (eg, ritonavir). CYP3A4/5 inhibitors (eg, ritonavir, ketoconazole, verapamil, diltiazem, cimetidine, troleandomycin, ciprofloxacin) may increase levels.

PREGNANCY: Category X, not for use in nursing.

MECHANISM OF ACTION: Selective type I and II 5α-reductase inhibitor (2nd generation); inhibits conversion of testosterone to dihydrotestosterone, the androgen primarily responsible for initial development and subsequent enlargement of the prostate gland.

PHARMACOKINETICS: Absorption: Absolute bioavailability (60%); T_{max}=2-3 hrs. **Distribution:** V_d=300-500L; plasma protein binding (99% albumin, 96.6% α-1 acid glycoprotein). **Metabolism:** Liver (extensive) via CYP3A4, 3A5; 4'-hydroxydutasteride, 1,2-dihydrodutasteride, 6-hydroxy-dutasteride (major active metabolites). **Elimination:** Feces (5% unchanged, 40% metabolites), urine (<1% unchanged); $T_{1/2}$=5 weeks.

NURSING CONSIDERATIONS

Assessment: Assess for urological conditions that may cause similar symptoms, previous hypersensitivity to the drug, and for possible drug interactions.

Monitoring: Monitor for signs/symptoms of prostate cancer and other urological diseases. Obtain new PSA baseline at least 3 months after starting treatment and monitor PSA periodically thereafter.

Patient Counseling: Inform of the importance of periodic PSA monitoring. Advise that therapy may increase risk of high-grade prostate cancer. Counsel that drug should not be handled by women who are pregnant or who could become pregnant, due to potential fetal risks; advise to wash area immediately with soap and water if contact is made. Instruct not to donate blood until at least 6 months after last dose.

Administration: Oral route. Swallow whole; do not chew or open. Take with or without food. **Storage:** 25°C (77°F); excursions permitted to 15-30°C (59-86°F).

AXERT
RX
almotriptan malate (Ortho-McNeil/Janssen)

THERAPEUTIC CLASS: 5-HT$_{1B/1D}$ agonist

INDICATIONS: Acute treatment of migraine attacks with a history of migraine with or without aura in adults. Acute treatment of migraine headache pain with a history of migraine attacks with or without aura usually lasting ≥4 hrs in adolescents 12-17 yrs of age.

DOSAGE: *Adults:* Initial: 6.25-12.5mg at onset of headache. May repeat after 2 hrs. Max: 25mg/day. Hepatic/Renal Impairment: 6.25mg at onset of headache. Max: 12.5mg/24 hrs. Elderly: Start at lower end of dosing range.
Pediatrics: 12-17 Yrs: Initial: 6.25-12.5mg at onset of headache. May repeat after 2 hrs. Max: 25mg/day. Hepatic/Renal Impairment: 6.25mg at onset of headache. Max: 12.5mg/24 hrs.

HOW SUPPLIED: Tab: 6.25mg, 12.5mg

CONTRAINDICATIONS: Ischemic heart disease, coronary artery vasospasm, other significant cardiovascular (CV) disease, cerebrovascular syndromes (eg, stroke, transient ischemic attacks [TIA]), peripheral vascular disease (eg, ischemic bowel disease), uncontrolled HTN, hemiplegic or basilar migraine. Avoid use within 24 hrs of another 5-HT$_1$ agonist (eg, triptans) or ergotamine-containing or ergot-type medications (eg, dihydroergotamine, ergotamine tartrate, methysergide).

WARNINGS/PRECAUTIONS: Confirm diagnosis. Supervise 1st dose and monitor cardiac function in those at risk of coronary artery disease (CAD). Monitor CV function with long-term intermittent use. Administration of 1st dose should be in physician's office or in a medically staffed and equipped facility as cardiac ischemia may occur in absence of clinical symptoms; ECG should be obtained immediately, during interval following administration, in those with risk factors. May cause vasospastic reactions or cerebrovascular events. Serotonin syndrome symptoms (eg, mental status changes, autonomic instability, neuromuscular aberrations, and GI symptoms) reported. Sensations of tightness, pain, pressure, and heaviness in the precordium, throat, neck, and jaw reported. May bind to melanin in the eye. Caution with renal or hepatic dysfunction. Caution with known hypersensitivity to sulfonamides. Caution in elderly.

ADVERSE REACTIONS: N/V, dizziness, somnolence, headache, paresthesia, coronary artery vasospasm, myocardial infarction (MI), ventricular tachycardia, ventricular fibrillation, transient myocardial ischemia, dry mouth.

INTERACTIONS: See Contraindications. Additive vasospastic reactions with ergotamines. SSRIs may cause weakness, hyperreflexia, and incoordination. Life-threatening serotonin syndrome reported with combined use of SSRIs or SNRIs. Clearance may be decreased by MAOIs. Increased levels possible with CYP3A4 inhibitors (eg, ketoconazole).

PREGNANCY: Category C, caution in nursing.

MECHANISM OF ACTION: Selective 5-HT$_{1B/1D}$ receptor agonist; binds with high affinity to 5-HT$_{1B/1D}$ receptors on extracerebral, intracranial blood vessels that become dilated during migraine attack and on nerve terminal in trigeminal system. Activation of these receptors results in cranial nerve constriction, inhibition of neuropeptide release, and reduced transmission in trigeminal pain pathways.

PHARMACOKINETICS: Absorption: Absolute bioavailability (70%); T_{max}=1-3 hrs. **Distribution:** V_d=180-200L; plasma protein binding (35%). **Metabolism:** MAO-mediated oxidative deamination and CYP450-mediated oxidation (major pathways), flavin monooxygenase (minor pathway); indoleacetic acid, gamma-aminobutyric acid (inactive metabolites). **Elimination:** Urine (75%, 40% unchanged), feces (13%, unchanged and metabolite); $T_{1/2}$=3-4 hrs.

NURSING CONSIDERATIONS

Assessment: Confirm diagnosis of migraine before therapy. Assess for cluster headache, ischemic heart disease (eg, angina pectoris, Prinzmetal's variant angina, MI or documented silent MI), HTN, hemiplegic or basilar migraine, presence of risk factors (eg, hypercholesterolemia, smoking, obesity, diabetes mellitus), ECG changes, hepatic/renal impairment, hypersensitivity to the drug and to sulfonamides, pregnancy/nursing status, and possible drug interactions.

Monitoring: Monitor for signs/symptoms of cardiac/cerebrovascular events, peripheral vascular ischemia, colonic ischemia with bloody diarrhea and abdominal pain, serotonin syndrome, ophthalmic effects, hypersensitivity reactions, and increased BP.

Patient Counseling: Inform about potential risks of therapy, especially if taken with SSRIs or SNRIs. Instruct to report adverse reactions to physician. Advise to take exactly ud. Counsel to use caution during hazardous tasks. Instruct to notify physician if pregnant/nursing or planning to become pregnant.

Administration: Oral route. **Storage:** 25°C (77°F); excursions permitted to 15-30°C (59-86°F).

AXIRON
testosterone (Lilly)

CIII

> Virilization reported in children secondarily exposed to topical testosterone. Children should avoid contact with unwashed or unclothed application sites in men using topical testosterone. Advise patients to strictly adhere to recommended instructions for use.

THERAPEUTIC CLASS: Androgen

INDICATIONS: Replacement therapy in males ≥18 yrs of age for conditions associated with a deficiency or absence of endogenous testosterone (congenital/acquired primary hypogonadism or hypogonadotropic hypogonadism).

DOSAGE: *Adults:* Initial: Apply 60mg (1 actuation of 30mg to each axilla) qam, to clean, dry, intact skin of axilla. Titrate: May adjust dose based on serum testosterone concentration from a single blood draw 2-8 hrs after application, and at least 14 days after starting treatment or following dose adjustment. If Serum Concentration <300ng/dL: May increase to 90mg or from 90mg to 120mg. If Serum Concentration >1050ng/dL: Decrease from 60mg to 30mg. D/C if consistently >1050ng/dL at lowest qd dose of 30mg. Refer to PI for application techniques.

HOW SUPPLIED: Sol: 30mg/actuation [110mL]

CONTRAINDICATIONS: Known/suspected prostate carcinoma or breast carcinoma in men, women who are or may become pregnant, or nursing mothers.

WARNINGS/PRECAUTIONS: Application site and dose are not interchangeable with other topical testosterone products. Patients with BPH may be at increased risk for worsening of signs/symptoms of BPH. May increase risk for prostate cancer; evaluate for prostate cancer before and 3-6 months after initiation of therapy. Increases in Hct and RBC mass may increase risk for thromboembolic events; consider lowering or discontinuing therapy. Not indicated for use in women. Suppression of spermatogenesis may occur at large doses. Edema with or without congestive heart failure (CHF) may occur in patients with preexisting cardiac, renal, or hepatic disease. Gynecomastia may develop and persist. May potentiate sleep apnea, especially with obesity or chronic lung disease. Changes in serum lipid profile reported; adjust dose or d/c therapy if necessary. Caution in cancer patients at risk of hypercalcemia and associated hyper-calciuria. May decrease concentrations of thyroxin-binding globulins, resulting in decreased total T4 and increased resin uptake of T3 and T4. Alcohol-based products are flammable; avoid fire, flame, or smoking until applied dose has dried.

ADVERSE REACTIONS: Application-site irritation, application-site erythema, headache, Hct increase, diarrhea, vomiting, prostate specific antigen (PSA) increase.

INTERACTIONS: May decrease blood glucose and insulin requirements. Changes in anticoagulant activity may occur; frequently monitor INR and PT in patients taking anticoagulants. May increase fluid retention with adrenocorticotropic hormone or corticosteroids.

PREGNANCY: Category X, not for use in nursing.

MECHANISM OF ACTION: Androgen; responsible for normal growth and development of male sex organs and for maintenance of secondary sex characteristics.

PHARMACOKINETICS: Absorption: Systemic. **Metabolism:** Estradiol, dihydrotestosterone (active metabolites). **Elimination:** (IM) Urine (90% glucuronic, sulfuric acid conjugates), feces (6% unconjugated); $T_{1/2}$=10-100 min.

NURSING CONSIDERATIONS

Assessment: Assess for conditions where treatment is contraindicated, prostate cancer, BPH, cardiac or renal/hepatic disease, obesity, chronic lung disease, and possible drug interactions. Assess Hct.

Monitoring: Monitor for signs/symptoms of prostate cancer, worsening of BPH, edema with or without CHF, gynecomastia, and sleep apnea. Periodically monitor Hct, Hgb, PSA, serum lipid profile, and serum testosterone levels. In cancer patients at risk for hypercalcemia, monitor serum Ca^{2+} levels.

Patient Counseling: Advise to strictly adhere to recommended instructions for use. Inform that men with known or suspected prostate/breast cancer should not use androgen therapy. Advise that children and women should avoid contact with application sites, and to report to physician any signs/symptoms of secondary exposure in these individuals. Instruct to apply only to axilla and not to any other part of the body, to wash hands immediately with soap and water after application, and to cover application site with clothing after waiting 3 min for the sol to dry. Instruct to wash application site with soap and water prior to direct skin-to-skin contact with others, and to immediately wash area of contact if unwashed/unclothed skin comes in direct contact with skin of another person. Inform of possible adverse reactions. Inform that antiperspirant or deodorant may be used before applying the medication. Counsel to avoid swimming or washing application site until 2 hrs following application. Advise to avoid splashing in the eyes; instruct to flush thoroughly with water in case of contact and to seek medical advice if irritation persists.

Administration: Topical route. Refer to PI for administration instructions. **Storage:** 25°C (77°F); excursions permitted to 15-30°C (59-86°F).

AZACTAM

RX

aztreonam (Bristol-Myers Squibb)

THERAPEUTIC CLASS: Monobactam

INDICATIONS: Treatment of complicated/uncomplicated urinary tract infections (UTIs) (eg, pyelonephritis and initial/recurrent cystitis), lower respiratory tract infections (eg, pneumonia, bronchitis), septicemia, skin and skin-structure infections (eg, postoperative wounds, ulcers, burns), intra-abdominal infections (eg, peritonitis), and gynecologic infections (eg, endometritis, pelvic cellulitis) caused by susceptible gram-negative microorganisms. Adjunctive therapy to surgery in the management of infections caused by susceptible organisms (eg, abscesses, hollow viscus perforation infections, cutaneous infections, infections of serous surfaces). Concurrent initial therapy with other antimicrobial agents before causative organism(s) is known in seriously ill patients who are also at risk of having gram-positive aerobic/anaerobic infection.

DOSAGE: *Adults:* Individualize dose. UTI: 500mg or 1g q8 or 12h. Max: 8g/day. Moderately Severe Systemic Infections: 1 or 2g q8 or 12h. Max: 8g/day. Severe Systemic/Life-Threatening Infections/ *Pseudomonas aeruginosa* Infection: 2g q6 or 8h. Max: 8g/day. Renal Impairment/Elderly: CrCl 10-30mL/min: Initial LD: 1g or 2g. Maint: 50% of dose. CrCl <10mL/min (eg, hemodialysis): Initial: 500mg, 1g, or 2g. Maint: 25% of initial dose given at fixed intervals of 6, 8, or 12 hrs. For serious/ life-threatening infections, in addition to the maintenance doses, give additional 1/8 of the initial dose after each hemodialysis session. Administer IV for single doses >1g or with bacterial septicemia, localized parenchymal abscess, peritonitis, or other severe systemic or life-threatening infections. Continue treatment for at least 48 hrs after the patient becomes asymptomatic or evidence of bacterial eradication has been obtained. Persistent infections may require treatment of several weeks.

Pediatrics: 9 Months-16 Yrs: Individualize dose. Mild-Moderate Infections: 30mg/kg IV q8h. Max: 120mg/kg/day. Moderate-Severe Infections: 30mg/kg IV q6 or 8h. Max: 120mg/kg/day. In patients with cystic fibrosis, higher doses may be warranted. Continue treatment for at least 48 hrs after the patient becomes asymptomatic or evidence of bacterial eradication has been obtained. Persistent infections may require treatment of several weeks.

HOW SUPPLIED: Inj: 1g, 2g; 1g/50mL, 2g/50mL [Galaxy]

WARNINGS/PRECAUTIONS: Hypersensitivity reactions may occur; d/c and institute appropriate supportive treatment. Caution with history of hypersensitivity to β-lactams (eg, penicillins, cephalosporins, carbapenems). *Clostridium difficile*-associated diarrhea (CDAD) reported; d/c if CDAD is suspected or confirmed. Toxic epidermal necrolysis (TEN) reported (rare) in patients undergoing bone marrow transplant with multiple risk factors (eg, sepsis, radiation therapy, concomitant drugs associated with TEN). May result in bacterial resistance with prolonged use in the absence of proven or suspected bacterial infection, or a prophylactic indication; take appropriate measures if superinfection develops. Caution with renal/hepatic impairment and in elderly.

ADVERSE REACTIONS: ALT/AST elevation, rash, eosinophilia, neutropenia, pain at inj site, increased SrCr, thrombocytosis.

INTERACTIONS: Avoid with β-lactamase inducing antibiotics (eg, cefoxitin, imipenem). Potential nephrotoxicity and ototoxicity with aminoglycosides; monitor renal function.

PREGNANCY: Category B, not for use in nursing.

MECHANISM OF ACTION: Monobactam; inhibits bacterial cell-wall synthesis. Has activity in the presence of some β-lactamases, both penicillinases and cephalosporinases, of gram-negative and gram-positive bacteria.

PHARMACOKINETICS: Absorption: Administration of variable doses resulted in different pharmacokinetic parameters. **Distribution:** Plasma protein binding (56%); V_d=12.6L; crosses placenta; found in breast milk. **Metabolism:** Ring hydrolysis. **Elimination:** Urine (60-70% unchanged and metabolites), (IV) feces (12% unchanged and metabolites); $T_{1/2}$=1.7 hrs.

NURSING CONSIDERATIONS

Assessment: Assess for drug hypersensitivity (eg, β-lactams), hypersensitivity to any allergens, hepatic/renal impairment, pregnancy/nursing status, and for possible drug interactions. Assess use in patients undergoing bone marrow transplant with multiple risk factors. Confirm diagnosis of causative organisms.

Monitoring: Monitor for signs/symptoms of hypersensitivity reactions, CDAD, superinfection, TEN in patients undergoing bone marrow transplant, and hepatic/renal function.

Patient Counseling: Inform that therapy should only be used to treat bacterial and not viral infections (eg, common cold). Advise to take exactly ud; inform that skipping doses or not completing full course may decrease effectiveness and increase resistance. Inform that diarrhea is a common problem caused by therapy and will usually end upon discontinuation of therapy. Inform that diarrhea may occur, even as late as ≥2 months after last dose of therapy; instruct to notify physician as soon as possible if watery/bloody stools (with or without stomach cramps and fever) occur.

Administration: IM/IV route. Refer to PI for preparation/administration instructions and compatibility information. **Storage:** Vial: Room temperature. Avoid excessive heat. Galaxy Container: ≤-20°C (-4°F). Thawed Sol: Stable for 14 days at 2-8°C (36-46°F) or 48 hrs at 25°C (77°F). Do not refreeze. Refer to PI for diluted/reconstituted sol storage information.

AZASITE   RX
azithromycin (Inspire)

THERAPEUTIC CLASS: Macrolide

INDICATIONS: Treatment of bacterial conjunctivitis caused by susceptible isolates of microorganisms.

DOSAGE: *Adults:* Instill 1 drop in the affected eye(s) bid, 8-12 hrs apart for the first 2 days, then 1 drop qd for the next 5 days.
Pediatrics: ≥1 Yr: Instill 1 drop in the affected eye(s) bid, 8-12 hrs apart for the first 2 days, then 1 drop qd for the next 5 days.

HOW SUPPLIED: Sol: 1% [2.5mL]

WARNINGS/PRECAUTIONS: Not for inj. Do not administer systemically, inject subconjunctivally, or introduce directly into the anterior chamber of the eye. Serious allergic reactions, including angioedema, anaphylaxis, and dermatologic reactions (eg, Stevens-Johnson syndrome, toxic epidermal necrolysis), rarely reported when administered systemically. May result in bacterial resistance with prolonged use; take appropriate measures if superinfection develops. Avoid wearing contact lenses if signs or symptoms of bacterial conjunctivitis exist.

ADVERSE REACTIONS: Eye irritation, blurred vision, burning/stinging upon instillation, contact dermatitis, corneal erosion, dry eye, eye pain, ocular discharge, dysgeusia, facial swelling, hives, nasal congestion, periocular swelling, rash.

PREGNANCY: Category B, caution in nursing.

MECHANISM OF ACTION: Macrolide; binds to the 50S ribosomal subunit of susceptible microorganisms and interferes with microbial protein synthesis.

NURSING CONSIDERATIONS

Assessment: Assess for hypersensitivity, proper diagnosis of causative organisms, use of contact lenses, and pregnancy/nursing status.

Monitoring: Monitor for hypersensitivity reactions, superinfection, eye irritation, and other adverse reactions.

Patient Counseling: Advise to avoid contaminating the applicator tip by allowing it to touch the eye, fingers, or other sources. Instruct to d/c and contact physician if any signs of allergic reaction occur. Instruct to use exactly ud; skipping doses or not completing full course may decrease effectiveness of treatment and increase bacterial resistance. Advise not to wear contact lenses if patient has signs/symptoms of bacterial conjunctivitis. Advise to wash hands thoroughly before instillation. Counsel on proper administration; shake bottle once before each use.

Administration: Ocular route. **Storage:** Unopened Bottle: 2-8°C (36-46°F). Opened Bottle: 2-25°C (36-77°F) for up to 14 days. Discard after 14 days.

Azilect   RX
rasagiline mesylate (Teva Neuroscience)

THERAPEUTIC CLASS: Monoamine oxidase inhibitor (type B)

INDICATIONS: Treatment of signs and symptoms of idiopathic Parkinson's disease as initial monotherapy and as adjunct therapy to levodopa.

DOSAGE: *Adults:* Monotherapy: 1mg qd. Adjunctive Therapy: Initial: 0.5mg qd. Titrate: May increase to 1mg qd if a sufficient clinical response is not achieved. May consider dosage reduction of concomitant levodopa based upon individual response. Mild Hepatic Impairment/Concomitant Ciprofloxacin or Other CYP1A2 Inhibitors: 0.5mg/day.

HOW SUPPLIED: Tab: 0.5mg, 1mg

CONTRAINDICATIONS: Concomitant use with any other MAOI, meperidine, tramadol, methadone, propoxyphene, dextromethorphan, St. John's wort, or cyclobenzaprine (a tricyclic muscle relaxant). At least 14 days should elapse between discontinuation of rasagiline and initiation of any MAOI or meperidine.

WARNINGS/PRECAUTIONS: Do not use in patients with moderate/severe hepatic impairment. Do not use at daily doses >1mg/day due to risks of hypertensive crisis and other adverse reactions associated with nonselective MAO inhibition. Patients with Parkinson's disease have a higher risk of developing melanoma; monitor for melanomas frequently and on a regular basis. May potentiate dopaminergic side effects, cause/exacerbate dyskinesia, cause postural hypotension, and increase incidence of a significant high BP, when used as an adjunct to levodopa. Hallucinations reported. May cause/exacerbate psychotic-like behavior; avoid in patients with a major psychotic disorder. A symptom complex resembling neuroleptic malignant syndrome reported with rapid dose reduction, withdrawal of, or changes in drugs that increase central dopaminergic tone.

ADVERSE REACTIONS: Arthralgia, dyspepsia, depression, fall, flu syndrome, dyskinesia, weight loss, postural hypotension, N/V, anorexia, abdominal pain, constipation, dry mouth, rash, abnormal dreams.

INTERACTIONS: See Contraindications and Dosage. Avoid with any antidepressant; severe CNS toxicity associated with hyperpyrexia reported. At least 14 days should elapse between discontinuation of therapy and initiation of an SSRI, SNRI, TCA, tetracyclic, or triazolopyridine antidepressant. At least 5 weeks (longer with chronic/high-dose fluoxetine) should elapse between discontinuation of fluoxetine and initiation of rasagiline due to the long $T_{1/2}$ of fluoxetine and its active metabolite. Ciprofloxacin and other CYP1A2 inhibitors may increase levels. Caution with sympathomimetics (eg, nasal/oral/ophthalmic decongestants, cold remedies). Hypertensive crisis/reactions reported with ephedrine or tyramine-rich foods; avoid foods containing a very large amount of tyramine (eg, aged cheese). Elevated BP reported with tetrahydrozoline ophthalmic drops. Many treatments for psychosis that decrease central dopaminergic tone may decrease effectiveness.

PREGNANCY: Category C, caution in nursing.

MECHANISM OF ACTION: MAOI (Type B); not established. Inhibits MAO type B, which causes an increase in extracellular dopamine levels in the striatum, subsequently increasing dopaminergic activity.

PHARMACOKINETICS: Absorption: Rapid. Absolute bioavailability (36%); T_{max}=1 hr. **Distribution:** V_d=87L; plasma protein binding (88-94%). **Metabolism:** Liver; N-dealkylation and/or hydroxylation via CYP1A2 (major); 1-aminoindan, 3-hydroxy-N-propargyl-1 aminoindan and 3-hydroxy-1-aminoindan (metabolites). **Elimination:** Urine (62% over 7 days, <1% unchanged), feces (7% over 7 days); $T_{1/2}$=3 hrs.

NURSING CONSIDERATIONS

Assessment: Assess for hepatic impairment, dyskinesia, major psychotic disorder, pregnancy/nursing status, and possible drug interactions.

Monitoring: Monitor for dyskinesia, postural hypotension, BP decrease/increase, hallucinations, psychotic-like behavior, and other adverse reactions. Monitor for melanomas frequently and on a regular basis.

Patient Counseling: Instruct to inform physician if taking or planning to take any prescription or OTC drugs, especially antidepressants, ciprofloxacin, and OTC cold medications. Instruct not to exceed 1mg/day and explain the risk of using higher daily doses; provide a brief description of the hypertensive/cheese reaction. Advise to avoid foods containing a very large amount of tyramine (eg, aged cheese) while on therapy. Advise to have periodic skin examinations. Inform of the possibility of developing dyskinesia with concomitant levodopa, increases in BP, hallucinations, or other manifestations of psychotic-like behavior. Inform that postural (orthostatic) hypotension may develop; caution against standing up rapidly after sitting or lying down for prolonged periods and at the initiation of treatment. Instruct to take drug as prescribed. Instruct to contact physician if discontinuation of therapy is desired, or if hallucinations, new/increased gambling urges, increased sexual urges, or other intense urges develop.

Administration: Oral route. May be administered with or without food. **Storage:** 25°C (77°F); excursions permitted to 15-30°C (59-86°F).

AZOPT   RX
brinzolamide (Alcon)

THERAPEUTIC CLASS: Carbonic anhydrase inhibitor

INDICATIONS: Treatment of elevated intraocular pressure (IOP) in patients with ocular HTN or open-angle glaucoma.

DOSAGE: *Adults:* 1 drop in the affected eye(s) tid. Space dosing by at least 10 min if using >1 topical ophthalmic drug.

HOW SUPPLIED: Sus: 1% [10mL, 15mL]

WARNINGS/PRECAUTIONS: Systemically absorbed. Fatalities occurred (rarely) due to severe reactions to sulfonamides including Stevens-Johnson syndrome, toxic epidermal necrolysis, fulminant hepatic necrosis, agranulocytosis, aplastic anemia, and other blood dyscrasias. Sensitization may recur when a sulfonamide is readministered irrespective of route. D/C if signs of serious reactions or hypersensitivity occur. Caution with low endothelial cell counts; increased potential for corneal edema. Not recommended with severe renal impairment (CrCl <30mL/min). Contains benzalkonium chloride, which may be absorbed by soft contact lenses; contact lenses should be removed during instillation, but may be reinserted 15 min after instillation.

ADVERSE REACTIONS: Blurred vision, bitter/sour/unusual taste, blepharitis, dermatitis, dry eye, foreign body sensation, headache, hyperemia, ocular discharge/discomfort/keratitis/pain/pruritus, rhinitis.

INTERACTIONS: Potential additive systemic effects with oral carbonic anhydrase inhibitors; coadministration is not recommended. Acid-base alterations reported with high-dose salicylate therapy in patients treated with oral carbonic anhydrase inhibitors.

PREGNANCY: Category C, not for use in nursing.

MECHANISM OF ACTION: Carbonic anhydrase II inhibitor; inhibits aqueous humor formation and reduces elevated IOP.

PHARMACOKINETICS: Absorption: Systemic. **Distribution:** Plasma protein binding (60%). **Metabolism:** N-desethyl brinzolamide (metabolite). **Elimination:** Urine (unchanged, metabolites); $T_{1/2}$=111 days (whole blood).

NURSING CONSIDERATIONS

Assessment: Assess for hypersensitivity to drug or to sulfonamides, low endothelial cell counts, renal impairment, contact lens use, pregnancy/nursing status, and possible drug interactions.

Monitoring: Monitor for sulfonamide/hypersensitivity reactions, and other adverse reactions.

Patient Counseling: Advise to d/c use and consult physician if serious or unusual ocular or systemic reactions or signs of hypersensitivity occur. Inform that vision may be temporarily blurred following administration; instruct to use caution in operating machinery or driving a motor vehicle. Instruct to avoid allowing the container tip to contact the eye or surrounding structures or other surfaces. Instruct to consult physician about the continued use of the present multidose container if undergoing ocular surgery or if an intercurrent ocular condition (eg, trauma, infection) develops. Instruct that if using >1 topical ophthalmic drug, to administer the drugs at least 10 min apart. Advise that contact lenses should be removed during instillation, but may be reinserted 15 min after instillation.

Administration: Ocular route. Shake well before use. **Storage:** 4-30°C (39-86°F).

AZOR   RX
olmesartan medoxomil - amlodipine (Daiichi Sankyo)

> D/C when pregnancy is detected. Drugs that act directly on the renin-angiotensin system (RAS) can cause death/injury to the developing fetus.

THERAPEUTIC CLASS: ARB/calcium channel blocker (dihydropyridine)

INDICATIONS: Treatment of HTN, alone or with other antihypertensive agents. Initial therapy in patients who are likely to need multiple antihypertensive agents to achieve their BP goals.

DOSAGE: *Adults:* Initial: 5mg-20mg qd. Titrate: May increase dose after 1-2 weeks to control BP. Max: 10mg-40mg qd. Replacement Therapy: May substitute for individually titrated components. When substituting for individual components, the dose of 1 or both components may be increased if BP is not adequately controlled. Add-On Therapy: May be used to provide additional BP lowering when not adequately controlled on amlodipine (or another dihydropyridine calcium channel blocker) or olmesartan (or another ARB) alone.

HOW SUPPLIED: Tab: (Amlodipine-Olmesartan) 5mg-20mg, 5mg-40mg, 10mg-20mg, 10mg-40mg

CONTRAINDICATIONS: Coadministration with aliskiren in patients with diabetes.

WARNINGS/PRECAUTIONS: Initial therapy is not recommended in patients ≥75 yrs of age or with hepatic impairment. May decrease Hct and Hgb levels. Amlodipine: Acute hypotension reported (rare); caution with severe aortic stenosis. May develop increased frequency, duration, or severity of angina or acute myocardial infarction (MI) with dosage initiation or increase, particularly in patients with severe obstructive coronary artery disease (CAD). May cause hepatic enzyme elevation. Caution with severe hepatic impairment and in elderly. Olmesartan: Symptomatic hypotension, especially in patients with an activated RAS (eg, volume- and/or salt-depleted patients treated with high doses of diuretics), may occur after initiation of treatment; initiate treatment under close medical supervision. May cause changes in renal function. Oliguria or progressive azotemia and (rarely) acute renal failure and/or death may occur in patients whose renal function may depend upon the activity of the RAS (eg, severe congestive heart failure [CHF]). May increase BUN or SrCr levels in patients with renal artery stenosis. Sprue-like enteropathy with symptoms of severe, chronic diarrhea with substantial weight loss reported; exclude other etiologies if these symptoms develop, and consider discontinuation in cases where no other etiology is identified. Hyperkalemia may occur.

ADVERSE REACTIONS: Edema, headache, palpitation, dizziness, flushing.

INTERACTIONS: See Contraindications. Amlodipine: May increase simvastatin exposure; limit simvastatin dose to 20mg/day. Olmesartan: Dual blockade of the RAS is associated with increased risks of hypotension, hyperkalemia, and changes in renal function (including acute renal failure); closely monitor BP, renal function, and electrolytes with concomitant agents that affect the RAS. Avoid with aliskiren in patients with renal impairment (GFR <60mL/min). NSAIDs, including selective COX-2 inhibitors, may deteriorate renal function and attenuate antihypertensive effect. Colesevelam may decrease levels; administer at least 4 hrs before colesevelam dose.

PREGNANCY: Category D, not for use in nursing.

MECHANISM OF ACTION: Amlodipine: Dihydropyridine calcium channel receptor blocker; inhibits transmembrane influx of Ca^{2+} ions into vascular smooth muscle and cardiac muscle. Acts directly on vascular smooth muscle to cause a reduction in peripheral vascular resistance and reduction in BP. Olmesartan: ARB; blocks the vasoconstrictor effects of angiotensin II by selectively blocking the binding of angiotensin II to the AT_1 receptor in vascular smooth muscle.

PHARMACOKINETICS: Absorption: Amlodipine: Absolute bioavailability (64-90%); T_{max}=6-12 hrs. Olmesartan: Absolute bioavailability (26%); T_{max}=1-2 hrs. **Distribution:** Amlodipine: Plasma protein binding (93%). Olmesartan: V_d=17L; plasma protein binding (99%). **Metabolism:** Amlodipine: Liver (extensive). Olmesartan: Ester hydrolysis. **Elimination:** Amlodipine: Urine (10% parent compound, 60% metabolites); $T_{1/2}$=30-50 hrs. Olmesartan: Urine (35-50%), feces; $T_{1/2}$=13 hrs.

NURSING CONSIDERATIONS

Assessment: Assess for severe obstructive CAD, CHF, severe aortic stenosis, volume/salt depletion, diabetes, renal/hepatic impairment, pregnancy/nursing status, and possible drug interactions.

Monitoring: Monitor for signs/symptoms of hypotension, sprue-like enteropathy, and other adverse reactions. Monitor for symptoms of angina or MI, particularly in patients with severe obstructive CAD, after dosage initiation or increase. Monitor for decrease in Hct/Hgb, increase in SrCr, BUN, K⁺ levels, and hepatic enzymes.

Patient Counseling: Inform about the consequences of exposure during pregnancy and of the treatment options in women if planning to become pregnant; instruct to report pregnancy to the physician as soon as possible.

Administration: Oral route. Take with or without food. **Storage:** 25°C (77°F); excursions permitted to 15-30°C (59-86°F).

AZULFIDINE   RX
sulfasalazine (Pharmacia & Upjohn)

THERAPEUTIC CLASS: 5-aminosalicylic acid derivative/sulfapyridine

INDICATIONS: Treatment of mild to moderate ulcerative colitis (UC). Adjunctive therapy in severe UC. To prolong remission period between acute attacks of UC.

DOSAGE: *Adults:* Individualize dose. Take preferably pc. Initial: 3-4g/day in evenly divided doses with intervals not >8 hrs. May initiate with a lower dose (eg, 1-2g/day) to reduce GI intolerance. Maint: 2g/day. When endoscopic examination confirms satisfactory improvement, reduce dose to a maintenance level. If diarrhea recurs, increase dose to previously effective levels. If symptoms of GI intolerance occur after 1st few doses, reduce daily dose by 1/2, then gradually increase over several days. If GI intolerance continues, d/c for 5-7 days, then reintroduce at a lower daily dose. Desensitization: Initial: 50-250mg/day. Titrate: Double every 4-7 days until desired therapeutic level is achieved. D/C if sensitivity recurs.
Pediatrics: ≥6 Yrs: Individualize dose. Take preferably pc. Initial: 40-60mg/kg/24 hrs divided into 3-6 doses. Maint: 30mg/kg/24 hrs divided into 4 doses. When endoscopic examination confirms satisfactory improvement, reduce dose to a maintenance level. If diarrhea recurs, increase dose to previously effective levels. If symptoms of GI intolerance occur after 1st few doses, reduce daily dose by 1/2, then gradually increase over several days. If GI intolerance continues, d/c for 5-7 days, then reintroduce at a lower daily dose. Desensitization: Initial: 50-250mg/day. Titrate: Double every 4-7 days until desired therapeutic level is achieved. D/C if sensitivity recurs.

HOW SUPPLIED: Tab: 500mg* *scored

CONTRAINDICATIONS: Intestinal or urinary obstruction, porphyria.

WARNINGS/PRECAUTIONS: Caution with hepatic/renal damage, blood dyscrasias, severe allergy, bronchial asthma, history of recurring/chronic infections, or with underlying conditions or concomitant drugs that may predispose patients to infections. Deaths reported from hypersensitivity reactions, agranulocytosis, aplastic anemia, other blood dyscrasias, renal and liver damage, irreversible neuromuscular and CNS changes, and fibrosing alveolitis. Perform CBC, including differential WBC count, and LFTs before starting therapy, every 2nd week for the first 3 months, monthly for the next 3 months, then every 3 months thereafter, and as clinically indicated; d/c while awaiting the results of blood tests. Monitor urinalysis and renal function periodically. Oligospermia and infertility reported in males. Serious infections (eg, fatal sepsis, pneumonia) reported. D/C if serious infection or toxic/hypersensitivity reactions develop. Closely monitor for signs and symptoms of infection during and after treatment; if a new infection develops, perform a prompt and complete diagnostic workup for infection and myelosuppression. Serious skin reactions, some fatal (eg, exfoliative dermatitis, Stevens-Johnson syndrome, toxic epidermal necrolysis), reported; d/c at 1st appearance of skin rash, mucosal lesions, or any other sign of hypersensitivity. Severe, life-threatening, systemic hypersensitivity reactions (eg, drug rash with eosinophilia and systemic symptoms) reported; evaluate immediately if signs/symptoms develop, and d/c if an alternative etiology cannot be established. Maintain adequate fluid intake to prevent crystalluria and stone formation. Closely monitor patients with G6PD deficiency for signs of hemolytic anemia. Do not attempt desensitization in patients who have a history of agranulocytosis, or who have experienced an anaphylactoid reaction with previous sulfasalazine (SSZ) therapy. Serum sulfapyridine (SP) levels >50mcg/mL appear to be associated with increased incidence of adverse reactions. Lab test interactions may occur.

ADVERSE REACTIONS: Anorexia, headache, N/V, gastric distress, reversible oligospermia.

INTERACTIONS: May reduce absorption of folic acid and digoxin.

PREGNANCY: Category B, caution in nursing.

MECHANISM OF ACTION: 5-aminosalicylic acid (5-ASA) derivative/SP; not established. May be related to anti-inflammatory and/or immunomodulatory properties, to its affinity for connective tissue, and/or to the relatively high concentration it reaches in serous fluids, the liver, and intestinal walls.

PHARMACOKINETICS: Absorption: SSZ: Absolute bioavailability (<15%); C_{max}=6mcg/mL; T_{max}=6 hrs. SP: Well absorbed from colon. Bioavailability (60%); T_{max}=10 hrs. 5-ASA: Much less well absorbed from GI tract. Bioavailability (10-30%); T_{max}=10 hrs. **Distribution:** Crosses placenta; found in breast milk. SSZ: V_d=7.5L (IV); plasma protein binding (>99.3%). SP: Plasma protein binding (70%, 90% [acetylsulfapyridine]). **Metabolism:** SSZ: Intestinal bacteria and liver to SP (active) and 5-ASA (metabolites). SP: Acetylation to acetylsulfapyridine (principal metabolite). 5-ASA: Liver and intestine to N-acetyl-5-ASA. **Elimination:** Urine, feces. SSZ: $T_{1/2}$=7.6 hrs (IV). SP: $T_{1/2}$=10.4 hrs (fast acetylators), 14.8 hrs (slow acetylators).

NURSING CONSIDERATIONS

Assessment: Assess for intestinal or urinary obstruction, porphyria, renal dysfunction, severe allergy, bronchial asthma, G6PD deficiency, pregnancy/nursing status, possible drug interactions, history of hypersensitivity to the drug, its metabolites, sulfonamides, or salicylates, history of recurring/chronic infections, and underlying conditions which may predispose patients to infections. Obtain CBC, including differential WBC count, and LFTs.

Monitoring: Monitor for GI intolerance, hypersensitivity/skin reactions, neuromuscular and CNS changes, fibrosing alveolitis, infection, signs of hemolytic anemia (in patients with G6PD deficiency), and other adverse reactions. Monitor CBC, including differential WBC count, and LFTs every 2nd week for the first 3 months, monthly for the next 3 months, then every 3 months thereafter, and as clinically indicated. Monitor urinalysis and renal function periodically, and serum SP levels. Monitor for diarrhea and/or bloody stools in infants fed milk from mothers taking SSZ. Monitor newborns for kernicterus.

Patient Counseling: Inform of possible adverse reactions and need for careful medical supervision. Instruct to seek medical advice if sore throat, fever, pallor, purpura, or jaundice occurs. Inform that UC rarely remits completely and that risk of relapse can be reduced by continued administration at a maintenance dosage. Advise that orange-yellow discoloration of urine or skin may occur.

Administration: Oral route. Take in evenly divided doses, preferably pc. **Storage:** 25°C (77°F); excursions permitted to 15-30°C (59-86°F).

AZULFIDINE EN-TABS   RX
sulfasalazine (Pharmacia & Upjohn)

THERAPEUTIC CLASS: 5-aminosalicylic acid derivative/sulfapyridine

INDICATIONS: Treatment of mild to moderate ulcerative colitis (UC). Adjunctive therapy in severe UC. To prolong remission period between acute attacks of UC. Treatment of rheumatoid arthritis (RA) or polyarticular-course juvenile RA that has responded inadequately to salicylates or other NSAIDs.

DOSAGE: *Adults:* Individualize dose. Take preferably pc. UC: Initial: 3-4g/day in evenly divided doses with intervals not >8 hrs. May initiate with lower dose (eg, 1-2g/day) to reduce GI intolerance. Maint: 2g/day. When endoscopic exam confirms satisfactory improvement, reduce dose to a maintenance level. If diarrhea recurs, increase dose to previously effective levels. If symptoms of GI intolerance occur after 1st few doses, reduce daily dose by 1/2, then gradually increase over several days. If GI intolerance continues, d/c for 5-7 days, then reintroduce at a lower daily dose. RA: 2g/day in 2 evenly divided doses. Initiate therapy with lower dose (eg, 0.5-1g/day) to reduce GI intolerance. May increase to 3g/day if clinical response after 12 weeks is inadequate; careful monitoring is recommended for doses >2g/day. Refer to PI for dosing schedule. Desensitization: Initial: 50-250mg/day. Titrate: Double every 4-7 days until desired therapeutic level is achieved. D/C if sensitivity recurs.
Pediatrics: ≥6 Yrs: Individualize dose. Take preferably pc. UC: Initial: 40-60mg/kg/24 hrs divided into 3-6 doses. Maint: 30mg/kg/24 hrs divided into 4 doses. When endoscopic exam confirms satisfactory improvement, reduce dose to a maintenance level. If diarrhea recurs, increase dose to previously effective levels. If symptoms of GI intolerance occur after 1st few doses, reduce daily dose by 1/2, then gradually increase over several days. If GI intolerance continues, d/c for 5-7 days, then reintroduce at a lower daily dose. Juvenile RA: 30-50mg/kg/day in 2 evenly divided doses. To reduce GI intolerance, initiate with 1/4 to 1/3 of planned maintenance dose and increase weekly until reaching maintenance dose at 1 month. Max: 2g/day. Desensitization: Initial: 50-250mg/day. Titrate: Double every 4-7 days until desired therapeutic level is achieved. D/C if sensitivity recurs.

HOW SUPPLIED: Tab, Delayed-Release: 500mg

CONTRAINDICATIONS: Intestinal or urinary obstruction, porphyria.

WARNINGS/PRECAUTIONS: Caution with hepatic/renal damage, blood dyscrasias, severe allergy, bronchial asthma, history of recurring/chronic infections, or with underlying conditions or

B

concomitant drugs that may predispose patients to infections. Deaths reported from hypersensitivity reactions, agranulocytosis, aplastic anemia, other blood dyscrasias, renal and liver damage, irreversible neuromuscular and CNS changes, and fibrosing alveolitis. Perform CBC, including differential WBC count, and LFTs before starting therapy, every 2nd week for the first 3 months, monthly for the next 3 months, then every 3 months thereafter, and as clinically indicated; d/c while awaiting the results of blood tests. Monitor urinalysis and renal function periodically. Oligospermia and infertility reported in males. Serious infections (eg, fatal sepsis, pneumonia) reported. D/C if serious infection or toxic/hypersensitivity reactions develop. Closely monitor for signs and symptoms of infection during and after treatment; if a new infection develops, perform a prompt/complete diagnostic workup for infection and myelosuppression. Serious skin reactions, some fatal (eg, exfoliative dermatitis, Stevens-Johnson syndrome, toxic epidermal necrolysis), reported; d/c at 1st appearance of skin rash, mucosal lesions, or any other sign of hypersensitivity. Severe, life-threatening, systemic hypersensitivity reactions (eg, drug rash with eosinophilia and systemic symptoms) reported; evaluate immediately if signs/symptoms develop, and d/c if an alternative etiology cannot be established. Maintain adequate fluid intake to prevent crystalluria and stone formation. Closely monitor patients with G6PD deficiency for signs of hemolytic anemia. Do not attempt desensitization in patients who have a history of agranulocytosis, or have experienced an anaphylactoid reaction with previous sulfasalazine (SSZ) therapy. Serum sulfapyridine (SP) levels >50mcg/mL appear to be associated with increased incidence of adverse reactions. D/C immediately if tabs pass without disintegrating. Lab test interactions may occur.

ADVERSE REACTIONS: Anorexia, headache, N/V, gastric distress, reversible oligospermia, dyspepsia, rash, abdominal pain, fever, dizziness, stomatitis, pruritus, abnormal LFTs, leukopenia.

INTERACTIONS: May reduce absorption of folic acid and digoxin. Increased incidence of GI adverse events (especially nausea) with methotrexate.

PREGNANCY: Category B, caution in nursing.

MECHANISM OF ACTION: 5-aminosalicylic acid (5-ASA) derivative/SP; not established. May be related to the anti-inflammatory and/or immunomodulatory properties, to its affinity for connective tissue, and/or to the relatively high concentration it reaches in serous fluids, liver, and intestinal walls.

PHARMACOKINETICS: Absorption: SSZ: Absolute bioavailability (<15%); C_{max}=6mcg/mL; T_{max}=6 hrs. SP: Well absorbed from colon. Bioavailability (60%); T_{max}=10 hrs. 5-ASA: Much less well absorbed from GI tract. Bioavailability (10-30%); T_{max}=10 hrs. **Distribution:** Crosses placenta; found in breast milk. SSZ: V_d=7.5L (IV); plasma protein binding (>99.3%). SP: Plasma protein binding (70%, 90% [acetylsulfapyridine]). **Metabolism:** SSZ: Intestinal bacteria and liver to SP (active) and 5-ASA (metabolites). SP: Acetylation to acetylsulfapyridine (principal metabolite). 5-ASA: Liver and intestine to N-acetyl-5-ASA. **Elimination:** Urine, feces. SSZ: $T_{1/2}$=7.6 hrs (IV). SP: $T_{1/2}$=10.4 hrs (fast acetylators), 14.8 hrs (slow acetylators).

NURSING CONSIDERATIONS

Assessment: Assess for intestinal or urinary obstruction, porphyria, renal dysfunction, severe allergy, bronchial asthma, G6PD deficiency, pregnancy/nursing status, possible drug interactions, history of hypersensitivity to the drug, its metabolites, sulfonamides, or salicylates, history of recurring/chronic infections, and underlying conditions which may predispose patients to infections. Obtain CBC, including differential WBC count, and LFTs.

Monitoring: Monitor for GI intolerance, hypersensitivity/skin reactions, neuromuscular and CNS changes, fibrosing alveolitis, infection, signs of hemolytic anemia (in patients with G6PD deficiency), and other adverse reactions. Monitor CBC, including differential WBC count, and LFTs every 2nd week for the first 3 months, monthly for the next 3 months, then every 3 months thereafter, and as clinically indicated. Monitor urinalysis and renal function periodically, and serum SP levels. Monitor for tabs passing without disintegrating. Monitor for diarrhea and/or bloody stools in infants fed milk from mothers taking SSZ. Monitor newborns for kernicterus.

Patient Counseling: Inform of possible adverse effects and need for careful medical supervision. Instruct to seek medical advice if sore throat, fever, pallor, purpura, or jaundice occurs. Advise that orange-yellow discoloration of urine or skin may occur. Inform that UC rarely remits completely and that risk of relapse can be substantially reduced by continued administration at a maintenance dosage. Inform that RA rarely remits; instruct to follow up with physician to determine the need for continued administration.

Administration: Oral route. Take in evenly divided doses, preferably pc. Swallow tabs whole. **Storage:** 25°C (77°F); excursions permitted to 15-30°C (59-86°F).

BACTROBAN NASAL   RX
mupirocin calcium (GlaxoSmithKline)

THERAPEUTIC CLASS: Bacterial protein synthesis inhibitor

INDICATIONS: Eradication of nasal colonization of methicillin-resistant *Staphylococcus aureus* (MRSA) in adults and healthcare workers in certain institutional settings during outbreaks of MRSA.

DOSAGE: *Adults:* Apply 1/2 of the single-use tube into each nostril bid for 5 days. Spread oint by pressing together and releasing the sides of the nose repetitively for 1 min. Do not reuse tube.
Pediatrics: ≥12 Yrs: Apply 1/2 of the single-use tube into each nostril bid for 5 days. Spread oint by pressing together and releasing the sides of the nose repetitively for 1 min. Do not reuse tube.

HOW SUPPLIED: Oint: 2% [1g pkt]

WARNINGS/PRECAUTIONS: Avoid eyes. D/C if sensitization or irritation occurs. May cause superinfection with prolonged use.

ADVERSE REACTIONS: Headache, rhinitis, respiratory disorder, pharyngitis, taste perversion.

INTERACTIONS: Avoid use with other intranasal products.

PREGNANCY: Category B, caution in nursing.

MECHANISM OF ACTION: Antibacterial agent; inhibits protein synthesis by reversibly and specifically binding to bacterial isoleucyl transfer-RNA synthetase.

PHARMACOKINETICS: Absorption: Significant in neonates and premature infants. **Elimination:** Urine.

NURSING CONSIDERATIONS

Assessment: Assess for drug hypersensitivity, high-risk healthcare workers during institutional outbreaks of MRSA, and for possible drug interactions.

Monitoring: Monitor for sensitization, severe local irritation, tearing, and for overgrowth of non-susceptible microorganisms (eg, fungi).

Patient Counseling: Instruct to avoid contact with eyes. Advise to consult physician if sensitization or severe irritation occurs.

Administration: Intranasal route. Apply approximately half of oint from single-use tube directly into 1 nostril and other half into other nostril; discard tube after using. Press sides of nose together and gently massage after application to spread oint throughout inside of nostril. **Storage:** 20-25°C (68-77°F); excursions permitted to 15-30°C (59-86°F). Do not refrigerate.

BACTROBAN TOPICAL   RX
mupirocin calcium (GlaxoSmithKline)

THERAPEUTIC CLASS: Bacterial protein synthesis inhibitor

INDICATIONS: (Oint) Topical treatment of impetigo due to *Staphylococcus aureus* and *Streptococcus pyogenes*. (Cre) Treatment of secondarily infected traumatic skin lesions (up to 10cm in length or 100cm² in area) due to *S. aureus* and *S. pyogenes*.

DOSAGE: *Adults:* Apply a small amount tid to the affected area. May be covered with gauze dressing if desired. Reevaluate if no response within 3-5 days. (Cre) Treat for 10 days.
Pediatrics: (Oint) 2 Months-16 Yrs/(Cre) 3 Months-16 Yrs: Apply a small amount tid to the affected area. May be covered with gauze dressing if desired. Reevaluate if no response within 3-5 days. (Cre) Treat for 10 days.

HOW SUPPLIED: Cre: 2% [15g, 30g]; Oint: 2% [22g]

WARNINGS/PRECAUTIONS: Avoid contact with the eyes; not for ophthalmic use. Prolonged use may result in overgrowth of nonsusceptible organism (including fungi). Not for use on mucosal surfaces. D/C and institute appropriate therapy if sensitivity or chemical irritation occurs. (Oint) Contains polyethylene glycol; avoid use in conditions where absorption of large quantities is possible, especially if there is evidence of moderate or severe renal impairment.

ADVERSE REACTIONS: (Cre) Headache, rash, nausea, burning at application site, pruritus, abdominal pain, bleeding secondary to eczema, hives. (Oint) Burning, stinging, pain, itching, rash, nausea, erythema.

PREGNANCY: (Cre) Category B, (Oint) Safety not known in pregnancy; (Oint/Cre) caution in nursing.

MECHANISM OF ACTION: Bacterial protein synthesis inhibitor; inhibits bacterial protein synthesis by reversibly and specifically binding to bacterial isoleucyl transfer-RNA synthetase. Active against a wide range of gram-positive bacteria, including methicillin-resistant *S. aureus*. Also active against certain gram-negative bacteria.

PHARMACOKINETICS: Absorption: (Cre) Minimal skin absorption. **Distribution:** Plasma protein binding (>97%). **Metabolism:** (Cre) Rapid once in systemic circulation. **Elimination:** Urine (metabolite); (IV) $T_{1/2}$=20-40 min.

NURSING CONSIDERATIONS

Assessment: Assess for hypersensitivity, area of skin infection, and pregnancy/nursing status.

Monitoring: Monitor for sensitivity or chemical irritation of the skin. In patients on prolonged therapy, monitor for possible overgrowth of nonsusceptible microorganisms, including fungi.

Patient Counseling: Instruct to use as prescribed. Inform that medication is for external use only and to avoid contact with eyes. Counsel that treated area can be covered with a gauze dressing. Advise to d/c medication and notify physician if any signs of local adverse reactions (eg, irritation, severe itching, rash) develop. Instruct to notify physician if no clinical improvement is seen within 3-5 days.

Administration: Topical route. **Storage:** (Cre) ≤25°C (77°F). Do not freeze. (Oint) 20-25°C (68-77°F).

BANZEL   RX
rufinamide (Eisai)

THERAPEUTIC CLASS: Triazole derivative

INDICATIONS: Adjunctive treatment of seizures associated with Lennox-Gastaut syndrome in adults and children ≥4 yrs of age.

DOSAGE: *Adults:* Initial: 400-800mg/day in two equally divided doses. Titrate: May increase by 400-800mg qod until max reached. Max: 3200mg/day. Hemodialysis: Consider dosage adjustment. With Valproate: Initiate dose lower than 400mg/day. Elderly: Start at lower end of dosing range.
Pediatrics: ≥4 Yrs: Initial: 10mg/kg/day in two equally divided doses. Titrate: May increase by 10mg/kg increments qod to target dose of 45mg/kg/day or 3200mg/day, whichever is less, given in two equally divided doses. With Valproate: Initiate dose lower than 10mg/kg/day.

HOW SUPPLIED: Sus: 40mg/mL [460mL]; Tab: 200mg*, 400mg* *scored

CONTRAINDICATIONS: Familial short QT syndrome.

WARNINGS/PRECAUTIONS: May increase risk of suicidal thoughts or behavior; monitor for emergence or worsening of depression, suicidal thoughts or behavior, and/or any unusual changes in mood or behavior. Associated with CNS-related adverse effects (eg, somnolence/fatigue, coordination abnormalities, dizziness, gait disturbances, and ataxia). QT interval shortening and leukopenia reported. Multiorgan hypersensitivity syndrome reported; d/c if suspected and start alternative treatment. Withdraw gradually to minimize risk of precipitating seizures, seizure exacerbation, or status epilepticus. If abrupt discontinuation is necessary, transition to other antiepileptic drugs should be made under close medical supervision. Not recommended in severe hepatic impairment. Caution with mild to moderate hepatic impairment and elderly.

ADVERSE REACTIONS: Somnolence, N/V, headache, fatigue, dizziness, tremor, nystagmus, nasopharyngitis, decreased appetite, rash, ataxia, diplopia, bronchitis, blurred vision.

INTERACTIONS: Carboxylesterase inducers may increase clearance; carboxylesterase inhibitors may decrease metabolism of rufinamide. Potent CYP450 inducers (eg, carbamazepine, phenytoin, primodone, phenobarbital) may increase clearance and decrease levels of rufinamide. Valproate may reduce clearance and increase levels of rufinamide. May increase phenytoin, phenobarbital, CYP2E1 substrates (eg, chlorzoxazone) levels. May decrease lamotrigine, carbamazapine, CYP3A4 substrates (eg, triazolam), or hormonal contraceptives levels. Additional forms of nonhormonal contraception are recommended during coadministration. Caution with other drugs that shorten QT interval.

PREGNANCY: Category C, not for use in nursing.

MECHANISM OF ACTION: Triazole derivative; mechanism not established. Suspected to modulate activity of Na+ channels and, in particular, prolongation of the inactive state of the channel. Slows Na+ channel recovery from inactivation after prolonged prepulse in cultured cortical neurons, and limited sustained repetitive firing of Na+-dependent action potentials.

PHARMACOKINETICS: Absorption: Well-absorbed, T_{max}=4-6 hrs. **Distribution:** Plasma protein binding (34%); V_d=50L (3200mg/day); likely to be excreted in breast milk. **Metabolism:** Extensive; via carboxylesterase mediated hydrolysis; CYP2E1 (weak inhibitor), CYP3A4 (weak inducer). **Elimination:** Urine (2%, unchanged; 66%, acid metabolite CGP 47292); $T_{1/2}$=6-10 hrs.

NURSING CONSIDERATIONS

Assessment: Assess for familial short QT syndrome, presence or history of depression, hepatic/renal impairment, pregnancy/nursing status, and for possible drug interactions.

Monitoring: Monitor for emergence or worsening of depression, suicidal thoughts, changes in behavior, CNS reactions (eg, somnolence, fatigue, coordination abnormalities, dizziness, gait disturbances, ataxia), QT interval shortening, multiorgan hypersensitivity syndrome, and leukopenia. Upon withdrawal of therapy, monitor for precipitation of seizures, exacerbation of seizures, and status epilepticus.

Patient Counseling: Inform patients, caregivers, and families of increased risk of suicidal thoughts/behavior and to be alert for emergence or worsening of signs/symptoms. Instruct to avoid alcohol and take only as prescribed. May develop somnolence or dizziness. Advise not to drive or operate machinery until gaining sufficient experience to gauge whether therapy adversely affects mental and/or motor performance. Encourage to enroll in North American Antiepileptic Drug (NAAED) Pregnancy Registry. Instruct to notify physician if rash associated with fever develops. Advise to take with food; tabs may be taken whole, cut in half, or crushed. Must shake suspension well before every administration.

Administration: Oral route. Take with food. Tab: May administer as whole, half, or crushed tab. Sus: Refer to PI for complete instructions. **Storage:** Tab/Sus: 25°C (77°F); excursions permitted to 15-30°C (59-86°F). Tab: Protect from moisture. Sus: Store in an upright position. Use within 90 days of first opening the bottle, discard any remainder.

BARACLUDE   RX

entecavir (Bristol-Myers Squibb)

> Severe acute exacerbations of hepatitis B reported upon discontinuation of therapy; monitor liver function for at least several months after discontinuation. If appropriate, may initiate antihepatitis B therapy. Potential for development of resistance to HIV nucleoside reverse transcriptase inhibitors if entecavir is used to treat chronic hepatitis B virus (HBV) infection in patients with untreated HIV infection. Not recommended for HIV/HBV coinfected patients not receiving highly active antiretroviral therapy (HAART). Lactic acidosis and severe hepatomegaly with steatosis, including fatal cases, have been reported with the use of nucleoside analogue inhibitors.

THERAPEUTIC CLASS: Guanosine nucleoside analogue

INDICATIONS: Treatment of chronic HBV infection in patients ≥2 yrs of age with evidence of active viral replication and either evidence of persistent elevations in serum aminotransferases (ALT/AST) or histologically active disease.

DOSAGE: *Adults:* Take on an empty stomach. Compensated Liver Disease: Nucleoside-Inhibitor-Treatment-Naive: 0.5mg qd. History of Hepatitis B Viremia While Receiving Lamivudine or Known Lamivudine- or Telbivudine-Resistant Substitutions: 1mg qd. Decompensated Liver Disease: 1mg qd. Refer to PI for renal impairment dosing.
Pediatrics: Take on an empty stomach. ≥16 Yrs: Compensated Liver Disease: Nucleoside-Inhibitor-Treatment-Naive: 0.5mg qd. History of Hepatitis B Viremia While Receiving Lamivudine or Known Lamivudine- or Telbivudine-Resistant Substitutions: 1mg qd. ≥2 Yrs: ≥10kg; refer to PI for dosing schedule. Refer to PI for renal impairment dosing.

HOW SUPPLIED: Sol: 0.05mg/mL [210mL]; Tab: 0.5mg, 1mg

WARNINGS/PRECAUTIONS: Dosage adjustment is recommended in renal dysfunction (CrCl <50mL/min), including patients on hemodialysis or continuous ambulatory peritoneal dialysis. May require HIV antibody testing prior to treatment. Caution with known risk factors for liver disease. D/C if lactic acidosis or pronounced hepatotoxicity occurs. Caution in elderly.

ADVERSE REACTIONS: Hepatitis B exacerbation, lactic acidosis, hepatomegaly, headache, fatigue, dizziness, nausea, ALT/lipase/total bilirubin elevation, hyperglycemia, glycosuria, hematuria.

INTERACTIONS: May increase levels of either entecavir or concomitant drugs that reduce renal function or compete for active tubular secretion; closely monitor for adverse events.

PREGNANCY: Category C, not for use in nursing.

MECHANISM OF ACTION: Guanosine nucleoside analogue; inhibits base priming, reverse transcription of negative strand from pregenomic mRNA, and synthesis of positive strand of HBV DNA.

PHARMACOKINETICS: Absorption: C_{max}=4.2ng/mL (0.5mg), 8.2ng/mL (1mg); T_{max}=0.5-1.5 hrs. **Distribution:** Serum protein binding (13%). **Metabolism:** Glucuronidation and sulfate conjugation. **Elimination:** Urine (62-73% unchanged); $T_{1/2}$=128-149 hrs.

NURSING CONSIDERATIONS

Assessment: Assess for hepatic/renal impairment, pregnancy/nursing status, and possible drug interactions. Perform HIV antibody testing before initiating therapy.

Monitoring: Monitor for signs/symptoms of lactic acidosis, hepatotoxicity, renal/hepatic impairment, and other adverse reactions.

Patient Counseling: Advise to remain under care of physician during therapy and report any new symptoms or concurrent medications. Advise that treatment has not been shown to reduce risk of transmission of HBV to others through sexual contact or blood contamination. Advise to take the missed dose as soon as remembered unless it is almost time for the next dose and not to take

2 doses at the same time. Inform that treatment may lower the amount of HBV in the body and improve the condition of the liver, but will not cure HBV. Counsel that it is not known whether treatment will reduce risk of liver cancer or cirrhosis. Inform that deterioration of liver disease may occur in some cases if treatment is discontinued, and to discuss any change in regimen with physician. Inform that drug may increase the chance of HIV resistance to HIV medication if HIV-infected patient is not receiving effective HIV treatment.

Administration: Oral route. Take on an empty stomach (at least 2 hrs pc and 2 hrs before the next meal). Sol: Hold dosing spoon in a vertical position and fill gradually to the mark corresponding to prescribed dose; refer to PI for further administration instructions. **Storage:** 25°C (77°F); excursions permitted between 15-30°C (59-86°F). Protect from light.

BAYER ASPIRIN   OTC
aspirin (Bayer Healthcare)

OTHER BRAND NAMES: Bayer Aspirin Children's (Bayer Healthcare) - Bayer Aspirin Regimen with Calcium (Bayer Healthcare) - Bayer Aspirin Regimen (Bayer Healthcare) - Genuine Bayer Aspirin (Bayer Healthcare)

THERAPEUTIC CLASS: Salicylate

INDICATIONS: To reduce the risk of death and nonfatal stroke with previous ischemic stroke or transient ischemia of the brain. To reduce risk of vascular mortality with suspected acute myocardial infarction (MI). To reduce risk of death and nonfatal MI with previous MI or unstable angina. To reduce risk of MI and sudden death in chronic stable angina pectoris. For patients who have undergone revascularization procedures with a preexisting condition for which ASA is indicated. Relief of signs of rheumatoid arthritis (RA), juvenile rheumatoid arthritis (JRA), osteoarthritis (OA), spondyloarthropathies, arthritis, and pleurisy associated with systemic lupus erythematosus (SLE). For minor aches and pains.

DOSAGE: *Adults:* Ischemic Stroke/TIA: 50-325mg qd. Suspected Acute MI: Initial: 160-162.5mg qd as soon as MI is suspected. Maint: 160-162.5mg qd for 30 days postinfarction, consider further therapy for prevention/recurrent MI. Prevention or Recurrent MI/Unstable Angina/Chronic Stable Angina: 75-325mg qd. CABG: 325mg qd, start 6 hrs postsurgery. Continue for 1 yr. PTCA: Initial: 325mg, 2 hrs presurgery. Maint: 160-325mg qd. Carotid Endarterectomy: 80mg qd to 650mg bid, start presurgery. RA: Initial: 3g qd in divided doses. Increase for anti-inflammatory efficacy to 150-300mcg/mL plasma salicylate level. Spondyloarthropathies: Up to 4g/day in divided doses. OA: Up to 3g/day in divided doses. Arthritis/SLE Pleurisy: Initial: 3g/day in divided doses. Increase for anti-inflammatory efficacy to 150-300mcg/mL plasma salicylate level. Pain: 325-650mg q4-6h. Max: 4g/day.
Pediatrics: JRA: Initial: 90-130mg/kg/day in divided doses. Increase for anti-inflammatory efficacy to 150-300mcg/mL plasma salicylate level. Pain: ≥12 Yrs: 325-650mg q4-6h. Max: 4g/day.

HOW SUPPLIED: Tab: (Genuine Bayer Aspirin) 325mg; Tab: (Bayer Aspirin Regimen with Calcium) 81mg; Tab, Chewable: (Bayer Aspirin Children's) 81mg; Tab, Delayed-Release: (Bayer Aspirin Regimen) 81mg, 325mg.

CONTRAINDICATIONS: NSAID allergy, viral infections in children or teenagers, syndrome of asthma, rhinitis, and nasal polyps.

WARNINGS/PRECAUTIONS: Increased risk of bleeding with heavy alcohol use (≥3 drinks/day). May inhibit platelet function; can adversely affect inherited (hemophilia) or acquired (hepatic disease, vitamin K deficiency) bleeding disorders. Monitor for bleeding and ulceration. Avoid in history of active peptic ulcer, severe renal failure, severe hepatic insufficiency, and Na⁺-restricted diets. Associated with elevated LFTs, BUN, and SrCr; hyperkalemia; proteinuria; and prolonged bleeding time. Avoid 1 week before and during labor.

ADVERSE REACTIONS: Fever, hypothermia, dysrhythmias, hypotension, agitation, cerebral edema, dehydration, hyperkalemia, dyspepsia, GI bleed, hearing loss, tinnitus, problems in pregnancy.

INTERACTIONS: Diminished hypotensive and hyponatremic effects of ACE inhibitors. May increase levels of acetazolamide or valproic acid. Increased bleeding risk with heparin, warfarin. Decreased levels of phenytoin. Decreased hypotensive effects of β-blockers. Decreased diuretic effects with renal or cardiovascular disease. Decreased methotrexate clearance; increased risk of bone marrow toxicity. Avoid NSAIDs. Increased effects of hypoglycemic agents. Antagonizes uricosuric agents.

PREGNANCY: Avoid in 3rd trimester of pregnancy and nursing.

MECHANISM OF ACTION: Provides temporary relief from arthritis pain and inflammation.

NURSING CONSIDERATIONS

Assessment: Assess for hypersensitivity, stomach problems, bleeding problems, ulcers, history of chickenpox or flu symptoms, and possible drug interactions.

Monitoring: Monitor for Reye's syndrome, allergic reactions including hives, facial swelling, or asthma (wheezing), and shock.

Patient Counseling: Instruct to immediately report worsening of any adverse effects.

Administration: Oral route. **Storage:** Room temperature.

BELVIQ   CIV
lorcaserin HCl (Eisai)

THERAPEUTIC CLASS: Serotonin 2C receptor agonist

INDICATIONS: Adjunct to a reduced-calorie diet and increased physical activity for chronic weight management in adults with an initial BMI of ≥30kg/m² (obese), or ≥27kg/m² (overweight) in the presence of at least 1 weight-related comorbid condition (eg, HTN, dyslipidemia, type 2 diabetes).

DOSAGE: *Adults:* Usual: 10mg bid. Do not exceed recommended dose. Evaluate response to therapy by Week 12; d/c therapy if patient has not lost at least 5% of baseline body weight.

HOW SUPPLIED: Tab: 10mg

CONTRAINDICATIONS: Pregnancy.

WARNINGS/PRECAUTIONS: Potentially life-threatening serotonin syndrome or neuroleptic malignant syndrome (NMS)-like reactions reported; monitor for emergence of serotonin syndrome or NMS-like signs/symptoms. Regurgitant cardiac valvular disease reported; evaluate and consider discontinuation of therapy if signs/symptoms of valvular heart disease develop. Caution with CHF. May impair mental/physical abilities. Monitor for emergence or worsening of depression, suicidal thoughts or behavior, and/or any unusual changes in mood or behavior; d/c in patients who experience suicidal thoughts or behaviors. Hypoglycemia reported; measure blood glucose levels prior to and during therapy in patients with type 2 diabetes. Caution in men who have conditions that might predispose them to priapism, or in men with anatomical deformation of the penis. Caution with bradycardia or history of heart block >1st degree, moderate renal impairment, and severe hepatic impairment. Not recommended with severe renal impairment or end stage renal disease. Decrease in WBCs and RBCs reported; consider monitoring CBC periodically during therapy. May elevate prolactin levels. May increase risk for pulmonary HTN.

ADVERSE REACTIONS: Nasopharyngitis, headache, constipation, diarrhea, hypoglycemia, cough, dizziness, fatigue, back pain, N/V, dry mouth, upper respiratory tract infection, peripheral edema, urinary tract infection, muscle spasms.

INTERACTIONS: Use extreme caution, particularly during initiation and dose increases, with drugs that may affect the serotonergic neurotransmitter system (eg, triptans, drugs that impair metabolism of serotonin including MAOIs [eg, linezolid], SSRIs, SNRIs, dextromethorphan, TCAs, bupropion, lithium, tramadol, tryptophan, St. John's Wort, antipsychotics, other dopamine antagonists); d/c lorcaserin and any concomitant serotonergic or antidopaminergic agents immediately if serotonin syndrome occurs. Consider decreasing dose of non-glucose dependent antidiabetic medications in order to mitigate risk of hypoglycemia. Caution with CYP2D6 substrates. Avoid with serotonergic and dopaminergic drugs that are potent 5-HT$_{2B}$ receptor agonists and are known to increase the risk for cardiac valvulopathy (eg, cabergoline). Caution with medications indicated for erectile dysfunction (eg, PDE-5 inhibitors).

PREGNANCY: Category X, not for use in nursing.

MECHANISM OF ACTION: Serotonin 2C receptor agonist; not established. Believed to decrease food consumption and promote satiety by selectively activating 5-HT$_{2C}$ receptors on anorexigenic pro-opiomelanocortin neurons located in the hypothalamus.

PHARMACOKINETICS: Absorption: T_{max}=1.5-2 hrs. **Distribution:** Plasma protein binding (70%). **Metabolism:** Liver (extensive); lorcaserin sulfamate (M1) (major circulating metabolite), N-carbamoyl glucuronide lorcaserin (major metabolite in urine). **Elimination:** Urine (92.3%), feces (2.2%); $T_{1/2}$= 11 hrs.

NURSING CONSIDERATIONS

Assessment: Assess for CHF, bradycardia or history of heart block >1st degree, renal/hepatic impairment, pregnancy/nursing status and possible drug interactions. Assess for conditions in men that might predispose them to priapism and assess for anatomical deformities of the penis in men. Assess baseline body weight and CBC. Assess baseline blood glucose levels in patients with type 2 diabetes.

Monitoring: Monitor for signs/symptoms of serotonin syndrome or NMS-like reactions, valvular heart disease, emergence or worsening of depression, suicidal thoughts or behavior and/or any unusual changes in mood or behavior, and other adverse reactions. Monitor CBC periodically during therapy. Monitor blood glucose levels in patients with type 2 diabetes. Evaluate response to treatment by Week 12 of therapy.

B

Patient Counseling: Inform about the risk and benefits of the drug. Inform that therapy is indicated for chronic weight management only in conjunction with a reduced-calorie diet and increased physical activity. Instruct to d/c therapy if patient has not achieved 5% weight loss by 12 weeks of therapy. Inform of the possibility of serotonin or NMS-like reactions. Instruct to use caution when operating hazardous machinery including automobiles, until aware of the effects of the medication. Instruct not to increase the dose. Instruct to notify physician if signs/symptoms of valvular heart disease, emergence or worsening of depression, suicidal thoughts or behavior, or if any unusual changes in mood or behavior develop. Instruct men who have an erection lasting >4 hrs to immediately d/c and seek emergency medical attention. Advise to avoid pregnancy/breastfeeding while on therapy and to inform physician if planning to get pregnant/breastfeed. Instruct to inform physician about all medications, nutritional supplements, and vitamins that patient is taking while on therapy.

Administration: Oral route. Take with or without food. **Storage:** 25°C (77°F); excursions permitted to 15-30°C (59-86°F).

BENICAR   RX
olmesartan medoxomil (Daiichi Sankyo)

> D/C when pregnancy is detected. Drugs that act directly on the renin-angiotensin system (RAS) can cause injury/death to the developing fetus.

THERAPEUTIC CLASS: Angiotensin II receptor antagonist

INDICATIONS: Treatment of HTN alone or in combination with other antihypertensives.

DOSAGE: *Adults:* Individualize dose. Monotherapy Without Volume Contraction: Initial: 20mg qd. Titrate: May increase to 40mg qd after 2 weeks if needed. May add diuretic if BP is not controlled. Intravascular Volume Depletion (eg, Treated With Diuretics, Particularly Those With Impaired Renal Function): Lower initial dose; monitor closely.
Pediatrics: 6-16 Yrs: Individualize dose. ≥35kg: Initial: 20mg qd. Titrate: May increase to 40mg qd after 2 weeks if needed. Max: 40mg qd. 20-<35kg: Initial: 10mg qd. Titrate: May increase to 20mg qd after 2 weeks if needed. Max: 20mg qd. Cannot Swallow Tab: Sus dose is same as tab.

HOW SUPPLIED: Tab: 5mg, 20mg, 40mg

CONTRAINDICATIONS: Coadministration with aliskiren in patients with diabetes.

WARNINGS/PRECAUTIONS: Symptomatic hypotension may occur in patients with an activated renin-angiotensin aldosterone system (RAAS) (eg, volume- and/or salt-depleted patients receiving high doses of diuretics) after treatment initiation; monitor closely. Changes in renal function may occur. Oliguria and/or progressive azotemia and (rarely) acute renal failure and/or death may occur in patients whose renal function may depend on the RAAS activity (eg, severe congestive heart failure [CHF]). May increase SrCr or BUN levels in patients with renal artery stenosis. Sprue-like enteropathy with symptoms of severe, chronic diarrhea with substantial weight loss reported; exclude other etiologies if these symptoms develop, and consider discontinuation in cases where no other etiology is identified.

ADVERSE REACTIONS: Dizziness.

INTERACTIONS: See Contraindications. NSAIDs, including selective COX-2 inhibitors, may attenuate antihypertensive effect and may deteriorate renal function. Dual blockade of the RAS is associated with increased risks of hypotension, hyperkalemia, and changes in renal function (including acute renal failure); closely monitor BP, renal function, and electrolytes with concomitant agents that affect the RAS. Avoid with aliskiren in patients with renal impairment (GFR <60mL/min). Reduced levels with colesevelam; administer at least 4 hrs before colesevelam dose.

PREGNANCY: Category D, not for use in nursing.

MECHANISM OF ACTION: Angiotensin II receptor antagonist; blocks the vasoconstrictor effects of angiotensin II by selectively blocking the binding of angiotensin II to the AT_1 receptor in vascular smooth muscle.

PHARMACOKINETICS: Absorption: Absolute bioavailability (26%); T_{max}=1-2 hrs. **Distribution:** V_d=17L; plasma protein binding (99%). **Metabolism:** Ester hydrolysis to olmesartan (active metabolite). **Elimination:** Urine (35-50%), feces; $T_{1/2}$=13 hrs.

NURSING CONSIDERATIONS

Assessment: Assess for diabetes, CHF, renal artery stenosis, volume/salt depletion, renal function, pregnancy/nursing status, and possible drug interactions.

Monitoring: Monitor for signs/symptoms of hypotension, renal dysfunction, sprue-like enteropathy, and other adverse reactions.

Patient Counseling: Inform females of childbearing potential of the consequences of exposure during pregnancy and of the treatment options for women planning to become pregnant. Instruct to report pregnancy to the physician as soon as possible.

Administration: Oral route. May be administered with or without food. Refer to PI for preparation of sus. Shake sus well before each use. **Storage:** (Tab) 20-25°C (68-77°F). (Sus) 2-8°C (36-46°F) for up to 4 weeks.

BENICAR HCT   RX
olmesartan medoxomil - hydrochlorothiazide (Daiichi Sankyo)

D/C when pregnancy is detected. Drugs that act directly on the renin-angiotensin system (RAS) can cause injury/death to the developing fetus.

THERAPEUTIC CLASS: Angiotensin II receptor antagonist/thiazide diuretic

INDICATIONS: Treatment of HTN.

DOSAGE: *Adults:* Begin combination therapy only after failure to achieve desired effect with monotherapy. Refer to PI for monotherapy dosing. Replacement Therapy: May be substituted for its titrated components. Uncontrolled BP on Olmesartan or HCTZ Alone: Switch to once-daily combination therapy. Individualize dose. Usual: 1 tab qd. Titrate: May adjust at intervals of 2-4 weeks. Max: 1 tab/day. May be administered with other antihypertensive agents. Elderly: Start at lower end of dosing range.

HOW SUPPLIED: Tab: (Olmesartan-HCTZ) 20mg-12.5mg, 40mg-12.5mg, 40mg-25mg

CONTRAINDICATIONS: Anuria, sulfonamide-derived drug hypersensitivity. Coadministration with aliskiren in patients with diabetes.

WARNINGS/PRECAUTIONS: Not indicated for initial therapy. Symptomatic hypotension may occur in patients with an activated RAS (eg, volume- or salt-depleted patients receiving high doses of diuretics) after treatment initiation; monitor closely. Sprue-like enteropathy with symptoms of severe, chronic diarrhea with substantial weight loss reported; exclude other etiologies if these symptoms develop, and consider discontinuation in cases where no other etiology is identified. Hypokalemia/hyperkalemia reported. Not recommended with severe renal impairment (CrCl ≤30mL/min). Oliguria and/or progressive azotemia and (rarely) acute renal failure and/or death may occur in patients whose renal function may depend on the renin-angiotensin aldosterone system activity (eg, severe congestive heart failure [CHF]). May increase SrCr or BUN levels in patients with renal artery stenosis. Caution with severe renal disease; may precipitate azotemia. Caution in elderly. HCTZ: Caution with hepatic impairment or progressive liver disease; may precipitate hepatic coma. May cause hypersensitivity reactions, exacerbation or activation of systemic lupus erythematosus (SLE), hyperuricemia or precipitation of frank gout, hyperglycemia, hypomagnesemia, hypercalcemia, and manifestations of latent diabetes mellitus (DM). May cause idiosyncratic reaction, resulting in acute transient myopia and acute angle-closure glaucoma; d/c as rapidly as possible. Observe for signs of fluid or electrolyte imbalance (eg, hyponatremia, hypochloremic alkalosis, hypokalemia). Hypokalemia may cause cardiac arrhythmia and may sensitize/exaggerate the response of the heart to toxic effects of digitalis. D/C before testing for parathyroid function. Enhanced effects in postsympathectomy patients. D/C or withhold if progressive renal impairment becomes evident. Increased cholesterol and TG levels reported.

ADVERSE REACTIONS: Dizziness, upper respiratory tract infection, hyperuricemia, nausea.

INTERACTIONS: See Contraindications. NSAIDs, including selective COX-2 inhibitors, may decrease effects of diuretics and angiotensin II receptor antagonists and may deteriorate renal function. Olmesartan: Dual blockade of the RAS is associated with increased risks of hypotension, hyperkalemia, and changes in renal function (including acute renal failure); closely monitor BP, renal function, and electrolytes with concomitant agents that affect the RAS. Avoid with aliskiren in patients with renal impairment (GFR <60mL/min). Reduced levels with colesevelam; administer at least 4 hrs before colesevelam dose. HCTZ: May increase risk of lithium toxicity; avoid concurrent use. Alcohol, barbiturates, or narcotics may potentiate orthostatic hypotension. Dose adjustment of antidiabetic drugs (eg, oral agents and insulin) may be required. Additive effect or potentiation with other antihypertensives. Anionic exchange resins (eg, cholestyramine, colestipol) may impair absorption. Corticosteroids and adrenocorticotropic hormone may intensify electrolyte depletion, particularly hypokalemia. May decrease response to pressor amines (eg, norepinephrine). May increase responsiveness to nondepolarizing skeletal muscle relaxants (eg, tubocurarine).

PREGNANCY: Category D, not for use in nursing.

MECHANISM OF ACTION: Olmesartan: Angiotensin II receptor antagonist; blocks the vasoconstrictor effects of angiotensin II by selectively blocking the binding of angiotensin II to the AT_1 receptor in vascular smooth muscle. HCTZ: Thiazide diuretic; not established. Affects renal tubular mechanisms of electrolyte reabsorption, directly increasing excretion of Na^+ and Cl^- in approximately equivalent amounts.

PHARMACOKINETICS: Absorption: Olmesartan: Absolute bioavailability (26%); T_{max}=1-2 hrs. **Distribution:** Olmesartan: V_d=17L; plasma protein binding (99%). HCTZ: Crosses placenta; found in breast milk. **Metabolism:** Olmesartan: Ester hydrolysis to olmesartan (active metabolite). **Elimination:** Olmesartan: Urine (35-50%), feces; $T_{1/2}$=13 hrs. HCTZ: Kidney (≥61% unchanged); $T_{1/2}$=5.6-14.8 hrs.

NURSING CONSIDERATIONS

Assessment: Assess for hypersensitivity to the drug and its components, anuria, sulfonamide-derived drug hypersensitivity, history of penicillin allergy, volume/salt depletion, SLE, DM, CHF, hepatic/renal impairment, postsympathectomy status, cirrhosis, renal artery stenosis, pregnancy/nursing status, and possible drug interactions.

Monitoring: Monitor for signs/symptoms of fluid/electrolyte imbalance, sprue-like enteropathy, exacerbation/activation of SLE, idiosyncratic reaction, latent DM, precipitation of gout, hypersensitivity reactions, and other adverse reactions. Monitor BP, serum electrolytes, cholesterol, and TG levels, and renal/hepatic function.

Patient Counseling: Inform females of childbearing potential of the consequences of exposure during pregnancy and of the treatment options for women planning to become pregnant. Instruct to report pregnancy to the physician as soon as possible. Counsel that lightheadedness may occur, especially during the 1st days of therapy; instruct to report to physician. Instruct to d/c therapy and consult physician if syncope occurs. Advise that inadequate fluid intake, excessive perspiration, diarrhea, or vomiting may lead to an excessive fall in BP, with the same consequences of lightheadedness and possible syncope.

Administration: Oral route. **Storage:** 20-25°C (68-77°F).

BENLYSTA   RX
belimumab (GlaxoSmithKline)

THERAPEUTIC CLASS: Monoclonal antibody/BLyS blocker

INDICATIONS: Treatment of adult patients with active, autoantibody-positive, systemic lupus erythematosus who are receiving standard therapy.

DOSAGE: *Adults:* 10mg/kg IV infusion over 1 hr at 2-week intervals for the first 3 doses and at 4-week intervals thereafter. Slow or interrupt infusion rate if infusion reaction develops. Consider premedication for prophylaxis against infusion and hypersensitivity reactions.

HOW SUPPLIED: Inj: 120mg [5mL], 400mg [20mL]

WARNINGS/PRECAUTIONS: Deaths reported; etiologies included infection, cardiovascular disease, and suicide. Serious and sometimes fatal infections reported; caution with chronic infections and interrupt treatment if new infection develops. JC virus-associated progressive multifocal leukoencephalopathy (PML) resulting in neurological deficits, including fatal cases reported. Consider diagnosis of PML in any patient presenting with new-onset or deteriorating neurological signs/symptoms. Consider stopping therapy in patients with confirmed PML. Malignancies, infusion reactions, psychiatric events (eg, depression) reported. Hypersensitivity reactions, including anaphylaxis and death, reported; onset may be delayed; d/c immediately if serious hypersensitivity reactions occur. Caution in elderly. Women of childbearing potential should use adequate contraception during treatment and for ≥4 months after the final treatment. Not recommended with severe active lupus nephritis or severe active CNS lupus.

ADVERSE REACTIONS: Serious infections, nausea, diarrhea, pyrexia, nasopharyngitis, bronchitis, insomnia, pain in extremity, depression, migraine, pharyngitis, cystitis, leukopenia, viral gastroenteritis.

INTERACTIONS: Not recommended with other biologics or IV cyclophosphamide. Live vaccines should not be given for 30 days before or concurrently; may interfere with the response to immunizations.

PREGNANCY: Category C, not for use in nursing.

MECHANISM OF ACTION: Monoclonal antibody/B lymphocyte stimulator protein (BLyS) blocker; blocks binding of soluble human BLyS to its receptors on B cells. Inhibits survival of B cells.

PHARMACOKINETICS: Absorption: AUC=3083mcg•day/mL; C_{max}=313mcg/mL. **Distribution:** V_d=5.29L; crosses placenta. **Elimination:** $T_{1/2}$=19.4 days.

NURSING CONSIDERATIONS

Assessment: Assess for chronic infection, PML, history of depression or other serious psychiatric disorders, previous anaphylaxis with the drug, history of multiple drug allergies or significant hypersensitivity, pregnancy/nursing status, and possible drug interactions.

Monitoring: Monitor for infusion and hypersensitivity reactions, infections, malignancy, psychiatric events, and other adverse reactions.

Patient Counseling: Advise that drug may decrease ability to fight infections. Instruct to notify physician if signs/symptoms of infection, allergic reaction, new or worsening depression, suicidal thoughts, or other mood changes develop, and if patients become pregnant or plan to breast-feed. Encourage pregnant patients to enroll in the pregnancy registry. Advise patients to contact physician if they experience new or worsening neurological symptoms. Inform about signs and symptoms of hypersensitivity reaction and instruct to seek medical care should reaction occur. Advise not to receive live vaccines while on therapy.

Administration: IV route. For IV infusion only; do not administer as an IV push or bolus. Reconstitute and dilute prior to administration; refer to PI for preparation and administration instructions. Dilute with 0.9% NaCl only. **Storage:** Unreconstituted/Reconstituted: 2-8°C (36-46°F). Do not freeze. Protect from light and store vials in original carton until use. Avoid exposure to heat. Diluted Sol: 2-8°C (36-46°F) or room temperature. Total time from reconstitution to completion of infusion should not exceed 8 hrs.

BENZACLIN
clindamycin phosphate - benzoyl peroxide (Valeant)

THERAPEUTIC CLASS: Antibacterial/keratolytic

INDICATIONS: Topical treatment of acne vulgaris.

DOSAGE: *Adults:* Apply bid (am and pm) or ud, to affected areas after the skin is gently washed, rinsed with warm water, and patted dry.
Pediatrics: ≥12 Yrs: Apply bid (am and pm) or ud, to affected areas after the skin is gently washed, rinsed with warm water, and patted dry.

HOW SUPPLIED: Gel: (Clindamycin-Benzoyl Peroxide) 1%-5% [25g, jar; 35g, 50g, pump]

CONTRAINDICATIONS: History of regional enteritis, ulcerative colitis (UC), or antibiotic-associated colitis.

WARNINGS/PRECAUTIONS: Severe colitis, which may result in death, reported following oral and parenteral clindamycin administration. Diarrhea, bloody diarrhea, and colitis (including pseudomembranous colitis) reported; d/c if significant diarrhea occurs. Not for ophthalmic use. May cause overgrowth of nonsusceptible organisms, including fungi; d/c use and take appropriate measures if this occurs. Avoid contact with eyes and mucous membranes.

ADVERSE REACTIONS: Dry skin, application-site reaction.

INTERACTIONS: Antiperistaltic agents (eg, opiates, diphenoxylate with atropine) may prolong and/or worsen colitis. Caution with concomitant topical acne therapy (eg, peeling, desquamating, or abrasive agents) because of possible cumulative irritancy effect. Do not use with erythromycin-containing products.

PREGNANCY: Category C, not for use in nursing.

MECHANISM OF ACTION: Antibacterial/keratolytic; individual components act against *Propionibacterium acnes*, an organism associated with acne vulgaris.

PHARMACOKINETICS: Absorption: Clindamycin: Systemic bioavailability (<1%). Benzoyl peroxide: Skin. **Distribution:** Clindamycin: (PO/Parenteral) Found in breast milk. **Metabolism:** Benzoyl peroxide: Converted to benzoic acid.

NURSING CONSIDERATIONS

Assessment: Assess for hypersensitivity to drug or to lincomycin, history of regional enteritis, UC, or antibiotic-associated colitis, pregnancy/nursing status, and possible drug interactions.

Monitoring: Monitor for signs/symptoms of diarrhea, colitis, overgrowth of nonsusceptible organisms, and other adverse reactions. For colitis, perform stool culture and assay for *Clostridium difficile* toxin. Consider large bowel endoscopy in cases of severe diarrhea.

Patient Counseling: Instruct to use externally ud and to avoid contact with eyes, and inside the nose, mouth, and all mucous membranes. Advise not to use for any disorder other than for which it was prescribed and not to use any other topical acne preparation unless otherwise directed by physician. Counsel to minimize or avoid exposure to natural or artificial sunlight (tanning beds or UVA/B treatment) while using medication; instruct to wear a wide-brimmed hat or other protective clothing, and use a sunscreen with SPF ≥15 to minimize exposure to sunlight. Instruct to report any signs of local adverse reactions to physician. Inform that drug may bleach hair or colored fabric.

Administration: Topical route. Wash skin gently, then rinse with warm water and pat dry before application. Reconstitute before dispensing; refer to PI for reconstitution instructions. **Storage:** Room temperature up to 25°C (77°F). Do not freeze. Discard product 3 months following reconstitution.

B

BEPREVE   RX
bepotastine besilate (Ista)

THERAPEUTIC CLASS: H$_1$-antagonist

INDICATIONS: Treatment of itching associated with signs and symptoms of allergic conjunctivitis.

DOSAGE: *Adults:* 1 drop into the affected eye(s) bid.
Pediatrics: ≥2 Yrs: 1 drop into the affected eye(s) bid.

HOW SUPPLIED: Sol: 1.5% [5mL, 10mL]

WARNINGS/PRECAUTIONS: For topical ophthalmic use only. Avoid touching the eyelids or surrounding areas with dropper tip of the bottle. Not for the treatment of contact lens-related irritation. Contains benzalkonium chloride, which may be absorbed by soft contact lenses; remove contact lenses prior to instillation and may reinsert 10 min after administration.

ADVERSE REACTIONS: Mild taste, eye irritation, headache, nasopharyngitis.

PREGNANCY: Category C, caution in nursing.

MECHANISM OF ACTION: H$_1$-antagonist; antagonizes H$_1$ receptor and inhibits release of histamine from mast cells.

PHARMACOKINETICS: Absorption: T$_{max}$=1-2 hrs; C$_{max}$=7.3ng/mL. **Distribution:** Plasma protein binding (55%). **Metabolism:** Liver via CYP450 (minimal). **Excretion:** Urine (75-90%, unchanged).

NURSING CONSIDERATIONS

Assessment: Assess for previous hypersensitivity to the drug, contact lens use, and pregnancy/nursing status.

Monitoring: Monitor for hypersensitivity and other adverse reactions.

Patient Counseling: Counsel that therapy is not for the treatment of lens-related irritation and advise not to instill while wearing contact lenses; inform that they may reinsert contact lenses 10 min after instillation. Advise not to touch the dropper tip to any surface, as this may contaminate the contents. Inform that sol is for topical ophthalmic use only.

Administration: Ocular route. **Storage:** 15-25°C (59-77°F). Keep bottle tightly closed when not in use.

BESIVANCE   RX
besifloxacin (Bausch & Lomb)

THERAPEUTIC CLASS: Fluoroquinolone

INDICATIONS: Treatment of bacterial conjunctivitis caused by susceptible isolates of bacteria.

DOSAGE: *Adults:* Instill 1 drop in affected eye(s) tid, 4-12 hrs apart for 7 days.
Pediatrics: ≥1 Yr: Instill 1 drop in affected eye(s) tid, 4-12 hrs apart for 7 days.

HOW SUPPLIED: Sus: 0.6% [5mL]

WARNINGS/PRECAUTIONS: For topical ophthalmic use only; should not be injected subconjunctivally, nor should it be introduced directly into the anterior chamber of the eye. May result in overgrowth of nonsusceptible organisms (eg, fungi) with prolonged use; d/c and institute alternative therapy if superinfection occurs. Avoid wearing contact lenses if signs or symptoms of bacterial conjunctivitis occur and avoid wearing contact lenses during the course of therapy.

ADVERSE REACTIONS: Conjunctival redness.

PREGNANCY: Category C, caution in nursing.

MECHANISM OF ACTION: Fluoroquinolone antibacterial; inhibits both bacterial DNA gyrase and topoisomerase IV. DNA gyrase is an essential enzyme required for replication, transcription, and repair of bacterial DNA. Topoisomerase IV is an essential enzyme required for partitioning of the chromosomal DNA during bacterial cell division.

PHARMACOKINETICS: Absorption: C$_{max}$=0.37ng/mL (Day 1), 0.43ng/mL (Day 6). **Elimination:** T$_{1/2}$=7 hrs.

NURSING CONSIDERATIONS

Assessment: Assess for previous hypersensitivity to the drug, use of contact lenses, and pregnancy/nursing status. Assess for proper diagnosis of causative organisms.

Monitoring: Monitor for superinfection; examine with magnification (eg, slit lamp biomicroscopy) and fluorescein staining, where appropriate. Monitor for hypersensitivity reactions and other adverse reactions.

Patient Counseling: Advise to avoid contaminating applicator tip with material from the eye, fingers, or other source. Advise to d/c use immediately and contact physician at first sign of a rash or allergic reaction. Instruct to use medication exactly ud. Inform that skipping doses or not completing the full course of therapy may decrease effectiveness and increase bacterial resistance. Advise to avoid wearing contact lenses if having signs or symptoms of bacterial conjunctivitis and avoid wearing during the course of therapy. Advise to thoroughly wash hands before use. Instruct to invert closed bottle and shake once before each use. Instruct to remove cap with bottle still in inverted position. Instruct to tilt head back, and with bottle inverted, gently squeeze bottle to instill 1 drop into the affected eye(s).

Administration: Ocular route. Invert closed bottle and shake once before use. **Storage:** 15-25°C (59-77°F). Protect from light.

BETAGAN   RX
levobunolol HCl (Allergan)

THERAPEUTIC CLASS: Nonselective beta-blocker

INDICATIONS: Treatment of elevated intraocular pressure (IOP) in chronic open-angle glaucoma and ocular HTN.

DOSAGE: *Adults:* (0.5%) 1-2 drops qd; bid for more severe or uncontrolled glaucoma. (0.25%): 1-2 drops bid.

HOW SUPPLIED: Sol: 0.25% [5mL, 10mL], 0.5% [2mL, 5mL, 10mL, 15mL]

CONTRAINDICATIONS: Bronchial asthma, chronic obstructive pulmonary disease (COPD), overt cardiac failure, sinus bradycardia, 2nd- and 3rd-degree atrioventricular block, cardiogenic shock.

WARNINGS/PRECAUTIONS: Caution with cardiac failure, diabetes mellitus (DM), COPD, cerebral insufficiency, pulmonary disease, bronchospastic disease, surgery, and hepatic impairment. May mask symptoms of hypoglycemia and thyrotoxicosis. Contains sodium metabisulfite. Follow with a miotic in angle-closure glaucoma. Potentiates muscle weakness (eg, diplopia, ptosis).

ADVERSE REACTIONS: Ocular burning, ocular stinging, decreased HR, decreased BP.

INTERACTIONS: Mydriasis with epinephrine. Additive effects with catecholamine-depleting drugs (eg, reserpine) and systemic β-blockers. AV conduction disturbance with Ca^{2+} antagonists and digitalis. Left ventricular failure and hypotension with Ca^{2+} antagonists. Additive hypotensive effects with phenothiazine-related drugs. Risk of hypoglycemia with insulin and oral hypoglycemic agents.

PREGNANCY: Category C, caution in nursing.

MECHANISM OF ACTION: Noncardioselective β-adrenoceptor blocking agent; equipotent at both β_1 and β_2 receptors. Responsible for reducing cardiac output, increasing airway resistance, and lowering elevated as well as normal IOP. Presumed to lower IOP through decreasing production of aqueous humor.

NURSING CONSIDERATIONS

Assessment: Assess for conditions where treatment may be contraindicated or cautioned. Assess for possible sulfite allergy prior to therapy. Assess use in patients who have DM, hyperthyroidism, diminished pulmonary function, cerebrovascular insufficiencies, patients undergoing major elective surgery, and in pregnant/nursing females. Assess that patients with angle-closure glaucoma are not using this drug as monotherapy. Assess for possible drug interactions.

Monitoring: Monitor for signs/symptoms of muscle weakness (eg, diplopia, ptosis), severe respiratory and cardiac reactions, and anaphylactic reactions. Monitor for occurrence of a thyroid storm in patients who have thyrotoxicosis and withdraw abruptly from medication. Monitor for signs/symptoms of acute hypoglycemia with DM.

Patient Counseling: Counsel to notify physician immediately if any signs of anaphylactic reaction, cardiac, or respiratory symptoms develop while on medication. Counsel patients with DM that medication may mask symptoms of hypoglycemia.

Administration: Ocular route. **Storage:** 15-25°C (59-77°F), protect from light.

BETAPACE   RX
sotalol HCl (Bayer Healthcare)

> To minimize risk of arrhythmia, for a minimum of 3 days, place patients initiated or reinitiated on therapy in a facility that can provide cardiac resuscitation and continuous ECG monitoring. Calculate CrCl prior to dosing. Not approved for atrial fibrillation or atrial flutter indication; do not substitute for Betapace AF.

OTHER BRAND NAMES: Sorine (Upsher-Smith)

B

THERAPEUTIC CLASS: Beta-blocker (group II/III antiarrhythmic)

INDICATIONS: Treatment of documented life-threatening ventricular arrhythmias (eg, sustained ventricular tachycardia).

DOSAGE: *Adults:* Individualize dose. Initial: 80mg bid. Titrate: May increase after appropriate evaluation to 240 or 320mg/day (120-160mg bid). Adjust dose gradually, allowing 3 days between dosing increments. Usual: 160-320mg/day in 2-3 divided doses. Refractory Ventricular Arrhythmia: 480-640mg/day when benefit outweighs risk. Renal Impairment: Refer to PI. Transfer to Betapace/Sorine: Withdraw previous antiarrhythmic therapy for a minimum of 2-3 plasma half-lives before initiating therapy. After discontinuation of amiodarone, do not initiate therapy until QT interval is normalized.
Pediatrics: Individualize dose. ≥2 Yrs: Initial: 30mg/m^2 tid (90mg/m^2 total daily dose). Titrate: Allow at least 36 hrs between dose increments. Guide titration by response, HR, and QTc. Max: 60mg/m^2. <2 Yrs: See dosing chart in PI. Reduce dose or d/c if QTc >550 msec. Renal Impairment: Lower doses or increase intervals between doses. Transfer to Betapace/Sorine: Withdraw previous antiarrhythmic therapy for a minimum of 2-3 plasma half-lives before initiating therapy. After discontinuation of amiodarone, do not initiate therapy until QT interval is normalized.

HOW SUPPLIED: Tab: (Betapace) 80mg*, 120mg*, 160mg*; (Sorine) 80mg*, 120mg*, 160mg*, 240mg* *scored

CONTRAINDICATIONS: Bronchial asthma, sinus bradycardia, 2nd- and 3rd-degree atrioventricular (AV) block (unless a functioning pacemaker is present), congenital or acquired long QT syndromes, cardiogenic shock, uncontrolled congestive heart failure (CHF).

WARNINGS/PRECAUTIONS: May provoke new or worsen ventricular arrhythmias (eg, sustained ventricular tachycardia or ventricular fibrillation). Torsades de pointes, QT interval prolongation, and new or worsened CHF reported. Anticipate proarrhythmic events upon initiation and every upward dose adjustment. Caution in patients with QTc >500 msec on-therapy and consider reducing dose or discontinuing therapy when QTc >550 msec. Avoid with uncorrected hypokalemia or hypomagnesemia. Give special attention to electrolyte and acid-base balance in patients with severe/prolonged diarrhea or with concomitant diuretic drugs. May cause further depression of myocardial contractility and precipitate more severe failure; caution with CHF controlled by digitalis and/or diuretics. Caution with left ventricular dysfunction, sick sinus syndrome associated with symptomatic arrhythmias, and renal impairment (especially with hemodialysis). Caution during the first 2 weeks post-myocardial infarction (MI); careful dose titration is especially important (eg, in patients with markedly impaired ventricular function). Exacerbation of angina pectoris, arrhythmias, and MI reported after abrupt discontinuation; reduce dose gradually over 1-2 weeks. May unmask latent coronary insufficiency in patients with arrhythmias. Avoid in patients with bronchospastic diseases; use lowest effective dose. Impaired ability of the heart to respond to reflex adrenergic stimuli may augment the risks of general anesthesia and surgical procedures; chronically administered therapy should not be routinely withdrawn prior to major surgery. Patients with a history of anaphylactic reaction to various allergens may have a more severe reaction on repeated challenge and may be unresponsive to usual doses of epinephrine. Caution in patients with diabetes (especially labile diabetes) or with a history of episodes of spontaneous hypoglycemia; may mask premonitory signs of acute hypoglycemia (eg, tachycardia). May mask certain clinical signs (eg, tachycardia) of hyperthyroidism.

ADVERSE REACTIONS: Torsades de pointes, dyspnea, fatigue, dizziness, bradycardia, chest pain, palpitation, asthenia, abnormal ECG, hypotension, headache, light-headedness, edema, N/V, pulmonary problems.

INTERACTIONS: Avoid with Class Ia (eg, disopyramide, quinidine, procainamide) and Class III (eg, amiodarone) antiarrhythmics. Additive Class II effects with other β-blockers. Proarrhythmic events were more common with digoxin. May increase risk of bradycardia with digitalis glycosides. Possible additive effects on AV conduction or ventricular function and BP with calcium-blocking agents. May produce excessive reduction of resting sympathetic nervous tone with catecholamine-depleting drugs (eg, reserpine, guanethidine). Hyperglycemia may occur; may require dose adjustment of insulin or antidiabetic agents. β$_2$-agonists (eg, salbutamol, terbutaline, isoprenaline) may need dose increase. May potentiate rebound HTN with clonidine withdrawal. Avoid administration within 2 hrs of antacids containing aluminum oxide and magnesium hydroxide; may reduce levels. Caution with drugs that prolong QT interval (eg, Class I and III antiarrhythmics, phenothiazines, TCAs, astemizole, bepridil, certain oral macrolides, certain quinolone antibiotics).

PREGNANCY: Category B, not for use in nursing.

MECHANISM OF ACTION: β-blocker (group II/III antiarrhythmic); has both β-adrenoreceptor blocking and cardiac action potential duration prolongation properties.

PHARMACOKINETICS: Absorption: Bioavailability (90-100%); T_{max}=2.5-4 hrs. **Distribution:** Crosses placenta; found in breast milk. **Elimination:** Urine (unchanged); $T_{1/2}$=12 hrs.

NURSING CONSIDERATIONS

Assessment: Assess for hypersensitivity to drug, bronchial asthma, sinus bradycardia, sick sinus syndrome, 2nd- and 3rd-degree AV block, pacemaker, long QT syndromes, cardiogenic shock, left ventricular dysfunction or uncontrolled CHF, recent MI, ischemic heart disease, hypokalemia or hypomagnesemia, bronchospastic disease, diabetes, episodes of hypoglycemia, upcoming major surgery, hyperthyroidism, renal impairment, any other conditions where treatment is contraindicated or cautioned, pregnancy/nursing status, and possible drug interactions.

Monitoring: Monitor for ECG changes, tachycardia, arrhythmias, depressed myocardial contractility, severe CHF, anaphylaxis, hypoglycemia, electrolyte imbalance, hyperthyroidism, and other adverse reactions.

Patient Counseling: Inform of the benefits/risks of therapy. Advise not to d/c therapy without consulting physician. Instruct to report any adverse reactions to physician.

Administration: Oral route. Refer to PI for preparation of extemporaneous oral sol. **Storage:** (Betapace) 25°C (77°F); excursions permitted to 15-30°C (59-86°F). (Sorine) 15-30°C (59-86°F). Sus: Stable for 3 months at 15-30°C (59-86°F) and ambient humidity.

BETAPACE AF   RX
sotalol HCl (Bayer Healthcare)

> To minimize risk of induced arrhythmia, for a minimum of 3 days, place patients initiated or reinitiated on therapy in a facility that can provide cardiac resuscitation, continuous ECG monitoring, and calculations of CrCl. Do not substitute Betapace for Betapace AF.

THERAPEUTIC CLASS: Beta-blocker (group II/III antiarrhythmic)

INDICATIONS: Maintenance of normal sinus rhythm in patients with symptomatic atrial fibrillation/atrial flutter who are currently in sinus rhythm.

DOSAGE: *Adults:* Individualize dose according to calculated CrCl. Start only if baseline QT interval is ≤450 msec. Initial: 80mg qd (CrCl 40-60mL/min) or bid (CrCl >60mL/min). Monitor QT interval 2-4 hrs after each dose. Reduce or d/c if QT interval prolongs to ≥500 msec. May discharge patient if QT <500 msec after at least 3 days. Alternatively, may increase dose to 120mg bid during hospitalization, and monitor for 3 days (monitor for 5 or 6 doses if receiving qd doses). If 120mg is inadequate, may increase to 160mg qd or bid depending on CrCl. Maint: Reduce dose if QT interval is ≥520 msec and monitor until QT returns to <520 msec. D/C if QT is ≥520 msec while on 80mg dose. If renal function deteriorates, reduce daily dose in 1/2 by administering the drug qd. Max: 160mg bid (CrCl >60mL/min). Transfer to Betapace AF: Withdraw previous antiarrhythmic therapy for a minimum of 2-3 plasma half-lives if patient's condition permits before initiating Betapace AF. After discontinuing amiodarone, do not initiate Betapace AF until QT interval is normalized.
Pediatrics: Individualize dose. ≥2 Yrs: Initial: 30mg/m² tid. Titrate: Wait ≥36 hrs between dose increases. Guide dose by response, HR, and QTc. Max: 60mg/m². <2 Yrs: See dosing chart in PI. Reduce dose or d/c if QTc >550 msec. Renal Impairment: Reduce dose or increase intervals between doses. Transfer to Betapace AF: Withdraw previous antiarrhythmic therapy for a minimum of 2-3 plasma half-lives if patient's condition permits before initiating Betapace AF. After discontinuing amiodarone, do not initiate Betapace AF until QT interval is normalized.

HOW SUPPLIED: Tab: 80mg*, 120mg*, 160mg* *scored

CONTRAINDICATIONS: Sinus bradycardia (<50bpm during waking hrs), sick sinus syndrome or 2nd- or 3rd-degree atrioventricular (AV) block (unless a functioning pacemaker is present), congenital or acquired long QT syndromes, baseline QT interval >450 msec, cardiogenic shock, uncontrolled heart failure (HF), hypokalemia (<4mEq/L), CrCl <40mL/min, bronchial asthma.

WARNINGS/PRECAUTIONS: May cause serious ventricular arrhythmias, primarily torsades de pointes. QT interval prolongation, bradycardia, and new/worsened congestive HF reported. Avoid with hypokalemia or hypomagnesemia; correct electrolyte imbalances before therapy. May cause depression of myocardial contractility and precipitate more severe failure in patients with congestive HF. Caution with HF controlled by digitalis and/or diuretics, left ventricular dysfunction, renal impairment, recent acute myocardial infarction (MI), and sick sinus syndrome associated with symptomatic arrhythmias. Exacerbation of angina pectoris, arrhythmias, and MI reported after abrupt discontinuation; reduce dose gradually over a period of 1-2 weeks. May unmask latent coronary insufficiency in patients with arrhythmias. Avoid in patients with bronchospastic diseases; use lowest effective dose. Impaired ability of heart to respond to reflex adrenergic stimuli may augment the risks of general anesthesia and surgical procedures; chronically administered therapy should not be routinely withdrawn prior to major surgery. Patients with a history of anaphylactic reaction to various allergens may have a more severe reaction on repeated challenge and may be unresponsive to usual doses of epinephrine. Caution in patients with diabetes (especially labile diabetes) or with a history of episodes of spontaneous hypoglycemia; may mask premonitory signs of acute hypoglycemia (eg, tachycardia). May mask certain clinical signs (eg, tachycardia) of hyperthyroidism.

ADVERSE REACTIONS: Bradycardia, dyspnea, fatigue, abnormal ECG, chest pain, abdominal pain, disturbance rhythm subjective, diarrhea, N/V, cough, hyperhidrosis, weakness, dizziness, headache, insomnia.

INTERACTIONS: Avoid with Class Ia (eg, disopyramide, quinidine, procainamide) and Class III (eg, amiodarone) antiarrhythmics. Not recommended with drugs that prolong the QT interval (eg, many antiarrhythmics, some phenothiazines, TCAs, bepridil, certain oral macrolides). Proarrhythmic events more common with digoxin. Increased risk of bradycardia with digitalis glycosides. Possible additive effects on AV conduction or ventricular function and BP with calcium-blocking agents. May produce an excessive reduction of resting sympathetic nervous tone with catecholamine-depleting drugs (eg, reserpine, guanethidine). Hyperglycemia may occur; may require dose adjustment of insulin or antidiabetic agents. β_2-agonists (eg, salbutamol, terbutaline, isoprenaline) may need dose increase. May potentiate rebound HTN with clonidine withdrawal. Avoid administration of therapy within 2 hrs of antacids containing aluminum oxide and magnesium hydroxide; may reduce levels.

PREGNANCY: Category B, not for use in nursing.

MECHANISM OF ACTION: β-blocker (group II/III antiarrhythmic); has both β-adrenoreceptor blocking and cardiac action potential duration prolongation properties.

PHARMACOKINETICS: Absorption: Bioavailability (90-100%); T_{max}=2.5-4 hrs. **Distribution:** Crosses placenta; found in breast milk. **Elimination:** Urine (unchanged); $T_{1/2}$=12 hrs.

NURSING CONSIDERATIONS

Assessment: Assess for hypersensitivity to drug, sinus bradycardia, sick sinus syndrome, 2nd- and 3rd-degree AV block, pacemaker, long QT syndromes, baseline QT interval >450 msec, cardiogenic shock, uncontrolled HF, hypokalemia, bronchial asthma, recent MI, ischemic heart disease, hypomagnesemia, bronchospastic disease, diabetes, hypoglycemia, upcoming major surgery, hyperthyroidism, renal impairment, or any other conditions where treatment is contraindicated or cautioned. Assess for pregnancy/nursing status and possible drug interactions.

Monitoring: Monitor for ECG changes, tachycardia, arrhythmias, depressed myocardial contractility, HF, anaphylaxis, hypoglycemia, electrolyte imbalance, hyperthyroidism, and other adverse reactions.

Patient Counseling: Inform of benefits/risks of therapy. Instruct to take exactly ud. Advise not to d/c therapy without consulting physician. Instruct to inform physician if taking any other medications, supplements, or OTC drugs and to report immediately if experiencing symptoms that may be associated with electrolyte imbalance. Instruct not to double next dose if a dose is missed and to take next dose at the usual time.

Administration: Oral route. Refer to PI for preparation of extemporaneous oral sol. **Storage:** 25°C (77°F); excursions permitted to 15-30°C (59-86°F). Sus: Stable for 3 months at 15-30°C (59-86°F) and ambient humidity.

BETHKIS

tobramycin (Cornerstone)

RX

THERAPEUTIC CLASS: Aminoglycoside

INDICATIONS: Management of cystic fibrosis patients with *Pseudomonas aeruginosa*.

DOSAGE: *Adults:* 300mg bid (as close to 12 hrs apart as possible; not <6 hrs apart) in repeated cycles of 28 days on drug, followed by 28 days off drug.
Pediatrics: ≥6 Yrs: 300mg bid (as close to 12 hrs apart as possible; not <6 hrs apart) in repeated cycles of 28 days on drug, followed by 28 days off drug.

HOW SUPPLIED: Sol, Inhalation: 300mg/4mL

WARNINGS/PRECAUTIONS: Ototoxicity (eg, tinnitus) may occur; caution with auditory or vestibular dysfunction. Nephrotoxicity may occur; caution with renal dysfunction. If nephrotoxicity occurs, d/c therapy until serum concentrations fall <2mcg/mL. If an increase in SrCr develops, closely monitor renal function. May aggravate muscle weakness; caution with muscular disorders (eg, myasthenia gravis, Parkinson's disease). Bronchospasm and wheezing reported. Consider an audiogram for patients with any evidence of or at increased risk for auditory dysfunction. May cause fetal harm.

ADVERSE REACTIONS: Decreased forced expiratory volume, rales, increased RBC sedimentation rate, dysphonia, wheezing, epistaxis, pharyngolaryngeal pain, bronchitis.

INTERACTIONS: Avoid concurrent and/or sequential use with other drugs with neurotoxic or ototoxic potential. Some diuretics may enhance toxicity by altering concentrations in serum and tissue; do not administer with ethacrynic acid, furosemide, urea, or mannitol.

PREGNANCY: Category D, not for use in nursing.

MECHANISM OF ACTION: Aminoglycoside; acts primarily by disrupting protein synthesis in the bacterial cell, which eventually leads to death of the cell.

PHARMACOKINETICS: Distribution: Crosses placenta. **Elimination:** Expectorated sputum (unabsorbed); $T_{1/2}$=4.4 hrs.

NURSING CONSIDERATIONS

Assessment: Assess for auditory, vestibular, or renal dysfunction, muscular disorders, drug hypersensitivity, pregnancy/nursing status, and possible drug interactions. Consider a baseline audiogram for patients at increased risk for auditory dysfunction.

Monitoring: Monitor for ototoxicity, nephrotoxicity, muscle weakness, bronchospasm, wheezing, and other adverse reactions. Consider an audiogram for patients who show any evidence of auditory dysfunction.

Patient Counseling: Instruct to take drug ud, and to complete a full 28-day course of therapy even if feeling better. Inform of the adverse reactions associated with therapy, such as ototoxicity, bronchospasm, nephrotoxicity, and neuromuscular disorders. Inform of the need to monitor hearing, serum concentrations, and renal function during treatment. Advise to inform physician if pregnant/nursing or planning to become pregnant. Counsel on proper storage of the drug.

Administration: Oral inhalation route. Administer by using a hand-held Pari LC Plus reusable nebulizer with a Pari Vios air compressor over approximately 15 min and until sputtering from the output of the nebulizer has occurred for at least 1 min. Refer to PI for further preparation and administration instructions. **Storage:** 2-8°C (36-46°F). Upon removal from the refrigerator, or if refrigeration is unavailable, may be stored at room temperature (up to 25°C [77°F]) for up to 28 days. Do not expose to intense light.

BETIMOL   RX
timolol (Vistakon)

THERAPEUTIC CLASS: Nonselective beta-blocker

INDICATIONS: Treatment of elevated intraocular pressure (IOP) in patients with open-angle glaucoma or ocular HTN.

DOSAGE: *Adults:* Initial: 1 drop 0.25% bid. May increase to max of 1 drop 0.5% bid. Maint: If adequate control, may try 1 drop 0.25-0.5% qd.

HOW SUPPLIED: Sol: 0.25%, 0.5% [2.5mL, 5mL, 10mL, 15mL]

CONTRAINDICATIONS: Bronchial asthma, history of bronchial asthma, severe chronic obstructive pulmonary disease (COPD), sinus bradycardia, 2nd- or 3rd-degree atrioventricular (AV) block, overt cardiac failure, cardiogenic shock.

WARNINGS/PRECAUTIONS: Caution with cardiac failure, diabetes mellitus (DM), or cerebrovascular insufficiency. Severe cardiac and respiratory reactions reported. May mask symptoms of hypoglycemia and hyperthyroidism. Bacterial keratitis reported with contaminated containers. May reinsert contacts 5 min after applying drops. Avoid with COPD or bronchospastic disease. Not for use alone in angle-closure glaucoma. May potentiate muscle weakness. D/C if cardiac failure develops. Withdrawal before surgery is controversial.

ADVERSE REACTIONS: Burning/stinging on instillation, dry eyes, itching, foreign body sensation, eye discomfort, eyelid erythema, conjunctival inj, headache.

INTERACTIONS: May potentiate systemic β-blockers and catecholamine-depleting drugs (eg, reserpine). Oral/IV Ca^{2+} antagonists can cause AV conduction disturbances, left ventricular failure, or hypotension. Digitalis can cause additive effects in prolonging AV conduction time. May antagonize epinephrine.

PREGNANCY: Category C, not for use in nursing.

MECHANISM OF ACTION: Nonselective β-adrenergic antagonist; blocks both $β_1$- and $β_2$-adrenergic receptors. Thought to reduce IOP through reducing production of aqueous humor.

PHARMACOKINETICS: Elimination: Urine (metabolites); $T_{1/2}$=4 hrs.

NURSING CONSIDERATIONS

Assessment: Assess for overt heart failure, cardiogenic shock, sinus bradycardia, 2nd- or 3rd-degree AV block, active or history of bronchial asthma, and severe COPD. Assess use in patients with cerebrovascular insufficiencies, undergoing elective surgery, with DM, with hyperthyroidism, and in pregnant/nursing females. Assess patients with angle-closure glaucoma who are not on monotherapy with this drug. Assess for possible drug interactions.

Monitoring: Monitor for signs/symptoms of reduced cerebral blood flow, cardiac failure, muscle weakness, bacterial keratitis when using multidose container, severe anaphylactic reactions, and hypoglycemia in patients with DM. Monitor for occurrence of thyroid storm in patients who abruptly withdraw from medication and have thyrotoxicosis.

Patient Counseling: Counsel to immediately notify physician if signs of cardiac, respiratory, or anaphylactic symptoms develop while on medication. Instruct patients with DM that this medication may mask signs of hypoglycemia. Instruct to avoid contaminating sol by not touching container tip to the eye or surrounding structures. Counsel that if taking concomitant topical ophthalmic medications, to separate dosing by at least 5 min. Instruct patients who wear soft contact lenses to wait at least 5 min after administration before reinserting.

Administration: Ocular route. **Storage:** 15-25°C (59-77°F). Do not freeze. Protect from light.

Betoptic S   RX
betaxolol HCl (Alcon)

THERAPEUTIC CLASS: Selective beta₁-blocker

INDICATIONS: Treatment of elevated intraocular pressure (IOP) in patients with chronic open-angle glaucoma or ocular HTN.

DOSAGE: *Adults:* Instill 1 drop in affected eyes bid.
Pediatrics: Instill 1 drop in affected eyes bid.

HOW SUPPLIED: Sus: 0.25% [2.5mL, 5mL, 10mL, 15mL]

CONTRAINDICATIONS: Sinus bradycardia, >1st-degree atrioventricular (AV) block, cardiogenic shock, overt cardiac failure.

WARNINGS/PRECAUTIONS: Do not use alone in treating angle-closure glaucoma. Absorbed systemically; severe respiratory/cardiac reactions reported. Caution with history of cardiac failure or heart block, diabetes mellitus, and cerebrovascular insufficiency. D/C on 1st sign of cardiac failure. May mask signs/symptoms of acute hypoglycemia and hyperthyroidism. Avoid abrupt withdrawal; may precipitate thyroid storm. May potentiate muscle weakness consistent with certain myasthenic symptoms. Withdrawal prior to major surgery is controversial. Caution in glaucoma patients with excessive restriction of pulmonary function; asthmatic attacks and pulmonary distress reported. May be more reactive to repeated challenge with history of atopy or severe anaphylactic reaction to variety of allergens; may be unresponsive to usual doses of epinephrine. Bacterial keratitis and choroidal detachment may occur.

ADVERSE REACTIONS: Transient ocular discomfort, blurred vision, corneal punctuate keratitis, foreign body sensation, photophobia, tearing, itching, dryness of eye, erythema, inflammation, discharge, ocular pain, decreased visual acuity, crusty lashes.

INTERACTIONS: Potential additive effects with oral β-blockers and catecholamine-depleting drugs (eg, reserpine). May produce hypotension and/or bradycardia with catecholamine-depleting drugs. Caution with adrenergic psychotropics and in patients receiving insulin or oral hypoglycemic agents. May augment risk of general anesthesia.

PREGNANCY: Category C, caution with nursing.

MECHANISM OF ACTION: Cardioselective (β-1-adrenergic) receptor inhibitor; reduces IOP through a reduction of aqueous production.

NURSING CONSIDERATIONS

Assessment: Assess for conditions where treatment is contraindicated or cautioned, hypersensitivity to the drug, pregnancy/nursing status, and possible drug interactions.

Monitoring: Monitor for signs/symptoms of cardiac/respiratory reactions, cardiac failure, muscle weakness, reduced cerebral blood flow, choroidal detachment, and hypersensitivity reactions. Monitor for development of bacterial keratitis in patients who are using multidose containers.

Patient Counseling: Instruct to avoid allowing tip of dispensing container to contact eye(s) or surrounding structures. Inform that ocular sol may become contaminated by bacteria that may cause ocular infections. Instruct to seek physician's advice if having an ocular surgery or if ocular condition (eg, trauma or infection) develops. Instruct to administer ≥10 min apart when receiving concomitant ophthalmic medications.

Administration: Ocular route. May be used alone or in combination with other IOP-lowering medications. Refer to PI for administration instructions. Shake well before use. **Storage:** 2-25°C (36-77°F). Store upright.

BEYAZ

levomefolate calcium - drospirenone - ethinyl estradiol (Bayer Healthcare)

> Cigarette smoking increases the risk of serious cardiovascular events from combination oral contraceptive (COC) use. Risk increases with age (>35 yrs) and with the number of cigarettes smoked. Should not be used by women who are >35 yrs of age and smoke.

THERAPEUTIC CLASS: Estrogen/progestogen combination

INDICATIONS: Prevention of pregnancy. Treatment of symptoms of premenstrual dysphoric disorder (PMDD). Treatment of moderate acne vulgaris in women ≥14 yrs of age who have achieved menarche and who desire an oral contraceptive for birth control. To raise folate levels for the purpose of reducing the risk of neural tube defect in a pregnancy conceived while taking the product or shortly after discontinuation.

DOSAGE: *Adults:* Contraception/Acne/PMDD: 1 tab qd for 28 days, then repeat. Start 1st Sunday after menses begin or 1st day of menses. Take at the same time each day, preferably pm pc or hs. *Pediatrics:* Postpubertal: Contraception/Acne (≥14 Yrs)/PMDD: 1 tab qd for 28 days, then repeat. Start 1st Sunday after menses begin or 1st day of menses. Take at the same time each day, preferably pm pc or hs.

HOW SUPPLIED: Tab: (Drospirenone [DRSP]-Ethinyl Estradiol [EE]-Levomefolate calcium) 3mg-0.02mg-0.451mg; Tab: (Levomefolate calcium) 0.451mg

CONTRAINDICATIONS: Renal impairment, adrenal insufficiency, high risk of arterial/venous thrombotic disease (eg, smoking if >35 yrs of age, history/presence of deep vein thrombosis/pulmonary embolism, cerebrovascular disease, coronary artery disease, thrombogenic valvular or thrombogenic rhythm diseases of the heart [eg, subacute bacterial endocarditis with valvular disease, atrial fibrillation], inherited/acquired hypercoagulopathies, uncontrolled HTN, diabetes mellitus [DM] with vascular disease, headaches with focal neurological symptoms or migraine with/without aura if >35 yrs of age), undiagnosed abnormal uterine bleeding, history/presence of breast or other estrogen-/progestin-sensitive cancer, benign/malignant liver tumors, liver disease, pregnancy.

WARNINGS/PRECAUTIONS: Increased risk of venous thromboembolism and arterial thromboses (eg, stroke, myocardial infarction). D/C if arterial/deep venous thrombotic events, unexplained loss of vision, proptosis, diplopia, papilledema, or retinal vascular lesions occur; evaluate for retinal vein thrombosis immediately. Caution in women with cardiovascular disease (CVD) risk factors. D/C at least 4 weeks before and through 2 weeks after major surgery or other surgeries known to have an elevated risk of thromboembolism. Avoid use in patients predisposed to hyperkalemia. May increase risk of breast cancer, cervical cancer, intraepithelial neoplasia, and gallbladder disease. Hepatic adenoma and increased risk of hepatocellular carcinoma reported; d/c if jaundice or acute/chronic disturbances of liver function occur. Cholestasis may occur with history of pregnancy-related cholestasis. Increased BP reported; d/c if BP rises significantly. May decrease glucose tolerance; monitor prediabetic and diabetic patients. Consider alternative contraception with uncontrolled dyslipidemia. Increased risk of pancreatitis with hypertriglyceridemia or family history thereof. May increase frequency/severity of migraine; d/c if new headaches that are recurrent, persistent, or severe develop. Unscheduled bleeding and spotting may occur; rule out pregnancies or malignancies. Caution with history of depression; d/c if depression recurs to serious degree. May change results of lab tests. Folate may mask vitamin B12 deficiency. May induce/exacerbate angioedema in patients with hereditary angioedema. Chloasma may occur, especially with history of chloasma gravidarum; avoid sun exposure or UV radiation. Women who do not breastfeed may start therapy no earlier than 4 weeks postpartum.

ADVERSE REACTIONS: Menstrual irregularities, N/V, headache/migraine, breast pain/tenderness, fatigue.

INTERACTIONS: Risk of hyperkalemia with ACE inhibitors, angiotensin II receptor antagonists, K⁺-sparing diuretics, K⁺ supplementation, heparin, aldosterone antagonists, and NSAIDs. Reduced effectiveness or increased breakthrough bleeding with enzyme inducers, including CYP3A4, (eg, phenytoin, barbiturates, carbamazepine, bosentan, felbamate, griseofulvin, oxcarbazepine, rifampicin, topiramate, St. John's wort). Significant changes (increase/decrease) in plasma estrogen and progestin levels with HIV/hepatitis C virus protease inhibitors or non-nucleoside reverse transcriptase inhibitors. Pregnancy reported with use of hormonal contraceptives and antibiotics. Increased levels with atorvastatin, ascorbic acid, acetaminophen, and CYP3A4 inhibitors (eg, itraconazole, ketoconazole). May decrease plasma concentrations of lamotrigine and reduce seizure control; adjust dose of lamotrigine. Increases thyroid-binding globulin; may need to increase dose of thyroid hormone in patients on thyroid hormone replacement therapy. May decrease pharmacological effect of antifolate drugs (eg, antiepileptics [phenytoin], methotrexate, pyrimethamine). Reduced folate levels via inhibition of dihydrofolate reductase enzyme (eg, methotrexate, sulfasalazine), reduced folate absorption (eg, cholestyramine), or unknown mechanism (eg, antiepileptics [carbamazepine, phenytoin, phenobarbital, primidone, valproic acid]).

B

PREGNANCY: Contraindicated in pregnancy, not for use in nursing.

MECHANISM OF ACTION: Estrogen/progestogen oral contraceptive; acts by primarily suppressing ovulation. Also causes cervical mucus changes that inhibit sperm penetration and endometrial changes that reduce the likelihood of implantation. (Levomefolate calcium) Folate supplementation.

PHARMACOKINETICS: Absorption: DRSP: Absolute bioavailability (76%); (Cycle 1/Day 21) C_{max}=70.3ng/mL; T_{max}=1.5 hrs; AUC=763ng•h/mL. EE: Absolute bioavailability (40%); (Cycle 1/Day 21) C_{max}=45.1pg/mL; T_{max}=1.5 hrs; AUC=220pg•h/mL. Levomefolate: T_{max}=0.5-1.5 hrs. **Distribution:** Found in breast milk; DRSP: V_d=4L/kg; serum protein binding (97%). EE: V_d=4-5L/kg; serum albumin binding (98.5%). **Metabolism:** DRSP: Liver, via CYP3A4 (minor). EE: Hydroxylation (via CYP3A4), conjugation with glucuronide and sulfate. **Elimination:** DRSP: Urine, feces; $T_{1/2}$=30 hrs. EE: Urine, feces; $T_{1/2}$=24 hrs. Levomefolate (L-5-methyl-THF): Urine, feces; $T_{1/2}$=4-5 hrs.

NURSING CONSIDERATIONS

Assessment: Assess for renal impairment, abnormal uterine bleeding, adrenal insufficiency, known or suspected pregnancy, and other conditions where treatment is cautioned or contraindicated. Assess use in women who are >35 yrs of age and smoke, have CVD and arterial/venous thrombosis risk factors, predisposition to hyperkalemia, pregnancy-related cholestasis, HTN, DM, uncontrolled dyslipidemia, history of hypertriglyceridemia, history of depression, hereditary angioedema, and history of chloasma. Assess for possible drug interactions.

Monitoring: Monitor for bleeding irregularities, venous/arterial thrombotic and thromboembolic events, cervical cancer or intraepithelial neoplasia, retinal vein thrombosis or any other ophthalmic changes, jaundice, acute/chronic disturbances in liver function, new/worsening headaches or migraines, serious depression, cholestasis with history of pregnancy-related cholestasis, and pancreatitis. Monitor K^+ levels, thyroid function if receiving thyroid replacement therapy, glucose levels in DM or prediabetes, lipids with dyslipidemia, and check BP annually.

Patient Counseling: Counsel that cigarette smoking increases the risk of serious CV events from COC use and to avoid use in women who are >35 yrs old and smoke. Inform that drug does not protect against HIV infection and other sexually transmitted diseases. Instruct to take at the same time every day, preferably pm pc or hs. Instruct on what to do if pills are missed or vomiting occurs within 3-4 hrs after taking tab. Inform that COCs may reduce breast milk production. Inform that amenorrhea may occur and pregnancy should be ruled out if amenorrhea occurs in ≥2 consecutive cycles. Counsel to report if taking folate supplements and advise to maintain folate supplementation upon discontinuation due to pregnancy. Advise to inform physician of preexisting medical conditions and/or drugs currently being taken. Counsel to use additional method of contraception when enzyme inducers are used with COCs. Counsel women who start COCs postpartum and have not yet had a period to use additional method of contraception until drug taken for 7 consecutive days. Instruct to d/c if pregnancy occurs during treatment.

Administration: Oral route. **Storage:** 25°C (77°F); excursions permitted to 15-30°C (59-86°F).

BIAXIN   RX
clarithromycin (AbbVie)

OTHER BRAND NAMES: Biaxin XL (AbbVie)

THERAPEUTIC CLASS: Macrolide

INDICATIONS: Treatment of the following mild to moderate infections caused by susceptible isolates of bacteria: (Tab, Sus) Pharyngitis/tonsillitis, acute maxillary sinusitis, community-acquired pneumonia (CAP), uncomplicated skin and skin structure infections (SSSI), and disseminated mycobacterial infections. *Mycobacterium avium* complex (MAC) prophylaxis in advanced HIV. Acute bacterial exacerbation of chronic bronchitis (ABECB) in adults. Acute otitis media in pediatric patients. (Tab) Combination therapy for *Helicobacter pylori* infection with duodenal ulcer disease (active or 5-yr history of duodenal ulcer) in adults. (XL) Acute maxillary sinusitis, CAP, and ABECB in adults.

DOSAGE: *Adults:* (Tab, Sus) Pharyngitis/Tonsillitis: 250mg q12h for 10 days. Sinusitis: 500mg q12h for 14 days. ABECB: 250-500mg q12h for 7-14 days. SSSI/CAP: 250mg q12h for 7-14 days. MAC Prophylaxis/Treatment: 500mg bid. CrCl <30mL/min: Reduce dose by 50%. *H. pylori:* Triple Therapy: 500mg + amoxicillin 1g + omeprazole 20mg, all q12h for 10 days (give additional omeprazole 20mg qd for 18 days for ulcer healing and symptom relief); or 500mg + amoxicillin 1g + lansoprazole 30mg, all q12h for 10-14 days. Dual Therapy: 500mg q8h + omeprazole 40mg qam for 14 days (give additional omeprazole 20mg qd for 14 days for ulcer healing and symptom relief); or 500mg q8h or q12h + ranitidine bismuth citrate 400mg q12h for 14 days (give additional ranitidine bismuth citrate 400mg bid for 14 days for ulcer healing and symptom relief). (XL) Sinusitis: 1000mg qd for 14 days. ABECB/CAP: 1000mg qd for 7 days. CrCl <30mL/min: Reduce dose by 50%.

Pediatrics: ≥6 Months: (Tab, Sus) Usual: 15mg/kg/day divided q12h for 10 days. MAC Prophylaxis/ Treatment: ≥20 Months: 7.5mg/kg bid, up to 500mg bid. CrCl <30mL/min: Reduce dose by 50%. Refer to PI for further pediatric dosage guidelines.

HOW SUPPLIED: Sus: 125mg/5mL, 250mg/5mL [50mL, 100mL]; Tab: 250mg, 500mg; Tab, Extended-Release (XL): 500mg

CONTRAINDICATIONS: History of cholestatic jaundice/hepatic dysfunction associated with prior use of clarithromycin. History of QT prolongation or ventricular cardiac arrhythmia, including torsades de pointes. Concomitant use with cisapride, pimozide, astemizole, terfenadine, ergotamine, or dihydroergotamine, and with HMG-CoA reductase inhibitors (statins) that are extensively metabolized by CYP3A4 (lovastatin or simvastatin). Concomitant use with colchicine in patients with renal/hepatic impairment.

WARNINGS/PRECAUTIONS: Avoid in pregnancy, except in clinical circumstances where no alternative therapy is appropriate. Hepatic dysfunction, including increased liver enzymes, and hepatocellular and/or cholestatic hepatitis, with or without jaundice, reported; d/c immediately if signs and symptoms of hepatitis occur. QT interval prolongation, arrhythmia (infrequent), and torsades de pointes reported; avoid with ongoing proarrhythmic conditions (eg, uncorrected hypokalemia or hypomagnesemia), and clinically significant bradycardia. *Clostridium difficile*-associated diarrhea (CDAD) reported; d/c if CDAD is suspected or confirmed. D/C therapy immediately and initiate prompt treatment if severe acute hypersensitivity reactions (eg, Stevens-Johnson syndrome, toxic epidermal necrolysis, drug rash with eosinophilia and systemic symptoms, Henoch-Schonlein purpura) occur. May result in bacterial resistance with prolonged use or use in the absence of a proven/suspected bacterial infection or a prophylactic indication. Exacerbation of symptoms of myasthenia gravis and new onset of symptoms of myasthenic syndrome reported. Caution in elderly.

ADVERSE REACTIONS: Diarrhea, N/V, abnormal taste, abdominal pain, rash, dyspepsia, headache.

INTERACTIONS: See Contraindications. Avoid Class IA (quinidine, procainamide) or Class III (dofetilide, amiodarone, sotalol) antiarrhythmic agents. Avoid doses of >1000mg/day with protease inhibitors. Concomitant use with phosphodiesterase inhibitors (sildenafil, tadalafil, vardenafil) is not recommended. Consider reduction of sildenafil dose. Ranitidine bismuth citrate is not recommended if CrCl <25mL/min or with history of acute porphyria. May increase serum theophylline, carbamazepine, omeprazole, digoxin, drugs metabolized by CYP3A, colchicine, saquinavir, and tolterodine levels. Concomitant use with itraconazole may increase levels of itraconazole and clarithromycin. Hypotension may occur with calcium channel blockers (CCBs) metabolized by CYP3A4 (eg, verapamil, amlodipine, diltiazem). Bradyarrhythmias and lactic acidosis observed with verapamil. May potentiate oral anticoagulant effects. Risk of serious hemorrhage and significant elevations in PT/INR with warfarin; monitor PT/INR frequently. Caution when prescribing with statins; if concomitant use with atorvastatin or pravastatin cannot be avoided, do not exceed atorvastatin dose of 20mg/day and pravastatin dose of 40mg/day; consider use of a statin that is not dependent on CYP3A metabolism (eg, fluvastatin); prescribe the lowest registered dose if concomitant use cannot be avoided. Significant hypoglycemia may occur with oral hypoglycemic agents (nateglinide, pioglitazone, repaglinide, rosiglitazone) and/ or insulin. Occurrence of torsades de pointes with quinidine or disopyramide reported; monitor for QT prolongation. CNS effects (eg, somnolence, confusion) may occur with concomitant use of triazolam; monitor for additive CNS effects. Caution and appropriate dose adjustments with alprazolam and triazolam required. May increase AUC of midazolam; dose adjustments may be necessary and possible prolongation and intensity of effect should be anticipated. Caution with other drugs known to be CYP3A enzyme substrates, especially if substrate has a narrow safety margin (eg, carbamazepine) and/or substrate is extensively metabolized by this enzyme. Increased levels with fluconazole and saquinavir. Decreased levels with CYP3A inducers (eg, efavirenz, nevirapine, rifampicin, rifabutin, rifapentine). Reduce dose by 50 or 75% for patients with CrCl 30-60mL/min or <30mL/min, respectively, if given with atazanavir or ritonavir. Reduce dose by 50% with concomitant atazanavir. Interaction may occur when concomitantly used with cyclosporine, tacrolimus, alfentanil, rifabutin, methylprednisolone, cilostazol, bromocriptine, vinblastine, hexobarbital, phenytoin, or valproate. (Tab) May decrease levels of zidovudine; separate zidovudine administration by at least 2 hrs.

PREGNANCY: Category C, caution in nursing.

MECHANISM OF ACTION: Semisynthetic macrolide antibiotic; exerts antibacterial action by binding to the 50S ribosomal subunit of susceptible microorganisms, resulting in inhibition of protein synthesis. Active against aerobic and anaerobic gram-positive and gram-negative microorganisms.

PHARMACOKINETICS: Absorption: Rapid; (250mg tab) Absolute bioavailability (50%). Administration of variable doses resulted in different parameters. **Metabolism:** 14-OH clarithromycin (primary metabolite). **Elimination:** Urine: 20% (250mg tab), 30% (500mg tab), 40% (250mg sus), 10-15% (14-OH). $T_{1/2}$=3-4 hrs (250mg tab), 5-7 hrs (500mg). 14-OH: $T_{1/2}$=5-6 hrs (250mg), 7-9 hrs (500mg).

NURSING CONSIDERATIONS

Assessment: Assess for history of cholestatic jaundice/hepatic dysfunction associated with prior use of clarithromycin, hepatic/renal impairment, history of QT prolongation, ongoing proarrhythmic conditions, clinically significant bradycardia, ventricular cardiac arrhythmia, torsades de pointes, myasthenia gravis, history of acute porphyria, pregnancy/nursing status, possible drug interactions, and hypersensitivity to the drug, any of its ingredients, erythromycin, or any of the macrolide antibiotics.

Monitoring: Monitor for development of drug-resistant bacteria, CDAD, hepatitis, QT prolongation, acute severe hypersensitivity reactions, exacerbation of myasthenia gravis, new onset of symptoms of myasthenic syndrome, and other adverse reactions. Monitor LFTs, INR/PT, and renal/hepatic function.

Patient Counseling: Inform about potential benefits/risks of therapy. Counsel that therapy should only be used to treat bacterial, not viral (eg, common cold), infections. Instruct to take exactly ud; inform that skipping doses or not completing full course may decrease effectiveness and increase antibiotic resistance. Instruct to notify physician if watery/bloody diarrhea (with/without stomach cramps) develops; inform that this may occur up to 2 or more months after treatment. Instruct to notify physician if pregnant/nursing and of all medications currently being taken.

Administration: Oral route. (Tab/Sus) Take with or without food, or with milk. (Sus) Shake well before each use. Refer to PI for constituting instructions. (XL) Take with food. Swallow whole; do not chew, crush, or break. **Storage:** (250mg tab) 15-30°C (59-86°F). Protect from light. (500mg tab) 20-25°C (68-77°F). (Sus) 15-30°C (59-86°F). Use within 14 days. Do not refrigerate. (XL) 20-25°C (68-77°F); excursions permitted 15-30°C (59-86°F).

BINOSTO   RX
alendronate sodium (Mission)

THERAPEUTIC CLASS: Bisphosphonate

INDICATIONS: Treatment of osteoporosis in postmenopausal women. Treatment to increase bone mass in men with osteoporosis.

DOSAGE: *Adults:* 1 tab once weekly. Take upon arising for the day and at least 30 min before the 1st food, beverage, or medication of the day. Avoid lying down for at least 30 min after taking the drug and until after 1st food of the day.

HOW SUPPLIED: Tab, Effervescent: 70mg

CONTRAINDICATIONS: Esophageal abnormalities that delay esophageal emptying (eg, stricture, achalasia), inability to stand or sit upright for at least 30 min, hypocalcemia, patients at increased risk of aspiration.

WARNINGS/PRECAUTIONS: Periodically reevaluate the need for continued therapy. Consider discontinuation after 3-5 yrs of use in patients at low-risk for fracture; periodically reevaluate risk for fracture in patients who d/c therapy. May cause local irritation of the upper GI mucosa; caution with active upper GI problems (eg, Barrett's esophagus, dysphagia, esophageal diseases, gastritis, duodenitis, ulcers). D/C if dysphagia, odynophagia, retrosternal pain, or new/worsening heartburn develops. Use therapy under appropriate supervision in patients who cannot comply with dosing instructions due to mental disability. Gastric and duodenal ulcers reported. Treat hypocalcemia and other disorders affecting mineral metabolism (eg, vitamin D deficiency) prior to therapy; monitor serum Ca^{2+} and for symptoms of hypocalcemia during therapy. Asymptomatic decreases in serum Ca^{2+} and phosphate may occur; ensure adequate Ca^{2+} and vitamin D intake. Severe and occasionally incapacitating bone, joint, and/or muscle pain reported; d/c if severe symptoms develop. Osteonecrosis of the jaw (ONJ) reported; risk may increase with duration of exposure to drug. If invasive dental procedures are required, discontinuation of treatment may reduce risk for ONJ. Consider discontinuation if ONJ develops. Atypical, low-energy, or low-trauma fractures of the femoral shaft reported; evaluate any patient with a history of bisphosphonate exposure who presents with thigh/groin pain to rule out incomplete femur fracture, and consider interruption of therapy. Not recommended with CrCl <35mL/min. Caution in patients who have Na^+-intake restrictions.

ADVERSE REACTIONS: Nausea, abdominal pain, musculoskeletal (bone/muscle/joint) pain, acid regurgitation, flatulence, dyspepsia, constipation, diarrhea.

INTERACTIONS: Ca^{2+} supplements, antacids, or oral medications containing multivalent cations will interfere with absorption; wait at least 1/2 hr after taking alendronate before taking any other oral medications. Increased incidence of upper GI adverse events in patients receiving concomitant therapy with daily doses of alendronate >10mg and aspirin-containing products. NSAID use is associated with GI irritation; use with caution. IV ranitidine may double bioavailability. Reduced bioavailability with coffee or orange juice.

PREGNANCY: Category C, caution in nursing.

MECHANISM OF ACTION: Bisphosphonate; binds to hydroxyapatite found in bone, and specifically inhibits the osteoclast-mediated bone resorption.

PHARMACOKINETICS: Absorption: Absolute bioavailability: Women (0.64%), men (0.59%). **Distribution:** V_d=at least 28L; plasma protein binding (78%). **Elimination:** (IV) Urine (50%), feces (little or none); $T_{1/2}$=>10 yrs.

NURSING CONSIDERATIONS

Assessment: Assess for esophageal abnormalities, ability to stand or sit upright for at least 30 min, hypocalcemia, risk for aspiration or ONJ, active upper GI problems, mental disability, Na+-intake restriction, renal impairment, drug hypersensitivity, any other conditions where treatment is contraindicated or cautioned, pregnancy/nursing status, and possible drug interactions.

Monitoring: Monitor for signs/symptoms of ONJ, atypical fractures, esophageal reactions, musculoskeletal pain, hypocalcemia, and other adverse events. Monitor serum Ca^{2+} levels. Periodically reevaluate the need for continued therapy.

Patient Counseling: Instruct to take supplemental Ca^{2+} and vitamin D if daily dietary intake is inadequate. Counsel to consider weight-bearing exercise along with modification of certain behavioral factors (eg, cigarette smoking, excessive alcohol use), if these factors exist. Instruct to follow all dosing instructions, and inform that failure to follow them may increase risk of esophageal problems. Advise to d/c and consult physician if symptoms of esophageal disease develop. Instruct that if a dose is missed, to take 1 dose on the am after they remember and to return to taking the dose, as originally scheduled on their chosen day; instruct not to take 2 doses on the same day. Inform patients on Na+-restricted diet that each tab contains 650mg Na+, equivalent to 1650mg NaCl.

Administration: Oral route. Dissolve effervescent tab in 4 oz. of room temperature plain water (not mineral water or flavored water). Wait at least 5 min after the effervescence stops and then stir the sol for 10 sec and ingest. Do not take at hs or before arising for the day. Refer to PI for further administration instructions. **Storage:** 20-25°C (68-77°F); excursions permitted to 15-30°C (59-86°F). Protect from moisture.

BONIVA   RX
ibandronate sodium (Genentech)

THERAPEUTIC CLASS: Bisphosphonate

INDICATIONS: Treatment of osteoporosis in postmenopausal women. (Tab) Prevention of osteoporosis in postmenopausal women.

DOSAGE: *Adults:* (Inj) 3mg IV over 15-30 sec every 3 months. Do not administer more frequently than once every 3 months. (Tab) 150mg once monthly on the same date each month. (Inj/Tab) Periodically reevaluate the need for continued therapy. Refer to PI for instructions for missed doses.

HOW SUPPLIED: Inj: 3mg/3mL [prefilled syringe]; Tab: 150mg

CONTRAINDICATIONS: Hypocalcemia. (Tab) Esophageal abnormalities that delay esophageal emptying (eg, stricture or achalasia), and inability to stand or sit upright for at least 60 min.

WARNINGS/PRECAUTIONS: Consider discontinuation after 3-5 yrs of use in patients at low-risk for fracture; periodically reevaluate risk for fracture in patients who d/c therapy. Hypocalcemia reported; treat hypocalcemia and other disturbances of bone and mineral metabolism before therapy, and ensure adequate Ca^{2+} and vitamin D intake. Osteonecrosis of the jaw (ONJ) reported; risk may increase with duration of exposure to drug. For patients requiring invasive dental procedures, discontinuation of treatment may reduce risk for ONJ. Consider discontinuation if ONJ develops. Severe and occasionally incapacitating bone, joint, and/or muscle pain reported; d/c if severe symptoms develop. Atypical, low-energy, or low-trauma fractures of the femoral shaft reported; evaluate any patient with a history of bisphosphonate exposure who presents with thigh/groin pain to rule out an incomplete femur fracture, and consider interruption of therapy. Anaphylaxis reported; d/c and initiate appropriate treatment if anaphylactic or other severe hypersensitivity/allergic reactions occur. Not recommended with severe renal impairment (CrCl <30mL/min). (Inj) Caution not to administer intra-arterially or paravenously as this could lead to tissue damage. (Tab) May cause local irritation of the upper GI mucosa; caution with active upper GI problems (eg, Barrett's esophagus, dysphagia, esophageal diseases, gastritis, duodenitis, ulcers). Esophageal reactions (eg, esophagitis, esophageal ulcers/erosions) reported; d/c if dysphagia, odynophagia, retrosternal pain, or new/worsening heartburn develops. Use therapy under appropriate supervision in patients who cannot comply with dosing instructions due to mental disability. Gastric and duodenal ulcers reported.

ADVERSE REACTIONS: Influenza, nasopharyngitis, abdominal pain, dyspepsia, constipation, arthralgia, back pain, pain in extremity, headache, diarrhea, urinary tract infection, myalgia.

INTERACTIONS: May interfere with the use of bone-imaging agents. (Tab) Products containing Ca^{2+} and other multivalent cations (eg, aluminum, Mg^{2+}, iron) may interfere with absorption; do not take these products within 60 min of dosing. Caution with aspirin or NSAIDs due to GI irritation.

PREGNANCY: Category C, caution in nursing.

MECHANISM OF ACTION: Bisphosphonate; has an affinity for hydroxyapatite, which is part of the mineral matrix of bone. Inhibits osteoclast activity and reduces bone resorption and turnover. In postmenopausal women, it reduces the elevated rate of bone turnover, leading to, on average, net gain in bone mass.

PHARMACOKINETICS: Absorption: (Tab) Bioavailability (0.6%); T_{max}=0.5-2 hrs. **Distribution:** V_d=at least 90L. (Inj) Plasma protein binding (86%). (Tab) Plasma protein binding (90.9-99.5% [2-10ng/mL concentration]; 85.7% [0.5-10ng/mL concentration]). **Elimination:** Kidney (50-60%, unchanged). (Inj) $T_{1/2}$=4.6-15.3 hrs (2mg), 5-25.5 hrs (4mg). (Tab) Feces (unchanged [unabsorbed drug]); $T_{1/2}$=37-157 hrs.

NURSING CONSIDERATIONS

Assessment: Assess for hypocalcemia, disturbances of bone and mineral metabolism, risk for ONJ, renal impairment, drug hypersensitivity, any other conditions where treatment is contraindicated or cautioned, pregnancy/nursing status, and possible drug interactions. (Inj) Obtain SrCr before each dose. Perform routine oral exam, and consider appropriate preventive dentistry in patients with history of concomitant risk factors for ONJ. (Tab) Assess for esophageal abnormalities, ability to stand or sit upright for at least 60 min, active upper GI problems, and mental disability.

Monitoring: Monitor for signs/symptoms of ONJ, musculoskeletal pain, hypocalcemia, atypical femoral fracture, and other adverse events. Monitor renal function and periodically reevaluate the need for continued therapy. (Tab) Monitor for esophageal reactions. (Inj) Monitor for severe hypersensitivity/allergic reactions.

Patient Counseling: Inform about benefits/risks of therapy. Instruct to take supplemental Ca^{2+} and vitamin D if dietary intake is inadequate. (Tab) Instruct to carefully follow dosing instructions and on what to do if doses are missed. Advise to d/c and seek medical attention if symptoms of esophageal irritation (eg, new/worsening dysphagia, pain on swallowing, retrosternal pain, or heartburn) develop. Instruct that drug should be taken at least 60 min before the 1st food or drink of the day other than water and advise not to eat, drink anything except plain water, or take other medications for at least 60 min after taking the drug. Advise to take with a full glass of plain water (6-8 oz.) and to avoid the use of water with supplements (eg, mineral water). Instruct to avoid lying down for 60 min after taking the drug.

Administration: IV/Oral route. (Inj) Do not mix with Ca^{2+}-containing sol or other IV administered drugs. (Tab) Take at least 60 min before the 1st food or drink of the day other than water, and before taking any oral medication or supplementation. Swallow whole; do not chew or suck the tab. **Storage:** 25°C (77°F); excursions permitted to 15-30°C (59-86°F).

BOOSTRIX   RX
diphtheria toxoid, reduced - acellular pertussis - tetanus toxoid (GlaxoSmithKline)

THERAPEUTIC CLASS: Toxoid/vaccine combination

INDICATIONS: Active booster immunization against tetanus, diphtheria, and pertussis as a single dose in individuals ≥10 yrs of age.

DOSAGE: *Adults:* 0.5mL IM into the deltoid muscle of the upper arm. Wound Management: May be given as a tetanus prophylaxis if no previous dose of any tetanus toxoid, reduced diphtheria toxoid and acellular pertussis vaccine, adsorbed (Tdap) has been administered.
Pediatrics: ≥10 Yrs: 0.5mL IM into the deltoid muscle of the upper arm. Wound Management: May be given as a tetanus prophylaxis if no previous dose of any Tdap has been administered.

HOW SUPPLIED: Inj: 0.5mL [vial, prefilled syringe]

CONTRAINDICATIONS: Encephalopathy (eg, coma, decreased level of consciousness, prolonged seizures) within 7 days of administration of a previous dose of a pertussis antigen-containing vaccine that is not attributable to another identifiable cause.

WARNINGS/PRECAUTIONS: Administer 5 yrs after last dose of recommended series of diphtheria and tetanus toxoids and acellular pertussis vaccine adsorbed and/or tetanus and diphtheria toxoids adsorbed for adult use vaccine. Tip caps of prefilled syringes may contain natural rubber latex; allergic reactions may occur in latex-sensitive individuals. May cause brachial neuritis and Guillain-Barre syndrome. Risk of Guillain-Barre syndrome may increase if Guillain-Barre syndrome occurred within 6 weeks of receipt of a prior tetanus toxoid-containing vaccine. Syncope may occur and can be accompanied by transient neurological signs (eg, visual disturbance, paresthesia, tonic-clonic limb movements). Defer vaccination in patients with progressive/unstable neurologic conditions (eg, cerebrovascular events, acute encephalopathic conditions). Avoid if experienced an Arthus-type hypersensitivity reaction following a prior dose of tetanus toxoid-containing vaccine unless at least 10 yrs have elapsed since last dose of tetanus toxoid-containing vaccine. Expected immune response may not be obtained in immunosuppressed persons. Review immunization history for possible vaccine sensitivity and previous vaccination-related adverse reactions; epinephrine and other appropriate agents should be immediately available for control of allergic reactions.

ADVERSE REACTIONS: Inj-site reactions (eg, pain, redness, swelling, increased arm circumference), headache, fatigue, fever, GI symptoms.

INTERACTIONS: Lower postvaccination geometric mean antibody concentrations (GMCs) to pertactin observed following concomitant administration with meningococcal conjugate vaccine as compared to Boostrix administered 1st. Lower GMCs for antibodies to the pertussis antigens filamentous hemagglutinin and pertactin observed when concomitantly administered with influenza virus vaccine as compared with Boostrix alone. Immunosuppressive therapies including irradiation, antimetabolites, alkylating agents, cytotoxic drugs, and corticosteroids (used in greater than physiologic doses), may reduce the immune response to vaccine.

PREGNANCY: Category B, caution in nursing.

MECHANISM OF ACTION: Vaccine/toxoid combination; develops neutralizing antibodies to tetanus, diphtheria, and pertussis.

NURSING CONSIDERATIONS

Assessment: Assess for history of encephalopathy, latex hypersensitivity, development of Guillain-Barre syndrome following a prior vaccine containing tetanus toxoid, progressive/unstable neurologic conditions, immunosuppression, pregnancy/nursing status, and for possible drug interactions. Review immunization history for possible vaccine sensitivity and previous vaccination-related adverse reactions.

Monitoring: Monitor for signs and symptoms of Guillain-Barre syndrome, brachial neuritis, allergic reactions, syncope, neurological signs, and other adverse reactions. Monitor immune response.

Patient Counseling: Inform about benefits/risks of immunization. Advise about the potential for adverse reactions. Instruct to notify physician if any adverse reactions occur, if pregnant, or plan to become pregnant. Encourage pregnant women receiving the vaccine to contact the pregnancy registry.

Administration: IM route. Shake well before use. Do not administer SQ, intradermally, or IV. Do not mix with any other vaccine in the same syringe or vial. **Storage:** 2-8°C (36-46°F). Do not freeze; discard if has been frozen.

BOSULIF   RX
bosutinib (Pfizer)

THERAPEUTIC CLASS: Tyrosine kinase inhibitor

INDICATIONS: Treatment of adults with chronic, accelerated, or blast phase Philadelphia chromosome-positive chronic myelogenous leukemia (CML) with resistance or intolerance to prior therapy.

DOSAGE: *Adults:* Usual: 500mg qd with food. Continue therapy until disease progression or patient intolerance. Titrate: Consider dose escalation to 600mg qd with food in patients who do not reach complete hematological response by week 8 or a complete cytogenetic response by week 12, who did not have Grade 3 or higher adverse reactions, and who are currently taking 500mg qd. Mild, Moderate, and Severe Hepatic Impairment: 200mg qd. Severe Renal Impairment (CrCl <30mL/min): 300mg qd. For patients with CrCl 30-50mL/min who cannot tolerate a 500mg dose, follow dose adjustment recommendations for toxicity. Refer to PI for dose adjustments for hematological and nonhematologic toxicities.

HOW SUPPLIED: Tab: 100mg, 500mg

WARNINGS/PRECAUTIONS: Diarrhea, N/V, and abdominal pain reported; monitor and manage patients using standards of care. Thrombocytopenia, anemia, and neutropenia reported; perform CBC weekly for the 1st month and then monthly thereafter, or as clinically indicated. Hepatic toxicity reported; perform monthly LFTs for the first 3 months of treatment and as clinically indicated, and, in patients with transaminase elevations, monitor LFTs more frequently. Fluid retention reported and may manifest as pericardial effusion, pleural effusion, pulmonary edema, and/or peripheral edema; monitor and manage patients using standards of care. May cause fetal harm.

ADVERSE REACTIONS: Diarrhea, N/V, thrombocytopenia, abdominal pain, rash, anemia, pyrexia, fatigue, neutropenia, edema, asthenia, respiratory tract infection, decreased appetite, headache, dyspnea.

B

INTERACTIONS: Avoid concomitant use with strong CYP3A inhibitors (eg, ritonavir, indinavir, nelfinavir, saquinavir, ketoconazole, boceprevir, telaprevir, itraconazole, voriconazole, posaconazole, clarithromycin, telithromycin, nefazodone, conivaptan), moderate CYP3A inhibitors (eg, fluconazole, darunavir, erythromycin, diltiazem, atazanavir, aprepitant, amprenavir, fosamprenavir, crizotinib, imatinib, verapamil, grapefruit products, ciprofloxacin), or P-glycoprotein (P-gp) inhibitors as increase in bosutinib concentration is expected. Avoid concomitant use with strong CYP3A inducers (eg, rifampin, phenytoin, carbamazepine, St. John's wort, rifabutin, phenobarbital) or moderate CYP3A inducers (eg, bosentan, nafcillin, efavirenz, modafinil, etravirine) as a large reduction in exposure is expected. Lansoprazole may decrease levels; consider using short-acting antacids or H_2-blockers instead of proton pump inhibitors, but separate dosing by >2 hrs. May increase concentrations of drugs that are P-gp substrates (eg, digoxin).

PREGNANCY: Category D, not for use in nursing.

MECHANISM OF ACTION: Tyrosine kinase inhibitor; inhibits the Bcr-Abl kinase that promotes CML. Also inhibits Src-family kinases, including Src, Lyn, and Hck.

PHARMACOKINETICS: Absorption: (500mg, Multiple-dose) C_{max}=200ng/mL; AUC=3650ng•hr/mL. (500mg, Single-dose) T_{max}=4-6 hrs (median). **Distribution:** Plasma protein binding (94%, in vitro; 96%, ex vivo [healthy]); (500mg, Single-dose) V_d=6080L. **Metabolism:** Via CYP3A4; oxydechlorinated bosutinib and N-desmethylated bosutinib (major metabolites). **Elimination:** Feces (91.3%), urine (3%) (healthy); (500mg, Single-dose) $T_{1/2}$=22.5 hrs.

NURSING CONSIDERATIONS

Assessment: Assess for hypersensitivity to drug, hepatic/renal impairment, pregnancy/nursing status, and possible drug interactions.

Monitoring: Monitor for signs/symptoms of GI toxicity, myelosuppression, hepatotoxicity, fluid retention, and other adverse reactions. Perform CBC weekly for the 1st month and then monthly thereafter, or as clinically indicated. Perform monthly LFTs for the first 3 months and as clinically indicated; monitor more frequently in patients with transaminase elevations.

Patient Counseling: Instruct to take medication exactly as prescribed and not to change the dose or d/c unless directed by physician. Instruct that if a dose is missed beyond 12 hrs, to skip the dose and take the usual prescribed dose on the following day. Advise to seek medical attention promptly if symptoms of GI problems (eg, diarrhea, N/V, abdominal pain, blood in stools) or fluid retention (eg, swelling, weight gain, SOB) develop, or if symptoms of other adverse reactions (eg, respiratory tract infections, rash, fatigue, loss of appetite, headache, dizziness, back pain, arthralgia, pruritus) are significant. Instruct to immediately report fever, any suggestion of infection, signs/symptoms of bleeding or easy bruising, or jaundice. Inform that drug may cause fetal harm; counsel females of reproductive potential to use effective contraceptive measures to prevent pregnancy during and for at least 30 days after completing treatment. Instruct to contact physician immediately if pregnancy occurs during treatment. Advise not to breastfeed or provide breast milk to infants while on therapy; if a patient wishes to restart breastfeeding after treatment, advise to discuss the appropriate timing with physician. Inform that drug and certain other medicines, including OTC drugs and herbal supplements (eg, St. John's wort), can interact with each other and may alter the effects of treatment.

Administration: Oral route. Take with food. Do not crush or cut tab; do not touch or handle crushed or broken tabs. **Storage:** 20-25°C (68-77°F); excursions permitted to 15-30°C (59-86°F).

BREO ELLIPTA   RX
fluticasone furoate - vilanterol (GlaxoSmithKline)

> Long-acting β_2-adrenergic agonists (LABAs) increase the risk of asthma-related death. Not indicated for the treatment of asthma.

THERAPEUTIC CLASS: Beta$_2$-agonist/corticosteroid

INDICATIONS: Long-term, once-daily, maintenance treatment of airflow obstruction in patients with chronic obstructive pulmonary disease (COPD), including chronic bronchitis and/or emphysema. To reduce exacerbations of COPD in patients with a history of exacerbations.

DOSAGE: *Adults:* 1 inh qd. Take at the same time every day. Do not use >1 time q24h.

HOW SUPPLIED: Powder, Inhalation: (Fluticasone Furoate-Vilanterol) 100mcg-25mcg/blister [14, 30 blisters]

CONTRAINDICATIONS: Severe hypersensitivity to milk proteins.

WARNINGS/PRECAUTIONS: Not indicated for the relief of acute bronchospasm. Treat acute symptoms with an inhaled short-acting β_2-agonist (SABA). Do not initiate during rapidly deteriorating or potentially life-threatening episodes of COPD. D/C regular use of oral/inhaled SABA when beginning treatment. Do not use more often or at higher doses than recommended; clinically significant cardiovascular (CV) effects and fatalities reported with excessive use.

Candida albicans infections of mouth and pharynx reported; treat and if needed, interrupt therapy. Increased incidence of pneumonia reported. Increased susceptibility to infections. May lead to serious/fatal course of chickenpox or measles; avoid exposure and if exposed, consider prophylaxis/treatment. Caution in patients with active/quiescent tuberculosis (TB), systemic fungal, bacterial, viral, or parasitic infections, or ocular herpes simplex. Deaths due to adrenal insufficiency reported during and after transfer from systemic to inhaled corticosteroids. Resume oral corticosteroids during periods of stress or a severe COPD exacerbation in patients previously withdrawn from systemic corticosteroids. Wean slowly from systemic corticosteroid use after transferring to therapy. Transferring from systemic to inhaled corticosteroid may unmask allergic conditions previously suppressed by systemic therapy (eg, rhinitis, conjunctivitis, eczema, arthritis, eosinophilic conditions). Monitor for systemic corticosteroid effects. Reduce dose slowly and consider other treatments if hypercorticism and adrenal suppression occur. May produce paradoxical bronchospasm; treat immediately, d/c therapy, and institute alternative therapy. Hypersensitivity reactions may occur. CV effects may occur; caution with CV disorders. Decreases in bone mineral density (BMD) reported with long-term use; caution with major risk factors for decreased bone mineral content, including chronic use of drugs that can reduce bone mass (eg, anticonvulsants, oral corticosteroids). Assess BMD prior to initiating therapy and periodically thereafter; if significant reductions in BMD are seen and therapy is still considered medically important, use medicine to treat or prevent osteoporosis. Glaucoma, increased intraocular pressure (IOP), and cataracts reported with long-term use. Caution with convulsive disorders or thyrotoxicosis, diabetes mellitus (DM), ketoacidosis, moderate/severe hepatic impairment, and in patients unusually responsive to sympathomimetic amines. May produce significant hypokalemia or transient hyperglycemia.

ADVERSE REACTIONS: Nasopharyngitis, upper respiratory tract infection, oropharyngeal candidiasis, headache, back pain, sinusitis, cough, oropharyngeal pain, arthralgia, HTN, influenza, pharyngitis, diarrhea, peripheral edema, pyrexia.

INTERACTIONS: Do not use with other medicines containing a LABA. Caution with long-term ketoconazole and other strong CYP3A4 inhibitors (eg, ritonavir, clarithromycin, conivaptan, indinavir, itraconazole, lopinavir, nefazodone, nelfinavir, saquinavir, telithromycin, troleandomycin, voriconazole); increased systemic corticosteroid and increased CV adverse effects may occur. Extreme caution with MAOIs, TCAs, or drugs known to prolong the QTc interval or within 2 weeks of discontinuation of such agents; effect on CV system may be potentiated by these agents. β-blockers may block pulmonary effects and produce severe bronchospasm in patients with reversible obstructive airways disease; if such therapy is needed, consider cardioselective β-blockers and use them with caution. ECG changes and/or hypokalemia that may result from non-K⁺-sparing diuretics (eg, loop or thiazide diuretics) may be acutely worsened; use with caution.

PREGNANCY: Category C, caution in nursing.

MECHANISM OF ACTION: Fluticasone: Corticosteroid; not established. Shown to have a wide range of actions on multiple cell types (eg, mast cells, eosinophils, neutrophils, macrophages, lymphocytes) and mediators (eg, histamine, eicosanoids, leukotrienes, cytokines) involved in inflammation. Vilanterol: LABA; attributable to stimulation of intracellular adenyl cyclase, the enzyme that catalyzes the conversion of adenosine triphosphate to cyclic-3',5'-adenosine monophosphate (cAMP). Increased cAMP levels cause relaxation of bronchial smooth muscle and inhibition of release of mediators of immediate hypersensitivity from cells, especially from mast cells.

PHARMACOKINETICS: Absorption: Fluticasone: Absolute bioavailability (15.2%); T_{max}=0.5-1 hr. Vilanterol: Absolute bioavailability (27.3%); T_{max}=10 min. **Distribution:** Fluticasone: V_d=661L (IV); plasma protein binding (99.6%). Vilanterol: V_d=165L (IV); plasma protein binding (93.9%). **Metabolism:** Fluticasone: Liver via CYP3A4. Vilanterol: Via CYP3A4. **Elimination:** Fluticasone: Feces (101% [PO], 90% [IV]), urine (1% [PO], 2% [IV]); $T_{1/2}$=24 hrs. Vilanterol: Urine (70%), feces (30%) (PO); $T_{1/2}$=21.3 hrs.

NURSING CONSIDERATIONS

Assessment: Assess for hypersensitivity to drug or to milk proteins, rapidly deteriorating COPD, active/quiescent TB, systemic infections, ocular herpes simplex, CV disorders, risk factors for decreased bone mineral content, convulsive disorders, thyrotoxicosis, DM, ketoacidosis, history of increased IOP, glaucoma, and/or cataracts, hepatic impairment, pregnancy/nursing status, and possible drug interactions. Assess use in patients unusually responsive to sympathomimetic amines. Assess BMD.

Monitoring: Monitor for deteriorating disease, localized oropharyngeal *C. albicans* infections, pneumonia, infections, systemic corticosteroid effects (eg, hypercorticism, adrenal suppression), paradoxical bronchospasm, hypersensitivity reactions, CV effects, glaucoma, cataracts, IOP, hypokalemia, hyperglycemia, and other adverse reactions. Periodically monitor BMD.

Patient Counseling: Inform that drug is not for treatment of asthma. Advise not to use to relieve acute COPD symptoms; inform that acute symptoms should be treated with a rescue inhaler (eg, albuterol). Instruct to notify physician immediately if experiencing worsening of symptoms, a need for more inhalations than usual of the rescue inhaler, or a significant decrease in lung function. Advise not to d/c therapy without physician guidance and not to use additional LABA. Instruct to contact physician if oropharyngeal candidiasis or symptoms of pneumonia develop. Advise to avoid exposure to chickenpox or measles, and, if exposed, to consult physician without delay. Inform about risk of immunosuppression, hypercorticism, adrenal suppression, reduction in BMD, ocular effects, and of adverse effects such as palpitations, chest pain, rapid HR, tremor, or nervousness. Inform that the inhaler is not reusable. Instruct not to take the inhaler apart.

Administration: Oral inhalation route. After inhalation, rinse mouth with water without swallowing. Take at the same time every day. **Storage:** 20-25°C (68-77°F); excursions permitted from 15-30°C (59-86°F). Store in a dry place away from direct heat or sunlight. Store inside the unopened moisture-protective foil tray and only remove from the tray immediately before initial use. Discard 6 weeks after opening the foil tray or when the counter reads "0" (after all blisters have been used), whichever comes 1st.

BREVIBLOC RX
esmolol HCl (Baxter)

THERAPEUTIC CLASS: Selective beta-blocker

INDICATIONS: Short-term use for rapid control of ventricular rate in patients with atrial fibrillation or atrial flutter in perioperative, postoperative, or other emergent circumstances, and for noncompensatory sinus tachycardia. Short-term treatment of tachycardia and HTN that occur during induction and tracheal intubation, during surgery, on emergence from anesthesia, and in the postoperative period.

DOSAGE: *Adults:* Supraventricular Tachycardia (SVT)/Noncompensatory Sinus Tachycardia: Administer by continuous IV infusion with or without LD. Additional LD and/or titration of maint infusion (step-wise dosing) may be necessary based on desired ventricular response. Step 1: Optional LD (500mcg/kg over 1 min), then 50mcg/kg/min for 4 min. Step 2: Optional LD if necessary, then 100mcg/kg/min for 4 min. Step 3: Optional LD if necessary, then 150mcg/kg/min for 4 min. Step 4: If necessary, increase dose to 200mcg/kg/min. Maint: 50-200mcg/kg/min. Max: 200mcg/kg/min. May continue maint infusions for up to 48 hrs. Intraoperative/Postoperative Tachycardia and HTN: Immediate Control: 1mg/kg bolus over 30 sec followed by 150mcg/kg/min infusion, if necessary. Adjust infusion rate as required to maintain desired HR and BP. Gradual Control: 500mcg/kg bolus over 1 min followed by maint infusion of 50mcg/kg/min for 4 min. Continue dosing as for SVT depending on response. Maint Infusion: Tachycardia: Max: 200mcg/kg/min. HTN: May require higher maint infusion dosages (250-300mcg/kg/min). Max: 300mcg/kg/min. Transition to Alternative Drugs: Reduce infusion rate by 50%, 30 min following 1st dose of alternative drug. After administration of 2nd dose of alternative drug, monitor response and if satisfactory control is maintained for 1st hr, d/c infusion. Elderly: Start at lower end of dosing range.

HOW SUPPLIED: Inj: 10mg/mL [10mL, vial; 250mL, premixed inj bag], 20mg/mL [100mL, double strength premixed inj bag]

CONTRAINDICATIONS: Severe sinus bradycardia, heart block >1st degree, sick sinus syndrome, decompensated heart failure, cardiogenic shock, pulmonary HTN, IV administration of cardiodepressant calcium channel antagonists (eg, verapamil) and esmolol in close proximity (eg, while cardiac effects from the other are still present).

WARNINGS/PRECAUTIONS: Not for prevention of intraoperative/postoperative tachycardia and/or HTN. Dose-related hypotension, loss of consciousness, cardiac arrest, and death may occur; monitor BP and reduce dose or d/c in case of an unacceptable drop in BP. Bradycardia, including sinus pause, heart block, and severe bradycardia, may occur; patients with 1st-degree atrioventricular (AV) block, sinus node dysfunction, or conduction disorders may be at increased risk. Monitor HR and rhythm during therapy; reduce dose or d/c if severe bradycardia develops. May cause cardiac failure and cardiogenic shock; d/c at 1st sign/symptom of impending cardiac failure and start supportive therapy. Monitor vital signs closely and titrate slowly in the treatment of patients whose BP is primarily driven by vasoconstriction associated with hypothermia. Should generally not be given to patients with reactive airways disease; titrate to lowest possible effective dose and d/c immediately in the event of bronchospasm. Caution in patients with hypoglycemia and in diabetics; may mask tachycardia occurring with hypoglycemia. Infusion-site reactions may develop; use an alternative infusion site and avoid extravasation if a local infusion-site reaction develops. Avoid infusions into small veins or through a butterfly-catheter. May exacerbate anginal attacks in patients with Prinzmetal's angina; do not use nonselective β-blockers. If used in the setting of pheochromocytoma, give in combination with an α-blocker, and only after α-blocker has been initiated; may cause a paradoxical increase in BP if administered alone. Can attenuate reflex tachycardia and increase risk of hypotension in hypovolemic patients. May aggravate peripheral circulatory disorders (eg, Raynaud's disease or syndrome, peripheral occlusive vascular disease). Severe exacerbations of angina, myocardial infarction, and ventricular arrhythmias reported upon abrupt discontinuation in patients with coronary artery disease (CAD); observe for signs of myocardial ischemia when discontinued. Hyperkalemia reported; increased risk in patients with renal impairment. Monitor serum electrolytes during therapy. May cause hyperkalemic renal tubular acidosis. May mask clinical signs of hyperthyroidism (eg, tachycardia). May precipitate thyroid storm with abrupt withdrawal; monitor for signs of thyrotoxicosis when withdrawing therapy. Patients at risk of anaphylactic reactions may be more reactive to allergen exposure (accidental, diagnostic, or therapeutic). Caution in elderly.

ADVERSE REACTIONS: Hypotension, dizziness, somnolence, nausea, infusion-site reactions.

INTERACTIONS: See Contraindications. May exaggerate effects on BP, contractility, and impulse propagation with other drugs that can lower BP, reduce myocardial contractility, or interfere with sinus node function or electrical impulse propagation in the myocardium. Concomitant use with digoxin may increase the risk of bradycardia and may increase digoxin levels. May prolong effects of succinylcholine-induced neuromuscular blockade. May moderately prolong effects and recovery index of mivacurium. Increased risk of clonidine-, guanfacine-, moxonidine-withdrawal rebound HTN; d/c β-blocker gradually 1st if antihypertensive therapy needs to be interrupted or discontinued. In patients with depressed myocardial function, use with cardiodepressant calcium channel antagonists (eg, verapamil) can lead to fatal cardiac arrests. Sympathomimetic drugs having β-adrenergic agonist activity will counteract effects. Do not use to control tachycardia in patients receiving drugs that are vasoconstrictive and have positive inotropic effects (eg, dopamine, epinephrine, norepinephrine) because of risk of reducing cardiac contractility in presence of high systemic vascular resistance. May be unresponsive to usual doses of epinephrine used to treat anaphylactic or anaphylactoid reactions. May enhance the effect of antidiabetic agents.

PREGNANCY: Category C, not for use in nursing.

MECHANISM OF ACTION: Selective β_1-blocker; inhibits β_1-receptors located chiefly in cardiac muscle, and at higher doses begins to inhibit β_2-receptors located chiefly in the bronchial and vascular musculature.

PHARMACOKINETICS: Distribution: Plasma protein binding (55%). **Metabolism:** Rapid through hydrolysis of the ester linkage in cytosol of RBCs to methanol and free acid. **Elimination:** Urine (73-88% acid metabolite, <2% unchanged); $T_{1/2}$=9 min (esmolol HCl), 3.7 hrs (acid metabolite).

NURSING CONSIDERATIONS

Assessment: Assess for severe sinus bradycardia, heart block >1st degree, sick sinus syndrome, decompensated heart failure, cardiogenic shock, pulmonary HTN, hypersensitivity, or any other conditions where treatment is contraindicated or cautioned. Assess pregnancy/nursing status and for possible drug interactions. Obtain baseline BP, HR and rhythm, and serum electrolytes.

Monitoring: Monitor for hypotension, bradycardia, signs/symptoms of impending cardiac failure, bronchospasm, infusion-site reactions, and other adverse reactions. Monitor for signs of thyrotoxicosis when withdrawing therapy in patients with hyperthyroidism. Monitor BP, HR and rhythm, and serum electrolytes.

Patient Counseling: Inform about benefits/risks of therapy. Instruct to report any adverse reactions to physician.

Administration: IV route. Refer to PI for administration and preparation instructions. **Storage:** 25°C (77°F); excursions permitted to 15-30°C (59-86°F). Protect from freezing. Avoid excessive heat. Ready to Use Bag: Use within 24 hrs once drug has been withdrawn; discard any unused portion. Do not use plastic containers in series connections. Do not remove unit from overwrap until time of use.

BRILINTA   RX
ticagrelor (AstraZeneca)

May cause significant, sometimes fatal, bleeding. Do not use in patients with active pathological bleeding or a history of intracranial hemorrhage. Do not start therapy in patients planned to undergo urgent coronary artery bypass graft surgery (CABG); when possible, d/c therapy at least 5 days prior to any surgery. Suspect bleeding in any patient who is hypotensive and has recently undergone coronary angiography, percutaneous coronary intervention (PCI), CABG, or other surgical procedures. If possible, manage bleeding without discontinuing therapy; stopping therapy increases the risk of subsequent cardiovascular (CV) events. Maintenance doses of aspirin (ASA) >100mg reduce the effectiveness and should be avoided; after any initial dose, use with ASA 75-100mg/day.

THERAPEUTIC CLASS: Platelet aggregation inhibitor

INDICATIONS: To reduce the rate of thrombotic CV events in patients with acute coronary syndrome (ACS) (unstable angina, non-ST elevation myocardial infarction [MI], or ST elevation MI).

DOSAGE: *Adults:* LD: 180mg with ASA (usually 325mg). Maint: 90mg bid with ASA (75-100mg/day). ACS patients who have received a LD of clopidogrel may be started on therapy. If a dose is missed, take one 90mg tab (next dose) at its scheduled time.

HOW SUPPLIED: Tab: 90mg

CONTRAINDICATIONS: History of intracranial hemorrhage, active pathological bleeding (eg, peptic ulcer, intracranial hemorrhage), severe hepatic impairment.

B

WARNINGS/PRECAUTIONS: Caution with risk factors for bleeding (eg, older age, history of bleeding disorders, performance of PCI procedures). Consider the risks and benefits of treatment, noting the probable increase in exposure, in patients with moderate hepatic impairment. Dyspnea reported; exclude underlying diseases that may require treatment if a patient develops new, prolonged, or worsened dyspnea. If dyspnea is determined to be related to therapy, no specific treatment is required; continue therapy without interruption. In the case of intolerable dyspnea requiring discontinuation of therapy, consider another antiplatelet agent. Avoid interruption of treatment; if it must be temporarily discontinued, restart it as soon as possible.

ADVERSE REACTIONS: Bleeding, dyspnea, headache, cough, dizziness, nausea, atrial fibrillation, HTN, noncardiac chest pain, diarrhea, back pain, hypotension, fatigue, chest pain.

INTERACTIONS: See Boxed Warning. Avoid with strong CYP3A inhibitors (eg, atazanavir, clarithromycin, indinavir, itraconazole, ketoconazole, nefazodone, nelfinavir, ritonavir, saquinavir, telithromycin, voriconazole). Avoid with potent CYP3A inducers (eg, rifampin, dexamethasone, phenytoin, carbamazepine, phenobarbital). May increase concentrations of simvastatin and lovastatin (CYP3A4 substrates); avoid simvastatin and lovastatin doses >40mg. Inhibits P-glycoprotein transporter; monitor digoxin levels with initiation of or any change in therapy. Increased risk of bleeding with anticoagulant and fibrinolytic therapy, higher doses of ASA, and chronic NSAIDs.

PREGNANCY: Category C, not for use in nursing.

MECHANISM OF ACTION: Platelet activation and aggregation inhibitor; reversibly interacts with the platelet $P2Y_{12}$ adenosine diphosphate receptor to prevent signal transduction and platelet activation.

PHARMACOKINETICS: Absorption: Absolute bioavailability (36%); T_{max} (median)=1.5 hrs, 2.5 hrs (AR-C124910XX). **Distribution:** V_d=88L; plasma protein binding (>99%). **Metabolism:** Liver via CYP3A4; AR-C124910XX (major active metabolite). **Elimination:** Urine (26%, <1% unchanged, <1% AR-C124910XX), feces (58%); $T_{1/2}$=7 hrs, 9 hrs (AR-C124910XX).

NURSING CONSIDERATIONS

Assessment: Assess for history of intracranial hemorrhage, active pathological bleeding, risk factors for bleeding, hepatic impairment, hypersensitivity to drug, pregnancy/nursing status, and possible drug interactions.

Monitoring: Monitor for bleeding, dyspnea, and other adverse reactions.

Patient Counseling: Instruct to take drug exactly as prescribed, not to d/c therapy without consulting physician, not to exceed 100mg/day ASA, and to avoid taking any other medications that contain ASA. Inform that patient will bleed and bruise more easily and will take longer than usual to stop bleeding. Advise to report any unanticipated, prolonged or excessive bleeding, or blood in stool or urine. Inform that drug can cause SOB; advise to contact physician if experiencing unexpected SOB, especially if severe. Instruct patients to inform physicians and dentists that they are taking the drug before any surgery or dental procedure, and to tell the physician performing any surgery or dental procedure to talk to the prescribing physician before stopping therapy. Advise patient to inform physician of all prescription/OTC medications or dietary supplements that he or she is taking or plans to take.

Administration: Oral route. Take with or without food. **Storage:** 25°C (77°F); excursions permitted to 15-30°C (59-86°F).

BRINTELLIX   RX
vortioxetine (Takeda)

> Antidepressants increased the risk of suicidal thoughts and behavior in children, adolescents, and young adults in short-term studies. Monitor closely for worsening and for emergence of suicidal thoughts and behaviors in patients who are started on antidepressant therapy. Not evaluated for use in pediatric patients.

THERAPEUTIC CLASS: Miscellaneous antidepressant

INDICATIONS: Treatment of major depressive disorder.

DOSAGE: *Adults:* Initial: 10mg/day. Titrate: Increase to 20mg/day, as tolerated. Max: 20mg/day. May consider decreasing dose to 5mg/day for patients who do not tolerate higher doses. Acute episodes of major depression should be followed by several months or longer of sustained therapy to decrease risk of recurrence. Discontinuation of Therapy: Decrease to 10mg/day for 1 week before full discontinuation of 15mg/day or 20mg/day. Switching to/from an MAOI for Psychiatric Disorders: Allow at least 14 days between discontinuation of an MAOI and initiation of treatment, and allow at least 21 days between discontinuation of treatment and initiation of an MAOI. Use with Other MAOIs (eg, Linezolid, IV Methylene Blue): Refer to PI. CYP2D6 Poor Metabolizers: Max: 10mg/day. Use with Strong CYP2D6 Inhibitors (eg, Bupropion, Fluoxetine, Paroxetine, Quinidine): Reduce dose by 1/2. Increase dose to original level when CYP2D6 inhibitor is discontinued. Use with Strong CYP Inducers (eg, rifampin, carbamazepine, phenytoin) for >14 Days: Consider increasing dose. Max: Not >3X original dose. Reduce dose to original level within 14 days when inducer is discontinued.

HOW SUPPLIED: Tab: 5mg, 10mg, 15mg, 20mg

CONTRAINDICATIONS: Use of an MAOI for psychiatric disorders either concomitantly or within 21 days of stopping treatment. Treatment within 14 days of stopping an MAOI for psychiatric disorders. Starting treatment in patients being treated with other MAOIs (eg, linezolid, IV methylene blue).

WARNINGS/PRECAUTIONS: May increase likelihood of precipitation of a mixed/manic episode in patients at risk for bipolar disorder. Screen patient to determine if at risk for bipolar disorder; not approved for treatment of bipolar depression. Serotonin syndrome reported; d/c immediately and initiate supportive symptomatic treatment. May increase risk of bleeding events. Activation of mania/hypomania reported; caution in patients with a history or family history of bipolar disorder, mania, or hypomania. Transient adverse reactions (eg, headache, muscle tension) reported following abrupt discontinuation of doses of 15mg/day or 20mg/day. Hyponatremia reported; caution in the elderly and in volume-depleted patients. D/C in patients with symptomatic hyponatremia and institute appropriate medical intervention. Not recommended with severe hepatic impairment.

ADVERSE REACTIONS: N/V, constipation, diarrhea, dry mouth, dizziness, flatulence, abnormal dreams, pruritus, sexual dysfunction.

INTERACTIONS: See Contraindications. May cause serotonin syndrome when coadministered with other serotonergic drugs (eg, SSRIs, SNRIs, triptans, TCAs, fentanyl, lithium, tramadol, tryptophan, buspirone, St. John's wort) and with drugs that impair metabolism of serotonin; d/c immediately if this occurs and initiate supportive symptomatic treatment. Increased risk of bleeding with aspirin (ASA), NSAIDs, warfarin, and other anticoagulants; monitor patients receiving other drugs that interfere with hemostasis when vortioxetine is initiated or discontinued. Increased risk of hyponatremia with diuretics. Reduce vortioxetine dose by one-half when coadministered with a strong CYP2D6 inhibitor (eg, bupropion, fluoxetine, paroxetine, quinidine). Consider increasing vortioxetine dose when coadministered with a strong CYP inducer (eg, rifampicin, carbamazepine, phenytoin). Coadministration with another drug that is highly protein bound may increase free concentrations of the other drug.

PREGNANCY: Category C, not for use in nursing.

MECHANISM OF ACTION: Antidepressant; has not been established. Thought to be related to its enhancement of serotonergic activity in the CNS through inhibition of the reuptake of serotonin (5-HT). Also has several other activities, including 5-HT3 receptor antagonism and 5-HT1A receptor agonism.

PHARMACOKINETICS: Absorption: Absolute bioavailability (75%); C_{max} =9, 18, and 33ng/mL following doses of 5, 10, 20mg/day, T_{max} =7-11 hrs. **Distribution:** V_d: 2600L. Plasma protein binding (98%). **Metabolism:** Extensive. Oxidation via CYP2D6 (primary), CYP3A4/5, CYP2C19, CYP2C9, CYP2A6, CYP2C8 and CYP2B6, and glucuronic acid conjugation. **Elimination:** Urine (59%), feces (26%); $T_{1/2}$ =66 hrs.

NURSING CONSIDERATIONS

Assessment: Assess for history or family history of bipolar disorder, mania, or hypomania. Assess for syndrome of inappropriate antidiuretic hormone secretion, volume depletion, hepatic dysfunction, pregnancy/nursing status, and for possible drug interactions.

Monitoring: Monitor for clinical worsening, suicidality, unusual changes in behavior, serotonin syndrome, abnormal bleeding, activation of mania/hypomania, hyponatremia, hypersensitivity reactions (eg, angioedema), and other adverse reactions. If discontinuing therapy (particularly if abrupt), monitor for discontinuation symptoms.

Patient Counseling: Inform of risks, benefits, and appropriate use of therapy. Advise patients and caregivers to look for the emergence of suicidality, especially early during treatment and when the dose is adjusted up or down. Inform that if taking 15mg/day or 20mg/day, patient may experience headache, muscle tension, mood swings, sudden outburst of anger, dizziness, and runny nose if therapy is abruptly discontinued; advise not to d/c without notifying physician. Advise to inform physician if taking or planning to take any prescription or OTC drugs. Caution about risk of bleeding with NSAIDs, ASA, warfarin, or other drugs that affect hemostasis. Advise to look for signs of activation of mania/hypomania. Inform of the greater risk of hyponatremia if treated with diuretics, if volume depleted, or if elderly. Inform that nausea is the most common adverse reaction, and is dose related. Instruct to notify physician if an allergic reaction (eg, rash, hives, swelling, difficulty breathing) occurs, if pregnant/planning to become pregnant, or if breastfeeding/planning to breastfeed.

Administration: Oral route. Take without regard to meals. **Storage:** 25°C (77°F); excursions permitted to 15-30°C (59-86°F).

BROMDAY   RX
bromfenac (Bausch & Lomb)

THERAPEUTIC CLASS: NSAID

INDICATIONS: Treatment of postoperative inflammation and reduction of ocular pain after cataract surgery.

DOSAGE: *Adults:* 1 drop qd in affected eye(s), starting 1 day prior to surgery, the day of surgery and continue for 2 weeks postsurgery.

HOW SUPPLIED: Sol: 0.09% [1.7mL]

WARNINGS/PRECAUTIONS: Contains sodium sulfite; may cause allergic-type reactions (eg, anaphylactic symptoms, asthmatic episodes). Sulfite sensitivity is seen more frequently in asthmatics. May slow or delay healing. Potential cross-sensitivity to acetylsalicylic acid, phenylacetic acid derivatives, and other NSAIDs. Caution when treating individuals who previously exhibited sensitivity to these drugs. May increase bleeding of ocular tissues (eg, hyphemas) in conjunction with ocular surgery. Caution in patients with known bleeding tendencies. May result in keratitis. Continued use may lead to sight-threatening epithelial breakdown, corneal thinning, corneal erosion, corneal ulceration, or corneal perforation; d/c if corneal epithelium breakdown occurs. Caution in patients with complicated ocular surgeries, corneal denervation, corneal epithelial defects, diabetes mellitus (DM), ocular surface diseases (eg, dry eye syndrome), rheumatoid arthritis (RA), or repeat ocular surgeries within a short period of time. Increased risk for occurrence and severity of corneal adverse events if used >24 hrs prior to surgery or use beyond 14 days postsurgery. Avoid use with contact lenses. Avoid use during late pregnancy because of the known effects on the fetal cardiovascular system (closure of ductus arteriosus).

ADVERSE REACTIONS: Abnormal sensation in eye, conjunctival hyperemia, eye irritation (burning/stinging), eye pain, eye pruritus, eye redness, headache, iritis.

INTERACTIONS: Concomitant use of topical NSAIDs and topical steroids may increase potential for healing problems. Caution with other medications that may prolong bleeding time.

PREGNANCY: Category C, caution in nursing.

MECHANISM OF ACTION: NSAID; thought to block prostaglandin synthesis by inhibiting cyclooxygenase 1 and 2.

NURSING CONSIDERATIONS

Assessment: Assess for hypersensitivity (eg, sodium sulfite) or cross-sensitivity (eg, aspirin) reactions, history of complicated or repeated ocular surgeries, corneal denervation, corneal epithelial defects, DM, ocular surface diseases (eg, dry eye syndrome), RA, bleeding tendencies, pregnancy/nursing status, and possible drug interactions.

Monitoring: Monitor for anaphylactic symptoms, severe asthma attacks, wound-healing problems, keratitis, corneal epithelial breakdown, corneal thinning/erosion/ulceration/perforation, increased bleeding time, and bleeding of ocular tissues (hyphemas) in conjunction with ocular surgery.

Patient Counseling: Advise not to wear contact lenses during therapy. Advise of the possibility of slow or delayed healing that may occur while using this product. Advise not to touch the dropper tip to any surface, as this may contaminate the contents. If >1 topical ophthalmic medication is used, instruct to administer 5 min apart.

Administration: Ocular route. May be used in conjunction with other topical ophthalmic medications (eg, α-agonists, β-blockers, carbonic anhydrase inhibitors, cycloplegics, mydriatics). Administer at least 5 min apart. **Storage:** 15-25°C (59-77°F).

BROVANA   RX
arformoterol tartrate (Sunovion)

> Long-acting β_2-adrenergic agonists (LABAs) increase the risk of asthma-related death. Contraindicated in asthma without use of a long-term asthma control medication.

THERAPEUTIC CLASS: Beta$_2$-agonist

INDICATIONS: Maintenance treatment of bronchoconstriction in patients with chronic obstructive pulmonary disease (COPD), including chronic bronchitis and emphysema.

DOSAGE: *Adults:* Usual: 15mcg bid (am and pm) by nebulization. Max: 30mcg/day (15mcg bid).

HOW SUPPLIED: Sol, Inhalation: 15mcg base/2mL [30^s, 60^s]

CONTRAINDICATIONS: Asthma without use of a long-term asthma control medication.

WARNINGS/PRECAUTIONS: Not indicated to treat asthma, acute deteriorations of COPD, or acute episodes of bronchospasm (eg, as rescue therapy). D/C regular use of inhaled short-acting β$_2$-agonist (SABA) when beginning treatment; use only for symptomatic relief of acute respiratory symptoms. Do not use more often or at higher doses than recommended; fatalities reported with excessive use. May produce paradoxical bronchospasm; d/c therapy immediately and institute alternative therapy. Cardiovascular (CV) effects may occur; d/c if such effects occur. Caution with CV disorders, convulsive disorders, thyrotoxicosis, diabetes mellitus (DM), ketoacidosis, hepatic impairment, and in patients unusually responsive to sympathomimetic amines. May produce significant hypokalemia or transient hyperglycemia. Immediate hypersensitivity reactions may occur.

ADVERSE REACTIONS: Pain, chest/back pain, diarrhea, sinusitis, leg cramps, dyspnea, rash, flu syndrome, peripheral edema.

INTERACTIONS: Do not use with other medications containing LABAs. Adrenergic drugs may potentiate sympathetic effects; use with caution. Methylxanthine (aminophylline, theophylline), steroids, or diuretics may potentiate hypokalemic effect. Increased HR and systolic BP with theophylline. ECG changes and/or hypokalemia that may result from non-K$^+$-sparing diuretics (eg, loop or thiazide diuretics) may be acutely worsened; use with caution. Extreme caution with MAOIs, TCAs, or drugs known to prolong the QTc interval; effect on CV system may be potentiated by these agents. Drugs known to prolong the QTc interval have an increased risk of ventricular arrhythmias. β-blockers and arformoterol may inhibit the effect of each other when administered concurrently. β-blockers may block therapeutic effects and produce severe bronchospasm in COPD patients; if such therapy is needed, consider cardioselective β-blockers and use with caution.

PREGNANCY: Category C, caution in nursing.

MECHANISM OF ACTION: LABA; stimulates intracellular adenyl cyclase, the enzyme that catalyzes the conversion of adenosine triphosphate to cAMP. Increased cAMP levels cause relaxation of bronchial smooth muscle and inhibition of release of mediators of immediate hypersensitivity from cells, especially from mast cells.

PHARMACOKINETICS: Absorption: C_{max}=4.3pg/mL; T_{max}=30 min (median); AUC_{0-12h}=34.5pg•hr/mL. **Distribution:** Plasma protein binding (52-65%). **Metabolism:** Glucuronidation (primary) via uridine diphosphoglucuronosyltransferase isozymes, and O-demethylation (secondary) via CYP2D6 and CYP2C19 (secondary). **Elimination:** (Within 48 hrs) Urine (63%), feces (11%); $T_{1/2}$=26 hrs.

NURSING CONSIDERATIONS

Assessment: Assess for asthma and use of control medication, acutely deteriorating COPD, CV disorders, convulsive disorders, thyrotoxicosis, DM, ketoacidosis, hepatic impairment, history of hypersensitivity to drug, pregnancy/nursing status, and possible drug interactions. Assess use in patients unusually responsive to sympathomimetic amines.

Monitoring: Monitor for deteriorating disease, paradoxical bronchospasm, CV effects, hypokalemia, hyperglycemia, immediate hypersensitivity reactions, and other adverse reactions.

Patient Counseling: Inform that drug is not for treatment of asthma. Advise not to use to relieve acute respiratory symptoms; inform that acute symptoms should be treated with an inhaled SABA. Instruct to seek medical attention if symptoms worsen despite recommended doses, if treatment becomes less effective, or if experiencing a need for more inhalations of a SABA than usual. Advise not to stop therapy unless directed by physician, not to inhale >1 dose at any 1 time, and not to exceed recommended daily dosage. Instruct to d/c the regular use of inhaled SABA (eg, levalbuterol) when beginning treatment. Counsel not to use with other inhaled medications containing LABA, and not to stop or change the dose of other concomitant COPD therapy without medical advice, even if symptoms improve after initiating treatment. Inform of the common adverse reactions with therapy. Instruct on how to properly use the medication. Advise to contact physician if pregnancy occurs, or if nursing.

Administration: Oral inhalation route. Administer via a standard jet nebulizer connected to an air compressor. Refer to PI for further administration instructions. **Storage:** 2-8°C (36-46°F). Store in the protective foil pouch. Protect from light and excessive heat. After opening the pouch, unused vials should be returned to, and stored in, the pouch. Use opened vial immediately; discard if solution is not colorless. Unopened foil pouches can also be stored at 20-25°C (68-77°F) for up to 6 weeks.

BUMETANIDE   RX
bumetanide (Various)

> May lead to profound diuresis with water and electrolyte depletion if given in excessive amounts; careful medical supervision required and dose and dosage schedule must be adjusted to individual patient's needs.

THERAPEUTIC CLASS: Loop diuretic

BUPRENEX

INDICATIONS: Treatment of edema associated with congestive heart failure (CHF), hepatic and renal disease, including nephrotic syndrome.

DOSAGE: *Adults:* Individualize dose. (Tab) Usual: 0.5-2mg/day as single dose. May give a 2nd or 3rd dose at 4- to 5-hr intervals if response is not adequate. Max: 10mg/day. Maint: Give on alternate days or for 3-4 days with rest periods of 1-2 days in between. Hepatic Failure: Give minimum dose, and if necessary, increase dose very carefully. (Inj) Initial: 0.5-1mg IV/IM. Give IV over 1-2 min. May give a 2nd or 3rd dose at 2- to 3-hr intervals if response is insufficient. Max: 10mg/day. Elderly: Start at lower end of dosing range.

HOW SUPPLIED: Inj: 0.25mg/mL [4mL, 10mL]; Tab: 0.5mg*, 1mg*, 2mg* *scored

CONTRAINDICATIONS: Anuria, hepatic coma, severe electrolyte depletion.

WARNINGS/PRECAUTIONS: Excessive doses may cause dehydration, blood volume reduction, and circulatory collapse with possible vascular thrombosis and embolism, particularly in elderly. Hypokalemia may occur; caution with hepatic cirrhosis and ascites, states of aldosterone excess with normal renal function, K^+-losing nephropathy, certain diarrheal states, other states where hypokalemia represents added risks, or in patients receiving digitalis and diuretics for CHF. Sudden alterations of electrolyte balance may precipitate hepatic encephalopathy and coma in patients with hepatic cirrhosis and ascites; initiate therapy in hospital. Ototoxicity, thrombocytopenia, hypocalcemia, hypomagnesemia, and hyperuricemia may occur. May affect glucose metabolism; monitor glucose levels in diabetics or suspected latent diabetes. Monitor for blood dyscrasias, hepatic damage, or idiosyncratic reactions. Caution with sulfonamide allergy. Reversible elevations of BUN and creatinine may occur; d/c if marked increase in BUN or creatinine occurs, or if oliguria develops in patients with progressive renal disease. Tab may be substituted at approximately a 1:40 ratio of bumetanide tabs to furosemide in patients allergic to furosemide.

ADVERSE REACTIONS: Muscle cramps, dizziness, hypotension, headache, nausea, encephalopathy, hyperuricemia, hypochloremia, hypokalemia, hyponatremia, hyperglycemia, azotemia, increased SrCr.

INTERACTIONS: Avoid with drugs known to have a nephrotoxic potential. Not recommended for use with indomethacin. High risk of lithium toxicity; avoid coadministration. Pretreatment with probenecid reduces effects; do not administer concurrently. May potentiate the effect of various antihypertensives; reduction in the dose of these drugs may be necessary. (Inj) Avoid with aminoglycosides (except in life-threatening situations).

PREGNANCY: Category C, not for use in nursing.

MECHANISM OF ACTION: Loop diuretic; inhibits Na^+ reabsorption in the ascending limb of the loop of Henle.

PHARMACOKINETICS: Absorption: T_{max}=15-30 min (IV), 1-2 hrs (PO). **Distribution:** Plasma protein binding (94-96%). **Metabolism:** Oxidation. **Elimination:** (PO) Urine (81%, 45% unchanged), bile (2%); $T_{1/2}$=1-1.5 hrs.

NURSING CONSIDERATIONS

Assessment: Assess for progressive renal disease, severe electrolyte depletion, anuria, diabetes or suspected latent diabetes, sulfonamide allergy, liver disease (hepatic coma), any other conditions where treatment is contraindicated or cautioned, pregnancy/nursing status, and possible drug interactions.

Monitoring: Monitor for ototoxicity, blood dyscrasias, liver damage or idiosyncratic reactions, hypersensitivity reactions, hyperuricemia, oliguria, thrombocytopenia, and other adverse reactions. Periodically monitor serum K^+, serum electrolytes, blood glucose, and renal function.

Patient Counseling: Inform of the risks/benefits of therapy. Advise to seek medical attention if adverse reactions occur.

Administration: Oral/IV/IM route. **Storage:** 20-25°C (68-77°F). Protect from light. (Inj) Excursions permitted to 15-30°C (59-86°F).

BUPRENEX   CIII
buprenorphine HCl (Reckitt Benckiser)

THERAPEUTIC CLASS: Opioid analgesic

INDICATIONS: Relief of moderate to severe pain.

DOSAGE: *Adults:* 0.3mg IM/IV q6h PRN. Repeat if needed, 30-60 min after initial dose and then PRN. High-Risk Patients/Concomitant CNS depressants: Reduce dose by approximately 50%. May use single doses ≤0.6mg IM if not at high risk.
Pediatrics: ≥13 Yrs: 0.3mg IM/IV q6h PRN. Repeat if needed, 30-60 min after initial dose and then PRN. High-Risk Patients/Concomitant CNS Depressants: Reduce dose by approximately 50%. May use single doses ≤0.6mg IM if not at high risk. 2-12 Yrs: 2-6mcg/kg IM/IV q4-6h.

HOW SUPPLIED: Inj: 0.3mg/mL

WARNINGS/PRECAUTIONS: Significant respiratory depression reported; caution with compromised respiratory function. May increase CSF pressure; caution with head injury, intracranial lesions. Caution with debilitated, BPH, biliary tract dysfunction, myxedema, hypothyroidism, urethral stricture, acute alcoholism, Addison's disease, CNS disease, coma, toxic psychoses, delirium tremens, elderly, pediatric patients, kyphoscoliosis or hepatic/renal/pulmonary impairment. May impair mental or physical abilities. May precipitate withdrawal in narcotic-dependence. May lead to psychological dependence.

ADVERSE REACTIONS: Sedation, N/V, dizziness, sweating, hypotension, headache, miosis, hypoventilation.

INTERACTIONS: Caution with MAOIs, CNS and respiratory depressants. Respiratory and cardiovascular collapse reported with diazepam. Increased CNS depression with other narcotic analgesics, general anesthetics, antihistamines, benzodiazepines, phenothiazines, other tranquilizers, sedative-hypnotics. Decreased clearance with CYP3A4 inhibitors (eg, macrolides, azole antifungals, protease inhibitors). Increased clearance with CYP3A4 inducers (eg, rifampin, carbamazepine, phenytoin).

PREGNANCY: Category C, not for use in nursing.

MECHANISM OF ACTION: Opioid analgesic; high affinity binding to μ-opiate receptors in CNS. Possesses slow rate of dissociation from its receptor. Also possesses narcotic antagonist activity.

PHARMACOKINETICS: Absorption: T_{max}=1 hr. **Distribution:** Found in breast milk. **Metabolism:** Liver. **Elimination:** $T_{1/2}$=1.2-7.2 hrs.

NURSING CONSIDERATIONS

Assessment: Assess for compromised respiratory function (eg, chronic obstructive pulmonary disease, hypoxia), head injury, intracranial lesions, hepatic/renal function, or any condition where treatment is cautioned, pregnancy/nursing status, and possible drug interactions.

Monitoring: Monitor for signs/symptoms of respiratory depression, CNS depression, elevation of CSF pressure, increased intracholedochal pressure, drug dependence, and withdrawal effects.

Patient Counseling: Inform that medication may impair mental/physical abilities; use caution when performing dangerous tasks (eg, operating machinery/driving). Advise to notify physician of all medications currently taken. Instruct to avoid use of other CNS depressants and alcohol during therapy. Advise that medication may lead to dependence. Counsel to not exceed prescribed dosage. Avoid abruptly discontinuing medication. Advise to contact physician if signs/symptoms of respiratory depression develop.

Administration: Deep IM or slow IV route. **Storage:** Avoid excessive heat (over 40°C or 104°F). Protect from prolonged exposure to light.

BUPRENORPHINE AND NALOXONE
naloxone HCl dihydrate - buprenorphine HCl (Various)

`CIII`

THERAPEUTIC CLASS: Partial opioid agonist/opioid antagonist

INDICATIONS: Maintenance treatment of opioid dependence and should be used as part of a complete treatment plan to include counseling and psychosocial support.

DOSAGE: *Adults:* Administer SL as a single daily dose in patients initially inducted using buprenorphine SL tab. Maint: Target Dose: 16mg-4mg/day as single dose. Titrate: Adjust dose progressively in increments/decrements of 2mg-0.5mg or 4mg-1mg to maintain treatment and suppress opioid withdrawal signs and symptoms. Range: 4mg-1mg to 24mg-6mg/day depending on the patient. Discontinuing Therapy: Should be made as part of a comprehensive treatment plan. Switching Between SL Film and SL Tab: Start on the same dose as the previously administered product. Dose adjustments may be necessary. Monitor for over-medication as well as withdrawal or other indications of underdosing. Hepatic Impairment: Adjust dose and observe for precipitated opioid withdrawal. Elderly: Start at lower end of dosing range.

HOW SUPPLIED: Tab, SL: (Buprenorphine-Naloxone) 2mg-0.5mg, 8mg-2mg

WARNINGS/PRECAUTIONS: Not appropriate as an analgesic. Hypersensitivity reactions, bronchospasm, angioneurotic edema, and anaphylactic shock reported. May precipitate opioid withdrawal signs and symptoms if administered before the agonist effects of the opioid have subsided. May impair mental/physical abilities. May produce orthostatic hypotension in ambulatory patients. Caution with debilitated patients, myxedema, hypothyroidism, adrenal cortical insufficiency (eg, Addison's disease), CNS depression or coma, toxic psychoses, prostatic hypertrophy or urethral stricture, acute alcoholism, delirium tremens, kyphoscoliosis, hepatic impairment, and in elderly. Buprenorphine: Potential for abuse. Significant respiratory depression reported; caution with compromised respiratory function. To manage overdose, higher than normal doses and repeated administration of naloxone may be necessary. Accidental pediatric exposure can cause severe, possibly fatal, respiratory depression. Chronic use produces physical dependence. Cytolytic hepatitis and hepatitis with jaundice reported; obtain LFTs prior to initiation and periodically thereafter. If a hepatic event is suspected, biological and etiological evaluation is recommended; careful discontinuation may be needed depending on the case. Caution with preexisting liver enzyme abnormalities, hepatitis B or C infection, use with other potentially hepatotoxic drugs, and ongoing injecting drug use. Neonatal withdrawal reported when used during pregnancy. May elevate CSF pressure; caution with head injury, intracranial lesions, and other circumstances when cerebrospinal pressure may be increased. May produce miosis and changes in consciousness level that may interfere with patient evaluation. May increase intracholedochal pressure; caution with biliary tract dysfunction. May obscure diagnosis or clinical course of patients with acute abdominal conditions.

ADVERSE REACTIONS: Headache, withdrawal syndrome, pain, N/V, insomnia, sweating, constipation, abdominal pain, vasodilation, chills, asthenia, infection, rhinitis, back pain, diarrhea.

INTERACTIONS: May cause respiratory depression, coma, and death with benzodiazepines or other CNS depressants (eg, alcohol); caution when used concurrently. May cause increased CNS depression with opioid analgesics, general anesthetics, benzodiazepines, phenothiazines, other tranquilizers, sedative/hypnotics, or other CNS depressants (eg, alcohol); consider dose reduction of 1 or both agents. Concomitant use with CYP3A4 inhibitors (eg, azole antifungals, macrolides, HIV protease inhibitors) should be monitored and may require dose reduction of 1 or both agents, Monitor for signs and symptoms of opioid withdrawal with CYP3A4 inducers (eg, efavirenz, phenobarbital, carbamazepine, phenytoin, rifampicin). Monitor dose if non-nucleoside reverse transcriptase inhibitors are added to treatment regimen. Atazanavir and atazanavir/ritonavir may increase levels; monitor and consider dose reduction of buprenorphine.

PREGNANCY: Category C, not for use in nursing.

MECHANISM OF ACTION: Buprenorphine: Partial agonist at the μ-opioid receptor and antagonist at the kappa-opioid receptor. Naloxone: Potent antagonist at μ-opioid receptors.

PHARMACOKINETICS: Absorption: Administration of variable doses resulted in different parameters. **Distribution:** Plasma protein binding (96%, buprenorphine; 45%, naloxone); found in breast milk (buprenorphine). **Metabolism:** Buprenorphine: N-dealkylation (by CYP3A4) and glucuronidation; norbuprenorphine (major metabolite). Naloxone: Glucuronidation, N-dealkylation, and reduction; naloxone-3-glucoronide (metabolite). **Elimination:** Buprenorphine: Urine (30%), feces (69%); $T_{1/2}$=24-42 hrs. Naloxone: $T_{1/2}$=2-12 hrs.

NURSING CONSIDERATIONS

Assessment: Assess for history of hypersensitivity reactions, debilitation, myxedema, hypothyroidism, acute alcoholism, adrenal cortical insufficiency (eg, Addison's disease), CNS depression or coma, toxic psychoses, prostatic hypertrophy, urethral stricture, delirium tremens, kyphoscoliosis, biliary tract dysfunction, hepatic impairment, compromised respiratory function, hepatitis B or C infection, head injury, intracranial lesions and other circumstances in which cerebrospinal pressure may be increased, acute abdominal conditions, pregnancy/nursing status, and possible drug interactions. Obtain baseline LFTs.

Monitoring: Monitor for hypersensitivity reactions, signs/symptoms of opioid withdrawal, impaired mental/physical ability, orthostatic hypotension, respiratory depression, drug abuse/dependence, cytolytic hepatitis, hepatitis with jaundice, elevation of CSF, miosis, changes in consciousness levels, and other adverse reactions. Monitor LFTs periodically. Monitor for overmedication as well as withdrawal or other indications of underdosing when switching between SL film and SL tab.

Patient Counseling: Warn patient on danger of self-administration of benzodiazepines and other CNS depressants, including alcohol, while on therapy. Advise that tabs contain an opioid that can be a target for abuse; instruct to keep tabs in safe place protected from theft and children. Instruct to seek medical attention immediately if a child is exposed to the drug. Caution that the drug may impair mental/physical abilities and cause orthostatic hypotension. Advise to take tab qd and not to change dose without consulting physician. Inform that treatment can cause dependence and withdrawal syndrome may occur upon discontinuation. Advise patients seeking to d/c treatment with buprenorphine for opioid dependence to work closely with physician on a tapering schedule, and apprise of the potential to relapse to illicit drug use associated with discontinuation of treatment. Advise to inform physician of all medications prescribed or currently being used. Advise women regarding possible effects during pregnancy and not to breastfeed. Advise to instruct family members that, in event of emergency, the treating physician or staff should be informed that patient is physically dependent on an opioid. Advise to dispose of unused drugs as soon as they are no longer needed by flushing the tabs down the toilet.

Administration: SL route. Refer to PI for further information on method of administration, clinical supervision, and unstable patients. **Storage:** 20-25°C (68-77°F); excursions permitted to 15-30°C (59-86°F).

BUSPIRONE

buspirone HCl (Various)

RX B

THERAPEUTIC CLASS: Atypical anxiolytic

INDICATIONS: Management of anxiety disorders or short-term relief of anxiety symptoms.

DOSAGE: *Adults:* Initial: 7.5mg bid. Titrate: May increase by 5mg/day at intervals of 2-3 days, PRN. Usual: 20-30mg/day in divided doses. Max: 60mg/day. With Potent CYP3A4 Inhibitor: Low dose given cautiously.

HOW SUPPLIED: Tab: 5mg*, 7.5mg*, 10mg*, 15mg*, 30mg* *scored

WARNINGS/PRECAUTIONS: May impair mental/physical abilities. Does not exhibit cross-tolerance with benzodiazepine or other common sedatives/hypnotics; withdraw patients gradually from these agents before starting therapy, especially with chronic CNS depressants. May cause acute and chronic changes in dopamine-mediated neurological function; syndrome of restlessness has been reported shortly after initiation. May interfere with urinary metanephrine/catecholamine assay; d/c therapy for at least 48 hrs prior to undergoing urine collection for catecholamines. Not recommended with severe hepatic/renal impairment. Periodically reassess usefulness of drug if used for extended periods.

ADVERSE REACTIONS: Dizziness, nausea, headache, nervousness, lightheadedness, excitement, drowsiness, fatigue, insomnia, dry mouth.

INTERACTIONS: Elevation of BP with MAOI reported; avoid concomitant use. Avoid with alcohol. Dizziness, headache, and nausea, and increased nordiazepam reported with diazepam. May increase serum concentrations of haloperidol. ALT elevations reported with trazodone. Caution with CNS-active drugs. Diltiazem, verapamil, erythromycin, grapefruit juice, itraconazole, nefazodone, and other CYP3A4 inhibitors (eg, ketoconazole, ritonavir) may increase concentrations; may require dose adjustment. Rifampin and other CYP3A4 inducers (eg, dexamethasone, phenytoin, phenobarbital, carbamazepine), including potent CYP3A4 inducers, may decrease concentrations; may require dose adjustment. Avoid with large amounts of grapefruit juice. May increase levels of nefazodone. Cimetidine may increase levels. Prolonged PT reported with warfarin. May displace less firmly bound drugs like digoxin.

PREGNANCY: Category B, not for use in nursing.

MECHANISM OF ACTION: Atypical anxiolytic; has not been established. Binds with high affinity to serotonin (5-HT1$_A$) receptors and moderate affinity for brain D$_2$-dopamine receptors; may have indirect effects on other neurotransmitter systems.

PHARMACOKINETICS: Absorption: Rapid. C_{max}=1-6ng/mL, T_{max}=40-90 min. **Distribution:** Plasma protein binding (86%). **Metabolism:** Liver (extensive), primarily by oxidation via CYP3A4, and by hydroxylation; 1-pyrimidinylpiperazine (active metabolite). **Elimination:** Urine (29-63%), feces (18-38%); $T_{1/2}$=2-3 hrs.

NURSING CONSIDERATIONS

Assessment: Assess for hypersensitivity to drug, hepatic/renal impairment, pregnancy/nursing status, and possible drug interactions.

Monitoring: Monitor for CNS effects, syndrome of restlessness, and other adverse reactions.

Patient Counseling: Instruct to inform physician about any medications, prescription or nonprescription, alcohol, or drugs being taken or planning to take, and if pregnant/breastfeeding, pregnancy occurs, or planning to become pregnant. Advise not to drive a car or operate potentially dangerous machinery until effects have been determined. Instruct to avoid drinking large amounts of grapefruit juice. Advise to take in a consistent manner with regard to timing and food.

Administration: Oral route. **Storage:** 20-25°C (68-77°F). (7.5mg) 25°C (77°F); excursions permitted between 15-30°C (59-86°F).

BUTRANS

buprenorphine (Purdue Pharmaceutical)

CIII

Exposes users to risks of addiction, abuse, and misuse, leading to overdose and death; assess each patient's risk prior to prescribing and monitor regularly for development of these behaviors/conditions. Serious, life-threatening, or fatal respiratory depression may occur; monitor during initiation or following a dose increase. Chewing, swallowing, snorting, or injecting buprenorphine extracted from the transdermal system will result in uncontrolled delivery and pose risk of overdose and death. Accidental exposure, especially in children, can result in a fatal overdose. Prolonged use during pregnancy can result in neonatal opioid withdrawal syndrome; advise pregnant women of the risk and ensure availability of appropriate treatment.

THERAPEUTIC CLASS: Opioid analgesic

B

INDICATIONS: Management of severe pain that requires daily, around-the-clock, long-term opioid treatment and for which alternative treatment options are inadequate.

DOSAGE: *Adults:* First Opioid Analgesic: Initial: 5mcg/hr. Titrate: Individualize dose. Minimum Titration Interval: 72 hrs; may adjust dose every 3 days. Dose adjustments may be made in 5mcg/hr or 10mcg/hr increments by using no more than 2 patches of the 5mcg/hr or 10mcg/hr systems. Max: 20mcg/hr. Cessation of Therapy: Use gradual downward titration every 7 days; consider introduction of an appropriate immediate-release opioid medication. Severe Hepatic Impairment: Consider use of an alternate analgesic that may permit more flexibility with dosing. Refer to PI for conversion from other opioids and further dosage information.

HOW SUPPLIED: Patch: 5mcg/hr, 10mcg/hr, 15mcg/hr, 20mcg/hr

CONTRAINDICATIONS: Significant respiratory depression, acute or severe bronchial asthma in an unmonitored setting or in the absence of resuscitative equipment, known or suspected paralytic ileus.

WARNINGS/PRECAUTIONS: Reserve use in patients for whom alternative treatment options are ineffective, not tolerated, or would be otherwise inadequate to provide sufficient management of pain. Should only be prescribed by healthcare professionals who are knowledgeable in the use of potent opioids for management of chronic pain. Doses of 10, 15, and 20mcg/hr are for opioid-experienced patients only. Life-threatening respiratory depression is more likely to occur in elderly, cachectic, or debilitated patients. Consider alternative nonopioid analgesics in patients with significant chronic obstructive pulmonary disease or cor pulmonale, and in patients who have a substantially decreased respiratory reserve, hypoxia, hypercapnia, or preexisting respiratory depression. QTc interval prolongation observed at dose of 40mcg/hr; caution with hypokalemia or clinically unstable cardiac disease. Avoid use with history/immediate family history of long QT syndrome. May cause severe hypotension, orthostatic hypotension, and syncope; increased risk in patients whose ability to maintain BP has already been compromised by a reduced blood volume or concurrent administration of certain CNS depressants. Monitor patients who may be susceptible to intracranial effects of carbon dioxide retention for signs of sedation and respiratory depression when initiating therapy. Therapy may obscure clinical course in patients with head injury. Avoid with impaired consciousness or coma. Obtain baseline liver enzyme levels and monitor periodically during treatment in patients at increased risk of hepatotoxicity (eg, history of excessive alcohol intake, IV drug abuse, liver disease). Application-site skin reactions with signs of marked inflammation reported; d/c if severe application-site reactions develop. Cases of acute and chronic hypersensitivity, bronchospasm, angioneurotic edema, and anaphylactic shock reported. Potential for temperature-dependent increases in drug release, resulting in possible overdose and death; avoid exposure of application site and surrounding area to direct external heat sources. If fever or increased core body temperature due to strenuous exertion develops, monitor for side effects and adjust dose if signs of respiratory/CNS depression occur. Avoid with GI obstruction. May cause spasm of sphincter of Oddi and increase in serum amylase; monitor patients with biliary tract disease. May aggravate convulsions and induce/aggravate seizures. May impair mental/physical abilities. Not approved for management of addictive disorders. Not for use during and immediately prior to labor. Caution in elderly.

ADVERSE REACTIONS: Respiratory depression, N/V, dizziness, headache, application-site pruritus/irritation/erythema/rash, constipation, somnolence, dry mouth, fatigue, hyperhidrosis, peripheral edema.

INTERACTIONS: Respiratory depression, hypotension, profound sedation, or coma may occur with alcohol and other CNS depressants (eg, sedatives, anxiolytics, neuroleptics); if coadministration is required, consider dose reduction of one or both agents. Monitor use in elderly, cachectic, and debilitated patients when coadministered with other drugs that depress respiration. Monitor closely with benzodiazepines. CYP3A4 inhibitors may increase levels and prolong opioid effects; these effects could be more pronounced with concomitant use of CYP2D6 and 3A4 inhibitors; if coadministration is necessary, monitor for respiratory depression and sedation at frequent intervals and consider dose adjustments. CYP3A4 inducers may decrease levels and cause lack of efficacy, or development of abstinence syndrome; if coadministration or discontinuation is necessary, monitor for signs of opioid withdrawal and consider dose adjustments. May enhance neuromuscular blocking action of skeletal muscle relaxants and increase respiratory depression. Avoid with Class IA antiarrhythmics (eg, quinidine, procainamide, disopyramide) or Class III antiarrhythmics (eg, sotalol, amiodarone, dofetilide). Anticholinergics or other drugs with anticholinergic activity may increase risk of urinary retention and/or severe constipation and lead to paralytic ileus.

PREGNANCY: Category C, not for use in nursing.

MECHANISM OF ACTION: Opioid analgesic; partial agonist at μ-opioid and ORL-1 (nociceptin) receptors, antagonist at kappa-opioid receptors, and agonist at delta-opioid receptors. Contributions of these actions to its analgesic profile are unclear.

PHARMACOKINETICS: Absorption: Absolute bioavailability (15%). Administration of variable doses resulted in different parameters. **Distribution:** Plasma protein binding (96%); found in breast milk; crosses placenta. (IV) V_d=430L. **Metabolism:** Liver; N-dealkylation via CYP3A4 to norbuprenorphine and glucuronidation by UGT-isoenzymes (mainly UGT1A1 and 2B7) to buprenorphine 3β-O-glucuronide; norbuprenorphine (active, major metabolite). **Elimination:** (2mcg/kg IM) Urine (27%), feces (70%). $T_{1/2}$=26 hrs.

NURSING CONSIDERATIONS

Assessment: Assess for abuse/addiction risk, pain intensity, prior opioid therapy, opioid tolerance, respiratory depression, drug hypersensitivity, pregnancy/nursing status, possible drug interactions, or any other conditions where treatment is contraindicated or cautioned. Obtain baseline liver enzyme levels in patients at increased risk of hepatotoxicity.

Monitoring: Monitor for respiratory depression (especially within first 24-72 hrs of initiation), hypotension, application-site skin reactions, seizures/convulsions, and other adverse reactions. Monitor BP and serum amylase levels. Regularly monitor for signs of misuse, abuse, and addiction. Periodically reassess the continued need for therapy. Monitor liver enzyme levels periodically in patients at increased risk of hepatotoxicity.

Patient Counseling: Inform that use of drug can result in addiction, abuse, and misuse; instruct not to share with others and to take steps to protect from theft or misuse. Inform patients about risk of respiratory depression. Advise to store securely and dispose unused patch by folding the patch in 1/2 and flushing down the toilet. Inform women of reproductive potential that prolonged use during pregnancy may result in neonatal opioid withdrawal syndrome and instruct to inform physician if pregnant or planning to become pregnant. Inform that potentially serious additive effects may occur when used with alcohol or CNS depressants, and not to use such drugs unless supervised by healthcare provider. Instruct about proper application, removal, and disposal instructions. Inform that drug may cause orthostatic hypotension, syncope, impair the ability to perform potentially hazardous activities; advise to not perform such tasks until patients know how they will react to medication. Advise of potential for severe constipation, including management instructions. Advise how to recognize anaphylaxis and when to seek medical attention.

Administration: Transdermal route. Each patch is intended to be worn for 7 days. Do not cut patch. Apply immediately after removal from individually sealed pouch. Apply to intact skin on upper outer arm, upper chest, upper back, or side of chest; rotate application site with a minimum of 21 days before reapplying to the same skin site. For use of 2 patches, remove current patch and apply the 2 new patches adjacent to one another at a different application site. Refer to PI for further administration and disposal instructions. **Storage:** 25°C (77°F); excursions permitted between 15-30°C (59-86°F).

BYDUREON RX
exenatide (Amylin)

> Causes an increased incidence in thyroid C-cell tumors at clinically relevant exposures in animal studies. It is unknown whether drug causes thyroid C-cell tumors (eg, medullary thyroid carcinoma [MTC]) in humans. Contraindicated in patients with a personal or family history of MTC and with multiple endocrine neoplasia syndrome type 2 (MEN 2). Routine serum calcitonin or thyroid ultrasound monitoring is of uncertain value in patients treated with exenatide. Counsel patients on the risk and symptoms of thyroid tumors.

THERAPEUTIC CLASS: Glucagon-like peptide-1 receptor agonist

INDICATIONS: Adjunct to diet and exercise to improve glycemic control in adults with type 2 diabetes mellitus (DM).

DOSAGE: *Adults:* Usual: 2mg/dose SQ once every 7 days, at any time of day. Changing Weekly Dosing Schedule: May change the day of weekly administration if necessary as long as the last dose was given ≥3 days before. Changing from Byetta to Bydureon: D/C Byetta. Prior treatment with Byetta is not required when initiating therapy.

HOW SUPPLIED: Inj, Extended-Release: 2mg [vial, pen]

CONTRAINDICATIONS: MEN 2, personal or family history of MTC.

WARNINGS/PRECAUTIONS: Not for IV or IM administration. Not recommended as 1st-line therapy with inadequate glycemic control on diet and exercise. Not a substitute for insulin; do not use in type 1 DM or for treatment of diabetic ketoacidosis. Not studied and cannot be recommended with insulin. Should not be used with other drugs containing the same active ingredient (eg, Byetta). Patients changing from Byetta may experience transient (approximately 2 weeks) elevations in blood glucose concentrations. Acute pancreatitis, including fatal and nonfatal hemorrhagic or necrotizing pancreatitis reported; observe for signs/symptoms of pancreatitis after initiation of therapy, d/c promptly if suspected, and do not restart therapy if confirmed. Not studied in patients with history of pancreatitis; consider other antidiabetic therapies. Refer patients with thyroid nodules and/or elevated calcitonin levels to an endocrinologist for further evaluation. Altered renal function, including increased SrCr, renal impairment, worsened chronic renal failure, and acute renal failure reported; avoid with severe renal impairment (CrCl <30mL/min) or end-stage renal disease. Caution with renal transplantation and moderate renal impairment (CrCl 30-50mL/min). Avoid with severe GI disease. May develop antibodies; consider alternative antidiabetic therapy if there is worsening glycemic control or failure to achieve targeted glycemic control. Serious hypersensitivity reactions (eg, anaphylaxis, angioedema) reported; d/c if a hypersensitivity reaction occurs. Caution in elderly.

ADVERSE REACTIONS: Constipation, diarrhea, dyspepsia, headache, N/V, inj-site nodule, fatigue, decreased appetite, inj-site pruritus, viral gastroenteritis, gastroesophageal reflux disease, inj-site erythema, inj-site hematoma.

INTERACTIONS: Increased risk of hypoglycemia with a sulfonylurea or other glucose-independent insulin secretagogues (eg, meglitinides); may require a lower dose of the sulfonylurea. May reduce the rate of absorption of orally administered drugs; caution with oral medications. May increase INR with warfarin, sometimes associated with bleeding; monitor INR more frequently after initiation of therapy.

PREGNANCY: Category C, not for use in nursing.

MECHANISM OF ACTION: Glucagon-like peptide-1 receptor agonist; enhances glucose-dependent insulin secretion by the pancreatic β-cell, suppresses inappropriately elevated glucagon secretion, and slows gastric emptying.

PHARMACOKINETICS: Absorption: T_{max}=2 weeks (initial peak), 6-7 weeks (second peak). **Distribution:** V_d=28.3L. **Elimination:** Kidney.

NURSING CONSIDERATIONS

Assessment: Assess for previous hypersensitivity reactions, MEN 2, personal or family history of MTC, history of pancreatitis, type of DM, diabetic ketoacidosis, renal impairment, severe GI disease, pregnancy/nursing status, and possible drug interactions. Assess glucose and HbA1c levels.

Monitoring: Monitor for signs/symptoms of thyroid tumor, pancreatitis, elevated serum calcitonin levels, hypoglycemia, GI events, immunogenicity, hypersensitivity reactions, and other adverse reactions. Monitor renal function, blood glucose levels, and HbA1c levels. Monitor INR more frequently after initiation of therapy in patients receiving warfarin.

Patient Counseling: Counsel on potential risks/benefits of therapy and alternative modes of therapy. Inform of importance of adhering to dietary instructions, regular physical activity, periodic blood glucose monitoring and HbA1c testing, recognition/management of hypoglycemia and hyperglycemia, and assessment for diabetes complications. Advise to report symptoms of thyroid tumors (eg, lump in the neck, hoarseness, dysphagia, dyspnea) to physician. Inform of potential risk for pancreatitis, worsening of renal function, and serious hypersensitivity reactions. Instruct to d/c therapy promptly and contact physician if persistent severe abdominal pain and/or symptoms of a hypersensitivity reaction occur. Instruct to never share a single-dose tray with another person, even if the needle is changed. Advise that if a dose is missed, administer as soon as noticed, provided that the next regularly scheduled dose is due at least 3 days later. Instruct to then resume the usual dosing schedule thereafter. Inform that if a dose is missed and the next regularly scheduled dose is due in 1 or 2 days, to not administer the missed dose and instead resume with the next regularly scheduled dose. Advise to inform physician if pregnant or intending to become pregnant. Inform about the importance of proper storage, injection technique, and dosing.

Administration: SQ route. Administer with or without meals. Inject in the abdomen, thigh, or upper arm region; use a different inj site each week when injecting in the same region. Administer immediately after powder is suspended in diluent. Refer to PI for further administration instructions. **Storage:** 2-8°C (36-46°F). May store at room temperature not exceeding 25°C (77°F) for ≤4 weeks. Do not freeze; do not use if product has been frozen. Protect from light.

BYETTA   RX
exenatide (Amylin)

THERAPEUTIC CLASS: Glucagon-like peptide-1 receptor agonist

INDICATIONS: Adjunct to diet and exercise to improve glycemic control in adults with type 2 diabetes mellitus (DM).

DOSAGE: *Adults:* Initial: 5mcg SQ bid, at any time within 60 min before am and pm meals (or before the 2 main meals of the day, approximately 6 hrs or more apart). Titrate: May increase to 10mcg bid after 1 month based on clinical response. CrCl 30-50mL/min: Caution when initiating or escalating doses from 5mcg to 10mcg.

HOW SUPPLIED: Inj: 5mcg/dose, 10mcg/dose [60-dose prefilled pen]

WARNINGS/PRECAUTIONS: Not a substitute for insulin; do not use for treatment of type 1 diabetes or diabetic ketoacidosis. Not studied and not recommended with prandial insulin. Evaluate dose of insulin if used in combination; consider dose reduction in patients at risk of hypoglycemia. Acute pancreatitis reported; observe for signs and symptoms after initiation and dose increases; d/c if suspected and do not restart if confirmed. Consider other antidiabetic therapies with history of pancreatitis. Altered renal function, including increased SrCr, renal impairment, worsened chronic renal failure, and acute renal failure, reported; avoid with severe renal impairment (CrCl <30mL/min) or end-stage renal disease. Caution with renal transplantation. Avoid with severe GI disease. May develop antibodies; consider alternative antidiabetic therapy if there is worsening glycemic control or failure to achieve targeted glycemic control. Serious hypersensitivity reactions (eg, anaphylaxis, angioedema) reported; d/c if any occur. No conclusive evidence of macrovascular risk reduction. Caution in elderly.

ADVERSE REACTIONS: Hypoglycemia, N/V, immunogenicity, dyspepsia, diarrhea, feeling jittery, dizziness, headache, constipation, asthenia.

INTERACTIONS: Caution with oral medications with narrow therapeutic index or that require rapid GI absorption. Drugs dependent on threshold concentrations for efficacy (eg, contraceptives, antibiotics) should be taken at least 1 hr before inj. May increase INR with warfarin, sometimes associated with bleeding; monitor PT more frequently after initiation or alteration of exenatide therapy. Sulfonylureas or other glucose-independent insulin secretagogues (eg, meglitinides) may increase the risk of hypoglycemia; may require lower dose of sulfonylurea. May alter levels of acetaminophen, digoxin, lovastatin, lisinopril, ethinyl estradiol, and levonorgestrel.

PREGNANCY: Category C, not for use in nursing.

MECHANISM OF ACTION: Glucagon-like peptide-1 receptor agonist; enhances glucose-dependent insulin secretion by the pancreatic β-cell, suppresses inappropriately elevated glucagon secretion, and slows gastric emptying.

PHARMACOKINETICS: Absorption: C_{max}=211pg/mL (10mcg), AUC=1036pg•h/mL (10mcg), T_{max}=2.1 hrs. **Distribution:** V_d=28.3L. **Elimination:** $T_{1/2}$=2.4 hrs.

NURSING CONSIDERATIONS

Assessment: Assess for type 1 diabetes, diabetic ketoacidosis, history of pancreatitis, renal impairment, severe GI disease, pregnancy/nursing status, drug hypersensitivity, and possible drug interactions.

Monitoring: Monitor for signs/symptoms of acute pancreatitis, hypoglycemia, GI events, immunogenicity, and for hypersensitivity reactions. Monitor renal function, glucose levels, and HbA1c levels.

Patient Counseling: Advise of the potential risks and benefits of therapy. Advise to never share inj pen. Inform about self-management practices (eg, proper storage of drug, inj technique, timing of dosage and concomitant oral drugs, adherence to meal planning, regular physical activity). Inform that pen needles are purchased separately and advise on proper needle selection and disposal. Advise not to reuse needle and not to transfer drug from pen to a syringe or vial. Advise not to mix with insulin in the same syringe or vial or administer after a meal. Inform that if a dose is missed, treatment regimen should be resumed as prescribed with the next scheduled dose. Instruct to inform physician if pregnant, intending to become pregnant, or if breastfeeding. Advise that treatment may result in reduction in appetite, food intake, and/or body weight, and that there is no need to modify the dosing regimen due to such effects. Inform that nausea, particularly upon initiation of therapy, may occur. Instruct to contact a physician if signs/symptoms suggestive of hypoglycemia, acute pancreatitis (eg, severe abdominal pain), renal dysfunction, or hypersensitivity develop.

Administration: SQ route. Inject into thigh, abdomen, or upper arm. Refer to PI for further information on administration and preparation. **Storage:** Prior to 1st use: 2-8°C (36-46°F). After 1st use: <25°C (77°F). Do not freeze. Do not use if has been frozen. Protect from light. Discard pen 30 days after the 1st use.

BYSTOLIC   RX
nebivolol (Forest)

THERAPEUTIC CLASS: Selective beta$_1$-blocker

INDICATIONS: Treatment of HTN alone or in combination with other antihypertensive agents.

DOSAGE: *Adults:* Individualize dose. Initial: 5mg qd. Titrate: May increase at 2-week intervals. Max: 40mg. Moderate Hepatic Impairment/Severe Renal Impairment (CrCl <30mL/min): Initial: 2.5mg qd; titrate up slowly if needed.

HOW SUPPLIED: Tab: 2.5mg, 5mg, 10mg, 20mg

CONTRAINDICATIONS: Severe bradycardia, heart block >1st degree, cardiogenic shock, decompensated cardiac failure, sick sinus syndrome (unless permanent pacemaker in place), severe hepatic impairment (Child-Pugh >B).

WARNINGS/PRECAUTIONS: Severe exacerbation of angina, myocardial infarction, and ventricular arrhythmias reported in patients with coronary artery disease (CAD) following abrupt discontinuation; taper over 1-2 weeks when possible. Restart therapy promptly, at least temporarily, if angina worsens or acute coronary insufficiency develops. Avoid with bronchospastic disease. Should generally continue therapy throughout perioperative period. Monitor patients closely with anesthetic agents that depress myocardial function (eg, ether, cyclopropane, trichloroeth-ylene). If discontinuing therapy prior to major surgery, impaired ability of heart to respond to reflex adrenergic stimuli may augment risks of general anesthesia and surgical procedures. May mask signs/symptoms of hypoglycemia or hyperthyroidism, particularly tachycardia. Abrupt withdrawal may be followed by exacerbation of the symptoms of hyperthyroidism or may pre-cipitate a thyroid storm. May precipitate/aggravate symptoms of arterial insufficiency in patients with peripheral vascular disease (PVD). Patients with history of severe anaphylactic reactions to variety of allergens may be more reactive to repeated accidental/diagnostic/therapeutic chal-lenge; may be unresponsive to usual doses of epinephrine. Initiate an α-blocker prior to use of any β-blocker in patients with known/suspected pheochromocytoma. Not recommended with severe hepatic impairment.

ADVERSE REACTIONS: Headache, fatigue, dizziness, diarrhea, nausea.

INTERACTIONS: Avoid with other β-blockers. D/C for several days before gradually tapering clonidine. CYP2D6 inhibitors (eg, quinidine, propafenone, paroxetine, fluoxetine) and cimetidine may increase levels. May decrease levels of sildenafil. Sildenafil may affect levels of nebivolol. May produce excessive reduction of sympathetic activity with catecholamine-depleting drugs (eg, reserpine, guanethidine). May increase risk of bradycardia with digitalis glycosides. May exacerbate effects of myocardial depressants/inhibitors of atrioventricular conduction (eg, antiarrhythmics, certain Ca^{2+} antagonists). May need to adjust dose with CYP2D6 inducers. May potentiate hypoglycemic effect of insulin and PO hypoglycemics. Monitor ECG and BP with vera-pamil and diltiazem.

PREGNANCY: Category C, not for use in nursing.

MECHANISM OF ACTION: Selective $β_1$-blocker; mechanism not established. Possible factors include decreased HR and myocardial contractility, diminution of tonic sympathetic outflow to the periphery from cerebral vasomotor centers, suppression of renin activity, vasodilation, and decreased peripheral vascular resistance.

PHARMACOKINETICS: Absorption: T_{max}=1.5-4 hrs. **Distribution:** Plasma protein binding (98%). **Metabolism:** Glucuronidation, N-dealkylation, and oxidation via CYP2D6. **Elimination:** Urine (38%, extensive metabolizers [EM]), (67%, poor metabolizers [PM]); feces (44%, EM), (13%, PM); $T_{1/2}$=12 hrs (EM), 19 hrs (PM).

NURSING CONSIDERATIONS

Assessment: Assess for CAD, bronchospastic disease, diabetes mellitus, hypoglycemia, hy-perthyroidism, PVD, pheochromocytoma, any conditions where treatment is contraindicated, hepatic/renal impairment, pregnancy/nursing status, and possible drug interactions.

Monitoring: Monitor for precipitation/aggravation of arterial insufficiency, hypersensitivity, and other adverse reactions. Monitor BP and serum glucose levels.

Patient Counseling: Inform of the risks and benefits of therapy. Advise to take drug regularly and continuously, ud, without regard to food. Instruct to take only the next scheduled dose (without doubling it) if a dose is missed, and not to d/c without consulting physician. Advise to consult physician if any difficulty in breathing occurs, or signs/symptoms of worsening congestive heart failure (eg, weight gain, increased SOB, excessive bradycardia) develop. Caution about operating automobiles, using machinery, or engaging in tasks requiring alertness. Caution patients subject to spontaneous hypoglycemia, or diabetic patients receiving insulin or PO hypoglycemics, that the drug may mask some of the manifestations of hypoglycemia, particularly tachycardia.

Administration: Oral route. **Storage:** 20-25°C (68-77°F).

CADUET   RX
atorvastatin calcium - amlodipine besylate (Pfizer)

THERAPEUTIC CLASS: Calcium channel blocker/HMG-CoA reductase inhibitor

INDICATIONS: Amlodipine: Treatment of HTN, alone or in combination with other antihyper-tensive agents. Treatment of chronic stable angina or confirmed or suspected vasospastic (Prinzmetal's/variant) angina, alone or in combination with other antianginals. To reduce the risk of hospitalization due to angina and to reduce risk of coronary revascularization procedures in patients with recently documented coronary artery disease (CAD) by angiography and without heart failure or ejection fraction <40%. Atorvastatin: To reduce the risk of myocardial infarc-tion (MI), stroke, revascularization procedures, and angina in adults without clinically evident coronary heart disease (CHD) but with multiple risk factors for CHD. To reduce the risk of MI and stroke in patients with type 2 diabetes, and without clinically evident CHD, but with multiple risk factors for CHD. To reduce the risk of nonfatal MI, fatal and nonfatal stroke, revascularization pro-cedures, hospitalization for congestive heart failure, and angina in patients with clinically evident CHD. Adjunct to diet for treatment of primary hypercholesterolemia (heterozygous familial and nonfamilial) and mixed dyslipidemia (Types IIa and IIb). Adjunct to diet for treatment of patients with elevated serum TG levels (Type IV). Treatment of primary dysbetalipoproteinemia (Type

III) inadequately responding to diet. Adjunct to other lipid-lowering treatments or if treatments are unavailable, for treatment of homozygous familial hypercholesterolemia (HoFH). Adjunct to diet for treatment of boys and postmenarchal girls, 10-17 yrs of age, with heterozygous familial hypercholesterolemia.

DOSAGE: *Adults:* Individualize dose. Amlodipine: HTN: Initial: 5mg qd. Titrate: Adjust dosage according to BP goals, generally every 7-14 days. Max: 10mg qd. Small/Fragile/Elderly/Hepatic Insufficiency/Concomitant Antihypertensive: 2.5mg qd. Chronic Stable Angina/Vasospastic Angina/CAD: Usual: 5-10mg qd. Elderly/Hepatic Insufficiency: Give lower dose. Atorvastatin: Hyperlipidemia/Mixed Dyslipidemia: Initial: 10mg or 20mg qd (or 40mg qd for LDL reduction >45%). Titrate: Upon titration, analyze lipid levels within 2 to 4 weeks and adjust dose accordingly. Usual: 10-80mg qd. HoFH: 10-80mg qd. Concomitant Lopinavir plus Ritonavir: Use lowest dose necessary. Concomitant Clarithromycin/Itraconazole/Saquinavir plus Ritonavir/Darunavir plus Ritonavir/Fosamprenavir/Fosamprenavir plus Ritonavir: Limit to 20mg; use lowest dose necessary. Concomitant Nelfinavir/Boceprevir: Limit to 40mg; use lowest dose necessary. Replacement Therapy: May substitute for individually titrated components.
Pediatrics: Amlodipine: 6-17 Yrs: HTN: Usual: 2.5-5mg qd. Max: 5mg qd. Atorvastatin: 10-17 Yrs: Individualize dose. Heterozygous Familial Hypercholesterolemia: Initial: 10mg/day. Titrate: Adjust dose at intervals of ≥4 weeks. Max: 20mg/day.

HOW SUPPLIED: Tab: (Amlodipine-Atorvastatin) 2.5mg-10mg, 2.5mg-20mg, 2.5mg-40mg, 5mg-10mg, 5mg-20mg, 5mg-40mg, 5mg-80mg, 10mg-10mg, 10mg-20mg, 10mg-40mg, 10mg-80mg

CONTRAINDICATIONS: Active liver disease, which may include unexplained persistent elevations in hepatic transaminases, women who are pregnant or may become pregnant, and nursing mothers.

WARNINGS/PRECAUTIONS: Caution in elderly. Amlodipine: Worsening angina and acute MI may develop after starting or increasing the dose, particularly with severe obstructive CAD. Symptomatic hypotension may occur, particularly in patients with severe aortic stenosis. Atorvastatin: Rare cases of rhabdomyolysis with acute renal failure secondary to myoglobinuria reported. Increased risk of rhabdomyolysis in patients with history of renal impairment; closely monitor for skeletal muscle effects. Myopathy (including immune-mediated necrotizing myopathy [IMNM]) reported; predisposing factor includes advanced age (≥65 yrs of age). D/C if markedly elevated CPK levels occur or if myopathy is diagnosed or suspected. Withhold or d/c if an acute, serious condition suggestive of a myopathy occurs or if there is a risk factor predisposing to development of renal failure secondary to rhabdomyolysis. Persistent increases in serum transaminases reported; perform LFTs prior to initiation and repeat as clinically indicated. Fatal and nonfatal hepatic failure (rare) reported; promptly interrupt therapy if serious liver injury with clinical symptoms and/or hyperbilirubinemia or jaundice occurs and do not restart if no alternate etiology found. Increases in HbA1c and FPG levels reported. May blunt adrenal and/or gonadal steroid production. Increased risk of hemorrhagic stroke in patients with recent stroke or transient ischemic attack (TIA).

ADVERSE REACTIONS: Edema, palpitations, dizziness, fatigue, nasopharyngitis, nausea, insomnia, diarrhea, arthralgia, pain in extremities, urinary tract infection, dyspepsia, myalgia.

INTERACTIONS: Amlodipine: Diltiazem increased systemic exposure in elderly hypertensive patients. Strong inhibitors of CYP3A4 (eg, ketoconazole, itraconazole, ritonavir) may increase plasma concentrations; monitor for symptoms of hypotension and edema with CYP3A4 inhibitors. Closely monitor BP if coadministered with CYP3A4 inducers. May increase cyclosporine levels in renal transplant patients. Atorvastatin: Avoid with cyclosporine, telaprevir, gemfibrozil, tipranavir plus ritonavir, and drugs that decrease levels or activity of endogenous steroid hormones (eg, ketoconazole, spironolactone, cimetidine). Increased risk of myopathy with fibric acid derivatives, erythromycin, lipid-modifying doses of niacin, strong CYP3A4 inhibitors, clarithromycin, combinations of HIV protease inhibitors, and azole antifungals; consider lower initial and maintenance doses. Strong CYP3A4 inhibitors (eg, clarithromycin, several combinations of HIV protease inhibitors, telaprevir, itraconazole, boceprevir) and grapefruit juice may increase levels. CYP3A4 inducers (eg, efavirenz, rifampin) may decrease levels; simultaneous coadministration with rifampin recommended. May increase digoxin levels; monitor appropriately. May increase area under the curve of norethindrone and ethinyl estradiol. Myopathy, including rhabdomyolysis, reported with colchicine; use with caution. OATP1B1 inhibitors (eg, cyclosporine) may increase bioavailability.

PREGNANCY: Category X, not for use in nursing.

MECHANISM OF ACTION: Amlodipine: Calcium channel blocker (dihydropyridine); inhibits transmembrane influx of calcium ions into vascular smooth muscle and cardiac muscle. Acts directly on vascular smooth muscle to cause a reduction in peripheral vascular resistance and reduction in BP. Atorvastatin: HMG-CoA reductase inhibitor; inhibits conversion of HMG-CoA to mevalonate (precursor of sterols, including cholesterol).

PHARMACOKINETICS: Absorption: Amlodipine: Absolute bioavailability (64-90%); T_{max}=6-12 hrs. Atorvastatin: Rapid; absolute bioavailability (14%); T_{max}=1-2 hrs. **Distribution:** Amlodipine: Plasma protein binding (93%). Atorvastatin: V_d=381L; plasma protein binding (≥98%). **Metabolism:** Amlodipine: Hepatic (extensive). Atorvastatin: CYP3A4 (extensive); ortho- and parahydroxylated

C

derivatives (active metabolites). **Elimination:** Amlodipine: Urine (10% parent compound; 60% metabolites); $T_{1/2}$=30-50 hrs. Atorvastatin: Bile (major), urine (<2%); $T_{1/2}$=14 hrs.

NURSING CONSIDERATIONS

Assessment: Assess for active liver disease, unexplained and persistent elevations in serum transaminase levels, history of renal impairment, risk factors for developing renal failure secondary to rhabdomyolysis, recent stroke or TIA, hypersensitivity to the drug, pregnancy/nursing status, and possible drug interactions. Obtain baseline lipid profile (total-C, LDL, HDL, TG), liver function (eg, AST, ALT) parameters, and BP.

Monitoring: Monitor for signs/symptoms of rhabdomyolysis, myopathy (including IMNM), worsening angina, MI, and other adverse reactions. Monitor lipid profile, and CPK levels. Monitor LFTs as clinically indicated, and for increases in HbA1c and FPG levels. Monitor BP.

Patient Counseling: Advise to adhere to medication, along with the National Cholesterol Education Program-recommended diet, a regular exercise program, and periodic fasting lipid panel testing. Inform of the substances that should not be taken concomitantly with the drug. Advise patients to inform other healthcare professionals that they are taking the drug. Inform of the risk of myopathy; instruct to report promptly any unexplained muscle pain, tenderness, or weakness, particularly if accompanied by malaise or fever, or if muscle signs and symptoms persist after discontinuation. Instruct to report promptly any symptoms that may indicate liver injury (eg, fatigue, anorexia, right upper abdominal discomfort, dark urine, jaundice). Instruct women of childbearing potential to use effective contraceptive methods to prevent pregnancy and to d/c therapy and contact physician if pregnancy occurs. Instruct not to use the drug if breastfeeding.

Administration: Oral route. Take with or without food. **Storage:** 25°C (77°F); excursions permitted to 15-30°C (59-86°F).

CALAN   RX
verapamil HCl (G.D. Searle)

THERAPEUTIC CLASS: Calcium channel blocker (nondihydropyridine)

INDICATIONS: Treatment of angina at rest including vasospastic (Prinzmetal's variant) angina and unstable (crescendo, pre-infarction) angina. Treatment of chronic stable angina (classic effort-associated angina). In association with digitalis, for the control of ventricular rate at rest and during stress in patients with chronic atrial flutter (A-flutter) and/or atrial fibrillation (A-fib). Prophylaxis of repetitive paroxysmal supraventricular tachycardia (PSVT). Treatment of essential HTN.

DOSAGE: *Adults:* Individualize dose by titration. Max: 480mg/day. HTN: Initial (Monotherapy): 80mg tid (240mg/day). Usual: 360-480mg/day; no evidence that dosages >360mg/day provided added effect. Consider beginning titration at 40mg tid in patients who might respond to lower doses (eg, elderly, people of small stature). Upward titration should be based on therapeutic efficacy, assessed at the end of the dosing interval. Angina: Usual: 80-120mg tid. Increased Response to Verapamil (eg, Decreased Hepatic Function, Elderly): 40mg tid may be warranted. Upward titration should be based on therapeutic efficacy and safety evaluated approximately 8 hrs after dosing. Titrate: May increase daily (eg, patients with unstable angina) or at weekly intervals until optimum response is obtained. Chronic A-Fib (Digitalized): Usual: 240-320mg/day in divided doses tid or qid. PSVT Prophylaxis (Non-Digitalized): Usual: 240-480mg/day in divided doses tid or qid. Max effects for any given dosage will be apparent during the first 48 hrs of therapy.

HOW SUPPLIED: Tab: 40mg, 80mg*, 120mg* *scored

CONTRAINDICATIONS: Severe left ventricular dysfunction, hypotension (systolic pressure <90mmHg) or cardiogenic shock, sick sinus syndrome or 2nd- or 3rd-degree atrioventricular (AV) block (except with functioning ventricular artificial pacemaker), A-fib/flutter and an accessory bypass tract (eg, Wolff-Parkinson-White, Lown-Ganong-Levine syndromes).

WARNINGS/PRECAUTIONS: Has negative inotropic effect; avoid with severe left ventricular dysfunction (eg, ejection fraction <30%) or moderate to severe symptoms of cardiac failure. Patients with milder ventricular dysfunction should, if possible, be controlled with optimum doses of digitalis and/or diuretics before treatment. May cause congestive heart failure (CHF), pulmonary edema, hypotension, asymptomatic 1st-degree AV block, transient bradycardia, and PR interval prolongation. Marked 1st-degree AV block or progressive development to 2nd- or 3rd-degree AV block requires dose reduction or, in rare instances, discontinuation and institution of appropriate therapy. Hepatocellular injury as well as elevated transaminases with or without concomitant elevations in alkaline phosphatase and bilirubin reported; monitor LFTs periodically. Sinus bradycardia, 2nd-degree AV block, pulmonary edema, severe hypotension, and sinus arrest reported in patients with hypertrophic cardiomyopathy. Caution with renal/hepatic impairment; monitor for abnormal PR interval prolongation or other signs of overdosage. 30% of normal dose should be given to patients with severe hepatic dysfunction. May decrease neuromuscular transmission in patients with Duchenne's muscular dystrophy and may cause worsening of myasthenia gravis; may be necessary to decrease dose when administered to patients with attenuated neuromuscular transmission. Caution in elderly.

ADVERSE REACTIONS: Constipation, dizziness.

INTERACTIONS: CYP3A4 inhibitors (eg, erythromycin, ritonavir) and grapefruit juice may increase levels. CYP3A4 inducers (eg, rifampin) may decrease levels. May cause myopathy/rhabdomyolysis with HMG-CoA reductase inhibitors that are CYP3A4 substrates and may increase levels of such drugs; limit dose of simvastatin to 10mg/day and lovastatin to 40mg/day, and lower starting/maintenance doses of other CYP3A4 substrates (eg, atorvastatin) may be required. Increased bleeding times with aspirin. Additive negative effects on HR, AV conduction, and/or cardiac contractility with β-blockers; monitor closely and avoid with any degree of ventricular dysfunction. Combined therapy with propranolol should usually be avoided in patients with AV conduction abnormalities and those with depressed left ventricular function. May produce asymptomatic bradycardia with a wandering atrial pacemaker with timolol eye drops. Decreased metoprolol and propranolol clearance and variable effect with atenolol reported. Chronic treatment may increase digoxin levels, which may result in digitalis toxicity; reduce maintenance and digitalization doses and monitor carefully to avoid over-/under-digitalization. May reduce total body/extrarenal clearance of digitoxin. Additive effects with other oral antihypertensives (eg, vasodilators, ACE inhibitors, diuretics); monitor appropriately. Coadministration with agents that attenuate α-adrenergic function (eg, prazosin) may excessively reduce BP. Avoid disopyramide within 48 hrs before or 24 hrs after administration. Coadministration with flecainide may result in additive negative inotropic effect and AV conduction prolongation. May counteract effects of quinidine on AV conduction and increase levels of quinidine; avoid concomitant use in patients with hypertrophic cardiomyopathy. Reduced or unchanged clearance with cimetidine. Increased sensitivity to effects of lithium (neurotoxicity) when used concomitantly; monitor carefully. May increase carbamazepine, theophylline, cyclosporine, and alcohol levels. Increased clearance with phenobarbital. Rifampin may reduce oral bioavailability. Titrate both verapamil and inhalation anesthetics carefully, in order to avoid excessive cardiovascular depression. May potentiate neuromuscular blockers (eg, curare-like and depolarizing); verapamil or both agents may need dose reduction. Hypotension and bradyarrhythmias reported with telithromycin. Sinus bradycardia resulting in hospitalization and pacemaker insertion reported with clonidine; monitor HR.

PREGNANCY: Category C, not for use in nursing.

MECHANISM OF ACTION: Calcium channel blocker (nondihydropyridine); modulates the influx of ionic Ca^{2+} across the cell membrane of the arterial smooth muscle, as well as in conductile and contractile myocardial cells.

PHARMACOKINETICS: Absorption: Bioavailability (20-35%); T_{max}=1-2 hrs. **Distribution:** Plasma protein binding (90%); crosses the placenta, found in breast milk. **Metabolism:** Liver (extensive); norverapamil (metabolite). **Elimination:** Urine (70% metabolites, 3-4% unchanged), feces (≥16%); $T_{1/2}$=4.5-12 hrs (repetitive dosing).

NURSING CONSIDERATIONS

Assessment: Assess for known hypersensitivity to the drug, cardiac failure, severe left ventricular dysfunction, hypertrophic cardiomyopathy, hepatic/renal impairment, attenuated neuromuscular transmission (eg, Duchenne's muscular dystrophy), any conditions where treatment is contraindicated or cautioned, pregnancy/nursing status, and possible drug interactions.

Monitoring: Monitor for CHF, hypotension, AV block, abnormal prolongation of the PR interval, transient bradycardia, and other adverse reactions. Monitor LFTs periodically.

Patient Counseling: Inform of the risks/benefits of therapy. Advise to seek medical attention if any adverse reactions occur.

Administration: Oral route. **Storage:** 15-25°C (59-77°F). Protect from light.

CALAN SR   RX
verapamil HCl (G.D. Searle)

THERAPEUTIC CLASS: Calcium channel blocker (nondihydropyridine)

INDICATIONS: Treatment of HTN.

DOSAGE: *Adults:* Individualize dose by titration. Initial: 180mg qam. Titrate: If response is inadequate, increase to 240mg qam, then 180mg bid (am and pm) or 240mg qam plus 120mg qpm, then 240mg q12h. Upward titration should be based on therapeutic efficacy and safety evaluated weekly and approximately 24 hrs after the previous dose. Switching from Immediate-Release Calan to Calan SR: Total daily dose in mg may remain the same. Increased Response to Verapamil (eg, Elderly, Small Stature): Initial: 120mg qam may be warranted.

HOW SUPPLIED: Tab, Extended-Release: 120mg, 180mg*, 240mg* *scored

C

CONTRAINDICATIONS: Severe left ventricular dysfunction, hypotension (systolic pressure <90mmHg) or cardiogenic shock, sick sinus syndrome or 2nd- or 3rd-degree atrioventricular (AV) block (except with functioning artificial ventricular pacemaker), atrial flutter/fibrillation and an accessory bypass tract (eg, Wolff-Parkinson-White, Lown-Ganong-Levine syndromes).

WARNINGS/PRECAUTIONS: Has negative inotropic effect; avoid with severe left ventricular dysfunction (eg, ejection fraction <30%) or moderate to severe symptoms of cardiac failure. Patients with milder ventricular dysfunction should, if possible, be controlled with optimum doses of digitalis and/or diuretics before treatment. May cause hypotension, congestive heart failure (CHF), pulmonary edema, asymptomatic 1st-degree AV block, transient bradycardia, and PR-interval prolongation. Marked 1st-degree AV block or progressive development to 2nd- or 3rd-degree AV block requires dose reduction, or in rare instances, discontinuation and institution of appropriate therapy. Sinus bradycardia, pulmonary edema, severe hypotension, 2nd-degree AV block, and sinus arrest reported in patients with hypertrophic cardiomyopathy. Hepatocellular injury as well as elevated transaminases with or without concomitant elevations in alkaline phosphatase and bilirubin reported; monitor LFTs periodically. Caution with renal/hepatic impairment; monitor for abnormal PR interval prolongation or other signs of overdosage. 30% of normal dose should be given to patients with severe hepatic dysfunction. May decrease neuromuscular transmission in patients with Duchenne's muscular dystrophy; may be necessary to decrease dose when administered to patients with attenuated neuromuscular transmission. Caution in elderly.

ADVERSE REACTIONS: Constipation, dizziness.

INTERACTIONS: May cause myopathy/rhabdomyolysis with HMG-CoA reductase inhibitors that are CYP3A4 substrates and may increase levels of such drugs; limit dose of simvastatin to 10mg/day or lovastatin to 40mg/day, and consider lower starting/maintenance doses of other CYP3A4 substrates (eg, atorvastatin). Additive negative effects on HR, AV conduction, and/or cardiac contractility with β-blockers; monitor closely and avoid with any degree of ventricular dysfunction. May produce asymptomatic bradycardia with a wandering atrial pacemaker with timolol eye drops. Decreased metoprolol and propranolol clearance and variable effect with atenolol reported. Additive effects with other oral antihypertensives (eg, vasodilators, ACE inhibitors, diuretics); monitor appropriately. Coadministration with agents that attenuate α-adrenergic function (eg, prazosin) may excessively reduce BP. May increase carbamazepine, theophylline, and cyclosporine levels. Chronic treatment may increase digoxin levels, which may result in digitalis toxicity; reduce maintenance and digitalization doses and monitor carefully to avoid over-/under-digitalization. May reduce total body/extrarenal clearance of digitoxin. Avoid disopyramide within 48 hrs before or 24 hrs after administration. Coadministration with flecainide may result in additive negative inotropic effect and AV conduction prolongation. May counteract effects of quinidine on AV conduction and increase levels of quinidine; avoid concomitant use in patients with hypertrophic cardiomyopathy. May increase ethanol concentrations that may prolong the intoxicating effects of alcohol. Increased sensitivity to effects of lithium (neurotoxicity) when used concomitantly; monitor carefully. Increased clearance with phenobarbital. Rifampin may reduce oral bioavailability. May potentiate neuromuscular blockers (eg, curare-like and depolarizing); verapamil or both agents may need dose reduction. Titrate both verapamil and inhalation anesthetics carefully to avoid excessive cardiovascular depression. Hypotension and bradyarrhythmias reported with telithromycin. Sinus bradycardia resulting in hospitalization and pacemaker insertion reported with clonidine; monitor HR. Reduced or unchanged clearance with cimetidine.

PREGNANCY: Category C, not for use in nursing.

MECHANISM OF ACTION: Calcium channel blocker (nondihydropyridine); modulates influx of ionic Ca^{2+} across the cell membrane of the arterial smooth muscle, as well as in conductile and contractile myocardial cells.

PHARMACOKINETICS: Absorption: (Fed) (240mg) T_{max}=7.71 hrs, C_{max}=79ng/mL, $AUC_{(0-24\ hr)}$ =841ng•hr/mL. (Fasted) T_{max}=5.21 hrs, C_{max}=164ng/mL, $AUC_{(0-24\ hr)}$=1478ng•hr/mL. **Distribution:** Plasma protein binding (90%); crosses placenta; found in breast milk. **Metabolism:** Liver (extensive); norverapamil (metabolite). **Elimination:** Urine (70% metabolites, 3-4% unchanged); feces (≥16%).

NURSING CONSIDERATIONS

Assessment: Assess for known hypersensitivity to drug, severe left ventricular dysfunction, attenuated neuromuscular transmission (eg, Duchenne's muscular dystrophy), cardiac failure, hypertrophic cardiomyopathy, hepatic/renal impairment, and for any other conditions where treatment is contraindicated or cautioned. Assess pregnancy/nursing status and for possible drug interactions.

Monitoring: Monitor for abnormal prolongation of PR-interval, hypotension, CHF, pulmonary edema, AV block, and transient bradycardia, and other adverse reactions. Monitor LFTs periodically.

Patient Counseling: Inform of the risks/benefits of therapy. Advise to seek medical attention if any adverse reactions occur.

Administration: Oral route. Take with food. **Storage:** 15-25°C (59-77°F). Protect from light and moisture.

CALDOLOR   RX   C
ibuprofen (Cumberland)

> NSAIDs increase risk of serious cardiovascular (CV) thrombotic events, myocardial infarction (MI), stroke, and serious GI adverse events including bleeding, ulceration, and perforation of the stomach and intestine. Contraindicated for the treatment of perioperative pain in the setting of coronary artery bypass graft (CABG) surgery.

THERAPEUTIC CLASS: NSAID

INDICATIONS: Management of mild to moderate pain and moderate to severe pain as an adjunct to opioid analgesics in adults. For reduction of fever in adults.

DOSAGE: *Adults:* Analgesia: 400-800mg IV q6h PRN. Infusion time must be no <30 min. Antipyretic: 400mg IV followed by 400mg q4-6h or 100-200mg q4h PRN. Infusion time must be no <30 min. Elderly: Start at lower end of dosing range.

HOW SUPPLIED: Inj: 100mg/mL

CONTRAINDICATIONS: Asthma, urticaria, or allergic-type reactions to aspirin or other NSAIDs. Treatment of perioperative pain in the setting of coronary artery bypass graft (CABG) surgery.

WARNINGS/PRECAUTIONS: Severe hepatic reactions (rare) reported (eg, jaundice, fulminant hepatitis, liver necrosis, and hepatic failure; d/c if signs/symptoms of liver disease develop or if systemic manifestations occur. May lead to onset of new HTN or worsening of preexisting HTN; monitor BP closely. Fluid retention and edema reported; caution in patients with fluid retention or heart failure (HF). Caution in patients with considerable dehydration. Renal papillary necrosis and other renal injury reported after long-term use. Caution with impaired renal function, HF, liver dysfunction, the elderly, and those taking diuretics and ACE inhibitors. Anaphylactoid reactions may occur. May cause serious skin adverse events (eg, exfoliative dermatitis, Stevens-Johnson syndrome [SJS], and toxic epidermal necrolysis [TEN]). Avoid in late pregnancy; may cause premature closure of ductus arteriosus. May mask signs of inflammation and fever. Anemia may occur; with long-term use, monitor Hgb/Hct if signs or symptoms of anemia develop. May inhibit platelet aggregation and prolong bleeding time; monitor with coagulation disorders. Infusion of drug product without dilution may cause hemolysis. Caution with preexisting asthma. Blurred or diminished vision, scotomata, and changes in color vision reported; d/c if such complaints develop. Aseptic meningitis with fever and coma reported in patients on oral ibuprofen therapy. Caution in elderly.

ADVERSE REACTIONS: N/V, flatulence, headache, hemorrhage, dizziness, urinary retention, peripheral edema, anemia, dyspepsia, eosinophilia, hypokalemia, hypoproteinemia, neutropenia.

INTERACTIONS: May increase adverse effects with aspirin. Synergistic effects on GI bleeding with warfarin. May decrease natriuretic effect of furosemide and thiazides; monitor for renal failure. May impair therapeutic response to ACE inhibitors, thiazides, or loop diuretics. Increased risk of renal effects with diuretics or ACE inhibitors. May increase lithium levels; monitor for toxicity. May enhance methotrexate toxicity; caution when coadministered. Increase GI bleeding with use of oral corticosteroids or anticoagulants and use of alcohol.

PREGNANCY: Category C (prior to 30 weeks gestation); Category D (starting 30 weeks gestation), not for use in nursing.

MECHANISM OF ACTION: NSAID; not established. May be related to prostaglandin synthetase inhibition. Possesses anti-inflammatory, analgesic, and antipyretic activity.

PHARMACOKINETICS: Absorption: (400mg) AUC=109.3mcg•h/mL, (800mg) AUC=192.8mcg•h/mL; (400mg) C_{max}=39.2mcg/mL, (800mg) C_{max}=72.6mcg/mL. **Distribution:** Plasma protein binding (>99%). **Elimination:** (400mg) $T_{1/2}$=2.22 hrs, (800mg) $T_{1/2}$=2.44 hrs.

NURSING CONSIDERATIONS

Assessment: Assess LFTs, CBC, and coagulation profile. Assess for history of asthma, urticaria or allergic-type reaction with previous use of NSAIDs, asthma, perioperative pain in setting of CABG surgery, cardiovascular disease (CVD) or risk factors for CVD, HTN, fluid retention or HF, ulcer disease or GI bleeding, coagulation disorders or anticoagulant therapy, renal/hepatic impairment, pregnancy/nursing status, possible drug interactions.

Monitoring: Monitor BP during initiation of therapy and thereafter. Monitor Hgb/Hct, coagulation profiles, LFTs, and renal function. Monitor for signs/symptoms of anaphylactic/anaphylactoid reactions, adverse skin events (eg, exfoliative dermatitis, SJS, TEN), eosinophilia, rash, GI bleeding/ulceration and perforation, anemia, CV thrombotic events, MI, stroke, new or worsening HTN, renal toxicity, renal papillary necrosis and other renal injury, ophthalmological effects and aseptic meningitis.

C

Patient Counseling: Counsel about potential CV, GI, hepatotoxic, and skin adverse events, as well as possible weight gain/edema. Inform of the signs of an anaphylactoid reaction and to d/c and initiate medical therapy if this occurs. Inform pregnant women to avoid use of the product starting at 30 weeks gestation. Counsel patients to be well hydrated prior to administration in order to reduce renal adverse reactions.

Administration: IV (infusion) route. Infusion time must be no <30 mins. Must be diluted prior to infusion. Refer to PI for preparation and administration. **Storage:** 20-25°C (68-77°F). Diluted sol are stable for up to 24 hrs at ambient temperature (approximately 20-25°C; 68-77°F) and room lighting.

CAMBIA   RX

diclofenac potassium (Nautilus Neurosciences)

> NSAIDs may cause an increased risk of serious cardiovascular (CV) thrombotic events, myocardial infarction (MI), stroke, and serious GI adverse events, including bleeding, ulceration, and perforation of the stomach or intestines that may be fatal. Contraindicated for the treatment of perioperative pain in the setting of coronary artery bypass graft (CABG) surgery.

THERAPEUTIC CLASS: NSAID

INDICATIONS: Acute treatment of migraine attacks with or without aura in adults ≥18 yrs of age.

DOSAGE: *Adults:* ≥18 Yrs: 1 pkt (50mg) in 1-2 oz. (30-60mL) water; mix well and drink immediately.

HOW SUPPLIED: Sol (Powder): 50mg/pkt

CONTRAINDICATIONS: Asthma, urticaria, or allergic reactions after taking aspirin (ASA) or other NSAIDs. Treatment of perioperative pain in the setting of CABG surgery.

WARNINGS/PRECAUTIONS: Use lowest effective dose for the shortest duration possible. May not be bioequivalent with other diclofenac PO formulation. Extreme caution with prior history of ulcer disease and/or GI bleeding. May cause elevations of LFTs; d/c immediately if liver disease develops or systemic manifestations occur. May lead to new onset or worsening of preexisting HTN; monitor BP closely. Fluid retention and edema reported; caution with fluid retention or heart failure. Caution when initiating treatment with considerable dehydration. Renal papillary necrosis and other renal injury reported after long-term use. Not recommended with advanced renal disease; if therapy must be initiated, closely monitor renal function. Anaphylactoid reactions may occur; avoid in patients with ASA-triad. May cause serious skin adverse reactions (eg, exfoliative dermatitis, Stevens-Johnson syndrome [SJS], and toxic epidermal necrolysis [TEN]). Avoid in pregnancy starting at 30 weeks gestation; may cause premature closure of ductus arteriosus. May diminish the utility of inflammation and fever in detecting complications of presumed noninfectious, painful conditions. Anemia may occur; monitor Hgb/Hct with long-term use. May inhibit platelet aggregation and prolong bleeding time; monitor platelet function in patients with coagulation disorders. Caution with preexisting asthma and avoid with ASA-sensitive asthma. Caution with phenylketonurics, elderly, and debilitated.

ADVERSE REACTIONS: Abdominal pain, constipation, diarrhea, dyspepsia, flatulence, anemia, edema, N/V, dizziness, headache, rashes, heartburn, pruritus, abnormal renal function.

INTERACTIONS: Increased adverse effects with ASA (eg, serious GI events); concomitant use not generally recommended. Synergistic effects on GI bleeding with anticoagulants (eg, warfarin). May diminish antihypertensive effect of ACE inhibitors. Patients taking thiazides and loop diuretics may have impaired response to these therapies. ACE inhibitors and diuretics may precipitate overt renal decompensation. May reduce natriuretic effect of furosemide and thiazides. May increase lithium levels; monitor for toxicity. May enhance methotrexate toxicity and increase nephrotoxicity of cyclosporine; caution with coadministration. May increase risk of GI bleeding with oral corticosteroids or anticoagulants, smoking, or alcohol use. Caution with potentially hepatotoxic drugs (eg, acetaminophen, certain antibiotics, antiepileptics); avoid taking nonprescription acetaminophen products. CYP2C9 inhibitors may affect pharmacokinetics.

PREGNANCY: Category C (prior to 30 weeks gestation) and D (starting at 30 weeks gestation); not for use in nursing.

MECHANISM OF ACTION: NSAID (benzeneacetic acid derivative); not known, suspected to inhibit prostaglandin synthetase.

PHARMACOKINETICS: Absorption: Absolute bioavailability (50%); T_{max}=0.25 hr. **Distribution:** V_d=1.3L/kg; plasma protein binding (>99%). **Metabolism:** Glucuronidation or sulfation via CYP2C8, 2C9, 3A4; 4'-hydroxydiclofenac (major metabolite), 5-hydroxy-, 3'-hydroxy-, 4',5-dihydroxy-, and 3'-hydroxy-4'-methoxy diclofenac (minor metabolites). **Elimination:** Urine (65%), bile (35%); $T_{1/2}$=2 hrs.

NURSING CONSIDERATIONS

Assessment: Assess for drug hypersensitivity, asthma, urticaria, or allergic-type reactions after taking ASA or other NSAIDs, risk factors for CV disease/GI adverse events, history of ulcer disease or GI bleeding, renal/hepatic function, any other conditions where treatment is contraindicated or cautioned, pregnancy/nursing status, and possible drug interactions.

Monitoring: Monitor for signs/symptoms of CV thrombotic events, MI, stroke, GI adverse events (eg, inflammation, bleeding, ulceration, perforation), hepatotoxicity, new/worsening HTN, fluid retention/edema, renal papillary necrosis or other renal injury, anaphylactoid reactions, serious skin reactions (eg, exfoliative dermatitis, SJS, TEN), anemia, and other adverse reactions. Monitor BP and renal function closely. Monitor LFTs (eg, AST, ALT), CBC, and chemistry profile periodically in patients receiving long-term therapy.

Patient Counseling: Advise patients to be alert for signs/symptoms of chest pain, SOB, weakness, slurring of speech, GI ulcerations/bleeding, epigastric pain, dyspepsia, melena, anaphylactoid reactions, skin rash and blisters, fever, or other signs of hypersensitivity (eg, itching) during therapy. Instruct to d/c therapy if any type of rash develops and to contact physician as soon as possible. Inform about signs/symptoms of hepatotoxicity; instruct to d/c and immediately seek medical therapy if any of these occur. Advise to notify physician if signs/symptoms of unexplained weight gain or edema occur. Advise women to avoid therapy starting at 30 weeks gestation. Inform phenylketonurics that the product contains aspartame equivalent to phenylalanine 25mg/pkt.

Administration: Oral route. Taking with food may reduce effectiveness compared to taking on empty stomach. **Storage:** 25°C (77°F); excursions permitted from 15-30°C (59-86°F).

CAMPATH   RX
alemtuzumab (Bayer Healthcare)

> Serious, including fatal, pancytopenia/marrow hypoplasia, autoimmune idiopathic thrombocytopenia, and autoimmune hemolytic anemia may occur; single doses >30mg or cumulative doses >90mg/week may increase incidence of pancytopenia. Serious, including fatal, infusion reactions may occur; monitor patients during infusion and withhold therapy for Grade 3/4 infusion reactions. Gradually escalate dose at initiation of therapy and if interrupted for ≥7days. Serious, including fatal, bacterial, viral, fungal, and protozoan infections can occur; administer prophylaxis against *Pneumocystis jiroveci* pneumonia (PCP) and herpes virus infections.

THERAPEUTIC CLASS: Monoclonal antibody/CD52-blocker

INDICATIONS: Treatment of B-cell chronic lymphocytic leukemia.

DOSAGE: *Adults:* Administer as IV infusion over 2 hrs. Initial: 3mg IV qd until infusion reactions are ≤Grade 2, then increase to 10mg IV qd. Continue until ≤Grade 2. Increase to maint dose of 30mg (usually takes 3-7 days). Maint: 30mg/day IV 3X/week on alternate days. Max: 30mg single dose or 90mg/week cumulative dose. Total duration of therapy is 12 weeks. Refer to PI for recommended concomitant medications and dose modifications for neutropenia or thrombocytopenia.

HOW SUPPLIED: Inj: 30mg/mL [1mL]

WARNINGS/PRECAUTIONS: Prolonged myelosuppression, pure red cell/bone marrow aplasia reported; withhold therapy for severe cytopenias and d/c for autoimmune cytopenias or recurrent/persistent severe cytopenias. Severe and prolonged lymphopenia with increased incidence of opportunistic infections reported; administer prophylactic therapy during and for a minimum of 2 months after therapy or until CD4+ count is ≥200 cells/μL. Monitor for cytomegalovirus (CMV) infection during and for ≥2 months after completion of treatment; withhold therapy for serious infections and during CMV infection treatment or confirmed CMV viremia. Administer only irradiated blood products to avoid transfusion-associated graft versus host disease unless emergent circumstances dictate immediate transfusion.

ADVERSE REACTIONS: Cytopenias, infusion reactions, CMV and other infections, immunosuppression, nausea, emesis, abdominal pain, insomnia, anxiety.

INTERACTIONS: Avoid live viral vaccines.

PREGNANCY: Category C, not for use in nursing.

MECHANISM OF ACTION: Monoclonal antibody/CD52-blocker; binds to CD52; proposed action is antibody-dependent cellular-mediated lysis following cell surface binding to the leukemic cells.

PHARMACOKINETICS: Distribution: V_d=0.18L/kg; crosses the placenta. **Elimination:** (1st dose) $T_{1/2}$=11 hrs. (Last dose) $T_{1/2}$=6 days.

NURSING CONSIDERATIONS

Assessment: Assess for pregnancy/nursing status and possible drug interaction. Obtain baseline CBC, CD4+, and platelet count.

Monitoring: Monitor CBC weekly and more frequently if worsening anemia, neutropenia, or thrombocytopenia occurs. Assess CD4+ counts after therapy until recovery to ≥200 cells/μL. Monitor for CMV infections during therapy and for ≥2 months following completion. Monitor for cytopenias, infusion reactions, immunosuppression, infection, and other adverse reactions.

Patient Counseling: Advise to seek medical attention if symptoms of bleeding, easy bruising, petechiae/purpura, pallor, weakness, fatigue, infusion reactions, or infections occur. Counsel patients of the need to take premedications and prophylactic anti-infectives as prescribed. Advise patients that irradiation of blood products is required. Inform to not be immunized with live vaccines if recently treated. Advise patients to use effective contraceptive methods during treatment and ≥6 months following therapy.

Administration: IV infusion. Do not administer as IV push or bolus. Refer to PI for preparation and administration instructions. Do not add or simultaneously infuse other drugs through the same IV line. **Storage:** 2-8°C (36-46°F). Do not freeze. If frozen, thaw at 2-8°C (36-46°F) before administration. Protect from direct sunlight. Diluted Sol: 2-8°C (36-46°F) or 15-30°C (59-86°F). Use ≤8 hrs. Protect from light.

CAMPTOSAR   RX
irinotecan HCl (Pharmacia & Upjohn)

Early and late forms of diarrhea can occur. Early diarrhea may be accompanied by cholinergic symptoms; may be prevented or ameliorated by atropine. Late diarrhea can be life-threatening; treat properly with loperamide. Monitor patients with diarrhea; give fluid/electrolytes PRN or institute antibiotic therapy if ileus, fever, or severe neutropenia develops. Interrupt therapy and reduce subsequent doses if severe diarrhea occurs. Severe myelosuppression may occur.

THERAPEUTIC CLASS: Topoisomerase I inhibitor

INDICATIONS: As a component of 1st-line therapy in combination with 5-fluorouracil (5-FU) and leucovorin (LV) for metastatic carcinoma of the colon or rectum, and for patients with metastatic carcinoma of the colon or rectum whose disease has recurred or progressed following initial 5-FU therapy.

DOSAGE: *Adults:* Combination Therapy: Administer as 90 min infusion followed by LV and 5-FU. Regimen 1 (6-Week Cycle with Bolus 5-FU/LV): 125mg/m² IV over 90 min on Days 1, 8, 15, and 22. Regimen 2 (6-Week Cycle with Infusional 5-FU/LV): 180mg/m² IV over 90 min on Days 1, 15, and 29. Both Regimens: Begin next cycle on Day 43. Refer to PI for doses of 5-FU/LV. Single Therapy: Regimen 1 (Weekly): 125mg/m² IV over 90 min on Days 1, 8, 15, and 22 followed by 2-week rest. Titrate: Subsequent doses may be adjusted to as high as 150mg/m² or to as low as 50mg/m² in 25-50mg/m² decrements, depending upon individual tolerance. Regimen 2 (Every 3 Weeks): 350mg/m² IV over 90 min once every 3 weeks. Titrate: Subsequent doses may be adjusted as low as 200mg/m² in 50mg/m² decrements, depending upon individual tolerance. Elderly (≥70 Yrs): Initial: 300mg/m² once every 3 weeks. Refer to PI for Dose Modifications for Combination and Single-Agent Schedules. All dose modifications should be based on worst preceding toxicity. Prior Pelvic or Abdominal Radiotherapy/Performance Status of 2/Increased Bilirubin: Consider reducing starting dose by one level. Reduced UGT1A1 Activity: Consider reducing starting dose by at least one level for patients known to be homozygous for the UGT1A1*28 allele. Subsequent dose modifications are based on individual tolerance; refer to PI.

HOW SUPPLIED: Inj: 20mg/mL [2mL, 5mL, 15mL]

WARNINGS/PRECAUTIONS: Not recommended in patients on dialysis or with bilirubin >2mg/dL. If late diarrhea occurs, delay subsequent weekly therapy until return of pretreatment bowel function for at least 24 hrs without antidiarrheals; decrease subsequent doses if late diarrhea is Grade 2, 3, or 4. Avoid diuretics or laxatives in patients with diarrhea. Deaths due to sepsis following severe neutropenia reported; d/c if neutropenic fever occurs, or if absolute neutrophil count <1000/mm³. Increased risk for neutropenia in patients homozygous for the UGT1A1*28 allele; consider reducing initial dose by at least one level. Severe anaphylactic/anaphylactoid reactions reported; d/c if anaphylactic reaction occurs. Renal impairment/acute renal failure reported, usually in patients who became volume depleted from severe vomiting and/or diarrhea. Interstitial pulmonary disease (IPD) events reported; d/c therapy if IPD is diagnosed and institute appropriate treatment. Should not be used with a regimen of 5-FU/LV administered for 4-5 consecutive days every 4 weeks due to increased toxicity. Increased toxicity in patients with performance status 2 at baseline. May cause fetal harm. Caution to avoid extravasation and monitor for inflammation at infusion site. Premedicate with antiemetics at least 30 min prior to therapy. Consider prophylactic/therapeutic administration of atropine if cholinergic symptoms develop. Caution in patients with deficient glucuronidation of bilirubin (eg, Gilbert's syndrome), renal/hepatic impairment, previous pelvic/abdominal irradiation, and in elderly. Avoid in unresolved bowel obstruction.

ADVERSE REACTIONS: N/V, diarrhea, neutropenia, abdominal pain, anemia, asthenia, anorexia, alopecia, fever, constipation, leukopenia, decreased body weight.

INTERACTIONS: Avoid concurrent irradiation therapy. Greater incidence of akathisia reported with prochlorperazine. Decreased levels with CYP3A4 enzyme-inducing anticonvulsants (eg, phenytoin, phenobarbital, carbamazepine) and St. John's wort reported; d/c St. John's wort at least 2 weeks prior to 1st cycle. Consider substituting nonenzyme-inducing anticonvulsants 2 weeks prior to treatment. Increased levels with ketoconazole; d/c ketoconazole at least 1 week prior to therapy. St. John's wort and ketoconazole are contraindicated during therapy. Increased systemic exposure of SN-38 (active metabolite) with atazanavir sulfate. May prolong neuromuscular-blocking effects of suxamethonium, and the neuromuscular blockade of nondepolarizing drugs may be antagonized.

PREGNANCY: Category D, not for use in nursing.

MECHANISM OF ACTION: Topoisomerase I inhibitor; binds to topoisomerase I-DNA complex and prevents religation of single-strand breaks.

PHARMACOKINETICS: Absorption: Irinotecan: C_{max}=1660ng/mL (125mg/m^2), 3392ng/mL (340mg/m^2); AUC_{0-24}=10,200ng•h/mL (125mg/m^2), 20,604ng•h/mL (340mg/m^2). SN-38: C_{max}=26.3ng/mL (125mg/m^2), 56ng/mL (340mg/m^2); AUC_{0-24}=229ng•h/mL (125mg/m^2), 474ng•h/mL (340mg/m^2). **Distribution:** Irinotecan: V_d=110L/m^2 (125mg/m^2), 234L/m^2 (340mg/m^2). Plasma protein binding (30-68%), (95%) [SN-38]. **Metabolism:** Liver via carboxyl esterase; SN-38 (active metabolite). **Elimination:** Irinotecan: Urine (11-20%); $T_{1/2}$=5.8 hrs (125mg/m^2), 11.7 hrs (340mg/m^2). SN-38: Urine (<1%); $T_{1/2}$=10.4 hrs (125mg/m^2), 21 hrs (340mg/m^2).

NURSING CONSIDERATIONS

Assessment: Assess for unresolved bowel obstruction, UGT1A1 status, deficient glucuronidation of bilirubin (Gilbert's syndrome), pelvic/abdominal irradiation, preexisting lung disease, renal/hepatic impairment, pregnancy/nursing status, and possible drug interactions. Obtain baseline CBC.

Monitoring: Monitor for diarrhea, signs/symptoms of neutropenia, neutropenic complications (eg, neutropenic fever), ileus, respiratory symptoms, inflammation and/or extravasation of infusion site, cholinergic symptoms, hypersensitivity reactions, and other adverse reactions. For patients with diarrhea, monitor for signs/symptoms of dehydration, electrolyte imbalance, ileus, fever, or severe neutropenia. Monitor CBC with differential.

Patient Counseling: Instruct to seek medical attention if experiencing diarrhea for 1st time during treatment, black or bloody stools, dehydration, inability to take fluids by mouth due to N/V, or inability to get diarrhea under control within 24 hrs. Inform about potential for dizziness or visual disturbances, which may occur within 24 hrs. Explain importance of routine blood cell counts. Instruct to report any occurrence of fever or infection. Inform that therapy may cause fetal harm and advise patients to avoid becoming pregnant while on therapy. Explain about the possibility of alopecia. Inform that the product contains sorbitol.

Administration: IV route. Refer to PI for preparation of infusion sol and safe handling instructions. **Storage:** 15-30°C (59-86°F). Protect from light. Keep in carton until time of use. Avoid freezing. Refer to PI for storage instructions for reconstituted sol.

CANASA   RX
mesalamine (Aptalis)

THERAPEUTIC CLASS: 5-aminosalicylic acid derivative

INDICATIONS: Treatment of mild to moderately active ulcerative proctitis.

DOSAGE: *Adults:* Usual: 1 sup rectally qhs for 3-6 weeks depending on symptoms and sigmoidoscopic findings. Retain sup for at least 1-3 hrs. Elderly: Start at lower end of dosing range.

HOW SUPPLIED: Sup: 1000mg

CONTRAINDICATIONS: Hypersensitivity to sup vehicle (saturated vegetable fatty acid esters).

WARNINGS/PRECAUTIONS: Renal impairment, including minimal change nephropathy, acute and chronic interstitial nephritis, and renal failure (rare), reported; evaluate renal function prior to initiation and periodically during therapy. Caution with known renal dysfunction or history of renal disease. Associated with acute intolerance syndrome (eg, cramping, acute abdominal pain and bloody diarrhea, fever, headache, rash); observe closely for worsening of these symptoms, and promptly d/c therapy if acute intolerance syndrome is suspected. Patients with sulfasalazine hypersensitivity may have similar reaction to therapy. Drug-induced cardiac hypersensitivity reactions (myocarditis, pericarditis) reported. Hepatic failure in patients with preexisting liver disease reported; caution with liver disease. Possible interference with measurements, by liquid chromatography, of urinary normetanephrine observed in patients exposed to sulfasalazine or its metabolite, mesalamine/mesalazine. Caution in elderly.

ADVERSE REACTIONS: Dizziness, rectal pain, fever, rash, acne, colitis, headache, flatulence, abdominal pain, diarrhea, nausea.

INTERACTIONS: Concurrent use with nephrotoxic agents (eg, NSAIDs) may increase risk of renal reactions. Concurrent use with azathioprine or 6-mercaptopurine may increase risk for blood disorders.

PREGNANCY: Category B, caution in nursing.

MECHANISM OF ACTION: 5-aminosalicylic acid (5-ASA) derivative; not established. Suspected to act topically rather than systemically.

PHARMACOKINETICS: Absorption: Variable. (500mg q8h) C_{max}=361ng/mL, 193-1304ng/mL (N-acetyl-5-ASA). **Distribution:** Found in breast milk. **Metabolism:** Extensive, mainly to N-acetyl-5-ASA (metabolite). **Elimination:** Urine (≤11% unchanged, 3-35% N-acetyl-5-ASA); $T_{1/2}$=7 hrs.

NURSING CONSIDERATIONS

Assessment: Assess for hypersensitivity to drug, sup vehicle, salicylates, or sulfasalazine. Assess renal/hepatic function, pregnancy/nursing status, and possible drug interactions.

Monitoring: Monitor for acute intolerance syndrome, hypersensitivity reactions (eg, myocarditis, pericarditis), hepatic failure, and other adverse reactions. Monitor renal function periodically. Monitor blood cell counts in elderly.

Patient Counseling: Instruct to notify physician of all medications being taken; if patient is allergic to sulfasalazine, salicylates, or mesalamine; experiences cramping, abdominal pain, bloody diarrhea, fever, headache, or rash; has a history of myocarditis/pericarditis or stomach blockage; has kidney/liver disease; is pregnant, intends to become pregnant, or is breastfeeding. Inform that sup will cause staining of direct contact surfaces (eg, fabrics, flooring, painted surfaces, marble, granite, vinyl, enamel).

Administration: Rectal route. **Storage:** <25°C (77°F). May be refrigerated. Keep away from direct heat, light, or humidity.

CANCIDAS RX
caspofungin acetate (Merck)

THERAPEUTIC CLASS: Echinocandin

INDICATIONS: In adults and pediatric patients (≥3 months of age) for empirical therapy for presumed fungal infections in febrile, neutropenic patients; treatment of candidemia and the *Candida* infections (intra-abdominal abscesses, peritonitis, and pleural space infections); treatment of esophageal candidiasis; and treatment of invasive aspergillosis in patients who are refractory to or intolerant of other therapies (eg, amphotericin B, lipid formulations of amphotericin B, itraconazole).

DOSAGE: *Adults:* ≥18 Yrs: Give by slow IV infusion over approximately 1 hr. Empirical Therapy: 70mg LD on Day 1, followed by 50mg qd thereafter. Continue until resolution of neutropenia. If fungal infection is found, treat for a minimum of 14 days; continue for at least 7 days after neutropenia and clinical symptoms are resolved. May increase to 70mg/day if 50mg dose is well tolerated but provides inadequate clinical response. Candidemia/Other *Candida* Infections: 70mg LD on Day 1, followed by 50mg qd thereafter. Continue for at least 14 days after the last positive culture. Persistently neutropenic patients may warrant a longer course of therapy pending resolution of neutropenia. Esophageal Candidiasis: 50mg qd for 7-14 days after symptom resolution. Consider suppressive oral therapy in patients with HIV infections due to risk of relapse. Invasive Aspergillosis: 70mg LD on Day 1, followed by 50mg qd thereafter. Duration of treatment should be based upon severity of underlying disease, recovery from immunosuppression, and clinical response. Moderate Hepatic Impairment (Child-Pugh 7-9): Usual: 35mg qd. May still administer 70mg LD on Day 1 if recommended. Concomitant Rifampin: 70mg qd. Concomitant Nevirapine/Efavirenz/Carbamazepine/Dexamethasone/Phenytoin: May require dose increase to 70mg qd. *Pediatrics:* 3 Months-17 Yrs: Give by slow IV infusion over approximately 1 hr. Dosing should be based on the patient's BSA. Usual: 70mg/m² LD on Day 1, followed by 50mg/m² qd thereafter. Max LD/Maint: 70mg/day. Individualize duration based on indication. May increase to 70mg/m²/day (not to exceed 70mg) if 50mg/m²/day dose is well tolerated but provides inadequate clinical response. Concomitant Inducers of Drug Clearance (eg, Rifampin, Efavirenz, Nevirapine, Phenytoin, Dexamethasone, Carbamazepine): Consider 70mg/m² qd (not to exceed 70mg).

HOW SUPPLIED: Inj: 50mg, 70mg

WARNINGS/PRECAUTIONS: Anaphylaxis reported; d/c and administer appropriate treatment if this occurs. Possible histamine-mediated adverse reactions (eg, rash, facial swelling, angioedema, pruritus, sensation of warmth, bronchospasm) reported and may require discontinuation and/or administration of appropriate treatment. Limit concomitant use with cyclosporine to patients for whom potential benefit outweighs potential risk. Abnormal LFTs reported; monitor patients who develop abnormal LFTs for evidence of worsening hepatic function and evaluate risk/benefit of continuing therapy. Isolated cases of significant hepatic dysfunction, hepatitis, and hepatic failure reported with multiple concomitant medications in patients with serious underlying conditions.

ADVERSE REACTIONS: Pyrexia, chills, hypokalemia, hypotension, diarrhea, increased blood alkaline phosphatase, increased ALT/AST, N/V, abdominal pain, peripheral edema, headache, rash, increased blood bilirubin, septic shock, pneumonia.

INTERACTIONS: Increased exposure and transient increases in ALT and AST reported with concomitant cyclosporine. Reduced levels of tacrolimus; monitor tacrolimus blood concentrations and adjust tacrolimus dosage appropriately. Inducers of drug clearance (eg, efavirenz, nevirapine, phenytoin, rifampin, dexamethasone, carbamazepine) may decrease levels.

PREGNANCY: Category C, caution in nursing.

MECHANISM OF ACTION: Echinocandin; inhibits the synthesis of β (1,3)-D-glucan, an essential component of the cell wall of susceptible *Aspergillus* and *Candida* species.

PHARMACOKINETICS: Absorption: Administration to different age groups resulted in different parameters. **Distribution:** Plasma protein binding (97%). **Metabolism:** Hydrolysis and N-acetylation. **Elimination:** Urine (41%, 1.4% unchanged), feces (35%); $T_{1/2}$=9-11 hrs.

NURSING CONSIDERATIONS

Assessment: Assess for drug hypersensitivity, hepatic function, pregnancy/nursing status, and possible drug interactions.

Monitoring: Monitor for anaphylaxis, histamine-mediated adverse reactions, resolution of neutropenia, and other adverse reactions. Monitor LFTs.

Patient Counseling: Inform that anaphylactic reactions have been reported; instruct to report signs/symptoms of hypersensitivity (eg, rash, facial swelling, angioedema, pruritus, sensation of warmth, bronchospasm) to physician. Inform that there have been isolated reports of serious hepatic effects.

Administration: IV route. Not for IV bolus administration. Refer to PI for preparation and reconstitution for administration. **Storage:** 2-8°C (36-46°F). Reconstituted: ≤25°C (77°F) for 1 hr prior to preparation of infusion sol. Diluted: ≤25°C (77°F) for 24 hrs or 2-8°C (36-46°F) for 48 hrs.

CAPRELSA   RX
vandetanib (AstraZeneca)

> May prolong the QT interval. Torsades de pointes and sudden death reported. Avoid with hypocalcemia, hypokalemia, hypomagnesemia, or long QT syndrome; correct hypocalcemia, hypokalemia, and/or hypomagnesemia prior to therapy. Monitor electrolytes periodically. Avoid drugs known to prolong QT interval. Only prescribers and pharmacies certified through the restricted distribution program are able to prescribe and dispense this therapy.

THERAPEUTIC CLASS: Multikinase inhibitor

INDICATIONS: Treatment of symptomatic or progressive medullary thyroid cancer in patients with unresectable locally advanced or metastatic disease.

DOSAGE: *Adults:* Usual: 300mg qd until disease progression or unacceptable toxicity occurs. Corrected QT Interval, Fridericia (QTcF) >500ms: Interrupt dosing until QTcF returns to <450ms, then resume at a reduced dose. Common Terminology Criteria for Adverse Events (CTCAE) Grade ≥3 Toxicities: Interrupt dosing until toxicity resolves or improves to CTCAE Grade 1, then resume at a reduced dose. For CTCAE Grade ≥3 toxicities, may reduce daily dose to 200mg (two 100mg tabs) and then to 100mg. Moderate (CrCl ≥30 to <50mL/min)/Severe (CrCl <30mL/min) Renal Impairment: Initial: 200mg qd. Take with or without food. Do not take a missed dose within 12 hrs of the next dose.

HOW SUPPLIED: Tab: 100mg, 300mg

CONTRAINDICATIONS: Congenital long QT syndrome.

WARNINGS/PRECAUTIONS: Caution in patients with indolent, asymptomatic, or slowly progressing disease. Do not start therapy with QTcF interval >450ms. Avoid with history of torsades de pointes, bradyarrhythmias, or uncompensated heart failure (HF). Severe skin reactions (eg, Stevens-Johnson syndrome) reported; consider permanent discontinuation if any develop. Photosensitivity reactions may occur during treatment and up to 4 months after discontinuation. Interstitial lung disease (ILD) or pneumonitis, reported; interrupt treatment for acute/worsening pulmonary symptoms and d/c if ILD is confirmed. Ischemic cerebrovascular events and serious hemorrhagic events, reported; d/c if severe. Avoid with recent history of hemoptysis of ≥1/2 tsp of red blood. HF reported; monitor for signs/symptoms of HF and consider discontinuation in patients with HF. Diarrhea of ≥Grade 3 reported; interrupt therapy for severe diarrhea and resume at a reduced dose upon improvement. HTN, including hypertensive crisis, may occur; monitor for HTN. Reduce dose or interrupt therapy if HTN occurs; do not restart therapy if BP cannot be controlled. Reversible posterior leukoencephalopathy syndrome (RPLS) reported; d/c in patients with RPLS. Not recommended for use in patients with moderate and severe hepatic impairment. May cause fetal harm. Women of childbearing potential should avoid pregnancy; use effective contraception during treatment and for at least 4 months following the last dose.

ADVERSE REACTIONS: QT interval prolongation, torsades de pointes, diarrhea/colitis, rash, acneiform dermatitis, HTN, N/V, headache, upper respiratory tract infections, decreased appetite, abdominal pain, fatigue, hypocalcemia, corneal abnormalities, proteinuria.

C

INTERACTIONS: See Boxed Warning. CYP3A4 inducers may decrease plasma concentrations. Avoid use with strong CYP3A4 inducers, St. John's wort, antiarrhythmic drugs (eg, amiodarone, disopyramide, procainamide, sotalol, dofetilide), and other drugs that may prolong QT interval (eg, chloroquine, clarithromycin, dolasetron, granisetron, haloperidol, methadone, moxifloxacin, pimozide). May require dose increase of thyroid replacement therapy; if signs or symptoms of hypothyroidism occur, examine thyroid hormone levels and adjust thyroid replacement therapy accordingly.

PREGNANCY: Category D, not for use in nursing.

MECHANISM OF ACTION: Multikinase inhibitor; inhibits the tyrosine kinase activity of the epidermal growth factor receptor and vascular endothelial growth factor receptor families, RET, BRK, TIE2, and members of the EPH receptor and Src kinase families, which are involved in both normal cellular function and pathologic processes such as oncogenesis, metastasis, tumor angiogenesis, and maintenance of the tumor microenvironment.

PHARMACOKINETICS: Absorption: Slow; T_{max}=6 hrs (median). **Distribution:** V_d=7450L; plasma protein binding (90% in vitro). **Metabolism:** Via CYP3A4; vandetanib N-oxide and N-desmethyl vandetanib (metabolites). **Elimination:** Urine (25%), feces (44%); $T_{1/2}$=19 days (median).

NURSING CONSIDERATIONS

Assessment: Assess for congenital long QT syndrome, history of torsades de pointes or hemoptysis, bradyarrhythmias, uncompensated HF, renal/hepatic impairment, pregnancy/nursing status, and possible drug interactions. Obtain baseline ECG, serum K^+, Ca^{2+}, Mg^{2+}, and TSH levels.

Monitoring: Monitor for QT interval prolongation, torsades de pointes, skin/photosensitivity reactions, ILD, ischemic cerebrovascular events, hemorrhage, HF, diarrhea, hypothyroidism, HTN, RPLS, and other adverse reactions. Monitor ECG, serum K^+, Ca^{2+}, Mg^{2+}, and TSH levels at 2-4 weeks and 8-12 weeks after initial therapy, every 3 months thereafter, and following any dose reduction for QT prolongation, or any dose interruptions >2 weeks. Monitor renal function.

Patient Counseling: Instruct to contact healthcare provider in the event of syncope, presyncopal symptoms, and cardiac palpitations. Inform patients that the healthcare provider will monitor electrolytes and ECGs during treatment. Advise to contact physician in the event of skin reactions or rash, sudden onset or worsening of breathlessness, persistent cough or fever, diarrhea, seizures, headaches, visual disturbances, confusion, or difficulty thinking. Advise patients of reproductive potential to use effective contraception during therapy and for at least 4 months after the last dose and to immediately contact physician if pregnancy is suspected or confirmed. Advise to d/c nursing while on therapy. Instruct to use appropriate sun protection due to the increased susceptibility to sunburn while on therapy and for at least 4 months after drug discontinuation.

Administration: Oral route. Take with or without food. Do not crush tabs. Refer to PI for administration instructions if unable to swallow tabs. **Storage:** 25°C (77°F); excursions permitted to 15-30°C (59-86°F).

CAPTOPRIL   RX
captopril (Various)

D/C when pregnancy is detected. Drugs that act directly on the renin-angiotensin system (RAS) can cause injury and death to the developing fetus.

THERAPEUTIC CLASS: ACE inhibitor

INDICATIONS: Treatment of HTN, alone or in combination with other antihypertensive agents (especially thiazide-type diuretics). Treatment of congestive heart failure (CHF), usually in combination with diuretics and digitalis. To improve survival following myocardial infarction (MI) in clinically stable patients with left ventricular dysfunction and to reduce the incidence of overt heart failure (HF) and subsequent hospitalizations for CHF in these patients. Treatment of diabetic nephropathy (proteinuria >500mg/day) in patients with type I diabetes mellitus and retinopathy.

DOSAGE: *Adults:* Individualize dose. Take 1 hr ac. HTN: If possible, d/c previous antihypertensive drug regimen for 1 week before starting therapy. Initial: 25mg bid or tid. Titrate: May increase to 50mg bid or tid if satisfactory BP reduction not achieved after 1 or 2 weeks. Add a modest dose of thiazide diuretic (eg, HCTZ, 25mg/day) if BP not controlled after 1-2 weeks at 50mg tid (and patient is not already receiving a diuretic). If further BP reduction required, may increase to 100mg bid or tid and then, if necessary, to 150mg bid or tid (while continuing the diuretic). Usual Range: 25-150mg bid or tid. Max: 450mg/day. Severe HTN: Continue diuretic but d/c other current antihypertensive medication. Initial: 25mg bid or tid. Titrate: May increase q24h or less under continuous supervision until satisfactory BP response is obtained or max dose is reached. May add a more potent diuretic (eg, furosemide). CHF: Initial: 25mg tid. Titrate: After a dose of 50mg tid is reached, delay further increases in dosage, where possible, for at least 2 weeks to determine if satisfactory response occurs. Usual: 50mg or 100mg tid. Max: 450mg/day. Diuretic-Treated/Hyponatremic/Hypovolemic Patients: Initial: 6.25mg or 12.5mg tid. Titrate: Adjust to the usual daily dosage within the next several days. Left Ventricular Dysfunction Post-MI: May initiate as early as 3 days following an MI. Initial: 6.25mg single dose, then 12.5mg tid. Titrate: Increase to 25mg tid during the next several days. Maint: 50mg tid. Diabetic Nephropathy: Usual: 25mg tid. Significant Renal Impairment: Reduce initial daily dosage, and titrate, using smaller increments, slowly (1- to 2-week intervals). Slowly back-titrate after desired therapeutic effect is achieved to determine minimal effective dose.

HOW SUPPLIED: Tab: 12.5mg*, 25mg*, 50mg*, 100mg* *scored

CONTRAINDICATIONS: History of ACE inhibitor-associated angioedema.

WARNINGS/PRECAUTIONS: Higher rate of angioedema in blacks than nonblacks. Head/neck angioedema reported; promptly institute appropriate therapy if this occurs. Intestinal angioedema reported; monitor for abdominal pain. Anaphylactoid reactions reported during desensitization with hymenoptera venom, dialysis with high-flux membranes, and LDL apheresis with dextran sulfate absorption; consider using a different type of dialysis membrane or a different class medication in patients undergoing hemodialysis with high-flux dialysis membranes. Neutropenia/agranulocytosis reported; risk of neutropenia is dependent on the clinical status of the patient. In patients with renal impairment, evaluate WBC and differential counts prior to starting treatment and at approximately 2-week intervals for about 3 months, then periodically. In patients with collagen vascular disease or who are exposed to other drugs known to affect the white cells or immune response, particularly with impaired renal function, use therapy only after an assessment of benefit and risk, and then with caution. Perform WBC count if infection is suspected. Withdraw therapy and closely follow patient's course if neutropenia (neutrophil count <1000/mm^3) is confirmed. Total urinary proteins >1g/day reported. Excessive hypotension may occur, most likely in patients with salt/volume depletion, HF, or undergoing renal dialysis; initiate therapy under very close medical supervision in these patients. Rarely, associated with syndrome that starts with cholestatic jaundice and progresses to fulminant hepatic necrosis and sometimes death; d/c if jaundice or marked elevations of hepatic enzymes develop. May increase BUN/SrCr in patients with severe renal artery stenosis or in HF patients on long-term treatment. Hyperkalemia and persistent nonproductive cough reported. Risk of decreased coronary perfusion in patients with aortic stenosis. Hypotension may occur with major surgery or during anesthesia. Lab test interactions may occur.

ADVERSE REACTIONS: Anemia, thrombocytopenia, pancytopenia, rash, diminution/loss of taste perception.

INTERACTIONS: Dual blockade of the RAS is associated with increased risks of hypotension, hyperkalemia, and changes in renal function (including acute renal failure); closely monitor BP, renal function and electrolytes with concomitant agents that also affect the RAS. Do not coadminister with aliskiren in patients with diabetes or renal impairment (GFR <60mL/min). NSAIDs, including selective COX-2 inhibitors, may cause deterioration of renal function and may attenuate antihypertensive effect; monitor renal function periodically. Precipitous BP reduction may occur with diuretics. Nitroglycerin, other nitrates, or drugs having vasodilator activity should, if possible, be discontinued before starting captopril; if resumed during captopril therapy, administer such agents cautiously, and perhaps at lower dosage. Antihypertensive agents that cause renin release may augment effect (eg, diuretics [eg, thiazides] may activate renin-angiotensin-aldosterone system [RAAS]). Caution with agents affecting sympathetic activity (eg, ganglionic-blocking agents, adrenergic neuron-blocking agents). Increased risk of hyperkalemia with K$^+$-sparing diuretics (eg, spironolactone, triamterene, amiloride), K$^+$ supplements, K$^+$-containing salt substitutes, or other drugs associated with increases in serum K$^+$; use with caution. Increased serum lithium levels and symptoms of lithium toxicity reported; use with caution and frequently monitor serum lithium levels. Nitritoid reactions reported with injectable gold.

PREGNANCY: Category D, not for use in nursing.

MECHANISM OF ACTION: ACE inhibitor; not established. Effects appear to result primarily from suppression of RAAS. Decreases plasma angiotensin II, which leads to decreased aldosterone secretion.

PHARMACOKINETICS: Absorption: Rapid. T_{max}=1 hr. **Distribution:** Plasma protein binding (25-30%); found in breast milk. **Elimination:** Urine (>95%; 40-50% unchanged); $T_{1/2}$=<3 hrs, <2 hrs (unchanged).

NURSING CONSIDERATIONS

Assessment: Assess for hypersensitivity to drug, history of ACE inhibitor-associated angioedema, collagen vascular disease, volume/salt depletion, HF, renal artery stenosis, risk factors for hyperkalemia, renal function, aortic stenosis, pregnancy/nursing status, and possible drug interactions. In patients with renal impairment, evaluate WBC and differential counts.

Monitoring: Monitor for angioedema, anaphylactoid reactions, neutropenia/agranulocytosis, hyperkalemia, and other adverse reactions. Monitor BP, LFTs, and renal function. In patients with renal impairment, evaluate WBC and differential counts during therapy at approximately 2-week intervals for about 3 months, then periodically.

Patient Counseling: Instruct to d/c therapy and to immediately report to physician any signs/symptoms of angioedema. Advise to report promptly any indication of infection (eg, sore throat, fever) or of progressive edema. Inform that excessive perspiration, dehydration, and other causes of volume depletion (eg, vomiting, diarrhea) may lead to excessive fall in BP; advise to consult with physician. Instruct not to use K⁺-sparing diuretics, K⁺ supplements, or K⁺-containing salt substitutes without consulting physician. Warn against interruption or discontinuation of medication unless instructed by physician. Caution HF patients against rapid increases in physical activity. Inform female patients of childbearing age about the consequences of exposure to therapy during pregnancy and discuss treatment options with women planning to become pregnant; instruct to report pregnancies to physician as soon as possible.

Administration: Oral route. Take 1 hr ac. **Storage:** 20-25°C (68-77°F). Protect from moisture.

CARBAGLU RX
carglumic acid (Orphan Europe)

THERAPEUTIC CLASS: Carbamoyl phosphate synthetase 1

INDICATIONS: Adjunctive therapy in pediatric and adult patients for the treatment of acute hyperammonemia due to deficiency of the hepatic enzyme N-acetylglutamate synthase (NAGS). Maintenance therapy in pediatric and adult patients for chronic hyperammonemia due to deficiency of NAGS.

DOSAGE: *Adults:* Acute Hyperammonemia: Initial: 100-250mg/kg/day. Titrate: Adjust dose based on individual plasma ammonia levels and clinical symptoms. Chronic Hyperammonemia: Maint: Usual: <100mg/kg/day. Titrate: Adjust to target normal plasma ammonia level for age. Divide total daily dose into 2-4 doses and round to the nearest 100mg.
Pediatrics: Acute Hyperammonemia: Initial: 100-250mg/kg/day. Titrate: Adjust dose based on individual plasma ammonia levels and clinical symptoms. Chronic Hyperammonemia: Maint: Usual: <100mg/kg/day. Titrate: Adjust to target normal plasma ammonia level for age. Divide total daily dose into 2-4 doses.

HOW SUPPLIED: Tab: 200mg* *scored

WARNINGS/PRECAUTIONS: Any episode of acute symptomatic hyperammonemia should be treated as a life-threatening emergency; treatment may require dialysis, preferably hemodialysis. Uncontrolled hyperammonemia can rapidly result in brain injury/damage or death; promptly use all therapies necessary to reduce plasma ammonia levels. Monitor plasma ammonia levels, neurological status, lab tests, and clinical responses during treatment. Maintain plasma ammonia levels within normal range for age via individual dose adjustment. Maintain complete protein restriction for 24-48 hrs and maximize caloric supplementation to reverse catabolism and nitrogen turnover.

ADVERSE REACTIONS: Vomiting, abdominal pain, pyrexia, tonsillitis, infection, anemia, ear infection, diarrhea, nasopharyngitis, headache, dysgeusia, asthenia, pneumonia, anorexia, somnolence.

PREGNANCY: Category C, not for use in nursing.

MECHANISM OF ACTION: Carbamoyl phosphate synthetase 1 (CPS 1) activator; a synthetic analog of N-acetylglutamate (NAG). Acts as a replacement for NAG in NAGS deficiency patients by activating CPS 1, the enzyme that converts ammonia into urea.

PHARMACOKINETICS: Absorption: T_{max}=3 hrs (median). **Distribution:** V_d=2657L. **Metabolism:** Via intestinal bacterial flora. **Elimination:** Urine (9%, unchanged), feces (up to 60%, unchanged), lungs; $T_{1/2}$=5.6 hrs (median).

NURSING CONSIDERATIONS

Assessment: Assess plasma ammonia levels and pregnancy/nursing status.

Monitoring: Monitor plasma ammonia levels, neurological status, lab tests, and clinical responses.

Patient Counseling: Advise that when plasma ammonia levels have normalized, dietary protein intake can usually be increased with the goal of unrestricted protein intake. Instruct not to breastfeed while on therapy. Inform of the most common adverse reactions.

Administration: Oral/NG route. Do not swallow whole or crush. Disperse tab in water immediately before use. Refer to PI for preparation for oral and NG tube administration. **Storage:** Before Opening: 2-8°C (36-46°F). After Opening: Do not refrigerate or store >30°C (86°F). Protect from moisture. Discard 1 month after 1st opening.

CARDENE IV   RX
nicardipine HCl (EKR)

THERAPEUTIC CLASS: Calcium channel blocker (dihydropyridine)

INDICATIONS: Short-term treatment of HTN when PO therapy is not feasible or not desirable.

DOSAGE: *Adults:* Individualize dose. Patients Not Receiving PO Nicardipine: Initial: 5mg/hr IV infusion. Titrate: May increase by 2.5mg/hr every 5 min (for rapid titration) to 15 min (for gradual titration). Max: 15mg/hr. Decrease rate to 3mg/hr after BP goal achieved with rapid titration. Equivalent PO Dose to IV Dose: 20mg q8h=0.5mg/hr; 30mg q8h=1.2mg/hr; 40mg q8h=2.2mg/hr. Transition to PO Nicardipine: Give 1st dose 1 hr prior to discontinuation of infusion. Hepatic Impairment/Reduced Hepatic Blood Flow: Consider lower dosages. Renal Impairment: Titrate gradually. Elderly: Start at low end of dosing range. (Cardene Premixed) Impending Hypotension/Tachycardia: D/C then restart at 3-5mg/hr when BP has stabilized and adjust to maintain desired BP.

HOW SUPPLIED: Inj: 2.5mg/mL [10mL], 0.1mg/mL [200mL], 0.2mg/mL [200mL]

CONTRAINDICATIONS: Advanced aortic stenosis.

WARNINGS/PRECAUTIONS: May induce or exacerbate angina in coronary artery disease (CAD) patients. Caution with heart failure (HF) or significant left ventricular dysfunction. To reduce possibility of venous thrombosis, phlebitis, local irritation, swelling, extravasation, and occurrence of vascular impairment, administer through large peripheral or central veins. Change IV site q12h to minimize risk of peripheral venous irritation. May occasionally produce symptomatic hypotension or tachycardia. Avoid systemic hypotension when administering in sustained acute cerebral infarction or hemorrhage. Caution in hepatic/renal impairment, reduced hepatic blood flow, and elderly.

ADVERSE REACTIONS: Headache, hypotension, tachycardia, N/V.

INTERACTIONS: Titrate slowly with β-blockers in HF or significant left ventricular dysfunction due to possible negative inotropic effects. Increased nicardipine levels when PO nicardipine is given with cimetidine. Elevated cyclosporine levels reported with PO nicardipine; closely monitor cyclosporine levels and reduce its dose accordingly.

PREGNANCY: Category C, not for use in nursing.

MECHANISM OF ACTION: Calcium channel blocker (dihydropyridine); inhibits transmembrane influx of Ca^{2+} ions into cardiac muscle and smooth muscles without changing serum Ca^{2+} concentrations.

PHARMACOKINETICS: Distribution: V_d=8.3L/kg; plasma protein binding (>95%); found in breast milk. **Metabolism:** Liver (extensive). **Elimination:** Urine (49%), feces (43%); $T_{1/2}$=14.4 hrs.

NURSING CONSIDERATIONS

Assessment: Assess for advanced aortic stenosis, HF, CAD, left ventricular dysfunction, sustained acute cerebral infarction or hemorrhage, hepatic/renal impairment, pregnancy/nursing status, and possible drug interactions.

Monitoring: Monitor BP and HR during administration. Monitor for symptomatic hypotension, tachycardia, induction or exacerbation of angina, and hepatic/renal function.

Patient Counseling: Advise to seek medical attention if adverse reactions occur.

Administration: IV route. Refer to PI for preparation and administration instructions. Cardene IV: Dilute before infusion. Cardene Premixed: No further dilution required. **Storage:** 20-25°C (68-77°F). Avoid elevated temperatures. Protect from light. Store in carton until ready to use. Diluted Sol: Stable at room temperature for 24 hrs. Premixed: Protect from freezing.

CARDENE SR   RX
nicardipine HCl (EKR)

THERAPEUTIC CLASS: Calcium channel blocker (dihydropyridine)

INDICATIONS: Treatment of HTN alone or in combination with other antihypertensives.

DOSAGE: *Adults:* Initial: 30mg bid. Titrate: Adjust according to BP response. Effective Dose Range: 30-60mg bid. Currently on Nicardipine Immediate-Release (IR): Titrate with SR starting at current total daily dose of IR; reexamine adequacy of BP control. Renal Impairment: Carefully titrate dose. Elderly: Start at lower end of dosing range.

HOW SUPPLIED: Cap, Sustained-Release (SR): 30mg, 60mg

CONTRAINDICATIONS: Advanced aortic stenosis.

WARNINGS/PRECAUTIONS: Increased frequency, duration, or severity of angina reported with nicardipine IR. Caution with congestive heart failure (CHF), particularly in combination with β-blocker and during dose titration. Not a β-blocker and therefore gives no protection against dangers of abrupt β-blocker withdrawal; reduce dose of β-blocker gradually (preferably over 8-10 days). May occasionally produce symptomatic hypotension. Avoid systemic hypotension when administering in patients who have sustained an acute cerebral infarction or hemorrhage. Measure BP 2-4 hrs after the 1st dose or dose increase and at the end of a dosing interval. Caution with hepatic/renal impairment, reduced hepatic blood flow, and in elderly.

ADVERSE REACTIONS: Headache, pedal edema, vasodilatation, dizziness, asthenia.

INTERACTIONS: May increase levels with cimetidine; monitor carefully. May elevate plasma cyclosporine levels; closely monitor cyclosporine levels and reduce its dose accordingly. May increase serum digoxin levels; evaluate serum digoxin levels after concomitant therapy is initiated. Caution with fentanyl anesthesia.

PREGNANCY: Category C, not for use in nursing.

MECHANISM OF ACTION: Calcium channel blocker (dihydropyridine); inhibits transmembrane influx of Ca^{2+} ions into cardiac muscle and smooth muscle without changing serum Ca^{2+} concentrations.

PHARMACOKINETICS: Absorption: Complete; bioavailability (35%); C_{max}=13.4ng/mL (30mg), 34ng/mL (45mg), 58.4ng/mL (60mg); T_{max}=1-4 hrs. **Distribution:** Plasma protein binding (>95%). **Metabolism:** Liver (extensive). **Elimination:** Urine (60%, <1% unchanged), feces (35%); $T_{1/2}$=8.6 hrs.

NURSING CONSIDERATIONS

Assessment: Assess for advanced aortic stenosis, angina, CHF, acute cerebral infarction or hemorrhage, hepatic/renal impairment, reduced hepatic blood flow, pregnancy/nursing status, and possible drug interactions.

Monitoring: Monitor for signs/symptoms of increased angina, symptomatic hypotension, and other adverse reactions. Monitor BP during the initiation and titration.

Patient Counseling: Inform of the risks/benefits of therapy. Advise to seek medical attention if adverse reactions occur.

Administration: Oral route. **Storage:** 15-30°C (59-86°F).

CARDIZEM   RX
diltiazem HCl (Valeant)

THERAPEUTIC CLASS: Calcium channel blocker (nondihydropyridine)

INDICATIONS: Management of chronic stable angina and angina due to coronary artery spasm.

DOSAGE: *Adults:* Initial: 30mg qid (before meals and hs). Titrate: Increase gradually (given in divided doses tid-qid) at 1- to 2-day intervals until optimum response obtained. Usual: 180-360mg/day. Elderly: Start at lower end of dosing range.

HOW SUPPLIED: Tab: 30mg, 60mg*, 90mg*, 120mg* *scored

CONTRAINDICATIONS: Sick sinus syndrome and 2nd- or 3rd-degree atrioventricular (AV) block (except with functioning ventricular pacemaker); hypotension (<90mmHg systolic); acute myocardial infarction (MI) and pulmonary congestion documented by x-ray on admission.

WARNINGS/PRECAUTIONS: May cause abnormally slow HR, particularly in patients with sick sinus syndrome. May cause 2nd- or 3rd-degree AV block. Periods of asystole reported in patients with Prinzmetal's angina. Caution in renal, hepatic, or ventricular dysfunction. Symptomatic hypotension may occur. Elevations in enzymes (eg, alkaline phosphatase, lactate dehydrogenase [LDH], AST, ALT) and other phenomena consistent with acute hepatic injury reported; reversible upon discontinuation. Monitor LFTs and renal function. Dermatologic reactions (eg, erythema multiforme, exfoliative dermatitis) may occur; d/c if a dermatologic reaction persists. Caution in elderly.

ADVERSE REACTIONS: Edema, headache, nausea, dizziness, rash, asthenia.

INTERACTIONS: May increase levels of propranolol, carbamazepine, quinidine, midazolam, triazolam, lovastatin, simvastatin; monitor closely. Increased levels with cimetidine. Monitor digoxin and cyclosporine levels if used concomitantly. Potentiates depression of cardiac contractility, conductivity, automaticity, and vascular dilation with anesthetics. Additive cardiac conduction effects with digitalis or β-blockers. Potential additive effects with agents known to affect cardiac contractility and/or conduction; caution and careful titration warranted. May have significant impact on efficacy and side effect profile with CYP450 3A4 substrates, inducers, and inhibitors. Avoid with CYP3A4 inducers (eg, rifampin). May enhance the effects and increase the toxicity of buspirone. Concomitant use with statins metabolized by CYP3A4 may increase the risk of myopathy and rhabdomyolysis. Sinus bradycardia resulting in hospitalization and pacemaker insertion reported with clonidine; monitor HR.

PREGNANCY: Category C, not for use in nursing.

MECHANISM OF ACTION: Calcium channel blocker; inhibits cellular influx of calcium ions during membrane depolarization of cardiac and vascular smooth muscle. Angina Due to Coronary Artery Spasm: A potent dilator of coronary arteries both epicardial and subendocardial; inhibits spontaneous and ergonovine-induced coronary artery spasm. Exertional Angina: Produces increases in exercise tolerance by its ability to reduce myocardial oxygen demand; accomplished via reduction in HR and systemic BP.

PHARMACOKINETICS: Absorption: Well-absorbed; Absolute bioavailability (40%); T_{max}=2-4 hrs. **Distribution:** Plasma protein binding (70-80%); found in breast milk. **Metabolism:** Liver (extensive). **Elimination:** Urine (2-4%, unchanged), bile. $T_{1/2}$=3-4.5 hrs.

NURSING CONSIDERATIONS

Assessment: Assess for sick sinus syndrome, 2nd- or 3rd-degree AV block, hypotension, acute MI, pulmonary congestion, congestive heart failure, ventricular dysfunction, hepatic/renal impairment, pregnancy/nursing status, and for possible drug interactions.

Monitoring: Monitor for slow HR, 2nd- or 3rd-degree AV block, hypotension, hepatic injury (eg, increased alkaline phosphatase, LDH, AST, ALT) and for dermatological events (eg, skin eruptions progressing to erythema multiforme and/or exfoliative dermatitis). Monitor liver and renal function regularly.

Patient Counseling: Inform about benefits/risks of therapy. Counsel to report any adverse reactions to physician and to notify physician if pregnant or nursing.

Administration: Oral route. **Storage:** 25°C (77°F); excursions permitted to 15-30°C (59-86°F). Avoid excessive humidity.

CARDIZEM CD   RX
diltiazem HCl (Valeant)

OTHER BRAND NAMES: Cartia XT (Watson) - Cardizem LA (AbbVie)

THERAPEUTIC CLASS: Calcium channel blocker (nondihydropyridine)

INDICATIONS: Treatment of HTN used alone or in combination with other antihypertensive medications. Management of chronic stable angina and (CD, Cartia XT) angina due to coronary artery spasm.

DOSAGE: *Adults:* Individualize dose. HTN: (CD, Cartia XT) Initial (Monotherapy): 180-240mg qd. Titrate: Adjust to individual patient needs (schedule accordingly). Usual: 240-360mg qd. Max: 480mg qd. (LA) Initial (Monotherapy): 180-240mg qd (am or hs). Titrate: Adjust to individual patient needs (schedule accordingly). Range: 120-540mg qd. Max: 540mg/day. Angina: (CD, Cartia XT) Initial: 120mg or 180mg qd. Titrate: Adjust to each patient's needs; may be carried out over a 7- to 14-day period when necessary. Max: 480mg qd. (LA) Initial: 180mg qd (am or pm). Titrate: Increase at 1- to 2-week intervals. Max: 360mg. Elderly: Start at lower end of dosing range.

HOW SUPPLIED: Cap, Extended-Release: (Cardizem CD, Cartia XT) 120mg, 180mg, 240mg, 300mg, (Cardizem CD) 360mg; Tab, Extended-Release: (Cardizem LA) 120mg, 180mg, 240mg, 300mg, 360mg, 420mg

CONTRAINDICATIONS: Sick sinus syndrome and 2nd- or 3rd-degree atrioventricular (AV) block (except with functioning ventricular pacemaker), hypotension (<90mmHg systolic), acute myocardial infarction (MI), and pulmonary congestion documented by x-rays on admission.

WARNINGS/PRECAUTIONS: Prolongs AV node refractory periods without significantly prolonging sinus node recovery time. Periods of asystole reported in a patient with Prinzmetal's angina. Worsening of congestive heart failure reported in patients with preexisting ventricular dysfunction. Symptomatic hypotension may occur. Mild transaminase elevation with or without concomitant alkaline phosphatase and bilirubin elevation reported. Significant enzyme elevations and other phenomena consistent with acute hepatic injury reported in rare instances. Caution with renal/hepatic dysfunction. Dermatologic reactions (eg, erythema multiforme, exfoliative dermatitis) may occur; d/c if such reaction persists. Caution in elderly.

ADVERSE REACTIONS: Dizziness, bradycardia, 1st-degree AV block. (CD, Cartia XT) Headache, edema. (LA) Edema lower limb, fatigue.

INTERACTIONS: May increase levels of propranolol, carbamazepine, quinidine, midazolam, triazolam, buspirone, and lovastatin. Increased levels with cimetidine. Monitor digoxin and cyclosporine levels. Depression of cardiac contractility, conductivity, automaticity, and vascular dilation potentiated with anesthetics. Additive cardiac conduction effects with digitalis or β-blockers. Potential additive effects with agents known to affect cardiac contractility and/or conduction; caution and careful titration warranted. May have significant impact on efficacy and side effect profile with CYP450 3A4 substrates, inducers, and inhibitors. Avoid with CYP3A4 inducers (eg, rifampin). (CD, LA) Sinus bradycardia resulting in hospitalization and pacemaker insertion reported with clonidine; monitor HR. Increased exposure of simvastatin; limit daily doses

C

of both agents. Risk of myopathy and rhabdomyolysis with statins metabolized by CYP3A4 may be increased; monitor closely.

PREGNANCY: Category C, not for use in nursing.

MECHANISM OF ACTION: Calcium channel blocker; inhibits cellular influx of calcium ions during membrane depolarization of cardiac and vascular smooth muscle. HTN: Relaxes vascular smooth muscle, resulting in decreased peripheral vascular resistance. Angina: Produces increases in exercise tolerance by its ability to reduce myocardial oxygen demand; accomplished via reduction in HR and systemic BP at submaximal and maximal work loads.

PHARMACOKINETICS: Absorption: Well-absorbed. Absolute bioavailability (40%); T_{max}=10-14 hrs (CD, Cartia XT), 11-18 hrs (LA). **Distribution:** Plasma protein binding (70-80%); found in breast milk. **Metabolism:** Liver (extensive). **Elimination:** Urine (2-4%, unchanged), bile. $T_{1/2}$=5-8 hrs (CD, Cartia XT), 6-9 hrs (LA).

NURSING CONSIDERATIONS

Assessment: Assess for sick sinus syndrome, 2nd- or 3rd-degree AV block, hypotension, acute myocardial infarction and pulmonary congestion, ventricular dysfunction, hepatic/renal impairment, pregnancy/nursing status, and possible drug interactions.

Monitoring: Monitor for bradycardia, AV block, symptomatic hypotension, and dermatological reactions. Perform regular monitoring of liver and renal function.

Patient Counseling: Counsel to report any adverse reactions to physician and to notify physician if pregnant or nursing. Instruct to swallow tab whole; do not chew or crush.

Administration: Oral route. (LA) Swallow whole; do not chew or crush. **Storage:** 25°C (77°F); excursions permitted to 15-30°C (59-86°F) (CD, LA); 20-25°C (68-77°F) (Cartia XT). Avoid excessive humidity and (LA) temperature >30°C (86°F).

CARDURA   RX
doxazosin mesylate (Roerig)

THERAPEUTIC CLASS: Alpha$_1$-blocker (quinazoline)

INDICATIONS: Treatment of HTN and of both the urinary outflow obstruction and obstructive and irritative symptoms associated with BPH.

DOSAGE: *Adults:* Individualize dose. HTN: Initial: 1mg qd (am or pm). Titrate: May increase to 2mg and thereafter if necessary to 4mg, 8mg, and 16mg qd depending on standing BP response. BPH: Initial: 1mg qd (am or pm). Titrate: May increase to 2mg and thereafter to 4mg, and 8mg qd in 1- to 2-week intervals, depending on urodynamics and BPH symptomatology. Max: 8mg qd. Elderly: Start at lower end of dosing range.

HOW SUPPLIED: Tab: 1mg*, 2mg*, 4mg*, 8mg* *scored

WARNINGS/PRECAUTIONS: May cause syncope and orthostatic hypotension (eg, dizziness, lightheadedness, vertigo), especially with 1st dose, dose increase, or if therapy is interrupted for more than a few days; restart using initial dosing regimen if therapy was discontinued for several days. Rule out carcinoma of the prostate prior to therapy. Priapism (rare) and leukopenia/neutropenia reported. Intraoperative floppy iris syndrome (IFIS) observed during cataract surgery. Caution with hepatic impairment and in the elderly.

ADVERSE REACTIONS: Dizziness, headache, fatigue/malaise, somnolence, edema, nausea, rhinitis.

INTERACTIONS: Caution with additional antihypertensive agents and drugs known to influence hepatic metabolism. Additive BP-lowering effects and symptomatic hypotension with PDE-5 inhibitors.

PREGNANCY: Category C, caution in nursing.

MECHANISM OF ACTION: α_1-blocker. BPH: Antagonizes phenylephrine (α_1-agonist)-induced contractions and binds with high affinity to the α1c adrenoreceptor in prostate. HTN: Competitively antagonizes the pressor effects of phenylephrine and the systolic pressor effect of norepinephrine.

PHARMACOKINETICS: Absorption: Bioavailability (65%); T_{max}=2-3 hrs. **Distribution:** Plasma protein binding (98%). **Metabolism:** Liver (extensive); O-demethylation or hydroxylation. **Elimination:** Feces (63%, 4.8% unchanged), urine (9%, trace amounts unchanged); $T_{1/2}$=22 hrs.

NURSING CONSIDERATIONS

Assessment: Assess for previous sensitivity to drug/quinazolines, hepatic impairment, prostate cancer, pregnancy/nursing status, and possible drug interactions.

Monitoring: Monitor for signs/symptoms of orthostatic hypotension, syncope, priapism, IFIS during cataract surgery, and other adverse reactions. Measure BP periodically, particularly 2-6 hrs after the 1st dose and with each increase in dose.

Patient Counseling: Inform of the possibility of syncopal and orthostatic symptoms, especially at the initiation of therapy; urge to avoid driving or hazardous tasks for 24 hrs after the 1st dose, dose increase, and interruption of therapy when treatment is resumed. Caution to avoid situations where injury could result should syncope occur. Advise to sit or lie down when symptoms of low BP occur. Instruct to report to physician if dizziness, lightheadedness, or palpitations are bothersome. Advise of possibility of priapism and to seek immediate medical attention if this occurs. Counsel to inform surgeon of drug use prior to cataract surgery.

Administration: Oral route. **Storage:** 25°C (77°F); excursions permitted to 15-30°C (59-86°F).

CARDURA XL RX
doxazosin mesylate (Pfizer)

THERAPEUTIC CLASS: Alpha$_1$-blocker (quinazoline)

INDICATIONS: Treatment of the signs and symptoms of BPH.

DOSAGE: *Adults:* Initial: 4mg qd with breakfast. Titrate: May increase to 8mg after 3-4 weeks based on symptomatic response and tolerability. Max: 8mg. If discontinued for several days, restart using 4mg qd dose. Switching from Cardura Immediate-Release to Cardura XL: Initial: 4mg qd. Final pm dose of Cardura should not be taken. Concomitant PDE-5 Inhibitors: Initiate PDE-5 inhibitor therapy at the lowest dose.

HOW SUPPLIED: Tab, Extended-Release: 4mg, 8mg

WARNINGS/PRECAUTIONS: Postural hypotension with or without symptoms (eg, dizziness) and syncope may develop; caution with symptomatic hypotension or patients who have hypotensive response to other medications. Intraoperative floppy iris syndrome has been observed during cataract surgery in some patients on, or previously treated with, α$_1$-blockers. Caution with preexisting severe GI narrowing (pathologic or iatrogenic). Prostate cancer causes many of the same symptoms associated with BPH; rule out prostate cancer prior to therapy. Caution with mild or moderate hepatic impairment; avoid with severe hepatic impairment. D/C if symptoms of worsening of or new onset angina pectoris develop.

ADVERSE REACTIONS: Dizziness, asthenia, headache, respiratory tract infection, dyspnea, somnolence, hypotension, postural hypotension.

INTERACTIONS: Caution with potent CYP3A4 inhibitors (eg, atazanavir, clarithromycin, indinavir, itraconazole, ketoconazole, nefazodone, nelfinavir, ritonavir, saquinavir, telithromycin, voriconazole). Additive BP-lowering effects and symptomatic hypotension with PDE-5 inhibitors. Caution with drugs known to influence hepatic metabolism. Drugs that reduce GI motility leading to markedly prolonged GI retention times may increase systemic exposure to doxazosin (eg, anticholinergics).

PREGNANCY: Category C, not for use in nursing.

MECHANISM OF ACTION: α$_1$-blocker; antagonizes α$_1$-agonist-induced contractions, decreasing urethral resistance, which may relieve BPH symptoms and improve urine flow.

PHARMACOKINETICS: Absorption: (4mg) C_{max}=10.1ng/mL, AUC=183ng•hr/mL, T_{max}=8 hrs. (8mg) C_{max}=25.8ng/mL, AUC=472ng•hr/mL, T_{max}=9 hrs. **Distribution:** Plasma protein binding (98%). **Metabolism:** Liver (extensive) via CYP3A4 (major) and CYP2D6, CYP2C19 (minor). **Elimination:** $T_{1/2}$=15-19 hrs.

NURSING CONSIDERATIONS

Assessment: Assess for hepatic impairment, symptomatic hypotension, history of hypotensive response to other medications, severe GI narrowing (chronic constipation), coronary insufficiency, and possible drug interactions. Rule out prostate cancer.

Monitoring: Monitor for signs/symptoms of postural hypotension and new onset or worsening of angina pectoris.

Patient Counseling: Instruct to take with breakfast, to swallow whole, and to not chew, divide, cut, or crush. Advise that symptoms related to postural hypotension (eg, dizziness, syncope) may occur; caution about driving, operating machinery, and performing hazardous tasks. Caution not to be alarmed if something that looks like a tab is occasionally noticed in the stool. Instruct to inform ophthalmologist of drug use prior to cataract surgery.

Administration: Oral route. **Storage:** 25°C (77°F); excursions permitted to 15-30°C (59-86°F).

CASODEX RX
bicalutamide (AstraZeneca)

THERAPEUTIC CLASS: Nonsteroidal antiandrogen

INDICATIONS: Treatment of stage D_2 metastatic carcinoma of the prostate in combination with a luteinizing hormone-releasing hormone (LHRH) analog.

DOSAGE: *Adults:* Usual: 50mg qd (am or pm) in combination with an LHRH analog. Take at the same time each day and start at the same time as treatment with an LHRH analog.

HOW SUPPLIED: Tab: 50mg

CONTRAINDICATIONS: Women, pregnancy.

WARNINGS/PRECAUTIONS: Cases of death or hospitalization due to severe liver injury (hepatic failure) reported. Hepatitis and marked increases in liver enzymes leading to drug discontinuation reported; measure serum transaminase levels prior to treatment, at regular intervals for the first 4 months, and periodically thereafter. Measure serum ALT immediately if signs/symptoms of liver dysfunction occur; d/c immediately with close follow-up of liver function if jaundice occurs or ALT rises >2X ULN. Reduction in glucose tolerance reported; monitor blood glucose. Regularly assess serum prostate-specific antigen (PSA) to monitor response; evaluate for clinical progression if PSA levels rise during therapy. For patients with objective disease progression with an elevated PSA, consider a treatment period free of antiandrogen while continuing the LHRH analog. Caution with moderate-severe hepatic impairment; monitor LFTs periodically on long-term therapy.

ADVERSE REACTIONS: Pain, hot flashes, HTN, constipation, nausea, diarrhea, anemia, peripheral edema, dizziness, dyspnea, rash, nocturia, hematuria, urinary tract infection, gynecomastia.

INTERACTIONS: Can displace coumarin anticoagulants from binding sites; monitor PT and consider anticoagulant dose adjustment. Caution with CYP3A4 substrates. May increase levels of midazolam.

PREGNANCY: Category X, not for use in nursing.

MECHANISM OF ACTION: Nonsteroidal antiandrogen; inhibits the action of androgens by binding to cytosol androgen receptors in target tissue.

PHARMACOKINETICS: Absorption: Well-absorbed; C_{max}=0.768µg/mL; T_{max}=31.3 hrs. **Distribution:** Plasma protein binding (96%). **Metabolism:** Liver via oxidation and glucuronidation. **Elimination:** Urine, feces; $T_{1/2}$=5.8 days.

NURSING CONSIDERATIONS

Assessment: Assess for drug hypersensitivity, diabetes, hepatic impairment, and possible drug interactions. Measure serum transaminase levels.

Monitoring: Measure serum transaminase levels at regular intervals for the first 4 months of treatment, then periodically thereafter. Measure serum ALT for signs/symptoms of liver dysfunction. Monitor LFT in hepatically impaired patients on long-term therapy. Regularly monitor serum PSA levels. Monitor for hypersensitivity reactions and blood glucose levels.

Patient Counseling: Advise not to interrupt or stop taking the medication without consulting physician. Inform that somnolence may occur; advise to use caution when driving or operating machinery. Advise to monitor blood glucose levels while on therapy.

Administration: Oral route. **Storage:** 20-25°C (68-77°F).

CATAFLAM   RX
diclofenac potassium (Novartis)

NSAIDs may cause an increased risk of serious cardiovascular (CV) thrombotic events, myocardial infarction (MI), stroke, and serious GI adverse events, including bleeding, ulceration, and perforation of the stomach or intestines. Contraindicated for the treatment of perioperative pain in the setting of coronary artery bypass graft (CABG) surgery.

THERAPEUTIC CLASS: NSAID

INDICATIONS: Relief of signs and symptoms of osteoarthritis (OA) and rheumatoid arthritis (RA). Treatment of primary dysmenorrhea and relief of mild to moderate pain.

DOSAGE: *Adults:* OA: 100-150mg/day in divided doses, 50mg bid or tid. RA: 150-200mg/day in divided doses, 50mg tid or qid. Pain/Primary Dysmenorrhea: Initial: 50mg tid or 100mg on 1st dose, then 50mg on subsequent doses.

HOW SUPPLIED: Tab: 50mg

CONTRAINDICATIONS: Aspirin (ASA) or other NSAID allergy that precipitates asthma, urticaria, or allergic reactions. Treatment of perioperative pain in the setting of CABG surgery.

WARNINGS/PRECAUTIONS: May lead to onset of new HTN or worsening of preexisting HTN; monitor BP closely. Fluid retention and edema reported; caution in patients with fluid retention or heart failure (HF). Caution with history of ulcer disease or GI bleeding. Caution in patients with considerable dehydration. Renal papillary necrosis and other renal injury reported after long-term use. Caution with impaired renal function, HF, liver dysfunction, and the elderly. Not recommended for use with advanced renal disease; if therapy must be initiated, monitor renal function. May cause elevations of LFTs; d/c if liver disease develops or systemic manifestations occur. Anaphylactoid reactions may occur. May cause serious skin adverse events (eg, exfoliative dermatitis, Stevens-Johnson syndrome, toxic epidermal necrolysis). Avoid in late pregnancy; may cause premature closure of ductus arteriosus. Not a substitute for corticosteroids or for the treatment of corticosteroid insufficiency. Anemia may occur; with long-term use, monitor Hgb/Hct if signs or symptoms of anemia develop. May inhibit platelet aggregation and prolong bleeding time; monitor with coagulation disorders. Caution with asthma and avoid with ASA-sensitive asthma.

ADVERSE REACTIONS: Dyspepsia, constipation, diarrhea, GI ulceration/perforation, N/V, flatulence, abnormal renal function, anemia, dizziness, edema, elevated liver enzymes, headache, increased bleeding time, rash, tinnitus.

INTERACTIONS: Avoid use with ASA. May enhance methotrexate toxicity; caution when coadministering. May increase nephrotoxicity of cyclosporine; caution when coadministering. May diminish antihypertensive effect of ACE inhibitors. May reduce natriuretic effect of furosemide and thiazides; monitor for renal failure. May increase lithium levels; monitor for toxicity. Synergistic effects on GI bleeding with warfarin. Caution with hepatotoxic drugs (eg, antibiotics, antiepileptics). Increased risk of GI bleeding with concomitant oral corticosteroids, anticoagulants, or alcohol. ACE inhibitors and diuretics may increase the risk of overt renal decompensation.

PREGNANCY: Category C, not for use in nursing.

MECHANISM OF ACTION: NSAID (benzeneacetic acid derivative); suspected to inhibit prostaglandin synthetase.

PHARMACOKINETICS: Absorption: Absolute bioavailability (55%), T_{max}=1 hr. **Distribution**: V_d=1.3L/kg; serum protein binding (>99%). **Metabolism**: Metabolites: 4'-hydroxy-, 5-hydroxy-, 3'-hydroxy-, 4',5-dihydroxy-, and 3'-hydroxy-4'-methoxy diclofenac. **Elimination:** Urine (65%), bile (35%); $T_{1/2}$=2 hrs.

NURSING CONSIDERATIONS

Assessment: Assess for history of a hypersensitivity reaction to ASA or other NSAIDS, asthma, cardiovascular disease (CVD) (eg, preexisting HTN, congestive heart failure) or risk factors for CVD, risk factors for a GI event (eg, prior history of ulcer disease or GI disease, smoking), fluid retention, renal/hepatic dysfunction, coagulation disorders, pregnancy/nursing status, and for possible drug interactions. Assess baseline LFTs, renal function, and CBC.

Monitoring: Monitor for signs/symptoms of CV thrombotic events, new onset or worsening of preexisting HTN, GI events (eg, inflammation, bleeding, ulceration, perforation), fluid retention and edema, renal effects (eg, renal papillary necrosis), hepatic effects (eg, jaundice, liver necrosis, liver failure), anaphylactoid reactions, skin reactions (eg, exfoliative dermatitis, Stevens-Johnson syndrome, toxic epidermal necrolysis), hematological effects (eg, anemia, prolongation of bleeding time), and for bronchospasm. Monitor BP. Perform periodic monitoring of CBC, renal function, and LFTs.

Patient Counseling: Instruct to seek medical attention for symptoms of hepatotoxicity (eg, nausea, fatigue, jaundice), anaphylactic reactions (eg, difficulty breathing, swelling of the face/throat), rash, CV events (eg, chest pain, SOB, weakness, slurring of speech), or if unexplained weight gain or edema occur. Inform of risks if used during pregnancy.

Administration: Oral route. **Storage:** Do not store >30°C (86°F). Dispense in tight container.

CATAPRES   RX
clonidine HCl (Boehringer Ingelheim)

OTHER BRAND NAMES: Catapres-TTS (Boehringer Ingelheim)

THERAPEUTIC CLASS: Alpha-adrenergic agonist

INDICATIONS: Treatment of HTN, alone or with other antihypertensives.

DOSAGE: *Adults:* (Patch) Apply to hairless area of intact skin of upper outer arm or chest once every 7 days. Apply each new patch on different skin site from previous location. Initial: Adjust according to individual therapeutic requirements, starting with TTS-1. Titrate: If inadequate reduction in BP after 1-2 weeks, increase dosage by adding another TTS-1 or changing to a larger system. No usual additional efficacy with dose increase above 2 TTS-3. When substituting for PO clonidine or other antihypertensives, gradually reduce prior drug dose; effect of patch may not commence until 2-3 days after initial application. Renal Impairment: May benefit from lower initial dose. (Tab) Adjust dose according to patient's individual BP response. Initial: 0.1mg bid (am and hs). Maint: May increase by 0.1mg/day at weekly intervals PRN until desired response is achieved. Usual: 0.2-0.6mg/day in divided doses. Max: 2.4mg/day. Elderly/Renal Impairment: May benefit from lower initial dose.

HOW SUPPLIED: Patch, Extended-Release (TTS): (TTS-1) 0.1mg, (TTS-2) 0.2mg, (TTS-3) 0.3mg; Tab: 0.1mg, 0.2mg, 0.3mg

C

WARNINGS/PRECAUTIONS: Sudden cessation of treatment may cause nervousness, agitation, headache, confusion, and tremor accompanied or followed by a rapid rise in BP and elevated catecholamine concentrations; if discontinuing therapy, reduce dose gradually over 2 to 4 days to avoid withdrawal symptoms. Rare instances of hypertensive encephalopathy, cerebrovascular accidents (CVA), and death reported after withdrawal. Continuation of clonidine transdermal system or substitution to PO may cause generalized skin rash and elicit an allergic reaction if with localized contact sensitization or allergic reaction to clonidine transdermal system. Monitor BP during surgery; additional measures to control BP should be available. No therapeutic effect can be expected in HTN caused by pheochromocytoma. May worsen sinus node dysfunction and atrioventricular (AV) block, especially with other sympatholytic drugs; patients with conduction abnormalities and/or taking other sympatholytic drugs may develop severe bradycardia. (Tab) Continue administration to within 4 hrs of surgery and resume as soon as possible thereafter. (Patch) Loss of BP control reported (rare). Do not remove during surgery. Remove before defibrillation or cardioversion due to potential for altered electrical conductivity, and before undergoing an MRI due to the occurrence of skin burns.

ADVERSE REACTIONS: Dry mouth, drowsiness, dizziness, constipation, sedation.

INTERACTIONS: May potentiate CNS depressive effects of alcohol, barbiturates, or other sedating drugs. Hypotensive effect may be reduced by TCAs; may need to increase clonidine dose. Neuroleptics may induce or exacerbate orthostatic regulation disturbances (eg, orthostatic hypotension, dizziness, fatigue). Monitor HR with agents that affect sinus node function or AV nodal conduction (eg, digitalis, calcium channel blockers, β-blockers). D/C concurrent β-blockers several days before the gradual withdrawal of clonidine. Reports of sinus bradycardia and pacemaker insertion with diltiazem or verapamil. High IV doses of clonidine may increase the arrhythmogenic potential (QT prolongation, ventricular fibrillation) of high IV doses of haloperidol as observed in patients in a state of alcoholic delirium.

PREGNANCY: Category C, caution in nursing.

MECHANISM OF ACTION: Centrally acting α-agonist; stimulates α-adrenoreceptors in brain stem, reducing sympathetic outflow from CNS and decreasing peripheral resistance, renal vascular resistance, HR, and BP.

PHARMACOKINETICS: Absorption: (Patch) Absolute bioavailability (60%); (Tab) absolute bioavailability (70-80%); T_{max}=1-3 hrs. **Distribution:** Crosses placenta; found in breast milk. **Metabolism:** Liver. **Elimination:** Urine (40-60%, unchanged); (Patch) $T_{1/2}$=20 hrs.

NURSING CONSIDERATIONS

Assessment: Assess for pheochromocytoma, renal impairment, allergic reactions/contact sensitization, pregnancy/nursing status, and for possible drug interactions.

Monitoring: Monitor BP and renal function periodically. Monitor for withdrawal signs/symptoms (eg, hypertensive encephalopathy, CVA), presence of generalized skin rash, and allergic reactions.

Patient Counseling: Caution patients against interrupting therapy without physician's advice and engaging in hazardous activities (eg, driving, operating appliances/machinery). Inform that sedative effect may be increased by concomitant use of alcohol, barbiturates, or other sedating drugs. Caution patients who wear contact lenses that drug may cause dryness of eyes. (Patch) Instruct to consult physician promptly about possible need to remove or replace patch if skin reactions develop. Inform that if patch begins to loosen, place adhesive cover directly over the patch to ensure adhesion for 7 days total. Advise to keep used and unused patch out of reach of children; instruct to fold in half with adhesive sides together and discard.

Administration: Oral/Transdermal route. **Storage:** (Patch) Below 30°C (86°F). (Tab) 25°C (77°F); excursions permitted to 15-30°C (59-86°F).

CAYSTON   RX
aztreonam (Gilead Sciences)

THERAPEUTIC CLASS: Monobactam

INDICATIONS: To improve respiratory symptoms in cystic fibrosis patients with *Pseudomonas aeruginosa*.

DOSAGE: *Adults:* 75mg tid via nebulizer for a 28-day course (followed by 28 days off therapy). Take doses at least 4 hrs apart. Use bronchodilator before administration.
Pediatrics: ≥7 Yrs: 75mg tid via nebulizer for a 28-day course (followed by 28 days off therapy). Take doses at least 4 hrs apart. Use bronchodilator before administration.

HOW SUPPLIED: Sol, Inh: 75mg/vial

WARNINGS/PRECAUTIONS: Severe allergic reactions reported; d/c and initiate treatment as appropriate if allergic reaction occurs. Caution with history of β-lactam allergy (eg, penicillins [PCNs], cephalosporins, carbapenems); cross-reactivity may occur. Treatment is associated with bronchospasm. Pulmonary exacerbations may occur after treatment course; consider baseline forced expiratory volume in 1 sec (FEV_1) measured prior to therapy and presence of other symptoms to evaluate if post-treatment changes in FEV_1 are caused by pulmonary exacerbations. May result in bacterial resistance with use in the absence of known *P. aeruginosa* infection.

ADVERSE REACTIONS: Cough, nasal congestion, wheezing, pharyngolaryngeal pain, pyrexia, chest discomfort, abdominal pain, vomiting, bronchospasm.

PREGNANCY: Category B, safe in nursing.

MECHANISM OF ACTION: Monobactam; binds to PCN-binding proteins of susceptible bacteria, which leads to inhibition of bacterial cell-wall synthesis and death of the cell.

PHARMACOKINETICS: Absorption: C_{max}=0.55mcg/mL, 0.67mcg/mL, 0.65mcg/mL (Days 0, 14, and 28, respectively). **Distribution:** Serum protein binding (56%); (IV) found in breast milk, crosses the placenta. **Metabolism:** Hydrolysis. **Elimination:** Urine (10%, unchanged), (IV) feces (12%); $T_{1/2}$=2.1 hrs.

NURSING CONSIDERATIONS

Assessment: Assess for previous hypersensitivity to the drug, history of β-lactam allergy, presence of other symptoms, and pregnancy/nursing status. Obtain baseline FEV_1.

Monitoring: Monitor for signs/symptoms of allergic reactions, bronchospasm, and other adverse reactions. Monitor for pulmonary exacerbations following the 28-day treatment cycle.

Patient Counseling: Instruct to take exactly ud; inform that skipping doses or not completing full course of therapy may decrease effectiveness and increase resistance. Advise that therapy is for inhalation use only using an Altera nebulizer system. Inform that if a dose is missed, all 3 daily doses should be taken as long as doses are at least 4 hrs apart. Advise to contact physician if allergic reaction or new/worsening symptoms develop. Inform that therapy should only be used to treat bacterial, not viral, infections. Advise to use a bronchodilator prior to administration. Instruct patients taking several medications to administer drugs in the following order: bronchodilator, mucolytics, and lastly, aztreonam.

Administration: Inhalation route. Administer only via Altera nebulizer system. Do not mix with any other drugs. Administer immediately after reconstitution. Refer to PI for reconstitution and administration instructions. **Storage:** 2-8°C (36-46°F). Once removed from refrigerator, store at up to 25°C (77°F) for up to 28 days. Protect from light.

CEFACLOR   RX
cefaclor (Various)

THERAPEUTIC CLASS: Cephalosporin (2nd generation)

INDICATIONS: Treatment of otitis media, pharyngitis, tonsillitis, and lower respiratory tract/urinary tract/skin and skin structure infections caused by susceptible strains of microorganisms.

DOSAGE: *Adults:* Usual: 250mg q8h. More Severe Infections (eg, Pneumonia)/Infections Caused by Less Susceptible Organisms: May double doses. Treat β-hemolytic streptococcal infections for at least 10 days.
Pediatrics: ≥1 Month: Usual: 20mg/kg/day q8h. More Serious Infections/Otitis Media/Infections Caused by Less Susceptible Organisms: Usual: 40mg/kg/day. Max: 1g/day. Treat β-hemolytic streptococcal infections for at least 10 days. (Sus) May administer q12h for otitis media and pharyngitis. Refer to PI for pediatric dosing charts.

HOW SUPPLIED: Cap: 250mg, 500mg; Sus: 125mg/5mL [75mL, 150mL], 187mg/5mL [50mL, 100mL], 250mg/5mL [75mL, 150mL], 375mg/5mL [50mL, 100mL]

WARNINGS/PRECAUTIONS: Caution in penicillin (PCN)-sensitive patients; cross-hypersensitivity among β-lactam antibiotics may occur. D/C if an allergic reaction occurs; serious acute hypersensitivity reactions may require treatment with epinephrine and other emergency measures as clinically indicated. *Clostridium difficile*-associated diarrhea (CDAD) (Sus)/Pseudomembranous colitis (Cap) reported. Consider CDAD/pseudomembranous colitis if diarrhea occurs. Institute appropriate fluid and electrolyte management, protein supplementation, antibiotic treatment of *C. difficile*, and surgical evaluation, as clinically indicated. Use in the absence of a proven or strongly suspected bacterial infection or prophylactic indication is unlikely to provide benefit and increases the risk of development of drug-resistant bacteria. May result in overgrowth of nonsusceptible organisms with prolonged use; take appropriate measures if superinfection develops. Lab test interactions may occur. Caution with markedly impaired renal function, history of GI disease particularly colitis, and in elderly. (Sus) If CDAD is suspected or confirmed, ongoing antibiotic use not directed against *C. difficile* may need to be discontinued.

ADVERSE REACTIONS: GI symptoms, hypersensitivity reactions, eosinophilia, genital pruritus, moniliasis, vaginitis, serum-sickness-like reactions.

INTERACTIONS: Renal excretion inhibited by probenecid. May increase anticoagulant effect of oral anticoagulants. (Cap) Concomitant use with warfarin may increase PT.

PREGNANCY: Category B, caution in nursing.

MECHANISM OF ACTION: Cephalosporin (2nd generation); bactericidal, inhibits cell-wall synthesis.

PHARMACOKINETICS: Absorption: Fasting: Well-absorbed; C_{max}=7mcg/mL (250mg), 13mcg/mL (500mg), 23mcg/mL (1g); T_{max}=30-60 min. **Distribution:** Found in breast milk. **Elimination:** Urine (60-85% unchanged); $T_{1/2}$=0.6-0.9 hrs (normal subjects), 2.3-2.8 hrs (anuria/complete absence of renal function).

NURSING CONSIDERATIONS

Assessment: Assess for hypersensitivity to cephalosporins/PCNs/other drugs, history of GI disease (particularly colitis), renal impairment, pregnancy/nursing status, and possible drug interactions. Perform appropriate culture and susceptibility tests to determine susceptible causative organisms.

Monitoring: Monitor for hypersensitivity reactions, CDAD/pseudomembranous colitis, development of superinfection or drug resistance, and other adverse reactions. Monitor renal function in the elderly and those with markedly impaired renal function. Monitor PT with warfarin.

Patient Counseling: Inform that drug only treats bacterial, not viral infections. Instruct to take exactly ud and that skipping doses or not completing full course of therapy may decrease effectiveness and increase the likelihood of bacterial resistance. (Sus) Instruct to contact physician as soon as possible if watery/bloody stools (with/without stomach cramps and fever) develop, even as late as 2 months after discontinuation.

Administration: Oral route. (Sus) Shake well before using. Refer to PI for mixing instructions. **Storage:** 20-25°C (68-77°F). Diluted Sol: Store in refrigerator after mixing. Discard unused portion after 14 days.

CEFACLOR ER   RX
cefaclor (Various)

THERAPEUTIC CLASS: Cephalosporin (2nd generation)

INDICATIONS: Treatment of the following mild to moderate infections: acute bacterial exacerbations of chronic bronchitis (ABECB), secondary bacterial infections of acute bronchitis, pharyngitis, tonsillitis, and uncomplicated skin and skin structure infections (SSSIs) caused by susceptible strains of microorganisms.

DOSAGE: *Adults:* ≥16 Yrs: ABECB/Acute Bronchitis: 500mg q12h for 7 days. Pharyngitis/Tonsillitis: 375mg q12h for 10 days. SSSI: 375mg q12h for 7-10 days. Take with meals.

HOW SUPPLIED: Tab, Extended-Release: 500mg

WARNINGS/PRECAUTIONS: Cross-sensitivity among β-lactam antibiotics reported; caution with penicillin (PCN) allergy. D/C if allergic reaction occurs and institute appropriate therapy. *Clostridium difficile*-associated diarrhea (CDAD) reported. May result in bacterial resistance with prolonged use or use in the absence of a proven/suspected bacterial infection or a prophylactic indication; take appropriate measures if superinfection develops. Lab test interactions may occur.

ADVERSE REACTIONS: Headache, rhinitis, diarrhea, nausea.

INTERACTIONS: Decreased absorption with magnesium or aluminum hydroxide-containing antacids. Renal excretion inhibited by probenecid. Concomitant use with warfarin may increase PT.

PREGNANCY: Category B, caution in nursing.

MECHANISM OF ACTION: Cephalosporin (2nd generation); bactericidal activity results from its inhibition of cell-wall synthesis.

PHARMACOKINETICS: Absorption: Fed: (375mg) C_{max}=3.7mcg/mL, T_{max}=2.7 hrs, AUC=9.9mcg•hr/mL. (500mg) C_{max}=8.2mcg/mL, T_{max}=2.5 hrs, AUC=18.1mcg•hr/mL. Fasting: (500mg) C_{max}=5.4mcg/mL, T_{max}=1.5 hrs, AUC=14.8mcg•hr/mL. **Distribution:** Found in breast milk. **Elimination:** $T_{1/2}$=1 hr.

NURSING CONSIDERATIONS

Assessment: Assess for hypersensitivity reactions to the drug, cephalosporins, PCNs, other drugs, pregnancy/nursing status, and possible drug interactions. Perform appropriate culture and susceptibility tests for diagnosis and identification of causative organisms.

Monitoring: Monitor for allergic reactions, CDAD, superinfection, and drug resistance.

Patient Counseling: Instruct to take ud and that skipping doses or not completing full course may decrease effectiveness and increase resistance. Inform that diarrhea may occur but that it usually ends once treatment is completed. Instruct to notify physician as soon as possible if watery and bloody stools (with/without stomach cramps and fever) develop, even as late as ≥2 months after taking last dose.

Administration: Oral route. Take with meals (within 1 hr of eating). Do not crush, cut, or chew tab.
Storage: 20-25°C (68-77°F). Store in a tight, light-resistant container.

CEFADROXIL

cefadroxil (Various)

RX

THERAPEUTIC CLASS: Cephalosporin (1st generation)

INDICATIONS: Treatment of urinary tract infections (UTIs), skin and skin structure infections (SSSIs), pharyngitis, and/or tonsillitis caused by susceptible strains of microorganisms.

DOSAGE: *Adults:* Uncomplicated Lower UTI (eg, Cystitis): Usual: 1 or 2g/day given qd or bid. Other UTI: Usual: 2g/day given bid. SSSI: Usual: 1g/day given qd or bid. Group A β-hemolytic Streptococcal Pharyngitis/Tonsillitis: 1g/day given qd or bid for 10 days. Renal Impairment: CrCl ≤50mL/min: Initial: 1g. Maint: CrCl 25-50mL/min: 500mg q12h; CrCl 10-25mL/min: 500mg q24h; CrCl 0-10mL/min: 500mg q36h.
Pediatrics: UTI/SSSI: Usual: 30mg/kg/day in divided doses q12h. Pharyngitis/Tonsillitis/Impetigo: Usual: 30mg/kg/day given qd or in equally divided doses q12h. β-hemolytic Streptococcal Infections: Give for at least 10 days. Refer to PI for daily dosage of PO sus.

HOW SUPPLIED: Cap: 500mg; Sus: 250mg/5mL [50mL, 100mL], 500mg/5mL [50mL, 75mL, 100mL]; Tab: 1000mg

WARNINGS/PRECAUTIONS: Caution in penicillin (PCN)-sensitive patients; cross-sensitivity among β-lactam antibiotics may occur. D/C if an allergic reaction occurs. *Clostridium difficile*-associated diarrhea (CDAD) reported; d/c if CDAD is suspected or confirmed. Caution with renal impairment (CrCl <50mL/min/1.73m^2); monitor prior to and during therapy. May result in bacterial resistance with prolonged use in the absence of a proven or suspected bacterial infection, or a prophylactic indication; take appropriate measures if superinfection develops. Caution with history of GI disease, particularly colitis. Positive direct Coombs' tests reported. D/C if seizure occurs. Caution in elderly.

ADVERSE REACTIONS: Diarrhea, allergies, hepatic dysfunction, genital moniliasis, vaginitis, moderate transient neutropenia, fever, toxic epidermal necrolysis, abdominal pain, superinfection, renal dysfunction, toxic nephropathy, aplastic anemia, hemolytic anemia, hemorrhage.

PREGNANCY: Category B, caution in nursing.

MECHANISM OF ACTION: Cephalosporin (1st generation); bactericidal activity results from its inhibition of cell-wall synthesis.

PHARMACOKINETICS: Absorption: Rapid. C_{max}=16mcg/mL (500mg), 28mcg/mL (1000mg).
Elimination: Urine (90% unchanged).

NURSING CONSIDERATIONS

Assessment: Assess for allergy to other cephalosporins, PCN, or to other drugs, renal impairment, history of GI disease, and pregnancy/nursing status. Initiate culture and susceptibility tests prior to therapy.

Monitoring: Monitor for signs/symptoms of an allergic reaction, CDAD, seizure, and superinfection. Carefully observe patients with known or suspected renal impairment.

Patient Counseling: Inform that therapy only treats bacterial, not viral, infections. Instruct to take exactly ud; skipping doses or not completing full course may decrease effectiveness and increase risk of bacterial resistance. Inform that diarrhea is a common problem that usually ends upon discontinuation. Instruct to notify physician as soon as possible if watery and bloody stools (with/without stomach cramps and fever) occur, even as late as 2 or more months after last dose.

Administration: Oral route. Take without regard to meals. (Sus) Shake well before use. Refer to PI for reconstitution directions. **Storage:** (Tab) 20-25°C (68-77°F). (Cap/Sus, Before Reconstitution) 25°C (77°F); excursions permitted to 15-30°C (59-86°F). (Sus, After Reconstitution) Store in refrigerator; discard unused portion after 14 days.

CEFAZOLIN

cefazolin (Various)

RX

THERAPEUTIC CLASS: Cephalosporin (1st generation)

INDICATIONS: Treatment of respiratory tract, urinary tract, skin and skin structure, biliary tract, bone and joint, and genital infections, septicemia, and endocarditis caused by susceptible strains of microorganisms. Perioperative prophylaxis for surgical procedures classified as contaminated or potentially contaminated.

DOSAGE: *Adults:* Moderate to Severe Infections: 500mg-1g IV/IM q6-8h. Mild Gram-Positive Cocci Infections: 250-500mg IV/IM q8h. Acute, Uncomplicated Urinary Tract Infection: 1g IV/

C

IM q12h. Pneumococcal Pneumonia: 500mg IV/IM q12h. Severe Life-Threatening Infections (eg, Endocarditis, Septicemia): 1-1.5g IV/IM q6h. Max: 12g/day (rare). Perioperative Prophylaxis: 1g IV/IM or 2g IV 0.5-1 hr before surgery. For Lengthy Procedures (eg, ≥2 Hrs): 500mg-1g IV/IM during surgery. Postoperative: 500mg-1g IV/IM q6-8h for 24 hrs. Continue for 3-5 days following the completion of surgery where occurrence of infection may be particularly devastating (eg, open-heart surgery, prosthetic arthroplasty). Renal Impairment: CrCl 35-54mL/min: Full dose q8h or longer. CrCl 11-34mL/min: 1/2 usual dose q12h. CrCl ≤10mL/min: 1/2 usual dose q18-24h. Apply reduced dosage recommendations after initial LD is given.

Pediatrics: >1 Month: Mild to Moderately Severe Infections: 25-50mg/kg/day IV/IM, given tid or qid. Titrate: May increase to 100mg/kg/day IV/IM for severe infections. Refer to PI for proper dosing guidelines. Renal Impairment: CrCl 41-70mL/min: 60% of usual dose given in equally divided doses q12h. CrCl 21-40mL/min: 25% of usual dose given in equally divided doses q12h. CrCl 5-20mL/min or less: 10% of usual dose given in equally divided doses q24h. Apply reduced dosage recommendations after an initial LD is given.

HOW SUPPLIED: Inj: 500mg, 1g

WARNINGS/PRECAUTIONS: Caution with penicillin (PCN)-sensitive patients; cross-hypersensitivity among β-lactam antibiotics may occur. D/C if an allergic reaction occurs. *Clostridium difficile*-associated diarrhea (CDAD) reported; d/c if CDAD suspected or confirmed. Institute appropriate fluid and electrolyte management, protein supplementation, antibacterial drug treatment of *C. difficile*, and surgical evaluation as clinically indicated. Use in the absence of a proven or strongly suspected bacterial infection or prophylactic indication is unlikely to provide benefit and increases the risk of the development of drug-resistant bacteria. May result in overgrowth of nonsusceptible microorganisms with prolonged use; take appropriate measures if superinfection develops. Lab test interactions may occur. Caution with renal impairment, overt/known subclinical diabetes mellitus (DM) or carbohydrate intolerance for any reason, and in elderly. Not recommended for premature infants and neonates.

ADVERSE REACTIONS: Diarrhea, oral candidiasis, N/V, stomach cramps, anorexia, anaphylaxis, leukopenia, thrombocytopenia, renal failure, hepatitis, pruritus, dizziness, fainting, confusion, weakness.

INTERACTIONS: Probenecid may decrease renal tubular secretion.

PREGNANCY: Category B, caution in nursing.

MECHANISM OF ACTION: Cephalosporin (1st generation); bactericidal agent that acts by inhibition of bacterial cell wall synthesis.

PHARMACOKINETICS: Absorption: (IV) C_{max}=185mcg/mL. **Distribution:** Crosses placenta; found in breast milk. **Elimination:** Urine (unchanged); $T_{1/2}$=2 hrs (IM), 1.8 hrs (IV).

NURSING CONSIDERATIONS

Assessment: Assess for hypersensitivity to cephalosporin class of antibacterial drugs/PCN/other β-lactams, DM, carbohydrate intolerance, renal impairment, pregnancy/nursing status, and possible drug interactions. Perform appropriate culture and susceptibility tests to determine susceptible causative organisms.

Monitoring: Monitor for hypersensitivity reactions, CDAD, development of superinfection, drug resistance, and other adverse reactions. Monitor renal function in elderly. Monitor for seizures in patients with renal dysfunction.

Patient Counseling: Advise that allergic reactions, including serious allergic reactions may occur and require immediate treatment and discontinuation of therapy. Instruct to notify physician of any previous allergic reactions to the drug, cephalosporins, PCNs, or other similar antibacterials. Advise that diarrhea is a common problem that usually ends when therapy is discontinued; however, if watery and bloody stools (with/without stomach cramps and fever) occur, even as late as 2 or more months after last dose, instruct to contact physician as soon as possible. Inform that therapy only treats bacterial, not viral (eg, common cold), infections. Instruct to take exactly as directed even if the patient feels better early in the course of therapy; skipping doses or not completing the full course of therapy may decrease effectiveness and increase risk of bacterial resistance.

Administration: IV/IM route. Shake well before use. Refer to PI for preparation of parenteral solution and administration instruction. **Storage:** Before Reconstitution: 20-25°C (68-77°F). Protect from light. After Reconstitution: Stable for 24 hrs at room temperature or for 10 days if stored under refrigeration (5°C [41°F]).

CEFDINIR   RX
cefdinir (Various)

THERAPEUTIC CLASS: Cephalosporin (3rd generation)

INDICATIONS: Community-acquired pneumonia (CAP), acute exacerbations of chronic bronchitis (AECB), acute maxillary sinusitis, pharyngitis/tonsillitis, and uncomplicated skin and skin structure infections (SSSIs) in adult and adolescent patients. Acute bacterial otitis media, pharyngitis/tonsillitis, and uncomplicated SSSIs in pediatric patients.

DOSAGE: *Adults:* (Cap) CAP/SSSI: 300mg q12h for 10 days. AECB/Pharyngitis/Tonsillitis: 300mg q12h for 5-10 days or 600mg q24h for 10 days. Acute Maxillary Sinusitis: 300mg q12h or 600mg q24h for 10 days. CrCl <30mL/min: 300mg qd. Hemodialysis: Initial: 300mg or 7mg/kg qod; give 300mg or 7mg/kg at the end of each hemodialysis session. Usual: 300mg or 7mg/kg qod. *Pediatrics:* (Cap) ≥13 Yrs: CAP/SSSI: 300mg q12h for 10 days. AECB/Pharyngitis/Tonsillitis: 300mg q12h for 5-10 days or 600mg q24h for 10 days. Acute Maxillary Sinusitis: 300mg q12h or 600mg q24h for 10 days. (Sus) ≥43 kg: Max dose: 600mg/day. 6 months-12 yrs: Otitis Media/Pharyngitis/Tonsillitis: 7mg/kg q12h for 5-10 days or 14mg/kg q24h for 10 days. Acute Maxillary Sinusitis: 7mg/kg q12h or 14mg/kg q24h for 10 days. SSSI: 7mg/kg q12h for 10 days. Refer to PI for pediatric dosage chart. CrCl <30mL/min/1.73m^2: 7mg/kg qd. Max: 300mg qd. Hemodialysis: Initial: 300mg or 7mg/kg qod; give 300mg or 7mg/kg at the end of each hemodialysis session. Usual: 300mg or 7mg/kg qod.

HOW SUPPLIED: Cap: 300mg; Sus: 125mg/5mL, 250mg/5mL [60mL, 100mL]

WARNINGS/PRECAUTIONS: Caution in penicillin (PCN)-sensitive patients; cross-hypersensitivity among β-lactam antibiotics may occur. D/C use if an allergic reaction occurs. Serious acute hypersensitivity reactions may require the use of SQ epinephrine and other emergency measures. *Clostridium difficile*-associated diarrhea (CDAD) reported. May result in bacterial resistance with prolonged use in the absence of a proven or suspected bacterial infection, or a prophylactic indication; take appropriate measures if superinfection develops. Reduce dose in patients with transient or persistent renal insufficiency (CrCl <30mL/min). Caution in patients with a history of colitis. Lab test interaction may occur.

ADVERSE REACTIONS: Diarrhea, vaginal moniliasis, nausea, rash.

INTERACTIONS: Iron-fortified foods (except iron-fortified infant formula), iron supplements, and aluminum- or magnesium-containing antacids reduce absorption; take dose at least 2 hrs before or after these medications. Inhibited renal excretion with probenecid. Reddish stools reported with iron-containing products. Possible interaction with diclofenac reported.

PREGNANCY: Category B, safe in nursing.

MECHANISM OF ACTION: Cephalosporin (3rd generation); bactericidal activity results from its inhibition of cell-wall synthesis.

PHARMACOKINETICS: Absorption: Cap: (300mg) C_{max}=1.60mcg/mL, T_{max}=2.9 hrs, AUC=7.05mcg•hr/mL. (600mg) C_{max}=2.87mcg/mL, T_{max}=3 hrs, AUC=11.1mcg•hr/mL. Sus: (7mg/kg) C_{max}=2.30mcg/mL, T_{max}=2.2 hrs, AUC=8.31mcg•hr/mL. (14mg/kg) C_{max}=3.86mcg/mL, T_{max}=1.8 hrs, AUC=13.4mcg•hr/mL. **Distribution:** V_d=0.35L/kg (adults), 0.67L/kg (pediatrics); plasma protein binding (60-70%). **Elimination:** (300mg) Urine (18.4% unchanged); (600mg) Urine (11.6% unchanged); $T_{1/2}$=1.7 hrs.

NURSING CONSIDERATIONS

Assessment: Assess for allergy to other cephalosporins, PCN, or to other drugs, history of colitis, renal impairment, and for possible drug interactions. Assess for diabetes if planning to use suspension formulation.

Monitoring: Monitor for signs/symptoms of hypersensitivity reactions, CDAD, and development of superinfection.

Patient Counseling: Inform that therapy only treats bacterial, not viral, infections (eg, common cold). Instruct to take as directed; skipping doses or not completing full course may decrease drug effectiveness and increase risk of bacterial resistance. Instruct to take dose at least 2 hrs before or after antacid or iron supplements. Inform diabetic patients and caregiver that suspension contains 2.86g of sucrose/tsp. Inform that diarrhea (watery/bloody stools) may be experienced as late as 2 months or more after last dose; contact physician as soon as possible if this occurs.

Administration: Oral route. Take without regard to meals. (Sus) Shake well before use. Refer to PI for preparation instructions. **Storage:** Cap: 25°C (77°F); excursions permitted to 15-30°C (59-86°F). Unsuspended Powder: 20-25°C (68-77°F). Reconstituted Sus: Can be stored at controlled room temperature for 10 days.

CEFOXITIN   RX
cefoxitin (Various)

THERAPEUTIC CLASS: Cephalosporin (2nd generation)

INDICATIONS: Treatment of lower respiratory tract/urinary tract/intra-abdominal/gynecological/skin and skin structure/bone and joint infections and septicemia caused by susceptible strains of microorganisms. Prophylaxis of infection in patients undergoing uncontaminated GI surgery, abdominal/vaginal hysterectomy, or cesarean section (CS).

DOSAGE: *Adults:* Usual: 1-2g IV q6-8h. Uncomplicated Infections: 1g IV q6-8h. Moderately Severe/Severe Infections: 1g IV q4h or 2g IV q6-8h. Gas Gangrene/Other Infections Requiring Higher Dose: 2g IV q4h or 3g IV q6h. Renal Impairment: LD: 1-2g IV. Maint: CrCl 30-50mL/min: 1-2g IV q8-12h. CrCl 10-29mL/min: 1-2g IV q12-24h. CrCl 5-9mL/min: 0.5-1g IV q12-24h. CrCl <5mL/min: 0.5-1g IV q24-48h. Hemodialysis: LD: 1-2g IV after each hemodialysis. Maint: See renal impairment maintenance dose above. Group A β-Hemolytic Streptococcal Infection: Maintain therapy ≥10 days. Prophylaxis: Uncontaminated GI Surgery/Vaginal or Abdominal Hysterectomy: 2g IV prior to surgery (1/2-1 hr before initial incision), then 2g IV q6h after 1st dose for ≤24 hrs. CS: 2g IV single dose as soon as umbilical cord is clamped, or 2g IV as soon as umbilical cord is clamped, followed by 2g IV at 4 and 8 hrs after initial dose. *Pediatrics:* ≥3 Months: 80-160mg/kg/day divided into 4-6 equal doses. More Severe/Serious Infections: Use higher doses. Max: 12g/day. Renal Impairment: Modify dosage and frequency of dosage consistent with recommendations for adults. Prophylaxis: Uncontaminated GI Surgery/Vaginal or Abdominal Hysterectomy: 30-40mg/kg IV prior to surgery (1/2-1 hr before initial incision), then 30-40mg/kg IV q6h after 1st dose for ≤24 hrs.

HOW SUPPLIED: Inj: 1g, 2g

WARNINGS/PRECAUTIONS: Caution with previous hypersensitivity to cephalosporins, penicillins (PCNs), or other drugs. D/C if allergic reaction occurs. *Clostridium difficile*-associated diarrhea (CDAD) reported; d/c if CDAD suspected or confirmed. May result in overgrowth of nonsusceptible organisms with prolonged use or use in the absence of a proven or strongly suspected bacterial infection or prophylactic indication; take appropriate measures if superinfection develops. Appropriate anti-chlamydial coverage should be added when used in the treatment of pelvic inflammatory disease and *Chlamydia trachomatis* is the suspected pathogen. Lab test interactions may occur. Caution with impaired renal function, history of GI disease (particularly colitis), and in elderly.

ADVERSE REACTIONS: Local reactions, rash, pruritus, fever, dyspnea, hypotension, diarrhea, pseudomembranous colitis, exacerbation of myasthenia gravis, eosinophilia, leukopenia, thrombocytopenia, bone marrow depression, elevated LFTs, SrCr elevation.

INTERACTIONS: Increased nephrotoxicity with aminoglycoside antibiotics.

PREGNANCY: Category B, caution in nursing.

MECHANISM OF ACTION: Cephalosporin (2nd generation); bactericidal, inhibits cell-wall synthesis.

PHARMACOKINETICS: Distribution: Found in breast milk. **Elimination:** Urine (85% unchanged); $T_{1/2}$=41-59 min.

NURSING CONSIDERATIONS

Assessment: Assess for previous hypersensitivity reactions to cephalosporins, PCNs, or other drugs, renal impairment, GI disease (eg, colitis), pregnancy/nursing status, and possible drug interactions. Perform appropriate culture and susceptibility studies to determine susceptible causative organisms.

Monitoring: Monitor for signs/symptoms of an allergic reaction, CDAD, development of superinfection or drug resistance, and other adverse reactions. Periodically monitor renal/hepatic/hematopoietic functions, especially with prolonged therapy.

Patient Counseling: Inform that drug only treats bacterial, not viral, infections. Instruct to take exactly ud; skipping doses or not completing full course of therapy may decrease effectiveness and increase the likelihood of bacterial resistance. Inform that diarrhea may occur and will usually end if therapy is discontinued. Instruct to contact physician as soon as possible if watery/bloody stools (with/without stomach cramps, fever) develop even as late as 2 or more months after discontinuation.

Administration: IV route. Refer to PI for preparation, administration procedures, and compatibility and stability instructions. **Storage:** Dry State: 2-25°C (36-77°F). Avoid >50°C (122°F). Reconstituted Sol: Maintains satisfactory potency at room temperature for 6 hrs or for 1 week under refrigeration (<5°C [41°F]). Further Diluted Sol: Room temperature for additional 18 hrs or additional 48 hrs under refrigeration.

CEFPODOXIME   RX
cefpodoxime proxetil (Various)

THERAPEUTIC CLASS: Cephalosporin (3rd generation)

INDICATIONS: Treatment of mild to moderate infections (acute otitis media, pharyngitis, tonsillitis, community-acquired pneumonia [CAP], acute bacterial exacerbation of chronic bronchitis [ABECB], acute uncomplicated urethral and cervical gonorrhea, acute uncomplicated anorectal infections in women, uncomplicated skin and skin structure infections [SSSIs], acute maxillary sinusitis, and uncomplicated urinary tract infections [UTIs] [cystitis]) caused by susceptible strains of microorganisms.

DOSAGE: *Adults:* Pharyngitis/Tonsillitis: 100mg q12h for 5-10 days. CAP: 200mg q12h for 14 days. Uncomplicated Gonorrhea (Men/Women)/Rectal Gonococcal Infections (Women): 200mg single dose. SSSI: 400mg q12h for 7-14 days. Acute Maxillary Sinusitis: 200mg q12h for 10 days. Uncomplicated UTI: 100mg q12h for 7 days. CrCl <30mL/min: Increase dosing intervals to q24h. Hemodialysis: Dose 3X/week after hemodialysis. (Tab) ABECB: 200mg q12h for 10 days. Take with food.
Pediatrics: ≥12 Yrs: Pharyngitis/Tonsillitis: 100mg q12h for 5-10 days. CAP: 200mg q12h for 14 days. Uncomplicated Gonorrhea (Men/Women)/Rectal Gonococcal Infections (Women): 200mg single dose. SSSI: 400mg q12h for 7-14 days. Acute Maxillary Sinusitis: 200mg q12h for 10 days. Uncomplicated UTI: 100mg q12h for 7 days. (Tab) ABECB: 200mg q12h for 10 days. 2 Months-12 Yrs: (Sus) Acute Otitis Media: 5mg/kg q12h (max 200mg/dose) for 5 days. Pharyngitis/Tonsillitis: 5mg/kg/dose q12h (max 100mg/dose) for 5-10 days. Acute Maxillary Sinusitis: 5mg/kg q12h (max 200mg/dose) for 10 days. (Sus/Tab) CrCl <30mL/min: Increase dosing intervals to q24h. Hemodialysis: Dose 3X/week after hemodialysis. (Tab) Take with food.

HOW SUPPLIED: Sus: 50mg/5mL, 100mg/5mL [50mL, 100mL]; Tab: 100mg, 200mg

WARNINGS/PRECAUTIONS: Cross hypersensitivity among β-lactam antibiotics reported; caution in patients with penicillin (PCN) sensitivity. D/C if an allergic reaction occurs. Serious acute hypersensitivity reactions may require treatment with epinephrine and other emergency measures. *Clostridium difficile*-associated diarrhea (CDAD) reported; d/c if CDAD is suspected or confirmed. Pseudomembranous colitis reported. May result in bacterial resistance with prolonged use or in the absence of proven or suspected bacterial infection, or a prophylactic indication; take appropriate measures if superinfection develops. Lab test interactions may occur.

ADVERSE REACTIONS: Diarrhea, nausea.

INTERACTIONS: High doses of antacids (sodium bicarbonate and aluminum hydroxide) or H_2 blockers reduce C_{max} and the extent of absorption. Oral anticholinergics (eg, propantheline) delay C_{max}. Probenecid inhibits renal excretion; monitor renal function with nephrotoxic agents. Caution with potent diuretics.

PREGNANCY: Category B, not for use in nursing.

MECHANISM OF ACTION: Cephalosporin (3rd generation); bactericidal agent that acts by inhibition of bacterial cell wall synthesis.

PHARMACOKINETICS: Absorption: (Tab) C_{max}=1.4mcg/mL (100mg), 2.3mcg/mL (200mg), 3.9mcg/mL (400mg); T_{max}=2-3 hrs. (Sus) C_{max}=1.5mcg/mL (100mg). **Distribution:** Plasma protein binding (21-29%); found in breast milk. **Metabolism:** Via deesterification; cefpodoxime (active metabolite). **Elimination:** Urine (29-33% unchanged). (Tab) $T_{1/2}$=2.09-2.84 hrs.

NURSING CONSIDERATIONS

Assessment: Assess for history of hypersensitivity to cephalosporins, PCNs, or other drugs, renal impairment, pregnancy/nursing status, and possible drug interactions. Perform culture and susceptibility testing.

Monitoring: Monitor for signs/symptoms of hypersensitivity reactions, CDAD, pseudomembranous colitis, development of superinfection, and other adverse reactions.

Patient Counseling: Inform that therapy should only be used to treat bacterial, not viral (eg, common cold), infections. Instruct to take exactly ud even if the patient feels better early in the course of therapy. Inform that skipping doses or not completing the full course of therapy may decrease effectiveness of immediate treatment and increase bacterial resistance. Inform that diarrhea is a common problem caused by therapy, which usually ends when therapy is discontinued. Instruct to immediately contact physician if watery and bloody stools (with or without stomach cramps and fever) occur, even as late as ≥2 months after the last dose. (Sus) Inform that drug contains phenylalanine.

Administration: Oral route. (Sus) May be given without regard to food. Shake well before using. Refer to PI for constitution directions. (Tab) Take with food. **Storage:** 20-25°C (68-77°F). (Sus) After Constitution: 2-8°C (36-46°F). Discard unused portion after 14 days.

CEFPROZIL   RX
cefprozil (Various)

THERAPEUTIC CLASS: Cephalosporin (2nd generation)

INDICATIONS: Treatment of mild to moderate pharyngitis/tonsillitis, otitis media, acute sinusitis, secondary bacterial infection of acute bronchitis, acute bacterial exacerbation of chronic bronchitis (ABECB), and uncomplicated skin and skin structure infections (SSSIs) caused by susceptible strains of microorganisms.

DOSAGE: *Adults:* Pharyngitis/Tonsillitis: 500mg q24h for 10 days. Acute Sinusitis: 250-500mg q12h for 10 days. ABECB/Acute Bronchitis: 500mg q12h for 10 days. SSSI: 250-500mg q12h or 500mg q24h for 10 days. CrCl <30mL/min: 50% of standard dose.
Pediatrics: ≥13 Yrs: Use adult dose. 2-12 Yrs: Pharyngitis/Tonsillitis: 7.5mg/kg q12h for 10 days. SSSI: 20mg/kg q24h for 10 days. 6 Months-12 Yrs: Otitis Media: 15mg/kg q12h for 10 days. Acute Sinusitis: 7.5-15mg/kg q12h for 10 days. Do not exceed adult dose. CrCl <30mL/min: 50% of standard dose.

HOW SUPPLIED: Sus: 125mg/5mL, 250mg/5mL [50mL, 75mL, 100mL]; Tab: 250mg, 500mg

WARNINGS/PRECAUTIONS: Caution with previous hypersensitivity to cephalosporins, penicillins (PCNs), or other drugs; cross-sensitivity may occur with history of PCN allergy. D/C if allergic reaction occurs. *Clostridium difficile*-associated diarrhea (CDAD) reported. May result in bacterial resistance with prolonged use or use in the absence of a proven/suspected bacterial infection or a prophylactic indication; take appropriate measures if superinfection develops. Caution with GI disease, particularly colitis. Caution with renal impairment and elderly. Lab test interactions may occur.

ADVERSE REACTIONS: Diarrhea, N/V, ALT/AST elevation, eosinophilia, genital pruritus, vaginitis, superinfection, diaper rash, dizziness, abdominal pain.

INTERACTIONS: Nephrotoxicity with aminoglycosides reported. Probenecid may increase plasma levels. Caution with potent diuretics.

PREGNANCY: Category B, caution in nursing.

MECHANISM OF ACTION: Cephalosporin (2nd generation); bactericidal activity results from its inhibition of cell-wall synthesis.

PHARMACOKINETICS: Absorption: C_{max}=6.1mcg/mL (250mg), 10.5mcg/mL (500mg), 18.3mcg/mL (1g); T_{max}=1.5 hrs (adults), 1-2 hrs (peds). Plasma concentration (peds) at 7.5, 15, and 30mg/kg doses similar to those observed within same time frame in normal adults at 250, 500, and 1000mg doses, respectively. **Distribution:** V_d=0.23L/kg; plasma protein binding (36%); found in breast milk. **Elimination:** Urine (60%); $T_{1/2}$=1.3 hrs (adults), 1.5 hrs (peds).

NURSING CONSIDERATIONS

Assessment: Assess for previous hypersensitivity reactions to PCNs/cephalosporins or other drugs, renal/hepatic function, GI disease, pregnancy/nursing status, and possible drug interactions. Perform appropriate culture and susceptibility studies to determine susceptible causative organisms.

Monitoring: Periodically monitor renal/hepatic/hematopoietic functions. Monitor for CDAD (may range from mild diarrhea to fatal colitis), development of superinfections or drug resistance, allergic reactions, and other adverse reactions.

Patient Counseling: Inform that the oral sus contains phenylalanine. Inform that drug only treats bacterial, not viral, infections. Instruct to take ud and that skipping doses or not completing full course may decrease effectiveness and increase resistance. Inform about potential benefits/risks. Notify physician if watery/bloody stools (with/without stomach cramps/fever) occur even ≥2 months after therapy. Notify if pregnant/nursing.

Administration: Oral route. Shake susp well before use. Refer to PI for reconstitution direction.
Storage: Tab/Dry Powder: 20-25°C (68-77°F). Reconstituted Sus: Refrigerate after mixing and discard unused portion after 14 days.

CEFTIN   RX
cefuroxime axetil (GlaxoSmithKline)

THERAPEUTIC CLASS: Cephalosporin (2nd generation)

INDICATIONS: Treatment of the following infections caused by susceptible strains of microorganisms: (Sus/Tab) Pharyngitis/tonsillitis and acute otitis media. (Sus) Impetigo. (Tab) Uncomplicated skin and skin structure infections (SSSIs), uncomplicated urinary tract infections (UTIs), uncomplicated gonorrhea, early Lyme disease, acute bacterial maxillary sinusitis, acute bacterial exacerbations of chronic bronchitis (ABECB), and secondary bacterial infections of acute bronchitis.

DOSAGE: *Adults:* (Tab) Pharyngitis/Tonsillitis/Sinusitis: 250mg bid for 10 days. ABECB/SSSI: 250-500mg bid for 10 days. Acute Bronchitis: 250-500mg bid for 5-10 days. UTI: 250mg bid for 7-10 days. Gonorrhea: 1000mg single dose. Lyme Disease: 500mg bid for 20 days.
Pediatrics: ≥13 Yrs: (Tab) Pharyngitis/Tonsillitis/Sinusitis: 250mg bid for 10 days. ABECB/SSSI: 250-500mg bid for 10 days. Acute Bronchitis: 250-500mg bid for 5-10 days. UTI: 250mg bid for 7-10 days. Gonorrhea: 1000mg single dose. Lyme Disease: 500mg bid for 20 days. 3 Months-12 Yrs: (Sus) Pharyngitis/Tonsillitis: 20mg/kg/day divided bid for 10 days. Max: 500mg/day. Otitis Media/Sinusitis/Impetigo: 30mg/kg/day divided bid for 10 days. Max: 1000mg/day. (Tab-If Can Swallow Whole) Otitis Media/Sinusitis: 250mg bid for 10 days.

HOW SUPPLIED: Sus: 125mg/5mL [100mL], 250mg/5mL [50mL, 100mL]; Tab: 250mg, 500mg

WARNINGS/PRECAUTIONS: Tabs are not bioequivalent to sus. Caution in patients with previous hypersensitivity to penicillins (PCNs) or other drugs; cross-sensitivity may occur in patients with a history of PCN allergy. D/C if an allergic reaction occurs. *Clostridium difficile*-associated diarrhea (CDAD) reported. May result in bacterial resistance with prolonged use or use in the absence of a proven/suspected bacterial infection or a prophylactic indication; take appropriate measures if superinfection develops. May cause fall in PT; those at risk include patients previously stable on anticoagulants, patients receiving protracted course of antibiotics, patients with renal/hepatic impairment, and patients in a poor nutritional state. Monitor PT and give vitamin K PRN. Lab test interactions may occur. (Sus) Contains phenylalanine.

ADVERSE REACTIONS: Diarrhea, N/V, vaginitis, (sus) dislike of taste, diaper rash.

INTERACTIONS: Probenecid increases plasma levels. Lower bioavailability with drugs that lower gastric acidity. Caution with agents causing adverse effects on renal function (diuretics). May lower estrogen reabsorption and reduce the efficacy of combined oral estrogen/progesterone contraceptives.

PREGNANCY: Category B, not for use in nursing.

MECHANISM OF ACTION: Cephalosporin (2nd generation); binds to essential target proteins and the resultant inhibition of cell-wall synthesis.

PHARMACOKINETICS: Absorption: Absolute bioavailability (37% before food), (52% after food). PO administration of variable doses resulted in different parameters. **Distribution:** Plasma protein binding (50%); found in breast milk. **Metabolism:** Rapid hydrolysis, via nonspecific esterases in the intestinal mucosa and blood. **Elimination:** Urine (50% unchanged).

NURSING CONSIDERATIONS

Assessment: Assess for previous hypersensitivity reactions to cephalosporins/PCNs or other drugs, renal/hepatic impairment, nutritional state, history of colitis, GI malabsorption, pregnancy/nursing status, and for possible drug interactions. For patients planning on using sus formulation, assess for phenylketonuria.

Monitoring: Monitor signs/symptoms of an allergic reaction, CDAD, and superinfection. Monitor PT and renal function.

Patient Counseling: Advise of potential benefits/risks of therapy. Inform that drug only treats bacterial, not viral, infections. Instruct to take exactly as directed; skipping doses or not completing full course may decrease effectiveness and increase resistance. Counsel to d/c and notify physician if an allergic reaction or if watery/bloody diarrhea (with/without stomach cramps or fever) develops. Instruct to notify physician if pregnant/nursing. Inform caregivers of pediatric patients that if the patient cannot swallow tab whole, they should receive oral sus. Advise that crushed tab has a strong/persistent bitter taste. Inform that tab may be administered without regard to meals but oral sus must be administered with food.

Administration: Oral route. Tab and sus are not bioequivalent and not substitutable on mg-per-mg basis. Refer to PI for reconstitution instructions for sus. Shake sus well before use. **Storage:** Tab: Store at 15-30°C (59-86°F). Sus Powder: Store at 2-30°C (36-86°F). Reconstituted Sus: Store at 2-8°C (36-46°F) in a refrigerator; discard after 10 days.

CEFTRIAXONE   RX
ceftriaxone sodium (Various)

OTHER BRAND NAMES: Rocephin (Genentech)

THERAPEUTIC CLASS: Cephalosporin (3rd generation)

INDICATIONS: Treatment of lower respiratory tract infections, acute bacterial otitis media, skin and skin structure infections (SSSIs), urinary tract infections, uncomplicated gonorrhea (cervical/urethral and rectal), pelvic inflammatory disease, bacterial septicemia, bone and joint infections, intra-abdominal infections, and meningitis caused by susceptible strains of microorganisms. Surgical prophylaxis during surgical procedures classified as contaminated or potentially contaminated and in surgical patients for whom infection at the operative site would present serious risk.

DOSAGE: *Adults:* Usual: 1-2g/day IV/IM given qd or in equally divided doses bid depending on the type and severity of infection. *Staphylococcus aureus* Infections: 2-4g/day. Max: 4g/day. Uncomplicated Gonococcal Infections: 250mg IM single dose. Surgical Prophylaxis: 1g IV single dose 1/2-2 hrs before surgery. Continue therapy for ≥2 days after signs and symptoms of infection have disappeared. Usual duration: 4-14 days; complicated infections may require longer therapy. *Streptococcus pyogenes* Infections: Continue therapy for ≥10 days. Hepatic Dysfunction and Significant Renal Disease: Max: 2g/day.
Pediatrics: SSSI: 50-75mg/kg/day IV/IM given qd or in equally divided doses bid. Max: 2g/day. Acute Bacterial Otitis Media: 50mg/kg (up to 1g) IM single dose. Serious Infections: 50-75mg/kg

IV/IM given q12h. Max: 2g/day. Meningitis: Initial: 100mg/kg (up to 4g) IV/IM, then 100mg/kg/day IV/IM given qd or in equally divided doses q12h for 7-14 days. Max: 4g/day.

HOW SUPPLIED: Inj: 250mg, 500mg, 1g, 2g; (Rocephin) 500mg, 1g

CONTRAINDICATIONS: Hyperbilirubinemic neonates (≤28 days), especially if premature; concurrent use of Ca^{2+}-containing IV solutions used in neonates.

WARNINGS/PRECAUTIONS: Caution in penicillin (PCN)-sensitive patients. D/C if an allergic reaction occurs; serious acute hypersensitivity reactions may require the use of SQ epinephrine and other emergency measures. Anaphylactic reactions reported. *Clostridium difficile*-associated diarrhea (CDAD) reported; d/c therapy if CDAD is suspected/confirmed. Severe cases of hemolytic anemia reported; consider and d/c until cause is determined. May result in overgrowth of nonsusceptible organisms with prolonged use or use in the absence of a proven or strongly suspected bacterial infection or prophylactic indication; take appropriate measures if superinfection develops. Transient BUN and SrCr elevations may occur. Caution in patients with both hepatic dysfunction and significant renal disease. Alterations in PT may occur rarely; monitor with impaired vitamin K synthesis or low vitamin K stores during treatment (eg, chronic hepatitis disease, malnutrition). Caution with history of GI disease, especially colitis. Gallbladder sonographic abnormalities reported; d/c if signs and symptoms of gallbladder disease develop. Pancreatitis reported rarely.

ADVERSE REACTIONS: Inj-site reactions (eg, warmth, tightness, induration), eosinophilia, thrombocytosis, AST/ALT elevation.

INTERACTIONS: See Contraindications.

PREGNANCY: Category B, caution in nursing.

MECHANISM OF ACTION: Cephalosporin (3rd generation); bactericidal agent that acts by inhibition of bacterial cell-wall synthesis.

PHARMACOKINETICS: Absorption: (IM) Complete; T_{max}=2-3 hrs. (Pediatrics) Bacterial meningitis: C_{max}=216mcg/mL (50mg/kg IV), 275mcg/mL (75mg/kg IV). Middle Ear Fluid: C_{max}=35mcg/mL; T_{max}=24 hrs. **Distribution:** Found in breast milk, crosses placenta; plasma protein binding (95%) (<25mcg/mL), (85%) (300mcg/mL); (Adults, healthy) V_d=5.78-13.5L. (Pediatrics) Bacterial Meningitis: V_d=338mL/kg (50mg/kg IV), 373mL/kg (75mg/kg IV). **Elimination:** Urine (33-67%, unchanged), feces. (Adults, healthy) $T_{1/2}$=5.8-8.7 hrs. (Pediatrics) Bacterial Meningitis: $T_{1/2}$=4.6 hrs (50mg/kg IV), 4.3 hrs (75mg/kg IV). Middle Ear Fluid: $T_{1/2}$=25 hrs.

NURSING CONSIDERATIONS

Assessment: Assess for hyperbilirubinemic neonates, especially if premature, hypersensitivity to cephalosporins/PCNs/other drugs, presence of both hepatic dysfunction and significant renal disease, impaired vitamin K synthesis or low vitamin K stores, history of GI disease (eg, colitis), pregnancy/nursing status, and possible drug interactions. Obtain appropriate specimens for isolation of the causative organism and for determination of susceptibility to the drug.

Monitoring: Monitor for signs/symptoms of hypersensitivity reactions, CDAD, overgrowth of nonsusceptible organisms (eg, superinfection), gallbladder disease, and pancreatitis. Periodically monitor BUN and SrCr levels. Monitor PT levels in patients with impaired vitamin K synthesis or low vitamin K stores (eg, chronic hepatic disease, malnutrition).

Patient Counseling: Inform that therapy only treats bacterial, not viral (eg, common cold), infections. Instruct to take exactly ud even if the patient is feeling better early in the course of therapy; skipping doses or not completing full course may decrease drug effectiveness and increase the likelihood of bacteria resistance. Instruct to contact physician as soon as possible if watery and bloody stools (with/without stomach cramps, fever) develop even as late as 2 or more months after having taken the last dose of therapy.

Administration: IV/IM route. Physically incompatible with vancomycin, amsacrine, aminoglycosides, and fluconazole; when administered concomitantly by intermittent IV infusion, give sequentially, with thorough flushing of the IV lines between administrations. Do not use diluents containing Ca^{2+} (eg, Ringer's sol or Hartmann's sol) to reconstitute or further dilute a reconstituted vial for IV administration. Avoid physically mixing with or piggybacking into sol containing other antimicrobial drugs. IV infusion should be administered over a period of 30 min. Refer to PI for reconstitution, compatibility, and stability directions. **Storage:** 20-25°C (68-77°F). Protect from light. Do not refreeze. Rocephin: ≤25°C (77°F).

CELEBREX

celecoxib (G.D. Searle)

> May increase risk of serious cardiovascular (CV) thrombotic events, myocardial infarction (MI), and stroke, which can be fatal; increased risk with duration of use and with CV disease (CVD) or risk factors for CVD. Increased risk of serious GI adverse events (eg, bleeding, ulceration, perforation of stomach/intestines) that can be fatal and occur anytime during use without warning symptoms; elderly patients are at a greater risk. Contraindicated for treatment of perioperative pain in the setting of coronary artery bypass graft (CABG) surgery.

THERAPEUTIC CLASS: COX-2 inhibitor

INDICATIONS: Relief of signs and symptoms of osteoarthritis (OA), rheumatoid arthritis (RA), and ankylosing spondylitis (AS). Management of acute pain (AP) in adults. Treatment of primary dysmenorrhea (PD). Relief of signs and symptoms of juvenile rheumatoid arthritis (JRA) in patients ≥2 yrs of age.

DOSAGE: *Adults:* OA: Usual: 200mg qd or 100mg bid. RA: Usual: 100-200mg bid. AS: Usual: 200mg qd or 100mg bid. Titrate: May increase to 400mg/day if no effect is observed after 6 weeks; consider alternative treatment if no effect is observed after 6 weeks on 400mg/day. AP/PD: Day 1: 400mg initially, then 200mg if needed. Maint: 200mg bid PRN. Moderate Hepatic Impairment (Child-Pugh Class B): Usual: Reduce daily dose by 50%. Poor Metabolizers of CYP2C9 Substrates: Initial: Consider half the lowest recommended dose. Elderly: <50kg: Initial: Lowest recommended dose.
Pediatrics: ≥2 Yrs: JRA: >25kg: Usual: 100mg bid. 10-25kg: Usual: 50mg bid. Moderate Hepatic Impairment (Child-Pugh Class B): Usual: Reduce daily dose by 50%. Poor Metabolizers of CYP2C9 Substrates: Consider using alternative management.

HOW SUPPLIED: Cap: 50mg, 100mg, 200mg, 400mg

CONTRAINDICATIONS: History of allergic-type reactions to sulfonamides, history of asthma, urticaria, or other allergic-type reactions with aspirin (ASA) or other NSAIDs, active GI bleeding. Treatment of perioperative pain in the setting of CABG surgery.

WARNINGS/PRECAUTIONS: Use lowest effective dose for the shortest duration possible. Not recommended with severe hepatic impairment. May lead to onset of new HTN or worsening of preexisting HTN; caution with HTN, and monitor BP closely. Fluid retention and edema reported; caution with fluid retention or heart failure (HF). Caution with history of ulcer disease, GI bleeding, and other risk factors for GI bleeding (eg, prolonged NSAID therapy, older age, poor general health status); monitor for GI ulceration/bleeding. May cause elevations of LFTs or severe hepatic reactions (eg, jaundice, fatal fulminant hepatitis, liver necrosis, hepatic failure); d/c if liver disease develops or systemic manifestations occur, or if abnormal LFTs persist/worsen. Renal injury reported with long-term use; increased risk with renal/hepatic impairment, HF, and in elderly. Not recommended with advanced renal disease; if therapy must be initiated, closely monitor renal function. D/C if abnormal renal tests persist/worsen. Anaphylactoid/anaphylactic reactions and angioedema reported. Caution with asthma and avoid with ASA-sensitive asthma and the ASA triad. May cause serious skin adverse events (eg, exfoliative dermatitis, Stevens-Johnson syndrome, toxic epidermal necrolysis); d/c at 1st appearance of skin rash or any other sign of hypersensitivity. Avoid in late pregnancy (starting at 30 weeks gestation); may cause premature closure of ductus arteriosus. Not a substitute for corticosteroids or for the treatment of corticosteroid insufficiency. Anemia reported; monitor Hgb/Hct if signs/symptoms of anemia or blood loss develop with long-term use. Caution in pediatric patients with systemic onset JRA due to risk of disseminated intravascular coagulation. Monitor CBC and chemistry profile periodically with long-term treatment. May mask signs of inflammation and fever. Caution with poor CYP2C9 metabolizers. Not a substitute for ASA for CV prophylaxis.

ADVERSE REACTIONS: CV thrombotic events, MI, stroke, GI adverse events, headache, HTN, diarrhea, fever, dyspepsia, upper respiratory infection, abdominal pain, N/V, cough, nasopharyngitis.

INTERACTIONS: Avoid with non-ASA NSAIDs. Caution with CYP2C9 inhibitors. Potential interaction with CYP2D6 substrates. Warfarin or similar agents may increase risk of bleeding complications; monitor anticoagulant activity. May increase lithium levels; monitor closely. ASA may increase rate of GI ulceration or other complications. May diminish the antihypertensive effect of ACE inhibitors and ARBs. Fluconazole may increase levels. May reduce the natriuretic effect of loop diuretics (eg, furosemide) and thiazides. Oral corticosteroids, anticoagulants, smoking, or alcohol may increase risk of GI bleeding. Risk of renal toxicity with diuretics, ACE inhibitors, and ARBs. Aluminum- and magnesium-containing antacids may reduce plasma concentrations.

PREGNANCY: Category C (<30 weeks gestation) and D (≥30 weeks gestation), caution in nursing.

MECHANISM OF ACTION: NSAID (COX-2 inhibitor); inhibits prostaglandin synthesis, primarily via inhibition of COX-2.

PHARMACOKINETICS: Absorption: C_{max}=705ng/mL, T_{max}=2.8 hrs (fasted, 200mg). **Distribution:** V_d=429L (fasted, 200mg); plasma protein binding (97%); found in breast milk. **Metabolism:** CYP2C9. **Elimination:** Feces (57%), urine (27%), urine and feces (<3% unchanged); $T_{1/2}$=11.2 hrs (fasted, 200mg).

NURSING CONSIDERATIONS

Assessment: Assess for history of allergic-type reactions to sulfonamides, history of asthma, urticaria, other allergic-type reactions with ASA or other NSAIDs, active GI bleeding, CVD, risk factors for CVD, renal/hepatic impairment, HTN, history of ulcer disease or GI bleeding, risk factors for GI bleeding, asthma, ASA triad, other conditions where treatment is contraindicated or cautioned, pregnancy/nursing status, and possible drug interactions.

Monitoring: Monitor for signs/symptoms of CV thrombotic events, GI events, anaphylactoid/hypersensitivity reactions, and other adverse reactions. Monitor BP, renal function, LFTs, CBC, and chemistry profile periodically. Monitor for development of abnormal coagulation tests in patients with systemic onset JRA.

Patient Counseling: Advise to seek medical attention if signs/symptoms of CV events (eg, chest pain, SOB, weakness, slurring of speech), GI ulceration/bleeding (eg, epigastric pain, dyspepsia, melena, hematemesis), hepatotoxicity (eg, nausea, fatigue, lethargy, pruritus, jaundice, right upper quadrant tenderness, and flu-like symptoms), skin/hypersensitivity reactions (eg, rash, blisters, fever, itching), unexplained weight gain or edema, or anaphylactoid reactions (eg, difficulty breathing, swelling of the face/throat) occur. Instruct to d/c the drug immediately if any type of rash, or if signs/symptoms of hepatotoxicity, occur. Instruct patients with preexisting asthma to seek immediate medical attention if asthma worsens after taking the medication. Inform that medication should be avoided in late pregnancy.

Administration: Oral route. May be given without regard to timing of meals. For patients with difficulty swallowing caps, contents may be added to applesauce and ingested immediately with water. **Storage:** 25°C (77°F); excursions permitted to 15-30°C (59-86°F). Sprinkled contents on applesauce are stable for up to 6 hrs at 2-8°C (35-45°F).

CELEXA   RX
citalopram HBr (Forest)

> Antidepressants increased the risk of suicidal thinking and behavior (suicidality) in children, adolescents, and young adults in short-term studies of major depressive disorder (MDD) and other psychiatric disorders. Monitor and observe closely for clinical worsening, suicidality, or unusual changes in behavior in patients who are started on antidepressant therapy. Not approved for use in pediatric patients.

THERAPEUTIC CLASS: Selective serotonin reuptake inhibitor

INDICATIONS: Treatment of depression.

DOSAGE: *Adults:* Initial: 20mg qd. Titrate: Increase dose to 40mg/day at an interval of no <1 week. Max: 40mg/day. Maint: Consider decreasing dose to 20mg/day if adverse reactions are bothersome. Discontinuation of Treatment: Consider resuming previously prescribed dose if intolerable symptoms occur following a decrease in dose or upon discontinuation of treatment. May continue decreasing the dose subsequently but at a more gradual rate. Elderly (>60 Yrs)/Hepatic Impairment/CYP2C19 Poor Metabolizers/Concomitant Cimetidine or Another CYP2C19 Inhibitor: Max: 20mg/day. Switching to/from an MAOI for Psychiatric Disorders: Allow at least 14 days between discontinuation of an MAOI and initiation of treatment, and allow at least 14 days between discontinuation of treatment and initiation of an MAOI. Use with Other MAOIs (eg, Linezolid, Methylene Blue): Refer to PI.

HOW SUPPLIED: Sol: 10mg/5mL [240mL]; Tab: 10mg, 20mg*, 40mg* *scored

CONTRAINDICATIONS: Use of an MAOI for psychiatric disorders either concomitantly or within 14 days of stopping treatment. Treatment within 14 days of stopping an MAOI for psychiatric disorders. Starting treatment in a patient being treated with MAOIs (eg, linezolid or IV methylene blue). Concomitant use with pimozide.

WARNINGS/PRECAUTIONS: Not approved for the treatment of bipolar depression. May cause dose-dependent QTc prolongation. Avoid in patients with congenital long QT syndrome, bradycardia, hypokalemia or hypomagnesemia, recent acute myocardial infarction (AMI), or uncompensated heart failure (HF); monitor ECG if therapy is needed. Correct hypokalemia and/or hypomagnesemia prior to initiation of therapy and monitor periodically. D/C therapy if found to have persistent QTc measurements >500 msec. May precipitate mixed/manic episode in patients at risk for bipolar disorder; screen for risk for bipolar disorder prior to initiating treatment. Serotonin syndrome reported; d/c immediately and initiate supportive symptomatic treatment. Avoid abrupt discontinuation; gradually reduce dose. May increase the risk of bleeding events. Hyponatremia may occur; caution in elderly and volume-depleted patients. Consider discontinuing in patients with symptomatic hyponatremia and institute appropriate medical intervention.

Activation of mania/hypomania reported; caution with history of mania. Seizures reported; caution with history of seizure disorder. Caution with hepatic impairment, severe renal impairment, and in pregnancy (3rd trimester). May impair mental/physical abilities.

ADVERSE REACTIONS: N/V, dyspepsia, diarrhea, dry mouth, somnolence, insomnia, increased sweating, ejaculation disorder, rhinitis, anxiety, anorexia, tremor, agitation, sinusitis.

INTERACTIONS: See Contraindications. Avoid with alcohol, other drugs that prolong the QTc interval (Class 1A [eg, quinidine, procainamide] or Class III [eg, amiodarone, sotalol] antiarrhythmic medications, antipsychotic medications [eg, chlorpromazine, thioridazine], antibiotics [eg, gatifloxacin, moxifloxacin], pentamidine, levomethadyl acetate, or methadone). Caution with other centrally acting drugs or TCAs (eg, imipramine). Risk of QT prolongation with CYP2C19 inhibitors (eg, cimetidine). May cause serotonin syndrome with other serotonergic drugs (eg, triptans, TCAs, fentanyl, lithium, tramadol, tryptophan, buspirone, St. John's wort) and with drugs that impair metabolism of serotonin; d/c immediately if this occurs. Increased risk of bleeding with aspirin (ASA), NSAIDs, warfarin, and other drugs that affect coagulation. Rare reports of weakness, hyperreflexia, and incoordination with sumatriptan. Possible increased clearance with carbamazepine. May decrease levels of ketoconazole. May increase levels of metoprolol. Increased risk of hyponatremia with diuretics.

PREGNANCY: Category C, not for use in nursing.

MECHANISM OF ACTION: SSRI; presumed to be linked to potentiation of serotonergic activity in the CNS, resulting from its inhibition of CNS neuronal reuptake of serotonin.

PHARMACOKINETICS: Absorption: T_{max}=4 hrs, absolute bioavailability (80%). **Distribution:** Plasma protein binding (80%); V_d=12L/kg; found in breast milk. **Metabolism:** Hepatic; N-demethylation via CYP3A4, 2C19; demethylcitalopram (DCT), didemethylcitalopram, citalopram-N-oxide, deaminated propionic acid derivative (metabolites). **Elimination:** (IV) Urine (10% unchanged, 5% DCT); $T_{1/2}$=35 hrs.

NURSING CONSIDERATIONS

Assessment: Assess for risk for bipolar disorder, history of mania, history of seizures, volume depletion, hypokalemia, hypomagnesemia, bradycardia, recent AMI, uncompensated HF, hepatic/renal impairment, drug hypersensitivity, congenital long QT syndrome, pregnancy/nursing status, and possible drug interactions. Obtain baseline serum K^+ and Mg^{2+} measurements for patients being considered for therapy who are at risk for significant electrolyte disturbances.

Monitoring: Monitor for signs/symptoms of clinical worsening (suicidality, unusual changes in behavior), serotonin syndrome, abnormal bleeding, hyponatremia, seizures, cognitive and motor impairment and other adverse reactions. Monitor electrolytes in patients with diseases or conditions that cause hypokalemia or hypomagnesemia. Monitor ECG in patients with cardiac conditions/disorders and in patients on concomitant QTc interval prolonging agents. If therapy is abruptly discontinued, monitor for discontinuation symptoms.

Patient Counseling: Inform about the benefits and risks of therapy. Counsel on the appropriate use of the drug. Advise to look for emergence of symptoms associated with an increased risk for suicidal thinking/behavior; instruct to report such symptoms, especially if severe, abrupt in onset, or not part of presenting symptoms. Caution about the concomitant use with triptans, tramadol, other serotonergic agents, ASA, NSAIDs, warfarin, or other drugs that affect coagulation. Instruct to notify physician if taking or planning to take any prescribed or OTC drugs. Inform that improvement may be noticed in 1-4 weeks; instruct to continue therapy ud. Caution against performing hazardous tasks (eg, operating machinery, driving). Instruct to avoid alcohol. Instruct to notify physician if pregnant, intending to become pregnant, or are breastfeeding.

Administration: Oral route. Administer qd, in am or pm, with or without food. **Storage:** 25°C (77°F); excursions permitted to 15-30°C (59-86°F).

CELLCEPT   RX
mycophenolate mofetil (Genentech)

Use during pregnancy is associated with increased risks of 1st trimester pregnancy loss and congenital malformations; counsel females of reproductive potential regarding pregnancy prevention and planning. Immunosuppression may lead to increased susceptibility to infection and possible development of lymphoma. Only physicians experienced in immunosuppressive therapy and management of renal, cardiac or hepatic transplant patients should prescribe mycophenolate mofetil. Manage patients in facilities equipped and staffed with adequate lab and supportive medical resources. Physician responsible for maintenance therapy should have complete information requisite for follow-up of the patient.

THERAPEUTIC CLASS: Inosine monophosphate dehydrogenase inhibitor

INDICATIONS: Prophylaxis of organ rejection in allogeneic renal, cardiac, or hepatic transplants; used concomitantly with cyclosporine and corticosteroids.

DOSAGE: *Adults:* Renal Transplant: 1g PO/IV bid. Cardiac Transplant: 1.5g PO/IV bid. Hepatic Transplant: 1.5g PO bid or 1g IV bid. Start PO dose as soon as possible after transplant. If unable to take PO medication, may alternatively start IV dose within 24 hrs after transplant and continue for up to 14 days; administer each dose over no <2 hrs. Switch to PO as soon as patient can tolerate PO therapy. Give PO on an empty stomach.

Pediatrics: 3 Months-18 Yrs: Renal Transplant: Usual: 600mg/m² sus bid. Max: 2g/10mL/day. BSA >1.5m²: 1g cap/tab bid. BSA 1.25m²-1.5m²: 750mg cap bid. Give PO on an empty stomach.

HOW SUPPLIED: Cap: 250mg; Inj: (HCl) 500mg/20mL; Sus: 200mg/mL; Tab: 500mg

WARNINGS/PRECAUTIONS: Do not administer IV dose by rapid or bolus inj. Limit exposure to sunlight and UV light due to increased risk for skin cancer. Activation of latent viral infections, including progressive multifocal leukoencephalopathy (PML) and BK virus-associated nephropathy (BKVAN), reported; consider reducing amount of immunosuppression if PML/BKVAN develops. Severe neutropenia reported; d/c or reduce dose if absolute neutrophil count (ANC) becomes <1.3 x 10³/μL. Cases of pure red cell aplasia (PRCA) reported when used with other immunosuppressive agents. Females of reproductive potential should have a pregnancy test immediately before starting therapy; repeat test after 8-10 days and during routine follow-up visits. Acceptable birth control must be used during therapy and for 6 weeks after discontinuation unless patient chooses abstinence. Consider alternative immunosuppressants with less potential for embryofetal toxicity in patients considering pregnancy. GI bleeding, ulceration, and perforation reported; caution with active serious digestive system disease. Avoid doses >1g bid in renal transplant patients with severe chronic renal impairment (GFR <25mL/min/1.73m²); caution with delayed renal graft function post-transplant. More reports of opportunistic/herpes virus infections in cardiac transplant patients in comparison with azathioprine. Avoid with rare hereditary deficiency of hypoxanthine-guanine phosphoribosyl-transferase (HGPRT) (eg, Lesch-Nyhan and Kelley-Seegmiller syndrome). Oral sus contains 0.56mg phenylalanine/mL; caution with phenylketonurics. Caution in elderly.

ADVERSE REACTIONS: Infection, diarrhea, leukopenia, sepsis, N/V, HTN, peripheral edema, abdominal pain, fever, headache, constipation, hyperglycemia, anemia, abnormal kidney function.

INTERACTIONS: Avoid with azathioprine, drugs that interfere with enterohepatic recirculation (eg, cholestyramine), and norfloxacin-metronidazole combination. Vaccinations may be less effective; avoid live attenuated vaccines. Decreased exposure with rifampin; concomitant use not recommended unless benefit outweighs risk. Increased levels of both drugs with drugs that compete with renal tubular secretion (eg, acyclovir/valacyclovir, ganciclovir/valganciclovir, probenecid). Oral ciprofloxacin and amoxicillin plus clavulanic acid may decrease levels. Mean mycophenolic acid (MPA) exposure may be 30-50% greater when mycophenolate mofetil is administered without cyclosporine compared to when coadministered with cyclosporine. May decrease levels and effectiveness of hormonal contraceptives; use with caution and must use additional barrier contraceptive methods. Drugs that alter GI flora may reduce levels available for absorption. Decreased levels with proton pump inhibitors (eg, lansoprazole, pantoprazole), Mg²⁺- and aluminum-containing antacids, and Ca²⁺ free phosphate binders (eg, sevelamer). Do not administer simultaneously with antacids containing aluminum and magnesium hydroxides. Do not administer Ca²⁺ free phosphate binders simultaneously; may give 2 hrs after intake.

PREGNANCY: Category D, not for use in nursing.

MECHANISM OF ACTION: Inosine monophosphate dehydrogenase inhibitor; inhibits the de novo pathway of guanosine nucleotide synthesis without incorporation into deoxyribonucleic acid.

PHARMACOKINETICS: Absorption: (PO) Rapid and complete; absolute bioavailability (94%). Refer to PI for parameters in different populations. **Distribution:** V_d=3.6L/kg (IV), 4L/kg (PO); plasma albumin binding (97%, MPA), (82%, phenolic glucuronide of MPA [MPAG]). **Metabolism:** MPA (active metabolite) metabolized by glucuronyl transferase to MPAG, which is converted to MPA via enterohepatic recirculation. **Elimination:** (PO) Urine (93%; <1% MPA, 87% MPAG), feces (6%); MPA: $T_{1/2}$=17.9 hrs (PO), 16.6 hrs (IV).

NURSING CONSIDERATIONS

Assessment: Assess for previous hypersensitivity to the drug or its components, hepatic/renal impairment, delayed renal graft function post-transplant, phenylketonuria, hereditary deficiency of HGPRT (eg, Lesch-Nyhan and Kelley-Seegmiller syndrome), active digestive disease, vaccination history, pregnancy/nursing status, and possible drug interactions.

Monitoring: Monitor for signs/symptoms of lymphomas, skin cancer and other malignancies, infections (eg, opportunistic/fatal infections, latent viral infections [eg, PML, BKVAN], herpes virus, sepsis), neutropenia, PRCA, and GI bleeding/perforation/ulceration. Monitor CBC weekly during the 1st month, twice monthly for the 2nd and 3rd months, and then monthly through the 1st year. Monitor pregnancy status by obtaining pregnancy test 8-10 days after initiation of therapy and repeatedly during follow-up visits.

Patient Counseling: Inform that use during pregnancy is associated with an increased risk of 1st trimester pregnancy loss and congenital malformations; discuss pregnancy testing, prevention (including acceptable contraception methods), and planning. Discuss appropriate alternative immunosuppressants with less potential for embryofetal toxicity in patients who are considering pregnancy. Advise of complete dosage instructions and inform about increased risk of

C

lymphoproliferative disease and certain other malignancies. Inform of the need for repeated appropriate lab tests during therapy. Instruct patients to report immediately to physician if any adverse reactions develop. Advise not to breastfeed during therapy. Encourage to enroll in the Mycophenolate Pregnancy Registry if patient becomes pregnant while on medication.

Administration: Oral/IV route. Sus may be given via NG route. Give PO dose on empty stomach. Administration of IV sol should be within 4 hrs from reconstitution and dilution; infuse over no <2 hrs. Refer to PI for reconstitution instructions of Sus and Inj. **Storage:** 25°C (77°F); excursions permitted to 15-30°C (59-86°F). Constituted Sus: Stable up to 60 days; may also be refrigerated at 2-8°C (36-46°F). Do not freeze.

CEPHALEXIN   RX
cephalexin (Various)

OTHER BRAND NAMES: Keflex (Shionogi)

THERAPEUTIC CLASS: Cephalosporin (1st generation)

INDICATIONS: Treatment of otitis media, skin and skin structure infection (SSSI), and bone, genitourinary tract (eg, prostatitis), and respiratory tract infections caused by susceptible strains of microorganisms.

DOSAGE: *Adults:* Range: 1-4g/day in divided doses. Usual: 250mg q6h. Streptococcal Pharyngitis/SSSI/Uncomplicated Cystitis (>15 Yrs): 500mg q12h. Treat cystitis for 7-14 days. May need larger doses in more severe infections or those caused by less susceptible organisms. If doses >4g/day are required, consider parenteral cephalosporins.
Pediatrics: Usual: 25-50mg/kg/day in divided doses. Streptococcal Pharyngitis (>1 Yr)/SSSI: May divide total daily dose and give q12h. Otitis Media: 75-100mg/kg/day in 4 divided doses. β-Hemolytic Streptococcal Infections: Administer for at least 10 days. May double the dosage in severe infections.

HOW SUPPLIED: Cap: 250mg, 500mg, (Keflex) 250mg, 500mg, 750mg; Sus: 125mg/5mL [100mL, 200mL], 250mg/5mL [100mL, 200mL]; Tab: 250mg*, 500mg* *scored

WARNINGS/PRECAUTIONS: Caution in penicillin (PCN)-sensitive patients; cross-hypersensitivity among β-lactam antibiotics may occur. D/C use if an allergic reaction occurs and institute appropriate therapy. *Clostridium difficile*-associated diarrhea (CDAD) reported; d/c if CDAD is suspected or confirmed. May result in bacterial resistance with prolonged use or use in the absence of a proven/suspected bacterial infection or a prophylactic indication; take appropriate measures if superinfection develops. Perform indicated surgical procedures in conjunction with antibiotic therapy. Caution in patients with markedly impaired renal function or history of GI disease, particularly colitis. May cause a fall in prothrombin activity; monitor PT in patients at risk (eg, hepatic/renal impairment, poor nutritional state, patients on protracted course of antimicrobial therapy, patients previously stabilized on anticoagulant therapy) and administer vitamin K as indicated. Lab test interactions may occur. Caution in elderly.

ADVERSE REACTIONS: Diarrhea, allergic reactions, dyspepsia, gastritis, abdominal pain.

INTERACTIONS: Probenecid inhibits renal excretion. Concomitant use with metformin may increase concentrations of metformin and produce adverse effects; monitor patient closely and adjust dose of metformin accordingly.

PREGNANCY: Category B, caution in nursing.

MECHANISM OF ACTION: Cephalosporin (1st generation); bactericidal activity results from its inhibition of cell-wall synthesis.

PHARMACOKINETICS: Absorption: Rapid. C_{max}=9μg/mL (250mg), 18μg/mL (500mg), 32μg/mL (1g); T_{max}=1 hr. **Distribution:** Found in breast milk. **Elimination:** Urine (90% unchanged).

NURSING CONSIDERATIONS

Assessment: Assess for previous hypersensitivity to cephalosporins, PCNs, or other drugs. Assess renal/hepatic function, for a history of GI disease, pregnancy/nursing status, and for possible drug interactions. Obtain baseline culture and susceptibility tests.

Monitoring: Monitor for signs/symptoms of hypersensitivity reactions, CDAD, superinfection, and other adverse reactions. Monitor PT and renal function when indicated. Perform culture and susceptibility tests.

Patient Counseling: Inform that drug only treats bacterial, not viral (eg, common cold), infections. Instruct to take exactly ud; inform that skipping doses or not completing full course of therapy may decrease effectiveness and increase bacterial resistance. Inform that diarrhea may be experienced as late as 2 or more months after last dose; counsel to contact physician if watery/bloody stools (with/without stomach cramps and fever) occur.

Administration: Oral route. Take without regard to meals. (Sus) Shake well before use. Refer to PI for directions for mixing. **Storage:** 20-25°C (68-77°F). (Sus) Store in refrigerator after mixing.

May be kept for 14 days without significant loss of potency. Keep tightly closed. (Keflex) 25°C (77°F); excursions permitted to 15-30°C (59-86°F).

C

Cervarix RX
human papillomavirus recombinant vaccine, bivalent (GlaxoSmithKline)

THERAPEUTIC CLASS: Vaccine

INDICATIONS: Prevention of cervical cancer, cervical intraepithelial neoplasia (CIN) Grade 2 or worse and adenocarcinoma in situ, and CIN Grade 1 caused by oncogenic human papillomavirus (HPV) types 16 and 18 in females 9-25 yrs of age.

DOSAGE: *Adults:* ≤25 Yrs: Give 3 separate doses of 0.5mL IM, preferably in the deltoid region of the upper arm at 0, 1, and 6 months.
Pediatrics: ≥9 Yrs: Give 3 separate doses of 0.5mL IM, preferably in the deltoid region of the upper arm at 0, 1, and 6 months.

HOW SUPPLIED: Inj: 0.5mL

WARNINGS/PRECAUTIONS: Does not provide protection against disease due to all HPV types or from vaccine and non-vaccine HPV types to which a woman has previously been exposed through sexual activity. May not result in protection in all vaccine recipients. Females should continue to adhere to recommended cervical cancer screening procedures. Syncope sometimes associated with falling with injury, tonic-clonic movements and other seizure-like activity reported; observe for 15 min after administration. Tip cap of prefilled syringe may contain natural rubber latex; may cause allergic reactions in latex-sensitive individuals. Review immunization history for possible vaccine hypersensitivity and previous vaccination-related adverse reactions; appropriate treatment and supervision must be available for possible anaphylactic reactions. Immunocompromised individuals may have diminished immune response.

ADVERSE REACTIONS: Local reactions (eg, pain, redness and swelling at the inj site), fatigue, headache, myalgia, GI symptoms, arthralgia, fever, rash, urticaria, nasopharyngitis, influenza.

INTERACTIONS: Immunosuppressive therapies (eg, irradiation, antimetabolites, alkylating agents, cytotoxic drugs, corticosteroids [used in greater than physiologic doses]), may reduce the immune response to vaccine.

PREGNANCY: Category B, caution in nursing.

MECHANISM OF ACTION: Vaccine; may be mediated by the development of immunoglobulin G-neutralizing antibodies directed against HPV-L1 capsid proteins generated as a result of vaccination.

NURSING CONSIDERATIONS

Assessment: Assess for latex hypersensitivity, immunosuppression, pregnancy/nursing status, and possible drug interactions. Review immunization history for possible vaccine hypersensitivity and for previous vaccination-related adverse reactions.

Monitoring: Monitor for syncope, tonic-clonic movements, seizure-like activity, anaphylactic reactions, and other adverse reactions.

Patient Counseling: Advise of the potential benefits and risks associated with vaccination. Inform that vaccine does not substitute for routine cervical cancer screening and advise women who receive the vaccine to continue to undergo cervical screening per standard of care. Counsel that vaccine does not protect against disease from HPV types to which a woman has previously been exposed through sexual activity. Inform that since syncope has been reported following vaccination in young females, observation for 15 min after administration is recommended. Instruct to report any adverse events to physician. Inform that vaccine is not recommended for use in pregnant women or women planning to become pregnant; advise to notify physician if pregnant or planning to become pregnant.

Administration: IM route. Do not administer IV, intradermally, or SQ. Do not mix with any other vaccine in the same syringe or vial. Shake well before withdrawal and use. **Storage:** 2-8°C (36-46°F). Do not freeze; discard if frozen.

Cesamet CII
nabilone (Meda)

THERAPEUTIC CLASS: Cannabinoid

INDICATIONS: Treatment of N/V associated with cancer chemotherapy in patients who have failed to respond adequately to conventional antiemetic treatments.

DOSAGE: *Adults:* Night Before Chemotherapy: May give 1 or 2 mg. Day of Chemotherapy: Start with a lower dose 1-3 hrs before the chemotherapy agent. Titrate: Increase PRN; may be given bid or tid during the entire course of each chemotherapy cycle and, PRN, for 48 hrs after the last dose of each cycle. Usual: 1 or 2mg bid. Max: 6mg/day in divided doses tid. Elderly: Start at the low end of dosing range.

HOW SUPPLIED: Cap: 1mg

WARNINGS/PRECAUTIONS: Not for use on PRN basis or as 1st antiemetic product prescribed. High potential for abuse. Adverse psychiatric reactions can persist for 48-72 hrs following discontinuation of treatment. May cause dizziness, drowsiness, euphoria, ataxia, anxiety, disorientation, depression, hallucinations, psychosis, tachycardia, and orthostatic hypotension. May alter mental states; keep patients under adult supervision, especially during initial use and dose adjustments. May impair mental/physical abilities. May elevate HR and cause postural hypotension. Caution with HTN, heart disease, elderly, current or previous psychiatric disorders (eg, manic depressive illness, depression, schizophrenia) and history of substance abuse. Caution in pregnant/nursing patients and pediatrics.

ADVERSE REACTIONS: Drowsiness, vertigo, dizziness, dry mouth, euphoria, ataxia, headache, concentration difficulties, dysphoria, sleep/visual disturbance, asthenia, anorexia, depression, hypotension.

INTERACTIONS: Avoid with alcohol, sedatives, hypnotics, or other psychoactive drugs. Additive HTN, tachycardia, and possible cardiotoxicity with sympathomimetics (eg, amphetamines, cocaine). Additive or super-additive tachycardia, and drowsiness with anticholinergics (eg, atropine, scopolamine, antihistamines). Additive tachycardia, HTN, and drowsiness with TCAs (eg, amitriptyline, amoxapine, desipramine). Additive drowsiness and CNS depression with CNS depressants (eg, barbiturates, benzodiazepines, ethanol). May result in hypomanic reaction with disulfiram and fluoxetine and increase theophylline metabolism in patients who smoked marijuana. May decrease clearance of antipyrine and barbiturates. Cross-tolerance and mutual potentiation with opioids. Enhanced tetrahydrocannabinol effects with naltrexone. Increase in the positive subjective mood effects of smoked marijuana with alcohol. Impaired psychomotor function with diazepam. May displace highly protein-bound drugs; monitor for dose requirement changes.

PREGNANCY: Category C, not for use in nursing.

MECHANISM OF ACTION: Cannabinoid; interacts with the cannabinoid receptor system, CB (1) receptor.

PHARMACOKINETICS: Absorption: Complete, C_{max}=2ng/mL, T_{max}=2 hrs. **Distribution:** V_d=12.5L/kg. **Metabolism:** Liver (extensive) via reduction and oxidation; CYP450. **Elimination:** Feces (60%), urine (24%); $T_{1/2}$=2 hrs (identified metabolites), 35 hrs (unidentified metabolites).

NURSING CONSIDERATIONS

Assessment: Assess for history of hypersensitivity to cannabinoids, heart disease, HTN, previous/current psychiatric disorders, history of substance abuse (eg, alcohol abuse/dependence, marijuana use), pregnancy/nursing status, and possible drug interactions.

Monitoring: Monitor for adverse psychiatric reactions or unmasking of symptoms of psychiatric disorders, signs/symptoms of CNS effects (eg, dizziness, drowsiness, euphoria, disorientation, depression, hallucinations, psychosis), postural hypotension. Monitor BP and HR. Monitor for signs of excessive use, abuse, and misuse. Monitor for signs/symptoms of hypersensitivity and other adverse reactions.

Patient Counseling: Inform about additive CNS depression effect if taken concomitantly with alcohol or other CNS depressants; advise to avoid this combination. Advise not to engage in hazardous activity (eg, operating machinery/driving). Inform of possible mood changes and other adverse behavioral effects that may occur during therapy. Instruct to remain under supervision of responsible adult during treatment.

Administration: Oral route. **Storage:** 25°C (77°F); excursions permitted to 15-30°C (59-86°F).

CHANTIX   RX
varenicline (Pfizer)

Serious neuropsychiatric events including, but not limited to, depression, suicidal ideation, suicide attempt, and completed suicide reported. Some reported cases may be complicated by nicotine withdrawal symptoms in patients who stopped smoking. Monitor for neuropsychiatric symptoms, including changes in behavior, hostility, agitation, depressed mood, and suicide-related events. Worsening of preexisting psychiatric illness and completed suicide reported in some patients attempting to quit smoking while on therapy. Advise patients and caregivers that the patient should stop taking therapy and contact a healthcare provider immediately if agitation, hostility, depressed mood, changes in behavior or thinking, suicidal ideation, or suicidal behavior occurs. Safety and efficacy not established in patients with serious psychiatric illness (eg, schizophrenia, bipolar disorder, major depressive disorder). Weigh risks against benefits of use.

THERAPEUTIC CLASS: Nicotinic acetylcholine receptor agonist

INDICATIONS: Aid to smoking cessation treatment.

DOSAGE: *Adults:* Set quit date and start 1 week before quit date. Alternatively, may begin therapy and then quit smoking between Days 8 and 35 of treatment. Days 1-3: 0.5mg qd. Days 4-7: 0.5mg bid. Day 8-End of Treatment: 1mg bid. Treat for 12 weeks. If patient has successfully stopped smoking at end of 12 weeks, additional course of 12-week treatment is recommended to ensure long-term abstinence. If not successful in stopping smoking during 12 weeks of initial therapy, or if relapse after treatment, should make another attempt once factors contributing to failed attempt are identified and addressed. Consider a temporary/permanent dose reduction in patients who cannot tolerate adverse effects. Severe Renal Impairment (CrCl <30mL/min): Initial: 0.5mg qd. Titrate: May titrate PRN to a max dose of 0.5mg bid. End-Stage Renal Disease with Hemodialysis: Max: 0.5mg qd if tolerated.

HOW SUPPLIED: Tab: 0.5mg, 1mg

WARNINGS/PRECAUTIONS: Hypersensitivity reactions, including angioedema, and rare but serious skin reactions (eg, Stevens-Johnson syndrome, erythema multiforme) reported; d/c if skin rash with mucosal lesions or any other signs of hypersensitivity develop. Cardiovascular (CV) events reported in patients with stable CV disease. Somnolence, dizziness, loss of consciousness, and difficulty concentrating reported; may impair physical/mental abilities. Nausea reported; consider dose reduction for patients with intolerable nausea. Caution in elderly.

ADVERSE REACTIONS: N/V, headache, insomnia, somnolence, abnormal dreams, flatulence, constipation, dysgeusia, fatigue, upper respiratory tract disorder, abdominal pain, dry mouth, dyspepsia, increased appetite.

INTERACTIONS: Nicotine replacement therapy (transdermal nicotine) may increase incidence of adverse events. Physiological changes resulting from smoking cessation may alter pharmacokinetics or pharmacodynamics of certain drugs (eg, theophylline, warfarin, insulin) for which dosage adjustment may be necessary.

PREGNANCY: Category C, not for use in nursing.

MECHANISM OF ACTION: Nicotinic acetylcholine receptor agonist; binds with high affinity and selectivity at α4β2 neuronal nicotinic acetylcholine receptors. The binding produces agonist activity while simultaneously preventing nicotine binding to these receptors.

PHARMACOKINETICS: Absorption: T_{max}=3-4 hrs. **Distribution:** Plasma protein binding (≤20%). **Metabolism:** Minimal. **Elimination:** Urine (92% unchanged); $T_{1/2}$=24 hrs.

NURSING CONSIDERATIONS

Assessment: Assess for preexisting psychiatric illness, CV disease, history of hypersensitivity to the drug, renal impairment, pregnancy/nursing status, and for possible drug interactions.

Monitoring: Monitor for neuropsychiatric symptoms or worsening of preexisting psychiatric illness, CV events, skin reactions, hypersensitivity reactions, nausea, somnolence, dizziness, loss of consciousness, difficulty concentrating, and for other adverse reactions. Monitor renal function.

Patient Counseling: Inform about risks and benefits of treatment. Instruct to set a date to quit smoking and initiate treatment 1 week before quit date. Encourage to continue to attempt to quit even with early lapses after quit day. Provide educational materials and necessary counseling to support attempt at quitting smoking. Instruct to notify physician if persistent nausea or insomnia develops. Advise to d/c and notify physician if agitation, hostility, depressed mood, or changes in behavior/thinking develop. Advise to notify physician prior to treatment of any history of psychiatric illness. Inform that quitting smoking may be associated with nicotine withdrawal symptoms or exacerbation of preexisting psychiatric illness. Instruct to d/c and seek immediate medical care if angioedema or a skin reaction occurs. Advise to notify physician if symptoms of new or worsening CV events develop and to seek immediate medical attention if signs/symptoms of a myocardial infarction or stroke are experienced. Advise to use caution when driving or operating machinery. Inform that vivid, unusual, or strange dreams may occur. If patient is pregnant, planning to become pregnant, or breastfeeding, advise about the risks of smoking, the potential risks of therapy, and the benefits of smoking cessation.

Administration: Oral route. Take pc and with a full glass of water. **Storage:** 25°C (77°F); excursions permitted to 15-30°C (59-86°F).

CIALIS   RX
tadalafil (Lilly)

THERAPEUTIC CLASS: Phosphodiesterase type 5 inhibitor

INDICATIONS: Treatment of erectile dysfunction (ED). Treatment of signs and symptoms of BPH. Treatment of ED and signs and symptoms of BPH (ED/BPH).

DOSAGE: *Adults:* PRN Use: ED: Initial: 10mg prior to sexual activity. Titrate: May increase to 20mg or decrease to 5mg, based on individual efficacy and tolerability. Max Dosing Frequency: Once/day. CrCl 30-50mL/min: Initial: 5mg qd. Max: 10mg/48 hrs. CrCl <30mL/min or Hemodialysis: Max: 5mg/72 hrs. Mild/Moderate Hepatic Impairment (Child-Pugh Class A/B) : Max: 10mg qd.

With α-Blockers: Initial: Use lowest recommended dose. With Potent CYP3A4 Inhibitors (eg, Ketoconazole, Ritonavir): Max: 10mg/72 hrs. Once-Daily Use: ED: Initial: 2.5mg qd at approximately the same time every day. Titrate: May increase to 5mg qd based on individual efficacy and tolerability. With α-Blockers: Initial: Use lowest recommended dose. BPH: 5mg qd at approximately the same time every day. BPH Initiated with Finasteride: 5mg qd at approximately the same time every day for ≤26 weeks. ED/BPH: 5mg qd at approximately the same time every day. BPH and ED/BPH with CrCl 30-50mL/min: Initial: 2.5mg. Titrate: May increase to 5mg based on individual response. With Potent CYP3A4 Inhibitors (eg, Ketoconazole, Ritonavir): Max: 2.5mg.

HOW SUPPLIED: Tab: 2.5mg, 5mg, 10mg, 20mg

CONTRAINDICATIONS: Any form of organic nitrate, either regularly and/or intermittently used.

WARNINGS/PRECAUTIONS: Cardiac risk associated with sexual activity may occur; avoid in men for whom sexual activity is inadvisable due to underlying cardiovascular (CV) status. May be sensitive to the action of vasodilators in patients with severely impaired autonomic control of BP and with left ventricular outflow obstruction (eg, aortic stenosis, idiopathic hypertrophic sub-aortic stenosis). Avoid with myocardial infarction (within last 90 days), unstable angina or angina occurring during sexual intercourse, NYHA Class 2 or greater heart failure (in the last 6 months), uncontrolled arrhythmias, hypotension (<90/50mmHg), uncontrolled HTN, and stroke (within the last 6 months). Mild systemic vasodilatory properties may result in transient decreases in BP. Prolonged erections (>4 hrs) and priapism (painful erections >6 hrs in duration) reported; caution in patients who have conditions predisposing to priapism (eg, sickle cell anemia, multiple myeloma, leukemia), or with anatomical deformation of the penis (eg, angulation, cavernosal fibrosis, Peyronie's disease). Non-arteritic anterior ischemic optic neuropathy (NAION) rarely reported; d/c if sudden loss of vision is experienced in one or both eyes. Sudden decrease or loss of hearing reported which may be accompanied by tinnitus and dizziness; d/c if this occurs. Avoid qd use in patients with CrCl <30mL/min or on hemodialysis. Avoid use with severe hepatic impairment (Child-Pugh Class C) and hereditary degenerative retinal disorders, including retinitis pigmentosa. Caution with mild to moderate hepatic impairment (Child-Pugh Class A/B), bleeding disorders, or significant active peptic ulceration. Consider other urological conditions that may cause similar symptoms prior to initiating treatment for BPH.

ADVERSE REACTIONS: Headache, dyspepsia, back pain, myalgia, nasal congestion, flushing, limb pain, nasopharyngitis, upper respiratory tract infection, gastroenteritis, cough, gastroesophageal reflux disease, HTN.

INTERACTIONS: See Contraindications. Avoid concomitant use with other PDE-5 inhibitors, including Adcirca. Avoid concomitant use with nitrates within 48 hrs. Caution with α-blockers. Concomitant use not recommended with α-blockers for the treatment of BPH. BP-lowering effects of each individual compound may be increased with alcohol. Additive hypotensive effects with selected antihypertensive medications (amlodipine, ARBs, bendrofluazide, enalapril, metoprolol). Antacids (magnesium hydroxide/aluminum hydroxide) may reduce the apparent rate of absorption. CYP3A4 inhibitors (eg, ketoconazole, erythromycin, itraconazole, grapefruit juice), and ritonavir and other HIV protease inhibitors may increase exposure. CYP3A4 inducers (eg, rifampin, carbamazepine, phenytoin, phenobarbital) may decrease exposure. A small increase in HR reported with theophylline.

PREGNANCY: Category B, not for use in nursing.

MECHANISM OF ACTION: PDE-5 inhibitor; increases amount of cGMP that causes smooth muscle relaxation and increased blood flow into the corpus cavernosum.

PHARMACOKINETICS: Absorption: T_{max}=2 hrs (median). **Distribution:** V_d=63L; plasma protein binding (94%). **Metabolism:** Liver, via CYP3A4 to a catechol metabolite, which undergoes extensive methylation and glucuronidation; methylcatechol glucuronide (major metabolite). **Elimination:** Urine (36%), feces (61%); $T_{1/2}$=17.5 hrs (healthy).

NURSING CONSIDERATIONS

Assessment: Assess for previous hypersensitivity to drug, CV disease, hereditary degenerative retinal disorders, bleeding disorders, significant active peptic ulceration, anatomical deformation of the penis or presence of conditions that would predispose to priapism, potential underlying causes of ED, other urological conditions, renal/hepatic impairment, pregnancy/nursing status, and possible drug interactions.

Monitoring: Monitor for hypersensitivity reactions, BP decrease, decrease/loss of hearing or vision, prolonged erection, priapism, and other adverse reactions.

Patient Counseling: Instruct to seek emergency medical attention if erection persists >4 hrs. Advise of potential BP-lowering effect of α-blockers, antihypertensive medications, and alcohol. Inform of the potential cardiac risk of sexual activity in patients with preexisting CV disease; instruct patients who experience symptoms upon initiation of sexual activity to refrain from further sexual activity and seek immediate medical attention. Counsel about the protective measures necessary to guard against sexually transmitted disease, including HIV, should be considered. Inform about contraindication with regular and/or intermittent use of organic nitrates and potential interactions with medications. Instruct to d/c and seek medical attention if sudden decrease or loss of vision or hearing occurs. Inform of the increased risk of NAION in individuals who have already experienced NAION in one eye. Counsel to take one tab at least 30 min before antici- pated sexual activity for PRN use in men with ED, and approximately the same time every day without regard to timing of sexual activity for qd use in men with ED, BPH, or ED/BPH.

Administration: Oral route. May be taken without regard to food. Do not split; entire dose should be taken. **Storage:** 25°C (77°F); excursions permitted to 15-30°C (59-86°F).

CILOXAN   RX
ciprofloxacin HCl (Alcon)

THERAPEUTIC CLASS: Fluoroquinolone

INDICATIONS: Treatment of bacterial conjunctivitis (sol/oint) and corneal ulcers (sol) caused by susceptible strains of microorganisms.

DOSAGE: *Adults:* (Oint) Bacterial Conjunctivitis: Apply 1/2-inch ribbon tid into conjunctival sac for 2 days, then bid for the next 5 days. (Sol) Bacterial Conjunctivitis: Instill 1-2 drops into conjunctival sac q2h while awake for 2 days, then 1-2 drops q4h while awake for the next 5 days. Corneal Ulcer: Instill 2 drops into the affected eye every 15 min for 1st 6 hrs, then 2 drops every 30 min for rest of Day 1, then 2 drops every hr on Day 2, then 2 drops q4h on Days 3-14. May con- tinue treatment after 14 days if reepithelialization has not occurred.
Pediatrics: (Oint) Bacterial Conjunctivitis: ≥2 Yrs: Apply 1/2-inch ribbon tid into conjunctival sac for 2 days, then bid for the next 5 days. (Sol) ≥1 Yr: Bacterial Conjunctivitis: Instill 1-2 drops into conjunctival sac q2h while awake for 2 days, then 1-2 drops q4h while awake for the next 5 days. Corneal Ulcer: Instill 2 drops into the affected eye every 15 min for first 6 hrs, then 2 drops every 30 min for rest of Day 1, then 2 drops every hr on Day 2, then 2 drops q4h on Days 3-14. May con- tinue treatment after 14 days if reepithelialization has not occurred.

HOW SUPPLIED: Oint: 0.3% [3.5g]; Sol: 0.3% [2.5mL, 5mL, 10mL]

WARNINGS/PRECAUTIONS: For topical ophthalmic use only; do not inject into eye. Serious and occasionally fatal hypersensitivity (anaphylactic) reactions reported in patients receiving systemic therapy; immediate emergency treatment with epinephrine and other resuscitation measures may be required as clinically indicated. Prolonged use may result in overgrowth of nonsusceptible organisms, including fungi; initiate appropriate therapy if superinfection occurs. D/C at 1st appearance of skin rash or other signs of hypersensitivity reaction. Remove contact lenses before use; avoid wearing contact lenses when signs/symptoms of bacterial conjunctivitis are present. (Oint) May retard corneal healing and cause visual blurring. (Sol) May form a white crystalline precipitate in the superficial portion of the corneal defect.

ADVERSE REACTIONS: Local discomfort, keratopathy, allergic reactions, corneal staining, for- eign body sensation. (Oint) Blurred vision, irritation, lid margin hyperemia. (Sol) Local burning, white crystalline precipitate formation, lid margin crusting, conjunctival hyperemia, crystals/ scales, itching, bad taste.

INTERACTIONS: Systemic quinolone therapy may increase theophylline levels, interfere with caffeine metabolism, enhance effects of warfarin and its derivatives, and elevate SrCr with cyclosporine.

PREGNANCY: Category C, caution in nursing.

MECHANISM OF ACTION: Fluoroquinolone; bactericidal, interferes with the enzyme DNA gyrase, which is needed for synthesis of bacterial DNA.

PHARMACOKINETICS: Absorption: (Sol) C_{max}=<5ng/mL.

NURSING CONSIDERATIONS

Assessment: Assess for previous hypersensitivity to the drug and other quinolones, use of con- tact lenses, pregnancy/nursing status, and possible drug interactions.

Monitoring: Monitor for signs/symptoms of hypersensitivity/anaphylactic reactions, and other adverse reactions. Monitor for superinfection; examine with magnification (eg, slit lamp biomi- croscopy) and fluorescein staining, where appropriate.

Patient Counseling: Instruct to use as prescribed. Instruct not to touch dropper tip to any surface because it may contaminate sol. Advise to contact physician if hypersensitivity reaction occurs (eg, rash). Instruct to remove contact lenses before use and not to wear contact lenses if signs/symptoms of bacterial conjunctivitis are present.

Administration: Ocular route. **Storage:** 2-25°C (36-77°F). (Sol) Protect from light.

CIMZIA

RX

certolizumab pegol (UCB)

C

Increased risk for developing serious infections (eg, active tuberculosis [TB], latent TB reactivation, invasive fungal infections, bacterial/viral and other opportunistic infections) leading to hospitalization or death, mostly with concomitant use with immunosuppressants (eg, methotrexate [MTX] or corticosteroids). D/C if serious infection or sepsis develops. Active TB/reactivation of latent TB may present with disseminated or extrapulmonary disease; test for latent TB before and during therapy and initiate treatment for latent TB prior to therapy. Invasive fungal infections reported; consider empiric antifungal therapy in patients at risk who develop severe systemic illness. Consider risks and benefits prior to therapy in patients with chronic or recurrent infection. Monitor patients for development of infection during and after treatment, including development of TB in patients who tested negative for latent TB infection prior to therapy. Lymphoma and other malignancies, some fatal, reported in children and adolescents.

THERAPEUTIC CLASS: TNF-blocker

INDICATIONS: Reduce signs/symptoms of Crohn's disease (CD) and maintain clinical response in adults with moderately to severely active disease who have had an inadequate response to conventional therapy. Treatment of adults with moderately to severely active rheumatoid arthritis (RA), with active psoriatic arthritis (PsA), or active ankylosing spondylitis (AS).

DOSAGE: *Adults:* CD: Initial: 400mg (given as 2 SQ inj of 200mg) initially, and at Weeks 2 and 4. Maint: 400mg every 4 weeks. RA/PsA: Initial: 400mg (given as 2 SQ inj of 200mg) initially and at Weeks 2 and 4, followed by 200mg every other week. Maint: Consider 400mg every 4 weeks. AS: Initial: 400mg (given as 2 SQ inj of 200mg) initially and at Weeks 2 and 4, followed by 200mg every 2 weeks or 400mg every 4 weeks.

HOW SUPPLIED: Inj: 200mg/mL [prefilled syringe, vial]

WARNINGS/PRECAUTIONS: May be used as monotherapy or concomitantly with non-biological disease modifying antirheumatic drugs (DMARDs). Do not initiate with an active infection. Increased risk of infection in elderly patients and in patients with comorbid conditions; consider the risks prior to therapy for those who have resided or traveled in areas of endemic TB or mycoses, and with any underlying conditions predisposing to infection. Postmarketing cases of aggressive and fatal hepatosplenic T-cell lymphoma (HSTCL) reported in patients with CD or ulcerative colitis and the majority were in adolescent and young adult males; almost all of these patients were treated concomitantly with azathioprine or 6-mercaptopurine (6-MP). Carefully consider the potential risk of HSTCL with the combination of azathioprine or 6-MP. Cases acute and chronic leukemia reported. Perform periodic skin examination, particularly in patients with risk factors for skin cancer. New onset and worsening of congestive heart failure (CHF) reported; caution in patients with heart failure (HF) and monitor carefully. Hypersensitivity reactions reported (rare); d/c and institute appropriate therapy if such reactions occur. Hepatitis B virus (HBV) reactivation reported; if reactivation occurs, d/c and initiate antiviral therapy with appropriate supportive treatment. Monitor patients closely and exercise caution when considering resumption of therapy. Associated with rare cases of new onset or exacerbation of clinical symptoms and/or radiographic evidence of CNS and peripheral demyelinating disease; caution with preexisting or recent-onset central or peripheral nervous system demyelinating disorders. Rare cases of neurological disorders (eg, seizure disorder, optic neuritis, peripheral neuropathy) reported. Hematological reactions (eg, leukopenia, pancytopenia, thrombocytopenia) reported; caution in patients with ongoing, or a history of, significant hematologic abnormalities, and consider discontinuation in patients with confirmed significant hematologic abnormalities. May result in the formation of autoantibodies and rarely, in the development of a lupus-like syndrome; d/c if lupus-like syndrome develops. Lab test interactions may occur. Caution in elderly.

ADVERSE REACTIONS: Infections, lymphoma and other malignancies, upper respiratory tract infections, rash, urinary tract infections, arthralgia, headache, HTN, nasopharyngitis, back pain, pyrexia, pharyngitis, acute bronchitis, fatigue.

INTERACTIONS: See Boxed Warning. Avoid concurrent use with live (eg, attenuated) vaccines. Concomitant administration with other biological DMARDs (eg, anakinra, abatacept, rituximab), other TNF blockers or natalizumab is not recommended; may increase risk of serious infections.

PREGNANCY: Category B, not for use in nursing.

MECHANISM OF ACTION: TNF-blocker; binds to and selectively neutralizes TNF-α, which has a central role in inflammatory processes.

PHARMACOKINETICS: Absorption: C_{max}=43-49mcg/mL (healthy); T_{max}=54-171 hrs; absolute bioavailability (80%). **Distribution:** V_d=6-8L. **Elimination:** $T_{1/2}$=14 days.

NURSING CONSIDERATIONS

Assessment: Assess for active/chronic/recurrent infection (eg, TB, HBV), TB exposure, history of an opportunistic infection, recent travel to areas of endemic TB or endemic mycoses, underlying conditions that may predispose to infection, HF, presence or history of significant hematologic abnormalities, neurologic disorders, risk factors for skin cancer, pregnancy/nursing status, and

C

possible drug interactions. Assess vaccination history in pediatric patients. Perform test for latent TB infection.

Monitoring: Monitor for sepsis, TB (active, reactivation, or latent), invasive fungal infections, bacterial/viral/other infections, lymphoma/other malignancies, new onset/worsening of CHF, active HBV infection, hematological events, hypersensitivity reactions, CNS demyelinating disorders, lupus-like syndrome, and other adverse reactions. Perform periodic skin examination, particularly in patients with risk factors for skin cancer and test for latent TB infection.

Patient Counseling: Advise of potential risks and benefits of therapy. Inform that therapy may lower the ability of the immune system to fight infections; instruct to immediately contact physician if any signs/symptoms of an infection develop, including TB and HBV reactivation. Counsel about the risks of lymphoma and other malignancies while on therapy. Advise to seek immediate medical attention if any symptoms of severe allergic reactions occur. Advise to report to physician signs of new or worsening medical conditions (eg, heart disease, neurological diseases, autoimmune disorders) and symptoms of a cytopenia (eg, bruising, bleeding, persistent fever). Instruct about proper administration techniques.

Administration: SQ route. Rotate inj sites; avoid areas where the skin is tender, bruised, red, or hard. When a 400mg dose is needed (given as 2 SQ inj of 200mg), inj should occur at separate sites in the thigh or abdomen. Refer to PI for further preparation and administration instructions. **Storage:** 2-8°C (36-46°F). Do not freeze. Protect sol from light. Reconstituted Sol: 2-8°C (36-46°F) for up to 24 hrs. Do not freeze.

CIPRO HC   RX
ciprofloxacin HCl - hydrocortisone (Alcon)

THERAPEUTIC CLASS: Antibacterial/corticosteroid combination

INDICATIONS: Treatment of acute otitis externa in adults and pediatric patients ≥1 yr caused by susceptible strains of microorganisms.

DOSAGE: *Adults:* 3 drops into affected ear bid for 7 days.
Pediatrics: ≥1 Yr: 3 drops into affected ear bid for 7 days.

HOW SUPPLIED: Sus: (Ciprofloxacin-Hydrocortisone) 0.2%-1% [10mL]

CONTRAINDICATIONS: Perforated tympanic membrane, viral infections of external ear canal, including varicella and herpes simplex infections.

WARNINGS/PRECAUTIONS: Not for inj and ophthalmic use. D/C at 1st appearance of skin rash or any other sign of hypersensitivity. Serious and occasionally fatal hypersensitivity (anaphylactic) reactions reported; may require immediate emergency treatment. May result in overgrowth of nonsusceptible organisms (eg, fungi). Reevaluate if no improvement after 1 week.

ADVERSE REACTIONS: Headache, pruritus.

PREGNANCY: Category C, not for use in nursing.

MECHANISM OF ACTION: Ciprofloxacin: Fluoroquinolone antibacterial; bactericidal action results from interference with the enzyme (DNA gyrase), which is needed for the synthesis of bacterial DNA. Hydrocortisone: Corticosteroid; aids in resolution of inflammatory response accompanying bacterial infection.

NURSING CONSIDERATIONS

Assessment: Assess for history of drug hypersensitivity, perforated tympanic membrane, viral infections of external ear canal, including varicella and herpes simplex infections, and pregnancy/nursing status.

Monitoring: Monitor for hypersensitivity reactions, overgrowth of nonsusceptible organisms (eg, fungi), and possible adverse reactions.

Patient Counseling: Instruct to d/c immediately and consult physician if rash or allergic reaction occurs. Advise not to use in the eyes. Advise to avoid contaminating the dropper with material from the ear, fingers, or other sources. Counsel to protect product from light. Instruct to shake well before using and to discard unused portion after therapy is completed.

Administration: Otic route. Shake well before use. Warm bottle in hand for 1-2 min to avoid dizziness (due to instillation of a cold sol in the ear canal). Lie with affected ear upward, then instill drops. Maintain position for 30-60 sec and repeat, if necessary, for the opposite ear. **Storage:** Below 25°C (77°F). Avoid freezing. Protect from light. Discard unused portion after therapy is completed.

CIPRO XR

RX

ciprofloxacin (Bayer Healthcare)

C

> Fluoroquinolones are associated with an increased risk of tendinitis and tendon rupture in all ages. Risk is further increased in patients >60 yrs of age, patients taking corticosteroids, and with kidney, heart, or lung transplants. May exacerbate muscle weakness with myasthenia gravis; avoid in patients with known history of myasthenia gravis.

THERAPEUTIC CLASS: Fluoroquinolone

INDICATIONS: Treatment of uncomplicated urinary tract infections (UTIs) (acute cystitis), complicated UTI, and acute uncomplicated pyelonephritis caused by susceptible strains of microorganisms.

DOSAGE: *Adults:* Uncomplicated UTI: 500mg q24h for 3 days. Complicated UTI/Acute Uncomplicated Pyelonephritis: 1000mg q24h for 7-14 days. CrCl ≤30mL/min: 500mg qd. Hemodialysis/Peritoneal Dialysis: Give after procedure is completed. Max: 500mg q24h. Continuous Ambulatory Peritoneal Dialysis: Max: 500mg q24h. May switch from ciprofloxacin IV to extended-release tab at discretion of physician.

HOW SUPPLIED: Tab, Extended-Release: 500mg, 1000mg

CONTRAINDICATIONS: Concomitant administration with tizanidine.

WARNINGS/PRECAUTIONS: Caution in patients with history of tendon disorders; d/c if pain, swelling, inflammation, or rupture of tendon occurs. Serious and occasionally fatal hypersensitivity reactions reported; d/c immediately and institute supportive measures if skin rash, jaundice, or hypersensitivity occurs. Severe hepatotoxicity, including hepatic necrosis, life-threatening hepatic failure, and fatal events, reported; d/c immediately if signs/symptoms of hepatitis occur. Convulsions, status epilepticus, increased intracranial pressure (including pseudotumor cerebri), toxic psychosis, and other CNS events reported; d/c and institute appropriate measures if CNS events occur. Caution with epilepsy and with CNS disorders (eg, severe cerebral arteriosclerosis, history of convulsion, reduced cerebral blood flow, altered brain structure, stroke) or other risk factors that may predispose to seizures or lower seizure threshold. *Clostridium difficile*-associated diarrhea (CDAD) reported; d/c if CDAD is suspected or confirmed. Cases of sensory or sensorimotor axonal polyneuropathy, resulting in paresthesias, hypoesthesias, dysesthesias, and weakness, reported; d/c immediately if symptoms of peripheral neuropathy occur. May prolong QT interval; avoid with known QT interval prolongation and with risk factors for QT prolongation/torsades de pointes (eg, congenital long QT syndrome, uncorrected hypokalemia/hypomagnesemia, cardiac disease). Crystalluria reported; maintain hydration and avoid alkalinity of urine. May cause photosensitivity/phototoxicity reactions; d/c if phototoxicity occurs. Avoid excessive exposure to sun/UV light. May result in bacterial resistance if used in the absence of a proven/suspected bacterial infection or a prophylactic indication. Caution in elderly and in patients with renal impairment. Not interchangeable with immediate-release tabs.

ADVERSE REACTIONS: Tendinitis, tendon rupture, nausea, headache.

INTERACTIONS: See Boxed Warning and Contraindications. May increase levels of CYP1A2 substrates (eg, theophylline, methylxanthines, tizanidine, caffeine, ropinirole, clozapine, olanzapine), pentoxifylline (oxpentifylline)-containing products, duloxetine, lidocaine, or sildenafil. Monitor for clozapine- or ropinirole-related side effects and adjust dose of clozapine or ropinirole during and shortly after coadministration with ciprofloxacin. Increased theophylline levels and its related adverse reactions; if use cannot be avoided, monitor theophylline levels and adjust dose. Multivalent cation-containing products (eg, Mg^{2+}/aluminum antacids, polymeric phosphate binders [eg, sevelamer, lanthanum carbonate], sucralfate, Videx [didanosine] chewable/buffered tab or pediatric powder, other highly buffered drugs, products containing Ca^{2+}, iron, or zinc) may substantially decrease absorption, resulting in serum and urine levels lower than desired; administer ≥2 hrs before or 6 hrs after these drugs. Avoid concomitant administration with dairy products alone, or with Ca^{2+}-fortified products. Omeprazole may decrease levels. May alter serum levels of phenytoin; monitor phenytoin therapy, including phenytoin levels during and shortly after coadministration. Caution with drugs that may lower seizure threshold. Hypoglycemia reported with oral antidiabetic agents, mainly sulfonylureas (eg, glyburide, glimepiride). Transient SrCr elevations with cyclosporine. May augment effects of oral anticoagulants (eg, warfarin); monitor PT and INR frequently. Probenecid may increase levels. May increase levels and toxic reactions of methotrexate. Avoid with Class IA (eg, quinidine, procainamide) and Class III (eg, amiodarone, sotalol) antiarrhythmics, TCAs, macrolides, and antipsychotics. Metoclopramide may significantly accelerate oral absorption. High-dose quinolones in combination with NSAIDs (not aspirin) may provoke convulsions.

PREGNANCY: Category C, not for use in nursing.

MECHANISM OF ACTION: Fluoroquinolone; inhibits the enzymes topoisomerase II (DNA gyrase) and topoisomerase IV (both Type II topoisomerases), which are required for bacterial DNA replication, transcription, repair, and recombination.

PHARMACOKINETICS: Absorption: (500mg) C_{max}=1.59mg/L; T_{max}=1.5 hrs; AUC_{0-24h}=7.97mg•h/L. (1000mg) C_{max}=3.11mg/L; T_{max}=2 hrs; AUC_{0-24h}=16.83mg•h/L. **Distribution:** V_d=2.1-2.7L/kg (IV); plasma protein binding (20-40%); found in breast milk. **Metabolism:** Oxociprofloxacin (M_3), sulfociprofloxacin (M_2) (primary metabolites). **Elimination:** Urine (35%, unchanged); $T_{1/2}$=6.6 hrs (500mg), 6.31 hrs (1000mg).

NURSING CONSIDERATIONS

Assessment: Assess for risk factors for developing tendinitis and tendon rupture, history of myasthenia gravis, drug hypersensitivity, epilepsy, CNS disorders or other risk factors that may predispose to seizures or lower seizure threshold, QT interval prolongation, uncorrected hypokalemia/hypomagnesemia, cardiac disease, renal/hepatic dysfunction, pregnancy/nursing status, and possible drug interactions. Obtain baseline culture and susceptibility tests.

Monitoring: Monitor for tendinitis or tendon rupture, signs/symptoms of hypersensitivity reactions, ECG changes (eg, QT interval prolongation), CNS events, CDAD, peripheral neuropathy, and photosensitivity/phototoxicity reactions. Monitor renal/hepatic function and perform periodic culture and susceptibility testing. Monitor PT and INR if coadministered with an oral anticoagulant (eg, warfarin).

Patient Counseling: Advise to notify physician if pain, swelling, or inflammation of a tendon, or weakness or inability to move joints develops; instruct to d/c therapy and rest/refrain from exercise. Instruct to notify physician if experiencing worsening muscle weakness or breathing problems, if sunburn-like reaction or skin eruption occurs, and of all medications and supplements currently being taken. Inform that drug treats only bacterial, not viral (eg, common cold), infections. Counsel to take exactly ud; inform that skipping doses or not completing full course of therapy may decrease effectiveness and increase bacterial resistance. Advise to take later in the day if dose at the usual time is missed, and not to take >1 tab/day. Advise to drink fluids liberally. Counsel to avoid concomitant use with dairy products (eg, milk, yogurt) or Ca^{2+}-fortified juices alone. Instruct to d/c and notify physician if allergic reaction, skin rash, or symptoms of peripheral neuropathy develop. Counsel to minimize or avoid exposure to natural/artificial sunlight (eg, tanning beds or UVA/B treatment). Inform that drug may cause dizziness and lightheadedness; advise to assess reaction to therapy before engaging in activities that require mental alertness or coordination. Advise to notify physician of any history of convulsions. Instruct to contact physician as soon as possible if watery and bloody stools (with/without stomach cramps and fever) develop.

Administration: Oral route. Swallow tab whole; do not split, crush, or chew. May take with or without meals. Administer ≥2 hrs before or 6 hrs after Mg^{2+}/aluminum-containing antacids, polymeric phosphate binders, sucralfate, Videx (didanosine) chewable/buffered tab or pediatric powder, other highly buffered drugs, or other products containing Ca^{2+}, iron, or zinc. Space Ca^{2+} intake (>800mg) by 2 hrs. **Storage:** 25°C (77°F); excursions permitted to 15-30°C (59-86°F).

CIPRODEX RX
dexamethasone - ciprofloxacin (Alcon)

THERAPEUTIC CLASS: Antibacterial/corticosteroid combination

INDICATIONS: Treatment of acute otitis media in pediatric patients (≥6 months of age) with tympanostomy tubes and treatment of acute otitis externa caused by susceptible organisms in pediatric patients (≥6 months of age), adults, and elderly patients.

DOSAGE: *Adults:* Acute Otitis Externa: 4 drops into the affected ear(s) bid for 7 days.
Pediatrics: Acute Otitis Media/Externa: ≥6 Months: 4 drops into the affected ear(s) bid for 7 days.

HOW SUPPLIED: Sus: (Ciprofloxacin-Dexamethasone) 0.3%-0.1% [7.5mL]

CONTRAINDICATIONS: Viral infections of external canal, including herpes simplex infections.

WARNINGS/PRECAUTIONS: For otic use only; not for ophthalmic use. D/C at 1st appearance of skin rash or any other sign of hypersensitivity. Serious and occasionally fatal hypersensitivity/anaphylactic reactions reported; may require immediate emergency treatment. May result in overgrowth of nonsusceptible organisms (eg, yeast, fungi); perform culture testing if infection is not improved after 1 week. If otorrhea persists after full course of therapy, or if ≥2 episodes of otorrhea occur within 6 months, evaluate to exclude underlying condition such as cholesteatoma, foreign body, or tumor.

ADVERSE REACTIONS: Ear discomfort/pain/precipitate/pruritus/debris/congestion, irritability, taste perversion, superimposed ear infection, erythema.

PREGNANCY: Category C, not for use in nursing.

MECHANISM OF ACTION: Ciprofloxacin: Fluoroquinolone antibacterial; bactericidal action results from interference with the enzyme (DNA gyrase), which is needed for the synthesis of bacterial DNA. Dexamethasone: Corticosteroid; aids in resolution of inflammatory response accompanying bacterial infection.

PHARMACOKINETICS: Absorption: Ciprofloxacin: C_{max}=1.39ng/mL; T_{max}=15 min-2 hrs. Dexamethasone: C_{max}=1.14ng/mL; T_{max}=15 min-2 hrs.

NURSING CONSIDERATIONS

Assessment: Assess for history of drug hypersensitivity, viral infection of the external canal (eg, herpes simplex virus infection), and pregnancy/nursing status.

Monitoring: Monitor for hypersensitivity/anaphylactic reactions, skin rash, overgrowth of non-susceptible organisms (eg, yeast, fungi), otorrhea, and other adverse reactions. Perform culture testing if infection is not improved after 1 week of treatment.

Patient Counseling: Inform that drug is for otic use only. Advise to avoid contaminating the tip with material from the ear, fingers, or other sources. Instruct to d/c immediately and consult physician if rash or allergic reaction occurs. Instruct to take as prescribed, even if symptoms improve. Advise to discard unused portion after therapy is completed.

Administration: Otic route. Warm bottle by holding in hand for 1 or 2 min prior to use and shake well before using. Lie with affected ear upward, and then instill drops. For otitis media, pump the tragus 5X by pushing inward to facilitate penetration of the drops into the middle ear. Maintain position for 60 sec and repeat, if necessary, for the opposite ear. **Storage:** 20-25°C (68-77°F); excursions permitted to 15-30°C (59-86°F). Avoid freezing. Protect from light.

CIPROFLOXACIN INJECTION   RX
ciprofloxacin (Various)

> Fluoroquinolones are associated with an increased risk of tendinitis and tendon rupture in all ages. Risk is further increased in patients >60 yrs of age, patients taking corticosteroids, and patients with kidney, heart, or lung transplants. May exacerbate muscle weakness with myasthenia gravis; avoid in patients with known history of myasthenia gravis.

OTHER BRAND NAMES: Cipro IV (Bayer Healthcare)

THERAPEUTIC CLASS: Fluoroquinolone

INDICATIONS: Treatment of urinary tract infections (UTIs), lower respiratory tract infections (LRTIs), acute exacerbations of chronic bronchitis, nosocomial pneumonia, skin and skin structure infections (SSSIs), bone and joint infections, complicated intra-abdominal infections (in combination with metronidazole), acute sinusitis, chronic bacterial prostatitis, and empirical therapy for febrile neutropenia (in combination with piperacillin sodium) in adults. Treatment of complicated UTIs and pyelonephritis in pediatric patients 1-17 yrs of age. To reduce the incidence or progression of postexposure inhalational anthrax in both adult and pediatric patients.

DOSAGE: *Adults:* Infuse IV over 60 min. UTIs: Mild/Moderate: 200mg q12h for 7-14 days. Severe/Complicated: 400mg q12h (or q8h) for 7-14 days. LRTIs/SSSIs: Mild/Moderate: 400mg q12h for 7-14 days. Severe/Complicated: 400mg q8h for 7-14 days. Nosocomial Pneumonia: 400mg q8h for 10-14 days. Bone and Joint Infections: Mild/Moderate: 400mg q12h for ≥4-6 weeks. Severe/Complicated: 400mg q8h for ≥4-6 weeks. Complicated Intra-Abdominal Infections (with Metronidazole): 400mg q12h for 7-14 days. Acute Sinusitis: Mild/Moderate: 400mg q12h for 10 days. Chronic Bacterial Prostatitis: Mild/Moderate: 400mg q12h for 28 days. Febrile Neutropenia (Empirical Therapy): Severe: 400mg q8h (with piperacillin 50mg/kg q4h; Max: 24g/day) for 7-14 days. Inhalational Anthrax (Postexposure): 400mg q12h for 60 days. CrCl 5-29mL/min: 200-400mg q18-24h. Refer to PI for conversion of IV to PO dosing. *Pediatrics:* Infuse IV over 60 min. Inhalational Anthrax (Postexposure): 10mg/kg q12h for 60 days. Max: 400mg/dose. 1-17 Yrs: Complicated UTIs/Pyelonephritis: 6-10mg/kg q8h for 10-21 days. Max: 400mg/dose.

HOW SUPPLIED: Inj: 200mg/100mL (0.2%); (Cipro) 400mg/200mL (0.2%)

CONTRAINDICATIONS: Concomitant administration with tizanidine.

WARNINGS/PRECAUTIONS: Caution in patients with history of tendon disorders; d/c if pain, swelling, inflammation, or rupture of tendon occurs. Serious and occasionally fatal hypersensitivity reactions reported; d/c immediately and institute supportive measures if skin rash, jaundice, or other signs of hypersensitivity occurs. Severe hepatotoxicity, including hepatic necrosis, life-threatening hepatic failure, and fatal events, reported; d/c immediately if symptoms of hepatitis occur. Convulsions, status epilepticus, increased intracranial pressure (including pseudotumor cerebri), toxic psychosis, and other CNS events reported; d/c and institute appropriate measures if CNS events occur. Caution with epilepsy and with CNS disorders (eg, severe cerebral arteriosclerosis, history of convulsion, reduced cerebral blood flow, altered brain structure, stroke) or other risk factors that may predispose to seizures or lower seizure threshold. *Clostridium difficile*-associated diarrhea (CDAD) reported; d/c if CDAD is suspected or confirmed. Cases of sensory or sensorimotor axonal polyneuropathy resulting in paresthesias, hypoesthesias, dysesthesias, and weakness reported; d/c immediately if symptoms of peripheral neuropathy occur. Increased incidence of musculoskeletal disorders in pediatric patients. May prolong QT interval; avoid with known QT interval prolongation and with risk factors for QT prolongation/torsades

C

de pointes (eg, congenital long QT syndrome, uncorrected hypokalemia/hypomagnesemia, cardiac disease). Local-site reactions reported. Crystalluria reported; maintain hydration and avoid alkalinity of urine. May cause photosensitivity/phototoxicity reactions; d/c if phototoxicity occurs. Avoid excessive exposure to sun/UV light. May result in bacterial resistance if used in the absence of a proven/suspected bacterial infection or a prophylactic indication. Caution in elderly and in patients with renal impairment.

ADVERSE REACTIONS: Tendinitis, tendon rupture, N/V, diarrhea, abdominal pain, neurological events, rhinitis, abnormal LFTs, rash, arthropathy.

INTERACTIONS: See Boxed Warning and Contraindications. May increase levels of CYP1A2 substrates (eg, theophylline, methylxanthines, tizanidine, caffeine, ropinirole, clozapine, olanzapine), pentoxifylline-containing products, duloxetine, lidocaine, or sildenafil. Monitor for clozapine- or ropinirole-related side effects and adjust dose of clozapine or ropinirole during and shortly after coadministration with ciprofloxacin. Increased theophylline levels and related adverse reactions; if concomitant use cannot be avoided, monitor theophylline levels and adjust dose. May reduce clearance of caffeine and prolong its $T_{1/2}$. May alter serum levels of phenytoin; monitor phenytoin therapy, including phenytoin levels, during and shortly after coadministration. High-dose quinolones in combination with NSAIDs (not aspirin) may provoke convulsions. Caution with drugs that may lower seizure threshold. Hypoglycemia reported with oral antidiabetic agents, mainly sulfonylureas (eg, glyburide, glimepiride). Probenecid may increase levels. Transient SrCr elevations with cyclosporine. May augment effects of oral anticoagulants (eg, warfarin); monitor PT and INR frequently. May increase levels and toxic reactions of methotrexate. Avoid with Class IA (eg, quinidine, procainamide) and Class III (eg, amiodarone, sotalol) antiarrhythmics, TCAs, macrolides, and antipsychotics. Mean serum concentration changes reported with piperacillin sodium 6-8 hrs after end of infusion.

PREGNANCY: Category C, not for use in nursing.

MECHANISM OF ACTION: Fluoroquinolone; inhibits the enzymes topoisomerase II (DNA gyrase) and topoisomerase IV (both Type II topoisomerases), which are required for bacterial DNA replication, transcription, repair, and recombination.

PHARMACOKINETICS: Absorption: Absolute bioavailability (PO) (70-80%). Administration of various doses resulted in different pharmacokinetic parameters. **Distribution:** Plasma protein binding (20-40%); found in breast milk. **Elimination:** Bile (<1%, unchanged), urine (50-70%, unchanged), feces (15%); $T_{1/2}$=5-6 hrs.

NURSING CONSIDERATIONS

Assessment: Assess for risk factors for developing tendinitis and tendon rupture, history of myasthenia gravis, drug hypersensitivity, epilepsy, CNS disorders or other risk factors that may predispose to seizures or lower seizure threshold, QT interval prolongation, uncorrected hypokalemia/hypomagnesemia, cardiac disease, renal/hepatic dysfunction, pregnancy/nursing status, and possible drug interactions. Obtain baseline culture and susceptibility tests.

Monitoring: Monitor for tendinitis or tendon rupture, signs/symptoms of hypersensitivity reactions, ECG changes (eg, QT interval prolongation), CNS events, CDAD, peripheral neuropathy, musculoskeletal disorders (pediatric patients), photosensitivity/phototoxicity reactions, and local-site reactions. Monitor renal/hepatic/hematopoietic function (with prolonged use), and perform periodic culture and susceptibility testing. Monitor PT and INR frequently if coadministered with an oral anticoagulant (eg, warfarin).

Patient Counseling: Advise to notify physician if pain, swelling, or inflammation of a tendon, or weakness or inability to move joints develops; instruct to d/c therapy and rest/refrain from exercise. Instruct to notify physician if experiencing worsening muscle weakness or breathing problems, sunburn-like reaction or skin eruption, and of all medications and supplements currently being taken. Inform that drug treats only bacterial, not viral (eg, common cold), infections. Counsel to take exactly ud; inform that skipping doses or not completing full course of therapy may decrease effectiveness and increase bacterial resistance. Instruct to d/c and notify physician if an allergic reaction, skin rash, or symptoms of peripheral neuropathy occur. Advise to minimize or avoid exposure to natural/artificial sunlight (tanning beds or UVA/B treatment). Inform that drug may cause dizziness and lightheadedness; advise to assess reaction to therapy before engaging in activities that require mental alertness or coordination. Instruct to notify physician of any history of convulsions. Instruct caregivers to inform physician if child has joint-related problems prior to, during, or after therapy. Advise to contact physician as soon as possible if watery and bloody stools (with/without stomach cramps and fever) develop even as late as ≥2 months after last dose.

Administration: IV route. Refer to PI for administration instructions. **Storage:** 5-25°C (41-77°F). Protect from light and freezing. Avoid excessive heat.

CIPROFLOXACIN ORAL   RX

ciprofloxacin (Various)

C

> Fluoroquinolones are associated with an increased risk of tendinitis and tendon rupture in all ages. Risk is further increased in patients >60 yrs of age, patients taking corticosteroids, and patients with kidney, heart, or lung transplants. May exacerbate muscle weakness with myasthenia gravis; avoid in patients with known history of myasthenia gravis.

OTHER BRAND NAMES: Cipro (Bayer Healthcare)

THERAPEUTIC CLASS: Fluoroquinolone

INDICATIONS: Treatment of urinary tract infections (UTIs), acute uncomplicated cystitis in females, chronic bacterial prostatitis, lower respiratory tract infections (LRTIs), acute exacerbations of chronic bronchitis, acute sinusitis, skin and skin structure infections (SSSIs), bone and joint infections, complicated intra-abdominal infections (in combination with metronidazole), infectious diarrhea, typhoid fever, and uncomplicated cervical and urethral gonorrhea caused by susceptible strains of microorganisms in adults. Treatment of complicated UTIs and pyelonephritis caused by susceptible strains of microorganisms in pediatric patients 1-17 yrs of age. To reduce the incidence or progression of postexposure inhalational anthrax in both adult and pediatric patients.

DOSAGE: *Adults:* Acute Uncomplicated UTIs: 250mg q12h for 3 days. Mild/Moderate UTIs: 250mg q12h for 7-14 days. Severe/Complicated UTIs: 500mg q12h for 7-14 days. Chronic Bacterial Prostatitis: Mild/Moderate: 500mg q12h for 28 days. LRTIs/SSSIs: Mild/Moderate: 500mg q12h for 7-14 days. Severe/Complicated: 750mg q12h for 7-14 days. Acute Sinusitis/Typhoid Fever: Mild/Moderate: 500mg q12h for 10 days. Bone and Joint Infections: Mild/Moderate: 500mg q12h for ≥4-6 weeks. Severe/Complicated: 750mg q12h for ≥4-6 weeks. Complicated Intra-Abdominal Infections (with Metronidazole): 500mg q12h for 7-14 days. Infectious Diarrhea: 500mg q12h for 5-7 days. Uncomplicated Urethral/Cervical Gonococcal Infections: 250mg single dose. Inhalational Anthrax (Postexposure): 500mg q12h for 60 days. CrCl 30-50mL/min: 250-500mg q12h. CrCl 5-29mL/min: 250-500mg q18h. Hemodialysis/Peritoneal Dialysis: 250-500mg q24h (after dialysis). Refer to PI for conversion of IV to PO dosing.
Pediatrics: Inhalational Anthrax (Postexposure): 15mg/kg q12h for 60 days. Max: 500mg/dose. 1-17 Yrs: Complicated UTIs/Pyelonephritis: 10-20mg/kg q12h for 10-21 days. Max: 750mg/dose.

HOW SUPPLIED: Sus: (Cipro) 250mg/5mL, 500mg/5mL [100mL]; Tab (HCl): 100mg, 750mg; (Cipro) 250mg, 500mg

CONTRAINDICATIONS: Concomitant administration with tizanidine.

WARNINGS/PRECAUTIONS: Caution in patients with history of tendon disorders; d/c if pain, swelling, inflammation, or rupture of tendon occurs. Serious and occasionally fatal hypersensitivity reactions reported; d/c immediately if signs of hypersensitivity occur. Severe hepatotoxicity, including hepatic necrosis, life-threatening hepatic failure, and fatal events, reported; d/c immediately if symptoms of hepatitis occur. Convulsions, status epilepticus, increased intracranial pressure (including pseudotumor cerebri), toxic psychosis, and other CNS events reported; d/c and institute appropriate measures if CNS events occur. Caution with epilepsy and with CNS disorders (eg, severe cerebral arteriosclerosis, history of convulsion, reduced cerebral blood flow, altered brain structure, stroke) or other risk factors that may predispose to seizures or lower the seizure threshold. *Clostridium difficile*-associated diarrhea (CDAD) reported; d/c if CDAD is suspected or confirmed. Cases of sensory or sensorimotor axonal polyneuropathy resulting in paresthesias, hypoesthesias, dysesthesias, and weakness reported; d/c immediately if symptoms of peripheral neuropathy occur. Increased incidence of musculoskeletal disorders in pediatric patients. May prolong QT interval; avoid with known QT interval prolongation and risk factors for QT prolongation/torsades de pointes. May mask or delay symptoms of incubating syphilis if used in high dose for short periods to treat gonorrhea. Crystalluria reported; maintain hydration and avoid alkalinity of urine. May cause photosensitivity/phototoxicity reactions; d/c if phototoxicity occurs. May result in bacterial resistance if used in the absence of a proven/suspected bacterial infection or a prophylactic indication. Caution in elderly and in patients with renal impairment.

ADVERSE REACTIONS: Tendinitis, tendon rupture, N/V, diarrhea, abdominal pain, neurological events, rhinitis, abnormal LFTs, rash, arthropathy.

INTERACTIONS: See Boxed Warning and Contraindications. May increase levels of CYP1A2 substrates (eg, theophylline, methylxanthines, tizanidine), pentoxifylline-containing products, duloxetine, lidocaine, or sildenafil. Monitor for clozapine- or ropinirole-related side effects and adjust dose of clozapine or ropinirole during and shortly after coadministration with ciprofloxacin. Increased theophylline levels and related adverse reactions; if concomitant use cannot be avoided, monitor theophylline levels and adjust dose. May decrease caffeine clearance and prolong its $T_{1/2}$. Multivalent cation-containing products (eg, Mg^{2+}/aluminum antacids, polymeric phosphate binders [eg, sevelamer, lanthanum carbonate], sucralfate, Videx [didanosine] chewable/buffered tab or pediatric powder, other highly buffered drugs, products containing Ca^{2+}, iron, or zinc) may substantially decrease absorption, resulting in serum and urine levels lower than desired; administer ≥2 hrs before or 6 hrs after these drugs. May alter serum levels of phenytoin; monitor phenytoin levels during and shortly after coadministration. Caution with drugs that may lower seizure threshold. High-dose quinolones in combination with NSAIDs (not aspirin) may provoke convulsions. Hypoglycemia reported with oral antidiabetic agents, mainly sulfonylureas. Transient SrCr elevations with cyclosporine. May augment effects of oral anticoagulants; monitor PT and INR frequently. Probenecid may increase levels. May increase levels and toxic reactions of methotrexate. Avoid with Class IA (eg, quinidine, procainamide) and Class III (eg, amiodarone, sotalol) antiarrhythmics, TCAs, macrolides, and antipsychotics. Metoclopramide may significantly accelerate oral absorption. Omeprazole may decrease levels.

PREGNANCY: Category C, not for use in nursing.

MECHANISM OF ACTION: Fluoroquinolone; inhibits the enzymes topoisomerase II (DNA gyrase) and topoisomerase IV (both Type II topoisomerases), which are required for bacterial DNA replication, transcription, repair, and recombination.

PHARMACOKINETICS: Absorption: T_{max}=1-2 hrs. (Tab) Rapid, well-absorbed. Absolute bioavailability (70%). Administration of various doses resulted in different pharmacokinetic parameters. **Distribution:** Plasma protein binding (20-40%); found in breast milk. **Elimination:** Urine (40-50%, unchanged), feces (20-35%), bile; $T_{1/2}$=4 hrs.

NURSING CONSIDERATIONS

Assessment: Assess for risk factors for developing tendinitis and tendon rupture, history of myasthenia gravis, drug hypersensitivity, epilepsy, CNS disorders or other risk factors that may predispose to seizures or lower seizure threshold, QT interval prolongation, renal/hepatic dysfunction, pregnancy/nursing status, and possible drug interactions. Obtain baseline culture and susceptibility tests. Perform serologic test for syphilis in patients with gonorrhea.

Monitoring: Monitor for tendinitis or tendon rupture, signs/symptoms of hypersensitivity reactions, ECG changes (eg, QT interval prolongation), CNS events, CDAD, peripheral neuropathy, musculoskeletal disorders (pediatric patients), and photosensitivity/phototoxicity reactions. Monitor renal/hepatic/hematopoietic function (with prolonged use), and perform periodic culture and susceptibility testing. Perform follow-up serologic test for syphilis after 3 months in patients with gonorrhea.

Patient Counseling: Advise to notify physician if pain, swelling, or inflammation of a tendon, or weakness or inability to move joints develops; instruct to d/c therapy and rest/refrain from exercise. Instruct to notify physician if experiencing worsening muscle weakness or breathing problems, sunburn-like reaction or skin eruption, and of all medications and supplements currently being taken. Inform that drug treats only bacterial, not viral (eg, common cold), infections. Counsel to take exactly ud; inform that skipping doses or not completing full course of therapy may decrease effectiveness and increase bacterial resistance. Advise to drink fluids liberally. Counsel to avoid concomitant use with dairy products or Ca²⁺-fortified juices alone. Instruct to d/c and notify physician if an allergic reaction, skin rash, or symptoms of peripheral neuropathy develop. Counsel to minimize or avoid exposure to natural/artificial sunlight (tanning beds or UVA/B treatment). Inform that drug may cause dizziness and lightheadedness; advise to assess reaction to therapy before engaging in activities that require mental alertness or coordination. Instruct to notify physician of any history of convulsions. Counsel caregiver to inform physician if child has joint-related problems prior to, during, or after therapy. Advise to contact physician as soon as possible if watery and bloody stools (with or without stomach cramps and fever) develop even as late as ≥2 months after last dose.

Administration: Oral route. May take with or without meals. Administer ≥2 hrs before or 6 hrs after multivalent cation-containing products. **Storage:** <30°C (86°F). (Reconstituted Sus) Store for 14 days and protect from freezing. Microcapsules and Diluent: <25°C (77°F). Protect from freezing.

CLARINEX   RX
desloratadine (Merck)

THERAPEUTIC CLASS: H₁-antagonist

INDICATIONS: Relief of nasal and non-nasal symptoms of seasonal allergic rhinitis in patients ≥2 yrs of age. Relief of nasal and non-nasal symptoms of perennial allergic rhinitis in patients ≥6 months of age. Symptomatic relief of pruritus and reduction in number and size of hives in patients ≥6 months of age with chronic idiopathic urticaria.

DOSAGE: *Adults:* Usual: 5mg or 10mL qd. Hepatic/Renal Impairment: Initial: 5mg tab qod. *Pediatrics:* ≥12 Yrs: 5mg or 10mL qd. 6-11 Yrs: 5mL qd. 12 Months-5 Yrs: 2.5mL qd. 6-11 Months: 2mL qd.

HOW SUPPLIED: Sol: 0.5mg/mL [4 oz., 16 oz.]; Tab: 5mg

WARNINGS/PRECAUTIONS: Hypersensitivity reactions (eg, rash, pruritus, urticaria, edema, dyspnea, anaphylaxis) reported; d/c therapy if any occur and consider alternative treatment. Caution in elderly patients.

ADVERSE REACTIONS: Pharyngitis, dry mouth, headache, N/V, fatigue, myalgia, fever, diarrhea, cough, upper respiratory tract infection, irritability, somnolence, bronchitis, otitis media, dizziness.

INTERACTIONS: CYP450 3A4 inhibitors (eg, ketoconazole, erythromycin, azithromycin), fluoxetine, and cimetidine may increase levels.

PREGNANCY: Category C, not for use in nursing.

MECHANISM OF ACTION: H_1-receptor antagonist; inhibits histamine release from human mast cells in vitro.

PHARMACOKINETICS: Absorption: (5mg tab) T_{max}=3 hrs, C_{max}=4ng/mL, AUC=56.9ng•hr/mL. **Distribution:** Plasma-protein binding (82-87%, 85-89% active metabolite); found in breast milk. **Metabolism:** Extensive; glucuronidation; 3-hydroxydesloratadine (active metabolite). **Elimination:** Urine and feces (87%); $T_{1/2}$=27 hrs.

NURSING CONSIDERATIONS

Assessment: Assess for hypersensitivity to drug, renal/hepatic impairment, pregnancy/nursing status, and possible drug interactions.

Monitoring: Monitor for hypersensitivity reactions and other adverse reactions.

Patient Counseling: Instruct to take ud; advise not to increase dose or dosing frequency.

Administration: Oral route. May take without regard to meals. (Sol) Administer age-appropriate dose of sol with a measuring dropper or syringe calibrated to deliver 2mL and 2.5mL. **Storage:** 25°C (77°F); excursions permitted to 15-30°C (59-86°F). (Tab) Avoid exposure at or >30°C (86°F). (Sol) Protect from light.

CLARINEX-D   RX
pseudoephedrine sulfate - desloratadine (Merck)

THERAPEUTIC CLASS: H_1-antagonist/sympathomimetic amine

INDICATIONS: Relief of nasal and non-nasal symptoms of seasonal allergic rhinitis, including nasal congestion, in adults and adolescents ≥12 yrs of age.

DOSAGE: *Adults:* (12 Hour) Usual/Max: 1 tab bid, approximately 12 hrs apart. (24 Hour) Usual/Max: 1 tab qd.
Pediatrics: ≥12 Yrs: (12 Hour) Usual/Max: 1 tab bid, approximately 12 hrs apart. (24 Hour) Usual/Max: 1 tab qd.

HOW SUPPLIED: Tab, Extended-Release: (Desloratadine-Pseudoephedrine) (12 Hour) 2.5mg-120mg, (24 Hour) 5mg-240mg

CONTRAINDICATIONS: Narrow-angle glaucoma, urinary retention, MAOI therapy or within 14 days of stopping an MAOI, severe HTN, or severe coronary artery disease (CAD).

WARNINGS/PRECAUTIONS: Can produce cardiovascular (CV) and CNS effects (eg, insomnia, dizziness, weakness, tremor, arrhythmias). CNS stimulation with convulsions or CV collapse with hypotension reported. Caution with CV disorders, diabetes, hyperthyroidism, prostatic hypertrophy, or increased intraocular pressure (IOP). Hypersensitivity reactions (eg, rash, pruritus, urticaria, edema, dyspnea, anaphylaxis) reported; d/c and consider alternative treatment if this occurs. Avoid in patients with hepatic/renal impairment. Caution in elderly patients.

ADVERSE REACTIONS: Dry mouth, headache, insomnia, fatigue, pharyngitis, somnolence, dizziness.

INTERACTIONS: See Contraindications. May reduce the antihypertensive effects of β-adrenergic blocking agents, methyldopa, and reserpine; use caution with these agents. Increased ectopic pacemaker activity may occur with concomitant digitalis; use caution with these agents.

PREGNANCY: Category C, not for use in nursing.

MECHANISM OF ACTION: Desloratadine: H_1-receptor antagonist; inhibits histamine release from human mast cells in vitro. Pseudoephedrine: Sympathomimetic amine; exerts a decongestant action on nasal mucosa.

PHARMACOKINETICS: Absorption: Desloratadine: (24 Hour) C_{max}=1.79ng/mL, T_{max}=6-7 hrs, AUC=61.1ng•hr/mL. (12 Hour) C_{max}=1.09ng/mL, T_{max}=4-5 hrs, AUC=31.6ng•hr/mL. Pseudoephedrine: (24 Hour) C_{max}=328ng/mL, T_{max}=8-9 hrs, AUC=6438ng•hr/mL. (12 Hour) C_{max}=263ng/mL, T_{max}=6-7 hrs, AUC=4588ng•hr/mL. **Distribution:** Desloratadine: Plasma protein binding (82-87%, 85-89% active metabolite); found in breast milk. Pseudoephedrine: Found in breast milk. **Metabolism:** Desloratadine: Extensive; 3-hydroxydesloratadine (active metabolite). Pseudoephedrine: Liver (incomplete), by N-demethylation. **Elimination:** Desloratadine: Urine and feces (87%); $T_{1/2}$=24 hrs (24 Hour), 27 hrs (12 Hour). Pseudoephedrine: Urine (55-96% unchanged); $T_{1/2}$=3-6 hrs (urinary pH=5), 9-16 hrs (urinary pH=8).

NURSING CONSIDERATIONS

Assessment: Assess for drug hypersensitivity, increased IOP, prostatic hypertrophy, CV disorders, diabetes, hyperthyroidism, narrow-angle glaucoma, urinary retention, HTN, CAD, hepatic/renal impairment, pregnancy/nursing status, and possible drug interactions.

Monitoring: Monitor for CV/CNS effects, hypersensitivity reactions, and other adverse reactions. Monitor for urinary retention and narrow-angle glaucoma in patients with prostatic hypertrophy or increased IOP.

Patient Counseling: Inform that CV or CNS effects may occur. Advise not to increase the dose or dosing frequency. Advise not to use with other antihistamines and/or decongestants. Advise not to use with an MAOI or within 14 days of stopping an MAOI. Advise patients with severe HTN or severe CAD, narrow-angle glaucoma, or urinary retention not to use this drug.

Administration: Oral route. Take with or without a meal. Swallow tab whole; do not break, chew, or crush. **Storage:** 25°C (77°F); excursions permitted to 15-30°C (59-86°F). Heat sensitive; avoid exposure at or >30°C (86°F). Protect from excessive moisture and light.

CLEOCIN   RX
clindamycin (Pfizer/Pharmacia & Upjohn)

> *Clostridium difficile*-associated diarrhea (CDAD) reported and may range in severity from mild diarrhea to fatal colitis. Due to association with severe colitis, reserve use for serious infections where less toxic agents are inappropriate. CDAD must be considered in all patients with diarrhea following antibiotic use. Careful medical history is necessary since CDAD has been reported to occur over 2 months after the administration of antibacterial agents. If CDAD is suspected or confirmed, ongoing antibiotic use not directed against *C. difficile* may need to be discontinued. Appropriate fluid and electrolyte management, protein supplementation, antibiotic treatment of *C. difficile* and surgical evaluation may be instituted as clinically indicated. Not for use with nonbacterial infections such as most upper respiratory infections.

OTHER BRAND NAMES: Cleocin Pediatric (Pfizer/Pharmacia & Upjohn)

THERAPEUTIC CLASS: Lincomycin derivative

INDICATIONS: Treatment of the following serious infections caused by susceptible strains of microorganisms: respiratory tract infections, skin and skin structure infections, septicemia, intra-abdominal infections, gynecological infections. (IV) Treatment of bone and joint infections and as adjunctive therapy in the surgical treatment of chronic bone and joint infections.

DOSAGE: *Adults:* Serious Infections: 150-300mg PO q6h or 600-1200mg/day IM/IV given bid, tid or qid. More Severe Infections: 300-450mg PO q6h or 1200-2700mg/day IM/IV given bid, tid or qid. (Inj) More Serious Infections: May increase dose. Life-Threatening Infections: May increase dose up to 4800mg/day IV. Max: 600mg/IM inj. Alternatively may administer as a single rapid infusion for the 1st dose followed by continuous IV infusion; refer to PI for dosing. Refer to PI for dilution and infusion rates. Treat β-hemolytic streptococcal infections for at least 10 days.
Pediatrics: PO: Serious Infections: (Cap) 8-16mg/kg/day (4-8mg/lb/day) given tid-qid or (Sol) 8-12mg/kg/day (4-6mg/lb/day) given tid-qid. Severe Infections: (Sol) 13-16mg/kg/day (6.5-8mg/lb/day) given tid-qid. More Severe Infections: (Cap) 16-20mg/kg/day (8-10mg/lb/day) given tid-qid or (Sol) 17-25mg/kg/day (8.5-12.5mg/lb/day) given tid-qid. ≤10kg: Minimum: 1/2 tsp (37.5mg) tid. IM/IV: 1 Month-16 Yrs: 20-40mg/kg/day given tid or qid; use the higher dose for more severe infections. Alternatively may give 350mg/m²/day for serious infections and 450mg/m²/day for more severe infections. <1 Month: 15-20mg/kg/day given tid-qid. Refer to PI for dilution and infusion rates. Treat β-hemolytic streptococcal infections for at least 10 days.

HOW SUPPLIED: Cap: (HCl) 75mg, 150mg, 300mg; Inj: (Phosphate) 150mg/mL [2mL, 4mL, 6mL vial]; 150mg/mL [4mL, 6mL] [ADD-Vantage vial]; 300mg/50mL, 600mg/50mL, 900mg/50mL [Galaxy plastic container]; (Pediatric) Sol: (Palmitate) 75mg/5mL [100mL]. Also available as a Pharmacy Bulk Package. Refer to individual package insert for more information.

WARNINGS/PRECAUTIONS: Reserve use for penicillin (PCN)-allergic patients or other patients for whom, a PCN is inappropriate. Perform indicated surgical procedures in conjunction with therapy. May increase bacterial resistance if used in the absence of a proven/strongly suspected bacterial infection or a prophylactic indication; take appropriate measures if superinfection develops. Not for treatment of meningitis. Caution with severe liver disease; perform periodic liver enzyme determinations. Caution with atopic patients, history of GI disease (eg, colitis), and in elderly. Perform periodic monitoring of blood counts, LFTs, and renal function tests with long-term use. (75mg/150mg Caps) Contains tartrazine, which may cause allergic-type reactions (eg, bronchial asthma); caution with aspirin hypersensitivity. (Inj) Do not inject IV undiluted as bolus. Contains benzyl alcohol; has been associated with "gasping syndrome" in premature infants.

ADVERSE REACTIONS: CDAD, abdominal pain, pseudomembranous colitis, N/V, maculopapular skin rash, pruritus, vaginitis, jaundice, abnormal LFTs, transient neutropenia, eosinophilia, drug reaction with eosinophilia and systemic symptoms, azotemia, oliguria, polyarthritis.

INTERACTIONS: Antagonism reported with erythromycin; avoid use concurrently. May enhance the action of neuromuscular blockers; use with caution.

PREGNANCY: Category B, not for use in nursing.

MECHANISM OF ACTION: Lincomycin-derivative antibiotic; inhibits bacterial protein synthesis by binding to the 50S subunit of the ribosome.

PHARMACOKINETICS: Absorption: Cap: Rapid, complete. C_{max}=2.5mcg/mL, T_{max}=45 min. Inj: T_{max}=3 hrs (Adults, IM), 1 hr (Peds, IM). Inj/Sol: Administration of variable doses resulted in different parameters. **Distribution:** Wide; distributed in body fluids, tissues, and bones; found in breast milk. **Elimination:** Cap: Urine (10%), feces (3.6%); $T_{1/2}$=2.4 hrs. Inj: $T_{1/2}$=3 hrs (Adults), 2.5 hrs (Peds). Sol: $T_{1/2}$=2 hrs.

NURSING CONSIDERATIONS

Assessment: Assess for history of hypersensitivity to drug or lincomycin, history of GI disease, presence of meningitis, hepatic function, pregnancy/nursing status, and for possible drug interactions. Assess use in atopic patients. Obtain baseline culture and susceptibility tests.

Monitoring: Monitor for CDAD, superinfection, allergic reactions, and other adverse reactions. Monitor for changes in bowel frequency in older patients. Consider culture and susceptibility information when modifying antibacterial therapy, if available. If on prolonged therapy, perform periodic LFTs, renal function tests, and blood counts. Perform periodic liver enzyme determinations in patients with severe liver disease.

Patient Counseling: Inform about potential benefits/risks of therapy. Inform that therapy only treats bacterial, not viral (eg, common cold), infections. Instruct to take exactly ud; skipping doses or not completing full course may decrease effectiveness and increase antibiotic resistance. Instruct to contact physician if an allergic reaction develops. Advise that watery and bloody stools may occur as late as 2 or more months after therapy; notify physician if occurs. Advise to notify physician if pregnant/nursing.

Administration: Oral/IM/IV route. (Cap) Take with full glass of water. (Sol/Inj) Refer to PI for preparation and administration instructions. (Inj) Refer to PI for compatibility info. **Storage:** 20-25°C (68-77°F). (Inj) Galaxy Container: 25°C (77°F); avoid temperatures >30°C (86°F). (Sol) Do not refrigerate the reconstituted solution; stable at room temperature for 2 weeks.

CLEVIPREX   RX
clevidipine (The Medicines Company)

THERAPEUTIC CLASS: Calcium channel blocker (dihydropyridine)

INDICATIONS: Reduction of BP in patients when PO therapy is not feasible or desirable.

DOSAGE: *Adults:* Individualize dose. Give by IV infusion. Initial: 1-2mg/hr. Titrate: May double the dose at 90-sec intervals initially. As BP approaches goal, increase in doses should be less than doubling and the time between dose adjustments should be lengthened to every 5-10 min. Maint: 4-6mg/hr. Max: 16mg/hr. Due to lipid load restrictions, no more than 1000mL or an average of 21mg/hr of infusion is recommended/24-hr period. Transition to PO Therapy: D/C or titrate downward until PO therapy is established. Consider the lag time of onset of the PO agent's effect when PO antihypertensive is instituted. Continue BP monitoring until desired effect is reached. Elderly: Start at the lower end of dosing range.

HOW SUPPLIED: Inj: 0.5mg/mL [50mL, 100mL]

CONTRAINDICATIONS: Allergies to soybeans, soy products, eggs, or egg products, severe aortic stenosis, defective lipid metabolism such as pathologic hyperlipemia, lipoid nephrosis, or acute pancreatitis if it is accompanied by hyperlipidemia.

WARNINGS/PRECAUTIONS: Systemic hypotension and reflex tachycardia may occur; decrease dose if either occurs. Lipid intake restrictions may be necessary with significant disorders of lipid metabolism; a reduction in the quantity of concurrently administered lipids may be necessary to compensate for the amount of lipid infused as part of the drug's formulation. May produce negative inotropic effects and exacerbation of heart failure (HF); monitor HF patients carefully. Does not reduce HR and does not protect against the effects of abrupt β-blocker withdrawal. Monitor for the possibility of rebound HTN for at least 8 hrs after discontinuation of infusion in patients who receive prolonged infusions and are not transitioned to other antihypertensive therapies. Caution in elderly.

ADVERSE REACTIONS: Atrial fibrillation, acute renal failure, headache, N/V, hypotension, reflex tachycardia.

PREGNANCY: Category C, safety not known in nursing.

MECHANISM OF ACTION: Calcium channel blocker (dihydropyridine); mediates the influx of Ca^{2+} during depolarization in arterial smooth muscle and reduces mean arterial BP by decreasing systemic vascular resistance; does not reduce cardiac filling pressure (preload).

PHARMACOKINETICS: Distribution: V_d=0.17L/kg; plasma protein binding (>99.5%). **Metabolism:** Hydrolysis of the ester linkage, glucuronidation or oxidation; carboxylic acid metabolite and formaldehyde (primary metabolites). **Elimination:** Urine (63-74%), feces (7-22%); $T_{1/2}$=15 min.

NURSING CONSIDERATIONS

Assessment: Assess for allergies to soybeans, eggs or soy/egg products, defective lipid metabolism, β-blocker usage, and pregnancy/nursing status. Obtain baseline parameters for BP, HR, and lipid profile.

Monitoring: Monitor for hypotension, reflex tachycardia, rebound HTN, HF exacerbation, and other adverse reactions. Monitor BP and HR during infusion, and until vital signs are stable.

Patient Counseling: Advise patients with underlying HTN that they require continued follow up for their medical condition, and, if applicable, to continue taking PO antihypertensive medication(s) ud. Instruct to report any signs of new hypertensive emergency (eg, neurological symptoms, visual changes, evidence of congestive HF) to a healthcare provider immediately.

Administration: IV route. Use aseptic technique. Refer to PI for administration and preparation instructions. **Storage:** 2-8°C (36-46°F). Do not freeze. Leave vials in cartons until use; may be transferred to 25°C (77°F) for a period not to exceed 2 months. Do not return to refrigerated storage after beginning room temperature storage. Discard any unused portion within 12 hrs of stopper puncture.

CLIMARA   RX
estradiol (Bayer Healthcare)

> Estrogens increase the risk of endometrial cancer. Perform adequate diagnostic measures, including endometrial sampling, to rule out malignancy with undiagnosed persistent or recurrent abnormal vaginal bleeding. Should not be used for the prevention of cardiovascular (CV) disease or dementia. Increased risks of myocardial infarction (MI), stroke, invasive breast cancer, pulmonary embolism (PE), and deep vein thrombosis (DVT) in postmenopausal women (50-79 yrs of age) reported. Increased risk of developing probable dementia in postmenopausal women ≥65 yrs of age reported. Should be prescribed at the lowest effective dose and for the shortest duration consistent with treatment goals and risks.

THERAPEUTIC CLASS: Estrogen

INDICATIONS: Treatment of moderate to severe vasomotor symptoms and/or vulvar/vaginal atrophy due to menopause. Treatment of hypoestrogenism due to hypogonadism, castration, or primary ovarian failure. Prevention of postmenopausal osteoporosis.

DOSAGE: *Adults:* Start therapy with 0.025mg/day applied to the skin once weekly. Vasomotor Symptoms/Vulvar and Vaginal Atrophy: D/C or taper dose at 3- to 6-month intervals. Hypoestrogenism Due to Hypogonadism/Castration/Primary Ovarian Failure: Adjust dose as necessary to control symptoms. Clinical response at lowest effective dose should be the guide for establishing administration, especially in women with an intact uterus.

HOW SUPPLIED: Patch: 0.025mg/day, 0.0375mg/day, 0.05mg/day, 0.06mg/day, 0.075mg/day, 0.1mg/day [4s]

CONTRAINDICATIONS: Undiagnosed abnormal genital bleeding, known/suspected/history of breast cancer, known/suspected estrogen-dependent neoplasia, active/history of DVT/PE, active/history of arterial thromboembolic disease (eg, stroke, MI), known liver impairment or disease, known protein C/protein S/antithrombin deficiency or other known thrombophilic disorders, known/suspected pregnancy.

WARNINGS/PRECAUTIONS: D/C immediately if stroke, DVT, PE, or MI occur or are suspected. Caution in patients with risk factors for arterial vascular disease and/or venous thromboembolism. If feasible, d/c at least 4 to 6 weeks before surgery of the type associated with an increased risk of thromboembolism, or during periods of prolonged immobilization. May increase risk of ovarian cancer and gallbladder disease. May lead to severe hypercalcemia in patients with breast cancer and bone metastases; d/c and take appropriate measures if hypercalcemia occurs. Retinal vascular thrombosis reported; d/c pending exam if sudden partial/complete loss of vision, sudden onset of proptosis, diplopia, or migraine occurs. D/C permanently if exam reveals papilledema or retinal vascular lesions. Consider addition of progestin for women with a uterus or with residual endometriosis post-hysterectomy. May elevate BP and thyroid-binding globulin levels. May elevate plasma TGs, leading to pancreatitis in patients with preexisting hypertriglyceridemia; consider discontinuation if pancreatitis occurs. Caution with impaired liver function and history of cholestatic jaundice associated with past estrogen use or with pregnancy; d/c in case of recurrence. May cause fluid retention; caution with cardiac/renal impairment. Caution with hypoparathyroidism; hypocalcemia may result. May exacerbate endometriosis, asthma, diabetes mellitus, epilepsy, migraine, porphyria, systemic lupus erythematosus, and hepatic hemangiomas; use with caution. May exacerbate symptoms of angioedema in women with hereditary angioedema. Conventional transdermal doses used in patients with normal renal function may be excessive for women with end-stage renal disease receiving maintenance hemodialysis. May affect certain endocrine and blood components in lab tests.

ADVERSE REACTIONS: Headache, arthralgia, edema, abdominal pain, flatulence, depression, breast pain, leukorrhea, upper respiratory tract infection, sinusitis, rhinitis, pruritus, nausea, pharyngitis, pain.

INTERACTIONS: CYP3A4 inducers (eg, St. John's wort preparations, phenobarbital, carbamazepine, rifampin) may decrease therapeutic effects and/or change uterine bleeding profile. CYP3A4 inhibitors (eg, erythromycin, ketoconazole, ritonavir, grapefruit juice) may increase levels, which may result in side effects. Patients concomitantly receiving thyroid hormone replacement therapy and estrogens may require increased doses of their thyroid replacement therapy; monitor thyroid function.

PREGNANCY: Contraindicated in pregnancy, not for use in nursing.

MECHANISM OF ACTION: Estrogen; binds to nuclear receptors in estrogen-responsive tissues. Circulating estrogen modulates pituitary secretion of gonadotropins, luteinizing hormone, and follicle-stimulating hormone, through negative feedback mechanism. Reduces elevated levels of these hormones in postmenopausal women.

PHARMACOKINETICS: Absorption: Transdermal administration of variable doses resulted in different parameters. **Distribution:** Largely bound to sex hormone-binding globulin and albumin; found in breast milk. **Metabolism:** Liver to estrone (metabolite), estriol (major urinary metabolite); sulfate and glucuronide conjugation (liver), biliary secretion of conjugates into the intestine, hydrolysis (intestine), reabsorption; CYP3A4 (partial metabolism). **Elimination:** Urine (parent compound and metabolites).

NURSING CONSIDERATIONS

Assessment: Assess for undiagnosed abnormal genital bleeding, presence or history of breast cancer, estrogen-dependent neoplasia, DVT, PE, arterial thromboembolic disease, liver impairment/disease, history of cholestatic jaundice, drug hypersensitivity, pregnancy/nursing status, any other conditions where treatment may be contraindicated or cautioned, need for progestin therapy, and possible drug interactions.

Monitoring: Monitor for signs/symptoms of CV disease, malignant neoplasms, dementia, gallbladder disease, hypercalcemia, visual abnormalities, BP and plasma TG elevations, pancreatitis, cholestatic jaundice, fluid retention, exacerbation of endometriosis and other conditions, and other adverse reactions. Perform annual breast exam; schedule mammography based on age, risk factors, and prior mammogram results. Periodically reevaluate (every 3-6 months) to determine need for therapy. Perform adequate diagnostic measures (eg, endometrial sampling) to rule out malignancies in cases of undiagnosed, persistent, or recurring abnormal genital bleeding. Regularly monitor thyroid function if on thyroid hormone replacement therapy.

Patient Counseling: Inform of the importance of reporting vaginal bleeding to physician as soon as possible. Inform of possible serious reactions of therapy including CV disorders, malignant neoplasms, and probable dementia. Inform of the possible less serious, but common adverse reactions of therapy (eg, headache, breast pain and tenderness, N/V).

Administration: Transdermal route. Apply immediately upon removal from the protective pouch. Refer to PI for proper application and removal of the system (patch). **Storage:** 20-25°C (66-77°F); excursions permitted between 15-30°C (59-86°F). Do not store >30°C (86°F). Do not store unpouched.

CLINDAGEL   RX
clindamycin phosphate (Galderma)

THERAPEUTIC CLASS: Lincomycin derivative

INDICATIONS: Acne vulgaris.

DOSAGE: *Adults:* Apply thin film qd.
Pediatrics: ≥12 Yrs: Apply thin film qd.

HOW SUPPLIED: Gel: 1% [40mL, 75mL]

CONTRAINDICATIONS: Hypersensitivity to lincomycin. History of regional enteritis, ulcerative colitis, or antibiotic-associated colitis.

WARNINGS/PRECAUTIONS: D/C if significant diarrhea occurs. Caution in atopic individuals.

ADVERSE REACTIONS: Peeling, pruritus, pseudomembranous colitis (rare).

INTERACTIONS: May potentiate neuromuscular blockers.

PREGNANCY: Category B, not for use in nursing.

MECHANISM OF ACTION: Lincomycin derivative; inhibits bacteria protein synthesis at ribosomal level by binding to the 50S ribosomal subunit and affecting the process of peptide chain initiation.

PHARMACOKINETICS: Absorption: $C_{max}=\le5.5$ng/mL. **Distribution:** Orally and parenterally administered clindamycin appears in breast milk. **Elimination:** Urine (<0.4% of total dose).

NURSING CONSIDERATIONS

Assessment: Assess for hypersensitivity to lincomycin, history of regional or ulcerative colitis, antibiotic-associated colitis, nursing status. Assess use in atopic individuals and for possible drug interactions.

Monitoring: Monitor for signs/symptoms of colitis (pseudomembranous colitis), diarrhea, and bloody diarrhea. In patients with diarrhea, consider stool culture for *Clostridium difficile* and stool assay for *C. difficile* toxin. In patients with significant diarrhea, consider large bowel endoscopy.

Patient Counseling: Instruct to notify physician of significant diarrhea during therapy or up to several weeks following end of therapy.

Administration: Topical application. **Storage:** Controlled room temperature, 20-25°C (68-77°F); excursions permitted to 15-30°C (59-86°F). Keep container tightly closed, out of direct sunlight.

CLINDESSE   RX
clindamycin phosphate (Ther-Rx)

THERAPEUTIC CLASS: Lincomycin derivative

INDICATIONS: Treatment of bacterial vaginosis in nonpregnant women.

DOSAGE: *Adults:* 1 applicatorful once intravaginally at any time of the day.
Pediatrics: Postmenarchal: 1 applicatorful once intravaginally at any time of the day.

HOW SUPPLIED: Cre: 2% [5g]

CONTRAINDICATIONS: Regional enteritis, ulcerative colitis, history of *Clostridium difficile*-associated diarrhea (CDAD).

WARNINGS/PRECAUTIONS: Not for ophthalmic, dermal, or oral use. CDAD reported; d/c if CDAD is suspected or confirmed. Contains mineral oil that may weaken latex or rubber products (eg, condoms, vaginal contraceptive diaphragms); use of such barrier contraceptives is not recommended concurrently or for 5 days following treatment.

ADVERSE REACTIONS: Fungal vaginosis, headache, back pain.

INTERACTIONS: Oral or IV clindamycin may enhance the action of other neuromuscular blockers; use with caution.

PREGNANCY: Category B, not for use in nursing.

MECHANISM OF ACTION: Lincomycin derivative; inhibits bacterial protein synthesis by binding preferentially to the 50S ribosomal subunit and affecting the process of peptide chain initiation.

PHARMACOKINETICS: Absorption: $C_{max}=6.6$ng/mL, $T_{max}=20$ hrs, AUC=175ng/mL•hr. **Distribution:** (PO/Parenteral) Found in breast milk.

NURSING CONSIDERATIONS

Assessment: Assess for history of hypersensitivity to the drug or other lincosamides, regional enteritis, ulcerative colitis, history of CDAD, pregnancy/nursing status, and possible drug interactions.

Monitoring: Monitor for CDAD and other adverse reactions.

Patient Counseling: Instruct not to engage in vaginal intercourse or use other vaginal products (eg, tampons, douches) during treatment. Inform that medication contains mineral oil that may weaken latex or rubber products (eg, condoms, vaginal contraceptive diaphragms); instruct not to use barrier contraceptives concurrently or for 5 days following treatment. Inform that vaginal fungal infection can occur and may require antifungal drug treatment. Inform that medication contains ingredients that cause burning and irritation of the eye; instruct to rinse eye with copious amounts of cool tap water and consult physician if accidental contact with eye occurs.

Administration: Intravaginal route. **Storage:** 20-25°C (68-77°F). Avoid heat >30°C (86°F).

CLONAZEPAM   CIV
clonazepam (Various)

OTHER BRAND NAMES: Klonopin (Genentech)

THERAPEUTIC CLASS: Benzodiazepine

INDICATIONS: Adjunct or monotherapy in the treatment of Lennox-Gastaut syndrome (petit mal variant) and of akinetic and myoclonic seizures. May be useful in patients with absence seizures (petit mal) who have failed to respond to succinimides. Treatment of panic disorder with or without agoraphobia.

DOSAGE: *Adults:* Seizure Disorders: Initial: Not to exceed 1.5mg/day divided into 3 doses. Titrate: May increase in increments of 0.5-1mg every 3 days until seizures are controlled or until side effects preclude any further increase. Maint: Individualize dose. Max: 20mg/day. Panic Disorder: Initial: 0.25mg bid. Titrate: May increase to target dose of 1mg/day after 3 days; for some, may increase in increments of 0.125-0.25mg bid every 3 days until panic disorder is controlled or until side effects make further increases undesired. Max: 4mg/day. D/C: Decrease by 0.125mg bid every 3 days. Elderly: Start at low end of dosing range. *Pediatrics:* Seizure Disorders: ≤10 Yrs or ≤30kg: Initial: 0.01-0.03mg/kg/day up to 0.05mg/kg/day given in 2 or 3 divided doses. Titrate: May increase by no more than 0.25-0.5mg every 3 days until maintenance dose is reached, unless seizures are controlled or until side effects preclude further increase. Maint: 0.1-0.2mg/kg/day divided into 3 doses.

HOW SUPPLIED: Tab: (Klonopin) 0.5mg*, 1mg, 2mg; Tab, Disintegrating (ODT): 0.125mg, 0.25mg, 0.5mg, 1mg, 2mg *scored

CONTRAINDICATIONS: Significant liver disease, untreated open-angle glaucoma, acute narrow-angle glaucoma.

WARNINGS/PRECAUTIONS: May impair mental/physical abilities. May increase risk of suicidal thoughts/behavior; monitor for the emergence of worsening of depression, suicidal thoughts/behavior, and/or any unusual changes in mood or behavior. Caution with use in pregnancy and women of childbearing potential; may increase risk of congenital malformations. Avoid use during the 1st trimester of pregnancy. May increase incidence or precipitate the onset of generalized tonic-clonic seizures in patients in whom several different types of seizure disorders coexist; addition of appropriate anticonvulsants or increase in their dosages may be required. Withdrawal symptoms reported after discontinuation of therapy. Avoid abrupt withdrawal; may precipitate status epilepticus. Caution with renal impairment. May produce an increase in salivation; caution with chronic respiratory diseases. Caution with addiction-prone individuals and elderly. (ODT) Contains phenylalanine.

ADVERSE REACTIONS: CNS depression, ataxia, drowsiness, abnormal coordination, depression, behavior problems, dizziness, upper respiratory tract infection, memory disturbance, dysmenorrhea, fatigue, influenza, nervousness, sinusitis.

INTERACTIONS: Decreased serum levels with CYP450 inducers (eg, phenytoin, carbamazepine, phenobarbital), and propantheline. Caution with CYP3A inhibitors (eg, oral antifungals). Alcohol, narcotics, barbiturates, nonbarbiturate hypnotics, antianxiety agents, phenothiazines, thioxanthene and butyrophenone antipsychotics, MAOIs, TCAs, other anticonvulsant drugs, and other CNS depressant drugs may potentiate CNS-depressant effects. May produce absence status with valproic acid.

PREGNANCY: Category D, not for use in nursing.

MECHANISM OF ACTION: Benzodiazepine; has not been established. Suspected to be related to its ability to enhance activity of gamma-aminobutyric acid, the major inhibitory neurotransmitter in the CNS.

PHARMACOKINETICS: Absorption: Rapid and complete. Absolute bioavailability (90%); T_{max}=1-4 hrs. **Distribution:** Plasma protein binding (85%). **Metabolism:** Liver via CYP450 (including CYP3A), acetylation, hydroxylation, and glucuronidation. **Elimination:** Urine (<2% unchanged); $T_{1/2}$=30-40 hrs.

NURSING CONSIDERATIONS

Assessment: Assess for history of sensitivity to benzodiazepines, acute narrow-angle glaucoma, untreated open-angle glaucoma, liver/renal impairment, mental depression, history of drug or alcohol addiction, chronic respiratory diseases, pregnancy/nursing status, and possible drug interactions.

Monitoring: Monitor for CNS depression, emergence or worsening of depression, suicidal thoughts/behavior, unusual changes in mood or behavior, and worsening of seizures. Periodically monitor blood counts and LFTs during prolonged therapy. Upon withdrawal, monitor for withdrawal symptoms.

Patient Counseling: Instruct to take medication as prescribed. Inform that therapy may produce physical and psychological dependence; instruct to consult physician before either increasing the dose or abruptly discontinuing the drug. Caution about operating hazardous machinery, including automobiles. Counsel that drug may increase risk of suicidal thoughts/behavior and advise of need to be alert for the emergence/worsening of symptoms of depression, any unusual changes in mood or behavior, or the emergence of suicidal thoughts/behavior, or thoughts of self-harm. Advise to notify physician if patient becomes pregnant or intends to become pregnant during therapy. Advise not to breastfeed while on therapy. Advise to inform physician if taking, or planning to take any prescription or OTC drugs and to avoid alcohol while on therapy. (ODT) Inform that drug contains phenylalanine.

Administration: Oral route. ODT: 1) Peel back foil on blister. Do not push tab through foil. 2) Using dry hands, remove tab and place it in mouth. Tab: Swallow whole with water. **Storage:** 20-25°C (68-77°F). (Klonopin) 25°C (77°F); excursions permitted to 15-30°C (59-86°F).

CLORPRES   RX

clonidine HCl - chlorthalidone (Mylan)

THERAPEUTIC CLASS: Alpha-agonist/monosulfamyl diuretic

INDICATIONS: Treatment of HTN. Not for initial therapy.

DOSAGE: *Adults:* Determine dose by individual titration. 0.1mg-15mg tab qd-bid. Max: 0.6mg-30mg/day.

HOW SUPPLIED: Tab: (Clonidine-Chlorthalidone) 0.1mg-15mg*, 0.2mg-15mg*, 0.3mg-15mg* *scored

CONTRAINDICATIONS: Anuria, sulfonamide hypersensitivity.

WARNINGS/PRECAUTIONS: Caution with severe renal disease, hepatic dysfunction, asthma, severe coronary insufficiency, recent myocardial infarction (MI), and cerebrovascular disease. May develop allergic reaction to oral clonidine if sensitive to clonidine patch. Avoid abrupt withdrawal. Continue therapy to within 4 hrs of surgery and resume after. Monitor for fluid/electrolyte imbalance. Hyperuricemia, hypokalemia, hyponatremia, hypochloremic alkalosis, and hyperglycemia may occur.

ADVERSE REACTIONS: Drowsiness, dizziness, constipation, sedation, fatigue, dry mouth, N/V, orthostatic symptoms.

INTERACTIONS: Potentiates other antihypertensives. May increase response to tubocurarine. May decrease arterial response to norepinephrine. Antidiabetic agents may need adjustment. Risk of lithium toxicity. TCAs may reduce effects of clonidine. Amitriptyline may enhance ocular toxicity. Enhanced CNS-depressive effects of alcohol, barbiturates, or other sedatives. Orthostatic hypotension aggravated by alcohol, barbiturates, narcotics. D/C β-blockers several days before the gradual withdrawal of clonidine in patients taking both.

PREGNANCY: (Clonidine) Category C, caution in nursing. (Chlorthalidone) Category B, not for use in nursing.

MECHANISM OF ACTION: Clonidine: Imidazoline derivative; stimulates α-adrenoceptor in brain stem, resulting in reduced sympathetic outflow from CNS and decrease in peripheral resistance, renal vascular resistance, HR, and BP. Chlorthalidone: Monosulfamyl diuretic; increases excretion of Na^+ and Cl^-; decreases extracellular fluid volume, plasma volume, cardiac output, total exchangeable Na^+, GFR, and renal plasma flow.

PHARMACOKINETICS: Absorption: Clonidine: T_{max}=3-5 hrs. **Distribution:** Chlorthalidone: Plasma protein binding (75%). **Metabolism:** Clonidine: Liver (50%). **Elimination:** Clonidine: Urine (40-60% unchanged); $T_{1/2}$=12-16 hrs; $T_{1/2}$ in severe renal impairment=41 hrs. Chlorthalidone: Urine (unchanged); $T_{1/2}$=40-60 hrs.

NURSING CONSIDERATIONS

Assessment: Assess for anuria, sulfonamide hypersensitivity, coronary insufficiency, recent MI, cerebrovascular disease, history of allergy or bronchial asthma, systemic lupus erythematosus (SLE), diabetes mellitus, renal/hepatic impairment, pregnancy/nursing status, and possible drug interactions. Perform and obtain serum and urine electrolytes.

Monitoring: Monitor BP. Periodically monitor serum and urine electrolytes, serum PBI level, serum K^+ levels, and renal function. Monitor for signs/symptoms of electrolyte imbalance, hypokalemia, possible exacerbation or activation of SLE, hyperglycemia, withdrawal symptoms, hyperuricemia or precipitation of gout, hypersensitivity reactions, renal/hepatic dysfunction.

Patient Counseling: Caution that drug may impair physical/mental abilities. Advise to avoid alcohol. Instruct not to interrupt or d/c therapy without consulting physician. Instruct to seek medical attention if symptoms of electrolyte imbalance (dry mouth, thirst, weakness), hypokalemia (thirst, tiredness, restlessness), withdrawal (nervousness, agitation, headaches), or hypersensitivity reactions occur.

Administration: Oral route. **Storage:** 15-30°C (59-86°F). Avoid excessive humidity.

CLOZAPINE

RX

clozapine (Various)

> Risk of potentially life-threatening agranulocytosis. Reserve use for severely ill patients with schizophrenia unresponsive to standard antipsychotic treatment or for patients with schizophrenia/schizoaffective disorder at risk for reexperiencing suicidal behavior. Obtain baseline WBC count and absolute neutrophil count (ANC) prior to therapy, regularly during treatment, and for at least 4 weeks after discontinuation. Seizures may occur and risk is dose related; caution with history of seizures or other predisposing factors. Increased risk of fatal myocarditis, especially during 1st month of therapy; d/c if suspected. Orthostatic hypotension, with or without syncope, can occur and is more likely during initial titration. Rare reports of profound collapse with respiratory and/or cardiac arrest reported; caution when initiating therapy in patients taking benzodiazepines or any other psychotropic drugs. Elderly patients with dementia-related psychosis treated with antipsychotic drugs are at an increased risk for death; most deaths appeared to be cardiovascular (CV) (eg, heart failure [HF], sudden death) or infectious (eg, pneumonia) in nature. Not approved for treatment of dementia-related psychosis.

OTHER BRAND NAMES: Clozaril (Novartis)

THERAPEUTIC CLASS: Dibenzapine derivative

INDICATIONS: Management of severely ill schizophrenic patients who fail to respond adequately to standard drug treatment for schizophrenia. Reduction of risk for recurrent suicidal behavior in patients with schizophrenia/schizoaffective disorder who are judged to be at chronic risk for reexperiencing suicidal behavior.

DOSAGE: *Adults:* Treatment-Resistant Schizophrenia: Initial: 12.5mg qd-bid. Titrate: Increase by 25-50mg/day, up to 300-450mg/day by end of 2 weeks, then increase once or twice weekly in increments not to exceed 100mg. Usual: 300-600mg/day on a divided basis. Titrate: May increase to 600-900mg/day. Max: 900mg/day. Maint: Lowest effective dose; periodically reassess need for maintenance treatment. To d/c, gradually reduce dose over 1-2 weeks. Reinitiation (≥2 days since last dose): Reinitiate with 12.5mg qd-bid. May titrate more quickly if initial dosing tolerated. Retitrate with extreme caution in patients who previously experienced cardiac/respiratory arrest with initial dose but were successfully titrated to therapeutic dose. Do not restart if discontinued for WBC count <2000/mm³ or ANC <1000/mm³. Reduction of Risk for Suicidal Behavior in Schizophrenia/Schizoaffective Disorder: May follow dosing recommendations for treatment-resistant schizophrenia. Range: 12.5-900mg/day (mean 300mg). To reduce the risk of suicidal behavior in patients who otherwise responded to therapy with another antipsychotic, treat for ≥2 yrs and then reevaluate. If risk for suicidal behavior is still present, continue treatment and reassess at regular intervals. If no longer at risk of suicidal behavior, d/c treatment. (Clozaril) Refer to PI if switching from a previous antipsychotic therapy.

HOW SUPPLIED: Tab: 25mg*, 50mg*, 100mg*, 200mg*; (Clozaril) 25mg*, 100mg* *scored

CONTRAINDICATIONS: Myeloproliferative disorders, uncontrolled epilepsy, paralytic ileus, history of clozapine-induced agranulocytosis or severe granulocytopenia, severe CNS depression, comatose states. Concomitant use with agents having potential to cause agranulocytosis or suppress bone marrow function.

WARNINGS/PRECAUTIONS: QT prolongation, ventricular arrhythmia, torsades de pointes, cardiac arrest, and sudden death may occur. Caution with history/family history of long QT syndrome, other conditions that may increase risk of QT prolongation (eg, recent acute myocardial infarction, uncompensated HF, cardiac arrhythmia), or CV disease. Caution in patients at risk for significant electrolyte disturbance, particularly hypokalemia; correct electrolyte abnormalities before initiation and monitor levels periodically. D/C if QTc interval >500 msec. Associated with metabolic changes (eg, hyperglycemia sometimes with ketoacidosis or hyperosmolar coma, dyslipidemia, weight gain) that may increase CV/cerebrovascular risk; monitor glucose/lipid levels and weight. Tachycardia and cardiomyopathy reported. D/C if cardiomyopathy is confirmed unless benefits outweigh risks. Neuroleptic malignant syndrome (NMS) reported; d/c therapy and institute symptomatic treatment. Transient fever may occur and may necessitate discontinuing treatment; rule out infection or agranulocytosis. Tardive dyskinesia (TD), deep vein thrombosis (DVT), pulmonary embolism (PE), impaired intestinal peristalsis, hepatitis, and ECG changes reported; consider discontinuation if TD or jaundice occurs and if LFT elevation is clinically relevant. Has potent anticholinergic effects; caution with prostatic enlargement and narrow-angle glaucoma. May impair mental/physical abilities. Caution with renal, cardiac, hepatic, or pulmonary disease. Increased risk of cerebrovascular adverse events; caution in patients with risk factors for stroke. Monitor for psychotic and cholinergic rebound symptoms if medical condition requires abrupt discontinuation (eg, leukopenia). Obtain WBC count and ANC at baseline, then weekly for first 6 months of therapy, then every 2 weeks for next 6 months, and then every 4 weeks thereafter if counts are acceptable (WBC count ≥3500/mm³ or ANC ≥2000/mm³). Refer to PI for frequency of monitoring based on stage of therapy, WBC count, and ANC. D/C treatment and do not rechallenge if WBC count <2000/mm³ or ANC <1000/mm³. Interrupt therapy if eosinophilia (>4000/mm³) develops until eosinophil count falls below 3000/mm³. Caution in elderly.

ADVERSE REACTIONS: Agranulocytosis, seizure, myocarditis, orthostatic hypotension, salivary hypersecretion, somnolence, drowsiness/sedation, weight increased, dizziness/vertigo, constipation, tachycardia, N/V, headache.

INTERACTIONS: See Contraindications and Boxed Warning. Avoid using epinephrine to treat clozapine-induced hypotension. Use with carbamazepine is not recommended. Caution with CNS-active drugs, general anesthesia, alcohol, paroxetine, fluoxetine, fluvoxamine, sertraline, drugs that inhibit clozapine metabolism, inhibitors/inducers, or in patients with reduced activity of CYP1A2, 2D6, 3A4. Consider dose reduction with paroxetine, fluoxetine, fluvoxamine, and sertraline. Dosage reduction may be needed with drugs metabolized by CYP2D6 (eg, antidepressants, phenothiazines, carbamazepine, Type 1C antiarrhythmics) or that inhibit this enzyme (eg, quinidine); use with caution. May potentiate hypotensive effects of antihypertensives and anticholinergic effects of atropine-type drugs. CYP450 inducers (eg, phenytoin, tobacco smoke, rifampin) may decrease plasma levels. CYP450 inhibitors (eg, cimetidine, caffeine, citalopram, ciprofloxacin, fluvoxamine, erythromycin) may increase plasma levels. NMS reported with lithium and other CNS-active drugs. May interact with other highly protein-bound drugs. Caution with drugs known to prolong the QTc interval, such as Class 1A antiarrhythmics (eg, quinidine, procainamide), Class III antiarrhythmics (eg, amiodarone, sotalol), antipsychotics (eg, ziprasidone, iloperidone, chlorpromazine, thioridazine, mesoridazine, droperidol, pimozide), certain antibiotics (eg, erythromycin, gatifloxacin, moxifloxacin, sparfloxacin), and other drugs known to prolong the QT interval (eg, pentamidine, levomethadyl acetate, methadone, halofantrine, mefloquine, dolasetron mesylate, probucol, tacrolimus). Caution with drugs that can cause electrolyte imbalance (eg, diuretics).

PREGNANCY: Category B, not for use in nursing.

MECHANISM OF ACTION: Tricyclic dibenzodiazepine derivative; atypical antipsychotic agent. Interferes with binding of dopamine at D_1, D_2, D_3, and D_5 receptors and has a high affinity for D_4 receptor. Also acts as an antagonist at the adrenergic, cholinergic, histaminergic, and serotonergic receptors.

PHARMACOKINETICS: Absorption: C_{max}=319ng/mL; T_{max}=2.5 hrs (100mg bid). **Distribution:** Plasma protein binding (97%). **Metabolism:** Demethylation, hydroxylation, N-oxidation. **Elimination:** Urine (50%), feces (30%); $T_{1/2}$=8 hrs (75mg single dose), $T_{1/2}$=12 hrs (100mg bid).

NURSING CONSIDERATIONS

Assessment: Assess previous course of standard therapy prior to treatment. Assess for myeloproliferative disorders, uncontrolled epilepsy, paralytic ileus, history of clozapine-induced agranulocytosis or severe granulocytopenia, severe CNS depression or comatose states, history of seizures or other predisposing factors, pregnancy/nursing status, possible drug interactions, and other conditions where treatment is cautioned or contraindicated. Obtain baseline WBC count, ANC, FPG levels in patients with diabetes mellitus (DM) or at risk for hyperglycemia/DM, serum K^+ and Mg^{2+} levels, and lipid evaluations.

Monitoring: Monitor for clinical response and need to continue treatment. Monitor for agranulocytosis, myocarditis, orthostatic hypotension, HF, tachycardia, severe respiratory effects, seizures, flu-like symptoms, infection, eosinophilia, fever, DVT, PE, NMS, TD, hepatitis, hyperglycemia, and other adverse reactions. Monitor WBC count and ANC during and for ≥4 weeks following discontinuation or until WBC count ≥3500/mm³ and ANC ≥2000/mm³. Monitor glucose control in patients with DM and check periodic FPG in patients at risk for hyperglycemia/DM. Obtain LFTs if patient develops N/V and/or anorexia. Monitor weight and electrolytes periodically.

Patient Counseling: Inform that drug is available only through a program designed to ensure the required blood monitoring schedule. Counsel on the significant risks of developing agranulocytosis. Advise to immediately report the appearance of lethargy, weakness, fever, sore throat, malaise, mucous membrane ulceration, flu-like complaints, or other possible signs of infection. Inform patients of the significant risk of seizure during treatment; advise to avoid driving and any other potentially hazardous activity while on treatment. Advise of the risk of orthostatic hypotension, especially during the period of initial dose titration. If dose was missed for >2 days, inform patients to not restart medication at same dose but to contact physician for dosing instructions. Instruct to notify physician if taking or planning to take any prescription or OTC drugs or alcohol. Instruct to notify physician if pregnant or intending to become pregnant. Advise not to breastfeed if taking the drug.

Administration: Oral route. Take with or without food. **Storage:** 20-25°C (68-77°F). (Clozaril) Should not exceed 30°C (86°F).

COARTEM   RX
lumefantrine - artemether (Novartis)

THERAPEUTIC CLASS: Artemisinin-based combination therapy

INDICATIONS: Treatment of acute, uncomplicated malaria infections due to *Plasmodium falciparum* in patients ≥5kg.

DOSAGE: *Adults:* >16 Yrs: ≥35kg: 4 tabs as a single initial dose, 4 tabs again after 8 hrs, and then 4 tabs bid (am and pm) for the following 2 days. <35kg: Refer to pediatric dosage. Take with food.
Pediatrics: ≥35kg: 4 tabs as a single initial dose, 4 tabs again after 8 hrs, and then 4 tabs bid (am and pm) for the following 2 days. 25-<35kg: 3 tabs as an initial dose, 3 tabs again after 8 hrs, and then 3 tabs bid (am and pm) for the following 2 days. 15-<25kg: 2 tabs as an initial dose, 2 tabs again after 8 hrs, and then 2 tabs bid (am and pm) for the following 2 days. 5-<15kg: 1 tab as an initial dose, 1 tab again after 8 hrs, and then 1 tab bid (am and pm) for the following 2 days. Take with food.

HOW SUPPLIED: Tab: (Artemether-Lumefantrine) 20mg-120mg* *scored

CONTRAINDICATIONS: Coadministration with strong CYP3A4 inducers (eg, rifampin, carbamazepine, phenytoin, St. John's wort).

WARNINGS/PRECAUTIONS: Not approved for prevention of malaria or for patients with severe or complicated *P. falciparum* malaria. May prolong the QT interval; avoid with congenital QT interval prolongation (eg, long QT syndrome) or any other clinical condition known to prolong the QT interval (eg, history of symptomatic cardiac arrhythmias, clinically relevant bradycardia, severe cardiac disease), family history of congenital QT interval prolongation or sudden death, or known disturbances of electrolyte balance (eg, hypokalemia, hypomagnesemia). Closely monitor patients who remain averse to food during treatment as risk of recrudescence may be greater; if recrudescent *P. falciparum* infection develops after treatment, treat patient with a different antimalarial drug. Caution with severe hepatic/renal impairment.

ADVERSE REACTIONS: Headache, dizziness, anorexia, asthenia, pyrexia, chills, fatigue, arthralgia, myalgia, N/V, abdominal pain, splenomegaly, hepatomegaly, cough.

INTERACTIONS: See Contraindications. Avoid with other medications that prolong the QT interval (eg, Class IA [quinidine, procainamide, disopyramide] or Class III [amiodarone, sotalol] antiarrhythmic agents, antipsychotics [pimozide, ziprasidone], antidepressants, certain antibiotics [macrolide/fluoroquinolone antibiotics, imidazole/triazole antifungal agents]); monitor ECG if concomitant use with a drug that prolongs the QT interval, including antimalarials such as quinine, is medically required. Avoid with medications metabolized by CYP2D6 that also have cardiac effects (eg, flecainide, imipramine, amitriptyline, clomipramine). Do not administer with halofantrine within 1 month of each other. Do not give with antimalarials, unless there is no other treatment option. Mefloquine administered immediately prior to therapy may lead to decreased exposure to lumefantrine. May decrease concentrations and efficacy of CYP3A4 substrates. CYP3A4 inhibitors (eg, grapefruit juice, ketoconazole) may increase concentrations and potentiate QT prolongation. CYP3A4 inducers may decrease concentrations and antimalarial efficacy. Caution with drugs that have a mixed effect on CYP3A4, especially antiretroviral drugs (eg, HIV protease inhibitors and non-nucleoside reverse transcriptase inhibitors), and those that have an effect on the QT interval. May reduce effectiveness of hormonal contraceptives; use an additional nonhormonal method of birth control. May increase concentrations of CYP2D6 substrates and increase risk of adverse effects.

PREGNANCY: Category C, caution in nursing.

MECHANISM OF ACTION: Artemether: Artemisinin derivative; antimalarial activity attributed to endoperoxide moiety. Lumefantrine: Antimalarial agent; not established. Suspected to inhibit the formation of β-hematin by forming a complex with hemin. Both artemether and lumefantrine inhibit nucleic acid and protein synthesis.

PHARMACOKINETICS: Absorption: Administration of variable doses resulted in different parameters. **Distribution:** Artemether: Plasma protein binding (95.4%, 47-76% dihydroartemisinin [DHA]). Lumefantrine: Plasma protein binding (99.7%). **Metabolism:** Artemether: Liver via CYP3A4/5 (major), CYP2B6, CYP2C9, CYP2C19 (minor); DHA (active metabolite). Lumefantrine: Liver via CYP3A4; desbutyl-lumefantrine (metabolite). **Elimination:** Artemether and DHA: $T_{1/2}$=2 hrs. Lumefantrine: $T_{1/2}$=3-6 days.

NURSING CONSIDERATIONS

Assessment: Assess for congenital QT interval prolongation or any other clinical condition known to prolong the QT interval, family history of congenital QT interval prolongation or sudden death, known disturbances of electrolyte balance, drug hypersensitivity, severe hepatic/renal impairment, pregnancy/nursing status, and possible drug interactions.

Monitoring: Monitor for QT interval prolongation, recrudescent *P. falciparum* infection, and other adverse reactions.

Patient Counseling: Instruct to inform physician of any personal/family history of QT prolongation or proarrhythmic conditions (eg, hypokalemia, bradycardia, recent myocardial ischemia), if taking any other medications, and if symptoms of QT interval prolongation (eg, prolonged heart palpitations, loss of consciousness) occur. Advise patients using hormonal contraceptives to use an additional nonhormonal method of birth control. Instruct to d/c therapy at the 1st sign of a skin rash, hives or other skin reactions, a rapid heartbeat, difficulty in swallowing or breathing, any swelling suggesting angioedema, or other symptoms of an allergic reaction.

Administration: Oral route. Take with food. Resume normal eating as soon as food can be tolerated. If unable to swallow tabs, may crush tabs and mix with small amount of water (1-2 tsp) in a clean container prior to administration; crushed tab preparation should be followed whenever possible by food/drink (eg, milk, formula, pudding, broth, porridge). If vomiting occurs within 1-2 hrs of administration, give a repeat dose. If the repeat dose is vomited, give an alternative antimalarial treatment. **Storage:** 25°C (77°F); excursions permitted to 15-30°C (59-86°F).

COLAZAL   RX
balsalazide disodium (Salix)

THERAPEUTIC CLASS: 5-aminosalicylic acid derivative

INDICATIONS: Treatment of mild to moderate active ulcerative colitis in patients ≥5 yrs.

DOSAGE: *Adults:* 3 caps tid for up to 8 weeks (or 12 weeks if needed). May open cap and sprinkle on applesauce.
Pediatrics: 5-17 Yrs: 1 or 3 caps tid for up to 8 weeks. May open cap and sprinkle on applesauce.

HOW SUPPLIED: Cap: 750mg

WARNINGS/PRECAUTIONS: May exacerbate symptoms of colitis. Prolonged gastric retention with pyloric stenosis. Caution with renal dysfunction or history of renal disease.

ADVERSE REACTIONS: Headache, abdominal pain, diarrhea, N/V, respiratory problems, arthralgia, rhinitis, insomnia, fatigue, rectal bleeding, flatulence, fever, dyspepsia.

INTERACTIONS: Oral antibiotics may interfere with the release of mesalamine in the colon.

PREGNANCY: Category B, caution in nursing.

MECHANISM OF ACTION: Not established; a prodrug enzymatically cleaved in colon to produce mesalamine (5-ASA), an anti-inflammatory drug that acts locally to block production of arachidonic acid metabolites in the colon.

PHARMACOKINETICS: Absorption: Different dosing conditions (fasted, fed, sprinkled) resulted in variable parameters. **Distribution:** Plasma protein binding (≥99%). **Metabolism:** Key metabolites: 5-ASA and N-acetyl-5-ASA. **Elimination:** Urine, feces.

NURSING CONSIDERATIONS

Assessment: Assess for pyloric stenosis, possible drug interactions, history of renal/hepatic disease.

Monitoring: Monitor renal function, LFTs, and CBC, and for signs/symptoms of prolonged gastric retention with pyloric stenosis, worsening of colitis symptoms, and hypersensitivity.

Patient Counseling: Inform that can be taken with/without food or sprinkled on applesauce; advise that teeth and/or tongue may get stained when using sprinkle form with food. Instruct to seek medical attention if diagnosed with pyloric stenosis or renal dysfunction, worsening of colitis symptoms occurs or if hypersensitivity (eg, anaphylaxis, bronchospasm, skin reaction) develops.

Administration: Oral route. **Storage:** 20-25°C (68-77°F); excursions permitted to 15-30°C (59-86°F).

COLCRYS   RX
colchicine (Takeda)

THERAPEUTIC CLASS: Miscellaneous gout agent

INDICATIONS: Prophylaxis and treatment of acute gout flares. Treatment of familial Mediterranean fever (FMF) in patients ≥4 yrs of age.

DOSAGE: *Adults:* Individualize dose. Gout Flare Prophylaxis: >16 Yrs: Usual: 0.6mg qd or bid. Max: 1.2mg/day. Severe Renal Impairment: Initial: 0.3mg/day. Titrate: Increase dose with close monitoring. Dialysis: Initial: 0.3mg twice a week with close monitoring. Severe Hepatic Impairment: Consider reducing dose. Gout Flare Treatment: Usual: 1.2mg at the 1st sign of the flare followed by 0.6mg 1 hr later. Max: 1.8mg over a 1-hr period. May be administered for treatment of a gout flare during prophylaxis at doses not to exceed 1.2mg at the 1st sign of the flare followed by 0.6mg one hr later; wait 12 hrs then resume prophylactic dose. Severe Renal/Hepatic Impairment: Do not repeat treatment course more than once every 2 weeks; consider alternate therapy if repeated treatment courses are required. Dialysis: Reduce to 0.6mg single dose. Do not repeat treatment course more than once every 2 weeks. FMF: Usual Range: 1.2-2.4mg/day in 1-2 divided doses. Titrate: Modify dose in increments of 0.3mg/day PRN to control disease or if with intolerable side effects. Max: 2.4mg/day. Mild (CrCl 50-80mL/min) to Moderate (CrCl 30-

50mL/min) Renal/Severe Hepatic Impairment: Consider reducing dose. Severe Renal Impairment (CrCl <30mL/min)/Dialysis: Initial: 0.3mg/day. Titrate: Increase dose with close monitoring. Refer to PI for dose modifications for coadministration of interacting drugs.
Pediatrics: Individualize dose. FMF: May be given qd or bid. >12 Yrs: 1.2-2.4mg/day. 6-12 Yrs: 0.9-1.8mg/day. 4-6 Yrs: 0.3-1.8mg/day. Mild (CrCl 50-80mL/min) to Moderate (CrCl 30-50mL/min) Renal/Severe Hepatic Impairment: Consider reducing dose. Severe Renal Impairment (CrCl <30mL/min)/Dialysis: Initial: 0.3mg/day. Titrate: Increase dose with close monitoring. Refer to PI for dose modifications for coadministration of interacting drugs.

HOW SUPPLIED: Tab: 0.6mg* *scored

CONTRAINDICATIONS: Concomitant use with P-glycoprotein (P-gp) or strong CYP3A4 inhibitors (this includes all protease inhibitors, except fosamprenavir) in patients with renal/hepatic impairment.

WARNINGS/PRECAUTIONS: Not an analgesic medication and should not be used to treat pain from other causes. Fatal overdoses (accidental/intentional), myelosuppression, leukopenia, granulocytopenia, thrombocytopenia, pancytopenia, and aplastic anemia reported. Drug-induced neuromuscular toxicity and rhabdomyolysis reported with chronic use; increased risk in elderly and in patients with renal dysfunction. Treatment of gout flare not recommended in patients with renal/hepatic impairment receiving prophylaxis. Caution with renal/hepatic impairment and in elderly.

ADVERSE REACTIONS: Diarrhea, pharyngolaryngeal pain, cramping, abdominal pain, N/V, fatigue, gout.

INTERACTIONS: See Contraindications. Significant increase in plasma levels reported with strong CYP3A4 inhibitors (eg, atazanavir, clarithromycin, darunavir/ritonavir, indinavir, itraconazole, tipranavir/ritonavir), moderate CYP3A4 inhibitors (eg, amprenavir, aprepitant, diltiazem, erythromycin, fluconazole, fosamprenavir) and P-gp inhibitors (eg, cyclosporine, ranolazine); see PI for dose adjustments. Fatal toxicity reported with clarithromycin and cyclosporine. Neuromuscular toxicity reported with diltiazem and verapamil. May potentiate the development of myopathy and rhabdomyolysis when used with HMG-CoA reductase inhibitors (eg, atorvastatin, simvastatin), gemfibrozil, and fibrates. May potentiate the development of myopathy when used with cyclosporine. Rhabdomyolysis reported with digoxin.

PREGNANCY: Category C, caution in nursing.

MECHANISM OF ACTION: Alkaloid; not established. May interfere with the intracellular assembly of the inflammasome complex present in neutrophils and monocytes that mediates activation of interleukin-1β in patients with FMF. Disrupts cytoskeletal functions through inhibition of β-tubulin polymerization into microtubules, consequently preventing the activation, degranulation, and migration of neutrophils thought to mediate some gout symptoms.

PHARMACOKINETICS: Absorption: Administration of variable doses resulted in different pharmacokinetic parameters. **Distribution:** V_d=5-8L/kg; plasma protein binding (39%). Crosses placenta; found in breast milk. **Metabolism:** CYP3A4; demethylation; 2-O-demethylcolchicine and 3-O-demethylcolchicine (primary metabolites); 10-O-demethylcolchicine (minor metabolite). **Elimination:** Urine (40-65%, unchanged); $T_{1/2}$=26.6-31.2 hrs.

NURSING CONSIDERATIONS

Assessment: Assess for renal/hepatic impairment, pregnancy/nursing status, and possible drug interactions.

Monitoring: Monitor for myelosuppression, leukopenia, granulocytopenia, thrombocytopenia, pancytopenia, aplastic anemia, neuromuscular toxicity, rhabdomyolysis, and other adverse reactions.

Patient Counseling: Inform about benefits and risks of therapy. Instruct to take medication ud. If a dose is missed for the treatment of a gout flare, instruct to take missed dose as soon as possible. If a dose is missed for the treatment of a gout flare during prophylaxis, instruct to take missed dose immediately, wait 12 hrs, then resume previous schedule. If a dose is missed for prophylaxis without treatment of gout flares or FMF, instruct to take the next dose as soon as possible, then return to normal dosing schedule, and not to double the next dose. Inform that fatal overdoses were reported. Counsel to avoid grapefruit/grapefruit juice consumption during treatment. Inform that bone marrow depression with agranulocytosis, aplastic anemia, and thrombocytopenia may occur. Advise to notify physician of all medications currently being taken and to notify physician before starting any new medications, particularly antibiotics. Advise to d/c therapy and notify physician if muscle pain/weakness, and/or tingling/numbness of fingers/toes occur.

Administration: Oral route. Take with or without food. **Storage:** 20-25°C (68-77°F). Protect from light.

COLESTID

RX

colestipol HCl (Pharmacia & Upjohn)

THERAPEUTIC CLASS: Bile acid sequestrant

INDICATIONS: Adjunct to diet, to reduce elevated serum total and LDL-C in primary hypercholesterolemia.

DOSAGE: *Adults:* Initial: Tab: 2g qd-bid. Granules: 1 pkt or 1 scoopful qd-bid. Titrate: Tab: Increase by 2g qd or bid at 1- to 2-month intervals. Granules: May increase at an increment of 1 dose/day (1 pkt or level tsp of granules) at 1- to 2-month intervals. Usual: 2-16g/day (tab) or 1-6 pkts or scoopfuls (granules) qd or in divided doses. Always mix granules with liquid. Take 1 tab at a time and swallow tabs whole with plenty of liquid.

HOW SUPPLIED: Granules: 5g/pkt [30^s 90^s], 5g/scoopful [300g, 500g]; Tab: 1g

WARNINGS/PRECAUTIONS: Exclude secondary causes of hypercholesterolemia and obtain a lipid profile prior to therapy. May interfere with normal fat absorption. Chronic use may increase bleeding tendency due to vitamin K deficiency. May cause hypothyroidism. May produce or worsen constipation. Avoid constipation with symptomatic coronary artery disease. Constipation associated with colestipol may aggravate hemorrhoids. May produce hyperchloremic acidosis with prolonged use. (Granules) Flavored form contains phenylalanine. Always mix granules with water or other fluids before ingesting.

ADVERSE REACTIONS: Constipation, abdominal discomfort, indigestion, musculoskeletal pain, headache, AST elevation, ALT elevation, alkaline phosphatase elevation, headache, chest pain, rash, anorexia, fatigue, tachycardia, SOB.

INTERACTIONS: May interfere with absorption of folic acid, fat-soluble vitamins (eg, A, D, K), oral phosphate supplements, and hydrocortisone. May delay or reduce absorption of concomitant oral medication; take other drugs 1 hr before or 4 hrs after colestipol. Reduces absorption of chlorothiazide, tetracycline, furosemide, penicillin G, HCTZ, and gemfibrozil. Caution with digitalis agents, propranolol.

PREGNANCY: Safety in pregnancy not known, caution in nursing.

MECHANISM OF ACTION: Bile acid sequestrant; binds bile acids in the intestine, forming a complex that is excreted in the feces, leading to increased fecal loss of bile acids and increased oxidation of cholesterol to bile acids, a decrease in β lipoprotein or LDL, and a decrease in serum cholesterol levels.

PHARMACOKINETICS: Elimination: Feces.

NURSING CONSIDERATIONS

Assessment: Assess for secondary causes of hypercholesterolemia (eg, hypothyroidism, diabetes mellitus, nephrotic syndrome, dysproteinemia, obstructive liver disease, alcoholism), preexisting constipation, pregnancy/nursing status, and for possible drug interactions. Determine baseline lipid profile.

Monitoring: Monitor for signs/symptoms of vitamin K deficiency (eg, tendency for bleeding), constipation, hypothyroidism, and for hyperchloremic acidosis. Monitor serum cholesterol, lipoprotein, and TG levels.

Patient Counseling: Instruct to take as prescribed. Advise to take other medications at least 1 hr before or 4 hrs after taking colestipol. Inform about benefits/risks of therapy. Instruct to report any adverse reactions to physician. (Tab) Instruct to take tab one at a time, with plenty of water. Counsel not to cut, crush, or chew tab. (Granules) Advise to mix with water or other fluids before ingesting.

Administration: Oral route. **Storage:** 20-25°C (68-77°F).

COMBIGAN

RX

timolol maleate - brimonidine tartrate (Allergan)

THERAPEUTIC CLASS: Alpha$_2$-agonist/beta-blocker

INDICATIONS: Reduction of elevated intraocular pressure (IOP) in patients with glaucoma or ocular HTN who require adjunctive or replacement therapy due to inadequately controlled IOP.

DOSAGE: *Adults:* 1 drop in affected eye(s) bid q12h. Space by at least 5 min if using >1 topical ophthalmic drug.
Pediatrics: ≥2 Yrs: 1 drop in affected eye(s) bid q12h. Space by at least 5 min if using >1 topical ophthalmic drug.

HOW SUPPLIED: Sol: (Brimonidine-Timolol) 0.2%-0.5% [5mL, 10mL]

CONTRAINDICATIONS: Bronchial asthma, history of bronchial asthma, severe chronic obstructive pulmonary disease (COPD), sinus bradycardia, 2nd- or 3rd-degree atrioventricular (AV) block, overt cardiac failure, cardiogenic shock, neonates, and infants (<2 yrs of age).

WARNINGS/PRECAUTIONS: Absorbed systemically; severe respiratory reactions in patients with asthma reported. May precipitate more severe failure in patients with diminished myocardial contractility; sympathetic stimulation may be essential for support of the circulation. D/C at the 1st sign/symptom of cardiac failure in patients without a history of cardiac failure. Avoid with bronchospastic disease, history of bronchospastic disease and/or mild to moderate COPD (eg, chronic bronchitis, emphysema). May potentiate syndromes associated with vascular insufficiency; caution with depression, cerebral or coronary insufficiency, Raynaud's phenomenon, orthostatic hypotension, or thromboangiitis obliterans. May increase reactivity to allergens. May potentiate muscle weakness consistent with certain myasthenic symptoms (eg, diplopia, ptosis, generalized weakness). May mask signs/symptoms of acute hypoglycemia; caution in patients subject to spontaneous hypoglycemia and in diabetic patients receiving insulin or hypoglycemic agents. May mask certain clinical signs of hyperthyroidism (eg, tachycardia); carefully manage patients suspected of developing thyrotoxicosis to avoid abrupt withdrawal that may precipitate a thyroid storm. Ocular hypersensitivity reactions reported. Bacterial keratitis reported with use of multiple-dose containers of topical ophthalmic products. May impair the ability of the heart to respond to β-adrenergically mediated reflex stimuli during surgery; gradual withdrawal of β-blocking agents is recommended in patients undergoing elective surgery.

ADVERSE REACTIONS: Allergic conjunctivitis, conjunctival folliculosis, conjunctival hyperemia, eye pruritus, ocular burning/stinging.

INTERACTIONS: May reduce BP; caution with antihypertensives and/or cardiac glycosides. Monitor for potentially additive effects, both systemic and on IOP with concomitant oral β-blockers; concomitant use of 2 topical β-blocking agents is not recommended. Possible AV conduction disturbances, left ventricular failure, and hypotension may occur with oral or IV calcium antagonists; use with caution and avoid use with impaired cardiac function. Closely observe patients receiving catecholamine-depleting drugs (eg, reserpine) because of possible additive effects and the production of hypotension and/or marked bradycardia. Possibility of additive or potentiating effect with CNS depressants (eg, alcohol, barbiturates, opiates, sedatives, anesthetics). Concomitant use of β-blockers with digitalis or calcium antagonists may have additive effects in prolonging AV-conduction time. Potentiated systemic β-blockade (eg, decreased HR, depression) reported with concomitant CYP2D6 inhibitors (eg, quinidine, SSRIs). May affect the metabolism and uptake of circulating amines with TCAs and/or MAOIs; caution with TCAs and MAOIs.

PREGNANCY: Category C, not for use in nursing.

MECHANISM OF ACTION: Decreases elevated IOP. Brimonidine: Selective α-2 adrenergic receptor agonist. Timolol: Nonselective β-blocker.

PHARMACOKINETICS: Absorption: Brimonidine: C_{max}=30pg/mL; T_{max}=1-4 hrs; AUC=128pg•hr/mL. Timolol: C_{max}=400pg/mL; T_{max}=1-3 hrs; AUC=2919pg•hr/mL. **Distribution:** Timolol: Plasma protein binding (60%); found in breast milk. **Metabolism:** Brimonidine: Liver (extensive). Timolol: Liver (partial). **Elimination:** Brimonidine: $T_{1/2}$=3 hrs. Timolol: $T_{1/2}$=7 hrs.

NURSING CONSIDERATIONS

Assessment: Assess for bronchial asthma, history of bronchial asthma, severe COPD, or any other conditions where treatment is contraindicated or cautioned. Assess for pregnancy/nursing status, and possible drug interactions.

Monitoring: Monitor for potentiation of respiratory reactions, vascular insufficiency, muscle weakness, increased reactivity to allergens, masking of signs/symptoms of hypoglycemia or hyperthyroidism, ocular hypersensitivity reactions, bacterial keratitis, and other adverse reactions.

Patient Counseling: Inform that ocular infections may occur if handled improperly or if the tip of dispensing container contacts the eye or surrounding structures. Advise that using contaminated sol may result in serious eye damage and subsequent loss of vision. Instruct to always replace cap after using. Advise not to use if sol changes color or becomes cloudy. Advise to immediately consult physician concerning continued use of multidose container if undergoing ocular surgery or if an intercurrent ocular condition (eg, trauma, infection) develops. Instruct to space dosing by at least 5 min apart if >1 topical ophthalmic drug is being used. Inform that drug contains benzalkonium chloride, which may be absorbed by soft contact lenses; instruct to remove contact lenses prior to administration and reinsert 15 min following administration. Inform that drug may cause fatigue and/or drowsiness in some patients; advise to use caution in engaging in hazardous activities because of the potential for a decrease in mental alertness.

Administration: Ocular route. **Storage:** 15-25°C (59-77°F). Protect from light.

COMBIPATCH   RX
norethindrone acetate - estradiol (Novartis)

> Should not be used for prevention of cardiovascular (CV) disease or dementia. Increased risk of myocardial infarction (MI), stroke, invasive breast cancer, pulmonary embolism (PE), and deep vein thrombosis (DVT) in postmenopausal women (50-79 yrs of age) reported. Increased risk of developing probable dementia in postmenopausal women ≥65 yrs of age reported. Increased risk of endometrial cancer in women with a uterus who use unopposed estrogens. Perform adequate diagnostic measures to rule out malignancy in postmenopausal women with undiagnosed persistent or recurrent abnormal vaginal bleeding. Should be prescribed at the lowest effective dose and for the shortest duration consistent with treatment goals and risks.

THERAPEUTIC CLASS: Estrogen/progestogen combination

INDICATIONS: Treatment of moderate to severe vasomotor symptoms and/or vulvar/vaginal atrophy due to menopause. Treatment of hypoestrogenism due to hypogonadism, castration, or primary ovarian failure.

DOSAGE: *Adults:* Continuous Combined Regimen: Apply 0.05mg-0.14mg patch on lower abdomen. Apply twice weekly during 28-day cycle. Continuous Sequential Regimen: Wear estradiol-only patch for first 14 days of 28-day cycle, replace twice weekly. Apply 0.05mg-0.14mg patch on the lower abdomen for remaining 14 days, replace twice weekly. For both regimens, use 0.05mg-0.25mg patch if greater progestin is required. Reevaluate at 3- to 6-month intervals.

HOW SUPPLIED: Patch: (Estradiol-Norethindrone Acetate) 0.05-0.14mg/day, 0.05-0.25mg/day [8*]

CONTRAINDICATIONS: Undiagnosed abnormal genital bleeding, known/suspected/history of breast cancer, known/suspected estrogen-dependent neoplasia, active/history of DVT/PE, active/history of arterial thromboembolic disease (eg, stroke, MI), known liver impairment or disease, known protein C/protein S/antithrombin deficiency or other known thrombophilic disorders, known/suspected pregnancy.

WARNINGS/PRECAUTIONS: D/C immediately if stroke, DVT, PE, or MI occurs or is suspected. Caution with risk factors for arterial vascular disease and/or venous thromboembolism. If feasible, d/c at least 4-6 weeks before surgery of the type associated with an increased risk of thromboembolism, or during periods of prolonged immobilization. May increase risk of ovarian cancer and gallbladder disease. May lead to severe hypercalcemia in patients with breast cancer and bone metastases; d/c and take appropriate measures if hypercalcemia occurs. Retinal vascular thrombosis reported; d/c pending exam if sudden partial/complete loss of vision or sudden onset of proptosis, diplopia, or migraine occurs. D/C permanently if exam reveals papilledema or retinal vascular lesions. May elevate BP and thyroid-binding globulin levels. May elevate plasma TGs leading to pancreatitis in patients with preexisting hypertriglyceridemia. Caution with history of cholestatic jaundice associated with past estrogen use or with pregnancy; d/c in case of recurrence. May cause fluid retention. Caution with hypoparathyroidism as estrogen-induced hypocalcemia may occur. May exacerbate symptoms of angioedema in women with hereditary angioedema. May exacerbate endometriosis, asthma, diabetes mellitus, epilepsy, migraine, porphyria, systemic lupus erythematosus, and hepatic hemangiomas. May affect certain endocrine and blood components in lab tests.

ADVERSE REACTIONS: Abdominal pain, back pain, asthenia, flu syndrome, headache, application-site reaction, diarrhea, nausea, nervousness, pharyngitis, respiratory disorder, breast pain, dysmenorrhea, menstrual disorder, vaginitis.

INTERACTIONS: CYP3A4 inducers (eg, St. John's wort preparations, phenobarbital, carbamazepine) may decrease levels and may decrease therapeutic effects and/or change uterine bleeding profile. CYP3A4 inhibitors (eg, erythromycin, clarithromycin, ketoconazole) may increase levels, which may result in side effects. Patients concomitantly receiving thyroid hormone replacement therapy and estrogens may require increased doses of their thyroid replacement therapy; monitor thyroid function.

PREGNANCY: Contraindicated in pregnancy, not for use in nursing.

MECHANISM OF ACTION: Estrogen/progestogen combination; estrogen binds to nuclear receptors in estrogen-responsive tissues. Circulating estrogens modulate pituitary secretion of the gonadotropins, luteinizing hormone, and follicle-stimulating hormone, through a negative feedback mechanism. Reduces elevated levels of these hormones in postmenopausal women.

PHARMACOKINETICS: Absorption: Transdermal administration of variable doses resulted in different parameters. **Distribution:** Found in breast milk. Estradiol: Largely bound to sex hormone-binding globulin (SHBG) and albumin. Norethindrone: 90% to SHBG and albumin. **Metabolism:** Estradiol: Liver to estrone (metabolite), estriol (major urinary metabolite); enterohepatic recirculation via sulfate and glucuronide conjugation in the liver, biliary secretion of conjugates into the intestine, hydrolysis in the intestine followed by reabsorption. Norethindrone: Liver. **Elimination:** Estradiol: Urine; $T_{1/2}$=2-3 hrs. Norethindrone: $T_{1/2}$=6-8 hrs.

NURSING CONSIDERATIONS

Assessment: Assess for undiagnosed abnormal genital bleeding, presence/history of breast cancer, estrogen-dependent neoplasia, active/history of DVT/PE/arterial thromboembolic disease, liver impairment/disease, thrombophilic disorders, drug hypersensitivity, pregnancy/nursing status, and for any other conditions where treatment is contraindicated or cautioned. Assess for possible drug interactions.

Monitoring: Monitor for signs/symptoms of CV disease, malignant neoplasms, dementia, gallbladder disease, hypercalcemia, visual abnormalities, BP and plasma TG elevations, pancreatitis, cholestatic jaundice, fluid retention, exacerbation of endometriosis and other conditions, and other adverse reactions. Perform annual breast exam; schedule mammography based on age, risk factors, and prior mammogram results. Periodically reevaluate (every 3-6 months) to determine need for therapy. Perform adequate diagnostic measures (eg, endometrial sampling) to rule out malignancies in cases of undiagnosed, persistent, or recurring abnormal genital bleeding. Regularly monitor thyroid function if on thyroid hormone replacement therapy.

Patient Counseling: Inform of the importance of reporting abnormal vaginal bleeding to physician as soon as possible. Inform of possible serious adverse reactions of therapy (eg, CV disorders, malignant neoplasms, probable dementia) and of possible less serious, but common adverse reactions (eg, headache, breast pain and tenderness, nausea). Instruct to have yearly breast exams by a healthcare provider and to perform monthly breast self-exams.

Administration: Transdermal route. Apply to a clean, dry area of the lower abdomen. Do not apply to or near the breasts. Refer to PI for for further administration instructions. **Storage:** Prior to Dispensing: 2-8°C (36-46°F). After Dispensing: 20-25°C (66-77°F) for up to 6 months. Store the systems in the sealed foil pouch. Do not store in areas where extreme temperatures may occur.

COMBIVENT RESPIMAT   RX

ipratropium bromide - albuterol (Boehringer Ingelheim)

THERAPEUTIC CLASS: Anticholinergic/beta$_2$-agonist

INDICATIONS: Treatment of patients with chronic obstructive pulmonary disease on a regular aerosol bronchodilator who continue to have evidence of bronchospasm and who require a 2nd bronchodilator.

DOSAGE: *Adults:* Usual: 1 inh qid. May take additional inh PRN. Max: 6 inh/24 hrs.

HOW SUPPLIED: Spray, Inhalation: (Albuterol-Ipratropium Bromide) 100mcg-20mcg/inh [4g]

CONTRAINDICATIONS: Hypersensitivity to atropine or any of its derivatives.

WARNINGS/PRECAUTIONS: May produce paradoxical bronchospasm; d/c and institute alternative therapy if this occurs. May produce significant cardiovascular (CV) effects (eg, ECG changes); d/c if symptoms occur. Caution with CV disorders (eg, coronary insufficiency, cardiac arrhythmias, HTN). Rare occurrences of myocardial ischemia reported. May increase intraocular pressure and result in precipitation/worsening of narrow-angle glaucoma. Avoid spraying in eyes; may cause acute eye pain/discomfort, temporary blurring of vision, mydriasis, visual halos, or colored images in association with red eyes from conjunctival or corneal congestion. May cause urinary retention; caution with prostatic hyperplasia or bladder-neck obstruction. Fatalities reported with excessive use of inhaled sympathomimetic drugs in patients with asthma. Hypersensitivity reactions may occur; d/c and consider alternative treatment if such a reaction occurs. Caution with convulsive disorders, hyperthyroidism, diabetes mellitus (DM), and in patients who are unusually responsive to sympathomimetic amines. May produce significant but usually transient hypokalemia.

ADVERSE REACTIONS: Nasopharyngitis, cough, headache, bronchitis, upper respiratory infection.

INTERACTIONS: Potential for an additive interaction with other anticholinergic-containing drugs; avoid coadministration. Increased risk of adverse CV effects with other sympathomimetic agents; use with caution. ECG changes and/or hypokalemia which may result from non-K$^+$-sparing diuretics (eg, loop or thiazide diuretics) may be acutely worsened; use with caution and consider monitoring K$^+$ levels. β-blockers and albuterol inhibit the effect of each other; use β-blockers with caution in patients with hyperreactive airways. Administration with MAOIs or TCAs, or within 2 weeks of discontinuation of such agents may potentiate the action of albuterol on CV system; use with extreme caution and consider alternative therapy.

PREGNANCY: Category C, not for use in nursing.

MECHANISM OF ACTION: Ipratropium: Anticholinergic bronchodilator; appears to inhibit vagally-mediated reflexes by antagonizing the action of acetylcholine. Prevents the increases in intracellular concentration of Ca^{2+}, which is caused by interaction of acetylcholine with the muscarinic receptors on bronchial smooth muscle. Albuterol: Selective β$_2$-adrenergic bronchodilator; activates β$_2$-receptors on airway smooth muscle resulting in activation of protein kinase, which inhibits phosphorylation of myosin and lowers intracellular ionic Ca^{2+} concentrations, resulting in relaxation.

PHARMACOKINETICS: Absorption: Ipratropium: Not readily absorbed. C_{max}=33.5pg/mL. **Distribution:** Ipratropium: Plasma protein binding (0-9%). **Metabolism:** Ipratropium: Partial; ester hydrolysis. Albuterol: Conjugation; albuterol 4'-O-sulfate (metabolite). **Elimination:** Ipratropium: $T_{1/2}$=2 hrs.

NURSING CONSIDERATIONS

Assessment: Assess for hypersensitivity to drug or to atropine or any of its derivatives, CV disorders, narrow-angle glaucoma, prostatic hyperplasia, bladder-neck obstruction, convulsive disorders, hyperthyroidism, DM, pregnancy/nursing status, and possible drug interactions. Assess if unusually responsive to sympathomimetic amines.

Monitoring: Monitor for signs/symptoms of hypersensitivity reactions, paradoxical bronchospasm, CV effects (measured by pulse rate and BP), hypokalemia, unexpected development of severe acute asthmatic crisis, hypoxia, and other adverse reactions.

Patient Counseling: Instruct to use caution to avoid spraying the product into eyes. Instruct to consult physician if ocular symptoms or difficulty with urination develop. Instruct to exercise caution when engaging in activities requiring balance and visual acuity (eg, driving a car, operating appliances/machinery). Instruct not to increase dose or frequency without consulting physician. Instruct to seek immediate medical attention if therapy lessens in effectiveness, symptoms worsen, and/or need to use product more frequently than usual. Counsel to take other inhaled drugs only ud by physician. Counsel to d/c if paradoxical bronchospasm occurs. Inform of possible adverse effects (eg, palpitations, chest pain, rapid HR, tremor, nervousness). Instruct to contact physician if pregnant/nursing.

Administration: Oral inhalation route. Refer to PI for administration instructions. **Storage:** 25°C (77°F); excursions permitted to 15-30°C (59-86°F). Avoid freezing.

COMBIVIR   RX
zidovudine - lamivudine (ViiV Healthcare)

> Lactic acidosis and severe hepatomegaly with steatosis, including fatal cases, reported with nucleoside analogues; suspend treatment if lactic acidosis or pronounced hepatotoxicity occurs. Lamivudine: Severe acute exacerbations of hepatitis B reported in patients coinfected with hepatitis B virus (HBV) upon discontinuation of therapy; closely monitor hepatic function for at least several months. If appropriate, initiation of anti-hepatitis B therapy may be warranted. Zidovudine: Associated with hematologic toxicity (eg, neutropenia, anemia), particularly with advanced HIV-1 disease. Symptomatic myopathy associated with prolonged use.

THERAPEUTIC CLASS: Nucleoside reverse transcriptase inhibitor

INDICATIONS: Treatment of HIV-1 infection in combination with other antiretrovirals.

DOSAGE: *Adults:* ≥30kg: CrCl ≥50mL/min: Usual: 1 tab bid.
Pediatrics: ≥30kg: CrCl ≥50mL/min: Usual: 1 tab bid.

HOW SUPPLIED: Tab: (Lamivudine-Zidovudine) 150mg-300mg* *scored

WARNINGS/PRECAUTIONS: Do not use in pediatrics weighing <30 kg, or patients requiring dosage adjustment (eg, renal impairment [CrCl <50mL/min], hepatic impairment, or those experiencing dose-limiting adverse reactions). Caution with history or known risk factors for pancreatitis; d/c if pancreatitis occurs. Immune reconstitution syndrome reported. Autoimmune disorders (eg, Graves' disease, polymyositis, Guillain-Barre syndrome) reported to occur in the setting of immune reconstitution and can occur many months after initiation of treatment. May cause redistribution/accumulation of body fat. Obesity and prolonged nucleoside exposure may be risk factors for lactic acidosis and hepatomegaly with steatosis. Caution with any known risk factors for liver disease and in elderly. Lamivudine: Emergence of lamivudine-resistant HBV reported. Zidovudine: Caution with granulocyte count <1000 cells/mm³ or Hgb <9.5g/dL; monitor blood counts frequently with advanced HIV-1 and periodically with other HIV-1 infected patients. Interrupt therapy if anemia or neutropenia develops.

ADVERSE REACTIONS: Lactic acidosis, severe hepatomegaly with steatosis, myopathy, hematologic toxicities, headache, malaise, fatigue, fever, chills, N/V, diarrhea, anorexia, insomnia, nasal signs and symptoms, cough.

INTERACTIONS: Avoid with other lamivudine-, zidovudine-, and/or emtricitabine-containing products. Lamivudine: Avoid with zalcitabine. Hepatic decompensation may occur in HIV/hepatitis C virus (HCV) coinfected patients receiving interferon-alfa with or without ribavirin. Nelfinavir and trimethoprim/sulfamethoxazole may increase levels. Zidovudine: Avoid with stavudine, doxorubicin, and nucleoside analogues affecting DNA replication (eg, ribavirin). May increase risk of hematologic toxicities with ganciclovir, interferon alfa, ribavirin, bone marrow suppressors, or cytotoxic agents. Atovaquone, fluconazole, methadone, probenecid, and valproic acid may increase levels. Clarithromycin, nelfinavir, rifampin, and ritonavir may decrease levels.

PREGNANCY: Category C, not for use in nursing.

MECHANISM OF ACTION: Nucleoside analogue combination; inhibits reverse transcriptase via DNA chain termination after incorporation of the nucleotide analogue.

PHARMACOKINETICS: Absorption: Lamivudine: Rapid; bioavailability (86%). Zidovudine: Rapid; bioavailability (64%). **Distribution:** Lamivudine: V_d=1.3L/kg; plasma protein binding (<36%); found in breast milk. Zidovudine: V_d=1.6L/kg; plasma protein binding (<38%); crosses the placenta; found in breast milk. **Metabolism:** Lamivudine: Trans-sulfoxide (metabolite). Zidovudine: Hepatic; 3'-azido-3'-deoxy-5'-O-β-D-glucopyranuronosylthymidine (GZDV) (major metabolite). **Elimination:** Lamivudine: (IV) Urine (70% unchanged); $T_{1/2}$=5-7 hrs. Zidovudine: Urine (14% unchanged, 74% GZDV); $T_{1/2}$=0.5-3 hrs.

NURSING CONSIDERATIONS

Assessment: Assess for advanced HIV disease, bone marrow compromise, liver function and risk factors for liver disease, hepatitis B infection, history of pancreatitis and risk factors for its development, renal function, hypersensitivity to drug, pregnancy/nursing status, and possible drug interaction. Obtain baseline weight and CBC.

Monitoring: Monitor signs/symptoms that suggest pancreatitis, lactic acidosis, hepatotoxicity, myopathy and myositis, immune reconstitution syndrome (eg, opportunistic infections), autoimmune disorders, and hypersensitivity reactions. Monitor CBC and renal/hepatic function.

Patient Counseling: Inform about risk for hematologic toxicities and advise on importance of close blood count monitoring while on therapy. Counsel about the possible occurrence of myopathy and myositis with pathological changes during prolonged use and that therapy may cause a rare but serious condition called lactic acidosis with liver enlargement (hepatomegaly). Inform that deterioration of liver disease has occurred in patients coinfected with HBV with treatment d/c. Instruct to discuss with physician any changes in regimen. Caution patients about the use of other medication and instruct to avoid use with other lamivudine-, zidovudine-, and/or emtricitabine-containing products. Inform that hepatic decompensation has been reported in patients coinfected with HCV receiving interferon alfa with or without ribavirin. Inform that fat redistribution/accumulation may occur. Inform that therapy is not a cure for HIV-1 infection and patients may continue to experience illnesses associated with HIV-1. Advise to avoid doing things that can spread HIV-1 infection to others (eg, sharing of needles/inj equipment/personal items that can have blood or body fluids on them, having sex without protection, breastfeeding). Advise to take exactly as prescribed.

Administration: Oral route. **Storage:** 2-30°C (36-86°F).

COMPLERA   RX
tenofovir disoproxil fumarate - emtricitabine - rilpivirine (Gilead)

> Lactic acidosis and severe hepatomegaly with steatosis, including fatal cases, reported with the use of nucleoside analogues. Not approved for the treatment of chronic hepatitis B virus (HBV) infection. Severe acute exacerbations of hepatitis B reported in patients coinfected with HBV upon discontinuation of therapy; closely monitor hepatic function for at least several months. If appropriate, initiation of anti-hepatitis B therapy may be warranted.

THERAPEUTIC CLASS: Non-nucleoside reverse transcriptase inhibitor/nucleoside analogue combination

INDICATIONS: For use as a complete regimen for the treatment of HIV-1 infection in adults with no antiretroviral treatment history and with HIV-1 RNA ≤100,000 copies/mL at the start of therapy, and in certain virologically-suppressed (HIV-1 RNA <50 copies/mL) adults on a stable antiretroviral regimen at start of therapy in order to replace current antiretroviral treatment regimen.

DOSAGE: *Adults:* ≥18 Yrs: 1 tab qd with food.

HOW SUPPLIED: Tab: (Emtricitabine-Rilpivirine-Tenofovir Disoproxil Fumarate [TDF]) 200mg-25mg-300mg

CONTRAINDICATIONS: Coadministration with CYP3A inducers or agents that increase gastric pH causing decreased plasma concentrations, which may result in loss of virologic response and possible resistance (eg, carbamazepine, oxcarbazepine, phenobarbital, phenytoin, rifabutin, rifampin, rifapentine, proton pump inhibitors [eg, dexlansoprazole, esomeprazole, lansoprazole, omeprazole, pantoprazole, rabeprazole], systemic dexamethasone [more than a single dose], St. John's wort).

WARNINGS/PRECAUTIONS: When considering replacing the current regimen in virologically-suppressed adults, patients should have no history of virologic failure, have been stably suppressed for at least 6 months prior to switching therapy, currently be on the 1st or 2nd antiretroviral regimen prior to switching therapy, and have no current/past history of resistance to any of the 3 drug components. Additional monitoring of HIV-1 RNA and regimen tolerability is recommended after replacing therapy to assess for potential virologic failure or rebound. Not

C

for patients requiring dose adjustment (eg, moderate or severe renal impairment [estimated CrCl <50mL/min]). Test for presence of chronic HBV prior to treatment. Immune reconstitution syndrome, autoimmune disorders (eg, Graves' disease, polymyositis, Guillain-Barre syndrome) in the setting of immune reconstitution, and redistribution/accumulation of body fat reported. Caution in elderly patients. Rilpivirine: Depressive disorders reported; immediate medical evaluation is recommended if severe depressive symptoms occur. Hepatic adverse events reported; increased risk for worsening/development of liver-associated test elevations in patients with underlying hepatitis B or C, or marked liver-associated test elevations prior to treatment; perform appropriate lab tests prior to therapy and monitor for hepatotoxicity during therapy. Consider liver-associated test monitoring for patients without preexisting hepatic dysfunction or other risk factors. TDF: Obesity and prolonged nucleoside exposure may be risk factors for lactic acidosis and severe hepatomegaly with steatosis. Caution with known risk factors for liver disease. D/C if lactic acidosis or pronounced hepatotoxicity occurs. Renal impairment, including cases of acute renal failure and Fanconi syndrome, reported; assess estimated CrCl prior to and during therapy. Decreased bone mineral density (BMD), increased biochemical markers of bone metabolism, and osteomalacia reported. Consider assessment of BMD in patients with history of pathologic bone fracture or other risk factors for osteoporosis or bone loss. Arthralgias and muscle pain/weakness reported in cases of proximal renal tubulopathy. Consider hypophosphatemia and osteomalacia secondary to proximal renal tubulopathy in patients at risk of renal dysfunction who present with persistent or worsening bone or muscle symptoms.

ADVERSE REACTIONS: Lactic acidosis, severe hepatomegaly with steatosis, nausea, headache, dizziness, depressive disorders, insomnia, abnormal dreams, rash, diarrhea, fatigue.

INTERACTIONS: See Contraindications. Avoid with concurrent or recent use of nephrotoxic agents (eg, high dose or multiple NSAIDs), other antiretrovirals, adefovir dipivoxil, or drugs containing any of the same active components or lamivudine. Rilpivirine: Caution with drugs that may reduce exposure or drugs with a known risk of torsades de pointes. Decreased levels, loss of virologic response, and possible resistance with CYP3A inducers or drugs increasing gastric pH (eg, antacids, H2-receptor antagonists [H2-RAs]). Administer antacids at least 2 hrs before or at least 4 hrs after dosing and H2-RAs at least 12 hrs before or at least 4 hrs after dosing. CYP3A inhibitors, azole antifungals, clarithromycin, erythromycin, or telithromycin may increase levels. May decrease levels of ketoconazole and methadone. Emtricitabine and TDF: Drugs that reduce renal function or compete for active tubular secretion (eg, acyclovir, adefovir dipivoxil, cidofovir, ganciclovir, valacyclovir, valganciclovir, aminoglycosides [eg, gentamicin], high-dose or multiple NSAIDs) may increase levels. Cases of acute renal failure after initiation of high dose or multiple NSAIDs reported in HIV-infected patients with risk factors for renal dysfunction who appeared stable on TDF; consider alternatives to NSAIDs, if needed.

PREGNANCY: Category B, not for use in nursing.

MECHANISM OF ACTION: Emtricitabine: Nucleoside analogue of cytidine; inhibits activity of HIV-1 reverse transcriptase (RT) by competing with natural substrate deoxycytidine 5'-triphosphate and incorporating into nascent viral DNA, resulting in chain termination. Rilpivirine: nonnucleoside reverse transcriptase inhibitor; inhibits HIV-1 replication by noncompetitive inhibition of HIV-1 RT. TDF: Acyclic nucleoside phosphonate diester analogue of adenosine monophosphate; inhibits activity of HIV-1 RT by competing with the natural substrate deoxyadenosine 5'-triphosphate and, after incorporation into DNA, by DNA chain termination.

PHARMACOKINETICS: Absorption: Emtricitabine: (Cap) Absolute bioavailability (93%), C_{max}=1.8mcg/mL, T_{max}=1-2 hrs, AUC=10mcg•hr/mL. Rilpivirine: T_{max}=4-5 hrs, AUC=2235ng•hr/mL. TDF: Bioavailability (25%, fasted), C_{max}=0.30mcg/mL, T_{max}=1 hr, AUC=2.29mcg•hr/mL. **Distribution:** Emtricitabine: Plasma protein binding (<4%); found in breast milk. Rilpivirine: Plasma protein binding (99.7%). TDF: Plasma protein binding (<0.7%); found in breast milk. **Metabolism:** Emtricitabine: 3'-sulfoxide diastereomers, glucuronic acid conjugate (metabolites). Rilpivirine: Oxidative metabolism by CYP3A system. **Elimination:** Emtricitabine: Feces (14%), urine (86%, 13% metabolites); $T_{1/2}$=10 hrs. Rilpivirine: Feces (85%, 25% unchanged), urine (6.1%, <1% unchanged); $T_{1/2}$=50 hrs. TDF: (IV) Urine (70-80% unchanged); $T_{1/2}$=17 hrs.

NURSING CONSIDERATIONS

Assessment: Assess for history of virologic failure, current/past history of resistance to any of the drug components, obesity, prolonged nucleoside exposure, liver dysfunction or risk factors for liver disease, renal impairment, HBV infection, pregnancy/nursing status, and possible drug interactions. Assess BMD in patients with a history of pathological bone fracture or with other risk factors for osteoporosis/bone loss. Assess estimated CrCl, serum P, urine glucose, and urine protein in patients at risk for renal dysfunction.

Monitoring: Monitor for signs/symptoms of lactic acidosis, severe hepatomegaly with steatosis, depressive symptoms, hepatotoxicity, decreased BMD, increased biochemical markers for bone metabolism, osteomalacia, fat redistribution/accumulation, immune reconstitution syndrome (eg, opportunistic infections), autoimmune disorders, renal impairment, and other adverse reactions. Monitor patients coinfected with HBV and HIV-1 with clinical and lab follow-up for acute exacerbations of hepatitis B for at least several months upon discontinuation of therapy. Monitor estimated CrCl, serum P, urine glucose, and urine protein periodically in patients at risk for renal dysfunction. Additional monitoring of HIV-1 RNA and regimen tolerability is recommended after replacing therapy to assess for potential virologic failure or rebound.

Patient Counseling: Inform that therapy is not a cure for HIV infection; continuous therapy is necessary to control HIV infection and decrease HIV-related illnesses. Advise to practice safe sex and use latex or polyurethane condoms. Instruct to never reuse or share needles. Advise not to breastfeed. Counsel to take on a regular dosing schedule with food and avoid missing doses. Inform that a protein drink is not a substitute for food. Counsel patients on missed dose instructions. Inform not to take more or less than the prescribed dose at any one time. Instruct to contact physician if symptoms of lactic acidosis or severe hepatomegaly with steatosis (eg, N/V, unusual stomach discomfort, weakness), depression, and any symptoms of infection occurs. Inform that hepatotoxicity has been reported during treatment. Inform that fat redistribution/accumulation, renal impairment, and decreases in BMD may occur. Advise to inform physician if taking any other prescription or nonprescription medications or herbal products (eg, St. John's wort).

Administration: Oral route. **Storage:** 25°C (77°F); excursions permitted to 15-30°C (59-86°F).

COMTAN RX
entacapone (Novartis)

THERAPEUTIC CLASS: COMT inhibitor

INDICATIONS: Adjunct to levodopa/carbidopa to treat patients with idiopathic Parkinson's disease who experience the signs and symptoms of end-of-dose "wearing-off."

DOSAGE: *Adults:* 200mg with each levodopa/carbidopa dose. Max: 1600mg/day. Consider levodopa dose adjustment.

HOW SUPPLIED: Tab: 200mg

WARNINGS/PRECAUTIONS: Orthostatic hypotension/syncope and hallucinations reported. Diarrhea and colitis reported; consider discontinuing and institute appropriate therapy if prolonged diarrhea is suspected to be related to therapy. May cause and/or exacerbate preexisting dyskinesia. Severe rhabdomyolysis and symptom complex resembling neuroleptic malignant syndrome (NMS) reported. Retroperitoneal fibrosis, pulmonary infiltrates, pleural effusion, and pleural thickening reported with ergot-derived dopaminergic agents. May increase risk of developing melanoma; monitor for melanomas frequently and on a regular basis and perform periodic skin exams. Caution with hepatic impairment (eg, biliary obstruction). Rapid withdrawal or abrupt dose reduction may lead to emergence of signs and symptoms of Parkinson's disease, and hyperpyrexia and confusion; when discontinuing, closely monitor patients and adjust other dopaminergic treatment PRN.

ADVERSE REACTIONS: Dyskinesia, hyperkinesia, hypokinesia, N/V, diarrhea, abdominal pain, urine discoloration, dizziness, constipation, dry mouth, fatigue, dyspnea, back pain.

INTERACTIONS: Avoid with nonselective MAOIs (eg, phenelzine, tranylcypromine). Caution with drugs metabolized by catechol-O-methyltransferase (COMT) (eg, isoproterenol, epinephrine, norepinephrine, dopamine, dobutamine, α-methyldopa, apomorphine, isoetharine, bitolterol); increased HR, possibly arrhythmias, and excessive BP changes may occur. Caution with drugs known to interfere with biliary excretion, glucuronidation, and intestinal β-glucuronidase (eg, probenecid, cholestyramine, some antibiotics [eg, erythromycin, rifampicin, ampicillin, chloramphenicol]). May potentiate dopaminergic side effects of levodopa.

PREGNANCY: Category C, caution in nursing.

MECHANISM OF ACTION: COMT inhibitor; inhibits COMT and alters the plasma pharmacokinetics of levodopa.

PHARMACOKINETICS: Absorption: Rapid, absolute bioavailability (35%); C_{max}=1.2μg/mL, T_{max}=1 hr. **Distribution:** Plasma protein binding (98%); (IV) V_d=20L. **Metabolism:** Isomerization to *cis*-isomer, and direct glucuronidation. **Elimination:** Urine (10%, 0.2% unchanged), feces (90%); $T_{1/2}$=0.4-0.7 hrs (β-phase); $T_{1/2}$=2.4 hrs (gamma-phase).

NURSING CONSIDERATIONS

Assessment: Assess for dyskinesia, biliary obstruction, hepatic function, history of hypotension, hypersensitivity to drug, pregnancy/nursing status, and possible drug interactions.

Monitoring: Monitor for signs/symptoms of orthostatic hypotension, diarrhea, hallucinations, dyskinesia, rhabdomyolysis, a symptom complex resembling NMS, retroperitoneal fibrosis, pulmonary infiltrates, pleural effusion, and pleural thickening. Monitor for melanoma frequently and on a regular basis; perform periodic skin exams.

Patient Counseling: Instruct to take drug only as prescribed. Inform that postural hypotension, hallucinations, nausea, diarrhea, increased dyskinesia, and change in urine color (brownish orange discoloration) may occur. Caution against rising rapidly after sitting or lying down for prolonged periods and during initiation of treatment. Instruct to avoid driving a car or operating other complex machinery until patient is aware of how medication affects their mental and/or motor performance. Advise to inform physician if experiencing new or increased gambling urges, sexual urges, or other intense urges while on therapy. Instruct to notify physician if intending to become or are pregnant/nursing.

Administration: Oral route. **Storage:** 25°C (77°F); excursions permitted to 15-30°C (59-86°F).

CONCERTA
methylphenidate HCl (Janssen)

> Caution with history of drug dependence or alcoholism. Chronic abusive use may lead to marked tolerance and psychological dependence with varying degrees of abnormal behavior. Frank psychotic episodes may occur, especially with parenteral abuse. Careful supervision is required during withdrawal from abusive use since severe depression may occur. Withdrawal following chronic use may unmask symptoms of underlying disorder that may require follow-up.

THERAPEUTIC CLASS: Sympathomimetic amine

INDICATIONS: Treatment of attention-deficit hyperactivity disorder in patients 6-65 yrs of age.

DOSAGE: *Adults:* 18-65 Yrs: New to Methylphenidate: Initial: 18mg or 36mg qam. Range: 18-72mg/day. Currently on Methylphenidate: Initial: 18mg qam if previous dose 5mg bid-tid; 36mg qam if previous dose 10mg bid-tid; 54mg qam if previous dose 15mg bid-tid; 72mg qam if previous dose 20mg bid-tid. Conversion dosage should not exceed 72mg/day. Titrate: May increase in 18mg increments at weekly intervals if optimal response is not achieved at a lower dose. Max: 72mg/day. Maint/Extended Treatment: Periodically reevaluate the long-term usefulness of the drug. Reduce dose or, if necessary, d/c if paradoxical aggravation of symptoms or other adverse events occur. D/C if no improvement observed after appropriate dosage adjustment over 1 month.
Pediatrics: New to Methylphenidate: 13-17 Yrs: Initial: 18mg qam. Range: 18-72mg/day not to exceed 2mg/kg/day. 6-12 Yrs: Initial: 18mg qam. Range: 18-54mg/day. Currently on Methylphenidate: ≥6 Yrs: Initial: 18mg qam if previous dose 5mg bid-tid; 36mg qam if previous dose 10mg bid-tid; 54mg qam if previous dose 15mg bid-tid; 72mg qam if previous dose 20mg bid-tid. Conversion dosage should not exceed 72mg/day. Titrate: May increase in 18mg increments at weekly intervals if optimal response is not achieved at a lower dose. Max: 13-17 Yrs: 72mg/day. 6-12 Yrs: 54mg/day. Maint/Extended Treatment: Periodically reevaluate the long-term usefulness of the drug. Reduce dose or, if necessary, d/c if paradoxical aggravation of symptoms or other adverse events occur. D/C if no improvement observed after appropriate dosage adjustment over 1 month.

HOW SUPPLIED: Tab, Extended-Release: 18mg, 27mg, 36mg, 54mg

CONTRAINDICATIONS: Marked anxiety, tension, agitation, glaucoma, motor tics, or family history or diagnosis of Tourette's syndrome. Treatment with MAOIs or within a minimum of 14 days following discontinuation of an MAOI.

WARNINGS/PRECAUTIONS: Avoid with known serious structural cardiac abnormalities, cardiomyopathy, serious heart rhythm abnormalities, coronary artery disease, or other serious cardiac problems. Sudden death reported in children and adolescents with structural cardiac abnormalities or other serious heart problems. Sudden deaths, stroke, and myocardial infarction (MI) reported in adults. May increase BP and HR; caution with conditions that might be compromised by increases in BP/HR (eg, preexisting HTN, heart failure, recent MI, ventricular arrhythmia). Prior to treatment, obtain medical history (including assessment for family history of sudden death or ventricular arrhythmia) and perform physical exam to assess for presence of cardiac disease. Promptly perform cardiac evaluation if symptoms of cardiac disease develop. May exacerbate symptoms of behavior disturbance and thought disorder in patients with preexisting psychotic disorder. Caution in patients with comorbid bipolar disorder; may induce mixed/manic episode. May cause treatment-emergent psychotic or manic symptoms (eg, hallucinations, delusional thinking, mania) in patients without prior history of psychotic illness or mania; consider discontinuation if such symptoms occur. Aggressive behavior or hostility reported. May lower convulsive threshold; d/c if seizures occur. Priapism reported; seek immediate medical attention if abnormally sustained or frequent and painful erections develop. Associated with peripheral vasculopathy, including Raynaud's phenomenon; carefully observe for digital changes. May cause long-term suppression of growth in children; monitor growth, and may need to interrupt treatment in patients not growing or gaining height or weight as expected. Difficulties with accommodation and blurring of vision reported. Tab is nondeformable and does not appreciably change in shape in the GI tract; avoid with preexisting severe GI narrowing (pathologic or iatrogenic).

ADVERSE REACTIONS: Decreased appetite, headache, dry mouth, nausea, insomnia, anxiety, dizziness, decreased weight, irritability, upper abdominal pain, hyperhidrosis, palpitations, tachycardia, depressed mood, nervousness.

INTERACTIONS: See Contraindications. Caution with vasopressor agents. May inhibit metabolism of coumarin anticoagulants, anticonvulsants (eg, phenobarbital, phenytoin, primidone), and some antidepressants (eg, TCAs, SSRIs); downward dose adjustment and monitoring of plasma drug concentrations (or coagulation times for coumarin) of these drugs may be necessary when initiating or discontinuing methylphenidate.

PREGNANCY: Category C, caution in nursing.

MECHANISM OF ACTION: Sympathomimetic amine; CNS stimulant. Has not been established; thought to block the reuptake of norepinephrine and dopamine into the presynaptic neuron and increase the release of these monoamines into the extraneuronal space.

PHARMACOKINETICS: Absorption: Readily absorbed. T_{max}=6-10 hrs. (Single-dose [18mg qd], Healthy Adults) AUC=41.8ng•hr/mL; C_{max}=3.7ng/mL. **Metabolism:** Via deesterification; α-phenyl-piperidine acetic acid [PPAA] (metabolite). **Elimination:** Urine (90%, 80% PPAA); $T_{1/2}$=3.5 hrs.

NURSING CONSIDERATIONS

Assessment: Assess for hypersensitivity to the drug, marked anxiety, tension, agitation, glaucoma, motor tics, family history or diagnosis of Tourette's syndrome, cardiovascular conditions, history of drug dependence or alcoholism, psychotic disorder, comorbid bipolar disorder, severe GI narrowing, any other conditions where treatment is contraindicated or cautioned, pregnancy/nursing status, and possible drug interactions.

Monitoring: Monitor for changes in HR and BP, signs/symptoms of cardiac disease, exacerbation of behavior disturbance and thought disorder, psychosis, mania, appearance of or worsening of aggressive behavior or hostility, seizures, priapism, peripheral vasculopathy (including Raynaud's phenomenon), visual disturbances, and other adverse reactions. In pediatric patients, monitor growth. Perform periodic monitoring of CBC, differential, and platelet counts during prolonged therapy. Periodically reevaluate long-term usefulness of drug.

Patient Counseling: Inform about risks, benefits, and appropriate use of the medication. Advise of the possibility of priapism; instruct to seek immediate medical attention in the event of priapism. Inform about the risk of peripheral vasculopathy, including Raynaud's phenomenon; instruct to report to physician any new numbness, pain, skin color change, sensitivity to temperature in fingers or toes, or any signs of unexplained wounds appearing on fingers/toes. Advise that the tab shell, along with insoluble core components, is eliminated from the body; inform not to be concerned if something that looks like a tab is noticed in the stool. Inform that therapy may impair mental/physical abilities; advise to use caution with hazardous tasks (eg, operating machinery, driving).

Administration: Oral route. Take with or without food. Swallow tab whole with the aid of liquids; do not chew, divide, or crush. **Storage:** 25°C (77°F); excursions permitted to 15-30°C (59-86°F). Protect from humidity.

COPAXONE   RX
glatiramer acetate (Teva Neuroscience)

THERAPEUTIC CLASS: Immunomodulatory agent

INDICATIONS: Treatment of relapsing forms of multiple sclerosis (MS).

DOSAGE: *Adults:* 20mg/mL: Administer SQ qd. 40mg/mL: Administer SQ 3X/week and at least 48 hrs apart.

HOW SUPPLIED: Inj: 20mg/mL, 40mg/mL

CONTRAINDICATIONS: Hypersensitivity to mannitol.

WARNINGS/PRECAUTIONS: 20mg/mL and 40mg/mL are not interchangeable. Immediate post-inj reaction (eg, flushing, chest pain, palpitations, anxiety, dyspnea, throat constriction, urticaria) reported. Transient chest pain reported. Localized lipoatrophy at inj sites and inj-site skin necrosis (rarely) may occur; follow proper inj technique and rotate inj sites with each inj. May interfere with immune functions. Continued alteration of cellular immunity due to chronic treatment may result in untoward effects.

ADVERSE REACTIONS: Inj-site reactions, vasodilatation, rash, dyspnea, chest pain, nasopharyngitis, infection, asthenia, pain, N/V, influenza, anxiety, back pain, palpitations, edema.

PREGNANCY: Category B, caution in nursing.

MECHANISM OF ACTION: Immunomodulatory agent; has not been established. Thought to act by modifying immune processes that are believed to be responsible for the pathogenesis of MS.

NURSING CONSIDERATIONS

Assessment: Assess for hypersensitivity to drug or mannitol, and pregnancy/nursing status.

Monitoring: Monitor for immediate post-inj reactions, chest pain, lipoatrophy, inj-site skin necrosis, and other adverse reactions.

Patient Counseling: Advise to inform physician if pregnant, planning to become pregnant, or breastfeeding. Inform that drug may cause various symptoms after inj (eg, flushing, chest pain, palpitations, anxiety, dyspnea, throat constriction, urticaria) that are generally transient and self-limited and do not require specific treatment; inform that these symptoms may occur early or may have their onset several months after treatment initiation. Inform that transient chest pain (either as part of the immediate post-inj reaction or in isolation) may occur; advise to seek medical attention if chest pain of unusual duration or intensity occurs. Instruct to follow proper inj technique and to rotate inj areas and sites with each inj to help minimize localized lipoatrophy and inj-site necrosis. Inform that 20mg/mL and 40mg/mL are not interchangeable. Caution to use aseptic technique. Caution against the reuse of needles or syringes. Inform of safe disposal procedures.

Administration: SQ route. Do not administer IV. Allow to stand at room temperature for 20 min before administration. Areas for SQ self-inj include arms, abdomen, hips, and thighs. **Storage:** 2-8°C (36-46°F). If needed, may store at 15-30°C (59-86°F) for up to 1 month, but refrigeration is preferred; avoid exposure to higher temperatures or intense light. Do not freeze; discard if frozen.

COPEGUS   RX
ribavirin (Genentech)

> Not for monotherapy treatment of chronic hepatitis C (CHC) virus infection. Primary toxicity is hemolytic anemia. Anemia associated with therapy may result in worsening of cardiac disease and lead to fatal and nonfatal myocardial infarctions. Avoid with history of significant or unstable cardiac disease. Contraindicated in women who are pregnant and male partners of pregnant women. Extreme care must be taken to avoid pregnancy during therapy and for 6 months after completion of therapy. Use at least 2 reliable forms of effective contraception during therapy and for 6 months after discontinuation.

THERAPEUTIC CLASS: Nucleoside analogue

INDICATIONS: In combination with Pegasys (peginterferon alfa-2a) for the treatment of patients ≥5 yrs of age with CHC virus infection who have compensated liver disease and have not been previously treated with interferon alfa.

DOSAGE: *Adults:* Take with food. Treat with Pegasys 180mcg SQ once weekly. CHC Monoinfection: Individualize dose. Usual: 800-1200mg/day in 2 divided doses. Genotypes 1 and 4: ≥75kg: 1200mg/day for 48 weeks. <75kg: 1000mg/day for 48 weeks. Genotypes 2 and 3: 800mg/day for 24 weeks. CHC with HIV Coinfection: Usual: 800mg/day for 48 weeks, regardless of genotype. Consider discontinuation if patient fails to demonstrate at least a 2 $\log_{10}$ reduction from baseline in hepatitis C virus (HCV) RNA by 12 weeks of therapy, or undetectable HCV RNA levels after 24 weeks of therapy. Refer to PI for dose modifications.
Pediatrics: ≥5 Yrs: Take with food. Treat with Pegasys 180mcg/1.73m² x BSA SQ once weekly, to a max of 180mcg. ≥75kg: 600mg qam and qpm. 60-74kg: 400mg qam and 600mg qpm. 47-59kg: 400mg qam and qpm. 34-46kg: 200mg qam and 400mg qpm. 23-33kg: 200mg qam and qpm. Genotypes 2 or 3: Treat for 24 weeks. Other Genotypes: Treat for 48 weeks. Maintain pediatric dosing through the completion of therapy in patients who initiate treatment prior to 18th birthday. Consider discontinuation if patient fails to demonstrate at least a 2 $\log_{10}$ reduction from baseline in HCV RNA by 12 weeks of therapy, or undetectable HCV RNA levels after 24 weeks of therapy. Refer to PI for dose modifications.

HOW SUPPLIED: Tab: 200mg

CONTRAINDICATIONS: Women who are or may become pregnant and men whose female partners are pregnant, hemoglobinopathies (eg, thalassemia major, sickle cell anemia), and in combination with didanosine. When used with Pegasys, refer to the individual monograph.

WARNINGS/PRECAUTIONS: Not for the treatment of adenovirus, respiratory syncytial virus, parainfluenza or influenza infections. Combination therapy is associated with significant adverse reactions (eg, severe depression and suicidal ideation, hemolytic anemia, suppression of bone marrow function, autoimmune/infectious/ophthalmologic/cerebrovascular disorders, pulmonary dysfunction, colitis, pancreatitis, diabetes). A negative pregnancy test is necessary prior to initiation. Caution with baseline risk of severe anemia (eg, spherocytosis, history of GI bleeding). Risk of hepatic decompensation and death in CHC patients with cirrhosis. Severe acute hypersensitivity reactions and serious skin reactions reported. D/C with hepatic decompensation, confirmed pancreatitis, severe hypersensitivity, or if signs/symptoms of severe skin reactions develop. Pulmonary disorders (eg, dyspnea, pulmonary infiltrates, pneumonitis, pulmonary HTN) reported; closely monitor and, if appropriate, d/c therapy if pulmonary infiltrates/function impairment develops. Caution with preexisting cardiac disease; d/c if cardiovascular status deteriorates. Delay in height and weight increase reported in pediatrics.

ADVERSE REACTIONS: Hemolytic anemia, fatigue, asthenia, neutropenia, headache, pyrexia, myalgia, irritability, anxiety, nervousness, insomnia, alopecia, rigors, N/V.

INTERACTIONS: See Contraindications. Closely monitor for toxicities (eg, hepatic decompensation) with nucleoside reverse transcriptase inhibitors; consider dose reduction or discontinuation. May reduce phosphorylation of lamivudine, stavudine, and zidovudine. Severe pancytopenia, bone marrow suppression, and myelotoxicity reported with azathioprine.

PREGNANCY: Category X, not for use in nursing.

MECHANISM OF ACTION: Nucleoside analogue; not established. Has direct antiviral activity in tissue culture against many RNA viruses; increases mutation frequency in the genomes of several RNA viruses and ribavirin triphosphate inhibits HCV polymerase in a biochemical reaction.

PHARMACOKINETICS: Absorption: C_{max}=2748ng/mL; T_{max}=2 hrs; AUC_{0-12hr}=25,361ng•hr/mL. **Elimination:** $T_{1/2}$=120-170 hrs.

NURSING CONSIDERATIONS

Assessment: Assess for hemoglobinopathies, autoimmune hepatitis, hepatic decompensation, baseline risk of severe anemia, history of or preexisting cardiac disease, renal impairment, hypersensitivity to drug, nursing status, and possible drug interactions. Conduct pregnancy test (including in female partners of male patients), standard hematological and biochemical lab tests, ECG in patients with preexisting cardiac abnormalities, thyroid function test, and CD4 count in HIV/AIDS patients.

Monitoring: Monitor for hepatic decompensation, pancreatitis, hypersensitivity/skin reactions, pulmonary infiltrates/function impairment, and other adverse reactions. Monitor growth in pediatrics, cardiac status, TSH, and HCV RNA. Perform hematological tests at Weeks 2 and 4 and biochemical tests at Week 4; perform additional testing periodically. Perform pregnancy testing monthly and for 6 months after discontinuation (including female partners of male patients).

Patient Counseling: Counsel on risks/benefits associated with treatment. Inform of pregnancy risks; instruct to use 2 forms of effective contraception during therapy and for 6 months after discontinuation of therapy (including female partners of male patients). Advise to notify physician in the event of pregnancy. Advise that lab evaluations are required prior to starting therapy and periodically thereafter. Advise to be well-hydrated, especially during the initial stages of treatment. Caution to avoid driving/operating machinery if dizziness, confusion, somnolence, or fatigue develops. Instruct not to drink alcohol; inform that alcohol may exacerbate CHC infection. Inform to take missed doses as soon as possible during the same day; advise not to double the next dose. Inform to take appropriate precautions to prevent HCV transmission or in the event of treatment failure.

Administration: Oral route. **Storage:** 25°C (77°F); excursions permitted between 15-30°C (59-86°F).

CORDARONE   RX
amiodarone HCl (Various)

> Use only in patients with the indicated life-threatening arrhythmias because of potentially fatal toxicities, including pulmonary toxicity (hypersensitivity pneumonitis or interstitial/alveolar pneumonitis). Liver injury is common, usually mild, and evidenced only by abnormal liver enzymes. Overt liver disease may occur, and has been fatal. May exacerbate arrhythmia. Significant heart block or sinus bradycardia reported. Patients must be hospitalized while LD is given, and a response generally requires at least 1 week, usually 2 or more. Maintenance-dose selection is difficult and may require dosage decrease or discontinuation of treatment.

OTHER BRAND NAMES: Amiodarone Tablet (Various)

THERAPEUTIC CLASS: Class III antiarrhythmic

INDICATIONS: Treatment of life-threatening recurrent ventricular fibrillation and recurrent hemodynamically unstable ventricular tachycardia when these have not responded to adequate doses of other available antiarrhythmics or when alternative agents could not be tolerated.

DOSAGE: *Adults:* Give LD in hospital. LD: 800-1600mg/day for 1-3 weeks. Give in divided doses with meals for total daily dose ≥1000mg or if GI intolerance occurs. After control is achieved or with prominent side effects, reduce to 600-800mg/day for 1 month. Maint: 400mg/day; up to 600mg/day. May be administered as a single dose, or in patients with severe GI intolerance, as a bid dose. Use lowest effective dose. Take consistently with regard to meals. Elderly: Start at the lower end of dosing range.

HOW SUPPLIED: Tab: 200mg* *scored

CONTRAINDICATIONS: Cardiogenic shock, severe sinus-node dysfunction causing marked sinus bradycardia, 2nd- or 3rd-degree atrioventricular (AV) block, when episodes of bradycardia have caused syncope (except when used with a pacemaker).

WARNINGS/PRECAUTIONS: D/C and institute steroid therapy if hypersensitivity pneumonitis occurs, or reduce dose if interstitial/alveolar pneumonitis occurs and institute appropriate treatment. In patients with implanted defibrillators or pacemakers, pacing and defibrillation thresholds should be assessed before and during treatment. Amiodarone-induced hyperthyroidism may result in thyrotoxicosis and/or the possibility of arrhythmia breakthrough or aggravation. D/C or reduce dose if LFTs are >3X normal or double in patients with elevated baseline. Optic neuropathy and/or optic neuritis usually resulting in visual impairment reported. May cause fetal harm in pregnancy and neonatal hypo/hyperthyroidism. May develop reversible corneal

C

microdeposits (eg, visual halos, blurred vision), photosensitivity, and peripheral neuropathy (rare). May cause either hypo/hyperthyroidism; monitor particularly in elderly and with history of thyroid nodules, goiter, or other thyroid dysfunction. Thyroid nodules/cancer reported. Hypotension reported upon discontinuation of cardiopulmonary bypass during open-heart surgery (rare). Adult respiratory distress syndrome (ARDS) reported with either cardiac or noncardiac surgery. Correct K^+ or Mg^{2+} deficiency before instituting and during therapy. Lab test interactions may occur. May be contraindicated with corneal refractive laser surgery devices. Caution with severe left ventricular dysfunction and in elderly.

ADVERSE REACTIONS: Pulmonary toxicity, arrhythmia exacerbation, liver injury, overt liver disease, heart block/sinus bradycardia, malaise, fatigue, involuntary movements, peripheral neuropathy, constipation, poor coordination and gait, N/V, anorexia, photosensitivity.

INTERACTIONS: Risk of interactions exists after discontinuation of therapy due to long and variable $T_{1/2}$. May increase sensitivity to myocardial depressant and conduction effects of halogenated inhalation anesthetics. CYP3A4 inhibitors increase serum levels (eg, protease inhibitors, loratadine, trazodone). Avoid with grapefruit juice. Consider monitoring for toxicity when used with protease inhibitors. QT interval prolongation and torsades de pointes reported with loratadine and trazodone. May cause QTc prolongation, with or without TdP, when used with disopyramide, fluoroquinolones, macrolides, and azoles. Inhibits P-glycoprotein, CYP1A2, CYP2C9, CYP2D6, and CYP3A4 and may increase levels of their substrates. Rhabdomyolysis/myopathy reported with HMG-CoA reductase inhibitors that are CYP3A4 substrates; limit simvastatin dose to 20mg/day, lovastatin to 40mg/day, and lower initial/maintenance doses of other CYP3A4 substrates (eg, atorvastatin) may be required. Elevated SrCr reported with cyclosporine. May increase levels of cyclosporine, quinidine, procainamide, flecainide, and phenytoin. May increase levels of digoxin; d/c or reduce dose by 50% upon amiodarone initiation. Quinidine and procainamide doses should be reduced by 1/3 if coadministered. Initiate added antiarrhythmic drug at a lower than usual dose with monitoring. Caution with β-blockers and calcium channel blockers; if necessary, amiodarone can continue to be used after insertion of a pacemaker in patients with severe bradycardia or sinus arrest. Reduce warfarin dose by 1/3-1/2 and monitor PT closely. Ineffective inhibition of platelet aggregation reported with clopidogrel. CYP3A4 inducers (eg, St. John's wort, rifampin) decrease levels. Fentanyl may cause hypotension, bradycardia, and decreased cardiac output. Sinus bradycardia reported with lidocaine; seizure associated with increased lidocaine concentrations reported with IV amiodarone. Cholestyramine increases enterohepatic elimination and may decrease levels and $T_{1/2}$. Hemodynamic and electrophysiologic interactions observed with propranolol, diltiazem, and verapamil. May impair metabolism of dextromethorphan, methotrexate, and phenytoin with chronic use (>2 weeks). Antithyroid drugs' action may be delayed in amiodarone-induced thyrotoxicosis. Radioactive iodine is contraindicated with amiodarone-induced hyperthyroidism. Caution with drugs that may induce hypokalemia and/or hypomagnesemia.

PREGNANCY: Category D, not for use in nursing.

MECHANISM OF ACTION: Class III antiarrhythmic; prolongs myocardial cell-action potential duration and refractory period, and causes noncompetitive α- and β-adrenergic inhibition.

PHARMACOKINETICS: Absorption: Slow and variable; bioavailability (50%); T_{max}=3-7 hrs (single dose). **Distribution:** V_d=60L/kg; plasma protein binding (96%); crosses the placenta, found in breast milk. **Metabolism:** Liver via CYP3A4, CYP2C8; desethylamiodarone (DEA) [major metabolite]. **Elimination:** Bile, urine. (Healthy) $T_{1/2}$=58 days, 36 days (DEA).

NURSING CONSIDERATIONS

Assessment: Assess for cardiogenic shock, severe sinus node dysfunction causing marked sinus bradycardia, 2nd- or 3rd-degree AV block, life-threatening arrhythmias, renal/hepatic impairment, thyroid dysfunction, hypersensitivity to the drug including iodine, presence of implanted defibrillators or pacemakers, pregnancy/nursing status, and possible drug interactions. Correct K^+ or Mg^{2+} deficiency prior to initiation. Obtain chest x-ray, pulmonary function tests (including diffusion capacity), and physical exam.

Monitoring: Monitor for pulmonary toxicities, worsened arrhythmia, sinus bradycardia, heart block, photosensitivity, and other adverse reactions. Perform history, physical exam, and chest x-ray every 3-6 months. Monitor LFTs and thyroid function tests. Peri- and postoperative monitoring for patients undergoing general anesthesia and ARDS recommended. Perform regular ophthalmic examination, including funduscopy and slit-lamp examination.

Patient Counseling: Inform about benefits and risks of therapy. Advise to report any adverse reactions to physician. Counsel to take as directed and not to take with grapefruit juice. Advise to avoid prolonged sunlight exposure and to use sun-barrier cre or protective clothing. Advise that corneal refractive laser surgery is contraindicated with concurrent use. Instruct to notify physician if pregnant/nursing.

Administration: Oral route. Administer consistently, either with or without food. **Storage:** 20-25°C (68-77°F). Protect from light.

CORDRAN   RX
flurandrenolide (Various)

THERAPEUTIC CLASS: Corticosteroid

INDICATIONS: Relief of the inflammatory and pruritic manifestations of corticosteroid-responsive dermatoses, (tape) particularly dry, scaling, localized lesions.

DOSAGE: *Adults:* (Cre) For moist lesions, apply a small quantity to affected area bid-tid and rub in gently. (Lot) Apply a small quantity to affected area bid-tid and rub in gently. (Cre/Lot) D/C when control is achieved. Reassess diagnosis if no improvement is seen within 2 weeks. Do not use with occlusive dressings unless directed by a physician. (Tape) Replace q12h, but may be left in place for 24 hrs if well tolerated and adheres satisfactorily. May be used at night only and removed during the day when necessary. If ends of tape loosen prematurely, may trim off and replace with fresh tape. May use occlusive dressings for psoriasis or recalcitrant conditions; d/c use of tape and other occlusive dressings and institute appropriate antimicrobial therapy if an infection develops.

Pediatrics: (Cre) For moist lesions, apply a small quantity to affected area bid-tid and rub in gently. (Lot) Apply a small quantity to affected area bid-tid and rub in gently. (Cre/Lot) D/C when control is achieved. Reassess diagnosis if no improvement is seen within 2 weeks. Do not use with occlusive dressings unless directed by a physician. (Tape) Replace q12h, but may be left in place for 24 hrs if well tolerated and adheres satisfactorily. May be used at night only and removed during the day when necessary. If ends of tape loosen prematurely, may trim off and replace with fresh tape. May use occlusive dressings for psoriasis or recalcitrant conditions; d/c use of tape and other occlusive dressings and institute appropriate antimicrobial therapy if an infection develops.

HOW SUPPLIED: Cre: 0.025% [30g, 60g, 120g], 0.05% [15g, 30g, 60g, 120g]; Lot: 0.05% [15mL, 60mL, 120mL]; Tape: 4mcg/cm^2 [60cm x 7.5cm, 200cm x 7.5cm]

CONTRAINDICATIONS: (Tape) Not recommended for lesions exuding serum or in intertriginous areas.

WARNINGS/PRECAUTIONS: Systemic absorption may produce reversible hypothalamic-pituitary-adrenal (HPA) axis suppression, manifestations of Cushing's syndrome, hyperglycemia, and glucosuria. Application of more potent steroids, use over large surface areas, prolonged use, and the addition of occlusive dressings may augment systemic absorption. Evaluate periodically for evidence of HPA-axis suppression when a large dose is applied to a large surface area or under an occlusive dressing; if noted, withdraw treatment, reduce frequency of application, or substitute with a less potent steroid. Infrequently, signs/symptoms of steroid withdrawal may occur, requiring supplemental systemic corticosteroids. Pediatric patients may be more susceptible to systemic toxicity. Chronic therapy may interfere with growth and development of children; use least amount effective for condition. D/C and institute appropriate therapy if irritation develops. Use appropriate antifungal or antibacterial agent in the presence of dermatologic infections; if favorable response does not occur promptly, d/c until infection has been adequately controlled.

ADVERSE REACTIONS: Burning, itching, irritation, dryness, folliculitis, hypertrichosis, acneiform eruptions, hypopigmentation, perioral dermatitis, allergic contact dermatitis, skin maceration, secondary infection, skin atrophy, striae, miliaria.

PREGNANCY: Category C, caution in nursing.

MECHANISM OF ACTION: Corticosteroid; possesses anti-inflammatory, antipruritic, and vasoconstrictive actions. Anti-inflammatory mechanism not established. May stabilize cellular and lysosomal membranes, thereby preventing release of proteolytic enzymes and consequently reducing inflammation.

PHARMACOKINETICS: Absorption: Percutaneous; extent of absorption is determined by the vehicle, integrity of epidermal barrier, and use of occlusive dressings. **Distribution:** Bound to plasma proteins in varying degrees; found in breast milk (systemically administered). **Metabolism:** Liver. **Elimination:** Kidney, bile.

NURSING CONSIDERATIONS

Assessment: Assess for drug hypersensitivity, dermatological infections, conditions that augment systemic absorption, and pregnancy/nursing status. (Tape) Assess for lesions exuding serum or intertriginous areas.

Monitoring: Monitor for signs/symptoms of HPA-axis suppression, Cushing's syndrome, hyperglycemia, glucosuria, skin irritation, systemic toxicity in pediatric patients, steroid withdrawal, and other adverse reactions. Periodically monitor for HPA-axis suppression using urinary free cortisol and adrenocorticotropic hormone stimulation tests.

Patient Counseling: Instruct to use externally ud and to avoid contact with eyes. Advise not to use for any disorder other than that for which it was prescribed. Counsel not to bandage, cover, or wrap treated skin areas unless directed by physician. Advise to report any signs of local

C

adverse reactions especially under occlusive dressing. Inform to avoid using tight-fitting diapers or plastic pants on a child being treated in the diaper area, as these garments may constitute occlusive dressings. (Cre/Lot) Instruct not to use on the face, underarms, or groin areas unless directed by physician. Instruct not to use other corticosteroid-containing products while on medication without first consulting physician. Advise to contact physician if no improvement is seen within 2 weeks.

Administration: Topical route. (Lot) Shake well before use. (Tape) Skin should be clean and dry before tape is applied; tape should always be cut, never torn. Refer to PI for further application and replacement instructions. **Storage:** (Cre/Lot) 20-25°C (68-77°F); excursions permitted to 15-30°C (59-86°F). Protect from light. (Lot) Do not freeze. (Tape) 20-25°C (68-77°F).

COREG CR   RX
carvedilol phosphate (GlaxoSmithKline)

OTHER BRAND NAMES: Coreg (GlaxoSmithKline)

THERAPEUTIC CLASS: Alpha₁/beta-blocker

INDICATIONS: Treatment of mild-to-severe chronic heart failure (HF) of ischemic or cardiomyopathic origin. Reduction of cardiovascular mortality in clinically stable patients who have survived the acute phase of a myocardial infarction (MI) and have a left ventricular ejection fraction of ≤40%. Management of essential HTN.

DOSAGE: *Adults:* Individualize dose and take with food. (Tab) HF: Minimize fluid retention prior to initiation. Initial: 3.125mg bid for 2 weeks. Titrate: May double dose over successive intervals of at least 2 weeks up to 25mg bid as tolerated. Maintain on lower doses if higher doses not tolerated. Max: 50mg bid if >85kg with mild-moderate HF. Reduce if HR <55 beats/min. HTN: Initial: 6.25mg bid. Titrate: May double dose every 7-14 days as tolerated and PRN. Max: 50mg/day. Left Ventricular Dysfunction (LVD) Post-MI: Start if hemodynamically stable and fluid retention has been minimized. Initial: 6.25mg bid. Titrate: May double dose every 3-10 days based on tolerability. Target dose: 25mg bid. May begin with 3.125mg bid and/or slow up-titration rate if clinically indicated. Maintain on lower doses if higher doses not tolerated. (Cap, ER) HF: Minimize fluid retention prior to initiation. Initial: 10mg qd for 2 weeks. Titrate: May double dose over successive intervals of at least 2 weeks up to 80mg qd as tolerated. Maintain on lower doses if higher doses not tolerated. Reduce dose if HR <55 beats/min. HTN: Initial: 20mg qd. Titrate: May double dose every 7-14 days as tolerated and PRN. Max: 80mg/day. LVD Post-MI: Start if hemodynamically stable and fluid retention has been minimized. Initial: 20mg qd. Titrate: May double dose every 3-10 days based on tolerability. Target dose: 80mg qd. May begin with 10mg qd and/or slow up-titration if clinically indicated. Maintain on lower doses if higher doses not tolerated. Elderly: Start at a lower dose (40mg) when switching from higher doses of immediate-release; may increase dose after an interval of at least 2 weeks as appropriate.

HOW SUPPLIED: Tab: 3.125mg, 6.25mg, 12.5mg, 25mg; Cap, Extended-Release: (Phosphate) 10mg, 20mg, 40mg, 80mg

CONTRAINDICATIONS: Bronchial asthma or related bronchospastic conditions, 2nd- or 3rd-degree atrioventricular (AV) block, sick sinus syndrome, severe bradycardia (without permanent pacemaker), cardiogenic shock, decompensated HF requiring IV inotropic therapy, severe hepatic impairment.

WARNINGS/PRECAUTIONS: Severe exacerbation of angina, MI, and ventricular arrhythmias reported with abrupt discontinuation; whenever possible, d/c over 1-2 weeks. Bradycardia reported. Hypotension, postural hypotension, and syncope reported, most commonly during up-titration period; avoid driving or hazardous tasks. Worsening HF or fluid retention may occur during up-titration. May mask signs of hypoglycemia and hyperthyroidism (eg, tachycardia). Caution with pheochromocytoma, peripheral vascular disease, Prinzmetal's variant angina, and in patients with bronchospastic disease who do not respond to, or cannot tolerate, other antihypertensives. Monitor renal function during up-titration in patients with low BP (systolic BP <100mmHg), ischemic heart disease, diffuse vascular disease, and/or underlying renal insufficiency. Chronically administered therapy should not be routinely withdrawn prior to major surgery. Patients with history of severe anaphylactic reaction to variety of allergens may be more reactive to repeated challenge; may be unresponsive to usual doses of epinephrine. Intraoperative floppy iris syndrome (IFIS) observed during cataract surgery.

ADVERSE REACTIONS: Bradycardia, fatigue, hypotension, dizziness, headache, diarrhea, N/V, hyperglycemia, weight increase, increased cough, asthenia, angina pectoris, syncope, edema.

INTERACTIONS: Potentially increased levels with potent CYP2D6 inhibitors (eg, quinidine, fluoxetine, paroxetine, propafenone). Monitor for hypotension and bradycardia with catecholamine-depleting agents (eg, reserpine, MAOIs). BP- and HR-lowering effects potentiated with clonidine. Reduced plasma levels with rifampin. Increased exposure with cimetidine. Conduction disturbances seen with diltiazem; monitor ECG and BP with verapamil and diltiazem. May enhance blood glucose-reducing effect of insulin and oral hypoglycemics; monitor blood glucose. May increase concentration of cyclosporine and digoxin; monitor levels of cyclosporine and digoxin. Caution with anesthetic agents that depress myocardial function (eg, ether, cyclopropane, trichloroethylene). Digitalis glycosides slow AV conduction and decrease HR; concomitant use can increase the risk of bradycardia. Amiodarone or other CYP2C9 inhibitors (eg, fluconazole) may enhance β-blocking properties, resulting in further slowing of the HR or cardiac conduction. Additive effects and exaggerated orthostatic component with diuretics.

PREGNANCY: Category C, not for use in nursing.

MECHANISM OF ACTION: Nonselective β-adrenergic and α₁ blocker.

PHARMACOKINETICS: Absorption: (Tab) Rapid and extensive; absolute bioavailability (25-35%). (Cap, ER) T_{max}=5 hrs. **Distribution:** Plasma protein binding (>98%); V_d=115L. **Metabolism:** Extensive by oxidation and glucuronidation; CYP2D6, 2C9 (primary); CYP3A4, 2C19, 1A2, 2E1 (minor). **Elimination:** Urine (<2% unchanged), feces; $T_{1/2}$=7-10 hrs.

NURSING CONSIDERATIONS

Assessment: Assess for coronary artery disease, hypotension, ischemic heart disease, diffuse vascular disease, hyperthyroidism, and any other conditions where treatment is contraindicated or cautioned. Assess for any upcoming surgery, history of serious hypersensitivity reaction, pregnancy/nursing status, and possible drug interactions. Obtain baseline blood glucose levels, LFTs, and renal function.

Monitoring: Monitor for bradycardia, signs/symptoms of cardiac failure, masking of hypoglycemia/hyperthyroidism, withdrawal symptoms, precipitation or aggravation of arterial insufficiency, hypotension, hypersensitivity reactions, and for IFIS during cataract surgery. Monitor blood glucose during initiation/dosage adjustments, and upon discontinuation of therapy. Monitor LFTs and renal function.

Patient Counseling: Instruct not to d/c therapy without consulting physician. Instruct patients with HF to consult physician if signs/symptoms of worsening HF occur. Inform that a drop in BP when standing, resulting in dizziness and, rarely, fainting, may occur; advise to sit or lie down if these symptoms occur. Advise to avoid driving or hazardous tasks if experiencing dizziness or fatigue, and to notify physician if dizziness or faintness occurs. Inform contact lens wearers that decreased lacrimation may be experienced, diabetic patients to report any changes in blood sugar levels, and to take drug with food. (Cap, ER) Advise not to divide, chew, or crush cap.

Administration: Oral route. Take with food. (Cap, ER) Take in am. Swallow caps whole or may open and sprinkle contents on applesauce; do not chew, crush, or divide. **Storage:** (Tab) <30°C (86°F). Protect from moisture. (Cap, ER) 25°C (77°F); excursions permitted to 15-30°C (59-86°F).

CORGARD   RX
nadolol (King)

> Hypersensitivity to catecholamines observed upon withdrawal; exacerbation of angina and, in some cases, myocardial infarction reported after abrupt discontinuation. When discontinuing chronically administered nadolol, particularly in patients with ischemic heart disease, reduce dose gradually over a period of 1-2 weeks and monitor carefully. If angina markedly worsens or acute coronary insufficiency develops, administration of therapy should be reinstituted promptly, at least temporarily, and other measures appropriate for the management of unstable angina should be taken. Warn against interruption or discontinuation of therapy without the physician's advice. Coronary artery disease (CAD) is common and may be unrecognized; it may be prudent not to d/c therapy abruptly even in patients treated only for HTN.

THERAPEUTIC CLASS: Nonselective beta-blocker

INDICATIONS: Long-term management of angina pectoris. Treatment of HTN alone or in combination with other antihypertensive agents, especially thiazide-type diuretics.

DOSAGE: *Adults:* Individualize dose. Angina Pectoris: Initial: 40mg qd. Titrate: May gradually increase in 40-80mg increments at 3- to 7-day intervals until optimum response is obtained or there is pronounced slowing of the HR. Maint: Usual: 40 or 80mg qd. Doses up to 160 or 240mg qd may be needed. Max: 240mg/day. Reduce gradually over a period of 1-2 weeks if treatment is to be discontinued. HTN: Initial: 40mg qd. Titrate: May gradually increase in 40-80mg increments until optimum BP reduction is achieved. Maint: Usual: 40 or 80mg qd. Doses up to 240 or 320mg qd may be needed. Renal Impairment: CrCl >50mL/min: Dose q24h. CrCl 31-50mL/min: Dose q24-36h. CrCl 10-30mL/min: Dose q24-48h. CrCl <10mL/min: Dose q40-60h.

HOW SUPPLIED: Tab: 20mg*, 40mg*, 80mg* *scored

CONTRAINDICATIONS: Bronchial asthma, sinus bradycardia and >1st degree conduction block, cardiogenic shock, overt cardiac failure.

WARNINGS/PRECAUTIONS: May precipitate more severe heart failure (HF) in patients with congestive heart failure (CHF); caution with history of well-compensated HF. May lead to cardiac failure in patients without a history of HF; digitalize and/or treat with diuretics at the first sign or symptom of HF and observe response closely or d/c. Avoid in patients with bronchospastic diseases. Chronically administered therapy should not be routinely withdrawn prior to major surgery. May prevent premonitory signs and symptoms of acute hypoglycemia (eg, tachycardia, BP changes). May mask certain clinical signs (eg, tachycardia) of hyperthyroidism. May precipitate thyroid storm with abrupt withdrawal. Caution in patients with renal impairment. Patients with a history of severe anaphylactic reaction to variety of allergens may be more reactive to repeated challenge and may be unresponsive to usual doses of epinephrine.

ADVERSE REACTIONS: Bradycardia, dizziness, fatigue, nausea, diarrhea, anorexia, abdominal discomfort, rash, pruritus, weight gain, blurred vision, peripheral vascular insufficiency, cardiac failure, hypotension, rhythm/conduction disturbances.

INTERACTIONS: Additive hypotension and/or bradycardia with catecholamine-depleting drugs (eg, reserpine); monitor closely. Increased risk of bradycardia with digitalis glycosides. Hyperglycemia or hypoglycemia may occur with antidiabetic drugs (oral agents and insulin); adjust dose of antidiabetic agents accordingly. May exaggerate hypotension induced by general anesthetics.

PREGNANCY: Category C, not for use in nursing.

MECHANISM OF ACTION: Nonselective β-blocker; has not been established. Inhibits β_1 and β_2 receptors, inhibiting chronotropic, inotropic, and vasodilator responses to β-adrenergic stimulation.

PHARMACOKINETICS: Absorption: T_{max}=3-4 hrs. **Distribution:** Plasma protein binding (30%); found in breast milk. **Elimination:** Urine (unchanged); $T_{1/2}$=20-24 hrs.

NURSING CONSIDERATIONS

Assessment: Assess for bronchial asthma, sinus bradycardia, AV heart block, cardiogenic shock, CHF, bronchospastic diseases, CAD, hyperthyroidism, diabetes, renal impairment, hypersensitivity to drug, pregnancy/nursing status, and possible drug interactions.

Monitoring: Monitor for signs/symptoms of CHF, hypoglycemia, thyrotoxicosis, withdrawal symptoms, renal dysfunction, hypersensitivity reactions, and other adverse reactions

Patient Counseling: Warn against interruption or discontinuation of therapy without consulting physician. Advise to consult physician at 1st sign/symptom of impending cardiac failure. Advise of proper course in the event of an inadvertently missed dose.

Administration: Oral route. May be administered without regard to meals. **Storage:** Room temperature; avoid excessive heat. Protect from light.

CORVERT   RX
ibutilide fumarate (Pharmacia & Upjohn)

> May cause potentially fatal arrhythmias, particularly sustained polymorphic ventricular tachycardia, usually in association with QT prolongation (torsades de pointes), but sometimes without documented QT prolongation. Administer in a setting of continuous ECG monitoring and by personnel trained in identification and treatment of acute ventricular arrhythmias. Patients with atrial fibrillation (A-fib) of >2-3 days' duration must be adequately anticoagulated, generally for ≥2 weeks. Patients should be carefully selected such that the expected benefits of maintaining sinus rhythm outweigh the immediate and maintenance therapy risks.

THERAPEUTIC CLASS: Class III antiarrhythmic

INDICATIONS: For rapid conversion of A-fib or atrial flutter of recent onset to sinus rhythm.

DOSAGE: *Adults:* ≥60kg: 1mg over 10 min. <60kg: 0.01mg/kg over 10 min. If arrhythmia still present within 10 min after the end of the initial infusion, repeat infusion 10 min after completion of 1st infusion. Elderly: Start at lower end of dosing range.

HOW SUPPLIED: Inj: 0.1mg/mL

WARNINGS/PRECAUTIONS: May induce/worsen ventricular arrhythmias. Not recommended in patients who have previously demonstrated polymorphic ventricular tachycardia (eg, torsades de pointes). Anticipate proarrhythmic events. Correct hypokalemia and hypomagnesemia before therapy. Reversible heart block reported. Caution in elderly.

ADVERSE REACTIONS: Sustained/nonsustained polymorphic ventricular tachycardia, nonsustained monomorphic ventricular tachycardia, bundle branch/atrioventricular block, ventricular/supraventricular extrasystoles, hypotension, bradycardia, headache, nausea, HTN, syncope, nodal arrhythmia, congestive heart failure.

INTERACTIONS: Avoid Class IA (eg, disopyramide, quinidine, procainamide) and other Class III (eg, amiodarone, sotalol) antiarrhythmics with or within 4 hrs postinfusion. Increased proarrhythmia potential with drugs that prolong the QT interval (eg, phenothiazines, TCAs, tetracyclic antidepressants, and antihistamine drugs [H_1-receptor antagonists]). Caution in patients with elevated or above the usual therapeutic range of plasma digoxin levels.

PREGNANCY: Category C, not for use in nursing.

MECHANISM OF ACTION: Class III antiarrhythmic agent; prolongs atrial and ventricular action potential duration and refractoriness. Delays repolarization by activation of a slow, inward current, rather than blocking outward K^+ currents.

PHARMACOKINETICS: Distribution: V_d=11L/kg; plasma protein binding (40%). **Metabolism:** Omega-oxidation and β-oxidation. **Elimination:** Urine (82%, 7% unchanged), feces (19%); $T_{1/2}$=6 hrs.

NURSING CONSIDERATIONS

Assessment: Assess for arrhythmia, bradycardia, polymorphic ventricular tachycardia, electrolyte imbalance, renal/hepatic function, pregnancy/nursing status, and for possible drug interactions. Perform ECG. Obtain baseline QTc.

Monitoring: Monitor for worsening of induction of new ventricular arrhythmia, torsades de pointes (polymorphic ventricular tachycardia), and any arrhythmic activity. Monitor ECG continuously for ≥4 hrs following infusion.

Patient Counseling: Inform about benefits/risks of therapy. Instruct to report any adverse reactions to physician.

Administration: IV route. Refer to PI for dilution instructions. **Storage:** Vial: 20-25°C (68-77°F). Admixture: 0.9% NaCl or D5W: Stable at 15-30°C (59-86°F) for 24 hrs; 2-8°C (36-46°F) for 48 hrs in polyvinyl chloride plastic or polyolefin bags.

COSOPT   RX
dorzolamide HCl - timolol maleate (Merck)

OTHER BRAND NAMES: Cosopt PF (Merck)

THERAPEUTIC CLASS: Carbonic anhydrase inhibitor/nonselective beta-blocker

INDICATIONS: Reduction of elevated intraocular pressure (IOP) in patients with ocular HTN or open-angle glaucoma who are insufficiently responsive to β-blockers.

DOSAGE: *Adults:* 1 drop in the affected eye(s) bid. Space dosing of drugs at least 10 min apart (Cosopt) or at least 5 min apart (Cosopt PF) if using >1 topical ophthalmic drug.
Pediatrics: ≥2 Yrs: 1 drop in the affected eye(s) bid. Space dosing of drugs at least 10 min apart (Cosopt) or at least 5 min apart (Cosopt PF) if using >1 topical ophthalmic drug.

HOW SUPPLIED: Sol: (Dorzolamide HCl-Timolol Maleate) (Cosopt) 2%-0.5% [10mL]; (Cosopt PF) 2%-0.5% [0.2mL, 60^{s}180^s]

CONTRAINDICATIONS: Bronchial asthma, history of bronchial asthma, severe chronic obstructive pulmonary disease, sinus bradycardia, 2nd- or 3rd-degree atrioventricular (AV) block, overt cardiac failure, cardiogenic shock.

WARNINGS/PRECAUTIONS: Absorbed systemically; severe respiratory/cardiac reactions in patients with asthma and death in association with cardiac failure reported. Rare reports of fatal sulfonamide hypersensitivity reactions reported; d/c if signs of hypersensitivity or other serious reactions occur. Sensitizations may recur if readministered irrespective of the route of administration. May precipitate more severe failure in patients with diminished myocardial contractility; sympathetic stimulation may be essential for support of the circulation. D/C at the 1st sign/symptom of cardiac failure in patients without a history of cardiac failure. Withdrawal before surgery is controversial; may augment the risk of general anesthesia in surgical procedures. Caution in diabetic patients (especially those with labile diabetes) who are receiving insulin or oral hypoglycemics, hepatic impairment, and patients suspected of developing thyrotoxicosis. May mask symptoms of acute hypoglycemia and hyperthyroidism. Avoid abrupt withdrawal; may precipitate thyroid storm. Not recommended in severe renal impairment (CrCl <30mL/min). May be more reactive to repeated challenge with history of atopy or severe anaphylactic reaction to variety of allergens; may be unresponsive to usual doses of epinephrine. Choroidal detachment after filtration procedures reported. May potentiate muscle weakness consistent with certain myasthenic symptoms. Caution in patients with low endothelial cell counts. (Cosopt) Bacterial keratitis with contaminated containers reported. Local ocular adverse effects (conjunctivitis and lid reactions) reported with chronic administration; d/c and evaluate before restarting therapy.

ADVERSE REACTIONS: Taste perversion, ocular burning/stinging, conjunctival hyperemia, blurred vision, superficial punctate keratitis, eye itching.

INTERACTIONS: Not recommended with PO carbonic anhydrase inhibitors and topical β-blockers. Caution with PO/IV calcium antagonists; avoid coadministration in patients with impaired cardiac function. Potentiated systemic β-blockade with CYP2D6 inhibitors (eg, quinidine, SSRIs) and oral β-blockers. Possible additive effects and the production of hypotension and/or marked bradycardia with catecholamine-depleting drugs (eg, reserpine); observe patient closely. May have additive effects in prolonging AV conduction time with digitalis and calcium antagonists. Caution with high-dose salicylates.

PREGNANCY: Category C, not for use in nursing.

MECHANISM OF ACTION: Carbonic anhydrase inhibitor/nonselective β-blocker; decreases elevated IOP, whether or not associated with glaucoma, by reducing aqueous humor secretion.
PHARMACOKINETICS: Absorption: Timolol: C_{max} =0.46ng/mL. **Distribution:** Dorzolamide: Plasma protein binding (33%). Timolol: Found in breast milk. **Elimination:** Dorzolamide: Urine (unchanged, metabolite).

NURSING CONSIDERATIONS

Assessment: Assess for hypersensitivity, severe renal impairment, conditions where the treatment is contraindicated or cautioned, pregnancy/nursing status, and for possible drug interactions.

Monitoring: Monitor for improvement in IOP, ocular HTN, serious reactions or hypersensitivity, and corneal edema in patients with low endothelial cell counts. Monitor serum electrolyte levels and blood pH levels. (Cosopt) Monitor for conjunctivitis and lid reactions with chronic therapy, and bacterial keratitis.

Patient Counseling: Instruct not to touch container tip to eye or surrounding structures. Advise to d/c use and contact physician if serious/unusual reactions or signs of hypersensitivity occurs. Advise to immediately contact physician concerning the continued use of the product if undergoing ocular surgery or an intercurrent ocular condition (eg, trauma, infection) develops. (Cosopt PF) Instruct to discard the remaining content immediately after administration. (Cosopt) Advise to remove contact lenses prior to administration; may be reinserted 15 min after. Instruct to d/c use and contact their physician if any ocular reactions (particularly conjunctivitis and lid reactions) develop.

Administration: Ocular route. Refer to PI for Instructions for Use. **Storage:** (Cosopt) 15-30°C (59-86°F). Protect from light. (Cosopt PF) 20-25°C (68-77°F). Do not freeze. Discard any unused containers 15 days after 1st opening the pouch.

COUMADIN RX
warfarin sodium (Bristol-Myers Squibb)

May cause major or fatal bleeding; monitor INR regularly. Drugs, dietary changes, and other factors affect INR levels achieved with therapy. Instruct patients about prevention measures to minimize risk of bleeding and to report signs/symptoms of bleeding.

OTHER BRAND NAMES: Jantoven (Upsher-Smith)
THERAPEUTIC CLASS: Vitamin K-dependent coagulation factor inhibitor
INDICATIONS: Prophylaxis and treatment of venous thrombosis and its extension, pulmonary embolism (PE), and thromboembolic complications associated with atrial fibrillation (A-fib) and/or cardiac valve replacement. To reduce risk of death, recurrent myocardial infarction (MI), and thromboembolic events, such as stroke or systemic embolization after MI.
DOSAGE: *Adults:* Individualize dose and duration of therapy. Adjust dose based on INR and condition being treated. (Coumadin) IV dose is the same as PO dose. CYP2C9 and VKORC1 Genotypes Unknown: Initial: 2-5mg qd. Maint: 2-10mg qd. Venous Thromboembolism (including deep vein thrombosis [DVT] and PE)/Non-Valvular A-fib: Target INR 2.5 (INR Range, 2-3). Mechanical/Bioprosthetic Heart Valve: Bileaflet Mechanical Valve/Medtronic Hall Tilting Disk Valve in the Aortic Position with Sinus Rhythm and without Left Atrial Enlargement: Target INR: 2.5 (INR Range, 2-3). Tilting Disk Valves and Bileaflet Mechanical Valves in the Mitral Position: Target INR: 3 (INR Range, 2.5-3.5). Caged Ball or Caged Disk Valve: Target INR 3 (INR Range, 2.5-3.5). Bioprosthetic Valves in the Mitral Position: Target INR: 2.5 (INR Range, 2-3) for the first 3 months after valve insertion. If additional risk factors for thromboembolism present, target INR 2.5 (INR Range, 2-3). Post-MI: INR 2-3 plus low-dose aspirin (ASA) (≤100mg/day) for at least 3 months after MI. Valvular Disease Associated with A-Fib/Mitral Stenosis/Recurrent Systemic Embolism of Unknown Etiology: INR 2-3. Elderly/Debilitated/Asians: Consider lower initial and maintenance doses. Refer to PI for recommended dosing durations, conversion from other anticoagulants (heparin), dosing recommendations with consideration of genotype, and for further dosing instructions.
HOW SUPPLIED: Inj: (Coumadin) 5mg; Tab: (Coumadin, Jantoven) 1mg*, 2mg*, 2.5mg*, 3mg*, 4mg*, 5mg*, 6mg*, 7.5mg*, 10mg* *scored
CONTRAINDICATIONS: Pregnancy, except in pregnant women with mechanical heart valves, who are at high risk of thromboembolism. Hemorrhagic tendencies or blood dyscrasias. Recent or contemplated surgery of the CNS, eye, or traumatic surgery resulting in large open surfaces. Bleeding tendencies associated with active ulceration or overt bleeding of GI/genitourinary/respiratory tract, CNS hemorrhage, cerebral aneurysms, dissecting aorta, pericarditis and pericardial effusions, or bacterial endocarditis. Threatened abortion, eclampsia, and preeclampsia. Unsupervised patients with conditions associated with potential high level of noncompliance.

C

Spinal puncture and other diagnostic/therapeutic procedures with potential for uncontrollable bleeding. Major regional, lumbar block anesthesia. Malignant HTN.

WARNINGS/PRECAUTIONS: Has no direct effect on established thrombus, nor does it reverse ischemic tissue damage. Some dental/surgical procedures may need interruption or change in the dose; determine INR immediately prior to procedure. Has a narrow therapeutic range (index) and its action may be affected by endogenous factors, other drugs, and dietary vitamin K; perform periodic INR monitoring. Risk of necrosis and/or gangrene of skin and other tissues; d/c if necrosis occurs and consider alternative therapy. May enhance the release of atheromatous plaque emboli, and systemic atheroemboli and cholesterol microemboli may occur. D/C if distinct syndrome resulting from microemboli to the feet ("purple toes syndrome") occurs. Do not use as initial therapy with heparin-induced thrombocytopenia (HIT) and with heparin-induced thrombocytopenia with thrombosis syndrome (HITTS); limb ischemia, necrosis, and gangrene reported when heparin was discontinued and warfarin started or continued. Can cause fetal harm in pregnant women. Increased risks of therapy in patients with hepatic impairment, infectious diseases/disturbances of intestinal flora, indwelling catheter, severe/moderate HTN, deficiency in protein C-mediated anticoagulant response, polycythemia vera, vasculitis, diabetes, and those undergoing eye surgery. Caution in elderly and hepatic impairment.

ADVERSE REACTIONS: Hemorrhage, necrosis of the skin and other tissues, systemic atheroemboli, cholesterol microemboli, hypersensitivity/allergic reactions, vasculitis, hepatitis, elevated liver enzymes, N/V, diarrhea, rash, dermatitis, tracheal/tracheobronchial calcifications, chills.

INTERACTIONS: May increase effect (increase INR) with CYP2C9, 1A2, and/or 3A4 inhibitors. May decrease effect (decrease INR) with CYP2C9, 1A2, and/or 3A4 inducers. Increased risk of bleeding with anticoagulants (argatroban, dabigatran, bivalirudin, desirudin, heparin, lepirudin), antiplatelet agents (ASA, cilostazol, clopidogrel, dipyridamole, prasugrel, ticlopidine), NSAIDs (celecoxib, diclofenac, diflunisal, fenoprofen, ibuprofen, indomethacin, ketoprofen, ketorolac, mefenamic acid, naproxen, oxaprozin, piroxicam, sulindac), serotonin reuptake inhibitors (eg, citalopram, desvenlafaxine, duloxetine, escitalopram, fluoxetine, fluvoxamine, milnacipran, paroxetine, sertraline, venlafaxine, vilazodone). Changes in INR reported with antibiotics or antifungals; closely monitor INR when starting or stopping any antibiotics or antifungals. Use caution with botanical (herbal) products. May potentiate anticoagulant effects with some botanicals (eg, garlic, *Ginkgo biloba*). May decrease effects with some botanicals (eg, coenzyme Q10, St. John's wort, ginseng). Some botanicals and foods can interact through CYP450 interactions (eg, *echinacea*, grapefruit juice, ginkgo, goldenseal, St. John's wort). Cholestatic hepatitis has been associated with coadministration of warfarin and ticlopidine.

PREGNANCY: Category D (with mechanical heart valves) or Category X (for other pregnant populations), caution in nursing.

MECHANISM OF ACTION: Vitamin K-dependent coagulation factor inhibitor; thought to interfere with clotting factor synthesis by inhibition of the C1 subunit of the vitamin K epoxide reductase enzyme complex, thereby reducing the regeneration of vitamin K1 epoxide.

PHARMACOKINETICS: Absorption: (PO) Complete; T_{max}=4 hrs. **Distribution:** V_d=0.14L/kg; plasma protein binding (99%); crosses placenta. **Metabolism:** Hepatic via CYP2C9, 2C19, 2C8, 2C18, 1A2, 3A4; hydroxylation (major), reduction. **Elimination:** Urine (≤92%, metabolites); $T_{1/2}$=1 week.

NURSING CONSIDERATIONS

Assessment: Assess for risk factors for bleeding (eg, age ≥65 yrs, history of highly variable INR, GI bleeding, HTN, cerebrovascular disease, malignancy, anemia, trauma, renal impairment, certain genetic factors), factors affecting INR (eg, diarrhea, hepatic disorders, poor nutritional state, steatorrhea, vitamin K deficiency, increased vitamin K intake, hereditary warfarin resistance), pregnancy/nursing status, other conditions where treatment is contraindicated or cautioned, and drug-drug/drug-disease interactions. Assess INR. Obtain platelet counts in patients with HIT or HITTS.

Monitoring: Monitor for signs/symptoms of bleeding, necrosis/gangrene of skin and other tissues, systemic atheroemboli, cholesterol microemboli, "purple toes syndrome," and other adverse reactions. Perform periodic INR testing.

Patient Counseling: Instruct to inform physician if patient falls often as this may increase risk for complications. Counsel to maintain strict adherence to dosing regimen. Advise not to start or stop other medications, including salicylates (eg, ASA, topical analgesics), OTC drugs, or herbal medications, except on advice of physician. Instruct to inform physician if pregnancy is suspected (to discuss pregnancy planning) or if considering breastfeeding. Counsel to avoid any activity or sport that may result in traumatic injury. Instruct that regular PT tests and visits to physician are required during therapy. Advise patient to carry ID card stating drug is being taken. Instruct to eat a normal, balanced diet to maintain consistent intake of vitamin K and to avoid drastic changes in diet, such as eating large amounts of leafy, green vegetables. Advise to take ud. Advise to immediately report unusual bleeding or symptoms or any serious illness, such as severe diarrhea, infection, or fever. Inform that anticoagulant effects may persist for about 2 to 5 days after discontinuation.

Administration: (Coumadin, Jantoven) Oral or (Coumadin) IV route. Inj: Reconstitute with 2.7mL sterile water for inj to yield 2mg/mL. Administer as slow bolus inj over 1-2 min into a peripheral vein. **Storage:** Tab: (Coumadin) 15-30°C (59-86°F). (Jantoven) 20-25°C (68-77°F); excursions permitted 15-30°C (59-86°F). Protect from light and moisture. Inj: (Coumadin) 15-30°C (59-86°F). Protect from light. Use reconstituted sol within 4 hrs. Do not refrigerate. Discard any unused sol.

COVERA-HS RX
verapamil HCl (G.D. Searle)

THERAPEUTIC CLASS: Calcium channel blocker (nondihydropyridine)

INDICATIONS: Management of HTN and angina.

DOSAGE: *Adults:* Individualize dose by titration. Initial: 180mg qhs. Titrate: If inadequate response with 180mg, increase to 240mg qhs, then 360mg (two 180mg tab) qhs, then 480mg (two 240mg tab) qhs. Severe Hepatic Dysfunction: Give 30% of normal dose. Elderly: Start at lower end of dosing range.

HOW SUPPLIED: Tab, Extended-Release: 180mg, 240mg

CONTRAINDICATIONS: Severe left ventricular dysfunction, hypotension or cardiogenic shock, sick sinus syndrome or 2nd/3rd-degree atrioventricular (AV) block (except with functioning artificial ventricular pacemaker), atrial fibrillation/flutter with an accessory bypass tract.

WARNINGS/PRECAUTIONS: Has negative inotropic effect; avoid with moderate to severe cardiac failure symptoms or any degree of ventricular dysfunction if taking a β-blocker. Patients with milder ventricular dysfunction should, if possible, be controlled with optimum doses of digitalis and/or diuretics before treatment. May cause congestive heart failure (CHF), pulmonary edema, hypotension, asymptomatic 1st-degree AV block, transient bradycardia, and PR interval prolongation. Marked 1st-degree block or progressive development to 2nd/3rd-degree AV block requires dose reduction, or discontinuation and institution of appropriate therapy (rare). Elevated transaminases with and without concomitant elevations in alkaline phosphatase and bilirubin reported; periodically monitor LFTs. Sinus bradycardia, 2nd-degree AV block, pulmonary edema, severe hypotension, and sinus arrest reported in patients with hypertrophic cardiomyopathy. Caution with preexisting severe GI narrowing. Caution with hepatic dysfunction; monitor for abnormal PR interval prolongation or other signs of excessive pharmacologic effects. May decrease neuromuscular transmission in patients with Duchenne's muscular dystrophy and cause worsening of myasthenia gravis; decrease dose with attenuated neuromuscular transmission. Caution with renal dysfunction; monitor for abnormal PR interval prolongation or other signs of overdosage. Caution in elderly.

ADVERSE REACTIONS: Constipation, dizziness, headache, edema, fatigue, sinus bradycardia, 2nd-degree AV block, upper respiratory infection.

INTERACTIONS: Increased levels with CYP3A4 inhibitors (eg, erythromycin, ritonavir) and grapefruit juice. Decreased levels with CYP3A4 inducers (eg, rifampin). May cause myopathy/rhabdomyolysis with HMG-CoA reductase inhibitors that are CYP3A4 substrates (eg, atorvastatin) and may increase levels of such drugs; limit dose of simvastatin to 10mg/day or lovastatin to 40mg/day. Increased bleeding times with aspirin. Additive negative effects on HR, AV conduction, and/or cardiac contractility with β-blockers. May produce asymptomatic bradycardia with a wandering pacemaker with timolol eye drops. Decreased metoprolol and propranolol clearance while variable effect with atenolol. Chronic treatment may increase digoxin levels, which may result in digitalis toxicity. May reduce clearance of digitoxin. Additive effect on lowering BP with other antihypertensives (eg, vasodilators, ACE inhibitors, diuretics, β-blockers). Excessive reduction in BP with prazosin. Avoid disopyramide within 48 hrs before or 24 hrs after therapy. Additive negative inotropic effects and AV conduction prolongation with flecainide. Avoid quinidine with hypertrophic cardiomyopathy. Reduced or unchanged clearance with cimetidine. Increased sensitivity to effects of lithium when used concomitantly; monitor carefully. May increase carbamazepine, theophylline, cyclosporine, and alcohol levels. Increased clearance with phenobarbital. Reduced oral bioavailability with rifampin. Titrate carefully with inhalation anesthetics to avoid excessive cardiovascular depression. May potentiate neuromuscular blockers (curare-like and depolarizing); both agents may need dose reduction. May cause hypotension and bradyarrhythmias with telithromycin. Sinus bradycardia resulting in hospitalization and pacemaker insertion with clonidine; monitor HR. Prolonged recovery from neuromuscular blocking agent vecuronium reported.

PREGNANCY: Category C, not for use in nursing.

MECHANISM OF ACTION: Calcium channel blocker (nondihydropyridine); selectively inhibits transmembrane influx of ionic Ca^{2+} into arterial smooth muscle and in conductile and contractile myocardial cells without altering serum Ca^{2+} concentrations.

PHARMACOKINETICS: Absorption: Administration of variable doses resulted in different pharmacokinetic parameters. T_{max}=11 hrs. (Immediate-release) Bioavailability (33-65%, R-verapamil),

C

(13-34%, S-verapamil). **Distribution:** Plasma protein binding (94% to albumin and 92% to α-1 acid glycoprotein, R-verapamil), (88% to albumin and 86% to α-1 acid glycoprotein, S-verapamil); crosses placenta, found in breast milk. **Metabolism:** Liver (extensive); norverapamil (active metabolite). **Elimination:** Urine (70% metabolites, 3-4% unchanged), feces (≥16%).

NURSING CONSIDERATIONS

Assessment: Assess for cardiac failure symptoms, ventricular dysfunction, preexisting severe GI narrowing, hypertrophic cardiomyopathy, hepatic/renal function, Duchenne's muscular dystrophy, attenuated neuromuscular transmission, any conditions where treatment is contraindicated, pregnancy/nursing status, and possible drug interactions.

Monitoring: Monitor for CHF, hypotension, AV block, abnormal PR interval prolongation, and worsening of myasthenia gravis. Periodically monitor LFTs and renal function.

Patient Counseling: Instruct to swallow tab whole and to not chew, break, or crush. Inform that outer shell of tab does not dissolve and may occasionally be observed in stool. Advise to seek medical attention if any adverse reactions occur. Counsel not to breastfeed and to report immediately if pregnant.

Administration: Oral route. Swallow whole; do not chew, break, or crush. **Storage:** 20-25°C (68-77°F).

COZAAR   RX
losartan potassium (Merck)

> D/C when pregnancy is detected. Drugs that act directly on the renin-angiotensin system (RAS) can cause injury/death to the developing fetus.

THERAPEUTIC CLASS: Angiotensin II receptor antagonist

INDICATIONS: Treatment of HTN, alone or with other antihypertensives, including diuretics. Reduce the risk of stroke in patients with HTN and left ventricular hypertrophy (LVH) (may not apply to black patients). Treatment of diabetic nephropathy with an elevated SrCr and proteinuria (urinary albumin to creatinine ratio ≥300mg/g) in patients with type 2 diabetes mellitus (DM) and a history of HTN.

DOSAGE: *Adults:* HTN: Individualize dose. Initial: 50mg qd. Intravascular Volume Depletion/History of Hepatic Impairment: Initial: 25mg qd. Usual Range: 25-100mg/day given qd or bid. HTN with LVH: Initial: 50mg qd. Add HCTZ 12.5mg qd and/or increase losartan to 100mg qd, followed by an increase in HCTZ to 25mg qd based on BP response. Diabetic Nephropathy: Initial: 50mg qd. Titrate: Increase to 100mg qd based on BP response. May be administered with insulin and other hypoglycemic agents.
Pediatrics: ≥6 Yrs: HTN: Initial: 0.7mg/kg qd (up to 50mg total) administered as a tab or sus. Adjust dose according to BP response. Max: 1.4mg/kg/day (or 100mg/day).

HOW SUPPLIED: Tab: 25mg, 50mg*, 100mg *scored

CONTRAINDICATIONS: Coadministration with aliskiren in patients with diabetes.

WARNINGS/PRECAUTIONS: Symptomatic hypotension may occur in patients who are intravascularly volume-depleted (eg, treated with diuretics); correct volume depletion before therapy or start therapy at a lower dose. Hypersensitivity, including angioedema, reported. Consider a lower dose in patients with hepatic dysfunction. Changes in renal function reported. Oliguria and/or progressive azotemia and (rarely) acute renal failure and/or death may occur in patients whose renal function is dependent on the RAS (eg, severe congestive heart failure [CHF]). May increase BUN and SrCr levels with renal artery stenosis. Electrolyte imbalances reported with renal impairment, with or without DM. Hyperkalemia reported in type 2 diabetics with proteinuria. Not recommended in pediatric patients with GFR <30mL/min.

ADVERSE REACTIONS: Dizziness, cough, upper respiratory infection, diarrhea, asthenia/fatigue, chest pain, hypotension, hypoglycemia, anemia, back pain, urinary tract infection, cataract, diabetic vascular disease, cellulitis, influenza-like disease.

INTERACTIONS: See Contraindications. Dual blockade of the RAS is associated with increased risks of hypotension, syncope, hyperkalemia, and changes in renal function (including acute renal failure); closely monitor BP, renal function, and electrolytes with concomitant agents that affect the RAS. Avoid with aliskiren in patients with renal impairment (GFR <60mL/min). May increase serum K^+ with K^+-sparing diuretics (eg, spironolactone, triamterene, amiloride), K^+ supplements, or salt substitutes containing K^+. May reduce lithium excretion; monitor lithium levels. NSAIDs, including selective COX-2 inhibitors, may attenuate antihypertensive effect and deteriorate renal function. Rifampin may decrease levels. Fluconazole may decrease levels of the active metabolite and increase levels of losartan.

PREGNANCY: Category D, not for use in nursing.

MECHANISM OF ACTION: Angiotensin II receptor antagonist; blocks vasoconstrictor and aldosterone-secreting effects of angiotensin II by selectively blocking the binding of angiotensin II to AT_1 receptor in many tissues (eg, vascular smooth muscle, adrenal gland).

PHARMACOKINETICS: Absorption: Well-absorbed. Bioavailability (33%); T_{max}=1 hr, 3-4 hrs (active metabolite). **Distribution:** V_d=34L, 12L (active metabolite); plasma protein binding (98.7%, 99.8% active metabolite). **Metabolism:** Liver via CYP2C9, 3A4; carboxylic acid (active metabolite). **Elimination:** Urine (35%, 4% unchanged, 6% active metabolite), feces (60%); $T_{1/2}$=2 hrs, 6-9 hrs (active metabolite).

NURSING CONSIDERATIONS

Assessment: Assess for history of hypersensitivity, volume depletion, CHF, DM, unilateral or bilateral renal artery stenosis, hepatic/renal impairment, pregnancy/nursing status, and possible drug interactions.

Monitoring: Monitor for signs/symptoms of electrolyte imbalance, hypotension, hypersensitivity reactions, oliguria, azotemia, hepatic dysfunction, and other adverse reactions. Monitor BP, serum electrolytes, and renal function periodically.

Patient Counseling: Inform of pregnancy risks and discuss treatment options with women planning to be pregnant; instruct to report pregnancy to their physician immediately. Instruct patients not to use K^+ supplements or salt substitutes containing K^+ without consulting physician.

Administration: Oral route. Take with or without food. Shake sus before use. Refer to PI for preparation of sus. **Storage:** (Tab) 25°C (77°F); excursions permitted to 15-30°C (59-86°F). Protect from light. (Sus) 2-8°C (36-46°F) for up to 4 weeks.

CREON   RX
pancrelipase (AbbVie)

THERAPEUTIC CLASS: Pancreatic enzyme supplement

INDICATIONS: Treatment of exocrine pancreatic insufficiency due to cystic fibrosis, chronic pancreatitis, pancreatectomy, or other conditions.

DOSAGE: *Adults:* Individualize dose based on clinical symptoms, degree of steatorrhea present, and fat content of diet. Start at the lowest recommended dose and increase gradually. Initial: 500 lipase U/kg/meal. Max: 2500 lipase U/kg/meal (or ≤10,000 lipase U/kg/day) or <4000 lipase U/g fat ingested/day. Half of the dose used for meals should be given with each snack. Reduce dose in older patients. Refer to PI for dosing limitations.
Pediatrics: Individualize dose based on clinical symptoms, degree of steatorrhea present, and fat content of diet. Start at the lowest recommended dose and increase gradually. ≥4 Yrs: Initial: 500 lipase U/kg/meal. Max: 2500 lipase U/kg/meal (or ≤10,000 lipase U/kg/day) or <4000 lipase U/g fat ingested/day. Half of the dose used for meals should be given with each snack. >12 Months-<4 Yrs: Initial: 1000 lipase U/kg/meal. Max: 2500 lipase U/kg/meal (or ≤10,000 lipase U/kg/day) or <4000 lipase U/g fat ingested/day. ≤12 Months: 3000 lipase U/120mL of formula or per breast-feeding. Administer immediately prior to each feeding. Refer to PI for dosing limitations.

HOW SUPPLIED: Cap, Delayed-Release: (Lipase-Protease-Amylase) 3000 U-9500 U-15,000 U; 6000 U-19,000 U-30,000 U; 12,000 U-38,000 U-60,000 U; 24,000 U-76,000 U-120,000 U; 36,000 U-114,000 U-180,000 U

WARNINGS/PRECAUTIONS: Not interchangeable with other pancrelipase products. Fibrosing colonopathy reported; monitor closely for progression to stricture formation. Caution with doses >2500 lipase U/kg/meal (or >10,000 lipase U/kg/day); use only if these doses are documented to be effective by 3-day fecal fat measures indicating significant improvement. Examine patients receiving >6000 lipase U/kg/meal; immediately decrease or titrate dose downward to a lower range. Ensure that no drug is retained in the mouth. Should not be crushed or chewed, or mixed in foods with pH >4.5; may disrupt enteric coating of cap, resulting in early release of enzymes, irritation of oral mucosa, and/or loss of enzyme activity. Caution in patients with gout, renal impairment, or hyperuricemia; may increase blood uric acid levels. Risk for transmission of viral diseases. Caution with known allergy to proteins of porcine origin; severe allergic reactions reported.

ADVERSE REACTIONS: Vomiting, flatulence, abdominal pain, headache, cough, dizziness, frequent bowel movements, abnormal feces, hyperglycemia, hypoglycemia, nasopharyngitis, decreased appetite, irritability.

PREGNANCY: Category C, caution in nursing.

MECHANISM OF ACTION: Pancreatic enzyme supplement; catalyzes the hydrolysis of fats to monoglyceride, glycerol, and free fatty acids, proteins into peptides and amino acids, and starches into dextrins and short-chain sugars (eg, maltose, maltriose) in the duodenum and proximal small intestine, thereby acting like digestive enzymes physiologically secreted by the pancreas.

NURSING CONSIDERATIONS

Assessment: Assess for known allergy to porcine proteins, gout, renal impairment, hyperuricemia, and pregnancy/nursing status.

Monitoring: Monitor for fibrosing colonopathy, stricture formation, oral mucosa irritation, viral diseases, and allergic reactions. Monitor serum uric acid levels.

Patient Counseling: Instruct to take ud and with food and fluids. Inform that if a dose is missed, take the next dose with the next meal/snack ud; instruct not to double doses. Inform that cap contents can also be sprinkled on soft acidic foods (eg, applesauce), if necessary. Instruct to notify physician if pregnant/breastfeeding or planning to become pregnant/breastfeed during treatment. Advise to contact physician immediately if allergic reactions develop.

Administration: Oral route. Take during meals or snacks, with sufficient fluid. Swallow whole; do not crush or chew caps/cap contents. Do not retain in mouth. Do not mix directly into formula or breast milk. Refer to PI for proper administration instructions. **Storage:** Room temperature up to 25°C (77°F); excursions permitted between 25-40°C (77-104°F) for up to 30 days. Discard if exposed to higher temperature and moisture conditions >70%. Protect from moisture. Store in original container.

CRESTOR   RX
rosuvastatin calcium (AstraZeneca)

THERAPEUTIC CLASS: HMG-CoA reductase inhibitor

INDICATIONS: Adjunct to diet to decrease total cholesterol, LDL, apolipoprotein B, and TG levels, and to increase HDL levels in primary hyperlipidemia or mixed dyslipidemia, hypertriglyceridemia, primary dysbetalipoproteinemia, heterozygous familial hypercholesterolemia (adolescent boys and girls, who are at least 1 yr postmenarche, 10-17 yrs of age), homozygous familial hypercholesterolemia (HoFH), slow progression of atherosclerosis, and for prevention of cardiovascular disease.

DOSAGE: *Adults:* Initial: 10-20mg qd. Range: 5-40mg qd. When initiating treatment or switching from another HMG-CoA reductase inhibitor, use the appropriate starting dose first, then titrate according to patient's response and individualized goal of therapy. Analyze lipid levels within 2-4 weeks and adjust dose accordingly. Use 40mg dose only if LDL goal is not achieved with 20mg dose. HoFH: Initial: 20mg qd. Asian Patients: Initial: 5mg qd. Concomitant Cyclosporine: Max: 5mg qd. Concomitant Lopinavir/Ritonavir or Atazanavir/Ritonavir or Gemfibrozil: Initial: 5mg qd. Max: 10mg qd. Severe Renal Impairment (CrCl <30mL/min) Not on Hemodialysis: Initial: 5mg qd. Max: 10mg qd.
Pediatrics: 10-17 Yrs: Individualize dose. HeFH: Usual: 5-20mg/day. Titrate: Adjust dose at intervals of ≥4 weeks. Max: 20mg/day. Asian Patients: Initial: 5mg qd. Concomitant Cyclosporine: Max: 5mg qd. Concomitant Lopinavir/Ritonavir or Atazanavir/Ritonavir or Gemfibrozil: Initial: 5mg qd. Max: 10mg qd. Severe Renal Impairment (CrCl <30mL/min) Not on Hemodialysis: Initial: 5mg qd. Max: 10mg qd.

HOW SUPPLIED: Tab: 5mg, 10mg, 20mg, 40mg

CONTRAINDICATIONS: Active liver disease including unexplained persistent elevations of hepatic transaminase levels, women who are pregnant or may become pregnant, nursing mothers.

WARNINGS/PRECAUTIONS: Myopathy (including immune-mediated necrotizing myopathy [IMNM]) and rhabdomyolysis reported with increased risk at 40mg; caution in patients with predisposing factors for myopathy (eg, age ≥65 yrs, inadequately treated hypothyroidism, renal impairment). D/C if markedly elevated CPK levels occur or myopathy is diagnosed or suspected. Temporarily withhold in any patient with an acute, serious condition suggestive of myopathy or predisposing to the development of renal failure secondary to rhabdomyolysis. Increases in serum transaminases reported; perform LFTs before initiation and if signs/symptoms of liver injury occur. Fatal and nonfatal hepatic failure reported (rare); promptly interrupt therapy if serious liver injury with clinical symptoms and/or hyperbilirubinemia or jaundice occurs, and do not restart if no alternate etiology found. Caution in patients who consume substantial quantities of alcohol and/or have a history of chronic liver disease, severe renal impairment, are Asian, or are elderly. Dipstick-positive proteinuria and microscopic hematuria reported; consider dose reduction for patients with unexplained persistent proteinuria and/or hematuria. Increases in HbA1c and FPG levels reported.

ADVERSE REACTIONS: Headache, myalgia, nausea, dizziness, arthralgia, constipation, increased CPK, asthenia, abdominal pain.

INTERACTIONS: Increased risk of myopathy with some other lipid-lowering therapies (fibrates or niacin), gemfibrozil, cyclosporine, lopinavir/ritonavir, atazanavir/ritonavir, organic anion transporting polyprotein 1B1 inhibitors, or breast cancer resistance protein inhibitors. Avoid with gemfibrozil. Caution with coumarin anticoagulants; determine INR before initiation and frequently during early therapy. May enhance the risk of skeletal muscle effects with ≥1g/day of niacin. Caution with drugs that may decrease levels or activity of endogenous steroid hormones (eg, ketoconazole, spironolactone, cimetidine), fenofibrates, or protease inhibitors in combination with ritonavir. Cyclosporine may increase levels. Caution with colchicine; cases of myopathy, including rhabdomyolysis, reported.

PREGNANCY: Category X, not for use in nursing.

MECHANISM OF ACTION: HMG-CoA reductase inhibitor; produces lipid-modifying effects by increasing the number of hepatic LDL receptors on the cell surface to enhance uptake and catabolism of LDL and by inhibiting hepatic synthesis of VLDL, which reduces the total number of VLDL and LDL particles.

PHARMACOKINETICS: Absorption: Absolute bioavailability (20%); T_{max}=3-5 hrs. **Distribution:** V_d=134L; plasma protein binding (88%). **Metabolism:** CYP2C9; N-desmethyl rosuvastatin (major metabolite). **Elimination:** Feces (90%); $T_{1/2}$=19 hrs.

NURSING CONSIDERATIONS

Assessment: Assess for active liver disease (including chronic alcohol liver disease), unexplained persistent elevations in serum transaminases, risk factors for developing myopathy or rhabdomyolysis, pregnancy/nursing status, and possible drug interactions. Obtain baseline lipid profile, LFTs, and evaluate renal function. Check INR with coumarin anticoagulants.

Monitoring: Monitor for signs/symptoms of myopathy (including IMNM), rhabdomyolysis, increases in serum transaminase levels, liver/endocrine dysfunction, proteinuria, hematuria, and other adverse reactions. Monitor lipid levels, CPK, and LFTs. Monitor INR with coumarin anticoagulants frequently during early therapy.

Patient Counseling: Advise to report promptly any unexplained muscle pain, tenderness, or weakness, particularly if accompanied by malaise or fever or if muscle signs and symptoms persist after discontinuing therapy. Advise to wait at least 2 hrs if taking an antacid containing a combination of aluminum and magnesium hydroxide. Inform of potential hazard to fetus if patient becomes pregnant while on therapy. Advise to report promptly any symptoms that may indicate liver injury (eg, fatigue, anorexia, right upper abdominal discomfort, dark urine, jaundice).

Administration: Oral route. Take with or without food. **Storage:** 20-25°C (68-77°F). Protect from moisture.

CRIXIVAN   RX
indinavir sulfate (Merck)

THERAPEUTIC CLASS: Protease inhibitor

INDICATIONS: Treatment of HIV infection in combination with other antiretroviral agents.

DOSAGE: *Adults:* 800mg (usually two 400mg caps) q8h. Mild to Moderate Hepatic Insufficiency Due to Cirrhosis: Reduce dosage to 600mg q8h. Nephrolithiasis/Urolithiasis: May temporarily interrupt (eg, 1-3 days) or d/c therapy. Take without food but with water 1 hr ac or 2 hrs pc. Refer to PI for dosing modifications when used with certain concomitant therapies.

HOW SUPPLIED: Cap: 200mg, 400mg

CONTRAINDICATIONS: Coadministration with CYP3A4 substrates for which elevated concentrations potentially cause serious or life-threatening reactions (eg, alfuzosin, amiodarone, dihydroergotamine, ergonovine, ergotamine, methylergonovine, cisapride, lovastatin, simvastatin, pimozide, sildenafil [for treatment of pulmonary arterial HTN], oral midazolam, triazolam, alprazolam).

WARNINGS/PRECAUTIONS: Nephrolithiasis/urolithiasis reported. Ensure adequate hydration in all patients. Acute hemolytic anemia, including cases resulting in death, reported; once a diagnosis is apparent, institute appropriate measures, including discontinuation of therapy. Hepatitis, including cases resulting in hepatic failure and death, reported. New onset or exacerbation of diabetes mellitus (DM), hyperglycemia, and diabetic ketoacidosis reported; initiation or dose adjustments of insulin or oral hypoglycemic agents may be required. Indirect hyperbilirubinemia reported frequently during treatment, and infrequently associated with increases in serum transaminases. Tubulointerstitial nephritis with medullary calcification and cortical atrophy observed in patients with asymptomatic severe leukocyturia (>100 cells/high power field); closely follow such patients and monitor frequently with urinalyses. Consider discontinuation of therapy in all patients with severe leukocyturia. Immune reconstitution syndrome reported. Autoimmune disorders (eg, Graves' disease, polymyositis, Guillain-Barre syndrome) reported in the setting of immune reconstitution and can occur many months after initiation of treatment. Spontaneous bleeding in patients with hemophilia A and B reported. Redistribution/accumulation of body fat reported. Caution in elderly.

ADVERSE REACTIONS: Nephrolithiasis/urolithiasis, hyperbilirubinemia, abdominal pain, headache, N/V, dizziness, pruritus, diarrhea, back pain.

INTERACTIONS: See Contraindications. Caution with atorvastatin, rosuvastatin, parenteral midazolam, sildenafil (for treatment of erectile dysfunction), tadalafil, or vardenafil. Do not coadminister with rifampin. Not recommended with St. John's wort, atazanavir, salmeterol, or fluticasone (when indinavir is coadministered with a potent CYP3A4 inhibitor [eg, ritonavir]). Avoid with colchicine in patients with renal/hepatic impairment. May increase levels of CYP3A4 substrates, ritonavir, saquinavir, antiarrhythmics, trazodone, colchicine, dihydropyridine calcium channel blockers, clarithromycin, bosentan, atorvastatin, rosuvastatin, immunosuppressants, salmeterol, fluticasone, parenteral midazolam, rifabutin, sildenafil, tadalafil, and vardenafil. CYP3A4 inducers, St. John's wort, efavirenz, nevirapine, anticonvulsants, rifabutin, and venlafaxine may decrease levels. CYP3A4 inhibitors, delavirdine, nelfinavir, ritonavir, clarithromycin, itraconazole, and ketoconazole may increase levels. Refer to PI for dosing modifications when used with certain concomitant therapies.

PREGNANCY: Category C, not for use in nursing.

MECHANISM OF ACTION: HIV-1 protease inhibitor; binds to the protease active site and inhibits the activity of the enzyme. This inhibition prevents cleavage of the viral polyproteins resulting in the formation of immature noninfectious viral particles.

PHARMACOKINETICS: Absorption: Rapid (fasted). C_{max}=12,617nM; T_{max}=0.8 hrs; AUC=30,691nM•hr. **Distribution:** Plasma protein binding (60%). **Metabolism:** Oxidation (via CYP3A4 [major]) and glucuronide conjugation. **Elimination:** Urine (<20%, unchanged); $T_{1/2}$=1.8 hrs.

NURSING CONSIDERATIONS

Assessment: Assess for hypersensitivity to drug, hepatic insufficiency, DM, severe leukocyturia, hemophilia, pregnancy/nursing status, and possible drug interactions.

Monitoring: Monitor for nephrolithiasis/urolithiasis, hemolytic anemia, hepatitis, new onset or exacerbation of DM, hyperglycemia, diabetic ketoacidosis, hyperbilirubinemia, serum transaminase elevations, immune reconstitution syndrome, autoimmune disorders, fat redistribution/accumulation, and other adverse reactions. Monitor patients with asymptomatic severe leukocyturia; monitor frequently with urinalyses. In patients with hemophilia, monitor for bleeding events.

Patient Counseling: Instruct to take drug ud. Inform that drug is not a cure for HIV-1 infection and that illnesses associated with HIV may continue. Advise to avoid doing things that can spread HIV to others. Instruct not to modify or d/c therapy without consulting physician. Instruct to report to physician the use of any other prescription, nonprescription medication, or herbal products (eg, St. John's wort). Inform that fat redistribution/accumulation may occur. Instruct to register in the Antiretroviral Pregnancy Registry. Instruct to d/c nursing if receiving therapy.

Administration: Oral route. Take without food but with water 1 hr ac or 2 hrs pc. Alternatively, may be administered with other liquids (eg, skim milk, juice, coffee, tea) or with a light meal (eg, dry toast with jelly, juice, and coffee with skim milk and sugar; or corn flakes, skim milk and sugar). Drink at least 1.5L of liquids during the course of 24 hrs to ensure adequate hydration. **Storage:** 15-30°C (59-86°F). Protect from moisture. Store in a tightly-closed container (original container).

CYCLOBENZAPRINE   RX
cyclobenzaprine HCl (Various)

THERAPEUTIC CLASS: Skeletal muscle relaxant (central-acting)

INDICATIONS: Adjunct to rest and physical therapy for relief of muscle spasm associated with acute, painful musculoskeletal conditions.

DOSAGE: *Adults:* Usual: 5mg tid. Titrate: May increase to 10mg tid. Use for periods longer than 2 or 3 weeks is not recommended. Mild Hepatic Impairment/Elderly: Consider less frequent dosing. Initial: 5mg dose. Titrate: Increase slowly.
Pediatrics: ≥15 Yrs: Usual: 5mg tid. Titrate: May increase to 10mg tid. Use for periods longer than 2 or 3 weeks is not recommended. Mild Hepatic Impairment: Consider less frequent dosing. Initial: 5mg dose. Titrate: Increase slowly.

HOW SUPPLIED: Tab: 5mg, 7.5mg, 10mg

CONTRAINDICATIONS: Concomitant use of MAOIs or within 14 days after their discontinuation. Arrhythmias, heart block or conduction disturbances, congestive heart failure (CHF), hyperthyroidism, acute recovery phase of myocardial infarction (MI).

WARNINGS/PRECAUTIONS: Not effective in the treatment of spasticity associated with cerebral or spinal cord disease or in children with cerebral palsy. May produce arrhythmias, sinus tachycardia, and conduction time prolongation leading to MI and stroke. Caution with history of urinary retention, angle-closure glaucoma, increased intraocular pressure (IOP), mild hepatic impairment, and in elderly. Not recommended with moderate to severe hepatic impairment.

Consider certain withdrawal symptoms; abrupt cessation after prolonged administration rarely may produce nausea, headache, and malaise.

ADVERSE REACTIONS: Drowsiness, dry mouth, fatigue, headache, dizziness.

INTERACTIONS: See Contraindications. Serotonin syndrome reported when used with SSRIs, SNRIs, TCAs, tramadol, bupropion, meperidine, verapamil, or MAOIs; d/c immediately if this occurs. Observe carefully, particularly during treatment initiation or dose increases, if concomitant use with other serotonergic drugs is warranted. May enhance effects of alcohol, barbiturates, and other CNS depressants. Caution with anticholinergics. May block the antihypertensive action of guanethidine and similarly acting compounds. May enhance seizure risk with tramadol.

PREGNANCY: Category B, caution in nursing.

MECHANISM OF ACTION: Skeletal muscle relaxant (central-acting); relieves skeletal muscle spasm of local origin without interfering with muscle function. Reduces tonic somatic motor activity, influencing both gamma and α motor systems.

PHARMACOKINETICS: Absorption: Oral bioavailability (33-55%); C_{max}=25.9ng/mL; AUC=177ng•hr/mL. **Metabolism:** Extensive; N-demethylation via CYP3A4, 1A2, and 2D6. **Elimination:** Kidney (glucuronides); $T_{1/2}$=18 hrs.

NURSING CONSIDERATIONS

Assessment: Assess for arrhythmias, heart block or conduction disturbances, CHF, hyperthyroidism, acute recovery phase of MI, history of urinary retention, angle-closure glaucoma, increased IOP, hepatic impairment, drug hypersensitivity, pregnancy/nursing status, and possible drug interactions.

Monitoring: Monitor for arrhythmias, sinus tachycardia, conduction time prolongation, stroke, withdrawal symptoms, and other adverse reactions.

Patient Counseling: Inform that the drug, especially when used with alcohol or other CNS depressants, may impair mental and/or physical abilities required to perform hazardous tasks (eg, operating machinery, driving). Caution about the risk of serotonin syndrome; instruct to seek medical care immediately if signs/symptoms occur.

Administration: Oral route. **Storage:** 20-25°C (68-77°F).

CYCLOPHOSPHAMIDE   RX
cyclophosphamide (Baxter)

THERAPEUTIC CLASS: Nitrogen mustard alkylating agent

INDICATIONS: Treatment of malignant lymphomas, Hodgkin's disease, lymphocytic lymphoma (nodular or diffuse), mixed-cell type lymphoma, histiocytic lymphoma, Burkitt's lymphoma, multiple myeloma, chronic lymphocytic leukemia, chronic granulocytic leukemia (usually ineffective in acute blastic crisis), acute myelogenous and monocytic leukemia, acute lymphoblastic (stem-cell) leukemia in children, mycosis fungoides (advanced disease), neuroblastoma (disseminated disease), ovarian adenocarcinoma, retinoblastoma, breast carcinoma. Treatment of selected cases of biopsy proven "minimal change" nephrotic syndrome in children, but not as primary therapy.

DOSAGE: *Adults:* Malignant Diseases (Without Hematologic Deficiency): (IV) Monotherapy: Initial: 40-50mg/kg in divided doses over 2-5 days, or 10-15mg/kg every 7-10 days, or 3-5mg/kg twice weekly. (PO) Initial/Maint: 1-5mg/kg/day. (IV/PO) Adjust dose according to evidence of antitumor activity and/or leukopenia. Elderly: Start at lower end of dosing range. *Pediatrics:* Malignant Diseases (Without Hematologic Deficiency): (IV) Monotherapy: Initial: 40-50mg/kg in divided doses over 2-5 days, or 10-15mg/kg every 7-10 days, or 3-5mg/kg twice weekly. (PO) Initial/Maint: 1-5mg/kg/day. (IV/PO) Adjust dose according to evidence of antitumor activity and/or leukopenia. Nephrotic Syndrome: (PO) 2.5-3mg/kg qd for 60-90 days.

HOW SUPPLIED: Inj: 500mg, 1g, 2g; Tab: 25mg, 50mg

CONTRAINDICATIONS: Severely depressed bone marrow function.

WARNINGS/PRECAUTIONS: Second malignancies (eg, urinary bladder, myeloproliferative, lymphoproliferative), cardiac dysfunction, and acute cardiac toxicity reported. May cause fetal harm. May cause sterility in both sexes. Amenorrhea, ovarian fibrosis, azoospermia, and oligospermia reported. Testicular atrophy may occur. Hemorrhagic cystitis and/or urinary bladder fibrosis may develop; d/c with severe hemorrhagic cystitis. May cause significant suppression of immune response; interrupt or reduce dose in patients who have or develop viral, bacterial, fungal, protozoan, or helminthic infections. Anaphylactic reactions and possible cross-sensitivity with other alkylating agents reported. Caution with leukopenia, thrombocytopenia, tumor cell infiltration of bone marrow, previous x-ray therapy or cytotoxic therapy, and hepatic/renal impairment; monitor for possible development of toxicity. May need to adjust dose in adrenalectomized patients. May interfere with normal wound healing. Caution in elderly.

ADVERSE REACTIONS: Sterility, syndrome of inappropriate antidiuretic hormone secretion, N/V, anorexia, alopecia, leukopenia, hemorrhagic ureteritis, interstitial pneumonitis, malaise, asthenia, renal tubular necrosis, infection.

INTERACTIONS: Chronic administration of high doses of phenobarbital increases rate of metabolism and leukopenic activity. Caution with other drugs (including other cytotoxic drugs) for possible combined drug actions (desirable or undesirable); may need to reduce dose, as well as that of the other drugs, when included in combined cytotoxic regimens. Potentiates succinylcholine chloride effects and doxorubicin-induced cardiotoxicity. Alert anesthesiologist if treated within 10 days of general anesthesia.

PREGNANCY: Category D, not for use in nursing.

MECHANISM OF ACTION: Nitrogen mustard alkylating agent; thought to involve cross-linking of tumor cell DNA.

PHARMACOKINETICS: Absorption: (PO) Well absorbed; bioavailability (>75%). (IV) T_{max}=2-3 hrs (metabolites). **Distribution:** Plasma protein binding (>60% as metabolites); found in breast milk. **Metabolism:** Liver by a mixed function microsomal oxidase system to active alkylating metabolites. **Elimination:** Urine (5-25%, unchanged); $T_{1/2}$=3-12 hrs.

NURSING CONSIDERATIONS

Assessment: Assess for drug hypersensitivity, immunosuppression, leukopenia, thrombocytopenia, tumor cell infiltration of bone marrow, previous x-ray therapy or cytotoxic therapy, hepatic/renal impairment, adrenalectomy, pregnancy/nursing status, and possible drug interactions.

Monitoring: Monitor for second malignancies, cardiac dysfunction, infections, anaphylactic reactions, toxicity, and other adverse reactions. Monitor hematologic profile (particularly neutrophils and platelets) and examine urine for red cells regularly.

Patient Counseling: Inform of the risks and benefits of therapy. Instruct to take exactly ud. Advise to avoid becoming pregnant while on therapy.

Administration: Oral/IV route. (IV) Refer to PI for procedures in preparation and handling of solution. **Storage:** ≤25°C (77°F). (Tab) Excursions permitted up to 30°C (86°F). (IV) After reconstitution (without further dilution) with 0.9% sterile NaCl or after reconstitution (with further dilution) with 0.45% sterile NaCl: Room temperature up to 24 hrs or refrigerated up to 6 days. After reconstitution (with further dilution) with D5W or D5W and 0.9% sterile NaCl: Room temperature up to 24 hrs or refrigerated up to 36 hrs. After dilution with aromatic elixir for PO administration: Under refrigeration in glass containers; use within 14 days.

CYMBALTA   RX
duloxetine HCl (Lilly)

Antidepressants increased the risk of suicidal thoughts and behavior in children, adolescents, and young adults in short-term studies. Monitor and observe closely for worsening, and for emergence of suicidal thoughts and behavior. Not approved for use in pediatric patients.

THERAPEUTIC CLASS: Serotonin and norepinephrine reuptake inhibitor

INDICATIONS: Treatment of major depressive disorder (MDD) and generalized anxiety disorder (GAD). Management of neuropathic pain associated with diabetic peripheral neuropathy (DPNP). Management of fibromyalgia (FM) and chronic musculoskeletal pain.

DOSAGE: *Adults:* MDD: Initial: 40mg/day (given as 20mg bid) to 60mg/day (given qd or as 30mg bid) or 30mg qd for 1 week before increasing to 60mg qd. Maint: 60mg qd. Reassess periodically to determine need for maint therapy and appropriate dose. Max: 120mg/day. GAD: Initial: 60mg qd or 30mg qd for 1 week before increasing to 60mg qd. Maint: 60-120mg qd. Dose increases to above 60mg qd should be in increments of 30mg qd. Reassess periodically to determine need for maint and appropriate dose. Max: 120mg/day. DPNP: Initial: 60mg qd. May lower starting dose if tolerability is a concern. Consider lower starting dose and gradual increase in renal impairment. Maint: Individualize dose. Treat for up to 12 weeks. Max: 60mg qd. FM: Initial: 60mg qd or 30mg qd for 1 week before increasing to 60mg qd. Maint: Based on patient's response. Max: 60mg qd. Chronic Musculoskeletal Pain: Initial: 60mg qd or 30mg qd for 1 week before increasing to 60mg qd. Maint: 60mg qd for up to 13 weeks. Max: 60mg/day. Elderly: Caution when increasing the dose.

HOW SUPPLIED: Cap, Delayed-Release: 20mg, 30mg, 60mg

CONTRAINDICATIONS: Use of an MAOI either concomitantly or within 5 days of stopping treatment. Treatment within 14 days of stopping an MAOI. Starting treatment in patients being treated with other MAOIs (eg, linezolid, IV methylene blue). Uncontrolled narrow-angle glaucoma.

WARNINGS/PRECAUTIONS: Not approved for use in treating bipolar depression. Hepatic failure (sometimes fatal) and cholestatic jaundice with minimal elevation of serum transaminases reported; d/c if jaundice or other evidence of hepatic dysfunction occurs. Avoid with substantial

C

alcohol use or evidence of chronic liver disease and/or hepatic insufficiency. Orthostatic hypotension and syncope reported; consider discontinuation if symptomatic orthostatic hypotension and/or syncope develop. Serotonin syndrome reported; monitor and d/c if signs/symptoms develop and initiate supportive symptomatic treatment. May increase risk of bleeding events. Severe skin reactions, including erythema multiforme and Stevens-Johnson syndrome (SJS) may occur; d/c if blisters, peeling rash, mucosal erosions, or if any other signs of hypersensitivity develop. Discontinuation should be gradual. Activation of mania or hypomania reported in patients with MDD. Caution with history of mania and/or seizure disorder. May increase BP; obtain baseline BP and monitor periodically throughout therapy. May cause hyponatremia; volume depletion may increase risk. D/C if symptomatic hyponatremia occurs and institute appropriate medical intervention. Urinary hesitation and retention reported. Caution with conditions that may slow gastric emptying and with controlled narrow-angle glaucoma, diabetes, and the elderly; glycemic control may be worsened in patients with diabetes. Avoid in end-stage renal disease/severe renal impairment (CrCl <30mL/min).

ADVERSE REACTIONS: Nausea, dry mouth, constipation, diarrhea, decreased appetite, fatigue, dizziness, somnolence, hyperhidrosis, headache, insomnia, abdominal pain.

INTERACTIONS: See Contraindications. Avoid use with thioridazine, potent CYP1A2 inhibitors (eg, fluvoxamine, cimetidine, some quinolone antibiotics), and substantial alcohol use. Increased levels with potent CYP2D6 inhibitors (eg, paroxetine, fluoxetine, quinidine). Caution with drugs metabolized by CYP2D6 having a narrow therapeutic index (eg, TCAs, phenothiazines, type 1C antiarrhythmics), and CNS-acting drugs; consider monitoring TCA plasma levels. May increase free concentrations of highly protein-bound drugs. Potential for interaction with drugs that affect gastric acidity. Potential increased risk for serotonin syndrome with other serotonergic drugs (eg, triptans, TCAs, fentanyl, lithium, tramadol, tryptophan, buspirone, St. John's wort) and with drugs that impair metabolism of serotonin. Caution with NSAIDs, aspirin (ASA), warfarin, or other drugs that affect coagulation due to potential increased risk of bleeding. Greater risk of hypotension with concomitant use of medications that induce orthostatic hypotension (eg, antihypertensives) and potent CYP1A2 inhibitors. Increased risk of hyponatremia with diuretics.

PREGNANCY: Category C, not for use in nursing.

MECHANISM OF ACTION: Selective SNRI; not established. Believed to be related to potentiation of serotonergic and noradrenergic activity in the CNS.

PHARMACOKINETICS: Absorption: Well-absorbed; T_{max}=6 hrs. **Distribution:** V_d=1640L; plasma protein binding (>90%); found in breast milk. **Metabolism:** Extensive, hepatic via CYP1A2, 2D6; oxidation and conjugation. **Elimination:** Urine (70% metabolites; <1% unchanged), feces (20%); $T_{1/2}$=12 hrs.

NURSING CONSIDERATIONS

Assessment: Assess for bipolar disorder risk, history of mania, chronic liver disease, substantial alcohol use, history of seizures, diseases/conditions that slow gastric emptying (eg, diabetes mellitus), narrow-angle glaucoma, risk factors for hyponatremia, history of urinary retention, pregnancy/nursing status, and possible drug interactions. Assess baseline BP, LFTs, BUN, SrCr, and blood glucose.

Monitoring: Monitor for signs/symptoms of clinical worsening (eg, suicidality, unusual changes in behavior), hepatotoxicity, serotonin syndrome, abnormal bleeding, skin reactions (eg, erythema multiforme, SJS), hyponatremia, seizures, orthostatic hypotension, worsened glycemic control, urinary hesitation/retention, and mydriasis. If abruptly discontinued, monitor for symptoms of dizziness, N/V, headache, paresthesia, fatigue, irritability, insomnia, diarrhea, anxiety, and hyperhidrosis. Periodically monitor BP, LFTs, SrCr, and BUN.

Patient Counseling: Inform about benefits/risks of therapy. Advise to avoid substantial alcohol use. Instruct to seek medical attention for clinical worsening (eg, suicidal ideation, unusual changes in behavior), signs/symptoms of manic reaction (eg, greatly increased energy, severe trouble sleeping, racing thoughts, reckless behavior, talking more or faster than usual, unusually grand ideas, excessive happiness or irritability), and symptoms of serotonin syndrome (eg, mental status changes, autonomic instability, neuromuscular changes, GI symptoms). Inform that abnormal bleeding (especially with the use of NSAIDs, ASA, warfarin, or other drugs that affect coagulation), orthostatic hypotension, syncope, hepatotoxicity, urinary hesitation/retention, seizures, or discontinuation symptoms (eg, irritability, agitation, dizziness, anxiety, headache, insomnia) may occur. Advise of the signs/symptoms of hyponatremia. Counsel to immediately seek consult if skin blisters, peeling rash, mouth sores, hives, or any other allergic reactions occur. Advise to inform physician if taking or planning to take any prescription or OTC medications, if pregnant, intending to become pregnant, or are breastfeeding. Inform that therapy may impair judgement, thinking, or motor skills; instruct to use caution with operating hazardous machinery, including automobiles. Inform that improvement may be noticed within 1-4 weeks; instruct to continue therapy ud. Advise not to alter dosing regimen, or d/c treatment without consulting physician.

Administration: Oral route. Swallow cap whole; do not chew, crush, nor open and sprinkle on food or mix with liquids. **Storage:** 25°C (77°F); excursions permitted to 15-30°C (59-86°F).

CYTOMEL
liothyronine sodium (King)

THERAPEUTIC CLASS: Thyroid replacement hormone

INDICATIONS: As replacement or supplemental therapy in patients with hypothyroidism of any etiology, except transient hypothyroidism during the recovery phase of subacute thyroiditis. In the treatment or prevention of various types of euthyroid goiters, including thyroid nodules, and Hashimoto's and multinodular goiter. As diagnostic agent in suppression tests to differentiate mild hyperthyroidism or thyroid gland autonomy.

DOSAGE: *Adults:* Individualize dose. Mild Hypothyroidism: Initial: 25mcg qd. Titrate: May increase by up to 25mcg qd every 1-2 weeks. Maint: 25-75mcg qd. Myxedema: Initial: 5mcg qd. Titrate: May increase by 5-10mcg qd every 1-2 weeks up to 25mcg qd, then increase by 5-25mcg qd every 1-2 weeks until desired response. Maint: 50-100mcg/day. Simple (Non-Toxic) Goiter: Initial: 5mcg/day. Titrate: May increase by 5-10mcg qd every 1-2 weeks up to 25mcg qd, then by 12.5-25mcg qd every 1-2 weeks. Maint: 75mcg qd. Elderly/Angina Pectoris/Coronary Artery Disease: Initial: 5mcg qd. Titrate: Increase by no more than 5mcg qd at 2-week intervals. Switch to Cytomel Tab from Thyroid, L-Thyroxine, or Thyroglobulin: D/C other medication and initiate Cytomel at low dose then increase gradually based on patient response. Thyroid Suppression Therapy: 75-100mcg qd for 7 days. Radioactive iodine uptake is determined before and after administration of the hormone.
Pediatrics: Congenital Hypothyroidism: Initial: 5mcg qd. Titrate: Increase by 5mcg qd every 3-4 days until desired response achieved. Maint: >3 yrs: 25-75mcg/day. 1-3 yrs: 50mcg qd. <1 yr: 20mcg.qd.

HOW SUPPLIED: Tab: 5mcg, 25mcg*, 50mcg* *scored

CONTRAINDICATIONS: Uncorrected adrenal cortical insufficiency and untreated thyrotoxicosis.

WARNINGS/PRECAUTIONS: Do not use in the treatment of obesity; larger doses in euthyroid patients can cause serious or life-threatening toxicity. Caution with cardiovascular (CV) disorders (eg, angina pectoris) and in the elderly; use lower doses. Use is unjustified for the treatment of male or female infertility unless accompanied by hypothyroidism. Rule out morphological hypogonadism and nephrosis prior to therapy. If hypopituitarism present, adrenal insufficiency must be corrected prior to starting therapy. Caution in myxedematous patients; start at very low dose and increase gradually. Severe and prolonged hypothyroidism can lead to adrenocortical insufficiency; supplement with adrenocortical steroids. May precipitate a hyperthyroid state or aggravate hyperthyroidism. Concurrent use with androgens, corticosteroids, estrogens, oral contraceptives containing estrogens, iodine-containing preparations, and salicylates may interfere with thyroid lab tests. May aggravate symptoms of diabetes mellitus (DM) or diabetes insipidus (DI) or adrenal cortical insufficiency. Add glucocorticoids with myxedema coma. Excessive doses may cause craniosynostosis in infants.

ADVERSE REACTIONS: Allergic skin reactions (rare).

INTERACTIONS: Coadministration of larger doses with sympathomimetic amines, such as those used for their anorectic effects, may cause serious or even life-threatening toxicity. Hypothyroidism decreases and hyperthyroidism increases sensitivity to oral anticoagulants; monitor PT. May cause increases in insulin and oral hypoglycemics requirements. Impaired absorption with cholestyramine; space dosing by 4-5 hrs. Estrogens increase thyroxine-binding globulin; increase in thyroid dose may be needed. Increased effects of both agents with TCAs (eg, imipramine). HTN and tachycardia may occur with ketamine. May potentiate digitalis toxicity. Increased adrenergic effects of catecholamines (eg, epinephrine, norepinephrine); caution with coronary artery disease (CAD).

PREGNANCY: Category A, caution in nursing.

MECHANISM OF ACTION: Synthetic thyroid hormone; mechanism not established. Suspected to enhance oxygen consumption by tissues and increase the basal metabolic rate and metabolism of carbohydrates, lipids, and proteins.

PHARMACOKINETICS: Distribution: Minimal amount found in breast milk. **Elimination:** $T_{1/2}$=2.5 days.

NURSING CONSIDERATIONS

Assessment: Assess thyroid status, CV disease (eg, CAD, angina pectoris), DM/DI, adrenal cortical insufficiency, thyrotoxicosis, myxedema, hypogonadism, nephrosis, pregnancy/nursing status, and for possible drug interactions.

Monitoring: Monitor thyroid function periodically. Monitor PT on oral anticoagulants, urinary glucose with DM and renal function. Monitor for signs/symptoms of precipitation of adrenocortical insufficiency, aggravation of DM/DI, hypoglycemia, hyperthyroidism, toxicity, and hypersensitivity reactions.

Patient Counseling: Inform that replacement therapy is taken for life. Warn that partial hair loss may be seen in pediatrics in 1st few months of therapy. Instruct to seek medical attention if symptoms of toxicity (eg, chest pain, increased HR, palpitations, excessive sweating, heat intolerance, nervousness), hypoglycemia, aggravation of DM/DI, or hypersensitivity reactions occur.

Administration: Oral route. **Storage:** 15-30°C (59-86°F).

D

DACOGEN RX
decitabine (Eisai)

THERAPEUTIC CLASS: DNA methyltransferase inhibitor

INDICATIONS: Treatment of myelodysplastic syndromes.

DOSAGE: *Adults:* Treat for a minimum of 4 cycles. May premedicate with standard antiemetic therapy. Treatment Option 1: 15mg/m^2 by continuous IV infusion over 3 hrs q8h for 3 days. Repeat cycle every 6 weeks. Adjust dose based on hematologic recovery and disease progression; see PI. Treatment Option 2: 20mg/m^2 by continuous IV infusion over 1 hr qd for 5 days. Repeat cycle every 4 weeks. Myelosuppression: Delay subsequent treatment cycles until hematologic recovery. Following the 1st cycle, do not restart treatment if SrCr ≥2mg/dL, SGPT/total bilirubin ≥2X ULN, and has an active or uncontrolled infection.

HOW SUPPLIED: Inj: 50mg

WARNINGS/PRECAUTIONS: Neutropenia and thrombocytopenia may occur; monitor CBC and platelets periodically (at minimum, before each dosing cycle). Myelosuppression and worsening neutropenia may occur more frequently in the 1st or 2nd treatment cycles; consider early institution of growth factors and/or antimicrobial agents. May cause fetal harm. Avoid pregnancy during and for 1 month after completion of treatment. Men should not father a child during and for 2 months after completion of treatment. Caution with renal and hepatic dysfunction.

ADVERSE REACTIONS: Neutropenia, thrombocytopenia, anemia, fatigue, pyrexia, N/V, cough, petechiae, constipation, diarrhea, hyperglycemia, anorexia, leukopenia, headache, insomnia.

PREGNANCY: Category D, not for use in nursing.

MECHANISM OF ACTION: DNA methyltransferase inhibitor; causes hypomethylation of DNA and cellular differentiation or apoptosis. In rapidly dividing cells, forms covalent adducts with DNA methyltransferase incorporated into DNA.

PHARMACOKINETICS: Absorption: (15mg/m^2) C_{max}=73.8ng/mL, AUC=163ng•h/mL; (20mg/m^2) C_{max}=147ng/mL, AUC=115ng•h/mL. **Metabolism:** Deamination in liver, granulocytes, intestinal epithelium, and blood. **Elimination:** $T_{1/2}$=0.62 hrs (15mg/m^2), 0.54 hrs (20mg/m^2).

NURSING CONSIDERATIONS

Assessment: Assess CBC and platelet counts, renal/hepatic function, and pregnancy/nursing status.

Monitoring: Monitor for signs/symptoms of neutropenia, thrombocytopenia, myelosuppression, hypersensitivity reactions, renal/hepatic function, infections and infestations, and other adverse reactions. Monitor CBC and platelet counts prior to each dosing cycle.

Patient Counseling: Advise women to avoid becoming pregnant during and for 1 month after completion of treatment, and men not to father a child during and for 2 months after completion of treatment; counsel to use effective contraception. Advise to monitor and report any symptoms of neutropenia, thrombocytopenia, or fever to physician as soon as possible.

Administration: IV route. Refer to PI for instructions for IV administration. **Storage:** Vial: 25°C (77°F); excursions permitted to 15-30°C (59-86°F). Reconstituted Sol: 2-8°C (36-46°F) for up to 7 hrs until administration.

DALIRESP RX
roflumilast (Forest)

THERAPEUTIC CLASS: Selective phosphodiesterase 4 (PDE4) inhibitor

INDICATIONS: Treatment to reduce the risk of chronic obstructive pulmonary disease (COPD) exacerbations in patients with severe COPD associated with chronic bronchitis and a history of exacerbations.

DOSAGE: *Adults:* 500mcg qd.

HOW SUPPLIED: Tab: 500mcg

CONTRAINDICATIONS: Moderate to severe liver impairment (Child-Pugh B or C).

WARNINGS/PRECAUTIONS: Not a bronchodilator; not indicated for the relief of acute bronchospasm. Psychiatric adverse reactions, including suicidality, reported; carefully evaluate the risks and benefits of treatment in patients with history of depression and/or suicidal thoughts or behavior, and of continuing treatment if such reactions occur. Weight loss reported; evaluate and consider discontinuation if unexplained or clinically significant weight loss occurs. Do not use during labor and delivery. Caution with mild liver impairment (Child-Pugh A).

ADVERSE REACTIONS: Diarrhea, weight loss, nausea, headache, back pain.

INTERACTIONS: Strong CYP450 inducers (eg, rifampicin, phenobarbital, carbamazepine, phenytoin) decrease exposure and may reduce therapeutic effectiveness; concomitant use is not recommended. CYP3A4 inhibitors or dual inhibitors that inhibit both CYP3A4 and CYP1A2 simultaneously (eg, erythromycin, ketoconazole, fluvoxamine, enoxacin, cimetidine) and oral contraceptives containing gestodene and ethinyl estradiol may increase exposure and may result in increased adverse reactions; use with caution.

PREGNANCY: Category C, not for use in nursing.

MECHANISM OF ACTION: Selective PDE-4 inhibitor; not established. Thought to be related to the effects of increased intracellular cAMP in lung cells.

PHARMACOKINETICS: Absorption: Absolute bioavailability (80%); T_{max}=1 hr, 8 hrs (roflumilast N-oxide). **Distribution:** V_d=2.9L/kg; plasma protein binding (99%, 97% roflumilast N-oxide). **Metabolism:** Extensive via Phase 1 (CYP450) and Phase 2 (conjugation) reactions; roflumilast N-oxide (major active metabolite). **Elimination:** Urine (70%); $T_{1/2}$=17 hrs, 30 hrs (roflumilast N-oxide).

NURSING CONSIDERATIONS

Assessment: Assess for liver impairment, history of depression and/or suicidal thoughts or behavior, pregnancy/nursing status, and possible drug interactions.

Monitoring: Monitor for psychiatric events (including suicidality), and other adverse reactions. Monitor weight regularly.

Patient Counseling: Inform that drug is not a bronchodilator and should not be used for the relief of acute bronchospasm. Advise of the need to be alert for the emergence or worsening of insomnia, anxiety, depression, suicidal thoughts, or other mood changes; instruct to contact physician if such changes occur. Counsel to monitor weight regularly, and to consult physician if unexplained or clinically significant weight loss occurs. Instruct to notify physician of all medications being taken.

Administration: Oral route. Take with or without food. **Storage:** 20-25°C (68-77°F); excursions permitted to 15-30°C (59-86°F).

DANTRIUM   RX
dantrolene sodium (JHP)

Has potential for hepatotoxicity. Symptomatic/overt hepatitis and liver dysfunction reported. Risk of hepatic injury greater in females, patients >35 yrs of age, and patients taking other medications. Monitor hepatic function. D/C if no benefit after 45 days. Lowest possible effective dose should be prescribed.

THERAPEUTIC CLASS: Direct acting skeletal muscle relaxant

INDICATIONS: To control manifestations of clinical spasticity from upper motor neuron disorders (eg, spinal cord injury, stroke, cerebral palsy, multiple sclerosis). Preoperatively to prevent or attenuate development of signs of malignant hyperthermia in known, or strongly suspected, malignant hyperthermia susceptible patients who require anesthesia and/or surgery.

DOSAGE: *Adults:* Chronic Spasticity: Individualize dose. Initial: 25mg qd for 7 days. Titrate: Increase to 25mg tid for 7 days, then 50mg tid for 7 days, then 100mg tid. Max: 100mg qid. If no further benefit at next higher dose, decrease to previous lower dose. Malignant Hyperthermia: Preop: 4-8mg/kg/day in 3 or 4 divided doses for 1-2 days before surgery; last dose given 3-4 hrs before scheduled surgery with a minimum of water. Adjust dose within recommended dose range to avoid incapacitation or excessive GI irritation (eg, nausea and/or vomiting). Postop Following Malignant Hyperthermia Crisis: 4-8mg/kg/day in 4 divided doses for 1-3 days. *Pediatrics:* ≥5 Yrs: Chronic Spasticity: Individualize dose. Initial: 0.5mg/kg qd for 7 days. Titrate: Increase to 0.5mg/kg tid for 7 days, then 1mg/kg tid for 7 days, then 2mg/kg tid. Max: 100mg qid. If no further benefit at next higher dose, decrease to previous lower dose.

HOW SUPPLIED: Cap: 25mg, 50mg, 100mg

CONTRAINDICATIONS: Active hepatic disease (eg, hepatitis and cirrhosis); where spasticity is utilized to sustain upright posture and balance in locomotion, or whenever spasticity is utilized to obtain or maintain increased function.

WARNINGS/PRECAUTIONS: Brief withdrawal for 2-4 days may exacerbate manifestations of spasticity. Obtain LFTs at baseline, then periodically thereafter. D/C if LFT abnormalities or jaundice appears. Caution with impaired pulmonary function (eg, obstructive pulmonary disease), severely impaired cardiac function due to myocardial disease, and history of liver disease/ dysfunction.

ADVERSE REACTIONS: Hepatotoxicity, hepatitis, liver dysfunction, drowsiness, dizziness, weakness, general malaise, fatigue, diarrhea.

INTERACTIONS: See Boxed Warning. Not recommended with calcium channel blockers during the management of malignant hyperthermia; cardiovascular collapse with concomitant verapamil reported (rare). Caution with estrogens; hepatotoxicity reported especially in women >35 yrs of age. May potentiate vecuronium-induced neuromuscular block. Increased drowsiness with CNS depressants (eg, sedatives, tranquilizers).

PREGNANCY: Category C, not for use in nursing.

MECHANISM OF ACTION: Direct-acting skeletal muscle relaxant; interferes with release of Ca^{2+} ions from the sarcoplasmic reticulum.

PHARMACOKINETICS: Absorption: Incomplete, slow. **Distribution:** Crosses placenta. **Metabolism:** Hepatic microsomal enzymes; 5-hydroxy and acetamido analog (major metabolites). **Elimination:** Urine; $T_{1/2}$=8.7 hrs.

NURSING CONSIDERATIONS

Assessment: Assess for active hepatic disease, if spasticity is used for upright posture and balance or increased function, history of liver disease/dysfunction, pulmonary dysfunction, impaired cardiac function due to myocardial disease, pregnancy/nursing status, and possible drug interactions. Perform baseline LFTs. Assess use in patients >35 yrs of age.

Monitoring: Monitor for liver disorders, jaundice, hepatotoxicity, and hepatitis. Monitor LFTs regularly.

Patient Counseling: Inform about risks and benefits of therapy. Caution against performing hazardous tasks (eg, operating machinery/driving). Caution about sunlight exposure; photosensitivity reactions may occur. Instruct to inform about other medications being taken. Notify if pregnant/nursing.

Administration: Oral route. **Storage:** 20-25°C (68-77°F).

DAYPRO   RX
oxaprozin (G.D. Searle)

> NSAIDs may increase risk of serious cardiovascular thrombotic events, myocardial infarction (MI), and stroke; increased risk with duration of use and with cardiovascular disease (CVD) or risk factors for CVD. Increased risk of serious GI adverse events (eg, bleeding, ulceration, stomach/intestinal perforation) that can be fatal and occur anytime during use without warning symptoms; elderly patients are at a greater risk. Contraindicated for treatment of perioperative pain in the setting of coronary artery bypass graft (CABG) surgery.

THERAPEUTIC CLASS: NSAID

INDICATIONS: Relief of signs and symptoms of osteoarthritis (OA), rheumatoid arthritis (RA), and juvenile rheumatoid arthritis (JRA).

DOSAGE: *Adults:* Individualize dose. RA/OA: 1200mg qd. Max: 1800mg/day in divided doses (not to exceed 26mg/kg/day). Low Body Weight/Severe Renal Impairment/Hemodialysis: Initial: 600mg qd. Titrate: May cautiously increase to 1200mg with close monitoring if insufficient relief of symptoms. See PI for larger LDs.
Pediatrics: 6-16 Yrs: JRA: ≥55kg: 1200mg qd. 32-54kg: 900mg qd. 22-31kg: 600mg qd.

HOW SUPPLIED: Tab: 600mg* *scored

CONTRAINDICATIONS: Active GI bleeding, patients who have experienced asthma, urticaria, or allergic reactions after taking aspirin (ASA) or other NSAIDs. Treatment of perioperative pain in the setting of CABG surgery.

WARNINGS/PRECAUTIONS: Use lowest effective dose for the shortest duration possible. May cause HTN or worsen preexisting HTN; monitor BP closely. Fluid retention and edema reported. Caution with prior history of ulcer disease, GI bleeding, or risk factors for GI bleeding; monitor for GI ulceration/bleeding, and d/c if serious GI event occurs. Renal injury reported with long-term use; increased risk with renal/hepatic impairment, heart failure (HF), and elderly. Not recommended with advanced renal disease; monitor renal function closely if therapy is initiated. Anaphylactoid reactions may occur. May cause serious skin adverse events (eg, exfoliative dermatitis, Stevens-Johnson syndrome, toxic epidermal necrolysis); d/c at 1st appearance of skin rash/hypersensitivity. Caution with asthma and avoid with ASA-sensitive asthma and the ASA-triad. Avoid in late pregnancy; may cause premature closure of ductus arteriosus. May cause elevated LFTs or severe hepatic reactions; d/c if liver disease or systemic manifestations occur, or if abnormal LFTs persist/worsen. Not a substitute for corticosteroids nor treatment for corticosteroid insufficiency; may mask signs of inflammation and fever. Rash and/or mild photosensitivity reactions reported. Anemia reported; monitor Hgb/Hct if anemia develops. May inhibit platelet aggregation and prolong bleeding time; monitor patients with coagulation disorders.

ADVERSE REACTIONS: Edema, abdominal pain/distress, anorexia, diarrhea, GI ulcers, gross bleeding/perforation, heartburn, LFT elevations, N/V, anemia, CNS inhibition, headache, rash, tinnitus, abnormal renal function.

INTERACTIONS: Not recommended with ASA. Coadministration with ACE inhibitors may result in deterioration of renal function and diminished antihypertensive effect. May reduce natriuretic effects of furosemide and thiazide diuretics. May increase lithium levels; monitor for lithium toxicity. May enhance methotrexate (MTX) toxicity; use caution and consider MTX dose reduction. Increased risk of GI bleeding with oral corticosteroids, anticoagulants (eg, warfarin), alcohol use, and smoking. Monitor blood glucose in the beginning phase of glyburide and oxaprozin cotherapy. Monitor BP levels when coadministered with β-blockers (eg, metoprolol).

PREGNANCY: Category C, not for use in nursing.

MECHANISM OF ACTION: NSAID; not established. May be related to prostaglandin synthetase inhibition.

PHARMACOKINETICS: Absorption: Administration of variable doses resulted in different pharmacokinetic parameters. **Distribution:** V_d=11-17L/70kg; plasma protein binding (99%). **Metabolism:** Liver via oxidation (65%) and glucuronic acid conjugation (35%). **Elimination:** Feces (35% metabolite), urine (5% unchanged, 65% metabolite).

NURSING CONSIDERATIONS

Assessment: Assess for history of asthma, urticaria, or allergic-type reaction with ASA or other NSAIDs, ASA triad, CVD, HTN, fluid retention, HF, history of ulcer disease, history of/risk factors for GI bleeding, general health status, renal/hepatic function, coagulation disorders, pregnancy/nursing status, and possible drug interactions. Assess use in elderly and debilitated patients.

Monitoring: Monitor BP, CBC, bleeding time, LFTs, renal function, and chemistry profile periodically. Monitor for GI bleeding/ulceration/perforation, CV thrombotic events, MI, stroke, HTN, renal/liver dysfunction, fluid retention, edema, skin/allergic reactions, hematological effects, bronchospasm, and other adverse reactions. Monitor patients receiving anticoagulants.

Patient Counseling: Instruct to seek medical advice if symptoms of CV events, GI ulceration/bleeding, skin/hypersensitivity reactions, unexplained weight gain or edema, hepatotoxicity, or anaphylactoid reactions occur. Instruct to avoid in late pregnancy.

Administration: Oral route. **Storage:** 25°C (77°F); excursions permitted to 15-30°C (59-86°F). Protect from light.

DAYTRANA CII
methylphenidate (Noven)

Caution with history of drug dependence or alcoholism. Chronic abuse may lead to marked tolerance and psychological dependence with varying degrees of abnormal behavior. Frank psychotic episodes may occur, especially with parenteral abuse. Careful supervision is required during withdrawal from abusive use since severe depression may occur. Withdrawal following chronic use may unmask symptoms of underlying disorder that may require follow-up.

THERAPEUTIC CLASS: Sympathomimetic amine

INDICATIONS: Treatment of attention-deficit hyperactivity disorder.

DOSAGE: *Pediatrics:* ≥6 Yrs: Individualize dose. Apply to hip area 2 hrs before effect is needed and remove 9 hrs after application. Titration Schedule: Week 1: 10mg/9 hrs. Week 2: 15mg/9 hrs. Week 3: 20mg/9 hrs. Week 4: 30mg/9 hrs. Maint/Extended Treatment: Periodically reevaluate long-term usefulness of drug for the individual patient with periods off medication. Dose/Wear Time Reduction and Discontinuation: May remove patch earlier than 9 hrs if a shorter duration of effect is desired or late day side effects appear; individualize wear time. Reduce dose/wear time or, if necessary, d/c if aggravation of symptoms or other adverse events occur.

HOW SUPPLIED: Patch: 10mg/9 hrs, 15mg/9 hrs, 20mg/9 hrs, 30mg/9 hrs [30s]

CONTRAINDICATIONS: Marked anxiety, tension, agitation, glaucoma, motor tics, or family history or diagnosis of Tourette's syndrome. Treatment with MAOIs or within a minimum of 14 days following discontinuation of an MAOI.

WARNINGS/PRECAUTIONS: Avoid with known serious structural cardiac abnormalities, cardiomyopathy, serious heart rhythm abnormalities, coronary artery disease, or other serious cardiac problems. Sudden death reported in children and adolescents with structural cardiac abnormalities or other serious heart problems. Sudden deaths, stroke, and myocardial infarction (MI) reported in adults. May increase BP and HR; caution with conditions that might be compromised by increases in BP/HR (eg, preexisting HTN, heart failure, recent MI, ventricular arrhythmia). Prior to treatment, obtain medical history (including assessment for family history of sudden death or ventricular arrhythmia) and perform physical exam to assess for presence of cardiac disease.

Promptly perform cardiac evaluation if symptoms of cardiac disease develop. May exacerbate symptoms of behavior disturbance and thought disorder in patients with preexisting psychotic disorder. Caution in patients with comorbid bipolar disorder; may induce mixed/manic episode. May cause treatment-emergent psychotic or manic symptoms (eg, hallucinations, delusional thinking, mania) in children and adolescents without prior history of psychotic illness or mania; consider discontinuation if such symptoms occur. Aggressive behavior or hostility reported in children and adolescents. May lower convulsive threshold; d/c if seizures occur. Priapism, sometimes requiring surgical intervention, reported. Associated with peripheral vasculopathy, including Raynaud's phenomenon; carefully observe for digital changes. May cause long-term suppression of growth in children; monitor growth, and may need to interrupt treatment in patients not growing or gaining height or weight as expected. Difficulties with accommodation and blurring of vision reported. May lead to contact sensitization; d/c if suspected. Patients who develop contact sensitization to therapy and require oral treatment with methylphenidate should be initiated on oral medication under close medical supervision. Avoid exposing application site to direct external heat sources while wearing the patch.

ADVERSE REACTIONS: Decreased appetite, headache, insomnia, N/V, decreased weight, irritability, tic, affect lability, anorexia, abdominal pain, dizziness.

INTERACTIONS: See Contraindications. Caution with pressor agents. May decrease effectiveness of drugs used to treat HTN. May inhibit metabolism of coumarin anticoagulants, anticonvulsants (eg, phenobarbital, phenytoin, primidone), and some TCAs (eg, imipramine, clomipramine, desipramine) and SSRIs; downward dose adjustments and monitoring of plasma drug concentrations (or coagulation times for coumarin) of these drugs may be necessary when initiating or discontinuing methylphenidate.

PREGNANCY: Category C, caution in nursing.

MECHANISM OF ACTION: Sympathomimetic amine; CNS stimulant. Has not been established; thought to block reuptake of norepinephrine and dopamine into presynaptic neuron and increase release of these monoamines into extraneuronal space.

PHARMACOKINETICS: Absorption: T_{max}=10 hrs (single application), 8 hrs (repeated applications). Administration of variable doses resulted in different parameters. **Metabolism:** Via deesterification; α-phenyl-piperidine acetic acid (ritalinic acid) (metabolite). **Elimination:** $T_{1/2}$=4-5 hrs (d-methylphenidate), 1.4-2.9 hrs (l-methylphenidate).

NURSING CONSIDERATIONS

Assessment: Assess for hypersensitivity to the drug, marked anxiety, tension, agitation, glaucoma, motor tics, family history or diagnosis of Tourette's syndrome, cardiovascular conditions, history of drug dependence or alcoholism, psychotic disorder, comorbid bipolar disorder, any other conditions where treatment is contraindicated or cautioned, pregnancy/nursing status, and possible drug interactions.

Monitoring: Monitor for changes in HR and BP, signs/symptoms of cardiac disease, exacerbation of behavior disturbance and thought disorder, psychosis, mania, appearance of or worsening of aggressive behavior or hostility, seizures, priapism, peripheral vasculopathy (including Raynaud's phenomenon), visual disturbances, contact sensitization, and other adverse reactions. In pediatric patients, monitor growth. Perform periodic monitoring of CBC, differential, and platelet counts during prolonged therapy. Periodically reevaluate long-term usefulness of drug.

Patient Counseling: Inform about the benefits and risks of therapy. Counsel on the appropriate use of the medication. Instruct to seek immediate medical attention in the event of priapism. Instruct to report to physician any new numbness, pain, skin color change, or sensitivity to temperature in fingers or toes; instruct to contact physician immediately with any signs of unexplained wounds appearing on fingers or toes while taking the drug. Advise to avoid exposing application site to direct external heat sources (eg, hair dryers, heating pads, electric blankets, heated water beds) while wearing the patch. Instruct to avoid touching the adhesive side of the patch during application, and to immediately wash hands after application if adhesive side is touched. Advise to take patch off earlier if there is an unacceptable duration of appetite loss or insominia in the pm. Counsel to not wear the patch and to consult physician if any swelling or blistering occurs. Instruct not to apply hydrocortisone or other sol, cre, oint, or emollients immediately prior to patch application. Caution against operating potentially hazardous machinery or vehicles until accustomed to effects of medication.

Administration: Transdermal route. Apply patch immediately upon removal from the individual protective pouch. Refer to PI for application, removal, and disposal instructions. **Storage:** 25°C (77°F); excursions permitted to 15-30°C (59-86°F). Do not store patches unpouched. Do not refrigerate or freeze patches. Once the sealed tray or outer pouch is opened, use contents within 2 months.

DEMEROL INJECTION
meperidine HCl (Hospira)

THERAPEUTIC CLASS: Opioid analgesic

INDICATIONS: For relief of moderate to severe pain. For preoperative medication, anesthesia support, and obstetrical analgesia.

DOSAGE: *Adults:* Pain: Usual: 50-150mg IM/SQ q3-4h PRN. Preop: Usual: 50-100mg IM/SQ 30-90 min before anesthesia. Anesthesia Support: Use repeated slow IV inj of fractional doses (eg, 10mg/mL) or continuous IV infusion of a more diluted sol (eg, 1mg/mL). Titrate PRN. Obstetrical Analgesia: Usual: 50-100mg IM/SQ when pain is regular, may repeat at 1- to 3-hr intervals. Elderly: Start at lower end of dosage range and observe. With Phenothiazines/Other Tranquilizers: Reduce dose by 25-50%. IM method preferred with repeated use. For IV inj: Reduce dose and administer slowly, preferably using diluted sol.
Pediatrics: Pain: Usual: 0.5-0.8mg/lb IM/SQ, up to 50-150mg, q3-4h PRN. Preop: Usual: 0.5-1mg/lb IM/SQ, up to 50-100mg, 30-90 min before anesthesia. With Phenothiazines/Other Tranquilizers: Reduce dose by 25-50%. IM method preferred with repeated use. For IV inj: Reduce dose and administer slowly, preferably using diluted sol.

HOW SUPPLIED: Inj: 25mg/mL, 50mg/mL, 75mg/mL, 100mg/mL

CONTRAINDICATIONS: During or within 14 days of MAOI use.

WARNINGS/PRECAUTIONS: May develop tolerance and dependence; abuse potential. Extreme caution with head injury, increased intracranial pressure, intracranial lesions, acute asthmatic attack, chronic obstructive pulmonary disease or cor pulmonale, decreased respiratory reserve, respiratory depression, hypoxia, and hypercapnia. Rapid IV infusion may result in increased adverse reactions. Caution with acute abdominal conditions, atrial flutter, supraventricular tachycardias. May aggravate convulsive disorders. Caution and reduce initial dose with elderly or debilitated, renal/hepatic impairment, hypothyroidism, Addison's disease, prostatic hypertrophy or urethral stricture. Severe hypotension may occur postop or if depleted blood volume. Orthostatic hypotension may occur. May impair mental/physical abilities. Not for use in pregnancy prior to labor. May produce depression of respiration and psychophysiologic functions in newborns when used as an obstetrical analgesic.

ADVERSE REACTIONS: Lightheadedness, dizziness, sedation, N/V, sweating, respiratory/circulatory depression.

INTERACTIONS: See Contraindications. Caution and reduce dose with other CNS depressants (eg, narcotics, anesthetics, phenothiazines, tranquilizers, sedative-hypnotics, TCAs, alcohol).

PREGNANCY: Safety in pregnancy and nursing not known.

MECHANISM OF ACTION: Narcotic analgesic; produces actions similar to morphine. Principal actions involve the CNS and organs composed of smooth muscle. Produces analgesic and sedative effects.

PHARMACOKINETICS: Distribution: Crosses placental barrier; found in breast milk.

NURSING CONSIDERATIONS

Assessment: Assess for pain intensity, or any other conditions where treatment is contraindicated or cautioned. Assess for pregnancy/nursing status, renal/hepatic function, and possible drug interactions.

Monitoring: Monitor for signs/symptoms of drug dependence (eg, psychic dependence, physical dependence), respiratory depression, circulatory depression (eg, hypotension), and convulsions.

Patient Counseling: Inform that medication may impair mental/physical abilities; use caution when performing hazardous tasks (eg, operating machinery/driving). Notify physician of all medications currently being taken. Avoid using other CNS depressants and alcohol. Advise about potential for dependence upon repeated administration.

Administration: SQ, IM, IV route. SQ route is suitable for occasional use, IM administration is preferred if repeated doses are required. IM inj should be injected well into the body of a large muscle. If IV route is required, dosage should be decreased and inj should be made very slowly, preferably using a diluted solution. Dosage should be adjusted according to severity of pain.
Storage: 20-25°C (68-77°F).

DENAVIR
penciclovir (Prestium Pharma)

RX

THERAPEUTIC CLASS: Nucleoside analogue

INDICATIONS: Treatment of recurrent herpes labialis (cold sores) in adults and children ≥12 yrs of age.

D

DOSAGE: *Adults:* Apply q2h during waking hours for a period of 4 days. Start treatment as early as possible (eg, during the prodrome or when lesions appear).
Pediatrics: ≥12 Yrs: Apply q2h during waking hours for a period of 4 days. Start treatment as early as possible (eg, during the prodrome or when lesions appear).

HOW SUPPLIED: Cre: 1% [1.5g, 5g]

WARNINGS/PRECAUTIONS: Should only be used on herpes labialis on the lips and face. Avoid application in mucous membranes and/or near the eyes. Evaluate for secondary bacterial infection if lesions worsen or do not improve on therapy. Effect has not been established in immunocompromised patients.

ADVERSE REACTIONS: Application-site reaction, hypesthesia, local anesthesia, taste perversion, rash (erythematous).

PREGNANCY: Category B, not for use in nursing.

MECHANISM OF ACTION: Nucleoside analogue; possesses inhibitory activity against herpes simplex virus (HSV) types 1 (HSV-1) and 2 (HSV-2). Inhibits HSV polymerase competitively with deoxyguanosine triphosphate. Consequently, herpes viral DNA synthesis and replication are selectively inhibited.

NURSING CONSIDERATIONS

Assessment: Assess for bacterial infection, drug hypersensitivity, and pregnancy/nursing status.

Monitoring: Monitor for clinical response and improvement of symptoms. Evaluate for secondary bacterial infection if lesions worsen or do not improve.

Patient Counseling: Inform that drug is not a cure for cold sores and not all patients respond to treatment. Instruct not to use if allergic to the drug or any of its ingredients. Instruct to notify physician if pregnant, planning to become pregnant, or breastfeeding. Instruct to use ud. Instruct to wash hands with soap and water before and after applying product. Inform that face should be clean and dry. Instruct to apply a layer to cover only the cold sore area or area of tingling before the cold sore appears, and to rub in the cream until it disappears. Inform of possible adverse effects (eg, application-site reactions, local anesthesia, taste perversion, rash).

Administration: Topical route. **Storage:** 20-25°C (68-77°F); excursions permitted to 15-30°C (59-86°F).

DEPAKENE   RX
valproic acid (AbbVie)

Fatal hepatic failure reported, usually during first 6 months of treatment. Serious/fatal hepatotoxicity may be preceded by nonspecific symptoms (eg, malaise, weakness, lethargy, facial edema, anorexia, vomiting) or loss of seizure control in patients with epilepsy; monitor closely. Monitor LFTs prior to therapy and at frequent intervals thereafter, especially during first 6 months of treatment. Increased risk of developing fatal hepatotoxicity in children <2 yrs of age, especially if on multiple anticonvulsants, with congenital metabolic disorders, severe seizure disorders with mental retardation, and organic brain disease; use with extreme caution and as a sole agent. Increased risk of drug-induced acute liver failure and resultant deaths in patients with hereditary neurometabolic syndromes caused by DNA mutations of the mitochondrial DNA Polymerase gamma (POLG) gene (eg, Alpers Huttenlocher Syndrome). Contraindicated in patients known to have mitochondrial disorders caused by POLG mutations and children <2 yrs of age who are clinically suspected of having a mitochondrial disorder. In patients >2 yrs of age who are clinically suspected of having a hereditary mitochondrial disease, drug should only be used after other anticonvulsants have failed; closely monitor for the development of acute liver injury with regular clinical assessments and serum liver testing. May cause major congenital malformations, particularly neural tube defects (eg, spina bifida). May cause decreased IQ scores following in utero exposure. Should only be used to treat pregnant women with epilepsy if other medications have failed to control their symptoms or are otherwise unacceptable. Do not administer to a woman of childbearing potential unless the drug is essential to the management of her medical condition; use effective contraception. Life-threatening pancreatitis reported; d/c if pancreatitis is diagnosed and initiate appropriate treatment.

THERAPEUTIC CLASS: Carboxylic acid derivative

INDICATIONS: Monotherapy and adjunctive therapy for treatment of simple and complex absence seizures, and complex partial seizures. Adjunctive therapy for multiple seizure types that include absence seizures.

DOSAGE: *Adults:* Simple/Complex Absence Seizure: Initial: 15mg/kg/day. Titrate: Increase weekly by 5-10mg/kg/day until seizures are controlled or side effects preclude further increases. Max: 60 mg/kg/day. If total dose exceeds 250mg/day, give in divided doses. Refer to PI for the initial daily dose guide. Complex Partial Seizure: Monotherapy/Conversion to Monotherapy/Adjunctive Therapy: Initial: 10-15mg/kg/day. Titrate: Increase by 5-10mg/kg/week until optimal response is achieved. If clinical response has not been achieved, measure plasma levels to determine whether or not they are in the usually accepted therapeutic range (50-100mcg/mL). Max: 60mg/kg/day. When converting to monotherapy, reduce concomitant antiepilepsy drug by 25% every 2 weeks, starting at initiation or delay by 1-2 weeks after start of therapy. For adjunctive therapy, if total dose exceeds 250mg/day, give in divided doses. Elderly: Reduce initial dose and titrate slowly.

Decrease dose or d/c in patients with decreased food or fluid intake or excessive somnolence. *Pediatrics:* Simple/Complex Absence Seizure: Initial: 15mg/kg/day. Titrate: Increase weekly by 5-10mg/kg/day until seizures are controlled or side effects preclude further increases. Max: 60 mg/kg/day. If total dose exceeds 250mg/day, give in divided doses. Refer to PI for the initial daily dose guide. ≥10 Yrs: Complex Partial Seizure: Monotherapy/Conversion to Monotherapy/Adjunctive Therapy: Initial: 10-15mg/kg/day. Titrate: Increase by 5-10mg/kg/week until optimal response is achieved. If clinical response has not been achieved, measure plasma levels to determine whether or not they are in the usually accepted therapeutic range (50-100mcg/mL). Max: 60mg/kg/day. When converting to monotherapy, reduce concomitant antiepilepsy drug by 25% every 2 weeks, starting at initiation or delay by 1-2 weeks after start of therapy. For adjunctive therapy, if total dose exceeds 250mg/day, give in divided doses.

HOW SUPPLIED: Cap: 250mg; Sol: 250mg/5mL

CONTRAINDICATIONS: Hepatic disease, significant hepatic dysfunction, known urea cycle disorders (UCD). Mitochondrial disorders caused by mutations in mitochondrial POLG (eg, Alpers-Huttenlocher syndrome) and children <2 yrs of age who are suspected of having a POLG-related disorder.

WARNINGS/PRECAUTIONS: Caution with prior history of hepatic disease. D/C immediately if significant hepatic dysfunction (suspected or apparent) occurs. Hyperammonemic encephalopathy reported in UCD patients; d/c and initiate treatment if symptoms develop. Prior to initiation of therapy, evaluate for UCD in high-risk patients (eg, history of unexplained encephalopathy, coma, etc.). Reversible and irreversible cerebral and cerebellar atrophy reported; routinely monitor motor and cognitive functions and evaluate continued use in the presence of suspected or apparent signs of brain atrophy. Cerebral atrophy reported in children exposed in utero. Increased risk of suicidal thoughts or behavior reported; monitor for the emergence/worsening of depression, suicidal thoughts or behavior, thoughts of self-harm, and/or any unusual changes in mood or behavior. Dose-related thrombocytopenia reported; monitor platelet and coagulation parameters before initiating therapy and periodically thereafter. Reduce dose or d/c if hemorrhage, bruising, or a disorder of hemostasis/coagulation occurs. Hyperammonemia reported and may be present despite normal LFTs. Measure ammonia levels if unexplained lethargy, vomiting, or mental status changes occur. Multiorgan hypersensitivity reactions (rare) and hypothermia reported; d/c and initiate alternative treatment if this reaction is suspected. Caution in the elderly; monitor fluid/nutritional intake, and for dehydration and somnolence. Altered thyroid function tests and urine ketone tests reported. May stimulate replication of HIV and cytomegalovirus. Avoid abrupt discontinuation.

ADVERSE REACTIONS: Hepatotoxicity, pancreatitis, N/V, somnolence, dizziness, abdominal pain, dyspepsia, rash, diarrhea, tremor, weight gain, back pain, alopecia, headache.

INTERACTIONS: Drugs that affect the level of expression of hepatic enzymes (eg, phenytoin, carbamazepine, phenobarbital, primidone) may increase valproate clearance. Concomitant use with aspirin decreases protein binding and inhibits metabolism of valproate; use with caution. Carbapenem antibiotics (eg, ertapenem, imipenem, meropenem) may reduce serum concentrations to subtherapeutic levels, resulting in loss of seizure control. Rifampin increases oral clearance; may require valproate dosage adjustment. Concomitant use with felbamate leads to an increase in valproate C_{max}; may require decrease in valproate dosage. Reduces the clearance of amitriptyline and nortriptyline. Induces metabolism of carbamazepine. Inhibits metabolism of diazepam, ethosuximide, phenobarbital, and phenytoin; monitor drug serum concentrations and adjust dose appropriately. Breakthrough seizures reported with concomitant phenytoin. Use with clonazepam may induce absence status in patients with absence seizures. Increases $T_{1/2}$ of lamotrigine; serious skin reactions reported. Concomitant use with topiramate associated with hypothermia and hyperammonemia, with or without encephalopathy. May displace protein-bound drugs (eg, phenytoin, carbamazepine, tolbutamide, warfarin); monitor coagulation tests when coadministered with warfarin. May decrease zidovudine clearance in HIV-seropositive patients.

PREGNANCY: Category D, caution in nursing.

MECHANISM OF ACTION: Carboxylic acid derivative; has not been established. Suggested to increase brain concentrations of gamma-aminobutyric acid.

PHARMACOKINETICS: Absorption: Depakote: (Tab) T_{max}=4 hrs (fasted), 8 hrs (fed); (Cap) T_{max}=3.3 hrs (fasted), 4.8 hrs (fed). **Distribution:** V_d=11L (total valproate), 92L (free valproate); found in breast milk, CSF. **Metabolism:** Liver; Mitochondrial β-oxidation (major), glucuronidation. **Elimination:** Urine (30-50% glucuronide conjugate, <3% unchanged); $T_{1/2}$=9-16 hrs (250-1000mg dose).

NURSING CONSIDERATIONS

Assessment: Assess for hepatic dysfunction, history of hepatic disease, UCD, pancreatitis, history of hypersensitivity to the drug, mitochondrial disorders caused by mutations in mitochondrial POLG and children <2 yrs of age who are suspected of having a POLG-related disorder, other conditions where treatment is contraindicated or cautioned, pregnancy/nursing status, and possible drug interactions. Assess LFTs, CBC with platelet counts, and coagulation parameters.

Monitoring: Monitor for hypersensitivity reactions, multiorgan hypersensitivity reactions, pancreatitis, hepatotoxicity, hyperammonemia, hypothermia, drug-induced acute liver failure, acute liver injury, brain atrophy, emergence/worsening of depression, suicidality or unusual changes in behavior, and other adverse reactions. Monitor LFTs frequently, especially during first 6 months. Monitor fluid/nutritional intake, ammonia levels, CBC with platelets, and coagulation parameters in patients on warfarin. Perform periodic plasma concentration determinations of valproate and concomitant drugs during the early course of therapy.

Patient Counseling: Instruct to take ud. Inform pregnant women and women of childbearing potential about the risk in pregnancy (eg, birth defects, decreased IQ); advise to use effective contraception while on therapy and counsel about alternative therapeutic options. Advise to read medication guide. Instruct to notify physician if pregnant or intend to become pregnant. Encourage patients to enroll in North American Antiepileptic Drug (NAAED) Pregnancy Registry. Advise to notify physician if depression, suicidal thoughts/behavior, or thoughts about self-harm emerge; instruct to report behaviors of concern. Counsel about signs/symptoms of pancreatitis, hepatotoxicity, hyperammonemia, or hyperammonemic encephalopathy; advise to notify physician if any symptoms or adverse effects occur. Advise not to engage in hazardous activities (eg, driving/operating machinery) until the effects of the drug are known. Instruct that a fever associated with other organ system involvement (eg, rash, lymphadenopathy) may be drug-related; instruct to report to physician.

Administration: Oral route. Swallow caps whole; do not chew. GI irritation: Take with food or slowly build up the dose from an initial low level. **Storage:** (Cap) 15-25°C (59-77°F). (Sol) Below 30°C (86°F).

DEPAKOTE   RX
divalproex sodium (AbbVie)

Fatal hepatic failure reported, usually during first 6 months of treatment. Serious/fatal hepatotoxicity may be preceded by nonspecific symptoms (eg, malaise, weakness, lethargy, facial edema, anorexia, vomiting) or loss of seizure control in patients with epilepsy; monitor closely. Monitor LFTs prior to therapy and at frequent intervals thereafter, especially during first 6 months of treatment. Increased risk of developing fatal hepatotoxicity in children <2 yrs of age, especially if on multiple anticonvulsants, with congenital metabolic disorders, severe seizure disorders with mental retardation, and organic brain disease; use with extreme caution and as a sole agent. Increased risk of drug-induced acute liver failure and resultant death in patients with hereditary neurometabolic syndromes caused by DNA mutations of the mitochondrial DNA Polymerase gamma (POLG) gene (eg, Alpers Huttenlocher Syndrome). Contraindicated in patients known to have mitochondrial disorders caused by POLG mutations and children <2 yrs of age who are clinically suspected of having a mitochondrial disorder. In patients >2 yrs of age who are clinically suspected of having a hereditary mitochondrial disease, drug should only be used after other anticonvulsants have failed; closely monitor for the development of acute liver injury with regular clinical assessments and serum liver testing. May cause major congenital malformations, particularly neural tube defects (eg, spina bifida). May cause decreased IQ scores following in utero exposure. Should only be used to treat pregnant women with epilepsy or bipolar disorder if other medications have failed to control their symptoms or are otherwise unacceptable. Do not administer to a woman of childbearing potential unless the drug is essential to the management of her medical condition; use effective contraception. Life-threatening pancreatitis reported; d/c if pancreatitis is diagnosed and initiate appropriate treatment.

OTHER BRAND NAMES: Depakote Sprinkle (AbbVie)

THERAPEUTIC CLASS: Valproate compound

INDICATIONS: Monotherapy and adjunctive therapy for treatment of simple and complex absence seizures, and complex partial seizures. Adjunctive therapy for multiple seizure types that include absence seizures. (Tab) Treatment of mania associated with bipolar disorder and migraine prophylaxis.

DOSAGE: *Adults:* Complex Partial Seizures: Monotherapy/Conversion to Monotherapy/Adjunctive Therapy: Initial: 10-15mg/kg/day. Titrate: Increase by 5-10mg/kg/week until optimal response is achieved. If clinical response has not been achieved, measure plasma levels to determine whether or not they are in the usually accepted therapeutic range (50-100mcg/mL). Max: 60mg/kg/day. When converting to monotherapy, reduce concomitant antiepilepsy drug by 25% every 2 weeks, starting at initiation or delay by 1-2 weeks after start of therapy. For adjunctive therapy, if total dose exceeds 250mg/day, give in divided doses. Simple/Complex Absence Seizures: Initial: 15mg/kg/day. Titrate: Increase weekly by 5-10mg/kg/day until seizures are controlled or side effects preclude further increases. Max: 60mg/kg/day. If total dose exceeds 250mg/day, give in divided doses. In epileptic patients previously receiving Depakene (valproic acid) therapy, initiate at the same daily dose and dosing schedule; a dosing schedule of bid or tid may be elected after the patient is stabilized. Elderly: Reduce initial dose and titrate slowly. Decrease dose or d/c in patients with decreased food/fluid intake or excessive somnolence. (Tab) Migraine: Initial: 250mg bid. Max: 1000mg/day. Mania: Initial: 750mg daily in divided doses. Titrate: Increase dose as rapidly as possible to achieve the lowest therapeutic dose that produces desired clinical effect or the desired range of plasma concentrations. Max: 60mg/kg/day. *Pediatrics:* Simple/Complex Absence Seizure: Initial: 15mg/kg/day. Titrate: Increase weekly by

5-10mg/kg/day until seizures are controlled or side effects preclude further increases. Max: 60mg/kg/day. If total dose exceeds 250mg/day, give in divided doses. ≥10 Yrs: Complex Partial Seizures: Monotherapy/Conversion to Monotherapy/Adjunctive Therapy: Initial: 10-15mg/kg/day. Titrate: Increase by 5-10mg/kg/week until optimal response is achieved. If clinical response has not been achieved, measure plasma levels to determine whether or not they are in the usually accepted therapeutic range (50-100mcg/mL). Max: 60mg/kg/day. When converting to monotherapy, reduce concomitant antiepilepsy drug by 25% every 2 weeks, starting at initiation or delay by 1-2 weeks after start of therapy. For adjunctive therapy, if total dose exceeds 250mg/day, give in divided doses.

HOW SUPPLIED: Cap: (Sprinkle) 125mg; Tab, Delayed-Release: 125mg, 250mg, 500mg

CONTRAINDICATIONS: Hepatic disease, significant hepatic dysfunction, known urea cycle disorders (UCD). Mitochondrial disorders caused by mutations in mitochondrial POLG (eg, Alpers-Huttenlocher syndrome) and children <2 yrs of age who are suspected of having a POLG-related disorder. (Tab) Prophylaxis of migraine headaches in pregnant women.

WARNINGS/PRECAUTIONS: Caution with prior history of hepatic disease. D/C immediately if significant hepatic dysfunction (suspected or apparent) occurs. Hyperammonemic encephalopathy reported in UCD patients; d/c and initiate treatment if symptoms develop. Prior to initiation of therapy, evaluate for UCD in high-risk patients (eg, history of unexplained encephalopathy, coma, etc.). Reversible and irreversible cerebral and cerebellar atrophy reported; routinely monitor motor and cognitive functions and evaluate continued use in the presence of suspected or apparent signs of brain atrophy. Cerebral atrophy reported in children exposed in utero. Increased risk of suicidal thoughts or behavior reported; monitor for the emergence/worsening of depression, suicidal thoughts or behavior, thoughts of self-harm, and/or any unusual changes in mood or behavior. Dose-related thrombocytopenia reported; monitor platelet and coagulation parameters before initiating therapy and periodically thereafter. Reduce dose or d/c if hemorrhage, bruising, or a disorder of hemostasis/coagulation occurs. Hyperammonemia reported and may be present despite normal LFTs. Measure ammonia levels if unexplained lethargy, vomiting, or mental status changes occur. Multiorgan hypersensitivity reactions (rare) and hypothermia reported; d/c and initiate alternative treatment if this reaction is suspected. Caution in the elderly; monitor fluid/nutritional intake, and for dehydration and somnolence. Altered thyroid function tests and urine ketone tests reported. May stimulate replication of HIV and cytomegalovirus. Avoid abrupt discontinuation. Medication residue in stool reported; checked valproate levels and monitor clinical condition, and consider alternative treatment if clinically indicated.

ADVERSE REACTIONS: Hepatotoxicity, pancreatitis, diarrhea, N/V, somnolence, dizziness, dyspepsia, thrombocytopenia, asthenia, abdominal pain, tremor, headache, anorexia, diplopia, blurred vision.

INTERACTIONS: Drugs that affect the level of expression of hepatic enzymes (eg, phenytoin, carbamazepine, phenobarbital, primidone) may increase or double valproate clearance. Concomitant use with aspirin decreases protein binding and inhibits metabolism of valproate; use with caution. Carbapenem antibiotics (eg, ertapenem, imipenem, meropenem) may reduce serum concentrations to subtherapeutic levels, resulting in loss of seizure control. Rifampin increases oral clearance; may require valproate dosage adjustment. Concomitant use with felbamate leads to an increase in valproate C_{max}; may require decrease in valproate dosage. Reduces the clearance of amitriptyline and nortriptyline. Induces metabolism of carbamazepine. Inhibits metabolism of diazepam, ethosuximide, phenobarbital, and phenytoin; monitor drug serum concentrations and adjust dose appropriately. Breakthrough seizures reported with concomitant use with phenytoin. Use with clonazepam may induce absence status in patients with absence seizures. Increases $T_{1/2}$ of lamotrigine; serious skin reactions reported. Concomitant use with topiramate associated with hypothermia and hyperammonemia, with or without encephalopathy. May displace protein-bound drugs (eg, phenytoin, carbamazepine, tolbutamide, warfarin); monitor coagulation tests when coadministered with warfarin. May decrease zidovudine clearance in HIV-seropositive patients.

PREGNANCY: Category D (for epilepsy and for manic episodes with bipolar disorder) or X (for prophylaxis of migraine headaches), caution in nursing.

MECHANISM OF ACTION: Anticonvulsant; has not been established. Suggested to increase brain concentrations of gamma-aminobutyric acid.

PHARMACOKINETICS: Absorption: T_{max}=4-8 hrs (tab), T_{max}=3.3-4.8 hrs (cap). **Distribution:** V_d=11L (total valproate), 92L (free valproate); found in breast milk, CSF. **Metabolism:** Liver; mitochondrial β-oxidation (major), glucuronidation. **Elimination:** Urine (30-50% glucuronide conjugate, <3% unchanged); $T_{1/2}$=9-16 hrs (250-1000mg dose).

NURSING CONSIDERATIONS

Assessment: Assess for hepatic dysfunction, history of hepatic disease, UCD, pancreatitis, history of hypersensitivity to the drug, mitochondrial disorders caused by mutations in mitochondrial POLG and children <2 yrs of age who are suspected of having a POLG-related disorder, other conditions where treatment is contraindicated or cautioned, pregnancy/nursing status, and possible drug interactions. Assess LFTs, CBC with platelet counts, and coagulation parameters.

Monitoring: Monitor for hypersensitivity reactions, multiorgan hypersensitivity reactions, pancreatitis, hepatotoxicity, hyperammonemia, hypothermia, drug-induced acute liver failure, acute liver injury, brain atrophy, emergence/worsening of depression, suicidality or unusual changes in behavior, medication residue in stool, and other adverse reactions. Monitor LFTs frequently, especially during first 6 months. Monitor fluid/nutritional intake, ammonia levels, CBC with platelets, and coagulation parameters in patients on warfarin. Perform periodic plasma concentration determinations of valproate and concomitant drugs during the early course of therapy.

Patient Counseling: Instruct to take ud. Inform pregnant women and women of childbearing potential about the risk in pregnancy (eg, birth defects, decreased IQ); advise to use effective contraception while on therapy and counsel about alternative therapeutic options. Advise to read medication guide. Notify physician if pregnant or intend to become pregnant. Encourage patients to enroll in North American Antiepileptic Drug (NAAED) Pregnancy Registry. Advise to notify physician if depression, suicidal thoughts/behavior, or thoughts about self-harm emerge; instruct to report behaviors of concern. Counsel about signs/symptoms of pancreatitis, hepatotoxicity, hyperammonemia, or hyperammonemic encephalopathy; advise to notify physician if any symptoms or adverse effects occur. Advise not to engage in hazardous activities (eg, driving/operating machinery) until the effects of the drug are known. Instruct that a fever associated with other organ system involvement (eg, rash, lymphadenopathy) may be drug-related; instruct to report to physician. Instruct patients to notify their healthcare provider if medication residue is noticed in the stool.

Administration: Oral route. GI irritation: Take with food or slowly build up the dose from an initial low level. (Cap) May be swallowed whole or the contents may be sprinkled on soft food. Swallow drug/food mixture immediately; avoid chewing. Refer to PI for administration guide. (Tab) Swallow whole; do cut crush or chew. **Storage:** (Cap) Below 25°C (77°F). (Tab) Below 30°C (86°F).

DEPAKOTE ER   RX
divalproex sodium (AbbVie)

> Fatal hepatic failure may occur, usually during first 6 months of treatment. Serious/fatal hepatotoxicity may be preceded by nonspecific symptoms such as malaise, weakness, lethargy, facial edema, anorexia, and vomiting, or loss of seizure control in patients with epilepsy. Monitor LFTs prior to therapy and at frequent intervals thereafter, especially during first 6 months of treatment. Increased risk of developing fatal hepatotoxicity in children <2 yrs of age, especially if on multiple anticonvulsants, with congenital metabolic disorders, severe seizure disorders with mental retardation, and organic brain disease; use with extreme caution and as a sole agent. Increased risk of drug-induced acute liver failure and resultant deaths in patients with hereditary neurometabolic syndromes caused by DNA mutations of the mitochondrial DNA Polymerase gamma (POLG) gene (eg, Alpers Huttenlocher Syndrome). Contraindicated in patients known to have mitochondrial disorders caused by POLG mutations and children <2 yrs of age who are clinically suspected of having a mitochondrial disorder. In patients >2 yrs of age who are clinically suspected of having a hereditary mitochondrial disease, drug should only be used after other anticonvulsants have failed; closely monitor for the development of acute liver injury with regular clinical assessments and serum liver testing. May cause major congenital malformations, particularly neural tube defects (eg, spina bifida). May cause decreased IQ scores following in utero exposure. Contraindicated in pregnant women treated for prophylaxis of migraine; should only be used to treat pregnant women with epilepsy or bipolar disorder if other medications have failed to control their symptoms or are otherwise unacceptable. Do not administer to a woman of childbearing potential unless the drug is essential to the management of her medical condition; use effective contraception. Life-threatening pancreatitis reported; d/c if pancreatitis is diagnosed and initiate appropriate treatment.

THERAPEUTIC CLASS: Valproate compound

INDICATIONS: Treatment of acute manic or mixed episodes associated with bipolar disorder, with or without psychotic features. In adults and children ≥10 yrs of age, monotherapy and adjunctive treatment of complex partial seizures, simple/complex absence seizures, and adjunct for multiple seizure types that include absence seizures. Migraine headache prophylaxis.

DOSAGE: *Adults:* Individualize dose. Migraine: Initial: 500mg qd for 1 week. Titrate: Increase to 1000mg qd. Mania: Initial: 25mg/kg/day given qd. Titrate: Rapidly increase dose to achieve clinical effect. Max: 60mg/kg/day. Complex Partial Seizures: Monotherapy/Conversion to Monotherapy/Adjunctive Therapy: Initial: 10-15mg/kg/day. Titrate: Increase by 5-10mg/kg/week until optimal response is achieved. Max: 60mg/kg/day. When converting to monotherapy, reduce concomitant antiepilepsy drug by 25% every 2 weeks, starting at initiation or delayed by 1-2 weeks after start of therapy. Simple/Complex Absence Seizures: Initial: 15mg/kg/day. Titrate: Increase weekly by 5-10mg/kg/day until optimal response is achieved. Max: 60mg/kg/day. Conversion from Depakote: Administer qd using a dose 8-20% higher than total daily dose of Depakote. Refer to PI for dose conversion. If total Depakote dose cannot be directly converted, consider increasing Depakote total daily dose to next higher dosage before converting to appropriate total daily Depakote ER dose. Elderly: Reduce initial dose and titrate slowly. Decrease dose or d/c in patients with decreased food or fluid intake or excessive somnolence.
Pediatrics: ≥10 Yrs: Individualize dose. Complex Partial Seizures: Monotherapy/Conversion to Monotherapy/Adjunctive Therapy: Initial: 10-15mg/kg/day. Titrate: Increase by 5-10mg/kg/week until optimal response is achieved. Max: 60mg/kg/day. When converting to monotherapy,

reduce concomitant antiepilepsy drug by 25% every 2 weeks, starting at initiation or delayed by 1-2 weeks after start of therapy. Simple/Complex Absence Seizures: Initial: 15mg/kg/day. Titrate: Increase weekly by 5-10mg/kg/day until optimal response is achieved. Max: 60mg/kg/day. Conversion from Depakote: Administer qd using a dose 8-20% higher than total daily dose of Depakote. Refer to PI for dose conversion. If total Depakote dose cannot be directly converted, consider increasing Depakote total daily dose to next higher dosage before converting to appropriate total daily Depakote ER dose.

HOW SUPPLIED: Tab, Extended-Release: 250mg, 500mg

CONTRAINDICATIONS: Hepatic disease, significant hepatic dysfunction, known urea cycle disorder (UCD). Mitochondrial disorders caused by mutations in mitochondrial POLG (eg, Alpers-Huttenlocher syndrome) and children <2 yrs of age who are suspected of having a POLG-related disorder. Prophylaxis of migraine headaches in pregnant women.

WARNINGS/PRECAUTIONS: D/C immediately if significant hepatic dysfunction (suspected or apparent) occurs. Reversible and irreversible cerebral and cerebellar atrophy reported; routinely monitor motor and cognitive functions and evaluate continued use in the presence of suspected or apparent signs of brain atrophy. Cerebral atrophy reported in children exposed in utero. Increased risk of suicidal thoughts or behavior reported; monitor for the emergence/worsening of depression, suicidal thoughts or behavior, thoughts of self-harm, and/or any unusual changes in mood or behavior. Dose-related thrombocytopenia reported; monitor platelet and coagulation parameters prior to therapy and periodically thereafter. Hyperammonemic encephalopathy reported in UCD patients; d/c and initiate treatment if symptoms develop. Prior to initiation of therapy, evaluate for UCD in high-risk patients (eg, history of unexplained encephalopathy, coma, etc.). Hyperammonemia reported and may be present despite normal LFTs. Measure ammonia levels if unexplained lethargy, vomiting, or mental status changes occur. Caution in the elderly; monitor fluid/nutritional intake, and for dehydration and somnolence. Altered thyroid function tests and urine ketone tests reported. Avoid abrupt discontinuation. May stimulate replication of HIV and cytomegalovirus. Multiorgan hypersensitivity reactions (rare) and hypothermia reported. Medication residue in stool reported; checked valproate levels and monitor clinical condition, and consider alternative treatment if clinically indicated.

ADVERSE REACTIONS: Hepatotoxicity, pancreatitis, N/V, somnolence, dizziness, abdominal pain, dyspepsia, rash, diarrhea, tremor, weight gain, back pain, alopecia, headache.

INTERACTIONS: Drugs that affect the level of expression of hepatic enzymes (eg, phenytoin, carbamazepine, phenobarbital, primidone) may increase valproate clearance. Concomitant use with aspirin decreases protein binding and inhibits metabolism of valproate. Carbapenem antibiotics (eg, ertapenem, imipenem, meropenem) may reduce serum concentrations to subtherapeutic levels, resulting in loss of seizure control. Rifampin increases oral clearance and may require valproate dosage adjustment. Concomitant use with felbamate leads to an increase in valproate C_{max} and may require decrease in valproate dosage. Reduces the clearance of amitriptyline, nortriptyline, and lorazepam. Induces metabolism of carbamazepine. Inhibits metabolism of diazepam, ethosuximide, phenobarbital, and phenytoin; monitor drug serum concentrations and adjust dose appropriately. Breakthrough seizures reported with concomitant use with phenytoin. Use with clonazepam may induce absence status in patients with absence seizures. Increases $T_{1/2}$ of lamotrigine; serious skin reactions reported. Concomitant use with topiramate associated with hyperammonemia, with or without encephalopathy, and hypothermia. Increased trough plasma levels reported with chlorpromazine. May displace protein-bound tolbutamide and warfarin; monitor coagulation tests when coadministered with warfarin. May decrease clearance of zidovudine in HIV-seropositive patients.

PREGNANCY: Category D (for epilepsy and for manic episodes with bipolar disorder) or X (for prophylaxis of migraine headaches), caution in nursing.

MECHANISM OF ACTION: Anticonvulsant; has not been established. Suggested to increase brain concentrations of gamma-aminobutyric acid.

PHARMACOKINETICS: Absorption: Bioavailability (90%); T_{max}=4-17 hrs (median). **Distribution:** Found in breast milk, CSF. (Free valproate) V_d=92L/1.73m^2. (Total valproate) V_d=11L/1.73m^2. **Metabolism:** Liver; glucuronidation, mitochondrial β-oxidation. **Elimination:** Urine (<3% unchanged); $T_{1/2}$=9-16 hrs.

NURSING CONSIDERATIONS

Assessment: Assess for hepatic dysfunction, history of hepatic disease, UCD, pancreatitis, history of hypersensitivity, mitochondrial disorders caused by mutations in mitochondrial POLG and children <2 yrs of age who are suspected of having a POLG-related disorders, pregnancy/nursing status, other diseases/conditions where treatment is contraindicated or cautioned, and possible drug interactions. Assess LFTs, CBC with platelet counts, and coagulation parameters.

Monitoring: Monitor for hypersensitivity reactions, multiorgan hypersensitivity reactions, pancreatitis, hepatotoxicity, hyperammonemia, hypothermia, drug-induced acute liver failure, acute liver injury, brain atrophy, emergence/worsening of depression, suicidality or unusual changes in behavior, medication residue in stool, and other adverse reactions. Monitor LFTs frequently, especially during first 6 months. Monitor fluid/nutritional intake, ammonia levels, CBC with plate-lets, and coagulation parameters in patients on warfarin.

Patient Counseling: Inform to take ud. Inform pregnant women and women of childbearing potential about the risk in pregnancy (eg, birth defects, decreased IQ); advise to use effective contraception while on therapy and counsel about alternative therapeutic options. Advise to read medication guide. Instruct to notify physician if pregnant or intending to become pregnant. Encourage patients to enroll in North American Antiepileptic Drug Pregnancy Registry. Advise to notify physician if depression, suicidal thoughts, behavior, or thoughts about self-harm emerge. Counsel about signs/symptoms of pancreatitis, hepatotoxicity, hyperammonemia, or hyperam-monemic encephalopathy; advise to notify physician if any symptoms or adverse effects occur. Advise not to engage in hazardous activities (eg, driving/operating machinery) until the effects of the drug are known. Instruct that a fever associated with other organ system involvement (eg, rash, lymphadenopathy) may be drug-related; instruct to report to physician. Instruct patients to notify their physician if medication residue is noticed in the stool.

Administration: Oral route. Swallow whole; do not crush or chew. **Storage:** 25°C (77°F); excur-sions permitted to 15-30°C (59-86°F).

DEPO-MEDROL   RX
methylprednisolone acetate (Pharmacia & Upjohn)

THERAPEUTIC CLASS: Glucocorticoid

INDICATIONS: Steroid-responsive disorders when oral therapy is not feasible.

DOSAGE: *Adults:* Individualize dose. Local Effect: Rheumatoid Arthritis/Osteoarthritis: Large Joint: 20-80mg. Medium Joint: 10-40mg. Small Joint: 4-10mg. Administer intra-articularly into synovial space. In chronic cases, may repeat inj at intervals ranging from 1-5 weeks or more, depending on relief. Ganglion/Tendinitis/Epicondylitis: 4-30mg. May repeat inj if necessary in recurrent or chronic conditions. Dermatologic Conditions: 20-60mg. In large lesions, may distribute 20-40mg dose by repeated inj (usually 1-4 inj). Systemic Effect: Temporary Substitute for Oral Therapy: Single IM inj during each 24-hr period equal to the total daily oral methylpred-nisolone dose. Prolonged Effect: Single IM inj equal to the weekly oral methylprednisolone dose. Adrenogenital Syndrome: 40mg IM single dose every 2 weeks. Rheumatoid Arthritis: Maint: 40-120mg IM weekly. Dermatologic Lesions: Usual: 40-120mg IM weekly for 1-4 weeks. Acute Severe Dermatitis (Poison Ivy): 80-120mg IM single dose. Chronic Contact Dermatitis: May repeat inj at 5- to 10-day intervals. Seborrheic Dermatitis: 80mg IM weekly. Asthma/Allergic Rhinitis: 80-120mg IM. If signs of stress are associated with the condition being treated, increase dose of sus. If a rapid hormonal effect of max intensity is required, the IV administration of highly soluble methylprednisolone sodium succinate is indicated. Acute Exacerbations of Multiple Sclerosis: 160mg/day for 1 week, then 64mg qod for 1 month. Elderly: Start at lower end of dosing range. *Pediatrics:* Individualize dose. Initial: 0.11-1.6mg/kg/day.

HOW SUPPLIED: Inj: 20mg/mL, 40mg/mL, 80mg/mL

CONTRAINDICATIONS: Idiopathic thrombocytopenic purpura (IM preparations), intrathecal administration, systemic fungal infections (except as an intra-articular inj for localized joint con-ditions), premature infants (formulations preserved with benzyl alcohol).

WARNINGS/PRECAUTIONS: May result in dermal and/or subdermal changes forming depres-sions in the skin at inj site. Multiple small inj into the area of lesion should be made whenever possible; caution against inj or leakage into dermis during intra-articular and IM inj. Avoid inj into deltoid muscle or into an infected site/previously infected joint. Anaphylactoid reactions may occur. May need to increase dose before, during, and after stressful situations. High systemic doses should not be used to treat traumatic brain injury. May cause elevation of BP, salt/water retention, and increased excretion of K+ and Ca2+; dietary salt restriction and K+ supplementation may be necessary. Caution with recent myocardial infarction; associated with left ventricular free wall rupture in these patients. Monitor for hypothalamic-pituitary-adrenal (HPA) axis suppres-sion, Cushing's syndrome, and hyperglycemia with chronic use. May produce reversible HPA-axis suppression with potential for glucocorticosteroid insufficiency after withdrawal of treatment; reduce dose gradually. May increase susceptibility to, mask signs of, or cause new infections; may exacerbate systemic fungal infections. Latent disease due to certain pathogens may be activated or intercurrent infections exacerbated. Rule out latent or active amebiasis before initiating therapy. Caution with *Strongyloides* infestation, latent tuberculosis (TB) or tuberculin reactivity, ocular herpes simplex, congestive heart failure (CHF), and renal insufficiency. May cause more serious/fatal course of chickenpox and measles. May produce posterior subcapsular cataracts, glaucoma with possible damage to optic nerves, and enhance the establishment of secondary ocular infections; systemic corticosteroids not recommended in the treatment of optic neuritis. Not for use in active ocular herpes simplex or in cerebral malaria. Sensitive to heat; should not be autoclaved when it is desirable to sterilize the exterior of the vial. Kaposi's sarcoma reported. Metabolic clearance is decreased in hypothyroidism and increased in hyperthyroidism; changes in thyroid status may necessitate dose adjustment. Caution with active or latent peptic ulcers, diverticulitis, fresh intestinal anastomoses, and nonspecific ulcerative colitis; may increase risk of perforation. Signs of peritoneal irritation following GI perforation may be minimal/absent. Intra-articularly injected corticosteroids may be systemically absorbed. Appropriate examination of any joint fluid present is necessary to exclude a septic process; institute appropriate antimicrobial therapy if septic arthritis occurs and diagnosis confirmed. May decrease bone formation and increase bone resorption, and may lead to inhibition of bone growth in pediatric patients and development of osteoporosis at any age; caution with increased risk of osteoporosis. Acute myopathy reported with high doses, most often in patients with disorders of neuromuscular transmission (eg, myasthenia gravis). Elevation of creatine kinase (CK) or intraocular pressure (IOP) may occur; monitor IOP if used >6 weeks. Psychic derangements may appear and existing emotional instability or psychotic tendencies may be aggravated. Caution in elderly. Formulations with preservative contain benzyl alcohol, which is potentially toxic to neural tissue. Excessive amounts of benzyl alcohol have been associated with toxicity, particularly in neonates.

ADVERSE REACTIONS: Allergic reactions, bradycardia, cardiac arrest, acne, allergic dermatitis, decreased carbohydrate/glucose tolerance, glycosuria, fluid retention, abdominal distention, bowel/bladder dysfunction, convulsions, depression, exophthalmoses, glaucoma, muscle weakness.

INTERACTIONS: Aminoglutethimide may lead to a loss of corticosteroid-induced adrenal suppression. May develop hypokalemia with K^+-depleting agents (eg, amphotericin B, diuretics). Cardiac enlargement and CHF reported following concomitant use of amphotericin B and hydrocortisone. Macrolide antibiotics may cause a significant decrease in clearance and cholestyramine may increase clearance. Concomitant use with anticholinesterase agents may produce severe weakness in patients with myasthenia gravis; d/c anticholinesterase agents at least 24 hrs before initiating therapy. May inhibit response to warfarin; frequently monitor coagulation indices. May increase blood glucose levels; dosage adjustments of antidiabetic agents may be required. May decrease serum levels of isoniazid. Increased activity of both drugs may occur with cyclosporine; convulsions reported with concurrent use. May increase risk of arrhythmias with digitalis glycosides. Estrogens, including oral contraceptives, may decrease hepatic metabolism and enhance effect. Drugs that induce CYP3A4 (eg, barbiturates, phenytoin, carbamazepine) may enhance metabolism and require corticosteroid dosage increase. Drugs that inhibit CYP3A4 (eg, ketoconazole, erythromycin, troleandomycin) may increase plasma levels. Ketoconazole may increase risk of corticosteroid side effects. Aspirin (ASA) or other NSAIDs may increase risk of GI side effects; caution with ASA in hypoprothrombinemia patients. May increase clearance of salicylates. May suppress reactions to skin tests. Administration of live or live, attenuated vaccines is contraindicated in patients receiving immunosuppressive doses. Killed or inactivated vaccines may be administered, although response is unpredictable. Acute myopathy reported with neuromuscular blocking drugs (eg, pancuronium).

PREGNANCY: Category C, not for use in nursing.

MECHANISM OF ACTION: Glucocorticoid; causes profound and varied metabolic effects and modifies the body's immune responses to diverse stimuli.

PHARMACOKINETICS: Distribution: Found in breast milk.

NURSING CONSIDERATIONS

Assessment: Assess for hypersensitivity to drug, traumatic brain injury, cerebral malaria, optic neuritis, ocular herpes simplex, CHF, renal insufficiency, systemic fungal infections, active or latent peptic ulcer, diverticulitis, ulcerative colitis, any other conditions where treatment is contraindicated or cautioned, pregnancy/nursing status, and possible drug interactions.

Monitoring: Monitor for anaphylactoid reactions, dermal and/or subdermal changes, cataracts, glaucoma, bone growth/development (in pediatric patients), osteoporosis, intestinal perforation, infections, psychic derangements, Kaposi's sarcoma, CK/IOP elevation, and other adverse reactions. Monitor for HPA-axis suppression, Cushing's syndrome, and hyperglycemia with chronic use. Frequently monitor coagulation indices with warfarin.

Patient Counseling: Warn not to d/c abruptly or without medical supervision. Instruct to seek medical advice at once if fever or other signs of infection develop. Warn to avoid exposure to chickenpox or measles; advise to report immediately if exposed.

Administration: IM/Intra-articular/Soft tissue or intralesional route. Do not dilute or mix with other sol. Refer to PI for preparation and administration instructions. **Storage:** 20-25°C (68-77°F).

DEPO-PROVERA   RX
medroxyprogesterone acetate (Pharmacia & Upjohn)

THERAPEUTIC CLASS: Progestogen

INDICATIONS: Adjunctive therapy and palliative treatment of inoperable, recurrent, and metastatic endometrial or renal carcinoma.

DOSAGE: *Adults:* Initial: 400-1000mg/week IM. If improvement is noted within a few weeks or months and the disease appears stabilized, may be possible to maintain improvement with as little as 400mg/month.

HOW SUPPLIED: Inj: 400mg/mL [2.5mL]

CONTRAINDICATIONS: Known or suspected pregnancy or as a diagnostic test for pregnancy, undiagnosed vaginal bleeding, known or suspected malignancy of the breast, active thrombophlebitis, current or past history of thromboembolic disorders or cerebral vascular disease, liver dysfunction or disease.

WARNINGS/PRECAUTIONS: D/C if early manifestations of thrombotic disorder (thrombophlebitis, cerebrovascular disorder, pulmonary embolism, retinal thrombosis) occurs or suspected. D/C, pending examination, if there is a sudden partial or complete loss of vision, or if sudden onset of proptosis, diplopia, or migraine. If examination reveals papilledema or retinal vascular lesions, withdraw therapy. Avoid contamination of multidose vials. Perform annual history and physical examination. Physical examination should include special reference to BP, breasts, abdomen and pelvic organs, including cervical cytology and relevant lab tests. In cases of undiagnosed, persistent, or recurrent vaginal bleeding, perform adequate diagnostic measures to rule out malignancies. Monitor women who have a family history of breast cancer and those who develop breast nodules. May cause fluid retention; caution with epilepsy, migraine, asthma, and cardiac/renal dysfunction. Perform adequate diagnostic measures in cases of breakthrough bleeding. Caution with history of psychic depression; d/c if depression recurs to a serious degree. May mask the onset of climacteric. Use with estrogen may produce adverse effects on carbohydrate and lipid metabolism. Decrease in glucose tolerance reported in patients on estrogen-progestin combination treatment; caution in diabetic patients on estrogen-progestin combination treatment. May affect certain endocrine, LFTs, and blood components in lab tests.

ADVERSE REACTIONS: Menstrual irregularities, nervousness, dizziness, edema, weight gain/loss and cervical erosion/secretion changes, cholestatic jaundice, breast tenderness, rash, alopecia, hirsutism, depression, pyrexia, fatigue, insomnia.

INTERACTIONS: Decreased levels with aminoglutethimide.

PREGNANCY: Contraindicated in pregnancy, safety not known in nursing.

MECHANISM OF ACTION: Progestogen; inhibits secretion of pituitary gonadotropins, preventing follicular maturation and ovulation. When given parenterally and in recommended doses, transforms proliferative endometrium into secretory endometrium in women with adequate endogenous estrogen.

PHARMACOKINETICS: Distribution: Found in breast milk.

NURSING CONSIDERATIONS

Assessment: Assess for drug hypersensitivity and for any other conditions where treatment is contraindicated or cautioned. Assess pregnancy/nursing status and for possible drug interactions.

Monitoring: Monitor for thrombotic disorders, loss of vision, proptosis, diplopia, migraine, papilledema, retinal vascular lesions, breakthrough bleeding, recurrence of depression, fluid retention, and other adverse reactions. Perform annual history and physical examination. If undiagnosed, persistent or recurrent abnormal vaginal bleeding occurs, take appropriate measures to rule out malignancy. Monitor for adverse effects on carbohydrate and lipid metabolism if used with estrogen therapy.

Patient Counseling: Inform of risks/benefits of treatment. Instruct to notify physician if pregnant, pregnancy occurs, or if any adverse reactions occur while on treatment.

Administration: IM route. Cleanse the vial top prior to aspiration of contents of multidose vial.
Storage: 20-25°C (68-77°F) in upright position.

DEPO-PROVERA CONTRACEPTIVE INJECTION   RX
medroxyprogesterone acetate (Pharmacia & Upjohn)

> May lose significant bone mineral density (BMD); greater with increasing duration of use and may not be completely reversible. Unknown if use during adolescence or early adulthood will reduce peak bone mass and increase risk for osteoporotic fractures in later life. Should not be used as long-term birth control (eg, >2 yrs) unless other birth control methods are considered inadequate.

THERAPEUTIC CLASS: Progestin contraceptive

INDICATIONS: Prevention of pregnancy.

DOSAGE: *Adults:* Usual: 150mg deep IM every 3 months (13 weeks) in the gluteal or deltoid muscle. Dosage does not need to be adjusted for body weight. Give the 1st inj only during the first 5 days of a normal menstrual period, only within the first 5 days postpartum if not breastfeeding, or only at the 6th postpartum week if exclusively nursing. If the interval between inj is >13 weeks, determine that patient is not pregnant before administering. Switching from Other Methods of Contraception: Give in a manner that ensures continuous contraceptive coverage based upon the mechanism of action of both methods (eg, switching from oral contraceptives should have the 1st inj on the day after the last active tab or at the latest, on the day following the final inactive tab). *Pediatrics:* Postmenarchal Adolescents: Usual: 150mg deep IM every 3 months (13 weeks) in the gluteal or deltoid muscle. Dosage does not need to be adjusted for body weight. Give the 1st inj only during the first 5 days of a normal menstrual period, only within the first 5 days postpartum if not breastfeeding, or only at the 6th postpartum week if exclusively nursing. If the interval between inj is >13 weeks, determine that patient is not pregnant before administering. Switching from Other Methods of Contraception: Give in a manner that ensures continuous contraceptive coverage based upon the mechanism of action of both methods (eg, switching from oral contraceptives should have the 1st inj on the day after the last active tab or at the latest, on the day following the final inactive tab).

HOW SUPPLIED: Inj: 150mg/mL [1mL, vial, prefilled syringe]

CONTRAINDICATIONS: Known or suspected pregnancy or as a diagnostic test for pregnancy, active thrombophlebitis, current or past history of thromboembolic disorders, cerebral vascular disease, known or suspected malignancy of the breast, significant liver disease, undiagnosed vaginal bleeding.

WARNINGS/PRECAUTIONS: May pose additional risk of BMD loss in patients with risk factors for osteoporosis (eg, metabolic bone disease, chronic alcohol and/or tobacco use, anorexia nervosa, strong family history of osteoporosis, chronic use of drugs that can reduce bone mass [eg, anticonvulsants, corticosteroids]); consider other birth control methods. Serious thrombotic events reported; d/c if thrombosis develops while on therapy unless there are no other acceptable options for birth control. Do not readminister therapy pending examination if there is sudden partial/complete loss of vision, or sudden onset of proptosis/diplopia/migraine; if examination reveals papilledema or retinal vascular lesions, do not readminister. May increase risk of breast cancer. Monitor women with family history of breast cancer or with breast nodules carefully. Be alert to possibility of ectopic pregnancy in patients who become pregnant or complain of severe abdominal pain. Anaphylaxis/anaphylactoid reactions reported; institute emergency medical treatment if an anaphylactic reaction occurs. D/C if jaundice or acute/chronic disturbances of liver function develop; do not resume use until markers of liver function return to normal and medroxyprogesterone acetate causation has been excluded. Convulsions and weight gain reported. Monitor patients who have history of depression; do not readminister if depression recurs. May cause disruption of menstrual bleeding patterns (eg, amenorrhea, irregular or unpredictable bleeding/spotting, prolonged spotting/bleeding, heavy bleeding); rule out possibility of organic pathology if abnormal bleeding persists or is severe, and institute appropriate treatment. Decrease in glucose tolerance reported; monitor diabetic patients carefully. May cause fluid retention; monitor patients with conditions that might be influenced by this condition (eg, epilepsy, migraine, asthma, cardiac/renal dysfunction). Return to ovulation and fertility after discontinuation of therapy may be delayed. Does not protect against HIV infection and other sexually transmitted diseases (STDs). Annual exam recommended for a BP check and for other indicated healthcare. May change results of some lab tests (eg, coagulation factors, lipids, glucose tolerance, binding proteins).

ADVERSE REACTIONS: BMD loss, menstrual irregularities, increased weight, abdominal pain/discomfort, dizziness, headache, asthenia/fatigue, nervousness, decreased libido, nausea, leg cramps.

INTERACTIONS: Drugs or herbal products that induce enzymes, including CYP3A4 that metabolize contraceptive hormones (eg, barbiturates, bosentan, carbamazepine, felbamate, griseofulvin, oxcarbazepine, phenytoin, rifampin, St. John's wort, topiramate) may decrease levels and effectiveness; use additional contraception or a different method of contraception. HIV protease inhibitors and non-nucleoside reverse transcriptase inhibitors may alter levels. Pregnancy reported with antibiotics.

PREGNANCY: Contraindicated in pregnancy, safety not known in nursing.

MECHANISM OF ACTION: Progestin contraceptive; inhibits secretion of gonadotropins which, in turn, prevents follicular maturation and ovulation, resulting in endometrial thinning.

PHARMACOKINETICS: Absorption: C_{max}=1-7ng/mL, T_{max}=3 weeks. **Distribution:** Plasma protein binding (86%); found in breast milk. **Metabolism:** Liver (extensive) via CYP450 enzymes; reduction, loss of the acetyl group and hydroxylation. **Elimination:** Urine; $T_{1/2}$=50 days.

NURSING CONSIDERATIONS

Assessment: Assess for active thrombophlebitis, current/past history of thromboembolic disorders or cerebral vascular disease, known or suspected malignancy of the breast, drug hypersensitivity, significant liver disease, undiagnosed vaginal bleeding, osteoporosis risk factors, family history of breast cancer, breast nodules, history of depression, diabetes mellitus (DM), conditions that may be influenced by fluid retention (eg, epilepsy, migraine, asthma, cardiac/renal dysfunction), pregnancy/nursing status, and possible drug interactions.

Monitoring: Monitor for thrombosis, loss of BMD, breast cancer, sudden/partial loss of vision, proptosis, diplopia, migraine, papilledema, retinal vascular lesions, anaphylaxis/anaphylactoid reactions, jaundice or acute/chronic disturbances in liver function, ectopic pregnancy, convulsions, weight gain, fluid retention, disruption of menstrual bleeding patterns, and other adverse reactions. Monitor patients with DM. Monitor for recurrence of depression with history of depression. Perform annual exam for a BP check and for other indicated healthcare.

Patient Counseling: Counsel about the risks/benefits of therapy. Advise at the beginning of treatment that the menstrual cycle may be disrupted and that irregular and unpredictable bleeding or spotting may occur; inform that this usually decreases to the point of amenorrhea as treatment continues without other therapy being required. Inform that drug does not protect against HIV infection and other STDs. Counsel to use a back-up method or alternative method of contraception when enzyme inducers are used with the drug. Advise to take adequate Ca^{2+} and vitamin D. Advise to have a yearly visit with healthcare provider for a BP check and for other indicated healthcare.

Administration: IM route. Shake vigorously before use. **Storage:** 20-25°C (68-77°F). Store vials upright.

Dᴇᴘᴏ-Tᴇsᴛᴏsᴛᴇʀᴏɴᴇ
testosterone cypionate (Pharmacia & Upjohn)

THERAPEUTIC CLASS: Androgen

INDICATIONS: Testosterone replacement in males with congenital or acquired primary hypogonadism or hypogonadotropic hypogonadism.

DOSAGE: *Adults:* Individualize dose. Give 50-400mg IM deep in the gluteal muscle every 2-4 weeks. Consider chronological and skeletal ages in determining initial dose and titration. Adjust according to response and adverse reactions.
Pediatrics: ≥12 Yrs: Individualize dose. Give 50-400mg IM deep in the gluteal muscle every 2-4 weeks. Consider chronological and skeletal ages in determining initial dose and titration. Adjust according to response and adverse reactions.

HOW SUPPLIED: Inj: 100mg/mL [10mL], 200mg/mL [1mL, 10mL]

CONTRAINDICATIONS: Serious cardiac, hepatic or renal disease. Males with carcinoma of the breast or known or suspected carcinoma of the prostate gland. Women who are or may become pregnant.

WARNINGS/PRECAUTIONS: May cause hypercalcemia in immobilized patients; d/c if this occurs. May develop hepatic adenomas, hepatocellular carcinoma, and peliosis hepatis with prolonged use of high doses. Caution in elderly; increased risk of prostatic hypertrophy and prostatic carcinoma. May develop gynecomastia. May accelerate bone maturation without linear growth. D/C with appearance of acute urethral obstruction, priapism, excessive sexual stimulation, or oligospermia; restart at lower doses. Caution with BPH and males with delayed puberty. Do not use interchangeably with testosterone propionate, for enhancement of athletic performance, or as IV. Contains benzyl alcohol.

ADVERSE REACTIONS: Gynecomastia, excessive frequency/duration of penile erections, male pattern baldness, increased/decreased libido, oligospermia, hirsutism, acne, nausea, hypercholesterolemia, clotting factor suppression, polycythemia, altered LFTs, priapism, anxiety, depression.

INTERACTIONS: May increase sensitivity to oral anticoagulants. Increased levels of oxyphenbutazone. May decrease insulin requirements in diabetic patients.

PREGNANCY: Category X, not for use in nursing.

MECHANISM OF ACTION: Endogenous androgen; responsible for normal growth and development of male sex organs and for maintenance of secondary sex characteristics.

PHARMACOKINETICS: Metabolism: Liver. **Elimination:** Urine (90%), feces (6%); $T_{1/2}$=8 days.

NURSING CONSIDERATIONS

Assessment: Assess males for known drug hypersensitivity, carcinoma of the breast, known or suspected carcinoma of the prostate gland, cardiac/hepatic/renal disease, delayed puberty, BPH, and possible drug interactions.

Monitoring: Periodically monitor Hgb and Hct. Monitor for signs/symptoms of hypersensitivity reactions, edema with/without congestive heart failure, gynecomastia, and hypercalcemia. Assess bone development every 6 months in males with delayed puberty.

Patient Counseling: Instruct to report to physician if N/V, changes in skin color, ankle swelling, or too frequent or persistent penile erections occur.

Administration: IM route. **Storage:** 20-25°C (68-77°F). Protect from light.

DETROL LA

RX

tolterodine tartrate (Pharmacia & Upjohn)

OTHER BRAND NAMES: Detrol (Pharmacia & Upjohn)

THERAPEUTIC CLASS: Muscarinic antagonist

INDICATIONS: Treatment of overactive bladder with symptoms of urge urinary incontinence, urgency, and frequency.

DOSAGE: *Adults:* (Cap, ER) Usual: 4mg qd. May be lowered to 2mg qd based on response and tolerability. Mild to Moderate Hepatic Impairment (Child-Pugh Class A or B)/Severe Renal Impairment (CrCl 10-30mL/min)/With Potent CYP3A4 Inhibitors (eg, ketoconazole, clarithromycin, ritonavir): Usual: 2mg qd. (Tab) Usual: 2mg bid. May be lowered to 1mg bid based on response and tolerability. Significantly Reduced Hepatic or Renal Function/With Potent CYP3A4 Inhibitors: Usual: 1mg bid.

HOW SUPPLIED: Cap, Extended-Release (ER): (Detrol LA) 2mg, 4mg; Tab: (Detrol) 1mg, 2mg

CONTRAINDICATIONS: Urinary/gastric retention, uncontrolled narrow-angle glaucoma, hypersensitivity to fesoterodine fumarate ER tab.

WARNINGS/PRECAUTIONS: Anaphylaxis/angioedema requiring hospitalization and emergency treatment occurred with 1st or subsequent doses; d/c and provide appropriate therapy if difficulty in breathing, upper airway obstruction, or fall in BP occurs. Risk of urinary retention; caution in patients with clinically significant bladder outflow obstruction. Risk of gastric retention; caution in patients with GI obstructive disorders (eg, pyloric stenosis). Caution with decreased GI motility (eg, intestinal atony), myasthenia gravis, known history of QT prolongation, hepatic/renal impairment, and in patients being treated for narrow-angle glaucoma. CNS anticholinergic effects (eg, dizziness, somnolence) reported; may impair physical/mental abilities. Monitor for signs of anticholinergic CNS effects (particularly after beginning treatment and increasing the dose); consider dose reduction or d/c if such effects occur. (Cap, ER) Not recommended with severe hepatic impairment (Child-Pugh Class C) or with CrCl <10mL/min.

ADVERSE REACTIONS: Dry mouth, dizziness, headache, abdominal pain, constipation.

INTERACTIONS: Caution with Class IA (eg, quinidine, procainamide) or Class III (eg, amiodarone, sotalol) antiarrhythmics. May aggravate dementia symptoms when initiating therapy in patients taking cholinesterase inhibitors. Increased concentrations with ketoconazole or other potent CYP3A4 inhibitors (eg, itraconazole, miconazole, clarithromycin). Increased levels with fluoxetine reported with immediate release tolterodine. May increase the frequency and/or severity of anticholinergic CNS effects with other anticholinergic (antimuscarinic) agents.

PREGNANCY: Category C, not for use in nursing.

MECHANISM OF ACTION: Muscarinic receptor antagonist; competitive antagonist of acetylcholine at postganglionic muscarinic receptors mediating urinary bladder contraction and salivation via cholinergic muscarinic receptors.

PHARMACOKINETICS: Absorption: Administration of variable doses resulted in different parameters in extensive metabolizers (EM) and poor metabolizers (PM) of CYP2D6. (Tab) Rapid. **Distribution:** Plasma protein binding (96.3%); (IV) V_d=113L. **Metabolism:** Liver (extensive); oxidation to 5-hydroxymethyl tolterodine (active metabolite) via CYP2D6; dealkylation via CYP3A4 (PM). **Elimination:** Urine (77%), feces (17%). (Tab) Single Dose: EM: $T_{1/2}$=2 hrs; PM: $T_{1/2}$=6.5 hrs. (Cap, ER) Single Dose: EM: $T_{1/2}$=8.4 hrs.

NURSING CONSIDERATIONS

Assessment: Assess for hypersensitivity to the drug or fesoterodine fumarate, urinary/gastric retention, bladder outflow obstruction, GI obstructive disorders, decreased GI motility, narrow-angle glaucoma, myasthenia gravis, history of QT prolongation, hepatic/renal impairment, pregnancy/nursing status, and possible drug interactions.

Monitoring: Monitor for anaphylaxis, angioedema, difficulty breathing, upper airway obstruction, fall in BP, urinary retention, gastric retention, CNS anticholinergic effects, QT prolongation, hypersensitivity reactions, and other adverse reactions.

Patient Counseling: Inform patients that drug may produce blurred vision, dizziness, or drowsiness. Advise to exercise caution against potentially dangerous activities until drug's effects have been determined.

Administration: Oral route. (Cap, ER) Take with water and swallow whole. **Storage:** (Tab): 25°C (77°F); excursions permitted to 15-30°C (59-86°F). (Cap, ER): 20-25°C (68-77°F); excursions permitted to 15-30°C (59-86°F). Protect from light.

DEXAMETHASONE OPHTHALMIC/OTIC RX
dexamethasone sodium phosphate (Bausch & Lomb)

THERAPEUTIC CLASS: Glucocorticoid

INDICATIONS: Treatment of steroid responsive inflammatory conditions of the palpebral and bulbar conjunctiva, cornea, and anterior segment of the globe, such as allergic conjunctivitis, acne rosacea, superficial punctate keratitis, herpes zoster keratitis, iritis, cyclitis, selected infective conjunctivitis when the inherent hazard of steroid use is accepted to obtain an advisable diminution in edema and inflammation. Treatment of corneal injury from chemical/thermal burns, or penetration of foreign bodies. Treatment of steroid responsive inflammatory conditions of the external auditory meatus, such as allergic otitis externa, selected purulent and nonpurulent infective otitis externa when the hazard of steroid use is accepted to obtain an advisable diminution in edema and inflammation.

DOSAGE: *Adults:* Eye: Initial: Instill 1 or 2 drops into the conjunctival sac qh (daytime) and q2h (nighttime). Titrate: Reduce dose to 1 drop q4h when a favorable response is observed. Maint: 1 drop tid or qid may suffice to control symptoms. Ear: Clean the aural canal thoroughly and sponge dry. Initial: Instill 3 or 4 drops directly into the aural canal bid or tid. Titrate: Reduce dose gradually and eventually d/c when a favorable response is obtained. If preferred, the aural canal may be packed with a gauze wick saturated with sol. Keep the wick moist with the preparation and remove from the ear after 12-24 hrs. May repeat PRN. Duration will vary with type of lesion and may extend from a few days to several weeks, according to therapeutic response. Relapses usually respond to retreatment.

HOW SUPPLIED: Sol: 0.1% [5mL]

CONTRAINDICATIONS: Epithelial herpes simplex keratitis (dendritic keratitis), acute infectious stages of vaccinia/varicella and many other viral diseases of the cornea and conjunctiva, mycobacterial infection of the eye, fungal diseases of ocular/auricular structures, and perforation of a drum membrane.

WARNINGS/PRECAUTIONS: Prolonged use may result in ocular HTN and/or glaucoma, with damage to the optic nerve, defects in visual acuity and fields of vision, and posterior subcapsular cataract formation. Persistent fungal infections of the cornea or suppression of the host response and increased hazard of secondary ocular infections may occur with prolonged use. May cause perforations in diseases causing thinning of the cornea or sclera. May mask infection or enhance existing infection in acute purulent conditions of the eye or ear. Routinely monitor intraocular pressure (IOP) if used for ≥10 days. Caution with herpes simplex; periodic slit-lamp microscopy is essential. Contains sodium bisulfite; allergic-type reactions may occur. Bacterial keratitis reported with the use of multiple dose containers contaminated by patients with concurrent corneal disease or disruption of ocular epithelial surface.

ADVERSE REACTIONS: Glaucoma with optic nerve damage, visual acuity and field defects, posterior subcapsular cataract formation, secondary ocular infection, globe perforation.

PREGNANCY: Category C, not for use in nursing.

MECHANISM OF ACTION: Glucocorticoid; not established. Suppresses the inflammatory response to a variety of agents and probably delays or slows healing.

NURSING CONSIDERATIONS

Assessment: Assess for hypersensitivity to the drug (including sulfites), diseases causing thinning of the cornea/sclera, acute purulent conditions of the eye/ear, herpes simplex, pregnancy/nursing status, and any other conditions where treatment is cautioned or contraindicated.

Monitoring: Monitor for allergic-type reactions, ocular HTN, glaucoma, optic nerve damage, defects in visual acuity and fields of vision, cataract formation, secondary ocular infections, fungal infections of the cornea, bacterial keratitis, and other adverse reactions. Routinely monitor IOP if used for ≥10 days.

Patient Counseling: Instruct to avoid allowing tip of the dispensing container to contact the eye or surrounding structures. Inform that ocular preparations, if handled improperly, can become contaminated by common bacteria known to cause ocular infections. Inform that serious damage to the eye and subsequent loss of vision may result from using contaminated sol. Advise to seek physician's advice immediately concerning the continued use of the present multidose container if an intercurrent ocular condition (eg, trauma, ocular surgery/infection) develops. Instruct patients wearing soft contact lenses to wait at least 15 min after instilling the sol before inserting their lenses.

Administration: Ocular/otic route. **Storage:** 15-25°C (59-77°F).

DEXAMETHASONE ORAL

RX

dexamethasone (Various)

THERAPEUTIC CLASS: Glucocorticoid

INDICATIONS: Treatment of steroid-responsive disorders.

DOSAGE: *Adults:* Individualize dose. Initial: 0.75-9mg/day depending on disease. Maint: Decrease in small amounts at appropriate time intervals to lowest effective dose. May need to increase dose for a period of time in stressful situations. Upon discontinuation after long-term therapy, withdraw gradually. Cushing's Syndrome Test: 1mg at 11pm; draw blood at 8 am next morning. Or, 0.5mg q6h for 48 hrs. Test to Distinguish Cushing's Syndrome Due to Pituitary Adrenocorticotropic Hormone (ACTH) Excess from Cushing's Syndrome Due to Other Causes: 2mg q6h for 48 hrs; obtain 24-hr urine collections. (Elixir) Less Severe Diseases: Doses <0.75mg may suffice. Severe Diseases: >9mg may be required. D/C and transfer to other therapy, if satisfactory clinical response does not occur. (Sol/Tab) Acute Exacerbations of Multiple Sclerosis: 30mg/day for 1 week, then 4-12mg qod for 1 month. Acute, Self-Limited Allergic Disorders/Acute Exacerbations of Chronic Allergic Disorders: Day 1: 1 or 2 mL of 4mg/mL dexamethasone sodium phosphate IM. Day 2-3: Four 0.75mg tabs in 2 divided doses. Day 4: Two 0.75mg tabs in 2 divided doses. Day 5-6: One 0.75mg tab/day. Day 7: No treatment. Day 8: Follow-up visit. Palliative Management of Recurrent or Inoperable Brain Tumors: Maint: 2mg bid or tid. Elderly: Start at lower end of dosing range.

Pediatrics: Individualize dose. (Sol/Tab) Initial: 0.02-0.3mg/kg/day in 3 or 4 divided doses (0.6-9mg/m²BSA/day) depending on the disease. Maint: Decrease in small amounts at appropriate time intervals to lowest effective dose. May need to increase dose for a period of time in stressful situations. Upon d/c after long-term therapy, withdraw gradually. Cushing's Syndrome Test: 1mg at 11 pm; draw blood at 8 am next morning. Or, 0.5mg q6h for 48 hrs. Test to Distinguish Cushing's Syndrome Due to Pituitary ACTH Excess from Cushing's Syndrome Due to Other Causes: 2mg q6h for 48 hrs; obtain 24-hr urine collections.

HOW SUPPLIED: Elixir: 0.5mg/5mL [237mL]; Sol: 0.5mg/5mL [240mL, 500mL], (Intensol) 1mg/mL [30mL]; Tab: 0.5mg*, 0.75mg*, 1mg*, 1.5mg*, 2mg*, 4mg*, 6mg* *scored

CONTRAINDICATIONS: Systemic fungal infections.

WARNINGS/PRECAUTIONS: May cause BP elevation, Na^+/water retention, and increased K^+ and Ca^{2+} excretion. May cause left ventricular free-wall rupture after a recent myocardial infarction; use with caution. May mask signs of current infection. May increase susceptibility to infections. Rule out latent or active amebiasis before initiating therapy. Use lowest possible dose to control treatment condition; reduce gradually if dosage reduction is possible. Caution with active/latent tuberculosis or tuberculin reactivity, active/latent peptic ulcers, diverticulitis, fresh intestinal anastomoses, nonspecific ulcerative colitis, HTN, and renal insufficiency. May have negative effects on pediatric growth; monitor growth and development of pediatric patients on prolonged use. May increase or decrease motility and number of spermatozoa in some patients. Enhanced effect in patients with cirrhosis. More serious/fatal course of chickenpox and measles reported; avoid exposure in patients who have not had these diseases. May produce posterior subcapsular cataracts, glaucoma with possible optic nerve damage, and enhance establishment of secondary ocular infections. Drug-induced secondary adrenocortical insufficiency may be minimized by gradual dose reduction. Psychic derangements, and emotional instability or psychotic tendencies aggravation may occur. Fat embolism reported. May suppress reactions to skin tests. False (-) dexamethasone suppression test results in patients being treated with indomethacin reported. (Elixir) Prolongation of coma and high incidence of pneumonia and GI bleeding in patients with cerebral malaria reported. Enhanced effect in patients with hypothyroidism. Caution with ocular herpes simplex, osteoporosis, myasthenia gravis. Withdrawal syndrome reported following prolonged use. (Sol/Tab) Anaphylactoid reactions may occur. Caution with congestive heart failure (CHF). May produce reversible hypothalamic-pituitary-adrenal axis suppression with the potential for corticosteroid insufficiency after withdrawal. Changes in thyroid status may necessitate dose adjustment. May activate latent disease or exacerbate intercurrent infections. May exacerbate systemic fungal infections; avoid use unless needed to control life-threatening drug reactions. May increase risk of GI perforation with certain GI disorders. Caution with known or suspected *Strongyloides* infestation and in the elderly. Not for use in cerebral malaria and active ocular herpes simplex. Not recommended in optic neuritis treatment. Kaposi's sarcoma reported. Acute myopathy reported with use of high doses. Creatinine kinase elevation may occur. May elevate intraocular pressure (IOP); monitor IOP if used for >6 weeks.

ADVERSE REACTIONS: Fluid retention, Na^+ retention, muscle weakness, osteoporosis, peptic ulcer, pancreatitis, ulcerative esophagitis, impaired wound healing, headache, psychic disturbances, growth suppression (pediatrics), glaucoma, weight gain, nausea, malaise.

INTERACTIONS: Live or live, attenuated vaccines are contraindicated with immunosuppressive doses. May diminish response to toxoids and live or inactivated vaccines. Observe closely for hypokalemia with K^+-depleting agents (eg, amphotericin B, diuretics). Dose adjustment of antidiabetic agents may be required. Barbiturates, phenytoin, and rifampin may enhance metabolism;

may need to increase corticosteroid dose. Caution with aspirin (ASA) in patients with hypo-prothrombinemia. Ephedrine may enhance metabolic clearance; may require an increase in corticosteroid dose. (Elixir) Phenobarbital may enhance the metabolic clearance; may require adjustment of corticosteroid dose. Monitor PT frequently with coumarin anticoagulants. (Sol/Tab) May potentiate replication of some organisms contained in live, attenuated vaccines. D/C anticholinesterase agents at least 24 hrs before start of therapy. Monitor coagulation indices with warfarin. Hepatic enzyme inducers (eg, carbamazepine) may enhance metabolism; may need to increase corticosteroid dose. CYP3A4 inhibitors may increase plasma concentrations. May decrease plasma concentrations of CYP3A4 substrates (eg, indinavir). Convulsions and increased activity of both drugs reported with cyclosporine. May increase risk of arrhythmias due to hypokalemia with digitalis glycosides. Estrogens and ketoconazole may decrease metabolism. ASA or other NSAIDs may increase risk of GI side effects. May increase clearance of salicylates. Acute myopathy reported with neuromuscular-blocking drugs (eg, pancuronium). May decrease concentrations of isoniazid. Cholestyramine may increase clearance. Cardiac enlargement and CHF reported when hydrocortisone is used with amphotericin B. Aminoglutethimide may diminish adrenal suppression. Macrolide antibiotics may decrease clearance. May increase and decrease levels of phenytoin, leading to alterations in seizure control. Caution with thalidomide; toxic epidermal necrolysis reported.

PREGNANCY: (Elixir) Safety not known in pregnancy, (Sol/Tab) Category C, not for use in nursing.

MECHANISM OF ACTION: Glucocorticoid; produces anti-inflammatory effects.

PHARMACOKINETICS: Distribution: Found in breast milk.

NURSING CONSIDERATIONS

Assessment: Assess for vaccination history, current infections, systemic fungal infections, thyroid status, latent/active amebiasis, cerebral malaria, ocular herpes simplex, cirrhosis, emotional instability or psychotic tendencies, any condition where treatment is cautioned, pregnancy/nursing status, and possible drug interactions.

Monitoring: Monitor for Na⁺/water retention, infections/secondary ocular infections, changes in thyroid status, posterior subcapsular cataracts, glaucoma, optic nerve damage, Kaposi's sarcoma, development of osteoporosis, acute myopathy, creatinine kinase elevation, psychic derangements, emotional instability or psychotic tendencies aggravation, and other adverse effects. Monitor IOP, BP, and serum K⁺ Ca²⁺ levels. Monitor bone growth and development in pediatric patients.

Patient Counseling: Instruct not to d/c therapy abruptly or without medical supervision. Advise to inform any medical attendants about current corticosteroid therapies. Instruct to seek medical advice if an acute illness including fever or other signs of infection develop. Advise to avoid exposure to chickenpox or measles; if exposed, instruct to seek medical advice without delay.

Administration: Oral route. (Intensol) Mixed with liquid or semi-solid food (eg, water, juices, soda or soda-like beverages. Use only calibrated dropper provided. Refer to PI for proper use. (Elixir) When large doses are given, take with meals and antacids in between meals to help prevent peptic ulcers. **Storage:** 20-25°C (68-77°F). (Tab) Protect from moisture. (Intensol) Do not freeze. Discard opened bottle after 90 days.

DEXILANT   RX
dexlansoprazole (Takeda)

THERAPEUTIC CLASS: Proton pump inhibitor

INDICATIONS: Healing of all grades of erosive esophagitis (EE) for up to 8 weeks. Maintenance of healed EE and relief of heartburn for up to 6 months. Treatment of heartburn associated with symptomatic nonerosive gastroesophageal reflux disease (GERD) for 4 weeks.

DOSAGE: *Adults:* Healing of EE: 60mg qd for up to 8 weeks. Maint of Healed EE/Relief of Heartburn: 30mg qd for up to 6 months. Symptomatic Nonerosive GERD: 30mg qd for 4 weeks. Moderate Hepatic Impairment (Child-Pugh Class B): Max: 30mg qd.

HOW SUPPLIED: Cap, Delayed-Release: 30mg, 60mg

WARNINGS/PRECAUTIONS: Symptomatic response does not preclude the presence of gastric malignancy. May increase risk of *Clostridium difficile*-associated diarrhea (CDAD), especially in hospitalized patients. May increase risk for osteoporosis-related fractures of the hip, wrist, or spine, especially with high-dose and long-term therapy. Use lowest dose and shortest duration appropriate to the conditions being treated. Hypomagnesemia reported and may require Mg²⁺ replacement and discontinuation of therapy; consider monitoring Mg²⁺ levels prior to and periodically during therapy with prolonged treatment.

ADVERSE REACTIONS: Diarrhea, abdominal pain, N/V, upper respiratory tract infection, flatulence.

INTERACTIONS: May substantially decrease atazanavir concentrations; avoid concurrent use. May interfere with the absorption of drugs where gastric pH is an important determinant of oral bioavailability (eg, ampicillin esters, digoxin, iron salts, ketoconazole, erlotinib). Monitor for increases in INR and PT with warfarin. May increase tacrolimus levels. Caution with digoxin or other drugs that may cause hypomagnesemia (eg, diuretics). May elevate and prolong levels of methotrexate (MTX) and/or its metabolite, possibly leading to toxicities; consider temporary withdrawal of therapy with high-dose MTX.

PREGNANCY: Category B, not for use in nursing.

MECHANISM OF ACTION: Proton pump inhibitor; suppresses gastric acid secretion by specific inhibition of the (H^+/K^+)-ATPase in the gastric parietal cell. Blocks the final step of acid production.

PHARMACOKINETICS: Absorption: C_{max}=658ng/mL (30mg), 1397ng/mL (60mg); AUC_{24}=3275ng•hr/mL (30mg), 6529ng•hr/mL (60mg); T_{max}=1-2 hrs (1st peak), 4-5 hrs (2nd peak). **Distribution:** V_d=40.3L; plasma protein binding (96.1-98.8%). **Metabolism:** Liver (extensive) via CYP3A4 (oxidation) and CYP2C19 (hydroxylation). **Elimination:** Urine (50.7%), feces (47.6%); $T_{1/2}$=1-2 hrs.

NURSING CONSIDERATIONS

Assessment: Assess for hypersensitivity to the drug, risk for osteoporosis-related fractures, hepatic impairment, pregnancy/nursing status, and possible drug interactions. Obtain baseline Mg^{2+} levels.

Monitoring: Monitor for signs/symptoms of CDAD, bone fractures, hypersensitivity reactions, and other adverse reactions. Monitor Mg^{2+} levels periodically. Monitor INR and PT when given with warfarin.

Patient Counseling: Instruct to watch for signs of an allergic reaction, as these could be serious and may require discontinuation. Advise to immediately report and seek care for diarrhea that does not improve, and for any cardiovascular/neurological symptoms (eg, palpitations, dizziness, seizures, tetany). Instruct to take ud and to inform physician of any other medication use.

Administration: Oral route. Take without regard to food. Swallow cap whole; do not chew. Refer to PI for alternate administration options. **Storage:** 25°C (77°F); excursions permitted to 15-30°C (59-86°F).

DiaBeta   RX
glyburide (Sanofi-Aventis)

THERAPEUTIC CLASS: Sulfonylurea (2nd generation)

INDICATIONS: Adjunct to diet and exercise to improve glycemic control in adults with type 2 diabetes mellitus (DM).

DOSAGE: *Adults:* Initial: 2.5-5mg qd with breakfast or 1st main meal; 1.25mg qd if more sensitive to hypoglycemic drugs. Titrate: Increase by ≤2.5mg at weekly intervals. Maint: 1.25-20mg/day as single dose or in divided doses. Max: 20mg/day. Transferring from Insulin: Insulin Dose: >40 U/day: Decrease insulin dose by 50% and start with 5mg qd; progressively withdraw insulin and increase dose in increments of 1.25-2.5mg every 2-10 days. 20-40 U/day: 5mg qd. <20 U/day: 2.5-5mg qd. Concomitant Colesevelam: Administer at least 4 hrs prior to colesevelam. Elderly/Debilitated/Malnourished/Renal or Hepatic Impairment: Initial/Maint: Dose conservatively.

HOW SUPPLIED: Tab: 1.25mg*, 2.5mg*, 5mg* *scored

CONTRAINDICATIONS: Type 1 DM or diabetic ketoacidosis, with or without coma. Coadministration with bosentan.

WARNINGS/PRECAUTIONS: Caution during the first 2 weeks of therapy if transferring from chlorpropamide. May be associated with increased cardiovascular (CV) mortality. May produce severe hypoglycemia; increased risk when caloric intake is deficient, after severe/prolonged exercise, with severe renal/hepatic insufficiency, adrenal/pituitary insufficiency, or in elderly, debilitated, or malnourished patients. Loss of glycemic control may occur when exposed to stress (eg, fever, trauma, infection, surgery); may be necessary to d/c therapy and administer insulin. Secondary failure may occur over a period of time. May cause hemolytic anemia; caution with G6PD deficiency and consider a non-sulfonylurea alternative. Caution in elderly. Not bioequivalent to Glynase PresTab and therefore not substitutable.

ADVERSE REACTIONS: Hypoglycemia, nausea, epigastric fullness, heartburn, hyponatremia, LFT abnormalities, photosensitivity reactions, leukopenia, agranulocytosis, thrombocytopenia, porphyria cutanea tarda, blurred vision, changes in accommodation, angioedema, arthralgia.

INTERACTIONS: See Contraindications and Dosage. Hypoglycemic effects may be potentiated by NSAIDs, ACE-inhibitors, disopyramide, fluoxetine, clarithromycin, fluoroquinolones, other highly protein-bound drugs, salicylates, sulfonamides, chloramphenicol, probenecid, MAOIs, and β-adrenergic blocking drugs; monitor closely for hypoglycemia during coadministration and for loss of glycemic control when such drugs are withdrawn. Increased risk of hypoglyce-mia with alcohol or use of >1 glucose-lowering drug. May be difficult to recognize hypoglyce-mia with β-adrenergic blocking drugs or other sympatholytics. Potential interaction leading to severe hypoglycemia reported with oral miconazole. Potentiates or weakens effects of coumarin derivatives. Rifampin may worsen glucose control. Thiazides and other diuretics, corticosteroids, phenothiazines, thyroid products, estrogens, oral contraceptives, phenytoin, nicotinic acid, sym-pathomimetics, calcium channel blockers, and isoniazid may produce hyperglycemia and may lead to loss of glycemic control; monitor closely for loss of control during coadministration and for hypoglycemia when such drugs are withdrawn. May increase cyclosporine plasma levels and toxicity; monitor and adjust dosage of cyclosporine. Colesevelam may decrease levels. Caution with inducers/inhibitors of CYP2C9.

PREGNANCY: Category C, not for use in nursing.

MECHANISM OF ACTION: Sulfonylurea (2nd generation); acts by stimulating insulin release from functioning pancreatic β-cells.

PHARMACOKINETICS: Absorption: T_{max}=4 hrs. **Distribution:** Plasma protein binding (extensive). **Metabolism:** 4-trans-hydroxy derivative (major metabolite). **Elimination:** Bile (50% metabolites), urine (50% metabolites); $T_{1/2}$=10 hrs.

NURSING CONSIDERATIONS

Assessment: Assess for previous hypersensitivity to drug or other sulfonamide derivatives, type of DM, risk factors of hypoglycemia, renal/hepatic impairment, G6PD deficiency, pregnancy/nursing status, and possible drug interactions. Obtain baseline FPG and HbA1c levels.

Monitoring: Monitor for CV effects, hypoglycemia, loss of glycemic control when exposed to stress, hypersensitivity reactions, secondary failure, hemolytic anemia, and other adverse reac-tions. Monitor FPG and HbA1c levels periodically.

Patient Counseling: Inform of the potential risks, benefits, and alternative modes of therapy. Counsel about importance of adherence to dietary instructions, regular exercise program, and regular testing of blood glucose. Inform about the symptoms, treatment, and predisposing con-ditions of hypoglycemia, as well as primary and secondary failure. During the insulin withdrawal period, instruct patients to test blood glucose and acetone in urine at least tid and report results to physician.

Administration: Oral route. Take with breakfast or 1st main meal. **Storage:** 25°C (77°F); excur-sions permitted to 15-30°C (59-86°F).

DICLEGIS   RX
pyridoxine HCl - doxylamine succinate (Duchesnay USA)

THERAPEUTIC CLASS: Antihistamine/vitamin B6 analog

INDICATIONS: Treatment of N/V of pregnancy in women who do not respond to conservative management.

DOSAGE: *Adults:* Take on an empty stomach with a glass of water. Initial: 2 tabs at hs (Day 1). Titrate: Continue taking 2 tabs/day at hs if dose adequately controls symptoms the next day. If symptoms persist into the afternoon of Day 2, take 2 tabs at hs that pm then take 3 tabs (1 tab in am and 2 tabs at hs) starting on Day 3. Continue taking 3 tabs/day if dose adequately controls symptoms, otherwise, take 4 tabs (1 tab in am, 1 tab mid-afternoon, and 2 tabs at hs) starting on Day 4. Max: 4 tabs/day (1 tab in am, 1 tab mid-afternoon, and 2 tabs at hs). Reassess for contin-ued need as pregnancy progresses.

HOW SUPPLIED: Tab, Delayed Release: (Doxylamine-Pyridoxine) 10mg-10mg

CONTRAINDICATIONS: Concomitant MAIOs.

WARNINGS/PRECAUTIONS: Not studied in women with hyperemesis gravidarum. May cause somnolence and impair physical/mental abilities. Caution with asthma, increased intraocular pressure (IOP), narrow-angle glaucoma, stenosing peptic ulcer, pyloroduodenal obstruction, and urinary bladder-neck obstruction.

ADVERSE REACTIONS: Somnolence, dyspnea, vertigo, visual disturbances, abdominal pain, fatigue, dizziness, anxiety, dysuria, pruritus, palpitation, constipation, malaise, paresthesia, rash.

INTERACTIONS: See Contraindications. Not recommended with alcohol and other CNS depres-sants (eg, hypnotic sedatives, tranquilizers).

PREGNANCY: Category A, not for use in nursing.

MECHANISM OF ACTION: Antihistamine and vitamin B6 analog combination; has not been established.

PHARMACOKINETICS: Absorption: GI tract, mainly jejunum. Administration of variable doses resulted in different pharmacokinetic parameters. **Distribution:** Found in breast milk. Pyridoxine: Plasma protein bound (60%). **Metabolism:** Doxylamine: Liver via N-dealkylation;

N-desmethyldoxylamine and N, N-didesmethyldoxylamine (principle metabolites). Pyridoxine: Liver; Pyridoxal 5'-phosphate (active metabolite). **Elimination:** Doxylamine: Kidney; $T_{1/2}$=12.5 hrs. Pyridoxine: $T_{1/2}$=0.5 hrs.

NURSING CONSIDERATIONS

Assessment: Assess for hypersensitivity reaction to the drug or to its components, hyperemesis gravidarum, asthma, IOP, narrow-angle glaucoma, stenosing peptic ulcer, pyloroduodenal obstruction, urinary bladder-neck obstruction, nursing status, and possible drug interactions.

Monitoring: Monitor for somnolence and other adverse reactions. Reassess for continued need as pregnancy progresses.

Patient Counseling: Instruct to avoid engaging in activities requiring complete mental alertness (eg, driving, operating heavy machinery), until cleared to do so. Inform of the importance of not taking the medication with alcohol or sedating medications including other antihistamines, opiates, and sleep aids.

Administration: Oral route. Take as a daily prescription and not PRN. Swallow tab whole; do not crush, chew, or split. **Storage:** 20-25°C (68-77°F); excursions permitted between 15-30°C (59-86°F). Protect from moisture.

DICLOXACILLIN   RX
dicloxacillin sodium (Sandoz)

THERAPEUTIC CLASS: Penicillin (penicillinase-resistant)

INDICATIONS: Treatment of infections caused by penicillinase-producing staphylococci or as initial therapy in suspected cases of resistant staphylococcal infections.

DOSAGE: *Adults:* Duration of therapy varies with type and severity of infection and clinical response. Take at least 1 hr ac or 2 hrs pc. Mild to Moderate Infections: 125mg q6h. Severe Infections: 250mg q6h; continue for at least 14 days. Continue therapy for at least 48 hrs after patient becomes afebrile, asymptomatic, and cultures are negative. Endocarditis/Osteomyelitis: May require longer term of therapy. May treat concurrently with probenecid if very high serum levels of penicillin (PCN) are necessary. Elderly: Start at lower end of dosing range.
Pediatrics: Duration of therapy varies with the type and severity of infection and clinical response. Take at least 1 hr ac or 2 hrs pc. ≥40kg: Mild to Moderate Infections: 125mg q6h. Severe Infections: 250mg q6h; continue for at least 14 days. <40kg: Mild to Moderate Infections: 12.5mg/kg/day in equally divided doses q6h. Severe Infections: 25mg/kg/day in equally divided doses q6h; continue for at least 14 days. Continue therapy for at least 48 hrs after patient becomes afebrile, asymptomatic, and cultures are negative. Endocarditis/Osteomyelitis: May require longer term of therapy. May treat concurrently with probenecid if very high serum levels of PCN are necessary.

HOW SUPPLIED: Cap: 250mg, 500mg

WARNINGS/PRECAUTIONS: Do not use in infections caused by PCN G-susceptible organisms and as initial therapy in serious, life-threatening infections. Serious and occasionally fatal hypersensitivity (anaphylactic shock with collapse) reactions reported; if an allergic reaction occurs, d/c unless condition being treated is life threatening and amenable only to PCN therapy, and institute supportive treatment. Caution with histories of significant allergies and/or asthma. *Clostridium difficile*-associated diarrhea (CDAD) reported; d/c if CDAD is suspected or confirmed. PO route should not be relied upon in patients with severe illness, or with N/V, gastric dilatation, cardiospasm, or intestinal hypermotility. May result in bacterial resistance if used in the absence of a proven/suspected bacterial infection or a prophylactic indication. Change to another active agent if culture tests fail to demonstrate the presence of staphylococci. Perform periodic urinalysis, BUN, and creatinine determinations; consider dosage alterations if these values become elevated. Monitor renal, hepatic, and hematopoietic functions periodically with prolonged therapy. If renal impairment is suspected or known to exist, reduce dose and monitor blood levels to avoid possible neurotoxic reactions. Monitor for possible liver function abnormalities. Not recommended for use in newborns. Caution in elderly. Lab test interactions may occur.

ADVERSE REACTIONS: Allergic reactions, N/V, diarrhea, stomatitis, black or hairy tongue, GI irritation.

INTERACTIONS: Tetracycline may antagonize effect; avoid concurrent use. Probenecid may increase and prolong serum levels. May reduce anticoagulant response to dicumarol and warfarin; carefully monitor PT and adjust anticoagulant dose as required. May inactivate aminoglycosides in vitro as PCNs are physically incompatible with aminoglycosides; avoid in vitro mixing and administer drugs separately.

PREGNANCY: Category B, caution in nursing.

MECHANISM OF ACTION: PCN (penicillinase-resistant); inhibits bacterial cell-wall biosynthesis.

D

PHARMACOKINETICS: Absorption: Rapid, incomplete. (500mg single dose) C_{max}=10-17mcg/mL, T_{max}=1-1.5 hrs. **Distribution:** Plasma protein binding (95-99%); found in breast milk. **Elimination:** Urine (unchanged); $T_{1/2}$=0.7 hrs.

NURSING CONSIDERATIONS

Assessment: Assess for hypersensitivity to drug and other PCNs, history of significant allergies and/or asthma, severe illness, N/V, gastric dilatation, cardiospasm, renal impairment, intestinal hypermotility, pregnancy/nursing status, and possible drug interactions. Perform culture and susceptibility testing to confirm diagnosis and sensitivity to drug. Obtain baseline blood cultures and WBC and differential cell counts.

Monitoring: Monitor for hypersensitivity reactions, CDAD, liver function abnormalities, and other adverse reactions. Monitor blood cultures, and WBC and differential cell counts at least weekly. Monitor BUN, urinalysis, creatinine, ALT, and AST periodically. Monitor renal, hepatic, and hematopoietic functions periodically with prolonged therapy. Carefully monitor PT if used with dicumarol or warfarin.

Patient Counseling: Counsel that drug treats only bacterial, not viral, infections. Advise to take exactly ud; inform that skipping doses or not completing full course may decrease effectiveness and increase bacterial resistance. Instruct not to take the drug if with previous PCN allergy and to inform physician of any allergies or previous allergic reactions to any drugs. Instruct patients who have previously experienced an anaphylactic reaction to PCN to wear a medical identification tag or bracelet. Instruct to take the entire course of therapy prescribed, even if fever and other symptoms develop. Advise to d/c and notify physician if SOB, wheezing, skin rash, mouth irritation, black tongue, sore throat, N/V, diarrhea, fever, swollen joints, or any unusual bleeding or bruising occur. Advise not to take additional medications, including nonprescription drugs (eg, antacids, laxatives, vitamins) without physician approval. Inform that diarrhea is a common problem caused by therapy and will usually end upon discontinuation of therapy. Instruct to immediately contact physician if watery and bloody stools (with or without stomach cramps and fever) occur, even as late as ≥2 months after discontinuation of therapy.

Administration: Oral route. Take at least 1 hr ac or 2 hrs pc with at least 4 fl. oz. (120mL) of water; do not take in supine position or immediately before going to bed. **Storage:** 20-25°C (68-77°F).

DICYCLOMINE HCl   RX
dicyclomine HCl (Various)

OTHER BRAND NAMES: Bentyl (Aptalis)

THERAPEUTIC CLASS: Anticholinergic

INDICATIONS: Treatment of functional bowel/irritable bowel syndrome.

DOSAGE: *Adults:* Individualize dose. (PO) Initial: 20mg qid. Titrate: May increase to 40mg qid after 1 week of initial dose, unless side effects limit dose escalation. D/C if efficacy not achieved within 2 weeks or side effects require doses below 80mg/day. (Inj) Initial: 10-20mg IM qid for 1-2 days if unable to take oral medication. Elderly: Start at lower end of dosing range.

HOW SUPPLIED: Sol: 10mg/5mL [473mL]; (Bentyl) Cap: 10mg; Inj: 10mg/mL; Tab: 20mg

CONTRAINDICATIONS: GI tract obstructive disease, obstructive uropathy, severe ulcerative colitis, reflux esophagitis, glaucoma, myasthenia gravis, unstable cardiovascular status in acute hemorrhage, nursing mothers, infants <6 months of age.

WARNINGS/PRECAUTIONS: Caution in conditions characterized by tachyarrhythmia (eg, thyrotoxicosis, congestive heart failure, in cardiac surgery). Caution with coronary heart disease; ischemia and infarction may worsen. Peripheral effects (eg, dryness of mouth with difficulty in swallowing/talking), CNS signs/symptoms (eg, confusional state, disorientation, amnesia) reported. Psychosis and delirium reported in sensitive individuals (eg, elderly patients and/or in patients with mental illness) given anticholinergic drugs. Heat prostration may occur in high environmental temperatures; d/c if symptoms occur and institute supportive measures. May impair mental abilities. Diarrhea may be the early symptom of incomplete intestinal obstruction, especially with ileostomy/colostomy patients; treatment would be inappropriate and possibly harmful. Caution with ulcerative colitis; large doses may suppress intestinal motility, produce paralytic ileus, and use of this drug may precipitate or aggravate the serious complication of toxic megacolon. Caution in patients with HTN, fever, autonomic neuropathy, prostatic enlargement, hepatic/renal impairment, and in the elderly. (Cap/Tab/Inj) Avoid with myasthenia gravis except to reduce adverse muscarinic effects of an anticholinesterase. Ogilvie's syndrome (colonic pseudo-obstruction) rarely reported. Caution with Salmonella dysentery; toxic dilation of intestine and intestinal perforation may occur. (Inj) For IM use only; inadvertent IV use may result in thrombosis, thrombophlebitis, and inj-site reactions. (Sol) Caution with hyperthyroidism and hiatal hernia.

ADVERSE REACTIONS: Dry mouth, dizziness, blurred vision, nausea, somnolence, asthenia, nervousness.

INTERACTIONS: May antagonize the effect of antiglaucoma agents and drugs that alter GI motility (eg, metoclopramide). Avoid concomitant use with corticosteroids in glaucoma patients. Potentiated by amantadine, Class I antiarrhythmics (eg, quinidine), antihistamines, antipsychotics (eg, phenothiazines), benzodiazepines, MAOIs, narcotic analgesics (eg, meperidine), nitrates/nitrites, sympathomimetics, TCAs, and other drugs with anticholinergic activity. Antacids may interfere with absorption; avoid simultaneous use. May affect GI absorption of various drugs by affecting GI motility; increased serum digoxin concentration may result with slowly dissolving forms of digoxin. Inhibiting effects on gastric hydrochloric acid secretion are antagonized by drugs used to treat achlorhydria and those used to test gastric secretion.

PREGNANCY: Category B, not for use in nursing.

MECHANISM OF ACTION: Anticholinergic and antispasmodic agent; relieves smooth muscle spasm of the GI tract.

PHARMACOKINETICS: Absorption: Rapid; T_{max}=60-90 min. **Distribution:** (20mg PO) V_d=approximately 3.65L/kg (extensive); found in breast milk. **Elimination:** Urine (79.5%), feces (8.4%); $T_{1/2}$=1.8 hrs.

NURSING CONSIDERATIONS

Assessment: Assess for cardiovascular conditions, myasthenia gravis, glaucoma, intestinal obstruction, psychosis, ulcerative colitis, tachycardia, or any other conditions where treatment is contraindicated or cautioned. Assess for history of hypersensitivity, pregnancy/nursing status, renal/hepatic dysfunction, and for possible drug interactions.

Monitoring: Monitor for increased HR, worsening of ischemia/infarction, heat prostration, drowsiness, blurred vision, confusion, disorientation, hallucinations, paralytic ileus with large doses, urinary retention, hypersensitivity reactions, and for other adverse reactions. Monitor renal function.

Patient Counseling: Counsel on proper administration. Advise not to breastfeed while on therapy and not to administer to infants <6 months of age. Advise not to engage in activities requiring mental alertness (eg, operating motor vehicle or other machinery) or to perform hazardous work while taking the drug. Inform of risk of heat prostration in high environmental temperature; instruct to d/c if symptoms occur and to consult a physician.

Administration: Oral, IM route. Refer to PI for preparation instructions for IM administration.

Storage: (Cap/Tab/Inj) Room temperature <30°C (86°F). Sol: 20-25°C (68-77°F). Inj: Protect from freezing. Tab: Avoid exposure to direct sunlight.

DIFFERIN   RX
adapalene (Galderma)

THERAPEUTIC CLASS: Naphthoic acid derivative (retinoid-like)

INDICATIONS: Topical treatment of acne vulgaris in patients ≥12 yrs of age.

DOSAGE: *Adults:* (Cre) Apply a thin film enough to cover the entire affected areas of the skin qhs. (0.1% Gel) Apply a thin film enough to cover the affected areas of the skin qpm after washing. (0.3% Gel) Apply a thin film enough to cover the entire face and other affected areas of the skin qpm after washing. Reevaluate if therapeutic results are not noticed after 12 weeks of treatment. (Lot) Apply a thin film to cover the entire face (3-4 actuations of pump) and other affected areas qd after washing.
Pediatrics: ≥12 Yrs: (Cre) Apply a thin film enough to cover the entire affected areas of the skin qpm. (0.1% Gel) Apply a thin film enough to cover the affected areas of the skin qhs after washing. (0.3% Gel) Apply a thin film enough to cover the entire face and other affected areas of the skin qpm after washing. Reevaluate if therapeutic results are not noticed after 12 weeks of treatment. (Lot) Apply a thin film to cover the entire face (3-4 actuations of pump) and other affected areas qd after washing.

HOW SUPPLIED: Cre: 0.1% [45g]; Gel: 0.1% [45g], 0.3% [45g]; Lot: 0.1% [2 oz.]

WARNINGS/PRECAUTIONS: Not for ophthalmic, oral, or intravaginal use. Avoid exposure to sunlight, including sunlamps; use sunscreen products and protective clothing over treated areas if exposure cannot be avoided. Caution in patients with high levels of sun exposure and those with inherent sensitivity to sun. Extreme weather (eg, wind, cold) may cause irritation. Local skin irritation (eg, erythema, dryness, scaling, burning, pruritus) may be experienced; depending on severity, may apply moisturizer, reduce frequency of application, or d/c use. Avoid contact with the eyes, lips, angles of the nose, and mucous membranes. Avoid application to cuts, abrasions, and eczematous or sunburned skin. (Cre/0.3% Gel/Lot) Avoid waxing as a depilatory method. (Cre/Gel) Apparent exacerbation of acne may occur. (Cre/0.1% Gel) D/C if reaction suggesting sensitivity or chemical irritation occurs. (Cre/0.3% Gel) A mild transitory sensation of warmth or slight stinging may occur shortly after application. (0.1% Gel) Avoid in patients with sunburn until fully recovered. (0.3% Gel) Reactions characterized by symptoms (eg, pruritus, face edema, eyelid edema, lip swelling) requiring medical treatment reported; d/c use if experiencing allergic or anaphylactoid/anaphylactic reactions during therapy.

ADVERSE REACTIONS: Skin erythema, scaling, dryness, burning/stinging sensation, pruritus. (0.3% Gel) Skin discomfort.

INTERACTIONS: Caution with preparations containing sulfur, resorcinol, or salicylic acid. (Cre/Gel) Caution with other potentially irritating topical products (eg, medicated/abrasive soaps and cleansers, soaps/cosmetics with strong drying effect, products with high concentrations of alcohol, astringents, spices, or limes); local irritation may occur. (Lot) Caution with concomitant topical acne therapy, especially with peeling, desquamating, or abrasive agents. Avoid with other potentially irritating topical products (abrasive soaps/cleansers, soaps/cosmetics with strong drying effect, products with high concentrations of alcohol, astringents, spices, or limes).

PREGNANCY: Category C, caution in nursing.

MECHANISM OF ACTION: Naphthoic acid derivative; not established. Binds to specific retinoic acid nuclear receptors and modulates cellular differentiation, keratinization, and inflammatory processes. (Cre/0.1% Gel) Suspected to normalize differentiation of follicular epithelial cells, resulting in decreased microcomedone formation.

PHARMACOKINETICS: Absorption: (0.3% Gel) C_{max}=0.553ng/mL, AUC=8.37ng•hr/mL. (Lot) Adolescent: C_{max}=0.128ng/mL, AUC=3.07ng•hr/mL. **Elimination:** (Cre/Gel) Bile. (0.3% Gel) $T_{1/2}$=17.2 hrs.

NURSING CONSIDERATIONS

Assessment: Assess use in patients with excessive sun exposure, sun sensitivity, hypersensitivity to any of the components of the drug, pregnancy/nursing status, and for possible drug interactions. Assess for presence of cuts, abrasions, eczematous, or sunburned skin at the treatment site.

Monitoring: Monitor for sensitivity or chemical irritation, cutaneous signs/symptoms (eg, erythema, dryness, scaling, burning/stinging, or pruritus), and other adverse reactions.

Patient Counseling: Advise to cleanse area with mild or soapless cleanser before applying the medication. Instruct to avoid or minimize exposure to sunlight and sunlamps and use sunscreen/protective clothing over treated areas when exposed. Instruct not to use more than the recommended amount. Instruct to avoid contact with eyes, lips, angles of the nose, and mucous membranes. Advise not to apply medication to cuts, abrasions, eczematous or sunburned skin. Counsel to avoid use of waxing as depilatory method. Advise to use moisturizers if necessary and to avoid products containing alpha hydroxyl or glycolic acids. Instruct to use externally and ud. Inform that an apparent exacerbation of acne may occur during the early weeks of therapy and should not be considered a reason for discontinuation of therapy. Instruct to contact the physician if signs of allergy or hypersensitivity develop.

Administration: Topical route. **Storage:** 20-25°C (68-77°F); excursions permitted to 15-30°C (59-86°F). Protect from freezing. (Lot) Do not refrigerate. Protect from light. Keep away from heat. Keep bottle tightly closed.

DIFICID   RX
fidaxomicin (Optimer)

THERAPEUTIC CLASS: Macrolide

INDICATIONS: Treatment of *Clostridium difficile*-associated diarrhea (CDAD) in adults ≥18 yrs of age.

DOSAGE: *Adults:* ≥18 Yrs: Usual: 200mg bid for 10 days.

HOW SUPPLIED: Tab: 200mg

WARNINGS/PRECAUTIONS: Not effective for treatment of systemic infections. Acute hypersensitivity reactions (dyspnea, rash, pruritus, angioedema) reported; d/c and institute appropriate therapy. May increase the risk of the development of drug resistant bacteria when prescribed in the absence of a proven or strongly suspected *C. difficile* infection.

ADVERSE REACTIONS: N/V, abdominal pain, GI hemorrhage, anemia, neutropenia.

PREGNANCY: Category B, caution in nursing.

MECHANISM OF ACTION: Macrolide; bactericidal against *C. difficile*, inhibiting RNA synthesis by RNA polymerases.

PHARMACOKINETICS: Absorption: Minimal; refer to PI for other pharmacokinetic parameters. **Metabolism:** Hydrolysis; OP-1118 (active metabolite). **Elimination:** Urine (0.59% OP-1118), feces (>92% fidaxomicin and OP-1118); $T_{1/2}$=11.7 hrs, 11.2 hrs (OP-1118).

NURSING CONSIDERATIONS

Assessment: Assess for hypersensitivity to the drug, macrolide allergy, and pregnancy/nursing status.

Monitoring: Monitor for development of drug resistant bacteria, hypersensitivity reactions, and other adverse reactions.

Patient Counseling: Inform that drug only treats CDAD infections, not other bacterial or viral infections. Instruct to take exactly ud; inform that skipping doses or not completing full course may decrease effectiveness and increase antibiotic resistance.

Administration: Oral route. Take with or without food. **Storage:** 20-25°C (68-77°F); excursions permitted 15-30°C (59-86°F).

DIFLUCAN ORAL   RX
fluconazole (Roerig)

THERAPEUTIC CLASS: Azole antifungal

INDICATIONS: Treatment of vaginal, oropharyngeal, and esophageal candidiasis; urinary tract infections (UTIs) and peritonitis caused by *Candida*; systemic *Candida* infections (eg, candidemia, disseminated candidiasis, pneumonia); and cryptococcal meningitis. To decrease the incidence of candidiasis in patients undergoing bone marrow transplantation who receive cytotoxic chemotherapy and/or radiation therapy.

DOSAGE: *Adults:* Single Dose: Vaginal Candidiasis: 150mg. Multiple Dose: Oropharyngeal Candidiasis: 200mg on the 1st day, followed by 100mg qd for ≥2 weeks. Esophageal Candidiasis: 200mg on the 1st day, followed by 100mg qd for a minimum of 3 weeks and for ≥2 weeks following resolution of symptoms; doses up to 400mg/day may be used. Systemic *Candida* Infections: Up to 400mg/day. UTIs/Peritonitis: 50-200mg/day. Cryptococcal Meningitis: 400mg on 1st day, followed by 200mg qd for 10-12 weeks after the CSF becomes culture negative; a dose of 400mg qd may be used. Suppression of Cryptococcal Meningitis Relapse in AIDS: 200mg qd. Prophylaxis in Bone Marrow Transplant: 400mg qd. Start prophylaxis several days before the anticipated onset of neutropenia in patients who are anticipated to have severe granulocytopenia; continue for 7 days after the neutrophil count rises >1000 cells/mm³. Renal Impairment (Multiple Doses): Initial LD: 50-400mg. Maint: CrCl ≤50mL/min (No Dialysis): Give 50% of recommended dose. Regular Dialysis: Give 100% of recommended dose after each dialysis.
Pediatrics: Oropharyngeal Candidiasis: 6mg/kg on the 1st day, followed by 3mg/kg qd for ≥2 weeks. Esophageal Candidiasis: 6mg/kg on the 1st day, followed by 3mg/kg qd for a minimum of 3 weeks and for ≥2 weeks following resolution of symptoms; doses up to 12mg/kg/day may be used. Systemic *Candida* Infections: 6-12mg/kg/day. Cryptococcal Meningitis: 12mg/kg on the 1st day, followed by 6mg/kg qd for 10-12 weeks after the CSF becomes culture negative; a dose of 12mg/kg qd may be used. Suppression of Cryptococcal Meningitis Relapse in AIDS: 6mg/kg qd. Renal Impairment (Multiple Doses): Initial LD: 50-400mg. Maint: CrCl ≤50mL/min (No Dialysis): Give 50% of recommended dose. Regular Dialysis: Give 100% of recommended dose after each dialysis.

HOW SUPPLIED: Sus: 10mg/mL, 40mg/mL [35mL]; Tab: 50mg, 100mg, 150mg, 200mg.

CONTRAINDICATIONS: Coadministration with terfenadine (with multiple doses ≥400mg of fluconazole), other drugs known to prolong the QT interval and which are metabolized via the enzyme CYP3A4 (eg, cisapride, astemizole, erythromycin, pimozide, quinidine).

WARNINGS/PRECAUTIONS: Associated with rare cases of serious hepatic toxicity; monitor for more severe hepatic injury if abnormal LFTs develop. D/C if clinical signs and symptoms consistent with liver disease develop. Rare cases of anaphylaxis and exfoliative skin disorders reported; closely monitor patients who develop rashes during treatment and d/c if lesions progress. If a rash develops in a patient treated for a superficial infection, d/c further therapy. Rare cases of QT prolongation and torsades de pointes reported; caution with potentially proarrhythmic conditions. Caution in elderly or with renal/hepatic dysfunction. May impair mental/physical abilities. (Sus) Contains sucrose; avoid with hereditary fructose, glucose/galactose malabsorption, and sucrase-isomaltase deficiency. (Tab) Consider risk versus benefits of single dose oral tab versus intravaginal agent therapy for the treatment of vaginal yeast infections.

ADVERSE REACTIONS: Headache, N/V, abdominal pain, diarrhea.

INTERACTIONS: See Contraindications. Avoid use of voriconazole. Risk of increased plasma concentration of compounds metabolized by CYP2C9 and CYP3A4; caution when coadministered and monitor patients carefully. May precipitate clinically significant hypoglycemia with oral hypoglycemics; monitor blood glucose and adjust dose of sulfonylurea as necessary. May increase PT with coumarin-type anticoagulants; monitor PT and, if necessary, adjust warfarin dose. May increase levels of phenytoin, cyclosporine, theophylline, rifabutin, oral tacrolimus, triazolam, celecoxib, halofantrine, flurbiprofen, racemic ibuprofen, methadone, saquinavir, sirolimus, vinca alkaloids (eg, vincristine, vinblastine), ethinyl estradiol, and levonorgestrel. May reduce the metabolism and increase levels of tolbutamide, glyburide, and glipizide. Monitor SrCr with cyclosporine. Rifampin may enhance metabolism. May increase levels and psychomotor effects of oral midazolam; consider dose reduction and monitor appropriately short-acting benzodiazepines metabolized by CYP450. May increase systemic exposure to tofacitinib; reduce tofacitinib dose when given concomitantly. HCTZ may increase levels. May reduce clearance/distribution volume and prolong $T_{1/2}$ of alfentanil, and increase effect of amitriptyline and nortriptyline. May increase levels of zidovudine; consider dose reduction. May potentially increase systemic exposure of other NSAIDs that are metabolized through CYP2C9 (eg, naproxen, lornoxicam, meloxicam, diclofenac), and calcium channel antagonists. Risk of carbamazepine toxicity. May increase serum bilirubin and SrCr with cyclophosphamide. May significantly delay elimination of fentanyl leading to respiratory depression. May increase risk of myopathy and rhabdomyolysis with HMG-CoA reductase inhibitors metabolized through CYP3A4 (eg, atorvastatin, simvastatin) or through CYP2C9 (eg, fluvastatin); monitor for symptoms and d/c statin if a marked increase in creatinine kinase is observed or myopathy/rhabdomyolysis is diagnosed or suspected. May inhibit the metabolism of losartan; monitor BP continuously. Acute adrenal cortex insufficiency reported after discontinuation of a 3-month therapy with fluconazole in liver-transplanted patients treated with prednisone. CNS-related undesirable effects reported with all-trans-retinoid acid (an acid form of vitamin A).

PREGNANCY: Category C (single 150mg tab use for vaginal candidiasis) and D (all other indications), caution in nursing.

MECHANISM OF ACTION: Triazole antifungal; selectively inhibits fungal CYP450 dependent enzyme lanosterol 14-α-demethylase, the enzyme that converts lanosterol to ergosterol. Subsequent loss of normal sterol correlates with the accumulation of 14-α-methyl sterols in fungi and may be responsible for the fungistatic activity.

PHARMACOKINETICS: Absorption: (PO) Rapid, almost complete; absolute bioavailability (>90%); C_{max}=6.72µg/mL (fasted, single 400mg dose); T_{max}=1-2 hrs (fasted). **Distribution:** Plasma protein binding (11-12%); found in breast milk. **Elimination:** Urine (80%, unchanged; 11%, metabolites); $T_{1/2}$=30 hrs (fasted). Refer to PI for pediatric and elderly pharmacokinetic parameters.

NURSING CONSIDERATIONS

Assessment: Assess for hypersensitivity to the drug, renal/hepatic impairment, AIDS, malignancies, risk factors for QT prolongation, any other conditions where treatment is cautioned or contraindicated, pregnancy/nursing status, and possible drug interactions. Obtain specimens for fungal culture and other relevant lab studies (serology, histopathology) to isolate and identify causative organisms. (Sus) Assess for hereditary fructose, glucose/galactose malabsorption, and sucrase-isomaltase deficiency.

Monitoring: Monitor for signs/symptoms of liver disease, rash, and other adverse reactions. Monitor LFTs, PT, renal function, blood glucose concentrations, SrCr, and BP.

Patient Counseling: Inform about risks/benefits of therapy. Advise to notify physician if pregnant/nursing and counsel about potential hazard to the fetus if pregnant or pregnancy occurs. Counsel to d/c if skin lesions progress. Instruct to inform physician of all medications currently being taken.

Administration: Oral route. Take with or without food. Shake sus well before using. Refer to PI for directions of mixing the oral sus. **Storage:** Tab: <30°C (86°F). Sus: Dry Powder: <30°C (86°F). Reconstituted: 5-30°C (41-86°F); discard unused portion after 2 weeks. Protect from freezing.

DIGOXIN ORAL   RX
digoxin (Various)

OTHER BRAND NAMES: Lanoxin (Covis)

THERAPEUTIC CLASS: Cardiac glycoside

INDICATIONS: Treatment of mild to moderate heart failure (HF) in adults; where possible, use in combination with a diuretic and an ACE inhibitor. Increases myocardial contractility in pediatric patients with HF. Control of ventricular response rate in adult patients with chronic atrial fibrillation (A-fib).

DOSAGE: *Adults:* Individualize dose. Dosing can be either initiated with LD followed by maintenance dosing if rapid titration is desired or initiated with maintenance dosing without LD. (Sol): LD: 10-15mcg/kg. Maint: (Normal Renal Function): 3-4.5mcg/kg/dose qd. Refer to PI for recommended maintenance dose based upon lean body weight and renal function. (Tab) Initial: Give 1/2 the total LD, then 1/4 the LD every 6-8 hrs, twice, with careful assessment of clinical response and toxicity before each dose. LD: 10-15mcg/kg. Maint (Normal Renal Function): 3.4-5.1mcg/kg/day qd. Titrate: May be increased every 2 weeks according to clinical response, serum drug levels, and toxicity. Refer to PI for recommended maintenance dose according to lean body weight and renal function and for information when switching from IV to PO.
Pediatrics: Individualize dose. Dosing can be either initiated with LD followed by maintenance

dosing if rapid titration is desired or initiated with maintenance dosing without LD. (Sol) LD (If needed): Give 1/2 the total as the 1st dose. Additional fractions of planned total dose may be given at 4- to 8-hr intervals, with careful assessment of clinical response before each additional dose. >10 Yrs: 10-15mcg/kg. 5-10 Yrs: 20-35mcg/kg. 2-5 Yrs: 30-45mcg/kg. 1-24 Months: 35-60mcg/kg. Full-Term Infants: 25-35mcg/kg. Premature Infants: 20-30mcg/kg. Maint: (Normal Renal Function): >10 Yrs: 3-4.5mcg/kg/dose qd. 5-10 Yrs: 2.8-5.6mcg/kg/dose bid. 2-5 Yrs: 4.7-6.6mcg/kg/dose bid. 1-24 Months: 5.6-9.4mcg/kg/dose bid. Full-Term Infants: 3.8-5.6mcg/kg/dose bid. Premature Infants: 2.3-3.9mcg/kg/dose bid. Refer to PI for recommended maintenance dose based upon lean body weight and renal function. (Tab) Initial: Give 1/2 the total LD, then 1/4 the LD every 6-8 hrs twice with careful assessment of clinical response and toxicity before each dose. LD: >10 Yrs: 10-15mcg/kg. 5-10 Yrs: 20-45mcg/kg. Maint (Normal Renal Function): >10 Yrs: 3.4-5.1mcg/kg/day qd. Titrate: May be increased every 2 weeks according to clinical response, serum drug levels, and toxicity. Refer to PI for recommended maintenance dose according to lean body weight and renal function. 5-10 Yrs: 3.2-6.4mcg/kg/dose bid. Refer to PI for recommended maintenance dose based upon lean body weight and renal function and for information when switching from IV to PO.

HOW SUPPLIED: Sol: 0.05mg/mL [60mL]; (Lanoxin) Tab: 62.5mcg, 125mcg*, 187.5mcg, 250mcg* *scored

CONTRAINDICATIONS: Ventricular fibrillation.

WARNINGS/PRECAUTIONS: Increased risk of ventricular fibrillation in patients with Wolff-Parkinson-White syndrome who develop A-fib. May cause severe sinus bradycardia or sinoatrial block with preexisting sinus node disease and may cause advanced or complete heart block in patients with preexisting incomplete atrioventricular (AV) block; consider insertion of a pacemaker before treatment. Avoid in patients with HF associated with preserved left ventricular ejection fraction (eg, restrictive cardiomyopathy, constrictive pericarditis, amyloid heart disease, acute cor pulmonale), idiopathic hypertrophic subaortic stenosis, and myocarditis. May be desirable to reduce dose or d/c therapy 1-2 days prior to electrical cardioversion of A-fib. If digitalis toxicity is suspected, delay elective cardioversion and if it is not prudent to delay cardioversion, select the lowest possible energy level to avoid provoking ventricular arrhythmias. Hypocalcemia may nullify the effects of treatment. Hypothyroidism may reduce the requirements for therapy. HF and/or atrial arrhythmias resulting from hypermetabolic or hyperdynamic states (eg, hyperthyroidism, hypoxia, arteriovenous shunt) are best treated by addressing the underlying condition. Signs/symptoms of digoxin toxicity may be mistaken for worsening symptoms of congestive heart failure. May increase myocardial oxygen demand and ischemia in patients with acute myocardial infarction (AMI); not recommended in patients with AMI. Caution with impaired renal function and in the elderly. Endogenous substances of unknown composition (digoxin-like immunoreactive substances) may interfere with standard radioimmunoassays for digoxin. (Sol) May result in potentially detrimental increases in coronary vascular resistance. (Tab) Avoid with acute cor pulmonale. Patients with low body weight, advanced age or impaired renal function, hypokalemia, hypercalcemia, or hypomagnesia may be predisposed to digoxin toxicity; assess serum electrolytes and renal function periodically. Patients with beri beri heart disease may fail to respond adequately to therapy if the underlying thiamine deficiency is not treated concomitantly.

ADVERSE REACTIONS: Cardiac arrhythmias, N/V, abdominal pain, intestinal ischemia, hemorrhagic necrosis of the intestines, headache, weakness, dizziness, apathy, mental disturbances.

INTERACTIONS: Potential to alter digoxin pharmacokinetics with drugs that induce/inhibit P-glycoprotein in the intestine/kidney. May increase risk of arrhythmias with rapid IV calcium administration, sympathomimetics (epinephrine, norepinephrine, dopamine), and succinylcholine. Increased digoxin dose requirement with thyroid supplements. Calcium channel blockers and β-adrenergic blockers produce additive effects on AV node conduction, which can result in bradycardia and advanced or complete heart block. Higher rate of torsades de pointes with dofetilide. Teriparatide transiently increases serum calcium. Increased levels with amiodarone, captopril, clarithromycin, erythromycin, itraconazole, nitrendipine, propafenone, quinidine, ranolazine, ritonavir, tetracycline, verapamil, carvedilol, diltiazem, indomethacin, nifedipine, propantheline, spironolactone, telmisartan, alprazolam, azithromycin, cyclosporine, diclofenac, diphenoxylate, epoprostenol, esomeprazole, ketoconazole, lansoprazole, metformin, omeprazole, rabeprazole. Decreased levels with acarbose, activated charcoal, albuterol, antacids, cholestyramine, colestipol, exenatide, kaolin-pectin, meals high in bran, metoclopramide, miglitol, neomycin, rifampin, St. John's wort, sucralfate, sulfasalazine. Proarrhythmic events reported to be more common in patients receiving concomitant therapy with sotalol. Refer to PI for dose adjustment information when used with certain concomitant therapies. (Sol) Increased PR interval and QRS duration reported with moricizine. Decreased levels with anti-cancer drugs, salbutamol. (Tab) Increased levels with dronedarone, gentamicin, atorvastatin, nefazodone, quinine, saquinavir, tolvaptan, trimethoprim, ibuprofen. Decreased levels with certain cancer chemotherapy or radiation therapy, penicillamine, and phenytoin. ACE inhibitors, ARBs, NSAIDs, and COX-2 inhibitors may impair digoxin excretion. Sudden death reported to be more common in patients receiving concomitant therapy with dronedarone.

PREGNANCY: Category C, caution in nursing.

MECHANISM OF ACTION: Cardiac glycoside; inhibits Na$^+$-K$^+$ ATPase, which is responsible for maintaining the intracellular milieu throughout the body by moving Na$^+$ ions out of and K$^+$ ions into cells.

PHARMACOKINETICS: Absorption: (Sol) Absolute bioavailability (70-85%); T$_{max}$=30-90 min. (Tab) Absolute bioavailability (60-80%); T$_{max}$=1-3 hrs. **Distribution:** V$_d$=475-500L; Plasma protein binding (25%); crosses placenta; found in breast milk. **Metabolism:** (Sol) 3 β-digoxigenin, 3-ketodigoxigenin (metabolites); (Tab) Hydrolysis, oxidation, and conjugation. **Elimination:** (Healthy, IV) Urine (50-70%, unchanged); T$_{1/2}$=(anuric patients) 3.5-5 days. (Sol) T$_{1/2}$=18-36 hrs (pediatrics), 36-48 hrs (adults). (Tab) T$_{1/2}$=(healthy) 1.5-2 days.

NURSING CONSIDERATIONS

Assessment: Assess for known hypersensitivity to the drug or other digitalis preparations, ventricular fibrillation, myocarditis, hypermetabolic or hyperdynamic states, sinus node disease, AV block, pregnancy/nursing status, possible drug interactions, and any other conditions where treatment is cautioned. Assess serum electrolytes and renal function. Obtain a baseline digoxin level.

Monitoring: Monitor for signs/symptoms of severe sinus bradycardia, sinoatrial block, advanced or complete heart block, digoxin toxicity, vasoconstriction, and other adverse reactions. Monitor serum electrolytes and renal function periodically. Obtain serum digoxin concentrations just before the next dose or at least 6 hours after the last dose. Monitor for clinical response.

Patient Counseling: Advise that therapy is a cardiac glycoside used to treat HF and heart arrhythmias. Instruct to take the drug ud by physician. Advise to notify physician if taking any OTC medications, including herbal medication, or if started on a new prescription. Inform that blood tests will be necessary to ensure the appropriate digoxin dose. Instruct to contact physician if N/V, persistent diarrhea, confusion, weakness, or visual disturbances occur. Advise parents or caregivers that symptoms of having too high doses may be difficult to recognize in infants and pediatric patients; symptoms such as weight loss, failure to thrive in infants, abdominal pain, and behavioral disturbances may be indications of digoxin toxicity. Suggest to monitor and record heart rate and BP daily. Instruct women of childbearing potential who become or are planning to become pregnant to consult physician prior to initiation or continuing therapy with digoxin. (Sol) Instruct to use calibrated dropper to measure the dose and to avoid less precise measuring tools (eg, tsp).

Administration: Oral route. (Sol) The calibrated dropper supplied with the 60mL bottle is not appropriate to measure doses <0.2mL. **Storage:** 25°C (77°F); excursions permitted to 15-30°C (59-86°F). Protect from light. (Tab) Store in dry place.

DILACOR XR   RX
diltiazem HCl (Watson)

OTHER BRAND NAMES: Diltia XT (Watson)

THERAPEUTIC CLASS: Calcium channel blocker (nondihydropyridine)

INDICATIONS: Treatment of HTN alone or in combination with other antihypertensives. Management of chronic stable angina.

DOSAGE: *Adults:* Individualize dose. Take in am on an empty stomach. Patients Treated with Other Diltiazem Formulations: May switch to nearest equivalent total daily dose. Titrate as clinically indicated. HTN: Initial: 180mg or 240mg qd. Titrate: Adjust PRN. Usual: 180-480mg qd. Max: 540mg qd. ≥60 Yrs: May respond to lower dose of 120mg qd. Angina: Initial: 120mg qd. Titrate: May titrate to doses up to 480mg qd. May be carried out over a 7 to 14 day period. Refer to PI for information regarding concomitant use with other cardiovascular agents.

HOW SUPPLIED: Cap, Extended-Release: (Dilacor XR) 240mg; (Diltia XT) 120mg, 180mg, 240mg

CONTRAINDICATIONS: Sick sinus syndrome and 2nd- or 3rd-degree atrioventricular (AV) block (except with functioning ventricular pacemaker), hypotension (<90mmHg systolic), acute myocardial infarction (AMI) and pulmonary congestion documented by x-ray.

WARNINGS/PRECAUTIONS: Prolongs AV node refractory periods without significantly prolonging sinus node recovery time. Periods of asystole reported in a patient with Prinzmetal's angina. Worsening of congestive heart failure (CHF) reported in patients with preexisting ventricular dysfunction. Decreases in BP may occasionally result in symptomatic hypotension. Mild transaminase elevation with or without concomitant alkaline phosphatase and bilirubin elevation reported. Significant elevations in alkaline phosphatase, LDH, AST, ALT, and other phenomena consistent with acute hepatic injury reported (rare). Caution with renal or hepatic impairment, and preexisting severe GI narrowing (pathologic or iatrogenic). Transient dermatological reactions and skin eruptions progressing to erythema multiforme and/or exfoliative dermatitis have been reported; d/c if a dermatologic reaction persists.

ADVERSE REACTIONS: Rhinitis, pharyngitis, increased cough, asthenia, headache, constipation.

INTERACTIONS: Additive cardiac conduction effects with digitalis or β-blockers. Potential additive effects with any agents known to affect cardiac contractility and/or conduction; caution and careful titration warranted. Competitive inhibition of metabolism with other agents that undergo biotransformation by CYP450 mixed function oxidase. May require dose adjustment of similarly metabolized drugs, particularly those of low therapeutic ratio (eg, cyclosporine), when initiating or stopping concomitantly administered diltiazem, especially in patients with renal and/or hepatic impairment. May increase levels of carbamazepine, resulting in toxicity. May increase levels of propranolol; adjust propranolol dose PRN. Increased levels with cimetidine; adjust diltiazem dose PRN. Monitor digoxin levels, especially when diltiazem therapy is initiated, adjusted, or discontinued. Potentiates depression of cardiac contractility, conductivity, and automaticity as well as vascular dilation with anesthetics; carefully titrate anesthetics and calcium channel blockers (CCBs) when used concomitantly. Additive antihypertensive effect when used concomitantly with other antihypertensive agents; dosage of diltiazem or the concomitant antihypertensives may need to be adjusted. Dilacor XR: Sinus bradycardia resulting in hospitalization and pacemaker insertion reported with clonidine; monitor HR. May increase simvastatin exposure; limit daily doses of simvastatin to 10mg and diltiazem to 240mg if coadministration is required. Risk of myopathy and rhabdomyolysis with statins metabolized by CYP3A4 may be increased. When possible, use a non-CYP3A4-metabolized statin; otherwise, consider dose adjustments for both agents and closely monitor for signs and symptoms of any statin-related adverse events.

PREGNANCY: Category C, not for use in nursing.

MECHANISM OF ACTION: CCB; inhibits influx of Ca^{2+} ions during membrane depolarization of cardiac and vascular smooth muscles. HTN: Relaxes vascular smooth muscle, resulting in decreased peripheral vascular resistance. Angina: Produces increases in exercise tolerance, probably due to its ability to reduce myocardial oxygen demand; accomplished via reductions in HR and systemic BP at submaximal and maximal workloads.

PHARMACOKINETICS: Absorption: Well-absorbed from GI tract; absolute bioavailability (41%); T_{max}=4-6 hrs. **Distribution:** Plasma protein binding (70-80%); found in breast milk. **Metabolism:** Liver (extensive). Desacetyldiltiazem (major metabolite). **Elimination:** Urine (2-4%, unchanged), bile; $T_{1/2}$=5-10 hrs.

NURSING CONSIDERATIONS

Assessment: Assess for sick sinus syndrome, 2nd- or 3rd-degree AV block, hypotension, AMI, pulmonary congestion, impairment of ventricular function, GI narrowing, renal/hepatic impairment, drug hypersensitivity, pregnancy/nursing status, and possible drug interactions.

Monitoring: Monitor for bradycardia, AV block, worsening of CHF, symptomatic hypotension, dermatological reactions, and other adverse reactions. Monitor laboratory parameters at regular intervals when given over prolonged periods. Monitor HR with clonidine.

Patient Counseling: Inform about benefits/risks of therapy. Instruct to take on an empty stomach and swallow cap whole; do not open, chew, or crush.

Administration: Oral route. Swallow whole; do not open, chew or crush. **Storage:** 20-25°C (68-77°F).

DILANTIN   RX
phenytoin sodium (Parke-Davis)

OTHER BRAND NAMES: Dilantin-125 (Parke-Davis) - Dilantin Infatabs (Parke-Davis)

THERAPEUTIC CLASS: Hydantoin

INDICATIONS: (Cap, Extended Release [ER]/Tab, Chewable) Control of generalized tonic-clonic (grand mal) and complex partial (psychomotor, temporal lobe) seizures. Prevention and treatment of seizures during or following neurosurgery. (Sus) Control of tonic-clonic (grand mal) and psychomotor (temporal lobe) seizures.

DOSAGE: *Adults:* Individualize dose. Do not change dose at intervals <7-10 days. May require dose adjustment when switching from product formulated with free acid to product formulated with Na^+ salt and vice versa. (Cap, ER) Divided Daily Dosing: Initial: 100mg tid. Maint: 100mg tid-qid. Titrate: May increase up to 200mg tid, if necessary. QD Dosing: May consider 300mg qd if seizure is controlled on divided doses of three 100mg caps daily. LD (Clinic/Hospital): Initial: 1g in 3 divided doses (400mg, 300mg, 300mg) at 2-hr intervals. Maint: Start maintenance dose 24 hrs after LD. Do not give PO loading regimen in patients with history of renal/liver disease. (Sus) Initial: 125mg (1 tsp) tid. Titrate: May increase to 625mg (5 tsp) daily. (Tab, Chewable) Initial: 100mg (2 tabs) tid. Maint: 300-400mg (6-8 tabs) daily. Titrate: May increase to 600mg (12 tabs) daily. Elderly: May require lower or less frequent dosing.

Pediatrics: Individualize dose. Do not change dose at intervals <7-10 days. Initial: 5mg/kg/day in 2 or 3 equally divided doses. Maint: 4-8mg/kg/day. Max: 300mg/day. >6 Yrs: May require the minimum adult dose (300mg/day). (Tab, Chewable) If daily dose cannot be divided equally, give larger dose before retiring.

HOW SUPPLIED: Cap, ER: (Sodium) 30mg, 100mg; (Dilantin-125) Sus: 125mg/5mL [237mL]; (Infatabs) Tab, Chewable: 50mg* *scored

CONTRAINDICATIONS: Coadministration with delavirdine.

WARNINGS/PRECAUTIONS: Caution in the interpretation of total phenytoin plasma concentrations with renal/hepatic disease, or in those with hypoalbuminemia. Avoid abrupt withdrawal; may precipitate status epilepticus. May increase risk of suicidal thoughts/behavior; monitor for emergence/worsening of depression, suicidal thoughts/behavior, and/or any unusual changes in mood/behavior. Serious and sometimes fatal dermatologic reactions, including toxic epidermal necrolysis (TEN) and Stevens-Johnson syndrome (SJS) reported; d/c at 1st sign of rash, unless the rash is clearly not drug-related. Do not resume therapy and consider alternative therapy if signs/symptoms suggest SJS/TEN. Avoid use as an alternative for carbamazepine in patients positive for HLA-B*1502. Drug reaction with eosinophilia and systemic symptoms (DRESS)/multiorgan hypersensitivity reported; evaluate immediately if signs and symptoms (eg, rash, fever, lymphadenopathy) are present and d/c if an alternative etiology cannot be established. Caution with history of hypersensitivity to structurally similar drugs (eg, carboxamides, barbiturates, succinimides, oxazolidinediones); consider alternatives to therapy. Acute hepatotoxicity (eg, acute hepatic failure) reported; d/c immediately and do not readminister. Hematopoietic complications and lymphadenopathy reported; extended follow-up observation is indicated and every effort should be made to achieve seizure control using alternative antiepileptic drugs in all cases of lymphadenopathy. Decreased bone mineral density and bone fractures reported during chronic use; consider screening and initiating treatment plans as appropriate. Caution with porphyria, hepatic impairment, and in elderly, or gravely ill patients. Bleeding disorder in newborns may occur; give vitamin K to mother before delivery and to neonate after birth. Check plasma levels immediately if early signs of dose-related CNS toxicity develop. Hyperglycemia reported; may increase serum glucose levels in diabetics. Not indicated for seizures due to hypoglycemia or other metabolic causes. Not effective for absence (petit mal) seizures; if tonic-clonic (grand mal) and absence (petit mal) seizures are present, combined drug therapy is needed. May produce confusional states at levels sustained above optimal range; reduce dose if plasma levels are excessive, or d/c if symptoms persist. Lab test interactions may occur. (Cap, ER) Do not use if discolored. (Tab, Chewable) Not for qd dosing.

ADVERSE REACTIONS: Rash, nystagmus, ataxia, slurred speech, decreased coordination, somnolence, mental confusion, dizziness, insomnia, transient nervousness, motor twitching, N/V, thrombocytopenia, altered taste sensation, Peyronie's disease.

INTERACTIONS: See Contraindications. Acute alcohol intake, amiodarone, antiepileptic agents (eg, ethosuximide, felbamate, oxcarbazepine, topiramate), azoles (eg, fluconazole, ketoconazole, itraconazole), capecitabine, chloramphenicol, chlordiazepoxide, diazepam, disulfiram, estrogens, fluorouracil, fluoxetine, fluvastatin, fluvoxamine, H_2-antagonists (eg, cimetidine), halothane, isoniazid, methylphenidate, omeprazole, phenothiazines, salicylates, sertraline, succinimides, sulfonamides (eg, sulfamethizole, sulfadiazine, sulfamethoxazole-trimethoprim), tacrolimus, ticlopidine, tolbutamide, trazodone, warfarin, miconazole, diltiazem, erythromycin, nifedipine, and phenylbutazone may increase levels. Anticancer drugs (eg, bleomycin, carboplatin, cisplatin, doxorubicin, methotrexate), carbamazepine, chronic alcohol abuse, folic acid, fosamprenavir, nelfinavir, reserpine, ritonavir, St. John's wort, sucralfate, vigabatrin, diazoxide, rifampin, and theophylline may decrease levels. Administration with preparations that increase gastric pH (eg, supplements or antacids containing calcium carbonate, aluminum hydroxide, and magnesium hydroxide) may affect absorption; do not take at the same time of day. Phenobarbital, sodium valproate, valproic acid, carbamazepine, ciprofloxacin, and diazepam may increase or decrease levels. May impair efficacy of azoles (eg, fluconazole, ketoconazole, voriconazole), corticosteroids, doxycycline, estrogens, furosemide, irinotecan, oral contraceptives, paclitaxel, paroxetine, quinidine, rifampin, sertraline, teniposide, theophylline, and vitamin D. Increased and decreased PT/INR responses reported with warfarin. May decrease levels of chlorpropamide, clozapine, diazoxide, methadone, nimodipine, verapamil, albendazole, certain HIV antivirals (eg, efavirenz, lopinavir/ritonavir, indinavir), anti-epileptic agents (eg, felbamate, topiramate, quetiapine), atorvastatin, cyclosporine, digoxin, fluvastatin, folic acid, mexiletine, nisoldipine, praziquantel, and simvastatin. May decrease levels of amprenavir (active metabolite) when given with fosamprenavir alone. May increase levels of amprenavir when given with the combination of fosamprenavir and ritonavir. Resistance to the neuromuscular blocking action of pancuronium, vecuronium, rocuronium, and cisatracurium reported in patients chronically administered phenytoin; monitor closely for more rapid recovery from neuromuscular blockade than expected, and higher infusion rate requirements. Avoid with enteral feeding preparations and/or nutritional supplements.

PREGNANCY: Category D, not for use in nursing.

MECHANISM OF ACTION: Hydantoin; inhibits seizure activity by promoting Na^+ efflux from neurons, stabilizing the threshold against hyperexcitability caused by excessive stimulation or environmental changes capable of reducing membrane Na^+ gradient. Reduces the maximal activity of the brain stem centers responsible for the tonic phase of tonic-clonic (grand mal) seizures.

PHARMACOKINETICS: Absorption: T_{max}=1.5-3 hrs (tab, chewable/sus), 4-12 hrs (cap, ER). **Distribution:** Plasma protein binding (high); found in breast milk. **Metabolism:** Liver (hydroxylation). **Elimination:** Bile (mostly as inactive metabolites), urine; $T_{1/2}$=22 hrs, 14 hrs (tab, chewable).

NURSING CONSIDERATIONS

Assessment: Assess for hypersensitivity to the drug, its inactive ingredients, or other hydantoins, alcohol use, hepatic/renal impairment, porphyria, grave illness, seizures due to hypoglycemia or other metabolic causes, absence seizures, any other conditions where treatment is contraindicated or cautioned, pregnancy/nursing status, and possible drug interactions.

Monitoring: Monitor for hypersensitivity reactions, dermatologic reactions, DRESS/multiorgan hypersensitivity, hepatotoxicity, hematopoietic complications, lymphadenopathy, decreased bone mineral density, bone fractures, exacerbation of porphyria, hyperglycemia, and other adverse reactions. Monitor for emergence/worsening of depression, suicidal thoughts/behavior, and/or any unusual changes in mood/behavior. Monitor serum levels when switching from Na⁺ salt to free acid form and vice versa.

Patient Counseling: Instruct to read medication guide and to take ud. Advise of the importance of adhering strictly to the prescribed dosage regimen, and of informing the physician of any clinical condition in which it is not possible to take the drug orally as prescribed (eg, surgery). Counsel about the early toxic signs and symptoms of potential hematologic, dermatologic, hypersensitivity, or hepatic reactions; instruct to immediately contact physician if these develop. Caution on the use of other drugs or alcoholic beverages without first seeking physician's advice. Stress the importance of good dental hygiene to minimize the development of gingival hyperplasia and its complications. Advise to notify physician immediately if depression, suicidal thoughts, behavior, or thoughts about self-harm emerge. Encourage patients to enroll in the North American Antiepileptic Drug Pregnancy Registry.

Administration: Oral route. (Tab, Chewable) May chew or swallow tab whole. (Sus) Use an accurately calibrated measuring device to ensure accurate dosing. **Storage:** 20-25°C (68-77°F). Protect from moisture. (Cap, ER) Preserve in tight, light-resistant containers. (Sus) Protect from freezing and light.

DILAUDID ORAL   `CII`
hydromorphone HCl (Purdue Pharma)

> Contains hydromorphone, a Schedule II controlled opioid agonist with the highest potential for abuse and risk of respiratory depression. Alcohol, other opioids, and CNS depressants (eg, sedative-hypnotics) potentiate respiratory depressant effects, increasing the risk of respiratory depression that may result in death.

THERAPEUTIC CLASS: Opioid analgesic

INDICATIONS: Management of pain in patients where an opioid analgesic is appropriate.

DOSAGE: *Adults:* Individualize dose. Periodically reassess after the initial dosing. (Sol) Usual: 2.5-10mg q3-6h ud by clinical situation. (Tab) Initial: 2-4mg q4-6h. Titrate: May increase gradually if analgesia is inadequate, as tolerance develops, or if pain severity increases. (Sol/Tab): Non-Opioid-Tolerant: Initial: 2-4mg q4h. Patients Taking Opioids: Base starting dose on prior opioid usage; refer to PI for conversion from prior opioid. Give only 1/2 to 2/3 of the estimated dose for the 1st few doses, then increase PRN according to response. Elderly: Start at lower end of dosing range. Hepatic/Renal Impairment: Start on a lower dose and closely monitor during titration; use oral liquid to adjust the dose. Chronic Pain: Administer dose around-the-clock. May give a supplemental dose of 5-15% of the total daily usage q2h PRN.

HOW SUPPLIED: Sol: 1mg/mL [473mL]; Tab: 2mg, 4mg, 8mg* *scored

CONTRAINDICATIONS: Respiratory depression in the absence of resuscitative equipment, status asthmaticus, obstetrical analgesia.

WARNINGS/PRECAUTIONS: Respiratory depression is more likely to occur in elderly, debilitated, and those suffering from conditions accompanied by hypoxia or hypercapnia; extreme caution with chronic obstructive pulmonary disease (COPD) or cor pulmonale, substantially decreased respiratory reserve, hypoxia, hypercapnia, or preexisting respiratory depression. May cause neonatal withdrawal syndrome. Respiratory depressant effects with carbon dioxide retention and secondary elevation of CSF pressure may be markedly exaggerated in the presence of head injury, other intracranial lesions, or preexisting increase in intracranial pressure (ICP). May produce effects on pupillary response and consciousness which can obscure the clinical course and neurologic signs of further increase in ICP in patients with head injuries. May cause severe hypotension; caution with circulatory shock. Contains sodium metabisulfite; may cause allergic-type reactions, including anaphylactic symptoms and life-threatening or less severe asthmatic episodes in certain susceptible people. Caution in elderly/debilitated and those with severe pulmonary/hepatic/renal impairment, myxedema/hypothyroidism, adrenocortical insufficiency (eg, Addison's disease), CNS depression or coma, toxic psychoses, prostatic hypertrophy, urethral

stricture, gallbladder disease, acute alcoholism, delirium tremens, kyphoscoliosis, or following GI surgery; reduce initial dose. May obscure the diagnosis or clinical course in patients with
acute abdominal conditions. May aggravate preexisting convulsions in patients with convulsive
disorders. Mild to severe seizures and myoclonus reported in severely compromised patients
administered high doses of parenteral hydromorphone. Caution with alcoholism and other drug
dependencies. May impair mental/physical abilities. May produce orthostatic hypotension in
ambulatory patients. May cause spasm of the sphincter of Oddi; caution in patients about to undergo biliary tract surgery. Physical dependence and tolerance may occur. Do not abruptly d/c.

ADVERSE REACTIONS: Respiratory depression, apnea, lightheadedness, dizziness, sedation,
N/V, sweating, flushing, dysphoria, euphoria, dry mouth, pruritus.

INTERACTIONS: See Boxed Warning. Concomitant use with other CNS depressants (eg, general
anesthetics, phenothiazines, tranquilizers) may produce additive depressant effects; use with
caution and in reduced dosages. Do not give with alcohol. May enhance action of neuromuscular
blocking agents and produce an excessive degree of respiratory depression. May cause severe
hypotension with phenothiazines or general anesthetics. Mixed agonist/antagonist analgesics
(pentazocine, nalbuphine, butorphanol, buprenorphine) may reduce the analgesic effect and/or
may precipitate withdrawal symptoms; use with caution.

PREGNANCY: Category C, not for use in nursing.

MECHANISM OF ACTION: Opioid analgesic; pure opioid agonist. Has not been established.
Believed to express pharmacologic effects by combining with specific CNS opiate receptors.

PHARMACOKINETICS: Absorption: Rapid. (Tab) Bioavailability (24%); C_{max}=5.5ng; T_{max}=0.74
hrs; AUC=23.7ng•hr/mL. (Sol) C_{max}=5.7ng; T_{max}=0.73 hrs; AUC=24.6ng•hr/mL. **Distribution:**
Plasma protein binding (8-19%); V_d=302.9L (IV bolus); crosses placenta; found in breast milk.
Metabolism: Liver (extensive) via glucuronidation; hydromorphone-3-glucuronide (metabolite).
Elimination: Urine; $T_{1/2}$=2.6 hrs (tab), 2.8 hrs (sol).

NURSING CONSIDERATIONS

Assessment: Assess for risk factors for drug abuse or addiction, pain type/severity, prior opioid
therapy, opioid tolerance, respiratory depression, COPD, cor pulmonale, decreased respiratory
reserve, hypoxia, hypercapnia, asthma, renal/hepatic impairment, pregnancy/nursing status, possible drug interactions, or any other conditions where treatment is contraindicated or
cautioned.

Monitoring: Monitor for respiratory depression, sedation, CNS depression, aggravation/induc-
tion of seizures/convulsions, increase in ICP, hypotension, tolerance, physical dependence, and
other adverse reactions. Routinely monitor for signs of misuse, abuse, and addiction.

Patient Counseling: Inform that medication may cause severe adverse effects (eg, respiratory
depression) if not taken ud. Instruct to report pain and adverse experiences occurring during
therapy. Advise not to adjust dose or combine with alcohol or other CNS depressants without
prescriber's consent. Inform that drug may impair mental/physical abilities; instruct to use caution when performing hazardous tasks (eg, operating machinery/driving). Advise to consult
physician if pregnant or planning to become pregnant. Inform that drug has potential for abuse;
instruct to protect it from theft and never to share with others. Advise to avoid abrupt withdrawal if taking medication for more than a few weeks and cessation of therapy is indicated. Instruct
to keep drug in a secure place, and to destroy unused tabs by flushing down toilet.

Administration: Oral route. Refer to PI for safety and handling instructions. **Storage:** 25°C
(77°F); excursions permitted to 15-30°C (59-86°F). Protect from light.

DILTIAZEM INJECTION   RX
diltiazem HCl (Various)

THERAPEUTIC CLASS: Calcium channel blocker (nondihydropyridine)

INDICATIONS: Temporary control of rapid ventricular rate in atrial fibrillation/flutter (A-fib/flut-
ter). Rapid conversion of paroxysmal supraventricular tachycardia (PSVT) to sinus rhythm.

DOSAGE: *Adults:* Bolus: 0.25mg/kg IV over 2 min. If no response after 15 min, may give 2nd dose
of 0.35mg/kg over 2 min. Continuous Infusion: 0.25-0.35mg/kg IV bolus, then 10mg/hr. Titrate:
Increase by 5mg/hr. Max: 15mg/hr and duration up to 24 hrs.

HOW SUPPLIED: Inj: 5mg/mL

CONTRAINDICATIONS: Sick sinus syndrome and 2nd- or 3rd-degree atrioventricular (AV) block
(except with functioning pacemaker), severe hypotension, cardiogenic shock, concomitant IV
β-blockers or within a few hrs of use, A-fib/flutter associated with accessory bypass tract (eg,
Wolff-Parkinson-White [WPW] syndrome, short PR syndrome), ventricular tachycardia.

WARNINGS/PRECAUTIONS: Initiate in setting with resuscitation capabilities. Caution if hemodynamically compromised, and with renal, hepatic, or ventricular dysfunction. Monitor ECG
continuously and BP frequently. Symptomatic hypotension, acute hepatic injury reported. D/C if

high-degree AV block occurs in sinus rhythm or if persistent rash occurs. Ventricular premature beats may be present on conversion of PSVT to sinus rhythm.

ADVERSE REACTIONS: Hypotension, inj-site reactions (eg, itching, burning), vasodilation (flushing), arrhythmias.

INTERACTIONS: See Contraindications. Caution with drugs that decrease peripheral resistance, intravascular volume, myocardial contractility or conduction. Increased area under the curve (AUC) of midazolam, triazolam, buspirone, quinidine, and lovastatin, which may require a dose adjustment due to increased clinical effects or increased adverse events. Elevates carbamazepine levels, which may result in toxicity. Cyclosporine may need dose adjustment. Potentiates the depression of cardiac contractility, conductivity, automaticity, and vascular dilation with anesthetics. Possible bradycardia, AV block, and contractility depression with oral β-blockers. Possible competitive inhibition of metabolism with drugs metabolized by CYP450. Avoid rifampin. Monitor for excessive slowing of HR and/or AV block with digoxin. Cimetidine increases peak diltiazem plasma levels and AUC.

PREGNANCY: Category C, not for use in nursing.

MECHANISM OF ACTION: Calcium channel blocker; inhibits influx of Ca^{2+} ions during membrane depolarization of cardiac and vascular smooth muscle. Has ability to slow AV nodal conduction time and prolong AV nodal refractoriness, which has therapeutic benefits on supraventricular tachycardia. Decreases peripheral resistance, resulting in decreased systolic and diastolic BP.

PHARMACOKINETICS: Distribution: V_d=305-391L; plasma protein binding (70-80%); found in breast milk. **Metabolism:** Liver (extensive) via CYP450; deacetylation, N-demethylation, O-demethylation, and conjugation; N-monodesmethyldiltiazem and desacetyldiltiazem (major metabolites). **Elimination:** Urine and bile; $T_{1/2}$=3.4 hrs (single IV inj), 4.1-4.9 hrs (constant IV infusion).

NURSING CONSIDERATIONS

Assessment: Assess for sick sinus syndrome and 2nd- or 3rd-degree AV block, presence of functioning pacemaker, severe hypotension, cardiogenic shock, A-fib/flutter associated with accessory bypass tract (eg, WPW syndrome, short PR syndrome), ventricular tachycardia, wide complex tachycardia, acute myocardial infarction, congestive heart failure, pulmonary congestion documented by x-ray, hypertrophic cardiomyopathy, renal/hepatic impairment, pregnancy/nursing status, and possible drug interactions.

Monitoring: Initiation of therapy should be done in setting with monitoring and resuscitation capabilities, including DC cardioversion/defibrillation. Monitor BP, HR, LFTs, and ECG. Monitor for hemodynamic deterioration, ventricular fibrillation, cardiac conduction abnormalities (eg, 2nd- or 3rd-degree AV block), ventricular premature beats, dermatologic events (erythema multiforme/exfoliative dermatitis), and acute hepatic injury.

Patient Counseling: Inform that initiation of therapy should be done in a setting with monitoring and resuscitation capabilities, including DC cardioversion/defibrillation. Inform of risks/benefits and instruct to report adverse reactions. Advise to notify physician if pregnant/nursing.

Administration: IV route. **Storage:** 2-8°C (36-46°F). Do not freeze. Room temperature for up to 1 month. Destroy after 1 month. Diluted Sol: D5W, 0.9% NaCl, or D5W & 0.45% NaCl: Stable at 20-25°C (68-77°F) or 2-8°C (36-46°F) for at least 24 hrs when stored in a glass or polyvinyl chloride bag.

DIOVAN   RX
valsartan (Novartis)

> D/C when pregnancy is detected. Drugs that act directly on the renin-angiotensin system (RAS) can cause injury/death to the developing fetus.

THERAPEUTIC CLASS: Angiotensin II receptor antagonist

INDICATIONS: Treatment of HTN alone or in combination with other antihypertensives. Treatment of heart failure (HF) (NYHA Class II-IV). Reduction of cardiovascular mortality in clinically stable patients with left ventricular failure/dysfunction following myocardial infarction (MI).

DOSAGE: *Adults:* HTN: Monotherapy without Volume Depletion: Initial: 80mg or 160mg qd. Titrate: May increase to a max of 320mg qd or add diuretic. Max: 320mg/day. HF: Initial: 40mg bid. Titrate: May increase to 80mg and 160mg bid (use highest dose tolerated). Consider dose reduction of concomitant diuretics. Max: 320mg/day in divided doses. Post-MI: Initial: 20mg bid as early as 12 hrs after MI. Titrate: May increase to 40mg bid within 7 days, with subsequent titrations to 160mg bid as tolerated. Maint: 160mg bid. Consider decreasing dose if develop symptomatic hypotension or renal dysfunction. May be given with other standard post-MI treatments, including thrombolytics, aspirin, β-blockers, and statins.
Pediatrics: 6-16 Yrs: HTN: Initial: 1.3mg/kg qd (up to 40mg total). Adjust dose according to BP response. Max: 2.7mg/kg (up to 160mg) qd. Use of a sus is recommended for children who cannot

D

swallow tabs, or if calculated dosage does not correspond to available tab strength. Adjust dose accordingly when switching dosage forms; exposure with sus is 1.6X greater than with tab.

HOW SUPPLIED: Tab: 40mg*, 80mg, 160mg, 320mg *scored

CONTRAINDICATIONS: Coadministration with aliskiren in patients with diabetes.

WARNINGS/PRECAUTIONS: Symptomatic hypotension may occur in patients with an activated RAS (eg, volume- and/or salt-depleted patients receiving high doses of diuretics); correct this condition prior to therapy. Caution when initiating therapy in patients with HF or post-MI. Renal function changes may occur; caution in patients whose renal function depend in part on the activity of the RAS (eg, renal artery stenosis, chronic kidney disease, severe CHF, volume deple-tion). Consider withholding or discontinuing therapy if clinically significant decrease in renal function develops. Increased K^+ in some patients with HF reported, and more likely to occur in patients with preexisting renal impairment; dose reduction and/or discontinuation of therapy may be required. Do not readminister to patients who have had angioedema. Caution with dosing in patients with hepatic or severe renal impairment.

ADVERSE REACTIONS: Headache, abdominal pain, cough, increased BUN, hyperkalemia, dizzi-ness, hypotension, SrCr elevation, viral infection, fatigue, diarrhea, arthralgia, back pain.

INTERACTIONS: See Contraindications. Dual blockade of the RAS is associated with increased risk of hypotension, hyperkalemia, and changes in renal function (including acute renal failure); closely monitor BP, renal function and electrolytes with concomitant agents that also affect the RAS. Avoid with aliskiren in patients with renal impairment (GFR <60mL/min). Inhibitors of the hepatic uptake transporter OATP1B1 (rifampin, cyclosporine) and the hepatic efflux transporter MRP2 (ritonavir) may increase exposure. Other agents that block the RAS, K^+-sparing diuretics, K^+ supplements, or salt substitutes containing K^+ may increase serum K^+ levels, and in HF pa-tients may increase SrCr; monitor serum K^+ levels. Greater antihypertensive effect with atenolol. NSAIDs, including selective COX-2 inhibitors may result in deterioration of renal function, includ-ing possible acute renal failure, and may attenuate antihypertensive effect. Increased lithium levels and lithium toxicity reported; monitor serum lithium levels during concomitant use.

PREGNANCY: Category D, not for use in nursing.

MECHANISM OF ACTION: Angiotensin II receptor antagonist; blocks vasoconstrictor and aldosterone-secreting effects of angiotensin II by selectively blocking the binding of angiotensin II to the AT_1 receptor in many tissues (eg, vascular smooth muscle, adrenal gland).

PHARMACOKINETICS: Absorption: Absolute bioavailability (25%); T_{max}=2-4 hrs. **Distribution:** Plasma protein binding (95%); (IV) V_d=17L. **Metabolism:** Via CYP2C9; valeryl 4-hydroxy valsartan (primary metabolite). **Elimination:** (Sol) Feces (83%), urine (13%). (IV) $T_{1/2}$=6 hrs.

NURSING CONSIDERATIONS

Assessment: Assess for hypersensitivity to the drug and its components, hepatic/renal impair-ment, volume/salt depletion, renal artery stenosis, HF, pregnancy/nursing status, and possible drug interactions.

Monitoring: Monitor for signs/symptoms of hypotension and other adverse reactions. Monitor electrolytes, BP, and renal function.

Patient Counseling: Counsel about the risk/benefits of therapy and possible adverse effects. Inform of consequences of exposure during pregnancy and discuss treatment options with wom-en planning to become pregnant. Instruct to report pregnancies to physician as soon as possible.

Administration: Oral route. Take with or without food. Refer to PI for instructions on preparation of oral sus. **Storage:** (Tab) 25°C (77°F); excursions permitted to 15-30°C (59-86°F). Protect from moisture. (Sus) <30°C (86°F) for up to 30 days or at 2-8°C (35-46°F) for up to 75 days.

DIOVAN **HCT**   RX
hydrochlorothiazide - valsartan (Novartis)

D/C when pregnancy is detected. Drugs that act directly on the renin-angiotensin system (RAS) can cause injury/death to the developing fetus.

THERAPEUTIC CLASS: Angiotensin II receptor antagonist/thiazide diuretic

INDICATIONS: Treatment of HTN alone or in combination with other antihypertensives. May be used in patients whose BP is not adequately controlled on monotherapy. May also be used as initial therapy in patients likely to need multiple drugs to achieve BP goals.

DOSAGE: *Adults:* Initial Therapy: 160mg-12.5mg qd. Titrate: May increase after 1-2 weeks of therapy. Max: 320mg-25mg qd. Add-On Therapy: Use if not adequately controlled with valsartan (or another ARB) alone or HCTZ alone. With dose-limiting adverse reactions to either component alone, may switch to therapy containing a lower dose of that component. Titrate: May increase after 3-4 weeks of therapy if BP uncontrolled. Max: 320mg-25mg. Replacement Therapy: May substitute for titrated components.

HOW SUPPLIED: Tab: (Valsartan-HCTZ) 80mg-12.5mg, 160mg-12.5mg, 160mg-25mg, 320mg-12.5mg, 320mg-25mg

CONTRAINDICATIONS: Anuria, sulfonamide-derived drug hypersensitivity. Coadministration with aliskiren in patients with diabetes.

WARNINGS/PRECAUTIONS: Not for initial therapy with intravascular volume depletion. Symptomatic hypotension may occur in patients with activated RAS (eg, volume- and/or salt-depleted patients receiving high doses of diuretics); correct this condition prior to therapy. Renal function changes may occur including acute renal failure; caution in patients whose renal function depend in part on the activity of the RAS (eg, renal artery stenosis, chronic kidney disease, severe congestive heart failure, or volume depletion). Consider withholding or discontinuing therapy if clinically significant decrease in renal function develops. May cause serum electrolyte abnormalities (eg, hyperkalemia, hypokalemia, hyponatremia, hypomagnesemia); correct hypokalemia and any coexisting hypomagnesemia prior to initiation of therapy and monitor periodically. D/C if hypokalemia is accompanied by clinical signs (eg, muscular weakness, paresis, ECG alterations). Increased K^+ in patients with heart failure (HF) reported; dose reduction or discontinuation of therapy may be required. Do not readminister to patients with angioedema. HCTZ: May cause hypersensitivity reactions and exacerbation or activation of systemic lupus erythematosus (SLE). May precipitate hepatic coma with hepatic impairment or progressive liver disease. May cause idiosyncratic reaction, resulting in acute transient myopia and acute angle-closure glaucoma; d/c as rapidly as possible. May alter glucose tolerance and increase serum cholesterol and TG levels. May cause or exacerbate hyperuricemia and precipitate gout in susceptible patients. May cause hypercalcemia.

ADVERSE REACTIONS: Dizziness, BUN elevations, hypokalemia, angioedema, dry cough, nasopharyngitis.

INTERACTIONS: See Contraindications. Increased lithium levels and lithium toxicity reported; monitor lithium levels during concomitant use. Valsartan: Dual blockade of the RAS is associated with increased risk of hypotension, hyperkalemia, and changes in renal function (including acute renal failure); closely monitor BP, renal function, and electrolytes with concomitant agents that also affect the RAS. Avoid with aliskiren in patients with renal impairment (GFR <60mL/min). Greater antihypertensive effect with atenolol. Inhibitors of the hepatic uptake transporter OATP1B1 (rifampin, cyclosporine) or the hepatic efflux transporter MRP2 (ritonavir) may increase exposure. NSAIDs, including selective COX-2 inhibitors, may result in deterioration of renal function, including possible acute renal failure, and may attenuate antihypertensive effect. Other agents that block the RAS, K^+-sparing diuretics, K^+ supplements, or salt substitutes containing K^+ may increase serum K^+ levels, and in HF patients may increase SrCr; monitor serum K^+ levels. HCTZ: Dosage adjustment of antidiabetic drugs (eg, oral agents, insulin) may be required. May lead to symptomatic hyponatremia with carbamazepine. Ion exchange resins (eg, cholestyramine, colestipol) may reduce exposure; space dosing at least 4 hrs before or 4-6 hrs after the administration of ion exchange resins. Cyclosporine may increase risk of hyperuricemia and gout-type complications.

PREGNANCY: Category D, not for use in nursing.

MECHANISM OF ACTION: Valsartan: Angiotensin II receptor antagonist; blocks vasoconstrictor and aldosterone-secreting effects of angiotensin II by selectively blocking binding of angiotensin II to AT_1 receptor. HCTZ: Thiazide diuretic; has not been established. Affects the renal tubular mechanisms of electrolyte reabsorption, directly increasing excretion of Na^+ and Cl^- in approximately equivalent amounts, and indirectly reducing plasma volume.

PHARMACOKINETICS: Absorption: Valsartan: (Cap) Absolute bioavailability (25%); T_{max}=2-4 hrs. HCTZ: Absolute bioavailability (70%); T_{max}=2-5 hrs. **Distribution:** Valsartan: Plasma protein binding (95%); (IV) V_d=17L. HCTZ: Albumin binding (40-70%); crosses placenta; found in breast milk. **Metabolism:** Valsartan: Via CYP2C9; valeryl 4-hydroxy valsartan (primary metabolite). **Elimination:** Valsartan: (Sol) Feces (83%), urine (13%); (IV) $T_{1/2}$=6 hrs. HCTZ: Urine (70%, unchanged); $T_{1/2}$=10 hrs.

NURSING CONSIDERATIONS

Assessment: Assess for hypersensitivity to the drug and its components, anuria, history of sulfonamide-derived hypersensitivity or penicillin allergy, renal/hepatic impairment, volume/salt depletion, risk for acute renal failure, SLE, electrolyte imbalances, pregnancy/nursing status, and possible drug interactions.

Monitoring: Monitor for signs/symptoms of hypotension, hypersensitivity/idiosyncratic reactions, exacerbation or activation of SLE, myopia, angle-closure glaucoma, precipitation of gout or hyperuricemia, and other adverse reactions. Monitor BP, serum electrolytes, cholesterol, TG levels, and renal function periodically.

Patient Counseling: Inform about the consequences of exposure during pregnancy and discuss treatment options in women planning to become pregnant. Instruct to report pregnancies to physician as soon as possible. Caution about lightheadedness, especially during the 1st days of therapy; instruct to d/c and consult physician if syncope occurs. Caution that inadequate fluid intake, excessive perspiration, diarrhea, and vomiting may lead to an excessive fall in BP with the same consequences of lightheadedness and possible syncope. Instruct to avoid use of K⁺ supplements or salt substitutes containing K⁺ without consulting a physician.

Administration: Oral route. Take with or without food. **Storage:** 25°C (77°F); excursions permitted to 15-30°C (59-86°F). Protect from moisture.

D

DIPHENHYDRAMINE INJECTION   RX
diphenhydramine HCl (Various)

THERAPEUTIC CLASS: Antihistamine

INDICATIONS: For amelioration of allergic reactions to blood or plasma, in anaphylaxis as an adjunct to epinephrine and other standard measures after the acute symptoms have been controlled, and for other uncomplicated allergic conditions of the immediate type when PO therapy is impossible or contraindicated. For active treatment of motion sickness when PO form is impractical. For parkinsonism when PO therapy is impossible or contraindicated.

DOSAGE: *Adults:* Individualize dose. Usual: 10-50mg IV at a rate ≤25mg/min, or deep IM. May use 100mg if required. Max: 400mg/day.
Pediatrics: Individualize dose. Usual: 5mg/kg/24 hrs or 150mg/m²/24 hrs in 4 divided doses. Administer IV at a rate ≤25mg/min, or deep IM. Max: 300mg/day.

HOW SUPPLIED: Inj: 50mg/mL [1mL]

CONTRAINDICATIONS: Neonates, premature infants, nursing, use as a local anesthetic.

WARNINGS/PRECAUTIONS: Caution with narrow-angle glaucoma, stenosing peptic ulcer, pyloroduodenal obstruction, symptomatic prostatic hypertrophy, or bladder-neck obstruction. May cause hallucinations, convulsions, or death in pediatrics, especially, in overdosage. May produce excitation and may diminish mental alertness in pediatrics. Increased risk of dizziness, sedation, and hypotension in elderly. Caution with a history of bronchial asthma, increased intraocular pressure (IOP), hyperthyroidism, lower respiratory disease (eg, asthma), cardiovascular disease (CVD), or HTN. Local necrosis reported with SQ or intradermal use of IV formulation.

ADVERSE REACTIONS: Sedation, sleepiness, dizziness, disturbed coordination, epigastric distress, thickening of bronchial secretions, drug rash, hypotension, hemolytic anemia, urinary frequency, headache, photosensitivity, agranulocytosis, insomnia, anorexia.

INTERACTIONS: Additive effects with alcohol and other CNS depressants (hypnotics, sedatives, tranquilizers). MAOIs prolong and intensify anticholinergic effects.

PREGNANCY: Category B, contraindicated in nursing.

MECHANISM OF ACTION: Antihistamine; appears to compete with histamine for cell receptor sites on effector cells.

PHARMACOKINETICS: Metabolism: Liver. **Elimination:** Urine.

NURSING CONSIDERATIONS

Assessment: Assess for narrow-angle glaucoma, stenosing peptic ulcer, pyloroduodenal obstruction, prostatic hypertrophy, bladder-neck obstruction, history of bronchial asthma, increased IOP, hyperthyroidism, CVD, lower respiratory disease, HTN, local anesthetic use, nursing status, and possible drug interactions.

Monitoring: Monitor for diminished mental alertness and for other adverse reactions. Monitor for dizziness, sedation, and hypotension in elderly. Monitor for hallucinations and convulsions in pediatric patients.

Patient Counseling: Advise that the drug may cause drowsiness and has an additive effect with alcohol. Warn about engaging in activities requiring mental alertness; inform that therapy may impair physical/mental abilities.

Administration: IV/IM route. **Storage:** 20-25°C (68-77°F); excursions permitted to 15-30°C (59-86°F). Protect from light.

DIVIGEL   RX
estradiol (Upsher-Smith)

Estrogens increase the risk of endometrial cancer in women with uterus. Perform adequate diagnostic measures (eg, endometrial sampling) to rule out malignancy with undiagnosed persistent or recurring abnormal genital bleeding. Should not be used for the prevention of cardiovascular disease (CVD) or dementia. Increased risk of myocardial infarction (MI), stroke, pulmonary embolism (PE), and deep vein thrombosis (DVT) in postmenopausal women (50-79 yrs) reported. May increase risk of invasive breast cancer. Increased risk of developing probable dementia in postmenopausal women ≥65 yrs reported. Should be prescribed at the lowest effective dose and for the shortest duration consistent with treatment goals and risks.

THERAPEUTIC CLASS: Estrogen

INDICATIONS: Treatment of moderate to severe vasomotor symptoms due to menopause.

DOSAGE: *Adults:* Initial: 0.25g qd applied on skin of right or left upper thigh. Reevaluate periodically.

HOW SUPPLIED: Gel: 0.1% [0.25g, 0.5g, 1g pkts]

CONTRAINDICATIONS: Undiagnosed abnormal genital bleeding, known/suspected/history of breast cancer, known/suspected estrogen-dependent neoplasia, active/history of DVT, PE, or arterial thromboembolic disease (eg, stroke, MI), liver impairment/disease, protein C/protein S/ antithrombin deficiency, or other known thrombophilic disorders, known/suspected pregnancy.

WARNINGS/PRECAUTIONS: D/C immediately if PE, DVT, stroke, or MI occurs or is suspected. Caution in patients with risk factors for arterial vascular disease and/or venous thromboembolism (VTE). If feasible, d/c at least 4-6 weeks before surgery of the type associated with increased risk of thromboembolism, or during periods of prolonged immobilization. May increase risk of gallbladder disease requiring surgery and ovarian cancer. Consider addition of progestin for women with a uterus or with residual endometriosis posthysterectomy. May lead to severe hypercalcemia in patients with breast cancer and bone metastases; d/c and take appropriate measures if this occurs. Retinal vascular thrombosis reported; d/c pending examination if sudden partial/complete loss of vision, sudden onset of proptosis, diplopia, or migraine occurs. D/C permanently if examination reveals papilledema or retinal vascular lesions. May elevate BP and thyroid-binding globulin levels. May elevate plasma TG levels (with preexisting hypertriglyceridemia); consider discontinuation if pancreatitis occurs. Caution with history of cholestatic jaundice; d/c in case of recurrence. May cause fluid retention; caution with cardiac or renal impairment. Caution with hypoparathyroidism; hypocalcemia may occur. May exacerbate symptoms of angioedema in women with hereditary angioedema. May exacerbate endometriosis, asthma, diabetes mellitus (DM), epilepsy, migraine, porphyria, systemic lupus erythematosus (SLE), and hepatic hemangiomas; use with caution. May affect certain endocrine, and blood components in lab tests. Alcohol-based gels are flammable; avoid fire, flame, or smoking until applied dose has dried. Occlusion of the application area with clothing or other barriers is not recommended until gel has completely dried. Potential for drug transfer following physical contact; cover application site after drying.

ADVERSE REACTIONS: Nasopharyngitis, upper respiratory tract infection, vaginal mycosis, breast tenderness, metrorrhagia.

INTERACTIONS: CYP3A4 inducers (eg, St. John's wort, phenobarbital, carbamazepine, rifampin) may decrease levels; may decrease therapeutic effects and/or change uterine bleeding profile. CYP3A4 inhibitors (eg, erythromycin, clarithromycin, ketoconazole, itraconazole, ritonavir, grapefruit juice) may increase levels; may result in side effects. Patients concomitantly receiving thyroid replacement therapy and estrogens may require increased doses of thyroid replacement therapy. May change systemic exposure with sunscreens.

PREGNANCY: Contraindicated in pregnancy, caution in nursing.

MECHANISM OF ACTION: Estrogen; binds to nuclear receptors in estrogen-responsive tissues. Circulating estrogens modulate pituitary secretion of gonadotropins, luteinizing hormone and follicle-stimulating hormone, through negative feedback mechanism. Reduces elevated levels of these hormones seen in postmenopausal women.

PHARMACOKINETICS: Absorption: Topical administration of variable doses resulted in different parameters. **Distribution:** Largely bound to sex hormone-binding globulin and albumin; found in breast milk. **Metabolism:** Liver to estrone (metabolite), estriol (major urinary metabolite); sulfate and glucuronide conjugation (liver); hydrolysis (intestine); CYP3A4 (partial metabolism). **Elimination:** Urine; $T_{1/2}$=10 hrs.

NURSING CONSIDERATIONS

Assessment: Assess for undiagnosed abnormal genital bleeding, liver impairment, presence/ history of breast cancer, estrogen-dependent neoplasia, DVT, PE, arterial thromboembolic disease, history of cholestatic jaundice, pregnancy/nursing status, any other conditions where treatment is contraindicated or cautioned, need for progestin therapy, and possible drug interactions. Assess for protein C, protein S, or antithrombin deficiency, or other known thrombophilic disorders.

Monitoring: Monitor for signs/symptoms of CVD, arterial vascular disease, VTE, malignant neoplasms, dementia, gallbladder disease, hypercalcemia, BP and plasma TG elevations, visual abnormalities, pancreatitis, cholestatic jaundice, hypothyroidism, fluid retention, exacerbation of endometriosis or other conditions. Perform annual breast exam; schedule mammography based on age, risk factors, and prior mammogram results. Monitor thyroid function in patients on thyroid replacement therapy. Perform adequate diagnostic measures (eg, endometrial sampling) in patients with undiagnosed persistent or recurrent genital bleeding. Perform periodic evaluation to determine treatment need.

Patient Counseling: Inform postmenopausal women of the importance of reporting vaginal bleeding as soon as possible and of possible serious adverse reactions of therapy and possible less serious but common adverse reactions. Advise to have yearly breast exams by a physician and to perform monthly self-breast exams. Instruct on the proper application and use. Inform that gel contains alcohol that is flammable; instruct to avoid fire, flame, or smoking until the gel has dried. Inform of potential for drug transfer from one individual to the other following physical contact; advise to avoid skin contact with other subjects until the gel is completely dried.

Administration: Topical route. Refer to PI for complete administration instructions. **Storage:** 20-25°C (68-77°F); excursions permitted to 15-30°C (59-86°F).

DOCETAXEL   RX
docetaxel (Various)

Increased treatment-related mortality reported with hepatic dysfunction, high-dose therapy, and in patients with non-small cell lung carcinoma (NSCLC) who had prior platinum-based chemotherapy with docetaxel at 100mg/m². Avoid if neutrophils <1500 cells/mm³, bilirubin >ULN, or AST/ALT >1.5X ULN with alkaline phosphatase >2.5X ULN; may increase risk for the development of Grade 4 neutropenia, febrile neutropenia, infections, severe thrombocytopenia, severe stomatitis, severe skin toxicity, and toxic death. Obtain LFTs before each treatment cycle and frequent blood counts to monitor for neutropenia. Severe hypersensitivity reactions reported with dexamethasone premedication; d/c immediately if symptoms occur. Contraindicated with history of severe hypersensitivity reactions to other drugs formulated with polysorbate 80. Severe fluid retention may occur despite dexamethasone premedication.

OTHER BRAND NAMES: Taxotere (Sanofi-Aventis)

THERAPEUTIC CLASS: Antimicrotubule agent

INDICATIONS: Treatment of locally advanced or metastatic breast cancer (BC) and NSCLC after failure of prior chemotherapy. In combination with doxorubicin and cyclophosphamide for adjuvant treatment of operable node-positive BC. In combination with cisplatin for treatment of unresectable, locally advanced or metastatic NSCLC in patients who have not previously received chemotherapy in this condition. In combination with prednisone for treatment of androgen-independent (hormone refractory) metastatic prostate cancer (HRPC). In combination with cisplatin and fluorouracil for treatment of advanced gastric adenocarcinoma (GC), including adenocarcinoma of the gastroesophageal junction, in patients who have not received prior chemotherapy for advanced disease. In combination with cisplatin and fluorouracil for induction treatment of locally advanced squamous cell carcinoma of the head and neck (SCCHN).

DOSAGE: *Adults:* Premedicate with oral corticosteroids. Premedicate patients receiving cisplatin with antiemetics and provide appropriate hydration. Refer to PI for dosage adjustments during treatment. BC: 60-100mg/m² IV over 1 hr every 3 weeks. Adjuvant to Operable Node-Positive BC: 75mg/m² 1 hr after doxorubicin 50mg/m² and cyclophosphamide 500mg/m² every 3 weeks for 6 courses. Granulocyte-colony stimulating factor may be given as prophylaxis. NSCLC: After Platinum Therapy Failure: 75mg/m² IV over 1 hr every 3 weeks. Chemotherapy-Naive: 75mg/m² IV over 1 hr followed by cisplatin 75mg/m² over 30-60 min every 3 weeks. HRPC: 75mg/m² IV over 1 hr every 3 weeks with prednisone 5mg bid. GC: 75mg/m² IV over 1 hr, followed by cisplatin 75mg/m² IV over 1-3 hrs (both on Day 1 only), followed by fluorouracil 750mg/m²/day IV over 24 hrs for 5 days, starting at end of cisplatin infusion. Repeat treatment every 3 weeks. SCCHN: Give prophylaxis for neutropenic infections. Induction Followed by Radiotherapy: 75mg/m² IV over 1 hr, followed by cisplatin 75mg/m² IV over 1 hr, on Day 1, followed by fluorouracil as a continuous IV infusion at 750mg/m²/day for 5 days. Administer every 3 weeks for 4 cycles. Induction Followed by Chemoradiotherapy: 75mg/m² IV over 1 hr on Day 1, followed by cisplatin 100mg/m² IV over 30 min to 3 hrs, followed by fluorouracil 1000mg/m²/day as a continuous IV infusion from Day 1 to Day 4. Administer every 3 weeks for 3 cycles.

HOW SUPPLIED: Inj: 10mg/mL [2mL, 8mL, 16mL], (Taxotere) 20mg/mL [1mL, 4mL, 8mL]

CONTRAINDICATIONS: Neutrophils <1500 cells/mm³.

WARNINGS/PRECAUTIONS: Avoid subsequent cycles until neutrophils recover to level >1500 cells/mm³ and platelets to >100,000 cells/mm³. Monitor from the 1st dose for possible exacerbation of preexisting effusions. Acute myeloid leukemia or myelodysplasia may occur in adjuvant therapy. Localized erythema of extremities with edema and desquamation reported; adjust dose if severe skin toxicity occurs. Severe neurosensory symptoms (eg, paresthesia, dysesthesia, pain) may develop; adjust dose if symptoms occur and d/c treatment if symptoms persist. Cystoid macular edema (CME) reported; d/c and initiate appropriate treatment if CME is diagnosed, and/or consider alternative non-taxane cancer treatment. Severe asthenia reported. May cause fetal harm. Caution in elderly.

ADVERSE REACTIONS: Myalgia, alopecia, N/V, diarrhea, nail disorders, skin reactions, fluid retention, thrombocytopenia, anemia, neutropenia, infections, hypersensitivity, neuropathy, dysgeusia, constipation.

INTERACTIONS: Avoid with CYP3A4 inhibitors; reduce dose by 50% if coadministered with strong CYP3A4 inhibitors (eg, ketoconazole, clarithromycin, atazanavir). CYP3A4 inducers and substrates may alter metabolism. Protease inhibitors (eg, ritonavir) may increase exposure.

Renal insufficiency and renal failure reported with concomitant nephrotoxic drugs. Rare cases of radiation pneumonitis reported in patients receiving concomitant radiotherapy.

PREGNANCY: Category D, not for use in nursing.

MECHANISM OF ACTION: Antimicrotubule agent; acts by disrupting the microtubular network in cells that is essential for mitotic and interphase cellular functions.

PHARMACOKINETICS: Distribution: V_d=113L; plasma protein binding (94%). **Metabolism:** CYP3A4. **Elimination:** Urine (6%, within 7 days), feces (75%, within 7 days); $T_{1/2}$=11.1 hrs.

NURSING CONSIDERATIONS

Assessment: Assess for history of severe hypersensitivity reactions to the drug or other drugs with polysorbate 80, preexisting effusion, hepatic impairment, pregnancy/nursing status, and possible drug interactions. Obtain baseline weight, CBC with platelets and differential count, and LFTs. Perform a comprehensive ophthalmologic examination in patients with impaired vision.

Monitoring: Monitor for fluid retention, acute myeloid leukemia, hematologic effects, skin toxicities, exacerbation of effusions, neurosensory symptoms, hepatic impairment, hypersensitivity reactions, asthenia, CME, and other adverse reactions. Monitor weight, CBC with platelets and differential count, and LFTs.

Patient Counseling: Inform about risks and benefits of therapy. Inform that drug may cause fetal harm; advise to avoid becoming pregnant and use effective contraceptives. Explain the significance of oral corticosteroid administration to help facilitate compliance; instruct to report if not compliant. Instruct to report signs of hypersensitivity reactions, fluid retention, myalgia, cutaneous, or neurologic reactions. Counsel about side effects that are associated with the drug. Explain the significance of routine blood cell counts. Instruct to monitor temperature frequently and immediately report any occurrence of fever.

Administration: IV route. Refer to PI for preparation and administration procedures/precautions. **Storage:** 20-25°C (68-77°F), (Taxotere) 2-25°C (36-77°F). Protect from light. After 1st use and following multiple needle entries and product withdrawals, multi-use vials are stable for up to 28 days when stored between 2°C and 8°C (36°F and 46°F) and protected from light. Reconstituted Sol: 0.9% NaCl or D5W: Stable at 2-25°C (36-77°F) for 4 hrs or (Taxotere) 6 hrs. Do not freeze infusion sol. (Taxotere) Infusion sol is stable in non-PVC bags up to 48 hrs at 2-8°C (36-46°F).

DOLOPHINE   CII
methadone HCl (Roxane)

> Contains methadone, an opioid agonist and Schedule II controlled substance with an abuse liability similar to other opioids, legal or illicit; assess each patient's risk for opioid abuse or addiction prior to prescribing. Increased risk in patients with a personal or family history of substance abuse (eg, drug/alcohol abuse/addiction) or mental illness (eg, major depressive disorder). Routinely monitor for signs of misuse, abuse, and addiction. Respiratory depression, including fatal cases, reported during initiation or even when used as recommended; proper dosing and titration are essential. Monitor for respiratory depression, especially during initiation or following a dose increase. QT interval prolongation and serious arrhythmia (torsades de pointes) occured; closely monitor for changes in cardiac rhythm during initiation and titration. Accidental ingestion, especially in children, can result in fatal overdose. For detoxification and maintenance of opioid dependence, methadone shall be dispensed only by certified opioid programs.

THERAPEUTIC CLASS: Opioid analgesic

INDICATIONS: Management of moderate to severe pain when a continuous, around-the-clock opioid analgesic is needed for an extended period of time. Detoxification treatment of opioid addiction (heroin or other morphine-like drugs). Maintenance treatment of opioid addiction (heroin or other morphine-like drugs), in conjunction with appropriate social and medical services.

DOSAGE: *Adults:* Pain: Initial: Refer to PI for factors to consider when selecting an initial dose. First Opioid Analgesic: Small doses no more than 2.5mg-10mg q8-12h. May require more frequent administration to maintain adequate analgesia. Conversion from Parenteral to PO Methadone: Use conversion ratio of 1:2mg. Refer to PI for conversion from other opioids. Titrate and Maint: Individually titrate to a dose that provides adequate analgesia and minimizes adverse reactions. May adjust dose every 1-2 days. Breakthrough Pain: May require dosage adjustment or rescue medication with a small dose of an immediate-release medication. If signs of excessive opioid-related adverse reactions observed, reduce next dose; adjust dose to obtain appropriate balance between management of pain and opioid-related adverse reactions. If intolerable opioid related adverse reactions develop, adjust dose or dosing interval. Discontinuation: Use gradual downward titration every 2-4 days; avoid abrupt d/c. Opioid Addiction Detoxification/ Maint: Initial: 20-30mg single dose. Max Initial Dose: 30mg. Evaluate after 2-4 hrs for same-day dosing adjustment. Give 5-10mg if withdrawal symptoms not suppressed or if symptoms reappear. Max on 1st Day of Treatment: 40mg/day. Use lower initial doses for expected low tolerance at treatment entry. Short-term Detoxification: Titrate to 40mg/day in divided doses. After 2-3 days of stabilization, gradually decrease dose on a daily basis or at 2-day intervals depending on tolerability level of withdrawal symptoms. Hospitalized patients may tolerate a daily reduction of

20% of the total daily dose; ambulatory patients may need a slower schedule. Titrate and Maint of Detoxification: Titrate to a dose at which opioid withdrawal symptoms are prevented for 24 hrs. Usual: 80-120mg/day. Medically Supervised Withdrawal After Maint Treatment: Reduce dose by <10% of the established tolerance or maint dose; 10-14 day intervals between dose reductions. Acute Pain During Methadone Maint Treatment: May require somewhat higher and/or more frequent doses than in nontolerant patients. Pregnancy: May need to increase dose or decrease dosing interval. Elderly: Start at lower end of dosing range.

HOW SUPPLIED: Tab: 5mg*, 10mg* *scored

CONTRAINDICATIONS: Significant respiratory depression, acute or severe bronchial asthma in unmonitored setting or in the absence of resuscitative equipment, and known or suspected paralytic ileus.

WARNINGS/PRECAUTIONS: Not for use as a PRN analgesic, for mild or acute pain, pain not expected to persist for an extended period of time, and postoperative pain. Patients tolerant to other opioids may be incompletely tolerant to methadone. Monitor patients with risk factors for prolonged QT interval (eg, cardiac hypertrophy, hypokalemia, hypomagnesemia) and a history of cardiac conduction abnormalities. Respiratory depression is more likely to occur in elderly, cachectic, or debilitated patients; monitor closely when initiating and titrating, and when given with drugs that depress respiration. Deaths reported during conversion from chronic, high dose treatment with other opioid agonists. Monitor for respiratory depression and consider alternative nonopioid analgesics in patients with significant chronic obstructive pulmonary disease (COPD) or cor pulmonale, and patients having a substantially decreased respiratory reserve, hypoxia, hypercapnia, or preexisting respiratory depression. May cause severe hypotension, especially in patients with compromised ability to maintain BP. Monitor for signs of sedation and respiratory depression in patients susceptible to the intracranial effects of carbon dioxide retention (eg, those with increased intracranial pressure or brain tumors). May obscure the clinical course in patients with head injury. Avoid with GI obstruction and impaired consciousness or coma. May cause spasm of sphincter of Oddi; monitor for worsening symptoms in patients with biliary tract disease including acute pancreatitis. May increase serum amylase. May aggravate convulsions in patients with convulsive disorders and may induce or aggravate seizures; monitor for worsened seizure control in patients with history of seizure disorder. May impair mental/physical abilities. Abrupt discontinuation may lead to opioid withdrawal symptoms. Infants born to opioid-dependent mothers may be physically dependent and may exhibit respiratory difficulties and withdrawal symptoms. Caution in elderly.

ADVERSE REACTIONS: Respiratory depression, QT prolongation, arrhythmia, systemic hypotension, lightheadedness, dizziness, sedation, sweating, N/V.

INTERACTIONS: CYP450 inducers (eg, rifampicin, phenytoin, phenobarbital, carbamazepine, St. John's wort) may precipitate withdrawal syndrome. CYP3A4 inhibitors (eg, ketoconazole, itraconazole, voriconazole, clarithromycin, erythromycin, telithromycin) and/or CYP2C9 inhibitors (eg, sertraline, fluvoxamine) may cause decreased clearance, which could increase or prolong adverse effects and may cause fatal respiratory depression. Antiretroviral drugs (eg, abacavir, amprenavir, darunavir + ritonavir, efavirenz, nelfinavir, nevirapine, ritonavir, telaprevir, lopinavir + ritonavir, saquinavir + ritonavir, tipranavir + ritonavir) may increase clearance or decrease plasma levels. May decrease levels of didanosine and stavudine. May increase area under the curve of zidovudine. CNS depressants (eg, sedatives, hypnotics, general anesthetics, antiemetics, phenothiazines, tranquilizers, alcohol, anxiolytics, neuroleptics, other opioids, and illicit drugs) may increase risk of respiratory depression, hypotension, profound sedation, or coma; reduce initial dose of 1 or both agents. Deaths reported when abused in conjunction with benzodiazepines. Monitor for cardiac conduction changes with drugs known to have potential to prolong QT interval. Pharmacodynamic interactions may occur with potentially arrhythmogenic agents (eg, Class I and III antiarrhythmics, neuroleptics, TCAs, calcium channel blockers). Monitor closely with drugs capable of inducing electrolyte imbalance that may prolong QT interval including diuretics, laxatives, mineralocorticoid hormones, and medications affecting cardiac conduction. May experience withdrawal symptoms and/or reduced analgesic effect with opioid antagonists, mixed agonist/antagonists, and partial agonists (eg, naloxone, naltrexone, pentazocine, nalbuphine, butorphanol, buprenorphine); avoid use. Severe reactions may occur with concurrent use or within 14 days of MAOIs use. May increase levels of desipramine. Anticholinergics may increase risk of urinary retention and/or severe constipation which may lead to paralytic ileus.

PREGNANCY: Category C, not for use in nursing.

MECHANISM OF ACTION: Synthetic opioid analgesic; mu-agonist. Produces actions similar to morphine; acts on CNS and organs composed of smooth muscle. May also act as an N-methyl-D-aspartate (NMDA) receptor antagonist.

PHARMACOKINETICS: Absorption: Bioavailability (36-100%); C_{max}=124-1255ng/mL; T_{max}=1-7.5 hrs. **Distribution:** V_d=1.0-8.0L/kg; plasma protein binding (85-90%). Found in breast milk; crosses placenta. **Metabolism:** Hepatic N-demethylation via CYP3A4, 2B6, 2C19 (major); 2C9, 2D6 (minor). **Elimination:** Urine, feces; $T_{1/2}$=8-59 hrs.

NURSING CONSIDERATIONS

Assessment: Assess for personal/family history or risk factors for drug abuse or addiction, general condition and medical status, opioid/experience/tolerance, pain type/severity, previous opioid daily dose, potency, and type of prior analgesics used, respiratory depression, cardiac conduction abnormalities, COPD or other respiratory complications, GI obstruction, paralytic ileus, hepatic/renal impairment, previous hypersensitivity to drug, pregnancy/nursing status, possible drug interactions, and any other conditions where treatment is contraindicated or cautioned.

Monitoring: Monitor for signs/symptoms of respiratory depression, QT prolongation and arrhythmias, orthostatic hypotension, syncope, symptoms of worsening biliary tract disease, aggravation/induction of seizure, tolerance, physical dependence, mental/physical impairment, and withdrawal syndrome, hypersensitivity reactions, and other adverse reactions. Monitor for signs of increased intracranial pressure with head injuries. Routinely monitor for signs of misuse, abuse, and addiction.

Patient Counseling: Inform that drug has potential for abuse; instruct not to share drug with others and to take steps to protect from theft or misuse. Discuss risks and how to recognize respiratory depression, orthostatic hypotension, and syncope. Instruct to seek medical attention immediately if they are experiencing breathing difficulties or symptoms suggestive of arrhythmia (eg, palpitations, near syncope, syncope). Advise patient to store drug securely; accidental exposure, especially in children, can result in fatal overdose. Inform about risks of concomitant use of alcohol and other CNS depressants; instruct not to consume alcoholic beverages, as well as prescription and OTC drug products containing alcohol. Advise to take drug as prescribed and not to d/c without 1st discussing with prescriber. Inform that drug may impair ability to perform potentially hazardous activities (eg, driving a car, operating heavy machinery). Advise about potential for severe constipation, including management instructions and when to seek medical attention. Inform that anaphylaxis may occur; advise how to recognize such a reaction and when to seek medical attention. Advise females that drug can cause fetal harm and to inform prescriber if pregnant or plan to become pregnant. Instruct nursing mothers to watch for signs of methadone toxicity in their infants (eg, increased sleepiness more than usual, difficulty breastfeeding, breathing difficulties, limpness); instruct to inform physician immediately if these signs occur.

Administration: Oral route. **Storage:** 25°C (77°F); excursions permitted to 15-30°C (59-86°F).

DONNATAL   RX

atropine sulfate - hyoscyamine sulfate - scopolamine hydrobromide - phenobarbital (PBM Pharmaceuticals)

THERAPEUTIC CLASS: Anticholinergic/barbiturate

INDICATIONS: Adjunct therapy for irritable bowel syndrome (irritable colon, spastic colon, mucous colitis), acute enterocolitis, and duodenal ulcers.

DOSAGE: *Adults:* Individualize dose. (Elixir/Tab) 1 or 2 tsp (5 or 10mL) or 1 or 2 tabs tid or qid according to conditions and severity of symptoms. (Extentabs) 1 tab q12h. May give 1 tab q8h if indicated. Hepatic Dysfunction: Use small initial doses.
Pediatrics: (Elixir) Individualize dose. May be dosed q4-6h. Initial: 45.4kg: 1 tsp (5mL) q4h or 1 1/2 tsp (7.5mL) q6h. 34kg: 3/4 tsp (3.75mL) q4h or 1 tsp (5mL) q6h. 22.7kg: 1/2 tsp (2.5mL) q4h or 3/4 tsp (3.75mL) q6h. 13.6kg: 1.5mL q4h or 2mL q6h. 9.1kg: 1mL q4h or 1.5mL q6h. 4.5kg: 0.5mL q4h or 0.75mL q6h. Hepatic Dysfunction: Use small initial doses.

HOW SUPPLIED: (Atropine-Hyoscyamine-Phenobarbital-Scopolamine) Elixir: 0.0194mg-0.1037mg-16.2mg-0.0065mg/5mL [4 fl. oz., 1 pint]; Tab: 0.0194mg-0.1037mg-16.2mg-0.0065mg; Tab, Extended-Release: (Extentabs) 0.0582mg-0.3111mg-48.6mg-0.0195mg

CONTRAINDICATIONS: Glaucoma, obstructive uropathy (eg, bladder-neck obstruction due to prostatic hypertrophy), obstructive GI disease (achalasia, pyloroduodenal stenosis, etc.), paralytic ileus, intestinal atony in elderly/debilitated, unstable cardiovascular status in acute hemorrhage, severe ulcerative colitis, especially if complicated by toxic megacolon, myasthenia gravis, hiatal hernia associated with reflux esophagitis, acute intermittent porphyria, and patients in whom phenobarbital produces restlessness and/or excitement.

WARNINGS/PRECAUTIONS: Heat prostration can occur with high environmental temperatures. Diarrhea may be an early symptom of incomplete intestinal obstruction, especially with ileostomy or colostomy; treatment would be inappropriate and possibly harmful. May impair physical/mental abilities. May be habit forming; avoid in patients prone to addiction or with history of physical and/or psychological drug dependence. Caution with autonomic neuropathy, hepatic/renal disease, hyperthyroidism, coronary heart disease, congestive heart failure (CHF), arrhythmias, tachycardia, and HTN. May delay gastric emptying. Curare-like action may occur with overdosage. Abrupt withdrawal may produce delirium or convulsions in patients habituated to barbiturates. (Tab/Elixir) Do not rely on the use of drug in the presence of biliary tract disease complications.

ADVERSE REACTIONS: Xerostomia, urinary hesitancy/retention, blurred vision, tachycardia, mydriasis, cycloplegia, increased ocular tension, loss of taste, headache, nervousness, drowsiness, weakness, dizziness, insomnia.

INTERACTIONS: Phenobarbital may decrease the effect of anticoagulants; may need larger doses of anticoagulant for optimal effect.

PREGNANCY: Category C, caution in nursing.

MECHANISM OF ACTION: Anticholinergic/barbiturate; provides peripheral anticholinergic/antispasmodic action and mild sedation.

NURSING CONSIDERATIONS

Assessment: Assess for previous hypersensitivity to the drug or any of its components, diarrhea, ileostomy, colostomy, history of physical and/or psychological drug dependence, biliary tract disease, hepatic dysfunction, pregnancy/nursing status, possible drug interactions, and any other conditions where treatment is contraindicated or cautioned.

Monitoring: Monitor for signs/symptoms of heat prostration, drowsiness, blurred vision, constipation, diarrhea, urinary hesitancy/retention, hypersensitivity reactions, and other adverse reactions.

Patient Counseling: Counsel about possible side effects and to report to a healthcare provider if any occur. Inform that the drug may be habit forming. If drowsiness or blurring of vision occurs, warn patients not to engage in activities requiring mental alertness (eg, operating a motor vehicle or other machinery) and not to perform hazardous work. Inform that treatment may decrease sweating, resulting in heat prostration, fever, or heat strokes.

Administration: Oral route. **Storage:** 20-25°C (68-77°F). Protect from light and moisture. (Elixir/Tab) Avoid freezing.

DORIBAX   RX
doripenem (Janssen)

THERAPEUTIC CLASS: Carbapenem

INDICATIONS: Treatment of complicated intra-abdominal and urinary tract infections (UTIs), including pyelonephritis, caused by susceptible microorganisms.

DOSAGE: *Adults:* ≥18 Yrs: Intra-Abdominal Infection: 500mg q8h by IV infusion over 1 hr for 5-14 days. Duration includes a possible switch to an appropriate PO therapy, after at least 3 days of parenteral therapy, once clinical improvement has been demonstrated. UTI: 500mg q8h by IV infusion over 1 hr for 10 days. Duration may be extended up to 14 days with concurrent bacteremia. Renal Impairment: CrCl ≥30 to ≤50mL/min: 250mg IV (over 1 hr) q8h. CrCl >10 to <30mL/min: 250mg IV (over 1 hr) q12h.

HOW SUPPLIED: Inj: 250mg, 500mg

WARNINGS/PRECAUTIONS: Serious and occasionally fatal hypersensitivity (anaphylactic) and serious skin reactions reported; d/c if an allergic reaction occurs. Seizures reported; higher risk in patients with preexisting CNS disorders (eg, stroke, history of seizures), patients with compromised renal function, and patients given doses >500mg q8h. *Clostridium difficile*-associated diarrhea (CDAD) reported; d/c if CDAD is suspected or confirmed. May result in bacterial resistance with use in the absence of a proven/strongly suspected bacterial infection. Do not administer via inhalation route; pneumonitis reported. Caution in elderly.

ADVERSE REACTIONS: Headache, nausea, diarrhea, rash, phlebitis, anemia, pruritus, hepatic enzyme elevation, oral candidiasis.

INTERACTIONS: May reduce serum valproic acid levels below the therapeutic concentrations, which may increase risk of breakthrough seizures; consider alternative antibacterial therapies in patients receiving valproic acid or sodium valproate, or if treatment with the drug is necessary, consider supplemental anticonvulsant therapy. Probenecid may increase levels; avoid coadministration.

PREGNANCY: Category B, caution in nursing.

MECHANISM OF ACTION: Carbapenem; exerts bactericidal activity by inhibiting bacterial cell-wall biosynthesis, resulting in cell death.

PHARMACOKINETICS: Absorption: C_{max}=23mcg/mL, AUC=36.3mcg•hr/mL. **Distribution:** V_d=16.8L (median); plasma protein binding (8.1%). **Metabolism:** Via dehydropeptidase-1; doripenem-M1 (inactive ring-opened metabolite). **Elimination:** Urine (71% unchanged, 15% metabolite), feces (<1%); $T_{1/2}$=1 hr.

NURSING CONSIDERATIONS

Assessment: Assess for CNS disorders (eg, stroke, history of seizures), renal impairment, pregnancy/nursing status, and possible drug interactions. Carefully assess for previous hypersensitivity reactions to drug, penicillin, cephalosporins, other β-lactams, and other allergens.

Monitoring: Monitor for hypersensitivity (anaphylactic) reactions, CDAD, seizures, and other adverse reactions. Monitor renal function in patients with moderate or severe renal impairment and in the elderly.

Patient Counseling: Advise that allergic reactions, including serious allergic reactions, could occur and that serious reactions may require immediate treatment. Advise to report any previous hypersensitivity reactions to the medication, other carbapenems, β-lactams, or other allergens. Counsel that therapy should only be used to treat bacterial, not viral (eg, common cold), infections . Instruct to take exactly ud; inform that skipping doses or not completing the full course of therapy may decrease effectiveness of treatment and increase bacterial resistance. Counsel to inform physician if patient has CNS disorders (eg, stroke, history of seizures) and if taking valproic acid or sodium valproate.

Administration: IV route. Do not mix with or physically add to sol containing other drugs. Refer to PI for further preparation instructions. **Storage:** 25°C (77°F); excursions permitted to 15-30°C (59-86°F). Refer to PI for storage information for constituted sol.

DORYX
doxycycline hyclate (Warner Chilcott)   **RX**

OTHER BRAND NAMES: Doxycycline Hyclate (Various)

THERAPEUTIC CLASS: Tetracycline derivative

INDICATIONS: Treatment of the following infections caused by susceptible microorganisms: Rocky Mountain spotted fever, typhus fever and the typhus group, Q fever, rickettsialpox, tick fevers, uncomplicated urethral/endocervical/rectal infections, nongonococcal urethritis, lymphogranuloma venereum, granuloma inguinale, uncomplicated gonorrhea, chancroid, respiratory tract infections, psittacosis (ornithosis), relapsing fever, plague, tularemia, cholera, *Campylobacter fetus* infections, brucellosis (in conjunction with streptomycin), bartonellosis, urinary tract infections (UTIs), trachoma, inclusion conjunctivitis, and anthrax (including inhalational anthrax [postexposure]). Treatment of infections caused by susceptible strains of *Escherichia coli*, *Enterobacter aerogenes*, *Shigella* species, and *Acinetobacter* species. When penicillin (PCN) is contraindicated, treatment of the following infections caused by susceptible microorganisms: syphilis, yaws, Vincent's infection, actinomycosis, and infections caused by *Clostridium* species. Adjunctive therapy in acute intestinal amebiasis and severe acne. Prophylaxis of malaria due to *Plasmodium falciparum* in short-term travelers (<4 months) to areas with chloroquine and/or pyrimethamine-sulfadoxine resistant strains.

DOSAGE: *Adults:* Initial: 100mg q12h on 1st day. Maint: 100mg qd or 50mg q12h. More Severe Infections (Chronic UTIs): 100mg q12h. Streptococcal Infections: Continue therapy for 10 days. Uncomplicated Urethral/Endocervical Infection: 100mg bid or 200mg qd for 7 days. Uncomplicated Rectal Infection or Nongonococcal Urethritis: 100mg bid for 7 days. Uncomplicated Gonococcal Infections (Except Anorectal Infections in Men): 100mg bid for 7 days or as an alternate single visit dose of 300mg stat followed in 1 hr by a second 300mg dose. Syphilis (Early): 100mg bid for 2 weeks. Syphilis (>1 Yr): 100mg bid for 4 weeks. Acute Epididymo-Orchitis: 100mg bid for at least 10 days. Malaria Prophylaxis: 100mg qd, beginning 1-2 days before travel, continuing daily during travel and for 4 weeks after departure from malarious area. Inhalational Anthrax (Postexposure): 100mg bid for 60 days.
Pediatrics: Inhalational Anthrax (Postexposure): ≥45kg: 100mg bid for 60 days. <45kg: 2.2mg/kg bid for 60 days. >8 Yrs: Malaria Prophylaxis: 2mg/kg qd up to 100mg qd, beginning 1-2 days before travel, continuing daily during travel and for 4 weeks after departure from malarious area. Infections: Usual: >45kg: Initial: 100mg q12h on 1st day. Maint: 100mg qd or 50mg q12h. More Severe Infections (Chronic UTIs): 100mg q12h. ≤45kg: 4.4mg/kg divided into 2 doses on 1st day, followed by 2.2mg/kg qd or as 2 divided doses, on subsequent days. More Severe Infections: Up to 4.4mg/kg. Streptococcal Infections: Continue therapy for 10 days.

HOW SUPPLIED: Tab, Delayed-Release: 100mg*, 150mg*, 200mg*; (generic) 75mg* *scored

WARNINGS/PRECAUTIONS: May cause permanent discoloration of the teeth (yellow-gray-brown) if used during tooth development (last half of pregnancy, infancy, and childhood to 8 yrs of age); do not use in this age group, except for anthrax. Enamel hypoplasia reported. *Clostridium difficile*-associated diarrhea (CDAD) reported; d/c if CDAD is suspected or confirmed. Photosensitivity, manifested by an exaggerated sunburn reaction, reported; d/c at the 1st evidence of skin erythema. May result in bacterial resistance if used in the absence of proven or suspected bacterial infection, or a prophylactic indication; take appropriate measures if superinfection develops. Bulging fontanels in infants and benign intracranial HTN in adults reported. May decrease fibula growth rate in prematures. May cause an increase in BUN. When used for malaria prophylaxis, patient may still transmit the infection to mosquitoes outside endemic areas. False elevations of urinary catecholamines may occur due to interference with the fluorescence test.

ADVERSE REACTIONS: N/V, diarrhea, bacterial vaginitis.

INTERACTIONS: Depresses plasma prothrombin activity; may require downward adjustment of anticoagulant dose. May interfere with bactericidal action of PCN; avoid concurrent use. Impaired absorption with bismuth subsalicylate, antacids containing aluminum, Ca^{2+}, or Mg^{2+}, and iron-containing preparations. May render oral contraceptives less effective. Decreased $T_{1/2}$ with barbiturates, carbamazepine, and phenytoin. Fatal renal toxicity reported with methoxyflurane.

PREGNANCY: Category D, not for use in nursing.

MECHANISM OF ACTION: Tetracycline; has bacteriostatic activity. Inhibits bacterial protein synthesis by binding to the 30S ribosomal subunit.

PHARMACOKINETICS: Absorption: Virtually complete. C_{max}=4.6mcg/mL (200mg single dose), 6.3mcg/mL (200mg multiple dose); T_{max}=3 hrs (median). **Distribution:** Found in breast milk. **Elimination:** Urine, feces; $T_{1/2}$=18-22 hrs.

NURSING CONSIDERATIONS

Assessment: Assess for hypersensitivity to drug, pregnancy/nursing status, and possible drug interactions. Perform culture and susceptibility testing.

Monitoring: Monitor for CDAD, photosensitivity, skin erythema, superinfection, benign intracranial HTN in adults, and other adverse reactions. In long-term therapy, perform periodic lab evaluation of organ systems, including hematopoietic, renal, and hepatic studies.

Patient Counseling: Apprise of the potential hazard to fetus if used during pregnancy. Inform that therapy does not guarantee protection against malaria; advise to use measures that help avoid contact with mosquitoes. Advise to avoid excessive sunlight or artificial UV light and to d/c therapy if phototoxicity (eg, skin eruptions) occurs. Inform that absorption of drug is reduced when taken with bismuth subsalicylate, antacids containing aluminum, Ca^{2+}, or Mg^{2+}, iron-containing preparations, and with foods, especially those that contain Ca^{2+}. Inform that drug may increase the incidence of vaginal candidiasis. Inform that diarrhea is a common problem caused by therapy and usually ends when therapy is discontinued. Instruct to immediately contact physician if watery and bloody stools (with or without stomach cramps and fever) occur, even as late as ≥2 months after the last dose. Counsel that therapy should only be used to treat bacterial, not viral (eg, common cold), infections. Instruct to take exactly ud. Inform that skipping doses or not completing the full course of therapy may decrease effectiveness of treatment and increase bacterial resistance.

Administration: Oral route. Administer with adequate amounts of fluid. May be given with food or milk if gastric irritation occurs. May breakup tab and sprinkle contents (delayed-release pellets) over applesauce; refer to PI for further instructions. May administer 200mg tab without regard to meals. **Storage:** 25°C (77°F); excursions permitted to 15-30°C (59-86°F). Protect from light. (Doryx) 20-25°C (68-77°F); excursions permitted to 15-30°C (59-86°F).

DOVONEX RX
calcipotriene (Leo Pharma)

THERAPEUTIC CLASS: Vitamin D3 derivative

INDICATIONS: Treatment of plaque psoriasis.

DOSAGE: *Adults:* Apply a thin layer to the affected skin bid and rub in gently and completely. Safety and efficacy demonstrated in patients treated for eight weeks.

HOW SUPPLIED: Cre: 0.005% [60g, 120g]

CONTRAINDICATIONS: Hypercalcemia, evidence of vitamin D toxicity. Do not use on the face.

WARNINGS/PRECAUTIONS: Transient irritation of both lesions and surrounding uninvolved skin may occur; d/c if irritation develops. Reversible elevation of serum Ca^{2+} reported; d/c until normal Ca^{2+} levels are restored. For external use only; not for ophthalmic, PO, or intravaginal use.

ADVERSE REACTIONS: Skin irritation, rash, pruritus, dermatitis, worsening of psoriasis.

PREGNANCY: Category C, caution in nursing.

MECHANISM OF ACTION: Vitamin D3 derivative.

PHARMACOKINETICS: Metabolism: Liver. **Elimination:** Bile.

NURSING CONSIDERATIONS

Assessment: Assess for history of hypersensitivity to any of the components of the preparation, hypercalcemia, evidence of vitamin D toxicity, and pregnancy/nursing status.

Monitoring: Monitor for serum Ca^{2+} elevation, irritation, and other adverse reactions.

Patient Counseling: Advise to use drug only ud by the physician. Inform that the medication is for external use only; instruct to avoid contact with face or eyes. Advise to wash hands after application. Counsel that the drug should not be used for any disorder other than for which it was prescribed. Instruct to report any signs of adverse reactions to the physician. Instruct patients who apply medication to the exposed portions of the body to avoid excessive exposure to either natural or artificial sunlight (eg, tanning booths, sun lamps). Instruct to keep out of the reach of children.

Administration: Topical route. Wash hands thoroughly after use. **Storage:** 15-25°C (59-77°F). Do not freeze.

DOXIL   RX
doxorubicin HCl liposome (Janssen)

> May lead to cardiac toxicity. Myocardial damage may lead to congestive heart failure when cumulative dose approaches 550mg/m²; include prior use of anthracyclines or anthracenediones in cumulative dose calculations. Cardiac toxicity may occur at lower cumulative doses with prior mediastinal irradiation or concurrent cyclophosphamide therapy. Acute infusion-related reactions reported. Severe myelosuppression may occur. Reduce dose with impaired hepatic function. Severe side effects reported with accidental substitution for doxorubicin HCl; do not substitute on a mg-per-mg basis.

THERAPEUTIC CLASS: Anthracycline

INDICATIONS: Treatment of ovarian cancer that has progressed or recurred after platinum-based chemotherapy. Treatment of AIDS-related Kaposi's sarcoma (KS) in patients after failure of/intolerance to prior systemic chemotherapy. In combination with bortezomib for the treatment of multiple myeloma (MM) in patients who have not previously received bortezomib and have received at least 1 prior therapy.

DOSAGE: *Adults:* Administer as IV infusion at initial rate of 1mg/min to minimize risk of infusion-related reactions; if no infusion-related adverse reactions, may increase rate of infusion to complete administration over 1 hr. Ovarian Cancer: 50mg/m² IV every 4 weeks (for as long as patient tolerates treatment, does not progress, and has no evidence of cardiotoxicity) for a minimum of 4 courses. Consider pretreatment with or concomitant antiemetics. KS: 20mg/m² IV every 3 weeks for as long as responding satisfactorily and tolerating treatment. MM: Give bortezomib 1.3mg/m² IV bolus on Days 1, 4, 8, and 11, every 3 weeks. Give doxorubicin 30mg/m² IV as a 1-hr IV infusion on Day 4 following bortezomib. May treat for up to 8 cycles until disease progression or occurrence of unacceptable toxicity. Hepatic Dysfunction: If serum bilirubin 1.2-3mg/dL, give 50% of normal dose. If serum bilirubin >3mg/dL, give 25% of normal dose. Adjust or delay dose based on toxicities; refer to PI for recommended dose modification guidelines.

HOW SUPPLIED: Inj: 2mg/mL [10mL, 25mL]

WARNINGS/PRECAUTIONS: Monitor cardiac function. Administer only when potential benefits outweigh the risks in patients with a history of cardiovascular disease (CVD). If hematologic toxicity occurs, dose reduction or delay/suspension of therapy may be required. Hand-foot syndrome (HFS) reported; may need to modify dose or d/c. Recall reaction reported after radiotherapy. May cause fetal harm. Avoid extravasation. Secondary oral cancers, primarily squamous cell carcinoma reported; examine at regular intervals for the presence of oral ulceration/discomfort.

ADVERSE REACTIONS: Cardiac toxicity, acute infusion-related reactions, myelosuppression, neutropenia, anemia, thrombocytopenia, stomatitis, fever, fatigue, N/V, asthenia, diarrhea, constipation, HFS, rash, anorexia.

INTERACTIONS: See Boxed Warning. May potentiate toxicity of other anticancer therapies. May exacerbate cyclophosphamide-induced hemorrhagic cystitis. May enhance hepatotoxicity of 6-mercaptopurine. May increase radiation-induced toxicity of the myocardium, mucosa, skin, and liver. Hematological toxicity may be more severe with agents that cause bone-marrow suppression.

PREGNANCY: Category D, not for use in nursing.

MECHANISM OF ACTION: Anthracycline topoisomerase inhibitor; suspected to bind DNA and inhibit nucleic acid synthesis.

PHARMACOKINETICS: Absorption: (10mg/m²) C_{max}=4.12mcg/mL, AUC=277mcg/mL•h. (20mg/m²) C_{max}=8.34mcg/mL, AUC=590mcg/mL•h. **Distribution:** (10mg/m²) V_d=2.83L/m²; (20mg/m²) V_d=2.72L/m². **Metabolism:** Doxorubicinol (major metabolite). **Elimination:** 1st Phase: $T_{1/2}$=4.7 hrs (10mg/m²); 5.2 hrs (20mg/m²). 2nd Phase: $T_{1/2}$=52.3 hrs (10mg/m²); 55 hrs (20mg/m²).

NURSING CONSIDERATIONS

Assessment: Assess for history of CVD, hepatic dysfunction, hypersensitivity, pregnancy/nursing status, history of drug/radiotherapy use, and possible drug interactions. Obtain baseline CBC and platelet counts.

Monitoring: Monitor for signs/symptoms of cardiotoxicity, infusion reactions, myelosuppression, radiation recall reaction, extravasation, HFS, and other adverse reactions. Monitor cardiac function (endomyocardial biopsy, echocardiography, multigated radionuclide scan). Obtain CBCs (including WBC, neutrophil, Hgb/Hct, platelets) frequently (at least once prior to each dose).

Patient Counseling: Inform that reddish-orange color may appear in urine and other bodily fluids. Advise of pregnancy risks. Instruct to notify physician if symptoms of HFS (eg, tingling, redness, flaking, bothersome swelling, small blisters), stomatitis (eg, painful redness, swelling, or sores in the mouth), fever of 100.5°F or higher, N/V, tiredness, weakness, rash, and mild hair loss occur.

Administration: IV route. Refer to PI for instructions on preparation, administration, handling, and disposal. **Storage:** 2-8°C (36-46°F). Administer diluted sol within 24 hrs. Avoid freezing.

DOXYCYCLINE IV RX
doxycycline hyclate (Bedford)

THERAPEUTIC CLASS: Tetracycline derivative

INDICATIONS: Treatment of rickettsiae, *Mycoplasma pneumoniae*, psittacosis, ornithosis, lymphogranuloma venereum, granuloma inguinale, relapsing fever, chancroid, *Pasteurella pestis*, *Pasteurella tularensis*, *Bartonella bacilliformis*, *Bacteroides* species, *Vibrio comma*, *Vibrio fetus*, *Brucella* species, *Escherichia coli*, *Enterobacter aerogenes*, *Shigella* species, *Mima* species, *Herellea* species, *Haemophilus influenzae*, *Klebsiella* species, *Streptococcus* species, *Diplococcus pneumoniae*, *Staphylococcus aureus*, anthrax, and trachoma. When penicillin (PCN) is contraindicated, treatment of *Neisseria gonorrhoeae*, *N. meningitis*, syphilis, yaws, *Listeria monocytogenes*, *Clostridium* species, *Fusobacterium fusiforme*, and *Actinomyces* species. Adjunct therapy for amebiasis.

DOSAGE: *Adults:* Usual: 200mg IV divided qd-bid on Day 1 then 100-200mg/day IV depending on severity, with 200mg administered in 1 or 2 infusions. Primary/Secondary Syphilis: 300mg/day IV for at least 10 days. Inhalational Anthrax (Postexposure): 100mg IV bid. Institute oral therapy as soon as possible and continue therapy for a total of 60 days.
Pediatrics: >8 Yrs: >100 lbs: Usual: 200mg IV divided qd-bid on Day 1 then 100-200mg/day IV depending on severity, with 200mg administered in 1 or 2 infusions. ≤100 lbs: 2mg/lb IV divided qd-bid on Day 1 then 1-2mg/lb/day IV divided qd-bid depending on severity. Inhalational Anthrax (Postexposure): <100 lbs: 1mg/lb IV bid. Institute oral therapy as soon as possible and continue therapy for total of 60 days.

HOW SUPPLIED: Inj: 100mg

WARNINGS/PRECAUTIONS: *Clostridium difficile*-associated diarrhea (CDAD) reported. May cause fetal harm during pregnancy. Permanent tooth discoloration during tooth development (last half of pregnancy and children <8 yrs of age) reported; avoid use in this age group except for anthrax treatment. Decreased bone growth in premature infants, bulging fontanels in infants and benign intracranial HTN in adults reported. May increase BUN. Photosensitivity, enamel hypoplasia reported. May result in bacterial resistance with prolonged use or use in the absence of a proven/suspected bacterial infection or a prophylactic indication; take appropriate measures if superinfection develops. Monitor hematopoietic, renal and hepatic labs periodically with long-term therapy. When coexistent syphilis is suspected, perform dark-field examination before treatment and repeat blood serology monthly for ≥4 months.

ADVERSE REACTIONS: GI effects, increased BUN, rash, hypersensitivity reactions, hemolytic anemia, thrombocytopenia.

INTERACTIONS: May decrease PT; adjust anticoagulants. Avoid use with bactericidal agents (eg, PCN).

PREGNANCY: Safety in pregnancy not known; not for use in nursing.

MECHANISM OF ACTION: Tetracycline derivative; thought to inhibit protein synthesis.

PHARMACOKINETICS: Absorption: Readily absorbed; C_{max}=2.5mcg/mL. **Elimination:** $T_{1/2}$=18-22 hrs.

NURSING CONSIDERATIONS

Assessment: Assess for pregnancy status, possible drug interactions, and renal impairment. Document indications for therapy, culture, and susceptibility testing. Perform incision and drainage in conjunction with antibiotic therapy when indicated.

Monitoring: Monitor for signs/symptoms of hypersensitivity reactions, photosensitivity, superinfection, CDAD, vaginal candidiasis, benign intracranial HTN, LFTs, renal function, and hematological manifestations. In venereal disease with suspected coexistent syphilis, perform dark field exam before treatment; repeat monthly for 4 months.

Patient Counseling: Inform of pregnancy risks and photosensitivity reactions (d/c at 1st sign of skin erythema). Advise to avoid excessive sunlight/UV light and to wear sunscreen or sunblock. Instruct to take ud and explain that skipping doses or not completing full course may decrease effectiveness and increase resistance. Inform that patient may experience diarrhea; instruct to contact physician if watery or bloody stools, hypersensitivity reactions, superinfections, photosensitivity, or benign intracranial HTN occurs.

Administration: IV route. **Storage:** Sol after reconstitution stable for 8 weeks when stored at -20°C (-4°F). If product warmed, care should be taken to avoid heating after thawing is complete.

DUETACT   RX
pioglitazone HCl - glimepiride (Takeda)

> Thiazolidinediones, including pioglitazone, cause or exacerbate congestive heart failure (CHF) in some patients. After initiation and dose increases, monitor carefully for signs and symptoms of heart failure (HF); manage accordingly and consider discontinuation or dose reduction if HF develops. Not recommended with symptomatic HF. Contraindicated with established NYHA Class III or IV HF.

THERAPEUTIC CLASS: Sulfonylurea/thiazolidinedione

INDICATIONS: Adjunct to diet and exercise to improve glycemic control in adults with type 2 diabetes mellitus (DM) already being treated with a thiazolidinedione and a sulfonylurea or who have inadequate glycemic control on a thiazolidinedione alone or sulfonylurea alone.

DOSAGE: *Adults:* Individualize dose. Administer qd with 1st main meal. Usual: 30mg-2mg or 30mg-4mg qd. Inadequately Controlled Glimepiride Monotherapy: Usual: 30mg-2mg or 30mg-4mg qd. Inadequately Controlled Pioglitazone Monotherapy: Usual: 30mg-2mg qd. Titrate: Gradually PRN, after assessing adequacy of response and tolerability. Changing from Combination Therapy of Pioglitazone Plus Glimepiride as Separate Tabs: Take at doses that are as close as possible to the dose of pioglitazone and glimepiride already being taken. Currently on Different Sulfonylurea Monotherapy or Switching from Combination Therapy of Pioglitazone Plus a Different Sulfonylurea (eg, Glyburide, Glipizide, Chlorpropamide, Tolbutamide, Acetohexamide): Usual: 30mg-2mg qd and adjust after assessing adequacy of therapeutic response. Observe for hypoglycemia for 1-2 weeks due to the potential overlapping drug effect. Patients with Systolic Dysfunction: Use lowest approved dose after titration from 15mg to 30mg of pioglitazone has been safely tolerated. Concomitant Insulin Secretagogue: Reduce insulin secretagogue dose if hypoglycemia occurs. Concomitant Use with an Insulin: Decrease insulin dose by 10-25% if hypoglycemia occurs; further insulin dose adjustment should be individualized based on glycemic response. Concomitant Use with Strong CYP2C8 Inhibitors (eg, Gemfibrozil): Max (Pioglitazone): 15mg qd. Concomitant Colesevelam: Administer at least 4 hrs prior to colesevelam. Renal Impairment/Elderly: Initial dosing, dose increments, and maintenance dosage should be conservative.

HOW SUPPLIED: Tab: (Pioglitazone-Glimepiride) 30mg-2mg, 30mg-4mg

CONTRAINDICATIONS: Established NYHA Class III or IV HF.

WARNINGS/PRECAUTIONS: Not for use in type 1 DM or for treatment of diabetic ketoacidosis. Caution with liver disease. Glimepiride: May produce severe hypoglycemia. May impair physical/mental abilities. Use caution when initiating and increasing dose in patients who may be predisposed to hypoglycemia (eg, elderly, renal impairment, other antidiabetic medications). Debilitated/malnourished patients and those with adrenal, pituitary, or hepatic impairment are particularly susceptible to hypoglycemia. Hypoglycemia is more likely to occur when caloric intake is deficient, or after severe/prolonged exercise. Early warning symptoms of hypoglycemia may be different or less pronounced with autonomic neuropathy, and in elderly. Hypersensitivity reactions (eg, anaphylaxis, Steven-Johnson syndrome) reported; promptly d/c therapy if hypersensitivity reaction is suspected. Increased risk of cardiovascular mortality. Hemolytic anemia reported in patients with G6PD deficiency; caution with G6PD deficiency and consider alternate non-sulfonylurea treatment. Pioglitazone: May cause dose-related fluid retention; d/c or reduce dose and manage according to current standards of care if CHF develops. Fatal and nonfatal hepatic failure reported. Obtain liver test panel before initiating therapy, and initiate with caution in patients with abnormal LFTs. Measure LFTs promptly in patients who report symptoms that may indicate liver injury. If abnormal LFTs (ALT >3X ULN) are reported, interrupt treatment and investigate for the probable cause, and do not restart therapy without another explanation for the LFT abnormalities. Patients who have serum ALT >3X the reference range with serum total bilirubin >2X the reference range without alternative etiologies are at risk for severe drug-induced liver injury, and should not be restarted on therapy. May use with caution in patients with lesser elevations of serum ALT/bilirubin and with an alternate probable cause. Not for use in patients with active bladder cancer; consider benefits versus risks for cancer recurrence in patients with a prior history of bladder cancer. New onset or worsening of edema reported. Caution in patients with edema and in patients at risk for CHF. Increased incidence of bone fracture reported in females; apply current standards of care for assessing and maintaining bone health. Macular edema reported; promptly refer patients who report any visual symptoms to an ophthalmologist. May result in ovulation in some premenopausal anovulatory women, which may increase risk for pregnancy; adequate contraception is recommended. Weight gain reported. May decrease Hgb and Hct.

ADVERSE REACTIONS: HF, hemolytic anemia, weight gain, dyspnea, edema, hypoglycemia, upper respiratory tract infection, accidental injury, headache, diarrhea, urinary tract infection, diarrhea, nausea, limb pain.

INTERACTIONS: Glimepiride: Hypoglycemia more likely to occur when alcohol is ingested. Severe hypoglycemia with oral miconazole reported. Early warning symptoms of hypoglycemia may be different or less pronounced with β-adrenergic blocking drugs or other sympatholytic agents. Decreased concentrations with colesevelam. May interact with inhibitors (eg, fluconazole) and inducers (eg, rifampicin) of CYP2C9. Pioglitazone: Concomitant use with other antidiabetic agents or insulin may cause fluid retention; d/c or reduce pioglitazone dose. Increased AUC levels with CYP2C8 inhibitors (eg, gemfibrozil). Decreased AUC levels with CYP2C8 inducers (eg, rifampin).

PREGNANCY: Category C, not for use in nursing.

MECHANISM OF ACTION: Pioglitazone: Thiazolidinedione; insulin-sensitizing agent that acts primarily by enhancing peripheral glucose utilization. Glimepiride: Sulfonylurea; insulin secretagogue that acts primarily by stimulating release of insulin from functioning pancreatic beta cells.

PHARMACOKINETICS: Absorption: Glimepiride: T_{max}=2-3 hrs (post-dose). Pioglitazone: T_{max}=2 hrs. **Distribution:** Pioglitazone: V_d=0.63L/kg, plasma protein binding (>99%). Glimepiride: (IV) V_d=8.8L, plasma protein binding (>99.5%). **Metabolism:** Pioglitazone: Extensive (hydroxylation & oxidation) via CYP2C8, CYP3A4, CYP1A1. M-II and M-IV (hydroxy derivatives) and M-III (keto derivatives) (active metabolites). Glimepiride: Complete. Oxidative biotransformation via CYP2C9. Cyclohexyl hydroxy methyl derivative (M1), carboxyl derivative (M2) (major metabolites). **Elimination:** Pioglitazone: Urine (15-30%), bile (unchanged), feces (metabolites); $T_{1/2}$=3-7 hrs (pioglitazone), 16-24 hrs (metabolites). Glimepiride: Urine (60%), feces (40%).

NURSING CONSIDERATIONS

Assessment: Assess for HF or risk of HF, previous hypersensitivity to the drug, type of DM, diabetic ketoacidosis, bone health, active/history of bladder cancer, G6PD deficiency, any other conditions where treatment is cautioned or contraindicated, pregnancy/nursing status, and possible drug interactions. Assess renal/liver and hematologic function.

Monitoring: Monitor for macular edema, bone fractures, hemolytic anemia, and other adverse reactions. Monitor for hypoglycemia and adverse reactions related to fluid retention and signs/symptoms of CHF after initiation or with dose increase. Monitor LFTs periodically in patients with liver disease. Perform regular eye exams in diabetes patients.

Patient Counseling: Inform patients that therapy is not recommended for patients with symptoms of HF; patients with severe HF (NYHA Class III or IV) cannot start therapy as the risks exceed the benefits in such patients. Advise on the importance of adherence to dietary instructions and regular testing of blood glucose and HbA1c, renal function, and hematologic parameters. Advise to seek medical advice promptly during periods of stress (eg, fever, trauma, infection, or surgery) as medication requirements may change. Instruct to promptly report any signs/symptoms of bladder cancer (eg, macroscopic hematuria, dysuria, urinary urgency), or HF (eg, unusually rapid increase in weight or edema, SOB). Inform that hypoglycemia may occur; explain the risks, symptoms, treatment and conditions that predispose to its development. Instruct to d/c use and seek medical consult if signs/symptoms of hepatotoxicity (eg, unexplained N/V, abdominal pain, fatigue, anorexia, dark urine) occur. Inform premenopausal anovulatory women to use adequate contraception during treatment. Advise to take a single dose qd with the 1st main meal and that any change in dosing should only be done if directed by physician.

Administration: Oral route. **Storage:** 25°C (77°F); excursions permitted to 15-30°C (59-86°F). Protect from moisture and humidity.

DUEXIS   RX
famotidine - ibuprofen (Horizon)

> NSAIDs may increase risk of serious cardiovascular (CV) thrombotic events, myocardial infarction (MI), and stroke; increased risk with duration of use and with CV disease (CVD) or risk factors for CVD. Increased risk of serious GI adverse reactions (eg, bleeding, ulceration, and perforation of stomach/intestines) that can be fatal and occur anytime during use and without warning symptoms; elderly patients are at greater risk. Contraindicated for the treatment of perioperative pain in the setting of coronary artery bypass graft (CABG) surgery.

THERAPEUTIC CLASS: H_2-blocker/NSAID

INDICATIONS: Relief of signs/symptoms of rheumatoid arthritis and osteoarthritis and to decrease the risk of developing upper GI ulcers (gastric and/or duodenal ulcer) in patients taking ibuprofen for those indications.

DOSAGE: *Adults*: 1 tab tid.

HOW SUPPLIED: Tab: (Ibuprofen-Famotidine) 800mg-26.6mg

CONTRAINDICATIONS: Patients who have experienced asthma, urticaria, or allergic reactions after taking aspirin (ASA) or other NSAIDs. Patients in the late stages of pregnancy. Treatment of perioperative pain in the setting of CABG surgery.

WARNINGS/PRECAUTIONS: Use for the shortest possible duration. Symptomatic response does not preclude the presence of gastric malignancy. D/C with active and clinically significant bleeding. Periodically monitor Hgb if initial Hgb ≤10g and long-term therapy is going to be received. D/C if visual disturbances occur and perform ophthalmologic exam. May mask signs of inflammation and fever. Ibuprofen: May cause HTN or worsen preexisting HTN; caution with HTN, and monitor BP closely. Fluid retention and edema reported; caution with fluid retention or heart failure (HF). Caution with history of ulcer disease or GI bleeding, or risk factors for GI bleeding (eg, prolonged NSAID therapy, older age, poor general health status); monitor for GI ulceration/bleeding, and d/c if serious GI adverse reaction occurs. May exacerbate inflammatory bowel disease (IBD). Renal injury reported with long-term use; increased risk with renal/hepatic impairment, HF, and in elderly. D/C if clinical signs and symptoms consistent with renal disease develop. Anaphylaxis may occur; avoid with ASA-triad. May cause serious skin adverse reactions; d/c at 1st appearance of skin rash or any sign of hypersensitivity. May cause elevated LFTs or severe hepatic reactions; d/c if liver disease or systemic manifestations occur. Anemia may occur; monitor Hgb/Hct if signs/symptoms of anemia develop with long-term use. May inhibit platelet aggregation and prolong bleeding time; monitor patients with coagulation disorders. Caution with preexisting asthma and avoid with ASA-sensitive asthma. Aseptic meningitis with fever and coma observed on rare occasions. Not a substitute for corticosteroids or for the treatment of corticosteroid insufficiency. Caution in elderly and debilitated. Famotidine: CNS adverse effects reported with moderate (CrCl <50mL/min) and severe renal insufficiency (CrCl <10mL/min); not recommended with CrCl <50mL/min.

ADVERSE REACTIONS: CV thrombotic events, MI, stroke, GI bleeding/ulceration/perforation, nausea, diarrhea, constipation, upper abdominal pain, headache, dyspepsia, upper respiratory tract infection, HTN.

INTERACTIONS: Increased risk of GI bleeding with oral corticosteroids, anticoagulants (eg, warfarin), antiplatelet drugs (including low-dose ASA), smoking, alcohol, and SSRIs. Risk of renal toxicity when coadministered with diuretics and ACE inhibitors. Avoid with other ibuprofen-containing products. Bleeding reported with coumarin-type anticoagulants. Increased risk of adverse events with ASA. May diminish effects of ACE inhibitors, thiazides, and loop (eg, furosemide) diuretics. May increase lithium levels; monitor for lithium toxicity. May enhance methotrexate toxicity; use with caution. Delayed absorption with cholestyramine.

PREGNANCY: Category C, not for use in nursing.

MECHANISM OF ACTION: Ibuprofen: NSAID; has not been established. Analgesic and antipyretic activity may be related to prostaglandin synthetase inhibition. Famotidine: H_2-receptor blocker; inhibits gastric secretion.

PHARMACOKINETICS: Absorption: Rapid. Ibuprofen: C_{max}=45mcg/mL, T_{max}=1.9 hrs. Famotidine: C_{max}=61ng/mL, T_{max}=2 hrs. **Distribution:** Famotidine: Plasma protein binding (15-20%); found in breast milk. **Metabolism:** Famotidine: S-oxide (metabolite). **Elimination:** Ibuprofen: Urine (45-79%, metabolites); $T_{1/2}$=2 hrs. Famotidine: Urine (25-30%, unchanged); $T_{1/2}$=4 hrs.

NURSING CONSIDERATIONS

Assessment: Assess for CABG surgery, CVD, a history of hypersensitivity to ASA or other NSAIDs, or any other conditions where treatment is contraindicated or cautioned. Assess for pregnancy/nursing status and for possible drug interactions. Obtain baseline BP, LFTs, CBC, and renal function.

Monitoring: Monitor for CV thrombotic events, GI events, active bleeding, anemia, anaphylaxis, skin reactions, visual disturbances, and other adverse reactions. Monitor BP, LFTs, renal function, CBC, and chemistry profiles.

Patient Counseling: Inform of possible serious CV and GI side effects. Advise to d/c drug immediately and contact physician if any type of rash develops. Instruct to d/c therapy and seek immediate medical therapy if nephrotoxicity, hepatotoxicity, or anaphylaxis occurs. Advise to report signs/symptoms of unexplained weight gain or edema to physician. Inform that medication should be avoided in late pregnancy. Instruct on what to do if a dose is missed.

Administration: Oral route. Swallow whole; do not cut, chew, divide, or crush. **Storage:** 25°C (77°F); excursions permitted to 15-30°C (59-86°F).

DULERA   RX
formoterol fumarate dihydrate - mometasone furoate (Merck)

> Long-acting β₂-adrenergic agonists (LABAs), such as formoterol, increase the risk of asthma-related death. LABAs may increase the risk of asthma-related hospitalization in pediatric patients and adolescents. Use only for patients not adequately controlled on a long-term asthma control medication (eg, inhaled corticosteroid) or whose disease severity clearly warrants initiation of treatment with both an inhaled corticosteroid and LABA. Do not use if asthma is adequately controlled on low- or medium-dose inhaled corticosteroids.

THERAPEUTIC CLASS: Beta₂-agonist/corticosteroid

INDICATIONS: Treatment of asthma in patients ≥12 yrs of age.

DOSAGE: *Adults:* 2 inh bid (am and pm). Max: 2 inh of 200mcg-5mcg bid. Previous Therapy: Inhaled Medium-Dose Corticosteroids: Initial: 2 inh of 100mcg-5mcg bid. Max: 400mcg-20mcg daily. Inhaled High-Dose Corticosteroids: Initial: 2 inh of 200mcg-5mcg bid. Max: 800mcg-20mcg daily. Do not use >2 inh bid of the prescribed strength. If inadequate response after 2 weeks of therapy, higher strength may provide additional asthma control.
Pediatrics: ≥12 Yrs: 2 inh bid (am and pm). Max: 2 inh of 200mcg-5mcg bid. Previous Therapy: Inhaled Medium-Dose Corticosteroids: Initial: 2 inh of 100mcg-5mcg bid. Max: 400mcg-20mcg daily. Inhaled High-Dose Corticosteroids: Initial: 2 inh of 200mcg-5mcg bid. Max: 800mcg-20mcg daily. Do not use >2 inh bid of the prescribed strength. If inadequate response after 2 weeks of therapy, higher strength may provide additional asthma control.

HOW SUPPLIED: MDI: (Mometasone furoate-Formoterol fumarate dihydrate) 100mcg-5mcg/inh, 200mcg-5mcg/inh [60 inhalations, 120 inhalations]

CONTRAINDICATIONS: Primary treatment of status asthmaticus or other acute episodes of asthma where intensive measures are required.

WARNINGS/PRECAUTIONS: Not indicated for the relief of acute bronchospasm; inhaled short-acting β₂-agonists (SABAs) (eg, albuterol) should be used. Do not initiate during rapidly deteriorating/potentially life-threatening asthma. D/C regular use of oral/inhaled SABA prior to treatment. Cardiovascular (CV) effects and fatalities reported with excessive use; do not use excessively or with other LABA. *Candida albicans* infections of mouth and pharynx reported; treat with antifungal therapy and, if needed, interrupt therapy. Increased susceptibility to infections. May lead to serious/fatal course of chickenpox or measles; avoid exposure and, if exposed, consider prophylaxis/treatment. Caution with active/quiescent tuberculosis (TB), untreated systemic fungal, bacterial, viral, or parasitic infections, or ocular herpes simplex. Deaths due to adrenal insufficiency reported with transfer from systemic to inhaled corticosteroids; if systemic corticosteroids required, wean slowly from systemic steroid after transferring to therapy. Resume oral corticosteroids during periods of stress or a severe asthma attack if patient previously withdrawn from systemic corticosteroid. Transferring from systemic to inhalation therapy may unmask previously suppressed allergic conditions (eg, rhinitis, conjunctivitis, eczema, arthritis, eosinophilic conditions). Observe for systemic corticosteroid withdrawal effects. Reduce dose slowly if hypercorticism and adrenal suppression appear. Inhalation induced bronchospasm with immediate increase in wheezing may occur; d/c immediately and institute alternative therapy. Immediate hypersensitivity reactions may occur. CV and CNS effects may occur. Caution with CV disorders (eg, coronary insufficiency, cardiac arrhythmias, HTN). Decreases in bone mineral density (BMD) reported; caution with major risk factors for decreased bone mineral content, including chronic use of drugs that can reduce bone mass (eg, anticonvulsants, corticosteroids). May reduce growth velocity in pediatric patients. Glaucoma, increased intraocular pressure (IOP), and cataracts reported. Caution in elderly and patients with aneurysm, pheochromocytoma, convulsive disorders, thyrotoxicosis, and in patients unusually responsive to sympathomimetic amines. May cause changes in blood glucose and serum K⁺ levels.

ADVERSE REACTIONS: Nasopharyngitis, sinusitis, headache, dysphonia.

INTERACTIONS: Do not use with other medications containing LABA (eg, salmeterol, formoterol fumarate, arformoterol tartrate); increased risk of CV effects. Caution with ketoconazole, other known strong CYP3A4 inhibitors (eg, ritonavir, atazanavir, clarithromycin, indinavir, itraconazole, nefazodone, nelfinavir, saquinavir, telithromycin), and non-K⁺-sparing diuretics (eg, loop or thiazide diuretics). Elevated risk of arrhythmias with concomitant anesthesia with halogenated hydrocarbons. Mometasone: Increased plasma concentration with oral ketoconazole and increased systemic exposure with CYP3A4 inhibitors. Formoterol: Potentiation of sympathetic effects with additional adrenergic drugs; use with caution. Potentiation of hypokalemic effect with xanthine derivatives and diuretics. Potentiation of CV effect with MAOIs, TCAs, or drugs known to prolong QTc interval. Caution with MAOIs, TCAs, macrolides, drugs known to prolong QTc interval or within 2 weeks of discontinuing such products. Use with β-blockers may block effects and produce severe bronchospasm in asthma patients; if needed, consider cardioselective β-blocker with caution.

PREGNANCY: Category C, not for use in nursing.

MECHANISM OF ACTION: Mometasone: Corticosteroid; not established. Shown to have inhibitory effects on multiple cell types (eg, mast cells, eosinophils, neutrophils, macrophages, lymphocytes) and mediators (eg, histamine, eicosanoids, leukotrienes, cytokines) involved in inflammation and asthmatic response. Formoterol: LABA; stimulates intracellular adenyl cyclase, which catalyzes conversion of ATP to cAMP, producing relaxation of bronchial smooth muscle and inhibition of release of mediators of immediate hypersensitivity from cells, especially from mast cells.

PHARMACOKINETICS: Absorption: (Single dose) Mometasone: C_{max}=20pg/mL; AUC=170pg•hr/mL; T_{max}=1-2 hrs. Formoterol: C_{max}=22pmol/L; AUC=125pmol•h/L; T_{max}=0.58-1.97 hrs. **Distribution:** Mometasone: V_d=152L (IV); plasma protein binding (98-99%). Formoterol: Plasma protein binding (61-64%). **Metabolism:** Mometasone: Liver (extensive) via CYP3A4. Formoterol: Direct glucuronidation, O-demethylation (via CYP2D6, 2C19, 2C9, 2A6), and conjugation. **Elimination:** Mometasone: Feces (74%); urine (8%); $T_{1/2}$=25 hrs. Formoterol: Urine (6.2-6.8%, unchanged); $T_{1/2}$=9.1-10.8 hrs (single dose), 9-11 hrs (multidose).

NURSING CONSIDERATIONS

Assessment: Assess use of long-term asthma control medication (eg, inhaled corticosteroid), status asthmaticus, acute asthma episodes, rapidly deteriorating asthma, bronchospasm, known hypersensitivity to any drug component, risk factors for decreased bone mineral content, CV or convulsive disorders, thyrotoxicosis, other conditions where treatment is contraindicated or cautioned, pregnancy/nursing status, and possible drug interactions. Obtain baseline BMD, eye exam, and lung function prior to therapy.

Monitoring: Monitor for localized oral *C. albicans* infections, worsening or acutely deteriorating asthma, development of glaucoma, increased IOP, cataracts, CV/CNS effects, hypercorticism, adrenal suppression, inhalation induced bronchospasm, hypokalemia, hyperglycemia, hypersensitivity reactions, and signs of increased drug exposure with hepatic impairment. Monitor BMD and lung function periodically. Perform periodic eye exams. Monitor growth in pediatric patients routinely. Monitor pulse rate, BP, ECG changes, blood glucose, and serum K+ levels.

Patient Counseling: Inform about increased risk of asthma-related hospitalization in pediatric patients/adolescents and asthma-related death. Instruct not to use to relieve acute asthma symptoms, if symptoms arise between doses, use an inhaled SABA for immediate relief. Instruct to seek medical attention if symptoms worsen, if lung function decreases, or if more inhalations than usual of a SABA are needed. If a dose is missed, instruct to take next dose at the same time patients normally do. Instruct not to d/c or reduce therapy without physician's guidance. Instruct not to use with other LABAs. Advise to avoid exposure to chickenpox or measles and, if exposed, consult physician without delay. Inform of potential worsening of existing TB, fungal, bacterial, viral, or parasitic infections, or ocular herpes simplex. Inform about risks of hypercorticism and adrenal suppression, decreased BMD, cataracts or glaucoma, oropharyngeal candidiasis, and reduced growth velocity in pediatric patients. Advise to taper slowly from systemic corticosteroids if transferring to treatment. Inform of adverse events associated with β_2-agonists (eg, palpitations, chest pain, rapid HR, tremor, or nervousness).

Administration: Oral inhalation. After inhalation, rinse mouth with water without swallowing. Shake well before use. Refer to PI for proper priming and administration. **Storage:** 20-25°C (68-77°F); excursions permitted to 15-30°C (59-86°F). Do not puncture. Do not use or store near heat or open flame. Discard inhaler when dose counter reads "0." 60-inhalation inhaler: Store with the mouthpiece down or in a horizontal position after priming.

DUONEB   RX
ipratropium bromide - albuterol sulfate (Dey)

THERAPEUTIC CLASS: Anticholinergic/beta$_2$-agonist

INDICATIONS: Treatment of bronchospasm associated with chronic obstructive pulmonary disease (COPD) in patients requiring >1 bronchodilator.

DOSAGE: *Adults:* 3mL qid via nebulizer. May give up to 2 additional 3mL doses/day, PRN.

HOW SUPPLIED: Sol, Inhalation: (Ipratropium Bromide-Albuterol Sulfate) 0.5mg-3mg/3mL

CONTRAINDICATIONS: History of hypersensitivity to atropine and its derivatives.

WARNINGS/PRECAUTIONS: Paradoxical bronchospasm may occur; d/c immediately and institute alternative therapy if occurs. Fatalities reported with excessive use of inhaled products containing sympathomimetic amines and with home use of nebulizers. May produce significant cardiovascular (CV) effects (eg, ECG changes). Immediate hypersensitivity reactions reported. Caution with CV disorders (eg, coronary insufficiency, cardiac arrhythmias, HTN), convulsive disorders, hyperthyroidism, diabetes mellitus (DM), narrow-angle glaucoma, prostatic hypertrophy, bladder-neck obstruction, hepatic/renal insufficiency, and in patients unusually responsive to sympathomimetic amines. Aggravation of preexisting DM and ketoacidosis reported with large doses of IV albuterol. May decrease serum K+.

ADVERSE REACTIONS: Lung disease, pharyngitis, pain, chest pain, diarrhea, dyspepsia, nausea, leg cramps, bronchitis, pneumonia, urinary tract infection, constipation, voice alterations.

INTERACTIONS: Additive effects with other anticholinergic drugs; use with caution. Other sympathomimetic agents may increase risk of adverse CV effects; use with caution. β-blockers and albuterol inhibit the effect of each other; use β-blockers with caution in patients with hyperreactive airways. ECG changes and/or hypokalemia that may result from non-K$^+$-sparing diuretics (eg, loop or thiazide diuretics) may be worsened by β-agonists; use with caution. Administration with MAOIs or TCAs, or within 2 weeks of discontinuation of such agents may potentiate the action of albuterol on CV system; use with extreme caution.

PREGNANCY: Category C, not for use in nursing.

MECHANISM OF ACTION: Albuterol: β$_2$-adrenergic bronchodilator; stimulates adenyl cyclase, enzyme that catalyzes formation of cAMP, and the cAMP formed mediates cellular response, resulting in relaxation of bronchial smooth muscle. Ipratropium: Anticholinergic bronchodilator; blocks muscarinic receptors of acetylcholine. Prevents the increases in intracellular concentration of cGMP, resulting from interaction of acetylcholine with the muscarinic receptors of bronchial smooth muscle.

PHARMACOKINETICS: Absorption: Albuterol: C$_{max}$=4.65mg/mL, T$_{max}$=0.8 hrs, AUC=24.2ng•hr/mL. **Distribution:** Ipratropium: Plasma protein binding (0-9%). **Metabolism:** Albuterol: Conjugation; albuterol 4'-O-sulfate (metabolite). Ipratropium: Ester hydrolysis. **Elimination:** Albuterol: urine (8.4% unchanged0); T$_{1/2}$=6.7 hrs. Ipratropium: urine (3.9% unchanged).

NURSING CONSIDERATIONS

Assessment: Assess for history of hypersensitivity to atropine and its derivatives, CV disorders, convulsive disorders, hyperthyroidism, DM, narrow-angle glaucoma, prostatic hypertrophy, bladder-neck obstruction, hepatic/renal insufficiency, pregnancy/nursing status, and possible drug interactions. Assess use in patients unusually responsive to sympathomimetic amines.

Monitoring: Monitor for signs/symptoms of hypersensitivity reactions, paradoxical bronchospasm, CV effects, and other adverse reactions. Monitor pulse rate and BP. Reassess therapy if signs of worsening COPD occur.

Patient Counseling: Advise not to exceed recommended dose or frequency without consulting physician. Instruct to contact physician if symptoms worsen. Instruct to avoid exposing eyes to this product as temporary pupillary dilation, blurred vision, eye pain, or precipitation/worsening of narrow-angle glaucoma may occur. Inform that proper nebulizer technique should be assured, particularly if a mask is used. Instruct to contact physician if pregnancy occurs or nursing is started while on therapy.

Administration: Inhalation route. Refer to PI for administration instructions. **Storage:** 2-25°C (36-77°F). Store in pouch until time of use. Protect from light.

DURAGESIC `CII`
fentanyl (Janssen)

Contains a Schedule II controlled substance with an abuse liability similar to other opioid agonists, legal or illicit; monitor for signs of misuse, abuse, or addiction. Respiratory depression and death may occur; monitor especially during the first 2 applications following initiation of dosing or an increase in dosage. Contraindicated for use as a PRN analgesic, use in nonopioid tolerant patients, acute pain, and postoperative pain. Death and serious medical problems have occurred following accidental exposure. Concomitant use with all CYP3A4 inhibitors may increase plasma concentrations and cause fatal respiratory depression. May increase absorption as a result of exposure to heat; avoid exposing application site and surrounding area to direct external heat source (eg, heating pads or electric blanket, heat or tanning lamps, sunbathing, hot baths, saunas, hot tubs, heated water beds). Increased risk of exposure in patients who develop fever or increased core body temperature due to strenuous exertion; dose adjustment may be required to avoid overdose and death.

THERAPEUTIC CLASS: Opioid analgesic

INDICATIONS: Management of persistent, moderate to severe chronic pain in opioid-tolerant patients ≥2 yrs of age when a continuous, around-the-clock opioid analgesic is required for an extended period, and the patient cannot be managed by other means (eg, nonsteroidal analgesics, opioid combination products, or immediate-release opioids).

DOSAGE: *Adults:* Determine dose based on opioid tolerance, previous analgesic requirement, and general condition/medical status of the patient. Minimum Initial: 25mcg/hr for 72 hrs. Titrate: May increase after 3 days; evaluate for further titrations after no less than two 3-day applications before any further increase in dosage is made. Dosage increments may be based on the daily dose of supplementary opioids using the ratio of 45mg/24 hrs of oral morphine to a 12mcg/hr increase in dose. Some patients may not achieve adequate analgesia and may require systems to be applied q48h rather than q72h; an increase in dose should be evaluated before changing the interval. Refer to PI for Dose Conversion Guidelines. Mild-Moderate Hepatic/Renal Impairment: Start with 1/2 of the usual dosage. Elderly: Start at lower end of the dosing range.
Pediatrics: ≥2 Yrs: Determine dose based on opioid tolerance, previous analgesic requirement,

and general condition/medical status of the patient. Minimum Initial: 25mcg/hr for 72 hrs. Titrate: May increase after 3 days; evaluate for further titrations after no less than two 3-day applications before any further increase in dosage is made. Dosage increments may be based on the daily dose of supplementary opioids using the ratio of 45mg/24 hrs of oral morphine to a 12mcg/hr increase in dose. Refer to PI for Dose Conversion Guidelines. Mild-Moderate Hepatic/Renal Impairment: Start with 1/2 of the usual dosage.

HOW SUPPLIED: Patch: 12mcg/hr, 25mcg/hr, 50mcg/hr, 75mcg/hr, 100mcg/hr [5ˢ]

CONTRAINDICATIONS: Opioid-nontolerant patients; management of acute or intermittent pain or in patients who require opioid analgesia for a short period; postoperative pain, including use after outpatient/day surgeries (eg, tonsillectomies) and mild pain; patients with significant respiratory compromise, especially if adequate monitoring and resuscitative equipment are not readily available; acute or severe bronchial asthma; diagnosis or suspicion of paralytic ileus.

WARNINGS/PRECAUTIONS: Monitor for respiratory depression after patch removal to ensure that patient's respiration has stabilized for at least 24-72 hrs or longer as clinical symptoms dictate. Increased risk of respiratory depression in elderly, cachectic, or debilitated patients. May decrease respiratory drive to the point of apnea in patients with significant chronic obstructive pulmonary disease or cor pulmonale, and patients having a substantially decreased respiratory reserve, hypoxia, hypercapnia, or preexisting respiratory depression; consider use of other nonopioid alternative if possible. Avoid in patients who may be susceptible to the intracranial effects of carbon dioxide retention (eg, increased intracranial pressure [ICP], impaired consciousness, or coma). May obscure clinical course of head injury and increase ICP; monitor patients with brain tumors. May produce bradycardia; closely monitor patients with bradyarrhythmias for changes in HR. Avoid use with severe hepatic/renal impairment. May cause spasm of the sphincter of Oddi; monitor patients with biliary tract disease (eg, acute pancreatitis). May cause increases in serum amylase concentration. Tolerance and physical dependence may occur. May impair mental/physical abilities. Withdrawal symptoms may occur (eg, N/V, diarrhea, anxiety, shivering); gradual reduction of dose is recommended.

ADVERSE REACTIONS: Respiratory depression, N/V, constipation, diarrhea, headache, pruritus, abdominal pain, dizziness, insomnia, somnolence, fatigue, anorexia.

INTERACTIONS: See Boxed Warning. Respiratory depression is more likely to occur when given with other drugs that depress respiration. Concomitant use with CNS depressants (eg, opioids, sedatives, hypnotics, tranquilizers, general anesthetics, phenothiazines, skeletal muscle relaxants, alcohol) may cause respiratory depression, hypotension, profound sedation, or potentially coma or death; closely monitor patients with CNS depressants and reduce dose of one or both agents. Coadministration with CYP3A4 inducers may lead to reduced efficacy of fentanyl. Avoid use within 14 days of an MAOI. Caution with CNS-active drugs.

PREGNANCY: Category C, not for use in nursing.

MECHANISM OF ACTION: Opioid analgesic; interacts predominantly with the opioid μ-receptor in the brain, spinal cord, and other tissues.

PHARMACOKINETICS: Absorption: T_{max}=20-72 hrs. Transdermal administration of variable doses resulted in different parameters. **Distribution:** V_d=6L/kg; found in breast milk; crosses placenta. **Metabolism:** Liver via CYP3A4; oxidative N-dealkylation to norfentanyl. **Elimination:** (IV) Urine (75%, <10% unchanged), feces (9% primarily metabolites); $T_{1/2}$=20-27 hrs.

NURSING CONSIDERATIONS

Assessment: Assess for degree of opioid tolerance, type and severity of pain, risks for opioid abuse or addiction, paralytic ileus, acute/bronchial asthma, history of hypersensitivity, cardiac/respiratory function, renal/hepatic function, debilitation, seizures, biliary tract disease, patient's general condition/medical status, any other conditions where treatment is contraindicated or cautioned, pregnancy/nursing status, and for possible drug interactions.

Monitoring: Monitor for signs/symptoms of respiratory depression; bradycardia; seizures; worsening of biliary tract disease; increases in ICP, serum amylase levels, and body temperature/fever; abuse; misuse; addiction; tolerance/physical dependence; overdose, especially when converting from another opioid; and other adverse reactions.

Patient Counseling: Inform that patch contains fentanyl, an opioid pain medicine that has a high potential for abuse that can cause serious breathing problems and therefore should be taken only as ud. Instruct to protect from theft or misuse, never give to anyone other than for whom it was prescribed, and to immediately notify physician if breathing problems occur. Advise never to change the dose or the number of patches applied to the skin unless instructed by the physician. Warn of the potential for temperature-dependent increases; instruct to avoid strenuous exertion that can increase body temperature and avoid exposing application site and surrounding area to direct external heat sources. Advise to keep patch in a secure place out of the reach of children. Instruct to immediately take the patch off if patch accidentally sticks to the skin of another person, and wash exposed area with water and seek medical attention. Inform of proper disposal of used and unneeded patch; advise to remove unused patch from pouch, fold, and flush them down the toilet. Counsel that medication may impair mental and/or physical ability; refrain from potentially hazardous tasks (eg, driving, operating machinery). Inform of pregnancy risk and instruct to notify physician if pregnant or planning to become pregnant. Advise to notify physician of all medications currently being taken and avoid using other CNS depressants and alcohol. Inform that severe constipation may develop. Advise to avoid abrupt withdrawal of medication.

Administration: Transdermal route. Refer to PI for further details on proper application and handling instructions. **Storage:** Up to 25°C (77°F); excursions permitted to 15-30°C (59-86°F). Store in original unopened pouch.

DURAMORPH   CII
morphine sulfate (Baxter)

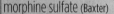

> Risk of severe adverse effects with epidural or intrathecal route; observe patients in a fully equipped and staffed environment for at least 24 hrs after initial dose. Naloxone inj and resuscitative equipment should be immediately available in case of life-threatening or intolerable side effects and whenever therapy is initiated. Intrathecal dosage is usually 1/10 that of epidural dosage. Remove any contaminated clothing and rinse affected area with water if accidental dermal exposure occurs. Associated with risk of overdosage, diversion, and abuse; special measures must be taken to control this product within the hospital/clinic. Do not use if color is darker than pale yellow, if it is discolored in any other way, or if it contains a precipitate.

THERAPEUTIC CLASS: Opioid analgesic

INDICATIONS: Management of pain unresponsive to non-narcotic analgesics.

DOSAGE: *Adults:* IV: Initial: 2-10mg/70kg. Epidural: Initial: 5mg in the lumbar region. Titrate: If adequate pain relief is not achieved within 1 hr, may give incremental doses of 1-2mg at intervals sufficient to assess effectiveness. Max: 10mg/24 hrs. Intrathecal: 0.2-1mg single dose; do not inject more than 2mL of the 0.5mg/mL ampul or 1mL of the 1mg/mL ampul in the lumbar area. Repeated intrathecal inj not recommended; if pain recurs, consider alternative routes of administration. May administer a constant IV infusion of 0.6mg/hr naloxone for 24 hrs after intrathecal inj to reduce incidence of potential side effects.

HOW SUPPLIED: Inj: 0.5mg/mL, 1mg/mL [10mL]

CONTRAINDICATIONS: Medical conditions that would preclude the administration of opioids by the IV route (acute bronchial asthma, upper airway obstruction).

WARNINGS/PRECAUTIONS: Not for use in continuous microinfusion devices. May be habit forming. Administration should be limited to use by those familiar with respiratory depression management. Rapid IV administration may result in chest-wall rigidity. Prior to any epidural or intrathecal administration, assess for patient conditions (eg, infection at the inj site, bleeding diathesis, anticoagulant therapy) which call for special evaluation of the benefit versus risk potential. Should be administered by or under the direction of a physician experienced in the techniques and familiar with the patient management problems associated with epidural or intrathecal administration. Severe respiratory depression up to 24 hrs following epidural/intrathecal administration reported. Unusual acceleration of neuraxial morphine requirements may occur, which may cause concern regarding systemic absorption and the hazards of large doses; patients may benefit from hospitalization and detoxification. Myoclonic-like spasm of the lower extremities reported with intrathecal doses of >20mg/day; after detoxification, may resume treatment at lower doses. Higher incidence of respiratory depression with intrathecal than epidural use. Seizures may result from high doses; caution with known seizure disorders. Extreme caution with head injury or increased intracranial pressure; pupillary changes (miosis) may obscure the existence, extent, and course of intracranial pathology. High neuraxial doses may produce myoclonic events. Maintain a high index of suspicion for adverse drug reactions when evaluating altered mental status or movement abnormalities. Caution with decreased respiratory reserve (eg, emphysema, severe obesity, kyphoscoliosis, paralysis of the phrenic nerve). Avoid with chronic asthma, upper airway obstruction, or in any other chronic pulmonary disorder. Use caution when administering epidurally to patients with reduced metabolic rates and with hepatic and/or renal dysfunction. Smooth muscle hypertonicity may result in biliary colic. Initiation of neuraxial opiate analgesia is frequently associated with micturition disturbances, especially in males with prostatic enlargement. Monitor patients with reduced circulating blood volume or impaired myocardial function for possible occurrence of orthostatic hypotension. May cause severe hypotension when ability to maintain BP has already been compromised by a depleted blood volume. Avoid abrupt withdrawal. Caution in elderly.

ADVERSE REACTIONS: Respiratory depression/arrest, convulsions, dysphoric reactions, toxic psychoses, pruritus, urinary retention, constipation, lumbar puncture-type headache.

INTERACTIONS: CNS depressants (eg, alcohol, sedatives, antihistaminics, psychotropic drugs) potentiate depressant effects. Neuroleptics may increase risk of respiratory depression. Monitor for possible occurrence of orthostatic hypotension in patients on sympatholytic drugs. May cause severe hypotension with concurrent administration of drugs such as phenothiazines or general anesthetics.

PREGNANCY: Category C, safety not known in nursing.

MECHANISM OF ACTION: Opioid analgesic; analgesia involves at least 3 anatomical areas of the CNS: the periaqueductal-periventricular gray matter, the ventromedial medulla, and the spinal cord. Interacts predominantly with μ-receptors distributed in the brain, spinal cord, and trigeminal nerve.

PHARMACOKINETICS: Absorption: (Epidural/Intrathecal) T_{max}=5-10 min (bolus). (Epidural) Rapid; C_{max}=33-40ng/mL; T_{max}=10-15 min. (Intrathecal) C_{max}<1-7.8ng/mL. **Distribution:** Plasma protein binding (36%); found in breast milk. (IV) V_d=1.0-4.7L/kg. **Metabolism:** Hepatic glucuronidation. **Elimination:** Urine (2-12% unchanged), feces (10%). (IV/IM) $T_{1/2}$=1.5-4.5 hrs. (Epidural) $T_{1/2}$=39-249 min.

NURSING CONSIDERATIONS

Assessment: Assess for patient's general condition and medical status, renal/hepatic impairment, hypersensitivity to drug, any other conditions where treatment is contraindicated or cautioned, pregnancy/nursing status, and possible drug interactions.

Monitoring: Monitor for signs/symptoms of respiratory depression, seizures, myoclonic events, biliary colic, urinary retention, orthostatic hypotension, drug abuse/dependence, and other adverse reactions.

Patient Counseling: Inform about risks and benefits of therapy. Inform of adverse reactions that may occur. Instruct to inform physician of other medications being taken. Inform that medication has potential for abuse and dependence.

Administration: IV/Epidural/Intrathecal route. Proper placement of a needle or catheter in the epidural space should be verified before therapy is injected. Limit administration by epidural/intrathecal routes to lumbar area. **Storage:** 20-25°C (68-77°F); excursions permitted to 15-30°C (59-86°F). Protect from light. Do not freeze. Do not heat-sterilize.

DYAZIDE   RX
hydrochlorothiazide - triamterene (GlaxoSmithKline)

> Abnormal elevation of serum K⁺ levels (≥5.5mEq/L) may occur with all K⁺-sparing diuretic combinations. Hyperkalemia is more likely to occur with renal impairment and diabetes (even without evidence of renal impairment), and in elderly or severely ill; monitor serum K⁺ levels at frequent intervals.

THERAPEUTIC CLASS: K⁺-sparing diuretic/thiazide diuretic

INDICATIONS: Treatment of HTN or edema if hypokalemia occurs on HCTZ alone, or when a thiazide diuretic is required and cannot risk hypokalemia. May be used alone or as an adjunct to other antihypertensives, such as β-blockers.

DOSAGE: *Adults:* 1-2 caps PO qd.

HOW SUPPLIED: Cap: (HCTZ-Triamterene) 25mg-37.5mg

CONTRAINDICATIONS: Anuria, acute and chronic renal insufficiency or significant renal impairment, sulfonamide hypersensitivity, preexisting elevated serum K⁺ (hyperkalemia), K⁺-sparing agents (eg, spironolactone, amiloride, or other formulations containing triamterene), K⁺ salt substitutes, K⁺ supplements (except with severe hypokalemia).

WARNINGS/PRECAUTIONS: Avoid in severely ill in whom respiratory or metabolic acidosis may occur; if used, frequent evaluations of acid/base balance and serum electrolytes are necessary. May cause idiosyncratic reaction, resulting in acute transient myopia and acute angle-closure glaucoma; d/c as rapidly as possible. Caution with diabetes; may cause hyperglycemia and glycosuria. Diabetes mellitus (DM) may become manifest. Caution with hepatic impairment; may precipitate hepatic coma with severe liver disease. Corrective measures must be taken if hypokalemia develops; d/c and initiate potassium chloride (KCl) supplementation if serious hypokalemia develops (serum K⁺ <3.0mEq/L). May potentiate electrolyte imbalance with heart failure, renal disease, or cirrhosis of the liver. May cause hypochloremia. Dilutional hyponatremia may occur in edematous patients in hot weather. Caution with history of renal stones. May increase BUN and SrCr. May decrease serum PBI levels. Decreased Ca^{2+} excretion reported. Changes in parathyroid glands with hypercalcemia and hypophosphatemia reported during prolonged therapy. May interfere with the fluorescent measurement of quinidine.

ADVERSE REACTIONS: Muscle cramps, N/V, pancreatitis, weakness, arrhythmia, impotence, dry mouth, jaundice, paresthesia, renal stones, anaphylaxis, acute renal failure, hyperkalemia, hyponatremia.

INTERACTIONS: See Contraindications. Increased risk of hyperkalemia with ACE inhibitors, blood from blood bank, and low-salt milk. Increased risk of severe hyponatremia with chlorpropamide. Possible interaction resulting in acute renal failure with indomethacin; caution with NSAIDs. Avoid with lithium due to risk of lithium toxicity. Decreased arterial responsiveness to norepinephrine. Amphotericin B, corticosteroids, and corticotropin may intensify electrolyte imbalance, particularly hypokalemia. Adjust dose of antigout drugs to control hyperuricemia and gout. May decrease effect of oral anticoagulants. May alter insulin requirements. Increased paralyzing effects of nondepolarizing muscle relaxants (eg, tubocurarine). Reduced K$^+$ levels with chronic or overuse of laxatives or use of exchange resins (eg, sodium polystyrene sulfonate). May reduce effectiveness of methenamine. May potentiate action of other antihypertensive drugs (eg, β-blockers).

PREGNANCY: Category C, not for use in nursing.

MECHANISM OF ACTION: Triamterene: K$^+$-sparing diuretic; exerts diuretic effect on distal renal tubules to inhibit the reabsorption of Na$^+$ in exchange for K$^+$ and hydrogen ions. HCTZ: thiazide diuretic; blocks reabsorption of Na$^+$ and Cl$^-$ ions and thereby increases the quantity of Na$^+$ transversing the distal tubule and the volume of water excreted.

PHARMACOKINETICS: Absorption: Well-absorbed. Triamterene: C_{max}=46.4ng/mL; T_{max}=1.1 hrs; AUC=148.7ng•hrs/mL. HCTZ: C_{max}=135.1ng/mL; T_{max}=2 hrs; AUC=834ng•hrs/mL. **Distribution:** Crosses placenta; found in breast milk.

NURSING CONSIDERATIONS

Assessment: Assess for anuria, renal/hepatic impairment, sulfonamide hypersensitivity, hyperkalemia, diabetes, history of renal stones, pregnancy/nursing status, and for possible drug interactions. Obtain baseline BUN, SrCr, and serum electrolytes.

Monitoring: Monitor for signs/symptoms of hyperkalemia, hypokalemia, hyperglycemia, hypochloremia, renal stones, and for electrolyte imbalance. Monitor for hepatic coma in patients with severe liver disease. Monitor serum K$^+$ levels, BUN, SrCr, and serum electrolytes.

Patient Counseling: Inform about risks/benefits of therapy. Advise to seek medical attention if symptoms of hyperkalemia (eg, paresthesias, muscular weakness, fatigue), hypokalemia, hyperglycemia, renal stones, electrolyte imbalance (eg, dry mouth, thirst, weakness), or hypersensitivity reactions occur.

Administration: Oral route. **Storage:** 20-25°C (68-77°F); excursions permitted to 15-30°C (59-86°F). Protect from light. Dispense in a tight, light-resistant container.

Dynacin   RX
minocycline HCl (Medicis)

THERAPEUTIC CLASS: Tetracycline derivative

INDICATIONS: Treatment of the following infections caused by susceptible microorganisms: Rocky Mountain spotted fever, typhus fever and the typhus group, Q fever, rickettsialpox, tick fevers, respiratory tract infections, lymphogranuloma venereum, psittacosis (ornithosis), trachoma, inclusion conjunctivitis, nongonococcal urethritis/endocervical/rectal infections (in adults), relapsing fever, chancroid, plague, tularemia, cholera, *Campylobacter fetus* infections, brucellosis (in conjunction with streptomycin), bartonellosis, granuloma inguinale, urinary tract infections, skin and skin structure infections. Treatment of infections caused by susceptible strains of *Escherichia coli*, *Enterobacter aerogenes*, *Shigella* species, and *Acinetobacter* species. When penicillin (PCN) is contraindicated, treatment of the following infections caused by susceptible microorganisms: uncomplicated urethritis in men due to *Neisseria gonorrhoeae* and for the treatment of other gonococcal infections, infections in women caused by *N. gonorrhoeae*, syphilis, yaws, listeriosis, anthrax, Vincent's infection, actinomycosis, infections caused by *Clostridium* species. Adjunctive therapy in acute intestinal amebiasis and severe acne. Treatment of asymptomatic carriers of *Neisseria meningitidis* to eliminate meningococci from the nasopharynx. Prophylaxis for situations in which the risk of meningococcal meningitis is high. Has been used successfully in the treatment of infections caused by *Mycobacterium marinum*.

DOSAGE: *Adults:* Initial: 200mg. Maint: 100mg q12h. Alternatively, if more frequent doses are preferred, two or four 50mg tabs may be given initially, followed by one 50mg tab qid. Uncomplicated Gonococcal Infections Other Than Urethritis and Anorectal Infections in Men: Initial: 200mg. Maint: 100mg q12h for a minimum of 4 days, with post-therapy cultures in 2-3 days. Uncomplicated Gonococcal Urethritis in Men: 100mg q12h for 5 days. Syphilis: Administer usual dosage for 10-15 days. Meningococcal Carrier State: 100mg q12h for 5 days. *M. marinum* Infections: 100mg q12h for 6-8 weeks. Uncomplicated Urethral/Endocervical/Rectal Infection Caused by *Chlamydia trachomatis* or *Ureaplasma urealyticum*: 100mg q12h for at least 7 days. Renal Impairment (CrCl <80mL/min): Max: 200mg/24 hrs. Elderly: Start at lower end of dosing range. Take with adequate amounts of fluids.
Pediatrics: >8 Yrs: Initial: 4mg/kg. Maint: 2mg/kg q12h, not to exceed usual adult dose. Take with adequate amounts of fluids.

HOW SUPPLIED: Tab: 50mg, 75mg, 100mg

WARNINGS/PRECAUTIONS: May cause fetal harm. May cause permanent discoloration of the teeth (yellow-gray-brown) if used during tooth development (last half of pregnancy, infancy, childhood to 8 yrs of age); do not use during tooth development. Enamel hypoplasia reported. May decrease fibula growth rate in premature infants. Drug rash with eosinophilia and systemic symptoms (DRESS), including fatal cases, reported; d/c immediately if this syndrome is recognized. May cause an increase in BUN; caution with renal impairment. Photosensitivity, manifested by an exaggerated sunburn reaction, reported. CNS side effects reported; may impair mental/physical abilities. *Clostridium difficile*-associated diarrhea (CDAD) reported; d/c if CDAD is suspected or confirmed. May result in bacterial resistance if used in the absence of proven or suspected bacterial infection, or if used in a prophylactic indication; take appropriate measures if superinfection develops. Associated with pseudotumor cerebri (benign intracranial HTN) in adults and bulging fontanels in infants. Hepatotoxicity reported; caution with hepatic dysfunction. Incision and drainage or other surgical procedures should be performed in conjunction with antibiotic therapy when indicated. False elevations of urinary catecholamine levels may occur due to interference with the fluorescence test. Caution in elderly. Not indicated for the treatment of meningococcal infection. Thyroid cancer reported; consider monitoring for signs of thyroid cancer when given over prolonged periods.

ADVERSE REACTIONS: Neutropenia, agranulocytosis, lupus-like syndrome, serum sickness-like syndrome, fever, N/V, diarrhea, increased liver enzymes, cough, anaphylaxis, exfoliative dermatitis, Stevens-Johnson syndrome, skin and mucous membrane pigmentation, headache.

INTERACTIONS: Caution with other hepatotoxic drugs. Depresses plasma prothrombin activity; may require downward adjustment of anticoagulant dosage. May interfere with bactericidal action of PCN; avoid concurrent use. Impaired absorption with antacids containing aluminum, Ca^{2+}, or Mg^{2+}, and iron-containing preparations. Fatal renal toxicity reported with methoxyflurane. May decrease effectiveness of oral contraceptives. Avoid isotretinoin shortly before, during, and shortly after therapy; each drug alone is associated with pseudotumor cerebri. Increased risk of ergotism with ergot alkaloids or their derivatives.

PREGNANCY: Category D, not for use in nursing.

MECHANISM OF ACTION: Tetracycline derivative; primarily bacteriostatic and thought to exert antimicrobial effect by inhibition of protein synthesis.

PHARMACOKINETICS: Absorption: Virtually complete. (100mg, Single-dose; Normal fasting adults) C_{max}=758.29ng/mL; T_{max}=1.71 hrs. **Distribution:** Crosses placenta; found in breast milk. **Elimination:** (Normal) Urine, feces; (100mg, Single-dose; Normal fasting adults) $T_{1/2}$=17.03 hrs.

NURSING CONSIDERATIONS

Assessment: Assess for hypersensitivity to drug or any tetracyclines, hepatic/renal impairment, pregnancy/nursing status, and possible drug interactions. Perform culture and susceptibility tests. In venereal disease when coexistent syphilis is suspected, perform a dark-field examination and blood serology.

Monitoring: Monitor for DRESS, photosensitivity, CNS effects, CDAD, superinfection, benign intracranial HTN in adults, and other adverse reactions. Perform periodic laboratory evaluations of organ systems, including hematopoietic, renal, and hepatic studies. In venereal disease when coexistent syphilis is suspected, repeat blood serology monthly for at least 4 months.

Patient Counseling: Apprise of the potential hazard to fetus if used during pregnancy; instruct to notify physician if pregnant. Inform that diarrhea is a common problem caused by therapy, which usually ends when therapy is discontinued. Instruct to immediately contact physician if watery and bloody stools (with or without stomach cramps and fever) occur, even as late as ≥2 months after having taken the last dose. Advise that photosensitivity manifested by an exaggerated sunburn reaction can occur; instruct to d/c treatment at the 1st evidence of skin erythema. Caution patients who experience CNS symptoms about driving vehicles or using hazardous machinery while on therapy. Inform that drug may render oral contraceptives less effective. Counsel that therapy should only be used to treat bacterial, not viral (eg, common cold), infections. Instruct to take exactly ud, even if patient feels better early in the course of therapy. Inform that skipping doses or not completing the full course of therapy may decrease effectiveness of treatment and increase bacterial resistance.

Administration: Oral route. May be taken with or without food. Take with adequate amounts of fluids. **Storage:** 20-25°C (68-77°F). Protect from light, moisture, and excessive heat.

DYRENIUM   RX
triamterene (WellSpring)

> Abnormal elevation of serum K+ levels (≥5.5mEq/L) can occur with all K+-sparing agents, including triamterene. Hyperkalemia is more likely to occur with renal impairment and diabetes (even without evidence of renal impairment), and in the elderly, or severely ill. Monitor serum K+ at frequent intervals.

THERAPEUTIC CLASS: K+-sparing diuretic

INDICATIONS: Treatment of edema associated with congestive heart failure (CHF), liver cirrhosis, and nephrotic syndrome. Treatment of steroid induced edema, idiopathic edema, and edema due to secondary hyperaldosteronism.

DOSAGE: *Adults:* Initial: 100mg bid pc. Max: 300mg/day. Titrate dose to the needs of the individual patient.

HOW SUPPLIED: Cap: 50mg, 100mg

CONTRAINDICATIONS: Anuria, severe or progressive kidney disease or dysfunction (except with nephrosis), severe hepatic disease, hyperkalemia, K⁺ supplements, K⁺ salts or K⁺-containing salt substitutes, K⁺-sparing agents (eg, spironolactone, amiloride).

WARNINGS/PRECAUTIONS: Check ECG if hyperkalemia occurs. Isolated reports of hypersensitivity reactions; monitor for possible occurrence of blood dyscrasias, liver damage, or other idiosyncratic reactions. In cirrhotics with splenomegaly, may contribute to megaloblastosis in cases where folic stores have been depleted; perform periodic blood studies and observe for exacerbation of liver disease. Monitor BUN periodically. Caution with gouty arthritis; may elevate uric acid levels. May aggravate or cause electrolyte imbalances in CHF, renal disease, or cirrhosis. Caution with history of renal stones.

ADVERSE REACTIONS: Hypersensitivity reactions, hyper- or hypokalemia, azotemia, renal stones, jaundice, thrombocytopenia, megaloblastic anemia, N/V, diarrhea, weakness, dizziness.

INTERACTIONS: See Contraindications. Increased risk of hyperkalemia with ACE inhibitors. Indomethacin may cause renal failure; caution with NSAIDs. Risk of lithium toxicity. Hyperkalemia may occur when used concomitantly with blood from blood bank, low-salt milk, or K⁺-containing medications (eg, parenteral penicillin G potassium). May cause hyperglycemia; adjust antidiabetic agents. Chlorpropamide may increase risk of severe hyponatremia. May potentiate nondepolarizing muscle relaxants, antihypertensives, other diuretics, preanesthetics, and anesthetics.

PREGNANCY: Category C, not for use in nursing.

MECHANISM OF ACTION: K⁺-sparing diuretic; inhibits reabsorption of Na⁺ ions in exchange for K⁺ and H⁺ ions at segment of distal tubule under control of adrenal mineralocorticoids.

PHARMACOKINETICS: Absorption: Rapid; C_{max}=30ng/mL, T_{max}=3 hrs. **Distribution:** Plasma protein binding (67%); crosses placental barrier. **Metabolism:** Hydroxytriamterene (metabolite). **Elimination:** Urine (21%).

NURSING CONSIDERATIONS

Assessment: Assess for anuria, CHF, diabetes mellitus, gout, hyperkalemia, history of kidney stones, liver/renal impairment, pregnancy/nursing status, and for possible drug interactions.

Monitoring: Monitor for signs/symptoms of electrolyte imbalance, exacerbation of gout, hypersensitivity reactions (eg, blood dyscrasias, liver damage), and for liver/renal dysfunction. Monitor for signs/symptoms of hyperkalemia and perform ECG if suspected. Monitor BUN, serum K⁺ levels, and CBC periodically.

Patient Counseling: Advise to take pc to avoid stomach upset. Inform that if single dose is prescribed, it may be preferable to take in am to minimize frequency of urination during nighttime sleep. Instruct not to take more than prescribed dose at next dosing interval if dose missed. Seek medical attention if symptoms of hyperkalemia, electrolyte imbalance, or hypersensitivity reactions occur.

Administration: Oral route. **Storage:** 25°C (77°F); excursions permitted to 15-30°C (59-86°F). Dispense in tight, light-resistant container.

EDARBI   RX
azilsartan medoxomil (Takeda)

D/C when pregnancy is detected. Drugs that act directly on the renin-angiotensin system (RAS) can cause injury/death to the developing fetus.

THERAPEUTIC CLASS: Angiotensin II receptor antagonist

INDICATIONS: Treatment of HTN alone or in combination with other antihypertensives.

DOSAGE: *Adults:* Usual: 80mg qd. With High Dose Diuretics: Initial: 40mg qd. May add other antihypertensives if BP is not controlled with monotherapy.

HOW SUPPLIED: Tab: 40mg, 80mg

CONTRAINDICATIONS: Coadministration with aliskiren in patients with diabetes.

WARNINGS/PRECAUTIONS: Symptomatic hypotension may occur in patients with an activated RAS (eg, volume- and/or salt-depleted patients, such as those receiving high doses of diuretics); correct this condition prior to therapy or start treatment at 40mg. Changes in renal function may occur. Oliguria or progressive azotemia and (rarely) acute renal failure and death may occur in patients whose renal function is dependent on the RAS (eg, severe congestive heart failure [CHF], renal artery stenosis, volume depletion). May increase SrCr or BUN in patients with renal artery stenosis.

ADVERSE REACTIONS: Dizziness, postural dizziness, diarrhea, nausea, asthenia, fatigue, muscle spasm, cough.

INTERACTIONS: See Contraindications. Dual blockade of the RAS is associated with increased risks of hypotension, hyperkalemia, and changes in renal function (including acute renal failure); closely monitor BP, renal function, and electrolytes with concomitant agents that also affect the RAS. Avoid with aliskiren in patients with renal impairment (GFR <60mL/min). May deteriorate renal function and attenuate antihypertensive effect with NSAIDs, including selective COX-2 inhibitors; monitor renal function periodically. Increases in SrCr may be larger with chlorthalidone or HCTZ.

PREGNANCY: Category D, not for use in nursing.

MECHANISM OF ACTION: Angiotensin II receptor antagonist; blocks the vasoconstrictor and aldosterone-secreting effects of angiotensin II by selectively blocking the binding of angiotensin II to AT_1 receptor in many tissues, such as vascular smooth muscle and adrenal glands.

PHARMACOKINETICS: Absorption: Absolute bioavailability (60%); T_{max}=1.5-3 hrs. **Distribution:** V_d=16L; plasma protein binding (>99%). **Metabolism:** Converted to azilsartan (active metabolite) in GI tract via hydrolysis, then in the liver via CYP2C9 by O-dealkylation and decarboxylation. **Elimination:** Urine (42%; 15% unchanged), feces (55%); $T_{1/2}$=11 hrs.

NURSING CONSIDERATIONS

Assessment: Assess for volume/salt depletion, renal impairment, CHF, renal artery stenosis, diabetes, pregnancy/nursing status, and possible drug interactions.

Monitoring: Monitor for signs/symptoms of hypotension, renal dysfunction, and other adverse reactions. Monitor BP.

Patient Counseling: Inform of pregnancy risks. Instruct to notify physician if pregnant or planning to become pregnant. Advise to seek medical attention if symptoms of hypotension or other adverse events occur.

Administration: Oral route. Take with or without food. **Storage:** 25°C (77°F); excursions permitted to 15-30°C (59-86°F). Protect from moisture and light.

EDARBYCLOR   RX
azilsartan medoxomil - chlorthalidone (Takeda)

D/C when pregnancy is detected. Drugs that act directly on the renin-angiotensin system (RAS) can cause injury/death to the developing fetus.

THERAPEUTIC CLASS: Angiotensin II receptor antagonist/thiazide diuretic

INDICATIONS: Treatment of HTN. May be used in patients whose BP is not adequately controlled on monotherapy. May also be used as initial therapy in patients likely to need multiple drugs to achieve BP goals.

DOSAGE: *Adults:* Initial: 40mg-12.5mg qd. Titrate: May increase to 40mg-25mg after 2-4 weeks PRN to achieve BP goals. Max: 40mg-25mg. Add-On Therapy: Use if not adequately controlled on ARBs or diuretic monotherapy. Replacement Therapy: May receive the corresponding dose of the titrated individual components. With Dose-Limiting Adverse Reaction on Chlorthalidone: Initially give with a lower dose of chlorthalidone.

HOW SUPPLIED: Tab: (Azilsartan-Chlorthalidone) 40mg-12.5mg, 40mg-25mg

CONTRAINDICATIONS: Anuria. Coadministration with aliskiren in patients with diabetes.

WARNINGS/PRECAUTIONS: Symptomatic hypotension may occur in patients with activated RAS (eg, volume- and/or salt-depleted patients); correct volume prior to therapy, particularly with renal impairment or if being treated with high doses of diuretics. Monitor for worsening of renal function in patients with renal impairment; withhold or d/c therapy if progressive renal impairment becomes evident. Azilsartan: Changes in renal function may occur. Oliguria and/or progressive azotemia and (rarely) acute renal failure and/or death may occur in patients whose renal function is dependent on the RAS (eg, severe congestive heart failure [CHF]). May increase BUN or SrCr in patients with renal artery stenosis. Chlorthalidone: May cause fetal/neonatal jaundice and thrombocytopenia. May precipitate azotemia with renal disease. May cause hypokalemia, hyperuricemia, and/or precipitate frank gout. May precipitate hepatic coma in patients with hepatic dysfunction or progressive liver disease.

ADVERSE REACTIONS: Dizziness, fatigue, hypotension, syncope, SrCr elevation.

INTERACTIONS: See Contraindications. May increase risk of symptomatic hypotension with high-dose diuretics. Azilsartan: Dual blockade of the RAS is associated with increased risks of hypotension, hyperkalemia, and changes in renal function (including acute renal failure); closely monitor BP, renal function, and electrolytes with concomitant agents that affect the RAS. Avoid with aliskiren in patients with renal impairment (GFR <60mL/min). May result in renal function deterioration or attenuate antihypertensive effects with NSAIDs, including selective COX-2 inhibitors. Chlorthalidone: May reduce lithium renal clearance and increase risk of lithium toxicity; monitor lithium levels. Coadministration with digitalis may exacerbate the adverse effect of hypokalemia.

PREGNANCY: Category D, not for use in nursing.

MECHANISM OF ACTION: Azilsartan: Angiotensin II receptor antagonist; blocks vasoconstrictor and aldosterone-secreting effects of angiotensin II on cardiac, vascular smooth muscle, adrenal, and renal cells by selectively blocking binding of angiotensin II to AT_1 receptor. Chlorthalidone: Thiazide-like diuretic; has not been established. Produces diuresis with increased excretion of Na^+ and Cl^- at the cortical diluting segment of the ascending limb of Henle's loop of the nephron.

PHARMACOKINETICS: Absorption: Azilsartan: Absolute bioavailability (60%), T_{max}=1.5-3 hrs. Chlorthalidone: T_{max}=1 hr. **Distribution:** Azilsartan: V_d=16L; plasma protein binding (>99%). Chlorthalidone: Plasma protein binding (75%); crosses the placenta; found in breast milk. **Metabolism:** Azilsartan: Via CYP2C9; O-dealkylation, decarboxylation; azilsartan (active metabolite), M-II (major metabolite), M-I (minor metabolite). **Elimination:** Azilsartan: Urine (42%, 15% as azilsartan), feces (55%); $T_{1/2}$=11-12 hrs. Chlorthalidone: Kidney; $T_{1/2}$=45 hrs.

NURSING CONSIDERATIONS

Assessment: Assess for anuria, volume/salt depletion, CHF, renal/hepatic function, renal artery stenosis, pregnancy/nursing status, and possible drug interactions. Obtain baseline BP.

Monitoring: Monitor for signs/symptoms of hypotension, oliguria, progressive azotemia, hypokalemia, hyperuricemia, precipitation of frank gout, and other adverse reactions. Monitor BP, serum electrolytes (eg, K^+), and hepatic/renal function.

Patient Counseling: Inform of the consequences of exposure during pregnancy in females of childbearing potential and of treatment options in women planning to become pregnant. Instruct to report pregnancy to the physician as soon as possible. Inform that if a dose is missed, take it later in the same day; do not double the dose on the following day. Instruct to report gout symptoms and occurrence of lightheadedness; advise to d/c and consult physician if syncope occurs. Inform that dehydration from excessive perspiration, vomiting, and diarrhea may lead to an excessive fall in BP; advise to consult physician if these occur. Advise patients with renal impairment to receive periodic blood tests while on therapy.

Administration: Oral route. Take with or without food. **Storage:** 25°C (77°F); excursions permitted to 15-30°C (59-86°F). Protect from moisture and light.

EDLUAR CIV
zolpidem tartrate (Meda)

THERAPEUTIC CLASS: Imidazopyridine hypnotic

INDICATIONS: Short-term treatment of insomnia, characterized by difficulties with sleep initiation.

DOSAGE: *Adults:* Individualize dose. 10mg SL qhs. Max: 10mg/day. Elderly/Debilitated Patients: 5mg SL qhs. Concomitant Use with CNS-Depressant Drugs: Require dose adjustment.

HOW SUPPLIED: Tab, SL: 5mg, 10mg

WARNINGS/PRECAUTIONS: Evaluate for primary psychiatric and/or medical illness if insomnia fails to remit after 7-10 days of treatment. Severe anaphylactic and anaphylactoid reactions reported; do not rechallenge if patient develops reactions. Visual/auditory hallucinations, complex behavior (eg, sleep-driving), abnormal thinking and behavior changes reported. Worsening of depression, including suicidal thoughts and actions have been reported in depressed patients. May impair mental/physical abilities. Caution with conditions that could affect metabolism or hemodynamic responses, sleep apnea, myasthenia gravis, and worsening depression. Signs and symptoms of withdrawal reported with abrupt discontinuation of sedative/hypnotics. Monitor elderly and debilitated patients for impaired motor and/or cognitive performance.

ADVERSE REACTIONS: Drowsiness, dizziness, diarrhea, headache, drugged feeling, dry mouth, back pain, allergy, sinusitis, pharyngitis.

INTERACTIONS: CNS-active drugs may potentially enhance effects. Additive effects on psychomotor performance with alcohol/chlorpromazine. Decreased alertness observed with imipramine/chlorpromazine. Ketoconazole may enhance sedative effects. May decrease effects with rifampin.

PREGNANCY: Category C, caution in nursing.

MECHANISM OF ACTION: Imidazopyridine, nonbenzodiazepine hypnotic; binds to GABA-BZ receptor complex at the α_1/α_5 subunits.

PHARMACOKINETICS: Absorption: Rapid; C_{max}=106ng/mL; T_{max}=82 min. **Distribution:** Plasma protein binding (92.5%). **Elimination:** Renal; (5mg) $T_{1/2}$=2.85 hrs, (10mg) $T_{1/2}$=2.65 hrs.

NURSING CONSIDERATIONS

Assessment: Assess for primary psychiatric and/or medical illness, preexisting respiratory impairment (eg, sleep apnea syndrome), myasthenia gravis, hypersensitivity reactions, hepatic impairment, history of alcohol, pregnancy/nursing status, and possible drug interactions.

Monitoring: Monitor for anaphylactic/anaphylactoid reactions, abnormal thinking, behavioral changes, complex behavior (eg, sleep-driving), hepatic impairment, and those on long-term treatment for drug abuse/dependence.

Patient Counseling: Instruct not to swallow or take with water. Inform that tab should be placed under the tongue. Advise that tab should not be taken with or immediately after a meal. Inform to take just before bedtime. Advise not to take with alcohol. Caution against hazardous tasks (eg, driving/operating machinery). Counsel about risks/benefits of use. Advise to seek medical attention if severe anaphylactic and anaphylactoid reactions occur. Advise to notify physician of all concomitant medications and any episodes of sleep-driving or complex behaviors.

Administration: Oral route. Tab should be placed under the tongue. **Storage:** 20-25°C (68-77°F). Protect from light and moisture.

EDURANT
rilpivirine (Janssen)

RX

THERAPEUTIC CLASS: Non-nucleoside reverse transcriptase inhibitor

INDICATIONS: Treatment of HIV-1 infection in combination with other antiretrovirals, in antiretroviral treatment-naive adults with HIV-1 RNA ≤100,000 copies/mL at the start of therapy.

DOSAGE: *Adults:* Usual: 1 tab qd with a meal.

HOW SUPPLIED: Tab: 25mg

CONTRAINDICATIONS: Concomitant use with carbamazepine, oxcarbazepine, phenobarbital, phenytoin, rifabutin, rifampin, rifapentine, proton pump inhibitors (eg, esomeprazole, lansoprazole, omeprazole, pantoprazole, rabeprazole), systemic dexamethasone (more than a single dose), and St. John's wort.

WARNINGS/PRECAUTIONS: Not recommended for patients <18 yrs of age. Depressive disorders reported; immediate medical evaluation is recommended if severe depressive symptoms occur. Hepatotoxicity reported; monitor liver enzymes before and during treatment with underlying hepatic disease and marked transaminase elevations; consider monitoring in patients without preexisting hepatic dysfunction/risk factors. Immune reconstitution syndrome, redistribution/accumulation of body fat, and autoimmune disorders (eg, Graves' disease, polymyositis, Guillain-Barre syndrome) in the setting of immune reconstitution reported. Caution with severe renal impairment or end-stage renal disease; monitor for adverse effects. Caution in elderly.

ADVERSE REACTIONS: Lab abnormalities (increased SrCr, AST/ALT, total bilirubin, total cholesterol, LDL), depressive disorders, insomnia, headache, rash.

INTERACTIONS: See Contraindications. Coadministration with CYP3A inducers or drugs that increase gastric pH may result in decreased plasma concentrations and loss of virologic response and possible resistance to rilpivirine. Not recommended with delavirdine and other non-nucleoside reverse transcriptase inhibitors. Concomitant didanosine should be given on an empty stomach and at least 2 hrs before or at least 4 hrs after dosing. Darunavir/ritonavir, lopinavir/ritonavir, unboosted protease inhibitors (PIs) or other boosted PIs (with ritonavir), may increase levels. Monitor for breakthrough fungal infections with azole antifungals. Increased levels with clarithromycin, erythromycin, or telithromycin; consider alternatives (eg, azithromycin) when possible. Administer antacids at least 2 hrs before or at least 4 hrs after dosing. Administer H$_2$-receptor antagonists at least 12 hrs before or at least 4 hrs after dosing. Clinical monitoring recommended as methadone maintenance therapy may need to be adjusted in some patients. Caution with drugs that have a known risk of torsades de pointes. Increased levels with CYP3A inhibitors.

PREGNANCY: Category B, not for use in nursing.

MECHANISM OF ACTION: Non-nucleoside reverse transcriptase inhibitor; inhibits HIV-1 replication by noncompetitive inhibition of HIV-1 reverse transcriptase.

PHARMACOKINETICS: Absorption: T_{max}=4-5 hrs. **Distribution:** Plasma protein binding (99.7%). **Metabolism:** Liver via CYP3A oxidation. **Elimination:** Feces (85%, 25% unchanged), urine (6.1%, <1% unchanged); $T_{1/2}$=50 hrs.

NURSING CONSIDERATIONS

Assessment: Assess for severe renal impairment or end-stage renal disease, hepatitis B or C, marked transaminase elevation, pregnancy/nursing status, and possible drug interactions.

Monitoring: Monitor for depressive disorders, immune reconstitution syndrome (eg, opportunistic infections), autoimmune disorders, fat redistribution/accumulation, hepatic events, and other adverse reactions.

Patient Counseling: Inform that product is not a cure for HIV infection; advise that continuous therapy is necessary to control HIV infection and decrease HIV-related illnesses. Advise to practice safer sex and to use latex or polyurethane condoms. Instruct never to reuse or share needles. Inform mothers to avoid nursing to reduce risk of transmission to their baby. Advise to take medication ud. Advise not to alter the dose or d/c therapy without consulting physician. If a dose is missed within 12 hrs of the time it is usually taken, instruct to take as soon as possible with a meal and then to take the next dose at the regular scheduled time. If dose is missed by >12 hrs of the time it is usually taken, instruct not to take the missed dose, but resume the usual dosing schedule. Advise to report to physician the use of any other prescription/nonprescription or herbal products (eg, St. John's wort). Instruct to seek medical evaluation if depressive symptoms are experienced. Inform that hepatotoxicity has been reported and redistribution or accumulation of body fat may occur.

Administration: Oral route. Take with food. **Storage:** 25°C (77°F); excursions permitted to 15-30°C (59-86°F). Protect from light.

EFFEXOR XR RX
venlafaxine HCl (Wyeth)

> Antidepressants increased the risk of suicidal thinking and behavior (suicidality) in children, adolescents, and young adults in short-term studies of major depressive disorder (MDD) and other psychiatric disorders. Monitor and observe closely for clinical worsening, suicidality, or unusual changes in behavior. Not approved for use in pediatric patients.

THERAPEUTIC CLASS: Serotonin and norepinephrine reuptake inhibitor

INDICATIONS: Treatment of MDD, generalized anxiety disorder (GAD), social anxiety disorder (SAD), and panic disorder (PD).

DOSAGE: *Adults:* MDD/GAD: Initial: 75mg qd, or 37.5mg qd for 4-7 days and then increase to 75mg qd. Titrate: May increase by increments of up to 75mg/day at ≥4-day intervals. Max: 225mg/day. PD: Initial: 37.5mg qd for 7 days. Titrate: May increase by increments of up to 75mg/day at ≥7-day intervals. Max: 225mg/day. SAD: 75mg/day. Switching from Effexor Immediate-Release Tab: Give the nearest equivalent dose (mg/day) qd. Individual dose adjustments may be necessary. Hepatic Impairment (Mild-Moderate)/Hemodialysis: Individualize dose. Reduce total daily dose by 50%. Renal Impairment: Individualize dose. Reduce total daily dose by 25-50%. Switching to/from an MAOI for Psychiatric Disorders: Allow at least 14 days between discontinuation of an MAOI and initiation of treatment, and allow at least 7 days between discontinuation of treatment and initiation of an MAOI. Use with Other MAOIs (eg, Linezolid or IV Methylene Blue): Refer to PI.

HOW SUPPLIED: Cap, Extended-Release: 37.5mg, 75mg, 150mg

CONTRAINDICATIONS: Use of an MAOI for psychiatric disorders either concomitantly or within 7 days of stopping treatment. Treatment within 14 days of stopping an MAOI for psychiatric disorders. Starting treatment in patients being treated with other MAOIs (eg, linezolid, IV methylene blue).

WARNINGS/PRECAUTIONS: Not approved for the treatment of bipolar depression. Avoid abrupt discontinuation; gradually reduce dose and monitor for withdrawal symptoms. Increased risk of bone fractures reported; mechanism leading to this risk is not fully understood. Serotonin syndrome reported; d/c immediately and initiate supportive symptomatic treatment. May cause sustained HTN; consider dose reduction or discontinuation. Mydriasis reported; monitor patients with raised intraocular pressure (IOP) or those at risk of angle-closure glaucoma. Treatment-emergent nervousness, insomnia, weight loss, anorexia, and activation of mania/hypomania reported. Hyponatremia may occur; caution in elderly and volume-depleted patients. Consider discontinuation in patients with symptomatic hyponatremia and institute appropriate medical intervention. May increase the risk of bleeding events. Elevation of cholesterol levels reported; consider measurement of serum cholesterol levels during long-term treatment. Caution with history of mania or seizures, conditions affecting hemodynamic responses or metabolism, conditions that may be compromised by increases in HR (eg, hyperthyroidism, heart failure, recent myocardial infarction [MI]), renal/hepatic impairment, and in elderly. D/C if seizures occur. Cases of QT prolongation, torsades de pointes (TdP), ventricular tachycardia and sudden death reported; caution with risk factors for QT prolongation. Interstitial lung disease and eosinophilic pneumonia rarely reported; consider discontinuation if symptoms occur. False (+) urine immunoassay screening tests for phencyclidine and amphetamines reported.

ADVERSE REACTIONS: Asthenia, sweating, headache, N/V, constipation, anorexia, dry mouth, dizziness, insomnia, nervousness, somnolence, abnormal ejaculation/orgasm, abnormal dreams, pharyngitis.

INTERACTIONS: See Contraindications. May cause serotonin syndrome with other serotonergic drugs (eg, triptans, TCAs, fentanyl, lithium, tramadol, tryptophan, buspirone, St. John's wort) and with drugs that impair metabolism of serotonin; d/c immediately if this occurs. Increased risk of bleeding with aspirin (ASA), NSAIDs, warfarin, and other anticoagulants or other drugs known to affect platelet function. Caution with cimetidine in elderly, patients with HTN, and hepatic dysfunction. May decrease clearance of haloperidol. May increase levels of metoprolol, risperidone, and desipramine. Increased levels with cimetidine and ketoconazole. May decrease levels of indinavir. May inhibit metabolism of CYP2D6 substrates. Caution with metoprolol, CYP3A4 inhibitors, and CNS-active drugs. Coadministration with weight-loss agents not recommended. Increased risk of hyponatremia with diuretics. Increased risk of QT prolongation and/or ventricular arrhythmias (eg, TdP) with other drugs that prolong the QT interval (eg, some antipsychotics and antibiotics).

PREGNANCY: Category C, not for use in nursing.

MECHANISM OF ACTION: SNRI; believed to be associated with its potentiation of neurotransmitter activity in CNS by inhibiting neuronal serotonin and norepinephrine reuptake.

PHARMACOKINETICS: Absorption: Venlafaxine: Well-absorbed. Absolute bioavailability (45%), C_{max}=150ng/mL, T_{max}=5.5 hrs. O-desmethylvenlafaxine (ODV) (metabolite): C_{max}=260ng/mL, T_{max}=9 hrs. **Distribution:** Venlafaxine: V_d=7.5L/kg; plasma protein binding (27%); found in breast milk. ODV: V_d=5.7L/kg; plasma protein binding (30%); found in breast milk. **Metabolism:** Extensive. Hepatic; ODV (major active metabolite). **Elimination:** Urine (5% unchanged, 29% unconjugated ODV, 26% conjugated ODV, 27% minor inactive metabolites); Venlafaxine: $T_{1/2}$=5 hrs. ODV: $T_{1/2}$=11 hrs.

NURSING CONSIDERATIONS

Assessment: Assess for bipolar disorder risk and history of mania, seizures, MI, unstable heart disease, HTN, hyperthyroidism, glaucoma, increased IOP, drug abuse, and attempted suicide. Assess for risk factors for QT prolongation, disease/condition that alters metabolism/hemodynamic response, volume depletion, hepatic/renal impairment, drug hypersensitivity, pregnancy/nursing status, and possible drug interactions. Obtain a detailed psychiatric history.

Monitoring: Monitor HR, BP, hepatic/renal function, height and weight, and ECG changes. Monitor for signs/symptoms of clinical worsening, suicidality, unusual behavior, serotonin syndrome, mydriasis, sustained HTN, lung disease, abnormal bleeding, hyponatremia, seizures, QT prolongation, bone fractures, and other adverse reactions. Measure serum cholesterol levels during long-term treatment. If discontinued abruptly, monitor for withdrawal symptoms (eg, dysphoric mood, confusion, agitation). Periodically reevaluate long-term usefulness of therapy.

Patient Counseling: Inform about the risks and benefits of therapy. Instruct to read the Medication Guide. Advise to look for emergence of suicidality, especially early during treatment and when the dose is adjusted up or down. Caution against operating hazardous machinery (including automobiles) until reasonably certain that therapy does not adversely affect ability to engage in such activities. Instruct to notify physician if taking or planning to take any prescription or OTC drugs, including herbal preparations and nutritional supplements. Advise to avoid alcohol. Caution about the risk of serotonin syndrome. Inform that concomitant use with ASA, NSAIDs, warfarin, or other drugs that affect coagulation may increase the risk of bleeding. Advise to notify physician if allergic phenomena (eg, rash, hives, swelling, difficulty breathing) develops, if pregnant, intending to become pregnant, or if breastfeeding.

Administration: Oral route. Take with food at same time each day, either in am or pm. Swallow whole with fluid and do not divide, crush, chew, or place in water. May administer by sprinkling contents of cap on spoonful of applesauce; swallow without chewing and follow with glass of water. **Storage:** 20-25°C (68-77°F).

EFFIENT   RX
prasugrel (Daiichi Sankyo/Eli Lilly)

May cause significant, sometimes fatal, bleeding; risk factors include <60kg body weight, propensity to bleed, and concomitant use of medications that increase risk of bleeding (eg, warfarin, heparin, fibrinolytic therapy, chronic use of NSAIDs). Do not use in patients with active pathological bleeding or a history of transient ischemic attack (TIA) or stroke. Not recommended in patients ≥75 yrs of age, due to increased risk of fatal and intracranial bleeding and uncertain benefit, except in high-risk situations (diabetes or history of prior myocardial infarction [MI]) where the effect appears to be greater and use may be considered. Do not start in patients likely to undergo urgent coronary artery bypass graft surgery (CABG); d/c at least 7 days prior to any surgery, when possible. Suspect bleeding in any patient who is hypotensive and has recently undergone coronary angiography, percutaneous coronary intervention (PCI), CABG, or other surgical procedures. If possible, manage bleeding without discontinuing the drug. Discontinuing, particularly in the 1st few weeks after acute coronary syndrome (ACS), increases the risk of subsequent cardiovascular (CV) events.

THERAPEUTIC CLASS: Platelet aggregation inhibitor

INDICATIONS: To reduce the rate of thrombotic CV events (including stent thrombosis) in patients with ACS who are to be managed with PCI as follows: patients with unstable angina or non-ST-elevation MI or patients with ST-elevation MI when managed with primary or delayed PCI.

DOSAGE: *Adults:* LD: 60mg as a single dose. Maint: 10mg qd. <60kg: Consider lowering the maintenance dose to 5mg qd. Take with aspirin (75-325mg/day).

HOW SUPPLIED: Tab: 5mg, 10mg

CONTRAINDICATIONS: Active pathological bleeding (eg, peptic ulcer, intracranial hemorrhage), history of prior TIA or stroke.

WARNINGS/PRECAUTIONS: Withholding a dose will not be useful in managing a bleeding event or the risk of bleeding associated with an invasive procedure. D/C for active bleeding, elective surgery, stroke, or TIA. Avoid therapy lapses; if temporary discontinuation is needed because of an adverse event(s), restart as soon as possible. Thrombotic thrombocytopenic purpura (TTP) reported; may occur after a brief exposure (<2 weeks) and requires urgent treatment (eg, plasmapheresis). Hypersensitivity including angioedema reported. Risk for bleeding with severe hepatic impairment or moderate to severe renal impairment.

ADVERSE REACTIONS: Bleeding, HTN, hypercholesterolemia/hyperlipidemia, headache, back pain, dyspnea, nausea, dizziness, cough, hypotension, fatigue, noncardiac chest pain.

INTERACTIONS: See Boxed Warning.

PREGNANCY: Category B, caution in nursing.

MECHANISM OF ACTION: Platelet aggregation inhibitor (thienopyridine class); inhibits platelet activation and aggregation through irreversible binding of its active metabolite to the $P2Y_{12}$ class of ADP receptors on platelets.

PHARMACOKINETICS: Absorption: Rapid. T_{max}=30 min (active metabolite). **Distribution:** (Active metabolite) Plasma protein binding (98%, albumin); V_d=44-68L (active metabolite). **Metabolism:** Hydrolysis in the intestine; converted to active metabolite via CYP3A4/2B6 (primary) and CYP2C9/2C19; then S-methylation or conjugation with cysteine. **Elimination:** Urine (68%, inactive metabolites), feces (27%, inactive metabolites); $T_{1/2}$=7 hrs (active metabolite).

NURSING CONSIDERATIONS

Assessment: Assess for active pathological bleeding, history of prior TIA or stroke, other risk factors for bleeding, hypersensitivity, pregnancy/nursing status, and possible drug interactions. Assess likelihood of undergoing urgent CABG.

Monitoring: Monitor for signs/symptoms of bleeding, TTP, hypersensitivity, stroke, TIA, and other adverse reactions.

Patient Counseling: Inform about the benefits and risks of treatment. Instruct to take exactly as prescribed and not to d/c without consulting the prescribing physician. Inform that patient may bruise and bleed more easily and that bleeding will take longer than usual to stop. Advise to report to physician any unanticipated, prolonged, or excessive bleeding, or blood in stool/urine. Inform that TTP, a rare but serious condition, has been reported; instruct to seek prompt medical attention if experiencing unexplained fever, weakness, extreme skin paleness, purple skin patches, yellowing of skin/eyes, or neurological changes. Inform that hypersensitivity reactions may occur. Instruct to notify physicians and dentists about therapy before scheduling any invasive procedure.

Administration: Oral route. May be administered with or without food. Do not break the tab.
Storage: 25°C (77°F); excursions permitted to 15-30°C (59-86°F).

EGRIFTA   RX
tesamorelin (EMD Serono)

THERAPEUTIC CLASS: Growth hormone-releasing factor

INDICATIONS: Reduction of excess abdominal fat in HIV-infected patients with lipodystrophy.

DOSAGE: *Adults:* 2mg SQ in the abdomen qd.

HOW SUPPLIED: Inj: 1mg

CONTRAINDICATIONS: Pregnancy, newly diagnosed or recurrent active malignancy, and disruption of hypothalamic-pituitary axis (HPA) due to hypophysectomy, hypopituitarism, pituitary tumor/surgery, head irradiation or head trauma.

WARNINGS/PRECAUTIONS: Carefully consider continuation of treatment in patients who do not show clear efficacy response. Not indicated for weight loss management. Caution with history of non-malignant neoplasms or treated and stable malignancies. Increases serum insulin growth factor-I (IGF-I); monitor IGF-I levels closely and consider discontinuation with persistent elevations. Fluid retention (eg, edema, arthralgia, carpal tunnel syndrome) may occur. May cause glucose intolerance and diabetes; evaluate glucose status prior to therapy then monitor periodically. May develop or worsen retinopathy in patients with diabetes. Hypersensitivity reactions may occur; d/c treatment immediately when reactions suspected. Rotate site of inj to different areas of abdomen to reduce inj-site reactions (eg, erythema, pruritus, pain, irritation, bruising). Consider discontinuation in critically ill patients; increased mortality reported in patients with acute critical illness after treatment with growth hormone (GH).

ADVERSE REACTIONS: Arthralgia, pain in extremity, myalgia, inj-site reactions (eg, erythema, pruritus, pain), peripheral edema, paresthesia, hypoesthesia, nausea, rash.

INTERACTIONS: GH may modulate CYP450 mediated antipyrine clearance; caution with CYP450 substrates (eg, corticosteroids, sex steroids, anticonvulsants, cyclosporine). May require an increase in maintenance or stress doses of glucocorticoids particularly in patients taking cortisone acetate and prednisone. Decreased absorption of simvastatin, simvastatin acid, and ritonavir.

PREGNANCY: Category X, not for use in nursing.

MECHANISM OF ACTION: Human growth hormone-releasing factor synthetic analog; acts on pituitary somatotroph cells to stimulate the synthesis and pulsatile release of endogenous GH, which is both anabolic and lipolytic.

PHARMACOKINETICS: Absorption: Absolute bioavailability (<4%, healthy); AUC=634.6pg•h/mL (healthy), 852.8pg•h/mL (HIV-infected); C_{max}=2874.6pg/mL (healthy), 2822.3pg/mL (HIV-infected); T_{max}=0.15 hr (healthy, HIV infected). **Distribution:** V_d=9.4L/kg (healthy), 10.5L/kg (HIV-infected). **Elimination:** $T_{1/2}$=26 min (healthy), 38 min (HIV-infected).

NURSING CONSIDERATIONS

Assessment: Assess for active malignancy, hypersensitivity to tesamorelin and/or mannitol, HPA disruption due to hypophysectomy, hypopituitarism, pituitary tumor/surgery, head irradiation or head trauma, history of nonmalignant neoplasms or treated and stable malignancies, glucose status, acute critical illness, pregnancy/nursing status, and possible drug interactions.

Monitoring: Monitor for response, IGF-I levels, HbA1c levels, changes in glucose metabolism, glucose intolerance, diabetes, worsening or development of retinopathy, and hypersensitivity reactions.

Patient Counseling: Advise that treatment may cause transient symptoms consistent with fluid retention (eg, edema, arthralgia, carpal tunnel syndrome) which resolve upon discontinuation. Instruct to seek medical attention and d/c therapy immediately when hypersensitivity reactions occur (eg, rash, urticaria). Advise to rotate the site of inj to different areas of abdomen to reduce incidence of inj-site reactions (eg, erythema, pruritus, pain, irritation, bruising). Counsel not to share syringe with another person, even if the needle is changed. Advise women to d/c treatment if pregnant and not to breastfeed; apprise of the potential hazard to the fetus.

Administration: SQ route. Recommended site is the abdomen. Do not inject into scar tissue, bruises, or the navel. Refer to Instructions For Use leaflet for reconstitution procedures. Reconstituted sol (1mg/mL) should be injected immediately. **Storage:** Unreconstituted: 2-8°C (36-46°F). Diluent/Syringes/Needles: 20-25°C (68-77°F). Protect from light. Keep in the original box until use.

ELIDEL   RX
pimecrolimus (Novartis)

> Rare cases of malignancy (eg, skin and lymphoma) reported with topical calcineurin inhibitors, including pimecrolimus, although causal relationship is not established. Avoid long-term use and application should be limited to areas of involvement with atopic dermatitis. Not indicated for children <2 yrs of age.

THERAPEUTIC CLASS: Macrolactam ascomycin derivative

INDICATIONS: Second-line therapy for the short-term and noncontinuous chronic treatment of mild to moderate atopic dermatitis in nonimmunocompromised patients ≥2 yrs of age who failed to respond adequately to other topical prescription treatments, or when those treatments are not advisable.

DOSAGE: *Adults:* Apply thin layer to the affected skin bid until signs and symptoms resolve. Reevaluate if signs and symptoms persist beyond 6 weeks.
Pediatrics: ≥2 Yrs: Apply thin layer to the affected skin bid until signs and symptoms resolve. Reevaluate if signs and symptoms persist beyond 6 weeks.

HOW SUPPLIED: Cre: 1% [30g, 60g, 100g]

WARNINGS/PRECAUTIONS: Long-term safety, beyond 1 yr of noncontinuous use, has not been established. Avoid with malignant or premalignant skin conditions, Netherton's syndrome, or other skin diseases that may increase the potential for systemic absorption. Avoid in immunocompromised patients. May cause local symptoms, such as skin burning (eg, burning sensation, stinging, soreness) or pruritus and may improve as the lesions of atopic dermatitis resolve. Resolve bacterial or viral infections at treatment sites before starting treatment. Increased risk of varicella zoster virus infection, herpes simplex virus infection, or eczema herpeticum. Skin papilloma/warts reported; consider discontinuation until complete resolution is achieved if skin papillomas worsen or are unresponsive to conventional treatment. Lymphadenopathy reported; monitor to ensure it resolves. D/C if lymphadenopathy of uncertain etiology or acute infectious mononucleosis occurs. Minimize or avoid natural or artificial sunlight exposure during treatment.

ADVERSE REACTIONS: Application-site burning, application-site reaction, upper respiratory tract infection, headache, nasopharyngitis, influenza, abdominal pain, diarrhea, sore throat, hypersensitivity, pyrexia, cough, rhinitis, N/V.

INTERACTIONS: Caution with CYP3A4 inhibitors (eg, erythromycin, itraconazole, ketoconazole, fluconazole, calcium channel blockers, cimetidine) in patients with widespread and/or erythrodermic disease. Skin flushing associated with alcohol use reported. Increased incidence of impetigo, skin infection, superinfection, rhinitis, and urticaria reported with topical corticosteroid administered sequentially.

PREGNANCY: Category C, not for use in nursing.

MECHANISM OF ACTION: Macrolactam ascomycin derivative; not fully established. Suspected to bind with high affinity to macrophilin-12 (FKBP-12) and inhibit the Ca^{2+}-dependent phosphatase, calcineurin. Consequently, this inhibits T-cell activation by blocking the transcription of early cytokines. In particular, pimecrolimus inhibits at nanomolar concentrations interleukin-2 (IL-2) and interferon gamma (Th1-type), and IL-4 and IL-10 (Th2-type) cytokine synthesis in human T cells. In addition, pimecrolimus prevents the release of inflammatory cytokines and mediators from mast cells in vitro after stimulation by antigen/IgE.

PHARMACOKINETICS: Absorption: C_{max}=1.4ng/mL (adults). **Distribution:** Plasma protein binding (99.5%). **Metabolism:** Liver via CYP3A; O-demethylation (metabolites). **Elimination:** Feces (78.4% metabolites, <1% unchanged).

NURSING CONSIDERATIONS

Assessment: Assess for malignant or premalignant skin conditions (eg, cutaneous-cell lymphoma), Netherton's syndrome or other skin diseases, viral or bacterial skin infections, generalized erythroderma, pregnancy/nursing status, and possible drug interactions.

Monitoring: Monitor for infections (eg, varicella virus infection, herpes simplex virus infection, eczema herpeticum), lymphomas, lymphadenopathy, skin malignancies, local symptoms such as skin burning (eg, burning sensation, stinging, soreness) or pruritus, and other adverse reactions.

Patient Counseling: Instruct to use as prescribed. Inform not to use drug continuously for long periods and to use only on areas of skin with eczema. Advise to d/c medication when signs/symptoms of eczema subside (eg, itching, rash, redness). Instruct to contact physician if symptoms get worse, a skin infection develops, if burning on skin lasts >1 week, or if symptoms do not improve after 6 weeks of treatment. Instruct to wash hands and dry skin before applying cre. Instruct not to bathe, shower, or swim after applying cre. Instruct to avoid natural or artificial sunlight exposure while on therapy. Instruct not to cover treated skin area with bandages, dressings, or wraps. Inform that the medication is for external use only; instruct to avoid contact with eyes, nose, mouth, vagina, or rectum (mucous membranes).

Administration: Topical route. **Storage:** 25°C (77°F); excursions permitted to 15-30°C (59-86°F). Do not freeze.

ELIGARD   RX
leuprolide acetate (Sanofi-Aventis)

THERAPEUTIC CLASS: Synthetic gonadotropin-releasing hormone analog

INDICATIONS: Palliative treatment of advanced prostate cancer.

DOSAGE: *Adults:* 7.5mg SQ monthly, 22.5mg SQ every 3 months, 30mg SQ every 4 months, or 45mg SQ every 6 months.

HOW SUPPLIED: Inj: 7.5mg, 22.5mg, 30mg, 45mg

CONTRAINDICATIONS: Women who are or may become pregnant.

WARNINGS/PRECAUTIONS: Transient increase in serum concentrations of testosterone and worsening of symptoms or onset of new signs/symptoms (eg, bone pain, neuropathy, hematuria) during the 1st few weeks of therapy may occur. Cases of ureteral obstruction and/or spinal cord compression reported; institute standard treatment if these complications occur. Closely monitor patients with metastatic vertebral lesions and/or urinary tract obstruction during 1st few weeks of therapy. Suppresses pituitary-gonadal system; may affect results of diagnostic tests of pituitary gonadotropic and gonadal functions conducted during and after therapy. Hyperglycemia and increased risk of developing diabetes, myocardial infarction, sudden cardiac death, and stroke reported.

ADVERSE REACTIONS: Hot flashes/sweats, inj-site reactions (eg, transient burning/stinging, pain, erythema, bruising, pruritus), malaise/fatigue, testicular atrophy, weakness, gynecomastia, myalgia, arthralgia, dizziness, decreased libido, clamminess, night sweats.

PREGNANCY: Category X, not for use in nursing.

MECHANISM OF ACTION: Synthetic gonadotropin-releasing hormone analog; acts as a potent inhibitor of gonadotropin secretion. Following an initial stimulation, chronic administration results in suppression of ovarian and testicular steroidogenesis.

PHARMACOKINETICS: Absorption: Administration of variable doses resulted in different parameters. **Distribution:** (IV bolus dose) V_d=27L; plasma protein binding (43-49%). **Metabolism:** Pentapeptide (M-1) metabolite (major metabolite). **Elimination:** (1mg IV bolus dose) $T_{1/2}$=3 hrs.

NURSING CONSIDERATIONS

Assessment: Assess for hypersensitivity to drug, metastatic vertebral lesions, urinary tract obstructions, and diabetes mellitus. Obtain baseline serum testosterone levels and prostate specific antigen (PSA) levels. Obtain baseline blood glucose and/or HbA1c levels.

Monitoring: Monitor for worsening/occurrence of signs/symptoms of prostate cancer, spinal cord compression, ureteral obstruction, suppression of pituitary-gonadal system, and signs/symptoms suggestive of cardiovascular disease development. Periodically monitor blood glucose, HbA1c, testosterone, and PSA levels.

Patient Counseling: Inform that hot flashes may be experienced. Inform that increased bone pain, difficulty in urinating, and onset or aggravation of weakness or paralysis may be experienced during the 1st few weeks of therapy. Notify physician if new or worsened symptoms develop after beginning treatment. Inform about inj-site related adverse reactions (eg, transient burning/stinging, pain, bruising, redness); notify physician if such reactions do not resolve. Contact physician immediately if an allergic reaction develops.

Administration: SQ route. Inj-site should be varied periodically. Refer to PI for mixing and administration procedures. **Storage:** 2-8°C (35.6-46.4°F). Once mixed, discard if not administered within 30 min.

ELIQUIS   RX
apixaban (Bristol-Myers Squibb)

Discontinuing therapy increases the risk of thrombotic events. Increased rate of stroke reported following discontinuation of therapy in patients with nonvalvular atrial fibrillation (A-fib). If therapy must be discontinued for a reason other than pathological bleeding, consider coverage with another anticoagulant. When neuraxial anesthesia (epidural/spinal anesthesia) or spinal puncture is employed, patients anticoagulated or scheduled to be anticoagulated with apixaban for prevention of thromboembolic complications are at risk of developing an epidural or spinal hematoma, which can result in long-term or permanent paralysis. Increased risk of epidural/spinal hematomas by the use of indwelling epidural catheters for administration of analgesia or by concomitant use of drugs affecting hemostasis (eg, NSAIDs, platelet aggregation inhibitors, or other anticoagulants). The risk also appears to be increased by traumatic or repeated epidural or spinal puncture. Monitor for signs/symptoms of neurologic impairment; urgent treatment is necessary if neurologic compromise is noted. Consider potential benefit vs risk before neuraxial intervention in patients anticoagulated or to be anticoagulated for thromboprophylaxis.

THERAPEUTIC CLASS: Selective factor Xa inhibitor

INDICATIONS: Reduce risk of stroke and systemic embolism in patients with nonvalvular A-fib. Prophylaxis of deep vein thrombosis (DVT), which may lead to pulmonary embolism, in patients who have undergone hip or knee replacement surgery.

DOSAGE: *Adults:* Reduction of Risk of Stroke and Systemic Embolism with Nonvalvular A-fib: Usual: 5mg bid. Prophylaxis of DVT: Usual: 2.5mg bid. Give initial dose 12-24 hrs after surgery. Treatment Duration: Hip Replacement Surgery: 35 days. Knee Replacement Surgery: 12 days. In Nonvalvular A-fib Patients with Any Two of the Following Characteristics: ≥80 Yrs, ≤60kg, or SrCr ≥1.5mg/dL: Usual: 2.5mg bid. Patients Receiving Apixaban 5mg BID with Strong Dual CYP3A4 and P-glycoprotein (P-gp) Inhibitors: Usual: Reduce to 2.5mg bid. If already taking 2.5mg bid, avoid coadministration with strong dual inhibitors of CYP3A4 and P-gp. Elective Surgery/Invasive Procedures: D/C at least 48 hrs prior to elective surgery or invasive procedures with moderate/high risk of unacceptable/clinically significant bleeding, or at least 24 hrs with a low risk of bleeding or where bleeding would be noncritical in location and easily controlled. Bridging anticoagulation during the 24-48 hrs after discontinuing therapy and prior to the intervention is not generally required. Restart therapy after the surgical or other procedures as soon as adequate hemostasis has been established. Switching from/to Warfarin or Anticoagulants Other Than Warfarin: Refer to PI. Nonvalvular A-fib Patients with End-Stage Renal Disease Maintained on Hemodialysis: Usual: 5mg bid. Reduce dose to 2.5mg bid (if patient is ≥80 yrs of age or ≤60kg).

HOW SUPPLIED: Tab: 2.5mg, 5mg

CONTRAINDICATIONS: Active pathological bleeding.

WARNINGS/PRECAUTIONS: Not recommended in patients with severe hepatic impairment or with prosthetic heart valves. May increase the risk of bleeding and cause serious, potentially fatal bleeding; d/c in patients with active pathological hemorrhage. In patients who receive both apixaban and neuraxial anesthesia, removal of indwelling epidural or intrathecal catheters should not be earlier than 24 hrs after the last administration of apixaban; next dose of apixaban should not be administered earlier than 5 hrs after the removal of the catheter. If traumatic spinal/epidural puncture occurs, delay administration of apixaban for 48 hrs.

ADVERSE REACTIONS: Bleeding.

INTERACTIONS: See Boxed Warning and Dosage. CYP3A4 and P-gp inhibitors may increase exposure and increase the risk of bleeding. CYP3A4 and P-gp inducers may decrease exposure and increase the risk of stroke. Avoid with strong dual inhibitors of CYP3A4 and P-gp (eg, ketoconazole, itraconazole, ritonavir, clarithromycin) in patients already taking 2.5mg apixaban bid. Avoid with strong dual inducers of CYP3A4 and P-gp (eg, rifampin, carbamazepine, phenytoin, St. John's wort). Increased risk of bleeding with drugs affecting hemostasis, including aspirin (ASA) and other antiplatelet agents, other anticoagulants, heparin, thrombolytics, SSRIs, SNRIs, NSAIDs, and fibrinolytics.

PREGNANCY: Category B, not for use in nursing.

MECHANISM OF ACTION: Selective factor Xa (FXa) inhibitor; inhibits free and clot-bound FXa, and prothrombinase activity. Has no direct effect on platelet aggregation, but indirectly inhibits platelet aggregation induced by thrombin. By inhibiting FXa, apixaban decreases thrombin generation and thrombus development. Does not require antithrombin III for antithrombotic activity.

PHARMACOKINETICS: Absorption: Absolute bioavailability (50% [doses up to 10mg]); T_{max}=3-4 hrs. **Distribution:** V_d=21L; plasma protein binding (87%). **Metabolism:** O-demethylation, hydroxylation via CYP3A4 (main contributor), CYP1A2, 2C8, 2C9, 2C19, and 2J2 (minor contributors). **Elimination:** Urine and feces (25%, metabolites); $T_{1/2}$=12 hrs.

NURSING CONSIDERATIONS

Assessment: Assess for drug hypersensitivity, active pathological bleeding, prosthetic heart valves, hepatic/renal impairment, pregnancy/nursing status, and possible drug interactions.

Monitoring: Monitor for active pathological hemorrhage and other adverse reactions. Monitor for thrombotic events in patients discontinuing therapy. In patients undergoing neuraxial anesthesia or spinal puncture, monitor for epidural or spinal hematomas and neurological impairment.

Patient Counseling: Instruct not to d/c without consulting physician. Inform that it may take longer than usual for bleeding to stop, and that patient may bruise/bleed more easily. Advise on how to recognize bleeding/symptoms of hypovolemia and of the urgent need to report any unusual bleeding to physician. Instruct to inform physicians and dentists if taking apixaban, and/or any other product known to affect bleeding (eg, nonprescription drugs such as ASA or NSAIDs), before any surgery/medical/dental procedure is scheduled and before any new drug is taken. Advise patients who had neuraxial anesthesia or spinal puncture, and particularly if they are taking concomitant medicinal products affecting hemostasis to watch for signs/symptoms of spinal/epidural hematoma (eg, numbness, weakness of legs, bowel/bladder dysfunction); instruct to contact physician immediately if symptoms occur. Advise to inform physician if pregnant or planning to become pregnant or breastfeeding or intend to breastfeed during treatment. If a dose is missed, instruct to take as soon as possible on the same day and bid administration should be resumed; instruct not to double the dose to make up for a missed dose.

Administration: Oral route. May crush and suspend tab in 60mL D5W and immediately delivered through a NG tube if unable to swallow tab whole. **Storage:** 20-25°C (68-77°F); excursions permitted to 15-30°C (59-86°F).

ELLA   RX
ulipristal acetate (Watson)

THERAPEUTIC CLASS: Emergency contraceptive kit

INDICATIONS: Prevention of pregnancy following unprotected intercourse or a known or suspected contraceptive failure.

DOSAGE: *Adults:* 1 tab as soon as possible within 120 hrs (5 days) after unprotected intercourse or a known or suspected contraceptive failure. Consider repeating the dose if vomiting occurs within 3 hrs of intake.
Pediatrics: Postpubertal: 1 tab as soon as possible within 120 hrs (5 days) after unprotected intercourse or a known or suspected contraceptive failure. Consider repeating the dose if vomiting occurs within 3 hrs of intake.

HOW SUPPLIED: Tab: 30mg

CONTRAINDICATIONS: Known or suspected pregnancy.

WARNINGS/PRECAUTIONS: Not for routine use as a contraceptive. Not indicated for termination of existing pregnancy. Exclude pregnancy prior to prescribing; perform pregnancy test if pregnancy cannot be excluded based on of history and/or physical examination. History of ectopic pregnancy is not a contraindication to use of therapy; however, consider possibility of ectopic pregnancy if lower abdominal pain or pregnancy occurs following use. For occasional use as emergency contraceptive only; should not replace regular method of contraception. Repeated use within the same menstrual cycle is not recommended. Rapid return of fertility may occur following treatment; continue or initiate routine contraception as soon as possible following use. After intake, menses sometimes occur earlier or later than expected by a few days; rule out pregnancy if there is a delay in the onset of expected menses beyond 1 week. Intermenstrual bleeding reported. Does not protect against HIV infection (AIDS) or other sexually transmitted infections.

ADVERSE REACTIONS: Headache, abdominal/upper abdominal pain, nausea, dysmenorrhea, fatigue, dizziness.

INTERACTIONS: Drugs or herbal products that induce enzymes, including CYP3A4 (eg, barbiturates, bosentan, carbamazepine, felbamate, griseofulvin, oxcarbazepine, phenytoin, rifampin, St. John's wort, topiramate), may decrease plasma concentrations and may decrease effectiveness. CYP3A4 inhibitors (eg, itraconazole, ketoconazole) may increase plasma concentrations. May reduce contraceptive action of regular hormonal contraceptive methods. May increase the concentration of P-glycoprotein (P-gp) substrates (eg, dabigatran etexilate, digoxin) due to inhibition of P-gp at clinically relevant concentrations.

PREGNANCY: Category X, not for use in nursing.

MECHANISM OF ACTION: Emergency contraceptive kit; synthetic progesterone agonist/antagonist. Postpones follicular rupture when taken immediately before ovulation. Likely primary mechanism of action is inhibition or delay of ovulation; alterations to endometrium that may affect implantation may also contribute to efficacy.

PHARMACOKINETICS: Absorption: (Healthy, Fasted) C_{max}=176ng/mL, 69ng/mL (monodemethyl-ulipristal acetate); T_{max} (median)=0.9 hr, 1 hr (monodemethyl-ulipristal acetate); AUC_{0-t}=548ng•hr/mL, 240ng•hr/mL (monodemethyl-ulipristal acetate); AUC_{0-inf}=556ng•hr/mL, 246ng•hr/mL (monodemethyl-ulipristal acetate). **Distribution:** Plasma protein binding (>94%). **Metabolism:** CYP3A4; monodemethyl-ulipristal acetate (active metabolite). **Elimination:** $T_{1/2}$=32.4 hrs, 27 hrs (monodemethyl-ulipristal acetate).

NURSING CONSIDERATIONS

Assessment: Assess pregnancy/nursing status and for possible drug interactions.

Monitoring: Monitor for ectopic pregnancy and effect on menstrual cycle. Perform follow-up physical/pelvic examination if in doubt concerning general health or pregnancy status.

Patient Counseling: Instruct to take as soon as possible and not >120 hrs after unprotected intercourse or a known or suspected contraceptive failure. Advise not to take if pregnancy is known or suspected and that drug is not indicated for termination of an existing pregnancy. Advise to contact physician immediately if vomiting occurs within 3 hrs of intake, if period is delayed after taking the drug by >1 week beyond expected date, or if experiencing severe lower abdominal pain 3-5 weeks after use. Advise not to use as routine contraception or repeatedly in the same menstrual cycle. Inform that therapy may reduce contraceptive action of regular hormonal contraceptive methods and to use a reliable barrier method of contraception after using medication, for any subsequent acts of intercourse that occur in that same menstrual cycle. Inform that drug does not protect against HIV infection (AIDS) and other sexually transmitted diseases/infections. Instruct not to use if breastfeeding.

Administration: Oral route. Can be taken at any time during the menstrual cycle, with or without food. **Storage:** 20-25°C (68-77°F). Keep blister in the outer carton to protect from light.

ELOCON   RX
mometasone furoate (Merck)

THERAPEUTIC CLASS: Corticosteroid

INDICATIONS: (Cre, Oint) Relief of inflammatory and pruritic manifestations of corticosteroid-responsive dermatoses in patients ≥2 yrs of age. (Lot) Relief of inflammatory and pruritic manifestations of corticosteroid-responsive dermatoses in patients ≥12 yrs of age.

DOSAGE: *Adults:* (Lot) Apply a few drops to affected skin areas qd and massage lightly until it disappears. (Cre/Oint) Apply a thin film to affected skin areas qd. (Cre/Lot/Oint) D/C therapy when control is achieved. Reassess diagnosis if no improvement seen within 2 weeks.
Pediatrics: (Lot) ≥12 Yrs: Apply a few drops to affected skin areas qd and massage lightly until it disappears. (Cre/Oint) ≥2 Yrs: Apply a thin film to affected skin areas qd. (Cre/Lot/Oint) D/C therapy when control is achieved. Reassess diagnosis if no improvement seen within 2 weeks.

HOW SUPPLIED: Cre: 0.1% [15g, 50g]; Lot: 0.1% [30mL, 60mL]; Oint: 0.1% [15g, 45g]

WARNINGS/PRECAUTIONS: Not for oral, ophthalmic, or intravaginal use. Avoid use on the face, groin, or axillae. Avoid use with occlusive dressings. Systemic absorption may produce reversible hypothalamic pituitary adrenal (HPA) axis suppression with the potential for glucocorticosteroid insufficiency, manifestations of Cushing's syndrome, hyperglycemia, and glucosuria. Periodically evaluate for HPA-axis suppression and, if noted, gradually withdraw drug, reduce frequency of application, or substitute a less potent corticosteroid. Factors predisposing to HPA-axis suppression include use of high-potency steroids, large treatment surface areas, prolonged use, use of occlusive dressings, altered skin barrier, liver failure, and young age. Glucocorticosteroid insufficiency may occur, requiring supplemental systemic corticosteroids. Pediatric patients may be more susceptible to systemic toxicity. D/C and institute appropriate therapy if irritation develops. Use appropriate antifungal or antibacterial agent if concomitant skin infections are present or develop; if favorable response does not occur promptly, d/c until infection is controlled. Caution in elderly. (Cre/Oint) Safety and efficacy of use in pediatric patients for >3 weeks have not been established.

ADVERSE REACTIONS: Burning, irritation, dryness, secondary infection, acneiform reaction, folliculitis, hypertrichosis, hypopigmentation, perioral dermatitis, allergic contact dermatitis, striae, miliaria, skin atrophy.

PREGNANCY: Category C, caution in nursing.

MECHANISM OF ACTION: Corticosteroid; not established. Possesses anti-inflammatory, antipruritic, and vasoconstrictive properties. Suspected to act by the induction of phospholipase A_2 inhibitory proteins called lipocortins, which control the biosynthesis of potent mediators of inflammation (eg, prostaglandins, leukotrienes) by inhibiting the release of arachidonic acid.

PHARMACOKINETICS: Absorption: Percutaneous; extent of absorption is determined by vehicle and integrity of the epidermal barrier. **Distribution:** Found in breast milk (systemically administered).

NURSING CONSIDERATIONS

Assessment: Assess for presence of concomitant skin infections, severity of dermatoses, factors that predispose to HPA-axis suppression, and pregnancy/nursing status.

Monitoring: Monitor for signs/symptoms of HPA-axis suppression, Cushing's syndrome, hyperglycemia, glucosuria, irritation, allergic contact dermatitis (eg, failure to heal), skin infections, and other adverse reactions. Perform periodic monitoring of HPA-axis suppression using adrenocorticotropic hormone stimulation test. Monitor for systemic toxicity (eg, adrenal suppression, intracranial HTN) in pediatric patients. Monitor response to therapy.

Patient Counseling: Instruct to use externally ud. Advise not to use on face, underarms, or groin areas. Instruct to avoid contact with eyes. Advise not to use for any disorder other than that for which it was prescribed. Inform not to bandage, cover, or wrap treated skin area unless directed by a physician. Instruct to report any signs of local adverse reactions to physician. Advise not to use medication for treatment of diaper dermatitis and not to apply to diaper area. Instruct to d/c use when control is achieved and to notify physician if no improvement seen within 2 weeks. Advise that other corticosteroid-containing products should not be used without first consulting with the physician.

Administration: Topical route. **Storage:** 25°C (77°F); excursions permitted to 15-30°C (59-86°F). (Cre) Avoid excessive heat.

ELOXATIN

RX

oxaliplatin (Sanofi-Aventis)

> Anaphylactic reactions reported and may occur within min of administration. Epinephrine, corticosteroids, and antihistamines have been employed to alleviate symptoms of anaphylaxis.

THERAPEUTIC CLASS: Organoplatinum complex

INDICATIONS: Treatment of advanced colorectal cancer and adjuvant treatment of stage III colon cancer in patients who have undergone complete resection of the primary tumor in combination with infusional 5-fluorouracil (5-FU) and leucovorin (LV).

DOSAGE: *Adults:* Premedicate with antiemetics, including 5-HT$_3$ blockers with or without dexamethasone. Day 1: 85mg/m² IV infusion and LV 200mg/m² IV infusion; give both over 120 min at the same time in separate bags using a Y-line, followed by 5-FU 400mg/m² IV bolus over 2-4 min, then 5-FU 600mg/m² IV infusion as a 22-hr continuous infusion. Day 2: LV 200mg/m² IV infusion over 120 min; followed by 5-FU 400mg/m² IV bolus over 2-4 min, then 5-FU 600mg/m² IV infusion as a 22-hr continuous infusion. Repeat cycle every 2 weeks. Advanced Colorectal Cancer: Continue treatment until disease progression or unacceptable toxicity. Adjuvant Therapy Stage III Colon Cancer: Treat for 6 months (12 cycles). Dose Modifications: Adjuvant Therapy Stage III Colon Cancer: Persistent Grade 2 Neurosensory Events: Consider reducing oxaliplatin to 75mg/m². Persistent Grade 3 Neurosensory Events: Consider discontinuing therapy. After Recovery from Grade 3/4 GI or Grade 4 Neutropenia or Grade 3/4 Thrombocytopenia: Reduce oxaliplatin to 75mg/m² and 5-FU to 300mg/m² bolus and 500mg/m² 22-hr infusion. Delay next dose until neutrophils ≥1.5 x 10⁹/L and platelets ≥75 x 10⁹/L. Advanced Colorectal Cancer: Persistent Grade 2 Neurosensory Events: Consider reducing oxaliplatin to 65mg/m². Persistent Grade 3 Neurosensory Events: Consider discontinuing therapy. The 5-FU/LV regimen need not be altered. After Recovery from Grade 3/4 GI or Grade 4 Neutropenia or Grade 3/4 Thrombocytopenia: Reduce oxaliplatin to 65mg/m^2 and 5-FU by 20% (300mg/m^2 bolus and 500mg/m^2 22-hr infusion). Delay next dose until neutrophils ≥1.5 x 10^9/L and platelets ≥75 x 10^9/L. Severe Renal Impairment: Initial: 65mg/m^2.

HOW SUPPLIED: Inj: 5mg/mL [50mg, 100mg]

WARNINGS/PRECAUTIONS: Should be administered under the supervision of a physician experienced in the use of cancer chemotherapeutic agents. Acute, reversible; and persistent (>14 days), primarily peripheral, sensory neuropathy reported. Cold temperature/objects may precipitate or exacerbate acute neurological symptoms; avoid ice for mucositis prophylaxis during infusion. Reversible posterior leukoencephalopathy syndrome (RPLS), also known as posterior reversible encephalopathy syndrome (PRES), reported. Potentially fatal pulmonary fibrosis reported. If unexplained respiratory symptoms develop, d/c until further pulmonary investigation excludes interstitial lung disease or pulmonary fibrosis. Hepatotoxicity observed; consider hepatic vascular disorders, and if appropriate, investigate in case of abnormal LFT results or portal HTN, which cannot be explained by liver metastases. May cause fetal harm. Caution with renal impairment.

ADVERSE REACTIONS: Anaphylactic reactions, peripheral sensory neuropathy, neutropenia, thrombocytopenia, anemia, N/V, increased transaminases/alkaline phosphatase, diarrhea, emesis, fatigue, stomatitis, abdominal pain, fever, skin disorder.

INTERACTIONS: Increased 5-FU plasma levels with doses of 130mg/m^2 oxaliplatin dosed every 3 weeks. Potentially nephrotoxic agents may decrease clearance. Prolonged PT and INR occasionally associated with hemorrhage reported in patients who concomitantly received oxaliplatin plus 5-FU/LV and anticoagulants; monitor patients requiring oral anticoagulants closely.

PREGNANCY: Category D, not for use in nursing.

MECHANISM OF ACTION: Organoplatinum complex; inhibits deoxyribonucleic acid replication and transcription.

PHARMACOKINETICS: Absorption: C_{max}=0.814mcg/mL. **Distribution:** V_d=440L; plasma protein binding (>90%). **Metabolism:** Rapid, extensive nonenzymatic biotransformation. **Elimination:** Urine (54%), feces (2%); $T_{1/2}$=391 hrs.

NURSING CONSIDERATIONS

Assessment: Assess for history of known allergy to the drug or other platinum compounds, renal impairment, pregnancy/nursing status, and possible drug interactions. Assess LFTs, WBC count with differential, Hgb, platelet count, and blood chemistries before each cycle.

Monitoring: Monitor for signs/symptoms of anaphylactic reactions, neurosensory toxicity, pulmonary toxicity, hepatotoxicity, portal HTN, RPLS, and other adverse reactions. Monitor patients with renal impairment closely. Monitor patients requiring oral anticoagulants closely.

Patient Counseling: Inform of pregnancy risks. Advise to expect side effects, particularly neurologic effects, both the acute, reversible effects and the persistent neurosensory toxicity. Inform that acute neurosensory toxicity may be precipitated or exacerbated by exposure to cold or cold objects. Instruct to avoid cold drinks and ice, and to cover exposed skin prior to exposure to cold temperature or cold objects. Inform of the risk of low blood cell counts and to contact physician immediately if fever, particularly if associated with persistent diarrhea, or evidence of infection develops. Advise to contact physician if persistent vomiting, diarrhea, fever, signs of dehydration, cough or breathing difficulties, or signs of an allergic reaction occur. Advise of the potential effects of vision abnormalities; instruct to use caution when driving and using machines.

Administration: IV route. Refer to PI for preparation of infusion sol. **Storage:** 25°C (77°F); excursions permitted to 15-30°C (59-86°F). Do not freeze and protect from light (keep in original outer carton).

EMEND CAPSULES   RX
aprepitant (Merck)

THERAPEUTIC CLASS: Substance P/neurokinin 1 receptor antagonist

INDICATIONS: Prevention of acute and delayed N/V associated with initial and repeat courses of highly emetogenic cancer chemotherapy, including high-dose cisplatin, in combination with other antiemetic agents. Prevention of N/V associated with initial and repeat courses of moderately emetogenic cancer chemotherapy in combination with other antiemetic agents. Prevention of postoperative N/V (PONV).

DOSAGE: *Adults:* Prevention of Chemotherapy-Induced N/V: Day 1: 125mg 1 hr prior to chemotherapy. Days 2 and 3: 80mg qam. Regimen should include a corticosteroid and a 5-hydroxytryptamine-3 (5-HT$_3$) antagonist; refer to PI for the specific dosing regimen. Prior to initiation of treatment, consult PI for the coadministered 5-HT$_3$ antagonist. Prevention of PONV: 40mg within 3 hrs prior to induction of anesthesia.

HOW SUPPLIED: Cap: 40mg, 80mg, 125mg

CONTRAINDICATIONS: Concomitant use with pimozide, terfenadine, astemizole, or cisapride.

WARNINGS/PRECAUTIONS: Not recommended for chronic continuous use for prevention of N/V. Caution with severe hepatic impairment (Child-Pugh score >9).

ADVERSE REACTIONS: Asthenia/fatigue, N/V, constipation, diarrhea, hiccups, anorexia, headache, dehydration, pruritus, dizziness, alopecia, hypotension, pyrexia.

INTERACTIONS: See Contraindications. May increase concentrations of CYP3A4 substrates (eg, vinblastine, vincristine, ifosfamide, dexamethasone, methylprednisolone, midazolam, alprazolam, triazolam); use with caution; refer to PI for dose adjustment recommendations for methylprednisolone and oral dexamethasone. May decrease concentrations of CYP2C9 substrates (eg, warfarin, tolbutamide, phenytoin). Coadministration with warfarin may decrease PT/INR; in patients on chronic warfarin therapy, closely monitor INR in the 2-week period, particularly at 7-10 days, following initiation of aprepitant with each chemotherapy cycle, or following administration of aprepitant for the prevention of PONV. May reduce efficacy of hormonal contraceptives; use alternative or back-up methods of contraception during treatment and for 1 month after the last dose. CYP3A4 inhibitors may increase concentrations; caution with strong inhibitors (eg, ketoconazole, itraconazole, nefazodone, troleandomycin, clarithromycin, ritonavir, nelfinavir) and moderate inhibitors (eg, diltiazem) of CYP3A4. CYP3A4 inducers (eg, rifampin, carbamazepine, phenytoin) may decrease concentrations and efficacy. May increase concentrations of diltiazem. Coadministration with paroxetine may decrease levels of both drugs.

PREGNANCY: Category B, not for use in nursing.

MECHANISM OF ACTION: Substance P/neurokinin 1 receptor antagonist; augments the antiemetic activity of the 5-HT$_3$ receptor antagonist ondansetron and the corticosteroid dexamethasone and inhibits both the acute and delayed phases of cisplatin-induced emesis.

PHARMACOKINETICS: Absorption: Administration of variable doses resulted in different parameters. **Distribution:** V_d=70L; plasma protein binding (>95%). **Metabolism:** Liver (extensive) by CYP3A4 (major), 1A2 and 2C19 (minor), via oxidation. **Elimination:** (IV) Urine (57%), feces (45%). $T_{1/2}$=9-13 hrs.

NURSING CONSIDERATIONS

Assessment: Assess for hypersensitivity to drug, severe hepatic impairment, pregnancy/nursing status, and possible drug interactions.

Monitoring: Monitor for hypersensitivity reactions and other adverse reactions. Monitor INR closely with warfarin.

Patient Counseling: Instruct to take drug dosing as prescribed. Instruct to d/c medication and contact physician immediately if patient experiences an allergic reaction. Advise to inform physician if using any other prescription, nonprescription medication, or herbal products. Inform that drug may reduce efficacy of hormonal contraceptives; advise to use alternative or back-up methods of contraception during therapy and for 1 month after the last dose.

Administration: Oral route. Take with or without food. **Storage:** 20-25°C (68-77°F).

EMEND FOR INJECTION
fosaprepitant dimeglumine (Merck)

RX

THERAPEUTIC CLASS: Substance P/neurokinin 1 receptor antagonist

INDICATIONS: Prevention of acute and delayed N/V associated with initial and repeat courses of highly emetogenic cancer chemotherapy (HEC), including high-dose cisplatin, in combination with other antiemetic agents. Prevention of N/V associated with initial and repeat courses of moderately emetogenic cancer chemotherapy (MEC) in adults in combination with other antiemetic agents.

DOSAGE: *Adults:* Prevention of N/V Associated with HEC: (Single-Dose Regimen) 150mg IV on Day 1 only as an infusion over 20-30 min initiated 30 min prior to chemotherapy. Prevention of N/V Associated with HEC/MEC: (3-Day Dosing Regimen) 115mg IV on Day 1 only as an infusion over 15 min initiated 30 min prior to chemotherapy. 125mg aprepitant cap may be substituted for 115mg fosaprepitant inj on Day 1. Give 80mg aprepitant cap on Days 2 and 3. Both regimens should include a corticosteroid and a 5-hydroxytryptamine-3 (5-HT$_3$) antagonist; refer to PI for specific dosing regimen. Prior to initiation of treatment, consult PI for the coadministered 5-HT$_3$ antagonist.

HOW SUPPLIED: Inj: 115mg, 150mg

CONTRAINDICATIONS: Concomitant use with pimozide or cisapride.

WARNINGS/PRECAUTIONS: Immediate hypersensitivity reactions reported; avoid reinitiating infusion if hypersensitivity occurs during 1st-time use. Not recommended for chronic continuous use for prevention of N/V. Caution with severe hepatic impairment (Child-Pugh score >9).

ADVERSE REACTIONS: Infusion-site reactions (erythema, pruritus, pain, induration), BP increased, thrombophlebitis.

INTERACTIONS: See Contraindications. May increase concentrations of CYP3A4 substrates (eg, vinblastine, vincristine, ifosfamide, dexamethasone, methylprednisolone, midazolam, alprazolam, triazolam); use with caution; refer to PI for dose adjustment recommendations for methylprednisolone and oral dexamethasone. May reduce efficacy of hormonal contraceptives; use alternative or back-up methods of contraception during treatment and for 1 month after the last dose. May decrease concentrations of CYP2C9 substrates (eg, warfarin, tolbutamide). Coadministration with warfarin may decrease PT/INR; in patients on chronic warfarin therapy, closely monitor INR in the 2-week period, particularly at 7-10 days, following initiation of fosaprepitant with each chemotherapy cycle. CYP3A4 inhibitors may increase concentrations; caution with strong inhibitors (eg, ketoconazole, itraconazole, nefazodone, troleandomycin, clarithromycin, ritonavir, nelfinavir) and moderate inhibitors (eg, diltiazem) of CYP3A4. CYP3A4 inducers (eg, rifampin, carbamazepine, phenytoin) may decrease concentrations and efficacy. May increase concentrations of diltiazem. Coadministration with paroxetine may decrease levels of both drugs.

PREGNANCY: Category B, not for use in nursing.

MECHANISM OF ACTION: Substance P/neurokinin 1 receptor antagonist; prodrug of aprepitant. Augments the antiemetic activity of the 5-HT$_3$ receptor antagonist ondansetron and the corticosteroid dexamethasone and inhibits both the acute and delayed phases of cisplatin-induced emesis.

PHARMACOKINETICS: Absorption: (Aprepitant, given as 115mg IV fosaprepitant) AUC=31.7mcg•hr/mL, C_{max}=3.27mcg/mL. (Aprepitant, given as 150mg IV fosaprepitant) AUC=37.38mcg•hr/mL, C_{max}=4.15mcg/mL. **Distribution:** (Aprepitant) V_d=70L; plasma protein binding (>95%). **Metabolism:** Rapidly converted to aprepitant in liver and extrahepatic tissues. (Aprepitant) Liver (extensive) by CYP3A4 (major), 1A2 and 2C19 (minor), via oxidation. **Elimination:** Urine (57%), feces (45%); (Aprepitant) $T_{1/2}$=9-13 hrs.

NURSING CONSIDERATIONS

Assessment: Assess for hypersensitivity to drug, severe hepatic impairment, pregnancy/nursing status, and possible drug interactions.

Monitoring: Monitor for hypersensitivity reactions and other adverse reactions. Monitor INR closely with warfarin.

Patient Counseling: Instruct to d/c medication and inform physician immediately if patient experiences an allergic reaction. Counsel patients who develop an infusion-site reaction (eg, erythema, edema, pain, thrombophlebitis) on how to care for the local reaction and when to seek further evaluation. Advise to inform physician if using any other prescription, nonprescription medication, or herbal products. Inform that drug may reduce efficacy of hormonal contraceptives; advise to use alternative or back-up methods of contraception during therapy and for 1 month after the last dose.

Administration: IV route. Do not mix or reconstitute with sol for which physical and chemical compatibility have not been established. Refer to PI for preparation instructions and incompatibility information. **Storage:** 2-8°C (36-46°F). Reconstituted Sol: Stable for 24 hrs at ambient room temperature ≤25°C (77°F).

EMLA

RX

lidocaine - prilocaine (APP Pharmaceuticals)

THERAPEUTIC CLASS: Acetamide local anesthetic

INDICATIONS: Topical anesthetic for use on normal intact skin. Topical anesthetic for genital mucous membranes for superficial minor surgery and as pretreatment for infiltration anesthesia.

DOSAGE: *Adults:* Apply thick layer of cre to intact skin and cover with occlusive dressing. Minor Dermal Procedure: Apply 2.5g over 20-25cm² of skin surface for at least 1 hr. Major Dermal Procedure: Apply 2g/10cm² of skin for 2 hrs. Adult Male Genital Skin: Apply 1g/10cm² of skin surface for 15 min. Female External Genitalia: Apply 5-10g for 5-10 min.
Pediatrics: 7-12 Yrs and >20kg: Max: 20g/200cm² for up to 4 hrs. 1-6 Yrs and >10kg: Max: 10g/100cm² for up to 4 hrs. 3-12 Months and >5kg: Max: 2g/20cm² for up to 4 hrs. 0-3 Months or <5kg: Max: 1g/10cm² for up to 1 hr. If >3 months and does not meet minimum weight requirement, max dose restricted to corresponding weight.

HOW SUPPLIED: Cre: (Lidocaine-Prilocaine) 2.5%-2.5%

WARNINGS/PRECAUTIONS: Application to larger areas or for longer than recommended times, may result in serious adverse effects. Should not be used where penetration or migration beyond the tympanic membrane into the middle ear is possible. Avoid with congenital or idiopathic methemoglobinemia and in infants <12 months of age receiving treatment with methemoglobin-inducing agents. Very young or patients with G6PD deficiency are more susceptible to methemoglobinemia. Reports of methemoglobinemia in infants and children following excessive applications. Monitor neonates and infants up to 3 months of age for Met-Hb levels before, during, and after application. Repeated doses may increase blood levels; caution in patients who may be more susceptible to systemic effects (eg, acutely ill, debilitated, elderly). Avoid eye contact and application to open wounds. Has been shown to inhibit viral and bacterial growth. Caution with severe hepatic disease and in patients with drug sensitivities.

ADVERSE REACTIONS: Erythema, edema, abnormal sensations, paleness (pallor or blanching), altered temperature sensations, burning sensation, itching, rash.

INTERACTIONS: Additive and potentially synergistic toxic effects with Class I antiarrhythmic drugs (eg, tocainide, mexiletine). May have additive cardiac effects with Class III antiarrhythmic drugs (eg, amiodarone, bretylium, sotalol, dofetilide). Avoid drugs associated with drug-induced methemoglobinemia (eg, sulfonamides, acetaminophen, acetanilid, aniline dyes, benzocaine, chloroquine, dapsone, naphthalene, nitrates/nitrites, nitrofurantoin, nitroglycerin, nitroprusside, phenobarbital, phenytoin, primaquine, pamaquine, para-aminosalicylic acid, phenacetin, quinine). Caution with other products containing lidocaine/prilocaine; consider the amount absorbed from all formulations.

PREGNANCY: Category B, caution in nursing.

MECHANISM OF ACTION: Amide-type local anesthetics; stabilizes neuronal membranes by inhibiting ionic fluxes required for initiation and conduction impulses, thereby affecting local anesthetic action.

PHARMACOKINETICS: Absorption: Lidocaine: (3 hrs 400cm^2) C_{max}=0.12mcg/mL, T_{max}=4 hrs; (24 hrs 400cm^2) C_{max}=0.28mcg/mL, T_{max}=10 hrs. Prilocaine: (3 hrs 400cm^2) C_{max}=0.07mcg/mL, T_{max}=4 hrs; (24 hrs 400cm^2) C_{max}=0.14mcg/mL, T_{max}=10 hrs. **Distribution:** (IV) V_d=1.5L/kg (lidocaine), 2.6L/kg (prilocaine); (Cre) plasma protein binding 70% (lidocaine), 55% (prilocaine). Crosses placental and blood-brain barrier; found in breast milk. **Metabolism:** Lidocaine: Liver (rapid); monoethylglycinexylidide and glycinexylidide (active metabolites). Prilocaine: Liver and kidneys by amidases; ortho-toluidine and N-n-propylalanine (metabolites). **Elimination:** (IV) Lidocaine: Urine (>98%); $T_{1/2}$=110 min. Prilocaine: $T_{1/2}$=70 min.

NURSING CONSIDERATIONS

Assessment: Assess for congenital or idiopathic methemoglobinemia, G6PD deficiency, hepatic disease, open wounds, presence of acute illness, presence of debilitation, history of drug sensitivities, pregnancy/nursing status, and for possible drug interactions. In neonates and infants ≤3 months of age, obtain Met-Hb levels prior to application.

Monitoring: Monitor for signs/symptoms of methemoglobinemia, ototoxicity, local skin reactions and for allergic/anaphylactoid reactions. Monitor Met-Hb levels in neonates and infants ≤3 months of age during and after application.

Patient Counseling: Inform about potential risks/benefits of drug. Advise to avoid inadvertent trauma to treated area. Instruct not to apply near eyes or on open wounds. Apply ud by physician. Advise to notify physician if pregnant/nursing or planning to become pregnant. Instruct to remove cre and consult physician if child becomes very dizzy, excessively sleepy, or develops duskiness on the face or lips after application.

Administration: Topical route. Not for ophthalmic use. **Storage:** 20-25°C (68-77°F). Keep tightly closed.

EMSAM   RX
selegiline (Mylan Specialty)

> Antidepressants increased the risk of suicidal thinking and behavior (suicidality) in short-term studies in children, adolescents, and young adults with major depressive disorder (MDD) and other psychiatric disorders. Monitor and observe closely for clinical worsening, suicidality, or unusual changes in behavior in patients who are started on antidepressant therapy. Not approved for use in pediatric patients.

THERAPEUTIC CLASS: Monoamine oxidase inhibitor (type B)

INDICATIONS: Treatment of MDD.

DOSAGE: *Adults:* Initial/Target Dose: 6mg/24 hrs. Titrate: May increase in increments of 3mg/24 hrs at intervals ≥2 weeks. Max: 12mg/24 hrs. Elderly: 6mg/24 hrs. Increase dose cautiously.

HOW SUPPLIED: Patch: 6mg/24 hrs, 9mg/24 hrs, 12mg/24 hrs [30^s]

CONTRAINDICATIONS: Pheochromocytoma. Concomitant use with SSRIs (eg, fluoxetine, sertraline, paroxetine), dual SNRIs (eg, venlafaxine, duloxetine), TCAs (eg, imipramine, amitriptyline), bupropion HCl, meperidine, analgesics (eg, tramadol, methadone, propoxyphene), dextromethorphan, St. John's wort, mirtazapine, cyclobenzaprine, PO selegiline or other MAOIs (eg, isocarboxazid, phenelzine, tranylcypromine), carbamazepine, oxcarbazepine, sympathomimetic amines including amphetamines, cold products and weight-reducing preparations that contain vasoconstrictors (eg, pseudoephedrine, phenylephrine, phenylpropanolamine, ephedrine), elective surgery requiring general anesthesia, cocaine, or local anesthesia containing sympathomimetic vasoconstrictors, (for patients receiving 9mg/24 hrs and 12mg/24 hrs) high tyramine-containing foods. D/C therapy at least 10 days prior to elective surgery.

WARNINGS/PRECAUTIONS: Not approved for treatment of bipolar depression. Postural hypotension may occur; monitor elderly for postural changes in BP, caution with preexisting orthostasis during dose increases, and consider dose adjustment if orthostatic symptoms occur. Activation of mania/hypomania may occur; caution with history of mania. Caution with disorders or conditions that can produce altered metabolism or hemodynamic responses.

ADVERSE REACTIONS: Headache, diarrhea, dyspepsia, insomnia, dry mouth, pharyngitis, sinusitis, application-site reaction, rash, low systolic BP, orthostatic hypotension, weight change.

INTERACTIONS: See Contraindications. Not recommended with buspirone HCl and alcohol. Approximately 1 week should elapse between discontinuation of SSRIs, SNRIs, TCAs, other MAOIs, meperidine, analgesics (eg, tramadol, methadone, propoxyphene), dextromethorphan, St. John's wort, mirtazapine, bupropion HCl, buspirone HCl, and start of therapy. At least 5 weeks should elapse between discontinuation of fluoxetine and start of therapy. At least 2 weeks should elapse after discontinuation of therapy before starting buspirone HCl or any contraindicated drug. Hypertensive crisis can occur with high tyramine-containing foods.

PREGNANCY: Category C, caution in nursing.

MECHANISM OF ACTION: MAOI (Type B); not established. Presumed to be linked to potentiation of monoamine neurotransmitter activity in the CNS resulting from its inhibition of MAO activity.

PHARMACOKINETICS: Absorption: AUC=46.2ng•hr/mL. **Distribution:** Plasma protein binding (90%). **Metabolism:** Extensive via N-dealkylation or N-depropargylation by CYP2B6, CYP2C9, CYP3A4/5 (major), CYP2A6 (minor); N-desmethylselegiline, R(-)-methamphetamine (metabolites). **Elimination:** Urine (10%, 0.1% unchanged), feces (2%); $T_{1/2}$=18-25 hrs (IV).

NURSING CONSIDERATIONS

Assessment: Assess for hypersensitivity to the drug, pheochromocytoma, risk of bipolar disorder, history of mania, preexisting orthostasis, diseases/conditions that alter metabolism or hemodynamic response, pregnancy/nursing status, and possible drug interactions.

Monitoring: Monitor for worsening of depression, emergence of suicidal ideation, unusual changes in behavior, hypertensive crisis, postural hypotension, activation of mania/hypomania, and other adverse reactions.

Patient Counseling: Counsel about benefits, risks, and appropriate use of therapy. Advise to report to physician if unusual changes in behavior, worsening of depression, suicidal ideation, or any acute symptoms (eg, severe headache, neck stiffness, heart racing or palpitations) occur. Advise to use caution when performing hazardous tasks (eg, operating machinery/driving). Counsel to avoid alcohol, tyramine-containing foods/supplements/beverages, and any cough medicine containing dextromethorphan, and to notify physician if taking or planning to take any prescription or OTC drugs. Instruct to use exactly as prescribed and avoid exposing application site to external sources of direct heat. Instruct not to cut patch into smaller portions. Advise to change position gradually if lightheaded, faint, or dizzy. Instruct to notify physician if pregnant, intend to become pregnant, or breastfeeding.

Administration: Transdermal route. Apply to dry, intact skin on the upper torso, upper thigh, or outer surface of upper arm. Apply immediately upon removal from the protective pouch. Refer to PI for further instructions. **Storage:** 20-25°C (68-77°F). Do not store outside of the sealed pouch.

EMTRIVA   RX
emtricitabine (Gilead)

> Lactic acidosis and severe hepatomegaly with steatosis, including fatal cases, reported with the use of nucleoside analogs alone or in combination with other antiretrovirals. Not approved for the treatment of chronic hepatitis B virus (HBV) infection. Severe acute exacerbations of hepatitis B reported in patients who have discontinued therapy. Closely monitor hepatic function with both clinical and lab follow-up for at least several months in patients who are coinfected with HIV-1 and HBV and d/c therapy. If appropriate, initiation of antihepatitis B therapy may be warranted.

THERAPEUTIC CLASS: Nucleoside reverse transcriptase inhibitor

INDICATIONS: Treatment of HIV-1 infection in combination with other antiretroviral agents.

DOSAGE: *Adults:* ≥18 Yrs: (Cap) 200mg qd. Renal Impairment: CrCl ≥50mL/min: 200mg qd. CrCl 30-49mL/min: 200mg q48h. CrCl 15-29mL/min: 200mg q72h. CrCl <15mL/min or on Hemodialysis: 200mg q96h. Give dose after dialysis if dosing on day of dialysis. (Sol) 240mg (24mL) qd. Renal Impairment: CrCl ≥50mL/min: 240mg q24h. CrCl 30-49mL/min: 120mg (12mL) q24h. CrCl 15-29mL/min: 80mg (8mL) q24h. CrCl <15mL/min or on Hemodialysis: 60mg (6mL) q24h. Give dose after dialysis if dosing on day of dialysis.
Pediatrics: 3 Months-17 Yrs: (Cap) >33kg: 200mg qd. (Sol) 6mg/kg qd. Max: 240mg (24mL) qd.

0-3 Months: (Sol) 3mg/kg qd. Renal Impairment: Consider reduction in the dose and/or increase in the dosing interval similar to adjustments for adults.

HOW SUPPLIED: Cap: 200mg; Sol: 10mg/mL [170mL]

WARNINGS/PRECAUTIONS: Obesity and prolonged nucleoside exposure may be risk factors for lactic acidosis and severe hepatomegaly with steatosis. Caution with known risk factors for liver disease. D/C if lactic acidosis or pronounced hepatotoxicity develops. Test for chronic HBV before initiating therapy. Reduce dose and closely monitor clinical response and renal function with renal impairment. Redistribution/accumulation of body fat and immune reconstitution syndrome reported. Autoimmune disorders (eg, Graves' disease, polymyositis, Guillain-Barre syndrome) in the setting of immune reconstitution reported. Caution in elderly.

ADVERSE REACTIONS: Lactic acidosis, severe hepatomegaly with steatosis, headache, diarrhea, nausea, fatigue, dizziness, depression, insomnia, abnormal dreams, rash, abdominal pain, asthenia, increased cough, rhinitis.

INTERACTIONS: Do not coadminister with emtricitabine- or lamivudine-containing products.

PREGNANCY: Category B, not for use in nursing.

MECHANISM OF ACTION: Nucleoside reverse transcriptase inhibitor; inhibits the activity of the HIV-1 reverse transcriptase by competing with the natural substrate deoxycytidine 5'-triphosphate and by being incorporated into nascent viral DNA, which results in chain termination.

PHARMACOKINETICS: Absorption: Rapid and extensive. T_{max}=1-2 hrs. (Cap) Absolute bioavailability (93%); C_{max}=1.8mcg/mL; AUC=10mcg•hr/mL. (Sol) Absolute bioavailability (75%). **Distribution:** Plasma protein binding (<4%); found in breast milk. **Metabolism:** Oxidation and conjugation; 3'-sulfoxide diastereomers and 2'-O-glucuronide (metabolites). **Elimination:** Urine (86%), feces (14%); $T_{1/2}$=10 hrs.

NURSING CONSIDERATIONS

Assessment: Assess for previous hypersensitivity, risk factors for lactic acidosis and liver disease, HBV infection, renal impairment, pregnancy/nursing status, and possible drug interactions.

Monitoring: Monitor for signs/symptoms of lactic acidosis, severe hepatomegaly with steatosis, hepatotoxicity, redistribution/accumulation of body fat, immune reconstitution syndrome, autoimmune disorders, and other adverse reactions. Closely monitor hepatic function with both clinical and lab follow-up for at least several months in patients who are coinfected with HIV-1 and HBV and d/c therapy. Closely monitor clinical response and renal function with renal impairment.

Patient Counseling: Inform that therapy is not a cure for HIV-1 infection and illnesses associated with HIV-1 infection, including opportunistic infections, may continue. Instruct not to breastfeed, and not to share needles or other injection equipment and personal items that can have blood or body fluids on them (eg, toothbrushes, razor blades). Advise to always practice safer sex by using a latex or polyurethane condom to lower the chance of sexual contact with semen, vaginal secretions, or blood. Inform that it is important to take drug with combination therapy on a regular dosing schedule to avoid missing doses. Instruct to notify physician if symptoms suggestive of lactic acidosis or pronounced hepatotoxicity (eg, N/V, unusual or unexpected stomach discomfort, weakness) develop.

Administration: Oral route. May be taken without regard to food. **Storage:** (Cap) 25°C (77°F); excursions permitted to 15-30°C (59-86°F). (Sol) 2-8°C (36-46°F). Use within 3 months if stored at 25°C (77°F).

ENABLEX   RX
darifenacin (Warner Chilcott)

THERAPEUTIC CLASS: Muscarinic antagonist

INDICATIONS: Treatment of overactive bladder with symptoms of urge urinary incontinence, urgency, and frequency.

DOSAGE: *Adults:* Initial: 7.5mg qd with water. Titrate: May increase to 15mg qd as early as 2 weeks after starting therapy based on individual response. Moderate Hepatic Impairment (Child-Pugh B)/Concomitant Potent CYP3A4 Inhibitors (eg, Ketoconazole, Ritonavir, Clarithromycin): Max: 7.5mg/day.

HOW SUPPLIED: Tab, Extended-Release: 7.5mg, 15mg

CONTRAINDICATIONS: Urinary retention, gastric retention, uncontrolled narrow-angle glaucoma, and in patients at risk for these conditions.

WARNINGS/PRECAUTIONS: Not recommended in patients with severe hepatic impairment (Child-Pugh C). Risk of urinary retention; caution with significant bladder outflow obstruction. Risk of gastric retention; caution with GI obstructive disorders. May decrease GI motility; caution with severe constipation, ulcerative colitis, and myasthenia gravis. Caution with moderate hepatic impairment and in patients being treated for narrow-angle glaucoma. Angioedema reported; d/c and institute appropriate therapy if involvement of the tongue, hypopharynx, or larynx occurs. CNS anticholinergic effects (eg, headache, confusion, hallucinations, somnolence) reported; monitor for signs of anticholinergic CNS effects (particularly after beginning treatment or increasing the dose) and d/c or reduce dose if this occurs.

ADVERSE REACTIONS: Dry mouth, constipation, dyspepsia, abdominal pain, nausea, urinary tract infection, headache, flu syndrome.

INTERACTIONS: Pharmacokinetics may be altered by CYP3A4 inducers and CYP2D6/CYP3A4 inhibitors. Caution with medications metabolized by CYP2D6 and which have a narrow therapeutic window (eg, flecainide, thioridazine, TCAs). May increase the frequency and/or severity of dry mouth, constipation, blurred vision, and other anticholinergic pharmacologic effects with other anticholinergic agents. May alter the absorption of some concomitantly administered drugs due to effects on GI motility. Increased concentration with cimetidine, erythromycin, fluconazole, or ketoconazole. May increase imipramine and desipramine (imipramine active metabolite) concentrations.

PREGNANCY: Category C, caution in nursing.

MECHANISM OF ACTION: Muscarinic receptor antagonist; inhibits cholinergic muscarinic receptors, which mediate contractions of urinary bladder smooth muscle and stimulation of salivary secretions.

PHARMACOKINETICS: Absorption: Variable doses resulted in different pharmacokinetic parameters in extensive metabolizers and poor metabolizers of CYP2D6. **Distribution:** V_d=163L; plasma protein binding (98%). **Metabolism:** Liver (extensive) via CYP2D6 and 3A4 (monohydroxylation, dihydrobenzofuran ring opening, N-dealkylation). **Elimination:** Urine (60%); feces (40%); unchanged, 3%. $T_{1/2}$=13-19 hrs.

NURSING CONSIDERATIONS

Assessment: Assess for urinary retention, gastric retention, narrow-angle glaucoma and risk for these conditions, bladder outflow obstruction, GI obstructive disorders, severe constipation, ulcerative colitis, myasthenia gravis, hepatic impairment, pregnancy/nursing status, and possible drug interactions.

Monitoring: Monitor for symptoms of urinary retention, gastric retention, decreased GI motility, and for angioedema (face, lips, tongue, hypopharynx, larynx). Monitor for signs of anticholinergic CNS effects (particularly after beginning treatment or increasing the dose).

Patient Counseling: Advise that dizziness or blurred vision may occur; instruct to exercise caution when engaging in potentially dangerous activities. Instruct to take qd with liquid. Instruct to swallow whole; advise to not chew, divide, or crush. Inform that symptoms of constipation, urinary retention, heat prostration when used in a hot environment, or angioedema may occur. Advise to d/c therapy and seek medical attention if edema of the tongue or laryngopharynx, or difficulty breathing occurs. Advise to read the patient information leaflet before starting therapy.

Administration: Oral route. Take with or without food. **Storage:** 25°C (77°F); excursions permitted to 15-30°C (59-86°F). Protect from light.

ENALAPRIL/HCTZ RX
enalapril maleate - hydrochlorothiazide (Various)

D/C when pregnancy is detected. Drugs that act directly on the renin-angiotensin system (RAS) can cause injury/death to developing fetus.

OTHER BRAND NAMES: Vaseretic (Valeant)

THERAPEUTIC CLASS: ACE inhibitor/thiazide diuretic

INDICATIONS: Treatment of HTN.

DOSAGE: *Adults:* BP Not Controlled with Enalapril or HCTZ Monotherapy: Initial: 5mg-12.5mg or 10mg-25mg qd. Titrate: Increase dose based on clinical response. May increase HCTZ dose after 2-3 weeks. Max: 20mg-50mg qd. Replacement Therapy: May substitute for titrated components. Elderly: Start at lower end of dosing range.

HOW SUPPLIED: Tab: (Enalapril-HCTZ) 5mg-12.5mg, 10mg-25mg*; (Vaseretic) 10mg-25mg* *scored

CONTRAINDICATIONS: Hereditary/idiopathic angioedema, anuria, hypersensitivity to other sulfonamide-derived drugs, history of ACE inhibitor-associated angioedema. Coadministration with aliskiren in patients with diabetes.

WARNINGS/PRECAUTIONS: Not for initial therapy. Avoid if CrCl ≤30mL/min. Caution in elderly. Enalapril: Excessive hypotension associated with oliguria and/or progressive azotemia, and rarely with acute renal failure and/or death has been observed in congestive heart failure (CHF) patients; monitor closely upon initiation and during first 2 weeks of therapy and when dose is increased. Head/neck angioedema reported; d/c and administer appropriate therapy. Intestinal angioedema reported; monitor for abdominal pain. More reports of angioedema in blacks than nonblacks. Anaphylactoid reactions reported during desensitization with hymenoptera venom, dialysis with high-flux membranes, and LDL apheresis with dextran sulfate absorption. Neutropenia/agranulocytosis reported; monitor WBCs in patients with collagen vascular disease and renal disease. Rarely, associated with syndrome that starts with cholestatic jaundice and progresses to fulminant hepatic necrosis and sometimes death; d/c if jaundice or marked elevations of hepatic enzymes occurs. Caution with left ventricular outflow obstruction. May cause changes in renal function. May increase BUN/SrCr in patients with renal artery stenosis or with no preexisting renal vascular disease; monitor renal function during the 1st few weeks of therapy in patients with renal artery stenosis. Hyperkalemia and persistent nonproductive cough reported. Hypotension may occur with major surgery or during anesthesia. HCTZ: May precipitate azotemia in patients with renal disease; caution with severe renal disease. Caution with hepatic impairment or progressive liver disease; may precipitate hepatic coma. Sensitivity reactions may occur. May exacerbate/activate systemic lupus erythematosus (SLE). May cause idiosyncratic reaction, resulting in acute transient myopia and acute angle-closure glaucoma; d/c as rapidly as possible. Observe for signs of fluid or electrolyte imbalance (eg, hyponatremia, hypochloremic alkalosis, hypokalemia). Hyperuricemia, gout precipitation, hyperglycemia, hypomagnesemia, hypercalcemia, and increased cholesterol and TG levels may occur. D/C before testing for parathyroid function. Enhanced effects in postsympathectomy patients.

ADVERSE REACTIONS: Dizziness, cough, fatigue, headache.

INTERACTIONS: See Contraindications. Dual blockade of the RAS is associated with increased risks of hypotension, hyperkalemia, and changes in renal function (including acute renal failure); closely monitor BP, renal function, and electrolytes with concomitant agents that affect the RAS. Avoid with aliskiren in patients with renal impairment (GFR <60mL/min). NSAIDs, including selective cyclooxygenase-2 inhibitors, may diminish effects of diuretics and ACE inhibitors, and may cause deterioration of renal function. Increased risk of lithium toxicity; avoid with lithium. Enalapril: Hypotension risk, and increased BUN/SrCr with diuretics. Antihypertensive agents that cause renin release (eg, diuretics) may augment effect. Increased risk of hyperkalemia with K^+-sparing diuretics, K^+ supplements, and/or K^+-containing salt substitutes. Nitritoid reactions reported with injectable gold. HCTZ: Potentiation of orthostatic hypotension may occur with alcohol, barbiturates, and narcotics. Dose adjustment of the antidiabetic drug (oral agents and insulin) may be required. Potentiation may occur with other antihypertensives. Cholestyramine and colestipol resins impair absorption. Corticosteroids and adrenocorticotropic hormone may intensify electrolyte depletion, particularly hypokalemia. May decrease response to pressor amines (eg, norepinephrine). May increase responsiveness to nondepolarizing skeletal muscle relaxants (eg, tubocurarine).

PREGNANCY: Category D, not for use in nursing.

MECHANISM OF ACTION: Enalapril: ACE inhibitor; decreases plasma angiotensin II, which leads to decreased vasopressor activity and decreased aldosterone secretion. HCTZ: Thiazide diuretic; has not been established. Affects distal renal tubular mechanism of electrolyte reabsorption. Increases excretion of Na^+ and Cl^-.

PHARMACOKINETICS: Absorption: Enalapril: T_{max}=1 hr, 3-4 hrs (enalaprilat). **Distribution:** Crosses placenta; found in breast milk. **Metabolism:** Enalapril: Hydrolysis to enalaprilat (active metabolite). **Elimination:** Enalapril: Urine and feces (94% as enalapril or enalaprilat); $T_{1/2}$=11 hrs (enalaprilat). HCTZ: Kidneys (at least 61% unchanged); $T_{1/2}$=5.6-14.8 hrs.

NURSING CONSIDERATIONS

Assessment: Assess for hereditary/idiopathic or history of ACE inhibitor-associated angioedema, anuria, hypersensitivity to the drug or sulfonamide-derived drugs, diabetes, CHF, left ventricular outflow obstruction, collagen vascular disease, SLE, risk factors for hyperkalemia, renal/hepatic function, pregnancy/nursing status, and possible drug interactions.

Monitoring: Monitor for signs/symptoms of angioedema, exacerbation/activation of SLE, idiosyncratic reaction, hyperglycemia, hypercalcemia, hypomagnesemia, hyperuricemia or precipitation of gout, sensitivity reactions, and other adverse reactions. Periodically monitor WBCs in patients with collagen vascular disease and renal disease. Monitor BP, serum electrolytes, renal/hepatic function, and cholesterol/TG levels.

Patient Counseling: Inform about fetal risks if taken during pregnancy and discuss treatment options in women planning to become pregnant; report pregnancy to physician as soon as possible. Instruct to d/c therapy and immediately report any signs/symptoms of angioedema (swelling of the face, extremities, eyes, lips, tongue; difficulty in swallowing or breathing). Instruct to report lightheadedness and to d/c therapy if actual syncope occurs. Inform that excessive perspiration, dehydration, and other causes of volume depletion (eg, diarrhea or vomiting) may lead to an excessive fall in BP. Instruct not to use salt substitutes containing K^+ without consulting physician, and to report promptly any signs/symptoms of infection.

Administration: Oral route. **Storage:** 20-25°C (68-77°F). Protect from moisture. (Vaseretic) 25°C (77°F); excursions permitted 15-30°C (59-86°F). Protect from moisture.

ENALAPRILAT RX
enalaprilat (Various)

> ACE inhibitors can cause death/injury to the developing fetus during 2nd and 3rd trimesters. D/C therapy if pregnancy detected.

THERAPEUTIC CLASS: ACE inhibitor

INDICATIONS: Treatment of HTN when oral therapy is not practical.

DOSAGE: *Adults:* Administer IV over a 5 min period. Usual: 1.25mg q6h for no longer than 48 hrs. Max: 20mg/day. Concomitant Diuretic: Initial: 0.625mg. May repeat after 1 hr if response is inadequate. May administer an additional dose of 1.25mg at 6 hr intervals. CrCl ≤30mL/min: Initial: 0.625mg. May repeat after 1 hr if response is inadequate. May administer an additional dose of 1.25mg at 6 hr intervals. Risk of Excessive Hypotension: Initial: 0.625mg over 5 min to 1 hr. IV to PO Conversion: Refer to PI.

HOW SUPPLIED: Inj: 1.25mg/mL [1mL, 2mL]

CONTRAINDICATIONS: History of ACE inhibitor-associated angioedema and hereditary or idiopathic angioedema.

WARNINGS/PRECAUTIONS: Excessive hypotension sometimes associated with oliguria or azotemia and (rarely) acute renal failure or death may occur; monitor closely whenever dose is adjusted and/or diuretic increased. May increase risk of angioedema in patients with history of angioedema unrelated to ACE inhibitor therapy. Angioedema of the face, extremities, lips, tongue, glottis, and larynx reported; d/c and administer appropriate therapy if this occurs. Higher incidence of angioedema reported in blacks than nonblacks. Anaphylactoid reactions reported during desensitization with hymenoptera venom, dialysis with high-flux membranes, and LDL apheresis with dextran sulfate absorption. Neutropenia or agranulocytosis and bone marrow depression reported; monitor WBCs in patients with renal disease and collagen vascular disease. Rarely, a syndrome that starts with cholestatic jaundice and progresses to fulminant hepatic necrosis and sometimes death reported; d/c if jaundice or marked elevations of hepatic enzymes develop. Caution with left ventricular outflow obstruction. May cause changes in renal function. Increases in BUN and SrCr reported with renal artery stenosis; monitor renal function during the 1st few weeks of therapy. Increases in BUN and SrCr reported with no preexisting renal vascular disease. Hyperkalemia may occur; risk factors include diabetes mellitus (DM) and renal insufficiency. Persistent nonproductive cough reported. Hypotension may occur with major surgery or during anesthesia; may be corrected by volume expansion.

ADVERSE REACTIONS: Hypotension, headache, nausea, angioedema, myocardial infarction, fatigue, dizziness, fever, rash, constipation, cough.

INTERACTIONS: Hypotension risk with diuretics. May increase BUN and SrCr with diuretics; may require dose reduction and/or discontinuation of diuretic and/or therapy. May further decrease renal dysfunction with NSAIDs. Increase risk of hyperkalemia with K+-sparing diuretics, K+-containing salt substitutes or K+ supplements. Antihypertensives that cause renin release (eg, thiazides) may augment antihypertensive effect. NSAIDs may diminish antihypertensive effect. Lithium toxicity reported with lithium; monitor serum lithium levels frequently. Nitritoid reactions (eg, facial flushing, N/V, hypotension) reported rarely with injectable gold.

PREGNANCY: Category C (1st trimester) and D (2nd and 3rd trimesters), not for use in nursing.

MECHANISM OF ACTION: ACE inhibitor; inhibition results in decreased plasma angiotensin II, which leads to decreased vasopressor activity and decreased aldosterone secretion.

PHARMACOKINETICS: **Absorption:** (PO) Poorly absorbed. **Distribution:** Crosses placenta (enalapril), found in breast milk. **Elimination:** (PO) Urine (>90% unchanged), $T_{1/2}$=11 hrs (enalaprilat).

NURSING CONSIDERATIONS

Assessment: Assess for history of angioedema, renal dysfunction/disease, collagen vascular disease, renal artery stenosis, left ventricular outflow obstruction, DM, pregnancy/nursing status, and possible drug interactions. Obtain baseline BP, WBC count, serum K+ levels, and renal function.

Monitoring: Monitor anaphylactoid reaction, angioedema, hypotension, hypersensitivity, and other adverse reactions. Monitor BP, renal function, WBC count, serum K+ levels.

Patient Counseling: Inform about the risks and benefits of therapy.

Administration: IV route. Should be administered as slow IV infusion as provided or diluted with up to 50mL of a compatible diluent. Refer to PI for list of compatible diluents. **Storage:** Below 30°C (86°F). (Diluted Sol) Stable for 24 hrs at room temperature.

ENBREL   RX
etanercept (Immunex)

> Increased risk for developing serious infections (eg, active tuberculosis [TB], latent TB reactivation, invasive fungal infec-
> tions, bacterial/viral infections, opportunistic infections) leading to hospitalization or death, mostly with concomitant
> use with immunosuppressants (eg, methotrexate [MTX], corticosteroids). D/C if serious infection or sepsis develops.
> Active/latent reactivation of TB may present with disseminated or extrapulmonary disease; test for latent TB before and
> during therapy and initiate treatment for latent TB prior to therapy. Consider empiric antifungal therapy in patients at risk
> for invasive fungal infections who develop severe systemic illness. Monitor for development of infection during and after
> treatment, including development of TB in patients who tested negative for latent TB infection prior to therapy. Lymphoma
> and other malignancies, some fatal, reported in children and adolescents.

THERAPEUTIC CLASS: TNF-blocker

INDICATIONS: Reduce signs/symptoms, induce major clinical response, inhibit progression of structural damage, and improve physical function in patients with moderately to severely active rheumatoid arthritis (RA); can be initiated in combination with MTX or used alone. Reduce signs/symptoms of moderately to severely active polyarticular juvenile idiopathic arthritis (JIA) in patients ≥2 yrs of age. Reduce signs/symptoms, inhibit progression of structural damage of active arthritis, and improve physical function in patients with psoriatic arthritis (PsA); can be used in combination with MTX in patients with inadequate response to MTX alone. Reduce signs/symptoms of active ankylosing spondylitis (AS). Treatment of adults (≥18 yrs of age) with chronic moderate to severe plaque psoriasis (PsO) who are candidates for systemic therapy or phototherapy.

DOSAGE: *Adults:* RA/AS/PsA: 50mg SQ weekly. May continue MTX, glucocorticoids, salicylates, NSAIDs, or analgesics during treatment. Max: 50mg/week. PsO: Initial: 50mg SQ twice weekly for 3 months; starting doses of 25mg or 50mg per week were also shown to be efficacious. Maint: 50mg once weekly.
Pediatrics: ≥2 Yrs: JIA: ≥63kg: 50mg SQ weekly. <63kg: 0.8mg/kg SQ weekly. May continue glucocorticoids, NSAIDs, or analgesics during treatment.

HOW SUPPLIED: Inj: 25mg [multiple-use vial, single-use prefilled syringe], 50mg [single-use prefilled syringe, single-use prefilled SureClick autoinjector]

CONTRAINDICATIONS: Sepsis.

WARNINGS/PRECAUTIONS: Do not initiate in patients with an active infection. Increased risk of infection in patients >65 yrs of age and in patients with comorbid conditions. New onset or exacerbation of CNS and peripheral nervous system demyelinating disorders, acute and chronic leukemia, new onset and worsening of congestive heart failure (CHF), melanoma and non-melanoma skin cancer, and Merkel cell carcinoma reported; consider periodic skin examinations for all patients at increased risk for skin cancer. Pancytopenia, including aplastic anemia, reported; consider discontinuation in patients with confirmed significant hematologic abnormalities. Reactivation of hepatitis B in patients who were previously infected with hepatitis B virus (HBV) reported; closely monitor for signs of active HBV infection during and for several months after therapy. Consider discontinuing therapy and initiating antiviral therapy with appropriate supportive treatment if HBV reactivation develops. Allergic reactions reported; d/c immediately and initiate appropriate therapy if an anaphylactic or other serious allergic reaction occurs. Needle cover of prefilled syringe and needle cover within the needle cap of autoinjector contain dry natural rubber, which may cause allergic reactions in latex-sensitive individuals. May result in the formation of autoantibodies and in the development of a lupus-like syndrome or autoimmune hepatitis; d/c and evaluate patient if a lupus-like syndrome or autoimmune hepatitis develops. Caution with moderate to severe alcoholic hepatitis and in the elderly. Patients with a significant exposure to varicella virus should temporarily d/c therapy and be considered for prophylactic treatment with varicella zoster immune globulin. Hypoglycemia reported following initiation of therapy in patients receiving antidiabetic medication; reduction in antidiabetic medication may be necessary.

ADVERSE REACTIONS: Infections, sepsis, malignancies, inj-site reactions, diarrhea, rash, pyrexia, pruritus.

INTERACTIONS: See Boxed Warning. Avoid with live vaccines; pediatric patients should be brought up-to-date with all immunizations in agreement with current immunization guidelines prior to initiating therapy. Not recommended with anakinra or abatacept; may increase risk of serious infections. Not recommended in patients with Wegener's granulomatosis receiving immunosuppressive agents; increased incidence of noncutaneous solid malignancies when added to standard therapy (eg, cyclophosphamide). Not recommended with cyclophosphamide. Mild decrease in mean neutrophil counts reported with sulfasalazine.

PREGNANCY: Category B, caution in nursing.

MECHANISM OF ACTION: TNF-blocker; inhibits binding of TNF-α and TNF-β (lymphotoxin alpha [LT-α]) to cell surface TNF-receptors, rendering TNF biologically inactive.

PHARMACOKINETICS: Absorption: C_{max}=2.4mcg/mL (50mg once weekly), 2.6mcg/mL (25mg twice weekly); T_{max}=69 hrs (single 25mg dose). **Distribution:** Found in breast milk; crosses the placenta. **Elimination:** $T_{1/2}$=102 hrs (single 25mg dose).

NURSING CONSIDERATIONS

Assessment: Assess for sepsis, active/chronic/recurrent infection, history of an opportunistic infection, recent travel in areas of endemic TB or endemic mycoses, underlying conditions that may predispose to infection, central or peripheral nervous system demyelinating disorders, CHF, history of significant hematologic abnormalities, latex sensitivity, alcoholic hepatitis, risk for skin cancer, pregnancy/nursing status, and possible drug interactions. Test for latent TB infection and for HBV infection. Assess immunization history in pediatric patients.

Monitoring: Monitor for development of infection during and after treatment. Monitor for sepsis, central or peripheral nervous system demyelinating disorders, malignancies, new or worsening CHF, hematologic abnormalities, HBV reactivation, allergic reactions, lupus-like syndrome, autoimmune hepatitis, and other adverse reactions. Periodically evaluate for TB infection. Consider periodic skin examinations for all patients at increased risk for skin cancer.

Patient Counseling: Advise of the potential risks and benefits of therapy. Inform that therapy may lower the ability of immune system to fight infections; instruct to contact physician if any symptoms of infection, TB, or HBV develop. Advise to report any signs of new/worsening medical conditions (eg, CNS demyelinating disorders, CHF, autoimmune disorders) or any symptoms suggestive of pancytopenia. Counsel about the risk of lymphoma and other malignancies. Instruct to seek immediate medical attention if any symptoms of a severe allergic reaction develop. Advise that the needle cover of prefilled syringe and the needle cover within the needle cap of the autoinjector contain dry natural rubber (a derivative of latex) that may cause allergic reactions in individuals sensitive to latex. Instruct in inj technique, as well as proper syringe and needle disposal, and caution against reuse of needles and syringes. Advise to inform physician if pregnant/breastfeeding.

Administration: SQ route. Refer to PI for preparation and administration instructions. **Storage:** 2-8°C (36-46°F). Do not shake. Protect from light or physical damage. Storage at room temperature for a max single period of 14 days is permissible, with protection from light, sources of heat, and (vial) humidity; once the product has been stored at room temperature, do not place back into the refrigerator. Discard if not used within 14 days at room temperature. Do not store in extreme heat or cold. Do not freeze. (Vial) Reconstituted Sol: Use immediately or may refrigerate for up to 14 days.

ENGERIX-B   RX
hepatitis B (recombinant) (GlaxoSmithKline)

THERAPEUTIC CLASS: Vaccine

INDICATIONS: Immunization against infection caused by all known hepatitis B virus (HBV) subtypes.

DOSAGE: *Adults:* ≥20 Yrs: Primary Immunization: 3-Dose Schedule: 1mL IM at 0, 1, 6 months. Booster: 1mL IM. Hemodialysis: Primary Immunization: 4-Dose Schedule: 2mL IM (given as a single 2-mL dose or two 1-mL doses) at 0, 1, 2, 6 months. Booster: 2mL IM when antibody levels decline <10 mIU/mL. Alternate Schedule: 1mL IM at 0, 1, 2, 12 months. Additional hepatitis B immune globulin (HBIG) should be given with known or presumed exposure to HBV.
Pediatrics: ≤19 Yrs: Primary Immunization: 3-Dose Schedule: 0.5mL IM at 0, 1, 6 months. Booster: 11-19 Yrs: 1mL IM. ≤10 Yrs: 0.5mL IM. Alternate Schedule: 11-19 Yrs: 1mL IM at 0, 1, 6 months or at 0, 1, 2, 12 months. 5-16 Yrs: 0.5mL IM at 0, 12, 24 months. ≤10 Yrs/Infants Born of Hepatitis B Surface Antigen (HBsAg)-Positive Mothers: 0.5mL IM at 0, 1, 2, 12 months. Additional HBIG should be given with known or presumed exposure to HBV.

HOW SUPPLIED: Inj: 10mcg/0.5mL, 20mcg/mL [vial, prefilled syringe]

CONTRAINDICATIONS: History of severe allergic reaction to yeast.

WARNINGS/PRECAUTIONS: Tip caps of prefilled syringes may contain natural rubber latex; allergic reactions may occur in latex-sensitive individuals. Syncope may occur and can be accompanied by transient neurological signs (eg, visual disturbance, paresthesia, tonic-clonic limb movements). Defer vaccine for infants weighing <2000g if mother is documented to be HBsAg negative at the time of infant's birth. Apnea in premature infants following IM administration observed; decisions about when to administer vaccine should be based on consideration of medical status, and the potential benefits and possible risks of vaccination. Review immunization history for possible vaccine sensitivity and previous vaccination-related adverse reactions; appropriate treatment must be available for possible anaphylactic reactions. Postpone vaccination with moderate or severe acute febrile illness unless at immediate risk of hepatitis B infection (eg, infants born of HBsAg-positive mothers). Immunocompromised persons may have a diminished immune response to vaccine. May not prevent hepatitis B infection in individuals who had an unrecognized hepatitis B infection at the time of vaccination. May not prevent infection in individuals who do not achieve protective antibody titers.

ADVERSE REACTIONS: Inj-site reactions (soreness, erythema, swelling, induration), fatigue, fever, headache, dizziness.

INTERACTIONS: May diminish immune response with immunosuppressant therapy.

PREGNANCY: Category C, caution in nursing.

MECHANISM OF ACTION: Vaccine; may produce immune response for protection against HBV infection.

NURSING CONSIDERATIONS

Assessment: Assess for hypersensitivity to yeast or latex, moderate or severe acute febrile illness, immunosuppression, unrecognized hepatitis B infection, weight of infants, pregnancy/nursing status, and for possible drug interactions. Review immunization history for possible vaccine sensitivity and previous vaccination-related adverse reactions.

Monitoring: Monitor for allergic and inj-site reactions, syncope, and other adverse reactions. Monitor immune response. Perform annual antibody testing in hemodialysis patients to assess the need for booster doses.

Patient Counseling: Inform of potential benefits/risks of immunization. Educate about potential side effects and instruct to notify physician if any side effects develop. Inform that vaccine contains noninfectious purified HBsAg and cannot cause hepatitis B infection.

Administration: IM route. Do not administer IV or intradermally. Do not administer in the gluteal region; anterolateral aspect of the thigh (<1 yr of age) and deltoid muscle (older children [whose deltoid is large enough for IM inj] and adults) is the preferred administration site. May give SQ if at risk of hemorrhage (eg, hemophiliacs). Shake well before use. Do not dilute to administer. Do not mix with any other vaccine or product in the same syringe or vial. **Storage:** 2-8°C (36-46°F). Do not freeze; discard if has been frozen.

Enjuvia

RX

conjugated estrogens (Teva)

> Estrogens increase the risk of endometrial cancer. Perform adequate diagnostic measures, including endometrial sampling, to rule out malignancy with undiagnosed persistent or recurrent abnormal vaginal bleeding. Should not be used for the prevention of cardiovascular disease (CVD) or dementia. Increased risks of myocardial infarction (MI), stroke, invasive breast cancer, pulmonary embolism (PE), and deep vein thrombosis (DVT) in postmenopausal women (50-79 yrs) reported. Increased risk of developing probable dementia in postmenopausal women ≥65 yrs reported. Should be prescribed at the lowest effective dose and for the shortest duration consistent with treatment goals and risks.

THERAPEUTIC CLASS: Estrogen

INDICATIONS: Treatment of moderate to severe vasomotor symptoms associated with menopause. Treatment of moderate to severe vaginal dryness and pain with intercourse, symptoms of vulvar and vaginal atrophy associated with menopause.

DOSAGE: *Adults:* Initial: 0.3mg qd. Adjust dose based on response. Reevaluate treatment need periodically (eg, 3- to 6-month intervals).

HOW SUPPLIED: Tab: 0.3mg, 0.45mg, 0.625mg, 0.9mg, 1.25mg

CONTRAINDICATIONS: Undiagnosed abnormal genital bleeding, known/suspected/history of breast cancer, known/suspected estrogen-dependent neoplasia, active or history of DVT/PE, active or recent arterial thromboembolic disease (eg, stroke, MI), liver dysfunction or disease, known/suspected pregnancy.

WARNINGS/PRECAUTIONS: Increased risk of CV events; d/c immediately if these occur or are suspected. Caution in patients with risk factors for arterial vascular disease and/or venous thromboembolism (VTE). If feasible, d/c at least 4-6 weeks before surgery of the type associated with an increased risk of thromboembolism, or during prolonged immobilization. May increase the risk of breast/endometrial/ovarian cancer and gallbladder disease. Consider addition of progestin for women with a uterus or with residual endometriosis posthysterectomy. May lead to severe hypercalcemia in patients with breast cancer and bone metastases; d/c and take appropriate measures if hypercalcemia occurs. Retinal vascular thrombosis reported; d/c pending examination if sudden partial/complete loss of vision, sudden onset of proptosis, diplopia, or migraine occurs. If examination reveals papilledema or retinal vascular lesions, d/c therapy permanently. May elevate BP, thyroid-binding globulin levels, plasma TGs leading to pancreatitis and other complications. Caution in patients with history of cholestatic jaundice; d/c in case of recurrence. May cause fluid retention; caution with cardiac/renal dysfunction. Caution with severe hypocalcemia. May exacerbate endometriosis, asthma, diabetes mellitus (DM), epilepsy, migraine or porphyria, systemic lupus erythematosus (SLE), and hepatic hemangiomas; use with caution. May affect certain endocrine, LFTs, and blood components in lab tests.

ADVERSE REACTIONS: Abdominal pain, flu syndrome, headache, pain, flatulence, nausea, dizziness, paresthesia, bronchitis, rhinitis, sinusitis, breast pain, dysmenorrhea, vaginitis.

INTERACTIONS: CYP3A4 inducers (eg, St. John's wort, phenobarbital, carbamazepine, rifampin) may decrease levels, which may decrease therapeutic effects and/or change uterine bleeding profile. CYP3A4 inhibitors (eg, erythromycin, clarithromycin, ketoconazole, itraconazole, ritonavir, grapefruit juice) may increase levels, which may result in side effects. Patients concomitantly receiving thyroid replacement therapy and estrogens may require increased doses of thyroid hormone.

PREGNANCY: Contraindicated in pregnancy, caution in nursing.

MECHANISM OF ACTION: Estrogen; binds to nuclear receptors in estrogen-responsive tissues. Circulating estrogens modulate pituitary secretion of the gonadotropins, luteinizing hormone and follicle-stimulating hormone, through a negative feedback mechanism. Reduces elevated levels of these hormones in postmenopausal women.

PHARMACOKINETICS: Absorption: Refer to PI for conjugated and unconjugated estrogen parameters. **Distribution:** Largely bound to sex hormone-binding globulin and albumin; found in breast milk. **Metabolism:** Liver to estrone (metabolite); estriol (major urinary metabolite); sulfate and glucuronide conjugation (liver), gut hydrolysis; CYP3A4 (partial metabolism). **Elimination:** Urine; $T_{1/2}$=14 hrs (estrone), 11 hrs (equilin).

NURSING CONSIDERATIONS

Assessment: Assess for undiagnosed abnormal genital bleeding, presence/history of breast cancer estrogen-dependent neoplasia, active/history of DVT/PE, active or recent (eg, within past yr) arterial thromboembolic disease (eg, stroke, MI), liver dysfunction/disease, pregnancy/nursing status, any other conditions where treatment is contraindicated or cautioned, need for progestin therapy, and possible drug interactions. Assess use in patient ≥65 yrs and in those with preexisting hypertriglyceridemia, history of cholestatic jaundice, presence of hypothyroidism, hypocalcemia, asthma, DM, epilepsy, migraine, porphyria, SLE, and for presence of hepatic hemangiomas.

Monitoring: Monitor for signs/symptoms of CV disorders (eg, stroke, MI), malignant neoplasms (eg, endometrial, breast/ovarian cancer), dementia, gallbladder disease, hypercalcemia, visual abnormalities, elevations in BP, fluid retention, elevations in serum TGs, pancreatitis, hypothyroidism, hypocalcemia, exacerbation of endometriosis and other conditions (eg, asthma, DM, epilepsy, migraine, SLE). Perform annual breast exam; schedule mammography based on age, risk factors, and prior mammogram results. Monitor BP, thyroid function in patients on thyroid replacement therapy, and periodically evaluate (every 3-6 months) to determine need for therapy. If undiagnosed, persistent, or recurring abnormal vaginal bleeding occurs, perform proper diagnostic testing (eg, endometrial sampling) to rule out malignancy.

Patient Counseling: Inform that therapy increases the risk for uterine cancer and may increase the chances of getting a heart attack, stroke, breast cancer, and blood clots. Advise to report breast lumps, unusual vaginal bleeding, dizziness or faintness, changes in speech, severe headaches, chest pain, SOB, leg pains, vision changes, or vomiting. Instruct to notify physician if taking other medications or if planning surgery or prolonged immobilization. Advise to have yearly breast examinations by a physician and to perform monthly breast self-examinations. Instruct to take exactly ud.

Administration: Oral route. **Storage:** 20-25°C (68-77°F).

ENTEREG   RX
alvimopan (Cubist)

> Potential risk of myocardial infarction with long-term use; for short-term hospital use only. Available only through a restricted program for short-term use (15 doses) under a Risk Evaluation and Mitigation Strategy called the Entereg Access Support and Education (E.A.S.E.) Program.

THERAPEUTIC CLASS: Opioid antagonist

INDICATIONS: To accelerate the time to upper and lower GI recovery following surgeries that include partial bowel resection with primary anastomosis.

DOSAGE: *Adults:* 12mg given 30 min to 5 hrs prior to surgery followed by 12mg bid beginning the day after surgery until discharge for a max of 7 days. Max: 15 doses.

HOW SUPPLIED: Cap: 12mg

CONTRAINDICATIONS: Patients who have taken therapeutic doses of opioids for >7 consecutive days immediately prior to therapy.

WARNINGS/PRECAUTIONS: Increased sensitivity to therapy and occurrence of GI adverse reactions (eg, abdominal pain, N/V, diarrhea) are expected with patients recently exposed to opioids; monitor patients receiving >3 doses of an opioid within the week prior to surgery for GI adverse reactions. Not recommended with severe hepatic impairment, end-stage renal disease, complete GI obstruction/surgery for correction of complete bowel obstruction, or pancreatic/gastric anastomosis. Closely monitor patients with mild-to-moderate hepatic impairment/mild-to-severe renal impairment and Japanese patients for possible adverse effects (eg, diarrhea, GI pain, cramping); d/c if adverse events occur.

ADVERSE REACTIONS: Dyspepsia.

INTERACTIONS: See Contraindications.

PREGNANCY: Category B, caution in nursing.

MECHANISM OF ACTION: Opioid antagonist; selective antagonist of μ-opioid receptor. Antagonizes the peripheral effects of opioids on GI motility and secretion by competitively binding to GI tract μ-opioid receptors.

PHARMACOKINETICS: Absorption: (Healthy) Absolute bioavailability (6%); T_{max}=2 hrs, 36 hrs (median) (metabolite); C_{max}=10.98ng/mL, 35.73ng/mL (metabolite); AUC_{0-12h}=40.2ng•hr/mL. **Distribution:** V_d=30L; plasma protein binding (80%, 94% [metabolite]). **Metabolism:** Intestinal flora; amide hydrolysis compound (active metabolite). **Elimination:** Feces, urine; $T_{1/2}$=10-17 hrs, 10-18 hrs (metabolite).

NURSING CONSIDERATIONS

Assessment: Assess for hepatic/renal impairment, complete GI obstruction/surgery for correction of complete bowel obstruction, pancreatic/gastric anastomosis, history of opioid use, and pregnancy/nursing status.

Monitoring: Monitor for GI adverse reactions, and other adverse effects.

Patient Counseling: Instruct to disclose long-term or intermittent opioid pain therapy, including any use of opioids in the week prior to receiving therapy; inform that recent use of opioids may increase susceptibility to adverse reactions, primarily those limited to the GI tract (eg, abdominal pain, N/V, diarrhea). Advise that therapy is for hospital use only for no more than 7 days after bowel resection surgery. Inform that dyspepsia may occur.

Administration: Oral route. **Storage:** 25°C (77°F); excursions permitted to 15-30°C (59-86°F).

Entocort EC   RX
budesonide (Prometheus)

THERAPEUTIC CLASS: Corticosteroid

INDICATIONS: Treatment of mild to moderate active Crohn's disease of the ileum and/or ascending colon. Maintenance of clinical remission of mild to moderate Crohn's disease of the ileum and/or ascending colon for up to 3 months.

DOSAGE: *Adults:* Usual: 9mg qd, in the am for up to 8 weeks. Recurring Episodes: Repeat therapy for 8 weeks. Maint: 6mg qd for 3 months, then taper to complete cessation. Moderate to Severe Hepatic Insufficiency/Concomitant CYP3A4 Inhibitors: Reduce dose. Swallow whole; do not chew or break.

HOW SUPPLIED: Cap: 3mg

WARNINGS/PRECAUTIONS: May reduce response of hypothalamic-pituitary-adrenal axis to stress. Supplement with systemic glucocorticosteroids if undergoing surgery or other stressful situations. Increased risk of infection; avoid exposure to varicella/varicella zoster and measles. Caution with tuberculosis (TB), HTN, diabetes mellitus (DM), osteoporosis, peptic ulcer, glaucoma, cirrhosis, cataracts, or family history of DM or glaucoma. Replacement of systemic glucocorticosteroids may unmask allergies. Chronic use may cause hypercorticism and adrenal suppression.

ADVERSE REACTIONS: Headache, respiratory infection, N/V, back pain, dyspepsia, dizziness, abdominal pain, diarrhea, flatulence, sinusitis, viral infection, arthralgia, benign intracranial HTN, signs/symptoms of hypercorticism.

INTERACTIONS: Ketoconazole caused an eight-fold increase of systemic exposure to oral budesonide. Increased levels with CYP3A4 inhibitors (eg, ketoconazole, saquinavir, erythromycin, grapefruit); monitor for increased signs and symptoms of hypercorticism and reduce budesonide dose if coadministered.

PREGNANCY: Category C, not for use in nursing.

MECHANISM OF ACTION: Glucocorticosteroid.

PHARMACOKINETICS: Absorption: C_{max}=5nmol/L; T_{max}=30-600 min; AUC=30nmol•hr/L. Bioavailability (9-21%). **Distribution:** V_d=2.2-3.9L/kg; plasma protein binding (85-90%). **Metabolism:** Liver; CYP3A4. **Elimination:** Urine (60%); $T_{1/2}$=2-3.6 hrs.

NURSING CONSIDERATIONS

Assessment: Assess for liver disease, history of chickenpox or measles, TB, HTN, osteoporosis, peptic ulcers, cataracts, history and/or family history of DM or glaucoma, and possible drug interactions. Obtain baseline LFTs.

Monitoring: Monitor LFTs periodically and for signs/symptoms of hypercorticism and hypersensitivity reactions.

Patient Counseling: Advise to swallow whole; do not chew or break. Instruct to avoid consumption of grapefruit and grapefruit juice during therapy. Caution to take particular care to avoid exposure to chickenpox or measles.

Administration: Oral route. **Storage:** 25° (77°F); excursions permitted to 15-30°C (59-86°F). Keep container tightly closed.

ENULOSE   RX
lactulose (Actavis)

OTHER BRAND NAMES: Generlac (Morton Grove)

THERAPEUTIC CLASS: Ammonium detoxicant

INDICATIONS: Prevention and treatment of portal-systemic encephalopathy, including stages of hepatic precoma and coma.

DOSAGE: *Adults:* Usual: 30-45mL tid-qid. Adjust dose every 1 or 2 days to produce 2-3 soft stools daily. May give hourly doses of 30-45mL to induce rapid laxation then reduce to usual dose after laxation achieved. Rectal Use: Reversal of Coma: Mix 300mL with 700mL of water or saline and retain for 30-60 min. May repeat q4-6h. Oral doses should be started before completely stopping enema.
Pediatrics: Older Children/Adolescents: 40-90mL/day in divided doses adjusted to produce 2-3 soft stools daily. Infants: 2.5-10mL in divided doses to produce 2-3 soft stools daily.

HOW SUPPLIED: Sol: 10g/15mL [473mL], Generlac [1892mL]

CONTRAINDICATIONS: Patients who require a low-galactose diet.

WARNINGS/PRECAUTIONS: Potential explosive reaction with electrocautery procedures during proctoscopy or colonoscopy; patients on therapy undergoing such procedures should have a thorough bowel cleansing with a non-fermentable solution. Contains galactose and lactose; caution with diabetes. May develop hyponatremia and dehydration in infants.

ADVERSE REACTIONS: Flatulence/belching, abdominal discomfort, diarrhea, N/V.

INTERACTIONS: May interfere the desired degradation and prevent the acidification of colonic contents with neomycin; closely monitor the status of the treated patients. Nonabsorbable antacids may decrease effects. Avoid use with other laxatives, especially during the initial phase of therapy.

PREGNANCY: Category B, caution in nursing.

MECHANISM OF ACTION: Osmotic laxative; bacterial degradation in the colon acidifies the colonic contents resulting in the retention of ammonia in the colon as ammonium ion; ammonia can be expected to migrate from the blood into the colon to form the ammonium ion; the acid colonic contents convert ammonia to the ammonium ion by trapping and preventing absorption; laxative action of the metabolites then expels the trapped ammonium ion from the colon.

PHARMACOKINETICS: Absorption: Poor. **Elimination:** Urine (≤3%).

NURSING CONSIDERATIONS

Assessment: Assess for diabetes, patients requiring a low-galactose diet, pregnancy/nursing status, and possible drug interactions. Assess use in electrocautery procedures during proctoscopy or colonoscopy.

Monitoring: Monitor for hyponatremia and dehydration in infants, diarrhea, vomiting, and other adverse reactions.

Patient Counseling: Inform about the risks and benefits of therapy. Instruct to take exactly ud. Advise to report any potential adverse effects.

Administration: Oral/Rectal route. **Storage:** Do not freeze. Prolonged exposure >30°C (86°F) or to direct light may cause extreme darkening and turbidity; do not use if this condition develops. Prolonged exposure to freezing temperature may cause change to a semi-solid, too viscous to pour; viscosity will return to normal upon warming to room temperature. (Enulose) 2-30°C (36-86°F). (Generlac) 20-25°C (68-77°F).

EPANED   RX
enalapril (Silvergate)

> D/C when pregnancy is detected. Drugs that act directly on the renin-angiotensin system (RAS) can cause injury/death to the developing fetus.

THERAPEUTIC CLASS: ACE inhibitor

INDICATIONS: Treatment of HTN, alone or with other antihypertensive agents (eg, thiazide-type diuretics).

DOSAGE: *Adults:* Initial: 5mg qd. Titrate: Increase dose PRN. Max: 40mg/day. Dose may be divided and administered bid if effect diminishes at the end of the dosing interval. May be administered with a low dose of diuretic if additional BP reduction is needed. Receiving Diuretics: Initial: 2.5mg/day. Moderate to Severe Renal Impairment (CrCl ≤30mL/min): Initial: 2.5mg/day. Dialysis Patients: Initial: 2.5mg/day on dialysis days. Adjust dosage on nondialysis days depending on BP response.
Pediatrics: >1 Month: Initial: 0.08mg/kg (up to 5mg) qd. Titrate: Adjust according to BP response. Max: 0.58mg/kg (or 40mg/day).

HOW SUPPLIED: Sol: 1mg/mL [150mL]

CONTRAINDICATIONS: Hereditary or idiopathic angioedema, history of ACE inhibitor-associated angioedema. Coadministration with aliskiren in patients with diabetes.

WARNINGS/PRECAUTIONS: Not recommended in neonates and in pediatric patients with GFR <30mL/min. Head/neck angioedema reported; d/c and administer appropriate therapy. Higher incidence of angioedema in blacks than nonblacks. Intestinal angioedema reported; monitor for abdominal pain. Anaphylactoid reactions reported during desensitization with hymenoptera venom, dialysis with high-flux membranes, and LDL apheresis with dextran sulfate absorption. May cause symptomatic hypotension, sometimes complicated by oliguria, progressive azotemia, acute renal failure, or death; closely monitor patients at risk of excessive hypotension (eg, those with heart failure with systolic BP <100mmHg, ischemic heart disease, cerebrovascular disease, hyponatremia, renal dialysis, or severe volume and/or salt depletion of any etiology) during first 2 weeks of therapy and whenever dose is increased. Symptomatic hypotension may occur in patients with severe aortic stenosis or hypertrophic cardiomyopathy. Hypotension may occur with major surgery or during anesthesia. Rarely, syndrome that starts with cholestatic jaundice and progresses to fulminant hepatic necrosis and (sometimes) death reported; d/c if jaundice or marked elevations of hepatic enzymes develop. May cause changes in renal function, including acute renal failure; consider withholding or discontinuing therapy if clinically significant decrease in renal function develops. May cause hyperkalemia.

ADVERSE REACTIONS: Fatigue.

INTERACTIONS: See Contraindications. Hypotension risk with high-dose diuretics. NSAIDs, including selective COX-2 inhibitors, may diminish antihypertensive effect and may cause deterioration of renal function. Dual blockade of the RAS is associated with increased risks of hypotension, hyperkalemia, and changes in renal function (including acute renal failure); closely monitor BP, renal function, and electrolytes with concomitant agents that also affect the RAS. Avoid with aliskiren in patients with renal impairment (GFR <60mL/min). Increased risk of hyperkalemia with K⁺-sparing diuretics (eg, spironolactone, triamterene, amiloride), K⁺-containing salt substitutes, or K⁺ supplements. Lithium toxicity reported; monitor serum lithium levels frequently. Nitritoid reactions reported with injectable gold.

PREGNANCY: Category D, not for use in nursing.

MECHANISM OF ACTION: ACE inhibitor; decreases plasma angiotensin II, which leads to decreased vasopressor activity and decreased aldosterone secretion.

PHARMACOKINETICS: Absorption: (Tab) T_{max}=1 hr, 3-4 hrs (enalaprilat). **Distribution:** Crosses placenta; found in breast milk. **Metabolism:** Hydrolysis to enalaprilat (active metabolite). **Elimination:** Urine and feces (94% [adults]); urine (68% [pediatric patients]). Enalaprilat: $T_{1/2}$=11 hrs (adults), 14 hrs (pediatric patients).

NURSING CONSIDERATIONS

Assessment: Assess for hereditary or idiopathic angioedema, diabetes, risk for excessive hypotension, severe aortic stenosis, hypertrophic cardiomyopathy, risk factors for hyperkalemia, renal impairment, history of ACE inhibitor-associated angioedema or hypersensitivity to drug, pregnancy/nursing status, and possible drug interactions.

Monitoring: Monitor for angioedema, anaphylactoid reactions, and other adverse reactions. Monitor BP, LFTs, renal function, and serum K⁺.

Patient Counseling: Inform about fetal risks if taken during pregnancy and discuss treatment options for women planning to become pregnant; instruct to report pregnancy to physician as soon as possible. Instruct to d/c therapy and to immediately report signs/symptoms of angioedema. Instruct to report lightheadedness, especially during the 1st few days of therapy; advise to d/c and consult with a physician if actual syncope occurs. Inform that excessive perspiration, dehydration, and other causes of volume depletion (eg, vomiting or diarrhea) may lead to an excessive fall in BP; advise to consult with physician. Advise not to use salt substitutes containing K⁺ without consulting physician.

Administration: Oral route. Refer to PI for preparation instructions. **Storage:** 25°C (77°F); excursions permitted to 15-30°C (59-86°F). Do not freeze. Protect from moisture. Discard 60 days after reconstitution.

EPIDUO

RX

benzoyl peroxide - adapalene (Galderma)

THERAPEUTIC CLASS: Antibacterial/keratolytic

INDICATIONS: Topical treatment of acne vulgaris in patients ≥9 yrs.

DOSAGE: *Adults:* Apply a thin film to affected areas of the face and/or trunk qd after washing. Use a pea-sized amount for each area of the face (eg, forehead, chin, each cheek).
Pediatrics: ≥9 Yrs: Apply a thin film to affected areas of the face and/or trunk qd after washing. Use a pea-sized amount for each area of the face (eg, forehead, chin, each cheek).

HOW SUPPLIED: Gel: (Adapalene-Benzoyl Peroxide) 0.1%-2.5% [45g]

WARNINGS/PRECAUTIONS: Not for oral, ophthalmic, or intravaginal use. Minimize exposure to sunlight and sunlamps; use sunscreen and protective apparel if exposure cannot be avoided. Exercise caution in patients with high levels of sun exposure and those with inherent sensitivity to sun. Extreme weather may cause irritation. Avoid contact with the eyes, lips, and mucous membranes. Avoid application to cuts, abrasions, eczematous, or sunburned skin. Erythema, scaling, dryness, stinging/burning, and irritant and allergic contact dermatitis may occur; depending on severity, may apply moisturizer, reduce frequency of application, or d/c use. Avoid waxing as a depilatory method on the treated skin.

ADVERSE REACTIONS: Local cutaneous reactions (eg, erythema, scaling, stinging/burning, dryness), contact dermatitis.

INTERACTIONS: Caution with concomitant topical acne therapy, especially with peeling, desquamating, or abrasive agents. Avoid with other potentially irritating topical products (medicated or abrasive soaps and cleansers, soaps and cosmetics that have strong skin-drying effect, and products with high concentrations of alcohol, astringents, spices, or limes).

PREGNANCY: Category C, caution in nursing.

MECHANISM OF ACTION: Adapalene: Naphthoic acid derivative; not established. Binds to specific retinoic acid nuclear receptors and modulates cellular differentiation, keratinization, and inflammatory processes. Benzoyl peroxide: Oxidizing agent with bactericidal and keratolytic effects.

PHARMACOKINETICS: Absorption: (Adapalene) C_{max}=0.21ng/mL; AUC_{0-24h}=1.99ng•h/mL. **Elimination:** (Adapalene) Bile. (Benzoyl peroxide) Urine.

NURSING CONSIDERATIONS

Assessment: Assess for presence of cuts, abrasions, eczematous, or sunburned skin at the treatment site. Assess for pregnancy/nursing status and possible drug interactions. Assess if patient has high levels of sun exposure or inherent sensitivity to the sun.

Monitoring: Monitor for irritation, erythema, scaling, dryness, stinging/burning, and other adverse reactions.

Patient Counseling: Advise to cleanse area with mild or soapless cleanser and to pat dry. Advise to avoid contact with the eyes, lips, and mucous membranes. Instruct not to use more than the recommended amount. Inform that drug may cause irritation and may bleach hair and colored fabric. Instruct to minimize exposure to sunlight and sunlamps. Recommend to use sunscreen products and protective apparel when exposure to sunlight cannot be avoided.

Administration: Topical route. **Storage:** 25°C (77°F); excursions permitted to 15-30°C (59-86°F). Keep tube tightly closed. Protect from light. Keep away from heat.

EPIFOAM

RX

pramoxine HCl - hydrocortisone acetate (Alaven)

THERAPEUTIC CLASS: Anesthetic/corticosteroid

INDICATIONS: Relief of the inflammatory and pruritic manifestations of corticosteroid-responsive dermatoses.

DOSAGE: *Adults:* Apply a small amount to the affected area tid-qid depending on severity of condition. May use occlusive dressings for management of psoriasis or recalcitrant conditions; d/c occlusive dressing if infection develops.
Pediatrics: Apply a small amount to the affected area tid-qid depending on severity of condition. May use occlusive dressings for management of psoriasis or recalcitrant conditions; d/c occlusive dressing if infection develops. Use least amount effective for the condition.

HOW SUPPLIED: Foam: (Hydrocortisone-Pramoxine) 1%-1% [10g]

WARNINGS/PRECAUTIONS: Not for prolonged use. D/C if redness, pain, irritation, or swelling persists. Systemic absorption may produce reversible hypothalamic-pituitary-adrenal (HPA) axis

E

suppression, manifestations of Cushing's syndrome, hyperglycemia, and glucosuria; evaluate periodically for evidence of HPA-axis suppression when large dose is applied to large surface areas or under an occlusive dressing. Withdraw treatment, reduce frequency of application, or substitute with a less potent steroid if HPA-axis suppression is noted. Application of more potent steroids, use over large surface areas, prolonged use, and the addition of occlusive dressings may augment systemic absorption. Signs and symptoms of steroid withdrawal may occur requiring supplemental systemic corticosteroids. D/C and institute appropriate therapy if irritation occurs. Use appropriate antifungal or antibacterial agent in the presence of dermatological infections; if favorable response does not occur promptly, d/c until infection is controlled. Pediatrics may be more susceptible to systemic toxicity. Chronic therapy may interfere with growth and development of pediatrics.

ADVERSE REACTIONS: Burning, itching, irritation, dryness, folliculitis, hypertrichosis, acneiform eruptions, hypopigmentation, perioral dermatitis, allergic contact dermatitis, maceration, secondary infection, skin atrophy, striae, miliaria.

PREGNANCY: Category C, caution in nursing.

MECHANISM OF ACTION: Hydrocortisone: Corticosteroid; possesses anti-inflammatory, anti-pruritic, and vasoconstrictive properties. Anti-inflammatory activity not established. Pramoxine: Local anesthetic.

PHARMACOKINETICS: Absorption: Percutaneous; inflammation, other disease processes in the skin, and occlusive dressings may increase absorption. **Distribution:** Plasma protein binding in varying degrees; found in breast milk (systemically administered). **Metabolism:** Liver. **Elimination:** Urine, feces.

NURSING CONSIDERATIONS

Assessment: Assess for previous hypersensitivity to any components of the drug, dermatological infections, and pregnancy/nursing status.

Monitoring: Monitor for signs/symptoms of reversible HPA-axis suppression, Cushing's syndrome, hyperglycemia, glucosuria, skin irritation, skin infections, systemic toxicity in pediatrics, hypersensitivity reactions, and other adverse reactions. When large dose is applied to large surface area or under occlusive dressings, monitor for HPA-axis suppression by using urinary free cortisol and adrenocorticotropic hormone stimulation tests. Monitor for signs/symptoms of steroid withdrawal following discontinuation.

Patient Counseling: Instruct to use externally and ud; instruct to avoid contact with eyes. Advise not to use for any disorder other than for which it was prescribed. Instruct not to bandage, cover, or wrap treated skin, unless directed by physician. Advise to report any signs of local adverse reactions, especially under occlusive dressing. Instruct not to use tight-fitting diapers or plastic pants on a child being treated in the diaper area, as these garments may constitute occlusive dressings.

Administration: Topical route. Shake container vigorously for 5-10 sec before each use. May also dispense a small amount to a pad and apply to affected areas. Rinse container and cap with warm water after use. Do not insert container into vagina or anus. **Storage:** 20-25°C (68-77°F). Store upright. Do not store at temperatures >120°F (49°C). Do not burn or puncture the aerosol container. Do not refrigerate.

EPIPEN RX

epinephrine (Mylan Specialty)

OTHER BRAND NAMES: EpiPen Jr. (Mylan Specialty)

THERAPEUTIC CLASS: Sympathomimetic catecholamine

INDICATIONS: Emergency treatment of allergic reactions (Type I), including anaphylaxis to stinging and biting insects, allergen immunotherapy, foods, drugs, diagnostic testing substances (eg, radiocontrast media), and other allergens, as well as idiopathic or exercise-induced anaphylaxis.

DOSAGE: *Adults:* Carefully assess each patient to determine the most appropriate dose. (EpiPen) ≥30kg: 0.3mg IM/SQ. (EpiPen Jr) 15-30kg: 0.15mg IM/SQ. Repeat injections may be necessary in patients with severe persistent anaphylaxis.
Pediatrics: Carefully assess each patient to determine the most appropriate dose. (EpiPen) ≥30kg: 0.3mg IM/SQ. (EpiPen Jr) 15-30kg: 0.15mg IM/SQ. Repeat injections may be necessary in patients with severe persistent anaphylaxis.

HOW SUPPLIED: Inj: (EpiPen Jr) 0.15mg/0.3mL, (EpiPen) 0.3mg/0.3mL

WARNINGS/PRECAUTIONS: Intended for immediate administration in patients at increased risk for anaphylaxis, including those with a history of anaphylactic reactions. Intended for immediate self-administration as emergency supportive therapy only and is not a substitute for immediate medical care. Do not inject into buttock; may not provide effective treatment of anaphylaxis. May result in loss of blood flow to the affected areas if accidentally injected into digits, hands, or feet. Not for IV use. Large doses or accidental IV use may cause cerebral hemorrhage due to sharp rise in BP; rapidly acting vasodilators can counteract this marked pressor effect. Contains sodium metabisulfite; may cause allergic-type reactions, including anaphylactic symptoms or life-threatening or less severe asthmatic episodes in certain susceptible persons. Caution in patients with heart disease, including cardiac arrhythmias, coronary artery or organic heart disease, or HTN. More than 2 sequential doses should only be administered under direct medical supervision. Higher risk of developing adverse reactions with hyperthyroidism, cardiovascular disease (CVD), HTN, diabetes mellitus (DM), in elderly, pregnant women, pediatric patients <30kg using EpiPen and <15kg using EpiPen Jr.

ADVERSE REACTIONS: Palpitations, sweating, N/V, respiratory difficulties, pallor, dizziness, weakness, tremor, headache, apprehensiveness, anxiety, restlessness.

INTERACTIONS: May precipitate/aggravate angina pectoris as well as produce ventricular arrhythmias with drugs that may sensitize the heart to arrhythmias (eg, digitalis, diuretics, quinidine). Coadministration with TCAs, MAOIs, levothyroxine sodium, and certain antihistamines, notably chlorpheniramine, tripelennamine, and diphenhydramine, may potentiate epinephrine effects. Cardiostimulating and bronchodilating effects antagonized by β-adrenergic blocking drugs (eg, propranolol). Vasoconstricting and hypertensive effects antagonized by α-adrenergic blocking drugs (eg, phentolamine). Ergot alkaloids may reverse pressor effects.

PREGNANCY: Category C, safety not known in nursing.

MECHANISM OF ACTION: Sympathomimetic catecholamine; acts on α-adrenergic receptors and lessens vasodilation and increased vascular permeability that occurs during anaphylaxis. Acts on β-adrenergic receptors, causing bronchial smooth muscle relaxation. Also alleviates pruritus, urticaria, and angioedema and may be effective in relieving GI and genitourinary symptoms associated with anaphylaxis.

NURSING CONSIDERATIONS

Assessment: Assess for risk of anaphylaxis, heart disease, HTN, DM, hyperthyroidism, pregnancy/nursing status, and for possible drug interactions.

Monitoring: Monitor for allergic-type reactions, angina pectoris, ventricular arrhythmias, cerebral hemorrhage, and for other adverse reactions. Monitor HR and BP.

Patient Counseling: Advise that therapy may produce signs and symptoms that include increased HR, sensation of more forceful heartbeat, palpitations, sweating, N/V, difficulty breathing, pallor, dizziness, weakness or shakiness, headache, apprehension, nervousness, or anxiety; advise that these signs and symptoms usually subside rapidly, especially with rest, quiet, and recumbency. Inform that more severe or persistent effects may develop if patient has HTN or hyperthyroidism. Inform that angina may be experienced if patient has coronary artery disease. Advise that patient may develop increased blood glucose levels following administration if patient has DM. Advise that a temporary worsening of symptoms may occur if patient has Parkinson's disease. Instruct to immediately go to the emergency room for further treatment of anaphylaxis and in case of accidental inj. Inform that the carrier tube is not waterproof.

Administration: IM/SQ route. Inject into the anterolateral aspect of the thigh, through clothing if necessary. **Storage:** 20-25°C (68-77°F); excursions permitted to 15-30°C (59-86°F). Store in the carrier tube provided. Protect from light. Do not refrigerate.

EPIQUIN MICRO   RX
hydroquinone (SkinMedica)

THERAPEUTIC CLASS: Depigmentation agent

INDICATIONS: Gradual treatment of UV-induced dyschromia and discoloration resulting from the use of oral contraceptives, pregnancy, hormone replacement therapy, or skin trauma.

DOSAGE: *Adults/Pediatrics:* >12 yrs: Apply to affected areas bid (am and hs) or ud.

HOW SUPPLIED: Cre: 4% [40g]

WARNINGS/PRECAUTIONS: May produce unwanted cosmetic effects if not used ud. Test for skin sensitivity prior to use; do not use if itching, vesicle formation, or excessive inflammatory response occurs. Avoid contact with eyes. D/C if no lightening effect observed after 2 months of therapy. Avoid sun exposure; use sunscreen (SPF 15 or greater) or protective clothing. Contains Na metabisulfite; may cause serious allergic reactions. D/C if blue-black darkening of the skin occurs. Limit treatment to small areas of the body at one time.

ADVERSE REACTIONS: Hypersensitivity (localized contact dermatitis).

PREGNANCY: Category C, caution in nursing.

MECHANISM OF ACTION: Depigmentation agent; produces a reversible depigmentation of the skin by inhibition of the enzymatic oxidation of tyrosine to 3-(3,4-dihydroxyphenyl) alanine (dopa) and suppresses other melanocyte metabolic processes.

NURSING CONSIDERATIONS

Assessment: Assess for drug hypersensitivity and pregnancy/nursing status.

Monitoring: Monitor for hypersensitivity reactions, blue-black darkening of the skin, and effectiveness for 2 months.

Patient Counseling: Advise to take as prescribed. Instruct to d/c and contact physician if a gradual blue-black darkening of skin occurs. Advise to avoid contact with eyes. Inform that sunscreen is essential during therapy; instruct to avoid exposure to sun and to wear protective clothing.

Administration: Topical route. **Storage:** 25°C (77°F); excursions permitted to 15-30°C (59-86°F).

EPIVIR RX
lamivudine (ViiV Healthcare)

> Lactic acidosis and severe hepatomegaly with steatosis, including fatal cases, reported with nucleoside analogues; suspend treatment if lactic acidosis or pronounced hepatotoxicity occurs. Severe acute exacerbations of hepatitis B reported in patients coinfected with hepatitis B virus (HBV) upon discontinuation of therapy; closely monitor hepatic function for at least several months. If appropriate, initiation of anti-hepatitis B therapy may be warranted. Epivir tabs and sol, used to treat HIV-1 infection, contain higher dose of lamivudine than Epivir-HBV tabs and sol, used to treat chronic HBV infection; only use appropriate dosing forms for HIV-1 treatment.

THERAPEUTIC CLASS: Nucleoside reverse transcriptase inhibitor

INDICATIONS: Treatment of HIV-1 infection in combination with other antiretrovirals.

DOSAGE: *Adults:* Usual: 150mg bid or 300mg qd. Renal Impairment (≥30kg): CrCl ≥50mL/min: 150mg bid or 300mg qd. CrCl 30-49mL/min: 150mg qd. CrCl 15-29mL/min: 150mg first dose, then 100mg qd. CrCl 5-14mL/min: 150mg first dose, then 50mg qd. CrCl <5mL/min: 50mg first dose, then 25mg qd.
Pediatrics: >16 Yrs: Usual: 150mg bid or 300mg qd. 3 Months-16 Yrs: (Sol) 4mg/kg bid. Max: 150mg bid. (Tab) ≥30kg: 1 tab (150mg) in am and pm. >21-<30kg: 1/2 tab (75mg) in am and 1 tab (150mg) in pm. 14-21kg: 1/2 tab (75mg) in am and pm. Renal Impairment (≥30kg): ≥16 Yrs: CrCl ≥50mL/min: 150mg bid or 300mg qd. CrCl 30-49mL/min: 150mg qd. CrCl 15-29mL/min: 150mg first dose, then 100mg qd. CrCl 5-14mL/min: 150mg first dose, then 50mg qd. CrCl <5mL/min: 50mg first dose, then 25mg qd. 3 Months-16 Yrs: Consider dose reduction and/or increase in dosing interval.

HOW SUPPLIED: Sol: 10mg/mL [240mL]; Tab: 150mg*, 300mg *scored

WARNINGS/PRECAUTIONS: Obesity and prolonged nucleoside exposure may be risk factors for lactic acidosis and severe hepatomegaly with steatosis. Caution with known risk factors for liver disease. Emergence of lamivudine-resistant HBV reported. Caution in pediatric patients with history of prior antiretroviral nucleoside exposure, history of pancreatitis, or other significant risk factors for development of pancreatitis; d/c if pancreatitis develops. Immune reconstitution syndrome reported. Autoimmune disorders (eg, Graves' disease, polymyositis, Guillain-Barre syndrome) reported to occur in the setting of immune reconstitution and can occur many months after initiation of treatment. Redistribution/accumulation of body fat may occur. Caution in elderly.

ADVERSE REACTIONS: Headache, malaise, fatigue, N/V, diarrhea, nasal signs/symptoms, neuropathy, insomnia, musculoskeletal pain, cough, fever, dizziness, lactic acidosis, severe hepatomegaly with steatosis.

INTERACTIONS: Avoid with other lamivudine-containing products, emtricitabine-containing products, and zalcitabine. Hepatic decompensation reported in HIV-1/hepatitis C virus coinfected patients receiving interferon-alfa with or without ribavirin; closely monitor for treatment-associated toxicities. Trimethoprim/Sulfamethoxazole may increase levels. Possible interaction with drugs whose main route of elimination is active renal secretion via the organic cationic transport system (eg, trimethoprim).

PREGNANCY: Category C, not for use in nursing.

MECHANISM OF ACTION: Nucleoside analogue; inhibits HIV-1 reverse transcriptase via DNA chain termination after incorporation of the nucleotide analogue into viral DNA.

PHARMACOKINETICS: **Absorption:** Rapid; absolute bioavailability (86% tab, 87% sol); C_{max}=1.5mcg/mL; T_{max}=0.9 hrs (fasting), 3.2 hrs (fed). **Distribution:** V_d=1.3L/kg (IV); plasma protein binding (<36%); found in breast milk. **Metabolism:** Trans-sulfoxide (metabolite). **Elimination:** Urine (71% unchanged [IV], 5.2% metabolite [PO]); $T_{1/2}$=5-7 hrs.

NURSING CONSIDERATIONS

Assessment: Assess for hepatic/renal impairment, risk factors for lactic acidosis, HIV-1 and HBV coinfection, previous hypersensitivity, pregnancy/nursing status, and possible drug interactions. In pediatric patients, assess for a history of prior antiretroviral nucleoside exposure, a history of pancreatitis, or risk factors for pancreatitis.

Monitoring: Monitor for signs/symptoms of pancreatitis, immune reconstitution syndrome (eg, opportunistic infections), autoimmune disorders, fat redistribution/accumulation, lactic acidosis, hepatomegaly with steatosis, hepatitis B exacerbation, hepatic/renal dysfunction, and hypersensitivity reactions. Monitor hepatic function closely for several months in patients with HIV/HBV coinfection who d/c therapy. Monitor CBC.

Patient Counseling: Inform that drug may rarely cause a serious condition called lactic acidosis with liver enlargement. Instruct to discuss any changes in regimen with physician. Instruct not to take concomitantly with emtricitabine- or other lamivudine-containing products. Advise parents or guardians of pediatric patients to monitor for signs and symptoms of pancreatitis. Inform that drug is not a cure for HIV-1 infection and that patient may continue to experience illnesses associated with HIV-1 infection. Inform that redistribution/accumulation of body fat may occur. Advise diabetic patients that each 15-mL dose of sol contains 3g of sucrose. Advise to avoid doing things that can spread HIV-1 to others. Inform to take all HIV medications exactly as prescribed.

Administration: Oral route. **Storage:** (Tab) 25°C (77°F); excursions permitted to 15-30°C (59-86°F). (Sol) 25°C (77°F).

EPIVIR-HBV   RX
lamivudine (GlaxoSmithKline)

> Lactic acidosis and severe hepatomegaly with steatosis, including fatal cases, reported with nucleoside analogues. Suspend treatment if lactic acidosis or pronounced hepatotoxicity occurs. Severe acute exacerbations of hepatitis B reported upon discontinuation of therapy; closely monitor hepatic function for at least several months. If appropriate, initiation of anti-hepatitis B therapy may be warranted. Not approved for treatment of HIV infection. Lamivudine dosage in Epivir-HBV is subtherapeutic and monotherapy is inappropriate for treatment of HIV infection. HIV-1 resistance may emerge in chronic hepatitis B-infected patients with unrecognized/untreated HIV infection. Offer HIV counseling and testing to all patients prior to therapy and periodically thereafter.

THERAPEUTIC CLASS: Nucleoside reverse transcriptase inhibitor

INDICATIONS: Treatment of chronic hepatitis B virus (HBV) infection associated with evidence of hepatitis B viral replication and active liver inflammation.

DOSAGE: *Adults:* Usual: 100mg qd. Renal Impairment: CrCl ≥50mL/min: 100mg qd. CrCl 30-49mL/min: 100mg 1st dose, then 50mg qd. CrCl 15-29mL/min: 100mg 1st dose, then 25mg qd. CrCl 5-14mL/min: 35mg 1st dose, then 15mg qd. CrCl <5mL/min: 35mg 1st dose, then 10mg qd. *Pediatrics:* 2-17 Yrs: 3mg/kg qd. Max: 100mg/day. Prescribe sol for patients requiring <100mg or if unable to swallow tab.

HOW SUPPLIED: Sol: 5mg/mL [240mL]; Tab: 100mg

WARNINGS/PRECAUTIONS: Consider initiation of treatment only when use of an alternative antiviral agent with a higher genetic barrier to resistance is not available/appropriate. Obesity and prolonged nucleoside exposure may be risk factors for lactic acidosis and severe hepatomegaly with steatosis. Caution with known risk factors for liver disease. Emergence of resistance-associated HBV substitutions reported; monitor ALT and HBV DNA levels if suspected. Not approved for patients dually infected with HBV and HIV. Epivir HBV contains a lower lamivudine dose than Epivir, Combivir, Epzicom, and Trizivir. If a decision is made to administer lamivudine to such coinfected patients, use the higher dosage indicated for HIV therapy as part of an appropriate combination regimen and refer to PI of such drugs. Caution in elderly patients.

ADVERSE REACTIONS: Lactic acidosis, severe hepatomegaly with steatosis, exacerbations of hepatitis B, ear/nose/throat infections, sore throat, diarrhea, serum lipase increase, CPK increase, ALT increase, thrombocytopenia.

INTERACTIONS: Avoid with other lamivudine- and emtricitabine-containing products. Possible interaction with other drugs whose main route of elimination is active renal secretion via the organic cationic transport system (eg, trimethoprim).

PREGNANCY: Category C, not for use in nursing.

MECHANISM OF ACTION: Nucleoside analogue; inhibits HBV reverse transcriptase via DNA chain termination after incorporation of the nucleotide analogue into viral DNA.

PHARMACOKINETICS: Absorption: Absolute bioavailability (86% tab, 87% sol); AUC=4.7mcg•hr/mL (repeated daily doses); C_{max}=1.28mcg/mL; T_{max}=0.5-2.0 hrs. **Distribution:** V_d=1.3L/kg (IV); plasma protein binding (<36%); found in breast milk. **Metabolism:** Trans-sulfoxide (metabolite). **Elimination:** Urine (unchanged); $T_{1/2}$=5-7 hrs.

NURSING CONSIDERATIONS

Assessment: Assess for hepatic/renal impairment, previous nucleoside exposure, risk factors for liver disease, HIV infection, hypersensitivity to drug, pregnancy/nursing status, and possible drug interactions. Perform HIV counseling and testing. Obtain baseline ALT and HBV DNA levels.

Monitoring: Monitor for renal/hepatic dysfunction, loss of therapeutic response (eg, persistent ALT elevation, increasing HBV DNA levels after an initial decline below assay limit, progression of clinical signs/symptoms of hepatic disease, worsening of hepatic necroinflammatory findings), signs/symptoms of lactic acidosis, hepatomegaly with steatosis, emergence of resistant HIV, hepatitis B exacerbation, and hypersensitivity reactions. Monitor hepatic function closely for several months in patients who d/c therapy.

Patient Counseling: Advise to remain under the care of a physician during therapy and to report any new symptoms or concurrent medications. Inform that drug is not a cure for hepatitis B and that long-term benefits and relationship of initial treatment response to outcomes (eg, hepatocellular carcinoma, decompensated cirrhosis) are unknown. Inform that liver disease deterioration may occur upon discontinuation. Instruct to discuss any changes in regimen with physician. Inform that emergence of resistant HBV and worsening of disease can occur; advise to report any new symptoms to physician. Counsel on importance of HIV testing to avoid inappropriate therapy and development of resistant HIV. Inform that drug contains a lower dose of lamivudine than Epivir, Combivir, Epzicom, and Trizivir; instruct not to take concurrently with these products. Instruct not to take concurrently with emtricitabine-containing products (eg, Atripla, Complera, Emtriva, Stribild, Truvada). Inform that therapy has not been shown to reduce the risk of HBV transmission through sexual contact/blood contamination. Instruct to avoid doing things that can spread HBV infection to others. Inform diabetics that each 20mL dose of oral sol contains 4g of sucrose.

Administration: Oral route. Take with or without food. Tab and sol may be used interchangeably; use solution for doses <100mg. **Storage:** Tab: 25°C (77°F); excursions permitted to 15-30°C (59-86°F). Sol: 20-25°C (68-77°F); store in tightly closed bottles.

EPOGEN   RX
epoetin alfa (Amgen)

> Increased risk of death, myocardial infarction (MI), stroke, venous thromboembolism (VTE), thrombosis of vascular access, and tumor progression or recurrence. Use the lowest dose sufficient to reduce/avoid the need for RBC transfusions. Chronic Kidney Disease (CKD): Greater risks for death, serious adverse cardiovascular (CV) reactions, and stroke when administered to target Hgb level >11g/dL. Cancer: Shortened overall survival and/or increased risk of tumor progression or recurrence in patients with breast, non-small cell lung, head and neck, lymphoid, and cervical cancers. Must enroll in and comply with the ESA APPRISE Oncology Program to prescribe and/or dispense drug to patients. Use only for anemia from myelosuppressive chemotherapy. Not indicated for patients receiving myelosuppressive chemotherapy when anticipated outcome is cure. D/C following completion of a chemotherapy course. Perisurgery: Due to increased risk of deep venous thrombosis (DVT), DVT prophylaxis is recommended.

THERAPEUTIC CLASS: Erythropoiesis stimulator

INDICATIONS: Treatment of anemia due to CKD, including patients on and not on dialysis; anemia due to zidovudine administered at ≤4200mg/week in HIV-infected patients with endogenous serum erythropoietin levels of ≤500 mU/mL; anemic patients with nonmyeloid malignancies where anemia is due to the effect of concomitant myelosuppressive chemotherapy, and upon initiation, there is a minimum of 2 additional months of planned chemotherapy. To reduce the need for allogeneic RBC transfusions among patients with perioperative Hgb >10-≤13g/dL who are at high risk for perioperative blood loss from elective, noncardiac, nonvascular surgery.

DOSAGE: *Adults:* CKD on Dialysis/Not on Dialysis: Initiate when Hgb is <10g/dL (see PI for additional parameters). Initial: 50-100 U/kg IV/SQ 3X weekly. IV route is recommended for hemodialysis patients. Titrate: Adjust dose based on Hgb levels; see PI. Zidovudine-Treated HIV-Infected Patients: Initial: 100 U/kg IV/SQ 3X weekly. Titrate: Adjust dose based on Hgb levels; see PI. Patients on Chemotherapy: Initiate when Hgb is <10g/dL (see PI for additional parameters). Initial: 150 U/kg SQ 3X weekly or 40,000 U SQ weekly until completion of a chemotherapy course. Titrate: Adjust dose based on Hgb levels; see PI. Surgery Patients: Usual: 300 U/kg/day SQ qd for 10 days before, on the day of, and for 4 days after surgery; or 600 U/kg SQ in 4 doses administered 21, 14, and 7 days before surgery and on the day of surgery. DVT prophylaxis is recommended. Elderly: Individualize dose selection and adjustment to achieve and maintain target Hgb.
Pediatrics: Initiate when Hgb is <10g/dL (see PI for additional parameters). 5-18 Yrs: Patients on Chemotherapy: Initial: 600 U/kg IV weekly until completion of a chemotherapy course. Titrate: Adjust dose based on Hgb levels; see PI. Max: 60,000 U weekly. 1 Month-16 Yrs: CKD on Dialysis: Initial: 50 U/kg IV/SQ 3X weekly. IV route is recommended for hemodialysis patients. Titrate: Adjust dose based on Hgb levels; see PI.

HOW SUPPLIED: Inj: 2000 U/mL, 3000 U/mL, 4000 U/mL, 10,000 U/mL, 40,000 U/mL [single-dose vial]; 10,000 U/mL [2mL], 20,000 U/mL [1mL] [multidose vial]

CONTRAINDICATIONS: Uncontrolled HTN, pure red cell aplasia (PRCA) that begins after treatment with epoetin alfa or other erythropoietin protein drugs. (Multidose Vials) Neonates, infants, pregnant women, and nursing mothers.

WARNINGS/PRECAUTIONS: Not indicated for use in patients with cancer receiving hormonal agents, biologic products, or radiotherapy, unless also receiving concomitant myelosuppressive chemotherapy; in patients scheduled for surgery who are willing to donate autologous blood; in patients undergoing cardiac/vascular surgery; or as a substitute for RBC transfusions in patients requiring immediate correction of anemia. Evaluate transferrin saturation and serum ferritin prior to and during treatment; administer supplemental iron when serum ferritin is <100mcg/L or serum transferrin saturation is <20%. Correct/exclude other causes of anemia (eg, vitamin deficiency, metabolic/chronic inflammatory conditions, bleeding) before initiating therapy. Hypertensive encephalopathy and seizures reported in patients with CKD. Appropriately control HTN prior to initiation of and during treatment; reduce/withhold therapy if BP becomes difficult to control. PRCA and severe anemia, with or without other cytopenias that arise following the development of neutralizing antibodies to erythropoietin, reported. Withhold and evaluate for neutralizing antibodies to erythropoietin if severe anemia and low reticulocyte count develop; d/c permanently if PRCA develops, and do not switch to other erythropoiesis-stimulating agents. Serious allergic reactions may occur; immediately and permanently d/c therapy. Contains albumin; may carry an extremely remote risk for transmission of viral diseases or Creutzfeldt-Jakob disease. Patients may require adjustments in their dialysis prescriptions after initiation of therapy, or require increased anticoagulation with heparin to prevent clotting of extracorporeal circuit during hemodialysis. Multidose vial contains benzyl alcohol; benzyl alcohol is associated with serious adverse events and death, particularly in pediatric patients.

ADVERSE REACTIONS: MI, stroke, VTE, thrombosis of vascular access, tumor progression/recurrence, pyrexia, N/V, HTN, cough, arthralgia, pruritus, rash, headache.

PREGNANCY: Category C, caution in nursing.

MECHANISM OF ACTION: Erythropoiesis-stimulating glycoprotein; stimulates erythropoiesis by the same mechanism as endogenous erythropoietin.

PHARMACOKINETICS: Absorption: Adults and Pediatrics with CKD: (SQ) T_{max}=5-24 hrs. Anemic Cancer Patients: (SQ) T_{max}=13.3 hrs (150 U/kg 3X weekly), 38 hrs (40,000 U weekly). **Elimination:** Adults and Pediatrics with CKD: (IV) $T_{1/2}$=4-13 hrs. Anemic Cancer Patients: (SQ) $T_{1/2}$=16-67 hrs.

NURSING CONSIDERATIONS

Assessment: Assess for uncontrolled HTN, previous hypersensitivity to the drug, causes of anemia, pregnancy/nursing status, and other conditions where treatment is contraindicated or cautioned. Obtain baseline Hgb levels, transferrin saturation, and serum ferritin.

Monitoring: Monitor for signs/symptoms of an allergic reaction, CV/thromboembolic events, stroke, premonitory neurologic symptoms, PRCA, severe anemia, progression/recurrence of tumor, and other adverse reactions. Monitor BP, transferrin saturation, and serum ferritin. Following initiation of therapy and after each dose adjustment, monitor Hgb weekly until Hgb is stable and sufficient to minimize need for RBC transfusion.

Patient Counseling: Inform of the risks and benefits of therapy, and of the increased risks of mortality, serious CV reactions, thromboembolic reactions, stroke, and tumor progression. Advise of the need to have regular lab tests for Hgb. Inform cancer patients that they must sign the patient-physician acknowledgment form prior to therapy. Instruct to undergo regular BP monitoring, adhere to prescribed antihypertensive regimen, and follow recommended dietary restrictions. Advise to contact physician for new-onset neurologic symptoms or change in seizure frequency. Instruct regarding proper disposal and caution against reuse of needles, syringes, or unused portions of single-dose vials.

Administration: IV/SQ route. IV route is recommended for hemodialysis patients. Do not shake. Do not dilute. Do not mix with other drug sol; refer to PI for admixing exceptions and for further preparation and administration instructions. **Storage:** 2-8°C (36-46°F). Do not freeze; do not use if it has been frozen. Protect from light. Discard unused portions of multidose vials 21 days after initial entry.

EPZICOM RX

abacavir sulfate - lamivudine (ViiV Healthcare)

> Lactic acidosis and severe hepatomegaly with steatosis, including fatal cases, reported with nucleoside analogues. Abacavir: Serious and sometimes fatal hypersensitivity reactions (multiorgan clinical syndrome) reported; d/c as soon as suspected and never restart therapy with any abacavir-containing product. Patients with HLA-B*5701 allele are at high risk for hypersensitivity; screen for HLA-B*5701 allele prior to therapy. Lamivudine: Severe acute exacerbations of hepatitis B reported in patients coinfected with hepatitis B virus (HBV) upon discontinuation of therapy; closely monitor hepatic function for at least several months. If appropriate, initiation of anti-hepatitis B therapy may be warranted.

THERAPEUTIC CLASS: Nucleoside reverse transcriptase inhibitor

INDICATIONS: Treatment of HIV-1 infection in combination with other antiretrovirals.

DOSAGE: *Adults:* CrCl ≥50mL/min: 1 tab qd.

HOW SUPPLIED: Tab: (Abacavir Sulfate-Lamivudine) 600mg-300mg

CONTRAINDICATIONS: Hepatic impairment.

WARNINGS/PRECAUTIONS: Obesity and prolonged nucleoside exposure may be risk factors for lactic acidosis and severe hepatomegaly with steatosis. Caution with known risk factors for liver disease; suspend therapy if clinical or lab findings suggestive of lactic acidosis or pronounced hepatotoxicity develop. Immune reconstitution syndrome reported. Autoimmune disorders (eg, Graves' disease, polymyositis, Guillain-Barre syndrome) reported to occur in the setting of immune reconstitution and can occur many months after initiation of treatment. Redistribution/accumulation of body fat may occur. Cross-resistance potential with nucleoside reverse transcriptase inhibitors reported. Not recommended with renal impairment (CrCl <50mL/min). Caution in elderly. Abacavir: Increased risk of myocardial infarction (MI) reported; consider the underlying risk of coronary heart disease when prescribing therapy. Lamivudine: Emergence of lamivudine-resistant HBV reported.

ADVERSE REACTIONS: Lactic acidosis, severe hepatomegaly with steatosis, hypersensitivity, insomnia, depression/depressed mood, headache/migraine, fatigue/malaise, dizziness/vertigo, nausea, diarrhea, rash, pyrexia.

INTERACTIONS: Avoid with other abacavir-, lamivudine-, and/or emtricitabine-containing products. Abacavir: Ethanol may decrease elimination causing an increase in overall exposure. May increase PO methadone clearance. Lamivudine: Hepatic decompensation may occur in HIV-1/hepatitis C virus (HCV) coinfected patients receiving interferon-alfa with or without ribavirin; closely monitor for treatment-associated toxicities. Trimethoprim/sulfamethoxazole and nelfinavir may increase levels.

PREGNANCY: Category C, not for use in nursing.

MECHANISM OF ACTION: Abacavir: Carbocyclic nucleoside analogue; inhibits HIV-1 reverse transcriptase (RT) activity by competing with natural substrate dGTP and incorporating into viral DNA. Lamivudine: Nucleoside analogue; inhibits RT via DNA chain termination after incorporation of the nucleotide analogue.

PHARMACOKINETICS: Absorption: Rapid. Abacavir: Bioavailability (86%), C_{max}=4.26mcg/mL, AUC=11.95mcg•hr/mL. Lamivudine: Bioavailability (86%), C_{max}=2.04mcg/mL, AUC=8.87mcg•hr/mL. **Distribution:** Abacavir: V_d=0.86L/kg; plasma protein binding (50%). Lamivudine: V_d=1.3L/kg; found in breast milk. **Metabolism:** Abacavir: Via alcohol dehydrogenase and glucuronyl transferase; 5'-carboxylic acid, 5'-glucuronide (metabolites). Lamivudine: Trans-sulfoxide (metabolite). **Elimination:** Abacavir: $T_{1/2}$=1.45 hrs. Lamivudine: Urine (70%, unchanged) (IV); $T_{1/2}$=5-7 hrs.

NURSING CONSIDERATIONS

Assessment: Assess medical history for prior exposure to any abacavir-containing product. Assess for HBV infection, history of hypersensitivity reactions, HLA-B*5701 status, hepatic/renal impairment, risk factors for coronary heart disease and lactic acidosis, pregnancy/nursing status, and possible drug interactions.

Monitoring: Monitor for signs/symptoms of hypersensitivity reactions, lactic acidosis, hepatomegaly with steatosis, immune reconstitution syndrome (eg, opportunistic infections), autoimmune disorders, fat redistribution/accumulation, and MI. Monitor hepatic and renal function. Closely monitor hepatic function for several months after discontinuing therapy.

Patient Counseling: Inform patients regarding hypersensitivity reactions with abacavir; instruct to contact physician immediately if symptoms develop and not to restart or replace with any other abacavir-containing products without medical consultation. Inform that the drug may cause lactic acidosis with liver enlargement (hepatomegaly). Inform patients coinfected with HIV-1 and HBV that deterioration of liver disease has occurred in some cases when treatment with lamivudine was discontinued; instruct to discuss any changes of regimen with the physician. Inform that hepatic decompensation has occurred in HIV-1/HCV coinfected patients with interferon alfa with or without ribavirin. Inform that redistribution/accumulation of body fat may occur. Advise that drug is not a cure for HIV-1 infection and that illnesses associated with HIV-1 may still be experienced. Advise to avoid doing things that can spread HIV-1 to others (eg, sharing needles/inj equipment/personal items that can have blood or body fluids on them, having sex without protection, breastfeeding). Inform patients to take all HIV medications exactly as prescribed.

Administration: Oral route. **Storage:** 25°C (77°F); excursions permitted to 15-30°C (59-86°F).

EQUETRO

carbamazepine (Validus)

RX

> Serious and fatal dermatologic reactions, including toxic epidermal necrolysis (TEN) and Stevens-Johnson syndrome (SJS) reported; increased risk with presence of HLA-B*1502 allele. Screen patients with ancestry in genetically at risk populations for the presence of HLA-B*1502 prior to initiation of therapy. Avoid in patients testing positive for the allele unless the benefit clearly outweighs the risk. D/C therapy if serious dermatologic reaction is suspected. Aplastic anemia and agranulocytosis reported; obtain CBC prior to treatment, and monitor periodically. Consider discontinuing therapy if significant bone marrow depression develops.

THERAPEUTIC CLASS: Carboxamide

INDICATIONS: Treatment of acute manic or mixed episodes associated with bipolar I disorder.

DOSAGE: *Adults:* Initial: 200mg bid. Titrate: May be increased by 200mg/day to achieve optimal clinical response. Max: 1600mg/day. When discontinuing treatment, reduce dose gradually and avoid abrupt discontinuation. Elderly: Start at lower end of dosing range.

HOW SUPPLIED: Cap, Extended-Release: 100mg, 200mg, 300mg

CONTRAINDICATIONS: Bone marrow depression, hypersensitivity to TCAs (eg, amitriptyline, desipramine, imipramine, protriptyline, and nortriptyline), coadministration with delavirdine or other non-nucleoside reverse transcriptase inhibitors (NNRTIs), nefazodone. Concomitant use of an MAOI or within 14 days after discontinuing an MAOI.

WARNINGS/PRECAUTIONS: Periodically reevaluate long-term risks and benefits of the drug if used for extended periods. Do not resume treatment if signs/symptoms suggest SJS/TEN. Drug reaction with eosinophilia and systemic symptoms (DRESS), also known as multiorgan hypersensitivity reported; evaluate and d/c therapy if an alternative etiology cannot be established. Hypersensitivity reactions reported. Increased risk of suicidal thoughts or behavior reported. May cause fetal harm. Avoid abrupt discontinuation, especially in patients with seizure disorder; may increase risk of developing seizure and status epilepticus with attendant hypoxia and threat to life. Hyponatremia may occur; consider discontinuing in patients with symptomatic hyponatremia. May impair mental/physical abilities. Avoid in patients with history of hepatic porphyria. Has mild anticholinergic activity; assess intraocular pressure (IOP) prior to therapy and periodically thereafter in patients with history of increased IOP. Consider reducing dose in patients with hepatic impairment. Caution in elderly patients.

ADVERSE REACTIONS: Dizziness, somnolence, N/V, ataxia, constipation, pruritus, dry mouth, rash, blurred vision, speech disorder, HTN, agranulocytosis, aplastic anemia, TEN, SJS.

INTERACTIONS: See Contraindications. CYP3A4 and/or epoxide hydrolase inhibitors (eg, acetazolamide, cimetidine, clarithromycin, protease inhibitors, valproate) may increase plasma levels. CYP3A4 inducers (eg, cisplatin, phenobarbital, rifampin, theophylline) may decrease plasma levels. May decrease levels of CYP1A2 and CYP3A4 substrates (eg, acetaminophen, bupropion, clonazepam, doxycycline). May increase plasma levels of clomipramine and primidone. May increase/decrease phenytoin plasma levels. May cause contraceptive failure or breakthrough bleeding with oral contraceptives. May reduce anticoagulant effect of warfarin. May increase risk of neurotoxic adverse reactions with lithium. Antimalarial drugs (eg, chloroquine, mefloquine) may antagonize carbamazepine activity. May increase risk of respiratory depression, profound sedation, hypotension, and syncope with other CNS depressants (eg, alcohol, opioid analgesics, benzodiazepines).

PREGNANCY: Category D, not for use in nursing.

MECHANISM OF ACTION: Carboxamide; not established. Modulates Na^+ and Ca^{2+} ion channels, receptor-mediated neurotransmitters, and intracellular signaling pathways in experimental preparations.

PHARMACOKINETICS: Absorption: C_{max}=1.9mcg/mL (single 200mg dose), 11mcg/mL (multiple 800mg dose), 3.2mcg/mL (400mg dose, fasted), 4.3mcg/mL (400mg dose, fed); T_{max}=19 hrs (single 200mg dose), 5.9 hrs (multiple 800mg dose), 24 hrs (400mg dose, fasted), 14 hrs (400mg dose, fed). **Distribution:** Plasma protein binding (76%); crosses placenta; found in breast milk. **Metabolism:** Liver via CYP3A4; carbamazepine-10,11-epoxide (metabolite). **Elimination:** Urine (72%; 3% unchanged), feces (28%); $T_{1/2}$=35-40 hrs (single dose), 12-17 hrs (multiple doses).

NURSING CONSIDERATIONS

Assessment: Assess for conditions where treatment is contraindicated or cautioned, pregnancy/nursing status, and possible drug interactions. Screen for HLA-B*1502 allele in suspected population. Obtain CBC, including platelets and differential counts. Assess IOP in patients with increased IOP.

Monitoring: Monitor for dermatological reactions, aplastic anemia, agranulocytosis, bone marrow depression, DRESS, emergence/worsening of depression, suicidal thoughts/behavior, unusual mood/behavior changes, seizures, or hyponatremia. Monitor CBC periodically. Closely monitor patients who exhibit low or decreased WBC or platelet count. Periodically monitor IOP in patients with increased IOP.

Patient Counseling: Inform to take drug as prescribed and to read Medication Guide. Inform about the risk of potentially fatal, serious skin reactions, agranulocytosis, and aplastic anemia; instruct to report immediately if signs and symptoms occur. Inform of the early toxic signs and symptoms of potential hematologic, dermatologic, hypersensitivity, or hepatic reactions. Counsel about the increased risk of suicidal thinking and behavior; advise to report behaviors of concern immediately. Advise women of childbearing potential that drug may cause fetal harm. Advise to notify physician if pregnant or planning to get pregnant; encourage patients to enroll in the North American Antiepileptic Drug Pregnancy Registry. Inform that abrupt discontinuation can cause seizures or an increase in seizure frequency; advise that the drug should be tapered when discontinued. Advise that drug may reduce serum Na$^+$ concentrations, especially if patient is taking other medications that lower Na$^+$; report symptoms of low Na$^+$. Advise to observe caution when operating machinery/automobiles or potentially dangerous tasks. Advise to exercise caution if taking alcohol. Inform to not take with delavirdine, NNRTIs, and any other medications containing carbamazepine.

Administration: Oral route. May take orally, or may open and sprinkle beads over food such as a tsp of applesauce. Do not crush or chew. Take with or without meals. **Storage:** 25°C (77°F); excursions permitted to 15-30°C (59-86°F). Protect from light and moisture.

ERAXIS   RX
anidulafungin (Pfizer)

THERAPEUTIC CLASS: Echinocandin

INDICATIONS: Treatment of candidemia and other forms of *Candida* infections (intra-abdominal abscess and peritonitis) and esophageal candidiasis.

DOSAGE: *Adults:* Rate of IV infusion should not exceed 1.1mg/min. Candidemia/Other *Candida* Infections (Intra-Abdominal Abscess and Peritonitis): Usual: 200mg LD on Day 1, followed by 100mg/day thereafter. Continue for at least 14 days after last positive culture. Esophageal Candidiasis: Usual: 100mg LD on Day 1, followed by 50mg/day thereafter. Treat for a minimum of 14 days and for at least 7 days following resolution of symptoms. Consider suppressive antifungal therapy after a course of treatment in patients with HIV infections, due to risk of relapse. *Pediatrics:* >16 Yrs: Rate of IV infusion should not exceed 1.1mg/min. Candidemia/Other *Candida* Infections (Intra-Abdominal Abscess and Peritonitis): Usual: 200mg LD on Day 1, followed by 100mg/day thereafter. Continue for at least 14 days after last positive culture. Esophageal Candidiasis: Usual: 100mg LD on Day 1, followed by 50mg/day thereafter. Treat for a minimum of 14 days and for at least 7 days following resolution of symptoms. Consider suppressive antifungal therapy after a course of treatment in patients with HIV infections, due to risk of relapse.

HOW SUPPLIED: Inj: 50mg, 100mg

WARNINGS/PRECAUTIONS: LFTs abnormalities reported; monitor for worsening of hepatic function and evaluate for risk/benefit of continuing therapy. Isolated cases of significant hepatic dysfunction, hepatitis, or hepatic failure reported. Anaphylactic reactions (eg, shock) reported; d/c and administer appropriate treatment if any occur. Infusion-related reactions (eg, rash, urticaria, flushing, pruritus, bronchospasm, dyspnea, hypotension), possibly histamine-mediated, reported; do not exceed the infusion rate of 1.1mg/min.

ADVERSE REACTIONS: Diarrhea, hypokalemia, pyrexia, bacteremia, N/V, hypotension, insomnia, urinary tract infection, dyspnea, HTN, hypomagnesemia, increased blood alkaline phosphatase, peripheral edema, pleural effusion.

INTERACTIONS: Significant hepatic abnormalities reported with multiple concomitant medications in patients with serious underlying medical conditions. Increased levels with cyclosporine.

PREGNANCY: Category B, caution in nursing.

MECHANISM OF ACTION: Echinocandin; inhibits glucan synthase, which results in inhibition of the formation of 1,3-β-D-glucan, an essential component of fungal cell walls.

PHARMACOKINETICS: Absorption: Administration of variable doses resulted in different parameters. **Distribution:** V_d=30-50L; plasma protein binding (>99%). **Elimination:** Urine (<1%), feces (30%, <10% intact drug); $T_{1/2}$=40-50 hrs.

NURSING CONSIDERATIONS

Assessment: Assess for hypersensitivity to the drug or other echinocandins, serious underlying medical conditions, hepatic function, pregnancy/nursing status, and possible drug interactions. Obtain specimens for fungal culture and other relevant lab studies (eg, histopathology) prior to therapy.

Monitoring: Monitor for hepatic dysfunction, hepatitis or hepatic failure, anaphylactic reactions, infusion-related reactions, and other adverse reactions. Monitor LFTs.

Patient Counseling: Inform about the risk of developing abnormal LFTs and/or hepatic dysfunction; advise that LFTs may be monitored during treatment. Inform that physician may d/c treatment if anaphylactic reactions (eg, shock) occur. Instruct to report to physician any symptoms of infusion-related reactions. Advise to notify physician if pregnant, intend to become pregnant, or plan to breastfeed during therapy.

Administration: IV route. Refer to PI for preparation for administration. **Storage:** 2-8°C (36-46°F); excursions permitted up to 25°C (77°F) for 96 hrs and can be returned to storage at 2-8°C (36-46°F). Do not freeze. Reconstituted: Up to 25°C (77°F) for up to 24 hrs. Infusion Sol: Up to 25°C (77°F) for up to 48 hrs or stored frozen for at least 72 hrs.

ERBITUX   RX
cetuximab (Bristol-Myers Squibb)

> Serious infusion reactions, some fatal, reported; immediately interrupt and permanently d/c infusion if these reactions occur. Cardiopulmonary arrest and/or sudden death occurred in patients with squamous cell carcinoma of the head and neck (SCCHN) treated with cetuximab in combination with radiation therapy or with European Union (EU)-approved cetuximab in combination with platinum-based therapy with 5-fluorouracil (5-FU); closely monitor serum electrolytes during and after therapy.

THERAPEUTIC CLASS: Epidermal growth factor receptor (EGFR) antagonist

INDICATIONS: In combination with radiation therapy for the initial treatment of locally/regionally advanced SCCHN. In combination with platinum-based therapy with 5-FU for the 1st-line treatment of recurrent locoregional disease/metastatic SCCHN. As monotherapy for treatment of patients with recurrent/metastatic SCCHN for whom prior platinum-based therapy has failed. Treatment of *KRAS* mutation negative (wild-type), EGFR-expressing, metastatic colorectal cancer in combination with FOLFIRI (irinotecan, 5-FU, leucovorin) for 1st-line treatment, in combination with irinotecan in patients who are refractory to irinotecan-based chemotherapy, and as monotherapy in patients who have failed oxaliplatin- and irinotecan-based chemotherapy or are intolerant to irinotecan.

DOSAGE: *Adults:* Premedication: H$_1$-antagonist (eg, 50mg diphenhydramine) IV 30-60 min prior to 1st dose; premedication for subsequent doses should be based on clinical judgment and presence/severity of prior infusion reactions. Max Infusion Rate: 10mg/min. SCCHN (with Radiation Therapy/Platinum-Based Therapy with 5-FU): Initial: 400mg/m^2 IV over 120 min, 1 week prior to initiation of a course of radiation therapy or on the day of initiation of platinum-based therapy with 5-FU. Complete administration 1 hr prior to platinum-based therapy with 5-FU. Maint: 250mg/m^2 IV over 60 min weekly for duration of radiation therapy (6-7 weeks) or until disease progression or unacceptable toxicity with platinum-based therapy with 5-FU. Complete administration 1 hr prior to radiation therapy/platinum-based therapy with 5-FU. SCCHN (Monotherapy)/Colorectal Cancer (Monotherapy/with Irinotecan or FOLFIRI): Initial: 400mg/m^2 IV over 120 min. Complete administration 1 hr prior to FOLFIRI. Maint: 250mg/m^2 IV over 60 min weekly until disease progression or unacceptable toxicity. Complete administration 1 hr prior to FOLFIRI. Dose Modifications Due to Infusion Reactions/Dermatologic Toxicity: Refer to PI.

HOW SUPPLIED: Inj: 2mg/mL [50mL, 100mL, vial]

WARNINGS/PRECAUTIONS: Monitor patients for 1 hr following infusions in a setting with resuscitation equipment and other agents necessary to treat anaphylaxis; monitor longer to confirm resolution of the event in patients requiring treatment for infusion reactions. Caution when used in combination with radiation therapy or platinum-based therapy with 5-FU in head and neck cancer patients with history of coronary artery disease (CAD), congestive heart failure (CHF), or arrhythmias. Interstitial lung disease (ILD) reported; interrupt for acute onset or worsening of pulmonary symptoms and permanently d/c if ILD is confirmed. Dermatologic toxicities (eg, acneiform rash, skin drying/fissuring, paronychial inflammation, infectious sequelae, hypertrichosis) reported; monitor for dermatologic toxicities and infectious sequelae; limit sun exposure during therapy. Addition of cetuximab to radiation and cisplatin in patients reported to increase incidence of Grade 3-4 mucositis, radiation recall syndrome, acneiform rash, cardiac events, and electrolyte disturbances compared to radiation and cisplatin alone; addition of cetuximab did not improve progression-free survival. Hypomagnesemia and electrolyte abnormalities reported; periodically monitor for hypomagnesemia, hypocalcemia, and hypokalemia, during and for at least 8 weeks following completion of therapy; replete electrolytes as necessary. Determine

KRAS mutation and EGFR-expression status in colorectal tumors using FDA-approved tests prior to treatment. Not effective for the treatment of *KRAS* mutation-positive colorectal cancer.

ADVERSE REACTIONS: Cutaneous reactions (eg, rash, pruritus, nail changes), headache, diarrhea, infection, infusion reactions, cardiopulmonary arrest, dermatologic toxicity, radiation dermatitis, sepsis, renal failure, ILD, pulmonary embolus.

PREGNANCY: Category C, not for use in nursing.

MECHANISM OF ACTION: EGFR antagonist (human/mouse chimeric monoclonal antibody); binds specifically to EGFR on both normal and tumor cells and competitively inhibits the binding of epidermal growth factor and other ligands, such as transforming growth factor-α.

PHARMACOKINETICS: Absorption: C_{max}=168-235mcg/mL. **Distribution:** V_d=2-3L/m²; may cross the placenta. **Elimination:** $T_{1/2}$=112 hrs.

NURSING CONSIDERATIONS

Assessment: Assess for history of CAD, CHF, arrhythmias, pulmonary disorders, pregnancy/nursing status, and possible drug interactions. Obtain serum electrolyte levels (Mg^{+2}, K^+, Ca^+). Determine *KRAS* mutation and EGFR-expression status in colorectal tumors using FDA-approved tests.

Monitoring: Monitor for signs/symptoms of infusion reactions, cardiopulmonary arrest, acute onset or worsening of pulmonary symptoms, dermatologic toxicities and infectious sequelae, and for other adverse reactions. Monitor patients for 1 hr after infusion, and for a longer period to confirm resolution of the event in patients requiring treatment for infusion reactions. Periodically monitor for hypomagnesemia, hypocalcemia, and hypokalemia during and for at least 8 weeks after therapy.

Patient Counseling: Advise to report to physician signs/symptoms of infusion reactions (eg, fever, chills, breathing problems). Inform of pregnancy/nursing risks; advise to use adequate contraception during and for 6 months after last dose for both males and females. Inform that nursing is not recommended during and for 2 months following last dose of therapy. Instruct to limit sun exposure (eg, use of sunscreen, wear hats) during and for 2 months after last dose of therapy.

Administration: IV route. Do not administer as IV push or bolus. Administer via infusion pump or syringe pump. Administer through low protein binding 0.22-μm in-line filter. Do not shake or dilute. **Storage:** Vials: 2-8°C (36-46°F). Do not freeze. Infusion Containers: Stable for up to 12 hrs at 2-8°C (36-46°F) and up to 8 hrs at 20-25°C (68-77°F). Discard unused portion of vial.

ERIVEDGE   RX
vismodegib (Genentech)

> May result in embryo-fetal death or severe birth defects. Verify pregnancy status prior to initiation of therapy. Advise male and female patients of these risks. Advise female patients of the need for contraception and advise male patients of the potential risk of exposure through semen.

THERAPEUTIC CLASS: Hedgehog pathway inhibitor

INDICATIONS: Treatment of adults with metastatic basal cell carcinoma, or with locally advanced basal cell carcinoma that has recurred following surgery or who are not candidates for surgery, and who are not candidates for radiation.

DOSAGE: *Adults:* 150mg qd until disease progression or until unacceptable toxicity.

HOW SUPPLIED: Cap: 150mg

WARNINGS/PRECAUTIONS: Do not donate blood or blood products while on therapy and for at least 7 months after the last dose.

ADVERSE REACTIONS: Muscle spasm, alopecia, dysgeusia, weight loss, fatigue, N/V, diarrhea, decreased appetite, constipation, arthralgia, ageusia.

INTERACTIONS: P-glycoprotein inhibitors (eg, clarithromycin, erythromycin, azithromycin) may increase systemic exposure and incidence of adverse events. Drugs that alter upper GI tract pH (eg, proton pump inhibitors, H_2-receptor antagonists, antacids) may alter solubility and reduce bioavailability.

PREGNANCY: Category D, not for use in nursing.

MECHANISM OF ACTION: Hedgehog pathway inhibitor; binds to and inhibits Smoothened, a transmembrane protein involved in Hedgehog signal transduction.

PHARMACOKINETICS: Absorption: Absolute bioavailability (31.8%). **Distribution:** V_d=16.4-26.6L; plasma protein binding (>99%). **Metabolism:** Oxidation, glucuronidation, and pyridine ring cleavage. **Elimination:** Feces (82%), urine (4.4%); $T_{1/2}$=4 days (continuous qd dosing), 12 days (single dose).

NURSING CONSIDERATIONS

Assessment: Assess pregnancy/nursing status, and for possible drug interactions.

Monitoring: Monitor for disease progression, toxicities, and other adverse reactions.

Patient Counseling: Inform that drug may cause embryo-fetal death or severe birth defects; instruct female patients of reproductive potential to use a highly effective form of contraception while on therapy and for at least 7 months after the last dose. Instruct male patients, even those with prior vasectomy, to use condoms with spermicide during sexual intercourse with female partners while on therapy and for at least 2 months after the last dose. Instruct to immediately contact physician if pregnancy occurs or is suspected following exposure to drug. Instruct to immediately report any pregnancy exposure to drug and encourage participation in the Erivedge pregnancy pharmacovigilance program. Inform female patients of the potential for serious adverse reactions in nursing infants. Advise not to donate blood or blood products while on therapy and for at least 7 months after the last dose.

Administration: Oral route. Take with or without food. Swallow caps whole; do not open or crush. **Storage:** 20-25°C (68-77°F); excursions permitted between 15-30°C (59-86°F).

ERY-TAB   RX
erythromycin (Arbor)

THERAPEUTIC CLASS: Macrolide

INDICATIONS: Treatment of mild to moderate upper/lower respiratory tract and skin and skin structure infections, listeriosis, pertussis, respiratory tract infections (*Mycoplasma pneumoniae*), diphtheria, erythrasma, intestinal amebiasis, acute pelvic inflammatory disease (PID) (*Neisseria gonorrhoeae*), primary syphilis (if penicillin [PCN]-allergic), chlamydial infections (eg, newborn conjunctivitis, pneumonia of infancy, urogenital infections during pregnancy, or urethral, endo-cervical, or rectal infections in adults when tetracyclines are contraindicated or not tolerated), nongonococcal urethritis (*Ureaplasma urealyticum*) when tetracyclines are contraindicated or not tolerated, and Legionnaires' disease caused by susceptible strains of microorganisms. Prophylaxis of initial attacks of rheumatic fever in PCN-allergic patients or recurrent attacks of rheumatic fever in PCN- and sulfonamide-allergic patients.

DOSAGE: *Adults:* Administer in the fasting state (at least 1/2 hr and preferably 2 hrs ac). Mild to Moderate Infections: Usual: 250mg q6h, 333mg q8h, or 500mg q12h. May increase up to 4g/day according to severity of infection. Do not take bid when dose is >1g/day. Streptococcal Upper Respiratory Tract Infections (URTIs) (eg, Tonsillitis, Pharyngitis): Treat for ≥10 days. Prophylaxis of Streptococcal URTIs for Prevention of Recurrent Attacks of Rheumatic Fever: 250mg bid. Urogenital Infections During Pregnancy: 500mg qid or two 333mg tabs q8h on an empty stom-ach for ≥7 days. If intolerable, reduce to 500mg q12h, 333mg q8h, or 250mg qid for ≥14 days. Uncomplicated Urethral/Endocervical/Rectal Infections and Nongonococcal Urethritis: 500mg qid or two 333mg tabs q8h for ≥7 days. Primary Syphilis: 30-40g in divided doses for 10-15 days. Acute PID: 500mg (erythromycin lactobionate) IV q6h for 3 days followed by 500mg PO q12h or 333mg PO q8h for 7 days. Intestinal Amebiasis: 500mg q12h, 333mg q8h, or 250mg q6h for 10-14 days. Pertussis: 40-50mg/kg/day in divided doses for 5-14 days. Legionnaires' Disease: 1-4g/day in divided doses. Preoperative Prophylaxis for Elective Colorectal Surgery: Refer to PI. *Pediatrics:* Administer in the fasting state (at least 1/2 hr and preferably 2 hrs ac). Mild to Moderate Infections: Usual: 30-50mg/kg/day in equally divided doses. Severe Infections: May double dose. Max: 4g/day. Streptococcal URTIs (eg, Tonsillitis, Pharyngitis): Treat for ≥10 days. Prophylaxis of Streptococcal URTIs for Prevention of Recurrent Attacks of Rheumatic Fever: 250mg bid. Conjunctivitis of Newborns and Pneumonia of Infancy: (Sus) 50mg/kg/day in 4 divided doses for ≥2 weeks and ≥3 weeks, respectively. Intestinal Amebiasis: 30-50mg/kg/day in divided doses for 10-14 days. Pertussis: 40-50mg/kg/day in divided doses for 5-14 days.

HOW SUPPLIED: Tab, Delayed-Release: 250mg, 333mg, 500mg

CONTRAINDICATIONS: Concomitant use of terfenadine, astemizole, cisapride, pimozide, ergot-amine, or dihydroergotamine.

WARNINGS/PRECAUTIONS: Hepatic dysfunction, including increased LFTs, and hepatocel-lular and/or cholestatic hepatitis, with or without jaundice, reported; caution with impaired hepatic function. Associated with QT interval prolongation and arrhythmia (infrequent); cases of torsades de pointes reported. Avoid with known QT interval prolongation and with ongoing proarrhythmic conditions (eg, uncorrected hypokalemia/hypomagnesemia, clinically significant bradycardia). Cardiovascular malformations reported when used during early pregnancy. Infants born to women treated during pregnancy for early syphilis should be treated with an appropri-ate PCN regimen. *Clostridium difficile*-associated diarrhea (CDAD) reported; d/c if CDAD is suspected or confirmed. Use in the absence of a proven or strongly suspected bacterial infection or prophylactic indication is unlikely to provide benefit and increases the risk of development of drug-resistant bacteria. Exacerbation of symptoms of myasthenia gravis, new onset of symptoms of myasthenic syndrome, and infantile hypertrophic pyloric stenosis (IHPS) reported. Prolonged and repeated use may result in an overgrowth of nonsusceptible bacteria or fungi; d/c and take appropriate measures if superinfection develops. Lab test interactions may occur. Caution in elderly.

ADVERSE REACTIONS: N/V, abdominal pain, diarrhea, anorexia.

INTERACTIONS: See Contraindications. Avoid with Class IA (quinidine, procainamide) or Class III (dofetilide, amiodarone, sotalol) antiarrhythmic agents. Serious adverse reactions reported with CYP3A4 substrates such as hypotension with calcium channel blockers (eg, verapamil, amlodipine, diltiazem). Monitor for colchicine toxicity with coadministration; starting dose of colchicine may need to be reduced, and max colchicine dose should be lowered. May increase theophylline levels and potential toxicity with high doses of theophylline; reduce theophylline dose in these cases. Decreased levels with theophylline. Hypotension, bradyarrhythmias, and lactic acidosis observed with verapamil. May elevate digoxin levels. May elevate concentrations that could increase or prolong both therapeutic and adverse effects of drugs primarily metabolized by CYP3A; closely monitor concentrations and consider dose adjustment. May increase the pharmacological effect of triazolam and midazolam. Increased systemic exposure of sildenafil; consider dose reduction of sildenafil. Increased anticoagulant effects of oral anticoagulants; may be more pronounced in elderly. Increased levels of HMG-CoA reductase inhibitors (eg, lovastatin, simvastatin); rhabdomyolysis (rare) reported. Carefully monitor for creatine kinase and serum transaminase levels with lovastatin. Interactions with drugs metabolized by CYP3A (eg, cyclosporine, carbamazepine, tacrolimus, alfentanil, disopyramide, rifabutin, quinidine, methylprednisolone, cilostazol, vinblastine, bromocriptine) and drugs not thought to be metabolized by CYP3A (eg, hexobarbital, phenytoin, valproate) reported.

PREGNANCY: Category B, caution in nursing.

MECHANISM OF ACTION: Macrolide; inhibits protein synthesis by binding 50S ribosomal subunits of susceptible organisms.

PHARMACOKINETICS: Absorption: Readily absorbed. **Distribution:** Largely bound to plasma proteins; crosses placenta, found in breast milk. **Elimination:** Bile, urine (<5%, active form).

NURSING CONSIDERATIONS

Assessment: Assess for hypersensitivity to drug, hepatic impairment, QT interval prolongation, ongoing proarrhythmic conditions, myasthenia gravis, pregnancy/nursing status, and possible drug interactions. Perform culture and susceptibility tests to confirm diagnosis of causative organism. Perform serologic test for syphilis (if treating gonorrhea) and spinal fluid exam (primary syphilis).

Monitoring: Monitor for hepatic dysfunction, CDAD, QT interval prolongation, arrhythmia, exacerbation of myasthenia gravis symptoms, new onset of symptoms of myasthenic syndrome, IHPS, superinfection, and other adverse reactions. Perform follow-up serologic test for syphilis (after 3 months) and spinal fluid exam (primary syphilis).

Patient Counseling: Inform that therapy should only be used to treat bacterial, not viral, infections. Instruct to take exactly ud. Inform that skipping doses or not completing full course may decrease effectiveness and increase bacterial resistance. Inform that diarrhea is a common problem caused by therapy and will usually end upon discontinuation of therapy. Instruct to immediately contact physician if watery and bloody stools (with or without stomach cramps and fever) occur, even as late as ≥2 months after discontinuation of therapy. Inform caregivers of infant patients to contact physician if vomiting or irritability with feeding occurs.

Administration: Oral route. **Storage:** <30°C (86°F).

ESTRACE   RX
estradiol (Warner Chilcott)

> Estrogens increase the risk of endometrial cancer. Perform adequate diagnostic measures, including endometrial sampling, to rule out malignancy with undiagnosed persistent or recurrent abnormal vaginal bleeding. Should not be used for the prevention of cardiovascular disease. Increased risk of myocardial infarction (MI), stroke, invasive breast cancer, pulmonary embolism (PE), and deep vein thrombosis (DVT) reported in postmenopausal women (50-79 yrs of age) reported. Increased risk of developing probable dementia in postmenopausal women ≥65 yrs of age reported. Should be prescribed at the lowest effective dose and for the shortest duration consistent with treatment goals and risks.

THERAPEUTIC CLASS: Estrogen

INDICATIONS: (Cre) Treatment of vulvar and vaginal atrophy. (Tab) Treatment of moderate to severe vasomotor symptoms associated with menopause. Treatment of moderate to severe symptoms of vulvar and vaginal atrophy associated with menopause. Treatment of hypoestrogenism due to hypogonadism, castration, or primary ovarian failure. Palliative treatment of breast cancer in appropriately selected women and men with metastatic disease, and advanced androgen-dependent prostate carcinoma. Prevention of osteoporosis.

DOSAGE: *Adults:* Reevaluate treatment need periodically (eg, 3- to 6-month intervals). (Cre) Vulvar or Vaginal Atrophy: Initial: 2-4g/day for 1-2 weeks, then gradually decrease to 1/2 initial dose for 1-2 weeks. Maint: 1g 1-3X/week. D/C or taper at 3- to 6-month intervals. (Tab) Vulvar or Vaginal Atrophy/Vasomotor Symptoms: Initial: 1-2mg/day. Titrate: Adjust as necessary to control presenting symptoms. Maint: Minimal effective dose should be determined by titration. Administer cyclically (eg, 3 weeks on and 1 week off). D/C or taper at 3- to 6-month intervals. Hypoestrogenism: Initial: 1-2mg/day. Titrate: Adjust as necessary to control presenting symptoms. Maint: Minimal effective dose should be determined by titration. Metastatic Breast Cancer: Usual: 10mg tid for at least 3 months. Prostate Carcinoma: Usual: 1-2mg tid. Osteoporosis Prevention: Use lowest effective dose.

HOW SUPPLIED: Cre: 0.01% [42.5g]; Tab: 0.5mg*, 1mg*, 2mg* *scored

CONTRAINDICATIONS: Undiagnosed abnormal genital bleeding, known/suspected/history of breast cancer, known/suspected estrogen-dependent neoplasia, active/history of DVT/PE, active or recent arterial thromboembolic disease (eg, stroke, MI), liver dysfunction or disease, known/suspected pregnancy.

WARNINGS/PRECAUTIONS: D/C immediately if stroke, DVT, PE, or MI occur or are suspected. Caution in patients with risk factors for arterial vascular disease and/or venous thromboembolism. If feasible, d/c at least 4-6 weeks before surgery of the type associated with an increased risk of thromboembolism, or during periods of prolonged immobilization. May increase the risk of gallbladder disease and ovarian cancer. May lead to severe hypercalcemia in patients with breast cancer and bone metastases; d/c and take appropriate measures if hypercalcemia occurs. Retinal vascular thrombosis reported; d/c pending exam if sudden partial/complete loss of vision, or sudden onset of proptosis, diplopia, or migraine occurs. D/C permanently if exam reveals papilledema or retinal vascular lesions. Consider addition of progestin for women with a uterus or with residual endometriosis post-hysterectomy. May elevate BP and thyroid-binding globulin levels. May elevate plasma TGs leading to pancreatitis in patients with preexisting hypertriglyceridemia. Caution with impaired liver function, and history of cholestatic jaundice associated with past estrogen use or with pregnancy; d/c in case of recurrence. May cause fluid retention; caution with cardiac/renal impairment. Caution with severe hypocalcemia. May exacerbate endometriosis, asthma, diabetes mellitus, epilepsy, migraine, porphyria, systemic lupus erythematosus, and hepatic hemangiomas; use with caution. May affect certain endocrine and blood components in lab tests. (Tab) 2mg tab contains tartrazine, which may cause allergic-type reactions (eg, bronchial asthma) in certain susceptible individuals.

ADVERSE REACTIONS: Vaginal bleeding pattern changes, vaginitis, breast tenderness, galactorrhea, N/V, thrombophlebitis, melasma, abdominal cramps, headache, mental depression, weight changes, edema, libido changes, MI, PE.

INTERACTIONS: CYP3A4 inducers (eg, St. John's wort preparations, phenobarbital, carbamazepine, rifampin) may decrease levels, which may decrease therapeutic effects and/or change uterine bleeding profile. CYP3A4 inhibitors (eg, erythromycin, ketoconazole, ritonavir, grapefruit juice) may increase levels, which may result in side effects. Patients concomitantly receiving thyroid replacement therapy and estrogens may require increased doses of thyroid replacement therapy; monitor thyroid function.

PREGNANCY: (Cre) Contraindicated in pregnancy, (Tab) Category X; caution in nursing.

MECHANISM OF ACTION: Estrogen; binds to nuclear receptors in estrogen-responsive tissues. Circulating estrogens modulate pituitary secretion of gonadotropins, luteinizing hormone, and follicle-stimulating hormone, through a negative feedback mechanism. Reduces elevated levels of these hormones in postmenopausal women.

PHARMACOKINETICS: Absorption: (Cre) Absorbed through skin, mucous membranes, and GI tract. **Distribution:** Largely bound to sex hormone-binding globulin and albumin; found in breast milk. **Metabolism:** Liver to estrone (metabolite); estriol (major urinary metabolite); sulfate and glucuronide conjugation (liver); biliary secretion of conjugates into the intestine; hydrolysis (gut); reabsorption; CYP3A4 (partial metabolism). **Elimination:** Urine (parent compound and metabolites).

NURSING CONSIDERATIONS

Assessment: Assess for undiagnosed abnormal genital bleeding, presence/history of breast cancer, estrogen-dependent neoplasia, active/history of DVT/PE/arterial thromboembolic disease, liver impairment/disease, history of cholestatic jaundice, drug hypersensitivity, pregnancy/nursing status, any other conditions where treatment is contraindicated or cautioned, need for progestin therapy, and possible drug interactions.

Monitoring: Monitor for signs/symptoms of CV events, malignant neoplasms, dementia, gallbladder disease, hypercalcemia, visual abnormalities, BP and serum TG elevations, pancreatitis, fluid retention, cholestatic jaundice, exacerbation of endometriosis and other conditions, and other adverse reactions. Perform annual breast exam; schedule mammography based on age, risk factors, and prior mammogram results. Monitor thyroid function in patients on thyroid hormone replacement therapy. Periodically evaluate (every 3-6 months) to determine need for therapy.

In cases of undiagnosed, persistent, or recurrent abnormal vaginal bleeding, perform adequate diagnostic measures (eg, endometrial sampling) to rule out malignancy.

Patient Counseling: Inform of the risks/benefits of therapy. Inform that medication increases risk for breast/uterine cancer. Advise to contact physician if breast lumps, unusual vaginal bleeding, dizziness or faintness, changes in speech, severe headaches, chest pain, SOB, leg pain, visual changes, or vomiting occur. Advise to have yearly breast exams by a physician and perform monthly breast self-exams. Advise to notify physician if pregnant/nursing.

Administration: (Cre) Intravaginal route. (Tab) Oral route. **Storage:** (Cre) Room temperature. Protect from temperatures in excess of 40°C (104°F). (Tab) 20-25°C (68-77°F).

ESTRADERM   RX
estradiol (Novartis)

> Estrogens increase the risk of endometrial cancer. Perform adequate diagnostic measures, including endometrial sampling, to rule out malignancy with undiagnosed persistent or recurrent abnormal vaginal bleeding. Should not be used for the prevention of cardiovascular disease (CVD) or dementia. Increased risk of myocardial infarction (MI), stroke, invasive breast cancer, pulmonary emboli (PE), and deep vein thrombosis (DVT) in postmenopausal women (50-79 yrs of age) reported. Increased risk of developing probable dementia in postmenopausal women ≥65 yrs of age reported. Should be prescribed at the lowest effective dose and for the shortest duration consistent with treatment goals and risks.

THERAPEUTIC CLASS: Estrogen

INDICATIONS: Treatment of moderate to severe vasomotor symptoms and vulvar/vaginal atrophy associated with menopause. Treatment of hypoestrogenism due to hypogonadism, castration, or primary ovarian failure. Prevention of postmenopausal osteoporosis.

DOSAGE: *Adults:* Vasomotor Symptoms/Vulvar/Vaginal Atrophy: Initial: Apply 0.05mg/day 2X weekly. Osteoporosis Prevention: Initial: 0.05mg/day as soon as possible after menopause and adjust dose if necessary. Currently Taking Oral Estrogen: Initiate 1 week after d/c oral hormonal therapy, or sooner if menopausal symptoms reappear in <1 week. May give continuously in patients with no intact uterus or cyclically (3 weeks on, 1 week off) with intact uterus. Reevaluate treatment need periodically (eg, 3-6 months interval).

HOW SUPPLIED: Patch: 0.05mg/day, 0.1mg/day [8^s]

CONTRAINDICATIONS: Undiagnosed abnormal genital bleeding, known/suspected/history of breast cancer, known/suspected estrogen-dependent neoplasia, active or history of DVT/PE, active or recent arterial thromboembolic disease (eg, stroke, MI), liver dysfunction or disease, known/suspected pregnancy.

WARNINGS/PRECAUTIONS: D/C immediately if stroke, DVT, PE, or MI occurs or is suspected. Caution in patients with risk factors for arterial vascular disease and/or venous thromboembolism (VTE). If feasible, d/c at least 4-6 weeks before surgery of the type associated with an increased risk of thromboembolism, or during periods of prolonged immobilization. May increase risk of breast/ovarian/endometrial cancer and gallbladder disease. Consider addition of progestin for women with a uterus or with residual endometriosis posthysterectomy. May lead to severe hypercalcemia in patients with breast cancer and bone metastases; d/c and take appropriate measures if hypercalcemia occurs. Retinal vascular thrombosis reported; if sudden partial or complete loss of vision, sudden onset of proptosis, diplopia, or migraine occurs, d/c pending examination. If examinations reveal papilledema or retinal vascular lesions, d/c permanently. May elevate BP, thyroid-binding globulin levels, and plasma TG levels leading to pancreatitis and other complications. Caution with history of cholestatic jaundice; d/c in case of recurrence. May cause fluid retention; caution with cardiac/renal dysfunction. Caution with impaired liver function and severe hypocalcemia. May exacerbate endometriosis, asthma, diabetes mellitus (DM), epilepsy, migraine, porphyria, systemic lupus erythematosus (SLE), and hepatic hemangiomas; use with caution. May affect certain endocrine and blood components in lab tests.

ADVERSE REACTIONS: Altered vaginal bleeding, vaginal candidiasis, breast tenderness/enlargement, N/V, chloasma, melasma, weight changes, VTE, pulmonary embolism, MI, stroke, application-site redness/irritation.

INTERACTIONS: CYP3A4 inducers (eg, St. John's wort, phenobarbital, carbamazepine, rifampin) may decrease levels, which may decrease therapeutic effects and/or change uterine bleeding profile. CYP3A4 inhibitors (eg, erythromycin, ketoconazole, ritonavir, grapefruit juice) may increase levels, which may result in side effects. Patients concomitantly receiving thyroid hormone replacement therapy and estrogens may require increased doses of their thyroid replacement therapy.

PREGNANCY: Contraindicated in pregnancy, caution in nursing.

MECHANISM OF ACTION: Estrogen; binds to nuclear receptors in estrogen-responsive tissues. Circulating estrogen modulates pituitary secretion of gonadotropins, luteinizing hormone and follicle-stimulating hormone, through negative feedback mechanism. Reduces elevated levels of these hormones in postmenopausal women.

PHARMACOKINETICS: Distribution: Largely bound to sex hormone-binding globulin and albumin; found in breast milk. **Metabolism:** Liver to estrone (metabolite); estriol (major urinary metabolite); sulfate and glucuronide conjugation (liver), gut hydrolysis; CYP3A4 (partial metabolism). **Elimination:** Urine (parent compound and metabolites); $T_{1/2}$=1 hr.

NURSING CONSIDERATIONS

Assessment: Assess for undiagnosed abnormal genital bleeding, presence/history of breast cancer, estrogen-dependent neoplasia, active or history of DVT/PE, active or recent (within past yr) arterial thromboembolic disease, liver dysfunction/disease, known/suspected pregnancy, any other conditions where treatment is contraindicated or cautioned, need for progestin therapy, and possible drug interactions. Assess use in women ≥65 yrs, nursing patients, and those with hypertriglyceridemia, hypothyroidism, DM, asthma, epilepsy, migraine or porphyria, SLE, and hepatic hemangiomas.

Monitoring: Monitor for signs/symptoms of CVD, malignant neoplasms, dementia, gallbladder disease, hypercalcemia, visual abnormalities, hypertriglyceridemia, pancreatitis, hypothyroidism, fluid retention, cholestatic jaundice, exacerbation of endometriosis and other conditions. Perform annual breast exam; schedule mammography based on age, risk factors, and prior mammogram results. Regularly monitor BP, thyroid function in patients on thyroid replacement therapy, and periodically evaluate (every 3-6 months) to determine need for therapy. In case of undiagnosed, persistent, or recurrent vaginal bleeding in women with uterus, perform adequate diagnostic testing measures (eg, endometrial sampling) to rule out malignancy.

Patient Counseling: Inform that therapy may increase the risk for uterine cancer and may increase chances of getting a heart attack, stroke, breast cancer, blood clots, and dementia. Instruct to report to physician any breast lumps, unusual vaginal bleeding, dizziness and faintness, changes in speech, severe headaches, chest pain, SOB, leg pains, changes in vision, or vomiting. Advise to notify physician if pregnant or nursing. Instruct to have annual breast examination by a physician and perform monthly breast self-examination. Instruct to place medication system on clean, dry skin on the trunk (including buttocks and abdomen); site should not be exposed to sunlight; area should not be oily, damaged, or irritated; and should not be applied on breasts or waistline. Counsel to rotate application sites with an interval of 1 week, and to apply immediately after opening pouch. Inform that if medication system falls off, reapply same system or apply new system PRN and continue with original treatment schedule.

Administration: Transdermal route. Apply immediately upon removal from the protective pouch. Refer to PI for application instructions. **Storage:** Do not store above 30°C (86°F). Do not store unpouched.

ESTROSTEP FE   RX

norethindrone acetate - ferrous fumarate - ethinyl estradiol (Warner Chilcott)

> Cigarette smoking increases the risk of serious cardiovascular (CV) side effects. Risk increases with age (>35 yrs) and with heavy smoking (≥15 cigarettes/day). Women who use oral contraceptives should be strongly advised not to smoke.

THERAPEUTIC CLASS: Estrogen/progestogen combination

INDICATIONS: Prevention of pregnancy. Treatment of moderate acne vulgaris in females ≥15 yrs who want contraception (for at least 6 months), have achieved menarche, and are unresponsive to topical acne agents.

DOSAGE: *Adults:* Contraception/Acne: 1 tab qd for 28 days, then repeat. Start 1st Sunday after menses begins or the 1st day of menses.
Pediatrics: Postpubertal: Contraception/Acne (≥15 Yrs): 1 tab qd for 28 days, then repeat. Start 1st Sunday after menses begins or the 1st day of menses.

HOW SUPPLIED: Tab: (Ethinyl Estradiol-Norethindrone) 0.035mg-1mg, 0.030mg-1mg, 0.020mg-1mg; Tab: (Ferrous Fumarate) 75mg

CONTRAINDICATIONS: Thrombophlebitis, thromboembolic disorders, history of deep vein thrombophlebitis or thromboembolic disorders, pregnancy, cerebrovascular disease, coronary artery disease, undiagnosed abnormal genital bleeding, cholestatic jaundice of pregnancy, jaundice with prior pill use, hepatic adenoma or carcinoma, breast carcinoma, carcinoma of the endometrium or other estrogen-dependent neoplasia.

WARNINGS/PRECAUTIONS: Increased risk of myocardial infarction (MI), vascular disease, thromboembolism, stroke, hepatic neoplasia and gallbladder disease. May increase risk of breast and cervical cancer. D/C if jaundice develops. Retinal thrombosis reported; d/c if unexplained partial or complete loss of vision, onset of proptosis or diplopia, papilledema, or retinal vascular lesions develop. Contact lens wearers who develop visual changes or changes in lens tolerance should be assessed by an ophthalmologist. Should not be used to induce withdrawal bleeding as a test for pregnancy, or to treat threatened or habitual abortion during pregnancy. May cause glucose intolerance; monitor prediabetic and diabetic patients. May cause fluid retention and increase BP; monitor closely with HTN and d/c if significant elevation of BP occurs. May elevate LDL levels or cause other lipid changes. May cause/exacerbate migraine or may develop headache with new pattern. Breakthrough bleeding and spotting reported; rule out malignancy or pregnancy. Perform annual physical exam. Monitor closely with depression and d/c if depression recurs to serious degree. Use before menarche is not indicated. May affect certain endocrine tests, LFTs, and blood components. Does not protect against HIV infection (AIDS) and other sexually transmitted diseases (STDs).

ADVERSE REACTIONS: Thrombophlebitis, arterial thromboembolism, pulmonary embolism, MI, cerebral hemorrhage, cerebral thrombosis, HTN, gallbladder disease, hepatic adenomas, benign liver tumors, N/V, breakthrough bleeding, spotting, amenorrhea.

INTERACTIONS: Reduced effects, increased breakthrough bleeding, and menstrual irregularities with rifampin, phenylbutazone and St. John's wort. Increased plasma levels with atorvastatin, ascorbic acid and acetaminophen (APAP). Decreased plasma levels of APAP. Increased clearance of temazepam, salicylic acid, morphine, and clofibric acid. Increased plasma levels of cyclosporine, prednisolone, and theophylline. Pregnancy reported when administered with antimicrobials, such as ampicillin, tetracycline, and griseofulvin. Reduced effects when used with anticonvulsants such as phenobarbital, phenytoin, and carbamazepine.

PREGNANCY: Category X, not for use in nursing.

MECHANISM OF ACTION: Estrogen/progestogen oral contraceptive; acts by suppressing gonadotropins, inhibiting ovulation, and causing other alterations, including changes in the cervical mucus (increasing difficulty of sperm entry into uterus) and the endometrium (reducing likelihood of implantation). Acne: not established; increases sex hormone-binding globulin and decreases free testosterone (reducing androgen stimulation of sebum production).

PHARMACOKINETICS: Absorption: Rapid and complete. Absolute bioavailability: Norethindrone (64%), ethinyl estradiol (43%); T_{max}=1-2 hrs. Refer to PI for dose specific parameters. **Distribution:** V_d=2-4L/kg; plasma protein binding (>95%). Excreted in breast milk. **Metabolism:** Norethindrone: Extensive; reduction, sulfate/glucuronide conjugation. Ethinyl estradiol: Extensive; oxidation via CYP3A4 and conjugation; 2-hydroxy ethinyl estradiol (major metabolite). **Elimination:** Urine, feces. Norethindrone: $T_{1/2}$=13 hrs. Ethinyl estradiol: $T_{1/2}$=19 hrs.

NURSING CONSIDERATIONS

Assessment: Assess for current or history of thrombophlebitis or thromboembolic disorders, cerebrovascular or coronary artery disease, known or suspected carcinoma of the breast, endometrium or other known or suspected estrogen-dependent neoplasia, undiagnosed abnormal genital bleeding, history of cholestatic jaundice of pregnancy or jaundice with previous pill use, hepatic adenomas or carcinomas, known or suspected pregnancy. Assess use in patients >35 yrs who smoke ≥15 cigarettes/day. Assess use in patients with HTN, hyperlipidemias, diabetes mellitus (DM), and obesity. Assess for conditions that might be aggravated by fluid retention, nursing status, and for possible drug interactions.

Monitoring: Monitor for venous and arterial thrombotic and thromboembolic events, hepatic neoplasia, gallbladder disease, ocular lesions, HTN, fluid retention, bleeding irregularities, and onset or exacerbation of headaches or migraines. Monitor blood glucose levels with history of DM or in prediabetic patients, BP with history of HTN, lipid levels with a history of hyperlipidemia. Monitor for signs/symptoms of liver toxicity, GI upset, and signs of worsening depression with previous history. Refer patients with contact lenses to ophthalmologist if ocular changes develop. Perform annual physical exam.

Patient Counseling: Counsel about possible side effects. Inform that medication does not protect against HIV and other STDs. Avoid smoking while on medication. Advise if spotting, light bleeding, or nausea develops during first 1-3 packs of pills, to continue taking medication, and to notify physician if symptoms do not subside. If N/V or diarrhea occurs, use backup birth control method until physician is contacted. Counsel to go for an annual physical, the appropriate way to use the pack and when to start. Take at the same time every day. See PI for detailed notes on administration regarding missed doses.

Administration: Oral route. **Storage:** Do not store above 25°C (77°F). Protect from light. Store tabs inside pouch when not in use.

ETODOLAC   RX
etodolac (Various)

NSAIDs may increase risk of serious cardiovascular thrombotic events, myocardial infarction (MI), stroke; increased risk with duration of use and with cardiovascular disease (CVD) or risk factors for CVD. Increased risk of serious GI adverse events (eg, bleeding, ulceration, stomach/intestinal perforation) that can be fatal and occur anytime during use without warning symptoms; elderly patients are at a greater risk. Contraindicated for the treatment of perioperative pain in the setting of coronary artery bypass graft (CABG) surgery.

THERAPEUTIC CLASS: NSAID

INDICATIONS: Acute and long-term use in the management of signs and symptoms of osteoarthritis (OA) and rheumatoid arthritis (RA). Management of acute pain.

DOSAGE: *Adults:* ≥18 yrs: Use lowest effective dose for the shortest duration consistent with individual patient treatment goals. After observing the response to initial therapy, adjust dose and frequency based on individual patient's need. Acute Pain: Usual: 200-400mg q6-8h. Max: 1000mg/day. OA/RA: Initial: 300mg bid-tid, or 400mg bid, or 500mg bid. May give a lower dose of 600mg/day for long-term use. Max: 1000mg/day. Elderly: Caution with dose selection.

HOW SUPPLIED: Cap: 200mg, 300mg; Tab: 400mg, 500mg

CONTRAINDICATIONS: History of asthma, urticaria, or other allergic-type reactions with aspirin (ASA) or other NSAIDs. Treatment of perioperative pain in the setting of CABG surgery.

WARNINGS/PRECAUTIONS: May cause HTN or worsen preexisting HTN; monitor BP closely. Fluid retention and edema reported; caution with fluid retention or heart failure (HF). Extreme caution with prior history of ulcer disease, GI bleeding, or risk factors for GI bleeding (eg, prolonged NSAID therapy, older age, poor general health status); monitor for GI ulceration/bleeding and d/c if serious GI event occurs. Renal papillary necrosis and other renal injury reported after long-term use; increased risk with renal/hepatic impairment, heart failure, and elderly. Caution with preexisting kidney disease. Not recommended for use with advanced renal disease; monitor renal function closely if therapy is initiated. Caution with mild to moderate renal impairment. Anaphylactoid reactions may occur. Avoid with ASA-triad. Caution with asthma and avoid with ASA-sensitive asthma. May cause serious skin adverse events (eg, exfoliative dermatitis, Stevens-Johnson syndrome, toxic epidermal necrolysis); d/c at 1st appearance of skin rash or any other signs of hypersensitivity. Avoid in late pregnancy; may cause premature closure of ductus arteriosus. Not a substitute for corticosteroids or for the treatment of corticosteroid insufficiency; may mask signs of inflammation and fever. May cause elevations of LFTs or severe hepatic reactions (eg, jaundice, fulminant hepatitis, liver necrosis, hepatic failure); d/c if liver disease or systemic manifestations occur, or if abnormal LFTs persist/worsen. Anemia reported; monitor Hgb/Hct if signs or symptoms of anemia develop. May inhibit platelet aggregation and prolong bleeding time; monitor patients with coagulation disorders. Caution in debilitated and elderly.

ADVERSE REACTIONS: Dyspepsia, abdominal pain, diarrhea, flatulence, N/V, constipation, anemia, pruritus, rashes, dizziness, increased bleeding time, GI ulcers, heartburn, abnormal renal function.

INTERACTIONS: Not recommended with phenylbutazone and ASA. Increased risk of GI bleeding with oral corticosteroids, anticoagulants, alcohol use, and smoking. May diminish antihypertensive effect of ACE inhibitors. May decrease peak concentration with antacids. May elevate cyclosporine, digoxin, and methotrexate levels. May enhance nephrotoxicity associated with cyclosporine. May enhance methotrexate toxicity; caution with concomitant use. May reduce natriuretic effect of furosemide and thiazides; monitor for signs of renal insufficiency or failure and diuretic efficacy. May impair response with thiazides or loop diuretics. Monitor for signs of lithium toxicity with lithium. Risk of renal toxicity with diuretics and ACE inhibitors. Caution with warfarin; prolonged PT, with or without bleeding, may occur with warfarin.

PREGNANCY: Category C, not for use in nursing.

MECHANISM OF ACTION: NSAID; has not been established. Suspected to inhibit prostaglandin synthetase.

PHARMACOKINETICS: Absorption: Well-absorbed. Bioavailability (100%); C_{max}=14-37µg/mL, T_{max}=80 min. Administration in various population resulted in different pharmacokinetic parameters. **Distribution:** V_d=390mL/kg; plasma protein binding (>99%). **Metabolism:** Liver (extensive); hydroxylation, glucuronidation; 6-, 7-, and 8- hydroxylated-etodolac, etodolac glucuronide (metabolites). **Elimination:** Urine (1% unchanged, 72% parent drug and metabolites), feces (16%); $T_{1/2}$=6.4 hrs.

NURSING CONSIDERATIONS

Assessment: Assess previous hypersensitivity to the drug, history of asthma, urticaria, or allergic-type reactions with ASA or other NSAIDs, ASA-triad, CVD, risk factors for CVD, HTN, fluid retention, HF, history of ulcer disease, history of/risk factors for GI bleeding, general health status, renal/hepatic impairment, coagulation disorders, pregnancy/nursing status, and possible drug interactions. Obtain baseline CBC and BP.

Monitoring: Monitor for bleeding time, GI bleeding/ulceration/perforation, CV thrombotic events, MI, HTN, stroke, fluid retention, edema, asthma, hypersensitivity, and other adverse reactions. Monitor for BP, LFTs, and renal function. Monitor for CBC and chemistry profile periodically with long-term use.

Patient Counseling: Inform to seek medical advice if symptoms of CV events, GI ulceration/bleeding, skin/hypersensitivity reactions, unexplained weight gain or edema, hepatotoxicity, or anaphylactoid reactions occur. Instruct to avoid use in late pregnancy.

Administration: Oral route. **Storage:** 20-25°C (68-77°F). (Cap) Protect from moisture. (Tab) Store in original container until ready to use.

ETOPOPHOS

RX

etoposide phosphate (Bristol-Myers Squibb)

> Administer under the supervision of a qualified physician experienced in use of cancer chemotherapeutic agents. Severe myelosuppression with resulting infection or bleeding may occur.

THERAPEUTIC CLASS: Podophyllotoxin derivative

INDICATIONS: Adjunct therapy for management of refractory testicular tumors. First-line combination therapy for management of small cell lung cancer (SCLC).

DOSAGE: *Adults:* Testicular Cancer: Usual: 50-100mg/m^2/day IV on Days 1-5 to 100mg/m^2/day on Days 1, 3, and 5. SCLC: 35mg/m^2/day IV for 4 days to 50mg/m^2/day for 5 days. Administer at infusion rates 5-210 min. After adequate recovery from any toxicity, repeat course for either therapy at 3-4 week intervals. CrCl 15-50mL/min: 75% of dose.

HOW SUPPLIED: Inj: 100mg

WARNINGS/PRECAUTIONS: Observe for myelosuppression during and after therapy. Withhold therapy if platelet count <50,000/mm^3 or if absolute neutrophil count (ANC) <500/mm^3. Risk of anaphylactic reaction, manifested by chills, fever, tachycardia, bronchospasm, dyspnea, and hypotension reported. Inj-site reactions may occur; monitor infusion site for possible infiltration during administration. May be carcinogenic in humans; acute leukemia with or without a preleukemic phase may occur. Caution with low serum albumin; increased risk of toxicity. May cause fetal harm in pregnancy. D/C or reduce dose if severe reactions occur. Dosage may be modified to account for other myelosuppressive drugs or the effects of prior x-ray or chemotherapy, which may have compromised bone marrow reserve. Do not give by bolus IV inj. Caution in elderly.

ADVERSE REACTIONS: Leukopenia, neutropenia, thrombocytopenia, anemia, constipation, diarrhea, leukopenia, dizziness, alopecia, N/V, mucositis, asthenia/malaise, chills, fever, anorexia.

INTERACTIONS: Caution with drugs known to inhibit phosphatase activities (eg, levamisole hydrochloride). High-dose cyclosporin A reduces clearance and increases exposure of oral etoposide. Prior use of cisplatin may decrease etoposide total body clearance in children. Displaced from protein binding sites by phenylbutazone, sodium salicylate, and aspirin.

PREGNANCY: Category D, not for use in nursing.

MECHANISM OF ACTION: Podophyllotoxin derivative; induces DNA strand breaks by interacting with DNA-topoisomerase II or formation of free radicals.

PHARMACOKINETICS: Absorption: Rapid, complete; Etopophos 150mg/m^2: AUC=168.3mcg•hr/mL, C$_{max}$=20mcg/mL. Refer to PI for pharmacokinetic parameters for VePesid, which is similar to Etopophos.

NURSING CONSIDERATIONS

Assessment: Assess for renal function, low serum albumin, pregnancy/nursing status, and possible drug interactions. Obtain platelet, Hgb, and WBC count with differential at start of therapy.

Monitoring: Monitor for signs/symptoms of anaphylactic reaction, severe myelosuppression, severe reactions, and renal dysfunction. Monitor for infusion-site reactions. Perform periodic CBC prior to each cycle of therapy and at appropriate intervals during and after therapy.

Patient Counseling: Inform of pregnancy risks; avoid pregnancy. Advise to seek medical attention if experiencing symptoms of severe myelosuppression (infection or bleeding) or anaphylactic reaction (chills, fever, tachycardia, bronchospasm, dyspnea, hypotension).

Administration: IV (infusion) route. Refer to PI for preparation and administration. **Storage:** 2-8°C (36-46°F); protect from light. Reconstituted and diluted vials stable for 7 days at 2-8°C (36-46°F) or 24 hrs at 20-25°C (68-77°F).

EVAMIST
estradiol (Ther-Rx)

Estrogens increase the risk of endometrial cancer. Perform adequate diagnostic measures, including endometrial sampling, to rule out malignancy with undiagnosed persistent or recurring abnormal vaginal bleeding. Should not be used for the prevention of cardiovascular disease (CVD) or dementia. Increased risk of myocardial infarction (MI), stroke, invasive breast cancer, pulmonary emboli (PE), and deep-vein thrombosis (DVT) in postmenopausal women (50-79 yrs of age) reported. Increased risk of developing probable dementia in postmenopausal women ≥65 yrs of age reported. Should be prescribed at the lowest effective dose for the shortest duration consistent with treatment goals and risks. Breast budding/masses in prepubertal females and gynecomastia and breast masses in prepubertal males following unintentional secondary exposure reported. Ensure that children do not come in contact with the application site. Advise to strictly adhere to recommended instructions for use.

THERAPEUTIC CLASS: Estrogen

INDICATIONS: Treatment of moderate to severe vasomotor symptoms due to menopause.

DOSAGE: *Adults:* Initial: 1 spray qd. Adjust dose based on response. Usual: 1-3 sprays qam to adjacent, non-overlapping areas on the inner surface of the forearm, starting near the elbow. Reevaluate treatment need periodically.

HOW SUPPLIED: Spray: 1.53mg/spray [8.1mL]

CONTRAINDICATIONS: Undiagnosed abnormal genital bleeding, known/suspected/history of breast cancer, known/suspected estrogen-dependent neoplasia, active or history of DVT/PE, active or recent arterial thromboembolic disease (eg, stroke, MI), liver dysfunction or disease, known/suspected pregnancy.

WARNINGS/PRECAUTIONS: Caution in patients with risk factors for arterial vascular disease and/or venous thromboembolism (VTE). If feasible, d/c at least 4-6 weeks before surgery of the type associated with an increased risk of thromboembolism, or during periods of prolonged immobilization. Application site should be covered with clothing if another person may come in contact with the site. Consider discontinuing if conditions of safe use cannot be met. May increase risk of gallbladder disease and ovarian cancer. Consider addition of progestin for women with a uterus or with residual endometriosis posthysterectomy. May lead to severe hypercalcemia in patients with breast cancer and bone metastases; d/c and take appropriate measures if hypercalcemia occurs. Retinal vascular thrombosis reported; d/c pending examination if sudden partial/complete loss of vision, sudden onset of proptosis, diplopia, or migraine occurs. If examination reveals papilledema or retinal vascular lesions, d/c therapy permanently. May elevate BP, thyroid-binding globulin levels, and plasma TGs with preexisting hypertriglyceridemia; consider discontinuing if pancreatitis occurs. Caution with history of cholestatic jaundice; d/c in case of recurrence. May cause fluid retention; caution with cardiac/renal dysfunction. Caution with severe hypocalcemia. May exacerbate endometriosis, asthma, diabetes mellitus (DM), epilepsy, migraine, porphyria, systemic lupus erythematosus (SLE), and hepatic hemangiomas. Avoid fire, flame, or smoking until spray has dried. May affect certain endocrine and blood components in lab tests.

ADVERSE REACTIONS: Breast tenderness, nipple pain, nausea, nasopharyngitis, back pain, arthralgia, headache.

INTERACTIONS: CYP3A4 inducers (eg, St. John's wort, phenobarbital, carbamazepine, rifampin) may decrease levels, which may decrease therapeutic effects and/or change uterine bleeding profile. CYP3A4 inhibitors (eg, erythromycin, ketoconazole, ritonavir, grapefruit juice) may increase levels, which may result in side effects. Patients concomitantly receiving thyroid replacement therapy may require increased doses of their thyroid replacement therapy. Decreased absorption with sunscreen applied 1 hr after estradiol application.

PREGNANCY: Contraindicated in pregnancy, not for use in nursing.

MECHANISM OF ACTION: Estrogen; binds to nuclear receptors in estrogen-responsive tissues. Circulating estrogens modulate pituitary secretion of the gonadotropins, luteinizing hormone, and follicle-stimulating hormone, through a negative feedback mechanism. Reduces elevated levels of these hormones in postmenopausal women.

PHARMACOKINETICS: Absorption: Topical administration of various doses resulted in different parameters. **Distribution:** Found in breast milk. Largely bound to sex hormone-binding globulin and albumin. **Metabolism:** Liver; estrone (metabolite); estriol (major urinary metabolite); sulfate and glucuronide conjugation (liver), gut hydrolysis; reabsorption. **Elimination:** Urine (parent and metabolites).

NURSING CONSIDERATIONS

Assessment: Assess for presence or history of breast cancer, estrogen-dependent neoplasia, abnormal genital bleeding, active or history of DVT/PE, active or recent (within past yr) arterial thromboembolic disease, pregnancy/nursing status, any other conditions where treatment is contraindicated or cautioned, need for progestin therapy, and possible drug interactions. Assess use in women ≥65 yrs, those with DM, asthma, epilepsy, migraines or porphyria, SLE, or hepatic hemangiomas.

Monitoring: Monitor for signs/symptoms of CVD, malignant neoplasms, dementia, gallbladder disease, hypercalcemia, visual abnormalities, BP elevations, fluid retention, elevations in plasma TGs, hypothyroidism, pancreatitis, exacerbation of endometriosis and other conditions (eg, asthma, DM, epilepsy, migraines, SLE, hepatic hemangiomas). Perform annual breast exam; schedule mammography based on age, risk factors, and prior mammogram results. Periodically monitor BP levels at regular intervals, thyroid function for patients on thyroid replacement therapy, and evaluate to determine treatment need. Perform proper diagnostic testing (eg, endometrial sampling) in patients with undiagnosed, persistent or recurring vaginal bleeding.

Patient Counseling: Instruct to contact physician if vaginal bleeding develops. Counsel about the possible side effects of therapy (eg, headache, breast pain and tenderness, N/V). Instruct to apply therapy ud and keep children from contacting exposed application site; if direct contact occurs, advise to thoroughly wash contact area with soap and water. Counsel to look for signs of unexpected sexual development (eg, breast mass or increased breast size) in prepubertal children; advise to have children evaluated by a physician if signs of unintentional secondary exposure are noticed and to d/c therapy until cause is identified. Instruct that before applying the 1st dose from a new applicator, the pump should be primed by spraying 3 sprays with cover on. Advise that medication contains alcohol; avoid fire, flame, or smoking until medication is dry. Inform to have yearly breast exams by a physician and perform monthly breast self-exams.

Administration: Topical route. Sprays should be allowed to dry for 2 min; do not wash site for 30 min. Should not be applied to skin surfaces other than the forearm. **Storage:** 25°C (77°F); excursions permitted to 15-30°C (59-86°F). Do not freeze.

EVISTA   RX
raloxifene HCl (Lilly)

> Increased risk of deep vein thrombosis (DVT) and pulmonary embolism (PE) reported. Avoid use in women with active or past history of venous thromboembolism (VTE). Increased risk of death due to stroke in postmenopausal women with documented coronary heart disease or at increased risk for major coronary events; consider risk-benefit balance in women at risk for stroke.

THERAPEUTIC CLASS: Selective estrogen receptor modulator

INDICATIONS: Treatment and prevention of osteoporosis in postmenopausal women. Reduction in risk of invasive breast cancer in postmenopausal women with osteoporosis and in postmenopausal women at high risk for invasive breast cancer.

DOSAGE: *Adults:* 60mg qd. Refer to PI for recommendations regarding Ca^{2+} and vitamin D supplementation.

HOW SUPPLIED: Tab: 60mg

CONTRAINDICATIONS: Active/past history of VTE (eg, DVT, PE, retinal vein thrombosis), pregnancy, women who may become pregnant, and in nursing mothers.

WARNINGS/PRECAUTIONS: VTE events, including superficial venous thrombophlebitis, reported. D/C at least 72 hrs prior to and during prolonged immobilization (eg, postsurgical recovery, prolonged bed rest); resume therapy only after patient is fully ambulatory. Caution in women at risk of thromboembolic disease for other reasons (eg, congestive heart failure, superficial thrombophlebitis, active malignancy). Should not be used for primary or secondary prevention of cardiovascular disease (CVD). Avoid use in premenopausal women. Monitor serum TG levels in women with history of hypertriglyceridemia in response to treatment with estrogen or estrogen plus progestin. Use in women with history of breast cancer has not been adequately studied. Caution with hepatic impairment or with moderate or severe renal impairment. Not recommended for use in men. Monitor for unexplained uterine bleeding and breast abnormalities.

ADVERSE REACTIONS: DVT, PE, hot flashes, leg cramps, infection, flu syndrome, headache, N/V, diarrhea, peripheral edema, arthralgia, vaginal bleeding, pharyngitis, sinusitis, cough increased.

INTERACTIONS: Avoid concomitant administration with cholestyramine, other anion exchange resins, and systemic estrogens. Monitor PT with warfarin and other warfarin derivatives. Caution with certain other highly protein-bound drugs (eg, diazepam, diazoxide, lidocaine).

PREGNANCY: Category X, not for use in nursing.

MECHANISM OF ACTION: Selective estrogen receptor modulator; binds to estrogen receptors. Binding results in activation of estrogenic pathways in some tissues and blockade of estrogenic pathways in others, depending on extent of recruitment of coactivators and corepressors to estrogen receptor target gene promoters. Acts as an estrogen agonist in bone; decreases bone resorption and bone turnover, increases bone mineral density, and decreases fracture incidence.

PHARMACOKINETICS: Absorption: Rapid; absolute bioavailability (2%). Single dose: C_{max}=0.5(ng/mL)/(mg/kg); AUC=27.2(ng•hr/mL)/(mg/kg). Multiple doses: C_{max}=1.36(ng/mL)/

(mg/kg); AUC=24.2(ng•hr/mL)/(mg/kg). **Distribution:** V_d=2348L/kg (single dose), 2853L/kg (multiple doses); plasma protein binding (95%). **Metabolism:** Extensive; glucuronidation; raloxifene-4'-glucuronide, raloxifene-6-glucuronide, raloxifene-6',4'-diglucuronide (metabolites). **Elimination:** Feces (primary), urine (<0.2% unchanged); $T_{1/2}$=27.7 hrs (single dose), 32.5 hrs (multiple doses).

NURSING CONSIDERATIONS

Assessment: Assess for active or history of VTE (eg, DVT, PE, retinal vein thrombosis), CVD, risk factors for stroke, history of breast cancer, history of hypertriglyceridemia, prolonged immobilization, renal/hepatic impairment, pregnancy/nursing status, and for possible drug interactions. Perform breast exams and mammograms prior to treatment.

Monitoring: Monitor for VTE (eg, DVT, PE, retinal vein thrombosis), stroke, unexplained uterine bleeding, breast abnormalities and other adverse reactions. Monitor serum TG levels with history of hypertriglyceridemia. Monitor PT with warfarin and other warfarin derivatives. Perform regular breast exams and mammograms after initial treatment.

Patient Counseling: For osteoporosis treatment/prevention, instruct to take supplemental Ca^{2+} and/or vitamin D if intake is inadequate. Counsel on weight-bearing exercise and modification of certain behavioral factors (eg, smoking, excessive alcohol consumption) for osteoporosis treatment/prevention. Advise to d/c therapy at least 72 hrs prior to and during prolonged immobilization. Instruct to avoid prolonged restrictions of movement during travel. Counsel that therapy may increase incidence of hot flashes or hot flashes may occur upon initiation of therapy. Inform that regular breast exams and mammography should be done before initiation of therapy and should continue during therapy.

Administration: Oral route. May be given at any time of day without regard to meals. **Storage:** 20-25°C (68-77°F); excursions permitted to 15-30°C (59-86°F).

EVOCLIN   RX
clindamycin phosphate (Stiefel)

THERAPEUTIC CLASS: Lincomycin derivative

INDICATIONS: Topical treatment of acne vulgaris in patients ≥12 yrs.

DOSAGE: *Adults*: Apply to affected areas qd. Use enough to cover the entire affected area. D/C if no improvement after 6-8 weeks or if condition worsens.
Pediatrics: ≥12 Yrs: Apply to affected areas qd. Use enough to cover the entire affected area. D/C if no improvement after 6-8 weeks or if condition worsens.

HOW SUPPLIED: Foam: 1% [50g, 100g]

CONTRAINDICATIONS: History of regional enteritis, ulcerative colitis, or antibiotic-associated colitis (including pseudomembranous colitis).

WARNINGS/PRECAUTIONS: Diarrhea, bloody diarrhea, and colitis (including pseudomembranous colitis) reported; d/c if significant diarrhea occurs. May cause irritation; d/c if irritation or dermatitis occurs. Avoid contact with eyes, mouth, lips, other mucous membranes, or areas of broken skin; rinse thoroughly with water if contact occurs. Caution in atopic individuals.

ADVERSE REACTIONS: Diarrhea, bloody diarrhea, colitis, headache, application-site burning.

INTERACTIONS: Antiperistaltic agents (eg, opiates, diphenoxylate with atropine) may prolong and/or worsen severe colitis. Avoid with topical/oral erythromycin-containing products due to possible antagonism to clindamycin. May enhance the action of other neuromuscular blockers; use with caution. Caution with concomitant topical acne therapy (eg, peeling, desquamating, or abrasive agents) due to possible cumulative irritancy effect.

PREGNANCY: Category B, not for use in nursing.

MECHANISM OF ACTION: Lincomycin derivative; not established. Binds to the 50S ribosomal subunits of susceptible bacteria and prevents elongation of peptide chains by interfering with peptidyl transfer, thereby suppressing protein synthesis. Shown to have in vitro activity against *Propionibacterium acnes*, which is associated with acne vulgaris.

PHARMACOKINETICS: Distribution: Orally and parenterally administered clindamycin found in breast milk. **Elimination:** Urine (<0.024% unchanged).

NURSING CONSIDERATIONS

Assessment: Assess for history of regional enteritis/ulcerative colitis or antibiotic-associated colitis (including pseudomembranous colitis), pregnancy/nursing status, and possible drug interactions. Assess use in atopic individuals.

Monitoring: Monitor for significant diarrhea, colitis, and irritation/dermatitis. For colitis, perform stool culture and assay for *Clostridium difficile* toxin.

Patient Counseling: Instruct to dispense foam directly into cap or onto cool surface, then apply enough to cover the face. Instruct to wash hands after application, and to avoid contact with eyes, mouth, lips, other mucous membranes, or areas of broken skin; instruct to rinse thoroughly with water if contact occurs. Inform that irritation (eg, erythema, scaling, itching, burning, stinging) may occur; advise to d/c if excessive irritancy or dermatitis occurs. Instruct to d/c and contact physician if experiencing severe diarrhea or GI discomfort. Inform that medication is flammable; avoid fire, flame, and/or smoking during and immediately following application.

Administration: Topical route. Not for oral, ophthalmic, or intravaginal use. Wash skin with mild soap and allow to fully dry before application. **Storage:** 20-25°C (68-77°F). Do not expose to heat or store at >49°C (120°F). Contents under pressure; do not puncture or incinerate.

EXALGO
hydromorphone HCl (Mallinckrodt)   CII

> Contains hydromorphone, an opioid agonist and Schedule II controlled substance with an abuse liability similar to other opioid agonists, legal or illicit; assess each patient's risk for opioid abuse or addiction prior to prescribing. Routinely monitor for signs of misuse, abuse, and addiction. Respiratory depression, including fatal cases, may occur even when used as recommended; proper dosing and titration are essential. Should only be prescribed by healthcare professionals who are knowledgeable in the use of potent opioids for the management of chronic pain. Monitor for respiratory depression, especially during initiation or following a dose increase. Crushing, dissolving, or chewing tab can cause rapid release and absorption of a potentially fatal dose. Accidental ingestion, especially in children, can result in a fatal overdose.

THERAPEUTIC CLASS: Opioid analgesic

INDICATIONS: Management of moderate to severe pain in opioid-tolerant patients requiring continuous, around-the-clock opioid analgesia for an extended period of time.

DOSAGE: *Adults:* >17 Yrs: Initial: Individualize dose. Administer q24h, approximately at the same time every day. D/C or taper all other ER opioids when beginning therapy. Conversion from Other Oral Hydromorphone Formulations: Initial: Dose equivalent to patient's total daily oral hydromorphone dose, taken qd. Conversion from Oral Opioids: Initial: Administer 50% of the calculated estimate of daily hydromorphone requirement. Refer to PI for conversion ratios to calculate the estimated daily hydromorphone requirement. Conversion from Transdermal Fentanyl: 12mg q24h for each 25mcg/hr fentanyl transdermal dose; initiate 18 hrs following removal of patch. Titrate: Determine dose that provides adequate analgesia and minimizes adverse reactions. Periodically reassess the continued need for the use of opioid analgesics during chronic therapy, especially for noncancer-related pain. May adjust dose every 3-4 days. May require dose adjustment or rescue medication in patients who experience breakthrough pain. Moderate Hepatic Impairment: Initial: 25% of dose for normal hepatic function. Closely monitor during dose initiation and titration. Severe Hepatic Impairment: Use alternate analgesic. Renal Impairment: Initial: Moderate Renal Impairment: 50% of dose for normal renal function. Severe Renal Impairment: 25% of dose for normal renal function; consider alternate analgesic. Closely monitor during dose initiation and titration. Discontinuation: Taper dose gradually by 25-50% every 2 or 3 days down to a dose of 8mg before discontinuation. Refer to PI for factors when selecting an initial dose.

HOW SUPPLIED: Tab, Extended-Release (ER): 8mg, 12mg, 16mg, 32mg

CONTRAINDICATIONS: Opioid-intolerant patients, significant respiratory depression, acute or severe bronchial asthma in unmonitored settings or in the absence of resuscitative equipment, known or suspected paralytic ileus, previous surgical procedures and/or underlying disease resulting in narrowing of the GI tract, or have "blind loops" of the GI tract or GI obstruction.

WARNINGS/PRECAUTIONS: Do not begin any patient on this drug as the 1st opioid. Not for use as PRN analgesic, for mild or acute pain, pain not expected to persist for an extended period of time, and postoperative pain. Respiratory depression more likely to occur in the elderly, cachectic, or debilitated; monitor closely, particularly during initiation, titration, and combination with other drugs that depress respiration. Monitor for respiratory depression in patients with significant chronic obstructive pulmonary disease (COPD) or cor pulmonale, and patients having a substantially decreased respiratory reserve, hypoxia, hypercapnia, or preexisting respiratory depression; consider alternative nonopioid analgesics if possible. May cause severe hypotension including orthostatic hypotension and syncope in ambulatory patients; monitor for signs of hypotension after dose initiation or titration. Monitor for signs of sedation and respiratory depression in patients susceptible to the intracranial effects of carbon dioxide retention (eg, those with increased intracranial pressure [ICP] or brain tumors). May obscure clinical course in patients with head injury. Avoid with impaired consciousness or coma. May cause spasm of the sphincter of Oddi; monitor for worsening of symptoms in patients with biliary tract disease (eg, acute pancreatitis). Contains sodium metabisulfite; may cause allergic-type reactions, including anaphylactic symptoms and life-threatening or less severe asthmatic episodes. May aggravate convulsions with convulsive disorders and may induce or aggravate seizures; monitor for worsened seizure control in patients with history of seizure disorders. Avoid abrupt discontinuation. May impair mental and/or physical abilities. Not recommended for use during and immediately prior to labor.

ADVERSE REACTIONS: Respiratory depression, constipation, N/V, somnolence, headache, asthenia, dizziness, diarrhea, insomnia, back pain, pruritus, anorexia, peripheral edema, hyperhidrosis.

INTERACTIONS: Avoid use with CNS depressants (eg, hypnotics, sedatives, antipsychotics, alcohol, phenothiazines) due to increased risk of respiratory depression, hypotension and profound sedation or coma; if coadministration is considered, start with a lower hydromorphone dose than usual and consider using a lower dose of concomitant CNS depressant. Avoid use with mixed agonist/antagonist analgesics (eg, buprenorphine, nalbuphine, pentazocine, butorphanol); may reduce analgesic effect and/or may precipitate withdrawal symptoms. Not recommended for use in patients who have received MAOIs within 14 days; if concurrent therapy is unavoidable, monitor patients for increased respiratory and CNS depression. Anticholinergics or other medications with anticholinergic activity may increase risk of urinary retention and/or severe constipation, which may lead to paralytic ileus.

PREGNANCY: Category C, not for use in nursing.

MECHANISM OF ACTION: Opioid analgesic; has not been established. Thought to be mediated through opioid-specific receptors located in the CNS.

PHARMACOKINETICS: Absorption: Single dose: (8mg) T_{max}=12 hrs, C_{max}=0.93ng/mL, AUC=18.1ng•hr/mL. Refer to PI for pharmacokinetic parameters for different dosages. **Distribution:** Plasma protein binding (27%); (IV) V_d=2.9L/kg; crosses placenta, found in breast milk. **Metabolism:** Liver (extensive) via glucuronidation; hydromorphone-3-glucuronide (metabolite). **Elimination:** Urine (75%, 7% unchanged), feces (1% unchanged); $T_{1/2}$=10.6 hrs (8mg).

NURSING CONSIDERATIONS

Assessment: Assess for risk factors for abuse/addiction, general condition and medical status, pain type/severity, prior opioid experience/tolerance, previous opioid dose and potency, COPD, cor pulmonale, decreased respiratory reserve, hypoxia, hypercapnia, asthma, GI obstruction, renal/hepatic impairment, any other conditions where treatment is contraindicated or cautioned, pregnancy/nursing status, and for possible drug interactions.

Monitoring: Monitor for respiratory depression, sedation, CNS depression, aggravation/induction of seizures/convulsions, increase in ICP, hypotension/syncope, symptoms of worsening biliary tract disease, physical dependence/tolerance, allergic-type reactions, and other adverse reactions. Routinely monitor for signs of misuse, abuse, and addiction.

Patient Counseling: Inform that the drug has potential for abuse; instruct not to share with others and to take steps to protect from theft or misuse. Discuss the risk of respiratory depression. Inform that accidental exposure may result in serious harm or death; advise to store securely, dispose unused tabs by flushing down toilet, or remit to authorities at a certified drug take-back program. Instruct not to consume alcoholic beverages or take prescription and OTC products that contain alcohol during treatment. Advise that patients with certain stomach or intestinal problems such as narrowing of the intestines or previous surgery may be at higher risk of developing a blockage; instruct to contact healthcare provider if symptoms develop, such as abdominal pain/distention, severe constipation, or vomiting. Inform that drug may cause orthostatic hypotension and syncope; instruct how to recognize symptoms of low BP and how to reduce the risk of serious consequences should hypotension occur (eg, sit or lie down, carefully rise from sitting or lying position). Inform that drug may impair the ability to perform potentially hazardous activities (eg, driving or operating heavy machinery); advise not to perform such tasks until they know how they will react. Advise of potential for severe constipation, including management instructions, and when to seek medical attention. Advise how to recognize anaphylaxis and when to seek medical attention. Inform female patients that drug can cause fetal harm; instruct to notify physician if pregnant or planning to become pregnant.

Administration: Oral route. Swallow tabs intact; do not crush, dissolve, or chew. Take with or without food. **Storage:** 25°C (77°F); excursions permitted to 15-30°C (59-86°F).

EXELON   RX
rivastigmine (Novartis)

THERAPEUTIC CLASS: Acetylcholinesterase inhibitor

INDICATIONS: Treatment of mild to moderate dementia associated with Alzheimer's disease (AD) and mild to moderate Parkinson's disease dementia (PDD). (Patch) Treatment of severe dementia of the Alzheimer's type.

DOSAGE: *Adults:* (PO) Take with meals in divided doses in am and pm. AD: Initial: 1.5mg bid. Titrate: May increase to 3mg bid, then 4.5mg bid, and 6mg bid after a minimum of 2 weeks at the previous dose, if well tolerated. Max: 12mg/day (6mg bid). PDD: Initial: 1.5mg bid. Titrate: May increase to 3mg bid, then 4.5mg bid and 6mg bid after a minimum of 4 weeks at the previous dose, if well tolerated. Max: 6mg bid (12mg/day). Interruption of Treatment: If not tolerated, d/c therapy for several doses and then restart at same or next lower dose. ≤3 Days' Interruption:

EXELON

Reinitiate with same or lower dose. >3 Days' Interruption: Restart with 1.5mg bid and titrate as above. (Patch) AD/PDD: Initial: Apply 4.6mg/24 hrs patch qd to skin. Titrate: Increase dose only after a minimum of 4 weeks at the previous dose, and if well tolerated. Effective Dose: Mild to Moderate AD/Mild to Moderate PDD: 9.5mg/24 hrs qd or 13.3mg/24 hrs qd. Severe AD: 13.3mg/24 hrs qd. Max: 13.3mg/24 hrs. Replace with a new patch q24h. Interruption of Treatment: ≤3 Days' Interruption: Restart with same or lower strength patch. >3 Days' Interruption: Restart with 4.6mg/24 hrs patch and titrate as above. Refer to PI for dose if switching to patch from caps/oral sol, and for dose modifications in patients with hepatic impairment or low body weight, or (PO) renal impairment.

HOW SUPPLIED: Cap: (Tartrate) 1.5mg, 3mg, 4.5mg, 6mg; Patch: 4.6mg/24 hrs, 9.5mg/24 hrs, 13.3mg/24 hrs [30*]; Sol: (Tartrate) 2mg/mL [120mL]

CONTRAINDICATIONS: Previous history of application-site reactions with rivastigmine transdermal patch suggestive of allergic contact dermatitis, (PO) in the absence of negative allergy testing.

WARNINGS/PRECAUTIONS: May cause dose-related GI adverse reactions, including significant N/V, diarrhea, anorexia/decreased appetite, and weight loss; always follow dosing guidelines. Disseminated skin hypersensitivity reactions irrespective of route of administration reported; d/c if these occur. In patients who develop application-site reactions suggestive of allergic contact dermatitis to patch and who still require therapy, switch to oral therapy only after negative allergy testing and under close medical supervision. May increase gastric acid secretion; monitor for symptoms of active/occult GI bleeding, especially those at increased risk of developing ulcers. May have vagotonic effect on HR (eg, bradycardia), which may be particularly important in sick sinus syndrome or supraventricular cardiac conduction conditions. May cause urinary obstruction and seizures. Caution in patients with asthma and obstructive pulmonary disease. May exacerbate or induce extrapyramidal symptoms and impair mental/physical abilities. Caution with mild or moderate hepatic impairment. Consider dosage adjustments in patients with high or low body weight. (PO) Syncopal episodes reported. Worsening of parkinsonian symptoms, particularly tremor, observed in patients treated with cap. Caution in patients with mild to moderate renal impairment. (Patch) Skin application-site reactions may occur. Allergic contact dermatitis should be suspected if application-site reactions spread beyond the patch size; d/c treatment if there is evidence of more intense local reaction (eg, increasing erythema, edema, papules, vesicles), and if symptoms do not significantly improve within 48 hrs after patch removal.

ADVERSE REACTIONS: N/V, anxiety, weight decreased, anorexia, headache, dizziness, fatigue, diarrhea, depression, asthenia, tremor, dyspepsia. (PO) Abdominal pain.

INTERACTIONS: May increase cholinergic effects of other cholinomimetics. May interfere with the activity of anticholinergics. May exaggerate succinylcholine-type muscle relaxation during anesthesia. Avoid with cholinomimetic and anticholinergic drugs unless clinically necessary.

PREGNANCY: Category B, not for use in nursing.

MECHANISM OF ACTION: Reversible cholinesterase inhibitor; has not been established, suspected to enhance cholinergic function by increasing concentration of acetylcholine through reversible inhibition of its hydrolysis by cholinesterase.

PHARMACOKINETICS: Absorption: (Patch) T_{max}=8-16 hrs. (PO) Rapid, complete; absolute bioavailability (36%) (3mg); T_{max}=1 hr. **Distribution:** V_d=1.8-2.7L/kg; plasma protein binding (40%). **Metabolism:** Rapid and extensive. Cholinesterase-mediated hydrolysis. **Elimination:** (PO) Urine (97%, 40% sulfate conjugate of decarbamylated metabolite), feces (0.4%); $T_{1/2}$=1.5 hrs. (Patch) Urine (>90%), feces (<1%); $T_{1/2}$=3 hrs after patch removal.

NURSING CONSIDERATIONS

Assessment: Assess for hypersensitivity to drug, history of GI ulcer disease, sick sinus syndrome, supraventricular cardiac conduction conditions, asthma or obstructive pulmonary disease, pregnancy/nursing status, and possible drug interactions. Assess body weight, for history of application-site reactions with rivastigmine patch suggestive of allergic contact dermatitis, and hepatic impairment. (PO) Assess for renal impairment.

Monitoring: Monitor for signs/symptoms of active or occult GI bleeding, hypersensitivity reactions, extrapyramidal symptoms, urinary obstruction, seizures, and GI adverse events. Routinely evaluate ability to continue driving or operating machinery. Closely monitor patients with high or low body weight. Monitor for toxicities (eg, excessive N/V) in patients with low body weight. (Patch) Monitor for skin reactions (allergic contact dermatitis).

Patient Counseling: Instruct caregivers to monitor for GI adverse reactions and to inform physician if these occur. Inform that allergic skin reactions have been reported regardless of formulation; instruct to consult physician immediately in case of skin reaction while on therapy. Instruct to d/c if disseminated skin hypersensitivity reaction occurs. Advise that therapy may exacerbate or induce extrapyramidal symptoms. (Patch) Instruct to rotate application site, not to use the same site within 14 days, to replace patch q24h at consistent time of day, and to wear only one patch at a time. Instruct to avoid exposure to external heat for long periods. Instruct on proper usage and discarding of patch. In case of accidental contact with eyes or if eyes become red after handling the patch, instruct to rinse immediately with plenty of water and seek medical advice if symptoms do not resolve. Advise not to take rivastigmine cap or oral sol, or other drugs with cholinergic effects while wearing patch. Instruct to inform physician if application-site reactions spread beyond the patch size, if there is evidence of more intense local reaction, and if symptoms do not significantly improve within 48 hrs after patch removal.

Administration: Oral/Transdermal route. (Cap/Sol) Take with meals in divided doses in am and pm. (Sol) Swallow directly from syringe or mix with small glass of water, cold fruit juice, or soda; stir mixture before drinking. (Patch) Refer to PI for administration instructions. **Storage:** 25°C (77°F); excursions permitted to 15-30°C (59-86°F). (Sol) Store in upright position and protect from freezing. Stable for up to 4 hrs at room temperature if combined with cold fruit juice or soda. (Patch) Keep in sealed pouch until use.

EXFORGE   RX
amlodipine - valsartan (Novartis)

> D/C when pregnancy is detected. Drugs that act directly on the renin-angiotensin system (RAS) can cause injury/death to the developing fetus.

THERAPEUTIC CLASS: ARB/calcium channel blocker (dihydropyridine)

INDICATIONS: Treatment of HTN alone or with other antihypertensive agents. May also be used as initial therapy in patients likely to need multiple drugs to achieve their BP goals.

DOSAGE: *Adults:* Initial: 5mg-160mg qd. Titrate: May increase after 1-2 weeks of therapy to control BP. Max: 10mg-320mg qd. Add-On Therapy: May be used if BP is not adequately controlled with amlodipine (or another dihydropyridine calcium channel blocker [CCB]) or valsartan (or another ARB) alone. Patients with dose-limiting adverse reactions to either component alone may be switched to therapy containing a lower dose of that component. Titrate: May increase dose if BP remains uncontrolled after 3-4 weeks of therapy. Max: 10mg-320mg qd. Replacement Therapy: May substitute for individually titrated components. Hepatic Impairment: Consider lower doses. Elderly: Start at lower end of dosing range.

HOW SUPPLIED: Tab: (Amlodipine-Valsartan) 5mg-160mg, 10mg-160mg, 5mg-320mg, 10mg-320mg

CONTRAINDICATIONS: Coadministration with aliskiren in patients with diabetes.

WARNINGS/PRECAUTIONS: Symptomatic hypotension may occur in patients with an activated RAS (eg, volume- and/or salt-depleted patients receiving high doses of diuretics); correct volume depletion prior to therapy. Caution when initiating therapy in patients with heart failure (HF) or recent myocardial infarction (MI), and in patients undergoing surgery/dialysis. Renal function changes may occur; caution in patients whose renal function depend in part on the activity of the RAS (eg, renal artery stenosis, severe heart failure (HF), post-myocardial infarction (MI), or volume depletion). Consider withholding or discontinuation if clinically significant decrease in renal function develops. Amlodipine: Caution with severe aortic stenosis. Worsening angina and acute MI may develop after starting or increasing dose, particularly with severe obstructive coronary artery disease (CAD). Valsartan: Increased K$^+$ in some patients with HF reported, and more likely to occur in patients with preexisting renal impairment; dose reduction and/or discontinuation of therapy may be required. Do not readminister to patients who have had angioedema. Caution in elderly and with liver disease.

ADVERSE REACTIONS: Increased BUN, peripheral edema, nasopharyngitis, hyperkalemia.

INTERACTIONS: See Contraindications. Amlodipine: May increase simvastatin exposure; limit simvastatin dose to 20mg/day. Increased systemic exposure with CYP3A4 inhibitors (moderate and strong) warranting dose reduction; monitor for symptoms of hypotension and edema to determine the need for dose adjustment. Monitor BP when coadministered with CYP3A4 inducers. Valsartan: Dual blockade of the RAS is associated with increased risks of hypotension, hyperkalemia, and changes in renal function (including acute renal failure); closely monitor BP, renal function, and electrolytes with concomitant agents that also affect the RAS. Avoid with aliskiren in patients with renal impairment (GFR <60mL/min). Greater antihypertensive effect with atenolol. Other agents that block the RAS, K$^+$-sparing diuretics, K$^+$ supplements, or salt substitutes containing K$^+$ may increase serum K$^+$ levels, and in HF patients may increase SrCr; monitor serum K$^+$ levels. NSAIDs, including selective COX-2 inhibitors may result in deterioration of renal function, including possible acute renal failure, and may attenuate antihypertensive effect. Inhibitors of the hepatic uptake transporter OATP1B1 (rifampin, cyclosporine) and the hepatic efflux transporter MRP2 (ritonavir) may increase exposure. Increases in lithium levels and lithium toxicity reported; monitor serum lithium levels during concomitant use.

PREGNANCY: Category D, not for use in nursing.

MECHANISM OF ACTION: Amlodipine: Dihydropyridine CCB; inhibits transmembrane influx of Ca^{2+} into vascular smooth muscle and cardiac muscle. Acts directly on vascular smooth muscle to cause a reduction in peripheral vascular resistance and reduction in BP. Valsartan: ARBs; blocks the vasoconstrictor and aldosterone-secreting effects of angiotensin II by selectively blocking the binding of angiotensin II to the AT_1 receptor in many tissues, such as vascular smooth muscle and the adrenal gland.

PHARMACOKINETICS: Absorption: Amlodipine: Absolute bioavailability (64-90%); T_{max}=6-12 hrs. Valsartan: Absolute bioavailability (25%); T_{max}=2-4 hrs. **Distribution:** Amlodipine: V_d=21L/kg; plasma protein binding (93%). Valsartan: (IV) V_d=17L; plasma protein binding (95%). **Metabolism:** Amlodipine: Hepatic (extensive). Valsartan: Via CYP2C9; valeryl 4-hydroxy valsartan (metabolite). **Elimination:** Amlodipine: Urine (10% unchanged, 60% metabolites); $T_{1/2}$=30-50 hrs. Valsartan: (Oral Sol) Feces (83%), urine (13%); (IV) $T_{1/2}$=6 hrs.

NURSING CONSIDERATIONS

Assessment: Assess for hypersensitivity to any component of the drug, volume/salt depletion, HF, recent MI, renal artery stenosis, severe aortic stenosis, severe obstructive CAD, renal/hepatic impairment, pregnancy/nursing status, and possible drug interactions.

Monitoring: Monitor for signs/symptoms of hypotension, hyperkalemia, hypersensitivity reactions, and other adverse reactions. Monitor for symptoms of angina or MI, particularly in patients with severe obstructive CAD, after dosage initiation or increase. Monitor BP, serum electrolytes (especially K^+), and renal function.

Patient Counseling: Counsel about risks/benefits of therapy and possible adverse effects. Inform of the consequences of exposure during pregnancy and the treatment options in women planning to become pregnant; instruct to report pregnancy to physician as soon as possible.

Administration: Oral route. Take with or without food. **Storage:** 25°C (77°F); excursions permitted to 15-30°C (59-86°F). Protect from moisture.

EXFORGE HCT   RX
hydrochlorothiazide - amlodipine - valsartan (Novartis)

> D/C when pregnancy is detected. Drugs that act directly on the renin-angiotensin system (RAS) can cause injury/death to the developing fetus.

THERAPEUTIC CLASS: ARB/calcium channel blocker (dihydropyridine)/thiazide diuretic

INDICATIONS: Treatment of HTN alone or with other antihypertensive agents.

DOSAGE: *Adults:* Usual: Dose qd. Titrate: May increase dose after 2 weeks. Max: 10mg-320mg-25mg qd. Add-On/Switch Therapy: May use for patients not adequately controlled on any 2 of the following: calcium channel blockers (CCBs), ARBs, and diuretics. Patients with dose-limiting adverse reactions to an individual component while on any dual combination of the components of therapy may be switched to a lower dose of that component. Replacement Therapy: May substitute for individually titrated components. Hepatic Impairment: Consider lower doses. Elderly: Consider lower initial doses.

HOW SUPPLIED: Tab: (Amlodipine-Valsartan-HCTZ) 5mg-160mg-12.5mg, 5mg-160mg-25mg, 10mg-160mg-12.5mg, 10mg-160mg-25mg, 10mg-320mg-25mg

CONTRAINDICATIONS: Anuria, sulfonamide-derived drug hypersensitivity. Coadministration with aliskiren in patients with diabetes.

WARNINGS/PRECAUTIONS: Not for initial therapy of HTN. Symptomatic hypotension may occur in patients with activated RAS (eg, volume- and/or salt-depleted patients receiving high doses of diuretics); correct this condition prior to therapy. Avoid with aortic or mitral stenosis or obstructive hypertrophic cardiomyopathy. Renal function changes including acute renal failure may occur; caution in patients whose renal function depend in part on the activity of the RAS (eg, renal artery stenosis, severe heart failure (HF), post-myocardial infarction (MI), or volume depletion). Consider withholding or discontinuing therapy if clinically significant decrease in renal function develops. May cause serum electrolyte abnormalities (eg, hyperkalemia, hypokalemia, hyponatremia, hypomagnesemia); correct hypokalemia and any coexisting hypomagnesemia prior to initiation of therapy and monitor periodically. D/C if hypokalemia is accompanied by clinical signs (eg, muscular weakness, paresis, ECG alterations). Do not readminister to patients who have had angioedema. Amlodipine: Worsening angina and acute MI may develop after starting or increasing dose, particularly in patients with severe obstructive coronary artery disease (CAD). Valsartan: Increased K^+ in some patients with HF reported, and more likely to occur in patients with preexisting renal impairment; dose reduction and/or discontinuation of diuretic and/or valsartan may be required. HCTZ: May cause hypersensitivity reactions and exacerbation or activation of systemic lupus erythematosus (SLE). Minor alterations of fluid and electrolyte balance may precipitate hepatic coma in patients with hepatic dysfunction or progressive liver disease. May cause idiosyncratic reaction, resulting in acute transient myopia and acute angle-closure glaucoma; d/c as rapidly as possible. May alter glucose tolerance and increase serum cholesterol and TG levels. May cause or exacerbate hyperuricemia and precipitate gout in susceptible patients. May cause hypercalcemia.

ADVERSE REACTIONS: Increased BUN, hypokalemia, dizziness, edema, headache.

INTERACTIONS: See Contraindications. Amlodipine: May increase simvastatin exposure; limit simvastatin dose to 20mg/day. Increased systemic exposure with CYP3A inhibitors (moderate and strong) warranting dose reduction; monitor for symptoms of hypotension and edema to determine the need for dose adjustment. Monitor BP when coadministered with CYP3A4 inducers. Valsartan: Dual blockade of the RAS is associated with increased risk of hypotension, hyperkalemia, and changes in renal function (including acute renal failure); closely monitor BP, renal function, and electrolytes with concomitant agents that also affect the RAS. Avoid with aliskiren in patients with renal impairment (GFR <60mL/min). Greater antihypertensive effect with atenolol. Other agents that block the RAS, K^+-sparing diuretics, K^+ supplements, or salt substitutes containing K^+ may lead to increases in serum K^+, and in HF patients to increases in SrCr; monitor serum K^+ levels. NSAIDs, including selective COX-2 inhibitors, may deteriorate renal function and attenuate antihypertensive effect. HCTZ: Dosage adjustment of antidiabetic drugs (eg, oral agents, insulin) may be required. May lead to symptomatic hyponatremia with carbamazepine. Ion exchange resins (eg, cholestyramine, colestipol) may reduce exposure; space dosing at least 4 hrs before or 4-6 hrs after the administration of resins. Cyclosporine may increase risk of hyperuricemia and gout-type complications. Valsartan-HCTZ: Increases in lithium levels and lithium toxicity reported; monitor serum lithium levels during concomitant use.

PREGNANCY: Category D, not for use in nursing.

MECHANISM OF ACTION: Amlodipine: Dihydropyridine CCB; inhibits transmembrane influx of Ca^{2+} into vascular smooth muscle and cardiac muscle, causing a reduction in peripheral vascular resistance and BP. Valsartan: ARB; blocks the vasoconstrictor and aldosterone-secreting effects of angiotensin II by selectively blocking the binding of angiotensin II to AT_1 receptor in many tissues (eg, vascular smooth muscle, adrenal gland). HCTZ: Thiazide diuretic; has not been established. Affects renal tubular mechanisms of electrolyte reabsorption directly increasing excretion of Na^+ and Cl^-, and indirectly reducing plasma volume.

PHARMACOKINETICS: Absorption: Amlodipine: Absolute bioavailability (64-90%); T_{max}=6-12 hrs. Valsartan: Absolute bioavailability (25%); T_{max}=2-4 hrs. HCTZ: Absolute bioavailability (70%); T_{max}=2-5 hrs. **Distribution:** Amlodipine: V_d=21L/kg; plasma protein binding (93%). Valsartan: (IV) V_d=17L; plasma protein binding (95%). HCTZ: Plasma protein binding (40-70%); crosses placenta; found in breast milk. **Metabolism:** Amlodipine: Hepatic (extensive). Valsartan: Via CYP2C9; valeryl-4-hydroxy valsartan (metabolite). **Elimination:** Amlodipine: Urine (10% unchanged, 60% metabolites), $T_{1/2}$=30-50 hrs. Valsartan: (Oral Sol) Feces (83%), urine (13%); (IV) $T_{1/2}$=6 hrs. HCTZ: Urine (70% unchanged), $T_{1/2}$=10 hrs.

NURSING CONSIDERATIONS

Assessment: Assess for hypersensitivity to the drug and its components, anuria, sulfonamide-derived drug or PCN hypersensitivity, history of allergy or bronchial asthma, renal/hepatic impairment, HF, aortic or mitral stenosis, renal artery stenosis, obstructive hypertrophic cardiomyopathy, SLE, volume/salt depletion, electrolyte imbalances, CAD, pregnancy/nursing status, and possible drug interactions.

Monitoring: Monitor for signs/symptoms of hypotension, hypersensitivity/idiosyncratic reactions, metabolic disturbances, myopia and angle-closure glaucoma, worsening angina or acute MI, fluid imbalance, exacerbation or activation of SLE, hyperglycemia, hyperuricemia or precipitation of gout, increases in cholesterol and TG levels, and other adverse reactions. Monitor BP, serum electrolytes, BUN, and renal function.

Patient Counseling: Inform of the consequences of exposure during pregnancy and the treatment options in women planning to become pregnant; instruct to report pregnancy to physician as soon as possible. Inform that lightheadedness may occur, especially during the 1st days of therapy; if syncope occurs, instruct to d/c therapy until physician has been consulted. Caution that inadequate fluid intake, excessive perspiration, diarrhea, or vomiting may lead to an excessive fall in BP, which may result in lightheadedness and possible syncope. Instruct to avoid K^+ supplements or salt substitutes containing K^+ without consulting prescribing physician.

Administration: Oral route. Take with or without food. **Storage:** 25°C (77°F); excursions permitted to 15-30°C (59-86°F). Protect from moisture.

EXTAVIA   RX
interferon beta-1b (Novartis)

THERAPEUTIC CLASS: Biological response modifier

INDICATIONS: Treatment of relapsing forms of multiple sclerosis to reduce the frequency of clinical exacerbations.

DOSAGE: *Adults:* Initial: 0.0625mg SQ qod. Titrate: Increase over 6 weeks to 0.25mg qod SQ. Refer to PI for dose titration schedule.

HOW SUPPLIED: Inj: 0.3mg

CONTRAINDICATIONS: Hypersensitivity to human albumin.

WARNINGS/PRECAUTIONS: Caution in patients with depression. Increased frequency of depression and suicide reported; consider discontinuing if depression develops. Inj-site necrosis reported; d/c if multiple lesions occur. Inj-site reactions reported. Anaphylaxis/allergic reactions (eg, dyspnea, bronchospasm, tongue edema, skin rash, urticaria), flu-like symptom complex, leukopenia, and hepatic enzyme elevation (ALT, AST) reported. Contains albumin; risk of viral disease transmission.

ADVERSE REACTIONS: Inj-site reactions/necrosis, flu-like symptom complex, headache, lymphopenia, hypertonia, asthenia, increased liver enzymes, skin disorder, insomnia, abdominal pain, incoordination, neutropenia, leukopenia, lymphadenopathy.

PREGNANCY: Category C, not for use in nursing.

MECHANISM OF ACTION: Biological response modifier; not established. Believed that interferon β-1b receptor binding induces expression of proteins that are responsible for pleiotropic bioactivities. Immunomodulatory effects include the enhancement of suppressor T cell activity, reduction of proinflammatory cytokine production, down-regulation of antigen presentation, and inhibition of lymphocyte trafficking into the CNS.

NURSING CONSIDERATIONS

Assessment: Assess for hypersensitivity to the drug or human albumin, depression, thyroid dysfunction, liver function, myelosuppression, and pregnancy/nursing status.

Monitoring: Monitor for anaphylaxis, depression, suicidal ideation, inj-site reactions, inj-site necrosis, and flu-like symptom complex. Monitor CBC, differential WBC count, platelet count, LFTs, and blood chemistry at regular intervals (1, 3, and 6 months) following introduction, then periodically thereafter. Perform thyroid function test every 6 months with history of thyroid dysfunction or as clinically indicated.

Patient Counseling: Inform about potential benefits/risks of therapy. Advise not to change dose or schedule of administration. Inform that depression and suicidal ideation, inj-site reactions, inj-site necrosis, allergic reactions, and anaphylaxis may occur; advise to d/c and notify physician if symptoms are experienced. Inform that antipyretics and analgesics are permitted for relief of flu-like symptoms, which are common following initiation of therapy. Advise to notify physician if pregnant or planning to become pregnant. Instruct on how to administer therapy.

Administration: SQ route. Rotate inj sites. Refer to PI for reconstitution instructions. **Storage:** 25°C (77°F); excursions permitted to 15-30°C (59-86°F). After reconstitution, if not used immediately, refrigerate and use within 3 hrs. Avoid freezing.

EXTINA   RX
ketoconazole (Stiefel)

THERAPEUTIC CLASS: Azole antifungal

INDICATIONS: Topical treatment of seborrheic dermatitis in immunocompetent patients ≥12 yrs of age.

DOSAGE: *Adults:* Apply to affected area(s) bid for 4 weeks.
Pediatrics: ≥12 Yrs: Apply to affected area(s) bid for 4 weeks.

HOW SUPPLIED: Foam: 2% [50g, 100g]

WARNINGS/PRECAUTIONS: Not for ophthalmic, oral, or intravaginal use. Safety and efficacy for the treatment of fungal infections not established. May cause contact sensitization, including photoallergenicity. Contents are flammable; avoid fire, flame, and/or smoking during and immediately following application. Hepatitis, lowered testosterone, and adrenocorticotropic hormone-induced corticosteroid serum levels reported with orally administered ketoconazole; not seen with topical ketoconazole.

ADVERSE REACTIONS: Application-site burning, application-site reactions (eg, dryness, erythema, irritation, paresthesia, pruritus, rash, warmth), photoallergenicity, contact sensitization.

PREGNANCY: Category C, caution in nursing.

MECHANISM OF ACTION: Azole antifungal; not established. Inhibits the synthesis of ergosterol, a key sterol in the cell membrane of *Malassezia furfur*.

NURSING CONSIDERATIONS

Assessment: Assess pregnancy/nursing status.

Monitoring: Monitor for contact sensitization and application-site reactions.

Patient Counseling: Instruct to use ud. Instruct to avoid fire, flame, and/or smoking during and immediately following application. Instruct not to apply directly to hands; apply to affected areas using the fingertips. Inform that skin irritation, and contact sensitization may occur; instruct to inform a physician if the area show signs of increased irritation, and to report any signs of adverse reactions. Instruct to wash hands after application.

Administration: Topical route. Refer to PI for proper administration techniques. **Storage:** 20-25°C (68-77°F). Do not store under refrigerated conditions or in direct sunlight. Do not expose containers to heat or store at temperatures above 49°C (120°F). Do not puncture and/or incinerate container.

EYLEA
aflibercept (Regeneron)

RX

THERAPEUTIC CLASS: Vascular endothelial growth factor (VEGF) inhibitor

INDICATIONS: Treatment of neovascular (wet) age-related macular degeneration (AMD), and macular edema following central retinal vein occlusion (CRVO).

DOSAGE: *Adults:* Neovascular (Wet) AMD: 2mg (0.05mL) by intravitreal inj every 4 weeks for the first 12 weeks, then every 8 weeks thereafter. Macular Edema Following CRVO: 2mg (0.05mL) by intravitreal inj every 4 weeks.

HOW SUPPLIED: Inj: 40mg/mL [0.05mL]

CONTRAINDICATIONS: Ocular/periocular infections, active intraocular inflammation.

WARNINGS/PRECAUTIONS: Endophthalmitis and retinal detachments may occur; always use proper aseptic inj technique. Acute increases in intraocular pressure (IOP) noted within 60 min of inj; IOP and perfusion of the optic nerve head should be monitored and managed appropriately. Potential risk of arterial thromboembolic events (ATEs) (eg, nonfatal stroke, nonfatal myocardial infarction, or vascular death).

ADVERSE REACTIONS: Conjunctival hemorrhage/hyperemia, eye pain, cataract, vitreous detachment/floaters, increased IOP, corneal erosion, retinal pigment epithelium detachment, inj-site pain, foreign body sensation in eyes, increased lacrimation.

PREGNANCY: Category C, not for use in nursing.

MECHANISM OF ACTION: VEGF inhibitor; acts as a soluble decoy receptor that binds VEGF-A and placental growth factor, and thereby can inhibit the binding and activation of these cognate VEGF receptors.

PHARMACOKINETICS: Absorption: C_{max}=0.02mcg/mL (wet AMD), 0.05mcg/mL (CRVO); T_{max}=1-3 days. **Distribution:** (IV) V_d=6L. **Metabolism:** Proteolysis. **Elimination:** (IV) $T_{1/2}$=5-6 days.

NURSING CONSIDERATIONS

Assessment: Assess for ocular/periocular infections, active intraocular inflammation, hypersensitivity to the drug, and pregnancy/nursing status.

Monitoring: Monitor IOP and perfusion of the optic nerve head. Monitor for signs/symptoms of endophthalmitis, retinal detachment, ATEs, and other adverse reactions.

Patient Counseling: Advise to seek immediate care from an ophthalmologist if eye becomes red, sensitive to light, painful, or develops a change in vision in the days following administration. Inform that temporary visual disturbances may be experienced after inj and the associated eye examinations; advise not to drive or use machinery until visual function has recovered sufficiently.

Administration: Intravitreal route. Refer to PI for preparation and administration instructions. **Storage:** 2-8°C (36-46°F). Do not freeze. Protect from light.

FACTIVE
gemifloxacin mesylate (Cornerstone)

RX

> Fluoroquinolones are associated with an increased risk of tendinitis and tendon rupture in all ages. Risk is further increased in patients >60 yrs, patients taking corticosteroids, and with kidney, heart, or lung transplants. May exacerbate muscle weakness with myasthenia gravis; avoid in patients with known history of myasthenia gravis.

THERAPEUTIC CLASS: Fluoroquinolone

INDICATIONS: Treatment of community-acquired pneumonia (CAP) and acute bacterial exacerbation of chronic bronchitis (ABECB) caused by susceptible strains of microorganisms.

DOSAGE: *Adults:* ≥18 Yrs: ABECB: 320mg qd for 5 days. CAP: 320mg qd for 5 days (*Streptococcus pneumoniae, Haemophilus influenzae, Mycoplasma pneumoniae,* or *Chlamydia pneumoniae*) or 7 days (multidrug resistant *S. pneumoniae, Klebsiella pneumoniae,* or *Moraxella catarrhalis*). CrCl ≤40mL/min or Dialysis: 160mg q24h.

HOW SUPPLIED: Tab: 320mg* *scored

WARNINGS/PRECAUTIONS: D/C if pain, swelling, inflammation, or rupture of a tendon occurs. May prolong QT interval; avoid with history of QTc interval prolongation or uncontrolled electrolyte disorders, and caution with proarrhythmic conditions. Serious and sometimes fatal hypersensitivity reactions reported; d/c if skin rash, jaundice, or any other sign of hypersensitivity appears and institute appropriate therapy. Rare cases of sensory or sensorimotor axonal polyneuropathy, resulting in paresthesias, hypoesthesias, dysesthesias, and weakness reported. CNS effects (infrequent) reported; caution with CNS diseases (eg, epilepsy or patients predisposed to convulsions), and d/c if CNS stimulation occurs. Convulsions, toxic psychoses, and increased intracranial pressure (including pseudotumor cerebri) reported. *Clostridium difficile*-associated diarrhea (CDAD) reported. May cause photosensitivity/phototoxicity reactions; d/c if photosensitivity/phototoxicity occurs. Avoid excessive exposure to source of light. Liver enzyme elevations reported. Caution in elderly and with renal impairment. Maintain adequate hydration. May result in bacterial resistance with prolonged use or use in the absence of a proven/suspected bacterial infection or a prophylactic indication; take appropriate measures if superinfection develops.

ADVERSE REACTIONS: Diarrhea, rash, N/V, headache, abdominal pain, dizziness.

INTERACTIONS: See Boxed Warning. Avoid Mg^{2+}- or aluminum-containing antacids, ferrous sulfate (iron), Videx (didanosine) chewable/buffered tab or pediatric powder for oral sol, and multivitamin preparations containing zinc or other metal cations, within 3 hrs before or 2 hrs after therapy and sucralfate within 2 hrs of therapy. Calcium carbonate may decrease levels. Reduced levels with oral estrogen/progesterone contraceptive product. Increased levels with cimetidine, omeprazole, probenecid. Avoid Class IA (eg, quinidine, procainamide) or Class III (eg, amiodarone, sotalol) antiarrhythmics. Caution with drugs that prolong the QTc interval (eg, erythromycin, antipsychotics, TCAs). Increased INR or PT and/or clinical episodes of bleeding reported with warfarin or its derivatives.

PREGNANCY: Category C, not for use in nursing.

MECHANISM OF ACTION: Fluoroquinolone; inhibits DNA synthesis through inhibition of both DNA gyrase and topoisomerase IV, which are essential for bacterial growth.

PHARMACOKINETICS: Absorption: Rapid. Absolute bioavailability (71%); AUC=8.36μg•hr/mL, C_{max}=1.61μg/mL, T_{max}=0.5-2 hrs. **Distribution:** V_d=4.18L/kg; plasma protein binding (55-73%). **Metabolism:** Liver. **Elimination:** Feces (61%), urine (36% unchanged); $T_{1/2}$=7 hrs.

NURSING CONSIDERATIONS

Assessment: Assess for hypersensitivity to drug, factors that increase the risk of tendon rupture, history of myasthenia gravis and QTc interval prolongation, uncontrolled electrolyte disorders, proarrhythmic conditions, CNS disease, pregnancy/nursing status, and possible drug interactions. Obtain baseline renal function and LFTs.

Monitoring: Monitor for signs/symptoms of tendinitis or tendon rupture, muscle weakness exacerbation, hypersensitivity and photosensitivity/phototoxicity reactions, peripheral neuropathy, CNS effects, and CDAD. Monitor renal function and LFTs.

Patient Counseling: Instruct to contact physician and advise to rest, refrain from exercise, and d/c therapy if pain, swelling, or inflammation of a tendon, or weakness or inability to move joints occur. Inform that drug may worsen myasthenia gravis symptoms; immediately contact physician if muscle weakness worsens or breathing problems occur. Inform that drug treats bacterial, not viral, infections. Instruct to take drug exactly ud, swallow whole, drink fluids liberally, and not to skip doses. Instruct to d/c therapy and notify physician if rash or other allergic reaction develops. Counsel to notify physician if watery and bloody stools, palpitations, sunburn-like reaction, or skin eruption occurs, and about medications taken concurrently. Instruct not to engage in activities requiring mental alertness and coordination if dizziness occurs, and to minimize or avoid sun/UV light exposure.

Administration: Oral route. Swallow whole with fluids. **Storage:** 25°C (77°F); excursions permitted to 15-30°C (59-86°F). Protect from light.

FAMOTIDINE RX
famotidine (Various)

OTHER BRAND NAMES: Pepcid (Various)

THERAPEUTIC CLASS: H_2-blocker

INDICATIONS: Short-term treatment of active duodenal ulcer (DU)/benign gastric ulcer (GU), gastroesophageal reflux disease (GERD), and esophagitis due to GERD, including erosive or ulcerative disease diagnosed by endoscopy. Maintenance therapy for DU after healing of an active ulcer. Treatment of pathological hypersecretory conditions (eg, Zollinger-Ellison syndrome, multiple endocrine adenomas). (Inj) Indicated in some hospitalized patients with pathological hypersecretory conditions or intractable ulcers, or as alternative for short-term use in patients who are unable to take oral medication.

DOSAGE: *Adults:* (IV) Usual: 20mg q12h. (PO) DU: Usual: 20mg bid or 40mg qhs for 4-8 weeks. Maint: 20mg qhs. Benign GU: Usual: 40mg qhs. GERD: Usual: 20mg bid for up to 6 weeks. GERD with Esophagitis: 20 or 40mg bid for up to 12 weeks. Pathological Hypersecretory Conditions: A higher starting dose may be required in some patients. Adjust dose to individual patient needs and continue as long as clinically indicated. (PO) Initial: 20mg q6h. Doses up to 160mg q6h have been administered to some patients with severe Zollinger-Ellison syndrome. Moderate (CrCl <50mL/min) or Severe (CrCl <10mL/min) Renal Insufficiency: May reduce to 1/2 dose, or may prolong dosing interval to 36-48 hrs based on response.
Pediatrics: Individualize dose based on response and/or gastric/esophageal pH determination and endoscopy. 1-16 Yrs: Peptic Ulcer: Initial: (PO) 0.5mg/kg/day qhs or divided bid. Max: 40mg/day. (IV) Initial: 0.25mg/kg over ≥2 min or as 15-min infusion q12h. Max: 40mg/day. GERD with or without Esophagitis: (PO) Initial: 1mg/kg/day divided bid. Max: 40mg bid. GERD: (PO) (Sus) 3 Months-<1 Yr: 0.5mg/kg/dose bid. <3 Months: 0.5mg/kg/dose qd for up to 8 weeks. Moderate or Severe Renal Impairment: Consider dose adjustment.

HOW SUPPLIED: Inj: 10mg/mL [2mL, 4mL, 20mL]; 20mg/50mL [50mL]; Sus: (Pepcid) 40mg/5mL [50mL]; Tab: (Pepcid) 20mg, 40mg

WARNINGS/PRECAUTIONS: Symptomatic response to therapy does not preclude presence of gastric malignancy. CNS adverse effects reported with moderate and severe renal insufficiency; may need to prolong dosing intervals or lower dose. Caution in elderly. (Inj) For IV use only. (Tab) Very rarely, prolonged QT interval reported in patients with impaired renal function whose dose/dosing interval may not have been adjusted appropriately.

ADVERSE REACTIONS: Headache, agitation.

PREGNANCY: Category B, not for use in nursing.

MECHANISM OF ACTION: Histamine H_2-receptor antagonist; inhibits both acid concentration and volume of gastric secretion.

PHARMACOKINETICS: Absorption: (PO) Incomplete; bioavailability (40-45%); T_{max}=1-3 hrs. **Distribution:** Plasma protein binding (15-20%); found in breast milk. **Metabolism:** S-oxide (metabolite). **Elimination:** Renal (65-70%; 25-30% unchanged [PO], 65-70% unchanged [IV]), metabolic (30-35%); $T_{1/2}$=2.5-3.5 hrs. Refer to PI for pediatric parameters.

NURSING CONSIDERATIONS

Assessment: Assess for hypersensitivity to the drug or to other H_2-receptor antagonists, renal insufficiency, gastric malignancy, pregnancy/nursing status, and possible drug interactions.

Monitoring: Monitor for hypersensitivity reactions and other adverse reactions. Monitor renal function in the elderly.

Patient Counseling: Inform of risks/benefits of therapy. Instruct to contact physician if hypersensitivity or other adverse reactions develop. Advise to avoid nursing while on medication.

Administration: IV/Oral route. May take with antacids if needed. Refer to PI for directions for preparation and administration instructions. (Sus) Shake vigorously for 5-10 sec prior to each use. **Storage:** (Inj) 2-8°C (36-46°F). Bring to room temperature if sol freezes. Diluted Sol: Stable at room temperature for 7 days. Refrigeration and use within 48 hrs is recommended if not used immediately after preparation. (Premixed Inj) 25°C (77°F); avoid exposure to excessive heat; brief exposure to temperatures ≤35°C (95°F) does not adversely affect product. (Sus) 25°C (77°F); excursions permitted to 15-30°C (59-86°F). Protect from freezing. Discard unused suspension after 30 days. (Tab) Controlled room temperature.

FAMVIR RX
famciclovir (Novartis)

THERAPEUTIC CLASS: Nucleoside analogue

INDICATIONS: Treatment of herpes zoster (shingles) and recurrent herpes labialis (cold sores) in immunocompetent adults. Treatment and chronic suppressive therapy of recurrent episodes of genital herpes in immunocompetent adults. Treatment of recurrent episodes of orolabial or genital herpes in HIV-infected adults.

DOSAGE: *Adults:* Immunocompetent Patients: Recurrent Herpes Labialis: 1500mg as a single dose; initiate at the 1st sign/symptom (eg, tingling, itching, burning, pain, or lesion). Genital Herpes: Recurrent Episodes: 1000mg bid for 1 day; initiate at the 1st sign/symptom. Suppressive Therapy: 250mg bid. Herpes Zoster: 500mg q8h for 7 days; initiate as soon as herpes zoster is diagnosed. HIV-Infected Patients: Recurrent Orolabial/Genital Herpes: 500mg bid for 7 days; initiate at the 1st sign/symptom. Refer to PI for dosage recommendations for renal impairment.

HOW SUPPLIED: Tab: 125mg, 250mg, 500mg

WARNINGS/PRECAUTIONS: Acute renal failure reported in patients with underlying renal disease who have received inappropriately high doses. Caution in elderly and with renal impairment.

ADVERSE REACTIONS: Headache, N/V, diarrhea, elevated lipase, ALT elevation, fatigue, flatulence, pruritus, rash, neutropenia, abdominal pain, dysmenorrhea, migraine.

INTERACTIONS: Probenecid or other drugs significantly eliminated by active renal tubular secretion may increase levels of penciclovir. Potential interaction with drugs metabolized by and/or inhibiting aldehyde oxidase. Raloxifene may decrease formation of penciclovir.

PREGNANCY: Category B, not for use in nursing.

MECHANISM OF ACTION: Nucleoside analogue; prodrug of penciclovir, which has demonstrated inhibitory activity against herpes simplex virus types 1 and 2 and varicella zoster virus.

PHARMACOKINETICS: Absorption: Penciclovir: Absolute bioavailability (77%). Oral administration of variable doses resulted in different parameters. **Distribution:** Penciclovir: (IV) V_d=1.08L/kg; plasma protein binding (<20%). **Metabolism:** Deacetylation and oxidation; famciclovir (prodrug) converted to penciclovir. **Elimination:** Urine (73%, 82% penciclovir, 7% 6-deoxy penciclovir), feces (27%); $T_{1/2}$=2.8 hrs (single dose, herpes zoster patients), 2.7 hrs (repeated doses, herpes zoster patients).

NURSING CONSIDERATIONS

Assessment: Assess for hypersensitivity to the drug, renal impairment, pregnancy/nursing status, and possible drug interactions.

Monitoring: Monitor renal function, and for adverse reactions.

Patient Counseling: Inform to take exactly ud. Advise to initiate treatment at earliest signs/symptoms of recurrence of cold sores, at the 1st sign/symptom of recurrent genital herpes if episodic therapy is indicated, and as soon as possible after a diagnosis of herpes zoster. Inform that drug is not a cure for cold sores or genital herpes. Advise to avoid contact with lesions or intercourse when lesions and/or symptoms are present to avoid infecting partners. Counsel to use safer sex practices. Instruct to refrain from driving or operating machinery if dizziness, somnolence, confusion, or other CNS disturbances occur. Inform that drug contains lactose; instruct to notify physician if with rare hereditary problems of galactose intolerance, a severe lactase deficiency, or glucose-galactose malabsorption.

Administration: Oral route. Take with or without food. **Storage:** 25°C (77°F); excursions permitted to 15-30°C (59-86°F).

FANAPT   RX
iloperidone (Novartis)

> Elderly patients with dementia-related psychosis treated with antipsychotic drugs are at an increased risk of death; most deaths appeared to be cardiovascular (CV) (eg, heart failure, sudden death) or infectious (eg, pneumonia) in nature. Not approved for the treatment of patients with dementia-related psychosis.

THERAPEUTIC CLASS: Benzisoxazole derivative

INDICATIONS: Treatment of adults with schizophrenia.

DOSAGE: *Adults:* Initial: 1mg bid. Titrate: Titrate slowly from a low starting dose. Dose increases may be made with daily dosage adjustments not to exceed 2mg bid (4mg/day) to reach the target range of 6-12mg bid (12-24mg/day). Max: 12mg bid (24mg/day). Concomitant use w/ Strong CYP2D6 Inhibitors or Strong CYP3A4 Inhibitors: Reduce dose by 50%. Increase to previous iloperidone dose upon withdrawal of strong CYP2D6 or strong CYP3A4 inhibitor. Poor CYP2D6 Metabolizers: Reduce dose by 50%. Maint: Responding patients may continue beyond acute response; periodically reassess need for maint treatment. Reinitiation of Treatment: Follow initiation titration schedule if have had an interval off for >3 days. Switching From Other Antipsychotics: Minimize overlapping period of antipsychotics.

HOW SUPPLIED: Tab: 1mg, 2mg, 4mg, 6mg, 8mg, 10mg, 12mg

WARNINGS/PRECAUTIONS: Not recommended in patients with hepatic impairment. QT prolongation reported; avoid with congenital long QT syndrome, history of cardiac arrhythmias, or history of significant CV illnesses. Obtain baseline measurements and periodically monitor K^+ and Mg^{2+} levels in patients at risk of electrolyte disturbances. D/C if persistent QTc measurements >500 msec occur. Risk of tardive dyskinesia (TD), especially in the elderly; consider d/c if signs/symptoms develop. Neuroleptic malignant syndrome (NMS) reported; immediately d/c and treat. May cause metabolic changes (eg, hyperglycemia, dyslipidemia, weight gain) that may increase CV and cerebrovascular risk. Hyperglycemia, in some cases extreme and associated with ketoacidosis or hyperosmolar coma or death reported; monitor for worsening of glucose control, and perform FPG testing at the beginning of therapy and periodically in patients at risk for diabetes mellitus (DM). Caution with a history of seizures, conditions that lower the seizure threshold, or in patients with reduced CYP2D6 activity. May induce orthostatic hypotension; caution with cardiovascular disease (CVD), cerebrovascular disease, or conditions that predispose to hypotension. Leukopenia, neutropenia, and agranulocytosis reported; d/c in cases of severe neutropenia (absolute neutrophil count <1000/mm³). Monitor CBC and d/c at 1st sign of decline in WBC if with preexisting low WBC count or history of drug-induced leukopenia/neutropenia and in the absence of other causative factors. May elevate prolactin levels. May disrupt body's ability to reduce core body temperature; caution in conditions that may elevate body core temperature. Esophageal dysmotility and aspiration reported; caution in patients at risk of aspiration pneumonia. Closely supervise high-risk patients for suicide attempt. Priapism reported. May impair mental/physical abilities. Evaluate for history of drug abuse; observe for drug misuse/abuse in these patients.

ADVERSE REACTIONS: Dizziness, somnolence, tachycardia, nausea, dry mouth, weight gain, nasal congestion, diarrhea, fatigue, extrapyramidal disorder, orthostatic hypotension, nasopharyngitis, arthralgia, tremor, upper respiratory tract infection.

INTERACTIONS: Caution with CYP3A4 (eg, ketoconazole, clarithromycin) or CYP2D6 (eg, fluoxetine, paroxetine) inhibitors; may increase levels and may augment effect on the QTc interval. Reduce dose by about 50% if administered concomitantly with both a CYP2D6 and CYP3A4 inhibitor. May increase total exposure of dextromethorphan with concomitant use. Avoid with Class IA (eg, quinidine, procainamide) or Class III (eg, amiodarone, sotalol) antiarrhythmics, antipsychotics (eg, chlorpromazine, thioridazine), antibiotics (eg, gatifloxacin, moxifloxacin), or other drugs known to prolong the QTc interval (eg, pentamidine, levomethadyl acetate, methadone). Caution with other centrally acting drugs and alcohol. May potentiate effects of antihypertensive agents. Concomitant use with medications with anticholinergic activity may contribute to an elevation in core body temperature. May increase levels of drugs that are predominantly eliminated by CYP3A4.

PREGNANCY: Category C, not for use in nursing.

MECHANISM OF ACTION: Piperidinyl-benzisoxazole derivative; not established. Proposed to be mediated through a combination of dopamine type 2 and serotonin type 2 antagonisms.

PHARMACOKINETICS: Absorption: Well-absorbed; T_{max}=2-4 hrs. **Distribution:** V_d=1340-2800L; plasma protein binding (95%). **Metabolism:** Liver via carbonyl reduction, hydroxylation (CYP2D6), O-demethylation (CYP3A4); P88, P95 (major metabolites). **Elimination:** Urine (58.2% extensive metabolizers [EM], 45.1% poor metabolizers [PM]), feces (19.9% EM, 22.1% PM); $T_{1/2}$= 18 hrs (iloperidone), 26 hrs (P88), 23 hrs (P95) (EM); 33 hrs (iloperidone), 37 hrs (P88), 31 hrs (P95) (PM).

NURSING CONSIDERATIONS

Assessment: Assess for known hypersensitivity to the drug, dementia-related psychosis, hepatic impairment, DM, risk factors for DM, CVD, cerebrovascular disease, congenital long QT syndrome, history of cardiac arrhythmias, conditions that predispose to hypotension, conditions that may contribute to an elevation in core body temperature, history of clinically significant low WBCs or drug-induced leukopenia/neutropenia, history of seizures, conditions that lower the seizure threshold, history of drug abuse, poor metabolizers of CYP2D6, risk for aspiration pneumonia, risk for suicide, pregnancy/nursing status, and possible drug interactions. Obtain baseline FPG in patients with DM or with risk factors for DM. Perform baseline CBC, orthostatic vital signs, serum K+ and Mg2+ levels.

Monitoring: Monitor for TD, NMS, priapism, extrapyramidal symptoms, esophageal dysmotility, aspiration, orthostatic hypotension, body temperature lability, seizures, weight gain, dyslipidemia, QT prolongation, cognitive/motor impairment, and other adverse effects. Monitor for signs of hyperglycemia; monitor FPG levels in patients with DM or at risk for DM. Monitor for suicide attempts. Monitor for drug misuse/abuse in patients with a history of drug misuse/abuse. Monitor for signs/symptoms of leukopenia, neutropenia, and agranulocytosis; frequently monitor CBC in patients with risk factors for leukopenia/neutropenia. Monitor serum K+ and Mg2+ levels, and orthostatic vital signs.

Patient Counseling: Advise to inform physician immediately if feeling faint, lose consciousness or have heart palpitations. Counsel to avoid drugs that cause QT interval prolongation and instruct to inform physician of all medications currently taking or plan to take (prescription or OTC drugs). Inform about the signs/symptoms of NMS, hyperglycemia, and DM. Counsel that weight gain may occur during treatment. Advise of risk of orthostatic hypotension, particularly at time of initiating/reinitiating treatment, or increasing the dose. Inform that the drug may impair judgment, thinking, or motor skills; advise to use caution against driving or operating hazardous machinery. Instruct to notify physician if pregnant or intend to become pregnant. Advise not to breastfeed. Instruct to avoid alcohol. Counsel about appropriate care to avoid overheating and dehydration.

Administration: Oral route. Take without regard to meals. **Storage:** 25°C (77°F); excursions permitted to 15-30°C (59-86°F). Protect from light and moisture.

FARXIGA RX
dapagliflozin (Bristol-Myers Squibb)

THERAPEUTIC CLASS: Sodium-glucose co-transporter 2 (SGLT2) inhibitor

INDICATIONS: Adjunct to diet and exercise to improve glycemic control in adults with type 2 diabetes mellitus (DM).

DOSAGE: *Adults:* Initial: 5mg qam. Titrate: May increase to 10mg qd in patients tolerating 5mg qd who require additional glycemic control.

HOW SUPPLIED: Tab: 5mg, 10mg

CONTRAINDICATIONS: Severe renal impairment, end-stage renal disease, patients on dialysis.

WARNINGS/PRECAUTIONS: Not recommended with type 1 DM or for treatment of diabetic ketoacidosis. Do not initiate in patients with an eGFR <60mL/min. Causes intravascular volume contraction. Symptomatic hypotension may occur, particularly in patients with renal impairment (eGFR <60mL/min), elderly patients, or patients on loop diuretics; correct volume status before initiating treatment in patients with ≥1 of these characteristics. Increases SrCr and decreases eGFR; caution in elderly patients and patients with renal impairment. Adverse reactions related to renal function may occur; evaluate renal function prior to initiation of therapy and periodically thereafter. D/C when eGFR is persistently <60mL/min. Increases risk of genital mycotic infections. Increases in LDL levels reported; monitor LDL levels and treat appropriately. Newly diagnosed cases of bladder cancer reported; do not use in patients with active bladder cancer and caution in patients with prior history of bladder cancer. Hypersensitivity reactions (eg, angioedema, urticaria, hypersensitivity) reported; d/c and treat if this occurs and monitor until signs/symptoms resolve. Caution in patients with severe hepatic impairment.

ADVERSE REACTIONS: Genital mycotic infections, nasopharyngitis, urinary tract infections (UTIs), back pain, increased urination.

INTERACTIONS: May increase risk of hypoglycemia when combined with insulin or an insulin secretagogue; a lower dose of insulin or insulin secretagogue may be required.

PREGNANCY: Category C, not for use in nursing.

MECHANISM OF ACTION: SGLT2 inhibitor; reduces reabsorption of filtered glucose and lowers the renal threshold for glucose, and thereby increases urinary glucose excretion.

PHARMACOKINETICS: Absorption: Absolute oral bioavailability (78%); T_{max}=2 hrs. **Distribution:** Plasma protein binding (91%). **Metabolism:** Extensive; O-glucuronidation by UGT1A9 (primary); CYP (minor). **Elimination:** (Single 50mg dose) Urine (75%, <2% unchanged), feces (21%, 15% unchanged). $T_{1/2}$=12.9 hrs.

NURSING CONSIDERATIONS

Assessment: Assess for diabetic ketoacidosis, type of DM, volume status, risk for genital mycotic infections, active/history of bladder cancer, drug hypersensitivity, pregnancy/nursing status, and possible drug interactions. Assess baseline renal/hepatic function, LDL levels, and BP.

Monitoring: Monitor for signs/symptoms of hypotension, genital mycotic infections, hypersensitivity reactions, and other adverse reactions. Monitor renal function and LDL levels.

Patient Counseling: Inform of the risks, benefits, and alternative modes of therapy. Advise about the importance of adherence to dietary instructions, regular physical activity, periodic blood glucose monitoring and HbA1c testing, recognition and management of hypoglycemia and hyperglycemia, and assessment of diabetes complications. Instruct to seek medical advice promptly during periods of stress (eg, fever, trauma, infection, surgery) as medication requirements may change. Instruct to immediately inform physician if pregnant, breastfeeding, planning to become pregnant or to breastfeed, or if experiencing signs/symptoms of hypotension or bladder cancer. Instruct to have adequate fluid intake. Counsel on the signs/symptoms of vaginal yeast infection, balanitis, balanoposthitis, and UTI; inform of treatment options and when to seek medical advice. Instruct to d/c therapy and consult physician if any signs/symptoms suggesting an allergic reaction or angioedema develop.

Administration: Oral route. Take in the am, with or without food. **Storage:** 20-25°C (68-77°F); excursions permitted between 15-30°C (59-86°F).

FASLODEX RX
fulvestrant (AstraZeneca)

THERAPEUTIC CLASS: Estrogen receptor antagonist

INDICATIONS: Treatment of hormone receptor positive metastatic breast cancer in postmenopausal women with disease progression following antiestrogen therapy.

DOSAGE: *Adults:* Administer on Days 1, 15, 29, and once monthly thereafter. Usual: 500mg IM into buttocks slowly (1-2 min/inj) as two 5-mL inj, one in each buttock. Moderate Hepatic Impairment (Child-Pugh Class B): Usual: 250mg IM into buttock slowly (1-2 min) as one 5-mL inj.

HOW SUPPLIED: Inj: 50mg/mL [5mL]

WARNINGS/PRECAUTIONS: Caution with bleeding diatheses and thrombocytopenia. Not studied in severe hepatic impairment (Child-Pugh Class C). May cause fetal harm during pregnancy.

ADVERSE REACTIONS: Inj-site pain, headache, back pain, diarrhea, N/V, bone pain, fatigue, pain in extremity, asthenia, hot flash, anorexia, musculoskeletal pain, cough, dyspnea.

INTERACTIONS: Caution with anticoagulant use.

PREGNANCY: Category D, not for use in nursing.

MECHANISM OF ACTION: Estrogen receptor antagonist; binds to estrogen receptor (ER) and downregulates ER protein in human breast cancer cells.

PHARMACOKINETICS: Absorption: (Single dose) C_{max}=25.1ng/mL; AUC=11,400ng•hr/mL. (Multiple dose) C_{max}=28ng/mL; AUC=13,100ng•hr/mL. **Distribution:** V_d=3-5L/kg; plasma protein binding (99%). **Metabolism:** CYP3A4 (oxidation), aromatic hydroxylation, conjugation. **Elimination:** Feces (90%), urine (<1%); $T_{1/2}$=40 days.

NURSING CONSIDERATIONS

Assessment: Assess for hypersensitivity to the drug, pregnancy/nursing status, bleeding diatheses, thrombocytopenia, hepatic impairment, and possible drug interactions.

Monitoring: Monitor for inj-site reactions, hepatic impairment, and other adverse reactions.

Patient Counseling: Inform to avoid pregnancy and breastfeeding while taking drug. Counsel on side effects and symptoms of an allergic reaction; instruct to seek medical attention if any develop.

Administration: IM route. Refer to PI for further administration instructions. **Storage:** 2-8°C (36-46°F). Protect from light. Store in original carton until time of use.

FAZACLO
clozapine (Jazz)

RX

> Risk of potentially life-threatening agranulocytosis. Reserve use for severely ill patients with schizophrenia unresponsive to standard antipsychotic treatment or for patients with schizophrenia/schizoaffective disorder at risk for re-experiencing suicidal behavior. Obtain baseline WBC count and absolute neutrophil count (ANC) prior to therapy, regularly during treatment, and for at least 4 weeks after d/c. Seizures associated with use and with greater likelihood at higher doses; caution with history of seizures or other predisposing factors. Increased risk of fatal myocarditis, especially during 1st month of therapy; d/c if suspected. Orthostatic hypotension, with or without syncope can occur. Rare reports of profound collapse with respiratory and/or cardiac arrest in patients taking benzodiazepines or any other psychotropic drugs. Elderly patients with dementia-related psychosis treated with atypical antipsychotic drugs are at an increased risk for death. Not approved for the treatment of dementia-related psychosis.

THERAPEUTIC CLASS: Dibenzapine derivative

INDICATIONS: Management of severely ill schizophrenic patients who fail to respond adequately to standard drug treatment for schizophrenia. Reduction of risk for recurrent suicidal behavior in patients with schizophrenia/schizoaffective disorder who are judged to be at chronic risk for re-experiencing suicidal behavior.

DOSAGE: *Adults:* Treatment-Resistant Schizophrenia: Initial: 12.5mg qd-bid. Titrate: Increase by 25-50mg/day, up to 300-450mg/day by end of 2 weeks; then increase by no more than once or twice weekly in increments not to exceed 100mg. Usual: 300-600mg/day given on a divided basis. Titrate: May increase to 600-900mg/day. Max: 900mg/day. Maint: Lowest effective dose. To d/c, gradually reduce dose over 1-2 weeks. Monitor for psychotic and cholinergic rebound symptoms if abrupt d/c warranted (eg, leukopenia). Reinitiation (even with brief interval off clozapine): Start with 12.5mg qd-bid; may titrate more quickly if initial dosing tolerated. Do not restart if d/c for WBC <2000/mm³ or absolute neutrophil count (ANC) <1000/mm³. Reduction of Risk of Recurrent Suicidal Behavior in Schizophrenia/Schizoaffective Disorder: May follow dosing recommendations for treatment-resistant schizophrenia or schizoaffective disorder. Range: 12.5-900mg/day (mean 300mg). Refer to PI for recommendations to reduce the risk of recurrent suicidal behavior who previously responded to treatment with another antipsychotic medication.

HOW SUPPLIED: Tab, Disintegrating: 12.5mg, 25mg, 100mg, 150mg, 200mg

CONTRAINDICATIONS: Myeloproliferative disorders, uncontrolled epilepsy, paralytic ileus, history of clozapine-induced agranulocytosis or severe granulocytopenia, severe CNS depression, comatose states. Concomitant use with agents with potential to cause agranulocytosis or suppress bone marrow function.

WARNINGS/PRECAUTIONS: QT prolongation, ventricular arrhythmia, torsades de pointes, cardiac arrest, and sudden death may occur. Caution with history or family history of long QT syndrome, history of or other conditions that may increase risk for QT prolongation, recent acute myocardial infarction, uncompensated heart failure (HF), cardiac arrhythmia, cardiovascular disease (CVD), risk for significant electrolyte disturbance (eg, hypokalemia, hypomagnesemia). D/C if QTc interval >500 msec. Hyperglycemia, sometimes with ketoacidosis, hyperosmolar coma or death, reported. Monitor for worsening of glucose control with diabetes mellitus (DM) and fasting blood glucose (FBG) levels with diabetes risk or symptoms of hyperglycemia. Tachycardia and cardiomyopathy reported. D/C if cardiomyopathy is confirmed unless benefits outweigh risk. Neuroleptic malignant syndrome (NMS), tardive dyskinesia (TD), impaired intestinal peristalsis, deep vein thrombosis (DVT), pulmonary embolism, and ECG changes reported. Fever reported; rule out infection or agranulocytosis. Consider NMS in the presence of high fever. Hepatitis reported. If N/V and/or anorexia develop, perform LFTs. D/C if symptoms of jaundice occur. Has potent anticholinergic effects; caution with prostatic enlargement and narrow-angle glaucoma. May impair mental/physical abilities. Caution with renal, cardiac, hepatic, or pulmonary disease. Increased risk of cerebrovascular adverse events; caution with risk factors for stroke. Obtain WBC and ANC at baseline, then weekly for 1st six months of therapy, then every 2 weeks for next 6 months, and then every 4 weeks thereafter if counts are acceptable (WBC ≥3500/mm^3 or ANC ≥2000/mm^3). Refer to PI for frequency of monitoring based on stage of therapy, WBC count, and ANC. Avoid treatment if WBC <3500/mm^3 or ANC <2000/mm^3. D/C treatment and do not rechallenge if WBC <2000/mm^3, ANC <1000/mm^3. Interrupt therapy if eosinophilia (>4000/mm^3) develops. Contains aspartame (of which phenylalanine is a component); caution with phenylketonurics. Not for use in infants. Caution in elderly.

ADVERSE REACTIONS: Agranulocytosis, seizure, myocarditis, orthostatic hypotension, salivary hypersecretion, somnolence, drowsiness/sedation, weight increased, dizziness/vertigo, constipation, insomnia, N/V, dyspepsia.

INTERACTIONS: See Contraindications and Boxed Warning. Avoid using epinephrine to treat clozapine-induced hypotension. Use with carbamazepine is not recommended. Caution with CNS-active drugs, general anesthesia, alcohol, paroxetine, fluoxetine, fluvoxamine, sertraline, or inhibitors/inducers of CYP1A2, 2D6, 3A4. Consider reduced dose with paroxetine, fluoxetine, fluvoxamine, and sertraline. Dosage reduction may be needed with drugs metabolized by CYP2D6 (eg, antidepressants, phenothiazines, carbamazepine, type 1C antiarrhythmics) or that inhibit this enzyme (eg, quinidine); use with caution. May potentiate hypotensive effects of antihypertensives and anticholinergic effects of atropine-type drugs. CYP450 inducers (eg, phenytoin, tobacco smoke, carbamazepine, rifampin) may decrease plasma levels. CYP450 inhibitors (eg, cimetidine, caffeine, citalopram, ciprofloxacin, fluvoxamine, erythromycin) may increase plasma levels. NMS reported with lithium and other CNS-active drugs. Concurrent psychopharmaceuticals may affect plasma clozapine levels. May interact with other highly protein-bound drugs. Caution with drugs known to prolong the QTc interval, such as Class 1A antiarrhythmics (eg, quinidine, procainamide), Class III antiarrhythmics (eg, amiodarone, sotalol), certain antipsychotics (eg, ziprasidone, iloperidone, chlorpromazine, thioridazine, mesoridazine, droperidol, pimozide), certain antibiotics (eg, erythromycin, gatifloxacin, moxifloxacin, sparfloxacin), and other drugs known to prolong the QT interval (eg, pentamidine, levomethadyl acetate, methadone, halofantrine, mefloquine, dolasetron mesylate, probucol, and tacrolimus). Caution with drugs that can cause electrolyte imbalance (eg, diuretics).

PREGNANCY: Category B, not for use in nursing.

MECHANISM OF ACTION: Tricyclic dibenzodiazepine derivative; atypical antipsychotic agent. Interferes with the binding of dopamine, specifically at the D_1, D_2, D_3, and D_5 receptors, and has a high affinity for D_4 receptor. Also acts as an antagonist at the adrenergic, cholinergic, histaminergic, and serotonergic receptors.

PHARMACOKINETICS: Absorption: C_{max}=413ng/mL, T_{max}=2.3 hrs (100mg bid). **Distribution:** Plasma protein binding (97%). **Metabolism:** Demethylation, hydroxylation, N-oxidation. Norclozapine (active metabolite). **Elimination:** Urine (50%), feces (30%); $T_{1/2}$=8 hrs (Single 75mg dose), 12 hrs (100mg bid).

NURSING CONSIDERATIONS

Assessment: Assess previous course of standard therapy prior to treatment. Assess for myeloproliferative disorders, paralytic ileus, history of clozapine-induced agranulocytosis or severe granulocytopenia, severe CNS depression or comatose states, history of seizures or other predisposing factors, pregnancy/nursing status, possible drug interactions, and other conditions where treatment is cautioned or contraindicated. Obtain baseline WBC count and ANC, baseline FBG levels in patients at risk for hyperglycemia/DM, and serum K$^+$ and magnesium levels.

Monitoring: Monitor for clinical response and need to continue treatment. Monitor for agranulocytosis, myocarditis, orthostatic hypotension, HF, tachycardia, severe respiratory effects, seizures, flu-like symptoms, infection, eosinophilia, fever, DVT, PE, NMS, TD, intestinal peristalsis impairment, hyperglycemia, or other adverse reactions. Monitor WBC counts and ANC during and for ≥4 weeks following d/c or until WBC ≥3500/mm^3 and ANC ≥2000/mm^3. Check periodic FBG levels if at risk for hyperglycemia and for signs/symptoms of hepatitis while on therapy. Obtain LFTs if patient develops N/V and/or anorexia. Monitor electrolytes and ECG periodically.

Patient Counseling: Inform that drug is available only through a program designed to ensure the required blood monitoring schedule. Counsel on the significant risks of developing agranulocytosis. Advise to immediately report the appearance of lethargy, weakness, fever, sore throat, malaise, mucous membrane ulceration, flu-like complaints, or other possible signs of infection. Inform patients of the significant risk of seizure during treatment; advise to avoid driving and any other potentially hazardous activity while on treatment. Inform phenylketonuric patients that drugs contain phenylalanine. Advise about the risk of orthostatic hypotension, especially during the period of initial dose titration. Inform patients to not restart medication at same dose but to contact physician for dosing instructions if they miss taking medication for >2 days. Notify physician if taking or planning to take any prescription or OTC drugs or alcohol. Instruct to notify physician if become pregnant or intend to become pregnant during therapy. Advise not to breast feed if taking the drug. Advise that tabs should remain in the original package until immediately before use.

Administration: Oral route. Allow to disintegrate in mouth and swallow with saliva or chew if desired. No water needed. **Storage:** 25°C (77°F); excursions permitted to 15-30°C (59-86°F). Protect from moisture.

FELBATOL RX
felbamate (Meda)

> Associated with increased incidence of aplastic anemia; d/c if any evidence of bone marrow depression occurs. Acute liver failure reported. Initiate treatment only in patients without active liver disease and with normal baseline serum transaminases. Obtain baseline and periodic monitoring of AST and ALT; d/c if AST or ALT increased ≥2X ULN or if clinical signs and symptoms suggest liver failure. Monitor blood count and LFTs routinely. Avoid with history of hepatic dysfunction.

THERAPEUTIC CLASS: Dicarbamate anticonvulsant

INDICATIONS: Monotherapy or adjunctive therapy in partial seizures, with and without generalization, in adults with epilepsy. Adjunctive therapy for partial and generalized seizures with Lennox-Gastaut syndrome in children. Use in patients who respond inadequately to alternative treatments and whose epilepsy is so severe that a substantial risk of aplastic anemia and/or liver failure is deemed acceptable.

DOSAGE: *Adults:* Monotherapy: Initial: 1200mg/day in divided doses (tid or qid). Titrate: Increase by 600mg every 2 weeks to 2400mg/day based on response and thereafter to 3600mg/day if indicated. Monotherapy Conversion: Initial: 1200mg/day in divided doses (tid or qid) while reducing present antiepileptic drugs (AEDs) (refer to PI). Titrate: Increase at Week 2 to 2400mg/day and at Week 3 up to 3600mg/day while reducing present AEDs (refer to PI) . Adjunctive Therapy: 1200mg/day in divided doses (tid or qid) while reducing present AEDs by 20%. Further reductions of AEDs dosage may be needed. Titrate: Increase by 1200mg/day increments at weekly intervals. Max: 3600mg/day. Renal Impairment: Initial/Maint: Reduce by 1/2. Adjunctive Therapy: May need further reductions in daily doses. Elderly: Start at lower end of dosing range. *Pediatrics:* ≥14 yrs: Monotherapy: Initial: 1200mg/day in divided doses (tid or qid). Titrate: Increase by 600mg every 2 weeks to 2400mg/day based on response and thereafter to 3600mg/day if indicated. Monotherapy Conversion: Initial: 1200mg/day in divided doses (tid or qid) while reducing present AEDs (refer to PI). Titrate: Increase at Week 2 to 2400mg/day and at Week 3 up to 3600mg/day while reducing present AEDs (refer to PI). Adjunctive Therapy: 1200mg/day in divided doses (tid or qid) while reducing present AEDs by 20%. Further reductions of AEDs dosage may be needed. Titrate: Increase by 1200mg/day increments at weekly intervals. Max: 3600mg/day. Renal Impairment: Initial/Maint: Reduce by 1/2. Adjunctive Therapy: May need further reductions in daily doses. 2-14 yrs: Lennox-Gastaut Adjunctive Therapy: Initial: 15mg/kg/day in divided doses (tid or qid) while reducing present AEDs by 20%. Further reductions of AEDs dosage may be needed. Titrate: Increase by 15mg/kg/day increments at weekly intervals to 45mg/kg/day.

HOW SUPPLIED: Sus: 600mg/5mL [8 oz., 32 oz.]; Tab: 400mg*, 600mg* *scored

CONTRAINDICATIONS: History of any blood dyscrasia or hepatic dysfunction.

WARNINGS/PRECAUTIONS: Not for 1st-line therapy. Avoid abrupt discontinuation; may increase seizure frequency. Weigh the risk of suicidal thought/behavior with the risk of untreated illness. Increased risk of suicidal thoughts or behavior; monitor for emergence or worsening of depression, suicidal thoughts/behavior, and any unusual changes in mood or behavior. Obtain full hematologic evaluations (eg, blood counts, including platelets and reticulocytes) and LFTs before, during, and after discontinuation. Encourage pregnant patients to enroll in North American Antiepileptic Drug Pregnancy Registry. Caution with renal impairment and in elderly.

ADVERSE REACTIONS: Aplastic anemia, acute liver failure, anorexia, upper respiratory tract infection, N/V, headache, fever, somnolence, dizziness, insomnia, fatigue, ataxia, constipation.

INTERACTIONS: Increases plasma concentrations of phenytoin, valproate, carbamazepine epoxide, and phenobarbital. Decreases carbamazepine concentration. Decreased felbamate levels with phenytoin, carbamazepine, and phenobarbital.

PREGNANCY: Category C, safety not known in nursing.

MECHANISM OF ACTION: Anticonvulsant; mechanism not established. Has weak inhibitory effects on gamma-aminobutyric acid receptor binding and benzodiazepine receptor binding. Acts as an antagonist at the strychnine-insensitive glycine recognition site of the N-methyl-D-aspartate receptor-ionophore complex.

PHARMACOKINETICS: Absorption: Well-absorbed. **Distribution:** V_d=756mL/kg (1200mg dose); plasma protein binding (22-25%); found in breast milk. **Metabolism:** Parahydroxyfelbamate, 2-hydroxyfelbamate, felbamate monocarbamate (metabolites). **Elimination:** Urine (90%, 40-50% unchanged); $T_{1/2}$=20-23 hrs.

NURSING CONSIDERATIONS

Assessment: Assess for known hypersensitivity, history of any blood dyscrasia, hepatic/renal function, depression, suicidal thoughts/behavior, pregnancy/nursing status, and possible drug interactions. Obtain baseline CBC (reticulocytes, platelets) and LFTs. Perform full hematologic evaluations prior to therapy.

Monitoring: Monitor for signs/symptoms of hepatic failure, renal impairment, aplastic anemia, bone marrow depression, seizures, emergence or worsening of depression, suicidal thoughts/behavior, and any unusual changes in mood or behavior. Monitor LFTs and CBC (platelets, reticulocytes) while on therapy and following treatment. Obtain hematologic evaluations frequently during and after treatment.

Patient Counseling: Inform of the need to obtain written, informed consent prior to therapy. Inform that use of drug is associated with aplastic anemia and hepatic failure. Advise to be alert for signs of infection, bleeding, easy bruising, or signs of anemia (fatigue, weakness, lassitude) and liver dysfunction (jaundice, anorexia, GI complaints, malaise) and to report immediately if any signs or symptoms appear. Advise to follow physician's directives for LFTs before and during therapy.

Administration: Oral route. (Sus) Shake well before using. **Storage:** 20-25°C (68-77°F).

FELODIPINE ER   RX
felodipine (Various)

THERAPEUTIC CLASS: Calcium channel blocker (dihydropyridine)

INDICATIONS: Treatment of HTN, alone or concomitantly with other antihypertensive agents, to lower BP.

DOSAGE: *Adults:* Initial: 5mg qd. Titrate: May decrease to 2.5mg qd or increase to 10mg qd at intervals of not <2 weeks, depending on the patient's response. Range: 2.5-10mg qd. Hepatic Impairment/Elderly: Initial: 2.5mg qd. Take regularly either without food or with a light meal.

HOW SUPPLIED: Tab, Extended-Release: 2.5mg, 5mg, 10mg

WARNINGS/PRECAUTIONS: May occasionally precipitate significant hypotension and, rarely, syncope. May lead to reflex tachycardia, which may precipitate angina pectoris. Caution with heart failure (HF) or compromised ventricular function, particularly in combination with a β-blocker. Closely monitor BP during dose adjustment in patients with hepatic impairment and in elderly. Peripheral edema reported. Caution in elderly.

ADVERSE REACTIONS: Peripheral edema, headache, asthenia, dyspepsia, dizziness, upper respiratory infection, flushing.

INTERACTIONS: CYP3A4 inhibitors (eg, ketoconazole, erythromycin, grapefruit juice, cimetidine) may increase plasma levels by several-fold. Decreased levels with long-term anticonvulsant therapy (eg, phenytoin, carbamazepine, phenobarbital); consider alternative antihypertensive therapy. May increase metoprolol and tacrolimus levels; monitor tacrolimus blood concentration and adjust tacrolimus dose if needed.

PREGNANCY: Category C, not for use in nursing.

MECHANISM OF ACTION: Calcium channel blocker (dihydropyridine); reversibly competes with nitrendipine and/or other calcium channel blockers for dihydropyridine binding sites and blocks voltage-dependent Ca^{2+} currents in vascular smooth muscle.

PHARMACOKINETICS: Absorption: Almost complete. Systemic bioavailability (20%); C_{max}=23nmol/L (20mg); T_{max}=2.5-5 hrs. **Distribution:** V_d=10L/kg; plasma protein binding (>99%). **Metabolism:** Extensive 1st-pass. **Elimination:** Urine (70%), feces (10%); $T_{1/2}$=11-16 hrs (immediate-release).

NURSING CONSIDERATIONS

Assessment: Assess for hypersensitivity to the drug, HF, compromised ventricular function, hepatic impairment, pregnancy/nursing status, and possible drug interactions.

Monitoring: Monitor for syncope, angina pectoris, peripheral edema, and other adverse reactions. Monitor BP.

Patient Counseling: Inform that mild gingival hyperplasia (gum swelling) has been reported and that good dental hygiene decreases its incidence and severity.

Administration: Oral route. Take regularly either without food or with a light meal. Swallow whole; do not crush or chew. **Storage:** 20-25°C (68-77°F). Protect from light.

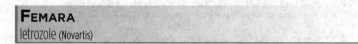

FEMARA RX
letrozole (Novartis)

THERAPEUTIC CLASS: Nonsteroidal aromatase inhibitor

INDICATIONS: Adjuvant treatment of postmenopausal women with hormone receptor positive early breast cancer. Extended adjuvant treatment of early breast cancer in postmenopausal women, who have received 5 yrs of adjuvant tamoxifen therapy. First-line treatment of postmenopausal women with hormone receptor positive or unknown, locally advanced or metastatic breast cancer. Treatment of advanced breast cancer in postmenopausal women with disease progression following antiestrogen therapy.

DOSAGE: *Adults:* 2.5mg qd. Adjuvant Early Breast Cancer: D/C at relapse. Advanced Breast Cancer: Continue until tumor progression is evident. Cirrhosis/Severe Hepatic Dysfunction: Usual: 2.5mg qod.

HOW SUPPLIED: Tab: 2.5mg

CONTRAINDICATIONS: Women who are or may become pregnant.

WARNINGS/PRECAUTIONS: May decrease bone mineral density (BMD); consider monitoring BMD. Bone fractures and osteoporosis reported. Hypercholesterolemia reported; consider monitoring serum cholesterol levels. Reduce dose by 50% with cirrhosis and severe hepatic impairment. May impair physical/mental abilities. Moderate decreases in lymphocyte counts and thrombocytopenia reported.

ADVERSE REACTIONS: Hypercholesterolemia, hot flushes, fatigue, edema, arthralgia/arthritis, myalgia, headache, dizziness, night sweats, nausea, back pain, bone fractures, weight increase, depression, osteopenia.

INTERACTIONS: Reduced plasma levels with coadministered tamoxifen.

PREGNANCY: Category X, not for use in nursing.

MECHANISM OF ACTION: Nonsteroidal aromatase inhibitor; inhibits the conversion of androgens to estrogens. Inhibits the aromatase enzyme by competitively binding to the heme of the CYP450 subunit of the enzyme, resulting in a reduction of estrogen biosynthesis in all tissues.

PHARMACOKINETICS: Absorption: Rapid and complete. **Distribution:** V_d=1.9L/kg. **Metabolism:** Liver via CYP3A4, CYP2A6. **Elimination:** Urine (75%, glucuronide of carbinol metabolite; 9%, unidentified metabolites; 6%, unchanged); $T_{1/2}$=2 days.

NURSING CONSIDERATIONS

Assessment: Assess for premenopausal endocrine status, cirrhosis or hepatic impairment, pregnancy/nursing status, and possible drug interactions.

Monitoring: Monitor for bone fractures, osteoporosis, fatigue, dizziness, somnolence, and other adverse reactions. Monitor BMD and serum cholesterol levels.

Patient Counseling: Inform that the drug is contraindicated in pregnant women and women of premenopausal endocrine status. Counsel perimenopausal and recently postmenopausal women to use contraception until postmenopausal status is fully established. Advise about possible fatigue, dizziness, and somnolence; caution against operating machinery/driving. Advise that BMD may be monitored while on therapy.

Administration: Oral route. Take without regard to meals. **Storage:** 25°C (77°F); excursions permitted to 15-30°C (59-86°F).

FEMCON FE RX
ethinyl estradiol - ferrous fumarate - norethindrone (Warner Chilcott)

> Cigarette smoking increases the risk of serious cardiovascular (CV) side effects from oral contraceptive use. Risk increases with age (>35 yrs) and with heavy smoking (≥15 cigarettes/day). Women who use oral contraceptives should be strongly advised not to smoke.

THERAPEUTIC CLASS: Estrogen/progestogen combination

INDICATIONS: Prevention of pregnancy.

DOSAGE: *Adults:* Take 1 white tab qd for 21 days, followed by 1 brown tab qd for 7 days. Begin next and all subsequent courses of tabs on the same day of the week 1st course began. Intervals between doses should not exceed 24 hrs. Start 1st Sunday after menses begin or the 1st day of menses. Take at the same time each day. Initiate no earlier than Day 28 postpartum in nonlactating mother.
Pediatrics: Postpubertal: Take 1 white tab qd for 21 days, followed by 1 brown tab qd for 7 days. Begin next and all subsequent courses of tablets on the same day of the week 1st course began. Intervals between doses should not exceed 24 hrs. Start 1st Sunday after menses begin or the 1st day of menses. Take at the same time each day. Initiate no earlier than Day 28 postpartum in nonlactating mother.

HOW SUPPLIED: Tab, Chewable: (Ethinyl Estradiol-Norethindrone) 0.035mg-0.4mg, Tab: (Ferrous Fumarate) 75mg

CONTRAINDICATIONS: Thrombophlebitis, current or history of thromboembolic disorders, history of deep vein thrombophlebitis, current or history of cerebral vascular disease or coronary artery disease (CAD), valvular heart disease with thrombogenic complications, uncontrolled HTN, diabetes mellitus (DM) with vascular involvement, headaches with focal neurological symptoms such as aura, major surgery with prolonged immobilization, known or suspected breast carcinoma (or personal history), carcinoma of the endometrium or other known or suspected estrogen-dependent neoplasia, undiagnosed abnormal genital bleeding, cholestatic jaundice of pregnancy or jaundice with prior hormonal contraceptive use, hepatic adenomas or carcinoma or active liver disease, and known or suspected pregnancy.

WARNINGS/PRECAUTIONS: Increased risk of venous and arterial thrombotic and thromboembolic events (eg, myocardial infarction, thromboembolism, stroke), vascular disease, hepatic neoplasia, gallbladder disease, and HTN. May increase risk of breast and cervical cancer. Retinal thrombosis reported; d/c if unexplained partial or complete loss of vision, onset of proptosis or diplopia, papilledema, or retinal vascular lesions develop. Should not be used to induce withdrawal bleeding as a test for pregnancy, or to treat threatened or habitual abortion during pregnancy. May cause glucose intolerance; monitor prediabetic and diabetic patients. May cause fluid retention and increase BP; monitor closely with HTN and d/c if significant elevation of BP occurs. D/C with onset or exacerbation of migraine or development of headache with new pattern that is persistent, recurrent, and severe. May cause breakthrough bleeding and spotting; if persistent or recurrent, rule out malignancy or pregnancy. Ectopic and intrauterine pregnancies may occur with contraceptive failures. Perform annual physical exam. Monitor closely with hyperlipidemias; may elevate LDL and/or plasma TGs. Caution with impaired liver function; d/c if jaundice develops. May cause depression; caution with history of depression and d/c if it recurs to serious degree. Visual changes or changes in lens tolerance may develop with contact lens use. May affect certain endocrine tests, LFTs, and blood components. Does not protect AIDS and other sexually transmitted disease.

ADVERSE REACTIONS: N/V, breakthrough bleeding, spotting, amenorrhea, migraine, depression, vaginal candidiasis, edema, weight changes.

INTERACTIONS: Reduced contraceptive effectiveness leading to unintended pregnancy or breakthrough bleeding with some anticonvulsants, other drugs that increase the metabolism of contraceptive steroids (eg, rifampin, phenytoin, carbamazepine, felbamate, griseofulvin). Contraceptive failure and breakthrough bleeding reported with antibiotics, such as ampicillin and tetracyclines. Anti-HIV protease inhibitors may increase or decrease levels. Reduced effectiveness with St. John's wort. Atorvastatin, ascorbic acid, acetaminophen, CYP3A4 inhibitors (eg, itraconazole, ketoconazole) may increase hormone levels. Increased plasma concentrations of cyclosporine, prednisolone, and theophylline. Decreased plasma concentrations of acetaminophen and increased clearance of temazepam, salicylic acid, morphine, and clofibric acid.

PREGNANCY: Category X, not for use in nursing.

MECHANISM OF ACTION: Estrogen/progestogen combination oral contraceptive; acts by suppressing gonadotropins. Primarily inhibits ovulation. Also causes changes in cervical mucus (increases difficulty of sperm entry into uterus) and endometrium (reduces likelihood of implantation).

PHARMACOKINETICS: Absorption: Rapid. Norethindrone: Absolute bioavailability (65%), C_{max}=4210.6pg/mL, T_{max}=1.24 hr, AUC=18034.9pg•h/mL. Ethinyl estradiol: Absolute bioavailability (43%), C_{max}=131.4pg/mL, T_{max}=1.44 hrs, AUC=1065.8pg•h/mL. **Distribution:** V_d=2-4L/kg; Norethindrone: Sex hormone-binding globulin (36%), albumin binding (61%). Ethinyl estradiol: Albumin binding (98.5%). **Metabolism:** Norethindrone: Reduction, sulfate, glucuronide conjugation. Ethinyl estradiol: CYP3A4, via oxidation (conjugation with sulfate and glucuronide), 2-hydroxy-ethinyl estradiol (primary oxidative metabolite). **Elimination:** Norethindrone: Urine (>50%), feces (20-40%); $T_{1/2}$=8.6 hrs. Ethinyl Estradiol: Urine, feces; $T_{1/2}$=17.1 hrs.

NURSING CONSIDERATIONS

Assessment: Assess for presence or history of breast cancer, estrogen dependent neoplasia, abnormal genital bleeding, active liver disease, and known/suspected pregnancy or any other conditions where treatment is cautioned or contraindicated. Assess use in patients who are

>35 yrs and heavy smokers (≥15 cigarettes/day); patients with HTN, hyperlipidemias, obesity, or DM; patients at increased risk for thrombosis; and assess for possible drug interactions.

Monitoring: Monitor bleeding irregularities, thromboembolic events, onset or exacerbation of headaches or migraines, and ectopic pregnancy. Monitor fasting blood glucose levels in DM and prediabetic patients, BP with history of HTN, lipid levels with a history of hyperlipidemia. Monitor for signs of liver dysfunction and signs of depression with previous history. Refer patients with contact lenses to an ophthalmologist if visual changes occur. Perform annual history and physical exam.

Patient Counseling: Advise about possible serious CV and respiratory effects. Inform that medication does not protect against HIV infection (AIDS) and other sexually transmitted diseases. Avoid smoking while on medication. Instruct to take medication at same time each day. Instruct if dose missed, take as soon as possible; take next pill at regularly scheduled time. If patient misses more than one dose, instruct to discuss with a pharmacist or physician, or refer to PI and to use back-up contraception. Inform that patient may have spotting, light bleeding, or stomach upset during first 1-3 packs of pills; advise not to d/c medication and if symptoms persist, notify physician. Vomiting, diarrhea, or concomitant medications may alter efficacy; use backup forms of contraception. Perform regular physical exams.

Administration: Oral route. **Storage:** 25° (77°F); excursions permitted to 15-30°C (59-86°F).

FENTANYL INJECTION `CII`
fentanyl citrate (Various)

THERAPEUTIC CLASS: Opioid analgesic

INDICATIONS: For analgesic action of short duration during the anesthetic periods, premedication, induction and maintenance, and in the immediate postoperative period (recovery room) as the need arises. For use as a narcotic analgesic supplement in general or regional anesthesia. For administration with a neuroleptic (eg, droperidol inj) as an anesthetic premedication, for the induction of anesthesia, and as an adjunct in the maintenance of general and regional anesthesia. For use as an anesthetic agent with oxygen in selected high-risk patients (eg, those undergoing open heart surgery, certain complicated neurological/orthopedic procedures).

DOSAGE: *Adults:* Individualize dose. Premedication: 50-100mcg IM 30-60 min prior to surgery. Adjunct to General Anesthesia: Low-Dose: Total Dose: 2mcg/kg for minor surgery. Maint: 2mcg/kg. Moderate Dose: Total Dose: 2-20mcg/kg for major surgery. Maint: 2-20mcg/kg or 25-100mcg IM or IV if surgical stress or lightening of analgesia. High-Dose: Total Dose: 20-50mcg/kg for open heart surgery, complicated neurosurgery, or orthopedic surgery. Maint: 20-50mcg/kg. Additional dosage selected must be individualized, especially if the anticipated remaining operative time is short. Adjunct to Regional Anesthesia: 50-100mcg IM or slow IV over 1-2 min. Postop: 50-100mcg IM, repeat q1-2h PRN. General Anesthetic: 50-100mcg/kg with oxygen and a muscle relaxant. Max: 150mcg/kg. Elderly/Debilitated: Reduce dose. *Pediatrics:* 2-12 Yrs: Individualize dose. Induction/Maint: 2-3mcg/kg.

HOW SUPPLIED: Inj: 50mcg/mL [5mL]

WARNINGS/PRECAUTIONS: Administer only by persons specifically trained in the use of IV anesthetics and management of the respiratory effects of potent opioids. An opioid antagonist, resuscitative and intubation equipment, and oxygen should be readily available. Fluids and other countermeasures to manage hypotension should be available when used with tranquilizers. Initial dose reduction recommended with narcotic analgesia for recovery. May cause muscle rigidity, particularly with muscles used for respiration. Adequate facilities should be available for postoperative monitoring and ventilation. May cause euphoria, miosis, bradycardia, and bronchoconstriction. Caution in respiratory depression-susceptible patients (eg, comatose patients with head injury or brain tumor); may obscure the clinical course of patients with head injury. Caution with chronic obstructive pulmonary disease, decreased respiratory reserve, potentially compromised respiration, liver/kidney dysfunction, and cardiac bradyarrhythmias. Monitor vital signs routinely.

ADVERSE REACTIONS: Respiratory depression, apnea, rigidity, bradycardia.

INTERACTIONS: Severe and unpredictable potentiation with MAOIs; appropriate monitoring and availability of vasodilators and β-blockers for HTN treatment is indicated. Additive or potentiating effects with other CNS depressants (eg, barbiturates, tranquilizers, narcotics, general anesthetics); reduce dose of other CNS depressants. Reports of cardiovascular (CV) depression with nitrous oxide. Alteration of respiration with certain forms of conduction anesthesia (eg, spinal anesthesia, some peridural anesthetics). Decreased pulmonary arterial pressure and hypotension with tranquilizers (eg, droperidol). May increase BP in patients with/without HTN with droperidol. May cause CV depression with diazepam.

PREGNANCY: Category C, caution in nursing.

MECHANISM OF ACTION: Narcotic analgesic; produces analgesic and sedative effects. Alters respiratory rate and alveolar ventilation, which may last longer than analgesic effects.

PHARMACOKINETICS: Distribution: V_d=4L/kg. **Metabolism:** Liver. **Elimination:** Urine (75%, <10% unchanged), feces (9%); $T_{1/2}$=219 min.

NURSING CONSIDERATIONS

Assessment: Assess level of pain intensity, patient's general condition and medical status, or any other conditions where treatment is contraindicated or cautioned. Assess for history of hypersensitivity, pregnancy/nursing status, renal/hepatic function, and possible drug interactions. Assess use in the elderly and debilitated patient.

Monitoring: Monitor for signs/symptoms of respiratory depression, muscle rigidity, medication abuse, and drug dependence. If given with nitrous oxide, monitor for CV depression. If administered with a tranquilizer, monitor for hypotension and hypovolemia. If combined with droperidol, monitor for increases in BP; perform ECG monitoring. Perform routine monitoring of vital signs.

Patient Counseling: Advise patient about the benefits and risks of the medication. Instruct to notify physician if any adverse reactions occur.

Administration: IM/IV route. **Storage:** 20-25°C (68-77°F); excursions permitted to 15-30°C (59-86°F). Protect from light.

FENTORA
fentanyl citrate (Cephalon)

Fatal respiratory depression may occur. Contraindicated in the management of acute or postoperative pain (eg, headache/migraine) and in opioid-nontolerant patients. Keep out of reach of children. Concomitant use with CYP3A4 inhibitors may increase plasma levels, and may cause fatal respiratory depression. Do not convert patients on a mcg-per-mcg basis from any other fentanyl products to Fentora. Do not substitute for any other fentanyl products; may result in fatal overdose. Contains fentanyl with abuse liability similar to other opioid analgesics. Available only through a restricted program called TIRF REMS Access program (Transmucosal Immediate Release Fentanyl Risk Evaluation Mitigation Strategy) due to risk of misuse, abuse, addiction, and overdose. Outpatients, healthcare professionals who prescribe to outpatients, pharmacies, and distributors must enroll in the program.

THERAPEUTIC CLASS: Opioid analgesic

INDICATIONS: Management of breakthrough pain in cancer patients ≥18 yrs who are already receiving and are tolerant to around-the-clock opioid therapy for their underlying persistent cancer pain.

DOSAGE: *Adults:* ≥18 Yrs: Initial: 100mcg. Titration >100mcg: Two 100mcg tabs (1 on each side of mouth in buccal cavity) with next breakthrough pain episode. Use two 100mcg tabs on each side of mouth (total of four 100mcg tabs) if dosage is not successful. Max: 2 doses/breakthrough pain episode; must wait at least 4 hrs before treating another episode of breakthrough pain. Titration >400mcg: 200mcg increments. Do not use >4 tabs simultaneously. Maint: Once titrated to an effective dose, use only 1 tab of the appropriate strength per breakthrough pain episode. May take only 1 additional dose of the same strength if not relieved after 30 min. Wait at least 4 hrs before treating another breakthrough pain episode. If >4 breakthrough pain episodes/day are experienced, reevaluate maint dose (around-the-clock) used for persistent pain. >65 Yrs: Titrate to slightly lower dose. Refer to PI for conversion directions for patients on Actiq.

HOW SUPPLIED: Tab, Buccal: 100mcg, 200mcg, 400mcg, 600mcg, 800mcg

CONTRAINDICATIONS: Opioid-nontolerant patients, management of acute or postoperative pain, including headache/migraine and dental pain.

WARNINGS/PRECAUTIONS: Increased risk of respiratory depression in patients with underlying respiratory disorders and in elderly/debilitated. May impair mental and/or physical abilities. Caution with chronic obstructive pulmonary disease or preexisting medical conditions predisposing to respiratory depression; may further decrease respiratory drive to the point of respiratory failure. Extreme caution in patients who may be susceptible to the intracranial effects of CO_2 retention (eg, with evidence of increased intracranial pressure or impaired consciousness). May obscure clinical course of head injuries. Application-site reactions (paresthesia, ulceration, bleeding) reported. Caution with bradyarrhythmias. Avoid use during labor and delivery. Caution with renal/hepatic impairment.

ADVERSE REACTIONS: Respiratory depression, headache, N/V, constipation, dizziness, dyspnea, somnolence, fatigue, anemia, asthenia, abdominal pain, dehydration, peripheral edema, diarrhea.

INTERACTIONS: See Boxed Warning. CYP3A4 inducers (eg, carbamazepine, efavirenz, modafinil, phenobarbital, pioglitazone, rifampin, St. John's wort) may decrease levels. Respiratory depression is more likely to occur when given with other drugs that depress respiration. Increased depressant effects with other CNS depressants (eg, sedatives, hypnotics, tranquilizers, skeletal muscle relaxants, sedating antihistamines, alcohol); adjust dose if warranted. Not recommended for use in patients who have received MAOIs within 14 days.

PREGNANCY: Category C, not for use in nursing.

MECHANISM OF ACTION: Opioid analgesic; has not been established. Known to be μ-opioid receptor agonist; specific CNS opioid receptors for endogenous compounds with opioid-like activity have been identified throughout the brain and spinal cord and play a role in analgesic effects.

PHARMACOKINETICS: Absorption: Readily absorbed. Absolute bioavailability (65%). Administration of variable doses resulted in different pharmacokinetic parameters. **Distribution:** V_d=25.4L/kg; plasma protein binding (80-85%); found in breast milk; crosses the placenta. **Metabolism:** Liver and intestinal mucosa via CYP3A4; norfentanyl (metabolite). **Elimination:** Urine (<7%, unchanged), feces (1%, unchanged). $T_{1/2}$=2.63 hrs (100mcg), 4.43 hrs (200mcg), 11.09 hrs (400mcg), 11.7 hrs (800mcg).

NURSING CONSIDERATIONS

Assessment: Assess for degree of opioid tolerance, previous opioid dose, level of pain intensity, type of pain, patient's general condition and medical status, or any other conditions where treatment is contraindicated or cautioned. Assess for hypersensitivity to drug, renal/hepatic function, pregnancy/nursing status, and possible drug interactions.

Monitoring: Monitor for signs/symptoms of respiratory depression, impairment of mental/physical abilities, application-site reactions, bradycardia, abuse/addiction, and other adverse reactions.

Patient Counseling: Advise to enroll in TIRF REMS Access program. Instruct to keep drug out of reach of children. Advise to take drug as prescribed and avoid sharing it with anyone else. Instruct to notify physician if breakthrough pain is not alleviated or worsens after taking the drug. Inform that drug may impair mental/physical abilities; caution against performing activities that require high level of attention (eg, operating machinery/driving). Advise not to combine with alcohol, sleep aids, or tranquilizers unless indicated by the physician. Instruct to notify physician if pregnant or planning to become pregnant. Inform of proper storage, administration, and disposal.

Administration: Buccal route. Refer to PI for proper administration. **Storage:** 20-25°C (68-77°F); excursions permitted to 15-30°C (59-86°F). Protect from freezing and moisture.

FETZIMA   RX
levomilnacipran (Forest)

> Antidepressants increased the risk of suicidal thoughts and behavior in children, adolescents, and young adults in short-term studies. Monitor and observe closely for worsening, and for emergence of suicidal thoughts and behaviors. Not approved for use in pediatric patients.

THERAPEUTIC CLASS: Serotonin and norepinephrine reuptake inhibitor

INDICATIONS: Treatment of major depressive disorder.

DOSAGE: *Adults:* Initial: 20mg qd for 2 days. Titrate: Increase to 40mg qd. Based on efficacy and tolerability, may then be increased in increments of 40mg at intervals of ≥2 days. Range: 40-120mg qd. Max: 120mg qd. Periodically reassess the need for maintenance treatment and the appropriate dose. Moderate Renal Impairment (CrCl 30-59mL/min): Max Maint: 80mg qd. Severe Renal Impairment (CrCl 15-29mL/min): Max Maint: 40mg qd. Switching to/from an MAOI for Psychiatric Disorders: Allow at least 14 days between discontinuation of an MAOI and initiation of treatment, and allow at least 7 days between discontinuation of treatment and initiation of an MAOI. Use with Other MAOIs (eg, Linezolid, IV Methylene Blue): Refer to PI. Use with Strong CYP3A4 Inhibitors (eg, Ketoconazole, Clarithromycin, Ritonavir): Max: 80mg qd.

HOW SUPPLIED: Cap, Extended-Release: 20mg, 40mg, 80mg, 120mg; (Titration Pack) 20mg [2s], 40mg [26s]

CONTRAINDICATIONS: Use of an MAOI for psychiatric disorders either concomitantly or within 7 days of stopping treatment. Treatment within 14 days of stopping an MAOI for psychiatric disorders. Starting treatment in patients being treated with other MAOIs (eg, linezolid, IV methylene blue). Uncontrolled narrow-angle glaucoma.

WARNINGS/PRECAUTIONS: Not approved for the management of fibromyalgia. Not recommended for patients with end-stage renal disease. Not approved for the treatment of bipolar depression. Serotonin syndrome reported; d/c immediately if symptoms occur and initiate supportive symptomatic treatment. Associated with increases in BP and HR; control preexisting HTN or treat preexisting tachyarrhythmias and other cardiac disease before initiating treatment. Caution with preexisting HTN, cardiovascular (CV) or cerebrovascular conditions that might be compromised by increases in BP. Consider discontinuation or other appropriate medical intervention if sustained increase in BP or HR occurs. May increase risk of bleeding events. Mydriasis reported; caution with controlled narrow-angle glaucoma, and monitor patients with raised intraocular pressure (IOP) or those at risk of acute narrow-angle glaucoma. May affect urethral resistance; caution in patients prone to obstructive urinary disorders. If symptoms of urinary hesitation, urinary retention, or dysuria develop, consider discontinuation or other appropriate medical intervention. Activation of mania/hypomania reported; caution with history or family history of bipolar disorder, mania, or hypomania. Seizures reported; caution in patients with a seizure disorder. Discontinuation symptoms may occur. Avoid abrupt discontinuation; reduce dose gradually whenever possible. Hyponatremia may occur; elderly and volume-depleted patients may be at greater risk. D/C in patients with symptomatic hyponatremia and institute appropriate medical intervention.

ADVERSE REACTIONS: N/V, constipation, hyperhidrosis, HR/BP increased, erectile dysfunction, tachycardia, palpitations, testicular pain, ejaculation disorder, urinary hesitation, hot flush, hypotension, HTN, decreased appetite.

INTERACTIONS: See Contraindications. May cause serotonin syndrome with other serotonergic drugs (eg, triptans, TCAs, fentanyl, lithium, St. John's wort) and with drugs that impair metabolism of serotonin; d/c immediately if serotonin syndrome occurs. Caution with NSAIDs, aspirin (ASA), warfarin, and other drugs that affect coagulation or bleeding due to potential increased risk of bleeding. Increased exposure with CYP3A4 inhibitor ketoconazole; dose adjustment is recommended when coadministered with strong CYP3A4 inhibitors. Caution with other CNS-active drugs, including those with a similar mechanism of action. Do not give with alcohol; pronounced accelerated drug release may occur. Caution with drugs that increase BP and HR. Increased risk of hyponatremia with diuretics.

PREGNANCY: Category C, not for use in nursing.

MECHANISM OF ACTION: SNRI; has not been established. Thought to be related to the potentiation of serotonin and norepinephrine in the CNS, through inhibition of reuptake at serotonin and norepinephrine transporters.

PHARMACOKINETICS: Absorption: C_{max}=341ng/mL; AUC=5196ng•hr/mL; T_{max}=6-8 hrs (median). **Distribution:** V_d=387-473L; plasma protein binding (22%). **Metabolism:** Desethylation (primarily via CYP3A4 with minor contribution by CYP2C8, 2C19, 2D6, and 2J2) and hydroxylation; further conjugation with glucuronide. **Elimination:** Urine (58% unchanged, 18% N-desethyl levomilnacipran); $T_{1/2}$=12 hrs.

NURSING CONSIDERATIONS

Assessment: Assess for narrow-angle glaucoma, risk for bipolar disorder, HTN, CV/cerebrovascular conditions that might be compromised by increases in BP, tachyarrhythmias, cardiac disease, raised IOP, risk for acute narrow-angle glaucoma, susceptibility to obstructive urinary disorders, history of mania/hypomania, seizure disorder, volume depletion, history of drug abuse, hypersensitivity to the drug, renal impairment, pregnancy/nursing status, and possible drug interactions.

Monitoring: Monitor for clinical worsening, suicidality, unusual changes in behavior, serotonin syndrome, bleeding events, mydriasis, urinary hesitation/retention, dysuria, activation of mania/hypomania, seizures, discontinuation symptoms, hyponatremia, and other adverse reactions. Monitor BP and HR periodically. Monitor patients with history of drug abuse for signs of misuse or abuse. Periodically reassess to determine the need for maintenance treatment and the appropriate dose for treatment.

Patient Counseling: Advise about the benefits and risks of therapy and counsel on its appropriate use. Counsel to look for the emergence of suicidality, especially early during treatment and when the dose is adjusted up or down. Caution about the risk of serotonin syndrome, particularly with the concomitant use with other serotonergic agents. Inform that concomitant use with ASA, NSAIDs, warfarin, or other drugs that affect coagulation may increase the risk of abnormal bleeding. Advise to have BP and HR monitored regularly, to observe for signs of activation of mania/hypomania, to avoid alcohol consumption, and not to d/c therapy without notifying physician. Caution against operating hazardous machinery until reasonably certain that therapy does not adversely affect ability to engage in such activities. Advise to notify physician if allergic reactions develop, if pregnant/intending to become pregnant, or if breastfeeding.

Administration: Oral route. Take at the same time each day, with or without food. Swallow cap whole; do not open, chew, or crush. **Storage:** 25°C (77°F); excursions permitted between 15-30°C (59-86°F).

FIBRICOR   RX
fenofibric acid (Caraco)

THERAPEUTIC CLASS: Fibric acid derivative

INDICATIONS: Adjunctive therapy to diet for treatment of severe hypertriglyceridemia (≥500mg/dL). Adjunctive therapy to diet to reduce elevated LDL, total cholesterol, TGs, and apolipoprotein B, and to increase HDL in patients with primary hypercholesterolemia or mixed dyslipidemia.

DOSAGE: *Adults:* Severe Hypertriglyceridemia: Initial: 35-105mg/day. Titrate: Adjust dose if necessary following repeat lipid determinations at 4- to 8-week intervals. Max: 105mg qd. Primary Hypercholesterolemia/Mixed Dyslipidemia: 105mg/day. Mild to Moderate Renal Impairment: Initial: 35mg qd. Titrate: Increase only after evaluation of effects on renal function and lipid levels. Elderly: Dose based on renal function. Consider reducing dose if lipid levels fall significantly below targeted range. D/C if no adequate response after 2 months of treatment with max dose.

HOW SUPPLIED: Tab: 35mg, 105mg

CONTRAINDICATIONS: Severe renal impairment (including dialysis), active liver disease (including primary biliary cirrhosis and unexplained persistent liver function abnormalities), preexisting gallbladder disease, and nursing mothers.

WARNINGS/PRECAUTIONS: Not shown to reduce coronary heart disease morbidity and mortality in patients with type 2 diabetes mellitus. Increased risk of myopathy and rhabdomyolysis; risk increased with diabetes, renal failure, hypothyroidism, and in elderly. D/C if marked CPK elevation occurs or myopathy/myositis is suspected or diagnosed. Increases in serum transaminases, hepatocellular, chronic active, and cholestatic hepatitis, and cirrhosis (rare) reported; perform baseline and regular periodic monitoring of LFTs, and d/c therapy if enzyme levels persist >3X the normal limit. Elevations in SrCr reported; monitor renal function in patients with renal impairment or at risk for renal insufficiency. May cause cholelithiasis; d/c if gallstones are found. Acute hypersensitivity reactions and pancreatitis reported. Mild to moderate decreases in Hgb, Hct, and WBCs, thrombocytopenia, and agranulocytosis reported; periodically monitor RBC and WBC counts during the first 12 months of therapy. May cause venothromboembolic disease. Severe decreases in HDL levels reported; check HDL levels within the 1st few months after initiation of therapy. If a severely depressed HDL level is detected, withdraw therapy, monitor HDL level until it has returned to baseline, and do not reinitiate therapy. Estrogen therapy, thiazide diuretics, and β-blockers may be associated with massive rises in plasma TGs; discontinuation of these drugs may obviate the need for specific drug therapy of hypertriglyceridemia.

ADVERSE REACTIONS: Abdominal pain, back pain, headache, abnormal LFTs, increased ALT/AST/CPK, respiratory disorder.

INTERACTIONS: Increased risk of rhabdomyolysis with HMG-CoA reductase inhibitors (statins); avoid combination unless benefit outweighs risk. May potentiate anticoagulant effects of coumarin anticoagulants; use with caution, reduce anticoagulant dosage, and monitor PT/INR frequently. Bile acid-binding resins may bind other drugs given concurrently; take at least 1 hr before or 4-6 hrs after the bile acid-binding resin. Immunosuppressants (eg, cyclosporine, tacrolimus) may produce nephrotoxicity; consider benefits and risks, use lowest effective dose, and monitor renal function with immunosuppressants and other potentially nephrotoxic agents. Cases of myopathy, including rhabdomyolysis, reported when coadministered with colchicine; caution when prescribing with colchicine.

PREGNANCY: Category C, not for use in nursing.

MECHANISM OF ACTION: Fibric acid derivative; activates peroxisome proliferator-activated receptor α. Increases lipolysis and elimination of TG-rich particles from plasma by activating lipoprotein lipase and reducing production of apoprotein C-III (lipoprotein lipase activity inhibitor). Also, induces an increase in the synthesis of apoproteins A-I, A-II, and HDL.

PHARMACOKINETICS: Absorption: T_{max}=2.5 hrs (median). **Distribution:** Plasma protein binding (99%). **Metabolism:** Conjugation with glucuronic acid. **Elimination:** Urine; $T_{1/2}$=20 hrs.

NURSING CONSIDERATIONS

Assessment: Assess for renal impairment, active liver disease, gallbladder disease, other medical conditions (eg, diabetes, hypothyroidism), hypersensitivity to the drug, pregnancy/nursing status, and possible drug interactions. Obtain baseline LFTs.

Monitoring: Monitor for myopathy, myositis, or rhabdomyolysis; measure CPK levels in patients reporting such symptoms. Monitor for cholelithiasis, pancreatitis, hypersensitivity reactions, pulmonary embolus, and deep vein thrombosis. Monitor renal function, LFTs, CBC, and lipid levels. Monitor PT/INR frequently with coumarin anticoagulants.

Patient Counseling: Advise of potential benefits and risks of therapy, and of medications to avoid during treatment. Instruct to follow appropriate lipid-modifying diet during therapy, and to take ud. Instruct to inform physician of all medications, supplements, and herbal preparations being taken, any changes in medical condition, development of muscle pain, tenderness, or weakness, and onset of abdominal pain or any other new symptoms. Advise to return for routine monitoring.

Administration: Oral route. May be taken without regard to meals. Swallow tab whole; do not crush, dissolve, or chew. **Storage:** 20-25°C (68-77°F).

FIORINAL

caffeine - aspirin - butalbital (Watson)

THERAPEUTIC CLASS: Analgesic/barbiturate

INDICATIONS: Relief of the symptom complex of tension (or muscle contraction) headache.

DOSAGE: *Adults:* 1-2 caps q4h. Max: 6 caps/day.

HOW SUPPLIED: Cap: (Butalbital-Aspirin [ASA]-Caffeine) 50mg-325mg-40mg

CONTRAINDICATIONS: Porphyria, peptic ulcer or other serious GI lesions, hemorrhagic diathesis (eg, hemophilia, hypoprothrombinemia, von Willebrand's disease, thrombocytopenia, thrombasthenia and other ill-defined hereditary platelet dysfunctions, severe vitamin K deficiency, severe liver damage). Syndrome of nasal polyps, angioedema, and bronchospastic reactivity to ASA or NSAIDs.

WARNINGS/PRECAUTIONS: Not for extended and repeated use. May be habit-forming. Caution in elderly, debilitated, with severe renal/hepatic impairment, hypothyroidism, urethral stricture, head injuries, elevated intracranial pressure, acute abdominal conditions, Addison's disease, prostatic hypertrophy, presence of peptic ulcer, and coagulation disorders. Therapeutic doses of ASA can lead to anaphylactic shock and severe allergic reactions. Significant bleeding possible with peptic ulcers, GI lesions, or bleeding disorders. Caution in children, including teenagers, with chickenpox or flu. Preoperative ASA may prolong bleeding time.

ADVERSE REACTIONS: Drowsiness, lightheadedness, dizziness, N/V, flatulence.

INTERACTIONS: Caution with anticoagulant therapy; may enhance bleeding. CNS effects enhanced by MAOIs. Additive CNS depression with alcohol, other narcotic analgesics, general anesthetics, tranquilizers (eg, chlordiazepoxide), sedatives/hypnotics, other CNS depressants. May cause hypoglycemia with oral antidiabetic agents and insulin. May cause bone marrow toxicity and blood dyscrasias with 6-mercaptopurine and methotrexate. Increased risk of peptic ulceration and bleeding with NSAIDs. Decreased effects of uricosuric agents (eg, probenecid, sulfinpyrazone). Withdrawal of corticosteroids may cause salicylism with chronic ASA use.

PREGNANCY: Category C, not for use in nursing.

MECHANISM OF ACTION: Butalbital: Short- to intermediate-acting barbiturate. ASA: Analgesic, antipyretic, and anti-inflammatory. Caffeine: CNS stimulant. Combines analgesic properties of ASA with anxiolytic and muscle relaxant properties of butalbital.

PHARMACOKINETICS: Absorption: ASA: (650mg dose) T_{max}=40 min, C_{max}=8.8mcg/mL. Butalbital: Well-absorbed; (100mg dose) C_{max}=2020ng/mL, T_{max}=1.5 hrs. Caffeine: Rapid; (80mg dose) C_{max}=1660ng/mL, T_{max}=<1 hr. **Distribution:** ASA: Found in fetal tissue, breast milk; Plasma protein binding (50-80%). Butalbital: Crosses placenta, found in breast milk; Plasma protein binding (45%). Caffeine: Found in fetal tissue, breast milk. **Metabolism:** ASA: Liver; salicyluric acid, phenolic/acyl glucuronides of salicylate, gentisic and gentisuric acid (major metabolites). Caffeine: Liver; 1-methylxanthine and 1-methyluric acid (metabolites). **Elimination:** ASA: Urine; $T_{1/2}$=12 min (ASA), 3 hrs (salicylic acid/total salicylates). Butalbital: Urine (59-88%); $T_{1/2}$=35 hrs. Caffeine: Urine (70%, 3% unchanged); $T_{1/2}$=3 hrs.

NURSING CONSIDERATIONS

Assessment: Assess for previous hypersensitivity to drug, renal/hepatic function, porphyria, peptic ulcer, other serious GI lesions, bleeding disorders, or any other conditions where treatment is cautioned or contraindicated. Assess for pregnancy/nursing status and possible drug interactions.

Monitoring: Serial monitoring of LFTs and/or renal function with severe hepatic/renal disease. Monitor for anaphylactoid/hypersensitivity reactions, drug abuse/dependence and bleeding.

Patient Counseling: Advise not to take if patient has ASA allergy. Instruct to take exactly as prescribed; instruct to avoid coadministration with alcohol or other CNS depressants. Advise to avoid hazardous tasks (eg, operating machinery/driving) while on therapy. Counsel that drug may be habit-forming.

Administration: Oral route. **Storage:** Below 25°C (77°F); tight container. Protect from moisture.

FLAGYL

RX

metronidazole (G.D. Searle)

Shown to be carcinogenic in mice and rats. Avoid unnecessary use. Should be reserved for the conditions for which it is indicated.

THERAPEUTIC CLASS: Nitroimidazole

INDICATIONS: Treatment of symptomatic/asymptomatic trichomoniasis, asymptomatic sexual partners, acute intestinal amebiasis, amebic liver abscess, and anaerobic bacterial infections caused by susceptible strains of microorganisms. Treatment of intra-abdominal, skin and skin structure, gynecologic, bone/joint (as adjunctive therapy), CNS, and lower respiratory tract infections, bacterial septicemia, and endocarditis caused by susceptible strains of microorganisms.

DOSAGE: *Adults:* Trichomoniasis: Female: Individualize dose. One-Day Treatment: (Tab) 2g given either as a single dose or in 2 divided doses of 1g each given in the same day. Seven-Day Course of Treatment: (Cap) 375mg bid or (Tab) 250mg tid for 7 consecutive days. When repeat courses are required, allow an interval of 4-6 weeks between courses, and reconfirm the presence of the trichomonad. Male: Individualize treatment as it is for the female. Acute Intestinal Amebiasis: 750mg tid for 5-10 days. Amebic Liver Abscess: (Tab) 500mg or (Cap/Tab) 750mg tid for 5-10 days. Anaerobic Bacterial Infections: IV therapy is usually administered initially in the treatment of most serious infections. Usual: 7.5mg/kg q6h (approximately 500mg for a 70-kg adult). Max: 4g/24 hrs. Usual Duration: 7-10 days; bone/joint, lower respiratory tract, and endocardium infections may require longer treatment. Severe Hepatic Impairment (Child-Pugh C): (Tab) Reduce dosage by 50%. (Cap) Reduce dosage in amebiasis by 50% and reduce dosage frequency for trichomoniasis from q12h to q24h. Hemodialysis: If administration cannot be separated from hemodialysis session, consider supplementation of dosage following the session, depending on patient's clinical situation. Elderly: May need to adjust dose based on serum levels.
Pediatrics: Amebiasis: 35-50mg/kg/24 hrs in 3 divided doses for 10 days.

HOW SUPPLIED: Cap: 375mg; Tab: 250mg, 500mg

CONTRAINDICATIONS: Disulfiram use within the last 2 weeks. Consumption of alcohol or products containing propylene glycol during and for at least 3 days after therapy. Use during the 1st trimester of pregnancy in trichomoniasis patients.

WARNINGS/PRECAUTIONS: Cases of encephalopathy and peripheral neuropathy (including optic neuropathy), convulsive seizures, and aseptic meningitis reported; promptly evaluate benefit/risk ratio of the continuation of therapy if abnormal neurologic signs/symptoms appear. Known or previously unrecognized candidiasis may present more prominent symptoms during therapy and requires treatment with a candidacidal agent. Caution with hepatic/renal impairment, evidence of or history of blood dyscrasia, and in the elderly. Mild leukopenia reported; monitor total and differential leukocyte counts before and after therapy. May result in bacterial/parasitic resistance if used in the absence of proven or suspected bacterial/parasitic infection, or a prophylactic indication. Lab test interactions may occur. (Tab) In pregnant patients for whom alternative treatment has been inadequate, the one-day course of therapy should not be used.

ADVERSE REACTIONS: Headache, syncope, dizziness, vertigo, incoordination, nausea, diarrhea, epigastric distress, abdominal cramping, constipation, unpleasant metallic taste, erythematous rash, pruritus, urticaria, dysuria.

INTERACTIONS: See Contraindications. May potentiate anticoagulant effect of warfarin and other oral coumarin anticoagulants, resulting in PT prolongation; carefully monitor PT and INR. May increase serum lithium, and may cause lithium toxicity; obtain serum lithium and SrCr levels several days after beginning metronidazole. May increase busulfan concentrations, which can result in increased risk for serious busulfan toxicity; avoid concomitant use, or, if coadministration is medically needed, frequently monitor busulfan concentration and adjust busulfan dose accordingly. Simultaneous administration of drugs that decrease microsomal liver enzyme activity (eg, cimetidine) may prolong $T_{1/2}$ and decrease clearance. Simultaneous administration of drugs that induce microsomal liver enzymes (eg, phenytoin, phenobarbital) may accelerate elimination, resulting in reduced levels. Impaired clearance of phenytoin reported.

PREGNANCY: Category B, not for use in nursing.

MECHANISM OF ACTION: Nitroimidazole antimicrobial; exerts antibacterial effects in an anaerobic environment. Upon entering the organism, the drug is reduced by intracellular electron transport proteins. Because of this alteration, a concentration gradient is maintained which promotes the drug's intracellular transport. Presumably, free radicals are formed which, in turn, react with cellular components, resulting in death of the bacteria.

PHARMACOKINETICS: Absorption: Well-absorbed. Administration of multiple doses resulted in different parameters. **Distribution:** Plasma protein binding (<20%); found in breast milk; crosses the placenta. **Metabolism:** Side-chain oxidation and glucuronide conjugation; 1-(β-hydroxyethyl)-2-hydroxymethyl-5-nitroimidazole and 2-methyl-5-nitroimidazole-1-yl-acetic acid (metabolites). **Elimination:** Urine (60-80%, 20% unchanged), feces (6-15%); (Healthy) $T_{1/2}$=8 hrs.

NURSING CONSIDERATIONS

Assessment: Assess for candidiasis, alcohol use, hepatic/renal impairment, evidence/history of blood dyscrasia, hypersensitivity to drug or other nitroimidazole derivatives, pregnancy/nursing status, and possible drug interactions. Obtain total and differential leukocyte counts.

Monitoring: Monitor for abnormal neurologic signs/symptoms, candidiasis, and other adverse reactions. Monitor total and differential leukocyte counts after therapy. Monitor PT and INR with oral coumarin anticoagulants (eg, warfarin).

Patient Counseling: Instruct to d/c consumption of alcoholic beverages or products containing propylene glycol while taking the drug and for at least 3 days afterward. Counsel that therapy should only be used to treat bacterial and parasitic, not viral (eg, common cold), infections. Instruct to take exactly ud. Inform that skipping doses or not completing the full course of therapy may decrease effectiveness of treatment and increase bacterial resistance.

Administration: Oral route. **Storage:** (Cap) 15-25°C (59-77°F). (Tab) <25°C (77°F). Protect from light.

FLAGYL ER   RX
metronidazole (G.D. Searle)

> Shown to be carcinogenic in mice and rats. Avoid unnecessary use. Should be reserved for the conditions for which it is indicated.

THERAPEUTIC CLASS: Nitroimidazole

INDICATIONS: Treatment of bacterial vaginosis in nonpregnant women.

DOSAGE: *Adults:* 750mg qd for 7 consecutive days. Take at least 1 hr ac or 2 hrs pc. Hemodialysis: If administration cannot be separated from hemodialysis session, consider supplementation of dosage following the session, depending on patient's clinical situation. Elderly: May need to adjust dose based on serum levels.
Pediatrics: Postmenarchal: 750mg qd for 7 consecutive days. Take at least 1 hr ac or 2 hrs pc. Hemodialysis: If administration cannot be separated from hemodialysis session, consider supplementation of dosage following the session, depending on patient's clinical situation.

HOW SUPPLIED: Tab, Extended-Release: 750mg

CONTRAINDICATIONS: Disulfiram use within the last 2 weeks. Consumption of alcohol or products containing propylene glycol during and for at least 3 days after therapy.

WARNINGS/PRECAUTIONS: Cases of encephalopathy and peripheral neuropathy (including optic neuropathy), convulsive seizures, and aseptic meningitis reported; promptly evaluate benefit/risk ratio of the continuation of therapy if abnormal neurologic signs/symptoms appear. Known or previously unrecognized candidiasis may present more prominent symptoms during therapy and requires treatment with a candidacidal agent. Do not administer to patients with severe (Child-Pugh C) hepatic impairment unless benefits outweigh risks. Caution with hepatic/renal impairment, evidence of or history of blood dyscrasia, and in the elderly. Mild leukopenia reported; monitor total and differential leukocyte counts before and after therapy. May result in bacterial resistance if used in the absence of proven or suspected bacterial infection, or a prophylactic indication. Lab test interactions may occur.

ADVERSE REACTIONS: Headache, vaginitis, nausea, metallic taste, bacterial infection, influenza-like symptoms, genital pruritus, abdominal pain, dizziness, diarrhea, upper respiratory tract infection, rhinitis, sinusitis, pharyngitis, dysmenorrhea.

INTERACTIONS: See Contraindications. May potentiate anticoagulant effect of warfarin and other oral coumarin anticoagulants, resulting in PT prolongation; carefully monitor PT and INR. May increase serum lithium, and may cause lithium toxicity; obtain serum lithium and SrCr levels several days after beginning metronidazole. May increase busulfan concentrations, which can result in increased risk for serious busulfan toxicity; avoid concomitant use, or, if coadministration is medically needed, frequently monitor busulfan concentration and adjust busulfan dose accordingly. Simultaneous administration of drugs that decrease microsomal liver enzyme activity (eg, cimetidine) may prolong $T_{1/2}$ and decrease clearance. Simultaneous administration of drugs that induce microsomal liver enzymes (eg, phenytoin, phenobarbital) may accelerate elimination, resulting in reduced levels. Impaired clearance of phenytoin reported.

PREGNANCY: Category B, not for use in nursing.

MECHANISM OF ACTION: Nitroimidazole antimicrobial; exerts antibacterial effects in an anaerobic environment. Upon entering the organism, the drug is reduced by intracellular electron transport proteins. Because of this alteration, a concentration gradient is maintained which promotes the drug's intracellular transport. Presumably, free radicals are formed which, in turn, react with cellular components, resulting in death of the bacteria.

PHARMACOKINETICS: Absorption: (Healthy adults) C_{max}=19.4mcg/mL (fed), 12.5mcg/mL (fasted); T_{max}=4.6 hrs (fed), 6.8 hrs (fasted); AUC=211mcg•hr/mL (fed), 198mcg•hr/mL (fasted). **Distribution:** Plasma protein binding (<20%); found in breast milk; crosses the placenta. **Metabolism:** Side-chain oxidation and glucuronide conjugation; 1-(β-hydroxyethyl)-2-hydroxymethyl-5-nitroimidazole and 2-methyl-5-nitroimidazole-1-yl-acetic acid (metabolites). **Elimination:** Urine (60-80%, 20% unchanged), feces (6-15%); (Healthy adults) $T_{1/2}$=7.4 hrs (fed), 8.7 hrs (fasted).

NURSING CONSIDERATIONS

Assessment: Assess for candidiasis, alcohol use, hepatic/renal impairment, evidence/history of blood dyscrasia, hypersensitivity to drug or other nitroimidazole derivatives, pregnancy/nursing status, and possible drug interactions. Obtain total and differential leukocyte counts.

Monitoring: Monitor for abnormal neurologic signs/symptoms, candidiasis, and other adverse reactions. Monitor total and differential leukocyte counts after therapy. Monitor PT and INR with oral coumarin anticoagulants (eg, warfarin).

Patient Counseling: Instruct to d/c consumption of alcoholic beverages or products containing propylene glycol while taking the drug and for at least 3 days afterward. Counsel that therapy should only be used to treat bacterial, not viral (eg, common cold), infections. Instruct to take exactly ud. Inform that skipping doses or not completing full course of therapy may decrease effectiveness of treatment and increase bacterial resistance.

Administration: Oral route. Take at least 1 hr ac or 2 hrs pc. Do not split, chew, or crush. **Storage:** 25°C (77°F); excursions permitted to 15-30°C (59-86°F). Store in a dry place.

FLAGYL IV   RX
metronidazole (Baxter)

Shown to be carcinogenic in mice and rats; reserve use for conditions for which it is indicated.

THERAPEUTIC CLASS: Nitroimidazole

INDICATIONS: Treatment of intra-abdominal (eg, peritonitis, intra-abdominal abscess, liver abscess), skin and skin structure, gynecologic (eg, endometritis, endomyometritis, tubo-ovarian abscess, postsurgical vaginal cuff infection), CNS (eg, meningitis, brain abscess), and lower respiratory tract (eg, pneumonia, empyema, lung abscess) infections, bacterial septicemia, endocarditis, and (as adjunctive therapy) bone and joint infections caused by susceptible strains of microorganisms (anaerobic bacteria). Prophylactic use to reduce incidence of postoperative infection in contaminated or potentially contaminated elective colorectal surgery. Effective against *Bacteroides fragilis* infections resistant to clindamycin, chloramphenicol, and penicillin.

DOSAGE: *Adults:* Anaerobic Infections: LD: 15mg/kg IV infusion over 1 hr (approximately 1g for a 70kg adult). Maint: 7.5mg/kg IV infusion over 1 hr q6h (approximately 500mg for a 70kg adult), starting 6 hrs after LD initiation. Usual Duration: 7-10 days; bone/joint, lower respiratory tract, and endocardium infections may require longer treatment. Max: 4g/24 hrs. Severe Hepatic Disease: Cautiously give doses below recommended; monitor plasma levels and for toxicity. Surgical Prophylaxis: Usual: 15mg/kg IV infusion over 30-60 min and completed 1 hr before surgery, then 7.5mg/kg IV infusion over 30-60 min at 6 and 12 hrs after initial dose. D/C within 12 hrs after surgery. Elderly: Adjust dose based on serum levels.

HOW SUPPLIED: Inj: 5mg/mL [100mL]

WARNINGS/PRECAUTIONS: Encephalopathy, peripheral neuropathy (including optic neuropathy), convulsive seizures, and aseptic meningitis reported; promptly evaluate benefit/risk ratio of continuation of therapy if abnormal neurologic signs/symptoms occur. Caution with severe hepatic disease. May cause Na$^+$ retention due to Na$^+$ content; caution in patients predisposed to edema. Known or previously unrecognized candidiasis may present more prominent symptoms during therapy; treat with candicidal agent. May result in bacterial resistance with prolonged use or use in the absence of a proven/suspected bacterial infection or a prophylactic indication; take appropriate measures if superinfection develops. Caution with evidence of or history of blood dyscrasias; mild leukopenia reported; monitor total and differential leukocyte counts before and after therapy. Lab test interactions may occur.

ADVERSE REACTIONS: Convulsive seizures, encephalopathy, aseptic meningitis, optic and peripheral neuropathy.

INTERACTIONS: Avoid with alcoholic beverages. Psychotic reactions reported with disulfiram in alcoholic patients; avoid in patients who have taken disulfiram within the last 2 weeks. May potentiate anticoagulant effect of warfarin and other oral coumarin anticoagulants, resulting in PT prolongation. Microsomal liver enzyme inducers (eg, phenytoin, phenobarbital) may accelerate elimination, resulting in reduced levels; impaired clearance of phenytoin reported. Microsomal liver enzyme inhibitors (eg, cimetidine) may prolong T$_{1/2}$ and decrease clearance. Caution with corticosteroids.

PREGNANCY: Category B, not for use in nursing.

MECHANISM OF ACTION: Nitroimidazole; active in vitro against most obligate anaerobes.

PHARMACOKINETICS: Absorption: C$_{max}$=25mcg/mL. **Distribution:** Plasma protein binding (<20%); found in breast milk; crosses the placenta. **Metabolism:** Side-chain oxidation and glucuronide conjugation; 2-hydroxymethyl metabolite (active). **Elimination:** Urine (60-80%, 20% unchanged), feces (6-15%); T$_{1/2}$=8 hrs.

NURSING CONSIDERATIONS

Assessment: Assess for history of hypersensitivity to drug, severe hepatic disease, predisposition to edema, candidiasis, evidence/history of blood dyscrasia, pregnancy/nursing status, and possible drug interactions. Obtain baseline total and differential leukocyte counts.

Monitoring: Monitor for abnormal neurologic signs/symptoms, Na⁺ retention, candidiasis, and other adverse reactions. Monitor total and differential leukocyte counts. Closely monitor plasma levels and for toxicity in patients with severe hepatic disease or in elderly.

Patient Counseling: Inform that drug treats only bacterial, not viral, infections. Instruct to take exactly ud; inform that skipping doses or not completing full course may decrease effectiveness and increase resistance.

Administration: IV route. Administer by slow IV drip infusion (either as continuous or intermittent) only. Do not introduce additives into drug sol. D/C primary sol during infusion if used with a primary IV fluid system. Do not use equipment containing aluminum (eg, needles, cannulae) that would come in contact with drug sol. **Storage:** 15-30°C (59-86°F). Protect from light. Do not remove unit from overwrap until ready for use.

FLECTOR   RX
diclofenac epolamine (King)

> NSAIDs may cause an increased risk of serious cardiovascular thrombotic events, myocardial infarction (MI), stroke, and serious GI adverse events including bleeding, ulceration, and perforation of the stomach or intestines that can be fatal. Patients with cardiovascular disease (CVD) or risk factors for CVD may be at greater risk. Elderly patients are at a greater risk for GI events. Contraindicated in the perioperative setting of coronary artery bypass graft (CABG) surgery.

THERAPEUTIC CLASS: NSAID

INDICATIONS: Topical treatment of acute pain due to minor strains, sprains, and contusions.

DOSAGE: *Adults:* Apply 1 patch to most painful area bid.

HOW SUPPLIED: Patch: 180mg (1.3%) [5ˢ]

CONTRAINDICATIONS: History of asthma, urticaria, or allergic-type reactions after taking aspirin (ASA) or other NSAIDs. Treatment of perioperative pain in the setting of CABG surgery. Use on non-intact or damaged skin.

WARNINGS/PRECAUTIONS: Use lowest effective dose for shortest duration possible. Extreme caution with history of ulcer disease/GI bleeding. Cases of severe hepatic reactions reported. May cause elevations of LFTs; d/c if abnormal LFTs persist or worsen, liver disease develops, or systemic manifestations occur. May lead to new onset or worsening of preexisting HTN; monitor BP closely. Fluid retention and edema reported; caution with fluid retention/heart failure (HF). Caution when initiating treatment in patients with considerable dehydration. Renal papillary necrosis and other renal injury reported after long-term use; increased risk with renal/hepatic impairment, HF, and elderly. Not recommended for use with advanced renal disease; if therapy must be initiated, monitor renal function. Anaphylactic reactions may occur; avoid in patients with aspirin (ASA)-triad. May cause serious skin adverse events (eg, exfoliative dermatitis, Stevens-Johnson syndrome [SJS], toxic epidermal necrolysis [TEN]); d/c at 1st appearance of skin rash or any other signs of hypersensitivity. Avoid starting at 30 weeks gestation; may cause premature closure of ductus arteriosus. Cannot replace corticosteroids or treat corticosteroid insufficiency. May diminish the utility of diagnostic signs in detecting complications of presumed noninfectious, painful conditions. Anemia may occur; monitor Hgb/Hct if signs/symptoms of anemia develop with long-term use. May inhibit platelet aggregation and prolong bleeding time; monitor patients with coagulation disorders. Caution with preexisting asthma and avoid with ASA-sensitive asthma. Avoid contact with eyes and mucosa. D/C if abnormal renal tests persist or worsen. Caution in elderly and debilitated patients.

ADVERSE REACTIONS: Cardiovascular thrombotic events, MI, stroke, GI adverse events, application-site reactions (eg, pruritus, dermatitis), headache, paresthesia, somnolence.

INTERACTIONS: Increased adverse effects with ASA; avoid use. May result in higher rate of hemorrhage, more frequent abnormal creatinine, urea, and Hgb with PO NSAIDs; avoid combination unless benefit outweighs risk. May diminish antihypertensive effect of ACE inhibitors. Patients taking thiazides or loop diuretics may have impaired response to these therapies. Increased risk of renal toxicity with diuretics and ACE inhibitors. May reduce natriuretic effect of furosemide and thiazides; monitor for signs of renal failure and diuretic efficacy. May increase lithium levels; monitor for toxicity. May enhance methotrexate toxicity and cyclosporine nephrotoxicity; caution with coadministration. Increased risk of GI bleeding with PO corticosteroids, anticoagulants (eg, warfarin), smoking, and alcohol. Synergistic effects on GI bleeding with anticoagulants (eg, warfarin). Caution with drugs known to be potentially hepatotoxic (eg, acetaminophen [APAP], certain antibiotics, antiepileptics).

PREGNANCY: Category C (<30 weeks gestation) and D (≥30 weeks gestation), not for use in nursing.

MECHANISM OF ACTION: NSAID; not established. May be related to prostaglandin synthesis inhibition.

PHARMACOKINETICS: Absorption: C_{max}=0.7-6ng/mL, T_{max}=10-20 hrs. **Distribution:** Serum albumin binding (>99%). **Metabolism:** CYP2C9, CYP2C8, CYP3A4, and UGT2B7; glucuronidation and sulfation; 4'-hydroxy-diclofenac (major metabolite). **Elimination:** Urine (65%), bile (35%); $T_{1/2}$=12 hrs.

NURSING CONSIDERATIONS

Assessment: Assess for history of asthma, urticaria, or allergic-type reactions with ASA or other NSAIDs, ASA-triad, risk factors for CVD, HTN, fluid retention, HF, history of ulcer disease, history of/risk factors for GI bleeding, general health status, history of renal/hepatic impairment, coagulation disorders, dehydration, tobacco/alcohol use, pregnancy/nursing status, and for possible drug interactions. Assess that skin at application site is intact and not damaged. Obtain baseline CBC and BP.

Monitoring: Monitor BP, CBC, LFTs, renal function, and chemistry profile periodically. Monitor for GI bleeding/ulceration/perforation, cardiovascular thrombotic events, MI, stroke, HTN, fluid retention, edema, skin/allergic reactions, and other adverse reactions.

Patient Counseling: Instruct only to use on intact skin. Advise to wash hands after applying, handling, or removing the patch. Instruct not to wear patch during bathing or showering. Instruct to avoid contact with eyes and mucosa; advise that if eye contact occurs, to wash out the eye with water or saline immediately and consult physician if irritation persists for >1 hr. Counsel to seek medical attention if symptoms of hepatotoxicity, anaphylactic reactions, skin and hypersensitivity reactions, cardiovascular events, GI ulceration and bleeding, bronchospasm, weight gain, or edema occurs. Inform of pregnancy risks. Instruct to tape down edges of patch if it begins to peel-off; if problems with adhesion persist, recommend to overlay the patch with a mesh netting sleeve. Advise to avoid coadministration with unprescribed APAP.

Administration: Transdermal route. **Storage:** 25°C (77°F); excursions permitted to 15-30°C (59-86°F). Keep sealed at all times when not in use.

FLOMAX   RX
tamsulosin HCl (Boehringer Ingelheim/Astellas Pharma)

THERAPEUTIC CLASS: Alpha$_1$-antagonist

INDICATIONS: Treatment of signs and symptoms of BPH.

DOSAGE: *Adults:* Usual: 0.4mg qd, 30 min after same meal each day. Titrate: May increase to 0.8mg qd after 2-4 weeks if response is inadequate. If therapy is discontinued or interrupted, restart with 0.4mg qd.

HOW SUPPLIED: Cap: 0.4mg

WARNINGS/PRECAUTIONS: Orthostasis/syncope may occur; caution to avoid situations in which injury could result should syncope occur. May cause priapism, which may lead to permanent impotence if not properly treated. Screen for presence of prostate cancer prior to treatment and at regular intervals afterward. Intraoperative floppy iris syndrome (IFIS) observed during cataract surgery; avoid initiation in patients who are scheduled for cataract surgery. Caution with sulfa allergy; allergic reaction has been rarely reported. Not for treatment of HTN, for use in women, or in pediatrics.

ADVERSE REACTIONS: Headache, abnormal ejaculation, rhinitis, dizziness, infection, asthenia, back pain, diarrhea, pharyngitis, cough increased, somnolence, nausea, sinusitis.

INTERACTIONS: Avoid with other α-adrenergic blockers. Caution with cimetidine and warfarin. Avoid with strong inhibitors of CYP3A4 (eg, ketoconazole); may increase plasma exposure. Caution with moderate inhibitors of CYP3A4 (eg, erythromycin), with strong (eg, paroxetine), or moderate (eg, terbinafine) inhibitors of CYP2D6; potential for significant increase in tamsulosin exposure. Caution with PDE-5 inhibitors; may cause symptomatic hypotension.

PREGNANCY: Category B, not for use in nursing.

MECHANISM OF ACTION: α$_1$-antagonist; selective blockade of α$_1$ receptors in the prostate results in relaxation of the smooth muscles of the bladder neck and prostate, improving urine flow and reducing symptoms.

PHARMACOKINETICS: Absorption: Complete. Bioavailability (>90%). **Distribution:** (IV) V_d=16L. Plasma protein binding (94-99%). **Metabolism:** Liver (extensive); CYP3A4, CYP2D6. **Elimination:** Urine (76%, <10% unchanged), feces (21%); $T_{1/2}$=14-15 hrs, 9-13 hrs (healthy).

NURSING CONSIDERATIONS

Assessment: Assess for BPH, known hypersensitivity, sulfa allergy, and possible drug interactions. Screen for the presence of prostate cancer prior to treatment.

Monitoring: Monitor for signs/symptoms of orthostasis (eg, postural hypotension, dizziness, vertigo), syncope, priapism, prostate cancer, IFIS during cataract surgery, and allergic/hypersensitivity reactions.

Patient Counseling: Inform about the possible occurrence of symptoms related to orthostatic hypotension (eg, dizziness); caution about driving, operating machinery, or performing hazardous tasks. Instruct not to crush or chew cap. Inform of the importance of screening for prostate cancer prior to therapy and at regular intervals afterwards. Advise to inform ophthalmologist of drug use if considering cataract surgery. Advise about the possibility of priapism and to seek immediate medical attention if it occurs.

Administration: Oral route. **Storage:** 25°C (77°F); excursions permitted to 15-30°C (59-86°F).

FLONASE

RX

fluticasone propionate (GlaxoSmithKline)

THERAPEUTIC CLASS: Corticosteroid

INDICATIONS: Management of the nasal symptoms of seasonal and perennial allergic and nonallergic rhinitis in adults and pediatric patients ≥4 yrs of age.

DOSAGE: *Adults:* Initial: 2 sprays/nostril qd or 1 spray/nostril bid. Maint: 1 spray/nostril qd. *Pediatrics:* ≥4 Yrs: Initial: 1 spray/nostril qd. Titrate: May increase to 2 sprays/nostril qd if response is inadequate, then return to initial dose once adequate control is achieved. Max: 2 sprays/nostril daily.

HOW SUPPLIED: Spray: 50mcg/spray [16g]

WARNINGS/PRECAUTIONS: Risk of adrenal insufficiency and withdrawal symptoms when replacing systemic corticosteroids with topical corticosteroids. May lead to serious/fatal course of chickenpox or measles; avoid exposure and if exposed, consider prophylaxis/treatment. May reduce growth velocity in pediatric patients. Rare hypersensitivity reactions or contact dermatitis may occur. Rare instances of wheezing, nasal septum perforation, cataracts, glaucoma, and increased intraocular pressure (IOP) reported. D/C slowly if hypercorticism or adrenal suppression occurs. *Candida albicans* infections of the nose and pharynx may occur; treat and, if needed, d/c therapy. Monitor for evidence of *Candida* infection or other signs of adverse effects on the nasal mucosa periodically during prolonged use. Caution with active or quiescent tuberculosis (TB), untreated local or systemic fungal or bacterial infections, systemic viral or parasitic infections, or ocular herpes simplex. Do not use until healing has occurred in patients with recent nasal septal ulcers, nasal surgery, or nasal trauma.

ADVERSE REACTIONS: Headache, pharyngitis, epistaxis, nasal burning/irritation, N/V, asthma symptoms, cough.

INTERACTIONS: Systemic corticosteroid effects including Cushing syndrome and adrenal suppression with ritonavir reported; avoid coadministration unless benefit outweighs the risk. Increased plasma exposure with ketoconazole; caution with ketoconazole and other known potent CYP3A4 inhibitors. Concomitant inhaled corticosteroids may increase the risk of hypercorticism and/or hypothalamic-pituitary-adrenal-axis suppression.

PREGNANCY: Category C, caution in nursing.

MECHANISM OF ACTION: Corticosteroid; not established. Shown to have wide range of effects on multiple cell types (eg, mast cells, eosinophils, neutrophils, macrophages, lymphocytes) and mediators (eg, histamine, eicosanoids, leukotrienes, cytokines) involved in inflammation.

PHARMACOKINETICS: Absorption: Absolute bioavailability (<2%). **Distribution:** (IV) V_d=4.2L/kg; plasma protein binding (91%). **Metabolism:** Liver via CYP3A4. **Elimination:** (PO) Urine (<5%, metabolites), feces (parent drug, metabolites); (IV) $T_{1/2}$=7.8 hrs.

NURSING CONSIDERATIONS

Assessment: Assess for drug hypersensitivity, active or quiescent TB, local/systemic infections, ocular herpes simplex, recent nasal ulcers/surgery/trauma, immunization status, pregnancy/nursing status, and possible drug interactions.

Monitoring: Monitor for acute adrenal insufficiency and withdrawal symptoms when replacing systemic corticosteroid with topical corticosteroid. Monitor for systemic corticosteroid effects (eg, hypercorticism, adrenal suppression), infections, nasal or pharyngeal *C. albicans* infections, hypersensitivity, contact dermatitis, and other adverse reactions. Monitor growth of pediatric patients routinely.

Patient Counseling: Instruct to take ud at regular intervals and not to increase prescribed dosage. Advise to contact physician if symptoms do not improve or if condition worsens. Warn to avoid exposure to chickenpox or measles; instruct to consult physician immediately if exposed. Counsel on the proper use of spray and instruct to avoid spraying in eyes.

Administration: Intranasal route. Shake gently before use. **Storage:** 4-30°C (39-86°F).

FLOVENT HFA
fluticasone propionate (GlaxoSmithKline)

RX

THERAPEUTIC CLASS: Corticosteroid

INDICATIONS: Maintenance treatment of asthma as prophylactic therapy in patients ≥4 yrs of age and for patients requiring oral corticosteroid therapy for asthma.

DOSAGE: *Adults:* Previous Bronchodilators Alone: Initial: 88mcg bid. Max: 440mcg bid. Previous Inhaled Corticosteroids: Initial: 88-220mcg bid. May consider starting doses >88mcg bid with poorer asthma control or previous high-dose inhaled corticosteroid requirement. Max: 440mcg bid. Previous Oral Corticosteroids: Initial: 440mcg bid. Max: 880mcg bid. Reduce oral prednisone no faster than 2.5-5mg/day on a weekly basis beginning after at least 1 week of fluticasone therapy. Titrate: Reduce to lowest effective dose once asthma stability is achieved. Higher dosages may provide additional asthma control if response to initial dose is inadequate after 2 weeks. *Pediatrics:* ≥12 Yrs: Previous Bronchodilators Alone: Initial: 88mcg bid. Max: 440mcg bid. Previous Inhaled Corticosteroids: Initial: 88-220mcg bid. May consider starting doses >88mcg bid with poorer asthma control or previous high-dose inhaled corticosteroid requirement. Max: 440mcg bid. Previous Oral Corticosteroids: Initial: 440mcg bid. Max: 880mcg bid. Reduce oral prednisone no faster than 2.5-5mg/day on a weekly basis beginning after at least 1 week of fluticasone therapy. 4-11 Yrs: Initial/Max: 88mcg bid. Titrate: Reduce to lowest effective dose once asthma stability is achieved. Higher dosages may provide additional asthma control if response to initial dose is inadequate after 2 weeks.

HOW SUPPLIED: MDI: 44mcg/inh, 110mcg/inh, 220mcg/inh [120 inhalations]

CONTRAINDICATIONS: Primary treatment of status asthmaticus or other acute episodes of asthma where intensive measures are required.

WARNINGS/PRECAUTIONS: Not indicated for rapid relief of bronchospasm. *Candida albicans* infections of mouth and pharynx reported; treat and/or interrupt therapy if needed. Increased susceptibility to infections. May lead to serious/fatal course of chickenpox or measles; avoid exposure, and if exposed, consider prophylaxis/treatment. Caution in patients with active/quiescent tuberculosis (TB), untreated systemic fungal, bacterial, viral, or parasitic infections, or ocular herpes simplex. Deaths due to adrenal insufficiency reported during and after transfer from systemic to inhaled corticosteroids; wean slowly from systemic corticosteroid use after transferring to therapy. Resume oral corticosteroids during periods of stress or a severe asthma attack in patients previously withdrawn from systemic corticosteroids. Transfer from systemic to inhaled corticosteroids may unmask conditions previously suppressed by systemic therapy (eg, rhinitis, conjunctivitis, eczema, arthritis, eosinophilic conditions). Monitor for systemic corticosteroid effects. Reduce dose slowly if hypercorticism and adrenal suppression/crisis occur. Hypersensitivity reactions may occur. Decreases in bone mineral density (BMD) reported with long-term use; caution with major risk factors for decreased bone mineral content, including chronic use of drugs that can reduce bone mass (eg, anticonvulsants, oral corticosteroids). May cause reduction in growth velocity in pediatric patients. Glaucoma, increased intraocular pressure (IOP), cataracts, rare cases of systemic eosinophilic conditions, and vasculitis consistent with Churg-Strauss syndrome reported. Paradoxical bronchospasm with immediate increase in wheezing may occur; d/c immediately, treat, and institute alternative therapy. Closely monitor patients with hepatic disease.

ADVERSE REACTIONS: Upper respiratory tract infection, throat irritation, sinusitis/sinus infection, upper respiratory inflammation, hoarseness/dysphonia, candidiasis, cough, bronchitis, headache.

INTERACTIONS: Not recommended with strong CYP3A4 inhibitors (eg, ritonavir, clarithromycin, nefazodone, ketoconazole); increased systemic corticosteroid adverse effects may occur. Ritonavir and ketoconazole may increase levels and reduce cortisol levels.

PREGNANCY: Category C, caution in nursing.

MECHANISM OF ACTION: Corticosteroid; possesses potent anti-inflammatory activity. Shown to inhibit multiple cell types (eg, mast cells, eosinophils, basophils, lymphocytes, macrophages, neutrophils) and mediator production or secretion (eg, histamine, eicosanoids, leukotrienes, cytokines) involved in the asthmatic response.

PHARMACOKINETICS: Absorption: Acts locally in the lung. **Distribution:** (IV) V_d=4.2L/kg; plasma protein binding (99%). **Metabolism:** Liver via CYP3A4; 17β-carboxylic acid derivative (metabolite). **Elimination:** (PO) Urine (<5% metabolites), feces; (IV) $T_{1/2}$=7.8 hrs.

NURSING CONSIDERATIONS

Assessment: Assess for hypersensitivity to drug, status asthmaticus, acute bronchospasm, active/quiescent TB, ocular herpes simplex, untreated systemic infections, risk factors for decreased bone mineral content, history of increased IOP, glaucoma, cataracts, hepatic impairment, pregnancy/nursing status, and possible drug interactions.

Monitoring: Monitor for signs of infection, systemic corticosteroid effects (eg, hypercorticism, adrenal suppression), hypersensitivity reactions, decreased BMD, glaucoma, increased IOP, cataracts, paradoxical bronchospasm, eosinophilic conditions, asthma instability, and other adverse reactions. Monitor growth in pediatric patients routinely (eg, via stadiometry). Monitor lung function, β-agonist use, and asthma signs/symptoms during oral corticosteroid withdrawal. Closely monitor patients with hepatic disease.

Patient Counseling: Advise that localized infections with *C. albicans* may occur in the mouth and pharynx. Inform that product is not intended for use as rescue medication for acute asthma exacerbations; instruct to contact physician immediately if deterioration of asthma occurs. Instruct to avoid exposure to chickenpox or measles and to consult physician without delay if exposed. Inform of potential worsening of existing TB, fungal, bacterial, viral, or parasitic infections, or ocular herpes simplex. Counsel about the risk of systemic corticosteroid effects, decreased BMD, and reduced growth velocity in pediatric patients. Inform that long-term use may increase risk of some eye problems. Instruct to d/c therapy if hypersensitivity reaction occurs. Instruct to use at regular intervals ud and not to stop use abruptly; advise to contact physician immediately if use is discontinued.

Administration: Oral inhalation route. Rinse mouth after inhalation. Shake well before use. Prime inhaler before use for the 1st time, if not used for >7 days, or if dropped. Avoid spraying in eyes. Refer to PI for further administration instructions. **Storage:** 25°C (77°F); excursions permitted to 15-30°C (59-86°F). Store with mouthpiece down. Contents under pressure; do not puncture, use/store near heat or open flame, or throw into fire/incinerator. Exposure to temperatures >49°C (120°F) may cause bursting. Discard when counter reads 000.

FLUDROCORTISONE   RX
fludrocortisone acetate (Various)

THERAPEUTIC CLASS: Corticosteroid

INDICATIONS: Partial replacement therapy for primary and secondary adrenocortical insufficiency in Addison's disease. Treatment of salt-losing adrenogenital syndrome.

DOSAGE: *Adults:* Dose depends on disease severity and patient response. Adjust dose during remission/exacerbations of the disease and stress (surgery, infection, trauma). Addison's Disease: Usual: 0.1mg/day; preferably administered with cortisone 10-37.5mg/day or hydrocortisone 10-30mg/day in divided doses. Range: 0.1mg 3X weekly to 0.2mg/day. If transient HTN develops, reduce to 0.05mg/day. Salt-Losing Adrenogenital Syndrome: Usual: 0.1-0.2mg/day.

HOW SUPPLIED: Tab: 0.1mg* *scored

CONTRAINDICATIONS: Systemic fungal infections.

WARNINGS/PRECAUTIONS: May mask signs of infection, and new infections may appear during therapy. There may be decreased resistance and inability to localize infection; promptly control infection with suitable antimicrobial therapy. Prolonged use may produce posterior subcapsular cataracts, glaucoma with possible damage to optic nerves, and secondary ocular infections due to fungi or viruses. May cause elevation of BP, salt and water retention, and increased K⁺ excretion; carefully monitor dosage and salt intake to avoid HTN, edema, or weight gain. Periodic serum electrolyte monitoring is advisable during prolonged therapy; dietary salt restriction and K⁺ supplementation may be necessary. May increase Ca²⁺ excretion. Use in patients with active tuberculosis (TB) should be restricted to fulminating or disseminated cases in conjunction with an appropriate antituberculous regimen. Reactivation of TB may occur; caution in patients with latent TB or tuberculin reactivity; patients on prolonged therapy should receive chemoprophylaxis. Avoid exposure to chickenpox or measles. Adverse effects may occur by too rapid withdrawal or by continued use of large doses. Enhanced effects with hypothyroidism and cirrhosis. To avoid drug-induced adrenal insufficiency, supportive dosage may be required in times of stress (eg, trauma, surgery, severe illness) both during treatment and for a yr afterwards. Use lowest possible dose; gradually reduce dosage when possible. Caution with ocular herpes simplex, nonspecific ulcerative colitis, HTN, diverticulitis, fresh intestinal anastomoses, active/latent peptic ulcer, renal insufficiency, osteoporosis, and myasthenia gravis. Psychic derangements may appear and existing emotional instability or psychotic tendencies may be aggravated. Lab test interactions may occur.

ADVERSE REACTIONS: HTN, congestive heart failure, edema, cardiac enlargement, K⁺ loss, hypokalemic alkalosis.

INTERACTIONS: Decreased pharmacologic effect and increased ulcerogenic effect of aspirin (ASA); monitor salicylate levels or therapeutic effect of ASA and adjust salicylate dosage accordingly if effect is altered. Caution with ASA in patients with hypoprothrombinemia. Enhanced hypokalemia with amphotericin B or K⁺-depleting diuretics (eg, benzothiadiazines, furosemide, ethacrynic acid) and enhanced possibility of arrhythmias or digitalis toxicity associated with hypokalemia with digitalis glycosides; monitor serum K⁺ levels and use K⁺ supplements if necessary. Rifampin, barbiturates, or phenytoin may diminish steroid effect; increase steroid dosage accordingly. Decreased PT response with oral anticoagulants; monitor prothrombin levels and adjust anticoagulant dosage accordingly. Diminished effect of oral hypoglycemics and insulin; monitor for symptoms of hyperglycemia and adjust dosage of antidiabetic drug upward if necessary. Enhanced tendency toward edema with anabolic steroids (particularly C-17 alkylated androgens [eg, oxymetholone, methandrostenolone, norethandrolone]); use with caution especially in patients with hepatic/cardiac disease. May require a reduction of corticosteroid dose when estrogen therapy is initiated, and may require increased amounts when estrogen is terminated. Avoid smallpox vaccination and other immunizations; possible hazards of neurologic complications and a lack of antibody response.

PREGNANCY: Category C, caution in nursing.

MECHANISM OF ACTION: Corticosteroid; acts on the distal tubules of the kidney to enhance reabsorption of Na$^+$ ions from tubular fluid into the plasma and increase urinary excretion of both K$^+$ and hydrogen ions.

PHARMACOKINETICS: Distribution: Found in breast milk. **Elimination:** T$_{1/2}$=18-36 hrs.

NURSING CONSIDERATIONS

Assessment: Assess for hypersensitivity to drug, systemic fungal infections, active/latent TB, HTN, renal insufficiency, psychotic tendencies, hypothyroidism, osteoporosis, myasthenia gravis, peptic ulcer, fresh intestinal anastomoses, ocular herpes simplex, diverticulitis, ulcerative colitis, other conditions where treatment is cautioned, pregnancy/nursing status, and possible drug interactions.

Monitoring: Monitor for infections, edema, weight gain, psychic derangement, cataracts, latent TB reactivation, and other adverse reactions. Monitor dosage, salt intake, serum electrolytes, and BP. Monitor for remission or exacerbations of disease and stress (surgery, infection, trauma). Monitor prothrombin levels if used with oral anticoagulants.

Patient Counseling: Advise to report any medical history of heart disease, high BP, and kidney/liver disease, and to report current use of any medicines. Instruct to avoid exposure to chickenpox or measles and, if exposed, to obtain medical advice. Inform of steroid-dependent status and of increased dosage requirement with stress; advise to carry medical identification indicating this dependence and, if necessary, instruct to carry an adequate supply of medication for emergency use. Inform of the importance of regular follow-up visits and the need to promptly notify physician of dizziness, severe or continuing headaches, swelling of feet or lower legs, or unusual weight gain. Instruct to take only ud, to take a missed dose as soon as possible, unless it is almost time for next dose, and not to double next dose.

Administration: Oral route. **Storage:** 15-30°C (59-86°F). Avoid excessive heat.

FLUTICASONE TOPICAL　　　　RX
fluticasone propionate (Various)

OTHER BRAND NAMES: Cutivate (PharmaDerm)

THERAPEUTIC CLASS: Corticosteroid

INDICATIONS: (Cre/Oint) Relief of the inflammatory and pruritic manifestations of corticosteroid-responsive dermatoses. (Lot) Relief of the inflammatory and pruritic manifestations of atopic dermatitis.

DOSAGE: *Adults:* Atopic Dermatitis: Apply a thin film to affected areas qd (lot) or qd-bid (cre). (Cre/Oint) Other Corticosteroid-Responsive Dermatoses: Apply a thin film to affected areas bid. (Cre/Oint/Lot) D/C when control is achieved. Reassess diagnosis if no improvement is seen within 2 weeks. Do not use with occlusive dressings.
Pediatrics: (Lot) ≥1 Yr: Atopic Dermatitis: Apply a thin film to affected areas qd. (Cre) ≥3 Months: Atopic Dermatitis: Apply a thin film to affected areas qd or bid. Other Corticosteroid-Responsive Dermatoses: Apply a thin film to affected areas bid. (Cre/Lot) D/C when control is achieved. Reassess diagnosis if no improvement is seen within 2 weeks. Do not use with occlusive dressings or apply in the diaper area.

HOW SUPPLIED: Cre: 0.05% [15g, 30g, 60g]; Oint: 0.005% [15g, 30g, 60g]; (Cutivate) Lot: 0.05% [60mL, 120mL]

WARNINGS/PRECAUTIONS: For dermatologic use only; not for ophthalmic use. Systemic absorption may produce reversible hypothalamic-pituitary-adrenal (HPA) axis suppression, manifestations of Cushing's syndrome, hyperglycemia, and glucosuria. Periodically evaluate for evidence of HPA axis suppression when applied to a large surface area or to areas under occlusion; if noted, withdraw the drug, reduce frequency of application, or substitute a less potent steroid. Infrequently, signs and symptoms of glucocorticosteroid insufficiency may occur, requiring supplemental systemic corticosteroids. Pediatric patients may be more susceptible to systemic toxicity. May cause local cutaneous adverse reactions. D/C if irritation develops. Allergic contact dermatitis may occur; confirm by patch testing. Use appropriate antifungal or antibacterial agent if concomitant skin infections are present or develop; if a favorable response does not occur promptly, d/c until infection has been adequately controlled. Do not use in the presence of preexisting skin atrophy and where infection is present at the treatment site. Do not use in the treatment of rosacea or perioral dermatitis. (Cre/Lot) Contains the excipient imidurea, which releases formaldehyde as a breakdown product; do not use in patients with hypersensitivity to formaldehyde, as it may prevent healing or worsen dermatitis. (Lot) Avoid excessive exposure to either natural or artificial sunlight (eg, sunbathing, tanning booths, sun lamps) if applied to exposed portions of the body.

ADVERSE REACTIONS: Pruritus, dryness of skin, telangiectasia, burning, hypertrichosis, erythema, skin irritation, folliculitis. (Lot) Common cold, upper respiratory tract infection, cough, fever.

PREGNANCY: Category C, caution in nursing.

MECHANISM OF ACTION: Corticosteroid; possesses anti-inflammatory, antipruritic, and vasoconstrictive properties. Anti-inflammatory mechanism not established; thought to act by the induction of phospholipase A_2 inhibitory proteins called lipocortins. Lipocortins control biosynthesis of potent mediators of inflammation (eg, prostaglandins, leukotrienes) by inhibiting release of their common precursor, arachidonic acid.

PHARMACOKINETICS: Absorption: Percutaneous; extent of absorption is determined by many factors (eg, vehicle, integrity of the epidermal barrier, use of occlusive dressings). **Distribution:** (IV) V_d=4.2L/kg; plasma protein binding (91%). Found in breast milk (systemically administered). **Metabolism:** Liver by CYP3A4-mediated hydrolysis of the 5-fluoromethyl carbothioate grouping. **Elimination:** (IV) $T_{1/2}$=7.2 hrs.

NURSING CONSIDERATIONS

Assessment: Assess for drug hypersensitivity, skin infections, presence of preexisting skin atrophy or of skin infection at treatment site, and pregnancy/nursing status. (Cre/Lot) Assess for hypersensitivity to formaldehyde.

Monitoring: Monitor for signs/symptoms of HPA axis suppression, Cushing's syndrome, hyperglycemia, glucosuria, irritation, allergic contact dermatitis, skin infections, and other adverse reactions. Following withdrawal of treatment, monitor for glucocorticosteroid insufficiency. Perform periodic monitoring for HPA axis suppression by using am plasma cortisol, urinary free cortisol, and adrenocorticotropic hormone stimulation tests. Reassess diagnosis if no improvement is seen within 2 weeks.

Patient Counseling: Instruct to use externally ud and to avoid contact with eyes. Advise not to use for any disorder other than for which it was prescribed. Instruct not to bandage, cover, or wrap the treated skin area unless directed by physician. Counsel to report to physician any signs of local adverse reactions. Advise not to use on the face, underarms, or groin areas unless directed by physician. Instruct to d/c therapy when control is achieved, and to contact physician if no improvement is seen within 2 weeks. (Cre/Lot) Advise not to use in the treatment of diaper dermatitis; instruct not to apply in the diaper areas as diapers or plastic pants may constitute occlusive dressings. Advise to notify physician if allergic to formaldehyde. (Lot) Counsel patients who apply product to exposed portions of the body to follow physician's advice and routine precautions to avoid excessive or unnecessary exposure to either natural or artificial sunlight.

Administration: Topical route. Rub in gently. **Storage:** (Cre) 2-30°C (36-86°F). (Oint) 20-25°C (68-77°F). (Lot) 15-30°C (59-86°F). Do not refrigerate.

FOCALIN CII
dexmethylphenidate HCl (Novartis)

> Caution with history of drug dependence or alcoholism. Chronic, abusive use may lead to marked tolerance and psychological dependence with varying degrees of abnormal behavior may occur with chronic abusive use. Frank psychotic episodes may occur, especially with parenteral abuse. Careful supervision is required during withdrawal from abusive use, since severe depression may occur. Withdrawal following chronic use may unmask symptoms of underlying disorder that may require follow-up.

THERAPEUTIC CLASS: Sympathomimetic amine

INDICATIONS: Treatment of attention-deficit hyperactivity disorder (ADHD).

DOSAGE: *Adults:* Individualize dose. Take bid, at least 4 hrs apart. Methylphenidate-Naive: Initial: 5mg/day (2.5mg bid). Titrate: May adjust weekly in 2.5-5mg increments. Max: 20mg/day (10mg bid). Currently on Methylphenidate: Initial: 1/2 of methylphenidate dose. Max: 20mg/day (10mg bid). Periodically reevaluate long-term usefulness of the drug. Reduce dose or d/c if paradoxical aggravation of symptoms or other adverse events occur. D/C if no improvement seen after appropriate dosage adjustment over a 1-month period.
Pediatrics: ≥6 Yrs: Individualize dose. Take bid, at least 4 hrs apart. Methylphenidate-Naive: Initial: 5mg/day (2.5mg bid). Titrate: May adjust weekly in 2.5-5mg increments. Max: 20mg/day (10mg bid). Currently on Methylphenidate: Initial: 1/2 of methylphenidate dose. Max: 20mg/day (10mg

bid). Periodically reevaluate long-term usefulness of the drug. Reduce dose or d/c if paradoxical aggravation of symptoms or other adverse events occur. D/C if no improvement seen after appropriate dosage adjustment over a 1-month period.

HOW SUPPLIED: Tab: 2.5mg, 5mg, 10mg

CONTRAINDICATIONS: Marked anxiety, tension, agitation, glaucoma, motor tics, or family history or diagnosis of Tourette's syndrome. Treatment with MAOIs or within a minimum of 14 days following discontinuation of an MAOI.

WARNINGS/PRECAUTIONS: Avoid in patients with known serious structural cardiac abnormalities, cardiomyopathy, serious heart rhythm abnormalities, coronary artery disease, or other serious cardiac problems. Sudden death reported in children and adolescents with structural cardiac abnormalities or other serious heart problems. Sudden death, stroke, and myocardial infarction (MI) reported in adults. May cause modest increase in average BP and HR; caution in patients whose underlying medical conditions might be compromised by increases in BP or HR (eg, preexisting HTN, heart failure, recent MI, ventricular arrhythmia). Prior to treatment, perform medical history (including assessment for family history of sudden death or ventricular arrhythmia) and physical exam to assess for presence of cardiac disease. Promptly perform cardiac evaluation if symptoms of cardiac disease develop during treatment. May exacerbate symptoms of behavior disturbance and thought disorder in patients with a preexisting psychotic disorder. Caution in patients with comorbid bipolar disorder; may induce mixed/manic episode. May cause treatment-emergent psychotic or manic symptoms (eg, hallucinations, delusional thinking, mania) at usual doses in children and adolescents without a prior history of psychotic illness or mania; discontinuation may be appropriate if such symptoms occur. Aggressive behavior or hostility reported in children and adolescents. May cause long-term suppression of growth in children; monitor growth and may need to interrupt treatment in patients not growing or gaining height or weight as expected. May lower convulsive threshold; d/c in the presence of seizures. Priapism reported; immediate medical attention should be sought if abnormally sustained or frequent and painful erections develop. Associated with peripheral vasculopathy, including Raynaud's phenomenon; monitor for digital changes. Difficulties with accommodation and blurring of vision reported. Periodically monitor CBC, differential, and platelet counts during prolonged therapy.

ADVERSE REACTIONS: Abdominal pain, fever, anorexia, nausea.

INTERACTIONS: See Contraindications. May decrease the effectiveness of drugs used to treat HTN. Caution with pressor agents. May inhibit metabolism of coumarin anticoagulants, anticonvulsants (eg, phenobarbital, phenytoin, primidone) and some antidepressants (eg, TCAs, SSRIs); downward dose adjustments and monitoring of plasma drug concentration (or coagulation times for coumarin) of these drugs may be necessary when initiating or discontinuing dexmethylphenidate.

PREGNANCY: Category C, caution in nursing.

MECHANISM OF ACTION: Sympathomimetic amine; CNS stimulant. Mechanism in ADHD has not been established; suspected to block the reuptake of norepinephrine and dopamine into the presynaptic neuron and increase the release of these monoamines into the extraneuronal space.

PHARMACOKINETICS: Absorption: Readily absorbed; T_{max}=2.9 hrs (fed), 1-1.5 hrs (fasted). **Metabolism:** Deesterification; d-ritalinic acid (primary metabolite). **Elimination:** Urine (90%, primarily as metabolite); $T_{1/2}$=2.2 hrs.

NURSING CONSIDERATIONS

Assessment: Assess for previous hypersensitivity to the drug, history of drug dependence or alcoholism, marked anxiety, agitation, tension, glaucoma, motor tics, family history or diagnosis of Tourette's syndrome, preexisting psychotic disorder, comorbid bipolar disorder, history of seizures, medical conditions that might be compromised by increases in BP or HR, any other conditions where treatment is contraindicated or cautioned, pregnancy/nursing status, and possible drug interactions. Perform a careful history (including assessment for a family history of sudden death or ventricular arrhythmia) and physical exam to assess for the presence of cardiac disease, and perform further cardiac evaluation if findings suggest such disease (eg, ECG, echocardiogram). Adequately screen patients with comorbid depressive symptoms to determine if they are at risk for bipolar disorder (eg, detailed psychiatric history, including a family history of suicide, bipolar disorder, and depression).

Monitoring: Monitor for signs/symptoms of cardiac disease, exacerbation of behavioral disturbance and thought disorder, psychosis, mania, appearance of or worsening of aggressive behavior or hostility, seizures, priapism, digital changes, visual disturbances, and other adverse reactions. Monitor BP and HR. During prolonged use, periodically evaluate usefulness of therapy and monitor CBC, differential, and platelet counts. In pediatric patients, monitor growth.

Patient Counseling: Inform about risks and benefits of treatment. Counsel on the appropriate use of the medication. Advise of the possibility of priapism; instruct to seek immediate medical attention in the event of priapism. Instruct to report to physician any new numbness, pain, skin color change, sensitivity to temperature in fingers or toes, or any signs of unexplained wounds appearing on the fingers or toes.

Administration: Oral route. Take with or without food. **Storage:** 25°C (77°F); excursions permitted to 15-30°C (59-86°F). Protect from light and moisture.

FOCALIN XR

CII

dexmethylphenidate HCl (Novartis)

> Caution with history of drug dependence or alcoholism. Marked tolerance and psychological dependence with varying degrees of abnormal behavior may occur with chronic abusive use. Frank psychotic episodes may occur, especially with parenteral abuse. Careful supervision is required during withdrawal from abusive use, since severe depression may occur. Withdrawal following chronic therapeutic use may unmask symptoms of underlying disorder that may require follow-up.

THERAPEUTIC CLASS: Sympathomimetic amine

INDICATIONS: Treatment of attention-deficit hyperactivity disorder (ADHD) in patients ≥6 yrs of age.

DOSAGE: *Adults:* Individualize dose. Methylphenidate-Naive: Initial: 10mg qam. Titrate: May adjust weekly in 10mg increments. Max: 40mg/day. Currently on Methylphenidate: Initial: 1/2 of methylphenidate total daily dose. Currently on Dexmethylphenidate Immediate-Release (IR): May switch to the same daily dose of the ER. Periodically reevaluate the long-term usefulness of the drug. Reduce dose or d/c if paradoxical aggravation of symptoms or other adverse events occur. D/C if no improvement seen after appropriate dosage adjustment over 1 month.
Pediatrics: ≥6 Yrs: Individualize dose. Methylphenidate-Naive: Initial: 5mg qam. Titrate: May adjust weekly in 5mg increments. Max: 30mg/day. Currently on Methylphenidate: Initial: 1/2 of methylphenidate total daily dose. Currently on Dexmethylphenidate IR: May switch to the same daily dose of the ER. Periodically reevaluate the long-term usefulness of the drug. Reduce dose or d/c if paradoxical aggravation of symptoms or other adverse events occur. D/C if no improvement seen after appropriate dosage adjustment over 1 month.

HOW SUPPLIED: Cap, Extended-Release (ER): 5mg, 10mg, 15mg, 20mg, 25mg, 30mg, 35mg, 40mg

CONTRAINDICATIONS: Marked anxiety, tension, agitation, glaucoma, motor tics or family history or diagnosis of Tourette's syndrome. Treatment with MAOIs or within a minimum of 14 days following discontinuation of an MAOI.

WARNINGS/PRECAUTIONS: Avoid in patients with known serious structural cardiac abnormalities, cardiomyopathy, serious heart rhythm abnormalities, coronary artery disease, or other serious cardiac problems. Sudden death reported in children and adolescents with structural cardiac abnormalities or other serious heart problems. Sudden death, stroke, myocardial infarction (MI) reported in adults. May cause modest increase in average BP and HR; caution with HTN, heart failure, recent MI, or ventricular arrhythmia. Prior to treatment, perform a medical history (including assessment for family history of sudden death or ventricular arrhythmia) and physical exam to assess for the presence of cardiac disease. Promptly perform cardiac evaluation if symptoms of cardiac disease develop during treatment. May exacerbate symptoms of behavior disturbance and thought disorder in patients with preexisting psychotic disorder. Caution in patients with comorbid bipolar disorder; may induce mixed/manic episodes. May cause treatment-emergent psychotic or manic symptoms (eg, hallucinations, delusional thinking, mania) in children and adolescents without prior history of psychotic illness or mania; discontinuation may be appropriate if such symptoms occur. Aggressive behavior or hostility reported in children and adolescents. May cause long-term suppression of growth in children; monitor growth, and may need to interrupt treatment in patients not growing or gaining height or weight as expected. May lower convulsive threshold; d/c in the presence of seizures. Priapism reported; seek immediate medical attention if abnormally sustained or frequent and painful erections develop. Associated with peripheral vasculopathy, including Raynaud's phenomenon; monitor for digital changes. Difficulties with accommodation and blurring of vision reported. Periodically monitor CBC, differential, and platelet counts during prolonged therapy.

ADVERSE REACTIONS: Dyspepsia, headache, anxiety, insomnia, anorexia, dry mouth, pharyngolaryngeal pain, feeling jittery, dizziness, decreased appetite, vomiting.

INTERACTIONS: See Contraindications. May decrease the effectiveness of drugs used to treat HTN. Caution with pressor agents. May inhibit metabolism of coumarin anticoagulants, anticonvulsants (eg, phenobarbital, phenytoin, primidone), and tricyclic drugs (eg, imipramine, clomipramine, desipramine); downward dose adjustments and monitoring of plasma drug concentration (or coagulation times for coumarin) of these drugs may be necessary when initiating or discontinuing therapy. Antacids or acid suppressants could alter drug release.

PREGNANCY: Category C, caution in nursing.

MECHANISM OF ACTION: Sympathomimetic amine; CNS stimulant. Mechanism in ADHD has not been established; suspected to block the reuptake of norepinephrine and dopamine into the presynaptic neuron and increase the release of these monoamines into the extraneuronal space.

PHARMACOKINETICS: Absorption: Absolute bioavailability (22-25%); T_{max}=1.5 hrs (1st peak), 6.5 hrs (2nd peak). **Distribution:** Plasma protein binding (12-15%, racemic methylphenidate); V_d=2.65L/kg. **Metabolism:** Deesterification; d-ritalinic acid (primary metabolite). **Elimination:** Urine (90%, racemic methylphenidate); (IV) $T_{1/2}$=2-4.5 hrs (healthy adults), 2-3 hrs (children).

NURSING CONSIDERATIONS

Assessment: Assess for previous hypersensitivity to the drug, history of drug dependence or alcoholism, marked anxiety, tension, agitation, glaucoma, motor tics, family history or diagnosis of Tourette's syndrome, preexisting psychotic disorder, comorbid bipolar disorder, cardiac disease, medical conditions that might be compromised by increases in BP and HR, any other conditions where treatment is cautioned, pregnancy/nursing status, and possible drug interactions.

Monitoring: Monitor BP, HR, and for signs/symptoms of cardiac disease (eg, exertional chest pain, unexplained syncope), exacerbation of behavioral disturbance and thought disorder, psychosis, mania, appearance of or worsening of aggressive behavior or hostility, seizures, priapism, digital changes, visual disturbances, and other adverse reactions. During prolonged use, periodically reevaluate usefulness of therapy and monitor CBC, differential, and platelet counts. In pediatric patients, monitor growth.

Patient Counseling: Inform about benefits and risks of treatment. Counsel on the appropriate use of the medication. Advise of the possibility of priapism; instruct to seek immediate medical attention in the event of priapism. Instruct to report to physician any new numbness, pain, skin color change, sensitivity to temperature in fingers or toes, or any signs of unexplained wounds appearing on fingers or toes.

Administration: Oral route. Swallow caps whole or sprinkle contents on a spoonful of applesauce. Do not crush, chew, or divide. Consume drug and applesauce mixture immediately; do not store for future use. **Storage:** 25°C (77°F); excursions permitted to 15-30°C (59-86°F).

FOLIC ACID

RX

folic acid (Various)

THERAPEUTIC CLASS: Erythropoiesis agent

INDICATIONS: Treatment of megaloblastic anemias due to folic acid deficiency and in anemias of nutritional origin, pregnancy, infancy, or childhood.

DOSAGE: *Adults:* Usual: Up to 1mg/day. Resistant cases may require larger doses. When clinical symptoms have subsided and the blood picture has become normal, a daily maintenance level should be used; refer to PI for recommended levels. With Alcoholism, Hemolytic Anemia, Anticonvulsant Therapy, or Chronic Infection: May need to increase maintenance level. *Pediatrics:* Usual: Up to 1mg/day. Resistant cases may require larger doses. When clinical symptoms have subsided and the blood picture has become normal, a daily maintenance level should be used; refer to PI for recommended levels. With Alcoholism, Hemolytic Anemia, Anticonvulsant Therapy, or Chronic Infection: May need to increase maintenance level.

HOW SUPPLIED: Tab: 1mg* *scored

WARNINGS/PRECAUTIONS: Folic acid alone is improper therapy for pernicious anemia and other megaloblastic anemias in which vitamin B12 is deficient. Folic acid >0.1mg/day may obscure pernicious anemia in that hematologic remission may occur while neurologic manifestations remain progressive; potential danger exists in administering folic acid to patients with undiagnosed anemia.

ADVERSE REACTIONS: Allergic sensitization.

INTERACTIONS: Antagonizes anticonvulsant action of phenytoin; increased doses may be required in a patient whose epilepsy is completely controlled by phenytoin. False low serum and red cell folate levels may occur with antibiotics (eg, tetracycline), which suppress the growth of *Lactobacillus casei*.

PREGNANCY: Category A, safe in nursing.

MECHANISM OF ACTION: Erythropoiesis agent; acts on megaloblastic bone marrow to produce normoblastic marrow. Required for nucleoprotein synthesis and maintenance of normal erythropoiesis. Precursor of tetrahydrofolic acid, which is involved as a cofactor for transformylation reactions in the biosynthesis of purines and thymidylates of nucleic acids.

PHARMACOKINETICS: Absorption: Rapid (small intestine). T_{max}=1 hr. **Distribution:** Found in breast milk. **Metabolism:** Liver via reduced diphosphopyridine nucleotide and folate reductase. **Elimination:** Urine, feces.

NURSING CONSIDERATIONS

Assessment: Assess for alcoholism, hemolytic anemia, chronic infection, pernicious anemia and other megaloblastic anemias, previous intolerance to the drug, pregnancy/nursing status, and possible drug interactions.

Monitoring: Monitor for allergic sensitization, and obtain CBC.

Patient Counseling: Inform of risks and benefits of therapy.

Administration: Oral route. **Storage**: 20-25°C (68-77°F).

FORADIL RX

formoterol fumarate (Merck)

> Long-acting β₂-adrenergic agonists (LABAs) may increase the risk of asthma-related death. Contraindicated in asthma without use of a long-term asthma control medication (eg, inhaled corticosteroid). Do not use if asthma is adequately controlled on low- or medium-dose inhaled corticosteroids. LABAs may increase risk of asthma-related hospitalization in pediatric patients and adolescents; ensure adherence with both long-term asthma control medication and LABAs.

THERAPEUTIC CLASS: Beta₂-agonist

INDICATIONS: Treatment of asthma and prevention of bronchospasm only as concomitant therapy with long-term asthma control medication (eg, inhaled corticosteroid) in adults and children ≥5 yrs of age with reversible obstructive airway disease, including nocturnal asthma. For acute prevention of exercise-induced bronchospasm (EIB) in adults and children ≥5 yrs of age on PRN basis; may use as single agent in patients without persistent asthma or use with long-term asthma control medication (eg, inhaled corticosteroid) in patients with persistent asthma. Long-term bid (am and pm) administration in the maintenance treatment of bronchoconstriction in patients with chronic obstructive pulmonary disease (COPD), including chronic bronchitis and emphysema.

DOSAGE: *Adults:* Asthma/COPD: One 12mcg cap q12h using Aerolizer Inhaler. Max: 24mcg/day. EIB: One 12mcg cap at least 15 min before exercise PRN; additional doses should not be used for 12 hrs after administration. Should not be used for prevention of EIB if already receiving bid dosing for asthma.
Pediatrics: ≥5 Yrs: Asthma: One 12mcg cap q12h using Aerolizer Inhaler. Max: 24mcg/day. EIB: One 12mcg cap at least 15 min before exercise PRN; additional doses should not be used for 12 hrs after administration. Should not be used for prevention of EIB if already receiving bid dosing for asthma.

HOW SUPPLIED: Cap, Inhalation: 12mcg [12ˢ, 60ˢ]

CONTRAINDICATIONS: Treatment of asthma without concomitant use of long-term asthma control medication (eg, inhaled corticosteroid). Primary treatment of status asthmaticus or other acute episodes of asthma or COPD where intensive measures are required. History of hypersensitivity to milk proteins.

WARNINGS/PRECAUTIONS: Not indicated for the relief of acute bronchospasm. Should not be initiated with significantly worsening, acutely deteriorating, or potentially life-threatening episodes of asthma or COPD. D/C regular use of inhaled, short-acting β₂-agonists (SABAs) when beginning treatment; use only for relief of acute asthma symptoms. Not a substitute for oral/inhaled corticosteroids. Do not use more often or at doses higher than recommended or with other LABAs (eg, salmeterol xinafoate, arformoterol tartrate). D/C if paradoxical bronchospasm or clinically significant cardiovascular (CV) effects occur. Caution in patients with CV disorders (eg, coronary insufficiency, cardiac arrhythmias, HTN, aneurysm, pheochromocytoma), convulsive disorders, thyrotoxicosis, preexisting diabetes mellitus (DM), and ketoacidosis. Caution in patients who are unusually responsive to sympathomimetic amines. ECG changes, immediate hypersensitivity reactions, significant hypokalemia, and changes in blood glucose may occur. Contains lactose; may cause allergic reactions in patients with severe milk protein allergy.

ADVERSE REACTIONS: Viral infection, upper respiratory tract infection, CV events, asthma exacerbations, bronchitis, back pain, pharyngitis, chest pain.

INTERACTIONS: Adrenergic drugs may potentiate sympathetic effects; use with caution. Xanthine derivatives or systemic corticosteroids may potentiate any hypokalemic effect. ECG changes or hypokalemia that may result from non-K⁺-sparing diuretics (eg, loop/thiazide diuretics) can be acutely worsened; use with caution. MAOIs, TCAs, macrolides, and drugs known to prolong the QTc interval may potentiate effect on CV system; use with extreme caution. Drugs known to prolong the QTc interval have an increased risk of ventricular arrhythmias. Use with β-blockers may block effects and produce severe bronchospasm in asthmatic patients; if needed, consider cardioselective β-blocker with caution. Elevated risk of arrhythmias with concomitant anesthesia with halogenated hydrocarbons.

PREGNANCY: Category C, caution in nursing.

MECHANISM OF ACTION: LABA; acts as a bronchodilator, stimulates intracellular adenyl cyclase, and increases cAMP levels, causing relaxation of bronchial smooth muscle and inhibition of release of mediators of immediate hypersensitivity from cells, especially from mast cells.

PHARMACOKINETICS: Absorption: Rapid; C$_{max}$=92pg/mL, T$_{max}$=5 min. **Distribution:** Plasma protein binding (61-64%). **Metabolism:** Direct glucuronidation, O-demethylation via CYP2D6, 2C19,

2C9, 2A6. **Elimination:** With Asthma: Urine (10%, unchanged; 15-18%, conjugates). With COPD: Urine (7%, unchanged; 6-9%, conjugates). $T_{1/2}$=10 hrs.

NURSING CONSIDERATIONS

Assessment: Assess for previous hypersensitivity to the drug or milk proteins, CV disorders, convulsive disorders, thyrotoxicosis, DM, ketoacidosis, pregnancy/nursing status, and possible drug interactions. Assess use in patients unusually responsive to sympathomimetic amines. Obtain baseline serum K$^+$ and blood glucose levels. In patients with asthma, assess for status asthmaticus or presence of an acute asthma episode and assess for use of long-term asthma control medication. In patients with COPD, assess for presence of an acute COPD episode.

Monitoring: Monitor for paradoxical bronchospasm, signs of worsening asthma, CV effects, hypersensitivity reactions, aggravation of DM, and ketoacidosis. Monitor pulse rate, BP, ECG changes, and serum K$^+$ and blood glucose levels.

Patient Counseling: Inform of the risks and benefits of therapy. Instruct not to use to relieve acute asthma symptoms or exacerbations of COPD. Advise to seek medical attention if symptoms worsen, if treatment becomes less effective, or if more than usual inhalations of SABA are needed. Instruct not to exceed prescribed dose, d/c, or reduce dose without first contacting physician. Inform that treatment may lead to palpitations, chest pain, rapid HR, tremor, or nervousness. Advise to administer only via the Aerolizer device, to always use the new device that comes with each refill, and not to use the device for other medications. Instruct not to use with a spacer and never to exhale into the device. Advise to avoid exposing caps to moisture and to handle with dry hands. Advise to strictly follow storage conditions, remove cap from blister only immediately before use, and pierce caps only once. Advise to contact physician if pregnant/nursing or if patient has severe milk protein allergy.

Administration: Oral inhalation route. Do not swallow cap. Refer to PI for further administration instructions. **Storage:** Prior to Dispensing: 2-8°C (36-46°F). After Dispensing: 20-25°C (68-77°F). Protect from heat and moisture. Always store caps in blister and only remove from blister immediately before use.

FORTAMET
metformin HCl (Shionogi)

RX

> Lactic acidosis reported (rare). May occur in association with other conditions such as diabetes mellitus (DM) with significant renal insufficiency, congestive heart failure (CHF), and conditions with risk of hypoperfusion and hypoxemia. Risk Increases with the degree of renal dysfunction and age. Avoid in patients ≥80 yrs unless renal function is normal. Avoid with clinical/lab evidence of hepatic disease. Temporarily d/c prior to IV radiocontrast studies or surgical procedures. Caution against excessive alcohol intake; may potentiate effects of metformin on lactate metabolism. Withhold in the presence of any condition associated with hypoxemia, dehydration, or sepsis. Regularly monitor renal function and use minimum effective dose to decrease risk. If lactic acidosis is suspected, immediately d/c and institute general supportive measures.

THERAPEUTIC CLASS: Biguanide

INDICATIONS: Adjunct to diet and exercise to improve glycemic control in type 2 DM.

DOSAGE: *Adults:* ≥17 Yrs: Take with pm meal. Initial: 500-1000mg qd. With Insulin: Initial: 500mg qd. Titrate: May increase by 500mg/week. Max: 2500mg/day. Decrease insulin dose by 10-25% if FPG <120mg/dL. Elderly/Debilitated/Malnourished: Dose conservatively; do not titrate to max.

HOW SUPPLIED: Tab, Extended-Release: 500mg, 1000mg

CONTRAINDICATIONS: Renal disease/dysfunction (eg, SrCr ≥1.5mg/dL [males], ≥1.4mg/dL [females], or abnormal CrCl), acute or chronic metabolic acidosis, including diabetic ketoacidosis with or without coma.

WARNINGS/PRECAUTIONS: Lactic acidosis may be suspected in diabetic patients with metabolic acidosis lacking evidence of ketoacidosis (ketonuria and ketonemia). Caution with concomitant medications that may affect renal function, result in significant hemodynamic change, or interfere with the disposition of metformin. Temporarily d/c prior to surgical procedures associated with restricted oral intake. Temporarily withhold drug before, during, and 48 hrs after radiologic studies with IV iodinated contrast materials; reinstitute only when renal function is normal. D/C in hypoxic states (eg, shock, CHF, acute myocardial infarction [MI]), dehydration, and sepsis. Avoid with hepatic impairment. May decrease vitamin B12 levels. Increased risk of hypoglycemia in elderly, debilitated/malnourished, adrenal or pituitary insufficiency, or alcohol intoxication. Temporarily withhold metformin and administer insulin if loss of glycemic control occurs due to stress; reinstitute metformin after acute episode is resolved.

ADVERSE REACTIONS: Lactic acidosis, infection, diarrhea, nausea, headache, dyspepsia, rhinitis, flatulence, abdominal pain.

INTERACTIONS: Furosemide, nifedipine, cimetidine, and cationic drugs (eg, amiloride, digoxin, morphine, procainamide, quinidine, quinine, ranitidine, triamterene, trimethoprim, vancomycin) may increase metformin levels. Thiazides, other diuretics, corticosteroids, phenothiazines, thyroid products, estrogens, oral contraceptives, phenytoin, nicotinic acid, sympathomimetics, calcium channel blockers, and isoniazid may cause hyperglycemia and loss of glycemic control. May decrease furosemide levels.

PREGNANCY: Category B, not for use in pregnancy or nursing.

MECHANISM OF ACTION: Biguanide; decreases hepatic production and intestinal absorption of glucose, and improves insulin sensitivity by increasing peripheral glucose uptake and utilization.

PHARMACOKINETICS: Absorption: C_{max}=2849ng/mL, T_{max}=6 hrs, AUC=26811ng•hr/mL. **Elimination:** Urine (90%); $T_{1/2}$=6.2 hrs (plasma), 17.6 hrs (blood).

NURSING CONSIDERATIONS

Assessment: Assess for hypoxic states (eg, acute CHF, acute MI, cardiovascular collapse), septicemia, acute/chronic metabolic acidosis, adrenal/pituitary insufficiency, alcoholism, pregnancy/nursing status, and possible drug interactions. Evaluate for other medical/surgical conditions and for possible drug interactions. Assess FPG, HbA1c, renal function, LFTs, and hematologic parameters (eg, Hgb/Hct, RBC indices).

Monitoring: Monitor for lactic acidosis, hypoglycemia, prerenal azotemia, hypoxic states, hypersensitivity reactions, and other adverse reactions. Monitor FPG, HbA1c, renal function (eg, SrCr), LFTs, and hematologic parameters (eg, Hgb/Hct, RBC indices).

Patient Counseling: Inform of the potential risks, benefits, and alternative modes of therapy. Inform about the importance of adherence to dietary instructions, regular exercise programs, and regular testing of blood glucose, HbA1c, renal function, and hematologic parameters. Inform of the risk of lactic acidosis with therapy and to contact physician if unexplained hyperventilation, myalgia, malaise, unusual somnolence, or other nonspecific symptoms occur. Counsel against excessive alcohol intake. Explain risks, symptoms, and conditions that predispose to the development of hypoglycemia when initiating combination therapy. Instruct that drug must be taken with food, swallowed whole with a full glass of water and should not be chewed, cut, or crushed, and that inactive ingredients may be eliminated in the feces as a soft mass.

Administration: Oral route. **Storage:** 20-25°C (68-77°F); excursions permitted to 15-30°C (59-86°F). Keep tightly closed. Protect from light and moisture. Avoid excessive heat and humidity.

FORTAZ   RX
ceftazidime (GlaxoSmithKline)

THERAPEUTIC CLASS: Cephalosporin (3rd generation)

INDICATIONS: Treatment of lower respiratory tract (eg, pneumonia), skin and skin structure (SSSI), bone/joint, gynecologic, CNS (eg, meningitis), intra-abdominal (eg, peritonitis), and urinary tract infections (UTIs); and bacterial septicemia caused by susceptible strains of microorganisms. Treatment of sepsis.

DOSAGE: *Adults:* Usual: 1g IM/IV q8-12h. Uncomplicated UTI: 250mg IM/IV q12h. Complicated UTI: 500mg IM/IV q8-12h. Bone and Joint infection: 2g IV q12h. Uncomplicated Pneumonia/Mild SSSI: 500mg-1g IM/IV q8h. Serious Gynecological and Intra-Abdominal/Meningitis/Severe Life-Threatening Infection: 2g IV q8h. Lung Infection Caused by *Pseudomonas* spp. in Cystic Fibrosis (Normal Renal Function): 30-50mg/kg IV q8h. Max: 6g/day. Renal Impairment: Refer to PI. *Pediatrics:* 1 Month-12 Yrs: 30-50mg/kg IV q8h. Max: 6g/day. Use higher doses for immunocompromised patients with cystic fibrosis or meningitis. Neonates (0-4 Weeks): 30mg/kg IV q12h. Renal Impairment: Refer to PI.

HOW SUPPLIED: Inj: 500mg, 1g, 2g; 1g, 2g [ADD-Vantage]; 1g/50mL, 2g/50mL [Galaxy]. Also available as a Pharmacy Bulk Package.

WARNINGS/PRECAUTIONS: Cross hypersensitivity among β-lactam antibiotics reported; caution with penicillin (PCN) sensitivity. D/C if allergic reaction occurs. *Clostridium difficile*-associated diarrhea (CDAD) reported. May result in bacterial resistance with prolonged use or use in the absence of a proven/suspected bacterial infection or a prophylactic indication; take appropriate measures if superinfection develops. Elevated levels with renal insufficiency may lead to seizures, encephalopathy, coma, asterixis, myoclonia, and neuromuscular excitability. Associated with fall in prothrombin activity; caution with renal/hepatic impairment, poor nutritional state, and protracted course of antimicrobial therapy. Caution with colitis, history of GI disease, and elderly. Distal necrosis may occur after inadvertent intra-arterial administration. Lab test interactions may occur.

ADVERSE REACTIONS: Allergic reactions, increased ALT/AST/GGT/LDH, eosinophilia, local/GI reactions.

INTERACTIONS: Nephrotoxicity reported with aminoglycosides or potent diuretics (eg, furosemide). Avoid with chloramphenicol. May reduce efficacy of combined oral estrogen/progesterone contraceptives.

PREGNANCY: Category B, caution in nursing.

MECHANISM OF ACTION: Cephalosporin (3rd generation); bactericidal, inhibits enzymes responsible for cell-wall synthesis.

PHARMACOKINETICS: Absorption: (IV/IM) Administration of variable doses resulted in different parameters. **Distribution:** Plasma protein binding (<10%); found in breast milk. **Elimination:** Urine (80-90%, unchanged); $T_{1/2}$=1.9 hrs (IV), 2 hrs (IM).

NURSING CONSIDERATIONS

Assessment: Assess for history of hypersensitivity to cephalosporins/PCNs, history of GI disease, colitis, renal/hepatic impairment, nursing status, and for possible drug interactions.

Monitoring: Monitor for signs and symptoms of hypersensitivity reactions, CDAD, LDH, LFTs, renal function, PT, hemolytic anemia, superinfection. Monitor for seizures, encephalopathy, coma, asterixis, neuromuscular excitability, and myoclonia with renal impairment. Perform periodic susceptibility testing.

Patient Counseling: Inform that therapy only treats bacterial, not viral (eg, common cold), infections. Instruct to take exactly ud; skipping doses or not completing full course may decrease effectiveness and increase resistance. Advise that patient may experience diarrhea; notify physician if watery/bloody stools (with/without stomach cramps and fever) occur.

Administration: IM/IV route. Refer to PI for administration, preparation of sol, use of frozen plastic container, compatibility and stability, and instructions for constitution of ADD-Vantage vials. **Storage:** 15-30°C (59-86°F), in dry state. Protect from light. Frozen as premixed sol should not be stored above -20°C.

FORTEO   RX
teriparatide, rdna origin (Lilly)

> Prescribe only when benefits outweigh risks; do not prescribe for patients who are at increased baseline risk for osteosarcoma (including those with Paget's disease of bone or unexplained alkaline phosphatase elevations, pediatric and young adult patients with open epiphyses, or prior external beam or implant radiation therapy involving the skeleton).

THERAPEUTIC CLASS: Recombinant human parathyroid hormone

INDICATIONS: Treatment of postmenopausal women with osteoporosis at high risk for fracture. To increase bone mass in men with primary or hypogonadal osteoporosis at high risk for fracture. Treatment of men and women with glucocorticoid-induced osteoporosis at high risk for fracture.

DOSAGE: *Adults:* 20mcg qd SQ into the thigh or abdominal wall.

HOW SUPPLIED: Inj: 250mcg/mL [2.4mL]

WARNINGS/PRECAUTIONS: Use for >2 yrs during a patient's lifetime is not recommended. Do not give in patients with bone metastases or history of skeletal malignancies, metabolic bone diseases other than osteoporosis, preexisting hypercalcemia, or underlying hypercalcemic disorder (eg, primary hyperparathyroidism). Transiently increases serum Ca^{2+}. Consider measurement of urinary Ca^{2+} excretion if active urolithiasis or preexisting hypercalciuria are suspected; caution in patients with active or recent urolithiasis. Transient episodes of symptomatic orthostatic hypotension reported with administration of initial doses; administer initially under circumstances where the patient can sit or lie down if symptoms of orthostatic hypotension occur.

ADVERSE REACTIONS: Pain, arthralgia, rhinitis, asthenia, N/V, dizziness, headache, HTN, increased cough, pharyngitis, constipation, dyspepsia, diarrhea, rash, insomnia.

INTERACTIONS: Hypercalcemia may predispose to digitalis toxicity; caution if taking digoxin concomitantly.

PREGNANCY: Category C, not for use in nursing.

MECHANISM OF ACTION: Recombinant human parathyroid hormone; binds to specific high-affinity cell-surface receptors. Stimulates new bone formation on trabecular and cortical (periosteal and/or endosteal) bone surfaces by preferential stimulation of osteoblastic activity over osteoclastic activity. Produces an increase in skeletal mass, markers of bone formation and resorption, and bone strength.

PHARMACOKINETICS: Absorption: Rapid. Absolute bioavailability (95%); T_{max}=30 min. **Distribution:** (IV) V_d=0.12L/kg. **Metabolism:** Liver (nonspecific enzymatic mechanisms). **Elimination:** Kidneys; $T_{1/2}$=1 hr.

NURSING CONSIDERATIONS

Assessment: Assess for increased baseline risk for osteosarcoma, bone metastases or history of skeletal malignancies, metabolic bone disease other than osteoporosis, hypercalcemia, hypercalcemic disorder, hypercalciuria, active or recent urolithiasis, hypersensitivity to drug, pregnancy/nursing status, and possible drug interactions. Consider measurement of urinary Ca^{2+} excretion if active urolithiasis or preexisting hypercalciuria are suspected.

Monitoring: Monitor for signs/symptoms of osteosarcoma, orthostatic hypotension, and other adverse reactions.

Patient Counseling: Inform of potential risk of osteosarcoma and encourage to enroll in the voluntary Forteo Patient Registry. Instruct to sit or lie down if lightheadedness or palpitations following inj develop; if symptoms persist or worsen, advise to consult physician before continuing treatment. Instruct to contact physician if persistent symptoms of hypercalcemia (eg, N/V, constipation, lethargy, muscle weakness) develop. Counsel on roles of supplemental Ca²⁺ and/or vitamin D, weight-bearing exercise, and modification of certain behavioral factors (eg, smoking, alcohol consumption). Instruct on proper use of delivery device (pen) and proper disposal of needles; advise not to share pen with other patients and not to transfer contents to a syringe.

Administration: SQ route. Inject into the thigh or abdominal wall. Administer initially under circumstances where the patient can sit or lie down if symptoms of orthostatic hypotension occur. **Storage:** 2-8°C (36-46°F). Recap pen when not in use. Minimize time out of the refrigerator during the use period; may deliver dose immediately following removal from the refrigerator. Do not freeze; do not use if it has been frozen. Discard after the 28-day use period.

FORTESTA
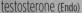
CIII

testosterone (Endo)

> Virilization reported in children secondarily exposed to testosterone gel. Children should avoid contact with unwashed or unclothed application sites in men using testosterone gel. Advise patients to strictly adhere to recommended instructions for use.

THERAPEUTIC CLASS: Androgen

INDICATIONS: Replacement therapy in males for conditions associated with a deficiency or absence of endogenous testosterone (congenital or acquired primary hypogonadism or hypogonadotropic hypogonadism).

DOSAGE: *Adults:* Initial: Apply 40mg qam to intact skin of the thighs. Titrate: May adjust between 10-70mg based on serum testosterone concentration from a single blood draw 2 hrs after application at 14 days, and 35 days after starting treatment or following dose adjustment. Max: 70mg. Total Serum Testosterone Concentration 2 Hrs Post Application: ≥2500ng/dL: Decrease daily dose by 20mg. ≥1250-<2500ng/dL: Decrease daily dose by 10mg. ≥500-<1250ng/dL: Continue on current dose. <500ng/dL: Increase daily dose by 10mg.

HOW SUPPLIED: Gel: 10mg/actuation [60g]

CONTRAINDICATIONS: Breast carcinoma or known/suspected prostate carcinoma in men; women who are or may become pregnant, or are breastfeeding.

WARNINGS/PRECAUTIONS: Application site and dose are not interchangeable with other topical testosterone products. Patients with BPH and geriatric patients may be at increased risk of worsening of signs/symptoms of BPH. May increase risk for prostate cancer. Risk of virilization in women due to secondary exposure; d/c until cause is identified. Not indicated for use in women. Increases in Hct/RBC mass may increase risk for thromboembolic events; may require dose reduction or discontinuation of therapy until Hct decreases to an acceptable concentration. Suppression of spermatogenesis may occur with large doses. Prolonged use of high doses may cause serious hepatic effects (eg, peliosis hepatis, hepatic neoplasms, cholestatic hepatitis, jaundice). Risk of edema with or without congestive heart failure (CHF) in patients with preexisting cardiac, renal, or hepatic disease. Gynecomastia may develop and persist. May potentiate sleep apnea, especially with risk factors such as obesity or chronic lung diseases. Changes in serum lipid profile may require dose adjustment or discontinuation of therapy. Caution in cancer patients at risk of hypercalcemia and associated hypercalciuria. May decrease levels of thyroxin-binding globulins, resulting in decreased total T4 serum levels and increased resin uptake of T3 and T4. Flammable; avoid fire, flame, or smoking until the gel has dried.

ADVERSE REACTIONS: Application-site reactions.

INTERACTIONS: Changes in insulin sensitivity or glycemic control may occur; may decrease blood glucose and, therefore, decrease insulin requirements in diabetic patients. Adrenocorticotropic hormone or corticosteroids may increase fluid retention; caution in patients with cardiac, renal, or hepatic disease. Changes in anticoagulant activity may occur; frequently monitor INR and PT in patients taking anticoagulants, especially at initiation and termination of androgen therapy.

PREGNANCY: Category X, contraindicated in nursing.

MECHANISM OF ACTION: Androgen; responsible for normal growth and development of male sex organs and for maintenance of secondary sex characteristics.

PHARMACOKINETICS: Distribution: Plasma protein binding (98%; 40% sex hormone-binding globulin). **Metabolism:** Estradiol and dihydrotestosterone (major active metabolites). **Elimination:** (IM) Urine (90% glucuronic and sulfuric acid conjugates), feces (6% unconjugated); $T_{1/2}$=10-100 min.

NURSING CONSIDERATIONS

Assessment: Assess for BPH, prostate cancer, cardiac/renal/hepatic disease, obesity, chronic lung disease, conditions where treatment is contraindicated or cautioned, and for possible drug interactions. Check Hct prior to therapy.

Monitoring: Monitor for prostate carcinoma, edema with or without CHF, gynecomastia, worsening of signs/symptoms of BPH, sleep apnea, and other adverse reactions. Perform periodic monitoring of Hgb, LFTs, prostate-specific antigen, and serum lipid profile. Obtain serum testosterone levels 14 days and 35 days after initiation of therapy or following dose adjustment. In cancer patients at risk for hypercalcemia, regularly monitor serum Ca^{2+} levels. Reevaluate Hct 3-6 months after start of therapy, then annually.

Patient Counseling: Inform that men with known or suspected prostate/breast cancer should not use androgen therapy. Advise to report signs/symptoms of secondary exposure in children (eg, penis/clitoris enlargement, premature development of pubic hair, increased erections) and in women (eg, changes in hair distribution, increase in acne) to the physician. Inform that children and women should avoid contact with unwashed or unclothed application sites of men using testosterone gel. Instruct to apply ud; instruct to cover application site with clothing after gel dries, and wash application site with soap and water prior to direct skin-to-skin contact with others. Inform about possible adverse reactions. Inform that drug is flammable; instruct to avoid fire, flame, or smoking until the gel has dried. Advise not to share the medication with anyone. Instruct to adhere to all the recommended monitoring, to wait 2 hrs before swimming or washing following application, and to report changes in their state of health.

Administration: Topical route. Prime canister pump in upright position, slowly and fully depress actuator 8 times. Refer to PI for further administration instructions. **Storage:** 20-25°C (68-77°F); excursions permitted to 15-30°C (59-86°F). Do not freeze. Discard used canisters in household trash in a manner that prevents accidental application or ingestion by children or pets.

FORTICAL   RX
calcitonin-salmon (rdna origin) (Upsher-Smith)

THERAPEUTIC CLASS: Hormonal bone resorption inhibitor

INDICATIONS: Treatment of postmenopausal osteoporosis in women >5 yrs postmenopause with low bone mass relative to healthy postmenopausal women; recommended in conjunction with an adequate Ca^{2+} and vitamin D intake.

DOSAGE: *Adults:* 200 IU qd intranasally. Alternate nostrils daily.

HOW SUPPLIED: Nasal Spray: 200 IU/activation

WARNINGS/PRECAUTIONS: Possibility of systemic allergic reactions (eg, anaphylaxis, anaphylactic shock). Allergic reactions should be differentiated from generalized flushing and hypotension. Consider skin testing if sensitivity suspected. Development of mucosal alterations or transient nasal conditions reported; perform periodic nasal exams. D/C if severe ulceration of nasal mucosa occurs (indicated by ulcers >1.5mm diameter or penetrating below mucosa, or associated with heavy bleeding). Incidence of rhinitis, irritation, erythema, and excoriation higher in geriatric patients.

ADVERSE REACTIONS: Rhinitis, nasal symptoms, back pain, arthralgia, epistaxis, headache, influenza-like symptoms, fatigue, erythematous rash, arthrosis, myalgia, sinusitis, bronchospasm, HTN, constipation.

INTERACTIONS: May reduce lithium levels; dose of lithium may need to be adjusted. Prior diphosphonate use appears to reduce the anti-resorptive response to calcitonin-salmon nasal spray in patients with Paget's disease.

PREGNANCY: Category C, not for use in nursing.

MECHANISM OF ACTION: Hormonal bone resorption inhibitor; actions on bone not fully established. Calcitonin receptors have been found in osteoclasts and osteoblasts. Initially causes a marked transient inhibition of the ongoing bone resorptive process. Prolonged use causes a smaller decrease in the rate of bone resorption. Associated with inhibition of osteoclast function and increased osteoblastic activity.

PHARMACOKINETICS: Absorption: T_{max}=13 min; Bioavailability (3%). **Elimination:** $T_{1/2}$=18 min.

NURSING CONSIDERATIONS

Assessment: Assess for previous allergy to calcitonin-salmon; perform skin testing if sensitivity suspected. Assess for pregnancy/nursing status and for possible drug interactions. Perform nasal and bone mineral density examination prior to treatment. Assess patient's intake of Ca^{2+} and vitamin D and recommend adequate intake (at least 1000mg/day elemental Ca^{2+} and 400 IU/day vitamin D) to retard progressive loss of bone mass.

Monitoring: Monitor for signs/symptoms of allergic reaction (eg, anaphylactic shock, anaphylaxis), nasal mucosal alterations, rhinitis, epistaxis, and sinusitis. Perform periodic nasal exams of nasal mucosa, turbinates, septum, and mucosal blood vessels. Perform periodic monitoring of urine sediment. Measure lumbar vertebral bone mass periodically to monitor for efficacy.

Patient Counseling: Counsel to notify physician of significant nasal irritation. Advise to seek emergency help if serious allergic reaction occurs (eg, troubled breathing, swelling of face, throat or tongue, rapid heartbeat, chest pain, feeling faint or dizzy). Advise to store new, unassembled medication in refrigerator away from light, and not to freeze. Instruct that before priming pump and using new medication, allow to reach room temperature. Inform that after opening, store at room temperature, in upright position; discard unused medication 30 days after 1st use. Recommend adequate intake of Ca^{2+} and vitamin D.

Administration: Intranasal route. To prime pump, hold bottle upright and depress the 2 white side arms of pump toward the bottle at least 5X until a full spray is produced. To administer, carefully place the nozzle into the nostril with the head in upright position and pump firmly depressed toward the bottle. Do not prime pump before each daily use. **Storage:** Unopened: 2-8°C (36-46°F). Protect from freezing. Opened: 20-25°C (68-77°F); excursions permitted to 15-30°C (59-86°F). Store in upright position. Discard 30 days after 1st use.

FOSAMAX PLUS D   RX
alendronate sodium - cholecalciferol (Merck)

THERAPEUTIC CLASS: Bisphosphonate/vitamin D analog

INDICATIONS: Treatment of osteoporosis in postmenopausal women. Treatment to increase bone mass in men with osteoporosis.

DOSAGE: *Adults:* 1 tab (70mg-2800 IU or 70mg-5600 IU) once weekly. Usual: 70mg-5600 IU once weekly. Periodically reevaluate the need for continued therapy. Refer to PI for recommendations for Ca^{2+} and vitamin D supplementation.

HOW SUPPLIED: Tab: (Alendronate-Cholecalciferol) 70mg-2800 IU, 70mg-5600 IU

CONTRAINDICATIONS: Esophageal abnormalities that delay esophageal emptying (eg, stricture or achalasia), inability to stand or sit upright for at least 30 min, hypocalcemia.

WARNINGS/PRECAUTIONS: Do not use alone to treat vitamin D deficiency. Consider discontinuation after 3-5 yrs of use in patients at low-risk for fracture; periodically reevaluate risk for fracture in patients who d/c therapy. Not recommended with CrCl <35mL/min. May cause local irritation of the upper GI mucosa; caution with active upper GI problems (eg, Barrett's esophagus, dysphagia, other esophageal diseases, gastritis, duodenitis, ulcers). Esophageal reactions (eg, esophagitis, esophageal ulcers/erosions) reported; d/c if dysphagia, odynophagia, retrosternal pain, or new/worsening heartburn develops. Use therapy under appropriate supervision in patients who cannot comply with dosing instructions due to mental disability. Gastric and duodenal ulcers reported. Treat hypocalcemia or other disorders affecting mineral metabolism (eg, vitamin D deficiency) prior to therapy; monitor serum Ca^{2+} and for symptoms of hypocalcemia during therapy. Asymptomatic decreases in serum Ca^{2+} and phosphate may occur. Severe and occasionally incapacitating bone, joint, and/or muscle pain reported; d/c if severe symptoms develop. Osteonecrosis of the jaw (ONJ) reported; risk may increase with duration of exposure to drug. If invasive dental procedures are required, discontinuation of treatment may reduce risk for ONJ. Consider discontinuation if ONJ develops. Atypical, low-energy, or low trauma fractures of the femoral shaft reported; evaluate any patient with a history of bisphosphonate exposure who presents with thigh/groin pain to rule out incomplete femur fracture, and consider interruption of therapy. Vitamin D3 supplementation may worsen hypercalcemia and/or hypercalciuria in patients with diseases associated with unregulated overproduction of 1,25-dihydroxyvitamin D (eg, leukemia, lymphoma, sarcoidosis); monitor urine and serum Ca^{2+}.

ADVERSE REACTIONS: Abdominal pain, musculoskeletal pain, nausea, dyspepsia, constipation, diarrhea.

INTERACTIONS: Ca^{2+} supplements, antacids, or oral medications containing multivalent cations will interfere with absorption of alendronate; wait at least 1/2 hr after dosing before taking any other oral medications. NSAID use is associated with GI irritation; use with caution. Alendronate: Increased incidence of upper GI adverse events in patients receiving concomitant therapy with daily doses of alendronate >10mg and aspirin-containing products. Cholecalciferol: Olestra, mineral oils, orlistat, and bile acid sequestrants (eg, cholestyramine, colestipol) may impair absorption; consider additional supplementation. Anticonvulsants, cimetidine, and thiazides may increase catabolism; consider additional supplementation.

PREGNANCY: Category C, caution in nursing.

MECHANISM OF ACTION: Alendronate: Bisphosphonate; binds to hydroxyapatite found in bone and specifically inhibits the osteoclast-mediated bone-resorption. Cholecalciferol: Vitamin D analog; increases intestinal absorption of both Ca^{2+} and phosphate. Regulates serum Ca^{2+}, renal Ca^{2+} and phosphate excretion, bone formation and bone resorption.

PHARMACOKINETICS: Absorption: Alendronate: Absolute bioavailability (0.64% in women), (0.59% in men). Cholecalciferol: (2800 IU) C_{max}=4ng/mL, T_{max}=10.6 hrs, AUC=120.7ng•hr/mL. Refer to PI. **Distribution:** Alendronate: V_d=at least 28L; plasma protein binding (78%). Cholecalciferol: Found in breast milk. **Metabolism:** Cholecalciferol: Liver (rapid) via hydroxylation to 25-hydroxyvitamin D3; subsequently metabolized in the kidney to 1,25-dihydroxyvitamin D3 (active metabolite). **Elimination:** Alendronate: (IV) Urine (50%); $T_{1/2}$>10 yrs. Cholecalciferol: (IV) Urine (2.4%), feces (4.9%); (PO) $T_{1/2}$=14 hrs.

NURSING CONSIDERATIONS

Assessment: Assess for esophageal abnormalities, ability to stand or sit upright for at least 30 min, hypocalcemia, risk for ONJ, active upper GI problems, mental disability, renal impairment, drug hypersensitivity, any other conditions where treatment is contraindicated or cautioned, pregnancy/nursing status, and possible drug interactions.

Monitoring: Monitor for signs/symptoms of ONJ, atypical fractures, esophageal reactions, musculoskeletal pain, hypocalcemia, and other adverse events. Monitor urine and serum Ca^{2+} in patients with diseases associated with unregulated overproduction of 1,25-dihydroxyvitamin D. Periodically reevaluate the need for continued therapy.

Patient Counseling: Instruct to take supplemental Ca^{2+} and vitamin D if dietary intake is inadequate. Counsel to consider weight-bearing exercise along with the modification of certain behavioral factors (eg, cigarette smoking, excessive alcohol consumption), if these factors exist. Instruct to take upon arising for the day and at least 1/2 hr before the 1st food, beverage, or other medication of the day with plain water only; advise to swallow tab with 6-8 oz. of water. Advise to avoid lying down for at least 30 min after taking the drug and until after 1st food of the day. Instruct to follow all dosing instructions and inform that failure to follow them may increase risk of esophageal problems. Advise to d/c and consult physician if symptoms of esophageal disease develop. Instruct that if a once-weekly dose is missed, to take 1 dose on the am after they remember and to return to taking 1 dose once a week, as originally scheduled on their chosen day; instruct not to take 2 doses on the same day.

Administration: Oral route. Take upon arising for the day. Take at least 1/2 hr before the 1st food, beverage, or medication of the day with plain water only. Do not chew or suck on the tab. **Storage:** 20-25°C (68-77°F); excursions permitted to 15-30°C (59-86°F). Protect from moisture and light.

FOSINOPRIL   RX
fosinopril sodium (Various)

> May cause injury and even death to the developing fetus during the 2nd and 3rd trimesters of pregnancy. D/C when pregnancy is detected.

THERAPEUTIC CLASS: ACE inhibitor

INDICATIONS: Treatment of HTN, alone or in combination with thiazide diuretics. Management of heart failure (HF) as adjunct therapy when added to conventional therapy including diuretics with or without digitalis.

DOSAGE: *Adults:* HTN: Not Receiving Diuretics: Initial: 10mg qd. Titrate: May adjust dosage based on BP response. Usual: 20-40mg qd. Some patients appear to have a further response to 80mg. Consider dividing daily dose if trough response is inadequate. Diuretic may be added if BP is not adequately controlled with therapy alone. Currently Treated with Diuretics: D/C diuretic 2-3 days prior to initiating therapy, if possible. May resume diuretic therapy if BP is not controlled with therapy alone. Initial: 10mg qd with careful monitoring until BP is stabilized. HF: Initial: 10mg qd. Monitor for hypotension or orthostasis for at least 2 hrs following administration, and if present, until BP stabilizes. HF with Moderate to Severe Renal Failure/Vigorous Diuresis: Initial: 5mg. Titrate: Increase over several weeks as tolerated. Usual: 20-40mg qd. Max: 40mg qd. Elderly: Start at lower end of dosing range.
Pediatrics: >50kg: HTN: 5-10mg qd.

HOW SUPPLIED: Tab: 10mg*, 20mg, 40mg *scored

CONTRAINDICATIONS: History of ACE inhibitor-associated angioedema.

WARNINGS/PRECAUTIONS: Head and neck angioedema reported; d/c and administer appropriate therapy if laryngeal stridor or angioedema of the face, lips, tongue, mucous membranes, glottis, or extremities occurs. More reports of angioedema in blacks than nonblacks. Intestinal angioedema reported; monitor for abdominal pain. Anaphylactoid reactions reported during desensitization with hymenoptera venom, dialysis with high-flux membranes, and LDL apheresis with dextran sulfate absorption. Symptomatic hypotension may occur, most likely in patients with volume and/or salt depletion; correct depletion prior to therapy. Excessive hypotension associated with oliguria, azotemia, and rarely acute renal failure and death may occur in patients with HF, with or without associated renal insufficiency; monitor closely during the first 2 weeks of treatment and whenever dose of therapy or diuretic is increased. May cause agranulocytosis and bone marrow depression; consider monitoring of WBC in patients with collagen-vascular disease, especially with renal impairment. Rarely, associated with syndrome that starts with cholestatic jaundice and progresses to fulminant hepatic necrosis and sometimes death; d/c if jaundice or marked elevation of hepatic enzymes occur. May cause renal function changes. May increase BUN and SrCr levels with renal artery stenosis or with no preexisting renal vascular disease; may need to reduce dose of therapy and/or d/c diuretic. Hyperkalemia reported; risk factors include diabetes mellitus (DM) and renal insufficiency. Hypotension may occur with surgery or during anesthesia. Persistent nonproductive cough reported. Caution in elderly.

ADVERSE REACTIONS: Dizziness, cough, hypotension, musculoskeletal pain.

INTERACTIONS: May increase lithium levels and symptoms of lithium toxicity; frequently monitor serum lithium levels. Hypotension risk with diuretics. Increased risk of hyperkalemia with K^+-sparing diuretics (eg, spironolactone, amiloride, triamterene), K^+-containing salt substitutes, or K^+ supplements; use with caution. Antacids may impair absorption; separate doses by 2 hrs. Nitritoid reactions reported rarely with injectable gold (sodium aurothiomalate).

PREGNANCY: Category C (1st trimester) and D (2nd and 3rd trimesters), not for use in nursing.

MECHANISM OF ACTION: ACE inhibitor; decreases plasma angiotensin II, which leads to decreased vasopressor activity and decreased aldosterone secretion.

PHARMACOKINETICS: Absorption: Slow. T_{max}=3 hrs (fosinoprilat). **Distribution:** (Fosinoprilat) Plasma protein binding (99.4%); found in breast milk. **Metabolism:** Hepatic; glucuronidation; fosinoprilat (active metabolite). **Elimination:** Urine (50% of the absorbed dose), feces. (Fosinoprilat) $T_{1/2}$=11.5 hrs (HTN), 14 hrs (HF).

NURSING CONSIDERATIONS

Assessment: Assess for history of angioedema, hypersensitivity to drug, volume/salt depletion, collagen vascular disease, DM, renal artery stenosis, HF, renal impairment, pregnancy/nursing status, and possible drug interactions.

Monitoring: Monitor for signs/symptoms of hypotension, anaphylactoid or hypersensitivity reactions, head/neck/intestinal angioedema, agranulocytosis, neutropenia, bone marrow depression, hyperkalemia, and other adverse reactions. Monitor BP and renal/hepatic function. Consider monitoring WBCs in patients with collagen vascular disease, especially if with renal impairment.

Patient Counseling: Instruct to d/c therapy and immediately report signs/symptoms of angioedema (eg, swelling of the face, eyes, lips, tongue, or extremities; difficulty swallowing/breathing). Caution about lightheadedness, especially during the 1st few days of therapy; advise to d/c therapy and consult physician if syncope occurs. Caution that inadequate fluid intake or excessive perspiration, diarrhea, or vomiting may lead to an excessive fall in BP resulting in lightheadedness or syncope. Instruct to avoid using K^+ supplements or salt substitutes-containing K^+ without consulting physician. Advise to report any symptoms of infection (eg, sore throat, fever). Inform of pregnancy risks during the 2nd or 3rd trimesters and instruct to report to physician as soon as possible if pregnant.

Administration: Oral route. **Storage:** 20-25°C (68-77°F). Protect from moisture.

FOSINOPRIL/HCTZ   RX
fosinopril sodium - hydrochlorothiazide (Various)

> D/C when pregnancy is detected. Drugs that act directly on the renin-angiotensin system (RAS) can cause injury/death to developing fetus.

THERAPEUTIC CLASS: ACE inhibitor/thiazide diuretic

INDICATIONS: Treatment of HTN.

DOSAGE: *Adults:* Not Controlled with Fosinopril/HCTZ Monotherapy: 10mg-12.5mg tab or 20mg-12.5mg tab qd. Titrate: Dosage must be guided by clinical response. Elderly: Start at lower end of dosing range.

HOW SUPPLIED: Tab: (Fosinopril-HCTZ) 10mg-12.5mg, 20mg-12.5mg* *scored

CONTRAINDICATIONS: Anuria and hypersensitivity to other sulfonamide-derived drugs.

WARNINGS/PRECAUTIONS: Not indicated for initial therapy. Caution in elderly and with severe renal disease. Avoid if CrCl <30mL/min. Caution with impaired hepatic function or progressive liver disease; may precipitate hepatic coma. Fosinopril: Angioedema reported; d/c and administer appropriate therapy if laryngeal stridor or angioedema of the face, tongue, or glottis occurs. Higher rate of angioedema in blacks than nonblacks. Intestinal angioedema reported; monitor for abdominal pain. Anaphylactoid reactions reported during desensitization with hymenoptera venom, dialysis with high-flux membranes, and LDL apheresis with dextran sulfate absorption. Symptomatic hypotension may occur, most likely in patients with volume and/or salt depletion; correct volume and/or salt depletion prior to therapy. Excessive hypotension associated with oliguria, azotemia, and rarely acute renal failure and/or death may occur in patients with conges-tive heart failure (CHF); monitor closely during the first 2 weeks of treatment and when dose is increased. May cause changes in renal function. May increase BUN and SrCr levels with renal artery stenosis and with no preexisting renal vascular disease; monitor renal function during 1st few weeks of therapy in patients with renal artery stenosis. May cause agranulocytosis and bone marrow depression; consider monitoring of WBCs in patients with collagen vascular disease and renal disease. Rarely, associated with syndrome that starts with cholestatic jaundice and progresses to fulminant necrosis and sometimes death; d/c if jaundice or marked hepatic enzyme elevations occur. Hyperkalemia and persistent nonproductive cough reported. Hypotension may occur with surgery or during anesthesia. HCTZ: May precipitate azotemia with severe renal dis-ease. May exacerbate or activate systemic lupus erythematosus (SLE). Dilutional hyponatremia may occur in edematous patients; institute appropriate therapy of water restriction rather than salt administration, except for life-threatening hyponatremia. May increase cholesterol, TGs, uric acid levels, and decrease glucose tolerance. Hyponatremia, hypokalemia, and hypochloremic alkalosis reported. Hypokalemia may sensitize or exaggerate the response of the heart to toxic effects of digitalis. Pathological changes in the parathyroid glands, with hypercalcemia and hy-pophosphatemia observed with prolonged therapy. May enhance effects in postsympathectomy patients. Neutropenia/agranulocytosis reported. Lab test interactions may occur.

ADVERSE REACTIONS: Headache, cough, fatigue, dizziness.

INTERACTIONS: Dual blockade of the RAS is associated with increased risks of hypotension, hyperkalemia, and changes in renal function (including acute renal failure); closely monitor BP, renal function, and electrolytes with concomitant agents that also affect the RAS. Avoid concomitant use of aliskiren in patients with diabetes and with renal impairment (GFR <60mL/min). Increased risk of hyperkalemia with K^+-sparing diuretics, K^+ supplements, or K^+-containing salt substitutes; use with caution and monitor serum K+ frequently. Caution with other antihy-pertensives. May alter insulin requirements in diabetic patients. May increase lithium levels and risk of toxicity; use with caution and monitor serum lithium levels frequently. Nitritoid reactions reported rarely with injectable gold (eg, sodium aurothiomalate). Fosinopril: Antacids (aluminum hydroxide, magnesium hydroxide, simethicone) may impair absorption; separate doses by 2 hrs. HCTZ: May potentiate action of other antihypertensives, especially ganglionic or peripheral adrenergic-blocking drugs. May decrease effectiveness of methenamine. May increase respon-siveness to tubocurarine. May decrease arterial responsiveness to norepinephrine. NSAIDs may decrease diuretic, natriuretic, and antihypertensive effects. Cholestyramine or colestipol resins reduce absorption. Increased risk of hypokalemia with corticosteroids and adrenocorticotropic hormone.

PREGNANCY: Category D, not for use in nursing.

MECHANISM OF ACTION: Fosinopril: ACE inhibitor; decreases plasma angiotensin II, which leads to decreased vasopressor activity and decreased aldosterone secretion. HCTZ: Thiazide diuretic; affects renal tubular mechanism of electrolyte reabsorption directly increasing excretion of Na^+ and Cl^- and indirectly reducing plasma volume.

PHARMACOKINETICS: Absorption: Fosinoprilat: T_{max}=3 hrs ; HCTZ: T_{max}=1-2.5 hrs . **Distribution:** Found in breast milk. Fosinoprilat: Plasma protein binding (95%). HCTZ: V_d=3.6-7.8L/kg; plasma protein binding (67.9%), crosses placenta. **Metabolism:** Fosinopril: Hepatic, glucuronidation; fosinoprilat (active metabolite). **Elimination:** Fosinoprilat: Urine, feces, $T_{1/2}$=11.5 hrs. HCTZ: Renal; $T_{1/2}$=5-15 hrs.

NURSING CONSIDERATIONS

Assessment: Assess for anuria, history of allergy or bronchial asthma, hypersensitivity to drug or to sulfonamides, volume/salt depletion, CHF, SLE, renal/hepatic function, collagen vascular disease, risk factors for hyperkalemia, pregnancy/nursing status, and possible drug interactions.

Monitoring: Monitor for signs/symptoms of angioedema, agranulocytosis, anaphylactoid/hyper-sensitivity reactions, hypotension, exacerbation/activation of SLE, and other adverse reactions. Monitor BP, serum electrolytes, serum uric acid levels, hepatic/renal function, cholesterol/TG levels, and glucose tolerance. Monitor WBCs in patients with collagen vascular disease and renal impairment.

Patient Counseling: Inform females of childbearing age of the consequences of exposure during pregnancy and of the treatment options for women planning to become pregnant; report preg-nancy to physician as soon as possible. Instruct to d/c therapy and immediately report signs/symptoms of angioedema (eg, swelling of face, eyes, lips, tongue, difficulty breathing). Caution that lightheadedness can occur, especially during the 1st days of therapy and advise to report to physician; instruct to d/c therapy and consult physician if syncope occurs. Caution that inad-equate fluid intake, excessive perspiration, diarrhea, or vomiting can lead to excessive fall in BP, resulting in lightheadedness or syncope. Instruct not to use salt substitutes containing K^+ or K^+ supplements without consulting physician. Instruct to promptly report any indication of infection (eg, sore throat, fever).

Administration: Oral route. **Storage:** 20-25°C (68-77°F). Protect from moisture.

FRAGMIN   RX
dalteparin sodium (Eisai)

Epidural or spinal hematomas may occur in patients anticoagulated with low molecular weight heparins or heparinoids and who are receiving neuraxial anesthesia or undergoing spinal puncture; long-term or permanent paralysis may result. Increased risk of developing epidural or spinal hematomas in patients using indwelling epidural catheters, concomitant use of other drugs that affect hemostasis (eg, NSAIDs, platelet inhibitors, other anticoagulants), history of traumatic or repeated epidural or spinal puncture, or a history of spinal deformity or spinal surgery. Monitor frequently for signs/symptoms of neurologic impairment; urgent treatment is necessary if neurologic compromise occurs. Consider benefits and risks before neuraxial intervention in patients anticoagulated or to be anticoagulated for thromboprophylaxis.

THERAPEUTIC CLASS: Low molecular weight heparin

INDICATIONS: Prophylaxis of ischemic complications in unstable angina and non-Q-wave myocardial infarction (MI) in conjunction with aspirin (ASA) therapy. Prophylaxis of deep vein thrombosis (DVT), which may lead to pulmonary embolism (PE), in hip replacement surgery, abdominal surgery in patients at risk for thromboembolic complications, and for those at risk for thromboembolic complications due to severely restricted mobility during acute illness. Extended treatment of symptomatic venous thromboembolism (VTE) (proximal DVT and/or PE) to reduce the recurrence of VTE in patients with cancer.

DOSAGE: *Adults:* Administer SQ. Prophylaxis of Ischemic Complications in Unstable Angina/Non-Q-Wave MI: 120 IU/kg q12h with PO ASA (75-165mg qd) until clinically stabilized. Usual Duration: 5-8 days. Max: 10,000 IU q12h. Prophylaxis of VTE Following Hip Replacement Surgery: Preop (Starting Day of Surgery): Usual: 2500 IU within 2 hrs preop, then 2500 IU 4-8 hrs postop. Preop (Starting PM Prior to Surgery): Usual: 5000 IU 10-14 hrs preop, then 5000 IU 4-8 hrs postop. Postop Start: Usual: 2500 IU 4-8 hrs postop. Maint (Pre/Postop): 5000 IU qd for 5-10 days postop (up to 14 days). Abdominal Surgery: Risk of Thromboembolic Complications: 2500 IU 1-2 hrs preop then qd for 5-10 days postop. Abdominal Surgery with High Thromboembolic Risk: 5000 IU pm preop then qd for 5-10 days postop. Abdominal Surgery with Malignancy: 2500 IU 1-2 hrs preop, followed by 2500 IU 12 hrs later, then 5000 IU qd for 5-10 days postop. Severely Restricted Mobility During Acute Illness: 5000 IU qd for 12-14 days. Treatment of Symptomatic VTE in Cancer Patients: 200 IU/kg qd for first 30 days, then 150 IU/kg qd for months 2-6. Max: 18,000 IU/day. Platelet Count 50,000-100,000/mm³: Reduce dose by 2500 IU until platelet count ≥100,000/mm³. Platelet Count <50,000/mm³: D/C therapy until platelet count >50,000/mm³. Severe Renal Impairment (CrCl <30mL/min): Monitor anti-Xa levels to determine appropriate dose.

HOW SUPPLIED: Inj: 2500 IU/0.2mL, 5000 IU/0.2mL, 7500 IU/0.3mL, 10,000 IU/0.4mL, 10,000 IU/1mL, 12,500 IU/0.5mL, 15,000 IU/0.6mL, 18,000 IU/0.72mL [Syringe]; 95,000 IU/3.8mL, 95,000 IU/9.5mL [Multi-Dose Vials]

CONTRAINDICATIONS: Active major bleeding, history of heparin-induced thrombocytopenia or heparin-induced thrombocytopenia with thrombosis, patients undergoing epidural/neuraxial anesthesia, as treatment for unstable angina/non-Q wave MI and for prolonged VTE prophylaxis, and hypersensitivity to pork products.

WARNINGS/PRECAUTIONS: Not for IM inj. Not indicated for acute treatment of VTE. Extreme caution in patients with increased risk of hemorrhage (eg, severe uncontrolled HTN, bacterial endocarditis, bleeding disorders, active ulceration, and angiodysplastic GI disease, hemorrhagic stroke, or shortly after brain, spinal, or ophthalmological surgery). Increased risk of bleeding with thrombocytopenia or platelet defects, severe liver/kidney insufficiency, hypertensive or diabetic retinopathy, and recent GI bleeding. May cause heparin-induced thrombocytopenia with or without thrombosis; d/c or reduce dose if platelet count <100,000/mm³. Multi-dose vials contain benzyl alcohol; caution in pregnant women. In premature infants, benzyl alcohol reported to be associated with fatal "gasping syndrome". Caution in elderly with low body weight (<45kg) and those predisposed to decreased renal function.

ADVERSE REACTIONS: Bleeding, inj-site pain, thrombocytopenia, elevation of serum transaminases (ALT, AST), inj-site hematoma.

INTERACTIONS: See Boxed Warning and Contraindications. Caution with oral anticoagulants, platelet inhibitors, and thrombolytic agents due to increased risk of bleeding.

PREGNANCY: Category B, caution in nursing.

MECHANISM OF ACTION: Low molecular weight heparin; enhances inhibition of factor Xa and thrombin by antithrombin, while only slightly affecting the activated PTT.

PHARMACOKINETICS: Absorption: Absolute bioavailability (87%); C_{max} =0.19 IU/mL (2500 IU), 0.41 IU/mL (5000 IU), 0.82 IU/mL (10,000 IU); T_{max} =4 hrs. **Distribution:** V_d =40-60mL/kg; found in breast milk. **Elimination:** $T_{1/2}$ =3-5 hrs.

NURSING CONSIDERATIONS

Assessment: Assess for risk factors for bleeding or developing epidural/spinal hematoma, active major bleeding, history of heparin-induced thrombocytopenia with or without thrombosis, if undergoing epidural/neuraxial anesthesia, known hypersensitivity to heparin or pork products, severe renal impairment, pregnancy/nursing status, possible drug interactions, or any other conditions where treatment is contraindicated or cautioned.

Monitoring: Monitor for signs/symptoms of neurological impairment, bleeding, thrombocytopenia, and allergic reactions. Monitor for signs/symptoms of spinal or epidural hematomas in patients receiving neuraxial anesthesia or undergoing spinal puncture. Perform periodic CBC with platelet count, blood chemistry, and stool occult blood tests. Monitor anti-Xa levels in patients with severe renal impairment or if abnormal coagulation parameters or bleeding occurs.

Patient Counseling: Inform patients who had neuraxial anesthesia/spinal puncture, particularly if taking concomitant NSAIDs, platelet inhibitors, or other anticoagulants to watch for signs/symptoms of spinal/epidural hematoma (eg, tingling, numbness, muscular weakness) and notify physician immediately if any of these occur. Instruct to d/c use of ASA or other NSAIDs prior to therapy. Counsel about injecting instructions if therapy is to continue after discharge from hospitals. Instruct to contact physician if any unusual bleeding, bruising, or signs of thrombocytopenia (eg, rash of dark red spots under skin) develop. Advise that it will take longer than usual to stop bleeding; may bruise and/or bleed more easily while on therapy. Advise to inform healthcare providers when taking medications known to affect bleeding before any surgery is scheduled or any new drug is taken. Instruct to inform physicians and dentists of all medications they are taking, including those obtained without prescription.

Administration: SQ route. Do not mix with other inj or infusions unless compatible. Refer to PI for proper administration technique. **Storage:** 20-25°C (68-77°F). MDV: Room temperature for ≤2 weeks after first penetration of the rubber stopper. Discard any unused sol after 2 weeks.

FROVA
frovatriptan succinate (Endo)

RX

THERAPEUTIC CLASS: 5-HT$_{1B/1D}$ agonist

INDICATIONS: Acute treatment of migraine with or without aura in adults.

DOSAGE: *Adults:* Usual: 2.5mg with fluids. May administer 2nd dose 2 hrs after 1st dose if migraine recurs after initial relief. Max: 7.5mg/day. Safety of treating >4 migraines/30 days not known.

HOW SUPPLIED: Tab: 2.5mg

CONTRAINDICATIONS: Ischemic coronary artery disease (CAD) (eg, angina pectoris, history of myocardial infarction (MI), documented silent ischemia) or coronary artery vasospasm (eg, Prinzmetal's angina), Wolff-Parkinson-White syndrome or arrhythmias associated with other cardiac accessory conduction pathway disorders, history of stroke, transient ischemic attack, or history of hemiplegic or basilar migraine, peripheral vascular disease, ischemic bowel disease, uncontrolled HTN. Recent use (within 24 hrs) of another 5-HT$_1$ agonist, an ergotamine-containing or ergot-type medication (eg, dihydroergotamine, methysergide).

WARNINGS/PRECAUTIONS: Use only if a clear diagnosis of migraine has been established. If no treatment response for the 1st migraine attack, reconsider diagnosis before treating any subsequent attacks. Not indicated for prevention of migraine attacks. Serious cardiac adverse reactions, including acute MI, reported. May cause coronary artery vasospasm (Prinzmetal's angina). Perform cardiovascular (CV) evaluation in triptan-naive patients who have multiple CV risk factors prior to therapy; consider administering 1st dose in a medically supervised setting and perform ECG immediately following administration in patients with a negative CV evaluation. Consider periodic CV evaluation in intermittent long-term users who have CV risk factors. Life-threatening cardiac rhythm disturbances (eg, ventricular tachycardia/fibrillation leading to death) reported; d/c if these occur. Sensations of pain, tightness, pressure, and heaviness reported in the chest, throat, neck, and jaw after treatment and are usually non-cardiac in origin; perform a cardiac evaluation if at high cardiac risk. Cerebral/subarachnoid hemorrhage, stroke, and other cerebrovascular events reported. Care should be taken to exclude other potentially serious neurological conditions before treatment. May cause noncoronary vasospastic reactions (eg, peripheral vascular ischemia, GI vascular ischemia, and infarction [presenting with abdominal pain and bloody diarrhea], splenic infarction, Raynaud's syndrome); rule out vasospastic reaction before using if experiencing signs/symptoms suggestive of noncoronary vasospasm reaction. Transient and permanent blindness and significant partial vision loss reported. Overuse of acute migraine drugs may lead to exacerbation of headache (medication overuse headache); detoxification, including withdrawal of the overused drugs, and treatment of withdrawal symptoms may be necessary. Serotonin syndrome may occur; d/c if serotonin syndrome is suspected. Significant elevation in BP, including hypertensive crisis with acute impairment of organ systems, reported; monitor BP. Anaphylaxis, anaphylactoid, and hypersensitivity reactions including angioedema reported; more likely to occur in patients with history of sensitivity to multiple allergens. Caution with severe hepatic impairment.

ADVERSE REACTIONS: Dizziness, fatigue, headache, paresthesia, flushing, dry mouth, hot or cold sensation, skeletal pain.

INTERACTIONS: See Contraindications. Serotonin syndrome reported with SSRIs, SNRIs, TCAs, and MAOIs.

PREGNANCY: Category C, not for use in nursing.

MECHANISM OF ACTION: 5-HT$_{1B/1D}$ agonist; binds with high affinity to 5-HT$_{1B/1D}$ receptors. Thought to be due to the agonist effects at the 5-HT$_{1B/1D}$ receptors on intracranial blood vessels (including the arterio-venous anastomoses) and sensory nerves of the trigeminal system resulting in cranial vessel constriction and inhibition of pro-inflammatory neuropeptide release.

PHARMACOKINETICS: Absorption: Absolute bioavailability: (20%) male, (30%) female; T_{max}=2-4 hrs. **Distribution:** V_d=(IV) 4.2L/kg (male), 3L/kg (female); plasma protein binding (15%). **Metabolism:** Via CYP1A2. **Elimination:** Feces (62%), urine (32%); $T_{1/2}$=26 hrs.

NURSING CONSIDERATIONS

Assessment: Assess for ischemic heart CAD, coronary artery vasospasm, uncontrolled HTN, neurological conditions, hepatic impairment, history of sensitivity to multiple allergens, drug hypersensitivity, any conditions where treatment is cautioned or contraindicated, pregnancy/nursing status, and possible drug interactions. Perform CV evaluation in triptan-naive patients prior to therapy who have multiple CV risk factors.

Monitoring: Monitor for cardiac adverse reactions, coronary artery vasospasm, cardiac rhythm disturbances, cerebrovascular event, noncoronary vasospastic reactions, serotonin syndrome, BP elevation, exacerbation of headache, anaphylactic/hypersensitivity reactions, ophthalmic changes, and other adverse events. Consider periodic CV evaluation in intermittent long-term users who have CV risk factors. Perform ECG immediately following administration in patients with a negative CV evaluation.

Patient Counseling: Inform that drug may cause serious CV side effects, to be alert for the signs/symptoms of chest pain, SOB, weakness, and slurring of speech, and to ask for medical advice when observing any indicative signs/symptoms. Inform that anaphylactic/anaphylactoid reactions have occurred and that they are more likely to occur in patients with history of sensitivity to multiple allergens. Inform that overuse (≥10 days/month) may lead to exacerbation of headache; encourage to record headache frequency and drug use. Caution about the risk of serotonin syndrome. Advise to notify physician if pregnant/nursing or planning to become pregnant.

Administration: Oral route. **Storage**: 25°C (77°F); excursions permitted to 15-30°C (59-86°F). Protect from moisture.

FULYZAQ   RX
crofelemer (Salix)

THERAPEUTIC CLASS: Antidiarrheal

INDICATIONS: Symptomatic relief of noninfectious diarrhea in patients with HIV/AIDS on antiretroviral therapy.

DOSAGE: *Adults:* 125mg bid.

HOW SUPPLIED: Tab, Delayed-Release: 125mg

WARNINGS/PRECAUTIONS: Not indicated for the treatment of infectious diarrhea; rule out infectious etiologies of diarrhea before initiating therapy.

ADVERSE REACTIONS: Upper respiratory tract infection, bronchitis, cough, flatulence, increased bilirubin.

PREGNANCY: Category C, not for use in nursing.

MECHANISM OF ACTION: Antidiarrheal; an inhibitor of both the cAMP-stimulated cystic fibrosis transmembrane conductance regulator Cl⁻ channel, and the Ca^{2+}-activated Cl⁻ channels at the luminal membrane of enterocytes. Blocks Cl⁻ secretion and accompanying high volume water loss in diarrhea, normalizing the flow of Cl⁻ and water in the GI tract.

NURSING CONSIDERATIONS

Assessment: Assess etiology of diarrhea and pregnancy/nursing status.

Monitoring: Monitor for adverse reactions.

Patient Counseling: Instruct to take ud.

Administration: Oral route. Take with or without food. Swallow whole; do not crush or chew. **Storage:** 20-25°C (68-77°F); excursions permitted between 15-30°C (59-86°F).

FUROSEMIDE
furosemide (Various)

OTHER BRAND NAMES: Lasix (Sanofi-Aventis)

THERAPEUTIC CLASS: Loop diuretic

INDICATIONS: Treatment of edema associated with congestive heart failure, cirrhosis of the liver, and renal disease, including nephrotic syndrome in adults and pediatric patients. (PO) Treatment of HTN alone or in combination with other antihypertensive agents in adults. (Inj) Adjunctive therapy for acute pulmonary edema.

DOSAGE: *Adults:* Individualize dose. (PO) Edema: Initial: 20-80mg as a single dose. Titrate: May repeat the same dose if needed or increase dose by 20mg or 40mg; give dose no sooner than 6-8 hrs after the previous dose until desired diuretic effect has been obtained. Give individually determined single dose qd or bid. Severe Edematous States: May carefully titrate dose up to 600mg/day. Consider giving on 2-4 consecutive days each week. Closely monitor when exceeding 80mg/day for prolonged periods. HTN: Initial: 40mg bid. Titrate: Adjust dose according to response. Add other antihypertensive agents if response is not satisfactory. Concomitant Antihypertensives: Reduce dose of other agents by at least 50%. May further reduce dose or d/c therapy of other antihypertensive drugs as BP falls. Elderly: Start at lower end of dosing range. (Inj) Edema: Initial: 20-40mg as a single dose IV/IM. Give IV dose slowly (1-2 min). Titrate: May repeat the same dose if needed or increase by 20mg not sooner than 2 hrs after the previous dose. Give individually determined single dose qd or bid. Acute Pulmonary Edema: Initial: 40mg IV slowly (over 1-2 min). Titrate: May increase to 80mg IV slowly (over 1-2 min), if satisfactory response does not occur within 1 hr. Additional therapy (eg, digitalis, oxygen) may be administered concomitantly if necessary. Elderly: Start at lower end of dosing range.
Pediatrics: Individualize dose. Edema: (PO) Initial: 2mg/kg as a single dose. Titrate: May increase by 1 or 2mg/kg no sooner than 6-8 hrs after the previous dose, if diuretic response is not satisfactory after the initial dose. Max: 6mg/kg. Maint: Adjust to the minimum effective level. (Inj) Initial: 1mg/kg IV/IM. Titrate: May increase by 1mg/kg not sooner than 2 hrs after the previous dose, if response is not satisfactory. Max: 6mg/kg. Premature Infants: Max: 1mg/kg/day.

HOW SUPPLIED: Inj: 10mg/mL [2mL, 4mL, 10mL]; Sol: 10mg/mL [60mL, 120mL], 40mg/5mL [500mL]; Tab: (Lasix) 20mg, 40mg*, 80mg *scored

CONTRAINDICATIONS: Anuria.

WARNINGS/PRECAUTIONS: May lead to profound diuresis with water and electrolyte depletion if given in excessive amounts; careful medical supervision required and dose and dose schedule must be adjusted to individual patient's needs. Initiate therapy in hospital with hepatic cirrhosis and ascites. Do not institute therapy until basic condition is improved in patients with hepatic coma and in states of electrolyte depletion. D/C if increasing azotemia and oliguria occur during treatment of severe progressive renal disease. Tinnitus, reversible or irreversible hearing impairment, and deafness reported. Ototoxicity is associated with rapid inj, severe renal impairment, use of higher than recommended doses, hypoproteinemia, or concomitant use with aminoglycoside antibiotics, ethacrynic acid, or other ototoxic drugs; control IV infusion rate if using high dose parenteral therapy. Excessive diuresis may cause dehydration, blood volume reduction with circulatory collapse, vascular thrombosis and embolism, particularly in elderly. Monitor for fluid/electrolyte imbalance (hyponatremia, hypochloremia alkalosis, hypokalemia, hypomagnesemia, or hypocalcemia), liver/kidney damage, blood dyscrasias, or other idiosyncratic reactions. Increased in blood glucose and alterations in glucose tolerance tests, and rarely, precipitation of diabetes mellitus (DM) reported. May cause acute urinary retention in patients with severe symptoms of urinary retention; monitor carefully, especially during the initial stages of treatment. May lead to a higher incidence of deterioration in renal function after receiving radiocontrast in patients at high risk for radiocontrast nephropathy. May potentiate ototoxicity and effect of therapy may be weakened in patients with hypoproteinemia. Asymptomatic hyperuricemia may occur and gout may rarely be precipitated. Caution in patients with sulfonamide allergy. May activate/exacerbate systemic lupus erythematosus (SLE). May precipitate nephrocalcinosis/nephrolithiasis in premature infants and children <4 yrs of age with no history of prematurity; monitor renal function and consider renal ultrasonography. May increase risk of persistence of patent ductus arteriosus in premature infants during the 1st weeks of life. May interfere with certain lab tests. Caution in elderly. (Inj) Use only in patients unable to take PO medication or in emergency situations; replace with PO therapy as soon as practical. May develop plasma level with potential toxic effects in premature infants with post conceptual age (gestational plus postnatal) <31 weeks receiving doses exceeding 1mg/kg/24 hrs. May cause hearing loss in neonates.

ADVERSE REACTIONS: Pancreatitis, jaundice, anorexia, paresthesias, diarrhea, N/V, dizziness, rash, urticaria, photosensitivity, fever, thrombophlebitis, restlessness, aplastic anemia, eosinophilia.

INTERACTIONS: May increase ototoxic potential of aminoglycoside antibiotics; avoid this combination, except in life-threatening situations. Avoid with ethacrynic acid and lithium. May experience salicylate toxicity at lower doses with concomitant high doses of salicylates for rheumatic disease. May antagonize skeletal muscle relaxing effect of tubocurarine. May potentiate action of succinylcholine. Potentiation of therapeutic effect of other antihypertensive drugs. Potentiation occurs with ganglionic or peripheral adrenergic blockers. May decrease arterial responsiveness to norepinephrine. Reduced CrCl in patients with chronic renal insufficiency with acetylsalicylic acid. Increased BUN, SrCr and K^+ levels, and weight gain reported with NSAIDs. Hypokalemia may develop with adrenocorticotropic hormone and corticosteroids. Reduced natriuretic and antihypertensive effects with indomethacin. Indomethacin may affect plasma renin levels, aldosterone excretion, and renin profile evaluation. Digitalis may exaggerate metabolic effects of hypokalemia. (Inj/Tab) Avoid with chloral hydrate. May enhance nephrotoxicity of nephrotoxic drugs (eg, cisplatin) if furosemide is not given in lower doses and with positive fluid balance. Severe hypotension and renal function deterioration including renal failure may occur; interruption or reduction in dose of furosemide, ACE inhibitors or ARBs may be necessary. Phenytoin interferes with renal action. Methotrexate and other drugs that undergo significant renal tubular secretion may reduce the effect of furosemide. May increase the risk of cephalosporin-induced nephrotoxicity. Increased risk of gouty arthritis with cyclosporine. Hypokalemia may develop with licorice in large amounts, or prolonged use of laxatives. (Tab/Sol) Reduced natriuretic and antihypertensive effects with sucralfate; separate intake by at least 2 hrs.

PREGNANCY: Category C, caution in nursing.

MECHANISM OF ACTION: Loop diuretic; primarily inhibits the absorption of Na^+ and Cl^- not only in the proximal and distal tubules but also in the loop of Henle.

PHARMACOKINETICS: Absorption: (Healthy) Bioavailability (64% tab), (60% sol). **Distribution:** (Healthy) Plasma protein binding (91-99%); found in breast milk. **Metabolism:** Biotransformation; furosemide glucuronide (major metabolite). **Elimination:** Urine; $T_{1/2}$=2 hrs.

NURSING CONSIDERATIONS

Assessment: Assess for anuria, sulfonamide/drug hypersensitivity, SLE, hepatic/renal impairment, hypoproteinemia, pregnancy/nursing status, and possible drug interactions.

Monitoring: Monitor for signs/symptoms of fluid/electrolyte imbalance, blood dyscrasias, hyperglycemia and alterations in glucose tolerance tests, hyperuricemia, precipitation of gout or DM, ototoxicity, dehydration, blood volume reduction with circulatory collapse, vascular thrombosis and embolism, acute urinary retention, and other adverse reactions. Monitor serum electrolytes, carbon dioxide, creatinine and BUN frequently during 1st few months of therapy, then periodically thereafter. Monitor urine and blood glucose periodically in diabetics. Monitor renal function and perform renal ultrasonography in pediatric patients.

Patient Counseling: Advise that patient may experience symptoms from excessive fluid and/or electrolyte losses. Advise that postural hypotension can be managed by getting up slowly. Inform patients with DM that drug may increase blood glucose levels and affect urine glucose tests. Advise that skin may be more sensitive to sunlight during therapy. Advise hypertensive patients to avoid medications that may increase BP, including OTC products for appetite suppression and cold symptoms.

Administration: Oral/IV/IM route. (Inj) Refer to PI for high dose parenteral therapy. **Storage:** Protect from light. (Inj) 20-25°C (68-77°F). (Tab/Sol) 25°C (77°F); excursions permitted to 15-30°C (59-86°F).

Fusilev   RX
levoleucovorin (Spectrum)

THERAPEUTIC CLASS: Cytoprotective agent

INDICATIONS: Rescue therapy after high-dose methotrexate (MTX) therapy in osteosarcoma. To diminish the toxicity and counteract the effects of impaired MTX elimination and of inadvertent overdosage of folic acid antagonists. For use in combination chemotherapy with 5-fluorouracil (5-FU) in the palliative treatment of patients with advanced metastatic colorectal cancer.

DOSAGE: *Adults:* Levoleucovorin Rescue: 7.5mg (5mg/m²) IV q6h for 10 doses starting 24 hrs after the beginning of MTX infusion. Continue therapy, hydration and urinary alkalinization until MTX level is <5 x 10⁻⁸M (0.05 micromolar). Refer to PI for guidelines on dosage adjustment and rescue extensions. Inadvertent MTX Overdosage: 7.5mg (5mg/m²) IV q6h until serum MTX is <10⁻⁸M. Titrate: Increase to 50mg/m² IV q3h until MTX level is <10⁻⁸M if 24-hr SrCr is 50% over baseline, or if 24-hr MTX level is >5 x 10⁻⁶M, or 48-hr level is >9 x 10⁻⁷M. Employ concurrent hydration (3L/day) and urinary alkalinization with Na bicarbonate; adjust bicarbonate dose to maintain urine pH at ≥7. Start rescue therapy as soon as possible after overdose and within 24 hrs of MTX administration when there is delayed excretion. Colorectal Cancer: 100mg/m² slow IV over a minimum of 3 min, followed by 370mg/m² 5-FU IV, daily for 5 days, or 10mg/m² IV, followed by 425mg/m² 5-FU IV, daily for 5 days. May repeat at 4-week intervals for 2 courses, then at 4- to 5-week intervals provided that the patient has completely recovered from the toxic effects of the prior treatment course. May increase 5-FU dose by 10% if no toxicity. Reduce 5-FU daily dose by 20% with moderate GI/hematologic toxicity and by 30% with severe toxicity.

HOW SUPPLIED: Inj: 50mg, 10mg/mL [17.5mL, 25mL]

WARNINGS/PRECAUTIONS: Do not inject >16mL/min. Do not administer intrathecally. Not approved for pernicious anemia and megaloblastic anemias secondary to the lack of vitamin B12; improper use may cause a hematologic remission while neurologic manifestations continue to progress. Do not initiate or continue therapy with 5-FU in patients with symptoms of GI toxicity until symptoms have completely resolved; caution in elderly and/or debilitated. Monitor patients with diarrhea until it has resolved, as rapid clinical deterioration leading to death can occur. Seizures and/or syncope reported in cancer patients, most commonly in those with CNS metastases or other predisposing factors.

ADVERSE REACTIONS: Stomatitis, N/V, diarrhea, dyspepsia, typhlitis, dyspnea, dermatitis, confusion, neuropathy, abnormal renal function, taste perversion.

INTERACTIONS: May enhance 5-FU toxicity. Seizures and/or syncope reported with fluoropyrimidine. Increased treatment failure and morbidity rates in trimethoprim-sulfamethoxazole-treated HIV patients with *Pneumocystis carinii* pneumonia. Folic acid in large amounts may counteract antiepileptic effect of phenobarbital, phenytoin, and primidone, and increase seizure frequency in children; use with caution when taken with anticonvulsants.

PREGNANCY: Category C, not for use in nursing.

MECHANISM OF ACTION: Folate analog; counteracts the therapeutic and toxic effects of folic acid antagonists, which act by inhibiting dihydrofolate reductase. Enhances therapeutic effects of fluoropyrimidines used in cancer therapy (eg, 5-FU).

PHARMACOKINETICS: Absorption: (Total-Tetrahydrofolate [THF]) C_{max}=1722ng/mL; (5-methyl-THF) C_{max}=275ng/mL, T_{max}=0.9 hrs. **Metabolism:** 5-methyl-THF (metabolite). **Elimination:** $T_{1/2}$=5.1 hrs (total-THF), 6.8 hrs (5-methyl-THF).

NURSING CONSIDERATIONS

Assessment: Assess for previous allergic reactions to folic acid or folinic acid, pernicious anemia and megaloblastic anemias secondary to the lack of vitamin B12, GI toxicity, third-space fluid accumulation (eg, ascites, pleural effusion), renal impairment, inadequate hydration, CNS metastases, pregnancy/nursing status, and possible drug interactions.

Monitoring: Monitor for GI toxicity, seizures, syncope, and hypersensitivity reactions. Monitor patients with diarrhea until it has resolved. Monitor fluid and electrolytes in patients with abnormalities in MTX excretion. Monitor SrCr and MTX levels at least qd.

Patient Counseling: Inform about risks and benefits of therapy. Advise to notify physician if any adverse reaction occurs. Instruct to inform physician if pregnant/nursing.

Administration: IV route. Do not administer with other agents in the same admixture. Administer 5-FU and levoleucovorin separately. Refer to PI for reconstitution and infusion instructions. **Storage:** (Powder) 25°C (77°F); excursions permitted from 15-30°C (59-86°F). Protect from light. Reconstitution/Dilution with 0.9% NaCl: Room temperature for ≤12 hrs. Dilution with D5W: Room temperature for ≤4 hrs. (Sol) 2-8°C (36-46°F). Protect from light. Dilution with 0.9% NaCl or D5W: Room temperature for ≤4 hrs.

FUZEON   RX
enfuvirtide (Genentech)

THERAPEUTIC CLASS: Fusion inhibitor

INDICATIONS: In combination with other antiretroviral agents for the treatment of HIV-1 infection in treatment-experienced patients with evidence of HIV-1 replication despite ongoing antiretroviral therapy.

DOSAGE: *Adults:* Usual: 90mg bid SQ into the upper arm, anterior thigh, or abdomen. *Pediatrics:* 6-16 Yrs: Usual: 2mg/kg bid SQ into the upper arm, anterior thigh, or abdomen. Max: 90mg SQ bid. Refer to PI for weight-based dosing chart.

HOW SUPPLIED: Inj: 90mg/mL

WARNINGS/PRECAUTIONS: Local inj-site reactions reported; monitor for signs/symptoms of cellulitis or local infection. Administration with Biojector 2000 may result in neuralgia and/or paresthesia, bruising, and hematomas. Patients with hemophilia or other coagulation disorders may have a higher risk of post-inj bleeding. May cause bacterial pneumonia; monitor for signs/symptoms of pneumonia, especially those predisposed to pneumonia (eg, low initial CD4 cell count, high initial viral load, IV drug use, smoking, prior history of lung disease). Associated with systemic hypersensitivity reactions; d/c immediately if signs/symptoms develop. May lead to anti-enfuvirtide antibody production, which cross-reacts with HIV gp41 and could result in false-positive HIV test with an ELISA assay. Immune reconstitution syndrome reported. Autoimmune disorders (eg, Graves' disease, polymyositis, Guillain-Barre syndrome) reported in the setting of immune reconstitution and can occur many months after initiation of treatment.

ADVERSE REACTIONS: Diarrhea, local inj-site reactions, fatigue, nausea, decreased weight, sinusitis, abdominal pain, cough, herpes simplex, decreased appetite, pancreatitis.

INTERACTIONS: May result in a higher risk of post-inj bleeding with anticoagulants.

PREGNANCY: Category B, not for use in nursing.

MECHANISM OF ACTION: Fusion inhibitor; interferes with the entry of HIV-1 into cells by inhibiting fusion of viral and cellular membranes; binds to the first heptad-repeat in the gp41 subunit of the viral envelope glycoprotein and prevents the conformational changes required for the fusion of viral and cellular membranes.

PHARMACOKINETICS: Absorption: Absolute bioavailability (84.3%); C_{max}=4.59mcg/mL; T_{max}=8 hrs; AUC=55.8mcg•hr/mL. **Distribution:** V_d=5.5L; plasma protein binding (92%). **Metabolism:** Liver via hydrolysis; M_3 (metabolite). **Elimination:** $T_{1/2}$=3.8 hrs.

NURSING CONSIDERATIONS

Assessment: Assess for risk factors for pneumonia (eg, history of lung disease, decreased CD4 cell count, increased viral load, IV drug use, smoking), infections, hemophilia, history of coagulation disorders, pregnancy/nursing status, and possible drug interactions.

Monitoring: Monitor for signs/symptoms of cellulitis or local inj-site reactions, pneumonia, immune reconstitution syndrome, autoimmune disorders, post-inj bleeding, nerve pain/paresthesia, hypersensitivity reactions, and other adverse reactions.

Patient Counseling: Inform that therapy is not a cure for HIV-1 infection and patients may continue to experience illnesses associated with HIV-1 infection, including opportunistic infections. Advise to avoid doing things that can spread HIV-1 infection to others (eg, sharing needles, other inj equipment, or personal items that can have blood fluids on them, having sex without protection, breastfeeding). Inform of risk for inj-site reactions; instruct to monitor for signs/symptoms of cellulitis and local infections. Advise to seek medical attention if experiencing signs/symptoms of pneumonia (eg, cough with fever, rapid breathing, SOB) and systemic hypersensitivity (eg, rash, fever, N/V, chills, rigors, hypotension). Advise that the drug must be taken as a part of a combination antiretroviral regimen. Advise to inform physician if pregnant, planning to become pregnant, or breastfeeding. Instruct not to change dosage or schedule without consulting physician.

Administration: SQ route. Do not inject into moles, scar tissue, bruises, navel, surgical scars, tattoos, burn sites, directly over a blood vessel, near areas where large nerves course close to the skin, into a preceding inj site, or a site with current inj-site reaction from an earlier dose. Refer to PI for administration instructions. **Storage:** Vial: 25°C (77°F); excursions permitted to 15-30°C (59-86°F). Reconstituted Sol: 2-8°C (36-46°F). Use within 24 hrs.

GABITRIL   RX
tiagabine HCl (Cephalon)

THERAPEUTIC CLASS: Nipecotic acid derivative

INDICATIONS: Adjunctive therapy in adults and children ≥12 yrs of age in the treatment of partial seizures.

DOSAGE: *Adults:* Induced (Patients Already Taking Enzyme-Inducing Antiepilepsy Drugs [AEDs]): Initial: 4mg qd. Titrate: May increase total daily dose by 4-8mg at weekly intervals until clinical response is achieved, or up to 56mg/day. Give total daily dose in divided doses (bid-qid). Refer to PI for Typical Dosing Titration Regimen. Non-Induced: Requires lower dose and slower dose titration. Hepatic Impairment: May require reduced initial/maint doses and/or longer dosing intervals.
Pediatrics: 12-18 Yrs: Induced: Initial: 4mg qd. Titrate: May increase total daily dose by 4mg at the beginning of Week 2, then may increase by 4-8mg at weekly intervals until clinical response is achieved, or up to 32mg/day. Give total daily dose in divided doses (bid-qid). Refer to PI for Typical Dosing Titration Regimen. Non-Induced: Requires lower dose and slower dose titration. Hepatic Impairment: May require reduced initial/maint doses and/or longer dosing intervals.

HOW SUPPLIED: Tab: 2mg, 4mg, 12mg, 16mg

WARNINGS/PRECAUTIONS: New-onset seizures and status epilepticus in patients without epilepsy reported; d/c therapy and evaluate for an underlying seizure disorder. Increased risk of suicidal thoughts or behavior may occur; monitor for emergence or worsening of depression, suicidal thoughts/behavior, and/or any unusual changes in mood or behavior. Avoid abrupt discontinuation; may increase seizure frequency. May affect thought processes (eg, impaired concentration, speech or language problems, confusion) and level of consciousness (eg, somnolence, fatigue). May exacerbate EEG abnormalities; caution with history of spike and wave discharges on EEG and adjust dosage. Sudden unexpected death in epilepsy reported. Moderately severe to incapacitating generalized weakness reported; weakness resolved after dose reduction or discontinuation. There may be a possibility of long-term ophthalmologic effects. Serious rash (eg, maculopapular, vesiculobullous, Stevens-Johnson syndrome) may occur. Caution with liver disease.

ADVERSE REACTIONS: Dizziness, asthenia, tremor, somnolence, N/V, nervousness, abdominal pain, pain, difficulty with concentration/attention, insomnia, confusion, pharyngitis, rash, diarrhea.

INTERACTIONS: May reduce valproate concentrations. Increased free concentration with valproate. Increased clearance with carbamazepine, phenytoin, and phenobarbital (primidone). Caution with drugs that may depress the nervous system (eg, ethanol, or triazolam); may cause possible additive depressive effects. Reports of new-onset seizures and status epilepticus in patients without epilepsy with concomitant drugs that lower the seizure threshold (antidepressants, antipsychotics, stimulants, narcotics). Potential interactions with drugs that induce or inhibit hepatic metabolizing enzymes. Use with highly protein-bound drugs may lead to higher free fractions of tiagabine or competing drugs.

PREGNANCY: Category C, caution in nursing.

MECHANISM OF ACTION: Nipecotic acid derivative; not established. Enhances activity of gamma-aminobutyric acid (GABA). Binds to recognition sites associated with the GABA uptake carrier, thereby blocking GABA uptake into presynaptic neurons, permitting more GABA to be available for receptor binding on the surfaces of postsynaptic cells.

PHARMACOKINETICS: Absorption: Rapid, well-absorbed; absolute bioavailability (90%); T_{max}=2.5 hrs (fed), T_{max}=45 min (fasting). **Distribution:** Plasma protein binding (96%). **Metabolism:** Liver via CYP3A; thiophene ring oxidation leading to formation of 5-oxo-tiagabine and glucuronidation. **Elimination:** Urine (25%), feces (63%); $T_{1/2}$=7-9 hrs (non-induced).

NURSING CONSIDERATIONS

Assessment: Assess for underlying seizure disorder, history of status epilepticus and spike and wave discharges on EEG, depression, suicidal thoughts/behavior, history of hypersensitivity reactions, hepatic impairment, pregnancy/nursing status, and possible drug interactions.

Monitoring: Monitor for occurrence of new-onset seizures and status epilepticus in patients without a previous history of epilepsy, withdrawal seizures, cognitive and neuropsychiatric events, EEG changes, rash, emergence or worsening of depression, suicidal thoughts/behavior, unusual changes in mood or behavior, generalized weakness, ophthalmologic changes, and other adverse reactions.

Patient Counseling: Inform patients, caregivers, and families about increased risk of suicidal thoughts and behavior and to alert for the emergence or worsening of symptoms of depression, any unusual changes in mood or behavior, or emergence of suicidal thoughts, behaviors, or thoughts of self-harm; instruct to report immediately to healthcare providers. Inform that dizziness, somnolence, and other symptoms/signs of CNS depression may occur; instruct to avoid driving/operating other complex machinery until adjusted to effects. Instruct to notify physician if pregnant, intending to become pregnant, or if breastfeeding. If multiple doses are missed, instruct to contact physician for possible retitration. Encourage pregnant patients to enroll in North American Antiepileptic Drug Pregnancy Registry.

Administration: Oral route. Take with food. **Storage:** 20-25°C (68-77°F). Protect from light and moisture.

GARDASIL

RX

human papillomavirus recombinant vaccine, quadrivalent (Merck)

THERAPEUTIC CLASS: Vaccine

INDICATIONS: Vaccination of girls and women 9-26 yrs of age for the prevention of cervical, vulvar, vaginal, and anal cancer caused by human papillomavirus (HPV) types 16 and 18, genital warts (condyloma acuminata) caused by HPV types 6 and 11, and cervical intraepithelial neoplasia (CIN) grade 2/3 and cervical adenocarcinoma in situ, CIN grade 1, vulvar intraepithelial neoplasia (VIN) grades 2 and 3, vaginal intraepithelial neoplasia (VaIN) grades 2 and 3, and anal intraepithelial neoplasia (AIN) grades 1, 2, and 3 caused by HPV types 6, 11, 16, and 18. Vaccination of boys and men 9-26 yrs of age for the prevention of anal cancer caused by HPV types 16 and 18, genital warts (condyloma acuminata) caused by HPV types 6 and 11, and AIN grades 1, 2, and 3 caused by HPV types 6, 11, 16, and 18.

DOSAGE: *Adults:* ≤26 Yrs: 0.5mL IM in the deltoid region of the upper arm or in the higher anterolateral area of the thigh at the following schedule: 0, 2 months, 6 months.
Pediatrics: ≥9 Yrs: 0.5mL IM in the deltoid region of the upper arm or in the higher anterolateral area of the thigh at the following schedule: 0, 2 months, 6 months.

HOW SUPPLIED: Inj: 0.5mL

CONTRAINDICATIONS: Hypersensitivity, including severe allergic reactions to yeast.

WARNINGS/PRECAUTIONS: Syncope may occur; observe for 15 min after administration. Appropriate medical treatment and supervision must be readily available in case of anaphylactic reactions. Women should continue to undergo cervical cancer screening. Recipients should not d/c anal cancer screening if it has been recommended by healthcare provider. Does not protect against disease from vaccine and non-vaccine HPV types to which a person has previously been exposed through sexual activity. Not intended for treatment of active external genital lesions; cervical, vulvar, vaginal, and anal cancers; CIN; VIN; VaIN; AIN. Vaccination may not result in protection in all vaccine recipients. Response to vaccine may be diminished in immunocompromised individuals.

ADVERSE REACTIONS: Inj-site pain/swelling/erythema/pruritus, pyrexia, nausea, dizziness, diarrhea, headache.

INTERACTIONS: Immunosuppressive therapies, including irradiation, antimetabolites, alkylating agents, cytotoxic drugs, and corticosteroids (used in greater than physiologic doses), may reduce the immune responses to vaccines.

PREGNANCY: Category B, caution in nursing.

MECHANISM OF ACTION: Vaccine; not established. May involve the development of humoral immune response.

NURSING CONSIDERATIONS

Assessment: Assess for hypersensitivity to yeast or the vaccine, immunocompromised conditions, pregnancy/nursing status, and possible drug interactions.

Monitoring: Monitor for syncope, anaphylactic reactions, and other adverse reactions.

Patient Counseling: Inform about benefits and risks associated with vaccine. Instruct women to continue to undergo cervical cancer screening per standard of care. Advise not to d/c anal cancer screening if recommended by physician. Inform that vaccine does not provide protection against disease from vaccine and non-vaccine HPV types to which a person has previously been exposed through sexual activity. Inform that syncope may occur following vaccination. Advise that vaccine is not recommended during pregnancy. Counsel about the importance of completing the immunization series unless contraindicated. Instruct to report any adverse reactions to physician.

Administration: IM route. Inject in the deltoid region of the upper arm or in the higher anterolateral area of the thigh. Shake well before use. Do not dilute or mix with other vaccines. Refer to PI for further administration instructions. **Storage:** 2-8°C (36-46°F). Do not freeze. Protect from light. Administer as soon as possible after being removed from refrigeration; can be out of refrigeration (≤25°C [77°F]) for a total time of not more than 72 hrs.

GAZYVA   RX
obinutuzumab (Genentech)

> Hepatitis B virus (HBV) reactivation may occur, in some cases resulting in fulminant hepatitis, hepatic failure, and death; screen all patients for HBV infection before treatment initiation. Monitor HBV positive patients during and after treatment. D/C therapy and concomitant medications in the event of HBV reactivation. Progressive multifocal leukoencephalopathy (PML), including fatal PML, may occur.

THERAPEUTIC CLASS: Monoclonal antibody/CD20-blocker

INDICATIONS: In combination with chlorambucil, for the treatment of patients with previously untreated chronic lymphocytic leukemia.

DOSAGE: *Adults:* Usual: 1000mg IV, with the exception of the 1st infusions in Cycle 1. Cycle 1: Day 1: 100mg IV. Day 2: 900mg IV. Days 8 and 15: 1000mg IV. Cycles 2-6: Day 1: 1000mg IV. Refer to PI for infusion rate information. Premedicate with a glucocorticoid, acetaminophen, and an antihistamine; refer to PI for further specifications. Consider treatment interruption, if patient experiences an infection, Grade 3 or 4 cytopenia, or a ≥Grade 2 nonhematologic toxicity. If a dose is missed, administer as soon as possible and adjust dosing schedule accordingly. If appropriate, patients who do not complete the Day 1 Cycle 1 dose may proceed to the Day 2 Cycle 1 dose.

HOW SUPPLIED: Inj: 25mg/mL [40mL]

WARNINGS/PRECAUTIONS: Only healthcare professionals with appropriate medical support to manage severe infusion reactions should administer Gazyva. Screen for HBV infection by measuring hepatitis B surface antigen and hepatitis B core antibody before initiating treatment. Consider diagnosis of PML in any patient with new onset or changes to preexisting neurologic manifestations; d/c therapy and consider discontinuation or reduction of any concomitant chemotherapy or immunosuppressive therapy in patients who develop PML. May cause severe and life-threatening infusion reactions; institute medical management for infusion reactions PRN. Stop infusion and permanently d/c therapy for patients with any Grade 4 infusion reaction (eg, anaphylaxis). Interrupt therapy for Grade 3 reactions until resolution of symptoms. Interrupt or reduce rate of infusion for Grade 1 or 2 reactions and manage symptoms. Monitor patients with preexisting cardiac/pulmonary conditions more frequently throughout infusion and postinfusion period. Hypotension may occur as part of an infusion reaction; consider withholding antihypertensive treatments for 12 hrs prior to, during each infusion, and for the 1st hr after administration until BP is stable. Acute renal failure, hyperkalemia, hypocalcemia, hyperuricemia, and/or hyperphosphatemia from tumor lysis syndrome (TLS) may occur within 12-24 hrs after the 1st infusion; caution with high tumor burden and/or high circulating lymphocyte count (>25 x 10⁹/L). Correct electrolyte abnormalities, monitor renal function, and fluid balance, and administer supportive care, including dialysis as indicated to treat TLS. Serious bacterial, fungal, and new/reactivated viral infections may occur during and following therapy; avoid in patients with active infection. Caution in patients with history of recurring/chronic infections. Grade 3 or 4 neutropenia reported; monitor patients with Grade 3-4 neutropenia frequently with regular laboratory tests until resolution. Anticipate, evaluate, and treat any signs/symptoms of developing infection. Thrombocytopenia reported; monitor platelet counts more frequently until resolution in patients with Grade 3 or 4 thrombocytopenia; transfusion of blood products may be necessary.

ADVERSE REACTIONS: HBV reactivation, fulminant hepatitis, hepatic failure, PML, infusion reactions, neutropenia, thrombocytopenia, anemia, pyrexia, cough, musculoskeletal disorders, leukopenia, lymphopenia, hypocalcemia, hyperkalemia.

INTERACTIONS: Immunization with live virus vaccines is not recommended during treatment and until B-cell recovery.

PREGNANCY: Category C, not for use in nursing.

MECHANISM OF ACTION: Monoclonal antibody/CD20-blocker; binds to CD20 antigen expressed on the surface of pre B- and mature B-lymphocytes, mediating B-cell lysis through engagement of immune effector cells, by directly activating intracellular death signaling pathways, and/or activation of the complement cascade.

PHARMACOKINETICS: Distribution: V_d=3.8L. **Elimination:** $T_{1/2}$=28.4 days.

NURSING CONSIDERATIONS

Assessment: Assess for HBV infection, active/history of chronic/recurring infection, preexisting cardiac/pulmonary conditions, or any other conditions where treatment is contraindicated or cautioned, pregnancy/nursing status, and possible drug interactions. Obtain baseline blood counts.

Monitoring: Monitor for signs/symptoms of bacterial/fungal/viral infections, PML, infusion reactions, TLS, neutropenia, thrombocytopenia, and other adverse reactions. Monitor blood counts at regular intervals. Closely monitor patients during each infusion. Monitor patients with evidence of current or prior HBV infection for clinical and lab signs of hepatitis or HBV reactivation during and for several months following treatment. Monitor patients with preexisting cardiac/pulmonary conditions more frequently throughout the infusion and the postinfusion period. Monitor renal function and fluid balance in patients with TLS.

Patient Counseling: Instruct to seek immediate medical attention for signs/symptoms of infusion reactions, symptoms of TLS, signs of infections, symptoms of hepatitis, and new or changes in neurological symptoms. Advise of the need for periodic monitoring of blood counts and to avoid vaccination with live viral vaccines. Inform patients with a history of HBV infection that they should be monitored and sometimes treated for their hepatitis.

Administration: IV route. Administer only as an IV infusion through a dedicated line; do not administer as an IV push/bolus. Do not mix with other drugs. Do not shake. Use diluted infusion immediately. Refer to PI for further preparation and administration instructions. **Storage:** 2-8°C (36-46°F). Do not freeze. Protect from light. Diluted Sol (in 0.9% NaCl at 0.4mg/mL-20mg/mL): Stable at 2-8°C (36-46°F) for 24 hrs followed by 48 hrs (including infusion time) at ≤30°C (86°F).

GEMCITABINE   RX
gemcitabine (Various)

OTHER BRAND NAMES: Gemzar (Lilly)

THERAPEUTIC CLASS: Nucleoside analogue antimetabolite

INDICATIONS: In combination with carboplatin for treatment of advanced ovarian cancer that has relapsed at least 6 months after completion of platinum-based therapy. In combination with paclitaxel for 1st-line treatment of metastatic breast cancer after failure of prior anthracycline-containing adjuvant chemotherapy, unless anthracyclines were clinically contraindicated. In combination with cisplatin for 1st-line treatment of inoperable, locally advanced (Stage IIIA or IIIB), or metastatic (Stage IV) non-small cell lung cancer (NSCLC). First-line treatment of locally advanced (nonresectable Stage II or Stage III) or metastatic (Stage IV) adenocarcinoma of the pancreas in patients previously treated with 5-fluorouracil.

DOSAGE: *Adults:* Ovarian Cancer: 1000mg/m^2 IV infusion over 30 min on Days 1 and 8 of each 21-day cycle, in combination with carboplatin area under the curve 4 IV after gemcitabine on Day 1 of each 21-day cycle. Breast Cancer: 1250mg/m^2 IV over 30 min on Days 1 and 8 of each 21-day cycle. Give paclitaxel at 175mg/m^2 on Day 1 as a 3-hr IV infusion before gemcitabine. NSCLC: Every 4-Week Schedule: 1000mg/m^2 IV over 30 min on Days 1, 8, and 15. Give cisplatin IV at 100mg/m^2 on Day 1 after gemcitabine infusion. Every 3-Week Schedule: 1250mg/m^2 IV over 30 min on Days 1 and 8. Give cisplatin IV at 100mg/m^2 on Day 1 after gemcitabine infusion. Pancreatic Cancer: 1000mg/m^2 IV over 30 min. Treatment Schedule: Weeks 1-8: Weekly dosing for the first 7 weeks followed by 1 week rest. After Week 8: Weekly dosing on Days 1, 8, and 15 of 28-day cycles. Refer to PI for dose modifications for myelosuppression and nonhematologic adverse reactions.

HOW SUPPLIED: Inj: 2g; (Gemzar) 200mg, 1g

WARNINGS/PRECAUTIONS: Prolongation of infusion time beyond 60 min or more frequent than weekly dosing resulted in an increased incidence of clinically significant hypotension, severe flu-like symptoms, myelosuppression, and asthenia. Myelosuppression manifested by neutropenia, thrombocytopenia, and anemia occurs with monotherapy; increased risk when combined with other cytotoxic drugs. Pulmonary toxicity (eg, interstitial pneumonitis, pulmonary fibrosis/edema, adult respiratory distress syndrome) reported; may lead to fatal respiratory failure despite discontinuation of therapy. D/C if unexplained dyspnea (with or without bronchospasm) or any evidence of pulmonary toxicity develops. Hemolytic-uremic syndrome (HUS) to include fatalities from renal failure or the requirement for dialysis may occur; consider the diagnosis of HUS if anemia with evidence of microangiopathic hemolysis, elevation of bilirubin/lactate dehydrogenase, reticulocytosis, severe thrombocytopenia, or evidence of renal failure (SrCr/BUN elevation) develops. Permanently d/c therapy in patients with HUS or severe renal impairment. Liver injury, including liver failure and death, reported alone or in combination with other potentially hepatotoxic drugs; administration in patients with concurrent liver metastases or a preexisting history of hepatitis, alcoholism, or liver cirrhosis may lead to exacerbation of the underlying hepatic insufficiency. D/C if severe liver injury develops. May cause fetal harm. Capillary leak syndrome (CLS) with severe consequences reported; d/c if CLS develops.

ADVERSE REACTIONS: N/V, anemia, increased ALT/AST/alkaline phosphatase, neutropenia, proteinuria, fever, hematuria, rash, thrombocytopenia, dyspnea, edema, diarrhea, hemorrhage, infection.

INTERACTIONS: Not indicated for use in combination with radiation therapy; life-threatening mucositis, especially esophagitis and pneumonitis occurred with concurrent thoracic radiation. Radiation recall reported when given after prior radiation.

PREGNANCY: Category D, not for use in nursing.

MECHANISM OF ACTION: Nucleoside analogue antimetabolite; kills cells undergoing DNA synthesis and blocks the progression of cells through the G1/S-phase boundary.

PHARMACOKINETICS: Distribution: V_d=50L/m^2. **Metabolism:** Via nucleoside kinases to diphosphate and triphosphate nucleosides; gemcitabine triphosphate (active metabolite). **Elimination:** Urine (92-98%, <10% unchanged); $T_{1/2}$=42-94 min.

NURSING CONSIDERATIONS

Assessment: Assess for hypersensitivity to drug, renal/hepatic dysfunction, pregnancy/nursing status, and possible drug interactions. Obtain CBC, including differential and platelet count, prior to each dose.

Monitoring: Monitor for signs/symptoms of myelosuppression, pulmonary toxicity, HUS, CLS, and other adverse reactions. Periodically monitor renal/hepatic function.

Patient Counseling: Inform of the risks and benefits of therapy. Advise of the potential need for blood transfusions and increased susceptibility to infections. Instruct to immediately contact physician if any signs/symptoms of infection, fever, prolonged/unexpected bleeding, bruising, SOB, wheezing, cough, changes in the color/volume of urine output, jaundice, or pain/tenderness in the right upper abdominal quadrant develops. Inform that drug may cause fetal harm; instruct to notify physician if pregnant or nursing.

Administration: IV route. Refer to PI for preparation and administration instructions. **Storage:** 20-25°C (68-77°F); excursions permitted between 15-30°C (59-86°F). Reconstituted Sol: 20-25°C (68-77°F) for 24 hrs. Do not refrigerate.

GEODON   RX
ziprasidone (Roerig)

THERAPEUTIC CLASS: Benzisoxazole derivative

INDICATIONS: (PO) Treatment of schizophrenia. As monotherapy for acute treatment of manic or mixed episodes associated with bipolar I disorder. Adjunct to lithium or valproate for maintenance treatment of bipolar I disorder. (IM) Treatment of acute agitation in schizophrenic patients for whom treatment with ziprasidone is appropriate and who need IM antipsychotic medication for rapid control of agitation.

DOSAGE: *Adults:* Schizophrenia: (PO) Initial: 20mg bid with food. Titrate: May subsequently be adjusted up to 80mg bid on the basis of individual clinical status; adjust dose at intervals of not <2 days if indicated. Max: 80mg bid. Reassess periodically to determine need for maintenance treatment. Bipolar Disorder: (PO) Initial: 40mg bid with food. Titrate: May increase to 60mg or 80mg bid on the 2nd day of treatment, and subsequently adjust based on tolerance and efficacy within the range 40-80mg bid. Maint (as Adjunct to Lithium/Valproate): Continue treatment at the same dose on which the patient was initially stabilized, within the range of 40-80mg bid. Reassess periodically to determine need for maintenance treatment. Agitation in Schizophrenia: (IM) Usual: 10mg IM q2h-20mg IM q4h. Max: 40mg/day. If long-term therapy is indicated, replace with PO ziprasidone HCl as soon as possible. Elderly: Start at lower end of dosing range.

HOW SUPPLIED: Cap: (HCl) 20mg, 40mg, 60mg, 80mg; Inj: (Mesylate) 20mg/mL [vial]

CONTRAINDICATIONS: Recent acute myocardial infarction (MI), uncompensated HF, or known history of QT prolongation (including congenital long QT syndrome). Concomitant dofetilide, sotalol, quinidine, other Class IA/III antiarrhythmics, mesoridazine, thioridazine, chlorpromazine, droperidol, pimozide, sparfloxacin, gatifloxacin, moxifloxacin, halofantrine, mefloquine, pentamidine, arsenic trioxide, levomethadyl acetate, dolasetron mesylate, probucol, tacrolimus, and other drugs that prolong QT interval.

WARNINGS/PRECAUTIONS: Avoid in patients with history of cardiac arrhythmias. D/C in patients with persistent QTc measurements >500 msec. Hypokalemia and/or hypomagnesemia may increase risk of QT prolongation and arrhythmia; replete those electrolytes before treatment. Initiate further evaluation if symptoms of torsades de pointes (eg, dizziness, palpitations, syncope) occur. Neuroleptic malignant syndrome (NMS) reported; d/c therapy and institute symptomatic treatment. May cause tardive dyskinesia (TD), especially in the elderly; d/c if this occurs. Hyperglycemia, in some cases extreme and associated with ketoacidosis or hyperosmolar coma or death, reported; monitor glucose control regularly in patients with diabetes mellitus (DM) and FPG in patients at risk for DM. Rash and/or urticaria reported; d/c upon appearance of rash. May induce orthostatic hypotension and syncope; caution with CV disease, cerebrovascular disease, or conditions that predispose to hypotension. Leukopenia, neutropenia, and agranulocytosis reported; d/c in patients with severe neutropenia (absolute neutrophil counts <1000/mm³) or at 1st sign of decline in WBCs. Seizures reported; caution with history of seizures or conditions that lower seizure threshold. May cause esophageal dysmotility and aspiration; caution in patients at risk for aspiration pneumonia. May elevate prolactin levels. May impair physical/mental abilities. Somnolence and priapism reported. May disrupt the body's ability to reduce core body temperature. Caution with those at risk for suicide and in elderly patients. Caution with renal impairment when administered IM. Concomitant use of IM and oral preparations in schizophrenic patients is not recommended.

ADVERSE REACTIONS: N/V, dyspepsia, diarrhea, somnolence, dizziness, headache, extrapyramidal symptoms, respiratory tract infection, akathisia, abnormal vision, asthenia.

INTERACTIONS: See Contraindications. Caution with centrally acting drugs and medications with anticholinergic activity. May enhance effects of certain antihypertensives. May antagonize effects of levodopa and dopamine agonists. Decreased levels with carbamazepine. Increased levels with CYP3A4 inhibitors (eg, ketoconazole). Periodically monitor serum electrolytes with diuretics.

PREGNANCY: Category C, not for use in nursing.

MECHANISM OF ACTION: Benzisoxazole derivative; not established. Proposed that efficacy in schizophrenia is mediated through a combination of dopamine type 2 and serotonin type 2 antagonism.

PHARMACOKINETICS: Absorption: (PO) Well-absorbed. Absolute bioavailability (60%); T_{max}=6-8 hrs. (IM) Absolute bioavailability (100%); T_{max}=60 min. **Distribution:** (PO) V_d=1.5L/kg; plasma protein binding (>99%). **Metabolism:** (PO) Liver (extensive) via aldehyde oxidase (primary), CYP3A4 and CYP1A2; benzisothiazole (BITP) sulphoxide, BITP-sulphone, ziprasidone sulphoxide, and S-methyl-dihydroziprasidone (major metabolites). **Elimination:** (PO) Urine (20%, <1% unchanged) and feces (66%, <4% unchanged); $T_{1/2}$=7 hrs. (IM) $T_{1/2}$=2-5 hrs.

NURSING CONSIDERATIONS

Assessment: Assess for history of QT prolongation, recent acute MI, uncompensated HF, dementia-related psychosis, and other conditions where treatment is cautioned. Assess for drug hypersensitivity, pregnancy/nursing status and possible drug interactions. Obtain baseline serum electrolytes (K⁺, Mg²⁺) in patients at risk for significant electrolyte disturbances. Obtain baseline FPG in patients with DM or at risk for DM. Obtain baseline CBC if at risk for leukopenia/neutropenia.

Monitoring: Monitor for QT prolongation, torsades de pointes, NMS, TD, rash, orthostatic hypotension, seizures, esophageal dysmotility, aspiration, suicidal ideation, hypokalemia, hypomagnesemia, and other adverse effects. Monitor CBC frequently in patients with preexisting low WBCs or history of drug-induced leukopenia/neutropenia. Monitor for fever or other signs/symptoms of infection in patients with neutropenia. Monitor FPG in patients with DM or at risk for DM. Reassess periodically to determine need for maintenance treatment.

Patient Counseling: Inform of the risks and benefits of therapy. Advise to inform healthcare providers of any history of QT prolongation, recent acute MI, uncompensated HF, risk for electrolyte abnormalities, history of cardiac arrhythmia, or if taking other QT prolonging drugs. Instruct to report conditions that increase risk for electrolyte disturbances (eg, hypokalemia, taking diuretics, prolonged diarrhea) and if dizziness, palpitations, or syncope occurs.

Administration: Oral/IM route. Take caps with food. (Inj) Refer to PI for preparation for administration instructions. **Storage:** (Cap) 25°C (77°F); excursions permitted to 15-30°C (59-86°F). (Inj) Dry form: 25°C (77°F); excursions permitted to 15-30°C (59-86°F). Protect from light. Reconstituted: 15-30°C (59-86°F) for up to 24 hrs when protected from light or refrigerated at 2-8°C (36-46°F) for up to 7 days.

GIAZO   RX
balsalazide disodium (Salix)

THERAPEUTIC CLASS: 5-aminosalicylic acid derivative

INDICATIONS: Treatment of mildly to moderately active ulcerative colitis in male patients ≥18 yrs of age.

DOSAGE: *Adults:* ≥18 Yrs: 3 tabs bid (6.6g/day) for up to 8 weeks.

HOW SUPPLIED: Tab: 1.1g

WARNINGS/PRECAUTIONS: Associated with acute intolerance syndrome (eg, cramping, acute abdominal pain and bloody diarrhea, fever, headache, and rash) that may be difficult to distinguish from exacerbation of ulcerative colitis; observe closely for worsening of symptoms and d/c therapy if acute intolerance syndrome is suspected. Renal impairment, including minimal change nephropathy, acute/chronic interstitial nephritis, and renal failure, reported; evaluate renal function prior to initiation and periodically while on therapy. Caution with known renal dysfunction or history of renal disease. Hepatic failure reported in patients with preexisting liver disease; use caution and consider LFTs in patients with liver disease. Caution in elderly; closely monitor blood cell counts during therapy.

ADVERSE REACTIONS: Headache, nasopharyngitis, anemia, diarrhea, fatigue, pharyngolaryngeal pain, urinary tract infection, GI disorders.

PREGNANCY: Category B, caution in nursing.

MECHANISM OF ACTION: 5-aminosalicylic acid (5-ASA) derivative; has not been established. Prodrug of mesalamine; action appears to be local to the colonic mucosa rather than systemic. Suspected to diminish inflammation by blocking production of arachidonic acid metabolites in the colon.

PHARMACOKINETICS: Absorption: Different dosing conditions (fed/fasted, single/repeated doses) resulted in different parameters. **Distribution:** Plasma protein binding (≥99% balsalazide, 43% 5-ASA, 78% N-Ac-5-ASA); crosses placenta. **Metabolism:** Bacterial azoreduction and acetylation; 5-ASA, N-Ac-5-ASA (metabolites). **Elimination:** Urine (23%, 0.16% unchanged); $T_{1/2}$=1.9 hrs (balsalazide), 9.5 hrs (5-ASA), 10.5 hrs (N-Ac-5-ASA).

NURSING CONSIDERATIONS

Assessment: Assess for hypersensitivity to salicylates, aminosalicylates, or their metabolites, and renal/hepatic function.

Monitoring: Monitor for signs/symptoms of acute intolerance syndrome, renal/hepatic impairment, and other adverse reactions. Monitor blood cell counts in elderly.

Patient Counseling: Instruct not to take drug if hypersensitive to salicylates (eg, aspirin). Advise patients who need to control Na⁺ intake that the recommended dosing of 6.6g/day provides about 756mg of Na⁺/day. Instruct to contact physician if worsening of ulcerative colitis symptoms is experienced. Instruct to inform physician if they have or are later diagnosed with renal dysfunction and/or liver disease.

Administration: Oral route. Take with or without food. **Storage:** 20-25°C (68-77°F); excursions permitted between 15-30°C (59-86°F).

GLEEVEC

RX

imatinib mesylate (Novartis)

THERAPEUTIC CLASS: Protein-tyrosine kinase inhibitor

INDICATIONS: Treatment of newly diagnosed patients with Philadelphia chromosome-positive (Ph+) chronic myeloid leukemia (CML) in chronic phase. *Adults:* Treatment of Ph+ CML in blast crisis, accelerated phase, or in chronic phase after failure of interferon-α therapy. Treatment of relapsed or refractory Ph+ acute lymphoblastic leukemia (ALL). Treatment of myelodysplastic/myeloproliferative diseases (MDS/MPD) associated with platelet-derived growth factor receptor (PDGFR) gene rearrangements. Treatment of aggressive systemic mastocytosis (ASM) patients without the D816V c-Kit mutation or with unknown c-Kit mutational status. Treatment of hypereosinophilic syndrome (HES) and/or chronic eosinophilic leukemia (CEL) patients who have the FIP1L1-PDGFRα fusion kinase (mutational analysis or FISH demonstration of CHIC2 allele deletion) and for patients with HES and/or CEL who are FIP1L1-PDGFRα fusion kinase-negative or unknown. Treatment of unresectable, recurrent, and/or metastatic dermatofibrosarcoma protuberans (DFSP). Treatment of patients with Kit (CD117)-positive unresectable and/or metastatic malignant GI stromal tumors (GIST). Adjuvant treatment of patients following complete gross resection of Kit (CD117)-positive GIST. *Pediatrics:* Treatment of newly diagnosed Ph+ ALL in combination with chemotherapy.

DOSAGE: *Adults:* CML: Chronic Phase: Usual: 400mg qd. Titrate: May increase to 600mg qd if conditions permit. See PI. Accelerated Phase/Blast Crisis: Usual: 600mg qd. Titrate: May increase to 400mg bid if conditions permit. See PI. Relapsed/Refractory Ph+ ALL: 600mg qd. MDS or MPD/ASM without D816V c-Kit Mutation or with Unknown c-Kit Mutational Status Not Responding Satisfactorily to Other Therapies/HES and/or CEL: 400mg qd. ASM with Eosinophilia/HES or CEL with FIP1L1-PDGFRα: Initial: 100mg qd. Titrate: May increase to 400mg qd in the absence of adverse reactions and presence of insufficient response. DFSP: 800mg/day (as 400mg bid). Unresectable and/or Metastatic Malignant GIST: Usual: 400mg qd. Titrate: May increase to 400mg bid if signs/symptoms of disease progression at a lower dose are clear and in the absence of severe adverse reactions. Adjuvant Treatment after Complete Gross Resection of GIST: 400mg qd for 3 yrs. Concomitant Strong CYP3A4 Inducers: Avoid concomitant use. If coadministration is necessary, increase dose by at least 50% and carefully monitor response. Severe Hepatic Impairment: Reduce dose by 25%. Moderate Renal Impairment (CrCl 20-39mL/min): Initial: Reduce dose by 50%. Titrate: Increase as tolerated. Max: 400mg. Mild Renal Impairment (CrCl 40-59mL/min): Max: 600mg. Severe Renal Impairment: Use with caution. Hepatotoxicity/Nonhematologic Adverse Reaction: If bilirubin >3X ULN or transaminases >5X ULN, withhold therapy until bilirubin <1.5X ULN and transaminases <2.5X ULN. Continue at reduced dose. Severe Nonhematologic Adverse Reaction: Withhold therapy until the event has resolved. Resume as appropriate, depending on initial severity of event. Neutropenia/Thrombocytopenia: See PI for dosage adjustments. Take with food and a large glass of water. *Pediatrics:* ≥1 Yr: Ph+ CML: Usual: 340mg/m² qd or split into 2 doses (am and pm). Max: 600mg. Ph+ ALL: Usual: 340mg/m² qd. Max: 600mg. Concomitant Strong CYP3A4 Inducers: Avoid concomitant use. If coadministration is necessary, increase dose by at least 50% and carefully monitor response. Severe Hepatic Impairment: Reduce dose by 25%. Moderate Renal Impairment (CrCl 20-39mL/min): Initial: Reduce dose by 50%. Titrate: Increase as tolerated. Max: 400mg. Mild Renal Impairment (CrCl 40-59mL/min): Max: 600mg. Severe Renal Impairment: Use with caution. Hepatotoxicity/Nonhematologic Adverse Reaction: If bilirubin >3X ULN or transaminases >5X ULN, withhold therapy until bilirubin <1.5X ULN and transaminases <2.5X ULN. Reduce dose to 260mg/m²/day. Severe Nonhematologic Adverse Reaction: Withhold therapy until the event has resolved. Resume as appropriate, depending on initial severity of event. Neutropenia/Thrombocytopenia: See PI for dosage adjustments. Take with food and a large glass of water.

HOW SUPPLIED: Tab: 100mg*, 400mg* *scored

WARNINGS/PRECAUTIONS: Edema and serious fluid retention reported. Hematologic toxicity (eg, anemia/neutropenia/thrombocytopenia) reported; monitor CBC weekly for 1st month, biweekly for 2nd month, and periodically thereafter as clinically indicated. Severe congestive heart failure (CHF) and left ventricular dysfunction reported; carefully monitor patients with cardiac disease or risk factors for cardiac failure or history of renal failure, and evaluate/treat any patient with cardiac or renal failure. Hepatotoxicity may occur; monitor LFTs before initiation of treatment and monthly, or as clinically indicated. Hemorrhages reported; monitor for GI symptoms at the start of therapy as GI tumor sites may be the source of GI hemorrhages. GI irritation/perforation reported. In patients with HES with occult infiltration of HES cells within the myocardium, cases of cardiogenic shock/left ventricular dysfunction have been associated with HES cell degranulation upon initiation of therapy; reversible with administration of systemic steroids, circulatory support measures, and temporarily withholding treatment. Consider performance of echocardiogram and determination of serum troponin in patients with HES/CEL, MDS/MPD or ASM associated with high eosinophil levels; if either is abnormal, consider prophylactic use of systemic steroids (1-2mg/kg) for 1-2 weeks concomitantly at initiation of therapy. Bullous dermatologic reactions, including erythema multiforme and Stevens-Johnson syndrome, reported. May cause fetal harm; sexually active female patients of reproductive potential should use highly effective contraception. Growth retardation reported in children and preadolescents; closely monitor growth. Tumor lysis syndrome (TLS) reported in patients with CML, GIST, ALL, and eosinophilic leukemia; caution in patients at risk of TLS (those with tumors with high proliferative rate or high tumor burden prior to treatment), and correct clinically significant dehydration and treat high uric acid levels prior to initiation of treatment. May impair mental/physical abilities.

ADVERSE REACTIONS: N/V, edema, muscle cramps, musculoskeletal pain, diarrhea, rash, fatigue, headache, asthenia, abdominal pain, hemorrhage, malaise, neutropenia, anemia, anorexia.

INTERACTIONS: See Dosage. Increased levels with CYP3A4 inhibitors; caution with strong CYP3A4 inhibitors (eg, ketoconazole, nefazodone, clarithromycin, itraconazole), and avoid with grapefruit juice. Decreased levels with rifampin, St. John's wort, and enzyme-inducing antiepileptic drugs (eg, carbamazepine, phenytoin, phenobarbital, primidone); consider alternative therapeutic agents with less enzyme induction potential in patients when CYP3A4 inducers are indicated. Increases levels of simvastatin, metoprolol, and CYP3A4 metabolized drugs (eg, dihydropyridine calcium channel blockers, triazolo-benzodiazepines, certain HMG-CoA reductase inhibitors); caution with CYP3A4/CYP2D6 substrates that have a narrow therapeutic window (eg, alfentanil, cyclosporine, dihydroergotamine, ergotamine, fentanyl, quinidine, sirolimus, tacrolimus, pimozide). Switch from warfarin to low molecular weight or standard heparin if anticoagulation is required during therapy. Inhibits acetaminophen O-glucuronidate pathway in vitro. When concomitantly used with chemotherapy, liver toxicity reported; monitor hepatic function. Hypothyroidism reported in thyroidectomy patients undergoing levothyroxine replacement; closely monitor TSH levels.

PREGNANCY: Category D, not for use in nursing.

MECHANISM OF ACTION: Protein-tyrosine kinase inhibitor; inhibits the bcr-abl tyrosine kinase, the constitutive abnormal tyrosine kinase created by the Philadelphia chromosome abnormality in CML. Inhibits proliferation and induces apoptosis in bcr-abl-positive cell lines as well as fresh leukemic cells from Ph+ CML. Inhibits the receptor tyrosine kinases for PDGF and stem cell factor (SCF), c-kit, and inhibits PDGF- and SCF-mediated cellular events. Inhibits proliferation and induces apoptosis in GIST cells, which express an activating c-Kit mutation, in vitro.

PHARMACOKINETICS: Absorption: Well-absorbed. Absolute bioavailability (98%); T_{max}=2-4 hrs. **Distribution:** Plasma protein binding (95%); found in breast milk. **Metabolism:** Liver via CYP3A4 (major), CYP1A2, CYP2D6, CYP2C9, CYP2C19 (minor); N-demethylated piperazine derivative (major active metabolite). **Elimination:** Feces (68%, 20% unchanged); urine (13%, 5% unchanged); (healthy) $T_{1/2}$=18 hrs (imatinib), 40 hrs (active metabolite).

NURSING CONSIDERATIONS

Assessment: Assess for cardiac disease, renal impairment, dehydration, high uric acid levels, pregnancy/nursing status, and possible drug interactions. Perform echocardiogram and determine troponin levels in patients with HES/CEL and with MDS/MPD or ASM associated with high eosinophil levels. Obtain CBC and LFTs.

Monitoring: Monitor for signs and symptoms of fluid retention, CHF, left ventricular dysfunction, hemorrhage, GI disorders, TLS, bullous dermatologic reactions, and other adverse events. Perform CBC weekly for the 1st month, biweekly for the 2nd month, and periodically thereafter. Monitor LFTs monthly or as clinically indicated. Monitor growth in children, and TSH levels in thyroidectomy patients undergoing levothyroxine replacement.

Patient Counseling: Instruct to take drug exactly as prescribed and not to change the dose or to stop taking medication unless told to do so by physician. Advise women of reproductive potential to avoid becoming pregnant and to notify physician if pregnant. Instruct sexually active females to use highly effective contraception. Instruct not to breastfeed while on therapy. Advise to contact physician if experiencing any side effects during therapy (eg, fever, SOB, blood in the stools, jaundice, sudden weight gain, symptoms of cardiac failure) or if patient has a history of cardiac disease or risk factors for cardiac failure. Counsel not to take any other medications, including OTC (eg, herbal products), without consulting physician. Advise that growth retardation has been reported in children and preadolescents, and that growth should be monitored. Inform that undesirable effects (eg, dizziness, blurred vision, somnolence) may occur; caution about driving a car or operating machinery.

Administration: Oral route. Take with food and a large glass of water. If unable to swallow tab, disperse in a glass of water or apple juice; required number of tab should be placed in the appropriate volume of beverage (approximately 50mL for 100mg tab and 200mL for 400mg tab); stir with a spoon and administer sus immediately after complete disintegration of tab. Do not crush tab. Avoid direct contact of crushed tab with the skin or mucous membranes; wash thoroughly as outlined in the references if contact occurs. Avoid exposure to crushed tab. **Storage:** 25°C (77°F); excursions permitted to 15-30°C (59-86°F). Protect from moisture.

GLUCAGON   RX
glucagon, rdna origin (Lilly)

THERAPEUTIC CLASS: Glucagon

INDICATIONS: Treatment for severe hypoglycemia. Diagnostic aid for radiologic examination of the stomach, duodenum, small bowel, and colon when diminished intestinal motility would be advantageous.

DOSAGE: *Adults:* Severe Hypoglycemia: ≥20kg: 1mg (1 U) SQ/IM/IV. After 15 min, may give additional dose if response is delayed, however seek an emergency aid so that parenteral glucose can be given. Give supplemental carbohydrate after the patient responds to treatment. Diagnostic Aid: Stomach/Duodenum/Small Bowel: 0.25-0.5mg (0.25-0.5 U) IV, or 1mg (1 U) IM, or 2mg (2 U) IV/IM before procedure. Colon Relaxation: 2mg (2 U) IM 10 min before procedure. Elderly: Start at lower end of dosing range.
Pediatrics: Severe Hypoglycemia: ≥20kg: 1mg (1 U) SQ/IM/IV. <20kg: 0.5mg (0.5 U) or dose equivalent to 20-30mcg/kg. After 15 min, may give additional dose if response is delayed, however seek an emergency aid so that parenteral glucose can be given. Give supplemental carbohydrate after the patient responds to treatment.

HOW SUPPLIED: Inj: 1mg/mL (1 U/mL)

CONTRAINDICATIONS: Pheochromocytoma.

WARNINGS/PRECAUTIONS: Caution with a history suggestive of insulinoma and/or pheochromocytoma. In patients with insulinoma, IV glucagon may produce an initial increase in blood glucose and then subsequently cause hypoglycemia. In the presence of pheochromocytoma, may cause the tumor to release catecholamines, which may result in a sudden and marked increase in BP. Generalized allergic reactions (eg, urticaria, respiratory distress, and hypotension) reported. Effective in treating hypoglycemia only if sufficient liver glycogen is present. Little or no help in states of starvation, adrenal insufficiency, or chronic hypoglycemia; treat with glucose.

ADVERSE REACTIONS: N/V, allergic reactions, urticaria, respiratory distress, hypotension.

INTERACTIONS: Addition of an anticholinergic during diagnostic examination may increase side effects.

PREGNANCY: Category B, caution in nursing.

MECHANISM OF ACTION: Glucagon; polypeptide hormone that increases blood glucose levels and relaxes smooth muscle of the GI tract.

PHARMACOKINETICS: Absorption: (SQ) C_{max}=7.9ng/mL, T_{max}=20 min; (IM) C_{max}=6.9ng/mL, T_{max}=13 min. **Distribution:** V_d=0.25L/kg (1mg dose). **Metabolism:** Extensively degraded in liver, kidneys, plasma. **Elimination:** $T_{1/2}$=8-18 min (1mg dose).

NURSING CONSIDERATIONS

Assessment: Assess if patient is in state of starvation, has adrenal insufficiency or chronic hypoglycemia. Assess for history suggestive of insulinoma and/or pheochromocytoma, pregnancy/nursing status, and possible drug interactions.

Monitoring: Monitor for signs/symptoms of an allergic reaction, HTN, and hypoglycemia. Monitor blood glucose levels in patients with hypoglycemia until asymptomatic.

Patient Counseling: Instruct patient and family members, in event of emergency, how to properly prepare and administer glucagon. Inform about measures to prevent hypoglycemia; including following a uniform regimen on a regular basis, careful adjustment of the insulin program, frequent testing of blood or urine for glucose, and routinely carrying hyperglycemic agents to quickly elevate blood glucose levels (eg, sugar, candy, readily absorbed carbohydrates). Inform about symptoms of hypoglycemia and how to treat it appropriately. Inform caregivers that if patient is hypoglycemic, patient should be kept alert and hypoglycemia should be treated as quickly as possible to prevent CNS damage. Advise to inform physician when hypoglycemia occurs.

Administration: IM/IV/SQ routes. Use immediately after reconstitution; discard any unused portion. Refer to PI for further instructions and directions for use. **Storage:** Before reconstitution: 20-25°C (68-77°F); excursions allowed between 15-30°C (59-86°F).

GLUCOPHAGE XR

RX

metformin HCI (Bristol-Myers Squibb)

Lactic acidosis reported (rare); increased risk with increased age, diabetes mellitus (DM), renal dysfunction, congestive heart failure (CHF), and conditions with risk of hypoperfusion and hypoxemia. Avoid use in patients ≥80 yrs of age unless renal function is normal. Withhold therapy in the presence of any condition associated with hypoxemia, dehydration, or sepsis. Avoid with clinical or lab evidence of hepatic disease. Caution against excessive alcohol intake; may potentiate the effects of metformin on lactate metabolism. Temporarily d/c prior to any IV radiocontrast study or surgical procedures. D/C use and institute appropriate therapy if lactic acidosis occurs.

OTHER BRAND NAMES: Glucophage (Bristol-Myers Squibb)

THERAPEUTIC CLASS: Biguanide

INDICATIONS: Adjunct to diet and exercise to improve glycemic control in type 2 DM.

DOSAGE: *Adults:* Individualize dose. (Tab) Initial: 500mg bid or 850mg qd with meals. Titrate: Increase by 500mg/week or 850mg every 2 weeks, up to a total of 2000mg/day given in divided doses, or may increase from 500mg bid to 850mg bid after 2 weeks. Patients Requiring Additional Glycemic Control: Max: 2550mg/day. With Insulin: Initial: 500mg qd. Titrate: Increase by 500mg/week. Max: 2500mg/day. Decrease insulin dose by 10-25% when FPG <120mg/dL. Give in 3 divided doses with meals if dose is >2g/day. (Tab, ER) Initial: ≥17 Yrs: 500mg qd with pm meal. Titrate: Increase by 500mg/week. Max: 2000mg/day. With Insulin: Initial: 500mg qd. Titrate: Increase by 500mg/week. Max: 2000mg/day. Decrease insulin dose by 10-25% when FPG <120mg/dL. Elderly/Debilitated/Malnourished: Dose conservatively; do not titrate to max. *Pediatrics:* 10-16 Yrs: (Tab) Individualize dose. Initial: 500mg bid with meals. Titrate: Increase by 500mg/week. Max: 2000mg/day, given in divided doses.

HOW SUPPLIED: Tab: (Glucophage) 500mg, 850mg, 1000mg; Tab, Extended-Release (ER): (Glucophage XR) 500mg, 750mg

CONTRAINDICATIONS: Renal disease/dysfunction (eg, SrCr ≥1.5mg/dL [males], ≥1.4mg/dL [females], or abnormal CrCl), acute or chronic metabolic acidosis, diabetic ketoacidosis with or without coma. D/C temporarily (48 hrs) for radiologic studies with intravascular iodinated contrast materials.

WARNINGS/PRECAUTIONS: D/C therapy if conditions associated with lactic acidosis and characterized by hypoxemia states (eg, acute CHF, cardiovascular [CV] collapse, acute myocardial infarction [MI]), or prerenal azotemia develop. D/C therapy if temporary loss of glycemic control occurs due to stress; temporarily give insulin and reinstitute after acute episode is resolved. May decrease serum vitamin B12 levels. Increased risk of hypoglycemia in elderly, debilitated/malnourished, with adrenal or pituitary insufficiency, or alcohol intoxication. Consider therapeutic alternatives, including initiation of insulin, if secondary failure occurs. Caution in elderly.

ADVERSE REACTIONS: Lactic acidosis, diarrhea, N/V, flatulence, asthenia, abdominal discomfort, hypoglycemia, dizziness, dyspnea, taste disorder, chest discomfort, flu syndrome, palpitations, indigestion.

INTERACTIONS: See Boxed Warning and Contraindications. May increase levels with furosemide, nifedipine, cimetidine, cationic drugs (eg, digoxin, amiloride, procainamide, quinidine, quinine, ranitidine, trimethoprim, vancomycin, triamterene, morphine). Observe for loss of glycemic control with thiazides, other diuretics, corticosteroids, phenothiazines, thyroid products, estrogens, oral contraceptives, phenytoin, nicotinic acid, sympathomimetics, calcium channel blockers, and isoniazid. May interact with highly protein-bound drugs (eg, salicylates, sulfonamides, chloramphenicol, probenecid). May decrease furosemide, glyburide levels. Caution with drugs that may affect renal function or result in significant hemodynamic change or may interfere with the disposition of metformin. Hypoglycemia may occur with concomitant use of other glucose-lowering agents (eg, sulfonylureas, insulin). May overlap drug effects when transferred from chlorpropamide. Hypoglycemia may be difficult to recognize with β-adrenergic blocking drugs.

PREGNANCY: Category B, not for use in nursing.

MECHANISM OF ACTION: Biguanide; decreases hepatic glucose production and intestinal absorption of glucose, and improves insulin sensitivity by increasing peripheral glucose uptake and utilization.

PHARMACOKINETICS: Absorption: (Tab) Absolute bioavailability (50-60%); (Tab, ER) T_{max}=7 hrs. Administration of different doses resulted in different parameters. **Distribution:** (Tab) V_d=654L. **Elimination:** Urine (90%); $T_{1/2}$=6.2 hrs (plasma), 17.6 hrs (blood).

NURSING CONSIDERATIONS

Assessment: Assess for renal/hepatic impairment, acute/chronic metabolic acidosis, presence of a hypoxic state (eg, acute CHF, acute MI, CV collapse), dehydration, sepsis, alcoholism, nutritional status, adrenal/pituitary insufficiency, pregnancy/nursing status, and for possible drug interactions. Assess baseline renal function, FPG, HbA1c, and hematological parameters (Hct, Hgb, RBC indices).

Monitoring: Monitor for lactic/metabolic acidosis, ketoacidosis, hypoglycemia, hypoxemia (eg, CV collapse, acute CHF, acute MI), prerenal azotemia, and for decreases in vitamin B12 levels. Monitor FPG, HbA1c, renal function (eg, SrCr, CrCl), and hematological parameters (eg, Hgb, Hct, RBC indices).

Patient Counseling: Inform of the potential risks and benefits of therapy. Inform about the importance of adherence to dietary instructions and a regular exercise program. Inform of the risk of developing lactic acidosis during therapy; advise to d/c therapy immediately and contact physician if unexplained hyperventilation, myalgia, malaise, unusual somnolence, or other nonspecific symptoms occur. Instruct to avoid excessive alcohol intake. Counsel to take tab with meals and tab ER with pm meal. Instruct that ER tab must be swallowed whole and not crushed or chewed.

Administration: Oral route. (Tab, ER) Must be swallowed whole; do not crush or chew. **Storage:** 20-25°C (68-77°F); excursions permitted to 15-30°C (59-86°F).

GLUCOTROL RX G
glipizide (Roerig)

THERAPEUTIC CLASS: Sulfonylurea (2nd generation)

INDICATIONS: Adjunct to diet and exercise to improve glycemic control in adults with type 2 diabetes mellitus (DM).

DOSAGE: *Adults:* Administer 30 min ac. Initial: 5mg qd; 2.5mg qd in elderly/with liver disease. Titrate: Adjust dose in increments of 2.5-5mg; several days should elapse between titration steps. May divide dose if response to single dose is not satisfactory. Maint: Doses >15mg/day should be divided and given ac of adequate caloric content. Max QD Dose: 15mg. Max Total Daily Dose: 40mg. Switching from Insulin: Insulin Dose: >20 U/day: Reduce insulin dose by 50% and begin therapy at usual dose. Subsequent insulin dose reductions should depend on individual patient response. ≤20 U/day: May d/c insulin and start therapy at usual dose. Coadministration with Colesevelam: Administer at least 4 hrs prior to colesevelam. Elderly/Debilitated/Malnourished/Renal or Hepatic Impairment: Initial/Maint: Dose conservatively.

HOW SUPPLIED: Tab: 5mg*, 10mg* *scored

CONTRAINDICATIONS: Type 1 DM or diabetic ketoacidosis, with or without coma.

WARNINGS/PRECAUTIONS: Caution during first 1-2 weeks of therapy if transferring from longer $T_{1/2}$ sulfonylureas (eg, chlorpropamide). Consider hospitalization during the insulin withdrawal period if patient has been receiving >40 U/day of insulin. May be associated with increased risk of cardiovascular mortality. May produce severe hypoglycemia; increased risk in the elderly, debilitated, or malnourished patients; with renal/hepatic impairment, or adrenal/pituitary insufficiency; when caloric intake is deficient; or after severe/prolonged exercise. Loss of glycemic control may occur when exposed to stress (eg, fever, trauma, infection, surgery); may be necessary to d/c therapy and administer insulin. Secondary failure may occur over time. May cause hemolytic anemia; caution with G6PD deficiency and consider a non-sulfonylurea alternative. Caution in elderly.

ADVERSE REACTIONS: Hypoglycemia, GI disturbances, dizziness, drowsiness, headache, porphyria cutanea tarda, photosensitivity reactions, leukopenia, agranulocytosis, thrombocytopenia, hemolytic anemia.

INTERACTIONS: See Dosage. Hypoglycemic effects may be potentiated by NSAIDs, some azoles, other highly protein-bound drugs, salicylates, sulfonamides, chloramphenicol, probenecid, coumarins, MAOIs, and β-blockers; monitor closely for hypoglycemia during coadministration and for loss of glycemic control when such drugs are withdrawn. Potential interaction leading to severe hypoglycemia reported with oral miconazole. Fluconazole may increase levels. Thiazides and other diuretics, corticosteroids, phenothiazines, thyroid products, estrogens, oral contraceptives, phenytoin, nicotinic acid, sympathomimetics, calcium channel blockers, and isoniazid may produce hyperglycemia and may lead to loss of glycemic control; monitor closely for loss of control during coadministration and for hypoglycemia when such drugs are withdrawn. Increased likelihood of hypoglycemia with alcohol and use of >1 glucose-lowering drug. May be difficult to recognize hypoglycemia with β-blockers. Caution with salicylate or dicumarol. Colesevelam may reduce levels.

PREGNANCY: Category C, not for use in nursing.

MECHANISM OF ACTION: Sulfonylurea (2nd generation); lowers blood glucose acutely by stimulating insulin release from pancreatic β cells.

PHARMACOKINETICS: **Absorption:** Rapid and complete. T_{max}=1-3 hrs. **Distribution:** Plasma protein binding (98-99%); (IV) V_d=11L. **Metabolism:** Liver (extensive). **Elimination:** Urine (<10% unchanged); $T_{1/2}$=2-4 hrs.

NURSING CONSIDERATIONS

Assessment: Assess for previous hypersensitivity to drug, renal/hepatic impairment, type of DM, diabetic ketoacidosis, risk factors for hypoglycemia, G6PD deficiency, pregnancy/nursing status, and possible drug interactions. Obtain baseline FPG and HbA1c levels.

Monitoring: Monitor for hypoglycemia, loss of glycemic control when exposed to stress, hypersensitivity reactions, secondary failure, hemolytic anemia, and other adverse reactions. Monitor blood/urine glucose and HbA1c levels periodically.

Patient Counseling: Inform of the risks, benefits, and alternative modes of therapy. Counsel about the importance of adherence to dietary instructions, regular exercise program, and regular testing of urine and/or blood glucose. Inform about the symptoms, treatment, and predisposing conditions of hypoglycemia, as well as primary and secondary failure. During the insulin withdrawal period, instruct to test for sugar and ketone bodies in urine at least tid and to contact physician immediately if these tests are abnormal.

Administration: Oral route. Take 30 min ac. **Storage:** <30°C (86°F).

GLUCOTROL XL RX
glipizide (Roerig)

THERAPEUTIC CLASS: Sulfonylurea (2nd generation)

INDICATIONS: Adjunct to diet and exercise to improve glycemic control in adults with type 2 diabetes mellitus (DM).

DOSAGE: *Adults:* Administer with breakfast. Initial: 5mg qd; may start at lower dose if sensitive to hypoglycemics. Titrate: Adjust dose based on laboratory measures of glycemic control. Maint: 5-10mg qd. Max: 20mg/day. Switching from Immediate-Release (IR) Glipizide: May give a qd dose at the nearest equivalent total daily dose or may titrate to ER starting with 5mg qd. Combination Therapy with Other Blood Glucose Lowering Agents: Initial: 5mg qd; may start at lower dose if sensitive to hypoglycemics. Titrate based on clinical judgment. Coadministration with Colesevelam: Administer at least 4 hrs prior to colesevelam. Switching from Insulin: Daily Insulin Requirement: >20 U/day: Reduce insulin dose by 50% and begin therapy at usual dose. Subsequent insulin dose reductions should depend on individual patient response. ≤20 U/day: May d/c insulin and start therapy at usual dose. Switching from Other Oral Hypoglycemics: No transition period necessary. Elderly/Debilitated/Malnourished/Renal or Hepatic Impairment: Initial/Maint: Dose conservatively.

HOW SUPPLIED: Tab, Extended-Release (ER): 2.5mg, 5mg, 10mg

CONTRAINDICATIONS: Type 1 DM, diabetic ketoacidosis, with or without coma.

WARNINGS/PRECAUTIONS: Patients being transferred from longer $T_{1/2}$ sulfonylureas (eg, chlorpropamide) may have overlapping drug effect; observe carefully (1-2 weeks) for hypoglycemia. Consider hospitalization during the insulin withdrawal period if patient has been receiving >40 U/day. May be associated with increased risk of cardiovascular mortality. Obstructive symptoms (rare) reported in patients with known strictures in association with ingestion of another non-deformable sustained release formulation; caution with preexisting severe GI narrowing (pathologic or iatrogenic). Markedly reduced GI retention times of the drug may influence clinical efficacy. May produce severe hypoglycemia; increased risk in the elderly, debilitated or malnourished patients; with renal/hepatic impairment, or adrenal/pituitary insufficiency; when caloric intake is deficient; or after severe/prolonged exercise. Loss of glycemic control may occur when exposed to stress (eg, fever, trauma, infection, surgery); may be necessary to d/c therapy and administer insulin. Secondary failure may occur over a period of time; assess adequacy of dose adjustment and adherence to diet. May cause hemolytic anemia; caution with G6PD deficiency and consider a non-sulfonylurea alternative.

ADVERSE REACTIONS: Hypoglycemia, asthenia, headache, dizziness, diarrhea, nervousness, tremor, flatulence.

INTERACTIONS: See Dosage. Hypoglycemic effects may be potentiated by NSAIDs and other highly protein-bound drugs, salicylates, sulfonamides, chloramphenicol, probenecid, coumarins, MAOIs, and β-blockers; monitor closely for hypoglycemia during coadministration and for loss of glycemic control during withdrawal of these drugs. Potential interaction leading to severe hypoglycemia reported with oral miconazole. Thiazides and other diuretics, corticosteroids, phenothiazines, thyroid products, estrogens, oral contraceptives, phenytoin, nicotinic acid, sympathomimetics, calcium channel blockers, and isoniazid may produce hyperglycemia and may lead to loss of glycemic control; monitor closely for loss of control during coadministration and for hypoglycemia during withdrawal of these drugs. Increased likelihood of hypoglycemia with alcohol and use of >1 glucose-lowering drug. May be difficult to recognize hypoglycemia with β-blockers. Caution with salicylate or dicumarol. Fluconazole may increase levels. Colesevelam may reduce levels.

PREGNANCY: Category C, not for use in nursing.

MECHANISM OF ACTION: Sulfonylurea (2nd generation); lowers blood glucose acutely by stimulating insulin release from pancreatic β cells. Also, increases insulin sensitivity and decreases hepatic glucose production.

PHARMACOKINETICS: Absorption: Rapid and complete (IR). (Single dose) Absolute bioavailability (100%); T_{max}=6-12 hrs. **Distribution:** V_d=10L; plasma protein binding (98-99%). **Metabolism:** Liver (primary); aromatic hydroxylation products (major metabolites); acetylamino-ethyl benzene derivative (minor metabolite). **Elimination:** Urine (80%, <10% unchanged), feces (10%, <10% unchanged); $T_{1/2}$=2-5 hrs.

NURSING CONSIDERATIONS

Assessment: Assess for previous hypersensitivity to drug, renal/hepatic impairment, type of DM, diabetic ketoacidosis, risk factors for hypoglycemia, severe GI narrowing, G6PD deficiency, pregnancy/nursing status, and for possible drug interactions. Obtain baseline FPG and HbA1c levels.

Monitoring: Monitor for hypoglycemia, loss of glycemic control when exposed to stress, hypersensitivity reactions, secondary failure, hemolytic anemia, and other adverse reactions. Monitor blood and urine glucose periodically and HbA1c levels every 3 months.

Patient Counseling: Inform of the risks, benefits, and alternative modes of therapy. Counsel not to be concerned if tab-like material is noticed in the stool. Inform about the importance of adherence to dietary instructions, of a regular exercise program, and of regular testing of urine and/ or blood glucose. Inform about the symptoms and treatment of hypoglycemia, the conditions that predispose to its development, as well as primary and secondary failure. During the insulin withdrawal period, instruct to test for sugar and ketone bodies in urine at least tid and to contact physician immediately if these tests are abnormal.

Administration: Oral route. Swallow tab whole; do not chew, divide, or crush. **Storage:** 15-30°C (59-86°F). Protect from moisture and humidity.

GLUCOVANCE   RX
metformin HCl - glyburide (Bristol-Myers Squibb)

> Lactic acidosis may occur due to metformin accumulation; risk increases with congestive heart failure (CHF), degree of renal dysfunction, and patient's age. Regularly monitor renal function and use the minimum effective dose of metformin. Do not initiate in patients ≥80 yrs of age unless measurement of CrCl demonstrates that renal function is not reduced. Promptly withhold therapy in the presence of any condition associated with hypoxemia, dehydration, or sepsis. Avoid with clinical or lab evidence of hepatic disease. Caution against excessive alcohol intake; alcohol potentiates the effects of metformin on lactate metabolism. Temporarily d/c therapy prior to any intravascular radiocontrast study and for any surgical procedure. D/C use immediately and promptly institute general supportive measures if lactic acidosis occurs. Prompt hemodialysis is recommended to correct the acidosis and remove the accumulated metformin.

THERAPEUTIC CLASS: Biguanide/sulfonylurea

INDICATIONS: Adjunct to diet and exercise to improve glycemic control in adults with type 2 diabetes mellitus.

DOSAGE: *Adults:* Individualize dose. Inadequate Glycemic Control on Diet and Exercise: Initial: 1.25mg-250mg qd with a meal; in patients with baseline HbA1c >9% or FPG >200mg/dL, may use 1.25mg-250mg bid with the am and pm meals. Titrate: Increase by 1.25mg-250mg/day every 2 weeks. Do not use 5mg-500mg as initial therapy. No experience with total doses >10mg-2000mg/day. Inadequate Glycemic Control on a Sulfonylurea and/or Metformin: Initial: 2.5mg-500mg or 5mg-500mg bid with the am and pm meals. Starting dose should not exceed the daily doses of glyburide (or equivalent dose of another sulfonylurea) or metformin already being taken. Titrate: Increase by no more than 5mg-500mg/day. Max: 20mg-2000mg/day. Addition of Thiazolidinediones to Therapy: A thiazolidinedione may be added to therapy if control is inadequate. Continue current dose of therapy, and initiate (and titrate if additional glycemic control is needed) thiazolidinedione as recommended; consider reducing dose of glyburide component if hypoglycemia develops, and adjust dosages of other components as clinically warranted. Coadministration with Colesevelam: Administer at least 4 hrs prior to colesevelam. Elderly: Initial/Maint: Dose conservatively. Elderly/Debilitated/Malnourished Patients: Do not titrate to max dose.

HOW SUPPLIED: Tab: (Glyburide-Metformin) 1.25mg-250mg, 2.5mg-500mg, 5mg-500mg

CONTRAINDICATIONS: Renal disease or dysfunction (eg, SrCr ≥1.5mg/dL [males], ≥1.4mg/dL [females], or abnormal CrCl), acute or chronic metabolic acidosis, including diabetic ketoacidosis, with or without coma. Coadministration with bosentan. Temporarily d/c in patients undergoing radiologic studies involving intravascular administration of iodinated contrast materials.

WARNINGS/PRECAUTIONS: May be associated with increased cardiovascular (CV) mortality. May cause hypoglycemia; increased risk when caloric intake is deficient, when strenuous exercise is not compensated by caloric supplementation, with renal/hepatic insufficiency, adrenal/pituitary insufficiency, alcohol intoxication, or in elderly, debilitated, or malnourished patients. Not recommended during pregnancy. Caution in elderly. Glyburide: May cause hemolytic anemia; caution with G6PD deficiency. Metformin: Assess renal function before initiation of therapy and at least annually thereafter; d/c with evidence of renal impairment. Temporarily d/c at the time of or prior to radiologic studies involving the use of intravascular iodinated contrast materials, withhold for 48 hrs subsequent to the procedure, and reinstitute only if renal function is normal. D/C promptly if CV collapse (shock), acute CHF, acute myocardial infarction, and other conditions characterized by hypoxemia occur. Temporarily suspend for any surgical procedure (except minor procedures not associated with restricted intake of food and fluids); restart when oral intake is resumed and renal function is normal. May decrease serum vitamin B12 levels; monitor hematological parameters annually. Caution in patients predisposed to developing subnormal vitamin B12 levels (eg, those with inadequate vitamin B12 or Ca^{2+} intake or absorption). Evaluate patients previously well controlled on therapy who develop laboratory abnormalities or clinical illness for evidence of ketoacidosis or lactic acidosis; d/c if acidosis occurs.

ADVERSE REACTIONS: Lactic acidosis, upper respiratory infection, N/V, abdominal pain, headache, dizziness, diarrhea.

INTERACTIONS: See Boxed Warning, Contraindications, and Dosage. Increased risk of hypoglycemia with other glucose-lowering agents or ethanol. May be difficult to recognize hypoglycemia with β-blockers. Thiazides and other diuretics, corticosteroids, phenothiazines, thyroid products, estrogens, oral contraceptives, phenytoin, nicotinic acid, sympathomimetics, calcium channel blockers, and isoniazid may produce hyperglycemia and may lead to loss of glycemic control; monitor closely for loss of control during coadministration and for hypoglycemia during withdrawal of these drugs. Weight gain observed with the addition of rosiglitazone to therapy. Monitor LFTs during coadministration with a thiazolidinedione. Metformin: Caution with drugs that may affect renal function or result in significant hemodynamic change or may interfere with the disposition of metformin (eg, cationic drugs eliminated by renal tubular secretion). Furosemide, nifedipine, and cimetidine may increase levels. May decrease furosemide levels. Cationic drugs that are eliminated by renal tubular secretion (eg, cimetidine, amiloride, digoxin, morphine, quinidine, vancomycin) may potentially produce an interaction; monitor and adjust dose of therapy and/or the interfering drug. Glyburide: Hypoglycemic effects may be potentiated by NSAIDs and other highly protein-bound drugs, salicylates, sulfonamides, chloramphenicol, probenecid, coumarins, MAOIs, and β-blockers; monitor closely for hypoglycemia during coadministration and for loss of glycemic control during withdrawal of these drugs. Possible interaction with ciprofloxacin (a fluoroquinolone antibiotic), resulting in potentiation of hypoglycemic action. Potential interaction leading to severe hypoglycemia reported with oral miconazole. Colesevelam may reduce levels.

PREGNANCY: Category B, not for use in nursing.

MECHANISM OF ACTION: Glyburide: Sulfonylurea; lower blood glucose acutely by stimulating release of insulin from the pancreas. Metformin: Biguanide; decreases hepatic glucose production, decreases intestinal absorption of glucose, and improves insulin sensitivity by increasing peripheral glucose uptake and utilization.

PHARMACOKINETICS: Absorption: Glyburide: T_{max}=4 hrs. Metformin: Absolute bioavailability (50-60%) (500mg); C_{max}=1.48mcg/mL (850mg single-dose); T_{max}=3.32 hrs (850mg single-dose). **Distribution:** Glyburide: plasma protein binding (extensive). Metformin: V_d=654L (850mg single-dose). **Metabolism:** Glyburide: metabolites: 4-trans-hydroxy derivative (major) and 3-cis hydroxy derivative. **Elimination:** Glyburide: Bile (50%, metabolites), urine (50%, metabolites); $T_{1/2}$=10 hrs. Metformin: Urine (90%); $T_{1/2}$=6.2 hrs (plasma), 17.6 hrs (blood).

NURSING CONSIDERATIONS

Assessment: Assess for metabolic acidosis, diabetic ketoacidosis, risk factors for lactic acidosis, renal/hepatic impairment, presence of malnourishment or debilitation, adrenal/pituitary insufficiency, alcoholism, G6PD deficiency, hypoxemia, inadequate vitamin B12 or Ca^{2+} intake/absorption, previous hypersensitivity to the drug, pregnancy/nursing status, and possible drug interactions. Assess if patient is planning to undergo any surgical procedure, or radiologic studies involving the use of intravascular iodinated contrast materials. Obtain baseline FPG and HbA1c levels, and hematologic parameters.

Monitoring: Monitor for signs/symptoms of lactic acidosis, CV effects, hypoglycemia, hemolytic anemia, and other adverse reactions. Monitor for changes in clinical status. Monitor renal function, especially in elderly, at least annually. Monitor hematological parameters annually. Perform routine serum vitamin B12 measurements at 2- to 3-yr intervals in patients predisposed to developing subnormal vitamin B12 levels. Monitor FPG and HbA1c levels periodically.

Patient Counseling: Inform of the risks, benefits, and alternative modes of therapy. Advise on the importance of adherence to dietary instructions, regular exercise program, and regular testing of blood glucose, HbA1c, renal function, and hematologic parameters. Inform of the risk of lactic acidosis; instruct to d/c therapy immediately and notify physician if unexplained hyperventilation, myalgia, malaise, unusual somnolence, or other nonspecific symptoms occur. Inform of the risk of hypoglycemia. Counsel against excessive alcohol intake.

Administration: Oral route. Take with meals. **Storage:** Up to 25°C (77°F).

GLUMETZA
metformin HCl (Depomed)

RX

> Lactic acidosis may occur due to metformin accumulation; increased risk with conditions such as sepsis, dehydration, excess alcohol intake, hepatic/renal impairment, and acute congestive heart failure (CHF). If acidosis is suspected, d/c and hospitalize patient immediately.

THERAPEUTIC CLASS: Biguanide

INDICATIONS: Adjunct to diet and exercise to improve glycemic control in adults with type 2 diabetes mellitus (DM).

DOSAGE: *Adults:* Individualize dose. Initial: 500mg qd. Titrate: May increase by 500mg no sooner than every 1-2 weeks if higher dose is needed and there are no GI adverse reactions. Max: 2000mg/day. Take with pm meal. Elderly: Start at lower end of dosing range.

HOW SUPPLIED: Tab, Extended-Release: 500mg, 1000mg

CONTRAINDICATIONS: Renal impairment (SrCr ≥1.5mg/dL [males], ≥1.4mg/dL [females], or abnormal CrCl), acute or chronic metabolic acidosis, including diabetic ketoacidosis.

WARNINGS/PRECAUTIONS: Not for treatment of type 1 diabetes or diabetic ketoacidosis. Verify renal function is normal prior to starting therapy and at least annually thereafter. Avoid use in patients ≥80 yrs unless renal function is not reduced. Avoid in hepatic impairment. D/C if conditions associated with hypoxemia, cardiovascular (CV) collapse, acute myocardial infarction (MI), acute CHF, or prerenal azotemia develop. Acute alteration of renal function and lactic acidosis reported with intravascular iodinated contrast materials (eg, IV urogram, IV cholangiography, angiography, and computed tomography); temporarily d/c at time of or prior to procedure, withhold for 48 hrs subsequent to procedure, and reinstitute only after renal function is normal. D/C prior to any surgical procedure necessitating restricted food/fluid intake; restart after oral intake resumed and renal function found to be normal. May decrease serum vitamin B12 levels; measure hematologic parameters annually. Increased risk of hypoglycemia in elderly, debilitated/malnourished, adrenal/pituitary insufficiency, and alcohol intoxication. Caution in elderly.

ADVERSE REACTIONS: Lactic acidosis (signs may include malaise, myalgia, respiratory distress, increasing somnolence, abdominal distress), hypoglycemia, diarrhea, nausea.

INTERACTIONS: Hypoglycemia may occur with other glucose-lowering agents (eg, sulfonylureas and insulin) or ethanol; may require lower doses of insulin secretagogues (eg, sulfonylurea) or insulin. Alcohol may potentiate effect on lactate metabolism; caution against excessive alcohol intake. Caution with medications that may affect renal function or result in significant hemodynamic change or may interfere with the disposition of metformin, such as cationic drugs (eg, amiloride, cimetidine, digoxin, morphine, procainamide, quinidine, quinine, ranitidine, triamterene, trimethoprim, or vancomycin) that are eliminated by renal tubular secretion; dosage adjustment recommended. Caution with topiramate or other carbonic anhydrase inhibitors (eg, zonisamide, acetazolamide or dichlorphenamide); may increase risk of lactic acidosis. Risk of hyperglycemia and loss of blood glucose control with thiazides and other diuretics, corticosteroids, phenothiazines, thyroid products, estrogens, oral contraceptives, phenytoin, nicotinic acid, sympathomimetics, calcium channel blockers, and isoniazid.

PREGNANCY: Category B, not for use in nursing.

MECHANISM OF ACTION: Biguanide; decreases hepatic glucose production, decreases intestinal absorption of glucose, and improves insulin sensitivity by increasing peripheral glucose uptake and utilization.

PHARMACOKINETICS: Absorption: T_{max}=7-8 hrs (1000mg, single dose). **Distribution:** V_d=654L (850mg immediate release, single dose). **Elimination:** Urine (90%, unchanged); $T_{1/2}$=6.2 hrs (plasma), 17.6 hrs (blood).

NURSING CONSIDERATIONS

Assessment: Assess for DM type, diabetic ketoacidosis, metabolic acidosis, sepsis, dehydration, excess alcohol intake, hepatic/renal impairment, CHF, hypoperfusion, hypoxemia, adequate vitamin B12 or Ca^{2+} intake/absorption, adrenal/pituitary insufficiency, caloric intake, general health status, pregnancy/nursing status, and possible drug interactions. Obtain baseline FPG, HbA1c, SrCr, CrCl, and LFTs. Evaluate for other medical/surgical conditions.

Monitoring: Monitor for hypoglycemia, lactic acidosis, malaise, myalgia, respiratory distress, somnolence, abdominal distress, hypoxemia, dehydration, sepsis, hypothermia, hypotension, resistant bradyarrhythmias, CV collapse, acute CHF, acute MI, or prerenal azotemia. Monitor renal/hepatic function, HbA1c, FPG, and hematologic parameters. Monitor serum vitamin B12 measurements at 2-3 yr intervals if inadequate B12 or Ca^{2+} intake/absorption.

Patient Counseling: Inform of the potential risks and benefits of the drug and of alternative modes of therapy. Counsel about the importance of adherence to dietary instructions, regular exercise program, regular testing of blood glucose, and HbA1c. Advise to seek medical advice during periods of stress (eg, fever, trauma, infection, surgery). Counsel about the risks/symptoms of, and conditions that predispose to the development of lactic acidosis. D/C and promptly seek medical attention if symptoms of unexplained hyperventilation, myalgia, malaise, unusual somnolence, or other nonspecific symptoms occur. Inform about the importance of regular testing of renal function and hematological parameters. Counsel against excessive alcohol intake, either acute or chronic, while on therapy. Inform that hypoglycemia may occur when used in conjunction with insulin secretagogues (eg, sulfonylureas and insulin). Instruct to swallow tab whole; do not crush or chew; if a dose is missed, do not take 2 doses of 2000mg the same day. Inactive ingredients may occasionally be eliminated in the feces as soft mass resembling the tab.

Administration: Oral route. Swallow whole; do not split, crush or chew. **Storage:** 20-25°C (68-77°F); excursions permitted to 15-30°C (59-86°F).

GLYNASE PRESTAB RX
glyburide (Pharmacia & Upjohn)

THERAPEUTIC CLASS: Sulfonylurea (2nd generation)

INDICATIONS: Adjunct to diet and exercise to improve glycemic control in adults with type 2 diabetes mellitus (DM).

DOSAGE: *Adults:* Determine the minimum effective dose. Initial: 1.5-3mg qd with breakfast or 1st main meal; 0.75mg qd if sensitive to hypoglycemic drugs. Maint: 0.75-12mg qd or in divided doses. Titrate: Increase in increments of ≤1.5mg at weekly intervals based on patient's response. Some patients receiving >6mg/day may have a more satisfactory response with bid dosage. Max: 12mg/day. Transfer from Other Oral Antidiabetic Agents: Retitrate. Initial: 1.5-3mg/day. Transfer from Chlorpropamide: Caution during the first 2 weeks of therapy. Switch from Insulin: Insulin Dose: >40 U/day: Decrease insulin dose by 50% and start with 3mg qd. Titrate: Progressively withdraw insulin and increase in increments of 0.75-1.5mg every 2-10 days. 20-40 U/day: 3mg qd. <20 U/day: 1.5-3mg qd. Concomitant Colesevelam: Administer at least 4 hrs prior to colesevelam. Concomitant Metformin: Add glyburide gradually to max dose of metformin monotherapy after 4 weeks. Titrate: Adjust dose of each drug to identify optimal dose to obtain desired glycemic control. Elderly/Debilitated/Malnourished/Renal or Hepatic Impairment: Initial/Maint: Dose conservatively.

HOW SUPPLIED: Tab: 1.5mg*, 3mg*, 6mg* *scored

CONTRAINDICATIONS: Type 1 DM, diabetic ketoacidosis with or without coma. Coadministration with bosentan.

WARNINGS/PRECAUTIONS: Associated with increased risk of cardiovascular (CV) mortality. No conclusive evidence of macrovascular risk reduction. May produce severe hypoglycemia; proper patient selection, dosage, and instructions are important to avoid hypoglycemic episodes. Increased risk of hypoglycemia in elderly, debilitated or malnourished patients, with renal/hepatic impairment, adrenal or pituitary insufficiency, deficient caloric intake, or after severe/prolonged exercise. Loss of glycemic control may occur when exposed to stress (eg, fever, trauma, infection, surgery); may be necessary to d/c therapy and administer insulin. Secondary failure may occur over time. May cause hemolytic anemia; caution with G6PD deficiency and consider a non-sulfonylurea alternative. Caution in elderly. 3mg tab is not bioequivalent to Micronase 5mg tab.

ADVERSE REACTIONS: Hypoglycemia, liver function abnormalities, nausea, epigastric distress, heartburn, leukopenia, agranulocytosis, thrombocytopenia, hemolytic anemia, aplastic anemia, pancytopenia, hyponatremia, changes in accommodation, blurred vision, allergic skin reactions.

INTERACTIONS: See Contraindications. Hypoglycemic effects may be potentiated by NSAIDs, other highly protein-bound drugs, salicylates, sulfonamides, chloramphenicol, probenecid, coumarins, MAOIs, and β-adrenergic blocking drugs; monitor closely for hypoglycemia during coadministration and for loss of glycemic control when such drugs are withdrawn. Severe hypoglycemia reported with oral miconazole. Increased risk of hypoglycemia with alcohol or use of >1 glucose-lowering drug. May be difficult to recognize hypoglycemia with β-adrenergic blocking drugs. Thiazides and other diuretics, corticosteroids, phenothiazines, thyroid products, estrogens, oral contraceptives, phenytoin, nicotinic acid, sympathomimetics, calcium channel blockers, and isoniazid may produce hyperglycemia and may lead to loss of glycemic control; monitor closely for loss of control during coadministration and for hypoglycemia when such drugs are withdrawn. Possible potentiation of hypoglycemic action with ciprofloxacin reported. Decreased levels with colesevelam.

PREGNANCY: Category B, not for use in nursing.

MECHANISM OF ACTION: Sulfonylurea (2nd generation); lowers blood glucose by stimulating insulin release from pancreatic β cells.

PHARMACOKINETICS: Absorption: (Single dose) C_{max}=106ng/mL (3mg); AUC=568ng•hr/mL (3mg); T_{max}=2-3 hrs. **Distribution:** Plasma protein binding (extensive). **Metabolism:** 4-trans-hydroxy derivative (major metabolite). **Elimination:** Bile (50% metabolites), urine (50% metabolites); $T_{1/2}$=4 hrs.

NURSING CONSIDERATIONS

Assessment: Assess for previous hypersensitivity to drug, type of DM, renal/hepatic impairment, diabetic ketoacidosis, risk factors for hypoglycemia, G6PD deficiency, pregnancy/nursing status, and possible drug interactions. Obtain baseline FPG and HbA1c levels.

Monitoring: Monitor for CV effects, hypoglycemia, loss of glycemic control when exposed to stress, hemolytic anemia, hypersensitivity reactions, secondary failure, and other adverse reactions. Monitor HbA1c levels and blood/urine glucose periodically.

Patient Counseling: Inform of the potential risks and advantages of therapy and alternative modes of therapy. Inform about importance of adherence to dietary instructions, of a regular exercise program, and of regular testing of urine and/or blood glucose. Inform about the symptoms, treatment and predisposing conditions of hypoglycemia as well as primary and secondary failure. During the insulin withdrawal period, instruct patient to test for glucose and acetone in urine at least tid and report results to physician.

Administration: Oral route. Take with breakfast or 1st main meal. **Storage:** 20-25°C (68-77°F). Keep container tightly closed.

GLYSET   RX
miglitol (Pharmacia & Upjohn)

THERAPEUTIC CLASS: Alpha-glucosidase inhibitor

INDICATIONS: Adjunct to diet and exercise to improve glycemic control in adults with type 2 diabetes mellitus.

DOSAGE: *Adults:* Individualize dose. Initial: 25mg tid at the start of each main meal. May start at 25mg qd to minimize GI side effects then gradually increase frequency to tid. Titrate: After 4-8 weeks of 25mg tid regimen, increase to 50mg tid for 3 months, then further to 100mg tid if HbA1c is not satisfactory. Maint: 50mg tid (although some may benefit from 100mg tid). Max: 100mg tid. If no further reduction in postprandial glucose or HbA1c levels is observed with 100mg tid, consider lowering the dose.

HOW SUPPLIED: Tab: 25mg, 50mg, 100mg

CONTRAINDICATIONS: Diabetic ketoacidosis, inflammatory bowel disease (IBD), colonic ulceration, partial intestinal obstruction or predisposition to it, and chronic intestinal diseases associated with marked disorders of digestion or absorption, or with conditions that may deteriorate as a result of increased gas formation in the intestine.

WARNINGS/PRECAUTIONS: Inhibits hydrolysis of sucrose to glucose and fructose; use oral glucose (dextrose) instead of sucrose (cane sugar) in the treatment of mild to moderate hypoglycemia. Temporary loss of blood glucose control may occur when patients are exposed to stress (eg, fever, trauma, infection, surgery); temporary insulin therapy may be necessary. Not recommended with significant renal dysfunction (SrCr >2mg/dL or CrCl <25mL/min). Pneumatosis cystoides intestinalis reported; d/c and perform appropriate diagnostic imaging if suspected.

ADVERSE REACTIONS: Flatulence, diarrhea, abdominal pain, skin rash, low serum iron.

INTERACTIONS: Coadministration with a sulfonylurea or insulin may increase risk of hypoglycemia; consider reducing the dose of the sulfonylurea or insulin. May reduce levels of glyburide, metformin, and digoxin. May reduce bioavailability of ranitidine and propranolol. Intestinal adsorbents (eg, charcoal) and digestive enzyme preparations containing carbohydrate-splitting enzymes (eg, amylase, pancreatin) may reduce effect; avoid concomitant use.

PREGNANCY: Category B, not for use in nursing.

MECHANISM OF ACTION: α-glucosidase inhibitor; reversibly inhibits membrane-bound intestinal α-glucosidase hydrolase enzymes.

PHARMACOKINETICS: Absorption: Complete (25mg), 50-70% (100mg). T_{max}=2-3 hrs. **Distribution:** V_d=0.18L/kg; plasma protein binding (<4%); found in breast milk. **Elimination:** Urine (>95%, unchanged) (25mg); $T_{1/2}$=2 hrs.

NURSING CONSIDERATIONS

Assessment: Assess for diabetic ketoacidosis, IBD, colonic ulceration, partial intestinal obstruction or predisposition to it, chronic intestinal diseases, renal function, drug hypersensitivity, pregnancy/nursing status, and possible drug interactions.

Monitoring: Monitor blood glucose and HbA1c levels. Monitor for signs/symptoms of pneumatosis cystoides intestinalis and other adverse reactions.

Patient Counseling: Inform about the importance of adhering to dietary instructions, a regular exercise program, and regular testing of urine and/or blood glucose. Counsel about the risk of hypoglycemia, its symptoms and treatment, and conditions that predispose to its development. Instruct to have a readily available source of glucose to treat symptoms of low blood sugar. Inform that side effects (GI effects such as flatulence, soft stools, diarrhea, abdominal discomfort) usually develop during the 1st few weeks of therapy, and generally diminish in frequency and intensity with time.

Administration: Oral route. **Storage:** 25°C (77°F); excursions permitted to 15-30°C (59-86°F).

GRALISE
gabapentin (Depomed)

RX

THERAPEUTIC CLASS: GABA analog

INDICATIONS: Management of postherpetic neuralgia.

DOSAGE: *Adults:* Take with pm meal. Initial: Day 1: 300mg qd. Titrate: Day 2: 600mg qd. Days 3-6: 900mg qd. Days 7-10: 1200mg qd. Days 11-14: 1500mg qd. Day 15: 1800mg qd. Dose Reduction/Discontinuation/Substitution: Gradually over ≥1 week. Renal Impairment: Initial: 300mg qd. Titrate: Follow the schedule listed above; individualize dose. CrCl ≥60mL/min: 1800mg qd. CrCl 30-60mL/min: 600-1800mg qd. CrCl <30mL/min/Hemodialysis: Do not administer.

HOW SUPPLIED: Tab: 300mg, 600mg

WARNINGS/PRECAUTIONS: Not interchangeable with other gabapentin products. Increased risk of suicidal thoughts or behavior; monitor for the emergence or worsening of depression, suicidal thoughts or behavior, and/or any unusual changes in mood or behavior. May have tumorigenic potential. Drug reaction with eosinophilia and systemic symptoms (DRESS)/multiorgan hypersensitivity reported; evaluate immediately if signs/symptoms are present, and d/c therapy if an alternative etiology cannot be established. Lab test interactions may occur.

ADVERSE REACTIONS: Dizziness, somnolence, headache, peripheral edema, diarrhea.

INTERACTIONS: Naproxen may increase absorption. May reduce levels of hydrocodone. Hydrocodone and morphine may increase area under the curve. Cimetidine may decrease oral clearance and CrCl. May increase C_{max} of norethindrone. Reduced bioavailability with an antacid containing aluminum hydroxide and magnesium hydroxide; take at least 2 hrs following the antacid.

PREGNANCY: Category C, caution in nursing.

MECHANISM OF ACTION: Gamma-aminobutyric acid analog; not established. Hypothesized to antagonize thrombospondin binding to α2delta-1 as a receptor involved in excitatory synapse formation. May function therapeutically by blocking new synapse formation.

PHARMACOKINETICS: Absorption: (1800mg qd) C_{max}=9585ng/mL; T_{max}=8 hrs; AUC_{0-24}=132,808ng•hr/mL. **Distribution:** Plasma protein binding (<3%); found in breast milk; (150mg IV) V_d=58L. **Elimination:** Renal (unchanged); (1200-3000mg/day) $T_{1/2}$=5-7 hrs.

NURSING CONSIDERATIONS

Assessment: Assess for preexisting tumors, depression, hypersensitivity to drug, renal function, pregnancy/nursing status, and possible drug interactions.

Monitoring: Monitor for emergence or worsening of depression, suicidal thoughts/behavior, and/or any unusual changes in mood/behavior, new or worsening tumors, DRESS, and other adverse reactions.

Patient Counseling: Advise that drug is not interchangeable with other formulations of gabapentin, and to take only as prescribed. Inform that drug may cause dizziness, somnolence, and other signs and symptoms of CNS depression; advise not to drive or operate machinery until sufficient experience on therapy is gained. Advise that if a dose is missed, to take drug with food as soon as remembered, or, if it is almost time for the next dose, to just skip the missed dose and take the next dose at the regular time; instruct not to take 2 doses at the same time. Inform that drug may increase the risk of suicidal thoughts and behavior; advise to report to physician any behaviors of concern.

Administration: Oral route. Swallow tabs whole; do not split, crush, or chew. **Storage:** 25°C (77°F); excursions permitted to 15-30°C (59-86°F).

GRANISETRON
granisetron HCl (Various)

RX

THERAPEUTIC CLASS: 5-HT$_3$ receptor antagonist

INDICATIONS: (Inj/PO) Prevention of N/V associated with initial and repeat courses of emetogenic cancer therapy (eg, high-dose cisplatin). (PO) Prevention of N/V associated with radiation (eg, total body irradiation and fractionated abdominal radiation).

DOSAGE: *Adults:* Emetogenic Chemotherapy: (PO) 2mg qd up to 1 hr before chemotherapy or 1mg tab bid up to 1 hr before chemotherapy and 12 hrs later. (IV) 10mcg/kg, undiluted over 30 sec or diluted (with 0.9% NaCl or D5W) over 5 min, within 30 min before chemotherapy. Prevention of N/V with Radiation: (PO) 2mg qd within 1 hr of radiation.
Pediatrics: 2-16 Yrs: Emetogenic Chemotherapy: 10mcg/kg IV within 30 min before chemotherapy.

HOW SUPPLIED: Inj: 0.1mg/mL [1mL], 1mg/mL [1mL, 4mL]; Tab: 1mg

WARNINGS/PRECAUTIONS: Does not stimulate gastric or intestinal peristalsis; do not use instead of nasogastric suction. May mask progressive ileus or gastric distension. QT prolongation reported; caution with preexisting arrhythmias, cardiac conduction disorders, cardiac disease, and electrolyte abnormalities. (Inj) Hypersensitivity reactions may occur in patients who exhibited hypersensitivity to other selective 5-HT$_3$ receptor antagonists.

ADVERSE REACTIONS: Headache, asthenia, somnolence, diarrhea, constipation, insomnia, fever, ALT/AST elevation.

INTERACTIONS: Hepatic CYP450 enzyme inducers or inhibitors may alter clearance and T$_{1/2}$. Caution with cardiotoxic chemotherapy, drugs known to prolong QT interval and/or arrhythmogenic drugs. May inhibit metabolism with ketoconazole. (Inj) Increased total plasma clearance with phenobarbital.

PREGNANCY: Category B, caution in nursing.

MECHANISM OF ACTION: 5-HT$_3$ receptor antagonist; blocks serotonin stimulation and subsequent vomiting after emetogenic stimuli.

PHARMACOKINETICS: Absorption: C$_{max}$=63.8ng/mL (IV, 40mcg/kg), 5.99ng/mL (PO).
Distribution: Plasma protein binding (65%). V$_d$=3.07L/kg (IV, 40mcg/kg). **Metabolism:** CYP3A; N-demethylation, aromatic ring oxidation, conjugation. **Elimination:** (PO) Urine (11% unchanged, 48% metabolites), feces (38% metabolites). (IV) Urine (12% unchanged, 49% metabolites), feces (34% metabolites); T$_{1/2}$=8.95 hrs (IV, 40mcg/kg).

NURSING CONSIDERATIONS

Assessment: Assess for preexisting arrhythmias, cardiac conduction disorders, cardiac disease, electrolyte abnormalities, previous hypersensitivity to drug, pregnancy/nursing status, and possible drug interactions.

Monitoring: Monitor for masking of progressive ileus and gastric distention, QT prolongation, and hypersensitivity reactions.

Patient Counseling: Inform about risks/benefits of therapy. Advise patients to report any adverse events to their healthcare provider.

Administration: Oral, IV route. Refer to PI for inj stability and compatibility. Undiluted IV should be administered over 30 sec. Diluted sol should be infused over 5 min. **Storage:** 20-25°C (68-77°F). Protect from light. Retain in carton until time of use. (Inj) Excursions permitted to 15-30°C (59-86°F). Diluted Sol: 0.9% NaCl or D5W: Stable at room temperature for 24 hrs under normal lighting conditions. Do not freeze. Once the multidose vial is penetrated, use within 30 days.

GRIS-PEG   RX
griseofulvin (Pedinol)

THERAPEUTIC CLASS: *Penicillium*-derived antifungal

INDICATIONS: Treatment of the following ringworm infections: tinea corporis, tinea pedis, tinea cruris, tinea barbae, tinea capitis, and tinea unguium when caused by one or more species of *Microsporum*, *Epidermophyton*, and *Trichophyton*.

DOSAGE: *Adults:* T. corporis/T. cruris/T. capitis: 375mg/day in single or divided doses. T. corporis: Treat for 2-4 weeks. T. capitis: Treat for 4-6 weeks. Difficult Fungal Infections to Eradicate/T. pedis/T.unguium: 750mg/day, given in a divided dose. T. pedis: Concomitant topical agents required. Treat for 4-8 weeks. T. unguium: Treat for at least 4 months (fingernails) and at least 6 months (toenails), depending on rate of growth.
Pediatrics: >2 Yrs: Usual: 3.3mg/lb/day. >60 lbs: 187.5-375mg/day. 35-60 lbs: 125-187.5mg/day. T. capitis: Treat for 4-6 weeks. T. corporis: Treat for 2-4 weeks. T. pedis: Treat for 4-8 weeks. T. unguium: Treat for at least 4 months (fingernail) and at least 6 months (toenails), depending on rate of growth.

HOW SUPPLIED: Tab: 125mg*, 250mg* *scored

CONTRAINDICATIONS: Porphyria, hepatocellular failure, pregnancy.

WARNINGS/PRECAUTIONS: Not for prophylactic use. Severe skin reactions (eg, Stevens-Johnson syndrome [SJS], toxic epidermal necrolysis) reported; d/c if these occur. Elevations in AST, ALT, bilirubin and jaundice reported; monitor for hepatic adverse events and d/c if warranted. Periodically organ system function including renal, hepatic, and hematopoietic functions, if on prolonged therapy; d/c if granulocytopenia occurs. Cross-sensitivity with penicillin (PCN) may exist. Photosensitivity reported. Lupus erythematosus or lupus-like syndromes reported. Clinical relapse may occur if therapy not continued until infecting organism eradicated.

ADVERSE REACTIONS: Hypersensitivity reactions (eg, skin rashes, urticaria, erythema multiforme-like reactions), granulocytopenia, oral thrush, N/V, epigastric distress, diarrhea, headache, dizziness, insomnia, mental confusion.

INTERACTIONS: Anticoagulants (warfarin-type) may require dosage adjustment. Decreased effect with barbiturates. Possible interaction with oral contraceptives. Increased alcohol effect, producing tachycardia and flush.

PREGNANCY: Contraindicated in pregnancy, safety not known in nursing.

MECHANISM OF ACTION: *Penicillium*-derived antifungal; fungistatic with in vitro activity against various species of *Microsporum*, *Epidermophyton*, and *Trichophyton*.

PHARMACOKINETICS: Absorption: (250mg unaltered tab) C_{max}=600.61ng/mL; T_{max}=4.04 hrs; AUC=8,618.89ng•hr/mL. (250mg physically altered tab [crushed and in applesauce]) C_{max}=672.61ng/mL; T_{max}=3.08 hrs; AUC=9,023.71ng•hr/mL.

NURSING CONSIDERATIONS

Assessment: Assess for identification of fungi responsible for infection (eg, cultures, microscopic exam). Assess for hepatocellular failure, porphyria, hypersensitivity to PCN, pregnancy/nursing status, and for possible drug interactions.

Monitoring: Monitor for signs/symptoms of serious skin reactions (eg, SJS, erythema multiforme), hepatotoxicity, photosensitivity reactions, and for lupus erythematosus or lupus-like syndromes. Perform periodic monitoring of organ system function, including renal, hepatic, and hematopoietic functions, in patients on prolonged therapy.

Patient Counseling: Inform of the importance of compliance with full course of therapy. Counsel to avoid intense natural or artificial sunlight while on medication. Instruct to take proper hygienic precautions to prevent spread of infection. Advise females to avoid pregnancy while on therapy. Instruct to notify physician if any adverse reactions occur.

Administration: Oral route. Swallow whole or crushed and sprinkled onto 1 tbsp of applesauce and swallow immediately without chewing. **Storage:** 15-30°C (59-86°F). Store in tight, light-resistant container.

HALAVEN   RX
eribulin mesylate (Eisai)

THERAPEUTIC CLASS: Antimicrotubule agent

INDICATIONS: Treatment of metastatic breast cancer in patients who have previously received at least 2 chemotherapeutic regimens for the treatment of metastatic disease. Prior therapy should have included an anthracycline and a taxane in either the adjuvant or metastatic setting.

DOSAGE: *Adults:* Administer IV over 2-5 min on Days 1 and 8 of a 21-day cycle. Usual: 1.4mg/m². Mild Hepatic Impairment (Child-Pugh A)/Moderate Renal Impairment (CrCl 30-50mL/min): Usual: 1.1mg/m². Moderate Hepatic Impairment (Child-Pugh B): Usual: 0.7mg/m². Refer to PI for dose modifications.

HOW SUPPLIED: Inj: 0.5mg/mL [2mL]

WARNINGS/PRECAUTIONS: Severe neutropenia (absolute neutrophil count <500/mm³) reported; monitor CBC prior to each dose and increase frequency of monitoring if Grade 3 or 4 cytopenias develop. Peripheral neuropathy reported; monitor closely for signs of peripheral motor and sensory neuropathy. May cause fetal harm during pregnancy. QT prolongation reported; monitor ECG in patients with congestive heart failure (CHF), bradyarrhythmias, and electrolyte abnormalities. Correct hypokalemia or hypomagnesemia prior to therapy and monitor these electrolytes periodically during therapy. Avoid with congenital long QT syndrome.

ADVERSE REACTIONS: Neutropenia, anemia, peripheral neuropathy, headache, asthenia, pyrexia, weight decreased, constipation, diarrhea, N/V, arthralgia, dyspnea, alopecia, anorexia, back pain.

INTERACTIONS: Monitor ECG with drugs known to prolong the QT interval (eg, Class IA and III antiarrhythmics).

PREGNANCY: Category D, not for use in nursing.

MECHANISM OF ACTION: Antimicrotubule agent; inhibits the growth phase of microtubules via a tubulin-based antimitotic mechanism leading to G_2/M cell-cycle block, disruption of mitotic spindles, and ultimately, apoptotic cell death after prolonged mitotic blockage.

PHARMACOKINETICS: Distribution: V_d=43-114L/m^2; plasma protein binding (49-65%). **Elimination:** Urine (9%, 91% unchanged), feces (82%, 88% unchanged); $T_{1/2}$=40 hrs.

NURSING CONSIDERATIONS

Assessment: Assess for renal/hepatic impairment, CHF, bradyarrhythmias, congenital long QT syndrome, electrolyte abnormalities, pregnancy/nursing status, and possible drug interactions. Assess for peripheral neuropathy and obtain CBC.

Monitoring: Monitor for severe neutropenia, and other adverse reactions. Monitor ECG in patients with CHF, bradyarrhythmias, and electrolyte abnormalities. Monitor K$^+$ and Mg^{2+} levels periodically. Evaluate for peripheral neuropathy and obtain CBC prior to each dose. Increase frequency of CBC monitoring if Grade 3 or 4 cytopenias develop.

Patient Counseling: Advise to contact physician for a fever ≥100.5°F or other signs/symptoms of infection (eg, chills, cough, or burning/pain on urination). Advise women of childbearing potential to avoid pregnancy and to use effective contraception during treatment.

Administration: IV route. Do not dilute in or administer through an IV line containing solutions with dextrose. Do not administer in the same IV line concurrent with the other medicinal products. Refer to PI for the preparation and administration instructions. **Storage:** 25°C (77°F); excursions permitted to 15-30°C (59-86°F). Do not freeze. Undiluted/Diluted Sol: Up to 4 hrs at room temperature or up to 24 hrs under refrigeration (4°C [40°F]).

HALCION

triazolam (Pharmacia & Upjohn)

THERAPEUTIC CLASS: Benzodiazepine

INDICATIONS: Short-term treatment of insomnia (generally 7-10 days).

DOSAGE: *Adults:* Individualize dose. Usual: 0.25mg at hs; 0.125mg may be sufficient for some patients. Max: 0.5mg. Elderly/Debilitated: Initial: 0.125mg. Range: 0.125-0.25mg. Max: 0.25mg. Use for more than 2-3 weeks requires complete reevaluation.

HOW SUPPLIED: Tab: 0.25mg* *scored

CONTRAINDICATIONS: Pregnancy. Coadministration with ketoconazole, itraconazole, nefazodone, HIV protease inhibitors, and medications that significantly impair the oxidative metabolism mediated by CYP3A.

WARNINGS/PRECAUTIONS: Initiate only after careful evaluation; failure of insomnia to remit after 7-10 days of treatment may indicate presence of a primary psychiatric and/or medical illness. Use lowest effective dose, especially in elderly. Complex behaviors (eg, sleep-driving) reported; consider discontinuation if sleep-driving occurs. Severe anaphylactic and anaphylactoid reactions reported; do not rechallenge if angioedema develops. Increased daytime anxiety reported; may d/c if observed. Abnormal thinking, behavior changes, anterograde amnesia, paradoxical reactions, traveler's amnesia, and dose-related side effects (eg, drowsiness, dizziness, lightheadedness, amnesia) reported. Worsening of depression, including suicidal thinking, reported in primarily depressed patients. May impair mental/physical abilities. Respiratory depression and apnea reported in patients with compromised respiratory function. Caution in patients with signs or symptoms of depression that could be intensified by hypnotic drugs, renal/hepatic impairment, chronic pulmonary insufficiency, and sleep apnea. Dependence and tolerance to drug may develop; caution with history of alcoholism, drug abuse, or with marked personality disorders, due to increased risk of dependence. Withdrawal symptoms reported following abrupt discontinuation; avoid abrupt discontinuation, and taper dose gradually in any patient taking more than the lowest dose for more than a few weeks or with history of seizure.

ADVERSE REACTIONS: Drowsiness, dizziness, lightheadedness, headache, nervousness, coordination disorders/ataxia, N/V.

INTERACTIONS: See Contraindications. Avoid with very potent CYP3A inhibitors (eg, azole-type antifungals). Caution and consider triazolam dose reduction with drugs inhibiting CYP3A to a lesser but significant degree. Macrolide antibiotics (eg, erythromycin, clarithromycin) and cimetidine may increase levels; use with caution and consider triazolam dose reduction. Isoniazid, oral contraceptives, grapefruit juice, and ranitidine may increase levels; use with caution. Additive CNS depressant effects with psychotropic medications, anticonvulsants, antihistamines, ethanol, and other CNS depressants. Increased risk of complex behaviors with alcohol and other CNS depressants. Caution with fluvoxamine, diltiazem, verapamil, sertraline, paroxetine, ergotamine, cyclosporine, amiodarone, nicardipine, and nifedipine.

PREGNANCY: Category X, not for use in nursing.

MECHANISM OF ACTION: Triazolobenzodiazepine hypnotic agent.

PHARMACOKINETICS: Absorption: C_{max}=1-6ng/mL; T_{max}=2 hrs. **Metabolism:** Hydroxylation via CYP3A. **Elimination:** Urine (79.9% metabolites); $T_{1/2}$=1.5-5.5 hrs.

NURSING CONSIDERATIONS

Assessment: Assess for physical and/or psychiatric disorder, depression, compromised respiratory function, renal/hepatic impairment, chronic pulmonary insufficiency, sleep apnea, history of seizures, alcoholism or drug abuse, marked personality disorders, hypersensitivity to the drug, pregnancy/nursing status, and possible drug interactions.

Monitoring: Monitor for complex behaviors, anaphylactic/anaphylactoid reactions, increased daytime anxiety, emergence of any new behavioral signs/symptoms of concern, tolerance, dependence, withdrawal symptoms, and other adverse reactions.

Patient Counseling: Inform of the risks and benefits of therapy. Caution against engaging in hazardous activities requiring complete mental alertness (eg, operating machinery, driving). Instruct to immediately report to physician if any adverse reactions (eg, sleep-driving, other complex behaviors) develop. Caution about the concomitant ingestion of alcohol and other CNS depressant drugs during treatment. Instruct to notify physician if pregnant, planning to become pregnant, or if nursing.

Administration: Oral route. **Storage:** 20-25°C (68-77°F).

HalfLytely

RX

polyethylene glycol 3350 - sodium bicarbonate - potassium chloride - sodium chloride - bisacodyl (Braintree)

THERAPEUTIC CLASS: Bowel cleanser/stimulant laxative

INDICATIONS: Colon cleansing prior to colonoscopy.

DOSAGE: *Adults:* Consume only clear liquids on day of preparation. Take 1 bisacodyl tab with water. Do not crush or chew tab. After 1st bowel movement (or max of 6 hrs) drink sol, at a rate of 8 oz. every 10 min. Drink all sol. Drink each portion at longer intervals or d/c sol temporarily if abdominal distension/discomfort occurs until symptoms improve.

HOW SUPPLIED: Kit: Tab, Delayed-Release: (Bisacodyl) 5mg. Sol: (Polyethylene Glycol 3350-Potassium Chloride-Sodium Bicarbonate-Sodium Chloride) 210g-0.74g-2.86g-5.6g [2000mL].

CONTRAINDICATIONS: Ileus, GI obstruction, gastric retention, bowel perforation, toxic colitis, toxic megacolon.

WARNINGS/PRECAUTIONS: Serious arrhythmias reported rarely; caution in patients at increased risk of arrhythmias (eg, history of prolonged QT, uncontrolled arrhythmias, recent myocardial infarction [MI], unstable angina, congestive heart failure [CHF], cardiomyopathy), and consider pre-dose and postcolonoscopy ECGs. Perform post-colonoscopy lab tests (electrolytes, creatinine, BUN) if patient develops vomiting or signs of dehydration. Hydrate patients adequately before, during, and after administration. Caution in patients with increased risk for seizure, renal impairment, and fluid and electrolyte disturbances. Correct electrolyte abnormalities prior to treatment. Caution in severe active ulcerative colitis (UC). Caution in patients with impaired gag reflex and patients prone to regurgitation/aspiration. Ischemic colitis reported; evaluate if severe abdominal pain or rectal bleeding develops. Generalized tonic-clonic seizures reported with the use of large volume (4L) polyethylene glycol-based colon preparation products; caution in patients with a history of seizures and patients at risk of seizure with known or suspected hyponatremia. Monitor closely with impaired water handling. Do not add additional ingredients other than flavor packs provided.

ADVERSE REACTIONS: N/V, abdominal fullness/cramping, overall discomfort.

INTERACTIONS: Oral medications taken within 1 hr of start of administration may not be absorbed from GI tract. Avoid bisacodyl delayed release tab within 1 hr of taking an antacid. Caution with drugs that lower the seizure threshold (eg, TCAs), in patients withdrawing from alcohol or benzodiazepines, drugs that increase the risk of electrolyte abnormalities (eg, diuretics); monitor baseline and postcolonoscopy lab tests (Na^+, K^+, Ca^{2+}, creatinine, BUN). Caution with drugs that may increase the risk of adverse events of arrhythmias and prolonged QT with fluid and electrolyte abnormalities. Caution with drugs that may affect renal function (eg, diuretics, ACE inhibitors, ARBs, NSAIDs); consider baseline and post colonoscopy labs (electrolytes, SrCr, BUN) in these patients.

PREGNANCY: Category C, caution in nursing.

MECHANISM OF ACTION: Polyethylene glycol-3350: Osmotic laxative; causes water to be retained within the GI tract. Bisacodyl: Simulant laxative; active metabolite acts directly on the colonic mucosa to produce colonic peristalsis. The stimulant laxative effect of bisacodyl, together with the osmotic effect of the unabsorbed PEG when ingested with a large volume of water, produces watery diarrhea.

PHARMACOKINETICS: Absorption: Polyethylene glycol-3350: Minimal. **Metabolism:** Bisacodyl: Hydrolysis by intestinal brush border enzymes and colonic bacteria to form bis-(p-hydroxyphenyl) pyridyl-2 methane (active metabolite).

NURSING CONSIDERATIONS

Assessment: Assess for GI obstruction, bowel perforation, electrolyte/fluid abnormalities, history of seizures, known or suspected hyponatremia, renal impairment, any other conditions where treatment is contraindicated or cautioned, hypersensitivity, pregnancy/nursing status, and possible drug interactions. Obtain baseline electrolytes, Na$^+$, K$^+$, Ca, SrCr, and BUN in patients at risk for seizures and patients with renal impairment. Perform baseline ECGs in patients at risk for arrhythmias.

Monitoring: Perform baseline and postcolonoscopy lab tests in patients with seizure risk (eg, known/suspected hyponatremia), and consider these tests in patients with impaired renal function. Monitor for hypersensitivity reactions, aspiration, cardiac arrhythmias, abdominal pain, rectal bleeding, ischemic colitis, and seizures.

Patient Counseling: Inform that oral medication administered within 1 hr of start of administration of sol may be flushed from GI tract-hence, not absorbed. Instruct to take exactly as directed. Advise not to take other laxatives while taking HalfLytely and Bisacodyl Tablet Bowel Prep Kit and to notify physician if they have trouble swallowing or are prone to regurgitation or aspiration. Instruct to slow or temporarily d/c administration if severe bloating, distention or abdominal pain occurs until symptoms abate and notify physician. Advise to d/c administration and contact physician if hives, rashes, allergic reaction or signs and symptoms of dehydration develop.

Administration: Oral route. **Storage:** 20-25°C (68-77°F); excursions permitted to 15-30°C (59-86°F). Refrigerate reconstituted sol and use within 48 hrs.

HALOPERIDOL   RX
haloperidol (Various)

Elderly patients with dementia-related psychosis treated with antipsychotic drugs are at an increased risk of death; most deaths appeared to be cardiovascular (CV) (eg, heart failure, sudden death) or infectious (eg, pneumonia) in nature. Not approved for the treatment of patients with dementia-related psychosis.

OTHER BRAND NAMES: Haldol (Ortho-McNeil)

THERAPEUTIC CLASS: Butyrophenone

INDICATIONS: (Inj) Treatment of schizophrenia and control of tics and vocal utterances of Tourette's disorder in adults. (Sol/Tab) Management of manifestations of psychotic disorders. Control of tics and vocal utterances of Tourette's disorder in children and adults. Treatment of severe behavior problems in children with combative, explosive, hyperexcitability and for short-term treatment of children with hyperactivity showing excessive motor activity accompanied by conduct disorders that failed to respond to psychotherapy and medications other than antipsychotics.

DOSAGE: *Adults:* Individualize dose. (PO) Initial: Moderate Symptoms/Elderly/Debilitated: 0.5-2mg bid or tid. Severe Symptoms/Chronic/Resistant: 3-5mg bid or tid. Doses up to 100mg/day may be needed to achieve optimal response. Doses >100mg/day have been used for severe resistant patients but safety on prolonged use not demonstrated. Refer to PI for dose adjustments/maint dosing. (Inj) 2-5mg IM for prompt control of acute agitation with moderately severe or very severe symptoms. May give subsequent doses as often as every hour, although 4- to 8-hr intervals may be satisfactory, depending on response. Refer to PI for switchover procedure. *Pediatrics:* 3-12 Yrs (15-40kg): (PO) Individualize dose. Initial: Lowest possible dose of 0.5mg/day. Increase by increments of 0.5mg/day at 5-7 day intervals until desired therapeutic effect obtained. May divide total dose to be given bid or tid. Psychotic Disorders: 0.05-0.15mg/kg/day. May require higher doses in severely disturbed psychotic children. Nonpsychotic Behavior Disorders/Tourette's Disorder: 0.05-0.075mg/kg/day. Short term treatment for severely disturbed nonpsychotic/hyperactive children with behavior disorders may suffice. Refer to PI for dose adjustments/maint dosing.

HOW SUPPLIED: Inj: 5mg/mL (Haldol); Sol: 2mg/mL [15mL, 120mL]; Tab: 0.5mg*, 1mg*, 2mg*, 5mg*, 10mg*, 20mg* *scored

CONTRAINDICATIONS: Severe toxic CNS depression or comatose states, Parkinson's disease.

WARNINGS/PRECAUTIONS: Risk of tardive dyskinesia (TD), especially in the elderly; consider discontinuation if signs/symptoms develop. Neuroleptic malignant syndrome (NMS) reported; d/c and treat immediately. Hyperpyrexia, heat stroke, and bronchopneumonia reported. Use only during pregnancy if benefit justifies risk to fetus. Caution with severe cardiovascular disease (CVD), history of seizures, EEG abnormalities, and known/history of allergic reactions to drugs.

May cause transient hypotension and/or anginal pain with severe CVD; treat hypotension with metaraminol, phenylephrine, or norepinephrine. May cause rapid mood swing to depression when used to control mania in cyclic disorders, severe neurotoxicity in patients with thyrotoxicosis, and increased prolactin levels. Caution in elderly. May impair mental/physical abilities. (Inj/Tab) Sudden death, QT prolongation, and torsades de pointes may occur. Caution with other QT-prolonging conditions (eg, electrolyte imbalance, underlying cardiac abnormalities, hypothyroidism, familial long QT-syndrome). Leukopenia, neutropenia, and agranulocytosis reported; d/c if severe neutropenia (absolute neutrophil count <1000/mm³) develops. Monitor CBC and d/c at 1st sign of decline in WBCs if with preexisting low WBC count or history of drug-induced leukopenia/neutropenia. (Inj) Not approved for IV administration.

ADVERSE REACTIONS: Extrapyramidal symptoms, TD, dystonia, ECG changes, ventricular arrhythmias, tachycardia, hypotension, HTN, N/V, constipation, diarrhea, dry mouth, blurred vision, urinary retention.

INTERACTIONS: Encephalopathic syndrome followed by irreversible brain damage may occur with lithium. Caution with anticonvulsants and anticoagulants (eg, phenindione). Anticholinergics, including antiparkinson agents, may increase intraocular pressure. May potentiate CNS depressants (eg, alcohol, anesthetics, opiates); avoid with alcohol. Avoid with epinephrine for hypotension treatment. (Inj/Tab) Caution with drugs prolonging QT interval or cause electrolyte imbalance. Rifampin may decrease levels. (Inj) Ketoconazole (400mg/day) and paroxetine (20mg/day) may increase QTc. CYP3A4 or CYP2D6 substrates/inhibitors may increase levels. Carbamazepine may decrease levels.

PREGNANCY: Safety not known in pregnancy, not for use in nursing.

MECHANISM OF ACTION: Butyrophenone; mechanism not established.

PHARMACOKINETICS: Distribution: (Inj) Found in breast milk.

NURSING CONSIDERATIONS

Assessment: Assess for history of dementia-related psychosis or any other conditions where treatment is cautioned or contraindicated. Assess for hypersensitivity to drug, pregnancy/nursing status, and possible drug interactions. Obtain baseline CBC, ECG, EEG, and serum electrolytes.

Monitoring: Monitor for signs/symptoms of NMS, TD, bronchopneumonia, hypersensitivity reactions, and other adverse reactions. Monitor for neurotoxicity in patients with thyrotoxicosis. Monitor vital signs, CBC, ECG, EEG, serum electrolytes, and cholesterol levels.

Patient Counseling: Inform about risks/benefits of therapy. Instruct to use caution in performing hazardous tasks (eg, operating machinery/driving). Instruct to avoid alcohol due to possible additive effects and hypotension. Advise to inform physician if nursing, pregnant, or planning to get pregnant.

Administration: Oral and IM route. (Inj) Inspect visually for particulate matter and discoloration prior to administration. Do not give IV. **Storage:** (Tab/Sol) 20-25°C (68-77°F). (Inj) 15-30°C (59-86°F). (Inj/Sol) Do not freeze. Protect from light.

HAVRIX   RX
hepatitis A vaccine (GlaxoSmithKline)

THERAPEUTIC CLASS: Vaccine

INDICATIONS: Active immunization against disease caused by hepatitis A virus (HAV) in persons ≥12 months of age.

DOSAGE: *Adults:* Single 1mL dose IM in the deltoid region, then 1mL IM booster dose anytime between 6-12 months later. Administer primary immunization at least 2 weeks prior to expected exposure to HAV.
Pediatrics: 12 Months-18 Yrs: Single 0.5mL dose IM in the anterolateral aspect of the thigh in young children or the deltoid muscle of the upper arm in older children, then 0.5mL IM booster dose anytime between 6-12 months later. Administer primary immunization at least 2 weeks prior to expected exposure to HAV.

HOW SUPPLIED: Inj: 720 EL.U./0.5mL, 1440 EL.U./mL [vial, prefilled syringe]

CONTRAINDICATIONS: History of severe allergic reaction to neomycin.

WARNINGS/PRECAUTIONS: Tip caps of prefilled syringes may contain natural rubber latex; may cause allergic reactions in latex-sensitive individuals. Syncope may occur and can be accompanied by transient neurological signs (eg, visual disturbance, paresthesia, tonic-clonic limb movements); procedures should be in place to avoid falling injury and to restore cerebral perfusion following syncope. Appropriate treatment and supervision must be available for possible anaphylactic reactions. Immunocompromised persons may have a diminished immune response to vaccine. May not prevent hepatitis A infection in individuals who have an unrecognized hepatitis

A infection at the time of vaccination. May not protect all individuals. Lower antibody response reported in patients with chronic liver disease.

ADVERSE REACTIONS: Inj-site reactions (eg, soreness, pain, redness, swelling, induration), headache, irritability, drowsiness, loss of appetite, fever, fatigue, malaise, anorexia, nausea.

INTERACTIONS: Immunosuppressive therapies, including irradiation, antimetabolites, alkylating agents, cytotoxic drugs, and corticosteroids (used in greater than physiologic doses), may reduce the immune response to vaccine.

PREGNANCY: Category C, caution in nursing.

MECHANISM OF ACTION: Vaccine; presence of antibodies to HAV confers protection against hepatitis A infection.

NURSING CONSIDERATIONS

Assessment: Assess for history of severe allergic reaction to hepatitis A vaccine or neomycin. Assess for latex sensitivity, immunosuppression, chronic liver disease, unrecognized hepatitis A infection, immunization status/vaccination history, pregnancy/nursing status, and possible drug interactions.

Monitoring: Monitor for allergic reactions, syncope, neurological signs, and other adverse reactions. Monitor immune response to vaccine.

Patient Counseling: Inform of the potential benefits and risks of immunization. Counsel about potential side effects and emphasize that the vaccine contains noninfectious killed viruses and cannot cause hepatitis A infection. Instruct to report any adverse events to physician.

Administration: IM route. Do not administer IV, intradermally, or SQ. Do not dilute; shake well before use. Do not administer in the gluteal region; administer in the anterolateral aspect of the thigh in young children or in the deltoid region in older children and adults. When concomitant administration of other vaccines or immune globulin is required, give with different syringes and at different inj sites. Do not mix with any other vaccine or product in the same syringe or vial. **Storage:** 2-8°C (36-46°F). Do not freeze; discard if vaccine has been frozen.

HECORIA   RX
tacrolimus (Novartis)

> Immunosuppression may lead to increased risk of lymphoma and other malignancies, particularly of the skin. Increased susceptibility to infections (bacterial, viral, fungal, protozoal, opportunistic). Should only be prescribed by physicians experienced in immunosuppressive therapy and management of organ transplant patients. Manage patients in facilities equipped and staffed with adequate laboratory and supportive medical resources. Physician responsible for maintenance therapy should have complete information requisite for patient follow-up.

THERAPEUTIC CLASS: Macrolide immunosuppressant

INDICATIONS: Prophylaxis of organ rejection in patients receiving allogeneic kidney, liver, or heart transplants with concomitant adrenal corticosteroids. In kidney or heart transplant patients, azathioprine or mycophenolate mofetil (MMF) coadministration is recommended.

DOSAGE: *Adults:* Initial: Administer no sooner than 6 hrs after liver/heart transplant. May administer within 24 hrs of kidney transplant, but should be delayed until renal function has recovered. Give daily doses as 2 divided doses, q12h. Adjunct therapy with adrenal corticosteroids is recommended early post-transplant. Kidney Transplant: 0.2mg/kg/day in combination with azathioprine or 0.1mg/kg/day in combination with MMF/interleukin-2 receptor antagonist. Liver Transplant: 0.1-0.15mg/kg/day. Heart Transplant: 0.075mg/kg/day. Titrate based on clinical assessments of rejection and tolerability. Maint: Lower dosages than the initial dosage may be sufficient. Black patients may require higher doses. If receiving tacrolimus IV infusion, give 1st oral dose 8-12 hrs after discontinuing the IV infusion. Refer to PI for therapeutic drug monitoring and dose adjustments in patients with renal/hepatic impairment. Elderly: Start at lower end of dosing range.
Pediatrics: Liver Transplant: Initial: 0.15-0.2mg/kg/day as 2 divided doses, q12h. Refer to PI for therapeutic drug monitoring and dose adjustments in patients with renal/hepatic impairment.

HOW SUPPLIED: Cap: 0.5mg, 1mg, 5mg

WARNINGS/PRECAUTIONS: Limit exposure to sunlight and UV light in patients at increased risk for skin cancer. Increased risk for polyoma virus infections, cytomegalovirus (CMV) viremia, and CMV disease. Polyoma virus-associated nephropathy (PVAN) reported; may lead to renal dysfunction and kidney graft loss. Progressive multifocal leukoencephalopathy (PML) reported; consider PML in differential diagnosis in patients reporting neurological symptoms and consider consultation with a neurologist. Consider reductions in immunosuppression if CMV viremia/disease, or evidence of PVAN or PML develops. May cause new-onset diabetes mellitus; closely monitor blood glucose concentrations. May cause acute/chronic nephrotoxicity; closely monitor patients with renal dysfunction. Consider changing to another immunosuppressive therapy in patients with persistent SrCr elevations unresponsive to dose adjustments. May cause neurotoxicity (eg, posterior reversible encephalopathy syndrome [PRES], delirium, coma); if PRES is suspected or diagnosed, maintain BP control and immediately reduce immunosuppression. Hyperkalemia and HTN reported. May prolong QT/QTc interval and may cause torsades de pointes; avoid in patients with congenital long QT syndrome and consider obtaining ECGs and monitoring electrolytes (Mg^{2+}, K^+, Ca^{2+}) periodically in patients with congestive heart failure (CHF), bradyarrhythmias, those taking certain antiarrhythmic medications or other medicinal products that lead to QT prolongation, and those with electrolyte disturbances. Myocardial hypertrophy reported; consider echocardiographic evaluation in patients who develop renal failure or clinical manifestations of ventricular dysfunction. Consider dose reduction or discontinuation if myocardial hypertrophy is diagnosed. Pure red cell aplasia (PRCA) reported; consider discontinuation if diagnosed. GI perforation reported; institute appropriate medical/surgical management promptly. Caution in elderly.

ADVERSE REACTIONS: Lymphoma, malignancies, infections, tremors, HTN, abnormal renal function, headache, insomnia, hyperglycemia, hyperkalemia, hypomagnesemia, diarrhea, N/V, paresthesia, anemia.

INTERACTIONS: Do not use simultaneously with cyclosporine; d/c tacrolimus or cyclosporine at least 24 hrs before initiating the other. Not recommended with sirolimus in liver and heart transplant; safety and efficacy with sirolimus in patients with kidney transplant. Increased whole blood concentrations with CYP3A4 inhibitors (eg, antifungals, calcium channel blockers [CCBs], macrolide antibiotics, lansoprazole, omeprazole, cimetidine), CYP3A inhibitors, and magnesium and aluminum hydroxide antacids. Decreased whole blood concentrations with CYP3A inducers. May increase mycophenolic acid (MPA) exposure after crossover from cyclosporine to tacrolimus in patients concomitantly receiving MPA-containing products. Avoid with grapefruit or grapefruit juice. Avoid with nelfinavir unless the benefits outweigh the risks. Monitor whole blood concentrations and adjust tacrolimus dose with concomitant protease inhibitors (eg, ritonavir, telaprevir, boceprevir), CCBs (eg, verapamil, diltiazem, nifedipine, nicardipine), erythromycin, clarithromycin, troleandomycin, chloramphenicol, rifampin, rifabutin, phenytoin, carbamazepine, phenobarbital, St. John's wort, magnesium and aluminum hydroxide antacids, bromocriptine, nefazodone, metoclopramide, danazol, ethinyl estradiol, amiodarone, or methylprednisolone. Monitor whole blood concentrations and adjust dose when concomitant use of antifungal drugs (eg, azoles, caspofungin) with tacrolimus is initiated or discontinued; initially reduce tacrolimus dose to 1/3 of the original dose when initiating voriconazole or posaconazole. May increase levels of phenytoin; monitor phenytoin levels and adjust phenytoin dose as needed. Additive/synergistic impairment of renal function with drugs that may be associated with renal dysfunction (eg, aminoglycosides, ganciclovir, amphotericin B, cisplatin, nucleotide reverse transcriptase inhibitors, protease inhibitors). Caution prior to use of other agents or antihypertensive agents associated with hyperkalemia (eg, K^+-sparing diuretics, ACE inhibitors, ARBs). Adjust tacrolimus dose and frequently monitor tacrolimus whole blood trough concentrations and for tacrolimus-associated adverse reactions when coadministered with CYP3A inhibitors/inducers or strong CYP3A4 inhibitors/inducers. Reduce tacrolimus dose, frequently monitor tacrolimus whole blood concentrations, and monitor for QT prolongation when coadministered with CYP3A4 substrates and/or inhibitors that also have the potential to prolong the QT interval. Amiodarone may increase whole blood concentrations with or without concurrent QT prolongation. Avoid live vaccines during therapy. Caution with concomitant immunosuppressants.

PREGNANCY: Category C, not for use in nursing.

MECHANISM OF ACTION: Macrolide immunosuppressant; not established. Inhibits T-lymphocyte activation. Binds to intracellular protein, FKBP-12, forming a complex of tacrolimus-FKBP-12, Ca^{2+}, calmodulin, and calcineurin and inhibiting phosphatase activity of calcineurin. This effect may prevent the dephosphorylation and translocation of nuclear factor of activated T-cells, a nuclear component thought to initiate gene transcription for the formation of lymphokines.

PHARMACOKINETICS: Absorption: Incomplete and variable. Administration of variable doses in different populations resulted in different pharmacokinetic parameters. **Distribution:** Plasma protein binding (99%); crosses placenta; found in breast milk. **Metabolism:** Liver (extensive), via CYP3A (demethylation and hydroxylation); 13-demethyl tacrolimus (major metabolite), 31-demethyl metabolite (active metabolite). **Elimination:** (PO) Feces (92.6%), urine (2.3%). Administration of variable doses in different populations resulted in different pharmacokinetic parameters.

NURSING CONSIDERATIONS

Assessment: Assess for congenital long QT syndrome, CHF, bradyarrhythmias, electrolyte disturbances, hypersensitivity to the drug, renal/hepatic impairment, pregnancy/nursing status, and possible drug interactions.

Monitoring: Monitor tacrolimus blood concentrations in conjunction with other laboratory and clinical parameters. Monitor for lymphomas and other malignancies, infections (including opportunistic infections), nephrotoxicity, neurotoxicity, HTN, QT prolongation, myocardial hypertrophy, PRCA, GI perforation, and other adverse reactions. Monitor serum K^+ and glucose concentrations.

Patient Counseling: Instruct to take caps at the same 12-hr intervals every day and not to eat grapefruit or drink grapefruit juice in combination with the drug. Advise to limit exposure to sunlight and UV light by wearing protective clothing and using sunscreen with high protection factor. Instruct to contact physician if any symptoms of infection, frequent urination, increased thirst or hunger, vision changes, deliriums, or tremors develop. Advise to attend all visits and complete all blood tests ordered by medical team. Instruct to inform physician if patient is planning to become pregnant or to breastfeed, or when patient starts or stops taking any medication (prescription and nonprescription, natural/herbal, nutritional supplements, vitamins).

Administration: Oral route. Take consistently either with or without food. **Storage:** 20-25°C (68-77°F).

HEPARIN SODIUM   RX
heparin sodium (Various)

THERAPEUTIC CLASS: Glycosaminoglycan

INDICATIONS: Prophylaxis and treatment of peripheral arterial embolism; in atrial fibrillation with embolization; treatment of acute and chronic consumptive coagulopathies (disseminated intravascular coagulation [DIC]); prevention of clotting in arterial and heart surgery. (Heparin Inj/Dextrose) Prophylaxis and treatment of pulmonary embolism (PE) and venous thrombosis and its extension. (Heparin Inj) Low-dose regimen for prevention of postoperative deep venous thrombosis and PE in patients undergoing major abdominothoracic surgery or who, for other reasons, are at risk of developing thromboembolic disease. Anticoagulant in blood transfusions. (Heparin Inj/IV) Anticoagulant in extracorporeal circulation and dialysis procedures. (Heparin in Dextrose) As a continuous IV infusion following an initial IV therapeutic dose of heparin sodium.

DOSAGE: *Adults:* Adjust dose according to coagulation test results. Refer to PI for details on converting to PO anticoagulant. Based on 68kg patient: (Heparin Inj) Deep SQ Inj: Initial: 5000 U IV, followed by 10,000-20,000 U SQ. Maint: 8000-10,000 U q8h or 15,000-20,000 U q12h. Use a different site for each inj. (Heparin Inj/IV) Intermittent IV Inj: Initial: 10,000 U IV. Maint: 5000-10,000 U q4-6h. Continuous IV Infusion: Initial: 5000 U IV. Maint: 20,000-40,000 U/24 hrs in 1000mL 0.9% (Inj) or 0.45% (IV) NaCl. (Heparin in Dextrose) Initial: 5000 U IV. Continuous IV infusion: 20,000-40,000 U/24 hrs. Elderly >60 yrs: May require lower doses of heparin. Refer to the PI for further dosing information.
Pediatrics: Initial: 75-100 U/kg (IV bolus over 10 min). Maint: Children >1 Yr: 18-20 U/kg/hr. Older children may require less heparin, similar to weight-adjusted adult dose. Infants: 25-30 U/kg/hr. Infants <2 Months: Have the highest requirements (average 28 U/kg/hr). Adjust heparin to maintain activated partial thromboplastin times of 60-85 sec, assuming this reflects an anti-factor Xa level of 0.35-0.70.

HOW SUPPLIED: Inj: (Heparin Inj) (Preservative-Free) 1000 U/mL [2mL], 5000 U/0.5mL [0.5mL]; (With Benzyl Alcohol) 5000 U/mL [10mL], 10,000 U/mL [4mL]; (With Parabens) 1000 U/mL [1mL, 10mL, 30mL], 5000 U/mL [1mL], 10,000 U/mL [1mL, 5mL], 20,000 U/mL [1mL]; (Heparin in Dextrose) 40 U/mL [500mL], 50 U/mL [500mL], 100 U/mL [250mL]; (Heparin IV) 100 U/mL [250mL], 50 U/mL [250mL, 500mL]

CONTRAINDICATIONS: Severe thrombocytopenia, if blood coagulation tests cannot be performed at appropriate intervals (with full-dose heparin), uncontrollable active bleeding state (except in DIC). (Heparin in Dextrose) Hypersensitivity to corn products.

WARNINGS/PRECAUTIONS: Not for IM use. Hemorrhage may occur at virtually any site; use with extreme caution in disease states with increased danger of hemorrhage. Thrombocytopenia, heparin-induced thrombocytopenia and thrombosis (HIT/HITT), and hyperaminotransferasemia reported. D/C if platelet count <100,000/mm³, recurrent thrombosis develops, coagulation tests unduly prolonged, or hemorrhage occurs. Avoid future use, especially within 3-6 months following diagnosis of HIT/HITT, and while positive for HIT antibodies. Do not use as a catheter lock flush product. Fatal hemorrhage reported in pediatrics due to medication errors (eg, confused with "catheter lock flush" vials). Excessive administration of K⁺-free solutions may result in significant hypokalemia. Increased heparin resistance with fever, thrombosis, thrombophlebitis, infections with thrombosing tendencies, myocardial infarction, cancer, and in postsurgical patients. Higher incidence of bleeding reported in women >60 yrs of age. Caution with congestive heart failure, severe renal insufficiency, and in clinical states in which there exists edema with Na⁺ retention. If given IV, may cause fluid and/or solute overload resulting in dilution of serum electrolyte concentrations, overhydration, congested states, or pulmonary edema. (Heparin Inj) Use preservative-free in neonates and infants; benzyl alcohol has been associated with serious adverse events and death in pediatrics. (Heparin in Dextrose) Sulfite sensitivity may occur; caution especially in asthmatics. Caution with overt or known subclinical diabetes mellitus, or carbohydrate intolerance.

ADVERSE REACTIONS: Thrombocytopenia, hemorrhage, local irritation, generalized hypersensitivity reactions, HIT/HITT.

INTERACTIONS: When taken with dicumarol or warfarin sodium, wait at least 5 hrs after last IV heparin dose or 24 hrs after last SQ heparin dose if a valid PT is to be obtained. Platelet inhibitors (eg, acetylsalicylic acid, dextran, phenylbutazone) may induce bleeding; use with caution. Digitalis, tetracyclines, nicotine, antihistamines, or IV nitroglycerin may partially counteract the anticoagulant action. Decreased PTT with IV nitroglycerin; monitor PTT and adjust heparin dose with concurrent use.

PREGNANCY: Category C, caution in nursing.

MECHANISM OF ACTION: Glycosaminoglycan; inhibits reactions that lead to the clotting of blood and the formation of fibrin clots. Acts at multiple sites in the normal coagulation system.

PHARMACOKINETICS: Absorption: (SQ) T_{max}=2-4 hrs. **Metabolism:** Liver and reticuloendothelial system. **Elimination:** $T_{1/2}$=10 min.

NURSING CONSIDERATIONS

Assessment: Assess for thrombocytopenia, HIT/HITT, uncontrollable active bleeding states, drug hypersensitivity, pregnancy/nursing status, and for any other conditions where treatment is contraindicated or cautioned. Assess for possible drug interactions. Obtain baseline platelet counts.

Monitoring: Monitor for signs/symptoms of hemorrhage, thrombocytopenia, heparin resistance, hypersensitivity reactions, hyperaminotransferasemia, and other adverse reactions. Perform periodic monitoring of platelet counts, Hct, and tests for occult blood in stool during entire therapy course, and frequent coagulation tests if given therapeutically. If given by continuous IV infusion, monitor coagulation time q4h in early stages of treatment. If given intermittently by IV inj, perform coagulation tests before each inj during the early stages of treatment and then at appropriate intervals thereafter. If given IV, monitor for fluid/solute overload.

Patient Counseling: Counsel about increased risk of bleeding tendencies while on medication. Instruct to notify physician if any type of unusual bleeding, hypersensitivity reaction, or any other adverse reaction occurs. Advise that periodic laboratory monitoring is required during treatment.

Administration: (Heparin Inj) IV/SQ routes. (Heparin IV/Dextrose) IV route. If given IV, avoid additives. Refer to PI for further administration instructions. **Storage:** (Heparin Inj/IV) 20-25°C (68-77°F). (Heparin in Dextrose) 25°C (77°F); brief exposure up to 40°C (104°F) does not adversely affect product. Avoid excessive heat. (Heparin IV/Dextrose) Protect IV from freezing.

HEPSERA   RX
adefovir dipivoxil (Gilead Sciences)

Lactic acidosis and severe hepatomegaly with steatosis, including fatal cases, reported with the use of nucleoside analogues alone or in combination with other antiretrovirals. Severe acute exacerbations of hepatitis reported in patients who have discontinued therapy. Closely monitor hepatic function with both clinical and laboratory follow-up for at least several months in patients who d/c therapy. If appropriate, resumption of antihepatitis B therapy may be warranted. Chronic use may result in nephrotoxicity in patients at risk of or having underlying renal dysfunction; monitor renal function and adjust dose if required. HIV resistance may occur in patients with unrecognized or untreated HIV infection.

THERAPEUTIC CLASS: Nucleotide analogue reverse transcriptase inhibitor

INDICATIONS: Treatment of chronic hepatitis B in patients ≥12 yrs of age with evidence of active viral replication and either evidence of persistent elevations in serum aminotransferases (ALT/AST) or histologically active disease.

DOSAGE: *Adults:* 10mg qd. Renal Impairment: CrCl 30-49mL/min: 10mg q48h. CrCl 10-29mL/min: 10mg q72h. Hemodialysis Patients: 10mg every 7 days following dialysis. *Pediatrics:* ≥12 Yrs: 10mg qd.

HOW SUPPLIED: Tab: 10mg

WARNINGS/PRECAUTIONS: Caution in adolescents with underlying renal dysfunction; monitor renal function closely. Offer HIV antibody testing before initiating therapy. Obesity and prolonged nucleoside exposure may be risk factors for lactic acidosis and severe hepatomegaly with steatosis. Caution with known risk factors for liver disease. D/C if findings suggestive of lactic acidosis or pronounced hepatotoxicity develop. Resistance to the drug can result in viral load rebound, which may result in exacerbation of hepatitis B, and in the setting of diminished hepatic function, lead to liver decompensation and possible fatal outcome. To reduce risk of resistance in patients with lamivudine-resistant hepatitis B virus (HBV), use adefovir dipivoxil in combination with lamivudine and not as monotherapy. To reduce risk of resistance in patients receiving monotherapy, consider modification of treatment if serum HBV DNA remains >1000 copies/mL with continued treatment. Caution in elderly.

ADVERSE REACTIONS: Nephrotoxicity, lactic acidosis, severe hepatomegaly with steatosis, asthenia, headache, abdominal pain, nausea, flatulence, diarrhea, dyspepsia.

INTERACTIONS: Avoid with tenofovir disoproxil fumarate (TDF) or TDF-containing products. Coadministration with drugs that reduce renal function or compete for active tubular secretion may increase levels of either adefovir and/or these coadministered drugs. Caution with nephrotoxic agents (eg, cyclosporine, tacrolimus, aminoglycosides, vancomycin, and NSAIDs).

PREGNANCY: Category C, not for use in nursing.

MECHANISM OF ACTION: Nucleotide analogue reverse transcriptase inhibitor; inhibits HBV DNA polymerase (reverse transcriptase) by competing with natural substrate deoxyadenosine triphosphate and by causing DNA chain termination after incorporation into viral DNA.

PHARMACOKINETICS: Absorption: Bioavailability (59%); C_{max}=18.4ng/mL; T_{max}=1.75 hrs (median); AUC=220ng•h/mL. Refer to PI for pharmacokinetic parameters in pediatric patients and in patients with varying degrees of renal function. **Distribution:** V_d=392mL/kg (IV, 1mg/kg/day), 352mL/kg (IV, 3mg/kg/day); plasma protein binding (≤4%). **Elimination:** Urine (45%); $T_{1/2}$=7.48 hrs.

NURSING CONSIDERATIONS

Assessment: Assess for renal dysfunction, risk factors for lactic acidosis and liver disease, hypersensitivity, pregnancy/nursing status, and possible drug interactions. Perform HIV antibody testing and assess CrCl.

Monitoring: Monitor for signs/symptoms of lactic acidosis, hepatotoxicity, nephrotoxicity, clinical resistance, and other adverse reactions. Monitor hepatic function (in patients who d/c therapy) and renal function.

Patient Counseling: Inform of risks, benefits, and alternative modes of therapy. Instruct to follow a regular dosing schedule to avoid missing doses. Advise to immediately report any severe abdominal pain, muscle pain, yellowing of the eyes, dark urine, pale stools, and/or loss of appetite. Instruct to notify physician if any unusual/known symptom develops, persists, or worsens. Advise not to d/c therapy without 1st informing physician. Advise that routine laboratory monitoring and follow-up is important during therapy. Inform of importance of obtaining HIV antibody testing prior to starting therapy. Counsel women of childbearing age about risks of drug exposure during pregnancy, and to notify physician if the patient becomes pregnant while on therapy. Inform pregnant patients about the pregnancy registry.

Administration: Oral route. Take without regard to food. **Storage:** 25°C (77°F); excursions permitted to 15-30°C (59-86°F).

HERCEPTIN   RX
trastuzumab (Genentech)

May result in cardiac failure; incidence and severity were highest with anthracycline-containing chemotherapy regimens. Evaluate left ventricular function prior to and during treatment; d/c in patients receiving adjuvant therapy and withhold in patients with metastatic disease for clinically significant decrease in left ventricular function. May result in serious and fatal infusion reactions and pulmonary toxicity; interrupt infusion for dyspnea or clinically significant hypotension, and monitor until symptoms completely resolve. D/C for anaphylaxis, angioedema, interstitial pneumonitis, or acute respiratory distress syndrome. Exposure during pregnancy may result in oligohydramnios and oligohydramnios sequence manifesting as pulmonary hypoplasia, skeletal abnormalities, and neonatal death.

THERAPEUTIC CLASS: Monoclonal antibody/HER2-blocker

INDICATIONS: Adjuvant treatment of human epidermal growth factor receptor 2 protein (HER2)-overexpressing node-positive or node-negative breast cancer as part of a treatment regimen consisting of doxorubicin, cyclophosphamide, and either paclitaxel or docetaxel, with docetaxel and carboplatin, or as single agent following multimodality anthracycline-based therapy. In combination with paclitaxel for 1st-line treatment of HER2-overexpressing metastatic breast cancer, or as single agent for treatment of HER2-overexpressing breast cancer in patients who have received ≥1 chemotherapy regimen for metastatic disease. In combination with cisplatin and capecitabine or 5-fluorouracil for treatment of patients with HER2-overexpressing metastatic gastric or gastroesophageal junction adenocarcinoma who have not received prior treatment for metastatic disease.

DOSAGE: *Adults:* Breast Cancer Adjuvant Treatment: Administer for 52 weeks. During and Following Paclitaxel, Docetaxel, or Docetaxel/Carboplatin: Initial: 4mg/kg IV infusion over 90 min, then at 2mg/kg IV infusion over 30 min weekly during chemotherapy for the first 12 weeks (paclitaxel or docetaxel) or 18 weeks (docetaxel/carboplatin). One week following the last weekly dose, give 6mg/kg IV infusion over 30-90 min every 3 weeks. As Single Agent Within 3 Weeks Following Completion of Multimodality Anthracycline-Based Chemotherapy Regimens: Initial: 8mg/kg IV infusion over 90 min. Maint: 6mg/kg IV infusion over 30-90 min every 3 weeks. Breast Cancer Metastatic Treatment: Initial: 4mg/kg as 90-min IV infusion. Maint: 2mg/kg once weekly as 30-min IV infusion until disease progression. Metastatic Gastric Cancer: Initial: 8mg/kg as 90-min IV infusion. Maint: 6mg/kg IV infusion over 30-90 min every 3 weeks until disease progression. Refer to PI for dose modifications.

HOW SUPPLIED: Inj: 440mg

WARNINGS/PRECAUTIONS: Patients with symptomatic intrinsic lung disease or extensive tumor involvement of the lungs, resulting in dyspnea at rest, may have more severe pulmonary toxicity. Detection of HER2 protein overexpression is necessary for appropriate patient selection; use FDA-approved tests for the specific tumor type to assess HER2 protein overexpression and HER2 gene amplification.

ADVERSE REACTIONS: Cardiac failure, infusion reactions, pulmonary toxicity, fever, N/V, headache, nasopharyngitis, diarrhea, infections, fatigue, anemia, neutropenia, rash, weight loss, increased cough.

INTERACTIONS: See Boxed Warning. Higher incidence of neutropenia with myelosuppressive chemotherapy. Paclitaxel may increase trough concentrations.

PREGNANCY: Category D, not for use in nursing.

MECHANISM OF ACTION: Monoclonal antibody (IgG1 kappa)/HER2 blocker; inhibits proliferation of human tumor cells that overexpress HER2.

PHARMACOKINETICS: Absorption: C_{max}=377mcg/mL (500mg), 123mcg/mL (4mg/kg initial, then 2mg/kg weekly), 216mcg/mL (8mg/kg initial, then 6mg/kg every 3 weeks). **Distribution:** V_d=44mL/kg. **Elimination:** $T_{1/2}$=2 days (10mg), 12 days (500mg), 6 days (4mg/kg initial, then 2mg/kg weekly), 16 days (8mg/kg initial, then 6mg/kg every 3 weeks).

NURSING CONSIDERATIONS

Assessment: Assess cardiac function, including history, physical exam, and baseline left ventricular ejection fraction (LVEF). Assess HER2 protein overexpression and HER2 gene amplification; should be performed by laboratories with demonstrated proficiency in the specific technology being utilized. Assess for symptomatic intrinsic lung disease or extensive tumor involvement of lungs, pregnancy/nursing status, and possible drug interactions.

Monitoring: Monitor for infusion reactions, pulmonary toxicity, neutropenia, and other adverse reactions. Monitor LVEF every 3 months during and upon completion of therapy, and every 6 months for at least 2 yrs following completion as a component of adjuvant therapy. Repeat LVEF measurement at 4-week intervals if therapy is withheld for significant left ventricular cardiac dysfunction.

Patient Counseling: Advise to contact physician immediately for new onset or worsening SOB, cough, swelling of ankles/legs/face, palpitations, weight gain of >5 lbs in 24 hrs, dizziness, or loss of consciousness. Inform that drug may cause fetal harm. Advise women of childbearing potential to use effective contraceptive methods during treatment and for a minimum of 6 months following therapy. Instruct not to breastfeed during treatment. Encourage women exposed to trastuzumab during pregnancy to enroll in MotHER- the Herceptin Pregnancy Registry.

Administration: IV route. Do not administer as IV push or bolus. Do not mix with other drugs. Refer to PI for preparation and administration instructions. **Storage:** 2-8°C (36-46°F). Reconstituted with Bacteriostatic Water for Inj: 2-8°C (36-46°F) for 28 days. Reconstituted with Unpreserved Sterile Water for Inj: Use immediately. Diluted in Polyvinylchloride or Polyethylene Bags Containing 0.9% NaCl Inj: 2-8°C (36-46°F) for no more than 24 hrs prior to use. Do not freeze following reconstitution/dilution.

HIBERIX   RX
haemophilus B conjugate - tetanus toxoid (GlaxoSmithKline)

THERAPEUTIC CLASS: Vaccine

INDICATIONS: Active immunization as a booster dose for the prevention of invasive disease caused by *Haemophilus influenza* type b in children 15 months-4 yrs (prior to 5th birthday).

DOSAGE: *Pediatrics:* 15 Months-4 Yrs: Single dose (0.5mL) IM into the anterolateral aspect of the thigh or deltoid.

HOW SUPPLIED: Inj: 0.5mL

WARNINGS/PRECAUTIONS: Use as a booster dose in children who have received a primary series with a *Haemophilus* b Conjugate Vaccine. Evaluate potential benefits and risks if Guillain-Barre syndrome occurs within 6 weeks of receipt of a prior tetanus toxoid-containing vaccine. Tip caps of prefilled syringe may contain natural rubber latex; allergic reactions may occur in latex-sensitive individuals. Syncope may occur and can be accompanied by transient neurological signs. Review immunization history for possible vaccine hypersensitivity; appropriate treatment should be available for possible anaphylactic reactions. Expected immune response may not be obtained in immunosuppressed children. Urine antigen detection may not have a diagnostic value within 1-2 weeks after receipt of vaccine. Not a substitute for routine tetanus immunization.

ADVERSE REACTIONS: Fever, fussiness, loss of appetite, restlessness, sleepiness, diarrhea, vomiting, inj-site reactions (eg, redness, pain, swelling).

INTERACTIONS: Immunosuppressive therapies, including irradiation, antimetabolites, alkylating agents, cytotoxic drugs, and corticosteroids (used in greater than physiologic doses) may reduce immune response to vaccine.

PREGNANCY: Category C, safety not known in nursing.

MECHANISM OF ACTION: Vaccine; protects against invasive disease due to *H. influenzae* type b.

NURSING CONSIDERATIONS

Assessment: Review immunization history, current health/medical status (eg, immunosuppression), and known allergic reaction to previous dose of any *H. influenzae* type b vaccination or tetanus toxoid-containing vaccine. Assess for latex hypersensitivity and possible drug interactions.

Monitoring: Monitor for allergic reactions, signs/symptoms of Guillian-Barre syndrome, inj-site reactions (eg, pain, redness, swelling), syncope, and for any other possible adverse events. Monitor immune response.

Patient Counseling: Inform patient's parents/guardians about benefits/risks of immunization. Counsel about the potential for adverse reactions; instruct to notify physician if any adverse reactions occur.

Administration: IM route. Do not administer SQ, intradermally, or IV. Do not mix with any other vaccine in the same syringe or vial. Refer to PI for reconstitution instructions. **Storage:** 2-8°C (36-46°F). Protect from light. Diluent: 2-8°C (36-46°F) or at 20-25°C (68-77°F). Do not freeze. After Reconstitution: 2-8°C (36-46°F). Do not freeze. Discard if not used within 24 hrs or if has been frozen.

H

HORIZANT
RX
gabapentin enacarbil (GlaxoSmithKline)

THERAPEUTIC CLASS: GABA analog

INDICATIONS: Treatment of moderate to severe primary restless legs syndrome (RLS) and management of postherpetic neuralgia (PHN) in adults.

DOSAGE: *Adults:* Take with food. RLS: Usual: 600mg qd at about 5 pm. Renal Impairment: CrCl 30-59mL/min: Initial: 300mg/day. Titrate: Increase to 600mg PRN. CrCl 15-29mL/min: 300mg/day. CrCl <15mL/min: 300mg qod. PHN: Initial: 600mg every am on Days 1-3. Titrate: Increase to 600mg bid (1200mg/day) on Day 4. Usual: 600mg bid. Refer to PI for dose modifications in PHN patients with renal impairment.

HOW SUPPLIED: Tab, Extended Release: 300mg, 600mg

WARNINGS/PRECAUTIONS: Not recommended for patients who are required to sleep during the day and remain awake at night or in RLS patients with CrCl <15mL/min on hemodialysis. May cause significant driving impairment, somnolence/sedation, and dizziness. Not interchangeable with other gabapentin products. Increases the risk of suicidal thoughts or behavior; monitor for the emergence or worsening of depression, suicidal thoughts/behavior, and/or any unusual changes in mood or behavior. Drug reaction with eosinophilia and systemic symptoms (DRESS)/ multiorgan hypersensitivity reported; evaluate immediately if signs/symptoms (eg, hypersensitivity, fever, lymphadenopathy) are present and d/c if alternative etiology cannot be established. For RLS patients, if recommended daily dose is exceeded, reduce dose to 600mg daily for 1 week prior to discontinuation to minimize potential for withdrawal seizure. For PHN patients receiving bid dose, reduce dose to qd for 1 week prior to d/c to minimize potential for withdrawal seizure. May have tumorigenic potential. Caution in elderly and with renal impairment.

ADVERSE REACTIONS: Somnolence/sedation, dizziness, headache, nausea, dry mouth, flatulence, fatigue, insomnia, irritability, feeling drunk/abnormal, peripheral edema, weight increase, vertigo.

INTERACTIONS: Drug is released faster from extended-release tab in the presence of alcohol; avoid alcohol consumption. Increased somnolence/sedation, dizziness, and nausea when taken in conjunction with morphine.

PREGNANCY: Category C, not for use in nursing.

MECHANISM OF ACTION: Gamma-aminobutyric acid analog; not established. Prodrug of gabapentin; binds with high affinity to the α2delta subunit of voltage-activated calcium channels.

PHARMACOKINETICS: Absorption: (PHN: 600mg bid) C_{max}=5.35μg/mL, AUC_{24}=109μg•hr/mL; bioavailability (75% [fed], 42-65% [fasted]); T_{max}=5 hrs (fasted), 7.3 hrs (fed). **Distribution:** Plasma protein binding (<3%); V_d=76L. **Metabolism:** Extensive 1st-pass hydrolysis to gabapentin (active form). **Elimination:** Kidney (unchanged); urine (94%), feces (5%); $T_{1/2}$=5.1-6 hrs.

NURSING CONSIDERATIONS

Assessment: Assess for preexisting tumors, history of depression, pregnancy/nursing status, renal function (CrCl), and possible drug interactions.

Monitoring: Monitor for withdrawal seizures with discontinuation, somnolence/sedation, dizziness, emergence or worsening of depression, suicidal thoughts/behavior, and/or any unusual changes in mood/behavior, DRESS, development or worsening of tumors, renal function, and hypersensitivity reactions.

Patient Counseling: Inform that therapy may cause significant driving impairment, somnolence, and dizziness; advise not to drive or operate dangerous machinery until sufficient experience on therapy is gained. Counsel that treatment may increase the risk of suicidal thoughts and behavior; advise to report to physician any behaviors of concern. Advise that multiorgan hypersensitivity reactions may occur; instruct to contact physician if experiencing any signs or symptoms of this condition. Advise not to interchange with other gabapentin products. If the dose is missed, instruct to take the next dose at the time of the next scheduled dose. Instruct about how to d/c therapy. Advise to avoid alcohol when taking the drug.

Administration: Oral route. Take with food. Swallow tab whole; do not cut, crush, or chew.
Storage: 25°C (77°F); excursions permitted to 15-30°C (59-86°F). Protect from moisture.

HUMALOG RX
insulin lispro, rdna origin (Lilly)

THERAPEUTIC CLASS: Insulin

INDICATIONS: To improve glycemic control in adults and children with diabetes mellitus.

DOSAGE: *Adults:* Individualize dose. Total Daily Insulin Requirement: Usual: 0.5-1 U/kg/day. (SQ) Give within 15 min ac or immediately pc. Use with an intermediate- or long-acting insulin. Continuous SQ Infusion by an External Pump: Initial: Based on the total daily insulin dose of the previous regimen. Usual: 50% of total dose given as meal-related boluses and the remainder given as a basal infusion. (IV) 0.1-1 U/mL in infusion systems containing 0.9% NaCl. Renal/Hepatic Impairment: May need to reduce dose.
Pediatrics: ≥3 Yrs: Individualize dose. Total Daily Insulin Requirement: Usual: 0.5-1 U/kg/day. (SQ) Give within 15 min ac or immediately pc. Use with an intermediate- or long-acting insulin. Continuous SQ Infusion by an External Pump: Initial: Based on the total daily insulin dose of the previous regimen. Usual: 50% of total dose given as meal-related boluses and the remainder given as a basal infusion. Renal/Hepatic Impairment: May need to reduce dose.

HOW SUPPLIED: Inj: 100 U/mL [3mL, cartridge, pen, KwikPen, vial; 10mL, vial]

CONTRAINDICATIONS: During episodes of hypoglycemia.

WARNINGS/PRECAUTIONS: Any change in insulin regimen should be made cautiously and under medical supervision. Changes in strength, manufacturer, type, or method of administration may result in the need for a change in dosage. Stress, major illness, or changes in exercise or meal patterns may alter insulin requirements. Hypoglycemia may occur and may impair ability to concentrate and react; caution in patients with hypoglycemia unawareness and in patients predisposed to hypoglycemia. Hypokalemia may occur; caution in patients who may be at risk. Severe, life-threatening, generalized allergy, including anaphylaxis, may occur. Frequent glucose monitoring and dose adjustments may be necessary with renal/hepatic impairment. Malfunction of the insulin pump or infusion set or insulin degradation can rapidly lead to hyperglycemia or ketosis; prompt identification and correction of the cause is necessary. Train patients using continuous SQ infusion pump therapy to administer by inj and have alternate insulin therapy available in case of pump failure. IV administration should be under medical supervision with close monitoring of blood glucose and K$^+$ levels.

ADVERSE REACTIONS: Flu syndrome, pharyngitis, rhinitis, headache, pain, cough increased, infection, diarrhea, nausea, fever, abdominal pain, asthenia, bronchitis, myalgia, urinary tract infection.

INTERACTIONS: May require dose adjustment and close monitoring with drugs that may increase blood glucose-lowering effect and susceptibility to hypoglycemia (oral antidiabetics, salicylates, sulfonamide antibiotics, MAOIs, fluoxetine, pramlintide, disopyramide, fibrates, propoxyphene, pentoxifylline, ACE inhibitors, ARBs, and somatostatin analogs [eg, octreotide]), drugs that may reduce blood glucose-lowering effect (corticosteroids, isoniazid, niacin, estrogens, oral contraceptives, phenothiazines, danazol, diuretics, sympathomimetic agents [eg, epinephrine, albuterol, terbutaline], somatropin, atypical antipsychotics, glucagon, protease inhibitors, and thyroid hormones), or drugs that may increase or reduce blood glucose-lowering effect (β-blockers, clonidine, lithium salts, and alcohol). Pentamidine may cause hypoglycemia, sometimes followed by hyperglycemia. Hypoglycemic signs may be reduced with β-blockers, clonidine, guanethidine, and reserpine. Caution with K$^+$-lowering drugs or drugs sensitive to serum K$^+$ concentrations. Observe for signs/symptoms of heart failure (HF) if treated concomitantly with a peroxisome proliferator-activated receptor (PPAR)-gamma agonist (eg, thiazolidinedione); consider discontinuation or dose reduction of the PPAR-gamma agonist if HF develops.

PREGNANCY: Category B, caution in nursing.

MECHANISM OF ACTION: Insulin lispro (rDNA origin); regulates glucose metabolism. Lowers blood glucose by stimulating peripheral glucose uptake by skeletal muscle and fat, and by inhibiting hepatic glucose production. Inhibits lipolysis and proteolysis, and enhances protein synthesis.

PHARMACOKINETICS: Absorption: (SQ, 0.1-0.2 U/kg) Absolute bioavailability (55-77%); (SQ, 0.1-0.4 U/kg) T_{max}=30-90 min. **Distribution:** (IV) V_d=1.55L/kg (0.1 U/kg), 0.72L/kg (0.2 U/kg). **Elimination:** (IV) $T_{1/2}$=0.85 hrs (0.1 U/kg), 0.92 hrs (0.2 U/kg); (SQ) $T_{1/2}$=1 hr.

NURSING CONSIDERATIONS

Assessment: Assess for predisposition to hypoglycemia, risk for hypokalemia, hypersensitivity, renal/hepatic impairment, pregnancy/nursing status, and possible drug interactions. Obtain baseline blood glucose and HbA1c levels.

Monitoring: Monitor for signs and symptoms of hypoglycemia, hypokalemia, allergic reactions, and other adverse effects. Monitor blood glucose levels, HbA1c levels, K^+ levels, and renal/hepatic function.

Patient Counseling: Instruct on self-management procedures (eg, glucose monitoring, proper inj technique, management of hypoglycemia/hyperglycemia). Advise on handling of special situations, such as intercurrent conditions (eg, illness, stress, emotional disturbances), inadequate or skipped doses, inadvertent administration of an increased dose, inadequate food intake, and skipped meals. Instruct diabetic women to inform physician if pregnant or contemplating pregnancy. Counsel to always check label before each inj to avoid medication errors, such as accidental mix-ups. Instruct on how to use external infusion pump.

Administration: IV/SQ route. Inject SQ in the abdominal wall, thigh, upper arm, or buttocks; rotate inj sites within the same region. Do not mix with any other insulins other than NPH insulin for SQ inj. Do not dilute or mix with any other insulins for use in an external SQ infusion pump. Refer to PI for further preparation and administration instructions. **Storage:** Refer to PI for storage conditions. Pump: Change the drug in the reservoir at least every 7 days, and the infusion sets and the infusion set insertion site at least every 3 days or after exposure to >37°C (98.6°F). Discard cartridge used in the D-Tron pumps after 7 days even if it still contains the drug. Diluted Humalog for SQ Inj: 5°C (41°F) for 28 days or 30°C (86°F) for 14 days. Do not dilute drug contained in a cartridge or drug used in an external insulin pump. IV Admixture: 2-8°C (36-46°F) for 48 hrs; may be used at room temperature for up to an additional 48 hrs.

HUMALOG MIX 75/25   RX

insulin lispro protamine, rdna origin - insulin lispro, rdna origin (Lilly)

THERAPEUTIC CLASS: Insulin

INDICATIONS: Treatment of patients with diabetes mellitus for the control of hyperglycemia.

DOSAGE: *Adults:* Individualize dose. Inject SQ within 15 min ac. Renal/Hepatic Impairment: May need to reduce/adjust dose.

HOW SUPPLIED: Inj: (Insulin Lispro Protamine-Insulin Lispro) 75 U-25 U/mL [3mL, Pen, KwikPen; 10mL, vial]

CONTRAINDICATIONS: During episodes of hypoglycemia.

WARNINGS/PRECAUTIONS: Any change of insulin should be made cautiously and only under medical supervision. Changes in strength, manufacturer, type, species, or method of manufacture may result in the need for a change in dosage. Hypoglycemia and hypokalemia may occur; caution in patients in whom such potential side effects might be clinically relevant (eg, patients who are fasting or have autonomic neuropathy). Lipodystrophy and hypersensitivity may occur. Dosage adjustment may be necessary if patient changes physical activity or usual meal plan. Illness, emotional disturbances, or other stress may alter insulin requirements. Careful glucose monitoring and dose adjustments may be necessary with hepatic/renal impairment. Inj-site reactions (eg, redness, swelling, itching) and severe, life-threatening, generalized allergy, including anaphylactic reactions, may occur. Contains metacresol as excipient; localized reactions and generalized myalgias reported with cresol-containing injectable products. Antibody production reported. Not for IV use.

ADVERSE REACTIONS: Hypoglycemia, allergic reactions, inj-site reactions, lipodystrophy, pruritus, rash.

INTERACTIONS: Drugs with hyperglycemic activity (eg, corticosteroids, isoniazid, certain lipid-lowering drugs [eg, niacin], estrogens, oral contraceptives, phenothiazines, thyroid replacement therapy) may increase insulin requirements. Drugs that increase insulin sensitivity or have hypoglycemic activity (eg, oral antidiabetic agents, salicylates, sulfa antibiotics, MAOIs, ACE inhibitors, ARBs, β-blockers, inhibitors of pancreatic function [eg, octreotide], alcohol) may decrease insulin requirements. β-blockers may mask symptoms of hypoglycemia. Caution with K^+-lowering drugs or drugs sensitive to serum K^+ levels. Observe for signs/symptoms of heart failure (HF) if treated concomitantly with a peroxisome proliferator-activated receptor (PPAR)-gamma agonist (eg, thiazolidinedione); d/c or reduce dose of the PPAR-gamma agonist if HF develops.

PREGNANCY: Category B, caution in nursing.

MECHANISM OF ACTION: Insulin; regulates glucose metabolism. In muscle and other tissues (except the brain), causes rapid transport of glucose and amino acids intracellularly, promotes anabolism, and inhibits protein catabolism. In the liver, promotes the uptake and storage of glucose in the form of glycogen, inhibits gluconeogenesis, and promotes the conversion of excess glucose into fat.

PHARMACOKINETICS: Absorption: T_{max}=30-240 min (0.3 U/kg). **Distribution:** V_d=0.26-0.36L/kg (insulin lispro).

NURSING CONSIDERATIONS

Assessment: Assess for presence of hypoglycemia or hypokalemia and for conditions where such potential side effects might be clinically relevant. Assess for hypersensitivity, renal/hepatic impairment, pregnancy/nursing status, and possible drug interactions. Obtain baseline blood glucose and HbA1c levels.

Monitoring: Monitor for signs and symptoms of hypoglycemia, hypokalemia, lipodystrophy, allergic reactions, antibody production, and other adverse effects. Monitor blood glucose levels, HbA1c levels, K^+ levels, and renal/hepatic function.

Patient Counseling: Inform of the potential risks and advantages of therapy and alternative therapies. Instruct not to mix drug with any other insulin. Inform of the importance of proper insulin storage, inj technique, timing of dosage, adherence to meal planning, regular physical activity, regular blood glucose monitoring, periodic HbA1c testing, recognition and management of hypo/hyperglycemia, and periodic assessment for diabetes complications. Advise to inform physician if pregnant or planning to become pregnant. Instruct if using insulin pen delivery device, how to properly use delivery device, prime the pen to a stream of insulin, and how to properly dispose of needles. Advise not to share insulin pen with others.

Administration: SQ route. **Storage:** Unopened: 2-8°C (36-46°F) until expiration date, or room temperature (<30°C [86°F]) for 28 days (vial) or 10 days (Pen, KwikPen). Do not freeze; do not use if frozen. Opened: <30°C (86°F) for 28 days (vial) or 10 days (Pen, KwikPen). Do not refrigerate Pen/KwikPen. Protect from direct heat and light.

HUMATROPE   RX
somatropin rdna origin (Lilly)

THERAPEUTIC CLASS: Recombinant human growth hormone

INDICATIONS: Treatment of pediatrics with growth failure due to inadequate secretion of endogenous growth hormone (GH), short stature associated with Turner syndrome (TS), idiopathic short stature (ISS), short stature or growth failure with short stature homeobox-containing gene (SHOX) deficiency, and for growth failure in children born small for gestational age (SGA) who fail to demonstrate catch-up growth by age 2-4 yrs. Replacement of endogenous GH in adults with adult-onset or childhood-onset growth hormone deficiency (GHD).

DOSAGE: *Adults:* GHD: Non-Weight Based: Initial: 0.2mg/day SQ (range, 0.15-0.30mg/day). Titrate: May increase gradually every 1-2 months by increments of 0.1-0.2mg/day based on response and insulin-like growth factor-I (IGF-I) concentrations. Maint: Individualize. Weight-Based: Initial: ≤0.006mg/kg/day (6mcg/kg/day) SQ. Titrate: May increase based on individual requirement. Max: 0.0125mg/kg/day (12.5mcg/kg/day). Estrogen Replete Women: May need higher doses than men. Elderly: Consider lower starting dose and smaller dose increments. *Pediatrics:* Individualize dose. The calculated weekly dose should be divided into equal doses given either 6 or 7 days/week. GHD: 0.026-0.043mg/kg/day SQ (0.18-0.30mg/kg/week). TS: ≤0.054mg/kg/day SQ (0.375mg/kg/week). ISS: ≤0.053mg/kg/day SQ (0.37mg/kg/week). SHOX Deficiency: 0.050mg/kg/day SQ (0.35mg/kg/week). SGA: ≤0.067mg/kg/day SQ (0.47mg/kg/week). Refer to PI for further details.

HOW SUPPLIED: Inj: 5mg [vial]; 6mg, 12mg, 24mg [cartridge]

CONTRAINDICATIONS: Acute critical illness due to complications following open heart surgery, abdominal surgery or multiple accidental trauma, or with acute respiratory failure. Pediatric patients with Prader-Willi syndrome (PWS) who are severely obese, have history of upper airway obstruction or sleep apnea, or have severe respiratory impairment. Pediatric patients who have growth failure due to genetically confirmed PWS. Active malignancy, evidence of progression or recurrence of an underlying intracranial tumor, or active proliferative or severe nonproliferative diabetic retinopathy. Pediatric patients with closed epiphyses.

WARNINGS/PRECAUTIONS: Increased mortality reported in patients with acute critical illnesses. Fatalities reported in patients with PWS; evaluate for signs of upper airway obstruction (eg, new/increased snoring) and sleep apnea and interrupt therapy if these signs occur. Implement effective weight control in patients with PWS. Examine for progression/recurrence of underlying disease in patients with preexisting tumors or GHD secondary to intracranial lesion. Monitor for malignant transformation of skin lesions. Undiagnosed impaired glucose tolerance and overt diabetes mellitus (DM) may be unmasked, and new-onset type 2 DM reported; monitor glucose levels. Intracranial HTN with papilledema, visual changes, headache, N/V reported; perform funduscopic exam before and during therapy, and d/c if papilledema occurs. Fluid retention in adults may occur. Monitor other hormonal replacement treatments in patients with hypopituitarism. Undiagnosed/untreated hypothyroidism may prevent optimal response. Hypothyroidism may become evident or worsen; perform periodic thyroid function tests. Slipped capital femoral epiphysis and progression of scoliosis may occur in pediatrics. Increased risk of ear/hearing and cardiovascular (CV) disorders in TS patients. Pancreatitis rarely reported; monitor for abdominal pain. Tissue atrophy may occur when administered at the same site over a long period; rotate inj site. Serum levels of inorganic P, alkaline phosphatase, parathyroid hormone, and IGF-I may increase. Caution in the elderly.

ADVERSE REACTIONS: Ear disorder, arthrosis, pain, edema, arthralgia, myalgia, HTN, paresthesia, gynecomastia, scoliosis, otitis media, hyperlipidemia, rhinitis, flu syndrome, headache.

INTERACTIONS: May inhibit 11β-hydroxysteroid dehydrogenase type 1, resulting in reduced serum cortisol concentrations; may need glucocorticoid replacement or dose adjustments of glucocorticoid therapy (eg, cortisone acetate, prednisone). Glucocorticoid therapy may attenuate growth-promoting effects in children; carefully adjust glucocorticoid replacement dosing. May increase clearance of antipyrine. May alter clearance of compounds metabolized by CYP450 liver enzymes (eg, corticosteroids, sex steroids, anticonvulsants, cyclosporine); monitor carefully. Oral estrogen replacement may increase dose requirements. May need to adjust dose of insulin and/or other hypoglycemic agents, and thyroid hormone replacement therapy.

PREGNANCY: Category C, caution in nursing.

MECHANISM OF ACTION: Recombinant human GH; binds to dimeric GH receptors located within the cell membranes of target tissue cells, resulting in intracellular signal transduction and subsequent induction of transcription and translation of GH-dependent proteins, including IGF-1, IGF BP-3, and acid labile subunit.

PHARMACOKINETICS: Absorption: Absolute bioavailability (75%); C_{max}=63.3ng/mL; AUC=585ng•hr/mL. **Distribution:** V_d=0.957L/kg. **Metabolism:** Liver and kidney (protein catabolism). **Elimination:** Urine. $T_{1/2}$=3.81 hrs.

NURSING CONSIDERATIONS

Assessment: Assess for preexisting DM or impaired glucose tolerance, hypothyroidism, hypopituitarism, history of scoliosis, hypersensitivity to drug/diluent/metacresol/glycerin, pregnancy/nursing status, possible drug interactions, and any other conditions where treatment is contraindicated or cautioned. Perform funduscopic exam.

Monitoring: Monitor for growth, clinical response, compliance, malignant transformation of skin lesions, slipped capital femoral epiphysis, progression of scoliosis in pediatrics, pancreatitis, fluid retention, weight control, respiratory status, and allergic reactions. Monitor patients with hypopituitarism who are on other hormone replacement therapy. Perform periodic thyroid function tests, funduscopic exam, and monitor glucose levels. In patients with TS, monitor for ear/hearing/CV disorders. In patients with preexisting tumors or GH deficiency secondary to an intracranial lesion, monitor for progression or recurrence of underlying disease process.

Patient Counseling: Inform of the potential benefits and risks of therapy, proper administration, usage and disposal, and caution against any reuse of needles and syringes.

Administration: SQ route. Refer to PI for reconstitution and general administration guidelines. Avoid use of cartridge if allergic to metacresol or glycerin. **Storage:** (Vial/Cartridge) Before Reconstitution: 2-8°C (36-46°F). Avoid freezing diluent. After Reconstitution: 2-8°C (36-46°F) for up to 14 days for vials and up to 28 days for cartridge. Avoid freezing. (Vial) After Reconstitution with Sterile Water: 2-8°C (36-46°F) for up to 24 hrs; use only one dose per vial and discard unused portion. After Reconstitution with Bacteriostatic Water for Inj: 2-8°C (36-46°F) for up to 14 days.

HUMIRA RX
adalimumab (AbbVie)

> Increased risk of serious infections (eg, active tuberculosis [TB] including latent TB reactivation, invasive fungal, bacterial, viral, and other infections due to opportunistic pathogens) leading to hospitalization or death, mostly with concomitant use of immunosuppressants (eg, methotrexate [MTX] or corticosteroids). D/C if serious infection or sepsis develops. Active/latent reactivation TB patients have frequently presented with disseminated or extrapulmonary disease; test for latent TB before and during therapy and initiate treatment for latent TB prior to adalimumab use. Invasive fungal infections reported; consider empiric antifungal therapy in patients at risk who develop severe systemic illness. Consider risks and benefits prior to therapy in patients with chronic or recurrent infection. Monitor patients closely for development of infection during and after treatment. Lymphoma and other malignancies, some fatal, reported in children and adolescents. Post marketing cases of aggressive and fatal hepatosplenic T-cell lymphoma (HSTCL) reported in patients with Crohn's disease (CD) or ulcerative colitis (UC) and the majority were in adolescent and young adult males; all of these patients were treated concomitantly with azathioprine or 6-mercaptopurine.

THERAPEUTIC CLASS: Monoclonal antibody/TNF-blocker

INDICATIONS: Reduce signs/symptoms, induce major clinical response, inhibit progression of structural damage, and improve physical function in adults with moderate to severe active rheumatoid arthritis (RA) with/without MTX or nonbiologic disease-modifying antirheumatic drugs (DMARDs). Reduce signs/symptoms of moderate to severe active polyarticular juvenile idiopathic arthritis (JIA) in pediatric patients ≥4 yrs of age with/without MTX. Reduce signs/symptoms in adults with active ankylosing spondylitis (AS). Reduce signs/symptoms, inhibit progression of structural damage, and improve physical function in adults with active psoriatic arthritis (PsA) with/without nonbiologic DMARDs. Reduce signs/symptoms and induce/maintain clinical remission in adults with moderate to severe active Crohn's disease (CD) with inadequate response to conventional therapy and lost response/intolerant to infliximab. Treatment of adults with moderate to severe chronic plaque psoriasis (Ps) who are candidates for systemic or phototherapy, and when other systemic therapies are medically less appropriate. Induce and sustain clinical remission in adults with moderate to severe active ulcerative colitis (UC) with inadequate response to immunosuppressants, such as corticosteroids, azathioprine, or 6-mercaptopurine (6-MP).

DOSAGE: *Adults:* RA/PsA/AS: 40mg SQ every other week. Some patients with RA not taking concomitant MTX may derive additional benefit from increasing to 40mg every week. CD/UC: Initial: 160mg SQ on Day 1 (given as four 40mg inj in 1 day or as two 40mg inj/day for 2 consecutive days); then 80mg after 2 weeks (Day 15). Maint: 40mg every other week beginning Week 4 (Day 29). UC: Continue only with evidence of clinical remission by 8 weeks (Day 57) of therapy. Ps: Initial: 80mg SQ followed by 40mg every other week starting 1 week after initial dose. *Pediatrics:* 4-17 Yrs: Polyarticular JIA: ≥30kg (66 lbs): 40mg SQ every other week. 15kg (33 lbs)-<30kg (66 lbs): 20mg SQ every other week.

HOW SUPPLIED: Inj: 20mg/0.4mL [prefilled syringe], 40mg/0.8mL [prefilled syringe, prefilled pen, vial]

WARNINGS/PRECAUTIONS: Do not initiate with an active infection. Increased risk of infection in patients >65 yrs of age and in patients with comorbid conditions; consider the risks prior to therapy for those who have resided or traveled in areas of endemic TB or mycoses, and with any underlying conditions predisposing to infection. Cases of acute and chronic leukemia and lymphoma in adults as well as other malignancies, including breast, colon, prostate, lung, melanoma and nonmelanoma skin cancer, reported. Carefully consider the potential risk of HSTCL with the combination of azathioprine or 6-MP. Anaphylaxis and angioneurotic edema reported; d/c immediately and institute appropriate therapy if anaphylactic or other serious allergic reaction occurs. May increase the risk of hepatitis B virus (HBV) reactivation in chronic carriers; closely monitor for signs of active HBV infection during and for several months after therapy termination. D/C if HBV reactivation develops and start effective antiviral therapy with appropriate supportive treatment. New onset or exacerbation of CNS demyelinating disease (eg, multiple sclerosis, optic neuritis) and peripheral demyelinating disease (eg, Guillain-Barre syndrome) reported; caution with preexisting or recent-onset CNS/peripheral nervous system demyelinating disorders. Hematologic system adverse reactions, including significant cytopenia (eg, thrombocytopenia, leukopenia), infrequently reported; consider discontinuation in patients with confirmed significant hematologic abnormalities. New onset or worsening of congestive heart failure (CHF) reported; caution and monitor patients who have heart failure. May result in autoantibody formation and development of a lupus-like syndrome; d/c if symptoms suggestive of a lupus-like syndrome develop. JIA patients should be brought up to date with all immunizations in agreement with current immunizations guidelines prior to initiating therapy, if possible. Needle cover of the prefilled syringe contains dry rubber (latex); avoid with patients sensitive to this substance. Caution in elderly.

ADVERSE REACTIONS: Serious infections, malignancies, upper respiratory infection, inj-site reaction, headache, rash, sinusitis, nausea, urinary tract infection, flu syndrome, abdominal pain, hyperlipidemia, hypercholesterolemia, back pain, hematuria.

INTERACTIONS: See Boxed Warning. Reduced clearance with MTX. Concomitant administration with other biologic DMARDs (eg, anakinra, abatacept) or other TNF blockers is not recommended due to possible increased risk for infections and other potential pharmacological interactions. Avoid with live vaccines. Upon initiation or discontinuation of adalimumab in patients being treated with CYP450 substrates with a narrow therapeutic index, monitor therapeutic effect (eg, warfarin) or drug concentration (eg, cyclosporine, theophylline) and adjust individual dose of the drug product as needed.

PREGNANCY: Category B, caution in nursing.

MECHANISM OF ACTION: Monoclonal antibody/TNF-α receptor blocker; binds specifically to TNF-α and blocks its interaction with p55 and p75 cell surface TNF receptors. Lyses surface TNF-expressing cells in vitro in the presence of complement. Modulates biological responses that are induced or regulated by TNF. In Ps, therapy may reduce the epidermal thickness and infiltration of inflammatory cells.

PHARMACOKINETICS: Absorption: (40mg SQ single dose) Absolute bioavailability (64%), C_{max}=4.7mcg/mL, T_{max}=131 hrs. **Distribution:** (0.25-10mg/kg IV dose) V_d=4.7-6L. **Elimination:** (0.25-10mg/kg IV dose) $T_{1/2}$=2 weeks.

NURSING CONSIDERATIONS

Assessment: Assess for active/latent infection, history of chronic/recurrent infection, infection risk, TB risk factors, HBV infection status, CNS/peripheral nervous system demyelinating disorders, known malignancy, CHF, hypersensitivity to the drug, latex allergy, pregnancy/nursing status, and possible drug interactions. Assess for recent travel to areas of endemic TB or endemic mycoses. Assess immunization history in pediatric patients. Perform test for latent TB. Perform a skin examination, particularly in patients with a medical history of prior prolonged immunosuppressant therapy or psoriasis patients with a history of PUVA treatment.

Monitoring: Monitor for serious infections, reactivation TB, malignancies (eg, lymphoma), hypersensitivity reactions, HBV reactivation, neurological reactions, hematological reactions, worsening/new-onset CHF, lupus-like syndrome, and other adverse reactions. Periodically evaluate for active TB and test for latent infection. Perform periodic skin examinations, particularly in patients with a medical history of prior prolonged immunosuppressant therapy or psoriasis patients with a history of PUVA treatment.

Patient Counseling: Inform about potential benefits/risks of therapy. Inform that therapy may lower the ability of immune system to fight infections; instruct to contact physician if any symptoms of infection, including TB, invasive fungal infections, and reactivation of HBV infections develop. Counsel about risk of malignancies. Advise to seek immediate medical attention if any symptoms of severe allergic reactions develop. Advise latex-sensitive patients that the needle cap of prefilled syringe contains latex. Advise to report any signs of new/worsening medical conditions (eg, CHF, neurological disease, autoimmune disorders) or any symptoms suggestive of a cytopenia (eg, bleeding, bruising, or persistent fever). Instruct on proper inj technique, as well as proper syringe and needle disposal.

Administration: SQ route. Rotate inj sites; avoid in areas where skin is tender, bruised, red, or hard. Refer to PI for general considerations for administration. **Storage:** 2-8°C (36-46°F). Do not freeze; do not use if frozen even if it has been thawed. Store in a cool carrier with an ice pack when traveling. Protect prefilled syringe from exposure to light. Store in original carton until time of administration.

HUMULIN 70/30   OTC
insulin human nph, rdna origin - insulin human, rdna origin (Lilly)

THERAPEUTIC CLASS: Insulin

INDICATIONS: To improve glycemic control in adults with diabetes mellitus.

DOSAGE: *Adults:* Individualize dose. Administer SQ 30-45 min ac.

HOW SUPPLIED: Inj: (Isophane-Regular) 70 U-30 U/mL [3mL, vial, pen, KwikPen; 10mL, vial]

CONTRAINDICATIONS: During episodes of hypoglycemia.

WARNINGS/PRECAUTIONS: Changes in strength, manufacturer, type, or method of administration may affect glycemic control and predispose to hypoglycemia/hyperglycemia; these changes should be made cautiously and under close medical supervision and the frequency of blood glucose monitoring should be increased. Hypoglycemia may occur; increase frequency of blood glucose monitoring in patients at higher risk for hypoglycemia and patients who have reduced symptomatic awareness of hypoglycemia. Hypoglycemia may impair concentration ability and reaction time. Severe, life-threatening, generalized allergy, including anaphylaxis, may occur; if hypersensitivity reactions occur, d/c therapy, treat per standard of care, and monitor until symptoms and signs resolve. May cause hypokalemia; monitor K^+ levels in patients at risk for hypokalemia if indicated. Patients with renal/hepatic impairment may require more frequent dose adjustment and blood glucose monitoring.

ADVERSE REACTIONS: Hypoglycemia, allergic reactions, peripheral edema, lipodystrophy, weight gain, immunogenicity.

INTERACTIONS: May require dose adjustment and increased frequency of glucose monitoring with drugs that may increase the risk of hypoglycemia (eg, antidiabetic agents, salicylates, sulfonamide antibiotics, MAOIs, fluoxetine, disopyramide, fibrates, propoxyphene, pentoxifylline, ACE inhibitors, ARBs, somatostatin analogs [octreotide]), drugs that may decrease the glucose-lowering effect (eg, corticosteroids, isoniazid, niacin, estrogens, oral contraceptives, phenothiazines, danazol, diuretics, sympathomimetic agents [eg, epinephrine, albuterol, terbutaline], somatropin, atypical antipsychotics, glucagon, protease inhibitors, thyroid hormones), or drugs that may increase or decrease glucose-lowering effect (eg, β-blockers, clonidine, lithium salts, alcohol). Pentamidine may cause hypoglycemia, sometimes followed by hyperglycemia. Signs and symptoms of hypoglycemia may be blunted with β-blockers, clonidine, guanethidine, and reserpine. Monitor K^+ levels with K^+-lowering medications or medications sensitive to serum K^+ concentrations. Observe for signs/symptoms of heart failure (HF) if treated concomitantly with a peroxisome proliferator-activated receptor (PPAR)-gamma agonist (eg, thiazolidinedione); consider discontinuation or dose reduction of the PPAR-gamma agonist if HF develops.

PREGNANCY: Category B, caution in nursing.

MECHANISM OF ACTION: Insulin; regulates glucose metabolism. Lowers blood glucose by stimulating peripheral glucose uptake by skeletal muscle and fat, and by inhibiting hepatic glucose production. Inhibits lipolysis and proteolysis, and enhances protein synthesis.

PHARMACOKINETICS: Absorption: (Healthy) T_{max} =2.2 hrs. **Metabolism:** Liver, kidney, muscle, and adipocytes.

NURSING CONSIDERATIONS

Assessment: Assess for risk of hypoglycemia or hypokalemia, hypersensitivity, renal/hepatic impairment, pregnancy/nursing status, and possible drug interactions. Obtain baseline FPG and HbA1c.

Monitoring: Monitor for signs and symptoms of hypoglycemia, hypokalemia, hypersensitivity reactions, and other adverse reactions. Monitor FPG, HbA1c, K^+ levels, and renal/hepatic function.

Patient Counseling: Instruct on self-management procedures, including glucose monitoring, proper inj technique, and management of hypoglycemia and hyperglycemia, and on handling of special situations, such as intercurrent conditions, inadequate or skipped insulin dose, inadvertent administration of an increased insulin dose, inadequate food intake, and skipped meals. Inform that hypoglycemia may impair ability to concentrate and react; advise to use caution when driving or operating machinery. Instruct to always check the label before each inj to avoid medication errors/accidental mix-ups. Inform on the symptoms of hypersensitivity reactions. Advise to inform physician if pregnant/contemplating pregnancy. Advise to use only if product contains no particulate matter and appears uniformly cloudy after mixing.

Administration: SQ route. Do not mix with any other insulins/diluents. Administer 30-45 min ac in the abdominal wall, thigh, upper arm, or buttocks; rotate the inj site within the same region from 1 inj to the next. Do not administer IV/IM and do not use in an insulin infusion pump. Refer to PI for preparation and administration instructions. **Storage:** Protect from heat and light. Do not freeze; do not use if it has been frozen. (Vial) Unopened: 2-8°C (36-46°F) until expiration date, or room temperature <30°C (86°F) for 31 days. Opened: 2-8°C (36-46°F) or room temperature <30°C (86°F) for 31 days. (Pen/KwikPen) Unopened: 2-8°C (36-46°F) until expiration date, or room temperature <30°C (86°F) for 10 days. Opened: Room temperature <30°C (86°F) for 10 days. Do not refrigerate.

HUMULIN N   OTC
insulin human nph, rdna origin (Lilly)

THERAPEUTIC CLASS: Insulin

INDICATIONS: To improve glycemic control in adults and pediatric patients with diabetes mellitus.

DOSAGE: *Adults:* Individualize dose. May need to adjust dosage based on metabolic needs, blood glucose monitoring results, and glycemic control goal.
Pediatrics: Individualize dose. May need to adjust dosage based on metabolic needs, blood glucose monitoring results, and glycemic control goal.

HOW SUPPLIED: Inj: 100 U/mL [3mL, vial, pen, KwikPen; 10mL, vial]

CONTRAINDICATIONS: During episodes of hypoglycemia.

WARNINGS/PRECAUTIONS: Changes in strength, manufacturer, type, or method of administration may affect glycemic control and predispose to hypoglycemia/hyperglycemia; these changes should be made cautiously and under close medical supervision and the frequency of blood glucose monitoring should be increased. Hypoglycemia may occur; increase frequency of blood glucose monitoring in patients at higher risk for hypoglycemia and in patients who have reduced symptomatic awareness of hypoglycemia. Hypoglycemia may impair concentration ability and reaction time. Severe, life-threatening, generalized allergy, including anaphylaxis, may occur; if hypersensitivity reactions occur, d/c therapy, treat per standard of care, and monitor until symptoms and signs resolve. May cause hypokalemia; monitor K⁺ levels in patients at risk for hypokalemia, if indicated. Patients with renal/hepatic impairment may require more frequent dose adjustment and blood glucose monitoring.

ADVERSE REACTIONS: Hypoglycemia, allergic reactions, peripheral edema, lipodystrophy, weight gain, immunogenicity.

INTERACTIONS: May require dose adjustment and increased frequency of glucose monitoring with drugs that may increase the risk of hypoglycemia (eg, antidiabetic agents, salicylates, sulfonamide antibiotics, MAOIs, fluoxetine, disopyramide, fibrates, propoxyphene, pentoxifylline, ACE inhibitors, ARBs, somatostatin analogs [eg, octreotide]), drugs that may decrease the glucose-lowering effect (eg, corticosteroids, isoniazid, niacin, estrogens, oral contraceptives, phenothiazines, danazol, diuretics, sympathomimetic agents [eg, epinephrine, albuterol, terbutaline], somatropin, atypical antipsychotics, glucagon, protease inhibitors, thyroid hormones), or drugs that may increase or decrease glucose-lowering effect (eg, β-blockers, clonidine, lithium salts, alcohol). Pentamidine may cause hypoglycemia, sometimes followed by hyperglycemia. Signs and symptoms of hypoglycemia may be blunted with β-blockers, clonidine, guanethidine, and reserpine. Monitor K⁺ levels with K⁺-lowering medications or medications sensitive to serum K⁺ concentrations. Observe for signs/symptoms of heart failure (HF) if treated concomitantly with a peroxisome proliferator-activated receptor (PPAR)-gamma agonist (eg, thiazolidinedione); consider discontinuation or dose reduction of the PPAR-gamma agonist if HF develops.

PREGNANCY: Category B, caution in nursing.

MECHANISM OF ACTION: Insulin; regulates glucose metabolism. Lowers blood glucose by stimulating peripheral glucose uptake by skeletal muscle and fat, and by inhibiting hepatic glucose production. Inhibits lipolysis and proteolysis, and enhances protein synthesis.

PHARMACOKINETICS: Absorption: (Healthy) T_{max}=4 hrs (median). **Metabolism:** Liver, kidney, muscle, and adipocytes. **Elimination:** (Healthy) $T_{1/2}$=4.4 hrs.

NURSING CONSIDERATIONS

Assessment: Assess for risk of hypoglycemia or hypokalemia, hypersensitivity, renal/hepatic impairment, pregnancy/nursing status, and possible drug interactions. Obtain baseline FPG and HbA1c.

Monitoring: Monitor for signs and symptoms of hypoglycemia, hypokalemia, hypersensitivity reactions, and other adverse reactions. Monitor FPG, HbA1c, K⁺ levels, and renal/hepatic function.

Patient Counseling: Instruct on self-management procedures, including glucose monitoring, proper inj technique, and management of hypoglycemia and hyperglycemia, and on handling of special situations, such as intercurrent conditions, inadequate or skipped insulin dose, inadvertent administration of an increased insulin dose, inadequate food intake, and skipped meals. Inform that hypoglycemia may impair ability to concentrate and react; advise to use caution when driving or operating machinery. Instruct to always check the label before each inj to avoid medication errors/accidental mix-ups. Educate on the symptoms of hypersensitivity reactions. Advise to inform physician if pregnant/contemplating pregnancy. Advise to use only if product contains no particulate matter and appears uniformly cloudy after mixing.

Administration: SQ route. Administer in the abdominal wall, thigh, upper arm, or buttocks; rotate the inj site within the same region from one inj to the next. Do not administer IV/IM and do not use in an insulin infusion pump. Refer to PI for preparation and administration instructions, and instructions for mixing with other insulins. **Storage:** Protect from heat and light. Do not freeze; do not use if it has been frozen. (Vial) Unopened: 2-8°C (36-46°F) until expiration date, or room temperature <30°C (86°F) for 31 days. Opened: 2-8°C (36-46°F) or room temperature <30°C (86°F) for 31 days. (Pen/KwikPen) Unopened: 2-8°C (36-46°F) until expiration date, or room temperature <30°C (86°F) for 14 days. Opened: Room temperature <30°C (86°F) for 14 days. Do not refrigerate.

HUMULIN R   OTC
insulin, human regular (rdna origin) (Lilly)

THERAPEUTIC CLASS: Insulin

INDICATIONS: Adjunct to diet and exercise to improve glycemic control in adults and children with type 1 and 2 diabetes mellitus.

DOSAGE: *Adults:* Individualize dose. SQ: ≥3X daily ac. Inj should be followed by a meal within 30 min. IV: 0.1-1 U/mL in infusion systems with 0.9% NaCl. Renal/Hepatic Impairment: May need to reduce dose.

Pediatrics: Individualize dose. SQ: ≥3X daily ac. Inj should be followed by a meal within 30 min. IV: 0.1-1 U/mL in infusion systems with 0.9% NaCl. Renal/Hepatic Impairment: May need to reduce dose.

HOW SUPPLIED: Inj: 100 U/mL [3mL, 10mL]

CONTRAINDICATIONS: Episodes of hypoglycemia.

WARNINGS/PRECAUTIONS: Any change in insulin should be made cautiously and only under medical supervision. Changes in strength, manufacturer, type, species, or method of administration may result in the need for a change in dosage. May require dosage adjustments with change in physical activity or usual meal plan. Stress, illness, or emotional disturbances may alter insulin requirements. Hypoglycemia may occur and may impair ability to concentrate and react; caution in patients with hypoglycemia unawareness and those predisposed to hypoglycemia (eg, pediatric population, those who fast or have erratic food intake). Hyperglycemia, diabetic ketoacidosis, or hyperosmolar coma may develop if taken less than needed. Hypokalemia may occur; caution in patients who may be at risk. Severe, life-threatening, generalized allergy, including anaphylaxis, may occur. Contains metacresol as excipient; localized reactions and generalized myalgia reported. May be administered IV under medical supervision; close monitoring of blood glucose and K^+ is required.

ADVERSE REACTIONS: Hypoglycemia, lipodystrophy, weight gain, peripheral edema.

INTERACTIONS: May require dose adjustment and close monitoring with drugs that may increase blood-glucose-lowering effect and susceptibility to hypoglycemia (eg, oral antihyperglycemics, salicylates, sulfa antibiotics, MAOIs, SSRIs, pramlintide, disopyramide, fibrates, fluoxetine, propoxyphene, pentoxifylline, ACE inhibitors, ARBs, inhibitors of pancreatic function [eg, octreotide]), drugs that may reduce blood-glucose-lowering effect (eg, corticosteroids, isoniazid, certain lipid-lowering drugs [eg, niacin], estrogens, oral contraceptives, phenothiazines, danazol, diuretics, sympathomimetic agents, somatropin, atypical antipsychotics, glucagon, protease inhibitors, thyroid replacement therapy), or drugs that may increase or decrease blood-glucose-lowering effect (eg, β-blockers, clonidine, lithium salts, alcohol). Pentamidine may cause hypoglycemia, which may sometimes be followed by hyperglycemia. β-blockers, clonidine, guanethidine, and reserpine may mask the signs of hypoglycemia. Caution with K^+-lowering medications or medications sensitive to serum K^+ concentrations. Observe for signs/symptoms of heart failure (HF) if treated concomitantly with a peroxisome proliferator-activated receptor (PPAR)-gamma agonist (eg, thiazolidinedione); consider discontinuation or dose reduction of the PPAR-gamma agonist if HF develops.

PREGNANCY: Category B, caution in nursing.

MECHANISM OF ACTION: Insulin; regulates glucose metabolism. Lowers blood glucose by stimulating peripheral glucose uptake by skeletal muscle and fat, and by inhibiting hepatic glucose production. Inhibits lipolysis, proteolysis, and gluconeogenesis, and enhances protein synthesis and conversion of excess glucose into fat.

NURSING CONSIDERATIONS

Assessment: Assess for risk of hypoglycemia or hypokalemia, hypersensitivity, renal/hepatic impairment, pregnancy/nursing status, and possible drug interactions. Obtain baseline FPG and HbA1c.

Monitoring: Monitor for signs and symptoms of hypoglycemia, hypokalemia, allergic reactions, and other adverse reactions. Monitor FPG, HbA1c, K^+ levels, and renal/hepatic function.

Patient Counseling: Advise to never share needles or syringes, to use the proper and correct syringe type, and to use disposable syringes and needles only once and then discard properly. Counsel on proper dose preparation and administration techniques. Instruct to always carry a quick source of sugar (eg, hard candy or glucose tabs). Counsel about signs/symptoms of hypoglycemia, importance of frequent monitoring of blood glucose levels, and need for a balanced diet and regular exercise. Advise to always keep an extra supply of insulin as well as a spare syringe and needle on hand, and always wear diabetic identification. Instruct to exercise caution when driving or operating machinery. Instruct to notify physician if pregnant/nursing, planning to become pregnant, or taking any other medications.

Administration: SQ/IV route. Inject SQ in the abdominal wall, thigh, gluteal region, or upper arm; rotate inj sites within the same region. Refer to PI for preparation and administration instructions. **Storage:** Unopened: 2-8°C (36-46°F). Do not freeze. Opened: <30°C (86°F). Protect from heat and light. Use within 31 days. Admixture: 2-8°C (36-46°F) for 48 hrs, then may use at room temperature for up to an additional 48 hrs.

HYALGAN   RX
sodium hyaluronate (Fidia Pharma)

THERAPEUTIC CLASS: Hyaluronan and derivatives

INDICATIONS: Treatment of pain in osteoarthritis of the knee in patients who have failed to respond adequately to conservative nonpharmacologic therapy and to simple analgesics (eg, acetaminophen).

DOSAGE: *Adults:* 2mL intra-articularly into the affected knee once a week for a total of 5 inj. Some patients may experience benefit with 3 inj given at weekly intervals.

HOW SUPPLIED: Inj: 10mg/mL [2mL]

CONTRAINDICATIONS: Intra-articular inj with presence of infections or skin diseases in the area of the inj site.

WARNINGS/PRECAUTIONS: Avoid use with disinfectants for skin preparation containing quaternary ammonium salts; may result in precipitate formation. Anaphylactoid and allergic reactions reported. Transient increases in inflammation in the injected knee reported in patients with inflammatory arthritis (eg, rheumatoid arthritis, gouty arthritis). Safety and effectiveness of use with other intra-articular injectables, or into the joints other than the knee have not been established. Caution with allergy to avian proteins, feathers, and egg products. Remove joint effusion if present, and inject SQ lidocaine or similar local anesthetic prior to treatment.

ADVERSE REACTIONS: GI complaints, inj-site pain, knee swelling/effusion, local skin reactions (eg, rash, ecchymosis), pruritus, headache.

PREGNANCY: Safety not known in pregnancy/nursing.

MECHANISM OF ACTION: Hyaluronan.

NURSING CONSIDERATIONS

Assessment: Assess for previous hypersensitivity to hyaluronate preparations; allergy to avian proteins, feathers, and egg products; infections or skin diseases in the area of inj site; use of disinfectants containing quaternary ammonium salts; and signs of acute inflammation prior to administration.

Monitoring: Monitor for anaphylactic and allergic reactions, transient increase of inflammation in inj site, and other adverse reactions.

Patient Counseling: Inform that transient pain/swelling of injected joint may occur after inj. Instruct to avoid strenuous activities or prolonged (>1 hr) weight-bearing activities (eg, jogging, tennis) within 48 hrs following therapy.

Administration: Intra-articular route. Use strict aseptic technique. Inject using 20-gauge needle. Use separate vial for each knee if treatment is bilateral. **Storage:** <25°C (77°F). Protect from light. Do not freeze. Discard any unused portions.

HYDROCHLOROTHIAZIDE   RX
hydrochlorothiazide (Various)

THERAPEUTIC CLASS: Thiazide diuretic

INDICATIONS: Management of HTN alone or in combination with other antihypertensives, and edema in pregnancy due to pathologic causes. (Tab) Adjunct therapy in edema associated with congestive heart failure, hepatic cirrhosis, corticosteroid and estrogen therapy, and renal dysfunction (eg, nephrotic syndrome, acute glomerulonephritis, chronic renal failure).

DOSAGE: *Adults:* (Cap) Initial: 12.5mg qd. Max: 50mg/day. Elderly: Initial: 12.5mg. Titrate: Increase by 12.5mg increments if needed. (Tab) Individualize dose according to response. Use lowest effective dose. Edema: Usual: 25-100mg daily as single or divided dose. May give qod or 3-5 days/week. HTN: Initial: 25mg qd. Titrate: May increase to 50mg daily as a single or in 2 divided doses.
Pediatrics: (Tab) Diuresis/HTN: 1-2mg/kg/day given as single or 2 divided doses. Max: 2-12 Yrs: 100mg/day. Infants up to 2 Yrs: 37.5mg/day. <6 Months: Up to 3mg/kg/day given in 2 divided doses may be required.

HOW SUPPLIED: Cap: 12.5mg; Tab: 12.5mg, 25mg*, 50mg* *scored

CONTRAINDICATIONS: Anuria, hypersensitivity to sulfonamide-derived drugs.

WARNINGS/PRECAUTIONS: Caution with severe renal disease. May precipitate azotemia and cumulative effects may develop with impaired renal function. Caution with impaired hepatic function or progressive liver disease; may precipitate hepatic coma. May cause idiosyncratic reaction, resulting in acute transient myopia and acute angle-closure glaucoma; d/c as rapidly as possible. Fluid or electrolyte imbalance (eg, hyponatremia, hypochloremic alkalosis, hypokalemia, hypomagnesemia) may develop; monitor serum electrolytes periodically. Hypokalemia may develop, especially with brisk diuresis, with severe cirrhosis, or after prolonged therapy; may use K$^+$-sparing diuretics, K$^+$ supplements, or foods high in K$^+$ to avoid or treat hypokalemia. Dilutional hyponatremia may occur in edematous patients in hot weather; appropriate therapy of water restriction rather than salt administration should be instituted except for life-threatening hyponatremia. Hyperuricemia may occur or acute gout may be precipitated. Hyperglycemia may occur. Latent diabetes mellitus (DM) may manifest. May decrease urinary Ca^{2+} excretion. D/C prior to parathyroid function tests. (Cap) Pathologic changes in parathyroid glands, with hypercalcemia and hypophosphatemia, observed on prolonged therapy. (Tab) Sensitivity reactions may occur. May exacerbate/activate systemic lupus erythematosus (SLE). Enhanced antihypertensive effects in postsympathectomy patients. Consider withholding or d/c therapy if progressive renal impairment becomes evident. May cause intermittent and slight elevation of serum Ca^{2+} in the absence of known disorders of calcium metabolism. May be associated with increases in cholesterol and TG levels.

ADVERSE REACTIONS: Weakness, hypotension (including orthostatic hypotension), pancreatitis, jaundice, diarrhea, vomiting, blood dyscrasias, rash, photosensitivity, electrolyte imbalance, impotence, renal dysfunction/failure, interstitial nephritis.

INTERACTIONS: Potentiation of orthostatic hypotension may occur with alcohol, barbiturates, and narcotics. Dosage adjustment of antidiabetic drugs (insulin or oral hypoglycemic agents) may be required. May potentiate or have an additive effect with other antihypertensives. Cholestyramine and colestipol resins may reduce absorption. Intensified electrolyte depletion, particularly hypokalemia, with concomitant corticosteroids and adrenocorticotropic hormone use. May decrease response to pressor amines (eg, norepinephrine). May increase responsiveness to nondepolarizing skeletal muscle relaxants (eg, tubocurarine). Increased risk of lithium toxicity; avoid concomitant use. NSAIDs may reduce diuretic, natriuretic, and antihypertensive effects. Hypokalemia and hypomagnesemia may sensitize or exaggerate the response of the heart to toxic effects of digitalis.

PREGNANCY: Category B, not for use in nursing.

MECHANISM OF ACTION: Thiazide diuretic; has not been established. Affects distal renal tubular mechanism of electrolyte reabsorption, increasing excretion of Na$^+$ and Cl$^-$.

PHARMACOKINETICS: Absorption: C$_{max}$=70-490ng/mL; T$_{max}$=1-5 hrs. **Distribution:** Plasma protein binding (40%-68%); crosses placenta; found in breast milk. **Elimination:** Urine (55%-77%, >95% unchanged [Cap]; ≥61% [Tab]); T$_{1/2}$=6-15 hrs (Cap), 5.6-14.8 hrs (Tab).

NURSING CONSIDERATIONS

Assessment: Assess for anuria, SLE, DM, sulfonamide or penicillin hypersensitivity, history of allergy or bronchial asthma, hepatic/renal impairment, pregnancy/nursing status, and possible drug interactions. Obtain baseline serum electrolytes.

Monitoring: Monitor serum electrolytes periodically. Monitor for signs/symptoms of fluid or electrolyte imbalance, exacerbation or activation of SLE, hyperglycemia, hyperuricemia or precipitation of gout, hypersensitivity reactions, myopia, angle-closure glaucoma, renal/hepatic dysfunction, and increases in cholesterol and TG levels.

Patient Counseling: Advise to seek medical attention if symptoms of electrolyte imbalance (eg, dry mouth, thirst, weakness) or hypersensitivity reactions occur. Counsel to take ud.

Administration: Oral route. **Storage:** 20-25°C (68-77°F). (Cap) Protect from light, moisture, freezing, -20°C (-4°F).

HYDROXYZINE HCl   RX
hydroxyzine HCl (Various)

THERAPEUTIC CLASS: Piperazine antihistamine

INDICATIONS: (PO) Symptomatic relief of anxiety and tension associated with psychoneurosis and adjunct in organic disease states in which anxiety is manifested. Sedative when used as premedication and following general anesthesia. Management of pruritus due to allergic conditions (eg, chronic urticaria, atopic/contact dermatitis) and in histamine-mediated pruritus. (Inj) Management of anxiety, tension, and psychomotor agitation in conditions of emotional stress. Useful in alleviating the manifestations of anxiety and tension as in the preparation for dental procedures and in acute emotional problems. Management of anxiety associated with organic disturbances (eg, certain types of heart disease) and as adjunctive therapy in alcoholism and allergic conditions with strong emotional overlay (eg, asthma, chronic urticaria, pruritus). Treatment of acutely disturbed or hysterical patients and acute/chronic alcoholic with anxiety withdrawal symptoms or delirium tremens. As pre- and postoperative and pre- and postpartum adjunctive medication to permit reduction in narcotic dosage, allay anxiety, and control emesis. To control N/V, excluding N/V of pregnancy.

DOSAGE: *Adults:* (PO) Anxiety/Tension: 50-100mg qid. Pruritus: 25mg tid or qid. Sedation: 50-100mg. Adjust dose according to response to therapy. When treatment is initiated by IM, subsequent doses may be administered PO. (Inj) Psychiatric/Emotional Emergencies (Including Acute Alcoholism): 50-100mg IM immediately and q4-6h PRN. N/V/Pre- and Postoperative Adjunctive Medication/Pre- and Postpartum Adjunctive Therapy: 25-100mg IM. Adjust dose according to response to therapy. Elderly: Start at lower end of dosing range.
Pediatrics: (PO) Anxiety/Tension/Pruritus: >6 yrs: 50-100mg/day in divided doses. <6 yrs: 50mg/day in divided doses. Sedation: 0.6mg/kg. Adjust dose according to response to therapy. When treatment is initiated IM, subsequent doses may be administered PO. (Inj) N/V/Pre- and Postoperative Adjunctive Medication: 0.5mg/lb IM. Adjust dose according to response to therapy.

HOW SUPPLIED: Inj: 25mg/mL [1mL], 50mg/mL [1mL, 2mL, 10mL]; Syrup: 10mg/5mL [118mL, 473mL]; Tab: 10mg, 25mg, 50mg

CONTRAINDICATIONS: Early pregnancy. (Inj) SQ, intra-arterial, or IV administration.

WARNINGS/PRECAUTIONS: Drowsiness may occur. May impair mental/physical abilities. Effectiveness for long-term use (>4 months) has not been established. Caution in elderly. (Inj) Should not be used as the sole treatment of psychosis or of clearly demonstrated cases of depression. Inadvertent SQ inj may result in significant tissue damage.

ADVERSE REACTIONS: Dry mouth, drowsiness, involuntary motor activity.

INTERACTIONS: Potentiated by CNS depressants (eg, narcotics, non-narcotic analgesics, barbiturates); reduce dose of CNS depressants when administered concomitantly. Modify use of meperidine and barbiturates, on an individualized basis, when used in preanesthetic adjunctive therapy. Effect of alcohol may be increased when used concomitantly. (Inj) Cardiac arrest and death reported with concomitant use of IM hydroxyzine and CNS depressants.

PREGNANCY: Contraindicated in early pregnancy; (PO) not for use in nursing, (Inj) safety not known in nursing.

MECHANISM OF ACTION: Piperazine antihistamine; believed to suppress activity in certain key regions of the subcortical area of the CNS and shown to have primary skeletal muscle relaxation, bronchodilator activity, antihistaminic, and analgesic effects. (Inj) Shown to have antispasmodic and antiemetic effects.

PHARMACOKINETICS: Absorption: (PO) Rapid.

NURSING CONSIDERATIONS

Assessment: Assess for hypersensitivity to drug, pregnancy/nursing status, and possible drug interactions.

Monitoring: Monitor for response to treatment. Monitor for drowsiness and other adverse reactions.

Patient Counseling: Inform about risks/benefits of therapy. Advise against simultaneous use of other CNS depressants and caution that the effect of alcohol may be increased. Advise that drowsiness may occur; instruct to use caution against driving or operating heavy machinery.

Administration: Oral/IM route. (Inj) May be administered without further dilution. Should be injected well into the body of a relatively large muscle. Refer to PI for further administration instructions. **Storage:** 20-25°C (68-77°F). (Syrup) Protect from freezing. (Inj) Excursions permitted to 15-30°C (59-86°F). Discard unused portion of the single dose vial. (Inj/Syrup) Protect from light.

HYZAAR

RX

losartan potassium - hydrochlorothiazide (Merck)

> D/C when pregnancy is detected. Drugs that act directly on the renin-angiotensin system (RAS) can cause injury/death to the developing fetus.

THERAPEUTIC CLASS: Angiotensin II receptor antagonist/thiazide diuretic

INDICATIONS: Treatment of HTN. Reduce the risk of stroke in patients with HTN and left ventricular hypertrophy (LVH) (may not apply to black patients).

DOSAGE: *Adults:* HTN: Individualize dose. Usual: 50mg-12.5mg qd. Max: 100mg-25mg qd. Uncontrolled BP on Losartan Monotherapy or HCTZ Alone/Uncontrolled BP on 25mg qd HCTZ/Controlled BP on 25mg qd HCTZ with Hypokalemia: Switch to 50mg-12.5mg qd. Titrate: If BP remains uncontrolled after about 3 weeks, increase to 100mg-25mg qd. Uncontrolled BP on 100mg Losartan Monotherapy: Switch to 100mg-12.5mg qd. Titrate: If BP remains uncontrolled after about 3 weeks, increase 100mg-25mg qd. Severe HTN: Initial: 50mg-12.5mg qd. Titrate: If inadequate response after 2-4 weeks, increase to 100mg-25mg qd. Max: 100mg-25mg qd. HTN with LVH: Initial: Losartan 50mg qd. If inadequate BP reduction, add 12.5mg HCTZ or substitute with losartan-HCTZ 50mg-12.5mg. If additional BP reduction needed, substitute with losartan 100mg and HCTZ 12.5mg or losartan-HCTZ 100mg-12.5mg, followed by losartan 100mg and HCTZ 25mg or losartan-HCTZ 100mg-25mg. Replacement Therapy: Combination may be substituted for titrated components.

HOW SUPPLIED: Tab: (Losartan-HCTZ) 50mg-12.5mg, 100mg-12.5mg, 100mg-25mg

CONTRAINDICATIONS: Anuria, sulfonamide-derived drug hypersensitivity. Coadministration with aliskiren in patients with diabetes.

WARNINGS/PRECAUTIONS: Not indicated for initial therapy of HTN. Symptomatic hypotension may occur in intravascularly volume-depleted patients (eg, treated with diuretics); correct volume depletion before therapy. Not recommended with hepatic impairment requiring losartan titration. Not recommended with severe renal impairment (CrCl ≤30mL/min). Angioedema reported (rare). HCTZ: Caution with impaired hepatic function or progressive liver disease; may precipitate hepatic coma. Hypersensitivity reactions may occur. May cause exacerbation or activation of systemic lupus erythematosus (SLE). May cause idiosyncratic reaction, resulting in acute transient myopia and acute angle-closure glaucoma; d/c as rapidly as possible. Observe for clinical signs of fluid or electrolyte imbalance (hyponatremia, hypochloremic alkalosis, and hypokalemia). Hypokalemia may develop, especially with brisk diuresis, severe cirrhosis, or after prolonged therapy. Hypokalemia may cause cardiac arrhythmia and may sensitize/exaggerate the response of the heart to the toxic effects of digitalis. Hyperuricemia may occur or frank gout may be precipitated. May cause hyperglycemia, hypomagnesemia, hypercalcemia, and manifestations of latent diabetes mellitus (DM). D/C prior to parathyroid function tests. Enhanced effects in postsympathectomy patients. Consider withholding or discontinuing therapy if progressive renal impairment becomes evident. Increased cholesterol and TG levels reported. May precipitate azotemia in patients with renal disease. Losartan: Oliguria and/or progressive azotemia and (rare) with acute renal failure and/or death may occur in patients whose renal function is dependent on the activity of the RAS (eg, severe congestive heart failure [CHF]). May increase SrCr and BUN levels in patients with renal artery stenosis.

ADVERSE REACTIONS: Hypokalemia, dizziness, upper respiratory infection.

INTERACTIONS: See Contraindications. NSAIDs, including selective COX-2 inhibitors, may decrease effects of diuretics and angiotensin II receptor antagonists and may deteriorate renal function. Clearance of lithium may be reduced. HCTZ: May increase risk of lithium toxicity; avoid concurrent use. Potentiation of orthostatic hypotension may occur with alcohol, barbiturates, or narcotics. Dose adjustment of antidiabetic drugs (oral agents, insulin) may be required. May cause additive effect or potentiation with other antihypertensives. Anionic exchange resins (eg, cholestyramine, colestipol) may impair absorption. Corticosteroids, adrenocorticotropic hormone, or glycyrrhizin (found in liquorice) may intensify electrolyte depletion, particularly hypokalemia. May decrease response to pressor amines (eg, norepinephrine). May increase response to nondepolarizing skeletal muscle relaxants (eg, tubocurarine). Losartan: Dual blockade of the RAS is associated with increased risks of hypotension, syncope, hyperkalemia, and changes in renal function (including acute renal failure); closely monitor BP, renal function, and electrolytes with concomitant agents that affect the RAS. Avoid with aliskiren in patients with renal impairment (GFR <60mL/min). Rifampin may reduce levels. Fluconazole may decrease levels of the active metabolite and increase levels of losartan. May increase serum K^+ with K^+-sparing diuretics (eg, spironolactone, triamterene, amiloride), K^+ supplements, or salt substitutes containing K^+.

PREGNANCY: Category D, not for use in nursing.

MECHANISM OF ACTION: Losartan: Angiotensin II receptor antagonist; blocks the vasoconstrictor and aldosterone-secreting effects of angiotensin II by selectively blocking the binding of angiotensin II to AT_1 receptor in many tissues (eg, vascular smooth muscle, adrenal gland). HCTZ: Thiazide diuretic; has not been established. Affects the renal tubular mechanisms of electrolyte reabsorption, directly increasing excretion of Na^+ and Cl^- in approximately equivalent amounts.

PHARMACOKINETICS: Absorption: Losartan: Well-absorbed. Systemic bioavailability (33%); T_{max}=1 hr, 3-4 hrs (active metabolite). **Distribution:** Losartan: V_d=34L, 12L (active metabolite); plasma protein binding (98.7%, 99.8% active metabolite). HCTZ: Crosses placenta; found in breast milk. **Metabolism:** Losartan: CYP2C9, 3A4; carboxylic acid (active metabolite). **Elimination:** Losartan: Urine (35%, 4% unchanged, 6% active metabolite), feces (60%); $T_{1/2}$=2 hrs, 6-9 hrs (active metabolite). HCTZ: Kidney (≥61% unchanged); $T_{1/2}$=5.6-14.8 hrs.

NURSING CONSIDERATIONS

Assessment: Assess for hypersensitivity to the drug and its components, anuria, sulfonamide-derived drug hypersensitivity, history of penicillin allergy, volume/salt depletion, SLE, DM, CHF, hepatic/renal function, postsympathectomy status, cirrhosis, renal artery stenosis, pregnancy/nursing status, and possible drug interactions. Obtain baseline BP.

Monitoring: Monitor for signs/symptoms of fluid/electrolyte imbalance, exacerbation/activation of SLE, idiosyncratic reaction, latent DM, precipitation of gout, hypersensitivity reactions, and other adverse reactions. Monitor BP, serum electrolytes, renal/hepatic function, cholesterol, and TG levels periodically.

Patient Counseling: Inform females of childbearing potential of the consequences of exposure during pregnancy and of the treatment options for women planning to become pregnant. Instruct to report pregnancy to the physician as soon as possible. Counsel that lightheadedness may occur, especially during the 1st days of therapy; instruct to report to physician. Instruct to d/c therapy and consult physician if syncope occurs. Caution that inadequate fluid intake, excessive perspiration, diarrhea, or vomiting may lead to an excessive fall in BP, with the same consequences of lightheadedness and possible syncope. Instruct not to use K⁺ supplements or salt substitutes containing K⁺ without consulting physician.

Administration: Oral route. Take with or without food. **Storage:** 25°C (77°F); excursions permitted to 15-30°C (59-86°F). Protect from light.

IMDUR   RX
isosorbide mononitrate (Schering Corporation)

THERAPEUTIC CLASS: Nitrate vasodilator

INDICATIONS: Prevention of angina pectoris due to coronary artery disease.

DOSAGE: *Adults:* Initial: 30mg (single tab or as 1/2 of a 60mg tab) or 60mg (single tab) qam on arising. Titrate: May increase to 120mg (single tab or as two 60mg tabs) qam after several days. Rarely, 240mg qam may be required. Elderly: Start at lower end of dosing range.

HOW SUPPLIED: Tab, Extended-Release: 30mg*, 60mg*, 120mg *scored

WARNINGS/PRECAUTIONS: Not useful in aborting acute anginal episode. Not recommended for use in patients with acute myocardial infarction (MI) or congestive heart failure; perform careful clinical or hemodynamic monitoring if used in these conditions. Severe hypotension, particularly with upright posture, may occur; caution in volume depleted, hypotensive, or elderly patients. Nitrate-induced hypotension may be accompanied by paradoxical bradycardia and increased angina pectoris. May aggravate angina caused by hypertrophic cardiomyopathy. May develop tolerance. Chest pain, acute MI, and sudden death reported during temporary withdrawal.

ADVERSE REACTIONS: Headache, dizziness, dry mouth, asthenia, cardiac failure, abdominal pain, earache, arrhythmia, hyperuricemia, arthralgia, purpura, anxiety, hypochromic anemia, atrophic vaginitis, bacterial infection.

INTERACTIONS: Sildenafil amplifies vasodilatory effects that can result in severe hypotension. Additive vasodilating effects with other vasodilators (eg, alcohol). Marked symptomatic orthostatic hypotension reported with calcium channel blockers; dose adjustments of either class of agents may be necessary.

PREGNANCY: Category B, caution in nursing.

MECHANISM OF ACTION: Nitrate vasodilator; relaxes vascular smooth muscle, producing dilatation of peripheral arteries and veins, especially the latter. Dilatation of the veins leads to reducing the left ventricular end-diastolic pressure and pulmonary capillary wedge pressure (preload). Arteriolar relaxation reduces systemic vascular resistance, systolic arterial pressure and mean arterial pressure (afterload). It also dilates the coronary artery.

PHARMACOKINETICS: Absorption: Single Dose (60mg): C_{max}=424-541ng/mL, T_{max}=3.1-4.5 hrs, AUC=5990-7452ng•hr/mL. Multiple Dose: C_{max}=557-572ng/mL (60mg), 1151-1180ng/mL (120mg); T_{max}=2.9-4.2 hrs (60mg), 3.1-3.2 hrs (120mg); AUC=6625-7555ng•hr/mL (60mg), 14,241-16,800ng•hr/mL (120mg). **Distribution:** V_d=0.6-0.7L/kg (IV); plasma protein binding (5%). **Metabolism:** Liver; denitration and glucuronidation. **Elimination:** Urine (96%, 2% unchanged), feces (1%); $T_{1/2}$=6.3-6.6 hrs (60mg single dose), 6.2-6.3 hrs (60mg multiple dose), 6.2-6.4 hrs (120mg multiple dose).

NURSING CONSIDERATIONS

Assessment: Assess for drug hypersensitivity, hypotension, volume depletion, angina caused by hypertrophic cardiomyopathy, pregnancy/nursing status, possible drug interactions, and any other conditions where treatment is cautioned or contraindicated.

Monitoring: Monitor for hypotension with paradoxical bradycardia and increased angina pectoris, tachycardia, aggravation of angina caused by hypertrophic cardiomyopathy, tolerance, manifestations of true physical dependence (eg, chest pain, acute MI), and other adverse reactions.

Patient Counseling: Inform about the risks and benefits of therapy. Counsel to carefully follow the prescribed schedule of dosing. Advise that daily headaches may accompany treatment and instruct to avoid altering schedule of treatment as the headaches are a marker of the activity of the medication and loss of headache may be associated with loss of antianginal efficacy. Inform that treatment may be associated with lightheadedness on standing, especially just after rising from a recumbent/seated position and may be more frequent with alcohol consumption.

Administration: Oral route. Swallow tab whole with a half-glassful of fluid; do not crush or chew. Do not break 30mg tab. **Storage:** 20-25°C (68-77°F).

IMITREX

RX

sumatriptan (GlaxoSmithKline)

THERAPEUTIC CLASS: 5-HT$_{1B/1D}$ agonist

INDICATIONS: Acute treatment of migraine attacks with or without aura in adults. (Inj) Acute treatment of cluster headache in adults.

DOSAGE: *Adults:* (Inj) Max Single Dose: 6mg SQ. Max Dose/24 hrs: Two 6mg inj separated by at least 1 hr. Consider a 2nd dose only if some response to 1st inj is observed. Migraine: Use lower doses (1-5mg) if side effects are dose limiting. (Spray) Usual: 5mg, 10mg, or 20mg single dose administered into 1 nostril; may repeat once after 2 hrs if migraine not resolved or returns after transient improvement. 10mg dose may be achieved by administering a single 5mg dose in each nostril. Max: 40mg/24 hrs. (Tab) Usual: 25mg, 50mg, or 100mg. May repeat after 2 hrs if migraine not resolved or returns after transient improvement. Max: 200mg/24 hrs. Use after Inj: If migraine returns after initial treatment with inj, may give additional single tabs (up to 100mg/day), with an interval of at least 2 hrs between tab doses. Mild to Moderate Hepatic Impairment: Max Single Dose: 50mg. (Spray, Tab) Safety of treating >4 headaches/30 days not known. Elderly: Start at lower end of dosing range.

HOW SUPPLIED: Inj: (Succinate) 4mg/0.5mL, 6mg/0.5mL; Spray: 5mg, 20mg [6^s]; Tab: (Succinate) 25mg, 50mg, 100mg

CONTRAINDICATIONS: Ischemic coronary artery disease (CAD) (eg, angina pectoris, history of myocardial infarction [MI], documented silent ischemia), coronary artery vasospasm, including Prinzmetal's angina, Wolff-Parkinson-White syndrome or arrhythmias associated with other cardiac accessory conduction pathway disorders, history of stroke or transient ischemic attack (TIA), history of hemiplegic/basilar migraine, peripheral vascular disease, ischemic bowel disease, uncontrolled HTN, and severe hepatic impairment. Use within 24 hrs of another 5-HT$_1$ agonist, or of ergotamine-containing or ergot-type medication (eg, dihydroergotamine, methysergide). Concurrent administration or recent use (within 2 weeks) of an MAO-A inhibitor.

WARNINGS/PRECAUTIONS: May cause coronary artery vasospasm. Perform a cardiovascular (CV) evaluation in triptan-naive patients with multiple CV risk factors (eg, diabetes, HTN, smoking, obesity, strong family history of CAD, increased age) prior to therapy; if negative, consider administering 1st dose under medical supervision and obtain ECG immediately following administration. Perform periodic CV evaluation in these patients if on long-term intermittent use. Evaluate patients with signs/symptoms suggestive of angina following inj for the presence of CAD or Prinzmetal's angina before receiving additional doses (Inj). Life-threatening cardiac rhythm disturbances (eg, ventricular tachycardia, ventricular fibrillation leading to death) reported (within a few hours following administration); d/c if these occur. Sensations of tightness, pain, pressure, and heaviness in the precordium, throat, neck, and jaw may occur. Cerebral/subarachnoid hemorrhage, stroke, other cerebrovascular events, noncoronary vasospasm reactions (eg, peripheral vascular ischemia, GI vascular ischemia/infarction, Raynaud's syndrome, splenic infarction) reported. Exclude other potentially serious neurologic conditions and noncoronary vasospasm reactions before therapy. May cause transient and permanent blindness and significant partial vision loss. Serotonin syndrome may occur; d/c if serotonin syndrome is suspected. Significant elevation in BP, including hypertensive crisis, reported rarely. Caution with controlled HTN. Hypersensitivity reactions may occur. Seizures reported; caution with history of epilepsy or conditions associated with a lowered seizure threshold. Reconsider the diagnosis of migraine or cluster headache before giving a 2nd dose if patient does not respond to the 1st dose of therapy. Overuse of acute migraine drugs may lead to exacerbation of headache; detoxification, including withdrawal of the overused drugs and treatment of withdrawal symptoms may be necessary. Not for prevention of migraine attacks. Should only be used where a clear diagnosis of migraine headache or (Inj) cluster headache has been established. Caution in elderly patients. (Inj) Avoid IM or intravascular delivery. (Spray) May cause irritation in the nose and throat.

ADVERSE REACTIONS: Atypical sensations, paresthesia, chest discomfort, neck pain/stiffness, N/V, warm/cold sensation, pressure sensation, (inj) tingling, burning sensation, feeling of tightness, numbness, flushing, inj-site reaction, dizziness (spray, tab) bad/unusual taste.

INTERACTIONS: See Contraindications. Serotonin syndrome reported with SSRIs, SNRIs, TCAs, or MAOIs.

PREGNANCY: Category C, (Spray/Tab) avoid breastfeeding for 12 hrs after administration; (Inj) not for use in nursing.

MECHANISM OF ACTION: Selective 5-HT$_{1B/1D}$ receptor agonist; thought to be due to the agonist effects at the 5-HT$_{1B/1D}$ receptors on intracranial blood vessels (including arteriovenous anastomoses) and sensory nerves of the trigeminal system, which result in cranial vessel constriction and inhibition of proinflammatory neuropeptide release.

PHARMACOKINETICS: Absorption: (Nasal Spray, 5mg) C$_{max}$=5ng/mL; (Nasal Spray, 20mg) C$_{max}$=16ng/mL; (PO, 25mg) C$_{max}$=18ng/mL; (PO, 100mg) C$_{max}$=51ng/mL; (SQ via manual inj, 6mg) (Healthy) Deltoid: C$_{max}$=74ng/mL, T$_{max}$=12 min. Thigh: (Autoinjector) C$_{max}$=52ng/mL, (Manual inj)

C_{max}=61ng/mL. (SQ) Absolute bioavailability (97%). **Distribution:** (Nasal Spray, Tab) V_d=2.7L/kg, (SQ, 6mg) V_d=50L; plasma protein binding (14-21%); found in breast milk. **Metabolism:** Via mono-amine oxidase-A; indole acetic acid (major metabolite). **Elimination:** (Nasal Spray) Urine (3%, unchanged; 42%, metabolite), $T_{1/2}$=2 hrs; (PO) Urine (60%), feces (40%), $T_{1/2}$=2.5 hrs; (SQ) Urine (22%, unchanged; 38%, metabolite), $T_{1/2}$=115 min.

NURSING CONSIDERATIONS

Assessment: Confirm diagnosis of migraine or (Inj) cluster headache and exclude other potentially serious neurologic conditions and noncoronary vasospasm reactions prior to therapy. Assess for CV disease, HTN, hemiplegic/basilar migraine, hypersensitivity to drug, and any other conditions where treatment is cautioned or contraindicated. Assess hepatic/renal function, pregnancy/nursing status, and possible drug interactions. Perform CV evaluation with multiple CV risk factors.

Monitoring: Monitor for signs/symptoms of cardiac events (eg, coronary vasospasm, acute MI, arrhythmia, ECG changes), cerebrovascular events (eg, hemorrhage, stroke, TIAs), peripheral vascular ischemia, GI vascular ischemia/infarction, serotonin syndrome, hypersensitivity reactions, HTN, and other adverse reactions. Perform periodic CV evaluation in patients on long-term intermittent use with risk factors for CAD.

Patient Counseling: Inform that therapy may cause CV side effects and anaphylactic/anaphylactoid reactions. Instruct to seek medical attention if signs/symptoms of chest pain, SOB, irregular heartbeat, significant rise in BP, weakness, and slurring of speech occur. Inform that use of acute migraine drugs for ≥10 days/month may lead to an exacerbation of headache; encourage to record headache frequency and drug use (eg, by keeping a headache diary). Inform about the risk of serotonin syndrome, particularly during combined use with SSRIs, SNRIs, TCAs, and MAOIs. Inform that drug may cause somnolence and dizziness; instruct to evaluate ability to perform complex tasks during migraine attacks and after administration of drug. Inform that medication should not be used during pregnancy and instruct to notify physician if breastfeeding or plan to breastfeed. (Inj) Instruct on proper use of autoinjector, to avoid IM or intravascular delivery, and to use inj sites with adequate skin and SQ thickness to accommodate length of needle. (Spray/Tab) Inform that use of medication within 24 hrs of another triptan or an ergot-type medication (eg, dihydroergotamine, methysergide) is contraindicated. (Spray) Inform that may experience local irritation of the nose and throat and that this will generally resolve in <2 hrs. Instruct on proper use of spray and to avoid spraying in eyes.

Administration: Oral, SQ, or nasal route. (Inj) Use the 6mg single dose vial for patients receiving doses other than 4mg or 6mg; do not use autoinjector. Avoid IM or intravascular delivery.
Storage: 2-30°C (36-86°F). (Spray, Inj) Protect from light.

INCIVEK
telaprevir (Vertex)

RX

> Fatal and nonfatal serious skin reactions, including Stevens-Johnson syndrome (SJS), drug reaction with eosinophilia and systemic symptoms (DRESS), and toxic epidermal necrolysis (TEN) reported. D/C combination therapy immediately if serious skin rash reactions, including rash with systemic symptoms or a progressive severe rash develop. Consider discontinuing other medications known to be associated with serious skin reactions. Promptly refer patients for urgent medical care.

THERAPEUTIC CLASS: HCV NS3/4A protease inhibitor

INDICATIONS: Treatment of genotype 1 chronic hepatitis C in combination with peginterferon alfa and ribavirin in adults with compensated liver disease, including cirrhosis, who are treatment-naive or who have previously been treated with interferon-based treatment.

DOSAGE: *Adults:* Combination Therapy with Peginterferon Alfa/Ribavirin: 1125mg (three 375mg tabs) bid (10-14 hrs apart) with food (not low fat) for 12 weeks. Monitor hepatitis C virus (HCV)-RNA levels at Weeks 4 and 12 to determine treatment duration and assess for treatment futility. To prevent treatment failure, dose of telaprevir should not be reduced or interrupted. Refer to PI for further information on treatment duration and discontinuation guidelines.

HOW SUPPLIED: Tab: 375mg

CONTRAINDICATIONS: Women who are or may become pregnant and men whose female partners are pregnant. Concomitant use with drugs that are highly dependent on CYP3A for clearance and for which elevated plasma concentrations are associated with serious and/or life-threatening reactions and with strong CYP3A inducers (eg, alfuzosin, carbamazepine, phenobarbital, phenytoin, rifampin, dihydroergotamine, ergonovine, ergotamine, methylergonovine, cisapride, St. John's wort, lovastatin, simvastatin, pimozide, sildenafil, or tadalafil when used for treatment of pulmonary arterial HTN, oral midazolam, triazolam). Refer to the individual monographs for peginterferon alfa and ribavirin.

WARNINGS/PRECAUTIONS: Monitor patients with mild to moderate rashes for progression of rash or development of systemic symptoms; d/c if rash becomes severe; peginterferon alfa and ribavirin may be continued; if improvement is not observed within 7 days of discontinuing telaprevir, consider sequential or simultaneous interruption or discontinuation of ribavirin and/ or peginterferon alfa. Female patients of childbearing potential and their male partners as well as male patients and their female partners must use 2 forms of effective nonhormonal contraception during treatment and for 6 months after all treatment has ended; female patients should have monthly pregnancy tests during this time. Anemia reported with peginterferon alfa and ribavirin therapy; addition of telaprevir to peginterferon alfa and ribavirin associated with an additional decrease in Hgb concentrations; monitor Hgb prior to and at least at weeks 2, 4, 8, and 12 during combination treatment and as clinically appropriate. Reduce ribavirin dose for the management of anemia. Do not reduce dose or restart telaprevir after discontinuing from either rash or anemia. Hematology evaluations (including Hgb, white cell differential, and platelet count) are recommended prior to and at weeks 2, 4, 8, and 12 and as clinically appropriate. Chemistry evaluations (including electrolytes, SrCr, uric acid, hepatic enzymes, bilirubin, and TSH) are recommended as frequently as hematology evaluations or as clinically appropriate. Caution in elderly. Must not be administered as monotherapy and must only be prescribed with both peginterferon alfa and ribavirin. Not recommended with moderate/severe hepatic impairment (Child-Pugh B or C, score ≥7) or with decompensated liver disease.

ADVERSE REACTIONS: Serious skin reactions, pruritus, anemia, N/V, hemorrhoids, diarrhea, anorectal discomfort, dysgeusia, fatigue, anal pruritus.

INTERACTIONS: See Contraindications. Dose adjustments of concomitant drugs made during treatment should be readjusted after completion of therapy. Avoid with colchicine in patients with renal/hepatic impairment; risk of toxicity. Not recommended with voriconazole; high doses of itraconazole or ketoconazole; rifabutin; systemic corticosteroids; salmeterol; darunavir, fosamprenavir, or lopinavir (all with ritonavir); and inhaled/nasal fluticasone or budesonide. Avoid use with atorvastatin. May increase levels of alfentanil, fentanyl, antiarrhythmics, statins, digoxin, clarithromycin, erythromycin, telithromycin, trazodone, azole antifungals, rifabutin, alprazolam, IV midazolam, amlodipine and other calcium channel blockers, corticosteroids, bosentan, atazanavir, tenofovir, colchicine, cyclosporine, sirolimus, tacrolimus, salmeterol, repaglinide, PDE5 inhibitors, CYP3A substrates, inhaled/nasal fluticasone or budesonide, and drugs that are substrates for P-glycoprotein (P-gp), OATP1B1, and OATP2B1 transport. May decrease levels of escitalopram, zolpidem, efavirenz, ethinyl estradiol, darunavir, fosamprenavir, and methadone. Use lowest digoxin dose initially with careful titration and monitoring of serum digoxin concentrations. May alter concentrations of warfarin; monitor INR. Clarithromycin, erythromycin, telithromycin, azoles, and CYP3A/P-gp inhibitors may increase levels. Rifabutin, systemic dexamethasone, HIV protease inhibitors, efavirenz, and CYP3A/P-gp inducers may decrease levels. Refer to PI for dosing modifications when used with certain concomitant therapies.

PREGNANCY: Category B, Category X when used with peginterferon alfa and ribavirin, not for use in nursing.

MECHANISM OF ACTION: HCV NS3/4A protease inhibitor; direct-acting antiviral agent against HCV.

PHARMACOKINETICS: Absorption: (750mg q8h) C_{max}=3510ng/mL; AUC_{8h}=22,300ng•hr/mL. (Single dose) T_{max}=4-5 hrs. **Distribution:** V_d=252L; plasma protein binding (59-76%). **Metabolism:** Liver (extensive) via CYP3A4; hydrolysis, oxidation, and reduction; R-diastereomer (major metabolite). **Elimination:** Urine (1%), feces (82%, 31.9% unchanged), exhaled air (9%); $T_{1/2}$=4-4.7 hrs.

NURSING CONSIDERATIONS

Assessment: Assess for hepatic impairment or decompensated liver disease, pregnancy/nursing status, men whose female partners are of childbearing potential, and for possible drug interactions. Perform baseline hematology evaluations (including Hgb, white cell differential, and platelet count) and chemistry evaluations (including electrolytes, SrCr, uric acid, hepatic enzymes, bilirubin, and TSH).

Monitoring: Monitor for SJS, DRESS, TEN, and other adverse reactions. Monitor HCV-RNA levels at Weeks 4, 12, and as clinically indicated. Perform hematology evaluations (including Hgb, white cell differential, and platelet count) at Weeks 2, 4, 8, and 12 and as clinically appropriate, and chemistry evaluations (including electrolytes, SrCr, uric acid, hepatic enzymes, bilirubin, and TSH) as frequently as hematology evaluations or as clinically appropriate. Perform a routine monthly pregnancy test in females during therapy and for 6 months after stopping treatment. Monitor INR when warfarin is coadministered.

Patient Counseling: Inform that drug must be used in combination with peginterferon alfa and ribavirin. Instruct female patients to notify physician immediately if pregnant and male patients if female partner is pregnant. Advise female patients of childbearing potential and their male partners as well as male patients and their female partners to use 2 nonhormonal methods of effective contraception during treatment and for 6 months after all treatment has ended. Inform that combination treatment may cause rash; advise to promptly report any skin changes or itching. Advise not to stop treatment due to rash unless instructed. Inform that the effect of treatment of hepatitis C on transmission is unknown and that appropriate precautions to prevent transmission should be taken. Inform about the importance of hydration and fluid intake. Instruct to recognize signs/symptoms of dehydration (eg, increased thirst, dry mouth, decreased urine output, and more concentrated urine); advise to notify physician if oral fluid intake is poor or if severe vomiting and/or diarrhea is experienced. If a dose is missed within 6 hrs of the time it is usually taken, instruct to take the prescribed dose with food as soon as possible and if >6 hrs has passed, instruct to not take the missed dose and to resume to the usual dosing schedule. Counsel to ingest food containing around 20g of fat within 30 min prior to dose.

Administration: Oral route. Swallow tab whole; do not chew, crush, break, cut, or dissolve.
Storage: 25°C (77°F); excursions permitted to 15-30°C (59-86°F).

INDERAL LA   RX
propranolol HCl (Akrimax)

THERAPEUTIC CLASS: Nonselective beta-blocker

INDICATIONS: Management of HTN. To decrease angina frequency and increase exercise tolerance with angina pectoris due to coronary atherosclerosis. Improves NYHA functional class in symptomatic patients with hypertrophic subaortic stenosis. Prophylaxis of common migraine headache.

DOSAGE: *Adults:* HTN: Initial: 80mg qd. Titrate: May increase to 120mg qd or higher until adequate BP control is achieved. Maint: 120-160mg qd. 640mg/day may be required. Angina: Initial: 80mg qd. Titrate: Increase gradually at 3- to 7-day intervals until optimal response is obtained. Maint: 160mg qd. Max: 320mg qd. Reduce dose gradually over a period of a few weeks if therapy is to be discontinued. Migraine: Initial: 80mg qd. Usual: 160-240mg qd. D/C gradually if a satisfactory response is not obtained within 4-6 weeks after reaching maximal dose. Hypertrophic Subaortic Stenosis: Usual: 80-160mg qd. Elderly: Start at lower end of dosing range.

HOW SUPPLIED: Cap, Extended-Release: 60mg, 80mg, 120mg, 160mg

CONTRAINDICATIONS: Cardiogenic shock, sinus bradycardia and >1st-degree block, bronchial asthma.

WARNINGS/PRECAUTIONS: Exacerbation of angina and myocardial infarction (MI) following abrupt discontinuation reported; when discontinuation is planned, reduce dose gradually over at least a few weeks. Reinstitute therapy if exacerbation of angina occurs upon interruption and take other measures for management of angina pectoris; follow same procedure in patients at risk of occult atherosclerotic heart disease who are given propranolol for other indication since coronary artery disease may be unrecognized. Hypersensitivity reactions (eg, anaphylactic/anaphylactoid reactions) and cutaneous reactions (eg, Stevens-Johnson syndrome, toxic epidermal necrolysis, exfoliative dermatitis, erythema multiforme, and urticaria) reported. May precipitate more severe failure in patients with congestive heart failure (CHF); avoid with overt CHF and caution in patients with history of heart failure (HF) who are well-compensated and are receiving diuretics PRN. Continued use in patients without history of HF may cause cardiac failure. Caution with bronchospastic lung disease, Wolff-Parkinson-White (WPW) syndrome, tachycardia, and hepatic/renal impairment. Chronically administered therapy should not be routinely withdrawn prior to major surgery; however, may augment risks of general anesthesia and surgical procedures. May prevent appearance of signs/symptoms of acute hypoglycemia. Caution with labile insulin-dependent diabetics; may be more difficult to adjust insulin dose. May mask certain clinical signs of hyperthyroidism; abrupt withdrawal may be followed by an exacerbation of symptoms of hyperthyroidism, including thyroid storm. May reduce intraocular pressure (IOP). Patients with history of severe anaphylactic reaction to a variety of allergens may be more reactive to repeated accidental/diagnostic/therapeutic challenge; may be unresponsive to usual doses of epinephrine. Lab test interactions may occur (eg, changes to thyroid function tests), including in patients with HTN/severe HF. Not for treatment of hypertensive emergencies. Caution in elderly.

ADVERSE REACTIONS: Bradycardia, CHF, hypotension, lightheadedness, mental depression, N/V, agranulocytosis, systemic lupus erythematosus, urticaria, alopecia.

INTERACTIONS: Administration with drugs that have an effect on CY2D6, 1A2 or C19 metabolic pathways may lead to clinically relevant drug interactions and changes on its efficacy and/or toxicity; use with caution. Alcohol may increase levels. Propafenone and amiodarone may cause additive effects. Quinidine may increase levels and may cause postural hypotension. Reduced clearance of lidocaine and lidocaine toxicity reported following coadministration. Caution with drugs that slow atrioventricular (AV) nodal conduction (eg, digitalis, lidocaine, calcium channel blocker); increased risk of bradycardia with digitalis. Bradycardia, HF, and cardiovascular collapse reported with verapamil. Bradycardia, hypotension, high-degree heart block, and HF reported with diltiazem. ACE inhibitors may cause hypotension particularly in the setting of acute MI. May antagonize effects of clonidine; administer cautiously to patients withdrawing from clonidine. May prolong 1st dose hypotension with prazosin. Postural hypotension reported with terazosin or doxazosin. May cause excessive reduction of resting sympathetic nervous activity with catecholamine-depleting drugs (eg, reserpine). May experience uncontrolled HTN with epinephrine. Effects can be reversed by β-receptor agonists (eg, dobutamine or isoproterenol). May reduce sensitivity to dobutamine stress echocardiography in patients undergoing evaluation for MI. May reduce efficacy with indomethacin and NSAIDs. May exacerbate hypotensive effects of MAOIs or TCAs. May depress myocardial contractility with methoxyflurane and trichloroethylene. May increase levels of warfarin; monitor PT. Hypotension and cardiac arrest reported with haloperidol. May lower T3 concentration with thyroxine.

PREGNANCY: Category C, caution in nursing.

MECHANISM OF ACTION: Nonselective β-adrenergic receptor blocker; has not been established. Thought to decrease cardiac output, inhibit renin release by the kidneys, and lessen tonic sympathetic nerve outflow from vasomotor centers in the brain.

PHARMACOKINETICS: Absorption: Almost complete; T_{max}=6 hrs. **Distribution:** V_d=4L/kg; plasma protein binding (90%); crosses placenta; found in breast milk. **Metabolism:** Liver (extensive); CYP2D6 (hydroxylation), CYP1A2, 2D6 (oxidation), N-dealkylation, glucuronidation; propranolol glucuronide, naphthyloxylactic acid, glucuronic acid, sulfate conjugates of 4-hydroxylpropranolol (major metabolites). **Elimination:** $T_{1/2}$=10 hrs.

NURSING CONSIDERATIONS

Assessment: Assess for cardiogenic shock, sinus bradycardia, AV heart block, bronchial asthma, CHF, bronchospastic lung disease, hyperthyroidism, diabetes, WPW syndrome, tachycardia, hepatic/renal impairment, history of HF, risk for occult atherosclerotic heart disease, hypersensitivity to drug, pregnancy/nursing status, and possible drug interactions.

Monitoring: Monitor for signs/symptoms of cardiac failure, hypoglycemia, decreased IOP, hyperthyroidism, withdrawal symptoms, hypersensitivity reactions, and other adverse reactions. Monitor PT with warfarin.

Patient Counseling: Inform of the risks/benefits of therapy. Instruct not to interrupt or d/c therapy without consulting physician. Inform that therapy may interfere with glaucoma screening test.

Administration: Oral route. **Storage:** 20-25°C (68-77°F); excursions permitted to 15-30°C (59-86°F). Protect from light, moisture, freezing, and excessive heat.

INDOMETHACIN   RX
indomethacin (Various)

> NSAIDs may cause an increased risk of serious cardiovascular (CV) thrombotic events, myocardial infarction (MI), stroke, and serious GI adverse events, including bleeding, ulceration, and perforation of the stomach or intestines. Contraindicated for the treatment of perioperative pain in the setting of coronary artery bypass graft (CABG) surgery.

OTHER BRAND NAMES: Indocin (Iroko)

THERAPEUTIC CLASS: NSAID

INDICATIONS: Management of moderate to severe rheumatoid arthritis (RA), including acute flares of chronic disease, ankylosing spondylitis (AS), and osteoarthritis (OA), acute painful shoulder (bursitis and/or tendinitis) and/or acute gouty arthritis.

DOSAGE: *Adults:* RA/AS/OA: Initial: 25mg (5mL) PO bid-tid. Titrate: May increase by 25mg (5mL) or 50mg (10mL) at weekly intervals. Max: 150-200mg (30-40mL) per day. Bursitis/Tendinitis: 75-150mg (15-30mL) per day given in 3 or 4 divided doses for 7-14 days. Acute Gouty Arthritis: 50mg (10mL) PO tid until pain is tolerable, then d/c.
Pediatrics: >14 Yrs: RA/AS/OA: Initial: 25mg (5mL) PO bid-tid. Titrate: May increase by 25mg (5mL) or 50mg (10mL) at weekly intervals. Max: 150-200mg (30-40mL) per day. Bursitis/Tendinitis: 75-150mg (15-30mL) per day given in 3 or 4 divided doses for 7-14 days. Acute Gouty Arthritis: 50mg (10mL) PO tid until pain is tolerable, then d/c.

HOW SUPPLIED: Cap: 25mg, 50mg; Sus: (Indocin) 25mg/5mL [237mL]

CONTRAINDICATIONS: Aspirin (ASA) or other NSAID allergy that precipitates acute asthmatic attack, urticaria, or rhinitis. Treatment of perioperative pain in the setting of CABG surgery.

WARNINGS/PRECAUTIONS: Not a substitute for corticosteroids or to treat corticosteroid insufficiency. May lead to onset of new HTN or worsening of preexisting HTN; monitor BP closely. Fluid retention and edema reported; caution with fluid retention or heart failure (HF). Renal papillary necrosis and other renal injury reported after long-term use. Not recommended for use with advanced renal disease; if therapy must be initiated, monitor renal function. Anaphylactoid reactions may occur; avoid in patient with ASA-triad. May cause serious skin adverse events (eg, exfoliative dermatitis, Stevens-Johnson syndrome [SJS], and toxic epidermal necrolysis [TEN]); d/c at the first appearance of skin rash or any other signs of hypersensitivity. Avoid in late pregnancy; may cause premature closure of ductus arteriosus. May cause elevations of LFTs; d/c if liver disease develops or systemic manifestations occur. Anemia may occur; with long-term use, monitor Hgb/Hct if signs or symptoms of anemia develop. May inhibit platelet aggregation and prolong bleeding time; monitor with coagulation disorders. Caution with preexisting asthma and avoid with ASA-sensitive asthma. Corneal deposits and retinal disturbances reported with prolonged therapy; d/c if such changes are observed. Blurred vision may be significant; perform eye exams at periodic intervals during prolonged therapy. May aggravate depression or other psychiatric disturbances, epilepsy, and parkinsonism; use with caution. D/C if severe CNS adverse reactions develop. May impair mental/physical abilities. Caution in elderly.

ADVERSE REACTIONS: Headache, dizziness, upper GI ulcers, GI bleeding, GI perforation, N/V, dyspepsia, heartburn, epigastric pain, indigestion.

INTERACTIONS: May diminish antihypertensive effect of ACE inhibitors (eg, captopril) and angiotensin II antagonists (eg, losartan). Avoid with ASA, salicylates, diflunisal, triamterene, and other NSAIDs. May reduce the diuretic, natriuretic, and antihypertensive effects of loop, K^+-sparing, and thiazide diuretics. Increased levels of digoxin reported. Reduced basal plasma renin activity (PRA), as well as those elevations of PRA induced by furosemide reported. May decrease lithium clearance; monitor for toxicity. Caution with methotrexate; may enhance methotrexate toxicity. May increase levels with probenecid. Caution with cyclosporine and anticoagulants. Blunting of the antihypertensive effects of β-blockers reported. May increase risk of serious GI bleeding when used concomitantly with oral corticosteroids or anticoagulants, alcohol, or smoking.

PREGNANCY: Category C, not for use in nursing.

MECHANISM OF ACTION: NSAID; not established; exhibits antipyretic, analgesic, and anti-inflammatory properties. Suspected to inhibit prostaglandin synthesis.

PHARMACOKINETICS: Absorption: Readily absorbed. (Cap) Bioavailability (100%); C_{max}=1-2mcg/mL; T_{max}=2 hrs. **Distribution:** Plasma protein binding (99%); crosses blood-brain barrier and placenta; found in breast milk. **Metabolism:** desmethyl, desbenzoyl, desmethyldesbenzoyl (metabolites). **Elimination:** Urine (60% as drug/metabolites), feces (33% as drug); $T_{1/2}$=4.5 hrs.

NURSING CONSIDERATIONS

Assessment: Assess for history of asthma, urticaria or allergic-type reaction after previous use of NSAIDs, history of ulcer disease or GI bleeding, coagulation disorders or anticoagulant therapy, concomitant use of corticosteroids, smoking, alcohol use, age, health status, anemia, renal/hepatic impairment, pregnancy/nursing status, any other conditions where treatment is cautioned or contraindicated, and possible drug interactions.

Monitoring: Monitor BP during initiation of therapy and thereafter. Monitor platelet function, CBCs, LFTs, dexamethasone suppression tests, renal function, and chemistry profile. Monitor signs/symptoms of anaphylactic/anaphylactoid reactions, adverse skin events (eg, exfoliative dermatitis, SJS, TEN), eosinophilia, rash, corneal deposits and retinal disturbances with periodic ophthalmic exam, CNS effects, aggravation of depression or other psychiatric disturbances, GI bleeding/ulceration and perforation, anemia, CV thrombotic events, MI, stroke, new or worsening HTN, renal toxicity, and hyperkalemia.

Patient Counseling: Inform about potential serious side effects (eg, CV side effects such as MI or stroke); seek medical attention if signs/symptoms of chest pain, SOB, weakness, slurred speech, skin rash, blisters or fever, GI effects, bleeding, ulceration and perforation, signs of anaphylactic/anaphylactoid reaction, or hepatic toxicity occurs. Advise to notify physician if weight gain/edema occurs. Inform of risks if used during pregnancy and to use caution while performing hazardous tasks (eg, operating machinery/driving).

Administration: Oral route. Take with food. **Storage:** (Cap) 20-25°C (68-77°F). Protect from light. Dispense in a tight, light-resistant container. (Sus) Below 30°C (86°F); avoid >50°C (122°F). Protect from freezing.

INFERGEN
RX
interferon alfacon-1 (Kadmon)

> May cause or aggravate fatal or life-threatening neuropsychiatric, autoimmune, ischemic, and infectious disorders. Monitor closely with periodic clinical and lab evaluations. D/C in patients with persistently severe or worsening signs/symptoms of these conditions. When used with ribavirin, refer to the individual monograph.

THERAPEUTIC CLASS: Biological response modifier

INDICATIONS: Treatment of chronic hepatitis C (CHC) in patients ≥18 yrs with compensated liver disease.

DOSAGE: *Adults:* Monotherapy: Initial: 9mcg SQ as a single inj 3X a week for 24 weeks. Tolerated Previous Interferon Therapy But Did Not Respond/Relapsed: 15mcg SQ as a single inj 3X a week for up to 48 weeks. Combination Treatment with Ribavirin: 15mcg SQ as a single inj with weight-based ribavirin at 1000mg-1200mg (<75kg and ≥75kg) PO in 2 divided doses for up to 48 weeks. Take ribavirin with food. D/C if patients failed to achieve at least a 2 $\log_{10}$ drop at 12 weeks or undetectable hepatitis C virus (HCV)-RNA levels at 24 weeks. Refer to PI for dose modifications and discontinuation.

HOW SUPPLIED: Inj: 9mcg/0.3mL, 15mcg/0.5mL

CONTRAINDICATIONS: Hepatic decompensation (Child-Pugh score >6 [Class B and C]), autoimmune hepatitis. When used with ribavirin, refer to the individual monograph.

WARNINGS/PRECAUTIONS: Use of monotherapy for the treatment of hepatitis C is not recommended unless a patient is unable to take ribavirin. Patients with response of <1 $\log_{10}$ drop HCV RNA on previous treatment, Genotype 1, high viral load (≥850,000 IU/mL), African American race, and/or presence of cirrhosis are less likely to benefit from retreatment with combination therapy. May cause severe psychiatric adverse events; extreme caution with history of depression. If patients develop psychiatric problems, monitor during treatment and in the 6-month follow-up period; d/c if psychiatric symptoms persist/worsen, or suicidal ideation/aggressive behavior towards others are identified. Cardiovascular (CV) events (eg, hypotension, arrhythmia, tachycardia, angina pectoris, cardiomyopathy, myocardial infarction [MI]) reported. Caution with CV disease; monitor with history of MI and arrhythmic disorder. Dyspnea, pulmonary infiltrates, pneumonia, bronchiolitis obliterans, interstitial pneumonitis, pulmonary HTN, and sarcoidosis, some resulting in respiratory failure and/or deaths, may be induced or aggravated; d/c if persistent or unexplained pulmonary infiltrates/pulmonary function impairment develops. Risk of hepatic decompensation in CHC patients with cirrhosis; d/c if symptoms of hepatic decompensation occur. Increases in SrCr levels, including renal failure, reported; evaluate renal function in all patients. Monitor for signs/symptoms of toxicity in patients with renal impairment. Ischemic and hemorrhagic cerebrovascular events reported. May suppress bone marrow function, resulting in severe cytopenias; d/c if severe decreases in neutrophil (<0.5 x 10^9/L) or platelet counts (<25 x 10^9/L). Caution with abnormally low peripheral blood cell counts and in transplantation or chronically immunosuppressed patients. Development or exacerbation of autoimmune disorders reported; caution with other autoimmune disorders. Hemorrhagic/ischemic colitis, pancreatitis, serious acute hypersensitivity reactions, and ophthalmologic disorders reported; d/c therapy if these occur. Caution with history of endocrine disorders. Perform periodic ophthalmologic exams in patients with preexisting ophthalmologic disorders (eg, diabetic retinopathy, hypertensive retinopathy). Hyperthyroidism/hypothyroidism occurrence/aggravation, hyperglycemia, and diabetes mellitus (DM) reported; d/c if uncontrollable. Neutropenia, thrombocytopenia, hypertriglyceridemia, and thyroid disorders reported; perform lab tests prior to therapy, 2 weeks after initiation, and periodically thereafter. Caution in elderly. Use with ribavirin: Caution in patients with low baseline neutrophil counts (<1500 cells/mm³). Avoid with history of significant/unstable cardiac disease.

ADVERSE REACTIONS: Neuropsychiatric/autoimmune/ischemic/infectious disorders, depression, insomnia, headache, fatigue, fever, myalgia, rigors, body pain, increased sweating, nausea, abdominal pain.

INTERACTIONS: Peripheral neuropathy reported with telbivudine. Caution with agents that are known to cause myelosuppression. When used with ribavirin, refer to the individual monograph.

PREGNANCY: Category C, Category X (with ribavirin); caution in nursing, not for use in nursing (with ribavirin).

MECHANISM OF ACTION: Type-I interferon; binds to the interferon cell-surface receptor leading to the production of several interferon-stimulated gene products.

NURSING CONSIDERATIONS

Assessment: Assess for hypersensitivity reactions, neuropsychiatric/autoimmune/ischemic/infectious disorders, cardiac/CV/pulmonary disease, transplantation or chronically immunosuppressed patients, autoimmune disorder, renal/hepatic dysfunction, preexisting ophthalmologic disorders, endocrine disorders, or any other condition where treatment is contraindicated or cautioned. Assess pregnancy/nursing status and for possible drug interactions. Obtain baseline CBC with platelet count, SrCr/CrCl, serum albumin, bilirubin, TSH/T4, and eye exam. Obtain electrocardiogram with preexisting cardiac abnormalities before combination therapy.

Monitoring: Monitor for occurrence or aggravation of neuropsychiatric/autoimmune/ischemic/infectious disorders, depression, psychiatric symptoms, CV events, persistent or unexplained pulmonary infiltrates, pulmonary function impairment, hepatic/renal impairment, ischemic/hemorrhagic cerebrovascular events, bone marrow suppression, development/exacerbation of autoimmune disorders, colitis, pancreatitis, serious acute hypersensitivity reactions, ophthalmologic disorders, neutropenia, thrombocytopenia, hypertriglyceridemia, thyroid disorders, DM, hyperglycemia, and other adverse reactions. Monitor for signs/symptoms of interferon toxicity, including increases in SrCr with impaired renal function. Perform periodic ophthalmologic exam in patients with preexisting ophthalmologic disorder. Monitor lab tests (eg, CBC with platelet count, SrCr/CrCl, serum albumin, bilirubin, TSH, T4) 2 weeks after initiation of therapy and periodically thereafter.

Patient Counseling: Inform about the benefits and risks associated with therapy. Instruct to avoid pregnancy during and for 6 months post-treatment with combination therapy; recommend monthly pregnancy tests during this period. Inform that therapy should only be initiated when a negative pregnancy test has been obtained. Inform that there are no data regarding whether therapy will prevent transmission of HCV infection to others. Inform of the most common/common adverse reactions occurring during therapy; inform that non-narcotic analgesics and bedtime administration may be used to prevent or lessen some of these symptoms. Advise to rule out other possible causes of persistent fever. Instruct about the importance of proper disposal procedures and caution against the reuse of needles, syringes, or re-entry of the vial. Advise to report signs/symptoms of depression or suicidal ideation to the physician. Inform that lab evaluations are required before and during therapy. Instruct patients to keep well hydrated.

Administration: SQ route. **Storage:** 2-8°C (36-46°F). Do not freeze; avoid vigorous shaking and exposure to direct sunlight. May allow to reach room temperature prior to inj. Discard unused portion.

INFUMORPH
morphine sulfate (West-Ward)

`CII`

Not recommended for single-dose IV, IM or SQ administration. Risk of severe adverse effects; observe patients in a fully equipped and staffed environment for at least 24 hrs after the initial (single) test dose, and as appropriate, for the 1st several days after catheter implantation. Improper or erroneous substitution of Infumorph 200 or 500 (10 or 25mg/mL, respectively) for regular Duramorph (0.5 or 1mg/mL) is likely to result in serious overdosage, leading to seizures, respiratory depression, and possibly, fatal outcome. Naloxone inj and resuscitative equipment should be immediately available for use in case of life-threatening or intolerable side effects and whenever therapy is initiated or manipulation/refilling of the reservoir system takes place. Remove any contaminated clothing and rinse affected area with water if accidental dermal exposure occurs. Associated with risk of overdosage, diversion and abuse; special measures must be taken to control this product within the hospital/clinic. Do not use if the sol in the unopened ampul contains a precipitate that does not disappear upon shaking. After removal, do not use unless the sol is colorless or pale yellow.

THERAPEUTIC CLASS: Opioid analgesic

INDICATIONS: Treatment of intractable chronic pain.

DOSAGE: *Adults:* Individualize starting dose based upon in-hospital evaluation of response to serial single-dose intrathecal/epidural bolus inj of regular Duramorph. Lumbar Intrathecal: Opioid-Intolerant: Initial: 0.2-1mg/day. Opioid-Tolerant: Range: 1-10mg/day. Individualize upper daily dosage limit for each patient. Epidural: Opioid-Intolerant: Initial: 3.5-7.5mg/day. Opioid-Tolerant: Initial: 4.5-10mg/day. Dosage requirements may increase to 20-30mg/day. Individualize upper daily dosage limit for each patient.

HOW SUPPLIED: Inj: 10mg/mL, 25mg/mL [20mL]

CONTRAINDICATIONS: (For neuraxial analgesia use) Infection at inj microinfusion site, concomitant anticoagulant therapy, uncontrolled bleeding diathesis, any other concomitant therapy or medical condition that would render epidural or intrathecal administration of medication especially hazardous.

WARNINGS/PRECAUTIONS: May be habit-forming. Developed for use in continuous microinfusion devices; not for single-dose neuraxial inj. Chronic neuraxial opioid analgesia is appropriate only when less invasive means of controlling pain failed and should only be undertaken by those experienced in applying this treatment in a setting where its complications can be managed adequately. Inflammatory masses (eg, granulomas) reported; monitor for new neurologic signs/symptoms in patients receiving continuous infusion via indwelling intrathecal catheter and further assessment or intervention should be based on the clinical condition of the patient. Unusual acceleration of neuraxial morphine requirement may occur, causing concern regarding systemic absorption and the hazards of large doses; may benefit from hospitalization/detoxification. Myoclonic-like spasm of the lower extremities reported with intrathecal doses of >20mg/day; may need detoxification. May resume treatment at lower doses after detoxification. High neuraxial doses may produce myoclonic events. Limit intrathecal route to lumbar area. Caution with head injury or increased intracranial pressure; pupillary changes (miosis) may obscure the existence, extent, and course of intracranial pathology. Caution with decreased respiratory reserve (eg, emphysema, severe obesity, kyphoscoliosis, paralysis of the phrenic nerve), hepatic/renal dysfunction, and in elderly. Avoid with chronic asthma, upper airway obstruction, or any other chronic pulmonary disorder. Smooth muscle hypertonicity may result in biliary colic. Initiation of neuraxial opiate analgesia is associated with micturition disturbances, especially in males with prostatic enlargement. Orthostatic hypotension may occur with reduced circulating blood volume and myocardial dysfunction. Avoid abrupt withdrawal.

ADVERSE REACTIONS: Respiratory depression, myoclonus, inflammatory mass formation, dysphoric reactions, pruritus, urinary retention, constipation, lumbar puncture-type headache, peripheral edema.

INTERACTIONS: See Contraindications. CNS depressants (eg, alcohol, sedatives, antihistamines, psychotropics) may potentiate depressant effects. Neuroleptics may increase risk of respiratory depression. Withdrawal symptoms may occur upon administration of a narcotic antagonist. Monitor for orthostatic hypotension in patients on sympatholytic drugs.

PREGNANCY: Category C, safety not known in nursing.

MECHANISM OF ACTION: Opioid analgesic; analgesia involves at least 3 anatomical areas of the CNS: the periaqueductal-periventricular gray matter, the ventromedial medulla, and the spinal cord. Interacts predominantly with μ-receptors distributed in the brain, spinal cord, and in the trigeminal nerve.

PHARMACOKINETICS: Absorption: (Epidural) Rapid absorption, C_{max}=33-40ng/mL. (Intrathecal) C_{max}=<1-7.8ng/mL. (Epidural/Intrathecal) T_{max}=5-10 min. **Distribution:** Plasma protein binding (36%); found in breast milk. (IV) V_d=1.0-4.7L/kg. **Metabolism:** Liver; glucuronidation to morphine-3-glucuronide. **Elimination:** Urine (2-12% unchanged), feces (10% conjugate); $T_{1/2}$=1.5-4.5 hrs (IM/IV), 39-249 min (epidural).

NURSING CONSIDERATIONS

Assessment: Assess for patient's general condition and medical status, any other conditions where treatment is contraindicated or cautioned, renal/hepatic impairment, pregnancy/nursing status, and possible drug interactions.

Monitoring: Monitor for signs/symptoms of respiratory depression, myoclonic events, biliary colic, urinary retention, orthostatic hypotension, drug abuse/dependence, and other adverse reactions.

Patient Counseling: Inform about risks and benefits of therapy. Inform of adverse reactions that may occur. Instruct to inform physician of other medications taken.

Administration: Epidural/Intrathecal route. Refer to PI for administration instructions. **Storage:** 20-25°C (68-77°F); excursions permitted to 15-30°C (59-86°F). Protect from light. Do not freeze. Discard any unused portion. Do not heat-sterilize.

INLYTA   RX
axitinib (Pfizer)

THERAPEUTIC CLASS: Kinase inhibitor

INDICATIONS: Treatment of advanced renal cell carcinoma after failure of one prior systemic therapy.

DOSAGE: *Adults:* Initial: 5mg bid (q12h). Moderate Hepatic Impairment (Child-Pugh Class B): Reduce dose by half. Titrate: Increase or decrease dose based on individual safety and tolerability. Normotensive/No Concomitant Antihypertensive/Tolerated for ≥2 Consecutive Weeks with No Adverse Reaction >Grade 2: May increase to 7mg bid, and further to 10mg bid. Adverse Reaction: May require temporary interruption or permanent discontinuation, and/or dose reduction to 3mg bid. May further reduce to 2mg bid if needed. Concomitant Strong CYP3A4/5 Inhibitor (eg, Ketoconazole, Itraconazole, Clarithromycin, Atazanavir, Indinavir, Nefazodone, Nelfinavir, Ritonavir, Saquinavir, Telithromycin, Voriconazole): Avoid coadministration, but if needed, decrease axitinib dose by half and increase or decrease subsequent doses based on individual safety and tolerability. Strong CYP3A4/5 Inhibitor Discontinuation: Allow 3-5 $T_{1/2}$ of CYP3A4/5 inhibitor to elapse after discontinuation before returning to dose used prior to coadministration.

HOW SUPPLIED: Tab: 1mg, 5mg

WARNINGS/PRECAUTIONS: HTN/Hypertensive crisis reported; control BP prior to treatment initiation. Monitor for HTN and treat as needed with standard antihypertensive therapy. Reduce dose if persistent HTN occurs despite antihypertensive therapy. D/C if HTN is severe and persistent or if hypertensive crisis develops. Caution with history of or risk for arterial thromboembolic events or venous thromboembolic events. Hemorrhagic events reported; do not use in patients with evidence of untreated brain metastasis or recent active GI bleeding. Temporarily interrupt treatment if any bleeding requiring medical intervention occurs. GI perforation/fistulas, hypothyroidism, and hyperthyroidism reported; monitor for symptoms periodically. Treat thyroid dysfunction according to standard medical practice to maintain euthyroid state. D/C treatment at least 24 hrs prior to surgery; resume therapy after surgery based on clinical judgment of adequate wound healing. D/C if reversible posterior leukoencephalopathy (RPLS) occurs. Proteinuria reported; reduce dose or interrupt temporarily if moderate to severe proteinuria develops. Increased ALT reported. Monitor ALT/AST/bilirubin levels, thyroid function, and for proteinuria before initiation and periodically throughout treatment. Caution with moderate hepatic impairment and with end-stage renal disease (CrCl <15mL/min). May cause fetal harm.

ADVERSE REACTIONS: Diarrhea, HTN, fatigue, decreased appetite, N/V, dysphonia, palmar-plantar erythrodysesthesia syndrome, weight decrease, asthenia, constipation, hypothyroidism, cough, mucosal inflammation, arthralgia, stomatitis.

INTERACTIONS: Avoid with CYP3A4/5 inhibitors (eg, ketoconazole, grapefruit, grapefruit juice, itraconazole, clarithromycin, atazanavir, indinavir, nefazodone, nelfinavir, ritonavir, saquinavir, telithromycin, voriconazole); if needed, reduce axitinib dose by half. Avoid with strong CYP3A4/5 inducers (eg, rifampin, dexamethasone, phenytoin, carbamazepine, rifabutin, rifapentine, phenobarbital, St. John's wort). Moderate CYP3A4/5 inducers (eg, bosentan, efavirenz, etravirine, modafinil, nafcillin) may reduce exposure; avoid use if possible.

PREGNANCY: Category D, not for use in nursing.

MECHANISM OF ACTION: Kinase inhibitor; inhibits receptor tyrosine kinases, including vascular endothelial growth factor receptors (VEGFR)-1, VEGFR-2, and VEGFR-3, resulting in inhibition of VEGF-mediated endothelial cell proliferation, cell survival, and tumor growth.

PHARMACOKINETICS: Absorption: (Single 5mg dose) Absolute bioavailability (58%); C_{max}=27.8ng/mL, AUC=265ng•hr/mL, T_{max}=2.5-4.1 hrs (median). **Distribution:** V_d=160L; plasma protein binding (>99%). **Metabolism:** Liver via CYP3A4/5 (primary), CYP1A2, 2C19, and UGT1A1 (lesser extent). **Elimination:** Feces (41%, 12% unchanged), urine (23%, metabolites); $T_{1/2}$=2.5-6.1 hrs.

NURSING CONSIDERATIONS

Assessment: Assess for HTN, risk for/history of arterial/venous thromboembolic events, untreated brain metastasis, recent active GI bleeding, thyroid dysfunction, proteinuria, renal/hepatic impairment, pregnancy/nursing status, and possible drug interactions. Obtain baseline AST, ALT, and bilirubin levels.

Monitoring: Monitor for HTN/hypertensive crisis, symptoms of GI perforation/fistula, thyroid dysfunction, RPLS, proteinuria, and other adverse events. Monitor AST, ALT, and bilirubin levels periodically.

Patient Counseling: Inform about benefits/risks of therapy. Inform that HTN may develop; instruct to have BP monitored regularly during treatment. Instruct to inform physician if experiencing symptoms suggestive of thromboembolic events, abnormal thyroid function, any bleeding episodes, or persistent/severe abdominal pain. Advise to inform physician if patient has an unhealed wound or has surgery scheduled. Advise to inform physician if patient has worsening of neurological function consistent with RPLS (eg, headache, seizure, lethargy, confusion, blindness, other visual and neurologic disturbances). Advise to avoid becoming pregnant while on therapy and counsel both male and female patients to use effective birth control. Instruct female patients not to breastfeed while receiving treatment. Advise to inform physician about all concomitant medications, vitamins, or dietary and herbal supplements. Instruct not to take additional dose if the patient vomits or misses a dose and to take the next dose at the usual time.

Administration: Oral route. Take with or without food. Swallow whole with a glass of water. **Storage:** 20-25°C (68-77°F); excursions permitted to 15-30°C (59-86°F).

INNOPRAN XL   RX
propranolol HCl (Akrimax)

> Exacerbation of angina pectoris and myocardial infarction (MI) reported following abrupt discontinuation. When discontinuing chronically administered drug, particularly in ischemic heart disease, gradually reduce dose over a period of 1-2 weeks and monitor patients. Promptly resume therapy at least temporarily and take other measures appropriate for the management of unstable angina if angina markedly worsens or acute coronary insufficiency develops. Caution against interruption or discontinuation of therapy without a physician's advice. Coronary artery disease (CAD) may be unrecognized; avoid abrupt discontinuation of therapy even in patient treated only for HTN.

THERAPEUTIC CLASS: Nonselective beta-blocker

INDICATIONS: Management of HTN.

DOSAGE: *Adults:* Individualize dose. Initial: 80mg qhs taken consistently, either on empty stomach or with food. May titrate to 120mg qhs PRN for BP control. Elderly: Start at lower end of dosing range.

HOW SUPPLIED: Cap, Extended-Release: 80mg, 120mg

CONTRAINDICATIONS: Cardiogenic shock or decompensated heart failure (HF), sinus bradycardia, sick sinus syndrome and >1st-degree heart block (unless a permanent pacemaker is in place), bronchial asthma.

WARNINGS/PRECAUTIONS: May cause depression of myocardial contractility and precipitate HF and cardiogenic shock; may be necessary to lower dose or d/c therapy. Avoid routine withdrawal prior to surgery. May mask tachycardia occurring with hypoglycemia and hyperthyroidism. Abrupt withdrawal may precipitate thyroid storm. Bradycardia including sinus pause, heart block, and cardiac arrest reported. Increased risk in patients with 1st-degree AV block, sinus node dysfunction, and conduction disorders (eg, Wolff-Parkinson-White). D/C or reduce dose if severe bradycardia occurs. Patients treated for severe anaphylactic reaction may be unresponsive to usual doses of epinephrine; consider other medications (eg, IV fluids, glucagon). Caution in elderly.

ADVERSE REACTIONS: Fatigue, dizziness, constipation.

INTERACTIONS: Increased concentrations with warfarin; monitor PT. Increased concentrations with propafenone. Increase levels with CYP2D6 inhibitors (eg, bupropion, fluoxetine, paroxetine, quinidine), CYP1A2 inhibitors (eg, ciprofloxacin, enoxamine, fluvoxamine), and CYP2C19 inhibitors (eg, fluconazole, fluvoxamine, ticlopidine). Decreased levels with CYP1A2 inducers (eg, phenytoin, montelukast, smoking) and CYP2C19 inducers (eg, rifampin), and cholestyramine and colestipol leading to loss of efficacy. May antagonize antihypertensive effects of clonidine; may result to rebound HTN if withdrawn abruptly. May prolong 1st dose hypotension and syncope with prazosin. May reduce sensitivity to dobutamine stress echocardiography in patients undergoing evaluation for myocardial ischemia. May exacerbate hypotensive effects of MAOIs or TCAs. NSAIDs may attenuate the antihypertensive effect of β-adrenoreceptor blocking agents. Increased risk of significant bradycardia with non-dihydropyridine calcium-channel blockers (eg, verapamil, diltiazem), digoxin or clonidine.

PREGNANCY: Category C, caution in nursing.

MECHANISM OF ACTION: Nonselective β-adrenergic receptor blocker; has not been established. Thought to decrease cardiac output, inhibit renin release by the kidneys, and diminish tonic sympathetic nerve outflow from vasomotor centers in the brain.

PHARMACOKINETICS: Absorption: Almost complete; T_{max}=12-14 hrs (fasted). **Distribution:** V_d=4L; plasma protein binding (90%); found in breast milk. **Metabolism:** Liver (extensive); CYP2D6 (aromatic hydroxylation), CYP1A2, 2D6 (oxidation), N-dealkylation, glucuronidation. Propranolol glucuronide, naphthyloxylactic acid, and glucuronic acid and sulfate conjugates of 4-hydroxy propranolol (major metabolites). **Elimination:** $T_{1/2}$=8 hrs.

NURSING CONSIDERATIONS

Assessment: Assess for cardiogenic shock, decompensated HF, sinus bradycardia, sick sinus syndrome, AV heart block, presence of pacemaker, bronchial asthma, hepatic or renal impairment, hyperthyroidism, hypoglycemia, history of anaphylactic reactions, possible drug interactions, and pregnancy/nursing status.

Monitoring: Monitor for signs/symptoms of HF, hyperthyroidism, hypoglycemia, anaphylactic reactions, and other adverse reactions. Monitor HR and PT.

Patient Counseling: Inform about risks and benefits of therapy. Instruct not to interrupt or d/c therapy without a physician's advice. Advise to contact physician if signs/symptoms of HF worsens (eg, weight gain or increasing SOB).

Administration: Oral route. **Storage:** 25°C (77°F); excursions permitted to 15-30°C (59-86°F).

INSPRA   RX
eplerenone (G.D. Searle)

THERAPEUTIC CLASS: Aldosterone blocker

INDICATIONS: To improve survival of stable patients with left ventricular systolic dysfunction (ejection fraction ≤40%) and clinical evidence of congestive heart failure (CHF) after an acute myocardial infarction (MI). Treatment of HTN, alone or in combination with other antihypertensive agents.

DOSAGE: *Adults:* CHF Post-MI: Initial: 25mg qd. Titrate: Increase to 50mg qd, preferably within 4 weeks as tolerated. Refer to PI for dose adjustment based on serum K⁺ level once treatment has begun. HTN: Initial: 50mg qd. Titrate: Increase to 50mg bid if BP response is inadequate. Max: 100mg/day. Hypertensive Patients Receiving Moderate CYP3A4 Inhibitors (eg, Erythromycin, Saquinavir, Verapamil, Fluconazole): Initial: 25mg qd.

HOW SUPPLIED: Tab: 25mg, 50mg

CONTRAINDICATIONS: All Patients: Serum K⁺ >5.5mEq/L at initiation, CrCl ≤30mL/min, concomitant administration of strong CYP3A4 inhibitors (eg, ketoconazole, itraconazole, nefazodone, troleandomycin, clarithromycin, ritonavir, nelfinavir). Patients Treated for HTN: Type 2 diabetes with microalbuminuria, SrCr >2mg/dL (males) or >1.8mg/dL (females), CrCl <50mL/min, concomitant administration of K⁺ supplements or K⁺-sparing diuretics (eg, amiloride, spironolactone, triamterene).

WARNINGS/PRECAUTIONS: Measure serum K⁺ before initiating therapy, within the 1st week, at 1 month after start of treatment or dose adjustment, and periodically thereafter. Minimize the risk of hyperkalemia with proper patient selection and monitoring; monitor for hyperkalemia until the effect of therapy is established. Caution in patients with CHF post-MI who have SrCr >2mg/dL (males) or >1.8mg/dL (females), or CrCl ≤50mL/min, or who are diabetic (especially those with proteinuria). Increased risk of hyperkalemia in patients with decreased renal function.

ADVERSE REACTIONS: Hyperkalemia, dizziness, increased SrCr/TGs.

INTERACTIONS: See Contraindications and Dosage. Monitor serum K$^+$ and SrCr in 3-7 days in patients who start taking a moderate CYP3A4 inhibitor. Increased risk of hyperkalemia with an ACE inhibitor and/or an ARB; closely monitor serum K$^+$ and renal function, especially in patients at risk for impaired renal function (eg, elderly). Monitor serum lithium levels frequently if coadministered with lithium. When used with NSAIDs, observe to determine whether the desired effect on BP is obtained and monitor for changes in serum K$^+$ levels.

PREGNANCY: Category B, not for use in nursing.

MECHANISM OF ACTION: Aldosterone blocker; binds to mineralocorticoid receptor and blocks the binding of aldosterone, a component of the renin-angiotensin-aldosterone-system.

PHARMACOKINETICS: Absorption: Absolute bioavailability (69%) (100mg tab); T_{max}=1.5 hrs. **Distribution:** V_d=43-90L; plasma protein binding (50%). **Metabolism:** CYP3A4. **Elimination:** Urine (67%, <5% unchanged), feces (32%, <5% unchanged); $T_{1/2}$=4-6 hrs.

NURSING CONSIDERATIONS

Assessment: Assess for type 2 diabetes with microalbuminuria/proteinuria, pregnancy/nursing status, and possible drug interactions. Assess serum K$^+$ levels and renal function (eg, CrCl, SrCr).

Monitoring: Monitor for signs/symptoms of hyperkalemia and other adverse reactions. Monitor serum K$^+$ within the 1st week, at 1 month after start of treatment or dose adjustment, and periodically thereafter. Monitor BP and renal function.

Patient Counseling: Advise not to use K$^+$ supplements or salt substitutes containing K$^+$ without consulting the prescribing physician. Instruct to contact physician if symptoms such as dizziness, diarrhea, vomiting, rapid or irregular heartbeat, lower extremity edema, or difficulty breathing occur. Inform that periodic monitoring of BP and serum K$^+$ is important.

Administration: Oral route. May be administered with or without food. **Storage:** 25°C (77°F); excursions permitted to 15-30°C (59-86°F).

INTEGRILIN
eptifibatide (Merck)

RX

THERAPEUTIC CLASS: Glycoprotein IIb/IIIa inhibitor

INDICATIONS: To decrease rate of a combined endpoint of death or new myocardial infarction (MI) in patients with acute coronary syndrome (ACS) (unstable angina/non-ST-elevation MI), including patients being managed medically and those undergoing percutaneous coronary intervention (PCI). To decrease rate of a combined endpoint of death, new MI, or need for urgent intervention in patients undergoing PCI, including those undergoing intracoronary stenting.

DOSAGE: *Adults:* ACS: 180mcg/kg IV bolus as soon as possible after diagnosis, followed by continuous infusion of 2mcg/kg/min (or 1mcg/kg/min, if CrCl is <50mL/min). Continue infusion until discharge or initiation of coronary artery bypass graft (CABG) surgery, up to 72 hrs. If undergoing PCI, continue infusion until discharge or for up to 18-24 hrs post-PCI, whichever comes first, allowing up to 96 hrs of therapy. PCI: 180mcg/kg IV bolus immediately before PCI, followed by continuous infusion of 2mcg/kg/min (or 1mcg/kg/min, if CrCl is <50mL/min) and a 2nd bolus of 180mcg/kg (given 10 min after 1st bolus). Continue infusion until discharge or for up to 18-24 hrs, whichever comes first; minimum of 12 hrs of infusion is recommended. In patients who undergo CABG surgery, d/c infusion prior to surgery. D/C therapy in patients requiring thrombolytic therapy. Refer to PI for concomitant aspirin (ASA) and heparin doses and dosing charts by weight.

HOW SUPPLIED: Inj: 0.75mg/mL [100mL vial], 2mg/mL [10mL, 100mL vial]

CONTRAINDICATIONS: History of bleeding diathesis or evidence of active abnormal bleeding within the previous 30 days, severe HTN (systolic BP >200mmHg or diastolic BP >110mmHg) not adequately controlled on antihypertensives, major surgery within preceding 6 weeks, history of stroke within 30 days or any history of hemorrhagic stroke, current or planned administration of another parenteral glycoprotein (GP) IIb/IIIa inhibitor, and renal dialysis dependency.

WARNINGS/PRECAUTIONS: Maintain activated PTT (aPTT) between 50-70 sec unless PCI is to be performed. Associated with an increase in major and minor bleeding. Minimize the use of arterial and venous punctures, IM inj, urinary catheters, nasotracheal intubation, and NG tubes. Avoid noncompressible sites (eg, subclavian or jugular veins) when obtaining IV access. Caution in patients undergoing PCI; d/c infusion and heparin immediately if bleeding at access site cannot be controlled with pressure. Both infusion and heparin should be discontinued and sheath hemostasis should be achieved at least 2-4 hrs before hospital discharge. Thrombocytopenia (immune-mediated and non-immune mediated) reported. D/C infusion and heparin if acute profound thrombocytopenia occurs or platelet count decreases to <100,000/mm³; monitor serial platelet counts, assess the presence of drug-dependent antibodies, and treat as appropriate.

ADVERSE REACTIONS: Bleeding, hypotension.

INTERACTIONS: See Contraindications. Increased risk of bleeding with antiplatelet agents, thrombolytics, heparin, ASA, chronic NSAID use, oral anticoagulants, and P2Y$_{12}$ inhibitors; monitor aPTT and activated clotting time (ACT) with heparin.

PREGNANCY: Category B, caution in nursing.

MECHANISM OF ACTION: GP IIb/IIIa inhibitor; reversibly inhibits platelet aggregation by preventing the binding of fibrinogen, von Willebrand factor, and other adhesive ligands to GP IIb/IIIa.

PHARMACOKINETICS: Distribution: Plasma protein binding (25%). **Elimination:** Urine; T$_{1/2}$=2.5 hrs.

NURSING CONSIDERATIONS

Assessment: Assess for drug hypersensitivity, history of bleeding diathesis or stroke, active abnormal bleeding within previous 30 days, severe HTN, major surgery within preceding 6 weeks, history of hemorrhagic stroke, dependency on renal dialysis, renal insufficiency, pregnancy/nursing status, and possible drug interactions. Obtain baseline Hgb, Hct, platelet count, SrCr, and PT/aPTT to identify preexisting hemostatic abnormalities. Measure ACT in patients undergoing PCI.

Monitoring: Monitor for signs/symptoms of bleeding, thrombocytopenia, and hypersensitivity reactions. Monitor platelet count in patients with low platelet counts.

Patient Counseling: Inform about the risks and benefits of therapy. Instruct to inform physician about any medical conditions, medications, and allergies.

Administration: IV route. Refer to PI for administration instructions. **Storage:** 2-8°C (36-46°F). May store at 25°C (77°F) for ≤2 months with excursions permitted to 15-30°C (59-86°F).

INTELENCE   RX
etravirine (Janssen)

THERAPEUTIC CLASS: Non-nucleoside reverse transcriptase inhibitor

INDICATIONS: Treatment of HIV-1 infection in combination with other antiretrovirals in antiretroviral treatment-experienced patients ≥6 yrs of age who have evidence of viral replication and HIV-1 strains resistant to a non-nucleoside reverse transcriptase inhibitor (NNRTI) and other antiretrovirals.

DOSAGE: *Adults:* Usual: 200mg (one 200mg tab or two 100mg tabs) bid pc. *Pediatrics:* 6-<18 Yrs: ≥30kg: 200mg bid pc. ≥25kg-<30kg: 150mg bid pc. ≥20kg-<25kg: 125mg bid pc. ≥16kg-<20kg: 100mg bid pc.

HOW SUPPLIED: Tab: 25mg*, 100mg, 200mg *scored

WARNINGS/PRECAUTIONS: Severe, potentially life-threatening, and fatal skin reactions (eg, erythema multiforme, toxic epidermal necrolysis, Stevens-Johnson syndrome), and hypersensitivity reactions including drug rash with eosinophilia and systemic symptoms (DRESS) reported; d/c immediately if these occur and initiate appropriate therapy. Immune reconstitution syndrome, autoimmune disorders (eg, Graves' disease, polymyositis, Guillain-Barre syndrome) in the setting of immune reconstitution, and redistribution/accumulation of body fat reported. Caution in elderly patients.

ADVERSE REACTIONS: Rash, peripheral neuropathy.

INTERACTIONS: May alter therapeutic effect and adverse reaction profile with drugs that induce, inhibit, or are substrates of CYP3A, CYP2C9, and CYP2C19, or are transported by P-glycoprotein. Avoid with other NNRTIs, delavirdine, rilpivirine, atazanavir (ATV) without low-dose ritonavir (RTV), ATV/RTV, fosamprenavir (FPV) without low-dose RTV, FPV/RTV, tipranavir/RTV, indinavir without low-dose RTV, nelfinavir without low-dose RTV, RTV (600mg bid), carbamazepine, phenobarbital, phenytoin, rifampin, rifapentine, and St. John's wort. Caution with digoxin; use lowest dose initially. May increase levels of nelfinavir without RTV, digoxin, warfarin (monitor INR), anticoagulants, 14-OH-clarithromycin, diazepam, fluvastatin, and pitavastatin. May increase maraviroc levels in the presence of a potent CYP3A inhibitor (eg, RTV boosted protease inhibitor). May decrease levels of maraviroc, antiarrhythmics, rifabutin, telaprevir, atorvastatin, lovastatin, simvastatin, immunosuppressant, and clopidogrel (active) metabolite. Fluconazole and voriconazole may increase exposure. Posaconazole, itraconazole, or ketoconazole may increase levels. May decrease clarithromycin exposure. Caution with artemether/lumefantrine. Efavirenz, nevirapine, rifabutin, and systemic dexamethasone may decrease levels. Darunavir/RTV, lopinavir/RTV, and saquinavir/RTV may decrease exposure. Consider alternatives to clarithromycin, such as azithromycin, for treatment of *Mycobacterium avium* complex. Monitor for withdrawal symptoms when coadministered with methadone, buprenorphine, buprenorphine/naloxone. May need to alter sildenafil dose. Refer to PI for additional drug interaction information.

PREGNANCY: Category B, not for use in nursing.

MECHANISM OF ACTION: Non-nucleoside reverse transcriptase inhibitor; binds directly to reverse transcriptase and blocks the RNA-dependent and DNA-dependent DNA polymerase activities by causing a disruption of the enzyme's catalytic site.

PHARMACOKINETICS: Absorption: T_{max}=2.5-4 hrs; AUC_{12h}=4522ng•hr/mL (adults), 3742ng•hr/mL (pediatric patients). **Distribution:** Plasma protein binding (99.9%). **Metabolism:** Liver via CYP3A, CYP2C9, and CYP2C19; methyl hydroxylation. **Elimination:** Feces (93.7%, 81.2-86.4% unchanged), urine (1.2%); $T_{1/2}$=41 hrs.

NURSING CONSIDERATIONS

Assessment: Assess treatment history, pregnancy/nursing status, and for possible drug interactions. Perform resistance testing where possible.

Monitoring: Monitor for signs/symptoms of severe skin/hypersensitivity reactions, body fat redistribution/accumulation, immune reconstitution syndrome (eg, opportunistic infections), autoimmune disorders, and other adverse reactions. Monitor clinical status, including liver transaminases.

Patient Counseling: Inform that product is not a cure for HIV and patients may continue to develop opportunistic infections and other complications associated with HIV disease. Advise to avoid doing things that can spread HIV-1 infection to others. Advise to take medication ud. Instruct to always use in combination with other antiretrovirals. Advise not to alter dose or d/c therapy without consulting physician. If a dose is missed within 6 hrs of time usually taken, instruct to take as soon as possible following a meal. If scheduled time exceeds 6 hrs, instruct not to take the missed dose and resume the usual dosing schedule. Advise to report to physician the use of any other prescription/nonprescription or herbal products (eg, St. John's wort). Counsel to d/c and notify physician if severe rash develops. Advise that redistribution or accumulation of body fat may occur.

Administration: Oral route. Swallow tab(s) whole with liquid. Tabs may be dispersed in glass of water if unable to swallow tab(s) whole. Refer to PI for further administration instruction. **Storage:** 25°C (77°F); excursions permitted to 15-30°C (59-86°F). Store in the original bottle. Protect from moisture.

INTERMEZZO
zolpidem tartrate (Purdue Pharma)

THERAPEUTIC CLASS: Imidazopyridine hypnotic

INDICATIONS: PRN treatment of insomnia when a middle-of-the-night awakening is followed by difficulty returning to sleep.

DOSAGE: *Adults:* Usual/Max: (Women) 1.75mg, (Men) 3.5mg once per night PRN if a middle-of-the-night awakening is followed by difficulty returning to sleep. Concomitant CNS Depressants/Elderly (>65 Yrs)/Hepatic Impairment: Use the 1.75mg dose.

HOW SUPPLIED: Tab, SL: 1.75mg, 3.5mg

WARNINGS/PRECAUTIONS: Not for use when patient has <4 hrs of bedtime before planning to awake. May cause CNS depressant effects; may be at risk for next-day driving and psychomotor impairment if taken with <4 hrs of bedtime remaining. Initiate only after careful evaluation; failure of insomnia to remit after 7-10 days of treatment may indicate presence of psychiatric and/or medical illness. Severe anaphylactic/anaphylactoid reactions reported; do not rechallenge if angioedema or anaphylaxis develops. Abnormal thinking, behavior changes, and visual/auditory hallucinations reported. Complex behaviors (eg, sleep-driving), reported. Worsening of depression, and suicidal thoughts and actions (including complete suicide) reported in depressed patients. Caution with compromised respiratory function; consider risk of respiratory depression in patients with respiratory impairment, including sleep apnea and myasthenia gravis. Withdrawal signs/symptoms reported following rapid dose decrease or abrupt d/c. Observe elderly patients closely for impaired motor/cognitive performance and for unusual sensitivity. Caution with hepatic impairment/insufficiency.

ADVERSE REACTIONS: Nervous system disorders, GI disorders, headache.

INTERACTIONS: May increase risk of CNS depression with other CNS depressants (eg, benzodiazepines, opioids, TCAs, alcohol). May have additive effects of decreased alertness and psychomotor performance with imipramine, chlorpromazine, and alcohol. Caution with chronic haloperidol administration. Sertraline and ketoconazole may increase exposure. May increase $T_{1/2}$ with multiple doses of fluoxetine. CYP3A inhibitors may increase exposure. Rifampin may reduce exposure and decrease efficacy.

PREGNANCY: Category C, safety not known in nursing.

MECHANISM OF ACTION: Imidazopyridine, nonbenzodiazepine hypnotic; binds with BZ1 receptor with a high affinity ratio of α_1/α_5 subunits.

PHARMACOKINETICS: Absorption: Rapid. T_{max}=35-75 min. Women: (3.5mg) C_{max}=77ng/mL, AUC=296ng•h/mL. (1.75mg) C_{max}=37ng/mL, AUC=151ng•h/mL. Men: (3.5mg) C_{max}=53ng/mL, AUC=198ng•h/mL. **Distribution:** Plasma protein binding (93%); found in breast milk. **Elimination:** (3.5mg) $T_{1/2}$=2.5 hrs.

NURSING CONSIDERATIONS

Assessment: Assess for known hypersensitivity, depression, chronic obstructive pulmonary disease, respiratory impairment, myasthenia gravis, hepatic dysfunction, pregnancy/nursing status, and possible drug interactions.

Monitoring: Monitor for signs/symptoms of withdrawal, tolerance, abuse, dependence, respiratory insufficiency, abnormal thinking, behavioral changes, agitation, depersonalization, visual/auditory hallucinations, complex behaviors (including "sleep-driving"), amnesia, anxiety, neuropsychiatric symptoms, worsening of depression, suicidal thoughts and actions, angioedema (tongue, glottis, or larynx), driving/psychomotor impairment, worsening of insomnia, thinking or behavioral abnormalities.

Patient Counseling: Inform about the benefits and risks of treatment. Instruct patient to take as prescribed. Counsel that medication has the potential to cause next-day impairment, and the risk is increased if dosing instructions are not carefully followed. Advise to wait at least 4 hrs after dosing and until they feel fully awake before driving or engaging in other activities requiring mental alertness. Inform that severe anaphylactic and anaphylactoid reactions may occur; notify physician immediately if signs/symptoms occur. Inform families that therapy has been associated with "sleep-driving" and other complex behaviors while not being fully awake; call healthcare providers immediately if symptoms develop. Instruct to report immediately for any suicidal thoughts. Advise not to take medication if alcohol has been taken on that day or before going to bed.

Administration: SL route. Take in bed. Allow to disintegrate under the tongue completely before swallowing; do not swallow whole. Do not administer with or immediately after a meal. **Storage:** 20-25°C (68-77°F); excursion permitted between 15-30°C (59-86°F). Protect from moisture. Do not remove blister from unit-dose pouch until time of use.

INTRON A   RX
interferon alfa-2b (Merck)

> May cause or aggravate fatal or life-threatening neuropsychiatric, autoimmune, ischemic, and infectious disorders. Monitor closely with periodic clinical and lab evaluations. D/C in patients with persistently severe or worsening signs/symptoms of these conditions.

THERAPEUTIC CLASS: Biological response modifier

INDICATIONS: (≥18 Yrs) Treatment of hairy cell leukemia. Adjuvant to surgical treatment in patients with malignant melanoma who are free of disease but at high risk for systemic recurrence, within 56 days of surgery. Initial treatment of clinically aggressive follicular non-Hodgkin's lymphoma with anthracycline-containing combination chemotherapy. Treatment of AIDS-related Kaposi's sarcoma and intralesional treatment of condylomata acuminata involving external surfaces of the genital and perianal areas in selected patients. Treatment of chronic hepatitis C in patients with compensated liver disease who have a history of blood or blood-product exposure and/or are hepatitis C virus (HCV) antibody positive. Treatment of chronic hepatitis C in patients (≥3 yrs) with compensated liver disease previously untreated with α-interferon therapy, and in patients (≥18 yrs) who have relapsed following α-interferon therapy, in combination with ribavirin; refer to ribavirin PI. Treatment of chronic hepatitis B in patients (≥1 yr) with compensated liver disease and those who are serum hepatitis B surface antigen (HBsAg) positive for at least 6 months and have evidence of hepatitis B virus replication (serum hepatitis B e antigen [HBeAg] positive) with elevated serum ALT.

DOSAGE: *Adults:* ≥18 Yrs: Hairy Cell Leukemia: 2 MIU/m² IM/SQ 3X/week for up to 6 months. Malignant Melanoma: Induction: 20 MIU/m² IV, over 20 min, 5 consecutive days/week for 4 weeks. Maint: 10 MIU/m² SQ 3X/week for 48 weeks. Follicular Lymphoma: 5 MIU SQ 3X/week for up to 18 months. Condylomata Acuminata: 1 MIU/lesion 3X/week alternating days for 3 weeks. Max: 5 lesions/course. An additional course may be administered at 12-16 weeks. AIDS-Related Kaposi's Sarcoma: 30 MIU/m²/dose IM/SQ 3X/week until disease progression or maximal response has been achieved after 16 weeks of treatment. Chronic Hepatitis C: 3 MIU IM/SQ 3X/week. In patients tolerating therapy with normalization of ALT at 16 weeks of treatment, extend therapy for 18-24 months. In patients who do not normalize their ALTs or have persistently high levels of HCV RNA after 16 weeks of therapy, consider discontinuing therapy. Chronic Hepatitis B: 5 MIU IM/SQ qd or 10 MIU IM/SQ 3X/week for 16 weeks. Refer to PI for dose adjustments, route of administration and dosage forms/strengths selection for each indication.
Pediatrics: ≥3 Yrs: Chronic Hepatitis C: 3 MIU IM/SQ 3X/week. In patients tolerating therapy with normalization of ALT at 16 weeks of treatment, extend therapy for 18-24 months. In patients

who do not normalize their ALTs or have persistently high levels of HCV RNA after 16 weeks of therapy, consider discontinuing therapy. ≥1 Yr: Chronic Hepatitis B: 3 MIU/m² SQ 3X/week for 1 week, then 6 MIU/m² SQ 3X/week for total therapy of 16-24 weeks. Max: 10 MIU/m² 3X/week. Refer to PI for dose adjustments, route of administration and dosage forms/strengths selection for each indication.

HOW SUPPLIED: Inj: 10 MIU, 18 MIU, 50 MIU [powder]; 18 MIU, 25 MIU [sol]

CONTRAINDICATIONS: Autoimmune hepatitis, decompensated liver disease. When used with Rebetol, refer to the individual monograph.

WARNINGS/PRECAUTIONS: Caution with coagulation disorders (eg, thrombophlebitis, pulmonary embolism), severe myelosuppression, debilitating medical conditions (eg, history of pulmonary disease, diabetes mellitus [DM] prone to ketoacidosis). Cardiovascular (CV) adverse experiences (eg, arrhythmia, cardiomyopathy, myocardial infarction [MI]), and ischemic and hemorrhagic cerebrovascular events reported; caution with history of CV disease (CVD). Depression and suicidal behavior reported. Monitor patients during treatment and in the 6-month follow-up period if psychiatric problems develop; d/c if severe, or if symptoms persist or worsen. Obtundation, coma, and encephalopathy may occur in some patients, usually in elderly, treated with higher doses. May suppress bone marrow function and may result in severe cytopenias; d/c if severe decreases in neutrophil (<0.5 x 10⁹/L) or platelet counts (<25 x 10⁹/L) occur. Ophthalmologic disorders may be induced or aggravated; conduct baseline eye exam and monitor periodically with preexisting ophthalmologic disorders. D/C if new or worsening ophthalmologic disorders develop. Thyroid abnormalities and DM reported; d/c if these conditions develop and cannot be normalized by medication. Hepatotoxicity and autoimmune disorders reported; monitor or d/c if appropriate. D/C if signs/symptoms of liver failure develop. Avoid in patients with a history of autoimmune disease and in patients who are immunosuppressed transplant recipients. Pulmonary disorders may be induced or aggravated. Closely monitor if the chest x-ray shows pulmonary infiltrates or there is evidence of pulmonary function impairment and d/c if appropriate. Powder formulation contains albumin; carries an extremely remote risk for transmission of viral diseases and Creutzfeldt-Jakob disease. Should not be used with rapidly progressive visceral disease. Acute serious hypersensitivity reactions reported; d/c immediately if an acute reaction develops. New or exacerbated sarcoidosis, exacerbated psoriasis, and hypertriglyceridemia reported. D/C if persistently elevated TG levels associated with symptoms of potential pancreatitis occur. Do not interchange brands. Caution in elderly.

ADVERSE REACTIONS: Neuropsychiatric/autoimmune/ischemic/infectious disorders, flu-like symptoms, fatigue, fever, chills, neutropenia, myalgia, anorexia, N/V, rigors, headache, GI disorders.

INTERACTIONS: May increase theophylline levels. Caution with other potentially myelosuppressive agents (eg, zidovudine). Higher incidence of neutropenia with zidovudine. Peripheral neuropathy reported when used in combination with telbivudine. Hemolytic anemia, dental, and periodontal disorders reported when used in combination with ribavirin.

PREGNANCY: Category C, Category X (with ribavirin); not for use in nursing.

MECHANISM OF ACTION: α-interferon; binds to specific membrane receptors on cell surface initiating induction of certain enzymes, suppression of cell proliferation, immunomodulating activities, and inhibition of virus replication in virus-infected cells.

PHARMACOKINETICS: Absorption: (IM/SQ) C_{max}=18-116 IU/mL, T_{max}=3-12 hrs; (IV) C_{max}=135-273 IU/mL. **Elimination:** (IM/SQ) $T_{1/2}$=2-3 hrs; (IV) $T_{1/2}$=2 hrs.

NURSING CONSIDERATIONS

Assessment: Assess for history of psychiatric disorders, CVD, autoimmune, and ophthalmologic disorders, hepatic/renal impairment, hypersensitivity reactions, or any other condition where treatment is contraindicated or cautioned. Assess pregnancy/nursing status and for possible drug interactions. Obtain baseline chest x-ray, standard hematologic tests (including Hgb, complete and differential WBC counts, and platelet count), blood chemistries (electrolytes, LFTs, and TSH), and eye exam. Perform ECG in patients with preexisting cardiac abnormalities and/or in advanced stages of cancer. Perform liver biopsy in patients with chronic hepatitis B and chronic hepatitis C. Test for presence of HCV antibody in patients with chronic hepatitis C.

Monitoring: Monitor for occurrence or aggravation of neuropsychiatric, autoimmune, ischemic, and infectious disorders; hypersensitivity reactions; exacerbation of preexisting psoriasis or sarcoidosis, development of new sarcoidosis; renal/hepatic dysfunction; and other adverse reactions. Closely monitor patients with a history of MI or arrhythmic disorder, liver/pulmonary function abnormalities, and WBC counts in myelosuppressed patients and in those receiving other myelosuppressive medications. Monitor LFTs, PT, alkaline phosphatase, albumin, and bilirubin levels periodically and at approximately 2-week intervals during ALT flare. Monitor TGs, LFTs, electrolytes, chest x-ray, complete and differential WBC count, and platelet count periodically. Perform ECG in patients with preexisting cardiac abnormalities and/or in advanced stages of cancer. Repeat TSH testing at 3 and 6 months during therapy. (Chronic hepatitis B) Monitor CBC, platelet counts, LFTs (including serum ALT, albumin, bilirubin) at treatment Weeks 1, 2, 4,

8, 12, and 16. Evaluate HBeAg, HBsAg, and ALT at the end of therapy, then at 3 and 6 months post-therapy. Monitor CBC and platelet counts at Weeks 1 and 2 following initiation of therapy and monthly thereafter. (Hepatitis C) Evaluate serum ALT at approximately 3-month intervals to assess response to treatment. Perform periodic ophthalmologic exams in patients who have a preexisting ophthalmologic disorder. Perform a prompt and complete eye exam if any ocular symptoms develop in any patient. If psychiatric problems develop, including clinical depression, monitor during treatment and in the 6 month follow-up period. (Malignant Melanoma) Monitor differential WBC counts and LFTs weekly during induction phase and monthly during maintenance phase of therapy.

Patient Counseling: Inform of risks/benefits associated with treatment. Instruct on proper use of product. Advise to seek medical attention if symptoms indicative of a serious adverse reaction associated with therapy develops (eg, suicidal ideation, chest pain, decrease in/or loss of vision, severe abdominal pain, high persistent fever, bruising, dyspnea). Inform that some side effects, such as fatigue and decreased concentration, may interfere with the ability to perform certain tasks. Advise to remain well hydrated during the initial stages of treatment; inform that use of an antipyretic may ameliorate some of the flu-like symptoms. Instruct self-administering patients on the importance of site selection and rotating inj site, proper disposal of needles/syringes, and caution against reuse of needles/syringes. Inform of the risks to the fetus when therapy is used in combination with ribavirin during pregnancy; encourage to report to Ribavirin Pregnancy Registry to monitor maternal-fetal outcomes. Instruct female patients and female partners of male patients to use 2 forms of birth control during treatment and for 6 months after therapy is discontinued. Instruct to brush teeth thoroughly bid and have regular dental exam. Inform that some patients may experience vomiting. Advise to rinse out the mouth thoroughly afterwards if vomiting occurs.

Administration: IM/SQ/IV/Intralesional route. Administer in the pm when possible. Refer to PI for preparation and further administration instructions. **Storage:** 2-8°C (36-46°F). (Powder) Use immediately after reconstitution; may store up to 24 hrs at 2-8°C (36-46°F). (Vial) Do not freeze. Keep away from heat.

INTUNIV   RX
guanfacine (Shire)

THERAPEUTIC CLASS: Alpha$_{2A}$-agonist

INDICATIONS: Treatment of attention-deficit hyperactivity disorder (ADHD) as monotherapy and as adjunctive therapy to stimulant medications.

DOSAGE: *Pediatrics:* 6-17 Yrs: Give qd, either in am or pm, at same time each day. Do not administer with high-fat meals. Non-Weight-Based: Initial: 1mg/day. Titrate: Adjust in increments of no more than 1mg/week. Maint: 1-4mg qd, depending on clinical response and tolerability. Max: 4mg/day. Weight-Based: Initial: 0.05-0.08mg/kg qd. Titrate: If well tolerated, may increase up to 0.12mg/kg qd. Consider dosing on a mg/kg basis to balance exposure-related potential benefits and risks of treatment. Switching from Immediate-Release (IR); D/C IR, and titrate with ER following the recommended schedule. Do not substitute for IR tabs on a mg-per-mg basis. Maint: Effectiveness for longer-term use (>9 weeks) has not been systematically evaluated; periodically reevaluate long-term usefulness if electing to use for extended periods. Discontinuation: Taper dose in decrements of no more than 1mg every 3-7 days. Missed Doses: When reinitiating to the previous maintenance dose after ≥2 missed consecutive doses, consider titration based on tolerability. Concomitant Use of Strong CYP3A4 Inhibitors/Inducers: Refer to PI. Significant Renal/Hepatic Impairment: May need to adjust dose.

HOW SUPPLIED: Tab, Extended-Release (ER): 1mg, 2mg, 3mg, 4mg

WARNINGS/PRECAUTIONS: May cause dose-dependent decreases in BP and HR. Orthostatic hypotension and syncope reported. Measure HR and BP prior to initiation of therapy, following dose increases, and periodically while on therapy. Caution in patients with history of hypotension, heart block, bradycardia, cardiovascular disease (CVD), or who have history of syncope or may have a condition that predisposes to syncope (eg, orthostatic hypotension, dehydration). Avoid becoming dehydrated or overheated. Somnolence and sedation commonly reported. May impair mental/physical abilities. Caution with significant renal/hepatic impairment.

ADVERSE REACTIONS: Somnolence/sedation, headache, fatigue, abdominal pain, hypotension, nausea, lethargy, dizziness, irritability, decreased appetite, dry mouth, constipation, insomnia, diarrhea.

INTERACTIONS: CYP3A4 inhibitors or inducers may affect plasma concentrations; adjust guanfacine dose if used concomitantly with strong CYP3A4 inhibitors (eg, boceprevir, clarithromycin, conivaptan, grapefruit juice, indinavir, itraconazole, ketoconazole, lopinavir/ritonavir, nefazodone, nelfinavir, posaconazole, ritonavir, saquinavir, telaprevir, telithromycin, voriconazole), or CYP3A4 inducers (eg, carbamazepine, phenytoin, rifampin, St. John's wort). Caution with antihypertensives or other drugs that can reduce BP/HR or increase the risk of syncope. Consider the potential for additive sedative effects before using with other centrally active depressants (eg, phenothiazines, barbiturates, benzodiazepines). Avoid with alcohol.

PREGNANCY: Category B, caution in nursing.

MECHANISM OF ACTION: Central alpha$_{2A}$-adrenergic agonist; mechanism in ADHD not established. Reduces sympathetic nerve impulses from the vasomotor center to the heart and blood vessels, resulting in decreased peripheral vascular resistance and reduction in HR.

PHARMACOKINETICS: Absorption: Readily absorbed. Children (6-12 yrs of age): C$_{max}$=10ng/mL; AUC=162ng•hr/mL. Adolescents (13-17 yrs of age): C$_{max}$=7ng/mL; AUC=116ng•hr/mL. Children and Adolescents: T$_{max}$=5 hrs. **Distribution:** Plasma protein binding (70%). **Metabolism:** CYP3A4. **Elimination:** T$_{1/2}$=18 hrs (1mg qd, adults).

NURSING CONSIDERATIONS

Assessment: Assess for history of hypotension, heart block, bradycardia, CVD, history of syncope, condition that predisposes to syncope, hypersensitivity to drug, renal/hepatic impairment, pregnancy/nursing status, and possible drug interactions. Assess HR and BP.

Monitoring: Monitor for hypotension, bradycardia, syncope, somnolence, sedation, and other adverse reactions. Monitor HR and BP following dose increases and periodically while on therapy. Observe human milk-fed infants for sedation and somnolence. Periodically reevaluate long-term usefulness if electing to use for extended periods.

Patient Counseling: Instruct caregiver to supervise the child or adolescent taking the drug. Counsel on how to properly taper the medication, if the physician decides to d/c treatment. Inform of the adverse reactions (eg, sedation, headache, abdominal pain) that may occur; advise to consult physician if any of these symptoms persist, or other symptoms occur. Caution against operating heavy equipment or driving until accustomed to effects of medication. Advise to avoid becoming dehydrated or overheated, and to avoid use with alcohol.

Administration: Oral route. Take either in am or pm, at same time each day. Swallow tabs whole with water, milk, or other liquid; do not crush, chew, or break. Do not administer with high-fat meals. **Storage:** 25°C (77°F); excursions permitted to 15-30°C (59-86°F).

INVANZ   RX
ertapenem (Merck)

THERAPEUTIC CLASS: Carbapenem

INDICATIONS: Treatment of adult and pediatric patients (≥3 months of age) with the following moderate to severe infections caused by susceptible isolates of microorganisms: complicated intra-abdominal infections; complicated skin and skin structure infections (cSSSIs), including diabetic foot infections without osteomyelitis; community-acquired pneumonia (CAP); complicated urinary tract infections (UTIs), including pyelonephritis; and acute pelvic infections, including postpartum endomyometritis, septic abortion, and postsurgical gynecological infections. Prevention of surgical-site infection following elective colorectal surgery in adults.

DOSAGE: *Adults:* 1g IV/IM qd. IM administration may be used as an alternative to IV administration in the treatment of those infections for which IM therapy is appropriate. Duration: Complicated Intra-Abdominal Infections: 5-14 days. cSSSIs: 7-14 days; patients with diabetic foot infections received up to 28 days of treatment (parenteral or parenteral plus oral switch therapy). CAP/Complicated UTIs: 10-14 days (includes a possible switch to an appropriate oral therapy, after at least 3 days of parenteral therapy, once clinical improvement has been demonstrated). Acute Pelvic Infections: 3-10 days. Prophylaxis of Surgical-Site Infection Following Colorectal Surgery: 1g as a single IV dose given 1 hr prior to surgical incision. Severe Renal Impairment (CrCl ≤30mL/min/1.73m²)/End-Stage Renal Disease (CrCl ≤10mL/min/1.73m²)/Hemodialysis: 500mg/day; if administered within 6 hrs prior to hemodialysis, give 150mg supplementary dose following hemodialysis session. May be administered by IV infusion for up to 14 days or IM inj for up to 7 days. Infuse IV over 30 min.
Pediatrics: ≥13 Yrs: 1g IV/IM qd. 3 Months-12 Yrs: 15mg/kg IV/IM bid (not to exceed 1g/day). IM administration may be used as an alternative to IV administration in the treatment of those infections for which IM therapy is appropriate. Duration: Complicated Intra-Abdominal Infections: 5-14 days. cSSSIs: 7-14 days. CAP/Complicated UTIs: 10-14 days (includes a possible switch to an appropriate oral therapy, after at least 3 days of parenteral therapy, once clinical improvement has been demonstrated). Acute Pelvic Infections: 3-10 days. May be administered by IV infusion for up to 14 days or IM inj for up to 7 days. Infuse IV over 30 min.

HOW SUPPLIED: Inj: 1g [vial]

CONTRAINDICATIONS: (IM) Hypersensitivity to amide-type local anesthetics.

WARNINGS/PRECAUTIONS: Serious and occasionally fatal hypersensitivity (anaphylactic) reactions reported; d/c immediately if an allergic reaction occurs. Seizures and other CNS adverse experiences reported; caution with known factors that predispose to convulsive activity, and continue anticonvulsant therapy with known seizure disorders. If focal tremors, myoclonus, or seizures occur, evaluate neurologically, place on anticonvulsant therapy if not already instituted, and reexamine dosage to determine whether it should be decreased or discontinued. *Clostridium difficile*-associated diarrhea (CDAD) reported; d/c if CDAD is suspected or confirmed. Use caution when administering IM to avoid inadvertent inj into a blood vessel. May result in bacterial resistance with prolonged use in the absence of proven or suspected bacterial infection, or a prophylactic indication; take appropriate measures if superinfection develops. Caution in elderly. Not recommended in the treatment of meningitis in the pediatric population.

ADVERSE REACTIONS: Diarrhea, infused vein complication, N/V, anemia, headache, edema/swelling, fever, abdominal pain, constipation, altered mental status, insomnia, vaginitis, infusion-site pain, infusion-site erythema.

INTERACTIONS: Increased plasma concentrations with probenecid; coadministration not recommended. May reduce concentrations of valproic acid, thereby increasing the risk of breakthrough seizures; concomitant use with valproic acid/divalproex sodium is generally not recommended, but if necessary, consider supplemental anticonvulsant therapy.

PREGNANCY: Category B, caution in nursing.

MECHANISM OF ACTION: Carbapenem; bactericidal activity results from the inhibition of cell wall synthesis and is mediated through ertapenem binding to penicillin (PCN)-binding proteins.

PHARMACOKINETICS: Absorption: (IM) Almost complete. Bioavailability (90%); T_{max}=2.3 hrs. **Distribution:** V_d=0.12L/kg (adults), 0.16L/kg (13-17 yrs of age), 0.2L/kg (3 months-12 yrs of age); plasma protein binding (85% [300mcg/mL plasma concentration], 95% [<100mcg/mL plasma concentration]); found in breast milk. **Metabolism:** Hydrolysis of the β-lactam ring; inactive ring-opened derivative (major metabolite). **Elimination:** (IV) Urine (80% [38% unchanged, 37% metabolite]), feces (10%); $T_{1/2}$=4 hrs (≥13 yrs of age), 2.5 hrs (3 months-12 yrs of age).

NURSING CONSIDERATIONS

Assessment: Assess for factors that predispose to convulsive activity, seizure disorders, renal impairment, pregnancy/nursing status, and possible drug interactions. Carefully assess for previous hypersensitivity reactions to drug, PCN, cephalosporins, other β-lactams, and other allergens. (IM) Assess for hypersensitivity to amide-type local anesthetics.

Monitoring: Monitor for hypersensitivity (anaphylactic) reactions, CNS effects (eg, focal tremors, myoclonus, seizures), CDAD, superinfection, and other adverse reactions. Periodically monitor organ system function (eg, renal, hepatic, and hematopoietic) during prolonged therapy.

Patient Counseling: Advise that allergic reactions, including serious allergic reactions, could occur, and that serious reactions may require immediate treatment. Advise to report any previous hypersensitivity reactions to the medication, other β-lactams, or other allergens. Counsel to inform physician if taking valproic acid or divalproex sodium. Counsel that therapy should only be used to treat bacterial, not viral (eg, common cold), infections. Instruct to take exactly ud. Inform that skipping doses or not completing the full course of therapy may decrease effectiveness of treatment and increase bacterial resistance. Inform that diarrhea is a common problem caused by therapy that usually ends when therapy is discontinued. Instruct to immediately contact physician if watery and bloody stools (with or without stomach cramps and fever) occur, even as late as ≥2 months after having taken the last dose.

Administration: IV/IM route. Do not mix or coinfuse with other medications. Do not use diluents containing dextrose. Refer to PI for preparation, reconstitution, and administration instructions. **Storage:** ≤25°C (77°F). Reconstituted and Infusion Sol: 25°C (77°F) and used within 6 hrs, or 5°C (41°F) for 24 hrs and used within 4 hrs after removal from refrigeration. Do not freeze sol.

INVEGA   RX
paliperidone (Janssen)

> Elderly patients with dementia-related psychosis treated with antipsychotic drugs are at an increased risk of death; most deaths appeared to be cardiovascular (CV) (eg, heart failure, sudden death) or infectious (eg, pneumonia) in nature. Not approved for the treatment of patients with dementia-related psychosis.

THERAPEUTIC CLASS: Benzisoxazole derivative

INDICATIONS: Treatment of schizophrenia in adults and adolescents. Treatment of schizoaffective disorder as monotherapy and an adjunct to mood stabilizers and/or antidepressant therapy in adults.

DOSAGE: *Adults:* Schizophrenia: 6mg qd. Titrate: If indicated may increase by 3mg/day; dose increases >6mg/day should be made at intervals >5 days. Usual: 3-12mg/day. Max: 12mg/day. Schizoaffective Disorder: 6mg qd. Titrate: If indicated, may increase by 3mg/day at intervals of >4 days. Usual: 3-12mg/day. Max: 12mg/day. Renal Impairment: Individualize dose. CrCl ≥50-<80mL/min: Initial: 3mg qd. Max: 6mg qd. CrCl ≥10-<50mL/min: Initial: 1.5mg qd. Max: 3mg qd. Elderly: Adjust dose according to renal function.

Pediatrics: 12-17 Yrs: Schizophrenia: Initial: 3mg qd. Titrate: If indicated, may increase by 3mg/day at intervals of >5 days. Max: <51kg: 6mg/day. ≥51kg: 12mg/day.

HOW SUPPLIED: Tab, Extended-Release: 1.5mg, 3mg, 6mg, 9mg

WARNINGS/PRECAUTIONS: Neuroleptic malignant syndrome (NMS) and tardive dyskinesia (TD) reported; d/c if these occur. May increase QTc interval; avoid with congenital long QT syndrome and history of cardiac arrhythmias. Hyperglycemia and diabetes mellitus (DM), in some cases extreme and associated with ketoacidosis or hyperosmolar coma or death reported; monitor for hyperglycemia and perform fasting blood glucose testing at the beginning of therapy, and periodically in patients at risk for DM. Undesirable alterations in lipids and weight gain reported. May elevate prolactin levels. Avoid with preexisting severe GI narrowing. May induce orthostatic hypotension and syncope; caution with known CV disease, cerebrovascular disease, or conditions that predispose to hypotension. Leukopenia, neutropenia, and agranulocytosis reported; d/c in cases of severe neutropenia (absolute neutrophil count <1000/mm³). Somnolence reported. May impair mental/physical abilities. Seizures reported; caution with history of seizures or conditions that lower the seizure threshold. May cause esophageal dysmotility and aspiration; caution with risk of aspiration pneumonia. May induce priapism; severe cases may require surgical intervention. May disrupt body's ability to reduce core body temperature; caution with conditions that may contribute to an elevated core body temperature. May have an antiemetic effect that may mask signs/symptoms of overdosage with certain drugs or of conditions (eg, intestinal obstruction, Reye's syndrome, brain tumor). Patients with Parkinson's disease or dementia with Lewy bodies may have increased sensitivity to therapy. Caution with suicidal tendencies, renal impairment, and in elderly. Not recommended with CrCl <10mL/min.

ADVERSE REACTIONS: Extrapyramidal symptoms, tachycardia, somnolence, akathisia, dyskinesia, dyspepsia, dizziness, nasopharyngitis, headache, nausea, hyperkinesia, constipation, weight gain, parkinsonism, tremors.

INTERACTIONS: Consider additive exposure with risperidone. Avoid with other drugs known to prolong QTc interval, including Class IA (eg, quinidine, procainamide) or Class III (eg, amiodarone, sotalol) antiarrhythmics, antipsychotics (eg, chlorpromazine, thioridazine), and antibiotics (eg, gatifloxacin, moxifloxacin). Caution with other centrally acting drugs, alcohol, and drugs with anticholinergic activity. May antagonize the effect of levodopa and other dopamine agonists. Additive effect may be observed with other agents that cause orthostatic hypotension. Carbamazepine may decrease levels. Paroxetine (a potent CYP2D6 inhibitor) may increase exposure in CYP2D6 extensive metabolizers. Divalproex sodium may increase levels; consider dose reduction with valproate.

PREGNANCY: Category C, not for use in nursing.

MECHANISM OF ACTION: Benzisoxazole derivative; not established. Proposed to be mediated through a combination of central dopamine type 2 (D_2) and serotonin type 2 ($5HT_{2A}$) receptor antagonism.

PHARMACOKINETICS: Absorption: Absolute bioavailability (28%); T_{max}=24 hrs. **Distribution:** Plasma protein binding (74%); V_d=487L; found in breast milk. **Metabolism:** CYP2D6, 3A4 (limited); (immediate-release) dealkylation, hydroxylation, dehydrogenation, and benzisoxazole scission. **Elimination:** (Immediate-release) Urine (80%; 59% unchanged), feces (11%); $T_{1/2}$=23 hrs.

NURSING CONSIDERATIONS

Assessment: Assess for dementia-related psychosis, congenital long QT syndrome, history of cardiac arrhythmias, DM, risk factors for DM, severe GI narrowing, history of clinically significant low WBCs or drug-induced leukopenia/neutropenia, Parkinson's disease, dementia with Lewy bodies, other conditions where treatment is contraindicated or cautioned, renal impairment, pregnancy/nursing status, and possible drug interactions. Obtain baseline FPG in patients at risk for DM.

Monitoring: Monitor for NMS, TD, QT prolongation, hyperprolactinemia, orthostatic hypotension, syncope, cognitive and motor impairment, seizures, esophageal dysmotility, aspiration, priapism, and disruption of body temperature. Monitor for signs of hyperglycemia; perform periodic monitoring of FPG levels in patients with DM or at risk for DM. Monitor for signs/symptoms of leukopenia/neutropenia; perform frequent monitoring of CBC in patients with history of clinically significant low WBC counts or drug-induced leukopenia/neutropenia. Monitor weight and renal function.

Patient Counseling: Inform of the risk of orthostatic hypotension during initiation/reinitiation or dose increases. Inform that therapy has the potential to impair judgment, thinking, or motor skills; advise to use caution when operating hazardous machinery (eg, automobiles). Advise to avoid alcohol during therapy. Instruct to notify physician of all prescription and nonprescription drugs currently taking, and if pregnant, intending to become pregnant, or breastfeeding. Counsel on appropriate care in avoiding overheating and dehydration. Inform that medication must be swallowed whole with liquids; advise not to chew, divide, or crush. Advise that tab shell, along with insoluble core components, may be found in stool.

Administration: Oral route. Swallow whole with liquids; do not crush, divide, or chew. **Storage:** Up to 25°C (77°F); excursions permitted to 15-30°C (59-86°F). Protect from moisture.

INVEGA SUSTENNA   RX
paliperidone palmitate (Janssen)

> Elderly patients with dementia-related psychosis treated with antipsychotic drugs are at an increased risk of death. Not approved for use in patients with dementia-related psychosis.

THERAPEUTIC CLASS: Benzisoxazole derivative

INDICATIONS: Treatment of schizophrenia in adults.

DOSAGE: *Adults:* Initial: 234mg IM on Day 1, then 156mg one week later (in deltoid muscle). Maint: Usual: 117mg/month (in deltoid or gluteal muscle). May adjust maint dose monthly based on tolerability and/or efficacy; some may benefit from lower or higher dose within the available strengths (39mg, 78mg, 156mg, 234mg). Reassess periodically to determine need for continued treatment. Mild Renal Impairment (CrCl ≥50-<80mL/min): Initial: 156mg IM on Day 1, then 117mg 1 week later (in deltoid muscle). Maint: 78mg/month (in deltoid or gluteal muscle). Concomitant Strong CYP3A4 Inducers (eg, carbamazepine, rifampin, St. John's wort): May need to increase dose when a strong CYP3A4 inducer is added. May need to decrease the dose when a strong CYP3A4 inducer is d/c. Switching from PO Antipsychotics: D/C PO antipsychotics then initiate as usual. Refer to PI for maint dose conversion from Invega to Invega Sustenna. Switching from Long-Acting Injectable Antipsychotics: Initiate in place of the next scheduled inj and continue with monthly maint dose. Refer to PI for instructions on missed doses.

HOW SUPPLIED: Inj, Extended-Release: 39mg, 78mg, 117mg, 156mg, 234mg

WARNINGS/PRECAUTIONS: Recommended to establish tolerability with PO paliperidone or PO risperidone prior to initiating treatment if have never taken PO paliperidone or PO or inj risperidone. Neuroleptic malignant syndrome (NMS) and tardive dyskinesia (TD) reported; d/c if these occur. May increase QTc interval; avoid with congenital long QT syndrome and history of cardiac arrhythmias. Hyperglycemia and diabetes mellitus (DM), in some cases extreme and associated with ketoacidosis or hyperosmolar coma or death, reported; monitor for symptoms of hyperglycemia and perform FPG testing at the beginning of therapy, and periodically in patients at risk for DM. Dyslipidemia, weight gain, and hyperprolactinemia reported. May induce orthostatic hypotension and syncope; caution with known cardiovascular/cerebrovascular disease or conditions that predispose to hypotension. Leukopenia, neutropenia, and agranulocytosis reported; d/c in cases of severe neutropenia (absolute neutrophil count <1000/mm³). Somnolence, sedation, and dizziness reported. May impair mental/physical abilities. Seizures reported; caution with history of seizures or conditions that lower the seizure threshold. May cause esophageal dysmotility and aspiration; caution with risk of aspiration pneumonia. May induce priapism; severe cases may require surgical intervention. May disrupt body's ability to reduce core body temperature; caution with conditions that may contribute to an elevated core body temperature. Patients with Parkinson's disease or dementia with Lewy bodies may have increased sensitivity to therapy. Caution with renal impairment and in elderly. Not recommended with CrCl <50mL/min.

ADVERSE REACTIONS: Upper abdominal pain, N/V, inj-site reactions, nasopharyngitis, weight gain, dizziness, akathisia, extrapyramidal disorder, headache, somnolence, agitation, anxiety, toothache, upper respiratory tract infection.

INTERACTIONS: Caution with other centrally acting drugs and alcohol. May antagonize the effect of levodopa and other dopamine agonists. An additive effect may be observed with other agents that also cause orthostatic hypotension. Avoid with other drugs known to prolong QTc interval, including Class 1A (eg, quinidine, procainamide) or Class III (eg, amiodarone, sotalol) antiarrhythmics, antipsychotics (eg, chlorpromazine, thioridazine), or antibiotics (eg, gatifloxacin, moxifloxacin). May be necessary to increase dose on initiation of strong CYP3A4 inducers (eg, carbamazepine, rifampin, or St. John's wort) and upon discontinuation of strong CYP3A4 inducers, may need to decrease dose. Carbamazepine may decrease levels. Additive exposure with PO paliperidone or PO/injectable risperidone. Caution with anticholinergics; may contribute to an elevated body temperature. Paroxetine (a potent CYP2D6 inhibitor) may increase exposure in CYP2D6 extensive metabolizers.

PREGNANCY: Category C, not for use in nursing.

MECHANISM OF ACTION: Benzisoxazole derivative; not established. Proposed to be mediated through a combination of central dopamine type 2 (D_2) and serotonin type 2 ($5HT_{2A}$) receptor antagonism.

PHARMACOKINETICS: Absorption: T_{max}=13 days. **Distribution:** V_d=391L; plasma protein binding (74%); found in breast milk. **Metabolism:** Dealkylation, hydroxylation, dehydrogenation, and benzisoxazole scission; CYP2D6, CYP3A4 (limited). **Elimination:** (39-234mg IM single-dose) $T_{1/2}$=25-49 days.

NURSING CONSIDERATIONS

Assessment: Assess for dementia-related psychosis, congenital long QT syndrome, history of cardiac arrhythmias, DM, risk factors for DM, history of clinically significant low WBCs or drug-induced leukopenia/neutropenia, Parkinson's disease, dementia with Lewy bodies, renal impairment, pregnancy/nursing status, possible drug interactions, or any other conditions where treatment is contraindicated or cautioned. Obtain baseline FPG in patients at risk for DM.

Monitoring: Monitor for NMS, TD, QT prolongation, hyperprolactinemia, orthostatic hypotension, syncope, cognitive and motor impairment, seizures, aspiration, priapism, and disruption of body temperature. Monitor for signs of hyperglycemia; perform periodic monitoring of FPG levels in patients with DM or at risk for DM. Monitor for signs/symptoms of leukopenia/neutropenia; perform frequent monitoring of CBC in patients with history of clinically significant low WBC counts or drug-induced leukopenia/neutropenia. Monitor weight and renal function.

Patient Counseling: Advise patients on risk of orthostatic hypotension. Caution about operating machinery/driving. Advise to avoid alcohol during therapy. Advise to avoid overheating and becoming dehydrated. Instruct to inform physician about any concomitant medications. Advise to notify physician if pregnancy occurs or is intended. Instruct not to breastfeed.

Administration: IM route. Inject slowly, deep into muscle. Avoid inadvertent inj into a blood vessel. Do not administer dose in divided inj. Refer to PI for proper instructions for use. **Storage:** 25°C (77°F); excursions permitted to 15-30°C (59-86°F).

INVIRASE   RX
saquinavir mesylate (Genentech)

THERAPEUTIC CLASS: Protease inhibitor

INDICATIONS: Treatment of HIV-1 infection in combination with ritonavir (RTV) and other antiretroviral agents in adults >16 yrs of age.

DOSAGE: *Adults:* >16 Yrs: Usual: 1000mg bid with RTV 100mg bid; take combination at the same time within 2 hrs pc. If administered with lopinavir/RTV 400/100 mg bid, no additional RTV is recommended.

HOW SUPPLIED: Cap: 200mg; Tab: 500mg

CONTRAINDICATIONS: Congenital long QT syndrome, refractory hypokalemia or hypomagnesemia, complete atrioventricular (AV) block without implanted pacemakers, high risk of complete AV block, severe hepatic impairment, and with drugs that both increase saquinavir plasma levels and prolong the QT interval. Coadministration with CYP3A substrates (eg, alfuzosin, amiodarone, bepridil, dofetilide, flecainide, lidocaine [systemic], propafenone, quinidine, trazodone, rifampin, dihydroergotamine, ergonovine, ergotamine, methylergonovine, cisapride, lovastatin, simvastatin, pimozide, sildenafil for treatment of pulmonary arterial HTN, triazolam, oral midazolam).

WARNINGS/PRECAUTIONS: Refer to the individual monograph of RTV. Interrupt therapy if serious or severe toxicity occurs until etiology identified or toxicity resolves. May prolong PR and QT intervals in a dose-dependent fashion. 2nd- or 3rd-degree AV block and torsades de pointes reported. Do not initiate if QT interval >450 msec. If therapy is initiated with QT interval <450 msec, monitor ECG after 3-4 days; d/c if QT interval >480 msec or increased >20 msec over pretreatment. Monitor ECG with preexisting conduction system abnormalities, certain heart diseases, electrolyte abnormalities, and hepatic impairment. Correct hypokalemia/hypomagnesemia prior to therapy and monitor periodically. New onset or exacerbation of diabetes mellitus (DM), hyperglycemia, diabetic ketoacidosis, immune reconstitution syndrome, autoimmune disorders (eg, Graves' disease, polymyositis, Guillain-Barre syndrome) in the setting of immune reconstitution, redistribution/accumulation of body fat, and spontaneous bleeding with hemophilia A and B reported. Worsening liver disease in patients with underlying hepatitis B or C, cirrhosis, chronic alcoholism, and/or other underlying liver abnormalities reported. Elevated cholesterol and/or TG levels observed; marked elevation in TGs is a risk factor for pancreatitis. Various degrees of cross-resistance observed. Caution with severe renal impairment, end-stage renal disease, and in elderly. Contains lactose; should not induce symptoms of intolerance.

ADVERSE REACTIONS: DM/hyperglycemia, lipodystrophy, N/V, diarrhea, abdominal pain, fatigue, fever, pneumonia, bronchitis, influenza, sinusitis, rash, pruritus.

INTERACTIONS: See Contraindications. Not recommended with garlic cap, fluticasone, salmeterol, ketoconazole or itraconazole >200mg/day, and tipranavir/RTV combination. Avoid with colchicine in patients with renal/hepatic impairment and tadalafil during initiation. Caution with drugs that prolong PR interval (eg, calcium channel blockers [CCBs], β-blockers, digoxin, atazanavir), lopinavir/RTV, ibutilide, sotalol, erythromycin, halofantrine, pentamidine, dexamethasone, methadone, proton pump inhibitors, neuroleptics, and anticonvulsants. Drugs that affect CYP3A and/or P-glycoprotein may modify pharmacokinetics. May increase levels of bosentan, maraviroc, warfarin (monitor INR), colchicine, ketoconazole, rifabutin, TCAs, benzodiazepines, IV midazolam, CCBs, digoxin, salmeterol, fluticasone, atorvastatin, immunosuppressants, clarithro-mycin, and PDE-5 inhibitors. May decrease levels of methadone and ethinyl estradiol. Delavirdine, atazanavir, indinavir, clarithromycin, and omeprazole may increase levels. Efavirenz, nevirapine, dexamethasone, St. John's wort, garlic cap, potent CYP3A inducers (eg, phenobarbital, pheny-toin, carbamazepine) may decrease levels. May require initiation or adjustments of insulin or oral hypoglycemics for treatment of DM. Refer to PI for dosing modifications when used with certain concomitant therapies.

PREGNANCY: Category B, not for use in nursing.

MECHANISM OF ACTION: HIV protease inhibitor; binds to the protease active site and inhibits activity of the enzyme, preventing cleavage of the viral polyproteins, and resulting in formation of immature, noninfectious virus particles.

PHARMACOKINETICS: Absorption: Administration of variable doses and combinations re-sulted in different parameters. **Distribution:** Plasma protein binding (98%). (12mg IV) V_d=700L. **Metabolism:** Hepatic via CYP3A4. **Elimination:** (600mg PO) Urine (1%), feces (88%). (10.5mg IV); Urine (3%), feces (81%).

NURSING CONSIDERATIONS

Assessment: Assess for conditions where treatment is contraindicated or cautioned, renal/hepatic impairment, drug hypersensitivity, pregnancy/nursing status, and possible drug in-teractions. Obtain serum K^+ and Mg^{2+}, TG and cholesterol levels, and ECG prior to initiation of treatment.

Monitoring: Periodically monitor ECG, serum K^+ and Mg^{2+} levels, TG and cholesterol levels, and hepatic/renal function. Monitor for signs/symptoms of AV block, PR/QT interval prolongation, cardiac conduction abnormalities, torsades de pointes, bleeding, immune reconstitution syn-drome, autoimmune disorders, fat redistribution/accumulation, new onset DM, and other adverse reactions.

Patient Counseling: Inform that therapy is not a cure for HIV-1 infection; opportunistic infections may still occur. Advise to avoid doing things that can spread HIV-1 infection to others. Inform that changes in the ECG (PR interval or QT interval prolongation) may occur; instruct to consult physician if experiencing dizziness, lightheadedness, or palpitations. Advise to report the use of any other prescription/nonprescription medications or herbal products (eg, St. John's wort). Inform that redistribution or accumulation of body fat may occur. Advise that therapy should be used in combination with ritonavir. Counsel about the importance of taking medication every day; instruct not to alter dose or d/c therapy without consulting physician.

Administration: Oral route. Take within 2 hrs pc. Refer to PI for administration instructions for patients unable to swallow cap. **Storage:** 25°C (77°F); excursions permitted to 15-30°C (59-86°F).

INVOKANA   RX
canagliflozin (Janssen)

THERAPEUTIC CLASS: Sodium-glucose co-transporter 2 (SGLT2) inhibitor

INDICATIONS: Adjunct to diet and exercise to improve glycemic control in adults with type 2 diabetes mellitus (DM).

DOSAGE: *Adults:* Initial: 100mg qd, taken before the 1st meal of the day. Titrate: May increase to 300mg qd in patients tolerating 100mg qd who have an eGFR ≥60mL/min and require ad-ditional glycemic control. Moderate Renal Impairment (eGFR 45-<60mL/min): Limit to 100mg qd. Concomitant Use with UDP-Glucuronosyl Transferase (UGT) Enzyme Inducers (eg, Rifampin, Phenytoin, Phenobarbital, Ritonavir): Consider increasing to 300mg qd in patients currently tolerating 100mg qd who have an eGFR ≥60mL/min and require additional glycemic control; consider another antihyperglycemic agent in patients with an eGFR of 45-<60mL/min.

HOW SUPPLIED: Tab: 100mg, 300mg

CONTRAINDICATIONS: Severe renal impairment (eGFR <30mL/min), end-stage renal disease, patients on dialysis.

WARNINGS/PRECAUTIONS: Not recommended with type 1 DM or for treatment of diabetic ketoacidosis. Do not initiate in patients with an eGFR <45mL/min. Causes intravascular volume contraction. Symptomatic hypotension may occur, particularly in patients with renal impairment (eGFR <60mL/min), elderly patients, patients on either diuretics or medications that interfere with the renin-angiotensin-aldosterone system (RAAS) (eg, ACE inhibitors, ARBs), or patients with low systolic BP; assess and correct volume status before initiating treatment in patients with ≥1 of these characteristics. Increases SrCr and decreases eGFR; caution in patients with hypo-volemia. Renal function abnormalities may occur; monitor renal function more frequently in pa-tients with an eGFR <60mL/min. D/C when eGFR is persistently <45mL/min. May lead to hyper-kalemia; increased risk in patients with moderate renal impairment who are taking medications that interfere with K^+ excretion (eg, K^+-sparing diuretics) or medications that interfere with the RAAS; monitor serum K^+ levels periodically in patients with renal impairment and in patients predisposed to hyperkalemia. Increases risk of genital mycotic infections; caution in patients with a history of genital mycotic infections and in uncircumcised males. Hypersensitivity reactions (eg, generalized urticaria), some serious, reported; d/c and treat if this occurs and monitor until signs/symptoms resolve. Dose-related increases in LDL levels reported; monitor LDL levels and treat appropriately. No conclusive evidence of macrovascular risk reduction. Not recommended in severe hepatic impairment.

ADVERSE REACTIONS: Genital mycotic infections, urinary tract infections (UTIs), increased urination, vulvovaginal pruritus, hypersensitivity reactions, hypoglycemia, increases in serum K^+ levels.

INTERACTIONS: See Dosage. May increase risk of hypoglycemia when combined with insulin or an insulin secretagogue; lower dose of insulin or insulin secretagogue may be required. Rifampin, a nonselective UGT enzyme inducer, decreased exposure. Increases levels/exposure of digoxin; monitor appropriately.

PREGNANCY: Category C, not for use in nursing.

MECHANISM OF ACTION: SGLT2 inhibitor; reduces reabsorption of filtered glucose and lowers the renal threshold for glucose, and thereby increases urinary glucose excretion.

PHARMACOKINETICS: Absorption: Absolute oral bioavailability (65%); T_{max}=1-2 hrs (median). **Distribution:** Plasma protein binding (99%); (IV, healthy) V_d=119L. **Metabolism:** O-glucuronidation (major) by UGT1A9 and UGT2B4; oxidation (minor) via CYP3A4. **Elimination:** (Healthy) Feces (41.5% unchanged), urine (33%, <1% unchanged); $T_{1/2}$=10.6 hrs (100mg), 13.1 hrs (300mg).

NURSING CONSIDERATIONS

Assessment: Assess for diabetic ketoacidosis, type of DM, volume status, predisposition to hyperkalemia, risk for genital mycotic infections, drug hypersensitivity, pregnancy/nursing status, and possible drug interactions. Assess baseline renal function, LDL levels, and BP.

Monitoring: Monitor for signs/symptoms of hypotension, genital mycotic infections, hypersensitivity reactions, and other adverse reactions. Monitor renal function, serum K^+ levels, and LDL levels.

Patient Counseling: Inform of the risks, benefits, and alternative modes of therapy. Advise about the importance of adherence to dietary instructions, regular physical activity, periodic blood glucose monitoring and HbA1C testing, recognition and management of hypoglycemia and hyperglycemia, and assessment for diabetes complications. Instruct to seek medical advice promptly during periods of stress (eg, fever, trauma, infection, surgery) as medication requirements may change. Instruct to report to physician if pregnant, nursing, or experiencing symptoms of hypotension. Instruct to have adequate fluid intake. Counsel on the signs/symptoms of UTI, vaginal yeast infection, balanitis, and balanoposthitis; inform of treatment options and when to seek medical advice. Instruct to d/c therapy and consult physician if any signs/symptoms suggesting an allergic reaction or angioedema develop.

Administration: Oral route. Take before the 1st meal of the day. **Storage:** 25°C (77°F); excursions permitted to 15-30°C (59-86°F).

ISENTRESS   RX
raltegravir (Merck)

THERAPEUTIC CLASS: HIV-integrase strand transfer inhibitor

INDICATIONS: Treatment of HIV-1 infection in combination with other antiretroviral agents in patients ≥4 weeks of age.

DOSAGE: *Adults:* (Tab) 400mg bid. Coadministration with Rifampin: 800mg bid.
Pediatrics: ≥4 Weeks: (Tab) ≥25kg: 400mg bid. (Tab, Chewable) ≥40kg: 300mg bid. 28-<40kg: 200mg bid. 20-<28kg: 150mg bid. (Sus/Tab, Chewable) 14-<20kg: 5mL (100mg) sus bid or one 100mg chewable tab bid. 11-<14kg: (80mg) sus bid or three 25mg chewable tabs bid. (Sus) 8-<11kg: 3mL (60mg) bid. 6-<8kg: 2mL (40mg) bid. 4-<6kg: 1.5mL (30mg) bid. 3-<4kg: 1mL (20mg) bid. Max: (Tab, Chewable) 300mg bid. (Sus) 100mg bid.

HOW SUPPLIED: Sus (Powder): 100mg/pkt; Tab: 400mg; Tab, Chewable: 25mg, 100mg* *scored

WARNINGS/PRECAUTIONS: Do not substitute chewable tabs or oral sus for the 400mg film-coated tab; not bioequivalent. Severe, potentially life-threatening, and fatal skin reactions (eg, Stevens-Johnson syndrome, toxic epidermal necrolysis), and hypersensitivity reactions reported; d/c therapy and other suspect agents immediately if signs/symptoms develop. Immune reconstitution syndrome reported. Autoimmune disorders (eg, Graves' disease, polymyositis, Guillain-Barre syndrome) reported in the setting of immune reconstitution and can occur many months after initiation of treatment. Caution in patients at increased risk of myopathy or rhabdomyolysis and in elderly. Avoid dosing before a dialysis session. (Tab, Chewable) Contains phenylalanine.

ADVERSE REACTIONS: Insomnia, headache, nausea, hyperglycemia, ALT/AST elevation, hyperbilirubinemia, low absolute neutrophil count, serum lipase/creatine kinase/pancreatic amylase increase, thrombocytopenia.

INTERACTIONS: See Dosage. UGT1A1 inhibitors (eg, atazanavir, atazanavir/ritonavir), drugs that increase gastric pH (eg, omeprazole), and telaprevir may increase levels. Rifampin (a strong UGT1A1 inducer), efavirenz, etravirine, tipranavir/ritonavir, and antacids containing divalent metal cations may decrease levels. Coadministration or staggered administration (by 2 hrs) with aluminum- and/or Mg^{2+}-containing antacids is not recommended.

PREGNANCY: Category C, not for use in nursing.

MECHANISM OF ACTION: HIV-1 integrase strand transfer inhibitor; inhibits the catalytic activity of HIV-1 integrase (an HIV-1 encoded enzyme required for viral replication) thus preventing the formation of HIV-1 provirus, resulting in the prevention of propagation of the viral infection.

PHARMACOKINETICS: Absorption: Adults: (Tab) T_{max}=3 hrs (fasted); AUC_{0-12h}=14.3μM•hr. **Pediatrics:** AUC_{0-12h}=14.1μM•hr (tab), 22.1μM•hr (tab, chewable; ≥25kg patient), 18.6μM•hr (tab, chewable; 11-<25kg patient), 24.5μM•hr (sus). **Distribution: Adults:** Plasma protein binding (83%). **Metabolism:** Glucuronidation via UGT1A1; raltegravir-glucuronide (metabolite). **Elimination: Adults:** Urine (9% unchanged, 23% raltegravir-glucuronide), feces (51% unchanged); $T_{1/2}$=9 hrs.

NURSING CONSIDERATIONS

Assessment: Assess for risk of myopathy or rhabdomyolysis, previous hypersensitivity to the drug, pregnancy/nursing status, and possible drug interactions. Assess if patient is undergoing dialysis session. (Tab, Chewable) Assess for phenylketonuria.

Monitoring: Monitor for signs/symptoms of severe skin/hypersensitivity reactions, immune reconstitution syndrome, autoimmune disorders, and other adverse reactions. If a severe skin reaction or hypersensitivity reaction develops, monitor clinical status, including liver aminotransferases.

Patient Counseling: Instruct to inform physician if any unusual symptom develops, or if any known symptom persists or worsens. Inform that drug is not a cure for HIV-1 infection and that illnesses associated with HIV-1 may still be experienced. Advise to avoid doing things that can spread HIV-1 to others. Instruct to always practice safe sex by using a latex or polyurethane condom. Instruct to immediately d/c therapy and seek medical attention if rash develops with signs/symptoms of a more serious skin reaction (eg, fever, extreme tiredness, muscle or joint aches). Instruct to immediately report to physician if any unexplained muscle pain, tenderness, or weakness occurs. Instruct to avoid taking aluminum- and/or Mg^{2+}-containing antacids. (Tab, Chewable) Inform patients with phenylketonuria that product contains phenylalanine. (Sus) Instruct to administer within 30 min of mixing.

Administration: Oral route. May be administered with or without food. If unable to swallow tab, consider chewable tab. (Tab) Swallow whole. (Tab, Chewable) Chew or swallow whole. (Sus) Refer to PI for preparation and administration instructions. **Storage:** 20-25°C (68-77°F); excursions permitted to 15-30°C (59-86°F). (Tab, Chewable) Protect from moisture. (Sus) Do not open foil pkt until ready for use.

ISONIAZID   RX
isoniazid (Various)

> Severe, fatal hepatitis may develop. Monitor LFTs monthly. D/C drug if signs and symptoms of hepatic damage occur. Patients with tuberculosis (TB) who have isoniazid-induced hepatitis should have appropriate treatment with alternative drugs. Defer preventive treatment in persons with acute hepatic disease.

THERAPEUTIC CLASS: Isonicotinic acid hydrazide

INDICATIONS: Prevention and treatment of TB.

DOSAGE: *Adults:* Active TB: 5mg/kg as a single dose. Max: 300mg qd or 15mg/kg 2 to 3 times/week. Max: 900mg/day. Use with other antituberculosis agents. Prevention: 300mg qd single dose.
Pediatrics: Active TB: 10-15mg/kg as a single dose. Max: 300mg qd or 20-40mg/kg 2 to 3 times/week. Max: 900mg/day. Use with other antituberculosis agents. Prevention: 10mg/kg qd single dose. Max: 300mg qd.

HOW SUPPLIED: Inj: 100mg/mL; Syrup: 50mg/5mL; Tab: 100mg, 300mg

CONTRAINDICATIONS: Severe hypersensitivity reactions, including drug-induced hepatitis, previous INH-associated hepatic injury, severe adverse effects (eg, drug fever, chills, arthritis), acute liver disease of any etiology.

WARNINGS/PRECAUTIONS: D/C if hypersensitivity occurs. Monitor closely with liver or renal disease, daily alcohol users, pregnancy, age >35, and concurrent chronic medications. Precaution with HIV seropositive patients. Take with vitamin B6 in malnourished and those predisposed to neuropathy.

ADVERSE REACTIONS: Peripheral neuropathy, N/V, anorexia, epigastric distress, elevated serum transaminases, bilirubinemia, jaundice, hepatitis, skin eruptions, pyridoxine deficiency.

INTERACTIONS: Alcohol is associated with hepatitis. May increase phenytoin, theophylline, and valproate serum levels. Do not take with food. Severe acetaminophen toxicity reported. Decreases carbamazepine metabolism and area under the curve of ketoconazole. Avoid tyramine- and histamine-containing foods.

PREGNANCY: Category C, caution in nursing.

MECHANISM OF ACTION: Isonicotinic acid hydrazide; inhibits mycolic acid synthesis and acts against actively growing tuberculosis bacilli.

PHARMACOKINETICS: Absorption: T_{max}=1-2 hrs. **Distribution:** Crosses placenta, found in breast milk. **Metabolism:** Acetylation and dehydrazination. **Elimination:** Urine (50-70%).

NURSING CONSIDERATIONS

Assessment: Assess for previous isoniazid-associated hepatic injury, acute liver disease, HIV status, pregnancy status, age, and drug interactions. Document reasons for therapy, culture, and susceptibility.

Monitoring: Prior to therapy and periodically thereafter, measure hepatic enzymes (AST, ALT). D/C at 1st sign of hypersensitivity reaction. Monitor for peripheral neuropathy, convulsions, N/V, agranulocytosis, hemolytic anemia, systemic lupus erythematosus-like syndrome, metabolic and endocrine reactions (hyperglycemia, pyridoxine deficiency, pellagra).

Patient Counseling: Instruct to immediately report signs/symptoms consistent with liver damage or other adverse events (unexplained anorexia, N/V, dark urine, icterus, rash, persistent paresthesias of the hands and feet, persistent fatigue, weakness or fever of >3 days duration, and/or abdominal tenderness). Instruct to take drug without food, and to take pyridoxine tabs if peripheral neuropathy develops.

Administration: Oral and IM route. **Storage:** Tab: 20-25°C (68-77°F). Syrup: 15-30°C (59-86°F). Protect from light and moisture. Dispense in tight, light-resistant container. Inj: 20-25°C (68-77°F). Protect from light. If vial contents crystallize, warm vial to room temperature to redissolve crystals before use.

ISOSORBIDE DINITRATE   RX
isosorbide dinitrate (Various)

OTHER BRAND NAMES: Isordil Titradose (Biovail)

THERAPEUTIC CLASS: Nitrate vasodilator

INDICATIONS: Prevention of angina pectoris due to coronary artery disease. (Tab, SL) Prevention and treatment of angina pectoris due to coronary artery disease.

DOSAGE: *Adults:* (Tab/Isordil Titradose) Initial: 5-20mg bid-tid. Maint: 10-40mg bid-tid. Allow a dose-free interval of ≥14 hrs. (Tab, ER) Refer to PI. (Tab, SL) Take 1 tab (2.5-5mg) 15 min before activity. Elderly: Start at lower end of dosing range.

HOW SUPPLIED: Tab, SL: 2.5mg, 5mg; Tab: 5mg*, 10mg*, 20mg*, 30mg*; (Isordil Titradose): 5mg*, 40mg*; Tab, Extended-Release (ER): 40mg* *scored.

WARNINGS/PRECAUTIONS: Severe hypotension, particularly with upright posture, may occur. Not for use with acute myocardial infarction (MI) or congestive heart failure (CHF); perform careful clinical or hemodynamic monitoring if used for these conditions. Hypotension may be accompanied by paradoxical bradycardia and increased angina pectoris. May aggravate angina caused by hypertrophic cardiomyopathy. Caution with volume depletion, hypotension, and elderly. May develop tolerance. Chest pain, acute MI, and sudden death reported during temporary withdrawal. (Tab, SL) Not the 1st drug of choice for abortion of acute anginal episode.

ADVERSE REACTIONS: Headache, lightheadedness, hypotension, syncope, crescendo angina, rebound HTN.

INTERACTIONS: Severe hypotension with sildenafil. Additive vasodilation with other vasodilators (eg, alcohol).

PREGNANCY: Category C, caution in nursing.

MECHANISM OF ACTION: Nitrate vasodilator; relaxes vascular smooth muscle and dilates peripheral arteries and veins; venous dilatation reduces left ventricular end diastolic pressure and pulmonary capillary wedge pressure (preload); arteriolar relaxation reduces systemic vascular resistance, systolic arterial pressure, and mean arterial pressure (afterload); dilates the coronary artery.

PHARMACOKINETICS: Absorption: Nearly complete (Tab/Isordil Titradose). Bioavailability (10-90%) (Tab/Isordil Titradose), (40-50%) (Tab, SL). T_{max}=1 hr (Tab/Isordil Titradose), 10-15 min (Tab, SL). **Distribution:** V_d=2-4L/kg. **Metabolism:** Liver; extensive 1st-pass metabolism (Tab/Tab, ER/Isordil Titradose); 2-mononitrate, 5-mononitrate (active metabolites). **Elimination:** $T_{1/2}$=1 hr; 5 hrs (5-mononitrate), 2 hrs (2-mononitrate).

NURSING CONSIDERATIONS

Assessment: Assess for drug hypersensitivity, hypotension, acute MI, CHF, volume depletion, hypertrophic cardiomyopathy, alcohol intake, pregnancy/nursing status, and possible drug interactions.

Monitoring: Careful clinical or hemodynamic monitoring for hypotension and tachycardia in patients with MI or CHF. Monitor for paradoxical bradycardia, increased angina pectoris, hypotension, hemodynamic rebound, decreased exercise tolerance, chest pain, acute MI, and other adverse reactions.

Patient Counseling: Counsel to carefully follow prescribed dosing regimen. Inform that headaches accompany therapy and are markers of drug activity; instruct not to alter schedule of therapy since loss of headache may be associated with simultaneous loss of anti-anginal efficacy. Inform that lightheadedness on standing may occur that may be more frequent with alcohol consumption.

Administration: Oral/SL route. **Storage:** (Isordil Titradose) 25°C (77°F); excursions permitted to 15-30°C (59-86°F). Protect from light. (Tab) 25°C (77°F). Protect from light. (Tab, SL/Tab, ER) 20-25°C (68-77°F). (Tab, SL) Protect from light and moisture.

IXEMPRA   RX
ixabepilone (Bristol-Myers Squibb)

> In combination with capecitabine, contraindicated in patients with AST/ALT >2.5X ULN or bilirubin >1X ULN due to increased risk of toxicity and neutropenia-related death.

THERAPEUTIC CLASS: Antimicrotubule agent

INDICATIONS: In combination with capecitabine for the treatment of patients with metastatic or locally advanced breast cancer resistant to treatment with an anthracycline and a taxane, or whose cancer is taxane-resistant and for whom further anthracycline therapy is contraindicated. As monotherapy for the treatment of metastatic or locally advanced breast cancer in patients whose tumors are resistant or refractory to anthracyclines, taxanes, and capecitabine.

DOSAGE: *Adults:* Usual: 40mg/m² IV over 3 hrs every 3 weeks. Doses for patients with BSA >2.2m² should be calculated based on 2.2m². Refer to PI for dose modifications based on toxicities. Retreatment: Do not begin a new cycle of treatment unless the neutrophil count is ≥1500 cells/mm³, the platelet count is ≥100,000 cells/mm³, and nonhematologic toxicities have improved to Grade 1 (mild) or resolved. Hepatic Impairment: Combination Therapy: AST and ALT ≤2.5X ULN and Bilirubin ≤1X ULN: 40mg/m². Monotherapy: First Course: Mild: AST and ALT ≤2.5X ULN and Bilirubin ≤1X ULN: 40mg/m². AST and ALT ≤10X ULN and Bilirubin ≤1.5X ULN: 32mg/m². Moderate: AST and ALT ≤10X ULN and Bilirubin >1.5X to ≤3X ULN: Initial: 20mg/m². Titrate: May escalate if tolerated. Max: 30mg/m². Subsequent Courses: Base further decreases on tolerance. Strong CYP3A4 Inhibitors: Avoid, or if must be coadministered, reduce dose to 20mg/m². If the strong inhibitor is discontinued, allow a washout period of approximately 1 week before adjusting the dose upward to the indicated dose. Strong CYP3A4 Inducers: Avoid, or if must be coadministered, gradually increase dose from 40mg/m² to 60mg/m², given as a 4-hr IV infusion. If the strong inducer is discontinued, return to the dose used prior to initiation of the strong inducer. Premedicate all patients approximately 1 hr before infusion with an H_1-antagonist (eg, diphenhydramine 50mg PO or equivalent) and an H_2-antagonist (eg, ranitidine 150-300mg PO or equivalent). Premedicate patients who experienced a hypersensitivity reaction to drug with corticosteroids (eg, dexamethasone 20mg IV, 30 min before infusion or PO, 60 min before infusion) in addition to pretreatment with H_1- and H_2-antagonists.

HOW SUPPLIED: Inj: 15mg, 45mg

CONTRAINDICATIONS: History of a severe (CTC Grade 3/4) hypersensitivity reaction to agents containing Cremophor EL or its derivatives (eg, polyoxyethylated castor oil). Neutrophil count <1500 cells/mm³ or platelet count <100,000 cells/mm³. In combination with capecitabine, patients with AST/ALT >2.5X ULN or bilirubin >1X ULN.

WARNINGS/PRECAUTIONS: Peripheral neuropathy reported; caution with diabetes mellitus (DM) or preexisting peripheral neuropathy. Myelosuppression, which is dose-dependent and primarily manifested as neutropenia, reported; frequently monitor peripheral blood cell counts. Monotherapy is not recommended in patients with AST/ALT >10X ULN or bilirubin >3X ULN, and should be used with caution in patients with AST/ALT >5X ULN. Observe for hypersensitivity reactions; d/c infusion and start aggressive supportive treatment if severe hypersensitivity reactions occur. May cause fetal harm. Cardiac adverse reactions (eg, myocardial ischemia, ventricular dysfunction) reported during combination therapy; caution with history of cardiac disease, and consider discontinuation of ixabepilone if cardiac ischemia or impaired cardiac function develops. Contains dehydrated alcohol USP; consider possibility of CNS and other effects of alcohol.

ADVERSE REACTIONS: Peripheral sensory neuropathy, fatigue/asthenia, myalgia/arthralgia, alopecia, N/V, stomatitis/mucositis, diarrhea, musculoskeletal pain, palmar-plantar erythrodysesthesia (hand-foot) syndrome, anorexia, abdominal pain, nail disorder, constipation, hematologic abnormalities.

INTERACTIONS: Strong CYP3A4 inhibitors (eg, ketoconazole, itraconazole, clarithromycin, atazanavir, grapefruit juice) may increase levels; avoid, or if must be coadministered, reduce dose of ixabepilone. Caution with mild/moderate CYP3A4 inhibitors (eg, erythromycin, fluconazole, verapamil). Monitor closely for acute toxicities in patients receiving CYP3A4 inhibitors during treatment. Strong CYP3A4 inducers (eg, rifampin, dexamethasone) may decrease levels; avoid, or if must be coadministered, consider gradual dose adjustment of ixabepilone. St. John's wort may decrease levels unpredictably; avoid concomitant use.

PREGNANCY: Category D, not for use in nursing.

MECHANISM OF ACTION: Microtubule inhibitor; semi-synthetic analog of epothilone B. Binds directly to β-tubulin subunits on microtubules, leading to suppression of microtubule dynamics. Blocks cells in the mitotic phase of the cell division cycle, leading to cell death.

PHARMACOKINETICS: Absorption: C_{max}=252ng/mL; T_{max}=3 hrs; AUC=2143ng•hr/mL. **Distribution:** V_d>1000L; plasma protein binding (67-77%). **Metabolism:** Liver (extensive); oxidation via CYP3A4. **Elimination:** Feces (65%, 1.6% unchanged), urine (21%, 5.6% unchanged); $T_{1/2}$=52 hrs.

NURSING CONSIDERATIONS

Assessment: Assess for history of a severe hypersensitivity reaction to Cremophor EL or its derivatives (eg, polyoxyethylated castor oil), DM, preexisting peripheral neuropathy, history of cardiac disease, pregnancy/nursing status, and possible drug interactions. Obtain CBC and LFTs.

Monitoring: Monitor for signs/symptoms of neuropathy, myelosuppression, hypersensitivity reactions, cardiac ischemia/impairment, and other adverse reactions. Perform periodic clinical observation and lab tests (eg, CBC, LFTs).

Patient Counseling: Advise to report to physician any numbness and tingling of the hands or feet, chest pain, difficulty breathing, palpitations, or unusual weight gain. Instruct to contact physician if a fever of ≥100.5°F or other evidence of potential infection (eg, chills, cough, burning or pain on urination) develops, or if experiencing urticaria, pruritus, rash, flushing, swelling, dyspnea, chest tightness, or other hypersensitivity-related symptoms following an infusion. Advise to use effective contraceptive measures to prevent pregnancy and to avoid nursing during treatment.

Administration: IV route. Refer to PI for preparation, proper handling, and administration instructions. **Storage:** 2-8°C (36-46°F). Protect from light. Constituted Sol: Dilute as soon as possible or store in the vial (not the syringe) for a max of 1 hr at room temperature and room light. Diluted with Infusion Fluid: Stable at room temperature and room light for a max of 6 hrs.

JALYN RX
tamsulosin HCl - dutasteride (GlaxoSmithKline)

THERAPEUTIC CLASS: 5-alpha reductase inhibitor/alpha antagonist

INDICATIONS: Treatment of symptomatic BPH in men with an enlarged prostate.

DOSAGE: *Adults:* Usual: 1 cap qd, 30 min after the same meal each day.

HOW SUPPLIED: Cap: (Dutasteride-Tamsulosin) 0.5mg-0.4mg

CONTRAINDICATIONS: Pregnancy, women of childbearing potential, pediatric patients.

WARNINGS/PRECAUTIONS: Not approved for the prevention of prostate cancer. Orthostatic hypotension/syncope may occur; avoid situations where syncope may result in an injury. May reduce serum prostate specific antigen (PSA) concentration during therapy; establish a new baseline PSA at least 3 months after starting therapy and monitor PSA periodically thereafter. Any confirmed increase from the lowest PSA value during treatment may signal the presence of prostate cancer and should be evaluated. May increase the risk of high-grade prostate cancer. Prior to initiating treatment, consideration should be given to other urological conditions that may cause similar symptoms; BPH and prostate cancer may coexist. Risk to male fetus; cap should not be handled by pregnant women or women who may become pregnant. May cause priapism; may lead to permanent impotence if not properly treated. Avoid blood donation until at least 6 months following the last dose. Intraoperative floppy iris syndrome (IFIS) reported during cataract surgery; initiation of therapy in patients for whom cataract surgery is scheduled is not recommended. Caution with sulfa allergy; allergic reaction rarely reported. Reduced total sperm count, semen volume, and sperm motility reported.

ADVERSE REACTIONS: Ejaculation disorders, impotence, decreased libido, breast disorders, dizziness.

INTERACTIONS: Avoid with strong inhibitors of CYP3A4 (eg, ketoconazole); may increase tamsulosin exposure. Caution with potent, chronic inhibitors of CYP3A4 (eg, ritonavir), moderate inhibitors of CYP3A4 (eg, erythromycin), strong (eg, paroxetine) or moderate (eg, terbinafine) inhibitors of CYP2D6; potential for significant increase in tamsulosin exposure. Potential for significant increase in tamsulosin exposure when coadministered with a combination of both CYP3A4 and CYP2D6 inhibitors. Caution with cimetidine and warfarin. Avoid with other α-adrenergic antagonists; may increase the risk of symptomatic hypotension. Caution with PDE-5 inhibitors; may cause symptomatic hypotension.

PREGNANCY: Category X, not for use in nursing.

MECHANISM OF ACTION: Dutasteride: Selective type I and II 5α-reductase inhibitor; inhibits conversion of testosterone to dihydrotestosterone, the androgen primarily responsible for the initial development and subsequent enlargement of the prostate gland. Tamsulosin: $α_{1A}$ antagonist; selective blockade of $α_1$ adrenoceptors in the prostate results in relaxation of the smooth muscles of the bladder neck and prostate, improving urine flow rate and reducing BPH symptoms.

PHARMACOKINETICS: Absorption: (Fed) Dutasteride: Absolute bioavailability (60%); C_{max}=2.14ng/mL, T_{max}=3 hrs, AUC=39.6ng•hr/mL. Tamsulosin: Complete; C_{max}=11.3ng/mL, T_{max}=6 hrs, AUC=187.2ng•hr/mL. **Distribution:** Dutasteride: V_d=300-500L, plasma protein binding (99% albumin, 96.6% α-1 acid glycoprotein). Tamsulosin: Plasma protein binding (94-99%); (IV) V_d=16L. **Metabolism:** Dutasteride: Extensive. CYP3A4/3A5; 4'-hydroxydutasteride, 1,2-dihydroxydutasteride, 6-hydroxydutasteride (major metabolites). Tamsulosin: Liver (extensive); CYP3A4, CYP2D6. **Elimination:** Dutasteride: Urine (<1% unchanged), feces (5% unchanged, 40% metabolites); $T_{1/2}$=5 weeks. Tamsulosin: Urine (76%, <10% unchanged), feces (21%); $T_{1/2}$=14-15 hrs, 9-13 hrs.

NURSING CONSIDERATIONS

Assessment: Assess for urological conditions that may cause similar symptoms, previous hypersensitivity to the drug, sulfa allergy, and possible drug interactions. Assess if patient is planning to undergo cataract surgery.

Monitoring: Monitor for signs/symptoms of prostate cancer, other urological diseases, orthostatic hypotension, syncope, priapism, IFIS, and allergic reactions. Obtain new baseline PSA at least 3 months after starting treatment and monitor PSA periodically thereafter.

Patient Counseling: Inform about the possible occurrence of symptoms related to orthostatic hypotension (eg, dizziness, vertigo) and the potential risk of syncope; instruct to avoid situations where injury may result if syncope occurs. Inform of an increase in high-grade prostate cancer reported. Inform females who are pregnant or who may become pregnant not to handle the drug due to potential risk to the fetus; instruct that if a pregnant woman or woman of childbearing potential comes in contact with a leaking cap to wash the area immediately with soap and water. Inform that cap may become deformed and/or discolored if kept at high temperatures; instruct to avoid use if this occurs. Advise about the possibility of priapism (rare) that may lead to permanent erectile dysfunction if not brought to immediate medical attention. Advise not to donate blood for at least 6 months following the last dose. If considering cataract surgery, advise to inform ophthalmologist of therapy.

Administration: Oral route. Swallow cap whole; do not chew, crush, or open. **Storage:** 25°C (77°F); excursions permitted to 15-30°C (59-86°F).

JANUMET   RX
metformin HCl - sitagliptin (Merck)

> Lactic acidosis may occur due to metformin accumulation; risk increases with conditions such as sepsis, dehydration, excess alcohol intake, hepatic/renal impairment, and acute congestive heart failure (CHF). If acidosis is suspected, d/c therapy and hospitalize patient immediately.

THERAPEUTIC CLASS: Biguanide/dipeptidyl peptidase-4 inhibitor

INDICATIONS: Adjunct to diet and exercise to improve glycemic control in adults with type 2 diabetes mellitus (DM) when treatment with both sitagliptin and metformin is appropriate.

DOSAGE: *Adults:* Individualize dose. Take bid with meals, with gradual dose escalation, to reduce GI side effects of metformin. Initial: Not Currently on Metformin: 50mg-500mg bid. On Metformin: 50mg bid (100mg/day) of sitagliptin and current metformin dose. On Metformin 850mg bid: 50mg-1000mg bid. Max: 100mg-2000mg/day. With Insulin Secretagogue (eg, Sulfonylurea)/Insulin: May require lower doses of insulin secretagogue or insulin.

HOW SUPPLIED: Tab: (Sitagliptin-Metformin) 50mg-500mg, 50mg-1000mg

CONTRAINDICATIONS: Renal impairment (eg, SrCr ≥1.5mg/dL [men], ≥1.4mg/dL [women], or abnormal CrCl), acute or chronic metabolic acidosis, including diabetic ketoacidosis.

WARNINGS/PRECAUTIONS: Not for use in type 1 DM or for treatment of diabetic ketoacidosis. Acute pancreatitis, including fatal and nonfatal hemorrhagic or necrotizing pancreatitis, reported; d/c if pancreatitis is suspected. Avoid in patients with clinical or laboratory evidence of hepatic disease. Worsening renal function, including acute renal failure, reported; assess renal function before initiation of therapy and at least annually thereafter; d/c with evidence of renal impairment. May decrease serum vitamin B12 levels; monitor hematologic parameters annually. Temporarily suspend for any surgical procedure (except minor procedures not associated with restricted food and fluid intake); restart when oral intake is resumed and renal function is normal. Evaluate patients previously well controlled on therapy who develop laboratory abnormalities or clinical illness for evidence of ketoacidosis or lactic acidosis; d/c if acidosis occurs. Caution in patients susceptible to hypoglycemic effects, such as elderly, debilitated/malnourished patients, and those with adrenal/pituitary insufficiency, or alcohol intoxication. Temporarily d/c at the time of or prior to radiologic studies involving the use of intravascular iodinated contrast materials, withhold for 48 hrs subsequent to the procedure, and reinstitute only if renal function is normal. D/C in hypoxic states (eg, acute CHF, shock, acute myocardial infarction). Temporary loss of glycemic control may occur when exposed to stress (eg, fever, trauma, infection, surgery); may be necessary to withhold therapy and temporarily administer insulin. Serious hypersensitivity reactions reported; if suspected, d/c therapy, assess for other potential causes, and institute alternative treatment for DM. Caution in patients with history of angioedema with another dipeptidyl peptidase-4 (DPP-4) inhibitor. No conclusive evidence of macrovascular risk reduction. Caution in elderly.

ADVERSE REACTIONS: Lactic acidosis, diarrhea, upper respiratory tract infection, headache, nausea, abdominal pain.

INTERACTIONS: Alcohol potentiates the effect of metformin on lactate metabolism; avoid excessive alcohol intake. Hypoglycemia may occur with other glucose-lowering agents (eg, sulfonylureas, insulin) or ethanol; may require a lower dose of sulfonylurea or insulin. Caution with drugs that may affect renal function or result in significant hemodynamic change or may interfere with the disposition of metformin (eg, cationic drugs eliminated by renal tubular secretion). Topiramate or other carbonic anhydrase inhibitors (eg, zonisamide, acetazolamide, dichlorphenamide) may induce metabolic acidosis; use with caution. Cationic drugs that are eliminated by renal tubular secretion (eg, cimetidine, amiloride, digoxin, morphine, procainamide, quinidine, quinine, ranitidine, triamterene, trimethoprim, vancomycin) may potentially produce an interaction; monitor and adjust dose of Janumet and/or the interfering drug. Observe for loss of glycemic control with thiazides and other diuretics, corticosteroids, phenothiazines, thyroid products, estrogens, oral contraceptives, phenytoin, nicotinic acid, sympathomimetics, calcium channel blockers, and isoniazid. Metformin: May be difficult to recognize hypoglycemia with β-adrenergic blocking drugs.

PREGNANCY: Category B, caution in nursing.

MECHANISM OF ACTION: Sitagliptin: DPP-4 inhibitor; slows inactivation of incretin hormones, thereby increasing insulin release and decreasing glucagon levels in the circulation in a glucose-dependent manner. Metformin: Biguanide; decreases hepatic glucose production, decreases intestinal absorption of glucose, and improves insulin sensitivity by increasing peripheral glucose uptake and utilization.

PHARMACOKINETICS: Absorption: Sitagliptin: Absolute bioavailability (87%). Metformin: Absolute bioavailability (50-60%) (fasted). **Distribution:** Sitagliptin: (IV) V_d=198L; plasma protein binding (38%). Metformin: V_d=654L. **Metabolism:** Sitagliptin: Via CYP3A4 (primary) and CYP2C8. **Elimination:** Sitagliptin: Feces (13%), urine (87%, 79% unchanged); $T_{1/2}$=12.4 hrs. Metformin: Urine (90%); $T_{1/2}$=6.2 hrs (plasma), 17.6 hrs (blood).

NURSING CONSIDERATIONS

Assessment: Assess for metabolic acidosis, risk factors for lactic acidosis, renal/hepatic impairment, previous hypersensitivity to the drug, history of pancreatitis, inadequate vitamin B12 or Ca^{2+} absorption, type of DM, diabetic ketoacidosis, alcoholism, hypoxemia, presence of malnourishment or debilitation, adrenal/pituitary insufficiency, history of angioedema with another DPP-4 inhibitor, pregnancy/nursing status, and possible drug interactions. Assess if patient is planning to undergo any surgical procedure, radiologic studies involving the use of intravascular iodinated contrast materials, or is under any form of stress. Obtain baseline FPG and HbA1c levels, and hematologic parameters.

Monitoring: Monitor for signs/symptoms of lactic acidosis, pancreatitis, hypoxic states, hypersensitivity reactions, and for other adverse reactions. Monitor for changes in clinical status. Monitor renal function, especially in elderly, at least annually. Monitor hematologic parameters annually. Perform routine serum vitamin B12 measurements at 2- to 3-yr intervals in patients predisposed to developing subnormal vitamin B12 levels. Monitor FPG and HbA1c levels, and hepatic function periodically.

Patient Counseling: Inform of the risks, benefits, and alternative modes of therapy. Advise on the importance of adherence to dietary instructions, regular physical activity, periodic blood glucose monitoring and HbA1c testing, recognition/management of hypoglycemia/hyperglycemia, and assessment of diabetic complications. Instruct to seek medical advice during periods of stress (eg, fever, trauma, infection, surgery) as medication needs may change. Inform of the risk of lactic acidosis; instruct to d/c therapy immediately and contact physician if unexplained hyperventilation, myalgia, malaise, unusual somnolence, dizziness, slow or irregular heartbeat, sensation of feeling cold (especially in the extremities), or other nonspecific symptoms occur. Counsel against excessive alcohol intake. Inform that GI symptoms and acute pancreatitis may occur; instruct to d/c therapy promptly and contact physician if persistent severe abdominal pain occurs. Inform that allergic reactions may occur; instruct to d/c therapy and seek medical advice promptly if symptoms occur. Counsel to inform physician if any bothersome or unusual symptom develops, or if any symptom persists or worsens.

Administration: Oral route. Take with meals. Do not split or divide tab before swallowing.
Storage: 20-25°C (68-77°F); excursions permitted to 15-30°C (59-86°F).

JANUMET **XR**   RX
metformin HCl - sitagliptin (Merck)

> Lactic acidosis may occur due to metformin accumulation; risk increases with conditions such as sepsis, dehydration, excess alcohol intake, hepatic/renal impairment, and acute congestive heart failure (CHF). If acidosis is suspected, d/c therapy and hospitalize patient immediately.

THERAPEUTIC CLASS: Biguanide/dipeptidyl peptidase-4 inhibitor

INDICATIONS: Adjunct to diet and exercise to improve glycemic control in adults with type 2 diabetes mellitus (DM) when treatment with both sitagliptin and metformin extended-release (ER) is appropriate.

DOSAGE: *Adults:* Individualize dose. Take qd with a meal, preferably in pm. Not Currently on Metformin: Initial: 100mg-1000mg/day; if metformin dose is inadequate to achieve glycemic control, titrate gradually (to reduce GI side effects of metformin) up to max recommended daily dose. On Metformin: Initial: 100mg/day of sitagliptin and previously prescribed metformin dose. On Metformin Immediate-Release (IR) 850mg bid or 1000mg bid: Initial: Two 50mg-1000mg tabs taken together qd. Max: 100mg-2000mg/day. Changing Between Janumet and Janumet XR: Maintain the same total daily dose of sitagliptin and metformin; if metformin dose is inadequate to achieve glycemic control, titrate gradually up to max recommended daily dose. With Insulin Secretagogue (eg, Sulfonylurea)/Insulin: May require lower doses of insulin secretagogue or insulin.

HOW SUPPLIED: Tab, ER: (Sitagliptin-Metformin ER) 50mg-500mg, 50mg-1000mg, 100mg-1000mg

CONTRAINDICATIONS: Renal impairment (eg, SrCr ≥1.5mg/dL [men], ≥1.4mg/dL [women], or abnormal CrCl), acute or chronic metabolic acidosis, including diabetic ketoacidosis.

WARNINGS/PRECAUTIONS: Not for use in type 1 DM or for treatment of diabetic ketoacidosis. Acute pancreatitis, including fatal and nonfatal hemorrhagic or necrotizing pancreatitis, reported; d/c if pancreatitis is suspected. Avoid in patients with clinical or laboratory evidence of hepatic disease. Worsening renal function, including acute renal failure, reported; assess renal function before initiation of therapy and at least annually thereafter; d/c with evidence of renal impairment. May decrease vitamin B12 levels; monitor hematologic parameters annually. Temporarily suspend for any surgical procedure (except minor procedures not associated with restricted food and fluid intake); restart when oral intake is resumed and renal function is normal. Evaluate patients previously well controlled on therapy who develop laboratory abnormalities or clinical illness for evidence of ketoacidosis or lactic acidosis; d/c if acidosis occurs. Caution in patients susceptible to hypoglycemic effects, such as elderly, debilitated/malnourished patients, and those with adrenal/pituitary insufficiency, or alcohol intoxication. Temporarily d/c at the time of or prior to radiologic studies involving the use of intravascular iodinated contrast materials, withhold for 48 hrs subsequent to the procedure, and reinstitute only if renal function is normal. D/C in hypoxic states (eg, acute CHF, shock, acute myocardial infarction). Temporary loss of glycemic control may occur when exposed to stress (eg, fever, trauma, infection, surgery); may be necessary to withhold therapy and temporarily administer insulin. Serious hypersensitivity reactions reported; if suspected, d/c therapy, assess for other potential causes, and institute alternative treatment for DM. Caution in patients with history of angioedema to another dipeptidyl peptidase-4 (DPP-4) inhibitor. Incompletely dissolved tabs being eliminated in the feces reported; assess adequacy of glycemic control if patient reports repeatedly seeing tabs in feces. Caution in elderly.

ADVERSE REACTIONS: Lactic acidosis, diarrhea, upper respiratory tract infection, headache, nausea, abdominal pain.

INTERACTIONS: Alcohol potentiates the effect of metformin on lactate metabolism; avoid excessive alcohol intake. Hypoglycemia may occur with other glucose-lowering agents (eg, sulfonylureas, insulin) or ethanol; may require a lower dose of sulfonylurea or insulin. Caution with drugs that may affect renal function or result in significant hemodynamic change or may interfere with the disposition of metformin (eg, cationic drugs eliminated by renal tubular secretion). Topiramate or other carbonic anhydrase inhibitors (eg, zonisamide, acetazolamide, dichlorphenamide) may induce metabolic acidosis; use with caution. Cationic drugs that are eliminated by renal tubular secretion (eg, cimetidine, amiloride, digoxin, morphine, procainamide, quinidine, quinine, ranitidine, triamterene, trimethoprim, vancomycin) may potentially produce an interaction; monitor and adjust dose of Janumet XR and/or the interfering drug. Observe for loss of glycemic control with thiazides and other diuretics, corticosteroids, phenothiazines, thyroid products, estrogens, oral contraceptives, phenytoin, nicotinic acid, sympathomimetics, calcium channel blockers, and isoniazid. Metformin: May be difficult to recognize hypoglycemia with β-adrenergic blocking drugs.

PREGNANCY: Category B, caution in nursing.

MECHANISM OF ACTION: Sitagliptin: DPP-4 inhibitor; slows the inactivation of incretin hormones, thereby increasing insulin release and decreasing glucagon levels in the circulation in a glucose-dependent manner. Metformin: Biguanide; decreases hepatic glucose production, decreases intestinal absorption of glucose, and improves insulin sensitivity by increasing peripheral glucose uptake and utilization.

PHARMACOKINETICS: Absorption: Sitagliptin: Absolute bioavailability (87%); (Healthy) T_{max}=3 hrs (median). Metformin ER: (Healthy) T_{max}=8 hrs (median). **Distribution:** Sitagliptin: (IV, Healthy) V_d=198L; plasma protein binding (38%). Metformin IR: V_d=654L. **Metabolism:** Sitagliptin: Via CYP3A4 (primary) and CYP2C8. **Elimination:** Sitagliptin: (Healthy) Feces (13%), urine (87%, 79% unchanged); $T_{1/2}$=12.4 hrs. Metformin: Urine (90%); $T_{1/2}$=6.2 hrs (plasma), 17.6 hrs (blood).

NURSING CONSIDERATIONS

Assessment: Assess for metabolic acidosis, risk factors for lactic acidosis, renal/hepatic impairment, previous hypersensitivity to the drug, history of pancreatitis, inadequate vitamin B12 or Ca^{2+} intake/absorption, type of DM, diabetic ketoacidosis, alcoholism, hypoxemia, presence of malnourishment or debilitation, adrenal/pituitary insufficiency, history of angioedema with another DPP-4 inhibitor, pregnancy/nursing status, and possible drug interactions. Assess if patient is planning to undergo any surgical procedure, radiologic studies involving the use of intravascular iodinated contrast materials, or is under any form of stress. Obtain baseline FPG and HbA1c levels, and hematologic parameters.

Monitoring: Monitor for signs/symptoms of lactic acidosis, pancreatitis, hypoxic states, hypersensitivity reactions, and other adverse reactions. Monitor for changes in clinical status. Monitor renal function, especially in elderly, at least annually. Monitor hematologic parameters annually. Perform routine serum vitamin B12 measurements at 2- to 3-yr intervals in patients predisposed to developing subnormal vitamin B12 levels. Monitor FPG and HbA1c levels, and hepatic function periodically.

Patient Counseling: Inform of the risks, benefits, and alternative modes of therapy. Advise on the importance of adherence to dietary instructions, regular physical activity, periodic blood glucose monitoring and HbA1c, renal function, and hematologic parameter testing, recognition/management of hypoglycemia/hyperglycemia, and assessment of diabetes complications. Instruct to seek medical advice during periods of stress (eg, fever, trauma, infection, surgery) as medication needs may change. Inform of the risk of lactic acidosis; instruct to d/c therapy immediately and notify physician if unexplained hyperventilation, myalgia, malaise, unusual somnolence, dizziness, slow or irregular heartbeat, sensation of feeling cold (especially in the extremities), or other nonspecific symptoms occur. Counsel against excessive alcohol intake. Inform that GI symptoms and acute pancreatitis may occur; instruct to d/c therapy promptly and contact physician if persistent severe abdominal pain occurs. Inform that allergic reactions may occur; instruct to d/c therapy and seek medical advice promptly if symptoms occur. Counsel to inform physician if any bothersome or unusual symptom develops, or if any known symptom persists or worsens. Inform that incompletely dissolved tabs may be eliminated in the feces; advise to report to physician if patient repeatedly see tabs in feces.

Administration: Oral route. Take qd with a meal, preferably in pm. Take 100mg-1000mg tab as a single tab qd. Patients using 2 tabs should take the 2 tabs together qd. Swallow tab whole; do not split, crush, or chew. **Storage:** 20-25°C (68-77°F); excursions permitted to 15-30°C (59-86°F). Store in a dry place.

JANUVIA RX

sitagliptin (Merck)

THERAPEUTIC CLASS: Dipeptidyl peptidase-4 inhibitor

INDICATIONS: Adjunct to diet and exercise to improve glycemic control in adults with type 2 diabetes mellitus (DM).

DOSAGE: *Adults:* Usual: 100mg qd. Renal Insufficiency: Moderate (CrCl ≥30-<50mL/min): 50mg qd. Severe (CrCl <30mL/min)/End-Stage Renal Disease Requiring Hemodialysis or Peritoneal Dialysis: 25mg qd. With Insulin/Insulin Secretagogue (eg, Sulfonylurea): May require lower dose of insulin secretagogue or insulin.

HOW SUPPLIED: Tab: 25mg, 50mg, 100mg

WARNINGS/PRECAUTIONS: Not for use with type 1 DM or for treatment of diabetic ketoacidosis. Acute pancreatitis reported; d/c if pancreatitis is suspected. Use caution to ensure that correct dose is prescribed with moderate/severe renal impairment. Worsening renal function, including acute renal failure, reported; assess renal function prior to therapy and periodically thereafter. Serious hypersensitivity reactions reported; if suspected, d/c therapy, assess for other potential causes, and institute alternative treatment. Caution in patients with a history of angioedema with another dipeptidyl peptidase-4 (DPP-4) inhibitor and in the elderly. No conclusive evidence of macrovascular risk reduction.

ADVERSE REACTIONS: Nasopharyngitis, upper respiratory tract infection.

INTERACTIONS: May slightly increase digoxin levels; monitor appropriately. Lower dose of insulin secretagogue (eg, sulfonylurea) or insulin may be required to reduce risk of hypoglycemia.

PREGNANCY: Category B, caution in nursing.

MECHANISM OF ACTION: DPP-4 inhibitor; slows inactivation of incretin hormones, thereby increasing insulin release and decreasing glucagon levels in the circulation in a glucose-dependent manner.

PHARMACOKINETICS: Absorption: Rapid. Absolute bioavailability (87%); T_{max}=1-4 hrs (median); AUC=8.52µM•hr; C_{max}=950nM. **Distribution:** (IV) V_d=198L; plasma protein binding (38%). **Metabolism:** Via CYP3A4 and CYP2C8. **Elimination:** Feces (13%), urine (87%, 79% unchanged); $T_{1/2}$=12.4 hrs.

NURSING CONSIDERATIONS

Assessment: Assess for previous hypersensitivity to the drug, type of DM, diabetic ketoacidosis, history of pancreatitis, history of angioedema with another DPP-4 inhibitor, pregnancy/nursing status, and possible drug interactions. Obtain baseline renal function, FPG, and HbA1c levels.

Monitoring: Monitor for pancreatitis, hypersensitivity reactions, and other adverse reactions. Monitor FPG, HbA1c, and renal function periodically.

Patient Counseling: Inform of risks, benefits, and alternative modes of therapy. Advise on the importance of adherence to dietary instructions, regular physical activity, periodic blood glucose monitoring, HbA1c testing, recognition/management of hypoglycemia/hyperglycemia, and assessment of diabetic complications. Instruct to seek medical advice during periods of stress (eg, fever, trauma, infection, surgery) as medication requirements may change. Instruct to d/c use and notify physician if signs and symptoms of pancreatitis or allergic reactions occur. Instruct to inform physician if any unusual symptom develops, or if any known symptom persists or worsens.

Administration: Oral route. May be taken with or without food. May be administered without regard to timing of dialysis. **Storage:** 20-25°C (68-77°F); excursions permitted to 15-30°C (59-86°F).

JENTADUETO   RX
metformin HCl - linagliptin (Boehringer Ingelheim)

> Lactic acidosis may occur due to metformin accumulation; risk increases with conditions such as sepsis, dehydration, excessive alcohol intake, hepatic/renal impairment, and acute congestive heart failure (CHF). If acidosis is suspected, d/c therapy and hospitalize patient immediately.

THERAPEUTIC CLASS: Biguanide/dipeptidyl peptidase-4 inhibitor

INDICATIONS: Adjunct to diet and exercise to improve glycemic control in adults with type 2 diabetes mellitus (DM) when treatment with both linagliptin and metformin is appropriate.

DOSAGE: *Adults:* Individualize dose. Take bid with meals. Initial: Not Currently on Metformin: 2.5mg-500mg bid. On Metformin: 2.5mg linagliptin and current metformin dose. On Individual Components: May be switched to strength containing the same doses of each component. Titrate: Increase gradually to reduce GI side effects of metformin. Max: 2.5mg-1000mg bid. With Insulin Secretagogue (eg, Sulfonylurea)/Insulin: May require lower dose of insulin secretagogue or insulin.

HOW SUPPLIED: Tab: (Linagliptin-Metformin) 2.5mg-500mg, 2.5mg-850mg, 2.5mg-1000mg

CONTRAINDICATIONS: Renal impairment (eg, SrCr ≥1.5mg/dL [men], ≥1.4mg/dL [women], or abnormal CrCl), acute or chronic metabolic acidosis, including diabetic ketoacidosis.

WARNINGS/PRECAUTIONS: Not for use in type 1 DM or for treatment of diabetic ketoacidosis. Acute pancreatitis, including fatal pancreatitis, reported; d/c if pancreatitis is suspected. Assess renal function before initiation of therapy and at least annually thereafter; d/c with evidence of renal impairment. Temporarily d/c at the time of or prior to radiologic studies involving the use of intravascular iodinated contrast materials, withhold for 48 hrs subsequent to the procedure, and reinstitute only if renal function is normal. Temporarily d/c for any surgical procedure (except minor procedures not associated with restricted food and fluid intake); restart when oral intake is resumed and renal function is normal. Avoid in patients with clinical or lab evidence of hepatic disease. Caution in patients susceptible to hypoglycemic effects, such as elderly, debilitated/ malnourished patients, and those with adrenal/pituitary insufficiency, or alcohol intoxication. May decrease serum vitamin B12 levels; monitor hematologic parameters annually. D/C in hypoxic states (eg, acute CHF, shock, acute myocardial infarction). No conclusive evidence of macrovascular risk reduction. Do not initiate in patients ≥80 yrs of age unless measurement of CrCl demonstrates that renal function is not reduced.

ADVERSE REACTIONS: Lactic acidosis, nasopharyngitis, diarrhea.

INTERACTIONS: Hypoglycemia may occur with other glucose-lowering agents (eg, insulin secretagogues [eg, sulfonylurea], insulin) or ethanol; may require a lower dose of insulin secretagogue or insulin. Observe for loss of glycemic control with thiazides and other diuretics, corticosteroids, phenothiazines, thyroid products, estrogens, oral contraceptives, phenytoin, nicotinic acid, sympathomimetics, calcium channel blockers, and isoniazid. Linagliptin: Strong P-glycoprotein or CYP3A4 inducers (eg, rifampin) may reduce efficacy; use alternative treatment. Metformin: Cationic drugs that are eliminated by renal tubular secretion (eg, cimetidine, amiloride, digoxin, morphine, procainamide, quinidine, quinine, ranitidine, triamterene, trimethoprim, vancomycin) may potentially produce an interaction; monitor and adjust dose of Jentadueto and/or the interfering drug. Topiramate or other carbonic anhydrase inhibitors (eg, zonisamide, acetazolamide, dichlorphenamide) may induce metabolic acidosis; use with caution. Caution with drugs that may affect renal function or result in significant hemodynamic change or interfere with the disposition of metformin. May be difficult to recognize hypoglycemia with β-adrenergic blocking drugs. Alcohol potentiates the effect of metformin on lactate metabolism; avoid excessive alcohol intake.

PREGNANCY: Category B, not for use in nursing.

MECHANISM OF ACTION: Linagliptin: Dipeptidyl peptidase-4 inhibitor; increases the concentrations of active incretin hormones, stimulating the release of insulin in a glucose-dependent manner and decreasing the levels of glucagon in the circulation. Metformin: Biguanide; decreases hepatic glucose production, decreases intestinal absorption of glucose, and improves insulin sensitivity by increasing peripheral glucose uptake and utilization.

PHARMACOKINETICS: Absorption: Linagliptin: Absolute bioavailability (30%). Metformin: Absolute bioavailability (50-60%) (fasted). **Distribution:** Linagliptin: V_d=1110L (IV); plasma protein binding (concentration-dependent). Metformin: V_d=654L; crosses placenta; found in breast milk. **Elimination:** Linagliptin: Enterohepatic (80%), urine (5%); $T_{1/2}$=12 hrs. Metformin: Urine (90%); $T_{1/2}$=6.2 hrs (plasma), 17.6 hrs (blood).

NURSING CONSIDERATIONS

Assessment: Assess for metabolic acidosis, risk factors for lactic acidosis, renal/hepatic impairment, previous hypersensitivity to the drug, history of pancreatitis, inadequate vitamin B12 or Ca^{2+} absorption, type of DM, diabetic ketoacidosis, alcoholism, hypoxemia, presence of malnourishment or debilitation, adrenal/pituitary insufficiency, pregnancy/nursing status, and possible drug interactions. Assess if patient is planning to undergo any surgical procedure or is under any form of stress. Obtain baseline FPG and HbA1c levels, and hematologic parameters.

Monitoring: Monitor for signs/symptoms of lactic acidosis, pancreatitis, hypoxic states, and for other adverse reactions. Monitor renal function, especially in elderly, at least annually. Monitor hematologic parameters annually. Perform routine serum vitamin B12 measurement at 2- to 3-yr intervals in patients predisposed to developing subnormal vitamin B12 levels. Monitor FPG and HbA1c levels, and hepatic function periodically.

Patient Counseling: Inform of the risks, benefits, and alternative modes of therapy. Advise on the importance of adherence to dietary instructions, regular physical activity, periodic blood glucose monitoring and HbA1c testing, recognition/management of hypo- or hyperglycemia, and assessment of diabetes complications. Instruct to seek medical advice promptly during periods of stress (eg, fever, trauma, infection, surgery) as medication needs may change. Inform of the risk of lactic acidosis; instruct to d/c therapy immediately and contact physician if unexplained hyperventilation, malaise, myalgia, unusual somnolence, slow or irregular heartbeat, sensation of feeling cold (especially in the extremities), or other nonspecific symptoms occur. Inform that GI symptoms and acute pancreatitis may occur; instruct to d/c therapy promptly and contact physician if persistent severe abdominal pain occurs. Counsel against excessive alcohol intake. Counsel to inform physician if any bothersome or unusual symptom develops, or if any symptom persists or worsens.

Administration: Oral route. Take with meals. **Storage:** 25°C (77°F); excursions permitted to 15-30°C (59-86°F). Protect from exposure to high humidity.

JEVTANA   RX
cabazitaxel (Sanofi-Aventis)

> Neutropenic deaths reported. Perform frequent blood cell counts to monitor for neutropenia. Avoid with neutrophil counts of ≤1500 cells/mm³. Severe hypersensitivity reactions may occur; d/c immediately if a severe hypersensitivity reaction occurs and administer appropriate therapy. Patients should receive premedication. Must not be given to patients who have a history of severe hypersensitivity reactions to cabazitaxel or other drugs formulated with polysorbate 80.

THERAPEUTIC CLASS: Antimicrotubule agent

INDICATIONS: In combination with prednisone for the treatment of hormone-refractory metastatic prostate cancer previously treated with a docetaxel-containing treatment regimen.

DOSAGE: *Adults:* Usual: 25mg/m² over 1-hr IV infusion every 3 weeks in combination with oral prednisone 10mg administered daily throughout treatment. Reduce dose to 20mg/m² if patient experiences prolonged Grade ≥3 neutropenia (>1 week) despite appropriate medication (including granulocyte-colony stimulating factor [G-CSF]), febrile neutropenia, or Grade ≥3 diarrhea or persisting diarrhea despite appropriate medication, fluid, and electrolyte replacement. Delay treatment until improvement or resolution of febrile neutropenia, diarrhea, and until neutrophil count is >1500 cells/mm³. Use G-CSF for secondary prophylaxis for neutropenia and febrile neutropenia. D/C treatment if patient continues to experience any of these reactions at 20mg/m². Premedicate at least 30 min prior to each dose with IV antihistamine (dexchlorpheniramine 5mg, or diphenhydramine 25mg or equivalent antihistamine), corticosteroid (dexamethasone 8mg or equivalent steroid), H₂-antagonist (ranitidine 50mg or equivalent H₂-antagonist). Antiemetic prophylaxis is recommended and can be given PO or IV PRN.

HOW SUPPLIED: Inj: 60mg/1.5mL

CONTRAINDICATIONS: Neutrophil counts ≤1500/mm³.

WARNINGS/PRECAUTIONS: Should only be administered under the supervision of a qualified physician and where adequate diagnostic and treatment facilities are readily available. G-CSF may be administered to reduce risks of neutropenia complications; consider primary prophylaxis with G-CSF in patients with high-risk clinical features (eg, age >65 yrs, poor performance status, previous episodes of febrile neutropenia, extensive prior radiation ports, poor nutritional status, or other serious comorbidities) that predispose them to increased complications from prolonged neutropenia. N/V and severe diarrhea may occur. Death related to diarrhea and electrolyte imbalance reported; may need to delay treatment or reduce dose with Grade ≥3 diarrhea. GI hemorrhage and perforation, ileus, colitis, including fatal outcome, reported; caution in patients at risk of developing GI complications (those with neutropenia, elderly, concomitant use of NSAIDs, anti-platelet therapy, or anti-coagulants, and prior history of pelvic radiotherapy, GI disease [eg, ulceration, GI bleeding]). Symptoms such as abdominal pain, fever, persistent constipation, diarrhea, with or without neutropenia, may be early manifestations of serious GI toxicity and should be evaluated and treated promptly; treatment delay or discontinuation may be necessary. Renal failure, including cases with fatal outcome, reported; identify causes and treat aggressively. Caution in the elderly. Caution with severe renal impairment (CrCl <30mL/min) and in patients with end-stage renal disease. Avoid with hepatic impairment (total bilirubin ≥ULN, or AST and/or ALT ≥1.5X ULN). May cause fetal harm if administered to a pregnant woman.

ADVERSE REACTIONS: Hypersensitivity reactions, neutropenia, anemia, leukopenia, thrombocytopenia, diarrhea, fatigue, N/V, constipation, asthenia, abdominal pain, anorexia, back pain, hematuria, dyspnea.

INTERACTIONS: Avoid with strong CYP3A inhibitors (eg, ketoconazole, itraconazole, clarithromycin, atazanavir, indinavir, nefazodone, nelfinavir, ritonavir, saquinavir, telithromycin, voriconazole), strong CYP3A inducers (eg, phenytoin, carbamazepine, rifampin, rifabutin, rifapentine, phenobarbital), and St. John's wort. Caution with moderate CYP3A inhibitors.

PREGNANCY: Category D, not for use in nursing.

MECHANISM OF ACTION: Antimicrotubule agent; binds to tubulin and promotes its assembly into microtubules while simultaneously inhibiting disassembly, which results in the inhibition of mitotic and interphase cellular functions.

PHARMACOKINETICS: Absorption: C_{max}=226ng/mL; AUC=991ng•hr/mL; T_{max}=1 hr. **Distribution:** V_d=4864L; plasma protein binding (89%-92%). **Metabolism:** Liver (extensive) via CYP3A4/5, and to a lesser extent, CYP2C8. **Elimination:** Urine (3.7%, 2.3% unchanged), feces (76%); $T_{1/2}$=95 hrs

NURSING CONSIDERATIONS

Assessment: Assess for history of drug hypersensitivity or hypersensitivity to other drugs formulated with polysorbate 80, hepatic/severe renal impairment, risk of developing GI complications, and possible drug interactions. Assess for high-risk clinical features that may predispose to increased complications from prolonged neutropenia. Obtain baseline CBC, including neutrophil count.

Monitoring: Monitor for signs/symptoms of neutropenia, infections, hypersensitivity reactions, severe diarrhea, dehydration, N/V, electrolyte imbalance, renal failure, serious GI toxicity, and other adverse reactions. Monitor CBC, including neutrophil count, on a weekly basis during Cycle 1 and before each treatment cycle thereafter.

Patient Counseling: Counsel about the risk of potential hypersensitivity; instruct to immediately report signs of a hypersensitivity reaction. Advise on the importance of routine blood cell counts. Instruct to immediately report to physician any occurrence of fever. Instruct to report to physician if not compliant with oral corticosteroid regimen. Counsel about side effects associated with exposure, such as severe and fatal infections, dehydration, and renal failure. Advise to report to physician significant vomiting or diarrhea, decreased urinary output, and hematuria. Advise to inform physician before taking any other medications. Inform elderly that certain side effects may be more frequent or severe.

Administration: IV route. Do not use PVC infusion containers or polyurethane infusions sets. Refer to PI for further preparation and administration instructions. **Storage:** Undiluted: 25°C (77°F); excursions permitted to 15-30°C (59-86°F). Do not refrigerate. Diluted First Sol: Use within 30 min. Discard any unused portion. Diluted Second Sol in 0.9% NaCl or D5W: Use within 8 hrs at ambient temperature (including the 1-hr infusion) or for a total of 24 hrs (including the 1-hr infusion) under refrigeration.

JUXTAPID   RX

lomitapide (Aegerion)

> May cause elevations in transaminases; measure ALT, AST, alkaline phosphatase, and total bilirubin prior to therapy, and then ALT/AST regularly as recommended. Adjust dose if ALT/AST is ≥3X ULN. D/C for clinically significant liver toxicity. May increase hepatic fat. Hepatic steatosis associated with lomitapide treatment may be a risk factor for progressive liver disease, including steatohepatitis and cirrhosis. Available only through a restricted program under a Risk Evaluation and Mitigation Strategy (REMS) because of the risk of hepatotoxicity.

THERAPEUTIC CLASS: Lipid-regulating agent

INDICATIONS: Adjunct to a low-fat diet and other lipid-lowering treatments, including LDL apheresis where available, to reduce LDL, total cholesterol, apolipoprotein B (Apo B), and non-HDL in patients with homozygous familial hypercholesterolemia.

DOSAGE: *Adults:* Prior to treatment, initiate a low-fat diet supplying <20% of energy from fat. Initial: 5mg qd. Titrate: Escalate gradually; refer to PI for recommended regimen for titrating dosage. Maint: Individualize dose. Max: 60mg qd. Concomitant Weak CYP3A4 Inhibitors: Max: 30mg/day. End-Stage Renal Disease Receiving Dialysis/Mild Hepatic Impairment (Child-Pugh A): Max: 40mg/day. Refer to PI for dose modification based on elevated transaminases. Take daily supplements containing 400 IU vitamin E and at least 200mg linoleic acid, 210mg alpha-linolenic acid, 110mg eicosapentaenoic acid, and 80mg docosahexaenoic acid.

HOW SUPPLIED: Cap: 5mg, 10mg, 20mg

CONTRAINDICATIONS: Pregnancy, moderate or severe hepatic impairment (based on Child-Pugh category B or C), active liver disease including unexplained persistent elevations of serum transaminases, concomitant moderate or strong CYP3A4 inhibitors.

WARNINGS/PRECAUTIONS: If baseline LFTs are abnormal, consider initiating therapy after an appropriate work-up and the baseline abnormalities are explained or resolved. May cause fetal harm; females of reproductive potential should have a negative pregnancy test before initiation of therapy and use effective contraception during therapy. May reduce absorption of fat-soluble nutrients, especially in patients with chronic bowel or pancreatic diseases that predispose to malabsorption; patients should take daily supplements. GI adverse reactions reported; absorption of concomitant oral medications may be affected in patients who develop diarrhea or vomiting. Avoid in patients with rare hereditary problems of galactose intolerance, Lapp lactase deficiency, or glucose-galactose malabsorption; may result in diarrhea and malabsorption. Caution in elderly.

ADVERSE REACTIONS: Hepatic steatosis, increased serum transaminases, diarrhea, N/V, dyspepsia, abdominal pain/discomfort/distention, weight loss, constipation, flatulence, chest pain, influenza, nasopharyngitis, fatigue.

INTERACTIONS: See Contraindications and Dosage. Not recommended with other LDL-lowering agents that can increase hepatic fat. Avoid grapefruit juice. Alcohol may increase levels of hepatic fat and induce/exacerbate liver injury; avoid consumption of >1 alcoholic drink/day. Caution with other medications known to have potential for hepatotoxicity (eg, isotretinoin, amiodarone, acetaminophen [>4g/day for ≥3 days/week]). Increased exposure with weak CYP3A4 inhibitors (eg, alprazolam, atorvastatin, cimetidine, oral contraceptives). May increase INR and plasma concentrations of both R(+)-warfarin and S(-)-warfarin; regularly monitor INR (particularly after any changes in lomitapide dosage) and adjust dose of warfarin as clinically indicated. May double the exposure of simvastatin; refer to simvastatin PI for dosing recommendations. May increase the exposure of lovastatin; consider reducing dose of lovastatin when initiating therapy. May increase the absorption of P-glycoprotein (P-gp) substrates (eg, aliskiren, colchicine, digoxin, sirolimus); consider dose reduction of the P-gp substrate. Separate dosing by at least 4 hrs with bile acid sequestrants.

PREGNANCY: Category X, not for use in nursing.

MECHANISM OF ACTION: Lipid-regulating agent; directly binds and inhibits microsomal TG transfer protein, which resides in the lumen of the endoplasmic reticulum, thereby preventing the assembly of Apo B-containing lipoproteins in enterocytes and hepatocytes. This inhibits the synthesis of chylomicrons and VLDL. The inhibition of the synthesis of VLDL leads to reduced levels of plasma LDL.

PHARMACOKINETICS: Absorption: Absolute bioavailability (7%); T_{max}=6 hrs. **Distribution:** V_d=985-1292L; plasma protein binding (99.8%). **Metabolism:** Liver (extensive) via oxidation, oxidative N-dealkylation, glucuronide conjugation, piperidine ring opening. CYP3A4; M1 and M3 (major metabolites). **Elimination:** Feces (33.4%-35.1%, mostly unchanged), urine (52.9%-59.5%, mostly M1); $T_{1/2}$=39.7 hrs.

NURSING CONSIDERATIONS

Assessment: Assess for active liver disease including unexplained persistent elevations of serum transaminases, bowel/pancreatic disease, galactose intolerance, renal dysfunction, pregnancy/ nursing status, and possible drug interactions. Measure ALT/AST, alkaline phosphatase, and serum bilirubin prior to therapy.

Monitoring: Monitor for hepatic steatosis, hepatotoxicity, and GI and other adverse reactions. Monitor renal/hepatic function. During the 1st yr, perform hepatic-related tests (eg, ALT, AST) prior to each increase in dose or monthly, whichever occurs 1st. After the 1st yr, perform these tests at least every 3 months and before any dose increase. Monitor INR with warfarin.

Patient Counseling: Encourage to participate in the registry to monitor/evaluate long-term effects and inform that participation is voluntary. Advise that medication is only available from certified pharmacies enrolled in the REMS program. Discuss the importance of liver-related tests before initiation, prior to each dose escalation, and periodically thereafter. Advise of the potential for increased risk of liver injury if alcohol is consumed and instruct to limit alcohol consumption to not >1 drink/day. Advise to report any symptoms of possible liver injury (eg, fever, jaundice, lethargy, flu-like symptoms). Advise females of reproductive potential to have a negative pregnancy test before starting treatment and to use effective contraception while on therapy. Discuss the importance of taking daily supplements. Inform that GI adverse reactions are common and that strict adherence to a low-fat diet (<20% of total calories from fat) may reduce these reactions. Inform that absorption of oral medications may be affected in patients who develop diarrhea or vomiting; instruct to seek physician's advice if symptoms develop. Instruct to omit grapefruit juice from diet; advise to inform physician about all medications, nutritional supplements, and vitamins taken. If a dose is missed, instruct to take the normal dose at the usual time the next day; if dose is interrupted for more than a week, advise to contact physician before restarting treatment.

Administration: Oral route. Take qd with a glass of water, without food, at least 2 hrs after pm meal. Swallow cap whole; do not open, crush, dissolve, or chew. **Storage:** 20-25°C (68-77°F); excursions permitted to 15-30°C (59-86°F). May tolerate brief exposure up to 40°C (104°F), provided the mean kinetic temperature does not exceed 25°C (77°F); however, such exposure should be minimized. Protect from moisture.

KADIAN `CII`
morphine sulfate (Actavis)

> Contains morphine, an opioid agonist and a Schedule II controlled substance with an abuse liability similar to other opioid agonists, legal or illicit; assess each patient's risk for opioid abuse or addiction prior to prescribing. Routinely monitor for signs of misuse, abuse, and addiction. Respiratory depression, including fatal cases, may occur even when used as recommended; proper dosing and titration are essential. Monitor for respiratory depression, especially during initiation or following a dose increase. Should only be prescribed by healthcare professionals who are knowledgeable in the use of potent opioids for the management of chronic pain. Swallow cap whole, or sprinkle contents of cap on applesauce and swallow without chewing; crushing, dissolving, or chewing the pellets within the cap can cause rapid release and absorption of a potentially fatal dose. Accidental consumption, especially in children, can result in fatal overdose.

THERAPEUTIC CLASS: Opioid analgesic

INDICATIONS: Management of moderate to severe pain when a continuous, around-the-clock opioid analgesic is needed for an extended period of time.

DOSAGE: *Adults:* Individualize dose. Administer either q24h or q12h. Refer to PI for the factors to consider when selecting an initial dose. First Opioid Analgesic: Initial: Begin treatment using immediate-release (IR) formulation. Conversion from Other PO Morphine: Initial: Give 1/2 total daily dose q12h or total daily dose q24h. Conversion from Parenteral Morphine: 2-6mg may be required to provide analgesia equivalent to 1mg of parenteral. Dose approximately 3X the daily parenteral requirement is typically sufficient. Conversion from Other PO or Parenteral Opioids: Initial: Give 1/2 of the estimated daily requirement. Supplement with IR morphine. May give 1st dose with the last dose of any IR opioid. Titrate and Maint: Individually titrate to a dose that provides adequate analgesia and minimizes adverse reactions. May adjust dose every 1-2 days. Breakthrough pain: May require dose adjustment or rescue medication with appropriate dose of IR medication. If experiencing inadequate analgesia with qd dosing, consider bid regimen. If signs of excessive opioid-related adverse reactions observed, reduce next dose; adjust dose to obtain appropriate balance between pain management and opioid related adverse reactions. Discontinuation: Use gradual downward titration every 2-4 days; avoid abrupt discontinuation.

HOW SUPPLIED: Cap, Extended-Release (ER): 10mg, 20mg, 30mg, 40mg, 50mg, 60mg, 70mg, 80mg, 100mg, 130mg, 150mg, 200mg

CONTRAINDICATIONS: Significant respiratory depression, acute or severe bronchial asthma in an unmonitored setting or in the absence of resuscitative equipment, and known or suspected paralytic ileus.

WARNINGS/PRECAUTIONS: Not for use as PRN analgesic, for acute or mild pain, pain not expected to persist for an extended period of time, and postoperative pain unless the patient is already receiving chronic opioid therapy prior to surgery, or if postoperative pain is expected to be moderate to severe and persist for an extended period of time. 100mg, 130mg, 150mg, and 200mg caps are only for use in opioid-tolerant patients. Conversion to the same total daily dose of another ER morphine product may lead to either excessive sedation at peak or inadequate analgesia at trough; monitor patients closely when initiating therapy and adjust dose PRN. Respiratory depression is more likely to occur in elderly, cachectic, or debilitated patients; monitor closely when initiating and titrating, and when given with drugs that depress respiration. Monitor for respiratory depression and consider nonopioid analgesics in patients with chronic obstructive pulmonary disease (COPD) or cor pulmonale, and patients having a substantially decreased respiratory reserve, hypoxia, hypercapnia, or preexisting respiratory depression. May cause severe hypotension, including orthostatic hypotension and syncope, in ambulatory patients; monitor for signs of hypotension after dose initiation or titration. Avoid with circulatory shock, impaired consciousness, coma, or GI obstruction. Monitor for signs of sedation and respiratory depression in patients susceptible to the intracranial effects of carbon dioxide retention (eg, those with increased intracranial pressure [ICP] or brain tumors). May obscure clinical course in patients with head injury. May cause spasm of sphincter of Oddi and increase in serum amylase; monitor for worsening of symptoms in patients with biliary tract disease (eg, acute pancreatitis). May aggravate convulsions in patients with convulsive disorders and may induce or aggravate seizures; monitor for worsened seizure control in patients with history of seizure disorders. May impair mental/physical abilities.

ADVERSE REACTIONS: Respiratory depression, drowsiness, dizziness, constipation, nausea, anxiety, confusion, dry mouth, diarrhea, anorexia, pain, dyspnea, peripheral edema, abdominal pain, rash.

INTERACTIONS: CNS depressants (eg, sedatives, hypnotics, general anesthetics, antiemetics, phenothiazines, tranquilizers, anxiolytics, neuroleptics, other opioids, illicit drugs, alcohol) may increase the risk of respiratory depression, hypotension, profound sedation, or coma; reduce initial dose of 1 or both agents. Concomitant use of alcohol may result in increased plasma levels and potentially fatal overdose. Mixed agonist/antagonist analgesics (eg, pentazocine, nalbuphine, butorphanol) may reduce analgesic effect and/or precipitate withdrawal symptoms; avoid coadministration. May enhance neuromuscular blocking action and produce increased respiratory depression with skeletal muscle relaxants. MAOIs may potentiate effects of morphine; avoid use or within 14 days of MAOI use. Confusion and severe respiratory depression in a patient undergoing hemodialysis reported when concurrently administered with cimetidine. May reduce efficacy of diuretics. Anticholinergics or other drugs with anticholinergic activity may increase risk of urinary retention and/or severe constipation, which may lead to paralytic ileus. P-glycoprotein inhibitors (eg, quinidine) may increase absorption/exposure by about 2-fold; monitor for signs of respiratory and CNS depression.

PREGNANCY: Category C, not for use in nursing.

MECHANISM OF ACTION: Opioid analgesic; acts as a full agonist, binds with and activates opioid receptors at sites in the periaqueductal and periventricular grey matter, the ventromedial medulla, and the spinal cord to produce analgesia.

PHARMACOKINETICS: Absorption: Various doses resulted in different parameters. **Distribution:** V_d=3-4L/kg; plasma protein binding (30-35%); crosses placenta, found in breast milk. **Metabolism:** Liver via glucuronidation and sulfation; (metabolites) morphine-3-glucuronide (M3G, about 50%), morphine-6-glucuronide (M6G, about 5-15%), morphine-3-etheral sulfate. **Elimination:** Urine (mostly M3G and M6G, 10% unchanged); bile; feces (7-10%); $T_{1/2}$=11-13 hrs.

NURSING CONSIDERATIONS

Assessment: Assess for personal/family history or risk factors for drug abuse or addiction, general condition and medical status, opioid experience/tolerance, pain severity/type, previous opioid daily dose, potency, and any prior opioid used, respiratory depression, COPD or other respiratory complications, GI obstruction, paralytic ileus, renal/hepatic impairment, pregnancy/nursing status, possible drug interactions, and any other conditions where treatment is contraindicated or cautioned.

Monitoring: Monitor for signs/symptoms of respiratory depression, orthostatic hypotension, syncope, symptoms of worsening biliary tract disease, increase in ICP, aggravation/induction of seizures, tolerance, physical dependence, mental/physical impairment, withdrawal syndrome, and other adverse reactions. Monitor serum amylase levels. Routinely monitor for signs of misuse, abuse, and addiction. Periodically reassess the continued need of therapy.

Patient Counseling: Inform that the drug has potential for abuse; instruct not to share with others and to take steps to protect from theft or misuse. Discuss the risk of respiratory depression, orthostatic hypotension, and syncope. Advise to store drug securely; accidental exposure, especially in children, can result in serious harm/death. Instruct to dispose unused cap by flushing down the toilet. Inform about risks of concomitant use of alcohol and other CNS depressants; advise not to use such drugs unless supervised by physician. Instruct on how to properly take the medication. Inform that therapy may impair the ability to perform potentially hazardous activities (eg, driving or operating heavy machinery); advise not to perform such tasks until they know how they will react to the medication. Advise of the potential for severe constipation, including management instructions, how to recognize anaphylaxis, and when to seek medical attention. Inform females that drug can cause fetal harm; notify physician if pregnant/plan to become pregnant.

Administration: Oral route. Swallow cap whole. Do not crush, dissolve, or chew. Refer to PI for alternative methods of administration. **Storage:** 25°C (77°F); excursions permitted to 15-30°C (59-86°F). Protect from light and moisture.

KALETRA
RX

ritonavir - lopinavir (AbbVie)

THERAPEUTIC CLASS: Protease inhibitor

INDICATIONS: Treatment of HIV-1 infection in adults and pediatric patients (14 days and older) in combination with other antiretrovirals.

DOSAGE: *Adults:* 400mg-100mg bid. <3 Lopinavir Resistance-Associated Substitutions: 800mg-200mg qd. Concomitant Therapy with Efavirenz, Nevirapine, or Nelfinavir: (Tab) 500mg-125mg bid; (Sol) 533mg-133mg bid. Refer to PI for dosing modifications when used with certain concomitant therapies.
Pediatrics: 6 Months-18 Yrs: (Sol) ≥15-40kg: 10mg-2.5mg/kg bid. <15kg: 12mg-3mg/kg bid. Max: 400mg-100mg bid. (Tab) >35kg: 400mg-100mg bid. >25-35kg: 300mg-75mg bid. 15-25kg: 200mg-50mg bid. 14 Days-6 Months: (Sol) 16mg-4mg/kg bid. Concomitant Therapy with Efavirenz, Nevirapine, or Nelfinavir: Treatment-Naive and Treatment-Experienced: 6 Months-18 Yrs: (Sol) ≥15-45kg: 11mg-2.75mg/kg bid. <15kg: 13mg-3.25mg/kg bid. Max: 533mg-133mg bid. (Tab) >45kg: 500mg-125mg bid. >30-45kg: 400mg-100mg bid. >20-30kg: 300mg-75mg bid. 15-20kg: 200mg-50mg bid. Refer to PI for BSA-based dosing and for dosing modifications when used with certain concomitant therapies.

HOW SUPPLIED: (Lopinavir-Ritonavir) Sol: 80mg-20mg/mL [160mL]; Tab: 100mg-25mg, 200mg-50mg

CONTRAINDICATIONS: Coadministration with CYP3A substrates for which elevated plasma concentrations are associated with serious and/or life-threatening reactions and with potent CYP3A inducers where significantly reduced lopinavir levels may be associated with the potential for loss of virologic response and possible resistance and cross-resistance (eg, alfuzosin, rifampin, dihydroergotamine, ergotamine, methylergonovine, St. John's wort, cisapride, lovastatin, simvastatin, sildenafil [when used to treat pulmonary arterial HTN], pimozide, triazolam, oral midazolam).

WARNINGS/PRECAUTIONS: Avoid sol in preterm neonates in the immediate postnatal period; preterm neonates may be at increased risk of propylene glycol-associated adverse events and other toxicities. Pancreatitis, including marked TG elevations, reported; evaluate and suspend therapy if clinically appropriate. Patients with underlying hepatitis B or C or marked serum transaminase elevations prior to treatment may be at increased risk for developing or worsening of transaminase elevations or hepatic decompensation; conduct appropriate lab testing prior to therapy and monitor closely during treatment. New onset or exacerbation of diabetes mellitus (DM), hyperglycemia, diabetic ketoacidosis, immune reconstitution syndrome, autoimmune disorders (eg, Graves' disease, polymyositis, Guillain-Barre syndrome) in the setting of immune reconstitution, redistribution/accumulation of body fat, lipid elevations, and increased bleeding with hemophilia A and B reported. PR and QT interval prolongation, torsades de pointes, and cases of 2nd- and 3rd-degree atrioventricular block reported; caution with underlying structural heart disease, preexisting conduction system abnormalities, ischemic heart disease, or cardiomyopathies. Avoid use with congenital long QT syndrome or hypokalemia and with other drugs that prolong QT interval. Once daily regimen not recommended for adults with ≥3 lopinavir resistance-associated substitutions or in pediatric patients <18 yrs. Caution with hepatic impairment and in elderly.

ADVERSE REACTIONS: Diarrhea, N/V, hypertriglyceridemia and hypercholesterolemia, dysgeusia, rash, decreased weight, insomnia.

INTERACTIONS: See Contraindications. Caution with drugs that prolong the PR interval (eg, calcium channel blockers [CCBs], β-adrenergic blockers, digoxin, atazanavir). Avoid with colchicine in patients with renal/hepatic impairment, tadalafil during initiation, tipranavir/ritonavir combination, and drugs that prolong the QT interval. Not recommended with voriconazole, high doses of itraconazole or ketoconazole, boceprevir, telaprevir, avanafil, and salmeterol. Not recommended with fluticasone or other glucocorticoids that are metabolized by CYP3A unless benefit outweighs the risk of systemic corticosteroid effects. Cushing's syndrome and adrenal suppression reported with budesonide and fluticasone propionate. May increase levels of CYP3A substrates, colchicine, fentanyl, tenofovir, indinavir, nelfinavir, saquinavir, maraviroc, antiarrhythmics, vincristine, vinblastine, dasatinib, nilotinib, trazodone, itraconazole, ketoconazole, rifabutin and rifabutin metabolite, clarithromycin in patients with renal impairment, IV midazolam, dihydropyridine CCB, bosentan, atorvastatin, rosuvastatin, immunosuppressants, salmeterol, rivaroxaban, glucocorticoids, sildenafil, tadalafil, and vardenafil. May decrease levels of methadone, phenytoin, bupropion, atovaquone, ethinyl estradiol, abacavir, zidovudine, lamotrigine, valproate, voriconazole, boceprevir, and amprenavir. Delavirdine and CYP3A inhibitors may increase levels. May alter concentrations of warfarin; monitor INR. Efavirenz, nevirapine, nelfinavir, carbamazepine, phenobarbital, and phenytoin may decrease levels; not for qd dosing regimen. Rifampin, fosamprenavir/ritonavir, systemic corticosteroids, and CYP3A inducers may decrease levels. May require initiation or dose adjustments of insulin or PO hypoglycemics for treatment of DM. (Sol) Contains alcohol; may produce disulfiram-like reactions with disulfiram or metronidazole. Didanosine should be given 1 hr before or 2 hrs after sol. Refer to PI for further information and dosing modifications when used with certain concomitant therapies.

PREGNANCY: Category C, not for use in nursing.

MECHANISM OF ACTION: Lopinavir: HIV-1 protease inhibitor; prevents cleavage of the Gag-Pol polyprotein, resulting in the production of immature, noninfectious viral particles. Ritonavir: HIV-1 protease inhibitor; CYP3A inhibitor that inhibits metabolism of lopinavir, increasing its plasma levels.

PHARMACOKINETICS: Absorption: Lopinavir: (400mg-100mg bid) C_{max}=9.8μg/mL, T_{max}=4 hrs, AUC=92.6μg•h/mL. Refer to PI for pediatric parameters. **Distribution:** Lopinavir: Plasma protein binding (98-99%). **Metabolism:** Lopinavir: Hepatic via CYP3A (extensive). Ritonavir: Induces own metabolism. **Elimination:** Unchanged lopinavir: Urine (2.2%), feces (19.8%).

NURSING CONSIDERATIONS

Assessment: Assess for history of hypersensitivity reactions, history of pancreatitis, hepatitis B or C, cirrhosis, DM or hyperglycemia, dyslipidemia, hemophilia type A or B, structural heart disease, preexisting conduction system abnormalities, ischemic heart disease or cardiomyopathies, congenital long QT syndrome, hypokalemia, renal/hepatic impairment, pregnancy/nursing status, and for possible drug interactions. Assess children for the ability to swallow intact tab.

Monitoring: Monitor for signs/symptoms of pancreatitis, hyperglycemia, hepatic dysfunction, immune reconstitution syndrome, autoimmune disorders, fat redistribution/accumulation, hypersensitivity reactions, and other adverse reactions. Monitor lipid profile, glucose levels, total bilirubin levels, ECG changes, serum lipase levels, and serum amylase levels. Monitor infants for increase in serum osmolality, SrCr, and other toxicities.

Patient Counseling: Instruct to take prescribed dose ud. Advise to inform physician if weight changes in children occur. Inform that if a dose is missed, take dose as soon as possible and return to normal schedule; instruct not to double the next dose. Advise that therapy is not a cure for HIV; opportunistic infections may still occur. Instruct to avoid doing things that can spread HIV-1 infection to others. Instruct not to have any kind of sex without protection; inform to always practice safe sex by using a latex or polyurethane condom to lower the chance of sexual contact with semen, vaginal secretions, or blood. Instruct to notify physician if using other prescription/OTC or herbal products, particularly St. John's wort. Inform that skin rashes, liver function changes, ECG changes, redistribution/accumulation of body fat, new onset or worsening of preexisting diabetes, and hyperglycemia may occur. Instruct to seek medical attention if symptoms of worsening liver disease (eg, loss of appetite, abdominal pain, jaundice, itchy skin), dizziness, abnormal heart rhythm, loss of consciousness, or any other adverse reactions develop.

Administration: Oral route. (Sol) Take with food. (Tab) Take with or without food. Swallow tabs whole; do not crush, break, or chew. **Storage:** (Tab) 20-25°C (68-77°F); excursions permitted to 15-30°C (59-86°F). (Sol) 2-8°C (36-46°F). Avoid exposure to excessive heat. If stored at room temperature up to 25°C (77°F), sol should be used within 2 months.

KALYDECO

RX

ivacaftor (Vertex)

THERAPEUTIC CLASS: CFTR potentiator

INDICATIONS: Treatment of cystic fibrosis (CF) in patients ≥6 yrs of age who have one of the following mutations in the cystic fibrosis transmembrane conductance regulator (*CFTR*) gene: *G551D, G1244E, G1349D, G178R, G551S, S1251N, S1255P, S549N,* or *S549R.*

DOSAGE: *Adults:* Usual: 150mg q12h. Moderate Hepatic Impairment (Child-Pugh Class B): 150mg qd. Severe Hepatic Impairment (Child-Pugh Class C): 150mg qd or less frequently. Concomitant Strong CYP3A Inhibitors (eg, ketoconazole): 150mg 2X/week. Concomitant Moderate CYP3A Inhibitors (eg, fluconazole): 150mg qd. Take with fat-containing food.
Pediatrics: ≥6 Yrs: Usual: 150mg q12h. Moderate Hepatic Impairment (Child-Pugh Class B): 150mg qd. Severe Hepatic Impairment (Child-Pugh Class C): 150mg qd or less frequently. Concomitant Strong CYP3A Inhibitors (eg, ketoconazole): 150mg 2X/week. Concomitant Moderate CYP3A Inhibitors (eg, fluconazole): 150mg qd. Take with fat-containing food.

HOW SUPPLIED: Tab: 150mg

WARNINGS/PRECAUTIONS: Elevated transaminases reported. Monitor closely if increased transaminase levels develop until abnormalities resolve and interrupt dosing with ALT or AST >5X ULN; consider benefits and risks of resuming dosing. Caution with severe hepatic impairment, severe renal impairment (CrCl ≤30mL/min), or end-stage renal disease. Use FDA-cleared CF mutation test to detect the presence of *CFTR* mutation followed by verification with bidirectional sequencing when recommended by the mutation test instructions for use. Not effective in patients with CF who are homozygous for the *F508del* mutation in the *CFTR* gene.

ADVERSE REACTIONS: Headache, oropharyngeal pain, upper respiratory tract infection, nasal congestion, abdominal pain, nasopharyngitis, diarrhea, rash, nausea, dizziness, rhinitis, arthralgia, bacteria in sputum, wheezing, acne.

INTERACTIONS: Not recommended with strong CYP3A inducers (eg, rifampin, rifabutin, phenobarbital, carbamazepine, phenytoin, St. John's wort); these drugs may substantially decrease exposure, which may reduce therapeutic effectiveness of therapy. Strong CYP3A inhibitors (eg, ketoconazole, itraconazole, posaconazole, voriconazole, telithromycin, clarithromycin), moderate CYP3A inhibitors (eg, fluconazole, erythromycin), and grapefruit juice may increase levels. Avoid food containing grapefruit or Seville oranges. May increase levels of CYP3A substrates (eg, midazolam) and CYP3A and/or P-glycoprotein substrates (eg, digoxin, cyclosporine, tacrolimus); use with caution and monitor appropriately.

PREGNANCY: Category B, caution in nursing.

MECHANISM OF ACTION: CFTR potentiator; facilitates increased chloride transport by potentiating the channel-open probability (or gating) of the CFTR protein.

PHARMACOKINETICS: Absorption: C_{max}=768ng/mL, AUC=10,600ng•hr/mL, T_{max}=4 hrs. **Distribution:** V_d=353L; plasma protein binding (99%). **Metabolism:** Extensive via CYP3A; M1 and M6 (major metabolites). **Elimination:** Feces (87.8%, 65% metabolites), urine; $T_{1/2}$=12 hrs.

NURSING CONSIDERATIONS

Assessment: Assess for renal/hepatic impairment, patients who are homozygous for the *F508del* mutation in the *CFTR* gene, other populations with CF, pregnancy/nursing status, and possible drug interactions. If genotype is unknown, perform FDA-cleared CF mutation test to detect the presence of the *CFTR* mutation followed by verification with bidirectional sequencing when recommended by the mutation test instructions for use.

Monitoring: Monitor ALT/AST levels every 3 months during the 1st year of therapy and annually thereafter. Monitor for other adverse reactions.

Patient Counseling: Inform that elevation in liver tests have occurred and LFTs will be performed prior to initiating therapy, every 3 months during the 1st year, and annually thereafter. Instruct to inform physician of all the medications patients are taking, including any herbal supplements or vitamins. Instruct to avoid food containing grapefruit or Seville oranges. Counsel that the drug is best absorbed when taken with fat-containing food, such as eggs, butter, peanut butter, or cheese pizza.

Administration: Oral route. Take with fat-containing food. **Storage:** 20-25°C (68-77°F); excursions permitted to 15-30°C (59-86°F).

KAPVAY

RX

clonidine HCl (Shionogi)

THERAPEUTIC CLASS: Alpha₂-agonist

INDICATIONS: Treatment of attention-deficit hyperactivity disorder as monotherapy and as adjunctive therapy to stimulant medications.

DOSAGE: *Pediatrics:* 6-17 Yrs: Individualize dose. Initial: 0.1mg at hs. Titrate: Adjust in increments of 0.1mg/day at weekly intervals until desired response is achieved. Doses should be taken bid, with either an equal or higher split dosage being given at hs. Refer to PI for dosing guidance. Max: 0.4mg/day. Maint: Periodically reevaluate the long-term usefulness for individual patient. Concomitant Psychostimulant: Adjust psychostimulant dose depending on response to clonidine. Renal Impairment: Give initial dosage based on degree of impairment. Titrate to higher doses cautiously. Discontinuation: Taper total daily dose in decrements of no more than 0.1mg every 3-7 days.

HOW SUPPLIED: Tab, Extended-Release: 0.1mg, 0.2mg

WARNINGS/PRECAUTIONS: Not intended for use in patients who exhibit symptoms secondary to environmental factors and/or other primary psychiatric disorders (eg, psychosis). Not interchangeable with the immediate-release formulation. Substitution for other clonidine products on mg-per-mg basis is not recommended. May cause dose-related decreases in BP and HR; measure HR and BP prior to initiation of therapy, following dose increases, and periodically while on therapy. Uptitrate slowly in patients with history of hypotension and those with underlying conditions that may be worsened by hypotension and bradycardia (eg, heart block, bradycardia, cardiovascular/vascular/cerebrovascular disease, chronic renal failure). Caution with a history of syncope or with a condition that predisposes to syncope (eg, hypotension, orthostatic hypotension, bradycardia, dehydration). Avoid becoming dehydrated or overheated. Somnolence and sedation reported. May impair mental/physical abilities. Gradually reduce dose when discontinuing. May elicit allergic reactions (eg, generalized rash, urticaria, angioedema) in patients who develop an allergic reaction from clonidine transdermal system. May worsen sinus node dysfunction and atrioventricular block; uptitrate slowly and monitor vital signs frequently in patients with cardiac conduction abnormalities.

ADVERSE REACTIONS: Somnolence, fatigue, upper respiratory tract infection, nausea, dizziness, nasal congestion, nightmare, throat pain, nasopharyngitis, insomnia, emotional disorder, headache, upper abdominal pain, irritability.

INTERACTIONS: May potentiate the CNS-depressive effects of alcohol, barbiturates, or other sedating drugs; avoid with alcohol. Decreased hypotensive effects with TCAs. Caution with agents known to affect sinus node function or atrioventricular nodal conduction (eg, digitalis, calcium channel blockers, β-blockers), antihypertensives, or other drugs that can reduce BP or HR or increase the risk of syncope. Avoid with other products containing clonidine. Consider the potential for additive sedative effects with other centrally active depressants (eg, phenothiazines, barbiturates, benzodiazepines). Uptitrate slowly and monitor vital signs frequently with other sympatholytics.

PREGNANCY: Category C, caution in nursing.

MECHANISM OF ACTION: α_2-agonist; not established. Stimulates α_2-adrenergic receptors in the brain.

PHARMACOKINETICS: Absorption: (Adults) C_{max}=235pg/mL (fed), 258pg/mL (fasted); AUC=6505pg•hr/mL (fed), 6729pg•hr/mL (fasted); T_{max}=6.80 hrs (fed), 6.50 hrs (fasted). **Distribution:** Found in breast milk. **Elimination:** (Adults) $T_{1/2}$=12.67 hrs (fed), 12.65 hrs (fasted).

NURSING CONSIDERATIONS

Assessment: Assess for drug hypersensitivity, history of hypotension, underlying conditions that may be worsened by hypotension and bradycardia, history of syncope or conditions that predispose to syncope, cardiac conduction abnormalities, renal dysfunction, pregnancy/nursing status, and for possible drug interactions. Obtain baseline HR and BP.

Monitoring: Monitor for somnolence, sedation, hypotension, bradycardia, allergic reactions, dehydration, overheating, and for other adverse reactions. Monitor BP and HR following dose increases and periodically while on therapy. Monitor vital signs frequently in patients with cardiac conduction abnormalities.

Patient Counseling: Inform about risks and benefits of therapy. Advise not to d/c abruptly and not to d/c therapy without consulting the physician. Advise patients who developed an allergic reaction from clonidine transdermal system that substitution of oral clonidine may also elicit an allergic reaction. Instruct to take ud. Advise to consult a physician if pregnant, nursing, or thinking of becoming pregnant while on therapy. If a dose is missed, instruct to skip the dose and take the next dose as scheduled; advise not to take more than the prescribed total daily amount in any 24-hr period. Advise to use caution when driving or operating hazardous machinery until they know how they will respond to treatment.

Administration: Oral route. Take with or without food. Swallow tab whole; do not crush, cut, or chew. **Storage:** 20-25°C (68-77°F).

KAZANO   RX
metformin HCl - alogliptin (Takeda)

> Lactic acidosis may occur due to metformin accumulation; risk increases with conditions such as sepsis, dehydration, excess alcohol intake, hepatic impairment, renal impairment, and acute congestive heart failure (CHF). If acidosis is suspected, d/c therapy and hospitalize patient immediately.

THERAPEUTIC CLASS: Biguanide/dipeptidyl peptidase-4 inhibitor

INDICATIONS: Adjunct to diet and exercise to improve glycemic control in adults with type 2 diabetes mellitus (DM) when treatment with both alogliptin and metformin is appropriate.

DOSAGE: *Adults:* Individualize dose. Take bid with food, with gradual dose escalation to reduce GI side effects of metformin. May adjust dose based on effectiveness and tolerability. Max: 25mg-2000mg/day.

HOW SUPPLIED: Tab: (Alogliptin-Metformin) 12.5mg-500mg, 12.5mg-1000mg

CONTRAINDICATIONS: Renal impairment (eg, SrCr ≥1.5mg/dL [men], ≥1.4mg/dL [women], or abnormal CrCl), acute or chronic metabolic acidosis, including diabetic ketoacidosis.

WARNINGS/PRECAUTIONS: Not for use in type 1 DM or for treatment of diabetic ketoacidosis. Acute pancreatitis reported; d/c if suspected and initiate appropriate management. Serious hypersensitivity reactions reported; d/c if suspected, assess for other potential causes, and institute alternative treatment for DM. Caution with history of angioedema to another dipeptidyl peptidase-4 (DPP-4) inhibitor. Fatal and nonfatal hepatic failure reported; interrupt therapy and investigate probable cause if liver enzymes are significantly elevated or if abnormal LFTs persist/worsen, and do not restart without another explanation for the liver tests abnormalities. Avoid in patients with clinical or lab evidence of hepatic disease. D/C if evidence of renal impairment is present and do not initiate in patients ≥80 yrs of age unless renal function is normal. Temporarily d/c at time of or prior to radiologic studies involving intravascular iodinated contrast materials, withhold for 48 hrs subsequent to the procedure, and reinstitute only if renal function is normal. Suspend temporarily for any surgical procedure (except minor procedures not associated with restricted food and fluid intake); restart when oral intake is resumed and renal function is normal. D/C in hypoxic states (eg, acute CHF, shock, acute myocardial infarction). May decrease vitamin B12 levels; monitor hematologic parameters annually. Caution in patients susceptible to hypoglycemic effects, such as elderly, debilitated/malnourished patients, and those with adrenal/pituitary insufficiency or alcohol intoxication. No conclusive evidence of macrovascular risk reduction.

ADVERSE REACTIONS: Lactic acidosis, upper respiratory tract infection, nasopharyngitis, diarrhea, HTN, headache, back pain, urinary tract infection, hypoglycemia.

INTERACTIONS: Topiramate or other carbonic anhydrase inhibitors (eg, zonisamide, acetazolamide, dichlorphenamide) may induce metabolic acidosis; use with caution. Hypoglycemia may occur with other glucose-lowering agents (eg, sulfonylureas, insulin) or ethanol; may require lower doses of sulfonylureas or insulin. Metformin: Cationic drugs that are eliminated by renal tubular secretion (eg, cimetidine, amiloride, digoxin, morphine, procainamide, quinidine, quinine, ranitidine, triamterene, trimethoprim, vancomycin) may potentially produce an interaction; monitor and adjust dose. Observe for loss of glycemic control with thiazides and other diuretics, corticosteroids, phenothiazines, thyroid products, estrogens, oral contraceptives, phenytoin, nicotinic acid, sympathomimetics, calcium channel blockers, and isoniazid. Alcohol may potentiate effect of metformin on lactate metabolism; avoid excessive alcohol intake. Caution with drugs that may affect renal function or result in significant hemodynamic change or may interfere with the disposition of metformin (eg, cationic drugs eliminated by renal tubular secretion). Hypoglycemia may be difficult to recognize with β-adrenergic blocking drugs.

PREGNANCY: Category B, caution in nursing.

MECHANISM OF ACTION: Alogliptin: DPP-4 inhibitor; slows inactivation of incretin hormones, thereby increasing their bloodstream concentrations and reducing fasting and postprandial glucose concentrations in a glucose-dependent manner. Metformin: Biguanide; decreases hepatic glucose production, decreases intestinal absorption of glucose, and improves insulin sensitivity by increasing peripheral glucose uptake and utilization.

PHARMACOKINETICS: Absorption: Alogliptin: Absolute bioavailability (100%). Metformin: Absolute bioavailability (50-60%) (fasting). **Distribution:** Alogliptin: V_d=417L (IV); plasma protein binding (20%). Metformin: V_d=654L. **Metabolism:** Alogliptin: Via CYP3A4 and CYP2D6; N-demethylated alogliptin, M-I (active metabolite) and N-acetylated alogliptin, M-II. **Elimination:** Alogliptin: Feces (13%), urine (60-71% unchanged). Metformin: Urine (90%); $T_{1/2}$=6.2 hrs (plasma), 17.6 hrs (blood).

NURSING CONSIDERATIONS

Assessment: Assess for metabolic acidosis, risk factors for lactic acidosis, renal/hepatic impairment, previous hypersensitivity to the drug, history of pancreatitis, inadequate vitamin B12 or calcium absorption, type of DM, diabetic ketoacidosis, history of angioedema with another DPP-4 inhibitor, pregnancy/nursing status, and possible drug interactions. Assess if patient is planning to undergo any surgical procedure. Obtain baseline FPG, HbA1c, and hematologic parameters.

Monitoring: Monitor for lactic acidosis, pancreatitis, hypoxic states, decreases in vitamin B12 levels, and hypersensitivity reactions. Monitor renal function, especially in patients in whom development of renal dysfunction is anticipated, at least annually. Monitor FPG, HbA1c, hepatic function, and hematologic parameters periodically.

Patient Counseling: Inform of risks and benefits of therapy. Advise of the risk of lactic acidosis; instruct to d/c therapy immediately and contact physician if unexplained hyperventilation, myalgia, malaise, unusual somnolence, or other nonspecific symptoms occur. Counsel against excessive alcohol intake. Inform that GI symptoms, acute pancreatitis, and hypoglycemia may occur. Advise to d/c and seek medical advice if signs/symptoms of allergic reactions, liver injury, or persistent severe abdominal pain occur. Inform about the importance of regular testing of renal function and hematological parameters during treatment. Counsel to inform physician if any unusual symptom develops, or if any known symptom persists or worsens. Instruct to take ud.

Administration: Oral route. Do not split tab before swallowing. **Storage:** 25°C (77°F); excursions permitted to 15-30°C (59-86°F). Keep container tightly closed.

KEPPRA XR
levetiracetam (UCB)

RX

THERAPEUTIC CLASS: Pyrrolidine derivative

INDICATIONS: Adjunct therapy in the treatment of partial onset seizures in patients ≥16 yrs of age with epilepsy.

DOSAGE: *Adults:* Initial: 1000mg qd. Titrate: Adjust dose in increments of 1000mg/day every 2 weeks. Max: 3000mg/day. Renal Impairment: Individualize dose. CrCl 50-80mL/min: 1000-2000mg q24h. CrCl 30-50mL/min: 500-1500mg q24h. CrCl <30mL/min: 500-1000mg q24h. End-Stage Renal Disease on Dialysis: Use immediate-release formulation.
Pediatrics: ≥16 Yrs: Initial: 1000mg qd. Titrate: Adjust dose in increments of 1000mg/day every 2 weeks. Max: 3000mg/day.

HOW SUPPLIED: Tab, Extended-Release: 500mg, 750mg

WARNINGS/PRECAUTIONS: Increased risk of suicidal thoughts or behavior. May cause behavioral abnormalities, somnolence, fatigue, and coordination difficulties. May impair mental/physical abilities. Serious dermatological reactions (eg, Stevens-Johnson syndrome [SJS], toxic epidermal necrolysis [TEN]) reported. Recurrence of serious skin reactions following rechallenge reported; d/c at the 1st sign of rash, unless the rash is clearly not drug-related. If signs/symptoms suggest SJS/TEN, do not resume therapy and consider alternative therapy. Withdraw gradually to minimize the potential of increased seizure frequency. Hematologic abnormalities may occur. Physiological changes may decrease plasma levels throughout pregnancy; monitor carefully during pregnancy and through the postpartum period especially if the dose was changed during pregnancy. Caution with renal impairment and in elderly.

ADVERSE REACTIONS: Nausea, influenza, nasopharyngitis, somnolence, dizziness, irritability.

PREGNANCY: Category C, not for use in nursing.

MECHANISM OF ACTION: Pyrrolidine derivative; not established. Inhibits burst firing without affecting normal neuronal excitability, suggesting that it may selectively prevent hypersynchronization of epileptiform burst firing and propagation of seizure activity.

PHARMACOKINETICS: Absorption: Almost complete; T_{max}=4 hrs. **Distribution:** Plasma protein binding (<10%); found in breast milk. **Metabolism:** Enzymatic hydrolysis of acetamide group; ucb L057 (metabolite). **Elimination:** Renal (66%, unchanged); $T_{1/2}$=7 hrs.

NURSING CONSIDERATIONS

Assessment: Assess for renal impairment, depression, and pregnancy/nursing status.

Monitoring: Monitor for emergence or worsening of depression, suicidal thoughts or behavior, and/or any unusual changes in mood or behavior, psychiatric reactions, somnolence and fatigue, coordination difficulties, serious dermatological reactions, and other adverse reactions. Monitor for hematologic abnormalities.

Patient Counseling: Inform that the drug may increase the risk of suicidal thoughts or behavior; instruct to report immediately to physician for the emergence or worsening of symptoms of depression, any unusual changes in mood/behavior, or suicidal thoughts, behavior, or thoughts about self-harm. Counsel that medication may cause changes in behavior (eg, irritability and aggression). Instruct to only take as prescribed. Inform that dizziness and somnolence may occur; advise not to drive or operate heavy machinery or engage in other hazardous activities until they have gained sufficient experience to gauge whether it adversely affects their performance of these activities. Advise that serious dermatological adverse reactions may occur; instruct to notify physician immediately if rash develops. Advise to notify physician if patient becomes pregnant or intends to become pregnant; encourage to enroll in the North American Antiepileptic Drug pregnancy registry.

Administration: Oral route. Swallow tabs whole; do not chew, break, or crush. **Storage:** 25°C (77°F); excursions permitted to 15-30°C (59-86°F).

KETEK   RX
telithromycin (Sanofi-Aventis)

> Contraindicated with myasthenia gravis. Fatal and life-threatening respiratory failure in patients with myasthenia gravis reported.

THERAPEUTIC CLASS: Ketolide antibiotic

INDICATIONS: Treatment of mild to moderate community-acquired pneumonia (CAP) due to susceptible strains of microorganisms in for patients ≥18 yrs of age.

DOSAGE: *Adults:* 800mg qd for 7-10 days. Severe Renal Impairment (CrCl <30mL/min): 600mg qd. Hemodialysis: 600mg qd, given after dialysis session on dialysis days. Severe Renal Impairment (CrCl <30mL/min) with Hepatic Impairment: 400mg qd.

HOW SUPPLIED: Tab: 300mg, 400mg

CONTRAINDICATIONS: Myasthenia gravis, history of hepatitis and/or jaundice associated with use of telithromycin or any macrolide antibiotic, hypersensitivity to macrolide antibiotics, concomitant use with cisapride or pimozide, and concomitant use with colchicine in patients with renal or hepatic impairment.

WARNINGS/PRECAUTIONS: Acute hepatic failure and severe liver injury, including fulminant hepatitis and hepatic necrosis, reported; monitor closely and d/c if any signs/symptoms of hepatitis occur. Permanently d/c if hepatitis or transaminase elevations combined with systemic symptoms occur. May prolong QTc interval leading to risk for ventricular arrhythmias, including torsades de pointes; avoid in patients with congenital prolongation of QTc interval, with ongoing proarrhythmic conditions (eg, uncorrected hypokalemia/hypomagnesemia), and in clinically significant bradycardia. Visual disturbances and loss of consciousness reported; minimize hazardous activities, such as driving and operating heavy machinery. *Clostridium difficile*-associated diarrhea (CDAD) reported. May result in bacterial resistance with prolonged use or use in the absence of a proven/suspected bacterial infection or a prophylactic indication; take appropriate measures if superinfection develops.

ADVERSE REACTIONS: Diarrhea, nausea, headache, dizziness.

INTERACTIONS: See Contraindications. Avoid with simvastatin, lovastatin, atorvastatin, rifampin, ergot alkaloid derivatives (eg, ergotamine, dihydroergotamine), Class IA (eg, quinidine, procainamide) or Class III (eg, dofetilide) antiarrhythmics. May increase levels of theophylline, midazolam, digoxin, simvastatin, metoprolol, levonorgestrel, substrates of OATP1 (B1, B3) family members, drugs metabolized by the CYP450 system (eg, cyclosporine, tacrolimus, sirolimus, hexobarbital), especially CYP3A4. May decrease levels of sotalol. Itraconazole and ketoconazole may increase levels. CYP3A4 inducers (eg, phenytoin, carbamazepine, phenobarbital, rifampin) may decrease levels. May potentiate effects of oral anticoagulants. Theophylline may worsen GI effects; take 1 hr apart from therapy. May cause hypotension, bradyarrhythmia, and loss of consciousness with calcium channel blockers metabolized by CYP3A4 (eg, verapamil, amlodipine, diltiazem). High levels of HMG-CoA reductase inhibitors increase risk of myopathy and rhabdomyolysis; monitor for signs and symptoms. Caution with benzodiazepines metabolized by CYP3A4 (eg, triazolam) and metoprolol in patients with heart failure.

PREGNANCY: Category C, caution in nursing.

MECHANISM OF ACTION: Ketolide antibiotic; blocks protein synthesis by binding to domains II and V of 23S rRNA of 50S ribosomal subunit and may also inhibit assembly of nascent ribosomal units.

PHARMACOKINETICS: Absorption: Absolute bioavailability (57%); C_{max}=1.9mcg/mL (single dose), 2.27mcg/mL (multiple dose); T_{max}=1 hr; $AUC_{(0-24)}$=8.25mcg•hr/mL (single dose), 12.5mcg•hr/mL (multiple dose). **Distribution:** V_d=2.9L/kg; plasma protein binding (60-70%). **Metabolism:** Via CYP3A4 dependent and independent pathways. **Elimination:** Urine (13% unchanged); feces (7% unchanged); $T_{1/2}$=7.16 hrs (single dose), 9.81 hrs (multiple dose).

NURSING CONSIDERATIONS

Assessment: Assess for myasthenia gravis, history of hepatitis and/or jaundice, previous hypersensitivity to telithromycin or macrolides, renal/hepatic impairment, LFTs, QTc prolongation risk (eg, congenital prolongation, proarrhythmic conditions, significant bradycardia), pregnancy/nursing status, and possible drug interactions. Perform culture and susceptibility testing.

Monitoring: Monitor LFTs and ECG for QTc prolongation. Monitor for visual disturbances, hepatitis, loss of consciousness associated with vagal syndrome, renal impairment, CDAD, pancreatitis, and allergic reactions (eg, angioedema, anaphylaxis).

Patient Counseling: Inform that therapy treats bacterial, not viral, infections. Advise against operating machinery or driving and inform to seek physician's advice if visual difficulties (eg, blurred vision, difficulty focusing, objects looking doubled), loss of consciousness, confusion, or hallucination is experienced. Advise that therapy is contraindicated with myasthenia gravis. Instruct to d/c and seek medical attention if signs and symptoms of liver injury develop (eg, nausea, fatigue, anorexia, jaundice, dark urine, light colored stools, pruritus, tender abdomen). Instruct to report any fainting during therapy and to inform physician of history of QTc prolongation, proarrhythmic conditions, or significant bradycardia. Advise to take ud; skipping doses or not completing full course may decrease effectiveness and increase antibiotic resistance. Advise to contact physician if diarrhea (watery/bloody stools) occurs. Advise to inform physician of any other medications taken concurrently with telithromycin.

Administration: Oral route. May give with or without food. **Storage:** 25°C (77°F); excursions permitted to 15-30°C (59-86°F).

KETOCONAZOLE TABLETS   RX
ketoconazole (Various)

> Serious hepatotoxicity, including cases with a fatal outcome or requiring liver transplantation, reported; monitor closely. Contraindicated with dofetilide, quinidine, pimozide, and cisapride; may cause elevated levels of these drugs and may prolong QT intervals, sometimes resulting in life-threatening ventricular dysrhythmias (eg, torsades de pointes). Should be used only when other effective antifungal therapy is not available or tolerated and potential benefits outweigh potential risks.

THERAPEUTIC CLASS: Azole antifungal

INDICATIONS: Treatment of the following systemic fungal infections in patients who have failed or who are intolerant to other therapies: blastomycosis, coccidioidomycosis, histoplasmosis, chromomycosis, and paracoccidioidomycosis.

DOSAGE: *Adults:* Initial: 200mg qd. Titrate: May be increased to 400mg qd if clinical responsiveness is insufficient within the expected time. Maint: Continue treatment until infection has subsided. Usual Duration: 6 months.
Pediatrics: >2 Yrs: 3.3-6.6mg/kg qd. Maint: Continue treatment until infection has subsided. Usual Duration: 6 months. Should not be used in pediatric patients unless the potential benefit outweighs the risks.

HOW SUPPLIED: Tab: 200mg* *scored

CONTRAINDICATIONS: Coadministration of CYP3A4 substrates. Acute or chronic liver disease.

WARNINGS/PRECAUTIONS: Cases of hepatitis reported in children. Monitor ALT weekly during treatment; interrupt therapy and obtain a full set of liver tests if ALT values increase to a level above the ULN or 30% above baseline, or if symptoms develop. Repeat liver tests to ensure normalization of values. Monitor frequently to detect any recurring liver injury, if oral ketoconazole is restarted. May prolong the QT interval. May decrease adrenal corticosteroid secretion at doses ≥400mg; do not exceed the recommended daily dose of 200-400mg. Monitor adrenal function in patients with adrenal insufficiency or with borderline adrenal function and in patients under prolonged periods of stress (eg, major surgery, intensive care). Not approved for treatment of advanced prostate cancer and Cushing's syndrome. Anaphylaxis and hypersensitivity reactions, including urticaria, reported. May lower serum testosterone levels. Penetrates poorly into the CSF; should not be used for fungal meningitis.

ADVERSE REACTIONS: Hepatotoxicity, anaphylactoid reaction, gynecomastia, anorexia, insomnia, headache, photophobia, orthostatic hypotension, epistaxis, N/V, abdominal pain, pruritus, myalgia, asthenia, thrombocytopenia.

INTERACTIONS: See Boxed Warning and Contraindications. Avoid with potentially hepatotoxic drugs. May elevate levels and potentiate/prolong hypnotic and sedative effects of alprazolam, oral midazolam, or oral triazolam, especially with repeated or chronic administration of these drugs; concomitant administration is contraindicated. Caution with parenteral midazolam; may prolong sedative effect. Not recommended with CYP3A4 inducers. Significantly increases systemic exposure of eplerenone, ergot alkaloids (eg, ergotamine, dihydroergotamine), and nisoldipine; concomitant administration is contraindicated. Increases systemic exposure of alfentanil, fentanyl, sufentanil, amlodipine, felodipine, nicardipine, nifedipine, bosentan, buspirone, busulfan, carbamazepine, cilostazol, cyclosporine, digoxin, docetaxel, paclitaxel, indinavir, saquinavir, methylprednisolone, oral anti-coagulants, rifabutin, sildenafil, sirolimus (coadministration not recommended), tacrolimus, telithromycin, tolterodine, trimetrexate, verapamil, and vinca alkaloids (eg, vincristine, vinblastine, vinorelbine); careful monitoring with possible dose adjustment of these drugs may be needed. Reduced systemic exposure with carbamazepine, gastric acid suppressants (eg, antacids, antimuscarinics, histamine H_2-blockers, proton pump inhibitors [eg, omeprazole, lansoprazole], sucralfate), nevirapine, phenytoin, rifampin, rifabutin, and isoniazid; concomitant use is not recommended. Increased systemic exposure with ritonavir; consider dose reduction of ketoconazole. May cause severe hypoglycemia with oral hypoglycemic agents. Disulfiram-like reactions to alcohol reported; avoid alcohol consumption while on treatment. Coadministration with CYP3A4-metabolized HMG-CoA reductase inhibitors (eg, simvastatin, lovastatin) may increase risk of skeletal muscle toxicity (eg, rhabdomyolysis); concomitant administration is contraindicated. May increase exposure and levels of loratadine. Refer to PI for further information on drug interactions.

PREGNANCY: Category C, not for use in nursing.

MECHANISM OF ACTION: Azole antifungal; blocks the synthesis of ergosterol, a key component of fungal cell membrane, through the inhibition of CYP450 dependent enzyme lanosterol 14α-demethylase responsible for the conversion of lanosterol to ergosterol in the fungal cell membrane.

PHARMACOKINETICS: Absorption: C_{max}=3.5mcg/mL; T_{max}=1-2 hrs. **Distribution:** Plasma protein binding (99%); found in breast milk. **Metabolism:** Via oxidation, degradation of imidazole and piperazine rings, oxidative O-dealkylation, and aromatic hydroxylation. **Elimination:** Biphasic. $T_{1/2}$=2 hrs (first 10 hrs), 8 hrs (thereafter); bile (major), urine (13%, 2-4% unchanged).

NURSING CONSIDERATIONS

Assessment: Assess for drug hypersensitivity, adrenal insufficiency, conditions where treatment is contraindicated or cautioned, pregnancy/nursing status, and possible drug interactions. Perform lab and clinical documentation of infection prior to therapy. Obtain lab tests (eg, GGT, alkaline phosphatase, ALT/AST, total bilirubin, PT, INR, testing for viral hepatitis) prior to therapy.

Monitoring: Monitor for signs/symptoms of hepatotoxicity, anaphylaxis/hypersensitivity reactions, and other adverse reactions. Monitor serum ALT weekly during treatment. Monitor adrenal function in patients with adrenal insufficiency or with borderline adrenal function and in patients under prolonged periods of stress.

Patient Counseling: Inform patients about risk of hepatotoxicity. Instruct to report any signs/symptoms of liver dysfunction (eg, unusual fatigue, anorexia, N/V, abdominal pain, jaundice, dark urine, pale stools) to physician. Advise against alcohol consumption while on treatment.

Administration: Oral route. **Storage:** 20-25°C (68-77°F). Protect from moisture.

KETOROLAC   RX
ketorolac tromethamine (Various)

For short-term (up to 5 days in adults) use only; total combined duration of oral and inj use should not exceed 5 days. Use tab only as continuation therapy following IV/IM dosing, if necessary. Not indicated for use in pediatric patients and not indicated for minor or chronic painful conditions. Increasing the dose beyond the label recommendations will not provide better efficacy but will increase risk of developing serious adverse events. May cause peptic ulcers, GI bleeding, and/or perforation of the stomach or intestines; contraindicated with active peptic ulcer disease, recent GI bleeding or perforation, and in patients with a history of peptic ulcer disease or GI bleeding. Elderly are at greater risk for serious GI events. May increase risk of serious cardiovascular (CV) thrombotic events, myocardial infarction (MI), and stroke; risk may increase with duration of use and with CV disease or risk factors for CV disease. Contraindicated for treatment of perioperative pain in the setting of coronary artery bypass graft (CABG) surgery, use as a prophylactic analgesic before any major surgery, with advanced renal impairment, in patients at risk for renal failure due to volume depletion, with suspected or confirmed cerebrovascular bleeding, with hemorrhagic diathesis, incomplete hemostasis, those at high risk of bleeding, use in labor and delivery, and in patients currently receiving aspirin (ASA) or NSAIDs. Adjust dosage for patients ≥65 yrs of age, <50kg (110 lbs), and with moderately elevated SrCr; doses of inj are not to exceed 60mg/day in these patients. (Inj) Hypersensitivity reactions reported and appropriate counteractive measures must be available when administering the 1st dose. Contraindicated in patients with previously demonstrated allergic manifestations to ASA or other NSAIDs, for intrathecal/epidural administration, and in nursing mothers.

THERAPEUTIC CLASS: NSAID

INDICATIONS: Short-term (≤5 days) management of moderately severe acute pain that requires analgesia at the opioid level, usually in postoperative setting. (Inj) Has been used concomitantly with morphine and meperidine.

DOSAGE: Adults: (Inj) May be given on a regular or PRN schedule. Single-Dose: (IM) ≥65 Yrs/Renal Impairment and/or <50kg (110 lbs): 30mg. <65 Yrs: 60mg. (IV) ≥65 Yrs/Renal Impairment and/or <50kg (110 lbs): 15mg. <65 Yrs: 30mg. Multiple-dose: (IM/IV) ≥65 Yrs/Renal Impairment and <50kg (110 lbs): Usual: 15mg q6h. Max: 60mg/day. <65 Yrs: Usual: 30mg q6h. Max: 120mg/day. Breakthrough Pain: Do not increase dose/frequency; consider low doses of opioids PRN unless otherwise contraindicated. (PO) Transition from IM/IV to PO: ≥65 Yrs/Renal Impairment and/or <50kg (110 lbs): 10mg once, then 10mg q4-6h PRN. Max: 40mg/day. 17-64 Yrs: 20mg once, then 10mg q4-6h PRN. Max: 40mg/day. Do not shorten interval of 4-6 hrs.

HOW SUPPLIED: Inj: 15mg/mL [1mL], 30mg/mL [1mL, 2mL, 10mL]; Tab: 10mg

CONTRAINDICATIONS: Active/history of peptic ulcer, recent/history of GI bleeding, recent GI perforation, advanced renal impairment or risk of renal failure due to volume depletion, labor and delivery, cerebrovascular bleeding, hemorrhagic diathesis, incomplete hemostasis, patients at high risk of bleeding. Patients who have experienced asthma, urticaria, or allergic reactions after taking ASA or other NSAIDs. Prophylactic analgesic before major surgery. Treatment of perioperative pain in the setting of CABG surgery. Current ASA or NSAIDs use. Concomitant use of probenecid and pentoxifylline. (Inj) Neuraxial (epidural or intrathecal) administration. Nursing mothers.

WARNINGS/PRECAUTIONS: Do not give oral formulation as an initial dose. Use lowest effective dose for the shortest duration possible. Increased risk for GI bleeding with longer duration of NSAID therapy, older age, and poor general health status. D/C and promptly initiate additional evaluation and treatment if a serious GI adverse event is suspected; consider alternate therapy that does not involve NSAIDs for high risk patients. May exacerbate inflammatory bowel disease (eg, ulcerative colitis, Crohn's disease). Renal papillary necrosis and other renal injury reported with long-term use. Renal toxicity reported; increased risk with renal/hepatic impairment, heart failure, and in the elderly. Acute renal failure, interstitial nephritis, and nephrotic syndrome reported. Caution with impaired renal function or history of kidney disease. May cause anaphylactoid reactions and serious skin adverse events (eg, exfoliative dermatitis, Stevens-Johnson syndrome, toxic epidermal necrolysis); d/c at 1st appearance of skin rash or any other signs of hypersensitivity. May lead to onset of new HTN or worsening of preexisting HTN; caution in patients with HTN. Monitor BP closely during initiation of therapy and throughout the course of therapy. Fluid retention, edema, retention of NaCl, oliguria, elevations of BUN and SrCr reported; caution with cardiac decompensation, HTN or similar conditions. Avoid in late pregnancy; may cause premature closure of the ductus arteriosus. Not a substitute for corticosteroids or for the treatment of corticosteroid insufficiency. May mask signs of inflammation. Caution with impaired hepatic function or history of liver disease; rare cases of severe hepatic reactions (eg, jaundice, fatal fulminant hepatitis, liver necrosis, hepatic failure) reported. Evaluate patients with signs/symptoms suggesting liver dysfunction, or abnormal LFTs for development of a more severe hepatic reaction; d/c if signs/symptoms of liver disease develop, or systemic manifestations (eg, eosinophilia, rash) occur. Anemia may occur; monitor Hgb or Hct if signs/symptoms of anemia develop with long-term use. May inhibit platelet aggregation and prolong bleeding time; caution with coagulation disorders and in postoperative setting when hemostasis is critical. Caution with preexisting asthma and avoid with ASA-sensitive asthma. Use with extreme caution in the elderly. Caution in debilitated patients. (Inj) Correct hypovolemia prior to administration.

ADVERSE REACTIONS: Hypersensitivity reactions, nausea, headache, dyspepsia, abdominal pain, edema, drowsiness, dizziness, abnormal renal function.

INTERACTIONS: See Boxed Warning and Contraindications. Binding reduced with concomitant use with salicylate. May increase risk of bleeding with drugs affecting hemostasis (eg, warfarin, dicumarol derivatives, heparin, dextrans). May increase risk of serious GI bleeding with oral corticosteroids, anticoagulants, SSRIs, smoking, and alcohol. May reduce natriuretic effect of furosemide and thiazide diuretics; observe closely for signs of renal failure and diuretic efficacy. May elevate plasma lithium levels and reduce renal lithium clearance; monitor for lithium toxicity. May enhance methotrexate toxicity; caution with concomitant use. Caution with ACE inhibitors and/or ARBs; may increase risk of renal impairment and diminish antihypertensive effect of ACE inhibitors and/or ARBs. Sporadic cases of seizures reported with concomitant use with antiepileptic drugs (eg, phenytoin, carbamazepine). Hallucinations reported with psychoactive drugs (eg, fluoxetine, thiothixene, alprazolam). (Inj) Apnea reported with nondepolarizing muscle relaxants.

PREGNANCY: Category C, (Inj) not for use in nursing, (Tab) caution in nursing.

MECHANISM OF ACTION: NSAID; has not been established. Suspected to inhibit prostaglandin synthetase.

PHARMACOKINETICS: Absorption: Absolute bioavailability (100%). Administration of variable doses/routes and in different populations resulted in different parameters. **Distribution:** V_d=13L; plasma protein binding (99.2%); found in breast milk. **Metabolism:** Liver; hydroxylation, conjugation. **Elimination:** Urine (92%; 40% metabolites, 60% unchanged), feces (6%); $T_{1/2}$=5-6 hrs (racemate), 2.5 hrs (S-enantiomer), 5 hrs (R-enantiomer).

NURSING CONSIDERATIONS

Assessment: Assess that use is not for perioperative pain in the setting of CABG surgery. Assess for previous hypersensitivity to drug, history of asthma, urticaria, or allergic-type reactions with ASA or other NSAIDs, CV disease, risk factors for GI events/CV disease, active/history of peptic ulcer, recent/history of GI bleeding, recent GI perforation, cerebrovascular bleeding, hemorrhagic diathesis, incomplete hemostasis, high risk of bleeding, renal/hepatic impairment, any other conditions where therapy is cautioned or contraindicated, pregnancy/nursing status, and for possible drug interactions. Obtain baseline BP.

Monitoring: Monitor for GI events, anaphylactoid/skin/hypersensitivity reactions, CV events, fluid retention, edema, hematological effects, and other adverse reactions. Monitor BP, LFTs, and renal function. Monitor CBC and chemistry profile periodically during long-term use.

K

Patient Counseling: Inform about potential risks/benefits of therapy. Advise not to give tab to other family members and to discard any unused drug. Instruct that the duration of use should not exceed 5 days. Inform that therapy is not indicated for use in pediatric patients. Instruct to seek medical attention for signs/symptoms of GI ulceration/bleeding (eg, epigastric pain, dyspepsia, melena, and hematemesis), CV events (eg, chest pain, SOB, weakness, slurring of speech), hepatotoxicity (eg, nausea, fatigue, lethargy, pruritus, jaundice, right upper quadrant tenderness, flu-like symptoms), skin reactions (eg, skin rash/blisters, fever or other signs of hypersensitivity such as itching), anaphylactoid reaction (eg, difficulty breathing, swelling of face/throat), or unexplained weight gain or edema. Instruct to avoid use in late pregnancy.

Administration: IM/IV/Oral route. (Inj) IV bolus must be given over ≥15 sec. Give IM doses slowly and deeply into muscle. Do not mix in a small volume (eg, in a syringe) with morphine sulfate, meperidine HCl, promethazine HCl or hydroxyzine HCl. **Storage:** 20-25°C (68-77°F). (Inj) Protect from light.

KLOR-CON M   RX
potassium chloride (Upsher-Smith)

OTHER BRAND NAMES: Klor-Con (Upsher-Smith)

THERAPEUTIC CLASS: K⁺ supplement

INDICATIONS: Treatment of hypokalemia with or without metabolic alkalosis, in digitalis intoxication, and in patients with hypokalemic familial periodic paralysis. Prevention of hypokalemia in patients at risk (eg, digitalized patients, cardiac arrhythmias).

DOSAGE: *Adults:* Individualize dose. Prevention: 20mEq/day. Hypokalemia: 40-100mEq/day. Divide dose if >20mEq. Elderly: Start at low end of dosing range. Take with meals and fluids. (Klor-Con ER Tab): Swallow tab whole; do not crush, chew, or suck. (Klor-Con M) May break Klor-Con M in half or mix with 4 oz. of water.

HOW SUPPLIED: (Klor-Con M) Tab, Extended-Release (ER): 10mEq, 15mEq, 20mEq; (Klor-Con) Pow: 20mEq, 25mEq; Tab, Extended-Release: 8mEq, 10mEq

CONTRAINDICATIONS: (Tab, ER) Hyperkalemia, cardiac patients with esophageal compression due to an enlarged left atrium. Structural, pathological (eg, diabetic gastroparesis) or pharmacological (eg, use of anticholinergic agents or other agents with anticholinergic properties) cause for arrest or delay through the GI tract with all solid dosage forms. (Powder) Hyperkalemia.

WARNINGS/PRECAUTIONS: (Tab, ER; Powder) Potentially fatal hyperkalemia and cardiac arrest may occur; monitor serum K⁺ levels and adjust dose appropriately. Extreme caution with acidosis and cardiac and renal disease; monitor ECG and electrolytes. Hypokalemia with metabolic acidosis should be treated with an alkalinizing K⁺ salt (eg, K⁺ bicarbonate, K⁺ citrate, K⁺ acetate, K⁺ gluconate). (Tab, ER) Solid oral dosage forms may produce ulcerative and/or stenotic lesions of the GI tract; d/c use if severe vomiting, abdominal pain, distention or GI bleeding occurs. Reserve use of ER preparations for those who cannot tolerate, cannot comply, or refuse to take liquid or effervescent preparations. Caution in elderly.

ADVERSE REACTIONS: Hyperkalemia, GI effects (eg, obstruction, bleeding, ulceration), N/V, abdominal pain/discomfort, flatulence, diarrhea.

INTERACTIONS: (Tab, ER) See Contraindications. Risk of hyperkalemia with ACE inhibitors (eg, captopril, enalapril). (Tab, ER; Powder) Risk of hyperkalemia with K⁺-sparing diuretics (eg, spironolactone, triamterene, amiloride).

PREGNANCY: Category C, (Tab, ER) Safety not known in nursing, (Powder) not for use in nursing.

MECHANISM OF ACTION: K⁺ supplement (electrolyte replenisher); participates in a number of essential physiological processes, including the maintenance of intracellular tonicity, the transmission of nerve impulses, the contraction of cardiac, skeletal, and smooth muscle, and the maintenance of normal renal function.

PHARMACOKINETICS: Absorption: (Klor-Con ER Tab) GI tract. **Elimination:** (Klor-Con ER Tab) Urine and feces.

NURSING CONSIDERATIONS

Assessment: Assess for hyperkalemia, chronic renal failure, systemic acidosis, cardiac patients, if patient cannot tolerate, refuses to take, or cannot comply with taking liquid or effervescent K⁺ preparations prior to administration of an ER tab formulation. Obtain baseline ECG, serum electrolyte levels, and renal function.

Monitoring: Monitor for signs/symptoms of hyperkalemia and other adverse events that may occur. In patients taking solid oral dosage forms, monitor for signs/symptoms of GI lesions. In patients with cardiac disease, acidosis, or renal disease, monitor acid-base balance and perform appropriate monitoring of serum electrolytes, ECG, renal function, and the clinical status of the patient.

Patient Counseling: Inform about benefits and risks of therapy. Instruct to report to physician if patient develops any type of GI symptoms (eg, tarry stools or other evidence of GI bleeding, vomiting, abdominal pain/distention) or if other adverse events occur. Instruct to contact physician if difficulty in swallowing develops or if the tablets are sticking in the throat. (Klor-Con): Instruct to swallow tablets whole and to take with meals and full glass of water or other liquid. Follow the frequency and amount prescribed by the physician, especially if also taking diuretics and/or digitalis preparations. (Klor-Con M): Instruct to take each dose with meals and with full glass of water or other liquid. Inform that may break tablets in half or make an oral aqueous suspension with tablets and 4 oz. of water (see PI for proper preparation). Inform that aqueous suspension not taken immediately should be discarded and use of other liquids for suspending is not recommended.

Administration: Oral route. (Klor-Con M) Refer to PI for preparation of aqueous suspension.
Storage: (Klor-Con): 15-30°C (59-86°F). (Klor-Con M): 20-25°C (68-77°F); excursions permitted to 15-30°C (59-86°F).

KOMBIGLYZE XR   RX
metformin HCl - saxagliptin (Bristol-Myers Squibb/ AstraZeneca)

> Lactic acidosis may occur due to metformin accumulation; risk increases with conditions such as sepsis, dehydration, excess alcohol intake, hepatic impairment, renal impairment, and acute congestive heart failure (CHF). If acidosis is suspected, d/c and hospitalize patient immediately.

THERAPEUTIC CLASS: Biguanide/dipeptidyl peptidase-4 inhibitor

INDICATIONS: Adjunct to diet and exercise to improve glycemic control in adults with type 2 diabetes mellitus (DM) when treatment with both saxagliptin and metformin is appropriate.

DOSAGE: *Adults:* Individualize dose. Take qd with evening meal, with gradual dose titration to reduce GI side effects of metformin. Patients on Metformin: Dose should provide metformin at the dose already being taken, or the nearest therapeutically appropriate dose. Adjust dose accordingly if switched from metformin immediate release (IR) to ER; monitor glycemic control. Patients Who Need 5mg Saxagliptin and Not Currently Treated with Metformin: Initial: 5mg-500mg qd. Patients Who Need 2.5mg Saxagliptin in Combination with Metformin ER: Initial: 2.5mg-1000mg qd. Patients Who Need 2.5mg Saxagliptin Who are Metformin Naive or Require >1000mg Metformin: Use individual components. Max: 5mg for saxagliptin and 2000mg for metformin ER. With Strong CYP3A4/5 Inhibitors: Max: 2.5mg-1000mg qd. With Insulin Secretagogue (eg, Sulfonylurea)/Insulin: May require lower doses of insulin secretagogue or insulin.

HOW SUPPLIED: Tab, Extended-Release (ER): (Saxagliptin-Metformin ER) 5mg-500mg, 5mg-1000mg, 2.5-1000mg

CONTRAINDICATIONS: Renal impairment (eg, SrCr ≥1.5mg/dL [men], ≥1.4mg/dL [women], or abnormal CrCl), acute or chronic metabolic acidosis, including diabetic ketoacidosis.

WARNINGS/PRECAUTIONS: Not for use for the treatment of type 1 DM or diabetic ketoacidosis. Not studied in patients with history of pancreatitis. Acute pancreatitis reported; d/c if pancreatitis is suspected. Assess renal function before initiation of therapy and at least annually thereafter; d/c with evidence of renal impairment. Avoid with hepatic disease/impairment. May decrease vitamin B12 levels; monitor hematological parameters annually. Suspend temporarily for any surgical procedure (except minor procedures not associated with restricted intake of foods and fluids); restart when oral intake is resumed and renal function is normal. Evaluate for evidence of ketoacidosis or lactic acidosis if laboratory abnormalities or clinical illness develops; d/c if acidosis occurs. Temporarily d/c at time of or prior to intravascular contrast studies with iodinated materials, withhold for 48 hrs subsequent to the procedure, and reinstitute only if renal function is normal. D/C in hypoxic states (eg, shock, acute CHF, acute myocardial infarction [MI]). Serious hypersensitivity reactions reported; d/c if suspected, assess for other potential causes, and institute alternative treatment for DM. Avoid in patients ≥80 yrs of age unless renal function is not reduced. Caution in patients susceptible to hypoglycemic effects, such as elderly, debilitated/malnourished patients, and those with adrenal/pituitary insufficiency or alcohol intoxication. Caution in patients with history of angioedema to another dipeptidyl peptidase-4 (DPP-4) inhibitor. No conclusive evidence of macrovascular risk reduction.

ADVERSE REACTIONS: Lactic acidosis, diarrhea, N/V, upper respiratory tract infection, urinary tract infection, headache, nasopharyngitis.

INTERACTIONS: Hypoglycemia may occur with other glucose-lowering agents (eg, sulfonylureas, insulin) or ethanol; may require lower dose of sulfonylurea or insulin. Metformin: Cationic drugs that are eliminated by renal tubular secretion (eg, cimetidine, amiloride, digoxin, morphine, procainamide, quinidine, quinine, ranitidine, triamterene, trimethoprim, or vancomycin) may potentially produce an interaction; monitor and adjust dose of Kombiglyze XR and/or cationic drug if necessary. Observe for loss of glycemic control with thiazides and other diuretics, corticosteroids, phenothiazines, thyroid products, estrogens, oral contraceptives, phenytoin, nicotinic acid, sympathomimetics, calcium channel blockers, and isoniazid. Alcohol may potentiate the

K

effect of metformin on lactate metabolism; avoid excessive alcohol intake. Caution with drugs that may affect renal function or result in significant hemodynamic change or may interfere with the disposition of metformin (eg, cationic drugs eliminated by renal tubular secretion). May be difficult to recognize hypoglycemia with β-adrenergic blocking drugs. Saxagliptin: Increased plasma concentrations with ketoconazole and other strong CYP3A4/5 inhibitors (eg, atazanavir, clarithromycin, indinavir, itraconazole, nefazodone, nelfinavir, ritonavir, saquinavir, and telithromycin); limit dose of saxagliptin to 2.5mg. Strong CYP3A4/5 inducers and inhibitors may alter pharmacokinetics of saxagliptin and its active metabolite.

PREGNANCY: Category B, caution in nursing.

MECHANISM OF ACTION: Metformin: Biguanide; decreases hepatic glucose production, decreases intestinal absorption of glucose, and improves insulin sensitivity by increasing peripheral glucose uptake and utilization. Saxagliptin: DPP-4 inhibitor; slows the inactivation of the incretin hormones, thereby increasing their bloodstream concentrations and reducing fasting and postprandial glucose concentrations in a glucose-dependent manner in type 2 DM.

PHARMACOKINETICS: Absorption: Saxagliptin: C_{max}=24ng/mL; AUC=78ng•hr/mL; T_{max}=2 hrs. 5-hydroxy saxagliptin: C_{max}=47ng/mL; AUC=214ng•hr/mL; T_{max}=4 hrs. Metformin: T_{max}=7 hrs (median). **Distribution:** Metformin IR: V_d=654L. **Metabolism:** Saxagliptin: Via CYP3A4/5; 5-hydroxy saxagliptin (active metabolite). **Elimination:** Saxagliptin: Feces (22%), urine (24% unchanged, 36% active metabolite); $T_{1/2}$=2.5 hrs (saxagliptin), 3.1 hrs (5-hydroxy saxagliptin). Metformin: Urine (90%); $T_{1/2}$=6.2 hrs (plasma), 17.6 hrs (blood).

NURSING CONSIDERATIONS

Assessment: Assess for metabolic acidosis, risk factors for lactic acidosis, renal/hepatic impairment, previous hypersensitivity to the drug, history of pancreatitis, inadequate vitamin B12 or Ca^{2+} absorption, type of DM, diabetic ketoacidosis, history of angioedema with another DPP-4 inhibitor, pregnancy/nursing status, and possible drug interactions. Assess if patient is planning to undergo any surgical procedure or is under any form of stress. Obtain baseline FPG and HbA1c levels, and hematological parameters.

Monitoring: Monitor for signs/symptoms of lactic acidosis, pancreatitis, hypoxic states, hypoglycemia, hypersensitivity reactions, and for other adverse reactions. Monitor for changes in clinical status. Monitor renal function, especially in elderly, at least annually. Perform routine serum vitamin B12 measurements at 2-3 yr intervals in patients predisposed to develop subnormal vitamin B12 levels. Monitor FPG and HbA1c levels, hepatic function, and hematologic parameters periodically.

Patient Counseling: Inform of the risks, benefits, and alternative modes of therapy. Advise on the importance of adherence to dietary instructions, regular physical activity, periodic blood glucose monitoring and HbA1c testing, recognition/management of hypoglycemia/hyperglycemia, and assessment of diabetes complications. Instruct to seek medical advice promptly during periods of stress (eg, fever, trauma, infection, surgery) as medication needs may change. Inform of the risk of developing lactic acidosis during therapy. Advise to d/c therapy and contact physician if symptoms of allergic reactions, unexplained hyperventilation, myalgia, malaise, unusual somnolence, dizziness, slow or irregular heartbeat, sensation of feeling cold (especially in the extremities) or other nonspecific symptoms occur. Counsel to inform physician if any unusual symptom develops, or if any known symptom persists or worsens. Counsel against excessive alcohol intake. Inform that inactive ingredients may be eliminated in the feces as a soft mass that may resemble the original tab.

Administration: Oral route. Swallow tab whole; do not cut, crush, or chew. Give with the evening meal. **Storage:** 20-25°C (68-77°F); excursions permitted to 15-30°C (59-86°F).

KRISTALOSE   RX
lactulose (Cumberland)

THERAPEUTIC CLASS: Osmotic laxative

INDICATIONS: Treatment of constipation.

DOSAGE: *Adults:* 10-20g/day. Max 40g/day. Dissolve pkt contents in 4oz. of water.

HOW SUPPLIED: Sol (Powder): 10g/pkt, 20g/pkt [1ˢ, 30ˢ]

CONTRAINDICATIONS: Patients who require a low galactose diet.

WARNINGS/PRECAUTIONS: Caution in diabetes mellitus (DM) due to galactose and lactose content. Monitor electrolytes periodically in elderly or debilitated if used for >6 months. Potential for explosive reaction with electrocautery procedures during proctoscopy or colonoscopy.

ADVERSE REACTIONS: Flatulence, intestinal cramps, diarrhea, N/V.

INTERACTIONS: Nonabsorbable antacids may decrease effects.

PREGNANCY: Category B, caution in nursing.

MECHANISM OF ACTION: Osmotic laxative; increases osmotic pressure and slight acidification of the colonic contents.

PHARMACOKINETICS: Absorption: Poorly absorbed from GI tract. **Elimination:** Urine (≤3%).

NURSING CONSIDERATIONS

Assessment: Assess for DM, patients requiring a low-galactose diet, pregnancy/nursing status, and possible drug interactions.

Monitoring: Monitor serum electrolytes (K$^+$, Na$^+$, Cl$^-$, carbon dioxide). Monitor for diarrhea, vomiting, and other adverse reactions.

Patient Counseling: Advise to report any potential adverse effects.

Administration: Oral route. Dissolve contents of pkt in 4 oz. of water. **Storage:** 15-30°C (59-86°F).

KRYSTEXXA   RX
pegloticase (Savient)

Anaphylaxis and infusion reactions reported during and after administration; delayed-type hypersensitivity reactions also reported. Should be administered in a healthcare setting and by a healthcare provider prepared to manage anaphylaxis and infusion reactions. Premedicate with antihistamines and corticosteroids. Closely monitor for an appropriate period of time for anaphylaxis after administration. Monitor serum uric acid levels prior to infusions and consider d/c treatment if levels increase to >6mg/dL, particularly when 2 consecutive levels >6mg/dL are observed.

THERAPEUTIC CLASS: Recombinant urate-oxidase enzyme

INDICATIONS: Treatment of chronic gout in adults refractory to conventional therapy.

DOSAGE: *Adults:* 8mg IV infusion every 2 weeks.

HOW SUPPLIED: Inj: 8mg/mL

CONTRAINDICATIONS: G6PD deficiency.

WARNINGS/PRECAUTIONS: Not recommended for the treatment of asymptomatic hyperuricemia. D/C oral urate-lowering medications before starting therapy, and do not institute oral urate-lowering agents while on therapy. Gout flares may occur after initiation of therapy; gout flare prophylaxis with an NSAID or colchicine is recommended starting at least 1 week before initiation of therapy and lasting at least 6 months, unless medically contraindicated or not tolerated. Congestive heart failure (CHF) exacerbation reported; caution with CHF and monitor closely following infusion. Risk of anaphylaxis and infusion reactions may increase during retreatment due to immunogenicity; carefully monitor patients receiving retreatment after a drug-free interval.

ADVERSE REACTIONS: Gout flares, infusion reactions, N/V, contusion/ecchymosis, nasopharyngitis, constipation, chest pain, anaphylaxis, delayed-type hypersensitivity reactions.

PREGNANCY: Category C, not for use in nursing.

MECHANISM OF ACTION: Recombinant urate-oxidase enzyme; catalyzes the oxidation of uric acid to allantoin, thereby lowering serum uric acid.

NURSING CONSIDERATIONS

Assessment: Assess for G6PD deficiency, CHF, and pregnancy/nursing status. Assess serum uric acid levels prior to infusion.

Monitoring: Monitor for signs/symptoms of anaphylaxis, infusion reactions, gout flares, and CHF exacerbation.

Patient Counseling: Inform that anaphylaxis and infusion reactions may occur while on therapy; counsel on the importance of adhering to any prescribed medications to help prevent or lessen the severity of these reactions. Advise to seek medical care immediately if patient experiences any symptoms of an allergic reaction during or at any time after therapy. Inform that gout flares may initially increase when starting therapy, and that medications to help reduce flares may need to be taken regularly for the 1st few months after therapy is started.

Administration: IV route. Do not administer as an IV push or bolus. Do not mix or dilute with other drugs. Refer to PI for further preparation and administration instructions. **Storage:** 2-8°C (36-46°F). Protect from light. Do not shake or freeze. Diluted Sol: Stable for 4 hrs at 2-8°C (36-46°F) and at 20-25°C (68-77°F).

KYPROLIS   RX
carfilzomib (Onyx)

THERAPEUTIC CLASS: Proteasome inhibitor

INDICATIONS: Treatment of multiple myeloma in patients who received at least 2 prior therapies, including bortezomib and an immunomodulatory agent and have demonstrated disease progression on or within 60 days of completion of the last therapy.

DOSAGE: *Adults:* Cycle 1: 20mg/m². Cycle 2: Escalate dose to 27mg/m² if dose in Cycle 1 is tolerated. Continue at 27mg/m² in subsequent cycles. Administer IV over 2-10 min, on 2 consecutive days, each week for 3 weeks (Days 1, 2, 8, 9, 15, 16), followed by a 12-day rest period (Days 17-28). Each 28-day period is 1 treatment cycle. Refer to PI for instructions on hydration, fluid monitoring, dexamethasone premedication, and dose modifications for toxicities.

HOW SUPPLIED: Inj: 60mg

WARNINGS/PRECAUTIONS: Death due to cardiac arrest has occurred within a day of administration. Cardiac failure events (eg, cardiac failure congestive, pulmonary edema, ejection fraction disease) reported; monitor for cardiac complications and manage promptly. Pulmonary arterial HTN (PAH) reported; withhold treatment until resolved or returned to baseline and consider whether to restart based on a benefit/risk assessment. Dyspnea reported; interrupt treatment until symptoms have resolved or returned to baseline. Infusion reactions (eg, fever, chills, vomiting, weakness, SOB, chest tightness) can occur immediately following or up to 24 hrs after treatment; administer dexamethasone prior to treatment to reduce the incidence and severity of reactions. Tumor lysis syndrome (TLS) may occur; interrupt treatment until TLS is resolved. May cause thrombocytopenia; reduce or interrupt dose as clinically indicated. Hepatic failure and elevations of serum transaminases and bilirubin reported; monitor liver enzymes frequently. May cause fetal harm; avoid becoming pregnant while on therapy.

ADVERSE REACTIONS: Fatigue, anemia, thrombocytopenia, dyspnea, diarrhea, pyrexia, upper respiratory tract infection, headache, cough, N/V, blood creatinine increased, lymphopenia, peripheral edema, constipation.

PREGNANCY: Category D, not for use in nursing.

MECHANISM OF ACTION: Proteasome inhibitor; irreversibly binds to the N-terminal threonine-containing active sites of the 20S proteasome, the proteolytic core particle within the 26S proteasome.

PHARMACOKINETICS: Absorption: (27mg/m²) AUC=379ng•hr/mL; C_{max}=4232ng/mL. **Distribution:** (20mg/m²) V_d=28L; plasma protein binding (97%). **Metabolism:** Rapid and extensive; peptidase cleavage and epoxide hydrolysis (major); CYP450 (minor). **Elimination:** $T_{1/2}$=≤1 hr.

NURSING CONSIDERATIONS

Assessment: Assess for dehydration, preexisting congestive heart failure, hepatic dysfunction, pregnancy/nursing status, and possible drug interactions. Obtain baseline CBC, LFTs, and SrCr.

Monitoring: Monitor for signs/symptoms of dehydration, cardiac failure events, PAH, dyspnea, TLS, and infusion reactions. Monitor CBC, LFTs, and SrCr.

Patient Counseling: Advise to contact physician if SOB, fever, chills, rigors, chest pain, cough, or swelling of the feet or legs develops. Instruct not to drive or operate machinery if fatigue, dizziness, fainting, and/or drop in BP are experienced. Advise regarding appropriate measures to avoid dehydration. Instruct female patients to use effective contraceptive measures to prevent pregnancy and instruct to inform physician immediately if pregnant. Instruct not to breastfeed while on therapy. Advise to notify physician if using or planning to take other prescription or OTC drugs.

Administration: IV route. Administer within 24 hrs after reconstitution. Refer to PI for further administration and preparation instructions. **Storage:** Unopened Vials: 2-8°C (36-46°F). Store in carton to protect from light. Reconstituted Sol: 2-8°C (36-46°F) for 24 hrs and 15-30°C (59-86°F) for 4 hrs.

LABETALOL   RX
labetalol HCl (Various)

THERAPEUTIC CLASS: Alpha₁ blocker/nonselective beta-blocker

INDICATIONS: (Tab) Management of hypertension. (Inj) Management of severe hypertension.

DOSAGE: *Adults:* (Tab) HTN: Initial: 100mg bid. Titrate: 100mg bid every 2-3 days. Maint: 200-400mg bid. Severe HTN: 1200-2400mg/day given bid-tid. Increments should not exceed 200mg bid for titration. (Inj) Severe HTN: Administer in supine position. Repeated IV Infusion: Initial: 20mg over 2 min. Titrate: Give additional 40mg or 80mg at 10-min intervals if needed. Max: 300mg. Slow Continuous Infusion: 200mg at rate of 2mg/min. Usual Dose Range: 50-200mg. Max: 300mg. May adjust dose according to BP. Switch to tabs when BP is stable while in hospital. Initial: 200mg, then 200-400mg 6-12 hrs later on Day 1. Titrate: May increase at 1-day interval.

HOW SUPPLIED: Inj: 5mg/mL; Tab: 100mg*, 200mg*, 300mg *scored

CONTRAINDICATIONS: Bronchial asthma, overt cardiac failure, >1st-degree heart block, cardiogenic shock, severe bradycardia, other conditions associated with severe and prolonged hypotension, history of obstructive airway disease.

WARNINGS/PRECAUTIONS: Severe hepatocellular injury reported; caution with hepatic dysfunction. Monitor LFTs periodically; d/c at 1st sign of liver injury or jaundice. Caution in well-compensated patients with a history of heart failure; congestive heart failure may occur. Avoid abrupt withdrawal; may exacerbate ischemic heart disease. Avoid with bronchospastic disease and in overt cardiac failure. Caution with pheochromocytoma; paradoxical HTN reported. Caution with diabetes mellitus (DM); may mask symptoms of hypoglycemia. Withdrawal before surgery is controversial. Several deaths reported during surgery. Caution when reducing severely elevated BP; cerebral infarction, optic nerve infarction, angina and ECG ischemic changes reported. Avoid inj with low cardiac indices and elevated systemic vascular resistance.

ADVERSE REACTIONS: Fatigue, dizziness, dyspepsia, N/V, nasal stuffiness, somnolence, ejaculation failure, postural hypotension, increased sweating, paresthesia.

INTERACTIONS: Increased tremors with TCAs. Potentiated by cimetidine; may need to reduce dose. Synergistic antihypertensive effects blunt the reflex tachycardia with nitroglycerin. Caution with calcium antagonists. May need to adjust dose of antidiabetic drugs. Antagonizes effects of β-agonists (bronchodilators). May block epinephrine effects. (Inj) Synergistic effects with halothane; do not use ≥3% halothane.

PREGNANCY: Category C, caution in nursing.

MECHANISM OF ACTION: α_1 and nonselective β-adrenergic receptor blocker; produces dose-related falls in BP without reflex tachycardia and significant reduction in heart rate.

PHARMACOKINETICS: Absorption: Complete; T_{max}=1-2 hrs. **Distribution:** Plasma protein binding (50%); found in breast milk; crosses placenta. **Metabolism:** Liver (conjugation and glucuronidation). **Elimination:** Urine (IV, 55-60% unchanged), feces; (Tab) $T_{1/2}$=6-8 hrs, (IV) $T_{1/2}$=5.5 hrs.

NURSING CONSIDERATIONS

Assessment: Assess for bronchospastic disease, heart block, severe bradycardia, cardiogenic shock, overt cardiac failure, DM, pheochromocytoma, ischemic heart disease, severe or prolonged hypotension, hepatic impairment, history of heart failure, and possible drug interactions.

Monitoring: Monitor LFTs periodically. Monitor for signs/symptoms of cardiac failure, HTN, exacerbation of ischemic heart disease following abrupt withdrawal, bronchospastic disease, hypoglycemia, hypersensitivity reactions, and hepatic dysfunction.

Patient Counseling: Instruct to remain supine during and immediately following (for up to 3 hrs) injection; advise on how to proceed gradually to become ambulatory. Instruct not to interrupt or d/c therapy without consulting physician. Instruct to report signs/symptoms of cardiac failure or hepatic dysfunction (eg, pruritus, dark urine, persistent anorexia, jaundice, right upper quadrant tenderness, or unexplained flu-like symptoms). Transient scalp itching may occur, usually when treatment with tabs is initiated.

Administration: Oral, IV route; refer to PI for administration technique. **Storage:** Tab: 15-30°C (59-86°F). IV: 20-25°C (68-77°F). Protect from light and freezing.

LAMICTAL

lamotrigine (GlaxoSmithKline)

RX

> Serious life-threatening rashes, including Stevens-Johnson syndrome, toxic epidermal necrolysis, and/or rash-related death reported. Serious rash occurs more often in pediatric patients than in adults. D/C at 1st sign of rash unless rash is clearly not drug related. Potential increased risk with concomitant valproate (including valproic acid and divalproex sodium) or exceeding the recommended initial dose/dose escalation.

OTHER BRAND NAMES: Lamictal ODT (GlaxoSmithKline)

THERAPEUTIC CLASS: Phenyltriazine

INDICATIONS: Adjunctive therapy in patients ≥2 yrs of age with partial seizures, primary generalized tonic-clonic seizures, and generalized seizures of Lennox-Gastaut syndrome. For conversion to monotherapy in adults (≥16 yrs of age) with partial seizures receiving a single antiepileptic drug (AED) (carbamazepine, phenytoin, phenobarbital, primidone, or valproate). Maintenance treatment of bipolar I disorder to delay the time to occurrence of mood episodes (depression, mania, hypomania, mixed episodes) in adults (≥18 yrs of age) treated for acute mood episodes with standard therapy.

DOSAGE: *Adults:* Epilepsy: Concomitant Valproate: Weeks 1 and 2: 25mg qod. Weeks 3 and 4: 25mg qd. Week 5 Onwards: Increase every 1-2 weeks by 25-50mg/day. Maint: 100-200mg/day with valproate alone or 100-400mg/day with valproate and other drugs inducing glucuronidation in 1 or 2 divided doses. Patients not Taking Carbamazepine, Phenytoin, Phenobarbital, Primidone, or Valproate: Weeks 1 and 2: 25mg qd. Weeks 3 and 4: 50mg qd. Week 5 Onwards:

Increase every 1-2 weeks by 50mg/day. Maint: 225-375mg/day in 2 divided doses. Concomitant Carbamazepine, Phenytoin, Phenobarbital, or Primidone, without Valproate: Weeks 1 and 2: 50mg/day. Weeks 3 and 4: 100mg/day in 2 divided doses. Week 5 Onwards: Increase every 1-2 weeks by 100mg/day. Maint: 300-500mg/day in 2 divided doses. Conversion to Monotherapy: Refer to PI. Bipolar Disorder: Patients not Taking Carbamazepine, Phenytoin, Phenobarbital, Primidone, or Valproate: Weeks 1 and 2: 25mg qd. Weeks 3 and 4: 50mg qd. Week 5: 100mg qd. Weeks 6 and 7: 200mg qd. Concomitant Valproate: Weeks 1 and 2: 25mg qod. Weeks 3 and 4: 25mg qd. Week 5: 50mg qd. Weeks 6 and 7: 100mg qd. Concomitant Carbamazepine, Phenytoin, Phenobarbital, or Primidone, without Valproate: Weeks 1 and 2: 50mg qd. Weeks 3 and 4: 100mg qd. Week 5: 200mg qd. Week 6: 300mg qd. Week 7: Up to 400mg qd. Weeks 3-7: Take in divided doses. Following Discontinuation of Psychotropic Drugs Excluding Carbamazepine, Phenytoin, Phenobarbital, Primidone, or Valproate: Maintain current dose. Following Discontinuation of Valproate with Current Dose of Lamotrigine 100mg qd: Week 1: 150mg qd. Week 2: 200mg qd. Week 3 Onward: 200mg qd. Following Discontinuation of Carbamazepine, Phenytoin, Phenobarbital, Primidone with Current Dose of Lamotrigine 400mg qd: Week 1: 400mg qd. Week 2: 300mg qd. Week 3 Onward: 200mg qd. Periodically reevaluate to determine the need for maintenance treatment. Concomitant/Starting/Stopping Estrogen-Containing Oral Contraceptives: Refer to PI. Hepatic Impairment: (Moderate/Severe): Reduce dose by 25%. (Severe with Ascites): Reduce dose by 50%. Adjust maint and escalation doses based on clinical response. Elderly: Start at lower end of dosing range.
Pediatrics: Epilepsy: ≥16 Yrs: Conversion to Monotherapy: Refer to PI. >12 Yrs: Same as in adults. 2-12 Yrs: Give in 1-2 divided doses, rounded down to the nearest whole tab. Concomitant Valproate: Weeks 1 and 2: 0.15mg/kg/day. Weeks 3 and 4: 0.3mg/kg/day. Week 5 Onwards: Increase every 1-2 weeks by 0.3mg/kg/day. Maint: 1-3mg/kg/day with valproate alone or 1-5mg/kg/day. Max: 200mg/day. Initial Weight-Based Dosing Guide (Weeks 1-4): Refer to PI. Patients not Taking Carbamazepine, Phenytoin, Phenobarbital, Primidone, or Valproate: Weeks 1 and 2: 0.3mg/kg/day. Weeks 3 and 4: 0.6mg/kg/day. Week 5 Onwards: Increase every 1-2 weeks by 0.6mg/kg/day. Maint: 4.5-7.5mg/kg/day. Max: 300mg/day. Concomitant Carbamazepine, Phenytoin, Phenobarbital, or Primidone, without Valproate: Weeks 1 and 2: 0.6mg/kg/day. Weeks 3 and 4: 1.2mg/kg/day. Week 5 Onwards: Increase every 1-2 weeks by 1.2mg/kg/day. Maint: 5-15mg/kg/day. Max: 400mg/day. <30kg: May increase maint dose by up to 50% based on clinical response.

HOW SUPPLIED: Tab: 25mg*, 100mg*, 150mg*, 200mg*; Tab, Chewable: 2mg, 5mg, 25mg; Tab, Disintegrating: (ODT) 25mg, 50mg, 100mg, 200mg *scored

WARNINGS/PRECAUTIONS: Drug reaction with eosinophilia and systemic symptoms (DRESS), also known as multiorgan hypersensitivity reactions, reported. Fatalities from acute multiorgan failure and various degrees of hepatic failure reported. Isolated liver failure without rash or involvement of other organs reported. D/C if alternative etiology for signs/symptoms of early manifestations of hypersensitivity cannot be established. Blood dyscrasias (eg, neutropenia, leukopenia) reported. Increased risk of suicidal thoughts or behavior; balance risk of suicidal thoughts or behavior with risk of untreated illness prior to therapy. Worsening of depressive symptoms and/or emergence of suicidal ideation and behaviors (suicidality) may be experienced in patients with bipolar disorder; consider discontinuation. Write prescriptions for smallest quantity of tabs consistent with good patient management to reduce risk of overdose. Increases risk of developing aseptic meningitis; evaluate for other causes of aseptic meningitis and treat appropriately. Avoid abrupt withdrawal due to risk of withdrawal seizures; taper dose over a period of at least 2 weeks (50% reduction/week). Treatment-emergent status epilepticus and sudden unexplained death in epilepsy reported. May cause toxicity in the eyes and other melanin-rich tissues due to melanin binding. Medication errors reported. Caution with renal/hepatic impairment and in elderly. Do not restart therapy in patients who discontinued due to rash associated with prior treatment unless potential benefits outweigh the risks. If restarting after discontinuation, assess the need to restart with initial dosing recommendations.

ADVERSE REACTIONS: Rash, dizziness, diplopia, infection, headache, ataxia, blurred vision, N/V, somnolence, fever, pharyngitis, rhinitis, diarrhea, abdominal pain, tremor.

INTERACTIONS: See Boxed Warning. Phenytoin, carbamazepine, phenobarbital/primidone, rifampin, and oral contraceptive preparations containing ethinyl estradiol and levonorgestrel may decrease levels. May decrease levels of levonorgestrel. Valproate may increase levels. May increase carbamazepine epoxide levels. May inhibit dihydrofolate reductase; caution with other medications that inhibit folate metabolism. May affect clearance with drugs known to induce or inhibit glucuronidation; may require dose adjustment.

PREGNANCY: Category C, caution in nursing.

MECHANISM OF ACTION: Phenyltriazine; has not been established. Suspected to inhibit voltage-sensitive Na^+ channels, thereby stabilizing neuronal membranes and consequently modulating presynaptic transmitter release of excitatory amino acids (eg, glutamate, aspartate).

PHARMACOKINETICS: Absorption: Rapid and complete. Absolute bioavailability (98%); T_{max}=1.4-4.8 hrs. **Distribution:** V_d=0.9-1.3L/kg; plasma protein binding (55%); found in breast milk. **Metabolism:** Liver via glucuronic acid conjugation; 2-N-glucuronide conjugate (major metabolite, inactive). **Elimination:** Urine (94%; 10% unchanged, 76% 2-N-glucuronide), feces (2%). Refer to PI for variable parameters with concomitant AEDs.

NURSING CONSIDERATIONS

Assessment: Assess for history of allergy/rash to other AEDs, renal/hepatic impairment, depression, systemic lupus erythematosus or other autoimmune diseases, hypersensitivity to drug, pregnancy/nursing status, and possible drug interactions.

Monitoring: Monitor for signs/symptoms of rash, DRESS, multiorgan failure, status epilepticus, blood dyscrasias, emergence/worsening of depression, suicidal thoughts or behavior, unusual mood/behavior changes, aseptic meningitis, ophthalmologic effects, and other adverse reactions. Monitor effectiveness of long-term use (>16 weeks) with bipolar disorder.

Patient Counseling: Inform that a rash or other signs/symptoms of hypersensitivity (eg, fever, lymphadenopathy) may herald a serious medical event; instruct to report such symptoms to physician immediately. Instruct to notify physician immediately if blood dyscrasias, DRESS, acute multiorgan failure, or aseptic meningitis occur. Inform about increased risk of suicidal thoughts and behavior; advise to be alert for emergence/worsening of symptoms of depression, any unusual changes in mood/behavior, suicidal thoughts/behavior, or thoughts about self-harm. Instruct to immediately report behaviors of concern to physician. Advise to notify physician if worsening of seizure control occurs. Inform that CNS depression may occur; advise to avoid operating machinery/driving until effects of the drug are known. Advise to notify physician if pregnant or intend to become pregnant, or breastfeeding. Encourage patients to enroll in the North American Antiepileptic Drug Pregnancy Registry. Instruct females to notify physician if they plan to start/stop use of oral contraceptives or other hormonal preparations. Advise to report changes in menstrual patterns and adverse reactions. Instruct to notify physician if medication is discontinued and not to resume therapy without consulting physician. Instruct to visually inspect tab to verify if correct drug/formulation was dispensed each time prescription is filled.

Administration: Oral route. Refer to PI for proper administration. **Storage:** (Tab/Tab, Chewable) 25°C (77°F); excursions permitted to 15-30°C (59-86°F) in a dry place. (Tab) Protect from light. (Tab, Disintegrating) 20-25°C (68-77°F); excursions permitted between 15-30°C (59-86°F).

LAMISIL   RX
terbinafine HCl (Novartis)

THERAPEUTIC CLASS: Allylamine antifungal

INDICATIONS: (Granules) Treatment of tinea capitis in patients ≥4 yrs of age. (Tab) Treatment of onychomycosis of toenail or fingernail due to dermatophytes (tinea unguium).

DOSAGE: *Adults:* (Tab) Onychomycosis: Fingernail: 250mg qd for 6 weeks. Toenail: 250mg qd for 12 weeks. (Granules) Tinea Capitis: Take qd with food for 6 weeks. >35kg: 250mg/day. 25-35kg: 187.5mg/day. <25kg: 125mg/day. (Tab) Elderly: Start at lower end of dosing range. *Pediatrics:* ≥4 Yrs: (Granules) Tinea Capitis: Take qd with food for 6 weeks. >35kg: 250mg/day. 25-35kg: 187.5mg/day. <25kg: 125mg/day.

HOW SUPPLIED: Granules: 125mg/pkt, 187.5mg/pkt; Tab: 250mg

WARNINGS/PRECAUTIONS: Cases of liver failure, some leading to liver transplant or death, reported in individuals with and without preexisting liver disease; d/c therapy if evidence of liver injury develops. Hepatotoxicity may occur. Not recommended for patients with chronic or active liver disease; perform LFTs prior to initiating therapy and periodically thereafter. D/C immediately in case of LFTs elevation or if any symptoms of persistent N/V, anorexia, fatigue, right upper abdominal pain, jaundice, dark urine, or pale stools occur. Taste/smell disturbance reported; d/c if symptoms occur. Depressive symptoms reported. Transient decreases in absolute lymphocyte counts and severe neutropenia reported; d/c and start supportive management if neutrophil count is ≤1000 cells/mm³. Consider monitoring CBCs in patients with known or suspected immunodeficiency if treatment continues for >6 weeks. Serious skin/hypersensitivity reactions (eg, Stevens-Johnson syndrome, toxic epidermal necrolysis, erythema multiforme, exfoliative/bullous dermatitis, drug reaction with eosinophilia and systemic symptoms (DRESS) syndrome) reported; d/c if progressive skin rash or signs/symptoms of DRESS occur. Precipitation and exacerbation of cutaneous and systemic lupus erythematosus reported; d/c in patients with clinical signs/symptoms suggestive of lupus erythematosus.

ADVERSE REACTIONS: Headache, diarrhea. (Granules) Nasopharyngitis, pyrexia, cough, vomiting, upper respiratory tract infection, upper abdominal pain. (Tab) Dyspepsia, nausea, rash, liver enzyme abnormalities, pruritus, taste disturbances.

INTERACTIONS: Coadministration with drugs predominantly metabolized by CYP2D6 (eg, TCAs, β-blockers, SSRIs, antiarrhythmics class 1C [eg, flecainide, propafenone], MAOIs type B, dextromethorphan) should be done with careful monitoring; may require dose reduction of the CYP2D6-metabolized drug. Increased dextromethorphan/dextrorphan metabolite ratio in urine in patients who are extensive metabolizers of dextromethorphan; may convert extensive CYP2D6 metabolizers to poor metabolizer status. Increased levels/exposure of desipramine. Increased clearance of cyclosporine. Decreased clearance of caffeine. Fluconazole may increase levels and exposure. May increase systemic exposure with other inhibitors of both CYP2C9 and CYP3A4 (eg, ketoconazole, amiodarone). Clearance increased by rifampin and decreased by cimetidine. Increased or decreased PT with warfarin.

PREGNANCY: Category B, not for use in nursing.

MECHANISM OF ACTION: Allylamine antifungal; acts by inhibiting squalene epoxidase, thus blocking biosynthesis of ergosterol, an essential component of fungal cell membrane.

PHARMACOKINETICS: Absorption: (Tab) Well-absorbed; bioavailability (40%); (250mg single dose) C_{max}=1mcg/mL, T_{max}=2 hrs, AUC =4.56mcg•hr/mL. **Distribution:** Plasma protein binding (>99%); found in breast milk. **Metabolism:** Extensive, (Granules) rapid. CYP2C9, CYP1A2, CYP3A4, CYP2C8, CYP2C19 (major). **Elimination:** Urine (70%). (Tab) $T_{1/2}$=200-400 hrs; (Granules) $T_{1/2}$=26.7 hrs (125mg dose), 30.5 hrs (187.5mg dose).

NURSING CONSIDERATIONS

Assessment: Assess for known hypersensitivity to the drug, active/chronic liver disease, immunodeficiency, lupus erythematosus, pregnancy/nursing status, and possible drug interactions. Confirm diagnosis of onychomycosis (potassium hydroxide preparation, fungal culture, or nail biopsy). Obtain baseline LFTs.

Monitoring: Monitor for signs/symptoms of hepatotoxicity, taste/smell disturbances, progressive skin rash, DRESS, depressive symptoms, lupus erythematosus, and other adverse reactions. Monitor CBC in patients with known or suspected immunodeficiency if therapy continues for >6 weeks, or if signs/symptoms of secondary infection occur. Monitor LFTs periodically.

Patient Counseling: Advise to d/c treatment and report immediately to physician if N/V, right upper abdominal pain, jaundice, dark urine, pale stools, taste/smell disturbance, anorexia, fatigue, depressive symptoms, hives, mouth sores, blistering and peeling of skin, swelling of face, lips, tongue, or throat, difficulty breathing/swallowing, fever, skin eruption, erythema, scaling, loss of pigment, unusual photosensitivity that can result in a rash, and lymph node enlargement occur. Instruct to minimize exposure to natural and artificial sunlight (tanning beds or UVA/B treatment) while on therapy. Advise to call physician if too many doses have been taken. If a dose is missed, advise to take tab as soon as remembered, unless it is <4 hrs before the next dose is due.

Administration: Oral route. (Granules) Take with food. Sprinkle contents of 1 pkt on a spoonful of pudding or other soft, nonacidic food (eg, mashed potatoes), and swallow entire spoonful (without chewing); do not use applesauce or fruit-based foods. Either the contents of both pkts may be sprinkled on 1 spoonful, or the contents of both pkts may be sprinkled on 2 spoonfuls of nonacidic food if 2 pkts are required/dose. (Tab) Take with or without food. **Storage:** (Tab) <25°C (77°F); in a tight container. Protect from light. (Granules) 25°C (77°F); excursions permitted to 15-30°C (59-86°F).

LANTUS   RX
insulin glargine, rdna origin (Sanofi-Aventis)

THERAPEUTIC CLASS: Insulin

INDICATIONS: To improve glycemic control in patients with type 1 diabetes mellitus (DM) and in adults with type 2 DM.

DOSAGE: *Adults:* Individualize dose. Inject SQ qd at same time every day. Type 1 DM: Initial: 1/3 of total daily insulin requirements. Use short-acting, premeal insulin to satisfy the remainder of daily insulin requirements. Type 2 DM not Currently Treated with Insulin: Initial: 10 U (or 0.2 U/kg) qd. Adjust according to blood glucose measurements. Switching from QD NPH Insulin: Initial: Same as NPH dose being discontinued. Switching from BID NPH Insulin: Initial: 80% of the total NPH dose being discontinued. Renal/Hepatic Impairment: May need to reduce dose. Elderly: Dose conservatively.
Pediatrics: ≥6 Yrs: Individualize dose. Inject SQ qd at same time every day. Type 1 DM: Initial: 1/3 of total daily insulin requirements. Use short-acting, premeal insulin to satisfy the remainder of daily insulin requirements. Adjust according to blood glucose measurements. Switching from QD NPH Insulin: Initial: Same as NPH dose being discontinued. Switching from BID NPH Insulin: Initial: 80% of the total NPH dose being discontinued. Renal/Hepatic Impairment: May need to reduce dose.

HOW SUPPLIED: Inj: 100 U/mL [3mL SoloStar, 10mL vial]

WARNINGS/PRECAUTIONS: Not recommended for the treatment of diabetic ketoacidosis. Must be used in regimens with short-acting insulin in patients with type 1 DM. Glucose monitoring is essential for all patients receiving insulin therapy. Changes to an insulin regimen should be made cautiously and only under medical supervision. Changes in insulin strength, manufacturer, type, or method of administration may result in need for a change in insulin dose or adjustment in concomitant oral antidiabetic treatment. Not for IV use or via an insulin pump. Do not share disposable or reusable insulin devices or needles between patients; may carry a risk for transmission of blood-borne pathogens. Hypoglycemia may occur; caution in patients with hypoglycemia unawareness and in patients who may be predisposed to hypoglycemia (eg, pediatric population, patients who fast or have erratic food intake). Hypoglycemia may impair ability to concentrate and react. Severe, life-threatening, generalized allergy, including anaphylaxis, may occur. Careful glucose monitoring and dose adjustments may be necessary with renal/hepatic impairment. Not recommended during periods of rapidly declining renal/hepatic function. Caution in elderly.

ADVERSE REACTIONS: Hypoglycemia, allergic reactions, upper respiratory tract infection, peripheral edema, HTN, influenza, sinusitis, cataract, bronchitis, arthralgia, infection, pain in extremities, back pain, cough, urinary tract infection.

INTERACTIONS: May require dose adjustment and close monitoring with drugs that may increase the blood-glucose-lowering effect and susceptibility to hypoglycemia (eg, oral antidiabetic drugs, pramlintide, ACE inhibitors, disopyramide, fibrates, fluoxetine, MAOIs, propoxyphene, pentoxifylline, salicylates, somatostatin analogs, sulfonamide antibiotics), drugs that may decrease the blood-glucose-lowering effect (eg, corticosteroids, niacin, danazol, diuretics, sympathomimetics [eg, epinephrine, albuterol, terbutaline], glucagon, isoniazid, phenothiazine derivatives, somatropin, thyroid hormones, estrogens, progestogens [eg, in oral contraceptives], protease inhibitors, atypical antipsychotics [eg, olanzapine, clozapine], or drugs that may either potentiate or weaken the blood-glucose-lowering effect (β-blockers, clonidine, lithium salts, alcohol). Pentamidine may cause hypoglycemia, sometimes followed by hyperglycemia. Signs of hypoglycemia may be reduced or absent with sympatholytics (eg, β-blockers, clonidine, guanethidine, reserpine). Fluid retention and heart failure (HF) can occur with concomitant use of thiazolidinediones; observe for signs/symptoms of HF and consider dose discontinuation/reduction of thiazolidinedione if HF develops.

PREGNANCY: Category C, caution in nursing.

MECHANISM OF ACTION: Insulin glargine (rDNA origin); regulates glucose metabolism. Lowers blood glucose by stimulating peripheral glucose uptake and by inhibiting hepatic glucose production. Inhibits lipolysis and proteolysis, and enhances protein synthesis.

PHARMACOKINETICS: Metabolism: M1 (21^A-Gly-insulin) and M2 (21^A-Gly-des-30^B-Thr-insulin) (active metabolites).

NURSING CONSIDERATIONS

Assessment: Assess for diabetic ketoacidosis, predisposition to hypoglycemia, hypersensitivity, renal/hepatic impairment, pregnancy/nursing status, and possible drug interactions. Obtain baseline blood glucose and HbA1c levels.

Monitoring: Monitor for signs/symptoms of hypoglycemia, allergic reactions, and other adverse reactions. Monitor blood glucose and HbA1c levels.

Patient Counseling: Inform about potential side effects (eg, lipodystrophy, weight gain, allergic reactions, hypoglycemia). Inform that hypoglycemia may impair ability to concentrate and react; advise to use caution when driving or operating machinery. Instruct to always check the label before each inj to avoid medication errors. Advise to use only if sol is clear and colorless with no particles visible. Advise not to share disposable or reusable insulin devices or needles with other patients. Instruct on self-management procedures, including glucose monitoring, proper inj technique, and management of hypoglycemia and hyperglycemia, and on handling of special situations, such as intercurrent conditions, inadequate or skipped dose, inadvertent administration of increased insulin dose, inadequate food intake, and skipped meals. Advise to inform physician if pregnant or contemplating pregnancy.

Administration: SQ route. Rotate inj sites within the same region (abdomen, thigh, or deltoid) from one inj to the next. Do not mix or dilute with any other insulin or sol. Refer to PI for further preparation, handling, and administration instructions. **Storage:** Do not freeze; discard if the vial has been frozen. Unopened: 2-8°C (36-46°F) until expiration date. Open (In-Use): 2-8°C (36-46°F) or ≤30°C (86°F) for vials and <30°C (86°F) for SoloStar. Discard after 28 days. Protect from direct heat and light. Do not refrigerate opened (in-use) SoloStar.

LASTACAFT   RX
alcaftadine (Allergan)

THERAPEUTIC CLASS: H$_1$-antagonist

INDICATIONS: Prevention of itching associated with allergic conjunctivitis.

DOSAGE: *Adults:* 1 drop in ou qd.
Pediatrics: ≥2 Yrs: 1 drop ou qd.

HOW SUPPLIED: Sol: 0.25% [3mL]

WARNINGS/PRECAUTIONS: For topical ophthalmic use only. Caution not to touch the dropper tip to eyelids or surrounding areas to minimize contamination. Do not wear contact lens if the eye is red. Not for treatment of contact lens-related irritation. Do not instill while wearing contact lenses; reinsert lenses after 10 min following administration.

ADVERSE REACTIONS: Eye irritation, burning and/or stinging upon instillation, eye redness, eye pruritus.

PREGNANCY: Category B, caution in nursing.

MECHANISM OF ACTION: H_1-receptor antagonist; inhibits release of histamine from mast cells, decreases chemotaxis, and inhibits eosinophil activation.

PHARMACOKINETICS: Absorption: C_{max}=60pg/mL, 3ng/mL (active metabolite); T_{max}=15 min (median), 1 hr after dosing (active metabolite). **Distribution:** Plasma protein binding (39.2%), (62.7%, active metabolite). **Metabolism:** non-CYP450 cytosolic enzymes; carboxylic acid metabolite (active metabolite). **Excretion:** Urine (unchanged); $T_{1/2}$=2 hrs (active metabolite).

NURSING CONSIDERATIONS

Assessment: Assess for contact lens-related irritation and pregnancy/nursing status.

Monitoring: Monitor for possible adverse reactions.

Patient Counseling: Advise to avoid touching the tip of dropper to any surface to avoid contamination. Advise not to wear contact lenses if the eye is red. Advise not to use to treat contact lens-related irritation. Advise to remove contact lenses prior to instillation, then reinsert lenses after 10 min following administration. Inform that the drug is for topical ophthalmic administration only.

Administration: Ocular route. **Storage:** 15-25°C (59-77°F). Keep bottle tightly closed when not in use.

LATISSE   RX
bimatoprost (Allergan)

THERAPEUTIC CLASS: Prostaglandin analog

INDICATIONS: Treatment of hypotrichosis of the eyelashes.

DOSAGE: *Adults:* 1 drop qpm using the supplied disposable sterile applicator. Apply evenly along the skin of upper eyelid margin at the base of eyelashes.

HOW SUPPLIED: Sol: 0.03% [3mL, 5mL]

WARNINGS/PRECAUTIONS: May lower intraocular pressure (IOP) when instilled directly to the eye. Increased iris pigmentation reported. May cause pigment changes (darkening) to periorbital pigmented tissues and eyelashes. May cause hair growth to occur in areas where sol comes in repeated contact. Caution with active intraocular inflammation (eg, uveitis); inflammation may be exacerbated. Macular edema, including cystoid macular edema, reported during treatment of elevated IOP; caution in aphakic patients, pseudophakic patients with torn posterior lens capsule, or patients at risk for macular edema. Avoid contact of bottle tip to any other surface. Use the accompanying sterile applicators on 1 eye, then discard; reuse of applicators increases the potential for contamination and infections. Bacterial keratitis associated with the use of multidose containers reported. Contact lenses should be removed prior to application and may be reinserted 15 min following administration.

ADVERSE REACTIONS: Eye pruritus, conjunctival hyperemia, skin hyperpigmentation, ocular irritation, dry eye symptoms, periorbital erythema.

INTERACTIONS: May interfere with the desired reduction in IOP with IOP-lowering prostaglandin analogs.

PREGNANCY: Category C, caution in nursing.

MECHANISM OF ACTION: Prostaglandin analog; has not been established. Believed that growth of eyelashes occur by increasing the percent of hairs in, and the duration of the anagen or growth phase.

PHARMACOKINETICS: Absorption: C_{max}=0.08ng/mL, AUC=0.09ng•hr/mL, T_{max}=10 min. **Distribution:** V_d=0.67L/kg. **Metabolism:** Oxidation, N-deethylation, and glucuronidation. **Elimination:** (IV) Urine (up to 67%), feces (25%); $T_{1/2}$=45 min.

NURSING CONSIDERATIONS

Assessment: Assess for active intraocular inflammation, aphakia, pseudophakia with a torn posterior lens capsule, risk for macular edema, pregnancy/nursing status, and possible drug interactions.

Monitoring: Monitor for IOP changes, increased iris pigmentation, pigment changes (darkening) to periorbital pigmented tissues and eyelashes, macular edema (eg, cystoid macular edema), bacterial keratitis, and other adverse reactions.

Patient Counseling: Instruct to apply medication every pm using only the accompanying sterile applicators, not to apply to lower eyelash line, and to blot any excess sol outside the upper eyelid margin with tissue or other absorbent material. Counsel that if any sol gets into the eye proper, it will not cause harm, and the eye should not be rinsed. Counsel that the effect is not permanent and can be expected to gradually return to original level upon d/c. Instruct to inform physician if using prostaglandin analogs for IOP reduction. Instruct that bottle must be maintained intact and to avoid contaminating the bottle tip or applicator. Advise to notify physician if patient has ocular surgery, or if new ocular condition (eg, trauma or infection) develops, sudden decrease in visual acuity occurs, or any ocular reactions (eg, conjunctivitis, eyelid reactions) develop. Advise about the potential for increased brown iris pigmentation (may be permanent), eyelid skin darkening, and unexpected hair growth or eyelash changes. Advise that contact lenses should be removed prior to application, and may be reinserted 15 min following its administration.

Administration: Ocular route. Refer to PI for further application instructions. **Storage:** 2-25°C (36-77°F).

LATUDA   RX
lurasidone HCl (Sunovion)

> Elderly patients with dementia-related psychosis treated with antipsychotic drugs are at an increased risk of death. Not approved for use in patients with dementia-related psychosis. Antidepressants increased the risk of suicidal thoughts and behavior in children, adolescents, and young adults in short-term studies. Monitor closely for worsening, and for emergence of suicidal thoughts and behaviors in patients who are started on antidepressant therapy.

THERAPEUTIC CLASS: Benzisothiazol derivative

INDICATIONS: Treatment of schizophrenia. As monotherapy or as adjunctive therapy with either lithium or valproate for the treatment of major depressive episodes associated with bipolar I disorder (bipolar depression).

DOSAGE: *Adults:* Schizophrenia: Initial: 40mg qd. Range: 40-160mg/day. Max: 160mg/day. Bipolar Depression: Initial: 20mg qd. Range: 20-120mg/day. Max: 120mg/day. Moderate (CrCl 30-<50mL/min) and Severe (CrCl <30mL/min) Renal Impairment/Moderate (Child-Pugh Score 7-9) Hepatic Impairment: Initial: 20mg/day. Max: 80mg/day. Severe (Child-Pugh Score 10-15) Hepatic Impairment: Initial: 20mg/day. Max: 40mg/day. Concomitant Moderate CYP3A4 Inhibitors (eg, Diltiazem, Atazanavir, Erythromycin, Fluconazole, Verapamil): Moderate CYP3A4 Inhibitor Added to Current Therapy with Lurasidone: Reduce lurasidone dose to 1/2 of the original dose level. Lurasidone Added to Current Therapy with a Moderate CYP3A4 Inhibitor: Initial: 20mg/day. Max: 80mg/day. Concomitant Moderate CYP3A4 Inducers: May need to increase lurasidone dose after chronic treatment (≥7 days) with the CYP3A4 inducer. Periodically reevaluate long-term usefulness for individual patient. Take with food (at least 350 calories).

HOW SUPPLIED: Tab: 20mg, 40mg, 60mg, 80mg, 120mg

CONTRAINDICATIONS: Concomitant use with strong CYP3A4 inhibitors (eg, ketoconazole, clarithromycin, ritonavir, voriconazole, mibefradil) or strong CYP3A4 inducers (eg, rifampin, avasimibe, St. John's wort, phenytoin, carbamazepine).

WARNINGS/PRECAUTIONS: Neuroleptic malignant syndrome (NMS) reported; d/c immediately and institute symptomatic treatment. May cause tardive dyskinesia (TD), especially in the elderly; d/c if this occurs. May cause metabolic changes (eg, hyperglycemia, dyslipidemia, weight gain) that may increase cardiovascular (CV)/cerebrovascular risk. Hyperglycemia, in some cases extreme and associated with ketoacidosis or hyperosmolar coma or death, reported; monitor glucose control regularly in patients with diabetes mellitus (DM) and FPG in patients at risk for DM. May elevate prolactin levels. Leukopenia, neutropenia, and agranulocytosis may occur; monitor CBC frequently during the 1st few months in patients with preexisting low WBC count or history of drug-induced leukopenia/neutropenia, and d/c at 1st sign of decline in WBC count without other causative factors. D/C therapy and follow WBC count until recovery in patients with severe neutropenia (absolute neutrophil count <1000/mm³). May cause orthostatic hypotension and syncope; consider using a lower starting dose/slower titration and monitor orthostatic vital signs in patients at increased risk of these reactions or at increased risk of developing complications from hypotension (eg, dehydration, hypovolemia, treatment with antihypertensives, history of CV/cerebrovascular disease, antipsychotic-naive patients). Caution with history of seizures or with conditions that lower the seizure threshold. May impair mental/physical abilities. May disrupt body's ability to reduce core body temperature; caution when prescribing for patients who will be experiencing conditions that may contribute to an elevation in core body temperature (eg, concomitant anticholinergics). Closely supervise patients at high risk of suicide. May increase risk of developing a manic or hypomanic episode, particularly in patients with bipolar disorder. May cause esophageal dysmotility and aspiration; caution in patients at risk for aspiration pneumonia.

Increased sensitivity reported in patients with Parkinson's disease or dementia with Lewy bodies. Evaluate for history of drug abuse; observe for drug misuse/abuse in these patients.

ADVERSE REACTIONS: Somnolence, akathisia, N/V, extrapyramidal symptoms, agitation, dyspepsia, back pain, dizziness, insomnia, anxiety, restlessness, diarrhea, dry mouth, nasopharyngitis.

INTERACTIONS: See Contraindications. Grapefruit/grapefruit juice may inhibit CYP3A4 and alter concentrations; avoid concomitant use. Adjust lurasidone dose when used in combination with moderate CYP3A4 inhibitors/inducers.

PREGNANCY: Category B, not for use in nursing.

MECHANISM OF ACTION: Benzisothiazol derivative; not established. Efficacy could be mediated through a combination of central dopamine type 2 and serotonin type 2 receptor antagonism.

PHARMACOKINETICS: Absorption: T_{max}=1-3 hrs. **Distribution:** (40mg) V_d=6173L; plasma protein binding (~99%). **Metabolism:** Mainly via CYP3A4; oxidative N-dealkylation, hydroxylation of norbornane ring, and S-oxidation; ID-14283 and ID-14326 (active metabolites), ID-20219 and ID-20220 (major metabolites). **Elimination:** Urine (9%), feces (80%); (40mg) $T_{1/2}$=18 hrs.

NURSING CONSIDERATIONS

Assessment: Assess for dementia-related psychosis, DM, renal/hepatic impairment, drug hypersensitivity, any other conditions where treatment is cautioned, pregnancy/nursing status, and possible drug interactions. Obtain baseline FPG in patients with DM or at risk for DM. Obtain baseline CBC if at risk for leukopenia/neutropenia.

Monitoring: Monitor for signs/symptoms of clinical worsening, suicidality, unusual changes in behavior, NMS, TD, hyperglycemia, hyperprolactinemia, orthostatic hypotension/syncope, cognitive/motor impairment, seizures, disruption of body temperature, manic/hypomanic episodes, esophageal dysmotility, aspiration, and other adverse reactions. Monitor FPG in patients with DM or at risk for DM, lipid profile, and weight. Monitor CBC frequently during the 1st few months in patients with preexisting low WBC count or history of drug-induced leukopenia/neutropenia. Monitor for fever or other signs/symptoms of infection in patients with neutropenia. Periodically reevaluate long-term usefulness for individual patient.

Patient Counseling: Advise to monitor for the emergence of suicidal thoughts and behavior, manic/hypomanic symptoms, irritability, agitation, or unusual changes in behavior and to report such symptoms to physician. Counsel about signs/symptoms of NMS (eg, hyperpyrexia, muscle rigidity, altered mental status, autonomic instability), hyperglycemia, and DM. Advise of the risk of dyslipidemia, weight gain, CV reactions, and orthostatic hypotension. Advise patients with preexisting low WBC count or history of drug-induced leukopenia/neutropenia to have their CBC monitored. Instruct to use caution when performing activities requiring mental alertness (eg, operating hazardous machinery, driving) until patients are reasonably certain that therapy does not affect them adversely. Instruct to notify physician if pregnant/intending to become pregnant, or if taking/planning to take any other medications. Advise to avoid alcohol while on treatment. Counsel regarding appropriate care in avoiding overheating and dehydration.

Administration: Oral route. Take with food (at least 350 calories). **Storage:** 25°C (77°F); excursions permitted to 15-30°C (59-86°F).

L<small>AZANDA</small>
fentanyl (Depomed)

> Fatal respiratory depression may occur. Contraindicated in the management of acute or postoperative pain (eg, headache/migraine) and in opioid-nontolerant patients. Keep out of reach of children. Concomitant use with CYP3A4 inhibitors may increase plasma levels, and may cause fatal respiratory depression. Do not convert patients on a mcg-per-mcg basis from any other fentanyl products to Lazanda. Do not substitute for any other fentanyl products; may result in fatal overdose. Contains fentanyl with abuse liability similar to other opioid analgesics. Available only through a restricted program called Transmucosal Immediate Release Fentanyl Risk Evaluation Mitigation Strategy (TIRF REMS) Access program, due to risk of misuse, abuse, addiction, and overdose. Outpatients, healthcare professionals who prescribe to outpatients, pharmacies, and distributors must enroll in this program.

THERAPEUTIC CLASS: Opioid analgesic

INDICATIONS: Management of breakthrough pain in cancer patients ≥18 yrs of age who are already receiving and who are tolerant to opioid therapy for their underlying persistent cancer pain. Patients must remain on around-the-clock opioids when taking Lazanda.

DOSAGE: *Adults:* ≥18 Yrs: Initial (Including Switching from Another Fentanyl Product): One 100mcg spray (1 spray in one nostril); if adequate analgesia is obtained within 30 min, treat subsequent episodes with this dose. Titrate: Individualize dose. If adequate analgesia is not achieved with the 1st 100mcg dose, escalate dose in a step-wise manner over consecutive episodes until adequate analgesia with tolerable side effects is achieved; wait at least 2 hrs before treating another episode. Refer to PI for titration steps. Max: 800mcg. Maint: Use the established dose for each subsequent episode; limit to ≤4 doses/day and wait at least 2 hrs before treating another episode. May use rescue medication if pain relief is inadequate after 30 min following dosing or if a separate episode occurs before the next dose is permitted (eg, within 2 hrs). Refer to PI for instructions on readjustment and discontinuation of therapy.

HOW SUPPLIED: Spray: 100mcg/spray, 400mcg/spray

CONTRAINDICATIONS: Opioid-nontolerant patients, management of acute or postoperative pain, including headache/migraine or dental pain.

WARNINGS/PRECAUTIONS: Increased risk of respiratory depression in patients with underlying respiratory disorders and in elderly/debilitated. May impair mental and/or physical abilities. Caution with chronic obstructive pulmonary disease or preexisting medical conditions predisposing to respiratory depression; may further decrease respiratory drive to the point of respiratory failure. Extreme caution in patients who may be susceptible to intracranial effects of CO_2 retention (eg, with evidence of increased intracranial pressure or impaired consciousness). May obscure the clinical course of head injuries. Avoid use during labor and delivery. Caution with renal/hepatic impairment, bradyarrhythmias, and in elderly.

ADVERSE REACTIONS: Respiratory depression, N/V, somnolence, dizziness, headache, constipation, pyrexia.

INTERACTIONS: See Boxed Warning. Not recomended with MAOIs or within 14 days of discontinuation of MAOIs. Increased depressant effects with other CNS depressants (eg, other opioids, sedatives/hypnotics, skeletal muscle relaxants); may require adjustment of fentanyl dose. CYP3A4 inducers (eg, barbiturates, carbamazepine, efavirenz) may decrease levels. Vasoconstrictive nasal decongestants such as oxymetazoline may decrease efficacy. Respiratory depression reported with other drugs that depress respiration.

PREGNANCY: Category C, not for use in nursing.

MECHANISM OF ACTION: Opioid analgesic; has not been established. Known to be mu-opioid receptor agonist; specific CNS opioid receptors for endogenous compounds with opioid-like activity have been identified throughout the brain and spinal cord and play a role in analgesic effects.

PHARMACOKINETICS: Absorption: Administration of various doses resulted in different parameters. **Distribution:** V_d=4L/kg; plasma protein binding (80-85%); crosses placenta; found in breast milk. **Metabolism:** Liver and intestinal mucosa via CYP3A4; norfentanyl (metabolite). **Elimination:** Urine (<7%, unchanged), feces (1%, unchanged); $T_{1/2}$=21.9 hrs (100mcg), 24.9 hrs (200mcg and 800mcg), 15 hrs (400mcg).

NURSING CONSIDERATIONS

Assessment: Assess for degree of opioid tolerance, previous opioid dose, level of pain intensity, type of pain, patient's general condition and medical status, and any other conditions where treatment is contraindicated or cautioned. Assess for hypersensitivity to the drug, renal/hepatic impairment, pregnancy/nursing status, and possible drug interactions.

Monitoring: Monitor for signs/symptoms of respiratory depression, impairment of mental/physical abilities, drug abuse/addiction, bradycardia, hypersensitivity reactions, and other adverse reactions.

Patient Counseling: Inform outpatients to enroll in the TIRF REMS Access program. Counsel that therapy may be fatal in children, in individuals for whom it was not prescribed, and in those who are not opioid tolerant. Counsel on proper administration and disposal. Advise to take drug as prescribed and to avoid sharing it with anyone else. Instruct not to take medication for acute or postoperative pain, pain from injuries, headache, migraine, or any other short-term pain. Instruct to notify physician if breakthrough pain is not alleviated or worsens after taking the drug. Inform that drug may impair mental/physical abilities; caution against performing activities that require high level of attention (eg, driving/using heavy machinery). Advise not to combine with alcohol, sleep aids, or tranquilizers, except if ordered by the physician. Instruct to notify physician if pregnant or planning to become pregnant.

Administration: Intranasal route. Refer to PI for proper administration and disposal instructions. **Storage:** Up to 25°C (77°F). Do not freeze. Protect from light.

LESCOL   RX
fluvastatin sodium (Novartis)

OTHER BRAND NAMES: Lescol XL (Novartis)

THERAPEUTIC CLASS: HMG-CoA reductase inhibitor

INDICATIONS: Adjunct to diet to decrease total cholesterol, LDL, apolipoprotein B, and TG levels, and to increase HDL levels in hypercholesterolemia and mixed dyslipidemia, heterozygous familial hypercholesterolemia (adolescent boys and girls who are at least 1 yr postmenarche, 10-16 yrs of age), and in secondary prevention of cardiovascular disease.

DOSAGE: *Adults:* Usual: 20-80mg/day. Do not take two 40mg cap at one time. LDL Reduction ≥25%: Initial: 40mg cap qpm or 80mg tab qd or 40mg cap bid. LDL Reduction <25%: Initial: 20mg cap qpm. Hypercholesterolemia/Mixed Dyslipidemia: Initial: 40mg cap qpm or 40mg cap bid or 80mg tab qd. Concomitant Cyclosporine/Fluconazole: Max: 20mg cap bid.
Pediatrics: 10-16 Yrs: Heterozygous Familial Hypercholesterolemia: Initial: One 20mg cap. Titrate: Adjust dose at 6-week intervals. Max: 40mg cap bid or 80mg tab qd. Concomitant Cyclosporine/Fluconazole: Max: 20mg cap bid.

HOW SUPPLIED: Cap: (Lescol) 20mg, 40mg; Tab, Extended-Release: (Lescol XL) 80mg

CONTRAINDICATIONS: Active liver disease or unexplained, persistent elevations of serum transaminases, women who are pregnant or may become pregnant, nursing mothers.

WARNINGS/PRECAUTIONS: Has not been studied in conditions where the major abnormality is elevation of chylomicrons, VLDL, or IDL (eg, hyperlipoproteinemia Types I, III, IV, or V). Rhabdomyolysis with acute renal failure secondary to myoglobinuria reported; caution in patients with predisposing factors to myopathy (eg, ≥65 yrs, renal impairment, and inadequately treated hypothyroidism). Myopathy (including immune-mediated necrotizing myopathy [IMNM]) reported; d/c if markedly elevated CPK levels occur or myopathy is diagnosed/suspected. Temporarily withhold in any patient experiencing an acute or serious condition predisposing to development of renal failure secondary to rhabdomyolysis. Increases in serum transaminases reported; perform LFTs before initiation and if signs/symptoms of liver injury occur. Fatal and nonfatal hepatic failure reported (rare); promptly interrupt therapy if serious liver injury and/or hyperbilirubinemia or jaundice occurs and do not restart if no alternate etiology found. Caution with heavy alcohol use or history of liver disease and in elderly. Increase in HbA1c and fasting serum glucose levels reported. May blunt adrenal and/or gonadal steroid hormone production. Evaluate if endocrine dysfunction develops. May cause CNS toxicity. Caution with severe renal impairment at doses >40mg.

ADVERSE REACTIONS: Dyspepsia, abdominal pain, headache, sinusitis, nausea, diarrhea, myalgia, flu-like symptoms, abnormal LFTs.

INTERACTIONS: Increased risk of myopathy and/or rhabdomyolysis with cyclosporine, erythromycin, fibrates, niacin, colchicine, and gemfibrozil; avoid with gemfibrozil, caution with colchicine and fibrates, and consider dose reduction with niacin. Caution with drugs that decrease levels of endogenous steroid hormones (eg, ketoconazole, spironolactone, cimetidine). Cyclosporine and fluconazole may increase levels. May increase levels of warfarin. Bleeding and/or increased PT reported with coumarin anticoagulants; monitor PT of patients on warfarin-type anticoagulants when therapy is initiated or dosage is changed. Increased glyburide and phenytoin levels.

PREGNANCY: Category X, not for use in nursing.

MECHANISM OF ACTION: HMG-CoA reductase inhibitor; inhibits conversion of HMG-CoA to mevalonate (precursor of sterols, including cholesterol). Inhibition of cholesterol biosynthesis reduces cholesterol in hepatic cells, which stimulates the synthesis of LDL receptors, thereby increasing uptake of LDL particles, resulting in reduction of plasma cholesterol concentration.

PHARMACOKINETICS: Absorption: Absolute bioavailability (24%); T_{max}=<1 hr. Tab: T_{max}=3 hrs (fasting), 2.5 hrs (low-fat meal), 6 hrs (high-fat meal). **Distribution:** V_d=0.35L/kg, plasma protein binding (98%). **Metabolism:** Liver via CYP2C9, 2C8, and 3A4 through hydroxylation, N-dealkylation, and β-oxidation pathways. **Elimination:** Feces (90% metabolites, <2% unchanged), urine (5%); $T_{1/2}$=3 hrs.

NURSING CONSIDERATIONS

Assessment: Assess for active liver disease or unexplained, persistent elevations in serum transaminases, pregnancy/nursing status, predisposing factors for myopathy, heavy alcohol intake, history of liver disease, and possible drug interactions. Obtain baseline lipid profile (total-C, LDL, HDL, TG) and LFTs.

Monitoring: Monitor for signs/symptoms of myopathy (including IMNM), rhabdomyolysis, liver/renal/endocrine dysfunction, CNS toxicity, and other adverse reactions. Perform periodic monitoring of lipid profile. Check PT with coumarin anticoagulants.

Patient Counseling: Inform of the substances that should not be taken concomitantly with the drug. Counsel to inform other healthcare professionals that they are taking the drug. Advise to report promptly unexplained muscle pain, tenderness, or weakness, particularly if accompanied by malaise or fever or if muscle signs/symptoms persist after discontinuation. Advise to report promptly any symptoms that may indicate liver injury (eg, fatigue, anorexia, right upper abdominal discomfort, dark urine, or jaundice). Inform women of childbearing age to use an effective method of birth control, stop taking drug if they become pregnant, and not to breastfeed while on therapy.

Administration: Oral route. Do not break, crush or chew tab, or open cap before administration. Take with or without food. **Storage:** 25°C (77°F); excursions permitted to 15-30°C (15-86°F). Protect from light.

LETAIRIS

RX

ambrisentan (Gilead Sciences)

> Do not administer to a pregnant female; may cause serious birth defects. Exclude pregnancy before initiation of treatment. Females of reproductive potential must use acceptable methods of contraception during and for 1 month after treatment; obtain monthly pregnancy tests during and 1 month after discontinuation of treatment. Females can only receive the drug through a restricted program called the Letairis Risk Evaluation and Mitigation Strategy (REMS) program.

THERAPEUTIC CLASS: Endothelin receptor antagonist

INDICATIONS: Treatment of pulmonary arterial HTN (World Health Organization [WHO] Group 1) to improve exercise ability and delay clinical worsening.

DOSAGE: *Adults:* Initial: 5mg qd. Titrate: May increase to 10mg qd if 5mg is tolerated. Max: 10mg qd.

HOW SUPPLIED: Tab: 5mg, 10mg

CONTRAINDICATIONS: Pregnancy, idiopathic pulmonary fibrosis (IPF), including IPF patients with pulmonary HTN (WHO Group 3).

WARNINGS/PRECAUTIONS: May cause peripheral edema; reported with greater frequency and severity in elderly patients. If clinically significant fluid retention develops, evaluate further to determine the cause and the possible need for specific treatment or discontinuation of therapy. If acute pulmonary edema develops during initiation of therapy, consider the possibility of pulmonary veno-occlusive disease (PVOD); d/c if confirmed. May decrease sperm count. Decreases in Hgb concentration and Hct reported and may result in anemia requiring transfusion; measure Hgb prior to initiation, at 1 month, and periodically thereafter. Not recommended with clinically significant anemia. Consider discontinuation if clinically significant Hgb decrease is observed and other causes have been excluded. Not recommended with moderate/severe hepatic impairment. Fully investigate the cause of liver injury if hepatic impairment develops; d/c if elevations of liver aminotransferases are >5X ULN or if elevations are accompanied by bilirubin >2X ULN, or by signs/symptoms of liver dysfunction and other causes are excluded.

ADVERSE REACTIONS: Peripheral edema, nasal congestion, flushing, sinusitis.

INTERACTIONS: Cyclosporine may increase exposure; limit dose of ambrisentan to 5mg qd when coadministered with cyclosporine.

PREGNANCY: Category X, not for use in nursing.

MECHANISM OF ACTION: Endothelin receptor antagonist; selective for endothelin type-A receptor, blocks the vasoconstriction and cell proliferation effects of endothelin-1 in the vascular smooth muscle and endothelium.

PHARMACOKINETICS: Absorption: T_{max}=2 hrs. **Distribution:** Plasma protein binding (99%). **Metabolism:** Liver via CYP3A, 2C19, and UGTs 1A9S, 2B7S, and 1A3S. **Elimination:** $T_{1/2}$=15 hrs.

NURSING CONSIDERATIONS

Assessment: Assess for IPF, anemia, hepatic impairment, pregnancy/nursing status, and possible drug interactions. Obtain baseline Hgb levels.

Monitoring: Monitor for fluid retention, pulmonary edema, PVOD, hepatic impairment, and other adverse reactions. Obtain monthly pregnancy tests in females of reproductive potential during therapy and 1 month after discontinuation of treatment. Measure Hgb at 1 month after initiating therapy and periodically thereafter.

Patient Counseling: Instruct on the risk of fetal harm when used in pregnancy and instruct to immediately contact physician if pregnancy is suspected. Inform female patients that drug is only available through a restricted program called the Letairis REMS program. Inform female patients that they must sign an enrollment form and that female patients of reproductive potential must comply with pregnancy testing and contraception requirements. Educate and counsel females of reproductive potential on the use of emergency contraception in the event of unprotected sex or known or suspected contraceptive failure. Advise prepubertal females to immediately report to physician any reproductive status changes. Instruct to contact physician if any symptoms of liver injury occur. Advise of the importance of Hgb testing and of other risks associated with therapy (eg, decreases in Hgb, Hct, and sperm count, fluid overload).

Administration: Oral route. May be taken with or without food. Do not split, crush, or chew tabs. **Storage:** 25°C (77°F); excursions permitted to 15-30°C (59-86°F).

LEUKERAN

RX

chlorambucil (GlaxoSmithKline)

> Can severely suppress bone marrow function. Potentially carcinogenic, mutagenic, and teratogenic. Produces infertility.

THERAPEUTIC CLASS: Nitrogen mustard alkylating agent

INDICATIONS: Treatment of chronic lymphatic (lymphocytic) leukemia, malignant lymphomas, including lymphosarcoma, giant follicular lymphoma, and Hodgkin's disease.

DOSAGE: *Adults:* Usual: 0.1-0.2mg/kg/day for 3-6 weeks as required. Adjust according to response; reduce with abrupt fall in WBC count. Hodgkin's Disease: Usual: 0.2mg/kg/day. Other Lymphomas/Chronic Lymphocytic Leukemia: Usual: 0.1mg/kg/day. Lymphocytic Infiltration of Bone Marrow/Hypoplastic Bone Marrow: Max: 0.1mg/kg/day. Maint: 2-4mg/day or less, depending on the status of blood counts. Hepatic Impairment: Reduce dose. Elderly: Start at the lower end of dosing range.

HOW SUPPLIED: Tab: 2mg

CONTRAINDICATIONS: Prior resistance to therapy.

WARNINGS/PRECAUTIONS: Should not be given for conditions other than chronic lymphatic leukemia or malignant lymphomas. Convulsions, leukemia, and secondary malignancies observed. Acute leukemia reported; risk increases with chronic treatment and large cumulative doses. Weigh benefit on an individual basis against possible risk of induction of secondary malignancy. Causes chromatid or chromosome damage and sterility. Rare instances of skin rash progressing to erythema multiforme, toxic epidermal necrolysis, or Stevens-Johnson syndrome reported; d/c if skin reactions develop. May cause fetal harm; women of childbearing potential should avoid becoming pregnant. Slowly progressive lymphopenia reported; lymphocyte count usually returns to normal upon completion of therapy. Caution with history of seizures, head trauma, or patients who are receiving other potentially epileptogenic drugs, hepatic impairment, and in elderly. Avoid live vaccines in the immunocompromised.

ADVERSE REACTIONS: Bone marrow suppression, anemia, leukopenia, neutropenia, thrombocytopenia, pancytopenia, infertility.

INTERACTIONS: Caution within 4 weeks of full course of radiation or chemotherapy because of the vulnerability of the bone marrow to damage; do not give at full dosages.

PREGNANCY: Category D, not for use in nursing.

MECHANISM OF ACTION: Nitrogen mustard alkylating agent; interferes with DNA replication and induces cellular apoptosis via the accumulation of cytosolic p53 and subsequent activation of Bax, an apoptosis promoter.

PHARMACOKINETICS: Absorption: Rapid and complete. (0.6-1.2 mg/kg) T_{max}=1 hr; (0.2mg/kg) C_{max}=492ng/mL, T_{max}=0.83 hrs, AUC=883ng•hr/mL; (Phenylacetic acid mustard [PAAM]) C_{max}=306ng/mL, T_{max}=1.9 hrs; AUC=1204ng•hr/mL. **Distribution:** V_d=0.31L/kg, plasma protein binding (99%). **Metabolism:** Liver (extensive); oxidative degradation to monohydroxy/dihydroxy derivatives; PAAM (major metabolite). **Elimination:** Urine (20-60%, <1% chlorambucil or PAAM); $T_{1/2}$=1.5 hrs (0.6-1.2mg/kg dose), 1.3 hrs (0.2mg/kg dose), 1.8 hrs (PAAM).

NURSING CONSIDERATIONS

Assessment: Assess for prior resistance, history of seizures or head trauma, hepatic impairment, pregnancy/nursing status, and possible drug interactions. Obtain baseline Hgb, WBC counts, and platelet count.

Monitoring: Monitor for signs/symptoms of bone marrow suppression, cross-hypersensitivity reactions, secondary malignancies, convulsions, infertility, leukemia, and skin reactions. Monitor Hgb levels, total and differential leukocyte counts, and quantitative platelet counts weekly. During first 3-6 weeks of therapy, blood counts should be made 3 or 4 days after each weekly CBC. Monitor for toxicity in patients with hepatic impairment.

Patient Counseling: Advise to avoid vaccinations with live vaccines. Inform that major toxicities are related to hypersensitivity, drug fever, myelosuppression, hepatotoxicity, infertility, seizures, GI toxicity, and secondary malignancies. Instruct not to take without medical supervision. Advise to consult a physician if skin rash, bleeding, fever, jaundice, persistent cough, seizures, N/V, amenorrhea, or unusual lumps/masses occur. Advise women of childbearing potential to avoid becoming pregnant.

Administration: Oral route. **Storage:** 2-8°C (36-46°F).

LEVAQUIN   RX
levofloxacin (Janssen)

> Fluoroquinolones are associated with an increased risk of tendinitis and tendon rupture in all ages. Risk is further increased with patients >60 yrs of age, patients taking corticosteroids, and with kidney, heart, or lung transplants. May exacerbate muscle weakness with myasthenia gravis; avoid in patients with known history of myasthenia gravis.

THERAPEUTIC CLASS: Fluoroquinolone

INDICATIONS: Treatment of uncomplicated and complicated skin and skin structure infections (cSSSIs), uncomplicated and complicated urinary tract infections (UTIs), acute bacterial sinusitis, acute bacterial exacerbation of chronic bronchitis (ABECB), community-acquired pneumonia (CAP), nosocomial pneumonia, chronic bacterial prostatitis, and acute pyelonephritis (AP), including cases with concurrent bacteremia caused by susceptible strains of microorganisms in adults ≥18 yrs of age. To reduce the incidence or progression of disease following anthrax exposure in adults and pediatric patients. Treatment of plague, including pneumonic and septicemic plague, and prophylaxis for plague in adults and pediatric patients ≥6 months of age.

DOSAGE: *Adults:* ≥18 Yrs: PO/IV: CAP: 750mg qd for 5 days or 500mg qd for 7-14 days. Acute Bacterial Sinusitis: 750mg qd for 5 days or 500mg qd for 10-14 days. ABECB: 500mg qd for 7 days. cSSSI/Nosocomial Pneumonia: 750mg qd for 7-14 days. Uncomplicated SSSI: 500mg qd for 7-10 days. Chronic Bacterial Prostatitis: 500mg qd for 28 days. Complicated UTI/AP: 750mg qd for 5 days or 250mg qd for 10 days. Uncomplicated UTI: 250mg qd for 3 days. Inhalational Anthrax: 500mg qd for 60 days. Plague: 500mg qd for 10-14 days. Refer to PI for dose adjustment with renal impairment (CrCl <50mL/min). IV: Infuse over 60 min q24h (250-500mg) or over 90 min q24h (750mg).
Pediatrics: ≥6 Months: PO/IV: Inhalational Anthrax: >50kg: 500mg q24h for 60 days. <50kg: 8mg/kg q12h for 60 days. Max: 250mg/dose. Plague: >50kg: 500mg q24h for 10-14 days. <50kg: 8mg/kg q12h for 10-14 days. Max: 250mg/dose. IV: Infuse over 60 min q24h (250-500mg).

HOW SUPPLIED: Inj: 25mg/mL [20mL, 30mL], 5mg/mL in 5% D5W [50mL, 100mL, 150mL]; Sol: 25mg/mL; Tab: 250mg, 500mg, 750mg

WARNINGS/PRECAUTIONS: D/C if patient experiences pain, swelling, inflammation, or rupture of a tendon. Serious and sometimes fatal hypersensitivity reactions reported; d/c if skin rash, jaundice, or any other sign of hypersensitivity appears and institute appropriate therapy. Severe hepatotoxicity, including acute hepatitis and fatal events, reported; d/c if signs and symptoms of hepatitis occur. Convulsions, toxic psychoses, and increased intracranial pressure (including pseudotumor cerebri) reported. CNS stimulation may occur; d/c and institute appropriate measures if CNS events occur. Caution with CNS disorders (eg, severe cerebral arteriosclerosis, epilepsy) or risk factors that may predispose to seizures or lower seizure threshold. Rare cases of sensory or sensorimotor axonal polyneuropathy resulting in paresthesias, hypoesthesias, dysesthesias, and weakness reported; d/c if symptoms of neuropathy occur. May prolong QT interval; avoid with known QT interval prolongation or uncorrected hypokalemia. Increased incidence of musculoskeletal disorders in pediatric patients. Blood glucose disturbances reported in diabetics; d/c if hypoglycemic reactions occur. May cause photosensitivity/phototoxicity reactions; avoid excessive exposure to sun/UV light and d/c if occurs. *Clostridium difficile*-associated diarrhea (CDAD) reported. May result in bacterial resistance with prolonged use or use in the absence of a proven/suspected bacterial infection or a prophylactic indication; take appropriate measures if superinfection develops. Crystalluria and cylindruria reported; maintain adequate hydration. Caution in elderly and with renal impairment.

ADVERSE REACTIONS: Tendinitis, tendon rupture, nausea, diarrhea, constipation, headache, insomnia, dizziness.

INTERACTIONS: See Boxed Warning. Caution with drugs that may lower the seizure threshold. May prolong QT interval; avoid with Class IA (eg, quinidine, procainamide) and Class III (eg, amiodarone, sotalol) antiarrhythmics. NSAIDs may increase risk of CNS stimulation and convulsive seizures. May enhance effects of warfarin; monitor PT and INR. May increase theophylline levels and increase risk of theophylline-related adverse reactions; monitor theophylline levels closely. Disturbances of blood glucose in diabetic patients receiving a concomitant antidiabetic agent reported; monitor glucose levels. Reduced renal clearance with either cimetidine or probenecid. (PO) Antacids containing magnesium, aluminum, as well as sucralfate, metal cations such as iron, and multivitamins containing zinc, or didanosine chewable/buffered tab or pediatric powder for PO sol may substantially interfere with the GI absorption and lower systemic concentrations; take at least 2 hrs before or 2 hrs after PO levofloxacin.

PREGNANCY: Category C, not for use in nursing.

MECHANISM OF ACTION: Fluoroquinolone; inhibits bacterial topoisomerase IV and DNA gyrase (both of which are type II topoisomerases), which are enzymes required for DNA replication, transcription, repair, and recombination.

PHARMACOKINETICS: Absorption: (PO) Rapid and complete; (Tab) absolute bioavailability (99%); administration of variable doses resulted in different parameters. **Distribution:** V_d=74-112L; plasma protein binding (24-38%); found in breast milk. **Metabolism:** Limited. **Elimination:** (PO) Urine (87% unchanged, <5% desmethyl and N-oxide metabolites), feces (<4%); $T_{1/2}$=6-8 hrs.

NURSING CONSIDERATIONS

Assessment: Assess for risk factors for developing tendinitis and tendon rupture, history of myasthenia gravis, drug hypersensitivity, CNS disorders or risk factors that may predispose to seizures or lower seizure threshold, QT interval prolongation, uncorrected hypokalemia, renal/hepatic function, pregnancy/nursing status, and possible drug interactions.

Monitoring: Monitor for ECG changes (eg, QT interval prolongation), anaphylactic reactions, hepatotoxicity, arrhythmias, CNS events, CDAD, peripheral neuropathy, musculoskeletal disorders (pediatric patients), tendon rupture, tendinitis, and for photosensitivity/phototoxicity reactions and superinfection. Monitor hydration status, blood glucose levels, and renal function. Monitor for muscle weakness in patients with myasthenia gravis. Monitor for evidence of bleeding, PT, and INR with warfarin.

Patient Counseling: Inform that drug treats only bacterial, not viral, infections. Advise to take as prescribed; inform that skipping doses or not completing the full course of therapy may decrease effectiveness and increase drug resistance. Advise to take PO sol 1 hr before or 2 hrs after eating, to take tab without regard to meals, to take medication at the same time each day, to drink fluids liberally, and that antacids, metal cations, and multivitamins should be taken at least 2 hrs before or 2 hrs after PO administration. Notify physician if symptoms of pain, swelling, or inflammation of a tendon, or weakness or inability to move joints develop. Notify physician of any history of convulsions, QT prolongation, or myasthenia gravis. D/C use and notify physician if allergic reaction, skin rash, signs/symptoms of liver injury or peripheral neuropathy occur. Caution in activities requiring mental alertness and coordination. Instruct to contact physician immediately if watery and bloody diarrhea (with or without stomach cramps and fever) develop. Inform physician if child has tendon or joint-related problems prior to, during, or after therapy. Advise to minimize or avoid exposure to natural or artificial sunlight. Instruct diabetic patients being treated with antidiabetic agents to d/c therapy and notify physician if hypoglycemia occurs. Advise to inform physician if taking warfarin.

Administration: IV, Oral route. (Sol) Give 1 hr before or 2 hrs after eating. (Inj) Refer to PI for administration, preparation, stability, compatibility, and thawing instructions. **Storage:** (Tab) 15-30°C (59-86°F). (Sol) 25°C (77°F); excursions permitted to 15-30°C (59-86°F). (Inj) Single-use Vials: Controlled room temperature and protected from light. Diluted in Plastic IV Container (5mg/mL): Stable at ≤25°C (77°F) for 72 hrs; 5°C (41°F) for 14 days; -20°C (-4°F) for 6 months. Premixed Sol: ≤25°C (77°F); brief exposure ≤40°C (104°F). Avoid excessive heat and protect from freezing and light.

LEVBID   RX
hyoscyamine sulfate (Alaven)

THERAPEUTIC CLASS: Anticholinergic

INDICATIONS: Adjunct treatment of peptic ulcer, irritable bowel syndrome, neurogenic bladder, and neurogenic bowel disturbances. Management of functional intestinal disorders (eg, mild dysenteries, diverticulitis, acute enterocolitis). To control gastric secretion, visceral spasm, and hypermotility in spastic colitis, spastic bladder, cystitis, pylorospasm, and associated abdominal cramps. Drying agent for symptomatic relief of acute rhinitis. Symptomatic relief of biliary and renal colic with concomitant morphine or other narcotics. To reduce rigidity and tremors and to control associated sialorrhea and hyperhidrosis in parkinsonism. Antidote for anticholinesterase poisoning.

DOSAGE: *Adults:* 1-2 tabs q12h. Max: 4 tabs/24 hrs. Elderly: Start at low end of dosing range. *Pediatrics:* ≥12 Yrs: 1-2 tabs q12h. Max: 4 tabs/24 hrs.

HOW SUPPLIED: Tab, Extended-Release: 0.375mg

CONTRAINDICATIONS: Glaucoma; obstructive uropathy; obstructive GI tract disease; paralytic ileus, intestinal atony of elderly/debilitated; unstable cardiovascular (CV) status in acute hemorrhage; severe ulcerative colitis; toxic megacolon complicating ulcerative colitis, myasthenia gravis.

WARNINGS/PRECAUTIONS: Risk of heat prostration with high environmental temperature. May impair physical/mental abilities. Caution with diarrhea, autonomic neuropathy, hyperthyroidism, coronary heart disease, congestive heart failure, cardiac arrhythmias, HTN, renal disease, and hiatal hernia associated with reflux esophagitis. Psychosis reported in sensitive patients.

ADVERSE REACTIONS: Anticholinergic effects, drowsiness, headache, nervousness, N/V, diarrhea.

INTERACTIONS: May have additive effects with other antimuscarinics, amantadine, haloperidol, phenothiazines, MAOIs, TCAs, and some antihistamines. Antacids may interfere with absorption.

PREGNANCY: Category C, caution in nursing.

MECHANISM OF ACTION: Belladonna alkaloid; inhibits action of acetylcholine on structures innervated by postganglionic cholinergic nerves and on smooth muscles that respond to acetylcholine but lack cholinergic innervation, inhibiting GI propulsive motility, decreasing gastric acid secretion, and controlling excess pharyngeal, tracheal, and bronchial secretions.

PHARMACOKINETICS: Absorption: Complete; T_{max}=4.2 hrs. **Distribution:** Crosses placenta; found in breast milk. **Metabolism:** Partial hydrolysis; tropic acid, tropine (metabolites). **Elimination:** Urine (unchanged); $T_{1/2}$=7.47 hrs.

NURSING CONSIDERATIONS

Assessment: Assess for glaucoma, obstructive uropathy, GI obstruction, paralytic ileus, intestinal atony, unstable CV status in acute hemorrhage, other conditions where treatment is contraindicated/cautioned, pregnancy/nursing status, and possible drug interactions.

Monitoring: Monitor for signs/symptoms of heat prostration, incomplete intestinal obstruction, blurred vision, psychosis, CNS events, diarrhea, and other adverse reactions. Monitor renal function.

Patient Counseling: Advise against engaging in activities requiring mental alertness (eg, operating a motor vehicle or other machinery) or performing hazardous work while on treatment. Inform that heat prostration may occur with drug use (fever and heat stroke due to decreased sweating); use caution if febrile, or exposed to high environmental temperatures.

Administration: Oral route. Do not crush or chew. **Storage:** 20-25°C (68-77°F); excursions permitted to 15-30°C (59-86°F).

LEVEMIR   RX
insulin detemir, rdna origin (Novo Nordisk)

THERAPEUTIC CLASS: Insulin

INDICATIONS: To improve glycemic control in adults and children with diabetes mellitus (DM).

DOSAGE: *Adults:* Individualize dose. Administer SQ. Administer qd dose with pm meal or at hs. If bid dosing is required, administer pm dose with pm meal, at hs, or 12 hrs after am dose. Type 2 DM Inadequately Controlled on Oral Antidiabetic Medications: Initial: 10 U (or 0.1-0.2 U/kg) qd or divided into bid. Type 2 DM Inadequately Controlled on Glucagon-Like Peptide (GLP)-1 Receptor Agonist: Initial: 10 U qd. Type 1 DM: Initial: 1/3 of total daily insulin requirements. Use rapid- or short-acting premeal insulin to satisfy remaining daily insulin requirements. Titrate: Adjust based on blood glucose measurements. Conversion from Insulin Glargine/NPH Insulin: Switch on a unit-to-unit basis. In converting from NPH insulin, some type 2 DM patients may require more units of therapy than NPH insulin. Hepatic/Renal Impairment: May need to adjust dose. Elderly: Dose conservatively.
Pediatrics: ≥2 Yrs: Type 1 DM: Individualize dose. Administer SQ. Administer qd dose with pm meal or at hs. If bid dosing is required, administer pm dose with pm meal, at hs, or 12 hrs after am dose. Initial: 1/3 of total daily insulin requirements. Use rapid- or short-acting premeal insulin to satisfy remaining daily insulin requirements. Titrate: Adjust based on blood glucose measurements. Conversion from Insulin Glargine/NPH Insulin: Switch on a unit-to-unit basis. Hepatic/Renal Impairment: May need to adjust dose.

HOW SUPPLIED: Inj: 100 U/mL [3mL, FlexPen, FlexTouch; 10mL, vial].

WARNINGS/PRECAUTIONS: Not recommended for treatment of diabetic ketoacidosis. Changes to an insulin regimen should be made cautiously and only under medical supervision. Changes in strength, manufacturer, type, or method of administration may result in the need for a change in dose or an adjustment of concomitant antidiabetic treatment. Not for IV/IM use or use in insulin infusion pumps. Hypoglycemia may occur; caution in patients with hypoglycemia unawareness and patients predisposed to hypoglycemia. Hypoglycemia may impair ability to concentrate and react. Severe, life-threatening, generalized allergy, including anaphylaxis, may occur. Careful glucose monitoring and dose adjustments may be necessary with renal/hepatic impairment.

ADVERSE REACTIONS: Hypoglycemia, upper respiratory tract infection, headache, pharyngitis, influenza-like illness, abdominal pain, back pain, gastroenteritis, bronchitis, pyrexia, cough, viral infection, N/V, rhinitis.

INTERACTIONS: May require insulin dose adjustment and close monitoring with drugs that may increase blood-glucose-lowering effect and susceptibility to hypoglycemia (eg, oral antidiabetic drugs, pramlintide acetate, ACE inhibitors, disopyramide, fibrates, fluoxetine, MAOIs, propoxyphene, pentoxifylline, salicylates, somatostatin analogs, sulfonamide antibiotics), drugs that may reduce blood-glucose-lowering effect (eg, corticosteroids, niacin, danazol, diuretics, sympathomimetic agents [eg, epinephrine, albuterol, terbutaline], glucagon, isoniazid, phenothiazine derivatives, somatropin, thyroid hormones, estrogens, progestogens [eg, in oral contraceptives], protease inhibitors, atypical antipsychotic medications [eg, olanzapine, clozapine]), or drugs that may either increase or decrease blood-glucose-lowering effect (eg, β-blockers, clonidine, lithium salts, alcohol). Pentamidine may cause hypoglycemia, sometimes followed by hyperglycemia. Signs of hypoglycemia may be reduced or absent with antiadrenergic drugs (eg, β-blockers, clonidine, guanethidine, reserpine). May need to lower or more conservatively titrate dose when used with a GLP-1 receptor agonist to minimize risk of hypoglycemia. Observe for signs/symptoms of heart failure (HF) if treated concomitantly with a peroxisome proliferator-activated receptor (PPAR)-gamma agonist (eg, thiazolidinedione); consider discontinuation or dose reduction of the PPAR-gamma agonist if HF develops.

PREGNANCY: Category B, caution in nursing.

MECHANISM OF ACTION: Insulin detemir (rDNA origin); regulates glucose metabolism. Lowers blood glucose by facilitating cellular uptake of glucose into skeletal muscle and adipose tissue and by inhibiting the output of glucose from the liver. Inhibits lipolysis in the adipocyte, inhibits proteolysis, and enhances protein synthesis.

PHARMACOKINETICS: Absorption: Absolute bioavailability (60%); T_{max}=6-8 hrs. **Distribution:** Plasma protein binding (>98%); V_d=0.1L/kg. **Elimination:** $T_{1/2}$=5-7 hrs.

NURSING CONSIDERATIONS

Assessment: Assess for diabetic ketoacidosis, predisposition to hypoglycemia, hypersensitivity, renal/hepatic impairment, pregnancy/nursing status, and possible drug interactions. Obtain baseline blood glucose and HbA1c levels.

Monitoring: Monitor for signs/symptoms of hypoglycemia, allergic reactions, and other adverse effects. Monitor blood glucose and HbA1c levels, and renal/hepatic function.

Patient Counseling: Inform about the potential side effects, including hypoglycemia, weight gain, and allergic reactions. Inform that hypoglycemia may impair ability to concentrate and react; advise to use caution when driving or operating machinery. Instruct to always check the label before each inj to avoid medication errors/accidental mix-ups. Advise to use only if solution is clear and colorless with no particles visible. Instruct on self-management procedures, including glucose monitoring, proper inj technique, and management of hypoglycemia and hyperglycemia, and on handling of special situations, such as intercurrent conditions, inadequate or skipped insulin dose, inadvertent administration of an increased insulin dose, inadequate food intake, and skipped meals. Advise to inform physician if pregnant/contemplating pregnancy. Counsel to never share a FlexPen or FlexTouch with another person, even if the needle is changed.

Administration: SQ route. Inject in the thigh, abdominal wall, or upper arm; rotate inj sites within the same region. Do not dilute or mix with any other insulin or solution. Refer to PI for further instructions on preparation, handling, and administration. **Storage:** Unopened: 2-8°C (36-46°F) until expiration date. If refrigeration is not possible, may be kept at room temperature <30°C (86°F) for 42 days. Do not freeze. Protect from direct heat and light. Opened: Vial: 2-8°C (36-46°F) or room temperature <30°C (86°F). Discard refrigerated vials 42 days after initial use and discard unrefrigerated vials 42 days after they are 1st kept out of the refrigerator. Do not freeze. Protect from direct heat and light. FlexPen/FlexTouch: Room temperature <30°C (86°F) for 42 days; do not refrigerate or store with the needle in place. Protect from direct heat and light.

LEVITRA   RX
vardenafil HCl (GlaxoSmithKline)

THERAPEUTIC CLASS: Phosphodiesterase type 5 inhibitor

INDICATIONS: Treatment of erectile dysfunction (ED).

DOSAGE: *Adults:* Initial: 10mg PRN, 60 min prior to sexual activity. Titrate: May decrease to 5mg or increase to max of 20mg based on efficacy and side effects. Max: 1 tab/day. Elderly: ≥65 Yrs: Initial: 5mg. Moderate Hepatic Impairment (Child-Pugh B): Initial: 5mg. Max: 10mg. Concomitant Ritonavir: Max: 2.5mg/72 hrs. Concomitant Indinavir/Saquinavir/Atazanavir/Clarithromycin/Ketoconazole (400mg/day)/Itraconazole (400mg/day): Max: 2.5mg/24 hrs. Concomitant Ketoconazole (200mg/day)/Itraconazole (200mg/day)/Erythromycin: Max: 5mg/24 hrs. Patients Stable on α-Blocker: Initial: 5mg; 2.5mg when used with certain CYP3A4 inhibitors. Consider a time interval between dosing.

HOW SUPPLIED: Tab: 2.5mg, 5mg, 10mg, 20mg

CONTRAINDICATIONS: Concomitant use (regularly or intermittently) with nitrates and nitric oxide donors.

WARNINGS/PRECAUTIONS: Avoid in men for whom sexual activity is not recommended due to underlying cardiovascular (CV) status, with severe hepatic impairment (Child-Pugh C), congenital QT prolongation, or in patients on renal dialysis. Patients with left ventricular outflow obstruction (eg, aortic stenosis, idiopathic hypertrophic subaortic stenosis) may be sensitive to vasodilation. Has vasodilatory properties resulting in transient decreases in supine BP. Not recommended with unstable angina, hypotension (resting SBP<90mmHg), uncontrolled HTN (>170/110mmHg), recent history of stroke, life-threatening arrhythmia, or myocardial infarction (within last 6 months), severe cardiac failure, or hereditary degenerative retinal disorders, including retinitis pigmentosa. Rare reports of prolonged erections >4 hrs and priapism. Caution with bleeding disorders, significant active peptic ulceration, anatomical deformation of the penis (eg, angulation, cavernosal fibrosis, Peyronie's disease) or conditions that predispose to priapism (eg, sickle cell anemia, multiple myeloma, leukemia). Non-arteritic anterior ischemic optic neuropathy (NAION) reported (rare); d/c therapy if sudden loss of vision occurs. Increased risk of NAION in patients who had NAION in one eye. Sudden decrease or loss of hearing accompanied by tinnitus and dizziness reported; d/c if this occurs. QT prolongation may occur.

ADVERSE REACTIONS: Headache, flushing, rhinitis, dyspepsia, sinusitis, flu syndrome.

INTERACTIONS: See Contraindications. Avoid with Class IA (eg, quinidine, procainamide) or Class III (eg, amiodarone, sotalol) antiarrhythmics and other agents for ED. Caution with medications known to prolong QT interval. Increased levels with CYP3A4 inhibitors (eg, ritonavir, ketoconazole, clarithromycin). Caution when coadministering α-blockers; additive effect on BP may be anticipated. CYP3A4/5 or CYP2C9 inhibitors may reduce clearance.

PREGNANCY: Category B, not for use in nursing.

MECHANISM OF ACTION: PDE-5 inhibitor; increases the amount of cGMP, triggering smooth muscle relaxation and allowing increased blood flow into the penis.

PHARMACOKINETICS: Absorption: Rapid. Absolute bioavailability (15%); (20mg dose, fasted) T_{max}=30 min-2 hrs. **Distribution:** V_d=208L; plasma protein binding (95%). **Metabolism:** Liver via CYP3A4, CYP3A5, CYP2C. M1 (major metabolite). **Elimination:** Feces (91-95%), urine (2-6%); $T_{1/2}$=4-5 hrs.

NURSING CONSIDERATIONS

Assessment: Assess for CV disease, left ventricular outflow obstruction, congenital or history of QT prolongation, hereditary degenerative retinal disorders, bleeding disorders, active peptic ulceration, anatomical deformation of the penis, conditions that predispose to priapism, renal/hepatic impairment, potential underlying causes of ED, any other conditions where treatment is contraindicated or cautioned, and for possible drug interactions. Obtain baseline BP.

Monitoring: Monitor for priapism, changes in vision/hearing, QT prolongation, and other adverse reactions.

Patient Counseling: Instruct to take ud. Inform that regular and/or intermittent use of nitrates may cause BP to suddenly drop to an unsafe level, resulting in dizziness, syncope, or even heart attack or stroke. Inform patients with preexisting CV risk factors of the potential cardiac risk of sexual activity. Inform that concomitant use of α-blockers may lower BP significantly, leading to symptomatic hypotension. Instruct to contact physician for dose modification if not satisfied with quality of sexual performance or in case of an unwanted effect. Instruct to seek immediate medical assistance if erection persists >4 hrs; inform that penile tissue damage and permanent loss of potency may result. Instruct to d/c and seek medical attention in the event of sudden loss of vision in 1 or both eyes; inform of the increased risk of NAION with history of NAION in 1 eye. Instruct to d/c treatment and seek prompt medical attention in the event of sudden decrease or loss of hearing which may be accompanied by tinnitus and dizziness. Counsel about protective measures necessary to guard against STDs, including HIV; inform that drug does not protect against STDs.

Administration: Oral route. Take with or without food. **Storage:** 25°C (77°F); excursions permitted to 15-30°C (59-86°F).

LEVOXYL   RX
levothyroxine sodium (King)

> Do not use for the treatment of obesity or weight loss; doses within range of daily hormonal requirements are ineffective for weight reduction in euthyroid patients. Serious or life-threatening manifestations of toxicity may occur when given in larger doses, particularly when given in association with sympathomimetic amines.

THERAPEUTIC CLASS: Thyroid replacement hormone

INDICATIONS: Replacement or supplemental therapy in congenital or acquired hypothyroidism of any etiology, except transient hypothyroidism during the recovery phase of subacute thyroiditis. Treatment or prevention of various types of euthyroid goiters, including thyroid nodules, subacute or chronic lymphocytic thyroiditis, multinodular goiter, and as an adjunct to surgery and radioiodine therapy for thyrotropin-dependent well-differentiated thyroid cancer.

DOSAGE: *Adults:* Individualize dose. Adjust dose based on periodic assessment of patient's clinical response and lab parameters. Take in the am on an empty stomach at least 30 min before food. Take at least 4 hrs apart from drugs that are known to interfere with its absorption. Hypothyroidism: Usual: 1.7mcg/kg/day. >200mcg/day seldom required. >50 Yrs/<50 Yrs with Cardiac Disease: Initial: 25-50mcg/day. Titrate: Increase by 12.5-25mcg increments every 6-8 weeks, PRN until euthyroid. Elderly with Cardiac Disease: Initial: 12.5-25mcg/day. Titrate: Increase by 12.5-25mg increments every 4-6 weeks until euthyroid. Severe Hypothyroidism: Initial: 12.5-25mcg/day. Titrate: Increase by 25mcg/day every 2-4 weeks until TSH level normalized. Secondary (Pituitary)/Tertiary (Hypothalamic) Hypothyroidism: Titrate until euthyroid and serum free-T4 level is restored to the upper half of the normal range. Pregnancy: May increase dose requirements. Subclinical Hypothyroidism: Lower doses may be adequate to normalize TSH level (eg, 1mcg/kg/day). TSH Suppression in Well-Differentiated Thyroid Cancer and Thyroid Nodules: Individualize dose based on the specific disease and the patient being treated. Refer to PI for further details.

Pediatrics: Individualize dose. Adjust dose based on periodic assessment of patient's clinical response and lab parameters. Take in the am on an empty stomach at least 30 min before food. Take at least 4 hrs apart from drugs that are known to interfere with absorption. Hypothyroidism: Growth/Puberty Complete: Usual: 1.7mcg/kg/day. >12 Yrs (Growth/Puberty Incomplete): 2-3mcg/kg/day. 6-12 Yrs: 4-5mcg/kg/day. 1-5 Yrs: 5-6mcg/kg/day. 6-12 Months: 6-8mcg/kg/day. 3-6 Months: 8-10mcg/kg/day. 0-3 Months: 10-15mcg/kg/day. Infants at Risk for Cardiac Failure: Use lower starting dose (eg, 25mcg/day). Titrate: Increase dose in 4-6 weeks PRN. Infants with Serum T4 <5mcg/dL: Initial: 50mcg/day. Chronic/Severe Hypothyroidism: Children: Initial: 25mcg/day. Titrate: Increase by 25mcg increments every 2-4 weeks until desired effect is achieved. Minimize Hyperactivity in Older Children: Initial: Give 1/4 of full replacement dose. Titrate: Increase on a weekly basis by an amount equal to 1/4 the full recommended replacement dose until the full recommended replacement dose is reached. May crush tab and mix with 5-10mL of water.

HOW SUPPLIED: Tab: 25mcg, 50mcg, 75mcg, 88mcg, 100mcg, 112mcg, 125mcg, 137mcg, 150mcg, 175mcg, 200mcg

CONTRAINDICATIONS: Untreated subclinical (suppressed serum TSH level with normal T3 level and T4 levels) or overt thyrotoxicosis of any etiology, acute myocardial infarction (MI), uncorrected adrenal insufficiency.

WARNINGS/PRECAUTIONS: Should not be used in the treatment of male or female infertility unless associated with hypothyroidism. Contraindicated in patients with nontoxic diffuse goiter or nodular thyroid disease, particularly in elderly or with underlying cardiovascular (CV) disease if serum TSH level is already suppressed; use with caution if TSH level is not suppressed and carefully monitor thyroid function. Has narrow therapeutic index; carefully titrate dose to avoid over- or under-treatment. May decrease bone mineral density (BMD) with long term use; give minimum dose necessary to achieve desired clinical and biochemical response. Caution with CV disorders and the elderly. If cardiac symptoms develop or worsen, reduce or withhold dose for 1 week and then restart at lower dose. Overtreatment may produce CV effects (eg, increase in HR, increase in cardiac wall thickness, increase in cardiac contractility, precipitation of angina or arrhythmias). Monitor patients with coronary artery disease (CAD) closely during surgical procedures; may precipitate cardiac arrhythmias. Caution in patients with diabetes mellitus (DM). Patients with concomitant adrenal insufficiency should be treated with replacement glucocorticoids prior to therapy.

ADVERSE REACTIONS: Fatigue, increased appetite, weight loss, heat intolerance, headache, hyperactivity, irritability, insomnia, palpitations, arrhythmias, dyspnea, hair loss, menstrual irregularities, pseudotumor cerebri (children), slipped capital femoral epiphysis (children).

INTERACTIONS: Concurrent sympathomimetics may increase effects of sympathomimetics or thyroid hormone; may increase risk of coronary insufficiency with CAD. Upward dose adjustments may be needed for insulin and oral hypoglycemic agents. May decrease absorption with soybean flour, cottonseed meal, walnuts, and dietary fiber. May increase oral anticoagulant activity; adjust dose of anticoagulant and monitor PT. May decrease levels and effects of digitalis glycosides. Transient reduction in TSH secretion with dopamine/dopamine agonists, glucocorticoids, octreotide. Decreased thyroid hormone secretion with aminoglutethimide, amiodarone, iodide (including iodine-containing radiographic contrast agents), lithium, methimazole, propylthiouracil (PTU), sulfonamides, and tolbutamide. May increase thyroid hormone secretion with amiodarone and iodide. May decrease T4 absorption with antacids (aluminum and magnesium hydroxides), simethicone, bile acid sequestrants (cholestyramine, colestipol), calcium carbonate, cation exchange resins (kayexalate), ferrous sulfate, orlistat, and sucralfate; administer at least 4 hrs apart. May increase serum thyroxine-binding globulin (TBG) concentrations with clofibrate, estrogen-containing oral contraceptives, oral estrogens, heroin/methadone, 5-fluorouracil, mitotane, and tamoxifen. May decrease serum TBG concentrations with androgens/anabolic steroids, asparaginase, glucocorticoids, and slow-release nicotinic acid. May cause protein-binding site displacement with furosemide (>80mg IV), heparin, hydantoins, NSAIDs (fenamates, phenylbutazone), and salicylates (>2g/day). May alter T4 and T3 metabolism with carbamazepine, hydantoins, phenobarbital, and rifampin. May decrease T4 5'-deiodinase activity with amiodarone, β-adrenergic antagonists (eg, propranolol >160mg/day), glucocorticoids (eg, dexamethasone >4mg/day), and PTU. Concurrent use with tricyclic (eg, amitriptyline) and tetracyclic (eg, maprotiline) antidepressants may increase the therapeutic and toxic effects of both drugs. Coadministration with sertraline in patients stabilized on levothyroxine may result in increased levothyroxine requirements. Interferon-α may cause development of antithyroid microsomal antibodies and transient hypothyroidism, hyperthyroidism, or both. Interleukin-2 has been associated with transient painless thyroiditis. Excessive use with growth hormones (eg, somatropin, somatrem) may accelerate epiphyseal closure. Ketamine may produce marked HTN and tachycardia. May reduce uptake of radiographic agents. Decreased theophylline clearance may occur in hypothyroid patients. Altered levels of thyroid hormone and/or TSH levels with choral hydrate, diazepam, ethionamide, lovastatin, metoclopramide, 6-mercaptopurine, nitroprusside, para-aminosalicylate sodium, perphenazine, resorcinol (excessive topical use), and thiazide diuretics.

PREGNANCY: Category A, caution in nursing.

MECHANISM OF ACTION: Thyroid replacement hormone; mechanism not established. Suspected that principal effects are exerted through control of DNA transcription and protein synthesis.

PHARMACOKINETICS: Absorption: Majority absorbed from jejunum and upper ileum. **Distribution:** Plasma protein binding (>99%); found in breast milk. **Metabolism:** Sequential deiodination and conjugation in liver (mainly), kidneys, and other tissues. **Elimination:** Urine, feces (approximately 20% unchanged); $T_{1/2}$=6-7days (T4), ≤2 days (T3).

NURSING CONSIDERATIONS

Assessment: Assess for untreated subclinical or overt thyrotoxicosis, acute MI, uncorrected adrenal insufficiency, CAD, CV disorders, nontoxic diffuse goiter, nodular thyroid disease, DM, hypersensitivity, pregnancy/nursing status, and possible drug interactions. In patients with secondary or tertiary hypothyroidism, assess for additional hypothalamic/pituitary hormone deficiencies. Assess TSH levels. In infants with congenital hypothyroidism, assess for other congenital anomalies.

Monitoring: Monitor for CV effects. In patients on long-term therapy, monitor for signs/symptoms of decreased BMD. In patients with nontoxic diffuse goiter or nodular thyroid disease, monitor for precipitation of thyrotoxicosis. In adults with primary hypothyroidism, perform periodic monitoring of serum TSH levels. In pediatric patients with congenital hypothyroidism, perform periodic monitoring of serum TSH levels and total or free T4 levels. In patients with secondary and tertiary hypothyroidism, perform periodic monitoring of serum free T4 levels. Refer to PI for TSH and T4 monitoring parameters. Closely monitor PT if coadministered with an oral anticoagulant.

Patient Counseling: Instruct to notify physician if allergic to any foods or medicines, pregnant or plan to become pregnant, breastfeeding or taking any other drugs, including prescriptions and OTC preparations. Instruct to notify physician of any other medical conditions, particularly heart disease, diabetes, clotting disorders, and adrenal or pituitary gland problems. Instruct not to stop or change dose unless directed by physician. Instruct to take on empty stomach, at least 1/2 hr before eating any food. Advise that partial hair loss may occur during the 1st few months of therapy, but is usually temporary. Instruct to notify physician or dentist prior to surgery about levothyroxine therapy. Inform that drug should not be used for weight control. Inform patients that tabs may rapidly swell and disintegrate resulting in choking, gagging, tab getting stuck in throat or difficulty swallowing; take with a full glass of water. Instruct to notify physician if rapid or irregular heartbeat, chest pain, SOB, leg cramps, headache, or any other unusual medical event occurs. Inform that dose may be increased during pregnancy. Inform that drug should not be administered within 4 hrs of agents such as iron/calcium supplements and antacids.

Administration: Oral route. Take with water. **Storage:** 20-25°C (68-77°F); excursions permitted to 15-30°C (59-86°F). Store away from heat, moisture, and light.

LEXAPRO   RX
escitalopram oxalate (Forest)

> Antidepressants increased the risk of suicidal thinking and behavior (suicidality) in children, adolescents, and young adults in short-term studies of major depressive disorder (MDD) and other psychiatric disorders. Monitor and observe closely for clinical worsening, suicidality, or unusual changes in behavior in patients who are started on antidepressant therapy. Not approved for use in pediatric patients <12 yrs of age.

THERAPEUTIC CLASS: Selective serotonin reuptake inhibitor

INDICATIONS: Acute and maintenance treatment of MDD in adults and adolescents 12-17 yrs. Acute treatment of generalized anxiety disorder (GAD) in adults.

DOSAGE: *Adults:* MDD: Initial: 10mg qd. Titrate: May increase to 20mg after ≥1 week. GAD: Initial: 10mg qd. Titrate: May increase to 20mg after ≥1 week. Efficacy >8 weeks not studied. Elderly/ Hepatic Impairment: 10mg qd. Periodically assess need for maint. Switching to/from an MAOI for Psychiatric Disorders: Allow at least 14 days between discontinuation of an MAOI and initiation of treatment and discontinuation of treatment and initiation of an MAOI. Use with Other MAOIs (eg, Linezolid, IV Methylene Blue): Refer to PI.
Pediatrics: 12-17 Yrs: MDD: Initial: 10mg qd. Titrate: May increase to 20mg after ≥3 weeks. Maint: Periodically assess need for maint. Hepatic Impairment: 10mg qd. Switching to/from an MAOI for Psychiatric Disorders: Allow at least 14 days between discontinuation of an MAOI and initiation of treatment and discontinuation of treatment and initiation of an MAOI. Use with Other MAOIs (eg, Linezolid, IV Methylene Blue): Refer to PI.

HOW SUPPLIED: Sol: 5mg/5mL [240mL]; Tab: 5mg, 10mg*, 20mg* *scored

CONTRAINDICATIONS: Use of an MAOI for psychiatric disorders either concomitantly or within 14 days of stopping treatment. Treatment within 14 days of stopping an MAOI for psychiatric disorders. Starting treatment in patients being treated with other MAOIs (eg, linezolid, IV methylene blue). Concomitant use with pimozide.

WARNINGS/PRECAUTIONS: Serotonin syndrome reported; d/c immediately and initiate supportive symptomatic treatment. Avoid abrupt discontinuation, gradually reduce dose whenever possible. May precipitate mixed/manic episode in patients at risk for bipolar disorder; screen for risk for bipolar disorder prior to initiating treatment. Activation of mania/hypomania reported; caution with history of mania. May increase the risk of bleeding events. Hyponatremia may occur; caution in elderly and volume-depleted patients. D/C in patients with symptomatic hyponatremia and institute appropriate medical intervention. Convulsions reported; caution with history of seizure disorder. Caution with conditions that alter metabolism or hemodynamic responses and in patients with severe renal impairment. May impair mental/physical abilities.

ADVERSE REACTIONS: N/V, insomnia, ejaculation disorder, increased sweating, somnolence, fatigue, diarrhea, dry mouth, headache, constipation, decreased appetite, neck/shoulder pain, decreased libido, anorgasmia.

INTERACTIONS: See Contraindications. May cause serotonin syndrome with other serotonergic drugs (eg, triptans, TCAs, fentanyl, lithium, tramadol, tryptophan, buspirone, St. John's wort) and with drugs that impair metabolism of serotonin; d/c immediately if serotonin syndrome occurs. Not recommended for use with alcohol. Caution with other centrally acting drugs, and drugs metabolized by CYP2D6 (eg, desipramine). Increased risk of bleeding with aspirin (ASA), NSAIDs, warfarin, and other drugs that affect coagulation. Rare reports of weakness, hyperreflexia, and incoordination with sumatriptan. May increase levels with cimetidine. May decrease levels of ketoconazole. May increase levels of metoprolol. Possible increased clearance with carbamazepine. Increased risk of hyponatremia with diuretics.

PREGNANCY: Category C, caution in nursing.

MECHANISM OF ACTION: SSRI; presumed to be linked to potentiation of serotonergic activity in the CNS, resulting from its inhibition of CNS neuronal reuptake of serotonin.

PHARMACOKINETICS: Absorption: T_{max}=5 hrs. **Distribution:** Plasma protein binding (56%); found in breast milk. **Metabolism:** Hepatic; N-demethylation via CYP3A4, 2C19. **Elimination:** Urine (8%); $T_{1/2}$=27-32 hrs.

NURSING CONSIDERATIONS

Assessment: Assess for risk for bipolar disorder, history of seizures, history of mania/hypomania, volume depletion, disease/condition that alters metabolism or hemodynamic response, hepatic/renal impairment, drug hypersensitivity, pregnancy/nursing status, and possible drug interactions. Obtain detailed psychiatric history.

Monitoring: Monitor for signs/symptoms of clinical worsening (suicidality, unusual changes in behavior), serotonin syndrome, abnormal bleeding, hyponatremia, seizures, cognitive and motor impairment, and other adverse reactions. Monitor hepatic/renal dysfunction. Regularly monitor weight and growth in pediatrics.

Patient Counseling: Advise to look for emergence of anxiety, agitation, panic attacks, insomnia, irritability, hostility, aggressiveness, impulsivity, akathisia, hypomania, mania, behavioral changes, worsening depression, or suicidal ideation; instruct to report such symptoms, especially if severe, abrupt in onset, or not part of presenting symptoms. Caution about risk of serotonin syndrome with other serotonergic agents (eg, triptans, buspirone, St. John's wort) and about risk of bleeding with ASA, warfarin, or other drugs that affect coagulation. Instruct to notify physician if taking or planning to take any prescribed or OTC drugs. Inform that may notice improvement in 1-4 weeks; continue therapy ud. Caution against performing hazardous tasks (eg, operating machinery and driving). Instruct to avoid alcohol. Instruct to notify physician if become pregnant, intend to become pregnant, or are breastfeeding. Inform of the need for comprehensive treatment program.

Administration: Oral route. Administer qd, in am or pm, with or without food. **Storage:** 25°C (77°F); excursions permitted to 15-30°C (59-86°F).

LIALDA   RX
mesalamine (Shire)

THERAPEUTIC CLASS: 5-aminosalicylic acid derivative

INDICATIONS: Induction of remission in patients with active, mild to moderate ulcerative colitis (UC) and for the maintenance of remission of UC.

DOSAGE: *Adults:* Induction of Remission: Usual: 2-4 tabs qd with a meal. Maintenance of Remission: Usual: 2 tabs qd with a meal. Elderly: Start at lower end of dosing range.

HOW SUPPLIED: Tab, Delayed-Release: 1.2g

WARNINGS/PRECAUTIONS: Renal impairment, including minimal change nephropathy, acute/chronic interstitial nephritis, and, rarely, renal failure reported; evaluate renal function prior to therapy and periodically thereafter. Caution with known renal impairment or history of renal disease. Has been associated with an acute intolerance syndrome that may be difficult to distinguish from an exacerbation of UC; observe closely for worsening of symptoms and d/c therapy if acute intolerance syndrome is suspected. Patients with sulfasalazine hypersensitivity may have similar reaction to therapy. Mesalamine-induced cardiac hypersensitivity reactions (eg, myocarditis, pericarditis) reported; caution with conditions that predispose to the development of myocarditis or pericarditis. Hepatic failure reported in patients with preexisting liver disease; caution with liver disease. Pyloric stenosis or other organic/functional obstruction in the upper GI tract may cause prolonged gastric retention of therapy, which could delay drug release in the colon. Caution with sulfasalazine hypersensitivity and in elderly. May interfere with lab tests.

ADVERSE REACTIONS: Headache, flatulence, UC, abnormal LFTs, abdominal pain.

INTERACTIONS: Nephrotoxic agents, including NSAIDs, may increase risk of renal reactions. Azathioprine or 6-mercaptopurine may increase risk for blood disorders.

PREGNANCY: Category B, caution in nursing.

MECHANISM OF ACTION: 5-aminosalicylic acid (5-ASA) derivative; has not been established. Suspected to diminish inflammation by blocking cyclooxygenase and inhibiting prostaglandin production in the colon.

PHARMACOKINETICS: Absorption: Administration of variable doses and different populations resulted in different parameters. **Distribution:** Plasma protein binding (43%); found in breast milk; crosses placenta. **Metabolism:** Liver and intestinal mucosa (acetylation); N-acetyl-5-ASA (major metabolite). **Elimination:** Urine (<8% unchanged, >13% N-acetyl-5-ASA); $T_{1/2}$=7-9 hrs (2.4g), 8-12 hrs (4.8g).

NURSING CONSIDERATIONS

Assessment: Assess for hypersensitivity to the drug, salicylates/aminosalicylates, or sulfasalazine, conditions that predispose to the development of myocarditis or pericarditis, pyloric stenosis or other organic/functional upper GI tract obstruction, hepatic impairment, pregnancy/nursing status, and possible drug interactions. Evaluate renal function prior to initiation of therapy.

Monitoring: Monitor for acute intolerance syndrome, hypersensitivity reactions, hepatic failure, and other adverse reactions. Perform periodic monitoring of renal function. Monitor blood cell counts in elderly.

Patient Counseling: Instruct not to take drug if hypersensitive to salicylates (eg, aspirin) or other mesalamines. Inform to notify physician of all medications being taken and if pregnant, planning to become pregnant, or breastfeeding. Instruct to inform physician if allergic to sulfasalazine, if taking NSAIDs or other nephrotoxic agents, azathioprine, or 6-mercaptopurine, and if experiencing cramping, abdominal pain, bloody diarrhea, fever, headache, or rash. Inform to notify physician of history of myocarditis/pericarditis or stomach blockage, and if patient has kidney/liver disease.

Administration: Oral route. Swallow tab whole. **Storage:** 15-25°C (59-77°F); excursions permitted to 30°C (86°F).

LIBRAX   RX
chlordiazepoxide HCl - clidinium bromide (Valeant)

THERAPEUTIC CLASS: Anticholinergic/benzodiazepine

INDICATIONS: Adjunctive therapy in the treatment of irritable bowel syndrome, acute enterocolitis, and peptic ulcer.

DOSAGE: *Adults:* Individualize dose. Usual/Maint: 1-2 caps tid-qid ac and hs. Elderly/Debilitated: Initial: Not more than 2 caps/day. Titrate: Increase gradually PRN.

HOW SUPPLIED: Cap: (Chlordiazepoxide-Clidinium) 5mg-2.5mg

CONTRAINDICATIONS: Glaucoma, prostatic hypertrophy, benign bladder neck obstruction.

WARNINGS/PRECAUTIONS: May impair mental/physical abilities. Risk of congenital malformations during 1st trimester of pregnancy; avoid use. Inhibition of lactation may occur. Paradoxical reactions (eg, excitement, stimulation, acute rage) reported in psychiatric patients. Caution in treatment of anxiety states with evidence of impending depression; suicidal tendencies may be present. Caution in elderly and with renal or hepatic dysfunction. Use lowest effective dose in debilitated patients. Avoid abrupt withdrawal after extended therapy; withdrawal symptoms reported following discontinuation.

ADVERSE REACTIONS: Drowsiness, ataxia, confusion, skin eruptions, edema, extrapyramidal symptoms, dry mouth, nausea, constipation, altered libido, blood dyscrasias, jaundice, hepatic dysfunction, blurred vision, urinary hesitancy.

INTERACTIONS: Additive effects with alcohol and CNS depressants. Coadministration with other psychotropic agents not recommended; caution with MAOIs and phenothiazines. Altered coagulation effects reported with oral anticoagulants. Constipation may occur when coadministered with other spasmolytic agents.

PREGNANCY: Not for use in pregnancy, safety not known in nursing.

MECHANISM OF ACTION: Chlordiazepoxide: Benzodiazepine; antianxiety agent. Clidinium: Anticholinergic; shown to have a pronounced antispasmodic and antisecretory effect on the GI tract.

NURSING CONSIDERATIONS

Assessment: Assess for glaucoma, prostatic hypertrophy, benign bladder neck obstruction, renal/hepatic dysfunction, alcohol intake, history of drug abuse, drug hypersensitivity, pregnancy/nursing status, and possible drug interactions.

Monitoring: Monitor for ataxia, oversedation, drowsiness, confusion, and other adverse reactions. Monitor for paradoxical reactions (eg, excitement, stimulation, acute rage) in psychiatric patients. Periodic blood counts and LFTs are advisable when treatment is protracted. Monitor for signs of impending depression, or any suicidal tendencies.

Patient Counseling: Inform that psychological and physical dependence may develop, and to consult physician before increasing dose or d/c abruptly. Advise to observe caution when performing hazardous tasks (eg, operating machinery/driving). Advise to notify physician if pregnant/breastfeeding or planning to become pregnant. Inform of potential additive effects with alcohol and other CNS depressants.

Administration: Oral route. **Storage:** 25°C (77°F); excursions permitted to 15-30°C (59-86°F).

LIBRIUM   CIV
chlordiazepoxide HCl (Valeant)

THERAPEUTIC CLASS: Benzodiazepine

INDICATIONS: Management of anxiety disorders and short-term relief of anxiety symptoms, withdrawal symptoms of acute alcoholism, and preoperative apprehension and anxiety.

DOSAGE: *Adults:* Individualize dose. Mild-Moderate Anxiety: 5-10mg tid-qid. Severe Anxiety: 20-25mg tid-qid. Alcohol Withdrawal: 50-100mg; repeat until agitation controlled. Max: 300mg/day. Preoperative Anxiety: 5-10mg tid-qid on days prior to surgery. Elderly/Debilitated: 5mg bid-qid. *Pediatrics:* ≥6 Yrs: Individualize dose. Usual: 5mg bid-qid. May increase to 10mg bid-tid.

HOW SUPPLIED: Cap: 5mg, 10mg, 25mg

WARNINGS/PRECAUTIONS: May impair mental/physical abilities, including mental alertness in children. Risk of congenital malformations during 1st trimester of pregnancy; avoid use. Paradoxical reactions (eg, excitement, stimulation, and acute rage) reported in psychiatric patients, and in hyperactive aggressive pediatric patients. Caution in treatment of anxiety states with evidence of impending depression; suicidal tendencies may be present. Caution with porphyria, renal or hepatic dysfunction. Use lowest effective dose in elderly and debilitated patients. Avoid abrupt withdrawal after extended therapy; withdrawal symptoms reported following d/c.

ADVERSE REACTIONS: Drowsiness, ataxia, confusion, skin eruptions, edema, nausea, constipation, extrapyramidal symptoms, libido changes, EEG changes.

INTERACTIONS: Additive effects with CNS depressants and alcohol. Coadministration with other psychotropic agents not recommended; caution with MAOIs and phenothiazines. Altered coagulation effects reported with oral anticoagulants.

PREGNANCY: Not for use in pregnancy, safety not known in nursing.

MECHANISM OF ACTION: Benzodiazepine; not established. Has antianxiety, sedative, appetite stimulating, and weak analgesic actions; blocks EEG arousal from stimulation of brain stem reticular formation.

PHARMACOKINETICS: Elimination: Urine (1-2% unchanged, 3-6% conjugates); $T_{1/2}$=24-48 hrs.

NURSING CONSIDERATIONS

Assessment: Assess for pregnancy status, hepatic/renal function, and possible drug interactions.

Monitoring: Monitor elderly/debilitated patients for ataxia and oversedation, drowsiness, confusion. Monitor for paradoxical reactions in psychiatric patients and in hyperactive aggressive pediatric patients. Periodic blood counts and LFTs are advisable when treatment is protracted. Monitor for signs of impending depression or any suicidal tendencies.

Patient Counseling: Inform that psychological/physical dependence may occur; advise to consult physician prior to increasing dose or abruptly discontinuing therapy. Advise to notify physician if patient becomes pregnant or plans to become pregnant. May impair mental/physical abilities; caution while operating machinery/driving. May impair mental alertness in children. Avoid alcohol and other CNS depressant drugs.

Administration: Oral route. **Storage:** 25°C (77°F); excursions permitted to 15-30°C (59-86°F).

LIDODERM PATCH

lidocaine (Endo)

RX

THERAPEUTIC CLASS: Acetamide local anesthetic

INDICATIONS: Relief of pain associated with post-herpetic neuralgia.

DOSAGE: *Adults:* Apply to intact skin to cover the most painful area. Apply up to 3 patches, only once for up to 12 hrs within 24-hr period. May cut patches into smaller sizes before removal of the release liner. Debilitated/Impaired Elimination: Treat smaller areas. Remove patch if irritation or burning occurs; may reapply when irritation subsides.

HOW SUPPLIED: Patch: 5% [30s]

WARNINGS/PRECAUTIONS: Serious adverse events may occur in children or pets if ingested; keep out of reach. Excessive dosing by applying to larger areas or for longer than the recommended wearing time may result in serious adverse effects. Increased risk of toxicity in patients with severe hepatic disease. Caution with history of drug sensitivities, smaller patients and patients with impaired elimination. Avoid broken or inflamed skin, placement of external heat (eg, heating pads, electric blankets) and eye contact.

ADVERSE REACTIONS: Application-site reactions (eg, erythema, edema, bruising, papules, vesicles, discoloration, depigmentation, burning sensation, pruritus, dermatitis, petechia, blisters, exfoliation, abnormal sensation).

INTERACTIONS: Additive toxic effects with concomitant Class I antiarrhythmics (eg, tocainide, mexiletine); use caution. Consider total amount absorbed from all formulations containing other local anesthetics.

PREGNANCY: Category B, caution in nursing.

MECHANISM OF ACTION: Local anesthetic; stabilizes neuronal membranes by inhibiting ionic fluxes required for initiation and conduction of impulses.

PHARMACOKINETICS: Absorption: C_{max}=0.13mcg/mL; T_{max}=11 hrs. **Distribution:** V_d=0.7-2.7L/kg (IV); Plasma protein binding (70%). Crosses placenta; found in breast milk. **Metabolism:** Liver (rapid); monoethylglycinexylidide, glycinexylidide (active metabolites). **Elimination:** Urine (<10%, unchanged); $T_{1/2}$=81-149 min (IV).

NURSING CONSIDERATIONS

Assessment: Assess for history of drug sensitivities to local anesthetics of the amide type and para-aminobenzoic acid derivatives, hepatic disease, pregnancy/nursing status, and for possible drug interactions.

Monitoring: Monitor for local skin reactions, allergic/anaphylactoid reactions, liver function, pain intensity, and pain relief periodically and other adverse reactions.

Patient Counseling: Instruct to remove patch and not to reapply if irritation or burning sensation occurs during application until irritation subsides. If eye contact occurs, immediately wash with water or saline and protect eye until sensation returns. Counsel to avoid application to larger areas and for longer than recommended wearing time. Avoid applying to broken or inflamed skin. Instruct to wash hands after handling patch and to fold used patches so adhesive side sticks to itself. Keep out of reach of children and pets.

Administration: Transdermal route. Refer to PI for proper handling and disposal. **Storage:** Store at 25°C (77°F); excursions permitted to 15-30°C (59-86°F).

LINZESS

linaclotide (Forest)

RX

> **Contraindicated in pediatric patients up to 6 yrs of age. Avoid use in pediatric patients 6-17 yrs of age.**

THERAPEUTIC CLASS: Guanylate cyclase-C agonist

INDICATIONS: Treatment of irritable bowel syndrome with constipation (IBS-C) and chronic idiopathic constipation (CIC) in adults.

DOSAGE: *Adults:* Take on empty stomach, at least 30 min prior to the 1st meal of the day. IBS-C: 290mcg qd. CIC: 145mcg qd.

HOW SUPPLIED: Cap: 145mcg, 290mcg

CONTRAINDICATIONS: Pediatric patients up to 6 yrs of age, known or suspected mechanical GI obstruction.

WARNINGS/PRECAUTIONS: Diarrhea commonly reported; consider discontinuation if severe diarrhea occurs.

ADVERSE REACTIONS: Diarrhea, abdominal pain, flatulence, abdominal distension, viral gastro-enteritis, headache, upper respiratory tract infection, sinusitis.

PREGNANCY: Category C, caution in nursing.

MECHANISM OF ACTION: Guanylate cyclase-C (GC-C) agonist; acts locally on the luminal surface of the intestinal epithelium by binding to and activating GC-C, resulting in an increase in both intracellular and extracellular cGMP levels. Elevation in intracellular cGMP stimulates secretion of Cl⁻ and bicarbonate into the intestinal lumen, resulting in increased intestinal fluid and accelerated transit.

PHARMACOKINETICS: Absorption: Minimal. **Metabolism:** GI tract. **Elimination:** Feces (5% [fasted], 3% [fed]).

NURSING CONSIDERATIONS

Assessment: Assess for known or suspected mechanical GI obstruction and pregnancy/nursing status.

Monitoring: Monitor for diarrhea and other adverse reactions.

Patient Counseling: Advise to seek medical attention if experiencing unusual or severe abdominal pain and/or severe diarrhea, especially if in combination with hematochezia or melena; instruct to stop treatment if severe diarrhea occurs. Instruct to skip dose if the dose is missed, and take next dose at the regular time; advise not to take 2 doses at the same time.

Administration: Oral route. Swallow cap whole; do not break apart or chew. **Storage:** 25°C (77°F); excursions permitted between 15-30°C (59-86°F). Keep cap in the original container. Do not subdivide or repackage. Protect from moisture. Do not remove desiccant from the container.

LIPITOR   RX
atorvastatin calcium (Parke-Davis/Pfizer)

THERAPEUTIC CLASS: HMG-CoA reductase inhibitor

INDICATIONS: Adjunct to diet to decrease total cholesterol, LDL, apolipoprotein B, and TG levels, and to increase HDL levels in primary hypercholesterolemia and mixed dyslipidemia, hypertriglyceridemia, primary dysbetalipoproteinemia, homozygous familial hypercholesterolemia, heterozygous familial hypercholesterolemia (boys and postmenarchal girls 10-17 yrs of age), and in prevention of cardiovascular disease.

DOSAGE: *Adults:* Individualize dose. Hyperlipidemia/Mixed Dyslipidemia: Initial: 10mg or 20mg qd (or 40mg qd for LDL reduction >45%). Titrate: Adjust dose accordingly at 2- to 4-week intervals. Usual: 10-80mg qd. HoFH: 10-80mg qd. Concomitant Lopinavir plus Ritonavir: Use lowest dose necessary. Concomitant Clarithromycin/Itraconazole/Fosamprenavir/Ritonavir plus Saquinavir, Darunavir, or Fosamprenavir: Limit to 20mg/day; use lowest dose necessary. Concomitant Nelfinavir or Boceprevir: Limit to 40mg/day; use lowest dose necessary. *Pediatrics:* 10-17 Yrs: Individualize dose. Heterozygous Familial Hypercholesterolemia: Initial: 10mg/day. Titrate: Adjust dose at intervals of ≥4 weeks. Max: 20mg/day.

HOW SUPPLIED: Tab: 10mg, 20mg, 40mg, 80mg

CONTRAINDICATIONS: Active liver disease, which may include unexplained persistent elevations in hepatic transaminases, women who are pregnant or may become pregnant, nursing mothers.

WARNINGS/PRECAUTIONS: Has not been studied in conditions where the major lipoprotein abnormality is elevation of chylomicrons (Fredrickson Types I and V). Rare cases of rhabdomyolysis with acute renal failure secondary to myoglobinuria reported. Increased risk of rhabdomyolysis with history of renal impairment; closely monitor for skeletal muscle effects. May cause myopathy (including immune-mediated necrotizing myopathy [IMNM]); d/c if markedly elevated CPK levels occur or if myopathy is diagnosed or suspected. Temporarily withhold or d/c if acute, serious condition suggestive of myopathy occurs or if with risk factor predisposing to development of renal failure secondary to rhabdomyolysis. Persistent increases in serum transaminases reported; obtain liver enzyme tests prior to initiation and repeat as clinically indicated. Fatal and nonfatal hepatic failure reported (rare); promptly interrupt therapy if serious liver injury with clinical symptoms and/or hyperbilirubinemia or jaundice occurs and do not restart if no alternate etiology found. Caution in patients who consume substantial quantities of alcohol and/or have history of liver disease. Increases in HbA1c and FPG levels reported. May blunt adrenal and/or gonadal steroid production. Increased risk of hemorrhagic stroke in patients with recent stroke or transient ischemic attack (TIA). Caution in elderly.

ADVERSE REACTIONS: Nasopharyngitis, arthralgia, diarrhea, diabetes, pain in extremity, urinary tract infection, dyspepsia, nausea, musculoskeletal pain, muscle spasms, myalgia, insomnia.

INTERACTIONS: Avoid with cyclosporine, telaprevir, gemfibrozil, or combination of tipranavir plus ritonavir. Caution with fibrates and drugs that decrease levels or activity of endogenous steroid hormones (eg, ketoconazole, spironolactone, cimetidine). Increased risk of myopathy with fibric acid derivatives, erythromycin, lipid-modifying doses of niacin, strong CYP3A4 inhibitors (eg, clarithromycin, HIV protease inhibitors), and azole antifungals; consider lower initial and maint doses. Strong CYP3A4 inhibitors (eg, clarithromycin, several combinations of HIV protease inhibitors, telaprevir, itraconazole) and grapefruit juice may increase levels. CYP3A4 inducers (eg, efavirenz, rifampin) may decrease levels; simultaneous coadministration with rifampin recommended. May increase digoxin levels; monitor appropriately. May increase area under the curve of norethindrone and ethinyl estradiol. Myopathy, including rhabdomyolysis, reported with colchicine; use with caution. OATP1B1 inhibitors (eg, cyclosporine) may increase bioavailability.

PREGNANCY: Category X, not for use in nursing.

MECHANISM OF ACTION: HMG-CoA reductase inhibitor; inhibits conversion of HMG-CoA to mevalonate (precursor of sterols, including cholesterol).

PHARMACOKINETICS: Absorption: Rapid; absolute bioavailability (14%); T_{max}=1-2 hrs. **Distribution:** V_d=381L; plasma protein binding (≥98%). **Metabolism:** CYP3A4 (extensive); ortho- and parahydroxylated derivatives (active metabolites). **Elimination:** Bile (major), urine (<2%); $T_{1/2}$=14 hrs.

NURSING CONSIDERATIONS

Assessment: Assess for active or history of liver disease, unexplained and persistent elevations in serum transaminase levels, pregnancy/nursing status, history of renal impairment, risk factors predisposing to the development of renal failure secondary to rhabdomyolysis, alcohol intake, recent stroke or TIA, hypersensitivity to the drug, and possible drug interactions. Obtain baseline LFTs.

Monitoring: Monitor for signs/symptoms of rhabdomyolysis and myopathy (including IMNM). Monitor lipid profile and CPK levels. Perform LFTs as clinically indicated.

Patient Counseling: Advise to adhere to the National Cholesterol Education Program-recommended diet, a regular exercise program, and periodic testing of a fasting lipid panel. Inform of the substances that should not be taken concomitantly with the drug. Advise to inform other healthcare professionals that they are taking the drug. Inform of the risk of myopathy; instruct to report promptly any unexplained muscle pain, tenderness, or weakness, particularly if accompanied by malaise or fever or if these muscle signs or symptoms persist after discontinuation. Inform that liver function will be checked prior to initiation and if signs or symptoms of liver injury occur; instruct to report promptly any symptoms that may indicate liver injury (eg, fatigue, anorexia, right upper abdominal discomfort, dark urine, jaundice). Instruct women of childbearing age to use effective method of birth control to prevent pregnancy. Advise to d/c therapy and contact physician if pregnancy occurs. Instruct not to use the drug if breastfeeding.

Administration: Oral route. Administer as a single dose at any time of the day, with or without food. **Storage:** 20-25°C (68-77°F).

LIPOFEN   RX
fenofibrate (Kowa)

THERAPEUTIC CLASS: Fibric acid derivative

INDICATIONS: Adjunctive therapy to diet to reduce elevated LDL, total cholesterol, TGs, and apolipoprotein B, and to increase HDL in adults with primary hypercholesterolemia or mixed dyslipidemia. Adjunctive therapy to diet for treatment of adults with severe hypertriglyceridemia.

DOSAGE: *Adults:* Primary Hypercholesterolemia/Mixed Dyslipidemia: 150mg qd. Severe Hypertriglyceridemia: Initial: 50-150mg/day. Titrate: Adjust dose if necessary following repeat lipid determination at 4- to 8-week intervals; individualize dose. Max: 150mg qd. Mild to Moderate Renal Impairment: Initial: 50mg/day. Titrate: Increase only after evaluation of the effects on renal function and lipid levels. Elderly: Dose based on renal function. Take with meals. Consider reducing dose if lipid levels fall significantly below the targeted range. D/C if no adequate response after 2 months of treatment with max dose.

HOW SUPPLIED: Cap: 50mg, 150mg

CONTRAINDICATIONS: Severe renal impairment (including dialysis), active liver disease (including primary biliary cirrhosis and unexplained persistent liver function abnormalities), preexisting gallbladder disease, nursing mothers.

WARNINGS/PRECAUTIONS: Not shown to reduce coronary heart disease morbidity and mortality in patients with type 2 diabetes mellitus. Increased risk of myopathy and rhabdomyolysis; increased risk with diabetes, renal insufficiency, hypothyroidism, and in elderly. D/C therapy if markedly elevated CPK levels occur or myopathy is diagnosed. Increases in serum transaminases, chronic active hepatocellular and cholestatic hepatitis, and cirrhosis (rare) reported; perform baseline and regular monitoring of LFTs, and d/c therapy if enzyme levels persist >3X the normal limit. Elevations in SrCr reported; monitor renal function in patients with renal impairment or at risk for renal insufficiency. May cause cholelithiasis; d/c if gallstones are found. Mild to moderate decreases in Hgb, Hct and WBCs, thrombocytopenia, and agranulocytosis reported; periodically monitor RBC and WBC counts during the first 12 months of therapy. Acute hypersensitivity reactions and pancreatitis reported. May cause venothromboembolic disease (eg, pulmonary embolus [PE], deep vein thrombosis [DVT]). Severe decreases in HDL levels reported; check HDL levels within the 1st few months after initiation of therapy. If a severely depressed HDL level is detected, withdraw therapy, monitor HDL level until it has returned to baseline, and do not reinitiate therapy. Estrogen therapy, thiazide diuretics and β-blockers may be associated with massive rises in plasma TGs; discontinuation of these drugs may obviate the need for specific drug therapy of hypertriglyceridemia.

ADVERSE REACTIONS: Abdominal pain, back pain, headache, abnormal LFTs, respiratory disorder, increased CPK/AST/ALT.

INTERACTIONS: Increased risk of rhabdomyolysis with HMG-CoA reductase inhibitors (statins); avoid combination unless benefits outweigh risks. May potentiate anticoagulant effects of coumarin anticoagulants; use with caution, adjust anticoagulant dose, and monitor PT/INR frequently. Immunosuppressants (eg, cyclosporine, tacrolimus) may impair renal function; use lowest effective dose and monitor renal function with immunosuppressants and other potentially nephrotoxic agents. Bile acid-binding resins may bind other drugs given concurrently; take at least 1 hr before or 4-6 hrs after the bile acid-binding resin. Cases of myopathy, including rhabdomyolysis, reported when coadministered with colchicine; caution when prescribing with colchicine. Changes in exposure/levels with atorvastatin, pravastatin, fluvastatin, glimepiride, metformin, and rosiglitazone.

PREGNANCY: Category C, not for use in nursing.

MECHANISM OF ACTION: Fibric acid derivative; activates peroxisome proliferator-activated receptor α. Increases lipolysis and elimination of TG-rich particles from plasma by activating lipoprotein lipase and reducing production of apoprotein C-III (lipoprotein lipase inhibitor). Also, induces an increase in the synthesis of apolipoproteins AI, AII, and HDL.

PHARMACOKINETICS: Absorption: Well-absorbed. T_{max}=5 hrs; (200mg single dose) AUC=40mcg/mL (fenofibrate), 204mcg/mL (fenofibric acid). **Distribution:** Plasma protein binding (99%). **Metabolism:** Rapid by ester hydrolysis to fenofibric acid (active metabolite); conjugation with glucuronic acid. **Elimination:** Urine (60%, fenofibric acid and its glucuronate conjugate), feces (25%); $T_{1/2}$=20 hrs (fenofibric acid).

NURSING CONSIDERATIONS

Assessment: Assess for renal impairment, active liver disease, preexisting gallbladder disease, other medical conditions (diabetes, hypothyroidism), hypersensitivity to the drug, pregnancy/nursing status, and possible drug interactions. Obtain baseline LFTs.

Monitoring: Monitor for signs/symptoms of myopathy or rhabdomyolysis; measure CPK levels in patients reporting such symptoms. Monitor for cholelithiasis, pancreatitis, hypersensitivity reactions, PE, and DVT. Monitor renal function, LFTs, CBC, and lipid levels. Monitor PT/INR frequently with coumarin anticoagulants.

Patient Counseling: Advise of the potential benefits and risks of therapy, and medications to be avoided during treatment. Instruct to continue to follow an appropriate lipid-modifying diet during therapy, and to take drug ud. Instruct to inform physician of all medications, supplements, and herbal preparations being taken, any changes in medical condition, development of muscle pain, tenderness, or weakness, onset of abdominal pain, or any other new symptoms. Advise to return to the physician's office for routine monitoring.

Administration: Oral route. Swallow cap whole; do not open, crush, dissolve, or chew. **Storage:** 15-30°C (59-86°F). Protect from moisture and light.

LIPTRUZET   RX
ezetimibe - atorvastatin (Merck)

THERAPEUTIC CLASS: Cholesterol absorption inhibitor/HMG-CoA reductase inhibitor

INDICATIONS: Adjunct to diet to reduce elevated total cholesterol (total-C), LDL-C, apolipoprotein B, TGs, and non-HDL-C, and to increase HDL-C in patients with primary hyperlipidemia or mixed hyperlipidemia, homozygous familial hypercholesterolemia (HoFH).

DOSAGE: *Adults:* Initial: 10mg-10mg/day or 10mg-20mg/day as a single dose at any time of the day; give 10mg-40mg/day if patient requires larger reduction in LDL-C (>55%). Range: 10mg-10mg/day to 10mg-80mg/day. Analyze lipid levels within 2 or more weeks after initiation and/or upon titration and adjust dose accordingly. HoFH: 10mg-40mg/day or 10mg-80mg/day. Coadministration with Bile Acid Sequestrants: Give either ≥2 hrs before or ≥4 hrs after bile acid sequestrant. Coadministration with Clarithromycin/Itraconazole/Saquinavir Plus Ritonavir/Darunavir Plus Ritonavir/Fosamprenavir/or Fosamprenavir Plus Ritonavir: Max: 10mg-20mg/day. Coadministration with Nelfinavir/Boceprevir: Max: 10mg-40mg/day.

HOW SUPPLIED: Tab: (Ezetimibe-Atorvastatin) 10mg-10mg, 10mg-20mg, 10mg-40mg, 10mg-80mg

CONTRAINDICATIONS: Active liver disease or unexplained persistent elevations in hepatic transaminase levels, women who are or may become pregnant, nursing mothers.

WARNINGS/PRECAUTIONS: Has not been studied in Fredrickson type I, III, IV, and V dyslipidemias. Myopathy (including immune-mediated necrotizing myopathy [IMNM]) and rhabdomyolysis reported; d/c if markedly elevated CPK levels occur or myopathy is diagnosed or suspected. Temporarily withhold or d/c therapy in any patient with an acute, serious condition suggestive of a myopathy or having a risk factor predisposing to development of renal failure secondary to rhabdomyolysis (eg, severe acute infection, hypotension, major surgery, trauma, severe metabolic/endocrine/electrolyte disorders, uncontrolled seizures). Liver enzyme elevations and fatal and nonfatal hepatic failure reported; obtain LFTs prior to initiating therapy and repeat as clinically indicated; promptly interrupt therapy if serious liver injury and/or hyperbilirubinemia or jaundice occurs and do not restart if no alternative etiology found. Caution in patients who consume substantial quantities of alcohol and/or have a history of liver disease. Increases in HbA1c and FPG levels reported. May blunt adrenal and/or gonadal steroid production. Increased risk of hemorrhagic stroke in patients with recent stroke or transient ischemic attack (TIA). Caution in elderly.

ADVERSE REACTIONS: Increased ALT/AST, musculoskeletal pain, abdominal pain, nausea, arthralgia.

INTERACTIONS: Avoid with gemfibrozil, cyclosporine, tipranavir plus ritonavir, and telaprevir. Caution with lopinavir plus ritonavir; use lowest dose necessary. Caution with drugs that decrease levels or activity of endogenous steroid hormones (eg, ketoconazole, spironolactone, cimetidine). Increased risk of myopathy with fibric acid derivatives, erythromycin, lipid-modifying doses of niacin, strong CYP3A4 inhibitors (eg, clarithromycin, HIV protease inhibitors), and azole antifungals; consider lower initial and maint doses. Monitor INR levels when used with warfarin. Atorvastatin: Strong CYP3A4 inhibitors, grapefruit juice, saquinavir plus ritonavir, diltiazem, and amlodipine may increase levels. Itraconazole may increase AUC. Myopathy, including rhabdomyolysis, reported with colchicine; use with caution. OATP1B1 inhibitors may increase bioavailability. May increase levels of digoxin; monitor appropriately. May increase AUC of norethindrone and ethinyl estradiol. CYP3A4 inducers (eg, efavirenz, rifampin) may decrease levels; simultaneous coadministration with rifampin is recommended. Ezetimibe: Cholestyramine may decrease levels.

PREGNANCY: Category X, not for use in nursing.

MECHANISM OF ACTION: Atorvastatin: HMG-CoA reductase inhibitor; lowers plasma cholesterol and lipoprotein levels by inhibiting HMG-CoA reductase and cholesterol synthesis in the liver and by increasing the number of hepatic LDL receptors on the cell-surface to enhance uptake and catabolism of LDL; also reduces LDL production and the number of LDL particles. Ezetimibe: Cholesterol absorption inhibitor; localizes at the brush border of the small intestine and inhibits absorption of cholesterol and decreases intestinal cholesterol delivery to the liver.

PHARMACOKINETICS: Absorption: Atorvastatin: Absolute bioavailability (14%); T_{max}=1-2 hrs. **Distribution:** Atorvastatin: V_d=381L; plasma protein binding (≥98%). Ezetimibe: Plasma protein binding (>90%). **Metabolism:** Atorvastatin: CYP3A4 (extensive); ortho- and parahydroxylated derivatives (active metabolites). Ezetimibe: Small intestine and liver via glucuronide conjugation; ezetimibe-glucuronide (active metabolite). **Elimination:** Atorvastatin: Bile (major), urine (<2%); $T_{1/2}$=14 hrs. Ezetimibe: Feces (78%, 69% unchanged drug), urine (11%, 9% metabolite); $T_{1/2}$=22 hrs.

NURSING CONSIDERATIONS

Assessment: Assess for history of or active liver disease, unexplained persistent elevations in hepatic transaminases, risk factors for developing myopathy (eg, advanced age, hypothyroidism, renal impairment), recent stroke or TIA, hypersensitivity to the drug, pregnancy/nursing status, and possible drug interactions. Assess use in patients who consume substantial quantities of alcohol. Obtain baseline lipid profile (total-C, LDL, HDL, TG) and LFTs (eg, AST, ALT).

Monitoring: Monitor for signs/symptoms of myopathy, rhabdomyolysis, liver dysfunction, and other adverse reactions. Analyze lipid levels within 2 or more weeks after initiation and/or upon titration. Monitor LFTs as clinically indicated, and for increases in HbA1c and FPG levels.

Patient Counseling: Advise to adhere to the National Cholesterol Education Program recommended diet, a regular exercise program, and periodic testing of a fasting lipid panel. Counsel about risk of myopathy and inform that consuming large quantities (>1L) of grapefruit juice may increase this risk. Advise to discuss with physician all medications, both prescription and OTC, currently taking. Instruct to report to physician any unexplained muscle pain, tenderness, or weakness, particularly if accompanied by malaise or fever, or if signs/symptoms persist after discontinuing therapy. Advise to report promptly any signs of liver injury, including fatigue, anorexia, right upper abdominal discomfort, dark urine, or jaundice. Counsel women of childbearing age to use an effective method of birth control while using the drug and to discuss future pregnancy plans; instruct to d/c therapy and contact physician if pregnancy occurs. Advise not to breastfeed during treatment.

Administration: Oral route. Take with or without food. Swallow tab whole; do not crush, dissolve, or chew. **Storage:** 20-25°C (68-77°F); excursions permitted to 15-30°C (59-86°F). Store in foil pouch until use. Protect from moisture and light and store in a dry place after the foil pouch is opened. Once a tab is removed, slide blister card back into case. Discard any unused tab 30 days after pouch is opened.

LITHIUM ER
lithium carbonate (Various)

RX

> Lithium toxicity is closely related to serum levels, and can occur at doses close to therapeutic levels. Facilities for prompt and accurate serum lithium determinations should be available before initiating therapy.

OTHER BRAND NAMES: Lithobid (Noven)

THERAPEUTIC CLASS: Antimanic agent

INDICATIONS: Treatment of manic episodes of bipolar disorder and maintenance treatment of bipolar disorder.

DOSAGE: *Adults:* Individualize dose. Acute Mania: 900mg bid or 600mg tid to achieve effective serum levels of 1-1.5mEq/L; monitor levels twice weekly until stabilized. Maint: 900-1200mg/day, given bid-tid to maintain serum levels of 0.6-1.2mEq/L; monitor levels every 2 months. Elderly: Start at lower end of dosing range.
Pediatrics: ≥12 Yrs: Individualize dose. Acute Mania: 900mg bid or 600mg tid to achieve effective serum levels of 1-1.5mEq/L; monitor levels twice weekly until stabilized. Maint: 900-1200mg/day, given bid-tid to maintain serum levels of 0.6-1.2 mEq/L; monitor levels every 2 months.

HOW SUPPLIED: Tab, Extended-Release: 300mg, 450mg*; (Lithobid) 300mg *scored

WARNINGS/PRECAUTIONS: Avoid with significant renal or cardiovascular disease (CVD), severe debilitation, dehydration, or Na⁺ depletion. Chronic therapy may be associated with diminution of renal concentrating ability; carefully manage to avoid dehydration with resulting lithium retention and toxicity. Morphologic changes with glomerular and interstitial fibrosis and nephron atrophy reported; assess kidney function prior to and during therapy. Decreased tolerance reported to ensue from protracted sweating or diarrhea; if this occurs, administer supplemental fluid and salt. Reduce dose or d/c with sweating, diarrhea, or infection with elevated temperatures. Caution with hypothyroidism; monitor thyroid function. May impair mental/physical abilities. May decrease Na⁺ reabsorption, which could lead to Na⁺ depletion; maintain normal diet, including salt and adequate fluid intake. Caution in elderly. May be associated with the unmasking of Brugada syndrome; avoid with Brugada syndrome.

ADVERSE REACTIONS: Fine hand tremor, polyuria, mild thirst, general discomfort, diarrhea, N/V, drowsiness, muscular weakness, lack of coordination, ataxia, giddiness, tinnitus, blurred vision, large output of diluted urine.

INTERACTIONS: Risk of encephalopathic syndrome (eg, weakness, lethargy, fever, tremulousness, confusion, extrapyramidal symptoms) followed by irreversible brain damage with haloperidol and other neuroleptics; monitor for evidence of neurological toxicity and d/c therapy if such signs appear. May prolong effects of neuromuscular blockers; use with caution. May increase risk of neurotoxic effects with calcium channel blockers or carbamazepine. Increased levels with indomethacin, piroxicam, and other NSAIDs (eg, COX-2 inhibitors); monitor levels closely when initiating or discontinuing NSAID use. Acetazolamide, urea, xanthine preparations, and alkalinizing agents (eg, sodium bicarbonate) may decrease levels. May produce hypothyroidism with iodide preparations. May provoke lithium toxicity with metronidazole; monitor closely. Risk of lithium toxicity with diuretics and ACE inhibitors due to reduced renal clearance; avoid concomitant use but if necessary, monitor levels closely and adjust dose. Fluoxetine may increase or decrease lithium levels; monitor closely. Caution with SSRIs. May interact with methyldopa or phenytoin.

PREGNANCY: Category D, not for use in nursing.

MECHANISM OF ACTION: Antimanic agent; not established. Alters Na⁺ transport in nerve and muscle cells and effects a shift toward intraneuronal metabolism of catecholamines.

PHARMACOKINETICS: Distribution: Found in breast milk. **Elimination:** Urine (primary), feces (insignificant). $T_{1/2}$ 24 hrs.

NURSING CONSIDERATIONS

Assessment: Assess for CVD, severe debilitation, dehydration, sodium depletion. Assess renal function (urinalysis, SrCr), thyroid function with history of thyroid disease, pregnancy/nursing status, and possible drug interactions. Assess for Brugada syndrome or patients with risk factors.

Monitoring: Monitor for diminution of renal concentrating ability (eg, nephrogenic diabetes insipidus), glomerular and interstitial fibrosis, and nephron atrophy in patients on long-term therapy, encephalopathic syndrome, renal function, thyroid function in patients with a history of hypothyroidism, serum lithium levels, signs of lithium toxicity, and other adverse effects. Monitor for unexplained syncope or palpitations.

Patient Counseling: Counsel about clinical signs of lithium toxicity (eg, diarrhea, vomiting, tremor, mild ataxia, drowsiness, muscle weakness); advise to d/c therapy and notify physician if any of these signs occur. Inform of the risks and benefits of therapy. Advise to seek immediate emergency assistance if fainting, lightheadedness, abnormal heartbeat, SOB, or other adverse reactions develop. Inform that lithium may impair mental/physical abilities; caution with activities requiring alertness.

Administration: Oral route. **Storage:** (Lithobid) 15-30°C (59-86°F). Protect from moisture. (300mg) 20-25°C (68-77°F) or (450mg) 25°C (77°F); excursions permitted to 15-30°C (59-86°F).

LIVALO   RX
pitavastatin (Kowa)

THERAPEUTIC CLASS: HMG-CoA reductase inhibitor

INDICATIONS: Adjunct to diet to reduce elevated total cholesterol, LDL, apolipoprotein B, TG, and to increase HDL in adults with primary hyperlipidemia or mixed dyslipidemia.

DOSAGE: *Adults:* Individualize dose. Initial: 2mg qd. Usual: 1-4mg qd. Max: 4mg qd. After initiation or upon titration, analyze lipid levels after 4 weeks and adjust dose accordingly. Moderate/ Severe Renal Impairment (GFR 30-59mL/min and GFR 15-29mL/min not receiving hemodialysis, respectively)/End-Stage Renal Disease Receiving Hemodialysis: Initial: 1mg qd. Max: 2mg qd. Concomitant Erythromycin: Max: 1mg qd. Concomitant Rifampin: Max: 2mg qd.

HOW SUPPLIED: Tab: 1mg, 2mg, 4mg

CONTRAINDICATIONS: Active liver disease, including unexplained persistent elevations of hepatic transaminase levels, women who are pregnant or may become pregnant, nursing mothers, and coadministration with cyclosporine.

WARNINGS/PRECAUTIONS: Increased risk for severe myopathy with doses >4mg qd. Myopathy (including immune-mediated necrotizing myopathy [IMNM]) and rhabdomyolysis with acute renal failure secondary to myoglobinuria reported. Caution with predisposing factors for myopathy (eg, advanced age [≥65 yrs], renal impairment, and inadequately treated hypothyroidism). D/C if markedly elevated creatine kinase (CK) levels occur or myopathy is diagnosed/suspected and temporarily withhold in any patient experiencing an acute or serious condition suggestive of myopathy or predisposing to the development of renal failure secondary to rhabdomyolysis (eg, sepsis, hypotension, dehydration). Increases in serum transaminases (eg, AST, ALT) reported; perform LFTs before the initiation of treatment and if signs or symptoms of liver injury occur. Fatal and nonfatal hepatic failure reported (rare); promptly interrupt therapy if serious liver injury with clinical symptoms and/or hyperbilirubinemia or jaundice occurs; do not restart if no alternative etiology found. Increases in HbA1c and fasting serum glucose levels reported. Caution with substantial alcohol consumption.

ADVERSE REACTIONS: Back pain, constipation, myalgia.

INTERACTIONS: See Contraindications. Erythromycin and rifampin may increase exposure. Due to an increased risk of myopathy/rhabdomyolysis, avoid coadministration with gemfibrozil and use caution when coadministered with fibrates and colchicine. May enhance risk of skeletal muscle effects with niacin; consider dose reduction with lipid-modifying doses of niacin. Monitor PT and INR with warfarin.

PREGNANCY: Category X, not for use in nursing.

MECHANISM OF ACTION: HMG-CoA reductase inhibitor; inhibits the rate-determining enzyme involved with biosynthesis of cholesterol so that it inhibits cholesterol synthesis in the liver.

PHARMACOKINETICS: Absorption: (Oral Sol) Absolute bioavailability (51%); T_{max}=1 hr. **Distribution:** Plasma protein binding (>99%); V_d=148L. **Metabolism:** CYP2C9, 2C8; lactone (major metabolite) via glucuronide conjugate by uridine 5'-diphosphate (UDP) glucuronosyltransferase (UGT1A3 and UGT2B7). **Elimination:** Urine (15%), feces (79%); $T_{1/2}$=12 hrs.

NURSING CONSIDERATIONS

Assessment: Assess for hepatic/renal impairment, inadequately treated hypothyroidism, substantial alcohol consumption, pregnancy/nursing status, possible drug interactions, and other conditions where treatment is cautioned/contraindicated. Obtain baseline lipid profile.

Monitoring: Monitor signs/symptoms of myopathy, rhabdomyolysis, IMNM, acute renal failure, hypersensitivity reactions, and other adverse reactions. Monitor for increases in HbA1c and fasting serum glucose levels. Perform periodic monitoring of lipid profile and CK levels. Analyze lipid levels 4 weeks after initiation/titration. Perform LFTs with signs or symptoms of liver injury. Monitor PT and INR when using warfarin.

Lo/Ovral

Patient Counseling: Advise to promptly notify physician of any unexplained muscle pain, tenderness, or weakness, particularly if accompanied by malaise or fever, or if these muscle signs/symptoms persist after discontinuing treatment. Advise to discuss all medications, both Rx and OTC, with physician. Counsel women of childbearing age to use effective method of birth control to prevent pregnancy during therapy. Instruct pregnant or breastfeeding women to d/c therapy and consult physician. Inform that liver enzymes will be checked before therapy and if signs/symptoms of liver injury occur (eg, fatigue, anorexia, right upper abdominal discomfort, dark urine, or jaundice). Advise to report promptly any symptoms that may indicate liver injury.

Administration: Oral route. Take at any time of the day with or without food. **Storage:** 15-30°C (59-86°F). Protect from light.

Lo/Ovral   RX
ethinyl estradiol - norgestrel (Wyeth)

Cigarette smoking increases the risk of serious cardiovascular (CV) side effects. Risk increases with age (>35 yrs) and with heavy smoking (≥15 cigarettes/day). Women who use oral contraceptives should be strongly advised not to smoke.

OTHER BRAND NAMES: Cryselle (Barr) - Low-Ogestrel (Watson)

THERAPEUTIC CLASS: Estrogen/progestogen combination

INDICATIONS: Prevention of pregnancy.

DOSAGE: *Adults:* 1 tab qd for 28 days, then repeat. Start 1st Sunday after menses begins or 1st day of menses. Take at the same time each day, (Cryselle) preferably after pm meal or at hs. (Lo/Ovral) Switching from 21-Day Regimen: Start 7 days after taking last dose. Switching from Progestin-Only Pill: Start the next day after last dose. Switching from Implant/Inj: Start on the day of implant removal or the day the next inj would be due. Use After Pregnancy/Abortion/Miscarriage: Start on Day 28 postpartum in nonlactating mother or after a 2nd-trimester abortion.
Pediatrics: Postpubertal: 1 tab qd for 28 days, then repeat. Start 1st Sunday after menses begins or 1st day of menses. Take at the same time each day, (Cryselle) preferably after pm meal or at hs. (Lo/Ovral) Switching from 21-Day Regimen: Start 7 days after taking last dose. Switching from Progestin-Only Pill: Start the next day after last dose. Switching from Implant/Inj: Start on the day of implant removal or the day the next inj would be due. Use After Pregnancy/Abortion/Miscarriage: Start on Day 28 postpartum in nonlactating mother or after a 2nd-trimester abortion.

HOW SUPPLIED: Tab: (Ethinyl Estradiol-Norgestrel) 0.03mg-0.3mg

CONTRAINDICATIONS: Thrombophlebitis, thromboembolic disorders, past history of deep vein thrombophlebitis or thromboembolic disorders, cerebrovascular or coronary artery disease (CAD), known or suspected carcinoma of the breast, carcinoma of the endometrium or other known or suspected estrogen-dependent neoplasia, undiagnosed abnormal genital bleeding, cholestatic jaundice of pregnancy or jaundice with prior pill use, known or suspected pregnancy, hepatic adenomas or carcinomas or (Low-Ogestrel) benign liver tumors. (Lo/Ovral) Active liver disease, valvular heart disease with thrombogenic complications, thrombogenic rhythm disorders, hereditary or acquired thrombophilias, major surgery with prolonged immobilization, diabetes with vascular involvement, headaches with focal neurological symptoms, uncontrolled HTN, past history of cerebrovascular or coronary artery disease, personal history of breast cancer.

WARNINGS/PRECAUTIONS: Increased risk of myocardial infarction (MI), vascular disease, thromboembolism, stroke, hepatic neoplasia, and gallbladder disease. Caution with CV disease risk factors. Increased risk of morbidity and mortality with HTN, hyperlipidemia, obesity, and diabetes. May increase risk of breast cancer and cancer of the reproductive organs. D/C at least 4 weeks prior to and for 2 weeks after elective surgery with an increased risk of thromboembolism during and following prolonged immobilization. Contact lens wearers who develop visual changes or changes in lens tolerance should be assessed by an ophthalmologist. Retinal thrombosis reported; d/c if there is unexplained partial or complete loss of vision, onset of proptosis or diplopia; papilledema; or retinal vascular lesions develop. May cause glucose intolerance; monitor prediabetic and diabetic patients. May elevate LDL levels and cause hypertriglyceridemia leading to pancreatitis; monitor closely with hyperlipidemias. May cause fluid retention and increased BP; monitor closely with HTN and d/c if significant BP elevation occurs. New onset/exacerbation of migraine or recurrent, persistent headache may develop; d/c if these occur. Breakthrough bleeding and spotting reported; rule out malignancies or pregnancy. D/C if jaundice develops. Caution with history of depression; d/c if depression recurs to serious degree. May affect certain endocrine function tests, LFTs, and blood components in laboratory tests. Should not be used to induce withdrawal bleeding as a test for pregnancy, or to treat threatened or habitual abortion during pregnancy. Not indicated before menarche. (Lo/Ovral) Diarrhea and/or vomiting may reduce hormone absorption, resulting in decreased serum concentrations. Ectopic and intrauterine pregnancy may occur in contraceptive failures. Increased risk of morbidity and mortality with certain inherited or acquired thrombophilias.

ADVERSE REACTIONS: N/V, breakthrough bleeding, spotting, amenorrhea, migraine, depression, vaginal candidiasis, edema, weight changes, abdominal cramps/bloating, menstrual flow changes, cervical erosion, and secretion changes.

INTERACTIONS: Reduced effectiveness and increased incidence of breakthrough bleeding and menstrual irregularities with rifampin, barbiturates, phenylbutazone, phenytoin, griseofulvin, ampicillin, and tetracyclines. (Lo/Ovral) Reduced effectiveness resulting in unintended pregnancy or breakthrough bleeding with antibiotics (eg, penicillins), anticonvulsants, and other drugs that increase the metabolism of contraceptive steroids (eg, rifabutin, primidone, dexamethasone, carbamazepine, felbamate, oxcarbazepine, topiramate, modafinil); consider back-up nonhormonal method of birth control. May reduce effectiveness and may also result in breakthrough bleeding with herbal products containing St. John's wort. Significant changes (increase or decrease) in plasma levels with anti-HIV protease inhibitors may occur. Atorvastatin, ascorbic acid, acetaminophen (APAP), and CYP3A4 inhibitors (eg, indinavir, itraconazole, ketoconazole, fluconazole, troleandomycin) may increase hormone levels. Increased risk of intrahepatic cholestasis with troleandomycin. Increased plasma concentrations of cyclosporine, prednisolone and other corticosteroids, and theophylline reported. Decreased plasma concentrations of APAP and increased clearance of temazepam, salicylic acid, morphine, and clofibric acid reported.

PREGNANCY: Category X, not for use in nursing.

MECHANISM OF ACTION: Estrogen/progestogen oral contraceptive; acts by suppression of gonadotropins. Primarily acts by inhibiting ovulation. Also produces alterations/changes in the cervical mucus (increases difficulty of sperm entry into uterus) and the endometrium (reduces likelihood of implantation).

PHARMACOKINETICS: Distribution: Found in breast milk.

NURSING CONSIDERATIONS

Assessment: Assess for breast cancer, estrogen-dependent neoplasia, abnormal genital bleeding, thrombophlebitis, thromboembolic disorders, past history of deep vein thrombophlebitis or thromboembolic disorders, cerebrovascular or CAD, or any other conditions where treatment is cautioned or contraindicated. Assess use in women who are >35 yrs and heavy smokers (≥15 cigarettes/day). Assess pregnancy/nursing status and for possible drug interactions.

Monitoring: Monitor for signs/symptoms of MI, bleeding irregularities, thromboembolism, onset or exacerbation of headaches or migraines, and other adverse reactions. Monitor serum glucose levels in diabetic and prediabetic patients, BP with history of HTN, lipid levels with history of hyperlipidemia, and for signs of worsening depression with previous history of the disorder. Refer contact lens wearers to an ophthalmologist if visual changes develop. Perform periodic history and physical exam.

Patient Counseling: Inform that drug does not protect against HIV infection (AIDS) and other sexually transmitted diseases. Counsel about potential adverse effects of the drug. Advise to avoid smoking. Instruct to take exactly ud at intervals not exceeding 24 hrs. Advise about risks of pregnancy if dose is missed; counsel to have a back-up nonhormonal birth control method at all times. Instruct that if one dose is missed, take as soon as possible and take next pill at regular scheduled time. Inform that spotting, light bleeding, or nausea may occur during the first 1-3 packs of pills; advise not to d/c medication and if symptoms persist, notify physician. Instruct to d/c if pregnancy is confirmed/suspected.

Administration: Oral route. **Storage:** (Cryselle) 15-30°C (59-86°F). (Lo/Ovral) 20-25°C (68-77°F). (Low-Ogestrel) 15-25°C (59-77°F).

LOESTRIN 21   RX
norethindrone acetate - ethinyl estradiol (Duramed)

> Cigarette smoking increases the risk of serious cardiovascular (CV) side effects. Risk increases with age (>35 yrs) and with heavy smoking (≥15 cigarettes/day). Women who use oral contraceptives should be strongly advised not to smoke.

OTHER BRAND NAMES: Junel 1.5/30 (Barr) - Junel 1/20 (Barr) - Microgestin 1.5/30 (Watson) - Microgestin 1/20 (Watson) - Loestrin 21 1.5/30 (Duramed) - Loestrin 21 1/20 (Duramed) - Gildess 1.5/30 (Qualitest) - Gildess 1/20 (Qualitest)

THERAPEUTIC CLASS: Estrogen/progestogen combination

INDICATIONS: Prevention of pregnancy.

DOSAGE: *Adults:* 1 tab qd for 21 days, stop 7 days, then repeat. Start 1st Sunday after menses begin or the 1st day of menses.
Pediatrics: Postpubertal: 1 tab qd for 21 days, stop 7 days, then repeat. Start 1st Sunday after menses begin or the 1st day of menses.

HOW SUPPLIED: Tab: (Ethinyl Estradiol-Norethindrone) (1/20) 20mcg-1mg, (1.5/30) 30mcg-1.5mg

CONTRAINDICATIONS: Thrombophlebitis, thromboembolic disorders, past history of deep vein thrombophlebitis or thromboembolic disorders, cerebrovascular or coronary artery disease (CAD), known or suspected carcinoma of the breast, carcinoma of the endometrium or other known or suspected estrogen-dependent neoplasia, undiagnosed abnormal genital bleeding, cholestatic jaundice of pregnancy or jaundice with prior pill use, hepatic adenomas or carcinomas, and pregnancy.

WARNINGS/PRECAUTIONS: Increased risk of myocardial infarction (MI), thromboembolism, stroke, hepatic neoplasia, gallbladder disease, and vascular disease. Increased risk of morbidity and mortality with HTN, hyperlipidemia, obesity, and diabetes. Caution in women with CV disease risk factors. Start use ≥4-6 weeks postpartum if not breastfeeding. May increase risk of breast cancer and cancer of the reproductive organs. Retinal thrombosis reported; d/c if unexplained partial or complete loss of vision occurs, onset of proptosis or diplopia, papilledema, or retinal vascular lesions develop. Should not be used to induce withdrawal bleeding as a test for pregnancy, or to treat threatened or habitual abortion during pregnancy. May cause glucose intolerance; monitor prediabetic and diabetic patients. May elevate BP; monitor closely and d/c use if significant BP elevation occurs. New onset/exacerbation of migraine, or recurrent, persistent, severe headache may develop; d/c therapy if these occur. Breakthrough bleeding and spotting reported; rule out malignancy or pregnancy. May cause serum TG or other lipid changes (eg, elevated LDL). May be poorly metabolized with impaired liver function; d/c if jaundice develops. May cause fluid retention; caution with conditions that aggravate fluid retention. Caution with history of depression; d/c if depression recurs to serious degree. May develop changes in vision or lens tolerance in contact lens wearers. Does not protect against HIV infection (AIDS) and other sexually transmitted diseases (STDs). Perform annual history and physical exam. Use before menarche is not indicated. May affect certain endocrine function tests, LFTs, and blood components in laboratory tests.

ADVERSE REACTIONS: N/V, breakthrough bleeding, spotting, amenorrhea, migraine, mental depression, vaginal candidiasis, edema, weight changes, abdominal cramps/bloating, menstrual flow changes, melasma.

INTERACTIONS: Reduced effects, increased breakthrough bleeding, and menstrual irregularities with rifampin and phenylbutazone. Increased metabolism and reduced contraceptive effectiveness with anticonvulsants (phenobarbital, phenytoin, carbamazepine). Pregnancy reported with antimicrobials (ampicillin, griseofulvin, and tetracyclines). Increased levels with atorvastatin, ascorbic acid, and acetaminophen (APAP). Increased plasma levels of cyclosporine, prednisolone, and theophylline. Decreased levels of APAP. Increased clearance of temazepam, salicylic acid, morphine, and clofibric acid. Reduced plasma levels with troglitazone resulting in reduced contraceptive effectiveness.

PREGNANCY: Category X, not for use in nursing.

MECHANISM OF ACTION: Estrogen/progestogen oral contraceptive; acts by suppressing gonadotropins, primarily inhibiting ovulation, and causing other alterations, including changes in cervical mucus (increases difficulty of sperm entry into uterus) and endometrium (reduces likelihood of implantation).

PHARMACOKINETICS: Absorption: Ethinyl Estradiol: Absolute bioavailability (43%). Norethindrone: Rapid and complete. Absolute bioavailability (64%). **Distribution:** V_d=2-4L/kg; plasma protein binding (>95%); found in breast milk. **Metabolism:** Ethinyl Estradiol: Extensive via CYP3A4; oxidation, sulfate/glucuronide conjugation; 2-hydroxy ethinyl estradiol (primary oxidative metabolite). Norethindrone: Extensive; reduction, sulfate/glucuronide conjugation. **Elimination:** Urine, feces.

NURSING CONSIDERATIONS

Assessment: Assess for presence or history of breast cancer, estrogen-dependent neoplasia, abnormal genital bleeding, active liver disease, and known/suspected pregnancy or any other conditions where treatment is cautioned or contraindicated. Assess use in patients who are >35 yrs and heavy smokers (≥15 cigarettes/day). Assess use with HTN, hyperlipidemias, obesity, DM, or in patients at increased risk for thrombosis. Assess for possible drug interactions.

Monitoring: Monitor for bleeding irregularities, thromboembolic events, onset or exacerbation of headaches or migraines, and ectopic pregnancy. Monitor fasting blood glucose levels in DM and prediabetic patients, BP with history of HTN, lipid levels with a history of hyperlipidemia. Monitor for signs of liver dysfunction (eg, jaundice) and signs of depression with previous history. Refer patients with contact lenses to an ophthalmologist if visual changes occur. Perform annual history and physical exam.

Patient Counseling: Counsel about potential adverse effects. Inform that drug does not protect against HIV infection and other STDs. Instruct to use additional method of protection until after the 1st week of administration in the initial cycle when utilizing the Sunday-Start Regimen. Instruct to take exactly as directed and at intervals not exceeding 24 hrs. Take drug regularly with meal or hs; if dose is missed, take as soon as remembered, then take next dose at regular scheduled time; continue regimen if spotting or breakthrough bleeding occurs; notify physician if bleeding persists. Avoid smoking while on medication.

Administration: Oral route. Refer to PI for special notes on administration. **Storage:** 20-25°C (68-77°F).

LOFIBRA
fenofibrate (Gate)

RX

THERAPEUTIC CLASS: Fibric acid derivative

INDICATIONS: Adjunct to diet for treatment of adults with hypertriglyceridemia (Fredrickson Types IV and V hyperlipidemia) and for the reduction of LDL, total cholesterol, TG, and apolipo-protein B in adults with primary hypercholesterolemia or mixed dyslipidemia (Fredrickson Types IIa and IIb). (Tab) Adjunct to diet to increase HDL in adults with primary hypercholesterolemia or mixed dyslipidemia (Fredrickson Types IIa and IIb).

DOSAGE: *Adults:* Primary Hypercholesterolemia/Mixed Hyperlipidemia: Initial: (Cap) 200mg/day. (Tab) 160mg/day. Hypertriglyceridemia: Individualize dose. Initial: (Cap) 67-200mg/day. (Tab) 54-160mg qd. Titrate: Adjust PRN after repeat lipid levels at 4-8 week intervals. Max: (Cap) 200mg/day. (Tab) 160mg/day. Renal Dysfunction: Initial: (Cap) 67mg/day. (Tab) 54mg/day. Increase only after evaluation of the effects on renal function and lipid levels at this dose. Elderly: Initial: (Cap) Limit to 67mg/day. (Tab) Limit to 54mg/day. Consider lowering dose if lipid levels fall significantly below targeted range.

HOW SUPPLIED: Cap: 67mg, 134mg, 200mg; Tab: 54mg, 160mg

CONTRAINDICATIONS: Hepatic or severe renal dysfunction (including primary biliary cirrhosis and unexplained persistent liver function abnormality), preexisting gallbladder disease.

WARNINGS/PRECAUTIONS: Hepatocellular, chronic active and cholestatic hepatitis and cirrhosis (rare) reported. Increases in serum transaminases (AST or ALT) reported; monitor LFTs regularly and d/c if enzyme level persists to >3X ULN. May cause cholelithiasis; d/c if gallstones found. May cause myositis, myopathy, or rhabdomyolysis; determine serum creatine kinase (CK) level if muscle pain, tenderness, or weakness occur; d/c if myopathy/myositis is suspected/diagnosed or marked CPK elevation occurs. Control lipids with appropriate diet, exercise, and weight loss in obese patients and control any medical problems (eg, diabetes mellitus, hypothyroidism) that are contributing to lipid abnormalities prior to therapy. Measure lipid levels prior to therapy and during initial treatment; d/c if inadequate response after 2 months on max dose of 200mg/day (Cap) or 145mg/day (Tab). Acute hypersensitivity reactions (rare) and pancreatitis reported. Mild to moderate decrease in Hgb, Hct, and WBCs reported; periodically monitor CBC during the first 12 months of therapy. Thrombocytopenia and agranulocytosis reported (rare). Caution in renally impaired elderly. (Tab) Pulmonary embolus, deep vein thrombosis, and elevated SrCr observed.

ADVERSE REACTIONS: Abnormal LFTs, abdominal pain, respiratory disorder, back pain, increases in ALT or AST, headache, increased CPK.

INTERACTIONS: Caution with anticoagulants due to potentiation of coumarin/coumarin-type anticoagulants; reduce anticoagulant dose to maintain desirable PT/INR. Avoid HMG-CoA reductase inhibitors unless benefits outweigh risks; rhabdomyolysis, markedly elevated CK levels, and myoglobinuria leading to acute renal failure reported. Bile acid sequestrants may impede absorption; take at least 1 hr before or 4-6 hrs after bile acid binding resin. Evaluate benefits/risks with immunosuppressants (eg, cyclosporine) and other nephrotoxic agents; use lowest effective dose. Prior to therapy, d/c or change if possible, medications that are known to exacerbate hypertriglyceridemia (eg, beta-blockers, thiazides, estrogens). (Tab) Increased plasma concentrations with pravastatin, glimepiride, and fluvastatin. Decreased plasma concentrations with atorvastatin.

PREGNANCY: Category C, not for use in nursing.

MECHANISM OF ACTION: Fibric acid derivative; activates peroxisome proliferator activated receptor α (PPARα), increasing lipolysis and elimination of TG-rich particles from plasma by activating lipoprotein lipase and reducing production of apoprotein C-III. Activation of PPARα induces an increase in the synthesis of apoproteins A-I, A-II, and HDL.

PHARMACOKINETICS: Absorption: Well-absorbed; T_{max}=6-8 hrs. **Distribution:** Plasma protein binding (99%). **Metabolism:** Rapid, via hydrolysis by esterases to fenofibric acid (active metabolite), conjugation. **Elimination:** Urine (60% metabolite), feces (25%); $T_{1/2}$=20 hrs.

NURSING CONSIDERATIONS

Assessment: Assess for hypersensitivity, hepatic/renal impairment, preexisting gallbladder disease, severe hypertriglyceridemia, pregnancy/nursing status, and possible drug interactions. Assess for body weight and alcohol intake. Obtain CPK, lipid levels, and LFTs prior to therapy.

Monitoring: Monitor for signs/symptoms of myositis, myopathy, and rhabdomyolysis; measure serum CK levels if myopathy is suspected. Monitor for signs/symptoms of increases in serum transaminases, hepatitis, and cirrhosis; perform periodic monitoring of LFTs. Monitor for signs/symptoms of cholelithiasis; perform gallbladder studies if cholelithiasis is suspected. Monitor for signs/symptoms of pancreatitis, hypersensitivity reactions, (Tab) PE and DVT. Periodically monitor blood counts (eg, Hgb, Hct, and WBC) and lipid levels.

Patient Counseling: Inform of risks/benefits of therapy. Advise to immediately notify physician if unexplained muscle pain, tenderness, or weakness, with malaise or fever occur. Recommend appropriate lipid-lowering diet.

Administration: Oral route. Take with meals. **Storage:** 20-25°C (68-77°F). Protect from moisture.

LOMOTIL
diphenoxylate HCl - atropine sulfate (Pfizer)

THERAPEUTIC CLASS: Anticholinergic/opioid

INDICATIONS: Adjunctive therapy for management of diarrhea.

DOSAGE: *Adults:* Initial: 2 tabs or 10mL qid. Titrate: Reduce dose after symptoms are controlled. Maint: 2 tabs or 10mL qd. Max: 20mg/day diphenoxylate. D/C if symptoms not controlled after 10 days at max dose of 20mg/day (diphenoxylate).
Pediatrics: 2-12 Yrs: Initial: 0.3-0.4mg/kg/day of solution in four divided doses. Titrate: Reduce dose after symptoms are controlled. Maint: May be as low as 25% of initial dose. D/C if no improvement within 48 hrs.

HOW SUPPLIED: (Diphenoxylate-Atropine) Sol: 2.5mg-0.025mg/5mL [60mL]; Tab: 2.5mg-0.025mg

CONTRAINDICATIONS: Obstructive jaundice, diarrhea associated with pseudomembranous enterocolitis or enterotoxin-producing bacteria.

WARNINGS/PRECAUTIONS: Avoid in children <2 yrs. Overdosage may result in severe respiratory depression and coma, leading to brain damage or death. Avoid use with severe dehydration or electrolyte imbalance until corrective therapy is initiated. May induce toxic megacolon with acute ulcerative colitis; d/c if abdominal distention occurs or untoward symptoms develop. May cause intestinal fluid retention. Avoid with diarrhea associated with organisms that penetrate the intestinal mucosa, and with pseudomembranous enterocolitis. Extreme caution with advanced hepatorenal disease and liver dysfunction. Caution in pediatrics, especially with Down's syndrome.

ADVERSE REACTIONS: Numbness of extremities, dizziness, anaphylaxis, drowsiness, toxic megacolon, N/V, urticaria, pruritus, anorexia, pancreatitis, paralytic ileus, euphoria, malaise/lethargy.

INTERACTIONS: MAOIs may precipitate hypertensive crisis. (Diphenoxylate) May potentiate barbiturates, tranquilizers, and alcohol. Potential to prolong $T_{1/2}$ of drugs for which the rate of elimination is dependent on the microsomal drug metabolizing enzyme system.

PREGNANCY: Category C, caution in nursing.

MECHANISM OF ACTION: Diphenoxylate: Antidiarrheal. Atropine: Anticholinergic.

PHARMACOKINETICS: Absorption: (4 tabs) C_{max}=163ng/mL; T_{max}=2 hrs. **Metabolism:** Rapid and extensive metabolism through ester hydrolysis to diphenoxylic acid (major metabolite). **Elimination:** Urine (14%), feces (49%). $T_{1/2}$=12-14 hrs (diphenoxylic acid).

NURSING CONSIDERATIONS

Assessment: Assess for hypersensitivity, obstructive jaundice, diarrhea associated with pseudomembranous enterocolitis or enterotoxin-producing bacteria, severe dehydration, electrolyte imbalance, hepatic dysfunction, hepatorenal disease, ulcerative colitis, Down's syndrome, diarrhea (caused by *Escherichia coli*, *Salmonella*, *Shigella*), pregnancy/nursing status, and possible drug interactions.

Monitoring: Monitor for severe dehydration, electrolyte imbalance, renal function, toxic megacolon in ulcerative colitis, abdominal distention, signs of atropinism, and other adverse reactions.

Patient Counseling: Instruct to take as directed and not to exceed the recommended dosage. Inform of consequences of overdosage, including severe respiratory depression and coma, possibly leading to permanent brain damage or death. Instruct to exercise caution while operating machinery/driving. Advise to avoid alcohol and other CNS depressants. Advise to keep medicines out of reach of children. Inform patient that drowsiness or dizziness may occur.

Administration: Oral route. Plastic dropper should be used when measuring liquid for administration to children. **Storage:** Dispense liquids in original container.

LOPID

RX

gemfibrozil (Parke-Davis)

THERAPEUTIC CLASS: Fibric acid derivative

INDICATIONS: Adjunctive therapy to diet for treatment of adults with very high elevations of serum TG levels (Types IV and V hyperlipidemia) who present a risk of pancreatitis and who do not respond adequately to diet. Adjunctive therapy to diet to reduce risk of developing coronary heart disease only in Type IIb patients without history of or symptoms of existing coronary heart disease who have had an inadequate response to weight loss, dietary therapy, exercise, and other pharmacologic agents and who have the triad of low HDL, elevated LDL, and elevated TG levels.

DOSAGE: *Adults:* 1200mg in 2 divided doses 30 min before am and pm meals.

HOW SUPPLIED: Tab: 600mg* *scored

CONTRAINDICATIONS: Severe renal dysfunction, hepatic dysfunction (including primary biliary cirrhosis), preexisting gallbladder disease, combination therapy with repaglinide or simvastatin.

WARNINGS/PRECAUTIONS: Cholelithiasis reported; perform gallbladder studies if cholelithiasis is suspected and d/c therapy if gallstones are found. May be associated with myositis; d/c if myositis is suspected/diagnosed. D/C if lipid response is inadequate after 3 months of therapy. Mild Hgb, Hct, and WBC decreases, and severe anemia, leukopenia, thrombocytopenia, and bone marrow hypoplasia reported; periodically monitor blood counts during the first 12 months of therapy. Abnormal LFTs reported; periodically monitor LFTs and d/c if abnormalities persist. Worsening renal insufficiency reported upon the addition of therapy in patients with baseline plasma creatinine >2mg/dL. Estrogen therapy is associated with massive rises in plasma TG; discontinuation of estrogen therapy may obviate the need for specific drug therapy of hypertriglyceridemia. Control any medical problems (eg, diabetes mellitus [DM], hypothyroidism) that contribute to lipid abnormalities before initiating therapy.

ADVERSE REACTIONS: Dyspepsia, abdominal pain, diarrhea, fatigue.

INTERACTIONS: See Contraindications. Caution with anticoagulants; reduce anticoagulant dose and frequently monitor prothrombin until it has been definitely determined that prothrombin level has stabilized. Increased risk of myopathy and rhabdomyolysis with HMG-CoA reductase inhibitors. Reduced exposure with resin-granule drugs (eg, colestipol); administer ≥2 hrs apart. May potentiate myopathy with colchicine; caution when prescribing with colchicine, especially in elderly patients or patients with renal dysfunction.

PREGNANCY: Category C, not for use in nursing.

MECHANISM OF ACTION: Fibric acid derivative; not established. Inhibits peripheral lipolysis and decreases hepatic extraction of free fatty acids, thus reducing hepatic TG production. Inhibits synthesis and increases clearance of VLDL carrier apolipoprotein B, leading to a decrease in VLDL production.

PHARMACOKINETICS: Absorption: Complete. T_{max}=1-2 hrs. **Distribution:** Plasma protein binding (highly bound). **Metabolism:** Oxidation to form a hydroxymethyl and a carboxyl metabolite. **Elimination:** Urine (70%, <2% unchanged), feces (6%).

NURSING CONSIDERATIONS

Assessment: Assess for hepatic/renal dysfunction, gallbladder disease, other medical conditions (eg, DM, hypothyroidism), hypersensitivity to drug, pregnancy/nursing status, and possible drug interactions. Obtain lipid levels.

Monitoring: Monitor for signs/symptoms of cholelithiasis, myositis, worsening renal insufficiency, and other adverse reactions. Periodically monitor serum lipids levels, CBC, and LFTs. Frequently monitor prothrombin with anticoagulants. Closely observe patients with significantly elevated TG during therapy.

Patient Counseling: Inform about potential risks/benefits of therapy. Advise to report to physician any muscle pain/tenderness/weakness, or other adverse reactions. Instruct to notify physician if pregnant/nursing or planning to become pregnant.

Administration: Oral route. Take 30 min before am and pm meals. **Storage:** 20-25°C (68-77°F). Protect from light and humidity.

LORAZEPAM ORAL

CIV

lorazepam (Various)

OTHER BRAND NAMES: Ativan (Valeant)

THERAPEUTIC CLASS: Benzodiazepine

INDICATIONS: Management of anxiety disorders or for short-term relief of the symptoms of anxiety or anxiety associated with depressive symptoms.

DOSAGE: *Adults:* Individualize dose, frequency, and duration. Anxiety: Initial: 2-3mg/day given bid or tid. Usual: 2-6mg/day in divided doses; take largest dose before hs. Increase dose gradually PRN; when higher dosage is indicated, increase pm dose before daytime doses. Dosage Range: 1-10mg/day. Insomnia: 2-4mg as a single dose qhs. Elderly/Debilitated: Initial: 1-2mg/day in divided doses; adjust PRN and as tolerated.

Pediatrics: ≥12 yrs: Individualize dose, frequency, and duration. Anxiety: Initial: 2-3mg/day given bid or tid. Usual Range: 2-6mg/day in divided doses; take largest dose before hs. Increase dose gradually PRN; when higher dosage is indicated, increase pm dose before daytime doses. Dosage Range: 1-10mg/day. Insomnia: 2-4mg as a single dose qhs.

HOW SUPPLIED: Sol: 2mg/mL; Tab: (Ativan) 0.5mg, 1mg*, 2mg* *scored

CONTRAINDICATIONS: Acute narrow-angle glaucoma.

WARNINGS/PRECAUTIONS: Effectiveness in long-term use (>4 months) has not been assessed; prescribe for short periods only (eg, 2-4 weeks) and periodically reassess usefulness of drug. Continuous long-term use is not recommended. Preexisting depression may emerge or worsen; not for use with primary depressive disorder or psychosis. May lead to potentially fatal respiratory depression. May impair mental/physical abilities. Use may lead to physical and psychological dependence; increased risk with higher doses, longer term use, and in patients with history of alcoholism/drug abuse, or with significant personality disorders. Withdrawal symptoms reported; avoid abrupt d/c and follow a gradual dosage-tapering schedule after extended therapy. May develop tolerance to sedative effects. Paradoxical reactions reported; d/c if these occur. May have abuse potential, especially with a history of drug and/or alcohol abuse. Possible suicide in patients with depression; do not use in such patients without adequate antidepressant therapy. Caution with compromised respiratory function (eg, chronic obstructive pulmonary disease, sleep apnea syndrome), impaired renal/hepatic function, hepatic encephalopathy, in elderly, and in debilitated patients. May worsen hepatic encephalopathy. Adjust dose with severe hepatic insufficiency; lower doses may be sufficient. Monitor frequently for symptoms of upper GI disease. Leukopenia and elevations of lactate dehydrogenase reported; perform periodic blood counts and LFTs with long-term therapy.

ADVERSE REACTIONS: Sedation, dizziness, weakness, unsteadiness.

INTERACTIONS: Increased CNS-depressant effects with other CNS depressants (eg, alcohol, barbiturates, antipsychotics, sedative/hypnotics, anxiolytics, antidepressants, narcotic analgesics, sedative antihistamines, anticonvulsants, anesthetics); may lead to potentially fatal respiratory depression. Concomitant use with clozapine may produce marked sedation, excessive salivation, hypotension, ataxia, delirium, and respiratory arrest. Increased plasma concentrations with valproate and more rapid onset or prolonged effect with probenecid; reduce dose by 50%. Decreased sedative effects with theophylline or aminophylline.

PREGNANCY: Not for use in pregnancy/nursing.

MECHANISM OF ACTION: Benzodiazepine; has a tranquilizing action on the CNS with no appreciable effect on the respiratory or cardiovascular systems.

PHARMACOKINETICS: Absorption: Readily absorbed. Absolute bioavailability (90%); (2mg) C_{max}=20ng/mL; T_{max}=2 hrs. **Distribution:** Plasma protein binding (85%); found in breast milk. **Metabolism:** Glucuronidation. **Elimination:** Urine; $T_{1/2}$=12 hrs.

NURSING CONSIDERATIONS

Assessment: Assess for acute narrow-angle glaucoma, primary depressive disorder, psychosis, personality disorders, compromised respiratory function, impaired renal/hepatic function, hepatic encephalopathy, history of alcohol/drug abuse, previous hypersensitivity to the drug, pregnancy/nursing status, and possible drug interactions.

Monitoring: Monitor for respiratory depression, physical/psychological dependence, withdrawal symptoms, tolerance, abuse, suicidal thinking, paradoxical reactions, symptoms of upper GI disease, and emergence/worsening of depression. Reassess usefulness of drug periodically. Monitor elderly/debilitated frequently and addiction-prone individuals carefully. Perform periodic blood counts and LFTs with long-term therapy.

Patient Counseling: Inform that psychological/physical dependence may occur; instruct to consult physician before increasing dose or abruptly d/c drug. Warn not to operate dangerous machinery or motor vehicles and that tolerance for alcohol and other CNS depressants will be diminished. Advise to consult physician if pregnancy occurs.

Administration: Oral route. (Sol) Dispense only in the bottle and only with the calibrated dropper provided. Mix with liquid or semi-solid food. Refer to PI for further instructions. **Storage:** (Sol) 2-8°C (36-46°F). Protect from light. Discard opened bottle after 90 days. (Tab) 25°C (77°F); excursions permitted to 15-30°C (59-86°F).

LOSEASONIQUE   RX
ethinyl estradiol - levonorgestrel (Teva)

> Cigarette smoking increases risk of serious cardiovascular (CV) events. Risk increases with age (>35 yrs of age) and with the number of cigarettes smoked. Should not be used by women who are >35 yrs of age and smoke.

OTHER BRAND NAMES: CamreseLo (Teva)

THERAPEUTIC CLASS: Estrogen/progestogen combination

INDICATIONS: Prevention of pregnancy.

DOSAGE: *Adults:* 1 tab qd at the same time every day for 91 days, then repeat. Start on the 1st Sunday after onset of menstruation. Use a nonhormonal back-up method of contraception (eg, condoms, spermicide) for the first 7 days of treatment. If patient does not immediately start the next pill pack, use a nonhormonal back-up method of contraception until patient has taken an orange tab qd for 7 consecutive days.
Pediatrics: Postpubertal: 1 tab qd at the same time every day for 91 days, then repeat. Start on the 1st Sunday after onset of menstruation. Use a nonhormonal back-up method of contraception (eg, condoms, spermicide) for the first 7 days of treatment. If patient does not immediately start the next pill pack, use a nonhormonal back-up method of contraception until patient has taken an orange tab qd for 7 consecutive days.

HOW SUPPLIED: Tab: (Levonorgestrel-Ethinyl Estradiol [EE]) 0.1mg-0.02mg; Tab: (EE) 0.01mg

CONTRAINDICATIONS: High risk of arterial/venous thrombotic diseases (eg, smoking if >35 yrs of age, history/presence of deep vein thrombosis/pulmonary embolism, cerebrovascular disease, coronary artery disease, thrombogenic valvular or thrombogenic rhythm diseases of the heart [eg, subacute bacterial endocarditis with valvular disease, or atrial fibrillation], hypercoagulopathies, uncontrolled HTN, diabetes with vascular disease, headaches with focal neurological symptoms or migraine with/without aura if >35 yrs of age), history/presence of breast or other estrogen-/progestin-sensitive cancer, benign/malignant liver tumors, liver disease, pregnancy.

WARNINGS/PRECAUTIONS: Increased risk of venous thromboembolism and arterial thrombosis (eg, stroke, myocardial infarction); d/c if an arterial/deep venous thrombotic event occurs. If feasible, d/c at least 4 weeks before and through 2 weeks after major surgery or other surgeries known to have an elevated risk of thromboembolism. Start therapy no earlier than 4 weeks postpartum in women who are not breastfeeding. D/C if there is unexplained loss of vision, proptosis, diplopia, papilledema, or retinal vascular lesions; evaluate for retinal vein thrombosis immediately. May increase risk of cervical cancer, intraepithelial neoplasia, and gallbladder disease. D/C if jaundice develops. Hepatic adenomas and increased risk of hepatocellular carcinoma reported. Cholestasis may occur in women with a history of pregnancy-related cholestasis. Increase in BP reported. Monitor BP in women with well-controlled HTN; d/c if BP rises significantly. May decrease glucose tolerance in a dose-related fashion; monitor prediabetic and diabetic women. Consider alternative contraception with uncontrolled dyslipidemias. If new headaches that are recurrent, persistent, or severe develop, evaluate the cause and d/c if indicated. Unscheduled bleeding and spotting may occur; rule out pregnancy or malignancies. Amenorrhea or oligomenorrhea may occur after discontinuing therapy. May change results of some laboratory tests (eg, coagulation factors, lipids, glucose tolerance, binding proteins).

ADVERSE REACTIONS: Headaches, irregular and/or heavy uterine bleeding, dysmenorrhea, N/V, back pain, breast tenderness.

INTERACTIONS: Agents that induce certain enzymes, including CYP3A4 (eg, barbiturates, carbamazepine, phenytoin), may decrease contraceptive efficacy or increase breakthrough bleeding; use additional or alternative contraceptive method. Significant changes (increase or decrease) in plasma estrogen and progestin levels reported with HIV protease inhibitors. Pregnancy reported with antibiotics. Atorvastatin may increase EE exposure; ascorbic acid and acetaminophen may increase EE levels. CYP3A4 inhibitors (eg, itraconazole, ketoconazole) may increase plasma hormone levels. May decrease concentrations of lamotrigine and reduce seizure control; dosage adjustments of lamotrigine may be needed. Increases thyroid-binding globulin; may need to increase dose of thyroid hormone in patients on thyroid hormone replacement therapy.

PREGNANCY: Contraindicated in pregnancy, not for use in nursing.

MECHANISM OF ACTION: Estrogen/progestogen combination oral contraceptive (COC); acts primarily by suppressing ovulation. Also causes cervical mucus changes that inhibit sperm penetration and endometrial changes that reduce the likelihood of implantation.

PHARMACOKINETICS: Absorption: Levonorgestrel: Rapid and complete. Bioavailability (nearly 100%). AUC=76.5ng•hr/mL; C_{max}=6ng/mL; T_{max}=1.6 hrs. EE: Rapid and almost complete. Systemic bioavailability (43%). AUC=1335.8pg•hr/mL; C_{max}=122.8pg/mL; T_{max}=1.8 hrs. **Distribution:** Found in breast milk. Levonorgestrel: V_d=1.8L/kg; plasma protein binding (97.5-99%). EE: V_d=4.3L/kg; plasma protein binding (95-97%, albumin). **Metabolism:** Levonorgestrel: Sulfate and glucuronide conjugation. EE: 1st-pass (gut wall); liver by hydroxylation via CYP3A4; methylation and/or conjugation. **Elimination:** Levonorgestrel: Urine (45%) (levonorgestrel and metabolites), feces (32%) (mostly metabolites); $T_{1/2}$=28.5 hrs. EE: Urine, feces (metabolites); $T_{1/2}$=17.5 hrs.

NURSING CONSIDERATIONS

Assessment: Assess for high risk of arterial or venous thrombotic diseases; benign or malignant liver tumors; liver disease; presence or history of breast cancer or other estrogen- or progestin-sensitive cancer; pregnancy; and any other conditions where treatment is contraindicated or cautioned. Assess nursing status and for possible drug interactions.

Monitoring: Monitor for arterial/deep venous thrombotic events; retinal vein thrombosis; cervical cancer or intraepithelial neoplasia; hepatic impairment; hepatic adenomas; gallbladder disease; new headaches that are recurrent, persistent, or severe; bleeding irregularities; and other adverse reactions. Monitor BP with history of HTN, glucose levels in diabetic or prediabetic women, lipid levels with dyslipidemia, and thyroid function if receiving thyroid replacement therapy. Conduct a yearly visit with patient for a BP check and for other indicated health care.

Patient Counseling: Counsel that cigarette smoking increases the risk of serious CV events, and that women who are >35 yrs of age and smoke should not use COCs. Inform that drug does not protect against HIV infection and other sexually transmitted diseases. Instruct on what to do if pills are missed. Counsel to use a back-up or alternative method of contraception when concomitantly using an enzyme inducer. Inform that COCs may reduce breast milk production. Counsel any patient who starts COCs postpartum, and who has not yet had a period, to use an additional method of contraception until patient has taken an orange tab for 7 consecutive days.

Administration: Oral route. Take at the same time every day. Refer to PI for further administration instructions. **Storage:** 20-25°C (68-77°F).

LOTEMAX SUSPENSION   RX
loteprednol etabonate (Bausch & Lomb)

THERAPEUTIC CLASS: Corticosteroid

INDICATIONS: Treatment of steroid responsive inflammatory conditions of the palpebral and bulbar conjunctiva, cornea and anterior segment of the globe such as allergic conjunctivitis, acne rosacea, superficial punctate keratitis, herpes zoster keratitis, iritis, cyclitis, selected infective conjuctivitides, when inherent hazard of steroid use is accepted to obtain an advisable diminution in edema and inflammation. Treatment of postoperative inflammation following ocular surgery.

DOSAGE: *Adults:* Steroid-Responsive Disease: 1-2 drops into the conjunctival sac of the affected eye(s) qid. May increase up to 1 drop qh, if necessary, during the initial treatment within the 1st week. Reevaluate if signs/symptoms fail to improve after 2 days. Postoperative Inflammation: 1-2 drops into the conjunctival sac of the operated eye(s) qid beginning 24 hrs after surgery and continuing throughout the first 2 weeks of the postoperative period.

HOW SUPPLIED: Sus: 0.5% [5mL, 10mL, 15mL]

CONTRAINDICATIONS: Most viral diseases of the cornea and conjunctiva (eg, epithelial herpes simplex keratitis [dendritic keratitis], vaccinia, varicella), mycobacterial infection of the eye, and fungal diseases of ocular structures.

WARNINGS/PRECAUTIONS: For ophthalmic use only. Prolonged use may result in glaucoma with damage to the optic nerve, defects in visual acuity and fields of vision, and in posterior subcapsular cataract formation; caution with glaucoma. Prolonged use may suppress host response and increase hazard of secondary ocular infections. Perforations reported with diseases causing thinning of cornea/sclera. May mask or enhance existing infection in acute purulent conditions of the eye. Caution with history of herpes simplex; may prolong course and exacerbate severity of many viral infections of the eye. May delay healing and increase incidence of bleb formation after cataract surgery. Initial prescription and renewal of medication order beyond 14 days should only be made after examination of the patient with aid of magnification (eg, slit lamp biomicroscopy) and, where appropriate, fluorescein staining. Monitor intraocular pressure (IOP) if used for ≥10 days. Fungal infections of the cornea may develop coincidentally with long-term use; consider fungal invasion in any persistent corneal ulceration and take fungal cultures when appropriate. For steroid-responsive diseases, caution not to d/c therapy prematurely. Should not be used for acute anterior uveitis in patients who require a more potent corticosteroid.

ADVERSE REACTIONS: Abnormal vision/blurring, burning on instillation, chemosis, discharge, dry eyes, epiphora, foreign body sensation, itching, photophobia, headache, rhinitis, pharyngitis.

PREGNANCY: Category C, caution in nursing.

MECHANISM OF ACTION: Corticosteroid; mechanism not been established. Thought to act by the induction of phospholipase A_2 inhibitory proteins which control the biosynthesis of potent mediators of inflammation such as prostaglandins and leukotrienes.

NURSING CONSIDERATIONS

Assessment: Assess for previous drug hypersensitivity, viral diseases of the cornea and conjunctiva, mycobacterial infection of the eye, fungal diseases of ocular structures, glaucoma, thinning of the cornea/sclera, history of herpes simplex, and pregnancy/nursing status. Perform examination of patient with the aid of magnification (eg, slit lamp biomicroscopy, fluorescein staining). Assess use in patients who have undergone recent cataract surgery.

Monitoring: Monitor for glaucoma and its complications, defects in visual acuity and fields of vision, posterior subcapsular cataract formation, perforation of the cornea/sclera, secondary ocular infections, fungal infections, masking of existing infections, and other adverse reactions. Reevaluate if signs/symptoms fail to improve after 2 days. Monitor IOP during prolonged use (≥10 days). Perform examination of patient with the aid of magnification (eg, slit lamp biomicroscopy, fluorescein staining) before renewal of medication order beyond 14 days.

Patient Counseling: Advise not to allow dropper tip to touch any surface to avoid contamination of sus. Instruct to consult physician if pain develops or if redness, itching, or inflammation becomes aggravated. Inform not to wear soft contact lenses during treatment.

Administration: Ocular route. Shake vigorously before use. **Storage:** 15-25°C (59-77°F); store upright. Do not freeze.

LOTENSIN   RX
benazepril HCl (Validus)

D/C when pregnancy is detected. Drugs that act directly on the renin-angiotensin system (RAS) can cause injury and death to the developing fetus.

THERAPEUTIC CLASS: ACE inhibitor

INDICATIONS: Treatment of HTN alone or in combination with thiazide diuretics.

DOSAGE: *Adults:* Not Receiving Diuretics: Initial: 10mg qd. Maint: 20-40mg/day as single dose or in 2 equally divided doses. Dosage adjustment should be based on measurement of peak (2-6 hrs after dosing) and trough responses. If no adequate trough response with qd regimen, consider an increase in dosage or divided administration. May add diuretic if BP is not controlled. Max: 80mg/day. Receiving Diuretics: D/C diuretic 2-3 days prior to therapy. Resume diuretic if BP is not controlled. If diuretic cannot be discontinued, give initial benazepril dose of 5mg. CrCl <30mL/min (SrCr >3mg/dL): Initial: 5mg qd. Titrate: May increase until BP is controlled. Max: 40mg/day.
Pediatrics: ≥6 Yrs: Initial: 0.2mg/kg qd. Max: 0.6mg/kg (or 40mg/day).

HOW SUPPLIED: Tab: 5mg, 10mg, 20mg, 40mg

CONTRAINDICATIONS: History of angioedema.

WARNINGS/PRECAUTIONS: Not recommended in pediatric patients with GFR <30mL/min. Head/neck angioedema reported; d/c and institute appropriate therapy immediately. Higher incidence of angioedema in blacks than nonblacks. Intestinal angioedema reported; monitor for abdominal pain. Anaphylactoid reactions reported during desensitization with hymenoptera venom, dialysis with high-flux membranes, and LDL apheresis with dextran sulfate absorption. Symptomatic hypotension may occur, most likely in patients with volume and/or salt depletion; correct depletion before initiating therapy. Excessive hypotension, which may be associated with oliguria or azotemia and, rarely, with acute renal failure and death, may occur in patients with congestive heart failure (CHF); monitor closely during first 2 weeks of therapy and whenever dose is increased. Rarely, syndrome that starts with cholestatic jaundice and progresses to fulminant hepatic necrosis and (sometimes) death reported; d/c if jaundice or marked hepatic enzyme elevations develop. May cause changes in renal function. Increases in BUN and SrCr reported in patients with renal artery stenosis or with no preexisting renal vascular disease; monitor renal function during the 1st few weeks of therapy, and may need to reduce dose and/or d/c the diuretic. Hyperkalemia and persistent nonproductive cough reported. Hypotension may occur with surgery or during anesthesia. Caution in elderly.

ADVERSE REACTIONS: Headache, dizziness.

INTERACTIONS: Hypotension risk and increased BUN and SrCr with diuretics. Increased risk of hyperkalemia with K⁺-sparing diuretics, K⁺-containing salt substitutes, or K⁺ supplements; use with caution and periodically monitor K⁺. Increased lithium levels and symptoms of lithium toxicity reported; monitor lithium levels. Nitritoid reactions reported with injectable gold. Hypoglycemia may develop with insulin or oral antidiabetics. NSAIDs, including selective COX-2 inhibitors, may attenuate antihypertensive effect and may cause deterioration of renal function. Dual blockade of the RAS is associated with increased risks of hypotension, hyperkalemia, and changes in renal function (including acute renal failure); closely monitor BP, renal function and electrolytes with concomitant agents that also affect the RAS. Do not coadminister with aliskiren in patients with diabetes. Avoid with aliskiren in patients with renal impairment (GFR <60mL/min).

L

PREGNANCY: Category D, safety not known in nursing.

MECHANISM OF ACTION: ACE inhibitor; decreases plasma angiotensin II, which leads to decreased vasopressor activity and aldosterone secretion.

PHARMACOKINETICS: Absorption: T_{max}=0.5-1 hr, 1-2 hrs (benazeprilat, fasting), 2-4 hrs (benazeprilat, nonfasting). **Distribution:** Plasma protein binding (96.7%, 95.3% benazeprilat); crosses placenta; found in breast milk. **Metabolism:** Liver, cleavage of ester group; benazeprilat (active metabolite). **Elimination:** Urine (trace amounts, unchanged; 20%, benazeprilat), bile (11-12%, benazeprilat); $T_{1/2}$=10-11 hrs (benazeprilat, adults), 5 hrs (benazeprilat, pediatric patients).

NURSING CONSIDERATIONS

Assessment: Assess for history of angioedema, volume/salt depletion, CHF, renal artery stenosis, risk factors for hyperkalemia, diabetes, drug hypersensitivity, renal dysfunction, pregnancy/nursing status, and possible drug interactions.

Monitoring: Monitor for angioedema, anaphylactoid reactions, hyperkalemia, and other adverse reactions. Monitor BP, LFTs, and renal function.

Patient Counseling: Inform about fetal risks if taken during pregnancy and discuss treatment options in women planning to become pregnant; instruct to report pregnancy as soon as possible. Instruct to d/c therapy and to immediately report signs/symptoms of angioedema. Instruct to report lightheadedness, especially during the 1st days of therapy; advise to d/c and consult with a physician if syncope occurs. Inform that inadequate fluid intake or excessive perspiration, diarrhea, or vomiting may lead to excessive fall in BP, with the same consequences of lightheadedness and possible syncope. Advise not to use K⁺ supplements or salt substitutes containing K⁺ without consulting physician. Consult to promptly report any indication of infection (eg, sore throat, fever).

Administration: Oral route. Refer to PI for preparation of sus instructions. Shake sus before each use. **Storage:** (Tab) ≤30°C (86°F). Protect from moisture. (Sus) 2-8°C (36-46°F) for up to 30 days.

Lᴏᴛᴇɴsɪɴ HCT   RX
benazepril HCl - hydrochlorothiazide (Validus)

> D/C when pregnancy is detected. Drugs that act directly on the renin-angiotensin system (RAS) can cause injury and death to the developing fetus.

THERAPEUTIC CLASS: ACE inhibitor/thiazide diuretic

INDICATIONS: Treatment of HTN.

DOSAGE: *Adults:* Usual: Dose qd. Titrate: May increase after 2-3 weeks PRN to help achieve BP goals. Max: 20mg-25mg. Uncontrolled BP on Benazepril Alone or HCTZ Alone: Initial: 10mg-12.5mg qd. Replacement Therapy: May be substituted for the titrated individual components.

HOW SUPPLIED: Tab: (Benazepril-HCTZ) 5mg-6.25mg*, 10mg-12.5mg*, 20mg-12.5mg*, 20mg-25mg* *scored

CONTRAINDICATIONS: Anuria, sulfonamide-derived drug hypersensitivity, history of angioedema.

WARNINGS/PRECAUTIONS: Not for initial therapy of HTN. Head/neck angioedema reported; d/c and institute appropriate therapy immediately. Higher incidence of angioedema in blacks than nonblacks. Intestinal angioedema reported; monitor for abdominal pain. Anaphylactoid reactions reported during desensitization with hymenoptera venom, dialysis with high-flux membranes, and LDL apheresis with dextran sulfate absorption. Symptomatic hypotension may occur, most likely in patients with volume and/or salt depletion; correct depletion before initiating therapy. Enhanced effects in postsympathectomy patients. Excessive hypotension, which may be associated with oliguria, azotemia, and (rarely) with acute renal failure and death, may occur in patients with congestive heart failure (CHF); monitor closely during first 2 weeks of therapy and whenever dose is increased. May cause changes in renal function; monitor renal function periodically and consider withholding or discontinuing therapy if clinically significant decrease in renal function develops. May increase BUN or SrCr in patients with renal artery stenosis. May cause agranulocytosis and bone marrow depression; consider monitoring of WBCs in patients with collagen vascular disease, especially if associated with renal impairment. Rarely, associated with syndrome that starts with cholestatic jaundice and progresses to fulminant hepatic necrosis and (sometimes) death; d/c if jaundice or marked hepatic enzyme elevations develop. May cause exacerbation or activation of systemic lupus erythematosus (SLE). May cause idiosyncratic reaction, resulting in acute transient myopia and acute angle-closure glaucoma; d/c as rapidly as possible. May cause serum electrolyte abnormalities (eg, hypokalemia, hyponatremia, hypomagnesemia, hyperkalemia); monitor serum electrolytes periodically. Persistent nonproductive cough reported. Hypotension may occur with surgery or during anesthesia. May decrease serum protein-bound iodine levels without signs of thyroid disturbance. D/C before testing for parathyroid function. HCTZ: May alter glucose tolerance and raise serum cholesterol and TG levels. May cause or exacerbate hyperuricemia and precipitate gout. May elevate serum Ca^{2+}; avoid with hypercalcemia. May precipitate hepatic coma in patients with hepatic impairment or progressive liver disease.

ADVERSE REACTIONS: Dizziness, fatigue, postural dizziness, headache.

INTERACTIONS: Caution with other antihypertensives. May affect K^+ levels with K^+ supplements and K^+-sparing diuretics; monitor K^+ periodically. Increased lithium levels and symptoms of lithium toxicity reported; monitor lithium levels. Dual blockade of the RAS is associated with increased risks of hypotension, hyperkalemia, and changes in renal function (including acute renal failure); closely monitor BP, renal function and electrolytes with concomitant agents that also affect the RAS. Do not coadminister with aliskiren in patients with diabetes. Avoid aliskiren in patients with renal impairment (GFR <60mL/min). NSAIDs, including selective COX-2 inhibitors, may attenuate antihypertensive effect and may cause deterioration of renal function. Benazepril: Nitritoid reactions reported with injectable gold. HCTZ: May potentiate action of other antihypertensives, especially ganglionic/peripheral adrenergic-blocking drugs. Cholestyramine and colestipol resins reduce absorption from GI tract; administer at least 4 hrs before or 4-6 hrs after administration of resins. Drug-induced hypokalemia or hypomagnesemia may predispose patient to digoxin toxicity. May increase responsiveness to skeletal muscle relaxants (eg, curare derivatives). Dosage adjustment of antidiabetic drugs may be required. May reduce renal excretion of cytotoxic agents (eg, cyclophosphamide, methotrexate) and enhance their myelosuppressive effects. Anticholinergics (eg, atropine, biperiden) may increase bioavailability due to decrease in GI motility and stomach emptying rate. Prokinetic drugs may decrease bioavailability. Increased risk of hyperuricemia and gout-type complications with cyclosporine. May potentiate orthostatic hypotension with alcohol, barbiturates, or narcotics. May reduce response to pressor amines (eg, noradrenaline).

PREGNANCY: Category D, not for use in nursing.

MECHANISM OF ACTION: Benazepril: ACE inhibitor; decreases plasma angiotensin II, which leads to decreased vasopressor activity and aldosterone secretion. HCTZ: Thiazide diuretic; has not been established. Affects renal tubular mechanisms of electrolyte reabsorption, directly increasing excretion of Na^+ and Cl^- in approximately equivalent amounts.

PHARMACOKINETICS: Absorption: Benazepril: T_{max}=0.5-1 hr, 1-2 hrs (benazeprilat, fasting), 2-4 hrs (benazeprilat, nonfasting). HCTZ: Absolute bioavailability (70%); T_{max}=2-5 hrs. **Distribution:** Found in breast milk; crosses placenta. Benazepril: Plasma protein binding (96.7%, 95.3% benazeprilat). HCTZ: Plasma protein binding (40-70%). **Metabolism:** Benazepril: Liver, cleavage of ester group; benazeprilat (active metabolite). **Elimination:** Benazepril: Urine (trace amounts, unchanged; 20%, benazeprilat), bile (11-12%, benazeprilat); $T_{1/2}$=10-11 hrs (benazeprilat). HCTZ: Urine (70%, unchanged); $T_{1/2}$=10 hrs.

NURSING CONSIDERATIONS

Assessment: Assess for anuria, sulfonamide-derived drug hypersensitivity, history of angioedema, allergy or asthma, volume/salt depletion, CHF, renal artery stenosis, collagen vascular diseases, SLE, hypercalcemia, diabetes, renal/hepatic function, postsympathectomy status, pregnancy/nursing status, and possible drug interactions.

Monitoring: Monitor for angioedema, anaphylactoid reactions, exacerbation/activation of SLE, myopia, angle-closure glaucoma, hyperuricemia or precipitation of gout, and other adverse reactions. Monitor BP, LFTs, renal function, serum electrolytes, cholesterol, and TG levels. Monitor WBCs in patients with collagen vascular disease.

Patient Counseling: Inform about fetal risks if taken during pregnancy and discuss treatment options in women planning to become pregnant; instruct to report pregnancy as soon as possible. Instruct to d/c therapy and to immediately report signs/symptoms of angioedema. Instruct to report lightheadedness, especially during the 1st days of therapy; advise to d/c and consult with a physician if syncope occurs. Inform that inadequate fluid intake, excessive perspiration, diarrhea, or vomiting may lead to excessive fall in BP, with the same consequences of lightheadedness and possible syncope. Advise not to use K^+ supplements or salt substitutes containing K^+ without consulting physician. Advise to promptly report any indication of infection (eg, sore throat, fever).

Administration: Oral route. **Storage:** ≤30°C (86°F). Protect from moisture and light.

LOTREL RX
benazepril HCl - amlodipine besylate (Novartis)

D/C when pregnancy is detected. Drugs that act directly on the renin-angiotensin system (RAS) can cause injury/death to the developing fetus.

THERAPEUTIC CLASS: ACE inhibitor/calcium channel blocker (dihydropyridine)

INDICATIONS: Treatment of HTN not adequately controlled on monotherapy with either agent.

DOSAGE: *Adults:* Initial: 2.5mg-10mg qd. Titrate: May increase up to 10mg-40mg qd if BP remains uncontrolled; individualize dose. Replacement Therapy: May substitute for titrated components. Elderly: Consider lower initial doses. Hepatic Impairment: Consider using lower doses.

HOW SUPPLIED: Cap: (Amlodipine-Benazepril) 2.5mg-10mg, 5mg-10mg, 5mg-20mg, 5mg-40mg, 10mg-20mg, 10mg-40mg

CONTRAINDICATIONS: History of angioedema. Coadministration with aliskiren in patients with diabetes.

WARNINGS/PRECAUTIONS: Symptomatic hypotension may occur, most likely in patients who have been volume- or salt-depleted as a result of diuretic therapy, dietary salt restriction, dialysis, diarrhea, or vomiting; correct volume and/or salt depletion before starting therapy. Not recommended with severe renal impairment (CrCl ≤30mL/min). May cause changes in renal function, including acute renal failure; consider withholding or d/c therapy if clinically significant decrease in renal function develops. Hyperkalemia reported. Benazepril: Head and neck angioedema reported; d/c and institute appropriate treatment if laryngeal stridor or angioedema of the face, tongue, or glottis occurs. More reports of angioedema in blacks than in nonblacks. Intestinal angioedema reported; monitor for abdominal pain. Anaphylactoid reactions reported during desensitization with hymenoptera venom, dialysis with high-flux membranes, and LDL apheresis with dextran sulfate absorption. Excessive hypotension, which may be associated with oliguria, azotemia, and (rare) acute renal failure or death, may occur in congestive heart failure (CHF) patients; monitor patients during first 2 weeks of therapy and whenever dose is increased or a diuretic is added/increased. Cholestatic hepatitis and acute liver failure rarely reported; d/c if jaundice or marked elevation of hepatic enzymes develops. Persistent nonproductive cough reported. Hypotension may occur with surgery or during anesthesia. Amlodipine: Worsening angina and acute myocardial infarction (MI) may develop after starting or increasing the dose, particularly in patients with severe obstructive coronary artery disease (CAD). Caution with aortic/mitral stenosis, or obstructive hypertrophic cardiomyopathy.

ADVERSE REACTIONS: Cough, headache, dizziness, edema, angioedema.

INTERACTIONS: See Contraindications. Dual blockade of the RAS is associated with increased risks of hypotension, hyperkalemia, and changes in renal function (including acute renal failure); closely monitor BP, renal function, and electrolytes with concomitant agents that also block the RAS. Avoid with aliskiren in patients with renal impairment (GFR <60mL/min). Benazepril: Coadministration with NSAIDs, including selective COX-2 inhibitors, may result in deterioration of renal function. Antihypertensive effect may be attenuated by NSAIDs. Diabetic patients receiving concomitant insulin or PO antidiabetics may develop hypoglycemia. K⁺ supplements, K⁺-sparing diuretics (eg, spironolactone, amiloride, triamterene), or K⁺-containing salt substitutes may increase risk of hyperkalemia; frequently monitor serum K⁺. Increased lithium levels and symptoms of lithium toxicity reported; frequently monitor lithium levels. Nitritoid reactions (eg, facial flushing, N/V, hypotension) reported with injectable gold. Amlodipine: May increase exposure of simvastatin; limit dose of simvastatin to 20mg daily. Increased systemic exposure with CYP3A inhibitors (moderate and strong) (eg, diltiazem); monitor for symptoms of hypotension and edema when coadministered with CYP3A4 inhibitors to determine the need for dose adjustment. Monitor BP when coadministered with CYP3A4 inducers. Strong CYP3A4 inhibitors (eg, ketoconazole, itraconazole, ritonavir) may increase concentrations to a greater extent.

PREGNANCY: Category D, not for use in nursing.

MECHANISM OF ACTION: Amlodipine: Calcium channel blocker (dihydropyridine); inhibits transmembrane influx of calcium ions into vascular smooth muscle and cardiac muscle. Acts directly on vascular smooth muscle to cause a reduction in peripheral vascular resistance and reduction in BP. Benazepril: ACE inhibitor; effects appear to result from suppression of renin-angiotensin-aldosterone system. Inhibition results in decreased plasma angiotensin II, which leads to decreased vasopressor activity and decreased aldosterone secretion.

PHARMACOKINETICS: Absorption: Amlodipine: Absolute bioavailability (64-90%); T_{max}=6-12 hrs. Benazepril: Bioavailability (≥37%); T_{max}=0.5-2 hrs, 1.5-4 hrs (benazeprilat). **Distribution:** Amlodipine: V_d=21L/kg; plasma protein binding (93%). Benazepril: V_d=0.7L/kg (benazeprilat); crosses the placenta; found in breast milk. **Metabolism:** Amlodipine: Liver (extensive). Benazepril: Liver (extensive) by enzymatic hydrolysis to benazeprilat (active metabolite). **Elimination:** Amlodipine: Urine (10% unchanged, 60% metabolites); $T_{1/2}$=30-50 hrs. Benazepril: Urine (<1% unchanged, 20% benazeprilat), bile; $T_{1/2}$=22 hrs (benazeprilat).

NURSING CONSIDERATIONS

Assessment: Assess for history of angioedema, diabetes, hypersensitivity to drug, aortic/mitral stenosis, obstructive hypertrophic cardiomyopathy, CHF, severe obstructive CAD, volume/salt depletion, hepatic/renal impairment, pregnancy/nursing status, and possible drug interactions.

Monitoring: Monitor for signs/symptoms of hypotension, anaphylactoid or hypersensitivity reactions, head/neck and intestinal angioedema, worsening angina or acute MI, and other adverse reactions. Monitor BP, hepatic/renal function, and serum K⁺ levels.

Patient Counseling: Inform of the consequences of exposure to the medication during pregnancy and of treatment options in women planning to become pregnant. Advise to report pregnancies as soon as possible. Advise diabetic patients about the possibility of hypoglycemic reactions when drug is used concomitantly with insulin or PO antidiabetics. Advise to seek medical attention if symptoms of hypotension, anaphylactoid or hypersensitivity reactions, angioedema (head/neck, intestinal), infection, trouble swallowing, breathing problems (eg, wheezing or asthma), and hepatic dysfunction (eg, itching, yellow eyes/skin, flu-like symptoms) occur.

Administration: Oral route. **Storage:** 25°C (77°F); excursions permitted to 15-30°C (59-86°F). Protect from moisture.

LOTRISONE   RX
betamethasone dipropionate - clotrimazole (Merck)

THERAPEUTIC CLASS: Azole antifungal/corticosteroid

INDICATIONS: Topical treatment of symptomatic inflammatory tinea pedis, tinea cruris, and tinea corporis due to *Epidermophyton floccosum, Trichophyton mentagrophytes,* and *Trichophyton rubrum* in patients ≥17 yrs of age.

DOSAGE: *Adults:* ≥17 Yrs: Gently massage sufficient amount into affected skin area(s) bid (am and pm). Do not use for >2 weeks for the treatment of tinea cruris and tinea corporis or for >4 weeks for the treatment of tinea pedis. Do not use >45g/week.

HOW SUPPLIED: Cre: (Betamethasone Dipropionate-Clotrimazole) 0.643mg-10mg [15g, 45g]

WARNINGS/PRECAUTIONS: Not for ophthalmic, oral, or intravaginal use. Not recommended in patients <17 yrs of age, with diaper dermatitis, or with occlusive dressing. Systemic absorption of corticosteroids may produce reversible hypothalamic-pituitary-adrenal (HPA) axis suppression, manifestations of Cushing's syndrome, hyperglycemia, and glucosuria; evaluate periodically for evidence of HPA-axis suppression if applying to large surface areas or under occlusion. Use over large surface areas, prolonged use, and use under occlusive dressings may augment systemic absorption. Withdraw drug, reduce frequency of application, or substitute a less potent corticosteroid if HPA axis suppression is noted. Infrequently, signs/symptoms of glucocorticosteroid insufficiency may occur, requiring supplemental systemic corticosteroids. Pediatric patients may be more susceptible to systemic toxicity. D/C and institute appropriate therapy if irritation develops. Review diagnosis if no clinical improvement seen after 1 week for tinea corporis or tinea cruris, and 2 weeks for tinea pedis.

ADVERSE REACTIONS: Paresthesia, rash, edema, secondary infection, itching, dryness, irritation, folliculitis, hypertrichosis, acneiform eruptions, hypopigmentation, erythema, stinging, blistering, peeling.

INTERACTIONS: Use with other corticosteroid-containing products may increase exposure.

PREGNANCY: Category C, caution in nursing.

MECHANISM OF ACTION: Azole antifungal agent/corticosteroid. Betamethasone: Corticosteroid; has been shown to have topical systemic pharmacologic and metabolic effects characteristic of this class of drugs. Clotrimazole: Imidazole antifungal agent; inhibits 14-α-demethylation of lanosterol in fungi by binding to one of the CYP450 enzymes.

PHARMACOKINETICS: Absorption: Betamethasone: Percutaneous; extent of absorption is determined by vehicle, integrity of epidermal barrier, and use of occlusive dressings. **Distribution:** Betamethasone: Bound to plasma proteins in varying degrees; found in breast milk (systemically absorbed). **Metabolism:** Betamethasone: Liver. **Elimination:** Betamethasone: Kidney, bile.

NURSING CONSIDERATIONS

Assessment: Assess for hypersensitivity to corticosteroids or imidazoles, conditions that augment systemic absorption, pregnancy/nursing status, and possible drug interactions.

Monitoring: Monitor for signs/symptoms of HPA-axis suppression, Cushing's syndrome, hyperglycemia, glucosuria, skin irritation, and other adverse reactions. Perform periodic monitoring for HPA-axis suppression using urinary free cortisol and adrenocorticotropic hormone stimulation tests. Review diagnosis if no clinical improvement seen after 1 week of treatment for tinea corporis or tinea cruris, and 2 weeks for tinea pedis.

Patient Counseling: Inform to use externally ud for fully prescribed treatment period. Advise to avoid intravaginal contact or contact with eyes and mouth. Instruct to notify physician if no improvement seen after 1 week of treatment for tinea cruris or tinea corporis, or 2 weeks for tinea pedis. Advise to use only for the disorder for which it was prescribed. Instruct not to bandage, cover, or wrap treated skin area. Advise not to use other corticosteroid-containing products without 1st consulting with physician. Instruct to report any signs of local adverse reactions to physician. Advise to avoid sources of infection or reinfection. When using in the groin area, counsel to use only for 2 weeks and apply the cream sparingly; advise to wear loose-fitting clothing and to notify physician if condition persists after 2 weeks.

Administration: Topical route. **Storage:** 25°C (77°F); excursions permitted to 15-30°C (59-86°F).

LOTRONEX   RX
alosetron HCl (Prometheus)

> Serious GI adverse events (eg, ischemic colitis, serious constipation complications) reported. Only prescribers enrolled in Prometheus Prescribing Program should prescribe this medication. Patients must read and sign the Patient Acknowledge Form before receiving initial prescription. D/C immediately if constipation or symptoms of ischemic colitis develop; do not resume therapy in patients with ischemic colitis. Indicated only for women with severe diarrhea-predominant irritable bowel syndrome (IBS) who have not responded adequately to conventional therapy.

THERAPEUTIC CLASS: 5-HT$_3$ receptor antagonist

INDICATIONS: Treatment for women with severe diarrhea-predominant IBS who have chronic symptoms (≥6 months), exclusion of anatomic or biochemical abnormalities of GI tract, failure to respond to conventional therapy.

DOSAGE: *Adults:* Initial: 0.5mg bid for 4 weeks. D/C if constipation occurs, then restart at 0.5mg qd if constipation resolves. D/C if constipation recurs at lower dose. Titrate: If tolerated and IBS symptoms are not adequately controlled, may increase to up to 1mg bid. D/C after 4 weeks if symptoms are not controlled on 1mg bid.

HOW SUPPLIED: Tab: 0.5mg, 1mg

CONTRAINDICATIONS: Current constipation. History of chronic/severe constipation or sequelae from constipation, intestinal obstruction, stricture, toxic megacolon, GI perforation/adhesions, ischemic colitis, impaired intestinal circulation, thrombophlebitis or hypercoagulable state, Crohn's disease, ulcerative colitis, diverticulitis, severe hepatic impairment. Inability to understand/comply with Patient Acknowledgment Form. Concomitant administration with fluvoxamine.

WARNINGS/PRECAUTIONS: Caution in elderly and debilitated patients; may be at greater risk for complications of constipation. Caution with mild/moderate hepatic impairment.

ADVERSE REACTIONS: Constipation, ischemic colitis, abdominal discomfort/pain, nausea, GI discomfort/pain.

INTERACTIONS: See Contraindications. Increased risk of constipation with medications that decrease GI motility. Inducers and inhibitors of CYP1A2, with minor contributions from CYP3A4 and CYP2C9, drug-metabolizing enzymes may alter clearance. Avoid with quinolone antibiotics and cimetidine. Caution with strong CYP3A4 inhibitors (eg, ketoconazole, clarithromycin, telithromycin, protease inhibitors, voriconazole, itraconazole).

PREGNANCY: Category B, caution in nursing.

MECHANISM OF ACTION: 5-HT$_3$ receptor antagonist; inhibits activation of nonselective cation channels, which results in the modulation of the enteric nervous system.

PHARMACOKINETICS: Absorption: Rapidly absorbed, absolute bioavailability (50-60%), 9ng/mL (young women); T_{max}=1 hr. **Distribution:** V_d=65-95L, plasma protein binding (82%). **Metabolism:** via liver (extensive). **Elimination:** Urine (74%, metabolites), feces (11%, <1% unchanged); $T_{1/2}$=1.5 hrs.

NURSING CONSIDERATIONS

Assessment: Assess for history of chronic or severe constipation or sequelae from constipation, intestinal obstruction or stricture, toxic megacolon, GI perforation or adhesion, ischemic colitis, impaired intestinal circulation, thrombophlebitis or hypercoagulable state, Crohn's disease or ulcerative colitis, diverticulitis, severe hepatic impairment, pregnancy/nursing status and possible drug interactions.

Monitoring: Monitor LFTs, signs/symptoms of ischemic colitis and serious complications of constipation, perforation, and other adverse reactions.

Patient Counseling: Counsel on the risk and benefits of the treatment. Review side effects and advise to report if any develop. Inform that tab may be taken with or without meals. Instruct to not start if patient is constipated; d/c and contact prescriber if constipation or symptoms of ischemic colitis develop, or if IBS symptoms are not controlled after 4 weeks of taking 1mg bid.

Administration: Oral route. **Storage:** 25°C (77°F); excursions permitted to 15-30°C (59-86°F).

LOVASTATIN   RX
lovastatin (Various)

OTHER BRAND NAMES: Mevacor (Merck)
THERAPEUTIC CLASS: HMG-CoA reductase inhibitor

INDICATIONS: Adjunct to diet to decrease total cholesterol and LDL levels in hypercholesterolemia, heterozygous familial hypercholesterolemia (boys and girls who are at least 1 yr postmenarche, 10-17 yrs of age), and in prevention and to slow progression of coronary heart disease.

DOSAGE: *Adults:* Individualize dose. Initial: 20mg qd with pm meal. Usual: 10-80mg/day in single or 2 divided doses. Max: 80mg/day. Requiring LDL Reduction of ≥20%: Initial: 20mg/day. May consider starting dose of 10mg if requiring smaller reductions. Titrate: Adjust at ≥4-week intervals. Consider dose reduction if cholesterol levels fall significantly below the targeted range. Concomitant Danazol, Diltiazem, Dronedarone, or Verapamil: Initial: 10mg/day. Max: 20mg/day. Concomitant Amiodarone: Max: 40mg/day. Severe Renal Insufficiency (CrCl <30mL/min): Carefully consider dosage increases >20mg/day; give cautiously if deemed necessary. *Pediatrics:* 10-17 Yrs: HeFH: Individualize dose. Usual: 10-40mg/day. Max: 40mg/day. Requiring LDL Reduction of ≥20%: Initial: 20mg/day. May consider starting dose of 10mg if requiring smaller reductions. Titrate: Adjust at ≥4-week intervals. Concomitant Danazol, Diltiazem, Dronedarone, or Verapamil: Initial: 10mg/day. Max: 20mg/day. Concomitant Amiodarone: Max: 40mg/day. Severe Renal Insufficiency (CrCl <30mL/min): Carefully consider dosage increases >20mg/day; give cautiously if deemed necessary.

HOW SUPPLIED: Tab: 10mg; (Mevacor) 20mg, 40mg

CONTRAINDICATIONS: Active liver disease or unexplained persistent elevations of serum transaminases, pregnancy, women of childbearing age who may become pregnant, and nursing mothers. Concomitant administration with strong CYP3A4 inhibitors (eg, itraconazole, ketoconazole, posaconazole, voriconazole, HIV protease inhibitors, boceprevir, telaprevir, erythromycin, clarithromycin, telithromycin, nefazodone, cobicistat-containing products).

WARNINGS/PRECAUTIONS: Myopathy (including immune-mediated necrotizing myopathy [IMNM]) and rhabdomyolysis reported; d/c if markedly elevated CPK levels occur or myopathy is diagnosed/suspected, and temporarily withhold in any patient experiencing acute or serious condition predisposing to development of renal failure secondary to rhabdomyolysis. Risk of myopathy/rhabdomyolysis is dose related. Persistent increases in serum transaminases reported; obtain LFTs prior to initiation and repeat as clinically indicated. Fatal and nonfatal hepatic failure (rare) reported; promptly interrupt therapy if serious liver injury with clinical symptoms and/or hyperbilirubinemia or jaundice occurs and do not restart if no alternate etiology found. Caution in patients who consume substantial quantities of alcohol and/or have history of liver disease. Increases in HbA1c and FPG levels reported. Evaluate patients who develop endocrine dysfunction. Caution in the elderly.

ADVERSE REACTIONS: Headache, constipation, flatulence, myalgia.

INTERACTIONS: See Contraindications and Dosage. Ranolazine may increase risk of myopathy/rhabdomyolysis; consider dose adjustment of lovastatin. Due to the risk of myopathy, avoid with gemfibrozil, cyclosporine, and grapefruit juice, and caution with fibrates, lipid-lowering doses (≥1g/day) of niacin, colchicine, danazol, diltiazem, dronedarone, verapamil, and amiodarone. Determine PT before initiation and frequently during therapy with coumarin anticoagulants. Caution with drugs that may decrease the levels or activity of endogenous steroid hormones (eg, spironolactone, cimetidine).

PREGNANCY: Category X, not for use in nursing.

MECHANISM OF ACTION: HMG-CoA reductase inhibitor; may involve both reduction of VLDL concentration and induction of LDL receptor, leading to reduced production and/or increased catabolism of LDL.

PHARMACOKINETICS: Absorption: T_{max}=2-4 hrs. **Distribution:** Plasma protein binding (>95%). **Metabolism:** Liver (extensive 1st pass), by hydrolysis via CYP3A4; β-hydroxyacid and 6'-hydroxy derivative (major active metabolites). **Elimination:** Feces (83%), urine (10%).

NURSING CONSIDERATIONS

Assessment: Assess for history of or active liver disease, unexplained persistent serum transaminase elevations, secondary causes for hypercholesterolemia, alcohol consumption, diabetes, drug hypersensitivity, pregnancy/nursing status, and possible drug interactions. Assess lipid profile, LFTs, and renal function.

Monitoring: Monitor for signs/symptoms of myopathy (including IMNM), rhabdomyolysis, liver/renal/endocrine dysfunction, increases in HbA1c and FPG levels, and other adverse reactions. Monitor lipid profile, creatine kinase, and LFTs. Check PT frequently with coumarin anticoagulants.

Patient Counseling: Advise about substances to be avoided and to report promptly any unexplained muscle pain, tenderness, or weakness, particularly if accompanied by malaise or fever or if muscle signs and symptoms persist after discontinuation. Inform that liver function will be checked prior to therapy and if signs/symptoms of liver injury occur; instruct to report promptly any symptoms that may indicate liver injury (eg, fatigue, anorexia, right upper abdominal discomfort, dark urine, jaundice). Instruct women of childbearing age to use an effective method of birth control, to stop taking drug if they become pregnant, and not to breastfeed while on

L

therapy. Advise patients to inform other physicians prescribing a new medication for them, that they are taking lovastatin.

Administration: Oral route. Take with meals. **Storage:** 20-25°C (68-77°F). Protect from light. Store in a dry place.

LOVAZA   RX
omega-3-acid ethyl esters (GlaxoSmithKline)

THERAPEUTIC CLASS: Lipid-regulating agent

INDICATIONS: Adjunct to diet to reduce TG levels in adults with severe (≥500mg/dL) hypertriglyceridemia.

DOSAGE: *Adults:* 4g/day (4 caps qd or 2 caps bid).

HOW SUPPLIED: Cap: 1g

WARNINGS/PRECAUTIONS: Increases in ALT levels without a concurrent increase in AST levels reported. Increased LDL-C levels reported; monitor LDL-C levels periodically during therapy. Contains ethyl esters of omega-3 fatty acids (eicosapentaenoic acid [EPA] and docosahexaenoic acid [DHA]), obtained from oil of several fish sources; caution with known hypersensitivity to fish and/or shellfish. Recurrent atrial fibrillation/flutter (A-fib/flutter) reported in patients with paroxysmal or persistent A-fib, particularly within the first 2-3 months of initiating therapy; not indicated for the treatment of A-fib/flutter. Assess TG levels carefully before initiating therapy and monitor TG levels periodically during therapy.

ADVERSE REACTIONS: Eructation, taste perversion, dyspepsia.

INTERACTIONS: Periodically monitor patients receiving concomitant treatment with an anticoagulant or other drugs affecting coagulation (eg, antiplatelet agents). D/C or change medications known to exacerbate hypertriglyceridemia (eg, β-blockers, thiazides, estrogens), if possible, prior to consideration of therapy.

PREGNANCY: Category C, caution in nursing.

MECHANISM OF ACTION: Lipid-regulating agent; not established. Potential mechanisms of action include inhibition of acyl CoA: 1,2-diacylglycerol acyltransferase, increased mitochondrial and peroxisomal β-oxidation in the liver, decreased lipogenesis in the liver, and increased plasma lipoprotein lipase activity. May reduce the synthesis of TG in the liver because EPA and DHA are poor substrates for the enzymes responsible for TG synthesis, and EPA and DHA inhibit esterification of other fatty acids.

PHARMACOKINETICS: Distribution: Found in breast milk.

NURSING CONSIDERATIONS

Assessment: Assess for hypersensitivity to drug, fish and/or shellfish, hepatic impairment, A-fib/flutter, pregnancy/nursing status, and possible drug interactions. Attempt to control serum lipids with appropriate diet, exercise, weight loss in obese patients, and control of any medical problems that are contributing to lipid abnormalities (eg, diabetes mellitus, hypothyroidism). Assess LDL-C and TG levels.

Monitoring: Monitor for allergic reactions and other adverse reactions. Periodically monitor ALT and AST levels in patients with hepatic impairment. Monitor LDL-C and TG levels periodically during therapy.

Patient Counseling: Instruct to notify physician if allergic to fish and/or shellfish. Advise that the use of lipid-regulating agents does not reduce the importance of adhering to diet. Advise not to alter caps in any way and to ingest intact caps only. Instruct to take as prescribed.

Administration: Oral route. Swallow whole; do not break open, crush, dissolve, or chew. **Storage:** 25°C (77°F); excursions permitted to 15-30°C (59-86°F). Do not freeze.

LOVENOX   RX
enoxaparin sodium (Sanofi-Aventis)

> Epidural or spinal hematomas resulting in long-term or permanent paralysis may occur in patients anticoagulated with low molecular weight heparins (LMWH) or heparinoids and are receiving neuraxial anesthesia or undergoing spinal puncture. Increased risk with indwelling epidural catheters, concomitant use of other drugs that affect hemostasis (eg, NSAIDs, platelet inhibitors, other anticoagulants), history of traumatic or repeated epidural or spinal punctures, a history of spinal deformity or spinal surgery, or when optimal timing between the administration of enoxaparin and neuraxial procedures is not known. Monitor frequently for signs/symptoms of neurological impairment; if neurological compromise noted, urgent treatment is necessary. Consider benefit and risks before neuraxial intervention in patients anticoagulated or to be anticoagulated for thromboprophylaxis.

THERAPEUTIC CLASS: Low molecular weight heparin

INDICATIONS: Prophylaxis of deep vein thrombosis (DVT) in patients undergoing abdominal surgery who are at risk for thromboembolic complications, undergoing hip replacement surgery during and following hospitalization, undergoing knee replacement surgery, or in medical patients who are at risk for thromboembolic complications due to severely restricted mobility during acute illness. Inpatient treatment of acute DVT with or without pulmonary embolism (PE) in conjunction with warfarin. Outpatient treatment of acute DVT without PE in conjunction with warfarin. Prophylaxis of ischemic complications of unstable angina and non-Q-wave myocardial infarction (MI) when administered with aspirin (ASA). Treatment of acute ST-segment elevation MI (STEMI) when administered with ASA in patients receiving thrombolysis and being managed medically or with percutaneous coronary intervention (PCI).

DOSAGE: *Adults:* DVT Prophylaxis: Abdominal Surgery: 40mg SQ qd with initial dose given 2 hrs prior to surgery for 7-10 days (up to 12 days in clinical trials). Hip/Knee Replacement Surgery: 30mg SQ q12h with initial dose given 12-24 hrs postop for 7-10 days (up to 14 days in clinical trials). Hip Replacement Surgery: 40mg SQ qd with initial dose 12 hrs prior to surgery for 7-10 days (up to 14 days in clinical trials). Continue prophylaxis with 40mg SQ qd for 3 weeks following initial phase. Acute Medical Illness: 40mg SQ qd for 6-11 days (up to 14 days in clinical trials). Acute DVT Treatment: Outpatient without PE: 1mg/kg SQ q12h for 7 days (up to 17 days in clinical trials). Inpatient with or without PE: 1mg/kg SQ q12h, or 1.5mg/kg SQ qd for 7 days (up to 17 days in clinical trials), administered at the same time daily. Initiate concomitant warfarin therapy when appropriate (usually within 72 hrs of enoxaparin). Continue treatment for a minimum of 5 days and until therapeutic oral anticoagulant effect has been achieved. Unstable Angina/Non-Q-Wave MI: 1mg/kg SQ q12h in conjunction with ASA therapy (100-325mg qd) for 2-8 days (up to 12.5 days in clinical trials). Treatment of Acute STEMI: <75 Yrs: 30mg single IV bolus plus a 1mg/kg SQ dose, followed by 1mg/kg SQ q12h. Max: 100mg for the first 2 doses only, followed by 1mg/kg dosing for the remaining doses. Continue therapy for 8 days or until hospital discharge, whichever comes first. ≥75 Yrs: Do not use initial IV bolus. Initial: 0.75mg/kg SQ q12h. Max: 75mg for the first 2 doses only, followed by 0.75mg/kg dosing for the remaining doses. Continue treatment for 8 days or until hospital discharge, whichever comes first. All patients should receive 75-325mg/day ASA as soon as they are identified as having STEMI. In Conjunction with Thrombolytic Therapy: Give enoxaparin dose between 15 min before and 30 min after start of fibrinolytic therapy. PCI: If last dose is given <8 hrs before balloon inflation, no additional dosing is needed. If last dose is given >8 hrs before balloon inflation, give an IV bolus of 0.3mg/kg. Refer to PI for dosage regimen with severe renal impairment (CrCl <30mL/min).

HOW SUPPLIED: Inj: (Multidose vial) 300mg/3mL; (Prefilled Syringe) 30mg/0.3mL, 40mg/0.4mL, 60mg/0.6mL, 80mg/0.8mL, 100mg/mL, 120mg/0.8mL, 150mg/mL

CONTRAINDICATIONS: Active major bleeding, thrombocytopenia associated with a positive in vitro test for antiplatelet antibody in the presence of enoxaparin sodium, hypersensitivity to heparin or pork products, hypersensitivity to benzyl alcohol (only with the multidose formulation).

WARNINGS/PRECAUTIONS: Consider pharmacokinetic profile of enoxaparin to reduce the potential risk of bleeding associated with concurrent use with epidural or spinal anesthesia/analgesia or spinal puncture. Placement or removal of catheter should be delayed for at least 12 hrs after administration of lower doses and at least 24 hrs after higher doses. Extreme caution with increased risk of hemorrhage (eg, bacterial endocarditis, congenital or acquired bleeding disorders) and with history of heparin-induced thrombocytopenia. Major hemorrhages, including retroperitoneal and intracranial bleeding, reported. To minimize the risk of bleeding following vascular instrumentation during treatment of unstable angina, non-Q-wave MI, and acute STEMI, adhere precisely to the intervals recommended between doses. Observe for signs of bleeding or hematoma formation at the site of the procedure. Caution in patients with bleeding diathesis, uncontrolled arterial HTN or history of recent GI ulceration, diabetic retinopathy, renal dysfunction, and hemorrhage. Thrombocytopenia reported; d/c if platelet count <100,000/mm^3. Cannot be used interchangeably (unit for unit) with heparin or other LMWH. Pregnant women with mechanical prosthetic heart valves may be at higher risk for thromboembolism and have a higher rate of fetal loss; monitor anti-factor Xa levels, and adjust dosage PRN. Multidose vial contains benzyl alcohol that crosses the placenta and has been associated with fatal "gasping syndrome" in premature neonates; use with caution or only when clearly needed in pregnant women. Periodic CBC, including platelet count and stool occult blood tests are recommended during course of treatment. Anti-factor Xa may be used to monitor anticoagulant activity in patients with significant renal impairment or if abnormal coagulation parameters or bleeding occur. Hyperkalemia reported in patients with renal failure. Increase in exposure with prophylactic dosages (non-weight adjusted) observed in low-weight women (<45kg) and low-weight men (<57kg). Higher risk for thromboembolism in obese patients; observe for signs/symptoms of thromboembolism. Caution with hepatic impairment.

ADVERSE REACTIONS: Epidural or spinal hematoma, hemorrhage, ecchymosis, anemia, peripheral edema, fever, dyspnea, nausea, ALT/AST elevations.

INTERACTIONS: See Boxed Warning. D/C agents that may enhance the risk of hemorrhage prior to therapy (eg, anticoagulants, platelet inhibitors, such as acetylsalicylic acid, salicylates, NSAIDs [including ketorolac tromethamine], dipyridamole, or sulfinpyrazone). If coadministration is essential, conduct close monitoring. May increase risk of hyperkalemia with K+-sparing drugs, and administration of K+.

PREGNANCY: Category B, not for use in nursing.

MECHANISM OF ACTION: LMWH; has antithrombotic properties.

PHARMACOKINETICS: Absorption: (SQ) Administration of variable doses resulted in different parameters. Absolute bioavailability (100%). (Anti-factor Xa/Antithrombin [Anti-factor IIa]) Max activity=3-5 hrs. **Distribution:** (Anti-factor Xa activity) V_d=4.3L. **Metabolism:** Liver; via desulfation and/or depolymerization. **Elimination:** Urine; (Anti-factor Xa activity) $T_{1/2}$=4.5-7 hrs.

NURSING CONSIDERATIONS

Assessment: Assess for presence of active major bleeding, thrombocytopenia, hypersensitivity to heparin or pork products, hypersensitivity to benzyl alcohol, renal dysfunction, obesity, any other conditions where treatment is cautioned, nursing/pregnancy status, and for possible drug interactions.

Monitoring: Monitor for signs/symptoms of hemorrhage, thrombocytopenia, hyperkalemia, thromboembolism and other adverse reactions. Monitor for epidural or spinal hematomas, and for neurological impairment if used concomitantly with spinal/epidural anesthesia or spinal puncture. Periodically monitor CBC, including platelet count, and stool occult blood tests. If bleeding occurs, monitor anti-factor Xa levels.

Patient Counseling: Inform of the benefits and risks of therapy. Inform to watch for signs/symptoms of spinal or epidural hematoma (tingling, numbness, muscular weakness) if patients have had neuraxial anesthesia or spinal puncture, particularly, if they are taking concomitant NSAIDs, platelet inhibitors, or other anticoagulants; contact physician if these occur. Advise to seek medical attention if unusual bleeding, bruising, signs of thrombocytopenia, or allergic reactions develop. Counsel that it will take longer than usual to stop bleeding; may bruise and/or bleed more easily when treated with enoxaparin. Inform of administration instructions if therapy is to continue after discharge. Instruct to notify physicians and dentists of enoxaparin therapy prior to surgery or taking a new drug.

Administration: SQ or IV (for multidose vial) route. Not for IM. Inspect visually for particulate matter and discoloration. Use tuberculin syringe or equivalent when using multidose vial. Refer to PI for administration techniques. (SQ) Do not mix with other inj or infusions. (IV) (eg, for treatment of acute STEMI), can be mix with normal saline solution (0.9%) or D5W. **Storage:** 25°C (77°F); excursions permitted to 15-30°C (59-86°F). Do not store multidose vials for >28 days after first use.

LUMIGAN   RX
bimatoprost (Allergan)

THERAPEUTIC CLASS: Prostaglandin analog

INDICATIONS: Reduction of elevated intraocular pressure (IOP) in patient with open-angle glaucoma or ocular HTN.

DOSAGE: *Adults:* Usual: 1 drop in affected eye(s) qd in pm. Max: Once-daily dosing. Space dosing with other ophthalmic drugs by at least 5 min.
Pediatrics: ≥16 Yrs: Usual: 1 drop in affected eye(s) qd in pm. Max: Once-daily dosing. Space dosing with other ophthalmic drugs by at least 5 min.

HOW SUPPLIED: Sol: 0.01%, 0.03% [2.5mL, 5mL, 7.5mL]

WARNINGS/PRECAUTIONS: Changes to pigmented tissues, including increased pigmentation of iris (may be permanent), eyelid, and eyelashes (may be reversible) reported. Regularly examine patients with noticeably increased iris pigmentation. May cause changes to eyelashes and vellus hair in the treated eye. Caution with active intraocular inflammation (eg, uveitis); inflammation may be exacerbated. Macular edema, including cystoid macular edema, reported; caution with aphakic patients, pseudophakic patients with torn posterior lens capsule, or patients at risk of macular edema. Bacterial keratitis reported with multidose container. Remove contact lenses prior to instillation; may reinsert 15 min after administration.

ADVERSE REACTIONS: Eyelash changes, conjunctival hyperemia, ocular pruritus/dryness/burning, visual disturbances, foreign body sensation, eye pain, periocular skin pigmentation, blepharitis, cataracts, periorbital erythema, eyelash darkening, superficial punctate keratitis, infections.

PREGNANCY: Category C, caution in nursing.

MECHANISM OF ACTION: Synthetic prostaglandin analog; selectively mimics the effects of naturally occurring substances, prostamides. Believed to lower IOP by increasing outflow of aqueous humor through both the trabecular meshwork and uveoscleral routes.

PHARMACOKINETICS: Absorption: (0.03%) C_{max}=0.08ng/mL, T_{max}=10 min, AUC=0.09ng•hr/mL. **Distribution:** (0.03%) V_d=0.67L/kg. **Metabolism:** Via oxidation, N-deethylation, and glucuronidation. **Elimination:** (IV) Urine (67%), feces (25%); $T_{1/2}$=45 min.

NURSING CONSIDERATIONS

Assessment: Assess for active intraocular inflammation (eg, uveitis), aphakic/pseudophakic patient with torn posterior lens capsule; angle-closure, inflammatory, or neovascular glaucoma; and pregnancy/nursing status.

Monitoring: Monitor for changes to pigmented tissue (eg, increased pigmentation of the iris, periorbital tissue [eyelid]), changes in eyelashes and vellus hair, exacerbation of intraocular inflammation, macular edema (eg, cystoid macular edema), and bacterial keratitis.

Patient Counseling: Inform about the potential for increased brown pigmentation of iris (may be permanent) and the possibility of darkening of eyelid skin (may be reversible after d/c). Inform about the possibility of eyelash and vellus hair changes in the treated eye during treatment. Advise to avoid touching tip of dispensing container to the eye, surrounding structures, fingers, or any other surface in order to avoid contamination of the solution. Advise to consult physician if having ocular surgery, or developed an intercurrent ocular condition (eg, trauma or infection) or ocular reaction. Instruct to remove contact lenses prior to instillation; reinsert 15 min after administration. Instruct to administer at least 5 min apart if using more than 1 topical ophthalmic drug.

Administration: Ocular route. **Storage:** 2-25°C (36-77°F).

LUNESTA

CIV

eszopiclone (Sunovion)

THERAPEUTIC CLASS: Nonbenzodiazepine hypnotic agent

INDICATIONS: Treatment of insomnia.

DOSAGE: *Adults:* Individualize dose. Initial: 2mg immediately before hs; may be initiated at 3mg if clinically indicated. Titrate: May be raised to 3mg if clinically indicated. Elderly: Difficulty Falling Asleep: Initial: 1mg immediately before hs. Titrate: May increase to 2mg if clinically indicated. Difficulty Staying Asleep: Usual: 2mg immediately before hs. Severe Hepatic Impairment: Initial: 1mg. Concomitant Potent CYP3A4 Inhibitors: Initial: Do not exceed 1mg. Titrate: May be raised to 2mg if needed. Concomitant CNS Depressants: Dosage adjustment may be necessary.

HOW SUPPLIED: Tab: 1mg, 2mg, 3mg

WARNINGS/PRECAUTIONS: Initiate only after careful evaluation; failure of insomnia to remit after 7-10 days of treatment may indicate presence of a primary psychiatric and/or medical illness that should be evaluated. Use the lowest possible effective dose, especially in elderly. Severe anaphylactic/anaphylactoid reactions reported; do not rechallenge if angioedema develops. Abnormal thinking and behavioral changes (eg, bizarre behavior, agitation, hallucinations, depersonalization) reported. Amnesia and other neuropsychiatric symptoms may occur unpredictably. Worsening of depression, including suicidal thoughts and actions (including completed suicides), reported in primarily depressed patients. Complex behaviors (eg, sleep-driving) reported; consider discontinuation if a sleep-driving episode occurs. Withdrawal signs/symptoms reported following rapid dose decrease or abrupt discontinuation. May impair mental/physical abilities. Should be taken immediately before hs; taking medications while still up and about may result in short-term memory impairment, hallucinations, impaired coordination, dizziness, and lightheadedness. Caution with severe hepatic impairment, elderly/debilitated patients, patients with diseases/conditions that could affect metabolism/hemodynamic responses, compromised respiratory function, history of alcohol/drug abuse, history of psychiatric disorders, and in patients exhibiting signs and symptoms of depression.

ADVERSE REACTIONS: Headache, unpleasant taste, somnolence, dry mouth, dizziness, infection, rash, pain, N/V, diarrhea, hallucinations, dyspepsia, nervousness, depression, anxiety.

INTERACTIONS: Increased risk of complex behaviors with alcohol and other CNS depressants. May produce additive CNS-depressant effects with other psychotropic medications, anticonvulsants, antihistamines, ethanol, and other drugs that produce CNS depression. Avoid with alcohol. Decreased digit symbol substitution test scores with olanzapine. Decreased exposure and effects with CYP3A4 inducers (eg, rifampicin). Increased exposure with ketoconazole and other strong CYP3A4 inhibitors (eg, itraconazole, clarithromycin, nefazodone, troleandomycin, ritonavir, nelfinavir); dose reduction needed.

PREGNANCY: Category C, safety not known in nursing.

MECHANISM OF ACTION: Nonbenzodiazepine hypnotic agent; not established. Effects believed to result from its interaction with GABA-receptor complexes at binding domains located close to or allosterically coupled to benzodiazepine receptors.

PHARMACOKINETICS: Absorption: Rapid. T_{max}=1 hr. **Distribution:** Plasma protein binding (52-59%). **Metabolism:** Liver (extensive) via oxidation and demethylation pathways by CYP3A4 and CYP2E1. (S)-zopiclone-N-oxide and (S)-N-desmethyl zopiclone (primary metabolites). **Elimination:** Urine (75% metabolites, <10% parent drug); $T_{1/2}$=6 hrs.

NURSING CONSIDERATIONS

Assessment: Assess for psychiatric or physical disorder, depression, severe hepatic impairment, diseases/conditions that could affect metabolism/hemodynamic responses, compromised respiratory function, history of alcohol/drug abuse, history of psychiatric disorders, drug hypersensitivity, pregnancy/nursing status, and possible drug interactions.

Monitoring: Monitor for complex behaviors, anaphylactic/anaphylactoid reactions, emergence of any new behavioral signs/symptoms, withdrawal symptoms, abnormal thinking, behavioral changes, and other adverse reactions.

Patient Counseling: Inform of the risks and benefits of therapy. Advise to seek medical attention immediately if any adverse reactions (eg, severe anaphylactic/anaphylactoid reactions, sleep-driving, and other complex behaviors) develop. Instruct to take immediately prior to hs and only if 8 hrs of sleep can be dedicated. Instruct not to take with alcohol or with other sedating medications. Advise to consult with physician if patients have history of depression, mental illness, suicidal thoughts, history of drug/alcohol abuse, or have liver disease. Advise to contact physician if pregnant, plan to become pregnant, or if nursing. Inform that taking with or immediately after a heavy, high-fat meal results in slower absorption and reduced effect on sleep latency.

Administration: Oral route. **Storage:** 25°C (77°F); excursions permitted to 15-30°C (59-86°F).

LUPRON DEPOT-PED   RX
leuprolide acetate (AbbVie)

THERAPEUTIC CLASS: Synthetic gonadotropin-releasing hormone analog

INDICATIONS: Treatment of children with central precocious puberty (CPP).

DOSAGE: *Pediatrics:* ≥2 Yrs: Individualize dose. D/C therapy at appropriate age of onset of puberty at discretion of physician. (1 Month) Administer single IM inj once a month. Initial: >37.5kg: 15mg. >25-37.5kg: 11.25mg. ≤25kg: 7.5mg. Titrate: May increase to next available higher dose (eg, 11.25mg or 15mg at the next monthly inj) if adequate hormonal and clinical suppression is not achieved. May also adjust dose with changes in body weight. Maint: Dose resulting in adequate hormonal suppression. (3 Month) 11.25mg or 30mg. Administer as a single IM inj every 3 months (12 weeks).

HOW SUPPLIED: Inj: (1 Month) 7.5mg, 11.25mg, 15mg; (3 Month) 11.25mg, 30mg

CONTRAINDICATIONS: Women who are or may become pregnant.

WARNINGS/PRECAUTIONS: Increase in clinical signs and symptoms of puberty may occur during the early phase of therapy due to initial rise in gonadotropins and sex steroids. Convulsions reported in patients with and without a history of seizures, epilepsy, cerebrovascular disorders, CNS anomalies or tumors, and in patients on concomitant medications that have been associated with convulsions (eg, bupropion, SSRIs). If noncompliant with drug regimen or dose is inadequate, gonadotropins and/or sex steroids may increase or rise above prepubertal levels. Suppresses pituitary-gonadal system; may affect diagnostic tests of pituitary gonadotropic and gonadal functions conducted during treatment and up to 6 months after discontinuation. Do not use partial syringes or combination of syringes to achieve a particular dose; each formulation and strength have different release characteristics.

ADVERSE REACTIONS: Inj-site reactions/pain, general pain, headache, acne/seborrhea, rash including erythema multiforme, emotional lability, vaginal bleeding/discharge/vaginitis, weight increase, mood altered.

PREGNANCY: Category X, not for use in nursing.

MECHANISM OF ACTION: Synthetic gonadotropin-releasing hormone (GnRH) analog; potent inhibitor of gonadotropin secretion. Following an initial stimulation of gonadotropins, chronic stimulation results in suppression and "downregulation" of these hormones and consequent suppression of ovarian and testicular steroidogenesis.

PHARMACOKINETICS: Absorption: (7.5mg in adults) C_{max}=20ng/mL, T_{max}=4 hrs; (11.25mg) C_{max}=19.1ng/mL; (30mg) C_{max}=52.5ng/mL; (11.5mg and 30mg) T_{max}=1 hr. **Distribution:** Plasma protein binding (43-49%), V_d=27L (IV). **Metabolism:** M-I (major metabolite). **Elimination:** (3.75mg) Urine (<5% as parent and M-1 metabolite); $T_{1/2}$=3 hrs (1mg IV).

NURSING CONSIDERATIONS

Assessment: Assess for history of seizures, cerebrovascular disorders, CNS anomalies or tumors. Assess for drug hypersensitivity and pregnancy status. Confirm clinical diagnosis of CPP by measuring blood concentrations of luteinizing hormone (LH) (basal or stimulated with a GnRH analog), sex steroids, and assessment of bone age versus chronological age. Obtain baseline evaluations of height and weight measurements, diagnostic imaging of the brain, pelvic/testicular/adrenal ultrasound, human chorionic gonadotropin levels, and adrenal steroid measurements to exclude congenital adrenal hyperplasia.

Monitoring: Monitor for convulsions and other adverse reactions. Monitor response with a GnRH stimulation test, basal LH or serum concentration of sex steroid levels; (1-Month) beginning 1-2 months following initiation of therapy, with changing doses, or potentially during therapy in order to confirm maintenance of efficacy or (3-Month) at months 2-3, month 6 and further as judged clinically appropriate, to ensure adequate suppression. (1-Month) Measure bone age for advancement every 6-12 months. (3-Month) Monitor height and bone age every 6-12 months.

Patient Counseling: Counsel about the potential risk to the fetus if inadvertently used during pregnancy, or if patient becomes pregnant while taking the drug. Counsel about the importance of continuous therapy and adherence to drug administration schedule. Inform that signs of puberty (eg, vaginal bleeding) may occur during 1st few weeks of therapy; instruct to notify physician if symptoms continue beyond 2nd month. Inform about the most common side effects related to treatment. Advise that some pain and irritation is expected after inj; instruct to report if more severe or any unusual signs or symptoms occur. Advise parents/caregivers to notify physician if new or worsened symptoms develop after beginning treatment.

Administration: IM route. Must be administered under physician's supervision. Inj-site should be varied periodically. Refer to PI for reconstitution and administration instructions. **Storage:** 25°C (77°F); excursions permitted to 15-30°C (59-86°F). Reconstituted Sus: Discard if not used within 2 hrs.

LUSEDRA CIV
fospropofol disodium (Eisai)

THERAPEUTIC CLASS: Anesthetic agent

INDICATIONS: For monitored anesthesia care (MAC) sedation in adult patients undergoing diagnostic or therapeutic procedures.

DOSAGE: *Adults:* Individualize dose. Standard Dosing Regimen: 18-<65 Yrs Who are Healthy or Patients with Mild Systemic Disease (ASA P1 or P2): Initial: 6.5mg/kg IV bolus. Supplemental: 1.6mg/kg IV as necessary. Max: 16.5mL (initial dose) and 4mL (supplemental dose). Modified Dosing Regimen: ≥65 yrs or Patients with Severe Systemic Disease (ASA P3 or P4): Initial/Supplemental: 75% of the standard dosing regimen. Give supplemental doses only when patients can demonstrate purposeful movement in response to verbal or light tactile stimulation and no more frequently than every 4 min. Refer to PI for specific information regarding standard and modified dosing regimens. Use supplemental oxygen in all patients undergoing sedation.

HOW SUPPLIED: Inj: 35mg/mL

WARNINGS/PRECAUTIONS: Only trained persons in general anesthesia administration and not involved in the conduct of the diagnostic or therapeutic procedure should administer fospropofol. Sedated patients should be continuously monitored and facilities for maintenance of patent airway, providing artificial ventilation, administration of supplemental oxygen, and instituting of cardiovascular resuscitation must be immediately available. Respiratory depression and hypoxemia reported. Hypotension reported; caution in patients with compromised myocardial function, reduced vascular tone, or reduced intravascular volume. May cause unresponsiveness or minimal responsiveness to vigorous tactile or painful stimulation. Caution in hepatic impairment.

ADVERSE REACTIONS: Paresthesia, pruritus, N/V, hypoxemia, hypotension.

INTERACTIONS: Concomitant use with other cardiorespiratory depressants (eg, benzodiazepines, sedative-hypnotics, narcotic analgesics) may produce additive cardiorespiratory effects.

PREGNANCY: Category B, not for use in nursing.

MECHANISM OF ACTION: Sedative-hypnotic agent. Prodrug of propofol; metabolized by alkaline phosphatases following IV injection.

PHARMACOKINETICS: Absorption: (Fospropofol) AUC=19mcg•h/mL. (Propofol) AUC=1.2mcg•h/mL. **Distribution:** (Fospropofol) V_d=0.33L/kg. (Propofol) V_d=5.8L/kg; plasma protein binding (98%). Crosses placenta, found in breast milk. **Metabolism:** Complete via alkaline phosphatases to propofol, formaldehyde, and phosphate; further metabolized to propofol glucuronide, quinol-4-sulfate, quinol-1-glucuronide, quinol-4-glucuronide (major metabolites). **Elimination:** (Fospropofol) $T_{1/2}$=0.88 hrs. (Propofol) $T_{1/2}$=1.13 hrs.

NURSING CONSIDERATIONS

Assessment: Assess for respiratory depression, hypotension or risk of hypotension (eg, compromised myocardial function, reduced vascular tone, reduced intravascular volume), hepatic impairment, pregnancy/nursing status, and for possible drug interactions.

Monitoring: Monitor continuously during sedation and recovery process for early signs of hypotension, apnea, airway obstruction, and/or oxygen desaturation. Monitor responsiveness to vigorous tactile or painful stimulation.

Patient Counseling: Inform that paresthesias (including burning, tingling, stinging) and/or pruritus are frequently experienced during the 1st inj and are typically mild to moderate in intensity, last a short time, and require no treatment. Counsel that a patient escort may be required after procedure. Instruct to avoid engaging in activities requiring complete alertness, coordination and/or physical dexterity (eg, operating hazardous machinery, signing legal documents, driving a motor vehicle) until physician has approved of performing such tasks.

Administration: IV route. **Storage:** 25°C (77°F); excursions permitted 15-30°C (59-86°F).

LUVOX CR

RX

fluvoxamine maleate (Jazz)

Antidepressants increased the risk of suicidal thinking and behavior (suicidality) in short-term studies in children, adolescents, and young adults with major depressive disorder (MDD) and other psychiatric disorders. Monitor and observe closely for clinical worsening, suicidality, or unusual changes in behavior in patients who are started on antidepressant therapy. Not approved for use in pediatric patients.

THERAPEUTIC CLASS: Selective serotonin reuptake inhibitor

INDICATIONS: Treatment of obsessive compulsive disorder (OCD) and social anxiety disorder (social phobia).

DOSAGE: *Adults:* Initial: 100mg qhs. Titrate: May increase by 50mg every week until maximum therapeutic response is achieved. Maint: 100-300mg/day. Max: 300mg/day. Maint/Continuation of Extended Treatment: Lowest effective dose. Periodically reassess need to continue. Switching to/from MAOI: Allow ≥14 days between d/c and initiation of therapy. Elderly/Hepatic Impairment: Titrate slowly. 3rd Trimester Pregnancy: Taper dose.

HOW SUPPLIED: Cap, Extended-Release: 100mg, 150mg

CONTRAINDICATIONS: Concomitant use of alosetron, tizanidine, thioridazine, or pimozide. Use during or within 14 days of MAOI therapy.

WARNINGS/PRECAUTIONS: Serotonin syndrome or neuroleptic malignant syndrome (NMS)-like reactions reported. May precipitate mixed/manic episode in patients at risk for bipolar disorder; screen for risk for bipolar disorder prior to initiating treatment. D/C should be gradual. May increase risk of bleeding events; caution with NSAIDs, aspirin (ASA), or other drugs that affect coagulation. Activation of mania/hypomania, syndrome of inappropriate antidiuretic hormone secretion, hyponatremia reported. Caution with history of mania or hepatic dysfunction, conditions that alter metabolism or hemodynamic responses. Caution with patients taking diuretics or who are volume depleted, especially the elderly; d/c if symptomatic hyponatremia occurs. Seizures reported; caution with history of convulsive disorders, avoid with unstable epilepsy and monitor patients with controlled epilepsy; d/c if seizures occur or seizure frequency increases. Consider potential risks and benefits of treatment during 3rd trimester of pregnancy. Decreased appetite and weight loss reported in children; monitor weight and growth.

ADVERSE REACTIONS: Headache, asthenia, nausea, diarrhea, anorexia, dyspepsia, insomnia, somnolence, nervousness, dizziness, anxiety, dry mouth, tremor, abnormal ejaculation.

INTERACTIONS: See Contraindications. Known potent inhibitor of CYP1A2, CYP3A4, CYP2C9, CYP2C19, and weak inhibitor of CYP2D6. Increased plasma concentrations of methadone, TCAs, propranolol, metoprolol, warfarin, alosetron, and alprazolam. Increased area under the curve (AUC), C_{max} of alprazolam, tacrine, ramelteon, and alosetron. Increased serum levels of clozapine; risk of adverse events may be higher. Increased levels of carbamazepine and symptoms of toxicity reported. Decreased clearance levels of mexiletine, theophylline, and benzodiazepines like alprazolam, midazolam, triazolam, and diazepam. Bradycardia reported; caution with diltiazem. Concomitant use of serotonergic drugs and with drugs that impair metabolism of serotonin may cause serotonin syndrome and NMS-like reactions. Caution with tryptophan; may enhance serotonergic effects and severe vomiting may occur. Weakness, hyperreflexia, incoordination with SSRIs and sumatriptan reported. Risk of seizures with lithium. Altered anticoagulation effects with warfarin. Diuretics may increase the risk of hyponatremia. A clinically significant interaction is possible with drugs having narrow therapeutic ratio such as pimozide, warfarin, theophylline, certain benzodiazepines, omeprazole, and phenytoin. Smoking increases metabolism. Avoid alcohol.

PREGNANCY: Category C, not for use in nursing.

MECHANISM OF ACTION: SSRI; inhibits neuronal uptake of serotonin.

PHARMACOKINETICS: Absorption: C_{max} (at doses 100mg, 200mg, 300mg) =47ng/mL, 161ng/mL, 319ng/mL. **Distribution:** V_d=25L/kg; plasma protein binding (80%); found in breast milk. **Metabolism:** Liver (extensive) via oxidative demethylation and deamination. **Elimination:** Urine (94%), $T_{1/2}$ =16.3 hrs.

NURSING CONSIDERATIONS

Assessment: Assess for MDD, risk for bipolar disorder, depressive symptoms, history of mania, seizures, suicide, drug abuse, disease/condition that alters metabolism or hemodynamic response, hepatic impairment, history of hypersensitivity to drug, pregnancy/nursing status and possible drug interactions. Obtain a detailed psychiatric history prior to therapy.

Monitoring: Monitor for signs/symptoms of clinical worsening (suicidality, unusual changes in behavior), serotonin syndrome, NMS-like reactions (muscle rigidity, hyperthermia, mental status changes), abnormal bleeding, hyponatremia, seizures, hepatic dysfunction, and other adverse reactions. If d/c therapy (particularly if abrupt), monitor for symptoms of dysphoric mood, irritability, agitation, dizziness, sensory disturbances, anxiety, confusion, headache, lethargy, emotional lability, insomnia, and hypomania.

Patient Counseling: Advise to avoid alcohol. Caution on risk of serotonin syndrome with concomitant use of triptans, tramadol, or other serotonergic agents. Seek medical attention for symptoms of serotonin syndrome (mental status changes, tachycardia, hyperthermia, N/V, diarrhea, incoordination), NMS, allergic reactions (rash, hives), abnormal bleeding (particularly if using NSAIDs or ASA), hyponatremia, activation of mania, seizures, clinical worsening (suicidal ideation, unusual changes in behavior), and discontinuation symptoms (eg, irritability, agitation, dizziness, anxiety, headache, insomnia). Instruct not to crush or chew; may be taken with or without food. Caution against hazardous tasks (eg, operating machinery and driving). Notify physician if pregnant, intend to become pregnant, or breastfeeding. Counsel about benefits and risks of therapy. Inform physician if taking or plan to take any over-the-counter medications.

Administration: Oral route. **Storage:** Store at 25°C (77°F); excursions permitted to 15-30°C (59-86°F). Avoid exposure to >30°C (86°F). Protect from high humidity. Keep out of reach of children.

Luxiq   RX   L
betamethasone valerate (Stiefel)

THERAPEUTIC CLASS: Corticosteroid

INDICATIONS: Relief of the inflammatory and pruritic manifestations of corticosteroid-responsive dermatoses of the scalp.

DOSAGE: *Adults:* Apply small amounts to affected scalp area bid (am and pm). Repeat until entire affected scalp area is treated. Reassess if no improvement within 2 weeks.

HOW SUPPLIED: Foam: 0.12% [50g, 100g]

WARNINGS/PRECAUTIONS: Systemic absorption may produce reversible hypothalamic-pituitary-adrenal (HPA) axis suppression, manifestations of Cushing's syndrome, hyperglycemia, and glucosuria. Evaluate periodically for evidence of HPA axis suppression when applying to large surface area or to areas under occlusion; d/c treatment, reduce frequency of application, or substitute a less potent steroid if HPA axis suppression is noted. D/C and institute appropriate therapy if irritation develops. Use appropriate antifungal or antibacterial agent in the presence of dermatological infections; if favorable response does not occur promptly, d/c until infection is controlled. Pediatric patients may be more susceptible to systemic toxicity from equivalent doses.

ADVERSE REACTIONS: Application-site burning/itching/stinging.

PREGNANCY: Category C, caution in nursing.

MECHANISM OF ACTION: Corticosteroid; possesses anti-inflammatory, antipruritic, and vasoconstrictive properties. Anti-inflammatory activity not established; thought to induce phospholipase A_2 inhibitory proteins, lipocortins, which control biosynthesis of potent mediators of inflammation (eg, prostaglandins, leukotrienes) by inhibiting release of their precursor, arachidonic acid.

PHARMACOKINETICS: Absorption: Percutaneous; occlusion, inflammation, and/or other disease processes in the skin may increase absorption. **Distribution:** Found in breast milk (systemically administered). **Metabolism:** Liver. **Elimination:** Kidney (major), bile.

NURSING CONSIDERATIONS

Assessment: Assess for hypersensitivity to the drug, dermatological infections, and pregnancy/nursing status.

Monitoring: Monitor for signs/symptoms of HPA axis suppression, Cushing's syndrome, hyperglycemia, glucosuria, skin irritation, allergic contact dermatitis, and other adverse reactions. Monitor for signs of glucocorticosteroid insufficiency after withdrawal. Monitor clinical improvement; if no improvement seen within 2 weeks, reassess diagnosis.

Patient Counseling: Advise to use externally and ud, to avoid contact with eyes, and not to use for any disorder other than that for which it was prescribed. Instruct not to bandage, cover, or wrap treated scalp area unless directed by physician. Advise to report any signs of local adverse reactions to physician. Advise to d/c use when control is achieved, and to notify physician if no improvement is seen within 2 weeks. Instruct to avoid fire, flame, or smoking during and immediately following application.

Administration: Topical route. Refer to PI for proper administration. **Storage:** 20-25°C (68-77°F). Do not expose to heat or store at >49°C (120°F).

LYRICA
pregabalin (Pfizer)

THERAPEUTIC CLASS: GABA analog

INDICATIONS: Management of neuropathic pain associated with diabetic peripheral neuropathy and/or spinal cord injury. Management of postherpetic neuralgia and fibromyalgia. Adjunctive therapy for adult patients with partial onset seizures.

DOSAGE: *Adults:* Neuropathic Pain Associated with Diabetic Peripheral Neuropathy: Initial: 50mg tid (150mg/day). Titrate: May increase to 300mg/day within 1 week PRN. Max: 100mg tid (300mg/day). Postherpetic Neuralgia: Initial: 75mg bid or 50mg tid (150mg/day). Titrate: May increase to 300mg/day within 1 week PRN. Max: 600mg/day divided bid or tid if no sufficient pain relief experienced following 2-4 weeks of treatment with 300mg/day. Partial-Onset Seizures: Initial: 150mg/day divided bid-tid. Titrate: May increase up to max dose of 600mg/day. Fibromyalgia: Initial: 75mg bid. Titrate: May increase to 150mg bid (300mg/day) within 1 week PRN. Max: 225mg bid (450mg/day). Neuropathic Pain Associated with Spinal Cord Injury: Initial: 75mg bid. Titrate: May increase to 150mg bid (300mg/day) within 1 week PRN. Max: 300mg bid (600mg/day) if no sufficient pain relief experienced following 2-3 weeks of treatment with 150mg bid. Refer to PI for dosage adjustment based on renal function. D/C: Taper over minimum of 1 week.

HOW SUPPLIED: Cap: 25mg, 50mg, 75mg, 100mg, 150mg, 200mg, 225mg, 300mg; Sol: 20mg/mL [16 fl. oz.]

WARNINGS/PRECAUTIONS: Angioedema reported; d/c immediately if symptoms of angioedema with respiratory compromise occurs. Caution in patients who had a previous episode of angioedema. Hypersensitivity reactions reported; d/c immediately if symptoms occur. Avoid abrupt withdrawal; gradually taper over a minimum of 1 week. Increased risk of suicidal thoughts/behavior; monitor for emergence or worsening of depression, suicidal thought/behavior, and/or unusual changes in mood/behavior. May cause weight gain and peripheral edema; caution with congestive heart failure (CHF). May cause dizziness and somnolence; may impair physical/mental abilities. New or worsening of preexisting tumors reported. Blurred vision, decreased visual acuity, visual field changes, and funduscopic changes reported. Creatine kinase (CK) elevations and rhabdomyolysis reported; d/c if myopathy is diagnosed or suspected or if markedly elevated CK levels occur. Associated with a decrease in platelet counts and PR interval prolongation. Caution in patients with renal impairment.

ADVERSE REACTIONS: Somnolence, dizziness, peripheral edema, ataxia, weight gain, dry mouth, fatigue, asthenia, blurred vision, diplopia, edema, nasopharyngitis, constipation, abnormal thinking, tremor.

INTERACTIONS: May increase risk of angioedema with other drugs associated with angioedema (eg, ACE inhibitors). Additive effects on cognitive and gross motor functioning with oxycodone, lorazepam, and ethanol. Caution with thiazolidinedione class of antidiabetic drugs; higher frequencies of weight gain and peripheral edema reported. Gabapentin reported to cause a small reduction in absorption rate. Reduced lower GI tract function (eg, intestinal obstruction, paralytic ileus, constipation) reported with medications that have the potential to produce constipation, such as opioid analgesics.

PREGNANCY: Category C, not for use in nursing.

MECHANISM OF ACTION: Gamma-aminobutyric acid derivative; not fully established; binds with high affinity to the α_2-delta site (an auxiliary subunit of voltage-gated calcium channels) in CNS tissues.

PHARMACOKINETICS: Absorption: Well-absorbed; T_{max}=1.5 hrs (fasting), 3 hrs (fed). **Distribution:** V_d=0.5L/kg. **Metabolism:** Negligible metabolism. N-methylated derivative (major metabolite). **Elimination:** Urine (90% unchanged); $T_{1/2}$=6.3 hrs.

NURSING CONSIDERATIONS

Assessment: Assess for hypersensitivity, renal impairment, preexisting tumors, history of drug abuse, history of depression, previous episode of angioedema, CHF, pregnancy/nursing status, and possible drug interactions. Obtain baseline weight.

Monitoring: Monitor for angioedema, hypersensitivity reactions, peripheral edema, weight gain, new tumors or worsening of preexisting tumors, ophthalmological effects, rhabdomyolysis, dizziness, somnolence, emergence or worsening of depression, suicidal thoughts or behavior, and/or changes in behavior. Monitor CK levels and platelet counts. Monitor ECG for PR interval prolongation.

Patient Counseling: Instruct to d/c therapy and seek medical attention if hypersensitivity reactions or symptoms of angioedema occur. Inform patients and caregivers to be alert for the emergence or worsening of depression, unusual changes in mood or behavior, or the emergence of suicidal thoughts or behavior; immediately report behaviors of concern to physician. Counsel that dizziness, somnolence, blurred vision, and other CNS signs and symptoms may occur; advise to use caution when operating machinery/driving. Inform that weight gain and edema may occur. Instruct not to abruptly/rapidly d/c therapy. Instruct to report unexplained muscle pain, tenderness, or weakness, particularly if accompanied by malaise or fever to physician. Instruct not to consume alcohol while on therapy. Instruct to notify physician if pregnant, intend to become pregnant, breastfeeding or intend to breastfeed. Inform men on therapy who plan to father a child of the potential risk of male-mediated teratogenicity. Instruct diabetic patients to pay attention to skin integrity while on therapy.

Administration: Oral route. **Storage:** 25°C (77°F); excursions permitted to 15-30°C (59-86°F).

MACROBID   RX
nitrofurantoin monohydrate - nitrofurantoin macrocrystals (Almatica)

THERAPEUTIC CLASS: Imidazolidinedione antibacterial

INDICATIONS: Treatment of acute uncomplicated urinary tract infections (acute cystitis) caused by susceptible strains of *Escherichia coli* or *Staphylococcus saprophyticus*.

DOSAGE: *Adults:* 100mg q12h for 7 days.
Pediatrics: >12 Yrs: 100mg q12h for 7 days.

HOW SUPPLIED: Cap: 100mg

CONTRAINDICATIONS: Anuria, oliguria, significant impairment of renal function (CrCl <60mL/min or clinically significant elevated SrCr), pregnancy at term (38-42 weeks' gestation), during labor and delivery or when onset of labor is imminent, and neonates <1 month of age, and previous history of cholestatic jaundice/hepatic dysfunction associated with nitrofurantoin.

WARNINGS/PRECAUTIONS: Not for treatment of pyelonephritis or perinephric abscesses. Many patients who undergo treatment are predisposed to persistence/reappearance of bacteriuria; if this occurs after treatment, select other therapeutic agents with broader tissue distribution. Acute, subacute, or chronic pulmonary reactions (diffuse interstitial pneumonitis, pulmonary fibrosis, or both) reported; d/c and take appropriate measures if these occur. Closely monitor pulmonary condition if on long-term therapy. Hepatic reactions (eg, hepatitis, cholestatic jaundice, chronic active hepatitis, hepatic necrosis) occur rarely. Monitor periodically for changes in biochemical tests that would indicate liver injury; withdraw immediately and take appropriate measures if hepatitis occurs. Peripheral neuropathy, which may become severe or irreversible, reported; risk may be enhanced with renal impairment, anemia, diabetes mellitus (DM), electrolyte imbalance, vitamin B deficiency, and debilitating disease. Monitor periodically for renal function changes with long-term therapy. Optic neuritis reported rarely. May induce hemolytic anemia of the primaquine-sensitivity type; d/c therapy if hemolysis occurs. *Clostridium difficile*-associated diarrhea (CDAD) reported; d/c therapy is CDAD is suspected/confirmed. Use in the absence of a proven or strongly suspected bacterial infection or prophylactic indication is unlikely to provide benefit and increases the risk of the development of drug-resistant bacteria. Lab test interactions may occur. Caution with impaired renal function and in elderly.

ADVERSE REACTIONS: Nausea, headache.

INTERACTIONS: Antacids containing magnesium trisilicate reduce both the rate and extent of absorption. Uricosuric drugs (eg, probenecid, sulfinpyrazone) may inhibit renal tubular secretion of nitrofurantoin; resulting increased nitrofurantoin serum levels may increase toxicity, and the decreased urinary levels could lessen its efficacy.

PREGNANCY: Category B, not for use in nursing.

MECHANISM OF ACTION: Imidazolidinedione/nitrofuran antimicrobial agent; inhibits the vital biochemical processes of protein synthesis, aerobic energy metabolism, and DNA, RNA, and cell-wall synthesis.

PHARMACOKINETICS: Absorption: C_{max}=<1mcg/mL. **Distribution:** Found in breast milk. **Elimination:** Urine (20-25% unchanged).

NURSING CONSIDERATIONS

Assessment: Assess for anuria, oliguria, significant renal impairment, history of cholestatic jaundice/hepatic dysfunction associated with nitrofurantoin, G6PD deficiency, DM, anemia, electrolyte imbalance, vitamin B deficiency, debilitating disease, drug hypersensitivity, pregnancy/nursing status, and possible drug interactions. Obtain urine specimens for culture and susceptibility testing prior to therapy.

Monitoring: Monitor for persistence or reappearance of bacteriuria, acute/subacute/chronic pulmonary reactions, hepatic reactions, peripheral neuropathy, optic neuritis, hematologic manifestations, and CDAD. Monitor LFTs periodically. Monitor renal and pulmonary function periodically during long-term therapy. Obtain urine specimens for culture and susceptibility testing after completion of therapy.

Patient Counseling: Inform of the potential risks and benefits of therapy. Advise to take with food (ideally breakfast and dinner) to further enhance tolerance and improve drug absorption. Instruct to complete the full course of therapy and advise to contact physician if any unusual symptoms occur during therapy. Advise not to take antacids containing magnesium trisilicate while on therapy. Inform that therapy treats bacterial, not viral, infections. Advise to take exactly ud; skipping doses or not completing full course may decrease effectiveness and increase drug resistance. Inform that diarrhea is a common problem that usually ends when antibiotic is discontinued. Inform that watery and bloody stools (with/without stomach cramps and fever) may develop even as late as 2 or more months after having taken the last dose; instruct to contact physician as soon as possible if this occurs.

Administration: Oral route. Take with food. **Storage:** 15-30°C (59-86°F).

MACRODANTIN   RX
nitrofurantoin macrocrystals (Almatica)

THERAPEUTIC CLASS: Imidazolidinedione antibacterial

INDICATIONS: Treatment of urinary tract infections due to susceptible strains of *Escherichia coli*, enterococci, *Staphylococcus aureus*, and certain susceptible strains of *Klebsiella* and *Enterobacter* species.

DOSAGE: *Adults:* 50-100mg qid for 1 week or for at least 3 days after sterility of the urine obtained. Long-term Suppressive Therapy: Reduce dose to 50-100mg qhs.
Pediatrics: ≥1 Month: 5-7mg/kg/day given in 4 divided doses for 1 week or for at least 3 days after sterility of the urine obtained. Long-term Suppressive Therapy: 1mg/kg/day given in a single dose or in 2 divided doses.

HOW SUPPLIED: Cap: 25mg, 50mg, 100mg

CONTRAINDICATIONS: Anuria, oliguria, significant impairment of renal function (CrCl <60mL/min or clinically significant elevated SrCr), pregnancy at term (38-42 weeks' gestation), during labor and delivery, or when the onset of labor is imminent, neonates <1 month of age, and previous history of cholestatic jaundice/hepatic dysfunction associated with nitrofurantoin.

WARNINGS/PRECAUTIONS: Not for the treatment of pyelonephritis or perinephric abscesses. Many patients who undergo treatment are predisposed to persistence/reappearance of bacteriuria; if this occurs after treatment, select other therapeutic agents with broader tissue distribution. Acute, subacute, or chronic pulmonary reactions (diffuse interstitial pneumonitis, pulmonary fibrosis, or both) reported; d/c and take appropriate measures if these occur. Closely monitor pulmonary condition if on long-term therapy. Hepatic reactions (eg, hepatitis, cholestatic jaundice, chronic active hepatitis, and hepatic necrosis) occur rarely. Monitor periodically for changes in biochemical tests that would indicate liver injury; withdraw immediately and take appropriate measures if hepatitis occurs. Peripheral neuropathy, which may become severe or irreversible, reported; risk may be enhanced with renal impairment, anemia, diabetes mellitus (DM), electrolyte imbalance, vitamin B deficiency, and debilitating disease. Monitor periodically for renal function changes with long-term therapy. Optic neuritis reported rarely. May induced hemolytic anemia of the primaquine-sensitivity type; d/c therapy if hemolysis occurs. *Clostridium difficile*-associated diarrhea (CDAD) reported; d/c therapy if CDAD is suspected/confirmed. Use in the absence of a proven or strongly suspected bacterial infection or prophylactic indication is unlikely to provide benefit and increases the risk of the development of drug-resistant bacteria. Lab test interactions may occur. Caution with impaired renal function and in elderly.

ADVERSE REACTIONS: Pulmonary hypersensitivity reactions, hepatic reactions, peripheral neuropathy, exfoliative dermatitis, erythema multiforme, lupus-like syndrome, nausea, emesis, anorexia, asthenia, vertigo, nystagmus, dizziness, headache, drowsiness.

INTERACTIONS: Antacids containing magnesium trisilicate reduce both the rate and extent of absorption. Uricosuric drugs (eg, probenecid, sulfinpyrazone) may inhibit renal tubular secretion of nitrofurantoin; resulting increased nitrofurantoin serum levels may increase toxicity, and the decreased urinary levels could lessen its efficacy.

PREGNANCY: Category B, not for use in nursing.

MECHANISM OF ACTION: Imidazolidinedione antibacterial. Nitrofuran antimicrobial agent; inhibits the vital biochemical processes of protein synthesis, aerobic energy metabolism, and DNA, RNA, and cell-wall synthesis.

PHARMACOKINETICS: Distribution: Found in breast milk. **Elimination:** Urine (100mg qid for 7 days: Day 1: 37.9%; Day 7: 35%).

NURSING CONSIDERATIONS

Assessment: Assess for anuria, oliguria, significant renal impairment, history of cholestatic jaundice/hepatic dysfunction associated with nitrofurantoin, G6PD deficiency, DM, anemia, electrolyte imbalance, vitamin B deficiency, debilitating disease, drug hypersensitivity, pregnancy/nursing status, and possible drug interactions. Obtain urine specimen for culture and susceptibility testing prior to therapy.

Monitoring: Monitor for persistence or reappearance of bacteriuria, acute/subacute/chronic pulmonary reactions, hepatic reactions, peripheral neuropathy, optic neuritis, hematologic manifestations, and CDAD. Monitor LFTs periodically. Monitor renal and pulmonary function periodically during long-term therapy. Obtain urine specimens for culture and susceptibility testing after completion of therapy.

Patient Counseling: Inform of the potential risks and benefits of therapy. Advise to take with food to further enhance tolerance and improve drug absorption. Instruct to complete full course of therapy and advise to contact physician if any unusual symptoms occur during therapy. Advise not to take antacid preparations containing magnesium trisilicate while on therapy. Inform that therapy treats bacterial, not viral, infections. Advise to take exactly ud; skipping doses or not completing full course may decrease effectiveness and increase drug resistance. Inform that diarrhea is a common problem that usually ends when antibiotic is discontinued. Inform that watery and bloody stools (with/without stomach cramps and fever) may develop even as late as ≥2 months after having taken the last dose; instruct to contact physician as soon as possible if this occurs.

Administration: Oral route. Take with food. **Storage:** 20-25°C (68-77°F).

MALARONE   RX
proguanil HCl - atovaquone (GlaxoSmithKline)

OTHER BRAND NAMES: Malarone Pediatric (GlaxoSmithKline)

THERAPEUTIC CLASS: Antiprotozoal agent/dihydrofolate reductase inhibitor

INDICATIONS: Prophylaxis of *Plasmodium falciparum* malaria, including in areas where chloroquine resistance has been reported. Treatment of acute, uncomplicated *P. falciparum* malaria.

DOSAGE: *Adults:* Prevention: 1 adult strength tab (250mg-100mg) qd. Start prophylactic treatment 1 or 2 days before entering a malaria-endemic area and continue daily during stay and for 7 days after return. Treatment: 4 adult strength tabs (1g-400mg) qd for 3 consecutive days. Take at the same time each day with food or a milky drink.
Pediatrics: Prevention: >40kg: 1 adult strength tab (250mg-100mg) qd. 31-40kg: 3 pediatric tabs (187.5mg-75mg) qd. 21-30kg: 2 pediatric tabs (125mg-50mg) qd. 11-20kg: 1 pediatric tab (62.5mg-25mg) qd. Start prophylactic treatment 1 or 2 days before entering a malaria-endemic area and continue daily during stay and for 7 days after return. Treatment: >40kg: 4 adult strength tabs (1g-400mg) qd. 31-40kg: 3 adult strength tabs (750mg-300mg) qd. 21-30kg: 2 adult strength tabs (500mg-200mg) qd. 11-20kg: 1 adult strength tab (250mg-100mg) qd. 9-10kg: 3 pediatric tabs (187.5mg-75mg) qd. 5-8kg: 2 pediatric tabs (125mg-50mg) qd. Treat for 3 consecutive days. Take at the same time each day with food or a milky drink.

HOW SUPPLIED: Tab: (Atovaquone-Proguanil) 250mg-100mg (adult), 62.5mg-25mg (pediatric)

CONTRAINDICATIONS: For prophylaxis in patients with severe renal impairment (CrCl <30mL/min).

WARNINGS/PRECAUTIONS: Reduced atovaquone absorption in patients with diarrhea or vomiting; monitor for parasitemia and consider use of an antiemetic if vomiting occurs. Alternative antimalarial therapy may be required in patients with severe or persistent diarrhea or vomiting. In mixed *P. falciparum* and *Plasmodium vivax* infections, *P. vivax* parasite relapse occurred commonly when patients were treated with atovaquone-proguanil alone. Treat with a different blood schizonticide in the event of recrudescent *P. falciparum* infections after treatment or failure of chemoprophylaxis. Elevated liver lab tests and cases of hepatitis and hepatic failure requiring liver transplantation reported with prophylactic use. Patients with severe malaria are not candidates for oral therapy. Caution for the treatment of malaria in patients with severe renal impairment. Caution in elderly.

ADVERSE REACTIONS: Abdominal pain, headache, N/V, diarrhea, asthenia, anorexia, dizziness, dreams, insomnia, oral ulcers, cough, pruritus.

INTERACTIONS: Atovaquone: Decreased levels with rifampin or rifabutin; not recommended with rifampin or rifabutin. Decreased levels with tetracycline; monitor for parasitemia. Reduced bioavailability with metoclopramide; use only if other antiemetics are not available. Decreased indinavir trough concentrations; use caution. Proguanil: May potentiate anticoagulant effect of warfarin and other coumarin-based anticoagulants; use caution when initiating or withdrawing in patients on continuous treatment with coumarin-based anticoagulants, and closely monitor coagulation tests with concomitant use.

PREGNANCY: Category C, caution in nursing.

MECHANISM OF ACTION: Atovaquone: Antiprotozoal; selective inhibitor of parasite mitochondrial electron transport. Proguanil: Dihydrofolate reductase inhibitor; disrupts deoxythymidylate synthesis.

PHARMACOKINETICS: Absorption: Atovaquone: Absolute bioavailability (23% with food). **Distribution:** Atovaquone: V_d=8.8L/kg; plasma protein binding (>99%). Proguanil: V_d=1617-2502L (patients >15 yrs of age with body weight 31-110kg), 462-966L (pediatric patients ≤15 yrs of age with body weight 11-56kg); plasma protein binding (75%); found in breast milk. **Metabolism:** Proguanil: via CYP2C19; cycloguanil and 4-chlorophenylbiguanide (metabolites). **Elimination:** Atovaquone: Feces (>94% unchanged), urine (<0.6%); $T_{1/2}$=2-3 days (adults), 1-2 days (pediatrics). Proguanil: Urine (40-60%); $T_{1/2}$=12-21 hrs (adults and pediatrics).

NURSING CONSIDERATIONS

Assessment: Assess for severity of malaria, drug hypersensitivity, renal dysfunction, diarrhea, vomiting, pregnancy/nursing status, and possible drug interactions.

Monitoring: Monitor for clinical response, N/V, diarrhea, hepatic/renal dysfunction, hypersensitivity, and other adverse reactions. Monitor parasitemia in patients who are vomiting. Monitor for relapse of infection when patients are treated with atovaquone-proguanil alone. Closely monitor coagulation tests when concomitant use with warfarin and other coumarin-based anticoagulants.

Patient Counseling: Instruct that if a dose is missed, to take a dose as soon as possible and then to return to normal dosing schedule. Advise not to double the next dose if a dose is skipped. Counsel about serious adverse events associated with therapy (eg, hepatitis, severe skin reactions, neurological and hematological events). Instruct to consult physician regarding alternative forms of prophylaxis if prophylaxis is prematurely discontinued for any reason. Inform that protective clothing, insect repellents, and bednets are important components of malaria prophylaxis. Instruct to seek medical attention for any febrile illness that occurs during or after return from a malaria-endemic area. Discuss with pregnant women anticipating travel to malarious areas about the risks/benefits of such travel.

Administration: Oral route. Take at the same time each day with food or a milky drink. Repeat dose in the event of vomiting within 1 hr after dosing. May crush and mix with condensed milk just prior to administration for patients who may have difficulty swallowing tabs. **Storage:** 25°C (77°F); excursions permitted to 15-30°C (59-86°F).

MARINOL
dronabinol (Abbott)

CIII

THERAPEUTIC CLASS: Cannabinoid

INDICATIONS: Treatment of anorexia associated with weight loss in AIDS patients and N/V associated with cancer chemotherapy in patients who have failed to respond adequately to conventional antiemetic treatments.

DOSAGE: *Adults:* Individualize dose. Appetite Stimulation: Initial: 2.5mg bid before lunch and supper. Titrate: Reduce dose to 2.5mg qpm or qhs if 5mg/day dose is intolerable. Max: 20mg/day in divided doses. Antiemetic: Initial: 5mg/m² 1-3 hrs before chemotherapy, then q2-4h after chemotherapy, for a total of 4-6 doses/day. Titrate: May increase dose by 2.5mg/m² increments. Max: 15mg/m²/dose.
Pediatrics: Antiemetic: Initial: 5mg/m² 1-3 hrs before chemotherapy, then q2-4h after chemotherapy, for a total of 4-6 doses/day. Titrate: May increase dose by 2.5mg/m² increments. Max: 15mg/m²/dose.

HOW SUPPLIED: Cap: 2.5mg, 5mg, 10mg

CONTRAINDICATIONS: Sesame oil hypersensitivity.

WARNINGS/PRECAUTIONS: May impair mental/physical abilities. Seizure and seizure-like activity reported; d/c immediately if seizures develop. Caution with history of seizure disorders, substance abuse, and cardiac disorders due to occasional hypotension, possible HTN, syncope, or tachycardia. Caution in patients with mania, depression, or schizophrenia; exacerbation of these illnesses may occur. Caution in elderly (particularly those with dementia), pregnancy, nursing, and pediatrics.

ADVERSE REACTIONS: Abdominal pain, N/V, dizziness, euphoria, paranoid reaction, somnolence, abnormal thinking.

INTERACTIONS: May displace highly protein-bound drugs; dose requirement changes may be needed. Additive or synergistic CNS effects with sedatives, hypnotics, or other psychoactive drugs. Additive HTN, tachycardia, and possible cardiotoxicity with sympathomimetics (eg,

amphetamines, cocaine). Additive or super-additive tachycardia, and drowsiness with anticholinergics (eg, atropine, scopolamine, antihistamines). Additive tachycardia, HTN, and drowsiness
with TCAs (eg, amitriptyline, amoxapine, desipramine). Additive drowsiness and CNS depression
with CNS depressants (eg, barbiturates, benzodiazepines, ethanol, lithium, opioids, buspirone,
antihistamines, muscle relaxants). May result in hypomanic reaction with disulfiram and fluoxetine
in patients who smoked marijuana. May decrease clearance of antipyrine and barbiturates. May
increase theophylline metabolism in patients who smoked marijuana/tobacco.

PREGNANCY: Category C, not for use in nursing.

MECHANISM OF ACTION: Cannabinoid; has complex effects on the CNS, including central sympathomimetic activity.

PHARMACOKINETICS: Absorption: Administration of variable doses resulted in different pharmacokinetic parameters. **Distribution:** V_d=10L/kg; plasma protein binding (97%); found in breast
milk. **Metabolism:** Liver via microsomal hydroxylation; 11-OH-delta-9-THC (active metabolite).
Elimination: Urine (10-15%), bile/feces (50%, <5% unchanged); $T_{1/2}$=25-36 hrs.

NURSING CONSIDERATIONS

Assessment: Assess for history of hypersensitivity to the drug and sesame oil, history of seizure
disorders, substance abuse (including alcohol abuse/dependence), cardiac disorders, mania,
depression, schizophrenia, pregnancy/nursing status, hepatic/renal impairment, and possible
drug interactions.

Monitoring: Monitor for psychiatric illness exacerbation, abdominal pain, N/V, dizziness, euphoria, paranoid reaction, somnolence, abnormal thinking, hypotension or HTN, syncope, tachycardia, for psychological and physiological dependence, and other adverse reactions.

Patient Counseling: Inform about additive CNS depression effect if taken concomitantly with
alcohol or other CNS depressants (eg, benzodiazepines, barbiturates). Advise to use caution
while performing hazardous tasks (eg, operating machinery/driving) until effect is well-tolerated.
Inform of mood changes and other behavioral effects that may occur during therapy. Advise that
patients must be under constant supervision of a responsible adult during initial use and following dosage adjustments. Instruct to immediately report to physician any adverse effects and
notify if pregnant or breastfeeding.

Administration: Oral route. **Storage:** 8-15°C (46-59°F). Protect from freezing.

M

MAVIK   RX
trandolapril (AbbVie)

> D/C when pregnancy is detected. Drugs that act directly on the renin-angiotensin system (RAS) can cause injury/death to
> the developing fetus.

THERAPEUTIC CLASS: ACE inhibitor

INDICATIONS: Treatment of HTN alone or in combination with other antihypertensives (eg,
HCTZ). For use in stable patients who have evidence of left-ventricular systolic dysfunction or
who are symptomatic from congestive heart failure (CHF) within the 1st few days after sustaining
acute myocardial infarction (MI).

DOSAGE: *Adults:* HTN: Not Receiving Diuretics: Initial: 1mg qd in nonblack patients; 2mg qd in
black patients. Titrate: Adjust dose at intervals of at least 1 week based on BP response. Usual:
2-4mg qd. Little clinical experience with doses >8mg. May treat with bid dosing if inadequately
treated with 4mg qd. May add diuretic if not adequately controlled. Receiving Diuretics: D/C diuretic 2-3 days prior to therapy if possible, then resume diuretic if BP is not controlled. If diuretic
cannot be discontinued, use initial dose of 0.5mg. Titrate to the optimal response as described
above. Heart Failure/Left-Ventricular Dysfunction Post-MI: Initial: 1mg qd. Titrate: Increase to
target dose of 4mg qd as tolerated; if not tolerated, continue with the greatest tolerated dose.
Renal Impairment (CrCl <30mL/min)/Hepatic Cirrhosis: Initial: 0.5mg qd. Titrate to optimal
response as described above.

HOW SUPPLIED: Tab: 1mg*, 2mg, 4mg *scored

CONTRAINDICATIONS: Hereditary/idiopathic angioedema, history of ACE inhibitor-associated
angioedema. Coadministration with aliskiren in patients with diabetes.

WARNINGS/PRECAUTIONS: Anaphylactoid reactions reported during desensitization with
hymenoptera venom, dialysis with high-flux membranes, and LDL apheresis with dextran sulfate
absorption. Angioedema reported; d/c, treat appropriately, and monitor until swelling disappears
if laryngeal stridor or angioedema of the face, tongue, or glottis occurs. Intestinal angioedema
reported; monitor for abdominal pain. Higher rate of angioedema in blacks than nonblacks.
Symptomatic hypotension may occur with volume and/or salt depletion, major surgery, or during anesthesia. Excessive hypotension associated with oliguria and/or azotemia, and rarely with
acute renal failure and/or death may occur in patients with CHF; monitor during first 2 weeks of

therapy and with dosage increases. Caution with ischemic heart disease, aortic stenosis, or cerebrovascular disease; avoid hypotension. Consider lower doses of drug or concomitant diuretic if transient hypotension occurs. May cause agranulocytosis and bone marrow depression; consider periodic monitoring of WBCs in patients with collagen vascular disease (eg, systemic lupus erythematosus, scleroderma) and/or renal disease. Rarely associated with syndrome of cholestatic jaundice, fulminant hepatic necrosis, and death; d/c if jaundice develops. May cause changes in renal function. Increases in BUN and SrCr reported; dosage reduction and/or discontinuation may be required. Hyperkalemia reported; caution with renal insufficiency and diabetes mellitus (DM). Persistent nonproductive cough reported.

ADVERSE REACTIONS: Cough, dizziness, hypotension, elevated serum uric acid, elevated BUN, dyspepsia, syncope, hyperkalemia, bradycardia, hypocalcemia, myalgia, elevated creatinine, gastritis, cardiogenic shock, intermittent claudication.

INTERACTIONS: See Contraindications. Dual blockade of the RAS is associated with increased risks of hypotension, hyperkalemia, and changes in renal function (including acute renal failure); closely monitor BP, renal function, and electrolytes with concomitant agents that also affect the RAS. Avoid with aliskiren in patients with renal impairment (GFR <60mL/min). Excessive BP reduction reported with diuretics. K⁺-sparing diuretics (spironolactone, triamterene, amiloride), K⁺ supplements, or K⁺-containing salt substitutes may increase risk of hyperkalemia; use with caution and monitor serum K⁺. May increase blood glucose lowering effect of antidiabetic medications (insulin, oral hypoglycemic agents). Increased lithium levels and symptoms of lithium toxicity reported; use with caution and frequently monitor serum lithium levels. Increased risk of lithium toxicity if a diuretic is also used. Coadministration with NSAIDs, including selective COX-2 inhibitors, may result in deterioration of renal function; monitor renal function periodically. Antihypertensive effect may be attenuated by NSAIDs. Nitritoid reactions (eg, facial flushing, N/V, hypotension) reported rarely with injectable gold. May enhance hypotensive effect of certain inhalation anesthetics.

PREGNANCY: Category D, not for use in nursing.

MECHANISM OF ACTION: ACE inhibitor; reduces angiotensin II formation, decreases vasoconstriction and aldosterone secretion, and increases plasma renin.

PHARMACOKINETICS: Absorption: Trandolapril: Absolute bioavailability (10%); T_{max}=1 hr. Trandolaprilat: Absolute bioavailability (70%); T_{max}=4-10 hrs. **Distribution:** V_d=18L; plasma protein binding (80% trandolapril; 65-94% trandolaprilat). **Metabolism:** Liver via glucuronidation and deesterification; trandolaprilat (active metabolite). **Elimination:** Urine (33%), feces (66%); $T_{1/2}$=6 hrs (trandolapril), 22.5 hrs (trandolaprilat).

NURSING CONSIDERATIONS

Assessment: Assess for hereditary/idiopathic angioedema, history of ACE inhibitor-associated angioedema, volume/salt depletion, CHF, ischemic heart disease, aortic stenosis, cerebrovascular disease, collagen vascular disease, DM, renal/hepatic impairment, hypersensitivity to the drug, pregnancy/nursing status, and possible drug interactions.

Monitoring: Monitor for anaphylactoid reactions, angioedema, hypotension, jaundice, hyperkalemia, cough, and other adverse reactions. Consider periodic monitoring of WBCs in patients with collagen vascular disease and/or renal disease. Monitor BP and renal/hepatic function.

Patient Counseling: Advise to d/c and consult physician if any signs/symptoms of angioedema (eg, swelling of the face, extremities, eyes, lips, or tongue, or difficulty in swallowing or breathing) develop or if syncope occurs. Inform that lightheadedness may occur, especially during the 1st days of therapy; instruct to report to physician if this occurs. Inform that inadequate fluid intake, excessive perspiration, diarrhea, or vomiting may lead to an excessive fall in BP with the same consequences of lightheadedness and possible syncope. Advise to inform physician of therapy prior to surgery and/or anesthesia. Advise not to use K⁺ supplements or salt substitutes containing K⁺ without consulting physician. Instruct to immediately report any signs/symptoms of infection (eg, sore throat, fever). Inform females of childbearing age about the consequences of exposure during pregnancy. Instruct to report pregnancies to physician as soon as possible.

Administration: Oral route. **Storage:** 20-25°C (68-77°F).

MAXAIR   RX
pirbuterol acetate (Medicis)

THERAPEUTIC CLASS: Beta₂-agonist

INDICATIONS: Prevention and reversal of bronchospasm in patients ≥12 yrs of age with reversible bronchospasm, including asthma, as monotherapy or with theophylline and/or corticosteroids.

DOSAGE: *Adults:* 2 inh (400mcg) q4-6h; 1 inh (200mcg) q4-6h may be sufficient for some patients. Max: 12 inh/day.

Pediatrics: ≥12 Yrs: 2 inh (400mcg) q4-6h; 1 inh (200mcg) q4-6h may be sufficient for some patients. Max: 12 inh/day.

HOW SUPPLIED: MDI: 200mcg/actuation [80, 400 inhalations]

WARNINGS/PRECAUTIONS: If a previously effective dose regimen fails to provide the usual relief or if more doses than usual are needed, this may be a marker of destabilization of asthma and may require reevaluation of the patient and treatment regimen; d/c immediately and institute alternative therapy if this develops. D/C if cardiovascular (CV) effects occur. ECG changes may occur. Caution with CV disorders (eg, coronary insufficiency, ischemic heart disease, HTN, arrhythmias), hyperthyroidism, diabetes mellitus (DM), convulsive disorders, and in patients unusually responsive to sympathomimetic amines. May cause significant BP changes and hypokalemia.

ADVERSE REACTIONS: Nervousness, tremor.

INTERACTIONS: Avoid with other short-acting β-adrenergic aerosol bronchodilators. Use extreme caution with MAOIs or TCAs, or within 2 weeks of discontinuation of such agents. ECG changes and/or hypokalemia caused by non-K⁺-sparing diuretics (eg, loop or thiazide diuretics) may be worsened; use with caution. Use with β-blockers may block pulmonary effects and produce severe bronchospasm in asthmatic patients; avoid concomitant use. If needed, consider cardioselective β-blockers and use with caution.

PREGNANCY: Category C, caution in nursing.

MECHANISM OF ACTION: β_2-agonist; stimulation through β_2-adrenergic receptors of intracellular adenyl cyclase, the enzyme which catalyzes the conversion of adenosine triphosphate to cyclic-3',5'-cAMP. Increased cAMP levels are associated with relaxation of bronchial smooth muscle and inhibition of release of mediators of immediate hypersensitivity from cells, especially from mast cells.

PHARMACOKINETICS: Elimination: Urine (51%); $T_{1/2}$=2 hrs (PO).

NURSING CONSIDERATIONS

Assessment: Assess for history of drug hypersensitivity, CV disorders, convulsive disorders, hyperthyroidism, DM, pregnancy/nursing status, and possible drug interactions. Assess use in patients unusually responsive to sympathomimetic amines.

Monitoring: Monitor for paradoxical bronchospasm, CV effects, hypokalemia, hypersensitivity reactions, deterioration of asthma, and other adverse effects. Monitor BP, HR, and ECG changes.

Patient Counseling: Counsel not to increase dose/frequency of doses without consulting physician. Advise to seek immediate medical attention if treatment becomes less effective for symptomatic relief, symptoms become worse, and/or there is a need to use the product more frequently than usual. Instruct to take concurrent inhaled drugs and other asthma medications only ud by physician. Inform of the common side effects (eg, chest pain, palpitations, rapid HR, tremor, nervousness). Instruct to contact physician if pregnant/nursing. Instruct not to use with any other inhalation aerosol canister or any other actuator.

Administration: Oral inhalation route. Shake well before use. Prime autohaler before use for the 1st time or if not used in 48 hrs by releasing 2 sprays into the air. Avoid spraying in eyes.

Storage: 15-30°C (59-86°F). Contents under pressure; do not puncture, use/store near heat or open flame, or throw container into fire/incinerator. Exposure to temperature >49°C (120°F) may cause bursting.

MAXALT   RX
rizatriptan benzoate (Merck)

OTHER BRAND NAMES: Maxalt-MLT (Merck)

THERAPEUTIC CLASS: 5-HT$_{1B/1D}$ agonist

INDICATIONS: Acute treatment of migraine with or without aura in adults and in pediatric patients 6-17 yrs of age.

DOSAGE: *Adults:* Usual: 5mg or 10mg single dose. Separate repeat doses by at least 2 hrs if migraine returns. Max: 30mg/24 hrs. Concomitant Propranolol: Usual: 5mg single dose. Max: 3 doses/24 hrs. Elderly: Start at lower end of dosing range.
Pediatrics: 6-17 Yrs: ≥40kg: Usual: 10mg single dose. <40kg: Usual: 5mg single dose. Concomitant Propranolol: ≥40kg: Usual: 5mg single dose. Max: 5mg/24 hrs.

HOW SUPPLIED: Tab: 5mg, 10mg; Tab, Disintegrating: (MLT) 5mg, 10mg

CONTRAINDICATIONS: Ischemic coronary artery disease (CAD) (angina pectoris, history of myocardial infarction [MI], or documented silent ischemia) or other significant underlying cardiovascular (CV) disease, coronary artery vasospasm (eg, Prinzmetal's angina), history of stroke or transient ischemic attack (TIA), peripheral vascular disease (PVD), ischemic bowel disease, uncontrolled HTN, hemiplegic/basilar migraine. Recent use (within 24 hrs) of another 5-hydroxytriptamine-1 (5-HT₁) agonist or ergotamine-containing/ergot-type medication (eg, dihydroergotamine, methysergide). Concurrent use or recent discontinuation (within 2 weeks) of an MAO-A inhibitor.

WARNINGS/PRECAUTIONS: Use only when diagnosis of migraine has been clearly established. If no response after the 1st migraine attack, reconsider diagnosis before treating subsequent attacks. Not indicated for prevention of migraine attacks. Serious cardiac adverse reactions, including acute MI, reported. May cause coronary artery vasospasm (Prinzmetal's angina). Perform CV evaluation prior to therapy with multiple CV risk factors; consider administering 1st dose in a medically-supervised setting and perform ECG immediately following administration in patients with a negative CV evaluation. Consider periodic CV evaluation in intermittent long-term users who have CV risk factors. Life-threatening cardiac rhythm disturbances (eg, ventricular tachycardia/fibrillation leading to death) reported; d/c if these occur. Sensations of tightness, pain, pressure, and heaviness in precordium, throat, neck, and jaw, usually of noncardiac origin, commonly occur after treatment; evaluate if cardiac origin is suspected. Cerebral/subarachnoid hemorrhage and stroke reported; d/c if cerebrovascular event occurs. Evaluate for other potentially serious neurological conditions before treatment. May cause noncoronary vasospastic reactions (eg, peripheral vascular ischemia, GI vascular ischemia, splenic infarction, Raynaud's syndrome); rule out before administering additional doses if experiencing signs/symptoms of noncoronary vasospasms. Transient and permanent blindness and significant partial vision loss reported. Overuse of acute migraine drugs may lead to exacerbation of headache (medication overuse headache); detoxification, including withdrawal of the overused drugs, and treatment of withdrawal symptoms may be necessary. Serotonin syndrome may occur; d/c if serotonin syndrome is suspected. Significant elevation in BP, including hypertensive crisis with acute impairment of organ systems, reported. Caution in elderly. (Tab, Disintegrating) Contains phenylalanine.

ADVERSE REACTIONS: Paresthesia, dry mouth, nausea, dizziness, somnolence, asthenia/fatigue, pain/pressure sensation.

INTERACTIONS: See Contraindications. Increased plasma area under the curve with propranolol; adjust dose. Serotonin syndrome reported with SSRIs, SNRIs, and TCAs.

PREGNANCY: Category C, caution in nursing.

MECHANISM OF ACTION: 5-HT₁B/₁D receptor agonist; binds with high affinity to human cloned 5-HT₁B/₁D receptors located on intracranial blood vessels and sensory nerves of the trigeminal system.

PHARMACOKINETICS: Absorption: Complete. Absolute bioavailability (45%) (tab); T_{max}=1-1.5 hrs (tab), delayed by up to 0.7 hr (tab, disintegrating). **Distribution:** V_d=140L (male), 110L (female); plasma protein binding (14%). **Metabolism:** Oxidative deamination by MAO-A; N-monodesmethyl-rizatriptan (active metabolite). **Elimination:** Urine (82%; 14% unchanged, 51% indole acetic acid metabolite), feces (12%); $T_{1/2}$=2-3 hrs.

NURSING CONSIDERATIONS

Assessment: Assess for ischemic CAD or other significant underlying CV disease, history of stroke or TIA, PVD, ischemic bowel disease, uncontrolled HTN, hemiplegic/basilar migraine, neurological conditions, phenylketonuria, drug hypersensitivity, pregnancy/nursing status, and possible drug interactions. Perform CV evaluation with multiple CV risk factors.

Monitoring: Monitor for coronary artery vasospasm, cardiac rhythm disturbances, cerebrovascular event, noncoronary vasospastic reactions, serotonin syndrome, BP elevation, and other adverse reactions. Consider periodic CV evaluation in intermittent long-term users who have CV risk factors.

Patient Counseling: Inform of possible serious CV side effects, including chest pain, SOB, weakness, and slurring of speech, and to seek medical advice in the presence of such symptoms. Caution about the risk of serotonin syndrome. Advise to notify physician if pregnant, breastfeeding, or planning to breastfeed. Instruct to evaluate their ability to perform complex tasks during migraine attacks and after administration. Inform that overuse (≥10 days/month) may lead to exacerbation of headache; encourage to record headache frequency and drug use. (Tab, Disintegrating) Inform phenylketonuric patients that tab contains phenylalanine.

Administration: Oral route. (Tab, Disintegrating) Do not remove blister from outer pouch until just prior to dosing. Peel open with dry hands and place tab on tongue, where it will dissolve and be swallowed with saliva. **Storage:** 15-30°C (59-86°F).

MAXIPIME   RX
cefepime HCl (Hospira)

THERAPEUTIC CLASS: Cephalosporin (4th generation)

INDICATIONS: Treatment of uncomplicated/complicated urinary tract infections (UTIs), including pyelonephritis, uncomplicated skin and skin structure infections (SSSIs), complicated intra-abdominal infections (in combination with metronidazole), pneumonia (moderate to severe), and empirical therapy for febrile neutropenia caused by susceptible strains of microorganisms.

DOSAGE: *Adults:* Moderate to Severe Pneumonia: 1-2g IV q12h for 10 days. Febrile Neutropenia: 2g IV q8h for 7 days or until neutropenia resolves. Reevaluate frequently the need for continued antimicrobial therapy in patients whose fever resolves but remain neutropenic for >7 days. Mild to Moderate UTI: 0.5-1g IM/IV q12h for 7-10 days. IM administration is indicated only for UTIs due to *Escherichia coli* when IM route is considered to be more appropriate route of administration. Severe UTI/Moderate to Severe Uncomplicated SSSI: 2g IV q12h for 10 days. Complicated Intra-Abdominal Infections: 2g IV q12h for 7-10 days. Renal Impairment: Refer to PI for recommended dosing schedule.
Pediatrics: 2 Months-16 Yrs: ≤40kg: UTI/Uncomplicated SSSI/Pneumonia: 50mg/kg/dose q12h. Severe UTI/Moderate to Severe Pneumonia/Moderate to Severe Uncomplicated SSSI: Give IV for 10 days. Mild to Moderate UTI: Give IM/IV for 7-10 days. IM administration is indicated only for UTIs due to *E. coli* when IM route is considered to be more appropriate route of administration. Febrile Neutropenia: 50mg/kg/dose IV q8h for 7 days or until neutropenia resolves. Reevaluate frequently the need for continued antimicrobial therapy in patients whose fever resolves but remain neutropenic for >7 days. Max: Do not exceed the recommended adult dose.

HOW SUPPLIED: Inj: 500mg, 1g, 2g

CONTRAINDICATIONS: Hypersensitivity to penicillins (PCNs) or other β-lactam antibiotics.

WARNINGS/PRECAUTIONS: Caution with PCN sensitivity; cross hypersensitivity among β-lactam antibiotics reported. D/C if an allergic reaction occurs. Caution with renal impairment; dose reduction may be needed. Encephalopathy, myoclonus, seizures, nonconvulsive status epilepticus reported. If neurotoxicity associated with therapy occurs, consider discontinuation of therapy or make appropriate dose adjustments in patients with renal impairment. *Clostridium difficile*-associated diarrhea (CDAD) reported; d/c if CDAD is suspected or confirmed. May result in overgrowth of nonsusceptible organisms with prolonged use; take appropriate measures if superinfection develops. Use in the absence of a proven or strongly suspected bacterial infection or prophylactic indication is unlikely to provide benefit and increases the risk of development of drug-resistant bacteria. May cause a fall in prothrombin activity. Caution in patients with renal/hepatic impairment, poor nutritional state, and in patients on a protracted course of antimicrobials; monitor PT and administer exogenous vitamin K as indicated. Caution with history of GI disease, particularly colitis. Lab test interactions may occur. Caution in elderly.

ADVERSE REACTIONS: Local reactions, rash, diarrhea, positive Coombs' test without hemolysis.

INTERACTIONS: Increased risk of nephrotoxicity and ototoxicity with high doses of aminoglycosides; monitor renal function. Nephrotoxicity with potent diuretics (eg, furosemide) reported.

PREGNANCY: Category B, caution in nursing.

MECHANISM OF ACTION: Cephalosporin (4th generation); bactericidal agent that acts by inhibiting cell-wall synthesis.

PHARMACOKINETICS: Absorption: Complete (IM). (IV/IM) Administration of variable doses resulted in different parameters. **Distribution:** V_d=18L; plasma protein binding (20%); found in breast milk. **Metabolism:** Metabolized to N-methylpyrrolidine (NMP), which is rapidly converted to the N-oxide (NMP-N-oxide). **Elimination:** Urine (85% unchanged, <1% NMP, 6.8% NMP-N-oxide, 2.5% epimer of cefepime); $T_{1/2}$=2 hrs.

NURSING CONSIDERATIONS

Assessment: Assess for hypersensitivity to cephalosporins, PCNs, or other β-lactam antibiotics, nutritional status, history of GI disease, renal/hepatic impairment, pregnancy/nursing status, and for possible drug interactions. Perform culture and susceptibility testing.

Monitoring: Monitor for signs/symptoms of hypersensitivity reactions (anaphylaxis), CDAD, superinfection, encephalopathy, myoclonus, seizures, nonconvulsive status epilepticus, and other adverse reactions. Monitor PT in patients with renal/hepatic impairment, poor nutritional state, and in patients on a protracted course of antimicrobials.

Patient Counseling: Counsel that drug treats only bacterial, not viral, infections (eg, common colds). Instruct to take ud; inform that skipping doses or not completing full course of therapy may decrease drug effectiveness and increase bacterial resistance. Inform that diarrhea (as late as ≥2 months after last dose), encephalopathy, myoclonus, seizures, and nonconvulsive status epilepticus may occur. Instruct to contact physician if watery/bloody stools (with/without stomach cramps and fever), hypersensitivity reactions, or neurological signs/symptoms (eg, confusion, hallucinations, stupor, or coma) occur.

Administration: IV/IM route. When giving IV, infuse over 30 min. Refer to PI for compatibility and instructions for use. **Storage:** 20-25°C (68-77°F). Protect from light. Refer to PI for stability information.

M

MAXITROL   RX
neomycin sulfate - polymyxin B sulfate - dexamethasone (Alcon)

THERAPEUTIC CLASS: Antibacterial/corticosteroid combination

INDICATIONS: For steroid-responsive inflammatory ocular conditions for which a corticosteroid is indicated and where bacterial infection or the risk of bacterial ocular infection exist.

DOSAGE: *Adults:* (Oint) Apply 1/2 inch in conjunctival sac(s) up to 3-4 times daily. Max: 8g for initial prescription. (Sus) Instill 1-2 drops in conjunctival sac(s) up to 4-6 times daily in mild disease and qh in severe disease. Taper to d/c as inflammation subsides. Max: 20mL for initial prescription.

HOW SUPPLIED: Oint: (Dexamethasone-Neomycin sulfate-Polymyxin sulfate) 0.1%-3.5mg-10,000 U/g [3.5g]; Sus: (Dexamethasone-Neomycin sulfate-Polymyxin sulfate) 0.1%-3.5mg-10,000 U/mL [5mL]

CONTRAINDICATIONS: Epithelial herpes simplex keratitis (dendritic keratitis), vaccinia, varicella, and other viral diseases of the cornea and conjunctiva, mycobacterial infection of the eye, fungal diseases of ocular structures.

WARNINGS/PRECAUTIONS: For topical ophthalmic use only. Prolonged use may cause glaucoma with damage to the optic nerve, defects in visual acuity and fields of vision, posterior subcapsular cataract formation, suppressed host response, increased risk of secondary ocular infections, or persistent corneal fungal infections. May cause perforations when used with diseases causing thinning of cornea or sclera. May mask infection or enhance existing infection in acute purulent conditions of the eye. Monitor intraocular pressure (IOP) if used for ≥10 days. May cause cutaneous sensitization. Caution in the treatment of herpes simplex. Perform eye exam prior to therapy and renewal of medication. (Sus) Usage after cataract surgery may delay healing and increase incidence of bleb formation. May prolong course and exacerbate severity of ocular viral infections (eg, herpes simplex). Do not inject subconjunctivally, nor directly introduce into anterior chamber of the eye. Reevaluate patient if no improvement seen after 2 days. Suspect fungal invasion in any persistent corneal ulceration during or after therapy; take fungal cultures when appropriate.

ADVERSE REACTIONS: Allergic sensitizations, elevated IOP, posterior subcapsular cataract formation, delayed wound healing, secondary infections.

PREGNANCY: Category C, caution in nursing.

MECHANISM OF ACTION: Antibacterial/corticosteroid combination. Dexamethasone: Corticosteroid; suppresses the inflammatory response to a variety of agents. May inhibit the body's defense mechanism against infection.

PHARMACOKINETICS: Distribution: (Systemically administered) found in breast milk.

NURSING CONSIDERATIONS

Assessment: Assess for active viral diseases of the cornea and conjunctiva, epithelial herpes simplex keratitis, vaccinia, varicella, mycobacterial infection of the eye, fungal disease of ocular structures, diseases causing thinning of sclera or cornea, acute purulent conditions, history of cataract surgery, hypersensitivity to the drug or its components, and pregnancy/nursing status. Perform eye exam (eg, slit lamp biomicroscopy, flourescein staining) prior to therapy.

Monitoring: Monitor for signs/symptoms of glaucoma, optic nerve damage, visual acuity and visual field defects, subcapsular cataract, ocular/corneal perforations, cutaneous sensitizations, bacterial, viral, fungal infections. Monitor IOP and perform eye exams (eg, slit lamp biomicroscopy, flourescein staining) prior to renewal of medication. (Sus) Monitor use after cataract surgery. Perform fungal cultures when fungal invasion is suspected.

Patient Counseling: Advise not to touch dropper tip to any surface; may contaminate drug. Instruct to keep out of reach of children. Instruct to use medication as prescribed. Inform that medication is for topical ophthalmic use only. Instruct to inform physician if pregnant or breast-feeding. (Oint) Advise not to wear contact lenses if signs and symptoms of bacterial ocular infection are present. Instruct not to use product if the imprinted carton seals have been damaged or removed. (Sus) Advise to d/c and consult physician if inflammation or pain persists >48 hrs or becomes aggravated. Warn that use of the same bottle by more than one person may spread infection. Instruct to shake well before use and keep bottle tightly closed when not in use.

Administration: Ocular route. (Oint) Tilt head back. Place finger on cheek just under the eye and gently pull down until a "V" pocket is formed between eyeball and lower lid. Place small amount of oint in the "V" pocket. Look downward before closing the eye. **Storage:** (Oint) 2-25°C (36-77°F). (Sus) 8-27°C (46-80°F). Store upright.

MAXZIDE   RX
hydrochlorothiazide - triamterene (Mylan Bertek)

> Abnormal elevation of serum K⁺ levels (≥5.5mEq/L) may occur with all K⁺-sparing diuretic combinations. Hyperkalemia is more likely to occur with renal impairment and diabetes (even without evidence of renal impairment), and in elderly or severely ill; monitor serum K⁺ levels at frequent intervals.

OTHER BRAND NAMES: Maxzide-25 (Mylan Bertek)

THERAPEUTIC CLASS: K⁺-sparing diuretic/thiazide diuretic

INDICATIONS: Treatment of HTN or edema if hypokalemia occurs on HCTZ alone, or when a thiazide diuretic is required and cannot risk hypokalemia. May be used alone or as an adjunct to other antihypertensives, such as β-blockers.

DOSAGE: *Adults:* (Maxzide-25) 1-2 tabs qd, given as a single dose or (Maxzide) 1 tab qd.

HOW SUPPLIED: Tab: (Triamterene-HCTZ) (Maxzide) 75mg-50mg*, (Maxzide-25) 37.5mg-25mg* *scored

CONTRAINDICATIONS: Elevated serum K⁺ (≥5.5mEq/L), anuria, acute or chronic renal insufficiency or significant renal impairment, sulfonamide hypersensitivity, K⁺-sparing agents (eg, spironolactone, amiloride, or other formulations containing triamterene), K⁺ supplements, K⁺ salt substitutes, K⁺-enriched diets.

WARNINGS/PRECAUTIONS: Obtain ECG if hyperkalemia is suspected. Avoid in severely ill in whom respiratory or metabolic acidosis may occur; if used, frequent evaluations of acid/base balance and serum electrolytes are necessary. May cause idiosyncratic reaction, resulting in acute transient myopia and acute angle-closure glaucoma; d/c as rapidly as possible. Monitor for fluid/electrolyte imbalances. May manifest latent diabetes mellitus (DM). Caution with hepatic impairment or progressive liver disease; minor alterations in fluid and electrolyte balance may precipitate hepatic coma. May cause hypochloremia. Dilutional hyponatremia may occur in edematous patients in hot weather. Caution with history of renal lithiasis. May increase BUN and SrCr; d/c if azotemia increases. May contribute to megaloblastosis in folic acid deficiency. Hyperuricemia may occur or acute gout may be precipitated. May decrease serum PBI levels. Decreased Ca²⁺ excretion reported. Changes in parathyroid glands with hypercalcemia and hypophosphatemia reported during prolonged use. Sensitivity reactions may occur. May exacerbate or activate systemic lupus erythematosus (SLE). May interfere with the fluorescent measurement of quinidine.

ADVERSE REACTIONS: Hyperkalemia, jaundice, pancreatitis, N/V, taste alteration, drowsiness, dry mouth, depression, anxiety, tachycardia, fluid/electrolyte imbalances.

INTERACTIONS: See Contraindications. Increased risk of hyperkalemia with ACE inhibitors. Hypokalemia may develop with corticosteroids, adrenocorticotropic hormone, or amphotericin B. Insulin requirements may be increased, decreased, or unchanged. May potentiate other antihypertensives (eg, β-blockers); dosage adjustments may be necessary. Avoid with lithium due to risk of lithium toxicity. Acute renal failure reported with indomethacin; caution with NSAIDs. May increase responsiveness to tubocurarine. May decrease arterial responsiveness to norepinephrine. Alcohol, barbiturates, or narcotics may aggravate orthostatic hypotension. May cause hypokalemia, which can sensitize or exaggerate the response of the heart to the toxic effects of digitalis (eg, increased ventricular irritability).

PREGNANCY: Category C, not for use in nursing.

MECHANISM OF ACTION: Triamterene: K⁺-sparing diuretic; exerts diuretic effect on distal renal tubule to inhibit the reabsorption of Na⁺ in exchange for K⁺ and H⁺. HCTZ: Thiazide diuretic; blocks renal tubular absorption of Na⁺ and Cl⁻ ions. This natriuresis and diuresis is accompanied by a secondary loss of K⁺ and bicarbonate.

PHARMACOKINETICS: Absorption: Well-absorbed. HCTZ: T_{max}=2 hrs. Triamterene: Rapid, T_{max}=1 hr. **Distribution:** Crosses placenta; found in breast milk. **Metabolism:** Triamterene: Sulfate conjugation; hydroxytriamterene (metabolite). **Elimination:** HCTZ: Urine (unchanged).

NURSING CONSIDERATIONS

Assessment: Assess for conditions where treatment is contraindicated or cautioned, DM, risk for respiratory or metabolic acidosis, SLE, pregnancy/nursing status, and for possible drug interactions. Obtain baseline BUN, SrCr, and serum electrolytes.

Monitoring: Monitor for signs/symptoms of hyperkalemia, idiosyncratic reaction, hypokalemia, azotemia, renal stones, hepatic coma, and for fluid/electrolyte imbalances. Monitor BUN, SrCr, and serum K⁺ and folic acid levels. Monitor serum and urine electrolytes if vomiting or receiving parenteral fluids.

Patient Counseling: Inform about risks/benefits of therapy. Advise to seek medical attention if symptoms of hyperkalemia (eg, paresthesias, muscular weakness, fatigue), hypokalemia, renal

M

stones, electrolyte imbalance (eg, dry mouth, thirst, weakness), or hypersensitivity reactions occur. Instruct to notify physician if pregnant/nursing.

Administration: Oral route. **Storage:** 20-25°C (68-77°F). Protect from light.

MEDROL

RX

methylprednisolone (Pharmacia & Upjohn)

THERAPEUTIC CLASS: Glucocorticoid

INDICATIONS: Steroid-responsive disorders.

DOSAGE: *Adults:* Individualize dose. Initial: 4-48mg/day, depending on disease and response. Maint: Decrease dose by small amounts to lowest effective dose. Withdraw gradually after long-term therapy. Acute Exacerbations of Multiple Sclerosis: 200mg/day for 1 week followed by 80mg qod for 1 month. Alternate Day Therapy (ADT): Twice the usual daily dose administered every other am. Refer to PI for detailed information on ADT.
Pediatric: Individualize dose. Initial: 4-48mg/day depending on disease and response. Maint: Decrease dose by small amounts to lowest effective dose. Withdraw gradually after long-term therapy. Acute Exacerbations of Multiple Sclerosis: 200mg/day for 1 week followed by 80mg qod for 1 month. ADT: Twice the usual daily dose administered every other am. Refer to PI for detailed information on ADT.

HOW SUPPLIED: Tab: 2mg*, 4mg*, 8mg*, 16mg*, 32mg*; (Dose-Pak) 4mg* [21ˢ] *scored

CONTRAINDICATIONS: Systemic fungal infections.

WARNINGS/PRECAUTIONS: May need to increase dose before, during, and after stressful situations. May mask signs of infection or cause new infections. Possible benefits should be weighed against potential hazards if used during pregnancy/nursing. Prolonged use may produce glaucoma, optic nerve damage, and secondary ocular infections. May cause BP elevation, increased K^+ excretion, and salt/water retention. More severe/fatal course of infections reported with chickenpox, measles. Caution with strongyloides, latent tuberculosis (TB), hypothyroidism, cirrhosis, ocular herpes simplex, HTN, diverticulitis, fresh intestinal anastomoses, ulcerative colitis, osteoporosis, myasthenia gravis, renal insufficiency, and peptic ulcer disease. Kaposi's sarcoma reported. Growth and development of children on prolonged therapy should be monitored. Monitor for psychic disturbances. Avoid abrupt withdrawal.

ADVERSE REACTIONS: Fluid and electrolyte disturbances, HTN, osteoporosis, muscle weakness, cushingoid state, menstrual irregularities, impaired wound healing, convulsions, ulcerative esophagitis, excessive sweating, increased intracranial pressure, glaucoma, abdominal distention, headache, decreased carbohydrate tolerance.

INTERACTIONS: Reduced efficacy with hepatic enzyme inducers (eg, phenobarbital, phenytoin, rifampin). Increases clearance of chronic high-dose aspirin (ASA). Caution with ASA in hypoprothrombinemia. Effects on oral anticoagulants are variable; monitor PT. Increased insulin and oral hypoglycemic requirements in diabetics. Avoid live vaccines with immunosuppressive doses. Possible decreased vaccine response with killed or inactivated vaccines with immunosuppressive doses. Mutual inhibition of metabolism with cyclosporine; convulsions reported. Potentiated by ketoconazole and troleandomycin. Concomitant administration with immunosuppressive agents may be associated with development of infections.

PREGNANCY: Safety in pregnancy and nursing not known.

MECHANISM OF ACTION: Anti-inflammatory glucocorticoid; causes profound and varied metabolic effects and modifies the body's immune responses to diverse stimuli.

PHARMACOKINETICS: Absorption: Readily absorbed from GI tract.

NURSING CONSIDERATIONS

Assessment: Assess for systemic fungal infections, current infections, active TB, vaccination history, ulcerative colitis, diverticulitis, peptic ulcer with impending perforation, renal/hepatic insufficiency, septic arthritis/unstable joint, HTN, osteoporosis, myasthenia gravis, thyroid status, psychotic tendencies, drug hypersensitivity and possible drug interactions.

Monitoring: Monitor for adrenocortical insufficiency, occurrence of infection, psychic derangement, cataracts, acute myopathy, Kaposi's sarcoma, and fluid retention. Monitor serum electrolytes, TSH, LFTs, intraocular pressure, and BP. Monitor urinalysis, blood sugar, weight, chest x-ray, and upper GI x-ray (if ulcer history) regularly during prolonged therapy. Monitor growth and development of infants and children on prolonged corticosteroids therapy.

Patient Counseling: Advise not to d/c abruptly or without medical supervision. Inform that susceptibility to infections may increase. Instruct to avoid exposure to chickenpox or measles and to seek medical advice immediately if exposed. Recommend dietary salt restriction and K^+ supplementation.

Administration: Oral route. **Storage:** 20-25°C (68-77°F).

MEFLOQUINE

RX

mefloquine HCl (Various)

THERAPEUTIC CLASS: Quinolinemethanol derivative

INDICATIONS: Treatment of mild to moderate acute malaria caused by susceptible strains of *Plasmodium falciparum* and/or *P. vivax*. Prophylaxis of *P. falciparum* and *P. vivax* malaria infections, including prophylaxis of chloroquine-resistant strains of *P. falciparum*.

DOSAGE: *Adults:* Treatment: 5 tabs (1250mg) single dose. If no improvement within 48 to 72 hrs, use alternative therapy. To avoid relapse after initial treatment of acute infection, subsequently treat with an 8-aminoquinoline derivative (eg, primaquine). Prophylaxis: 250mg once weekly. Take subsequent weekly doses regularly, always on the same day of each week, after the main meal. Start 1 week before arrival in endemic area and continue for additional 4 weeks after leaving.
Pediatrics: Treatment: ≥6 Months: 20-25mg/kg in 2 divided doses taken 6-8 hrs apart. Max: 1250mg. If no improvement within 48 to 72 hours, use alternative therapy. If vomiting occurs <30 min after dose, give a 2nd full dose. If vomiting occurs 30-60 min after dose, give additional half-dose. If vomiting recurs, consider alternative treatment if no improvement within a reasonable period of time. Prophylaxis: 5mg/kg once weekly. >45kg: 1 tab/week. 30-45kg: 3/4 tab once weekly. 20-30kg: 1/2 tab once weekly.

HOW SUPPLIED: Tab: 250mg* *scored

CONTRAINDICATIONS: For prophylaxis in patients with active or recent history of depression, generalized anxiety disorder, psychosis, schizophrenia, or other major psychiatric disorders, or with a history of convulsions.

WARNINGS/PRECAUTIONS: Do not use for curative treatment if previous prophylaxis has failed. High risk of relapse seen with acute *P. vivax*; after initial treatment, subsequently treat with 8-aminoquinoline (eg, primaquine). Use IV antimalarials in life-threatening, serious, or overwhelming malaria infection due to *P. falciparum*; may give tab after completion of IV treatment. May cause neuropsychiatric adverse reactions; monitor these symptoms, especially in nonverbal children. Psychiatric symptoms (eg, anxiety, depression) and suicidal ideation/suicide may occur. During prophylactic use, psychiatric symptoms suggest a risk for more serious psychiatric disturbances or neurologic adverse reactions; d/c therapy and substitute alternative medication. Neurological symptoms (eg, dizziness, vertigo, tinnitus, loss of balance) reported; d/c therapy and substitute alternative medication if these occur during prophylactic use. May impair mental/ physical abilities. Increased risk of convulsions in epileptic patients; use only for curative treatment if there are compelling reasons in such patients. Hypersensitivity reactions reported. Higher risk of adverse reactions in patients with liver dysfunction. Periodically perform ophthalmic exams with long-term use. Transitory and clinically silent ECG alterations reported. Geographical drug resistance patterns of *P. falciparum* occur and the preferred choice of malaria prophylaxis might be different from one area to another. Agranulocytosis and aplastic anemia reported. Caution in elderly.

ADVERSE REACTIONS: Cardiopulmonary arrest, N/V, myalgia, fever, dizziness, headache, chills, diarrhea, abdominal pain, fatigue, tinnitus, loss of appetite, skin rash.

INTERACTIONS: Do not administer with halofantrine or ketoconazole within 15 weeks of the last dose of mefloquine tab; may prolong QT interval. Increased plasma concentration and $T_{1/2}$ with ketoconazole. Concomitant administration with other related antimalarial compounds may cause ECG abnormalities and increase risk of convulsions; delay mefloquine dose at least 12 hrs after last dose of these drugs. Cardiopulmonary arrest, with full recovery, reported when used concomitantly with a β-blocker (eg, propranolol). Coadministration of drugs known to alter cardiac conduction (eg, anti-arrhythmic, calcium channel blockers, antihistamines, TCAs, and phenothiazines) may contribute to QT interval prolongation. May reduce seizure control by lowering plasma levels of anticonvulsants; monitor levels of anticonvulsant medication and adjust dosage accordingly. Complete vaccinations with live, attenuated vaccines (eg, typhoid vaccine) at least 3 days before 1st dose of therapy. Caution with rifampin. Evaluate diabetics and patients on anticoagulants prior to departure. CYP3A4 inhibitors may increase plasma concentrations, and CYP3A4 inducers may decrease plasma concentrations; use with caution when administered concomitantly.

PREGNANCY: Category B, caution in nursing.

MECHANISM OF ACTION: Quinolinemethanol derivative; has not been established. Suspected to act as blood schizonticide.

PHARMACOKINETICS: **Absorption:** C_{max}=1000-2000mcg/L (250mg/week); T_{max}=17 hrs (median, single dose), 7-10 weeks (250mg/week). **Distribution:** V_d=20L/kg; plasma protein binding (98%); crosses placenta; found in breast milk. **Metabolism:** Extensive. Liver via CYP3A4; 2,8-bis-trifluoromethyl-4-quinoline carboxylic acid. **Elimination:** Bile/feces, urine (9% unchanged, 4% metabolite); $T_{1/2}$=3 weeks.

NURSING CONSIDERATIONS

Assessment: Assess for active/history of depression, generalized anxiety disorder, psychosis, schizophrenia, other major psychiatric disorders, epilepsy, liver dysfunction, cardiac disease, pregnancy status/nursing, drug hypersensitivity, and possible drug interactions.

Monitoring: Monitor for neurologic/psychiatric symptoms, hypersensitivity reactions, convulsions, ECG alterations, agranulocytosis, and aplastic anemia. Periodically evaluate LFTs, neuropsychiatric effects, and perform ophthalmic exams.

Patient Counseling: Instruct to read Medication Guide. Inform that malaria can be a life-threatening infection and that drug is prescribed to help prevent/treat this serious infection. Inform that dizziness, vertigo, or loss of balance may occur, and it may be necessary to change medications. Inform that insomnia may occur. Instruct to take 1st dose one week prior to arrival in an endemic area if used as prophylaxis. Inform that if psychiatric symptoms occur, therapy should be discontinued and an alternative medication should be substituted. Advise that no chemoprophylactic regimen is 100% effective; use of protective clothing, insect repellants, and bed nets are important components of malaria prophylaxis. Instruct to seek medical attention for any febrile illness that occurs after return from a malaria area and to inform physician that they may have been exposed to malaria.

Administration: Oral route. Do not take on empty stomach and administer with ample water (at least 8 oz. (240mL) in adults). May crush and suspend tab in small amount of water, milk, or other beverages for small children/other persons unable to swallow tab whole. **Storage:** 20-25°C (68-77°F).

MEGACE ES   RX
megestrol acetate (Par)

OTHER BRAND NAMES: Megace (Bristol-Myers Squibb)

THERAPEUTIC CLASS: Progesterone

INDICATIONS: Treatment of anorexia, cachexia, or an unexplained, significant weight loss in AIDS patients.

DOSAGE: *Adults:* (Megace) Initial: 800mg/day (20mL/day). Effective Dose Range: 400-800mg/day. (Megace ES) Initial: 625mg/day (5mL/day).

HOW SUPPLIED: Sus: (Megace) 40mg/mL [240mL]; (Megace ES) 125mg/mL [150mL]

CONTRAINDICATIONS: Known or suspected pregnancy.

WARNINGS/PRECAUTIONS: May cause fetal harm when administered to a pregnant woman. Not for prophylactic use to avoid weight loss. New onset or exacerbation of preexisting diabetes mellitus (DM) and overt Cushing's syndrome reported with chronic use; may increase insulin requirements in patients with DM. Adrenal insufficiency reported in patients receiving or being withdrawn from chronic therapy; laboratory evaluation for adrenal insufficiency and consideration of replacement or stress doses of a rapidly acting glucocorticoid are strongly recommended. Caution with history of thromboembolic disease and in elderly. Institute only after treatable causes of weight loss are sought and addressed. Breakthrough bleeding reported in women.

ADVERSE REACTIONS: Diarrhea, impotence, rash, flatulence, nausea, HTN, asthenia, insomnia, anemia, fever, decreased libido, dyspepsia, headache, hyperglycemia.

INTERACTIONS: (Megace ES) May decrease exposure of indinavir; consider higher dose of indinavir.

PREGNANCY: Category X, not for use in nursing.

MECHANISM OF ACTION: Progesterone; has not been established; has appetite-enhancing property.

PHARMACOKINETICS: Absorption: (800mg/day) C_{max}=753ng/mL, AUC=10,476ng•hr/mL, T_{max}=5 hrs (median). (750mg/day) C_{max}=490ng/mL, AUC=6779ng•hr/mL, T_{max}=3 hrs (median). **Elimination:** Urine (66.4%, 5%-8% metabolites), feces (19.8%); (Megace ES) $T_{1/2}$=20-50 hrs.

NURSING CONSIDERATIONS

Assessment: Assess for preexisting DM, history of thromboembolic disease, hypersensitivity to drug, pregnancy/nursing status, and for possible drug interactions.

Monitoring: Monitor for new/worsening DM, Cushing's syndrome, vaginal bleeding, and adrenal insufficiency.

Patient Counseling: Instruct to use ud. Inform about product differences to avoid overdosing or underdosing. Advise to report any adverse reactions. Advise to use contraception in woman capable of becoming pregnant and to notify physician if they become pregnant while on therapy.

Administration: Oral route. Shake well before use. **Storage:** 15-25°C (59-77°F). Protect from heat.

MENACTRA   RX
meningococcal polysaccharide diphtheria toxoid conjugate vaccine (Sanofi Pasteur)

THERAPEUTIC CLASS: Vaccine

INDICATIONS: Active immunization to prevent invasive meningococcal disease caused by *Neisseria meningitidis* serogroups A, C, Y, and W-135 for persons 9 months-55 yrs.

DOSAGE: *Adults:* ≤55 Yrs: 0.5mL IM.
Pediatrics: ≥2 Yrs: 0.5mL IM. 9-23 months: 0.5mL IM and repeat after 3 months.

HOW SUPPLIED: Inj: 0.5mL

WARNINGS/PRECAUTIONS: Guillain-Barre syndrome (GBS) reported; may be at increased risk if previously diagnosed with GBS. Review immunization history for possible vaccine hypersensitivity and previous vaccination-related adverse reactions. Epinephrine and other appropriate agents must be immediately available for possible acute anaphylactic reactions. Immunocompromised persons may have diminished immune response to therapy. May not protect all recipients.

ADVERSE REACTIONS: Inj-site reactions, headache, fatigue, malaise, arthralgia, anorexia, chills, fever, diarrhea, drowsiness, irritability, rash, vomiting.

INTERACTIONS: Immunosuppressive therapies (eg, irradiation, antimetabolites, alkylating agents, cytotoxic drugs, and corticosteroids [used in greater than physiologic doses]) may reduce immune response to vaccine. Tetanus and diphtheria toxoids vaccine may increase serum bactericidal assay titer to meningococcal serogroups A, C, Y, and W-135; higher rate of systemic adverse events with concomitant use. Pneumococcal antibody responses to some serotypes in pneumococcal conjugate vaccine 7 (PCV7) were decreased following coadministration with PCV7.

PREGNANCY: Category C, caution in nursing.

MECHANISM OF ACTION: Vaccine; leads to production of bactericidal antibodies directed against the capsular polysaccharides of serogroups A, C, Y, and W-135.

NURSING CONSIDERATIONS

Assessment: Assess current health and immune status, for history of GBS, pregnancy/nursing status, and possible drug interactions. Review immunization history for possible vaccine sensitivity and previous vaccination-related adverse reactions.

Monitoring: Monitor for GBS, allergic/anaphylactic reactions, and other potential adverse effects.

Patient Counseling: Inform of the potential benefits/risks of immunization therapy. Instruct to report any adverse reactions to physician.

Administration: IM route. Do not mix with any other vaccine in the same syringe. **Storage:** 2-8°C (35-46°F). Do not freeze.

MENVEO   RX
meningococcal (groups A, C, Y, and W-135) oligosaccharide diphtheria crm 197 conjugate (Novartis)

THERAPEUTIC CLASS: Vaccine

INDICATIONS: Active immunization to prevent invasive meningococcal disease caused by *Neisseria meningitidis* serogroups A, C, Y, and W-135 for persons 2 months through 55 yrs of age.

DOSAGE: *Adults:* ≤55 Yrs: Single 0.5mL IM dose.
Pediatrics: ≥11 Yrs: Single 0.5mL IM dose. 2-5 Yrs: Single 0.5mL IM dose; may administer a 2nd dose 2 months after the 1st dose if at continued high risk of meningococcal disease. 7-23 Months: 2-dose series with the 2nd dose administered in 2nd yr of life and at least 3 months after 1st dose. 2 Months: 4-dose series at 2, 4, 6, and 12 months of age.

HOW SUPPLIED: Inj: 0.5mL

WARNINGS/PRECAUTIONS: Appropriate medical treatment must be available should an acute allergic reaction, including an anaphylactic reaction, occur. Syncope resulting in falling injury associated with seizure-like movements reported; observe for at least 15 min after administration to prevent and manage syncopal reactions. Expected immune response may not be obtained in immunocompromised persons. Guillain-Barre syndrome (GBS) reported; caution with history of GBS. Apnea reported in premature infants; consider individual infant's medical status, and the potential benefits and possible risks.

ADVERSE REACTIONS: Inj-site reactions (eg, pain, tenderness, erythema, induration), irritability, sleepiness, change in eating, diarrhea, headache, myalgia, malaise, N/V, rash, fever, chills.

INTERACTIONS: Immunosuppressive therapies (eg, irradiation, antimetabolites, alkylating agents, cytotoxic drugs, and corticosteroids [used in greater than physiologic doses]) may reduce immune response to vaccine. Lower geometric mean antibody concentrations for antibodies to the pertussis antigens filamentous hemagglutinin and pertactin observed when coadministered with Tdap and HPV as compared with Tdap alone.

PREGNANCY: Category B, caution in nursing.

MECHANISM OF ACTION: Vaccine; leads to production of bactericidal antibodies directed against the capsular polysaccharides of serogroups A, C, Y, and W-135.

NURSING CONSIDERATIONS

Assessment: Assess for previous hypersensitivity to vaccine or other vaccines containing similar components, immune system status, *N. meningitidis* serogroup B infections, history of GBS, infant's medical status, pregnancy/nursing status, and possible drug interactions. Assess children 2-5 yrs of age for continued high risk of meningococcal disease. Review immunization history for possible vaccine sensitivity and previous vaccination-related adverse reactions.

Monitoring: Monitor for allergic reactions, syncope, seizure-like activity, GBS, apnea in premature infants, and other adverse reactions. Monitor immune response.

Patient Counseling: Inform about the potential benefits/risks of immunization therapy, importance of completing the immunization series, and potential adverse reactions temporally associated with the vaccine. Instruct to report any side effects to the physician. Inform about the pregnancy registry, as appropriate.

Administration: IM route. Do not mix with any other vaccine or diluent in the same syringe or vial. Administer preferably into the anterolateral aspect of the thigh in infants or into the deltoid muscle (upper arm) in toddlers, adolescents, and adults. Refer to PI for reconstitution instructions. **Storage:** 2-8°C (36-46°F); maintain at 2-8°C (36-46°F) during transport. Do not freeze or use frozen/previously frozen product. Protect from light. Use reconstituted vaccine immediately, but may be held at or below 25°C (77°F) for up to 8 hrs.

MEPERIDINE ORAL CII
meperidine HCl (Roxane)

OTHER BRAND NAMES: Demerol (Sanofi-Aventis)

THERAPEUTIC CLASS: Opioid analgesic

INDICATIONS: Relief of moderate to severe pain.

DOSAGE: *Adults:* Usual: 50-150mg q3-4h PRN. Concomitant Phenothiazines/Other Tranquilizers: Reduce dose by 25-50%.
Pediatrics: Usual: 1.1-1.8mg/kg, up to the adult dose, q3-4h PRN. Concomitant Phenothiazines/Other Tranquilizers: Reduce dose by 25-50%.

HOW SUPPLIED: Sol: 50mg/5mL; Tab: 50mg*, 100mg*; (Demerol) Tab: 50mg*, 100mg *scored

CONTRAINDICATIONS: During or within 14 days of MAOI use. (Demerol) Severe respiratory insufficiency.

WARNINGS/PRECAUTIONS: May be habit forming. Not for chronic pain; may increase risk of toxicity (eg, seizures) with prolonged use. Respiratory depressant effects and elevation of CSF pressure may be exaggerated in the presence of head injury, other intracranial lesions, or preexisting increase in intracranial pressure. May obscure diagnosis or clinical course of head injuries or acute abdominal conditions. Extreme caution with acute asthmatic attack, chronic obstructive pulmonary disease or cor pulmonale, or other respiratory conditions. May cause severe hypotension in postoperative patients or individuals whose ability to maintain BP has been compromised by depleted blood volume. May impair mental/physical abilities. May produce orthostatic hypotension in ambulatory patients. Not recommended during labor. Caution in elderly, debilitated, patients with atrial flutter or other supraventricular tachycardias, and other special risk patients; refer to PI. May aggravate preexisting convulsions. Caution with alcoholism or other drug dependencies; may develop tolerance, dependence, addiction, or abuse. Avoid abrupt discontinuation.

ADVERSE REACTIONS: Lightheadedness, dizziness, sedation, N/V, sweating, respiratory/circulatory depression.

INTERACTIONS: See Contraindications. Additive effects with alcohol, other opioids, or illicit drugs that cause CNS depression. Caution and consider dose reduction with other CNS depressants (eg, sedatives or hypnotics, general anesthetics, phenothiazines, other tranquilizers, alcohol); may result in respiratory depression, hypotension, profound sedation, or coma. Caution with agonist/antagonist analgesics (eg, pentazocine, nalbuphine, butorphanol, buprenorphine); may reduce the analgesic effect and/or precipitate withdrawal symptoms. Acyclovir may increase levels. Cimetidine may reduce clearance and V_d; caution with coadministration. Phenytoin may enhance hepatic metabolism; use caution. Avoid with ritonavir; may increase levels of active metabolite. May enhance neuromuscular-blocking action of skeletal muscle relaxants. May result in severe hypotension with phenothiazines or certain anesthetics.

PREGNANCY: Category C, not for use in nursing.

MECHANISM OF ACTION: Narcotic analgesic; produces actions similar to morphine most prominently involving the CNS and organs composed of smooth muscle. Produces analgesic and sedative effects.

PHARMACOKINETICS: Metabolism: Liver; normeperidine (metabolite). **Distribution:** Crosses placental barrier; found in breast milk.

NURSING CONSIDERATIONS

Assessment: Assess for intensity/type of pain, patient's general condition and medical status, any other conditions where treatment is contraindicated or cautioned, renal/hepatic dysfunction, pregnancy/nursing status, and possible drug interactions.

Monitoring: Monitor for signs/symptoms of tolerance or dependence, misuse or abuse, increase in CSF pressure, hypotension, respiratory depression, convulsions, and toxicity.

Patient Counseling: Advise to report pain or adverse events occurring during treatment. Instruct not to adjust dose or abruptly d/c therapy without consulting physician. Counsel that drug may impair mental and/or physical ability required for driving, operating heavy machinery, or other potentially hazardous tasks. Instruct not to drink alcohol or take other CNS depressants (eg, sleep aids, tranquilizers). Advise women who become or are planning to become pregnant about the effects of the drug in pregnancy. Inform that medication has potential for drug abuse; counsel to protect from theft and use by anyone other than the prescribed patient. Instruct to keep medication in a secure place and flush unused tab if no longer needed.

Administration: Oral route. (Sol) Take each dose in 1/2 glass of water. **Storage:** 25°C (77°F); excursions permitted to 15-30°C (59-86°F).

MERREM   RX
meropenem (AstraZeneca)

THERAPEUTIC CLASS: Carbapenem

INDICATIONS: Treatment of intra-abdominal infections (complicated appendicitis and peritonitis) and complicated skin and skin structure infections (cSSSIs) in adult and pediatric patients ≥3 months of age, and of bacterial meningitis in pediatric patients ≥3 months of age caused by susceptible microorganisms. Useful as presumptive therapy in the indicated conditions prior to identification of causative organisms.

DOSAGE: *Adults:* Usual: cSSSIs: 500mg q8h. cSSSIs Caused by *Pseudomonas aeruginosa*/ Intra-Abdominal Infections: 1g q8h. Renal Impairment: CrCl >25-50mL/min: Give usual dose q12h. CrCl 10-25mL/min: Give 1/2 usual dose q12h. CrCl <10mL/min: Give 1/2 usual dose q24h. Administer by IV infusion over approximately 15-30 min; doses of 1g may also be given as an IV bolus inj (5-20mL) over approximately 3-5 min.
Pediatrics: ≥3 Months: >50kg: cSSSIs: 500mg q8h. cSSSIs Caused by *P. aeruginosa*/Intra-Abdominal Infections: 1g q8h. Meningitis: 2g q8h. ≤50kg: cSSSIs: 10mg/kg q8h. Max: 500mg q8h. cSSSIs Caused by *P. aeruginosa*/Intra-Abdominal Infections: 20mg/kg q8h. Max: 1g q8h. Meningitis: 40mg/kg q8h. Max: 2g q8h. Administer as IV infusion over approximately 15-30 min or as an IV bolus inj (5-20mL) over approximately 3-5 min.

HOW SUPPLIED: Inj: 500mg, 1g

WARNINGS/PRECAUTIONS: Serious and occasionally fatal hypersensitivity (anaphylactic) reactions reported; d/c immediately if an allergic reaction occurs. Seizures and other adverse CNS effects reported; caution in patients with CNS disorders (eg, brain lesions, history of seizures) or with bacterial meningitis and/or compromised renal function. Continue anticonvulsant therapy in patients with known seizure disorders. If focal tremors, myoclonus, or seizures occur, evaluate neurologically, place on anticonvulsant therapy if not already instituted, and reexamine dosage to determine whether it should be decreased or discontinued. *Clostridium difficile*-associated diarrhea (CDAD) reported; d/c if CDAD is suspected or confirmed. May result in bacterial resistance if used in the absence of proven or suspected bacterial infection, or a prophylactic indication; take appropriate measures if superinfection develops. Thrombocytopenia reported in patients with renal impairment. Inadequate information on use in patients on hemodialysis or peritoneal dialysis. May impair mental/physical abilities. Caution in elderly.

ADVERSE REACTIONS: Diarrhea, N/V, headache, constipation, diarrhea, anemia, pain.

INTERACTIONS: Increased plasma concentrations with probenecid; coadministration not recommended. May reduce concentrations of valproic acid, thereby increasing the risk of breakthrough seizures; concomitant use with valproic acid or divalproex sodium is generally not recommended, but if necessary, consider supplemental anticonvulsant therapy.

PREGNANCY: Category B, caution in nursing.

MECHANISM OF ACTION: Carbapenem; bactericidal activity results from the inhibition of cell-wall synthesis.

PHARMACOKINETICS: Absorption: 30-min IV Infusion (Single Dose): C_{max}=23mcg/mL (500mg); 49mcg/mL (1g). 5-min IV Bolus Inj: C_{max}=45mcg/mL (500mg); 112mcg/mL (1g). **Distribution:** Plasma protein binding (2%); found in breast milk. **Elimination:** Urine (70% unchanged, 28% inactive metabolite), feces (2%); $T_{1/2}$=1 hr, 1.5 hrs (pediatric patients 3 months-2 yrs of age).

NURSING CONSIDERATIONS

Assessment: Assess for CNS/seizure disorders, factors that predispose to convulsive activity, renal impairment, pregnancy/nursing status, and possible drug interactions. Carefully assess for previous hypersensitivity reactions to drug, penicillins, cephalosporins, other β-lactams, and other allergens.

Monitoring: Monitor for hypersensitivity reactions, CNS effects (eg, focal tremors, myoclonus, seizures), CDAD, superinfection, and other adverse reactions. Periodically monitor organ system functions including renal, hepatic, and hematopoietic, during prolonged therapy.

Patient Counseling: Counsel that therapy should only be used to treat bacterial, not viral, infections. Instruct to take exactly ud, even if patient feels better early in the course of therapy. Inform that skipping doses or not completing the full course of therapy may decrease effectiveness of treatment and increase bacterial resistance. Inform that diarrhea is a common problem caused by therapy, which usually ends when therapy is discontinued. Instruct to immediately contact physician if watery and bloody stools (with or without stomach cramp and fever) occur, even as late as ≥2 months after the last dose. Counsel to inform physician if taking valproic acid or divalproex sodium. Advise that adverse events (eg, seizures, headaches, and/or paresthesias) may develop that could interfere with mental alertness and/or cause motor impairment; instruct not to operate machinery or motorized vehicles until it is reasonably well established that therapy is well tolerated.

Administration: IV route. Do not mix with or physically add to solutions containing other drugs. Refer to PI for further preparation and administration instructions. **Storage:** 20-25°C (68-77°F). Constituted Sol: Do not freeze. Refer to PI for further stability and storage information.

METADATE CD CII
methylphenidate HCl (UCB)

> Caution with history of drug dependence or alcoholism. Chronic abuse may lead to marked tolerance and psychological dependence with varying degrees of abnormal behavior. Frank psychotic episodes may occur, especially with parenteral abuse. Careful supervision is required during withdrawal from abusive use since severe depression may occur. Withdrawal following chronic use may unmask symptoms of underlying disorder that may require follow-up.

THERAPEUTIC CLASS: Sympathomimetic amine

INDICATIONS: Treatment of attention-deficit hyperactivity disorder.

DOSAGE: *Pediatrics:* ≥6 Yrs: Individualize dose. Administer qam before breakfast. Initial: 20mg qam. Titrate: May adjust in weekly 10-20mg increments, depending upon tolerability and degree of efficacy observed. Max: 60mg/day. Maint/Extended Treatment: Periodically reevaluate long-term usefulness of drug for the individual patient with trials off medication. Reduce dose or, if necessary, d/c if paradoxical aggravation of symptoms or other adverse events occur. D/C if no improvement seen after appropriate dosage adjustment over 1 month.

HOW SUPPLIED: Cap, Extended-Release: 10mg, 20mg, 30mg, 40mg, 50mg, 60mg

CONTRAINDICATIONS: Marked anxiety, tension, agitation, glaucoma, motor tics, family history or diagnosis of Tourette's syndrome, severe HTN, angina pectoris, cardiac arrhythmias, heart failure, recent myocardial infarction (MI), hyperthyroidism, or thyrotoxicosis. Rare hereditary problems of fructose intolerance, glucose-galactose malabsorption, or sucrase-isomaltase insufficiency. On the day of surgery. Treatment with MAOIs or within a minimum of 14 days following discontinuation of an MAOI.

WARNINGS/PRECAUTIONS: Avoid with known serious structural cardiac abnormalities, cardiomyopathy, serious heart rhythm abnormalities, coronary artery disease, or other serious cardiac problems. Sudden death reported in children and adolescents with structural cardiac abnormalities or other serious heart problems. Sudden deaths, stroke, and MI reported in adults. May increase BP and HR; caution with conditions that might be compromised by increases in BP/HR. Prior to treatment, obtain medical history (including assessment for family history of sudden death or ventricular arrhythmia) and perform physical exam to assess for presence of cardiac disease. Promptly perform cardiac evaluation if symptoms of cardiac disease develop. May exacerbate symptoms of behavior disturbance and thought disorder in patients with preexisting psychotic disorder. Caution in patients with comorbid bipolar disorder; may induce mixed/manic episodes. May cause treatment-emergent psychotic or manic symptoms (eg, hallucinations, delusional thinking, mania) in children and adolescents without prior history of psychotic illness or mania; consider discontinuation if such symptoms occur. Aggressive behavior or hostility reported in children and adolescents. May cause long-term suppression of growth in children; monitor growth, and may need to interrupt treatment in patients not growing or gaining height or weight as expected. May lower convulsive threshold; d/c if seizures occur. Priapism, sometimes requiring surgical intervention, reported. Associated with peripheral vasculopathy, including Raynaud's phenomenon; carefully observe for digital changes. Difficulties with accommodation and blurring of vision reported. May produce a positive result during drug testing.

ADVERSE REACTIONS: Headache, abdominal pain, anorexia, insomnia.

INTERACTIONS: See Contraindications. Caution with pressor agents. May inhibit metabolism of coumarin anticoagulants, anticonvulsants (eg, phenobarbital, phenytoin, primidone), phenylbutazone, and some antidepressants (eg, TCAs, SSRIs); downward dose adjustment and monitoring of plasma drug concentrations (or coagulation times for coumarin) of these drugs may be necessary when initiating or discontinuing methylphenidate. Clearance might be affected by urinary pH, either being increased with acidifying agents or decreased with alkalinizing agents; caution with agents that alter urinary pH. Avoid with alcohol.

PREGNANCY: Category C, caution in nursing.

MECHANISM OF ACTION: Sympathomimetic amine; CNS stimulant. Has not been established; thought to block reuptake of norepinephrine and dopamine into presynaptic neuron and increase release of these monoamines into extraneuronal space.

PHARMACOKINETICS: Absorption: Readily absorbed. Administration of variable doses resulted in different parameters. **Metabolism:** Via deesterification; α-phenyl-piperidine acetic acid (ritalinic acid) (metabolite). **Elimination:** (Healthy) $T_{1/2}$=6.8 hrs.

NURSING CONSIDERATIONS

Assessment: Assess for hypersensitivity to the drug, hereditary problems of fructose intolerance, glucose-galactose malabsorption, or sucrase-isomaltase insufficiency, marked anxiety, tension, agitation, glaucoma, motor tics, family history or diagnosis of Tourette's syndrome, cardiovascular conditions, history of drug dependence or alcoholism, psychotic disorder, comorbid bipolar disorder, any other conditions where treatment is contraindicated or cautioned, pregnancy/nursing status, and possible drug interactions.

Monitoring: Monitor for changes in HR and BP, signs/symptoms of cardiac disease, exacerbation of behavior disturbance and thought disorder, psychosis, mania, appearance of or worsening of aggressive behavior or hostility, seizures, priapism, peripheral vasculopathy (including Raynaud's phenomenon), visual disturbances, and other adverse reactions. In pediatric patients, monitor growth. Perform periodic monitoring of CBC, differential, and platelet counts during prolonged therapy. Periodically reevaluate long-term usefulness of drug.

Patient Counseling: Advise to avoid alcohol while taking the drug. Inform about the benefits and risks of therapy. Counsel on the appropriate use of the medication. Instruct to seek immediate medical attention in the event of priapism. Instruct to report to physician any new numbness, pain, skin color change, or sensitivity to temperature in fingers or toes; instruct to contact physician immediately with any signs of unexplained wounds appearing on fingers or toes while taking the drug.

Administration: Oral route. May be swallowed whole with the aid of liquids, or alternatively, cap may be opened and cap contents sprinkled onto a small amount (tbsp) of applesauce and given immediately, and not stored for future use. Drinking some fluids (eg, water) should follow the intake of the sprinkles with applesauce. Do not crush or chew cap and cap contents. **Storage:** 25°C (77°F); excursions permitted to 15-30°C (59-86°F).

METADATE ER
methylphenidate HCl (UCB)

`CII`

Caution with history of drug dependence or alcoholism. Chronic abusive use may lead to marked tolerance and psychological dependence with varying degrees of abnormal behavior. Frank psychotic episodes may occur, especially with parenteral abuse. Careful supervision is required during withdrawal from abusive use since severe depression may occur. Withdrawal following chronic use may unmask symptoms of underlying disorder that may require follow-up.

THERAPEUTIC CLASS: Sympathomimetic amine

INDICATIONS: Treatment of attention-deficit hyperactivity disorder (ADHD) and narcolepsy.

DOSAGE: *Adults:* Individualize dose. (Immediate-Release [IR] Methylphenidate) 10-60mg/day given in divided doses bid-tid 30-45 min ac. Take last dose before 6 pm if unable to sleep. (Tab, ER) May be used in place of the IR tabs when the 8-hr dosage corresponds to the titrated 8-hr dosage of the IR tabs.
Pediatrics: ≥6 Yrs: Individualize dose. Initiate in small doses, with gradual weekly increments. Max: 60mg/day. D/C if no improvement seen after appropriate dosage adjustment over 1 month. (IR Methylphenidate) Initial: 5mg bid before breakfast and lunch. Titrate: Increase gradually by

5-10mg weekly. (Tab, ER) May be used in place of the IR tabs when the 8-hr dosage corresponds to the titrated 8-hr dosage of the IR tabs. Reduce dose or, if necessary, d/c if paradoxical aggravation of symptoms or other adverse effects occur. Periodically d/c to assess child's condition. Drug treatment should not and need not be indefinite and usually may be discontinued after puberty.

HOW SUPPLIED: Tab, Extended-Release: 20mg

CONTRAINDICATIONS: Marked anxiety, tension, agitation, glaucoma, motor tics, family history or diagnosis of Tourette's syndrome, severe HTN, angina pectoris, cardiac arrhythmias, heart failure, recent myocardial infarction (MI), hyperthyroidism, or thyrotoxicosis. Rare hereditary problems of galactose intolerance, the Lapp lactase deficiency, or glucose-galactose malabsorption. On the day of surgery. Treatment with MAOIs or within a minimum of 14 days following discontinuation of an MAOI.

WARNINGS/PRECAUTIONS: Avoid with known serious structural cardiac abnormalities, cardiomyopathy, serious heart rhythm abnormalities, coronary artery disease, or other serious cardiac problems. Sudden death reported in children and adolescents with structural cardiac abnormalities or other serious heart problems. Sudden deaths, stroke, and MI reported in adults. May increase BP and HR; caution with conditions that might be compromised by increases in BP/HR. Prior to treatment, obtain medical history (including assessment for family history of sudden death or ventricular arrhythmia) and perform physical exam to assess for presence of cardiac disease. Promptly perform cardiac evaluation if symptoms of cardiac disease develop. May exacerbate symptoms of behavior disturbance and thought disorder in patients with preexisting psychotic disorder. Caution in patients with comorbid bipolar disorder; may induce mixed/manic episodes. May cause treatment-emergent psychotic or manic symptoms (eg, hallucinations, delusional thinking, mania) in children and adolescents without prior history of psychotic illness or mania; consider discontinuation if such symptoms occur. Aggressive behavior or hostility reported in children and adolescents. May cause long-term suppression of growth in children; monitor growth, and may need to interrupt treatment in patients not growing or gaining height or weight as expected. May lower convulsive threshold; d/c if seizures occur. Difficulties with accommodation and blurring of vision reported. Patients with an element of agitation may react adversely; d/c if necessary. May produce a positive result during drug testing.

ADVERSE REACTIONS: Nervousness, insomnia, hypersensitivity reactions, anorexia, nausea, dizziness, palpitations, headache, dyskinesia, drowsiness, BP and pulse changes, tachycardia, angina, cardiac arrhythmia, abdominal pain.

INTERACTIONS: See Contraindications. Caution with pressor agents. May decrease effectiveness of drugs used to treat HTN. May inhibit metabolism of coumarin anticoagulants, anticonvulsants (eg, phenobarbital, phenytoin, primidone), phenylbutazone, and TCAs (eg, imipramine, clomipramine, desipramine); downward dose adjustment and monitoring of plasma drug concentration (or coagulation times for coumarin) of these drugs may be necessary when initiating or discontinuing methylphenidate. Clearance might be affected by urinary pH, either being increased with acidifying agents or decreased with alkalinizing agents; caution with agents that alter urinary pH.

PREGNANCY: Category C, caution in nursing.

MECHANISM OF ACTION: Sympathomimetic amine; mild CNS stimulant. Has not been established; suspected to activate the brain stem arousal system and cortex to produce its stimulant effect.

PHARMACOKINETICS: Absorption: (Children) T_{max}=4.7 hrs (sustained-release tab), 1.9 hrs (IR tab).

NURSING CONSIDERATIONS

Assessment: Assess for hypersensitivity to the drug, hereditary problems of galactose intolerance, the Lapp lactase deficiency, glucose-galactose malabsorption, marked anxiety, tension, agitation, glaucoma, motor tics, family history or diagnosis of Tourette's syndrome, cardiovascular conditions, history of drug dependence or alcoholism, psychotic disorder, comorbid bipolar disorder, any other conditions where treatment is contraindicated or cautioned, pregnancy/nursing status, and possible drug interactions.

Monitoring: Monitor for changes in HR and BP, signs/symptoms of cardiac disease, exacerbation of behavior disturbance and thought disorder, psychosis, mania, appearance of or worsening of aggressive behavior or hostility, seizures, visual disturbances, and other adverse reactions. In pediatric patients, monitor growth. Perform periodic monitoring of CBC, differential, and platelet counts during prolonged therapy.

Patient Counseling: Inform about the benefits and risks of therapy. Counsel on the appropriate use of the medication.

Administration: Oral route. Swallow tabs whole; do not crush or chew. **Storage:** 20-25°C (68-77°F); excursions permitted to 15-30°C (59-86°F). Protect from moisture.

METHADONE ORAL SOLUTION AND SUSPENSION `CII`
methadone HCl (Roxane)

> Contains methadone, an opioid agonist and Schedule II controlled substance with an abuse liability similar to other opioids, legal or illicit; assess each patient's risk for opioid abuse or addiction prior to prescribing. Increased risk in patients with a personal or family history of substance abuse (eg, drug/alcohol abuse/addiction) or mental illness (eg, major depressive disorder). Routinely monitor for signs of misuse, abuse, and addiction. Respiratory depression, including fatal cases, reported during initiation or even when used as recommended; proper dosing and titration are essential. Monitor for respiratory depression, especially during initiation or following a dose increase. QT interval prolongation and serious arrhythmia (torsades de pointes) reported; closely monitor for changes in cardiac rhythm during initiation and titration. Accidental ingestion, especially in children, can result in fatal overdose. For detoxification and maintenance of opioid dependence, methadone shall be dispensed only by certified opioid programs.

THERAPEUTIC CLASS: Opioid analgesic

INDICATIONS: Detoxification treatment of opioid addiction (heroin or other morphine-like drugs). Maintenance treatment of opioid addiction (heroin or other morphine-like drugs), in conjunction with appropriate social and medical services. (Oral Concentrate, Sol) Management of moderate to severe pain when a continuous, around-the-clock opioid analgesic is needed for an extended period of time.

DOSAGE: *Adults*: Refer to PI for conversion from other opioids. Opioid Addiction Detoxification/ Maint: Initial: 20-30mg single dose. Max Initial Dose: 30mg. Evaluate after 2-4 hrs for same-day dosing adjustment. Give 5-10mg if withdrawal symptoms not suppressed or if symptoms reappear. Max on 1st Day of Treatment: 40mg/day. Use lower initial doses for expected low tolerance at treatment entry. Short-Term Detoxification: Titrate to 40mg/day in divided doses. After 2-3 days of stabilization, gradually decrease dose on a daily basis or at 2-day intervals depending on tolerability level of withdrawal symptoms. Hospitalized patients may tolerate a daily reduction of 20% of the total daily dose; ambulatory patients may need a slower schedule. Titrate and Maint of Detoxification: Titrate to a dose at which symptoms are prevented for 24 hrs. Usual: 80-120mg/day. Medically Supervised Withdrawal After Maint Treatment: Reduce dose by <10% of the established tolerance or maint dose; 10-14 day intervals between dose reductions. Acute Pain During Methadone Maint Treatment: May require somewhat higher and/or more frequent doses than in nontolerant patients. Pregnancy: May need to increase dose or decrease dosing interval. Elderly: Start at lower end of dosing range. (Oral Concentrate, Sol) Pain: Initial: Refer to PI for factors to consider when selecting an initial dose. First Opioid Analgesic: Small doses no more than 2.5mg-10mg q8-12h. May require more frequent administration to maintain adequate analgesia. Conversion From Parenteral to PO Methadone: Use conversion ratio of 1:2mg. Titrate and Maint: Individually titrate a dose that provides adequate analgesia and minimizes adverse reactions. Re-assess the need for continued use, especially for noncancer-related pain. May adjust dose every 1-2 days. Breakthrough Pain: May require dosage adjustment or rescue medication with a small dose of an immediate-release medication. If signs of excessive opioid-related adverse reactions observed, reduce next dose; adjust dose to obtain appropriate balance between management of pain and opioid-related adverse reactions. If intolerable opioid related adverse reactions develop, adjust dose or dosing interval. Discontinuation: Use gradual downward titration every 2-4 days; avoid abrupt d/c.

HOW SUPPLIED: Oral Concentrate: 10mg/mL [30mL]; Sol: 5mg, 10mg [5mL]; Tab, Dispersible: 40mg* *scored

CONTRAINDICATIONS: Significant respiratory depression, acute or severe bronchial asthma in unmonitored setting or in the absence of resuscitative equipment, and known or suspected paralytic ileus.

WARNINGS/PRECAUTIONS: For oral administration only. Preparation must not be injected. Patients tolerant to other opioids may be incompletely tolerant to methadone. Closely monitor patients with risk factors for prolonged QT interval (eg, cardiac hypertrophy, hypokalemia, hypomagnesemia) and a history of cardiac conduction abnormalities. Respiratory depression is more likely to occur in elderly, cachectic, or debilitated patients; monitor closely when initiating and titrating, and when given with drugs that depress respiration. Deaths reported during conversion from chronic, high dose treatment with other opioid agonists. Monitor for respiratory depression and consider alternative nonopioid analgesics in patients with significant chronic obstructive pulmonary disease (COPD) or cor pulmonale, and in patients having a substantially decreased respiratory reserve, hypoxia, hypercapnia, or preexisting respiratory depression. May cause severe hypotension especially in patients with compromised ability to maintain BP; monitor for signs of hypotension after initiation or titration. Monitor for signs of sedation and respiratory depression in patients susceptible to the intracranial effects of carbon dioxide retention (eg, those with increased intracranial pressure or brain tumors). May obscure clinical course in patients with head injury. Avoid with GI obstruction and impaired consciousness or coma. May cause spasm of the sphincter of Oddi; monitor for worsening symptoms in patients with biliary tract disease including acute pancreatitis. May increase serum amylase. May aggravate convulsions in patients with convulsive disorders and may induce or aggravate seizures; monitor for worsened seizure control

M

in patients with history of seizure disorder. May impair mental/physical abilities. Abrupt discontinuation may lead to opioid withdrawal symptoms. Infants born to opioid-dependent mothers may be physically dependent and may exhibit respiratory difficulties and withdrawal symptoms. Caution in elderly. (Oral Concentrate, Sol) Avoid as PRN analgesic, for mild or acute pain, pain not expected to persist for an extended period of time, and postoperative pain.

ADVERSE REACTIONS: Respiratory depression, QT prolongation, arrhythmia, systemic hypotension, lightheadedness, dizziness, sedation, N/V, sweating.

INTERACTIONS: CYP450 inducers (eg, rifampicin, phenytoin, phenobarbital, carbamazepine, St. John's wort) may precipitate withdrawal syndrome. CYP3A4 inhibitors (eg, ketoconazole, itraconazole, voriconazole, clarithromycin, erythromycin, telithromycin) and/or CYP2C9 inhibitors (eg, sertraline, fluvoxamine) may cause decreased clearance, which could increase or prolong adverse effects and may cause fatal respiratory depression. Antiretroviral drugs (eg, abacavir, amprenavir, darunavir + ritonavir, efavirenz, nelfinavir, nevirapine, ritonavir, telaprevir, lopinavir + ritonavir, saquinavir + ritonavir, tipranavir + ritonavir) may increase clearance or decrease plasma levels. May decrease levels of didanosine and stavudine. May increase area under the curve of zidovudine. CNS depressants (eg, sedatives, hypnotics, general anesthetics, antiemetics, phenothiazines, tranquilizers, alcohol, anxiolytics, neuroleptics, other opioids, and illicit drugs) may increase risk of respiratory depression, hypotension, profound sedation, or coma; reduce initial dose of 1 or both agents. Deaths reported when abused in conjunction with benzodiazepines. Monitor for cardiac conduction changes with drugs known to have potential to prolong QT interval. Pharmacodynamic interactions may occur with potentially arrhythmogenic agents (eg, Class I and III antiarrhythmics, neuroleptics, TCAs, calcium channel blockers). Monitor closely with drugs capable of inducing electrolyte imbalance that may prolong QT interval including diuretics, laxatives, mineralocorticoid hormones, and medications affecting cardiac conduction. May reduce analgesic effect or experience withdrawal symptoms with opioid antagonists, mixed agonist/antagonists, and partial agonists (eg, naloxone, naltrexone, pentazocine, nalbuphine, butorphanol, buprenorphine); avoid use. Severe reactions may occur with concurrent use or within 14 days of MAOIs use. May increase levels of desipramine. Anticholinergics may increase risk of urinary retention and/or severe constipation which may lead to paralytic ileus.

PREGNANCY: Category C, caution in nursing.

MECHANISM OF ACTION: Synthetic opioid analgesic; mu-agonist. Produces actions similar to morphine; acts on CNS and organs composed of smooth muscle. May also act as an N-methyl-D-aspartate (NMDA) receptor antagonist.

PHARMACOKINETICS: Absorption: Bioavailability (36-100%); C_{max}=124-1255ng/mL; T_{max}=1-7.5 hrs. **Distribution:** V_d=1-8L/kg; plasma protein binding (85-90%); found in breast milk. **Metabolism:** Hepatic N-demethylation via CYP3A4, 2B6, 2C19 (major); 2C9, 2D6 (minor). **Elimination:** Urine, feces; $T_{1/2}$=8-59 hrs.

NURSING CONSIDERATIONS

Assessment: Assess for personal/family history or risk factors for drug abuse or addiction, general condition and medical status, opioid/experience/tolerance, pain type/severity, previous opioid daily dose, potency, and type of prior analgesics used, respiratory depression, cardiac conduction abnormalities, COPD or other respiratory complications, GI obstruction, paralytic ileus, hepatic/renal impairment, previous hypersensitivity to drug, pregnancy/nursing status, possible drug interactions, and any other conditions where treatment is contraindicated or cautioned.

Monitoring: Monitor for signs/symptoms of respiratory depression, QT prolongation and arrhythmias, orthostatic hypotension, syncope, symptoms of worsening biliary tract disease, aggravation/induction of seizure, tolerance, physical dependence, mental/physical impairment and withdrawal syndrome, hypersensitivity reactions, and other adverse reactions. Monitor for signs of increased intracranial pressure with head injuries. Routinely monitor for signs of misuse, abuse, and addiction.

Patient Counseling: Inform that drug has potential for abuse; instruct not to share drug with others and to take steps to protect from theft or misuse. Discuss risks and how to recognize respiratory depression, orthostatic hypotension, and syncope. Instruct to seek medical attention immediately if they are experiencing breathing difficulties or symptoms suggestive of arrhythmia (eg, palpitations, near syncope, syncope). Advise patient to store drug securely; accidental exposure, especially in children, can result in fatal overdose. Inform about risks of concomitant use of alcohol and other CNS depressants; instruct not to consume alcoholic beverages, as well as prescription and OTC drug products containing alcohol. Advise to take drug as prescribed and not to d/c without 1st discussing with prescriber. Inform that drug may impair ability to perform potentially hazardous activities (eg, driving a car, operating heavy machinery). Advise about potential for severe constipation, including management instructions and when to seek medical attention. Inform that anaphylaxis may occur; advise how to recognize such a reaction and when to seek medical attention. Advise females that drug can cause fetal harm and to inform prescriber if pregnant or plan to become pregnant. Instruct nursing mothers to watch for signs of methadone toxicity in their infants (eg, increased sleepiness, difficulty breastfeeding, breathing difficulties, limpness); instruct to inform physician immediately if these signs occur. Inform patients treated for opioid dependence that discontinuation may lead to relapse of illicit drug use. Reassure that dose of methadone will hold for longer periods of time as treatment progresses after initiation. Advise patients to dispose of unused methadone by flushing the drug down the toilet.

Administration: Oral route. **Storage:** 25°C (77°F); excursions permitted to 15-30°C (59-86°F). (Oral Concentrate) Protect from light.

METHOTREXATE INJECTION RX
methotrexate (Various)

Should be used only by physicians with knowledge and experience in the use of antimetabolite therapy. Use only in life-threatening neoplastic diseases, or in patients with psoriasis or rheumatoid arthritis (RA) with severe, recalcitrant, disabling disease not adequately responsive to other forms of therapy. Deaths reported in the treatment of malignancy, psoriasis, and RA. Closely monitor for bone marrow, liver, lung, and kidney toxicities. Patients should be informed of the risks involved and be under physician's care throughout therapy. Use of high-dose regimens recommended for osteosarcoma requires meticulous care. Formulations and diluents containing preservatives must not be used for intrathecal or high-dose therapy. Fetal death and/or congenital anomalies reported; not recommended for women of childbearing potential unless benefits outweigh risks. Contraindicated in pregnant women with psoriasis or RA. Reduced elimination with impaired renal function, ascites, or pleural effusions; monitor for toxicity and reduce dose or d/c in some cases. Unexpectedly severe (sometimes fatal) bone marrow suppression, aplastic anemia, and GI toxicity reported with coadministration of therapy (usually high dosage) with some NSAIDs. Causes hepatotoxicity, fibrosis, and cirrhosis (generally only after prolonged use); perform periodic liver biopsies in psoriatic patients on long-term therapy. Acutely, liver enzyme elevations frequently seen. Drug-induced lung disease (eg, acute/chronic interstitial pneumonitis) may occur acutely at any time during therapy and reported at low doses. Interrupt therapy if pulmonary symptoms (especially a dry, nonproductive cough), diarrhea, or ulcerative stomatitis occurs. Malignant lymphomas, which may regress following withdrawal of treatment, may occur with low-dose therapy and, thus, may not require cytotoxic treatment; d/c therapy 1st and, if lymphoma does not regress, institute appropriate treatment. May induce tumor lysis syndrome in patients with rapidly growing tumors; may be prevented/alleviated with appropriate supportive and pharmacologic measures. Severe, occasionally fatal, skin reactions reported. Potentially fatal opportunistic infections, especially *Pneumocystis carinii* pneumonia, may occur. Concomitant use with radiotherapy may increase risk of soft tissue necrosis and osteonecrosis.

THERAPEUTIC CLASS: Dihydrofolic acid reductase inhibitor

INDICATIONS: Treatment of gestational choriocarcinoma, chorioadenoma destruens, and hydatidiform mole. Prophylaxis of meningeal leukemia and maintenance therapy in combination with other chemotherapeutic agents in acute lymphocytic leukemia. Treatment of meningeal leukemia. Treatment of breast cancer, epidermoid cancers of the head and neck, advanced mycosis fungoides (cutaneous T-cell lymphoma), and lung cancer, particularly squamous cell and small cell types, alone or in combination with other anticancer agents. Treatment of advanced stage non-Hodgkin's lymphomas in combination with other chemotherapeutic agents. Effective in prolonging relapse-free survival in patients with nonmetastatic osteosarcoma who have undergone surgical resection or amputation for the primary tumor when used in high doses followed by leucovorin rescue in combination with other chemotherapeutic agents. Symptomatic control of severe, recalcitrant, disabling psoriasis not adequately responsive to other forms of therapy, but only when the diagnosis has been established, as by a biopsy and/or after dermatologic consultation. Management of selected adults with severe, active RA (American College of Rheumatology criteria), or children with active polyarticular-course juvenile RA, who have had insufficient therapeutic response to, or are intolerant of, an adequate trial of 1st-line therapy including full-dose NSAIDs.

DOSAGE: *Adults:* Choriocarcinoma and Similar Trophoblastic Diseases: 15-30mg/day IM for a 5-day course. Repeat such courses for 3-5X as required, with rest periods of ≥1 week interposed between courses, until manifesting toxic symptoms subside. Acute Lymphoblastic Leukemia: Induction: 3.3mg/m²/day with prednisone 60mg/m²/day. Remission Maint: 30mg/m²/week IM given 2X weekly or 2.5mg/kg IV every 14 days. If and when relapse occurs, repeat the initial induction regimen to obtain reinduction of remission. Meningeal Leukemia: Prophylaxis/Treatment: 12mg intrathecally. Treatment: May be given at 2- to 5-day intervals; administer until CSF cell count returns to normal, then give one additional dose. Burkitt's Tumor: Stages I-II: 10-25mg/day PO for 4-8 days. Lymphosarcoma: Stage III: 0.625-2.5mg/kg/day with other antitumor agents. Treatment in all stages usually consists of several courses with 7- to 10-day rest periods. Mycosis Fungoides: Early Stage: 5-50mg once weekly, or 15-37.5mg 2X weekly if response is poor to weekly therapy. Dose reduction/cessation is guided by response and hematologic monitoring. Advanced Stages: Combination chemotherapy regimens that include IV methotrexate administered at higher doses with leucovorin rescue have been utilized. Osteosarcoma: Initial: 12g/m² IV as 4-hr infusion. Titrate: May increase to 15g/m² in subsequent treatments if initial dose is not sufficient to produce a peak serum concentration of 1000 micromolar at the end of the infusion. Refer to PI for doses and schedule of chemotherapeutic agents, and guidelines for methotrexate therapy with leucovorin rescue. RA: Initial: 7.5mg PO as single dose once weekly, or 2.5mg PO at 12-hr intervals for 3 doses given as a course once weekly. Titrate: May adjust gradually to achieve optimal response. Max: 20mg/week. Psoriasis: Initial: 10-25mg IM/IV as single weekly dose until adequate response is achieved, or 2.5mg PO at 12-hr intervals for 3 doses. Titrate: May adjust

617

gradually to achieve optimal response. Max: 30mg/week. Maint: Reduce each dosage schedule to lowest possible amount and to longest possible rest period. Elderly: Consider relatively low doses and closely monitor for early signs of toxicity.

Pediatrics: Acute Lymphoblastic Leukemia: Induction: $3.3mg/m^2$/day with prednisone $60mg/m^2$/day. Remission Maint: $30mg/m^2$/week IM given 2X weekly or 2.5mg/kg IV every 14 days. If and when relapse occurs, repeat the initial induction regimen to obtain reinduction of remission. Meningeal Leukemia: Prophylaxis/Treatment: Administer intrathecally. ≥3 Yrs: 12mg. 2 Yrs: 10mg. 1 Yr: 8mg. <1 Yr: 6mg. Treatment: May be given at 2- to 5-day intervals; administer until CSF cell count returns to normal, then give one additional dose. Osteosarcoma: Refer to PI. Juvenile RA: 2-16 Yrs: Initial: $10mg/m^2$ once weekly. Titrate: May adjust gradually to achieve optimal response. Max: $30mg/m^2$/week.

HOW SUPPLIED: Inj: 25mg/mL [2mL, 4mL, 8mL, 10mL], 1g

CONTRAINDICATIONS: Pregnant women with psoriasis or RA (should be used in treatment of pregnant women with neoplastic diseases only when potential benefit outweighs risk to the fetus), nursing mothers. Psoriasis or RA patients with alcoholism, alcoholic liver disease, chronic liver disease, immunodeficiency syndromes, or preexisting blood dyscrasias (eg, bone marrow hypoplasia, leukopenia, thrombocytopenia, significant anemia).

WARNINGS/PRECAUTIONS: Toxic effects may be related to dose/frequency of administration; if toxicity occurs, reduce dose or d/c therapy and take appropriate corrective measures, which may include use of leucovorin calcium and/or acute, intermittent hemodialysis with high-flux dialyzer, if necessary. If therapy is reinstituted, carry it out with caution, with adequate consideration of further need for the drug and increased alertness as to possible recurrence of toxicity. Caution in elderly/debilitated. Avoid pregnancy if either partner is receiving therapy (during and for a minimum of 3 months after therapy for male patients, and during and for at least 1 ovulatory cycle after therapy for female patients). May impair mental/physical abilities. May cause multiple organ system toxicities (eg, GI, hematologic). May cause impairment of fertility, oligospermia, and menstrual dysfunction during and for a short period after cessation of therapy.

ADVERSE REACTIONS: Bone marrow/liver/lung/kidney toxicities, diarrhea, ulcerative stomatitis, malignant lymphomas, tumor lysis syndrome, skin reactions, opportunistic infections, nausea, abdominal distress, malaise, undue fatigue, chills.

INTERACTIONS: See Boxed Warning. Do not administer NSAIDs prior to or concomitantly with high doses of therapy (eg, treatment of osteosarcoma); elevated and prolonged levels reported with concomitant NSAIDs. Caution when NSAIDs or salicylates are administered concomitantly with lower doses of therapy. Toxicity may be increased due to displacement by salicylates, phenylbutazone, phenytoin, and sulfonamides. Renal tubular transport diminished by probenecid. In the treatment of patients with osteosarcoma, exercise caution if high-dose therapy is administered with a potentially nephrotoxic chemotherapeutic agent (eg, cisplatin). Increases levels of mercaptopurine; may require dose adjustment. Oral antibiotics (eg, tetracycline, chloramphenicol, nonabsorbable broad spectrum) may decrease intestinal absorption or interfere with enterohepatic circulation. Penicillins may reduce renal clearance; hematologic and GI toxicity observed. Closely monitor for increased risk of hepatotoxicity with hepatotoxins (eg, azathioprine, retinoids, sulfasalazine). May decrease theophylline clearance; monitor theophylline levels. Vitamin preparations containing folic acid or its derivatives may decrease responses to drug; high doses of leucovorin may reduce the efficacy of intrathecally administered drug. Trimethoprim/sulfamethoxazole may increase bone marrow suppression by decreasing tubular secretion and/or additive antifolate effect. Proton pump inhibitors (PPIs) (eg, omeprazole, esomeprazole, pantoprazole) may elevate and prolong levels, possibly leading to toxicities; use caution when administering high-dose therapy with PPIs. Immunization may be ineffective when given during therapy; immunization with live virus vaccines is generally not recommended. Disseminated vaccinia infections after smallpox immunizations reported. Combined use with gold, penicillamine, hydroxychloroquine, sulfasalazine, or cytotoxic agents may increase incidence of adverse effects.

PREGNANCY: Category X, not for use in nursing.

MECHANISM OF ACTION: Dihydrofolic acid reductase inhibitor; interferes with DNA synthesis, repair, and cellular replication. Mechanism in RA not established; may affect immune function.

PHARMACOKINETICS: Absorption: Complete. T_{max}=30-60 min (IM). **Distribution:** Plasma protein binding (50%); found in breast milk. (IV) V_d=0.18L/kg (initial), 0.4-0.8L/kg (steady state). **Metabolism:** Hepatic and intracellular to polyglutamated forms (active); 7-hydroxymethotrexate (metabolite). **Elimination:** $T_{1/2}$=3-10 hrs (psoriasis/RA/low-dose antineoplastic therapy), 8-15 hrs (high dose). (IV) Urine (80-90%, unchanged), bile (≤10%).

NURSING CONSIDERATIONS

Assessment: Assess for alcoholism, alcoholic/chronic liver disease, immunodeficiency, blood dyscrasias, ascites, pleural effusions, tumors, hypersensitivity to drug, pregnancy/nursing status, any other condition where treatment is cautioned or contraindicated, and possible drug interactions. Obtain baseline CBC with differential and platelet counts, hepatic enzymes, renal function tests, liver biopsy, and chest x-ray.

Monitoring: Monitor for toxicities of bone marrow, liver, lung, kidney, and GI, diarrhea, ulcerative stomatitis, malignant lymphoma, tumor lysis syndrome, skin reactions, opportunistic infections, and other adverse reactions. Monitor hematology at least monthly and renal/hepatic function every 1-2 months during therapy of RA/psoriasis and more frequently during antineoplastic therapy, during initial/changing doses, or during periods of increased risk of elevated drug levels (eg, dehydration). If drug-induced lung disease is suspected, perform pulmonary function tests.

Patient Counseling: Inform of the early signs/symptoms of toxicity, the need to see physician promptly if they occur, and the need for close follow-up, including periodic lab tests to monitor toxicity. Emphasize that the recommended dose is taken weekly in RA and psoriasis, and that mistaken daily use of recommended dose has led to fatal toxicity. Counsel about risks/benefits of therapy, and effects on reproduction.

Administration: IM/IV/Intra-arterial/Intrathecal route. Consider procedures for proper handling and disposal. Refer to PI for reconstitution/dilution instructions. **Storage:** 20-25°C (68-77°F). Protect from light.

METHYLIN
methylphenidate HCl (Shionogi)

`CII`

> Caution with history of drug dependence or alcoholism. Chronic abuse may lead to marked tolerance and physiological dependence with varying degrees of abnormal behavior. Frank psychotic episodes may occur, especially with parenteral abuse. Careful supervision required during withdrawal from abusive use since severe depression may occur. Withdrawal following chronic use may unmask symptoms of underlying disorder that may require follow-up.

THERAPEUTIC CLASS: Sympathomimetic amine

INDICATIONS: Treatment of attention deficit disorders and narcolepsy.

DOSAGE: *Adults:* Individualize dose. 10-60mg/day given in divided doses bid or tid 30-45 min ac. Last dose should be taken before 6 pm if patient is unable to sleep as a result of taking medication late in the day.
Pediatrics: ≥6 Yrs: Individualize dose. Initial: 5mg bid before breakfast and lunch. Titrate: Increase gradually in increments of 5-10mg weekly. Max: 60mg/day. Reduce dose or d/c if paradoxical aggravation of symptoms or other adverse effects occur. D/C if no improvement seen after appropriate dosage adjustment over 1 month. D/C drug periodically to assess the child's condition; therapy should not be indefinite.

HOW SUPPLIED: Sol: 5mg/5mL [500mL], 10mg/5mL [500mL]; Tab, Chewable: 2.5mg, 5mg, 10mg* *scored

CONTRAINDICATIONS: Marked anxiety, tension, agitation, glaucoma, motor tics, or family history or diagnosis of Tourette's syndrome. Treatment with MAOIs or within a minimum of 14 days following discontinuation of an MAOI.

WARNINGS/PRECAUTIONS: Avoid with known serious structural cardiac abnormalities, cardiomyopathy, serious heart rhythm abnormalities, coronary artery disease or other serious cardiac problems. Sudden death reported in children and adolescents with structural cardiac abnormalities or other serious heart problems. Sudden death, stroke, and myocardial infarction (MI) reported in adults. May cause modest increase in average BP and HR; caution with conditions that might be compromised by increases in BP/HR (eg, preexisting HTN, heart failure, recent MI, ventricular arrhythmias). Prior to treatment, obtain medical history (including assessment for family history of sudden death or ventricular arrhythmia) and perform physical exam to assess for presence of cardiac disease. Promptly perform cardiac evaluation if symptoms suggestive of cardiac disease develop. May exacerbate symptoms of behavior disturbance and thought disorder in patients with a preexisting psychotic disorder. Caution in patients with comorbid bipolar disorder; may induce mixed/manic episode. May cause treatment-emergent psychotic or manic symptoms (eg, hallucinations, delusional thinking, mania) in children and adolescents without prior history of psychotic illness or mania; discontinuation may be appropriate if such symptoms occur. Aggressive behavior or hostility reported in children and adolescents. May lower convulsive threshold; d/c if seizures occur. Priapism, sometimes requiring surgical intervention, reported. May cause long-term suppression of growth in children; monitor growth and may need to interrupt treatment in patients not growing or gaining height or weight as expected. Associated with peripheral vasculopathy, including Raynaud's phenomenon; monitor for digital changes. Difficulties with accommodation and blurring of vision reported. Patients with an element of agitation may react adversely; d/c therapy if necessary. Periodically monitor CBC, differential, and platelet counts during prolonged therapy. Not indicated in all cases of this behavioral syndrome, and in symptoms associated with acute stress reactions. Long-term effects in children not well established.

ADVERSE REACTIONS: Nervousness, insomnia, hypersensitivity, anorexia, nausea, dizziness, palpitations, headache, dyskinesia, drowsiness, BP and pulse changes, tachycardia, weight loss, abdominal pain, loss of appetite.

INTERACTIONS: See Contraindications. May decrease hypotensive effect of guanethidine. Caution with pressor agents. May inhibit metabolism of coumarin anticoagulants, anticonvulsants (eg, phenobarbital, diphenylhydantoin, primidone), phenylbutazone, and TCAs (eg, imipramine, clomipramine, desipramine); may require downward dose adjustments of these drugs.

PREGNANCY: Safety not known in pregnancy and nursing.

MECHANISM OF ACTION: Sympathomimetic amine; CNS stimulant. Has not been established; thought to block the reuptake of norepinephrine and dopamine into the presynaptic neuron and increase the release of monoamines into the extraneuronal space. Presumably activates the brain stem arousal system and cortex to produce stimulant effect.

PHARMACOKINETICS: Absorption: T_{max}=1-2 hrs. (Tab, Chewable) C_{max}=10ng/mL (20mg). (Sol) C_{max}=9ng/mL (20mg). **Metabolism:** Deesterification to α-phenyl-piperidine acetic acid (major metabolite). **Elimination:** Urine (90%; 80% metabolite). (Sol) $T_{1/2}$=2.7 hrs (20mg, healthy). (Tab, Chewable) $T_{1/2}$=3 hrs (20mg, healthy).

NURSING CONSIDERATIONS

Assessment: Assess for previous hypersensitivity to the drug, history of drug dependence or alcoholism, marked anxiety, tension, agitation, glaucoma, motor tics, family history or diagnosis of Tourette's syndrome, preexisting psychotic disorder, comorbid bipolar disorder, cardiac disease, any other conditions where treatment is cautioned or contraindicated, pregnancy/nursing status, and possible drug interactions.

Monitoring: Monitor BP/HR, signs/symptoms of cardiac disease, exacerbations of behavior disturbances and thought disorders, psychosis, mania, appearance of or worsening of aggressive behavior or hostility, seizures, priapism, digital changes, visual disturbances and other adverse reactions. Monitor growth in children. Perform periodic monitoring of CBC, differential, and platelet counts during prolonged therapy.

Patient Counseling: Inform patients/families/caregivers about risks, benefits, and appropriate use of treatment. Instruct to read the Medication Guide. Instruct to seek immediate medical attention in the event of priapism. Instruct to report to physician if any new numbness, pain, skin color change, sensitivity to temperature in fingers or toes, or any signs of unexplained wounds appearing on fingers or toes develop. (Tab, Chewable) Advise not to take the drug if have difficulty swallowing. Seek medical attention if experience chest pain, vomiting, or difficulty in swallowing or breathing after taking the drug. Inform that drug contains phenylalanine.

Administration: Oral route. (Tab, Chewable) Take with at least 8 oz. (full glass) of water or other fluid. **Storage:** 20-25°C (68-77°F). (Tab, Chewable) Protect from moisture.

METOCLOPRAMIDE
metoclopramide (Various)

RX

> May cause tardive dyskinesia (TD); d/c if signs/symptoms of TD develop. Avoid use for >12 weeks of therapy unless benefit outweighs risk.

OTHER BRAND NAMES: Reglan Injection (Baxter) - Reglan Tablets (ANI)

THERAPEUTIC CLASS: Dopamine antagonist/prokinetic

INDICATIONS: (PO) Short-term therapy (4-12 weeks) for adults with symptomatic, documented gastroesophageal reflux disease (GERD) who fail to respond to conventional therapy. (PO, Inj) Relief of symptoms associated with acute and recurrent diabetic gastric stasis in adults. (Inj) Prevention of postoperative N/V (PONV) or chemotherapy-induced N/V. Facilitates small bowel intubation in adults and pediatric patients in whom the tube does not pass the pylorus with conventional maneuvers. Stimulates gastric emptying and intestinal transit of barium in cases where delayed emptying interferes with radiological examination of the stomach and/or small intestine.

DOSAGE: *Adults:* (PO) GERD: 10-15mg up to qid 30 min ac and hs. Intermittent Symptoms: Up to 20mg as single dose prior to the provoking situation. Sensitive to Metoclopramide/Elderly: 5mg/dose. Esophageal Lesions Present: 15mg/dose qid. Max: 12 weeks of therapy. (PO, Inj) Diabetic Gastroparesis: 10mg PO 30 min ac and hs for 2-8 weeks. If severe, begin with IM or IV (may give 10mg IV slowly over 1-2 min); may need inj for up to 10 days before symptoms subside, at which time PO administration may be instituted. (Inj) Antiemetic: (PONV) 10-20mg IM near end of surgery. (Chemotherapy-Induced N/V) 1-2mg/kg IV infusion over a period of ≥15 min, 30 min before chemotherapy, then q2h for 2 doses, then q3h for 3 doses. Give the 2mg/kg dose for highly emetogenic drugs for the initial 2 doses. Small Bowel Intubation/Radiological Exam: 10mg IV single dose (undiluted) given slowly over 1-2 min. Renal Impairment: CrCl <40mL/min: Initial: 1/2 of recommended dose. May adjust as appropriate. Elderly: Start at lower end of dosing range. *Pediatrics:* (Inj) Small Bowel Intubation: Administer single dose (undiluted) IV slowly over 1-2 min. >14 Yrs: 10mg. 6-14 Yrs: 2.5-5mg. <6 Yrs: 0.1mg/kg. Renal Impairment: CrCl <40mL/min: Initial: 1/2 of recommended dose. May adjust as appropriate.

HOW SUPPLIED: Inj (Reglan): 5mg/mL [2mL, 10mL, 30mL]; Sol: 5mg/5mL [473mL]; Tab (Reglan): 5mg, 10mg* *scored

CONTRAINDICATIONS: When GI motility stimulation is dangerous (eg, GI hemorrhage, mechanical obstruction, perforation), pheochromocytoma, epilepsy, and concomitant drugs that cause extrapyramidal symptoms (EPS).

WARNINGS/PRECAUTIONS: Mental depression may occur; caution with prior history of depression. EPS, primarily as acute dystonic reactions, may occur. May cause parkinsonian-like symptoms; caution with preexisting Parkinson's disease. May suppress signs of TD; do not use for symptomatic control of TD. Neuroleptic malignant syndrome reported; d/c, monitor, and institute intensive symptomatic treatment. Risk of developing fluid retention and volume overload, especially in patients with cirrhosis or congestive heart failure (CHF); d/c if these occur. Caution with HTN, renal impairment, and/or in elderly. May increase risk of developing methemoglobinemia and/or sulfhemoglobinemia with NADH-cytochrome b_5 reductase deficiency. May experience withdrawal symptoms after discontinuation. (Inj) Undiluted IV inj should be given slowly since rapid administration may cause anxiety, restlessness, and drowsiness. May increase pressure on suture lines after a gut anastomosis or closure; use caution with PONV.

ADVERSE REACTIONS: TD, restlessness, drowsiness, fatigue, lassitude.

INTERACTIONS: See Contraindications. GI motility effect antagonized by anticholinergics and narcotic analgesics. Additive sedation with alcohol, sedatives, hypnotics, narcotics, or tranquilizers. Caution with MAOIs. May diminish absorption of drugs from stomach (eg, digoxin) and increase rate and/or extent of absorption of drugs from small bowel (eg, acetaminophen, tetracycline, levodopa, ethanol, cyclosporine). Insulin dose or timing of dose may require adjustment. Rare cases of hepatotoxicity reported with drugs with hepatotoxic potential. Inhibits central and peripheral effects of apomorphine.

PREGNANCY: Category B, caution in nursing.

MECHANISM OF ACTION: Dopamine antagonist/prokinetic; not established. Appears to sensitize tissues to the action of acetylcholine; stimulates motility of upper GI tract without stimulating gastric, biliary, or pancreatic secretions and accelerates gastric emptying and intestinal transit. Also increases resting tone of the lower esophageal sphincter. Antiemetic; antagonizes central and peripheral dopamine receptors, thereby blocking stimulation of chemoreceptor trigger zone.

PHARMACOKINETICS: Absorption: Rapid and well-absorbed; (PO) absolute bioavailability (80%); (PO) T_{max}=1-2 hrs; IV administration resulted in varying parameters. **Distribution:** Plasma protein binding (30%); V_d=3.5L/kg; found in breast milk. **Elimination:** (PO) Urine (85%; 50% free or conjugated); $T_{1/2}$=5-6 hrs.

NURSING CONSIDERATIONS

Assessment: Assess for conditions when GI motility stimulation is dangerous, pheochromocytoma, epilepsy, sensitivity or tolerance to the drug, CHF, cirrhosis, history of depression, Parkinson's disease, HTN, NADH-cytochrome b_5 reductase and G6PD deficiency, diabetes mellitus, renal impairment, pregnancy/nursing status, and possible drug interactions.

Monitoring: Monitor for signs/symptoms of depression, EPS, parkinsonian-like symptoms, TD, NMS, HTN, fluid retention/volume overload, withdrawal symptoms, hypersensitivity reactions, and other adverse reactions.

Patient Counseling: Inform that drug may impair mental and physical abilities; advise to use caution while operating machinery/driving. Discuss the risks and benefits of treatment.

Administration: Oral, IV/IM route. Refer to PI for IV administration, preparation, and compatibility instructions. **Storage:** 20-25°C (68-77°F). (Inj) If diluted with NaCl, may be stored frozen for up to 4 weeks. Diluted sol may be stored up to 48 hrs (without freezing) if protected from light; 24 hrs in normal lighting conditions.

METOPROLOL   RX
metoprolol tartrate (Various)

OTHER BRAND NAMES: Lopressor (Novartis)

THERAPEUTIC CLASS: Selective beta$_1$-blocker

INDICATIONS: Treatment of hemodynamically stable patients with definite or suspected acute myocardial infarction (MI) to reduce cardiovascular mortality. (Tab) Treatment of HTN alone or in combination with other antihypertensives. Long-term treatment of angina pectoris.

DOSAGE: *Adults:* HTN: Individualize dose. Initial: 100mg/day PO in single or divided doses given alone or with a diuretic. Titrate: May increase at weekly (or longer) intervals until optimum BP reduction is achieved. Effective Range: 100-450mg/day. Max: 450mg/day. Angina Pectoris: Individualize dose. Initial: 100mg/day PO in 2 divided doses. Titrate: Gradually increase at weekly intervals until optimum clinical response is achieved or pronounced slowing of HR. Effective Range: 100-400mg/day. Max: 400mg/day. Upon discontinuation, taper gradually over 1-2 weeks.

MI (Early Phase): 5mg IV bolus every 2 min for 3 doses (monitor BP, HR, and ECG). Patients Who Tolerate Full IV Dose (15mg): Give 50mg PO q6h, 15 min after last IV dose and continue for 48 hrs. Maint: 100mg PO bid. Patients Who Cannot Tolerate Full IV Dose: Give either 25 or 50mg PO q6h (depending on the degree of intolerance) 15 min after the last IV dose or as soon as clinical condition allows. D/C if with severe intolerance. MI (Late Phase): 100mg PO bid for ≥3 months. Hepatic Impairment: Initiate at low doses with cautious gradual dose titration according to clinical response. Elderly: Start at lower end of dosing range. Take tab with or immediately following meals.

HOW SUPPLIED: Tab: 25mg*, 50mg*, 100mg*; (Lopressor) Inj: 1mg/mL [5mL]; Tab: 50mg*, 100mg* *scored

CONTRAINDICATIONS: HR <45 beats/min, 2nd- and 3rd-degree heart block, significant 1st-degree heart block, systolic BP <100mmHg, moderate to severe cardiac failure. (Tab) Sinus bradycardia, >1st-degree heart block, cardiogenic shock, overt cardiac failure, sick sinus syndrome, severe peripheral arterial circulatory disorders.

WARNINGS/PRECAUTIONS: May cause depression of myocardial contractility and may precipitate heart failure and cardiogenic shock. If signs/symptoms of heart failure develop, treat patient according to recommended guidelines; lower dose or d/c if necessary. Avoid abrupt discontinuation in patients with coronary artery disease (CAD). Severe exacerbation of angina, MI, and ventricular arrhythmias reported in patients with coronary artery disease following abrupt discontinuation. When discontinuing chronic therapy, particularly with coronary heart disease, reduce dose over 1-2 weeks with careful monitoring. If angina markedly worsens or acute coronary insufficiency develops, reinstate promptly, at least temporarily, and take other measures for the management of unstable angina. Chronically administered therapy should not be routinely withdrawn prior to major surgery; impaired ability of the heart to respond to reflex adrenergic stimuli may augment the risks of general anesthesia and surgical procedures. Bradycardia, including sinus pause, heart block, and cardiac arrest reported; increased risk in patients with 1st degree atrioventricular block, sinus node dysfunction, or conduction disorders. Reduce or d/c if severe bradycardia develops. Avoid with bronchospastic diseases, may be used in patients with bronchospastic disease who do not respond to, or cannot tolerate other antihypertensive treatment. May mask tachycardia occurring with hypoglycemia; other manifestations (eg, dizziness, sweating) may not be significantly affected. If used in the setting of pheochromocytoma, should be given in combination with an α-blocker, and only after the α-blocker has been initiated; may cause a paradoxical increase in BP if administered alone. May mask certain clinical signs (eg, tachycardia) of hyperthyroidism. Avoid abrupt withdrawal; may precipitate thyroid storm. Patients with a history of severe anaphylactic reaction to variety of allergens may be more reactive to repeated challenge and may be unresponsive to usual doses of epinephrine.

ADVERSE REACTIONS: Bradycardia, tiredness, dizziness, depression, SOB, diarrhea, pruritus, rash, heart block, heart failure, hypotension.

INTERACTIONS: Additive effects with catecholamine-depleting drugs (eg, reserpine). May increase risk of bradycardia with digitalis glycosides; monitor HR and PR interval. May produce an additive reduction in myocardial contractility with calcium channel blockers. May increase levels with potent CYP2D6 inhibitors (eg, antidepressants, antipsychotics, antiarrhythmics, antiretrovirals, antihistamines, antimalarials, antifungals). Hydralazine may inhibit presystemic metabolism, leading to increased levels. May potentiate antihypertensive effects of α-blockers (eg, guanethidine, betanidine, reserpine, α-methyldopa, or clonidine). May potentiate the postural hypotensive effect of 1st dose of prazosin. May potentiate hypertensive response to withdrawal of clonidine; when given concomitantly with clonidine, d/c several days before clonidine is withdrawn. May enhance vasoconstrictive action of ergot alkaloids. Withhold therapy before dipyridamole testing, with careful monitoring of HR following the dipyridamole inj. (Inj) May enhance cardiodepressant effect with some inhalational anesthetics.

PREGNANCY: Category C, safety not known in nursing.

MECHANISM OF ACTION: Selective β₁-blocker; has not been established. Proposed to competitively antagonize catecholamines at peripheral adrenergic-neuronal sites; has central effect, leading to reduced sympathetic outflow to periphery and suppression of renin activity.

PHARMACOKINETICS: Absorption: Oral Bioavailability (50%). **Distribution:** V_d=3.2-5.6L/kg. Plasma serum albumin binding (10%); crosses placenta and found in breast milk. **Metabolism:** CYP2D6 (oxidation). **Elimination:** Urine (95%; [PO] <5% unchanged, [IV] <10% unchanged); $T_{1/2}$=3-4 hrs, 7-9 hrs (poor metabolizers).

NURSING CONSIDERATIONS

Assessment: Assess for sinus bradycardia, heart block, cardiogenic shock, heart failure, CAD, bronchospastic diseases, hypoglycemia, hyperthyroidism, hypersensitivity to the drug, hepatic function, any other conditions where treatment is contraindicated or cautioned, pregnancy/nursing status, and possible drug interactions. Obtain baseline ECG.

Monitoring: Monitor BP, HR, ECG, and hemodynamic status. Monitor for signs/symptoms of heart failure, cardiogenic shock, thyrotoxicosis, hypotension, hypersensitivity reactions, and other adverse reactions.

Patient Counseling: Advise to take regularly and continuously, ud, with or immediately following meals. If a dose is missed, instruct to take only the next scheduled dose (without doubling) and to not interrupt or d/c without consulting a physician. Advise to avoid operating automobiles and machinery or engaging in other tasks requiring alertness until response to therapy has been determined. Advise to contact physician if difficulty in breathing or other adverse reactions occur, and to inform physician/dentist of metoprolol therapy before undergoing any type of surgery.

Administration: Oral, IV route. (Tab) Swallow unchewed with a glass of water. Always take in standardized relation with meals; continue taking with the same schedule during the course of therapy. (Inj) Inspect for particulate matter and discoloration prior to administration. Parenteral administration should be done in a setting with intensive monitoring. **Storage:** 20-25°C (77°F). Protect from moisture. (Lopressor) 25°C (77°F); excursions permitted to 15-30°C (59-86°F). Protect from moisture, heat, and light.

METOPROLOL/HCTZ   RX
metoprolol tartrate - hydrochlorothiazide (Various)

Exacerbation of angina and, in some cases, myocardial infarction (MI) reported following abrupt discontinuation. When discontinuing therapy, avoid abrupt withdrawal even without overt angina pectoris. Caution patients against interruption of therapy without physician's advice.

OTHER BRAND NAMES: Lopressor HCT (Novartis)

THERAPEUTIC CLASS: Selective beta$_1$-blocker/thiazide diuretic

INDICATIONS: Management of HTN.

DOSAGE: *Adults:* Individualize dose. Combination Therapy: Metoprolol: 100-200mg/day given qd or in divided doses. HCTZ: 25-50mg/day given qd or in divided doses. Max: 50mg/day. May gradually add another antihypertensive when necessary, beginning with 50% of the usual recommended starting dose. Elderly: Start at lower end of dosing range.

HOW SUPPLIED: Tab: (Metoprolol-HCTZ) 50mg-25mg*, 100mg-25mg*, 100mg-50mg*; (Lopressor HCT) 50mg-25mg*, 100mg-25mg* *scored

CONTRAINDICATIONS: Sinus bradycardia, >1st-degree heart block, cardiogenic shock, overt cardiac failure, sick sinus syndrome, severe peripheral arterial circulatory disorders, anuria, hypersensitivity to sulfonamide-derived drugs.

WARNINGS/PRECAUTIONS: Not for initial therapy. Caution with hepatic dysfunction and in elderly. Metoprolol: May cause/precipitate heart failure; d/c if cardiac failure continues despite adequate treatment. Avoid with bronchospastic diseases, but may use with caution if unresponsive to/intolerant of other antihypertensives. Avoid withdrawal of chronically administered therapy prior to major surgery; however, may augment risks of general anesthesia and surgical procedures. Caution with diabetic patients; may mask tachycardia occurring with hypoglycemia. Paradoxical BP increase reported with pheochromocytoma; give in combination with and only after initiating α-blocker therapy. May mask hyperthyroidism. Avoid abrupt withdrawal in suspected thyrotoxicosis; may precipitate thyroid storm. HCTZ: Caution with severe renal disease; may precipitate azotemia. If progressive renal impairment becomes evident, d/c therapy. May precipitate hepatic coma in patients with liver dysfunction/disease. Sensitivity reactions are more likely to occur with history of allergy or bronchial asthma. May exacerbate/activate systemic lupus erythematosus (SLE). May cause idiosyncratic reaction, resulting in acute transient myopia and acute angle-closure glaucoma; d/c HCTZ as rapidly as possible. Fluid/electrolyte imbalance (eg, hyponatremia, hypochloremic alkalosis, hypokalemia) may develop. May cause hyperuricemia and precipitation of frank gout. Latent diabetes mellitus (DM) may manifest during therapy. Enhanced effects seen in postsympathectomy patients. D/C prior to parathyroid function test. Decreased Ca^{2+} excretion observed. Altered parathyroid gland, with hypercalcemia and hypophosphatemia observed with prolonged therapy. May increase urinary excretion of Mg^{2+}, resulting in hypomagnesemia.

ADVERSE REACTIONS: Fatigue, lethargy, dizziness, vertigo, flu syndrome, drowsiness, somnolence, hypokalemia, headache, bradycardia.

INTERACTIONS: Metoprolol: May exhibit additive effect with catecholamine-depleting drugs (eg, reserpine). Digitalis glycosides may increase risk of bradycardia. Some inhalation anesthetics may enhance cardiodepressant effect. May be unresponsive to usual doses of epinephrine. Potent CYP2D6 inhibitors (eg, certain antidepressants, antipsychotics, antiarrhythmics, antiretrovirals, antihistamines, antimalarials, antifungals, stomach ulcer drugs) may increase levels. Increased risk for rebound HTN following clonidine withdrawal; d/c metoprolol several days before withdrawing clonidine. Effects can be reversed by β-agonists (eg, dobutamine, isoproterenol). HCTZ: Hypokalemia can sensitize/exaggerate cardiac response to toxic effects

M

of digitalis. Risk of hypokalemia with steroids or adrenocorticotropic hormone. Insulin requirements may change in diabetic patients. May decrease arterial responsiveness to norepinephrine. May increase responsiveness to tubocurarine. May increase risk of lithium toxicity. Rare reports of hemolytic anemia with methyldopa. NSAIDs may reduce diuretic, natriuretic, and antihypertensive effects. Impaired absorption reported with cholestyramine and colestipol. Alcohol, barbiturates, and narcotics may potentiate orthostatic hypotension. May potentiate other antihypertensive drugs (eg, ganglionic or peripheral adrenergic blocking drugs).

PREGNANCY: Category C, not for use in nursing.

MECHANISM OF ACTION: Metoprolol: β_1-adrenergic receptor blocker; not established. Proposed to competitively antagonize catecholamines at peripheral adrenergic-neuron sites, have central effect leading to reduced sympathetic outflow to periphery, and suppress renin activity. HCTZ: Thiazide diuretic; not established. Affects renal tubular mechanism of electrolyte reabsorption and increases excretion of Na^+ and Cl^-.

PHARMACOKINETICS: Absorption: Metoprolol: Rapid and complete. HCTZ: Rapid; T_{max}=1-2.5 hrs. **Distribution:** Found in breast milk. Metoprolol: Plasma protein binding (12%); found in CSF. HCTZ: V_d=3.6-7.8L/kg; plasma protein binding (67.9%); crosses the placenta. **Metabolism:** Metoprolol: Liver (extensive) via CYP2D6 (oxidation). **Elimination:** Metoprolol: Urine (<5%, unchanged); $T_{1/2}$=2.8 hrs (extensive metabolizers), 7.5 hrs (poor metabolizers). HCTZ: Urine (72-97%); $T_{1/2}$=10-17 hrs.

NURSING CONSIDERATIONS

Assessment: Assess for history of heart failure, sulfonamide hypersensitivity, SLE, hyperthyroidism, DM, pheochromocytoma, hepatic/renal impairment, any other conditions where treatment is contraindicated/cautioned, pregnancy/nursing status, and possible drug interactions. Obtain baseline serum electrolytes.

Monitoring: Monitor for signs/symptoms of cardiac failure, hypoglycemia, thyrotoxicosis, electrolyte imbalance, exacerbation/activation of SLE, hyperuricemia or precipitation of gout, hypersensitivity reactions, hepatic/renal dysfunction, myopia, angle-closure glaucoma, and other adverse reactions. Monitor serum electrolytes.

Patient Counseling: Instruct to take regularly and continuously, ud, with or immediately following meals. Inform that if dose is missed, advise to take next dose at scheduled time (without doubling the dose) and not to d/c without consulting physician. Instruct to avoid driving, operating machinery, or engaging in tasks requiring alertness until response to therapy is determined. Advise to contact physician if difficulty in breathing or other adverse reactions occur, and to inform physician/dentist of drug therapy before undergoing any type of surgery.

Administration: Oral route. **Storage:** (Lopressor HCT) 25°C (77°F); excursions permitted to 15-30°C (59-86°F). (Metoprolol-HCTZ) 20-25°C (68-77°F). Protect from moisture.

METROGEL-VAGINAL   RX
metronidazole (Medicis)

THERAPEUTIC CLASS: Nitroimidazole

INDICATIONS: Treatment of bacterial vaginosis.

DOSAGE: *Adults:* Usual: 1 applicatorful intravaginally qd or bid for 5 days. For qd dosing, administer at hs.

HOW SUPPLIED: Gel: 0.75% [70g]

WARNINGS/PRECAUTIONS: Not for ophthalmic, dermal, or PO use. Convulsive seizures and peripheral neuropathy reported; d/c promptly if abnormal neurologic signs appear. Caution with CNS diseases and severe hepatic disease. Known or previously unrecognized vaginal candidiasis may present more prominent symptoms during therapy. May develop symptomatic *Candida* vaginitis during or immediately after therapy. Contains ingredients that may cause burning and irritation of the eye; rinse with copious amounts of cool tap water in the event of accidental contact. May interfere with certain types of serum chemistry values (eg, AST, ALT, LDH, TG, glucose hexokinase).

ADVERSE REACTIONS: Symptomatic *Candida* cervicitis/vaginitis, vaginal discharge, pelvic discomfort, N/V, headache, vulva/vaginal irritation, GI discomfort.

INTERACTIONS: May potentiate anticoagulant effect of warfarin and other coumarin anticoagulants, resulting in prolongation of PT. Elevation of serum lithium levels and signs of lithium toxicity may occur in short-term therapy with high doses of lithium. Cimetidine may prolong $T_{1/2}$ and decrease plasma clearance. May cause disulfiram-like reaction with alcohol. May cause psychotic reactions in alcoholic patients using disulfiram concurrently; do not administer within 2 weeks of discontinuation of disulfiram.

PREGNANCY: Category B, not for use in nursing.

MECHANISM OF ACTION: Nitroimidazole; intracellular targets of action on anaerobes unknown. Reduced by metabolically active anaerobes and the reduced form of the drug interacts with bacterial DNA.

PHARMACOKINETICS: Absorption: C_{max}=214ng/mL (Day 1), 294ng/mL (Day 5); T_{max}=6-12 hrs; AUC=4977ng•hr/mL. **Distribution:** Found in breast milk (PO); crosses the placenta.

NURSING CONSIDERATIONS

Assessment: Assess for hypersensitivity to drug, CNS/severe hepatic diseases, vaginal candidiasis, alcohol intake, nursing status, and possible drug interactions. Assess for clinical diagnosis of bacterial vaginosis.

Monitoring: Monitor for convulsive seizures, peripheral neuropathy, *Candida* vaginitis, and other adverse reactions.

Patient Counseling: Caution about drinking alcohol while on therapy. Instruct not to engage in vaginal intercourse during treatment. Inform to avoid contact with eyes and instruct to rinse with copious amounts of cool tap water in the event of accidental contact.

Administration: Intravaginal route. Refer to PI for administration instructions. **Storage:** 15-30°C (59-86°F). Protect from freezing.

MIACALCIN   RX
calcitonin-salmon (Novartis)

THERAPEUTIC CLASS: Hormonal bone resorption inhibitor

INDICATIONS: Treatment of postmenopausal osteoporosis in females >5 yrs postmenopause. (Inj) Treatment of Paget's disease of bone and hypercalcemia.

DOSAGE: *Adults:* (Inj) Paget's Disease: Initial: 100 IU SQ/IM qd. SQ is preferred for outpatient self-administration. 50 IU IM/SQ qd or qod may be sufficient in some patients; maintain higher dose with serious deformity and neurological involvement. Hypercalcemia: Initial: 4 IU/kg SQ/IM q12h. Titrate: May increase to 8 IU/kg q12h after 1-2 days if response is unsatisfactory. If response remains unsatisfactory after 2 more days, may be further increased to a max of 8 IU/kg q6h. Postmenopausal Osteoporosis: (Inj) Usual: 100 IU SQ/IM qod. If >2mL, use IM inj (preferably) and multiple inj sites. Take with supplemental Ca^{2+} (1.5g calcium carbonate/day) and vitamin D (400 IU/day). (Spray) Usual: 1 spray (200 IU) qd intranasally, alternating nostrils daily.

HOW SUPPLIED: Inj: 200 IU/mL [2mL]; Spray: 200 IU/actuation [3.7mL]

WARNINGS/PRECAUTIONS: Serious allergic-type reactions (eg, bronchospasm, swelling of the tongue or throat, anaphylactic shock) reported. Consider skin testing prior to treatment with suspected sensitivity to calcitonin. Urinary casts reported; monitor urine sediment periodically. (Inj) May lead to possible hypocalcemic tetany; provisions for parenteral Ca^{2+} administration should be available during the 1st several administrations of calcitonin. (Spray) Perform periodic nasal exams. D/C if severe ulceration (ulcers >1.5mm diameter, penetrating below mucosa or if with heavy bleeding) of the nasal mucosa occurs.

ADVERSE REACTIONS: N/V, flushing. (Inj) Local inflammatory reactions. (Spray) Nasal symptoms, rhinitis, back pain, epistaxis, headache, and arthralgia.

INTERACTIONS: May reduce plasma lithium concentrations; adjust lithium dose. (Spray) In patients with Paget's disease, prior use of diphosphonate appears to reduce the antiresorptive response to therapy.

PREGNANCY: Category C, not for use in nursing.

MECHANISM OF ACTION: Hormonal bone resorption inhibitor; actions on bone has not been fully established. Single inj cause a marked transient inhibition of the ongoing bone resorptive process. Prolonged use causes a smaller decrease in the rate of bone resorption, which is associated with a decreased number of osteoclasts as well as decrease in their resorptive activity.

PHARMACOKINETICS: Absorption: (Inj) Absolute bioavailability (66% IM), (71% SQ); T_{max}=23 min (SQ). (Spray) T_{max}=13 min. **Distribution:** V_d=0.15-0.3L/kg. **Metabolism:** Kidneys, blood, peripheral tissues. **Elimination:** (Inj) Urine; $T_{1/2}$=58 min (IM), $T_{1/2}$=59-64 min (SQ). (Spray) $T_{1/2}$=18 min.

NURSING CONSIDERATIONS

Assessment: Assess for hypersensitivity to drug, pregnancy/nursing status, and possible drug interactions. Consider skin testing for patients with suspected sensitivity to calcitonin. (Inj) For treatment of osteoporosis, obtain baseline measurement of biochemical markers of bone resorption/turnover and bone mineral density (BMD). (Spray) Obtain baseline nasal exam (eg, visualization of the nasal mucosa, turbinates, septum, and mucosal blood vessel status).

Monitoring: Monitor for signs/symptoms of serious allergic reactions (eg, bronchospasm, swelling of the tongue or throat, anaphylactic shock). Perform periodic exams of urine sediment. (Inj) Monitor for hypocalcemic tetany. For treatment of Paget's disease, perform periodic

M

measurement of serum alkaline phosphatase and 24-hr urinary hydroxyproline. For treatment of osteoporosis, monitor biochemical markers of bone resorption/turnover and BMD. (Spray) Monitor for nasal mucosal alterations, transient nasal conditions, and ulceration of nasal mucosa; perform periodic nasal exams. Perform periodic measurements of lumbar vertebral bone mass.

Patient Counseling: (Inj) Instruct about sterile inj technique. (Spray) Instruct how to assemble and prime pump, and introduce medication in the nasal passages. Advise to contact physician if allergic reaction or nasal irritation occurs. Inform that new, unassembled bottles should be refrigerated and protected from freezing. Instruct to allow medication to reach room temperature before priming pump and using a new bottle. Inform that after 30 doses, each spray may not deliver correct amount of medication; instruct to keep track of number of doses used.

Administration: Intranasal/IM/SQ routes. **Storage:** (Spray) Unopened: 2-8°C (36-46°F). Protect from freezing. Used: 15-30°C (59-86°F) for up to 35 days. (Inj) 2-8°C (36-46°F).

MICARDIS RX
telmisartan (Boehringer Ingelheim)

D/C when pregnancy is detected. Drugs that act directly on the renin-angiotensin system (RAS) can cause injury/death to the developing fetus.

THERAPEUTIC CLASS: Angiotensin II receptor antagonist

INDICATIONS: Treatment of HTN alone or in combination with other antihypertensives. Reduction of risk of myocardial infarction, stroke, or death from cardiovascular (CV) causes in patients ≥55 yrs of age at high risk of developing major CV events who are unable to take ACE inhibitors.

DOSAGE: *Adults:* HTN: Individualize dose. Initial: 40mg qd. Usual: 20-80mg/day. If additional BP reduction is required beyond that achieved with the 80mg dose, a diuretic may be added. CV Risk Reduction: Usual: 80mg qd. Monitor BP and adjust dose of medications that lower BP if needed. Biliary Obstructive Disorders/Hepatic Insufficiency: Start at low doses and titrate slowly.

HOW SUPPLIED: Tab: 20mg, 40mg, 80mg

CONTRAINDICATIONS: Coadministration with aliskiren in patients with diabetes.

WARNINGS/PRECAUTIONS: May develop orthostatic hypotension in patients on dialysis. Symptomatic hypotension may occur in patients with an activated RAS (eg, volume- and/or salt-depleted patients receiving high doses of diuretics); correct this condition before therapy or monitor closely. Hyperkalemia may occur, particularly in patients with advanced renal impairment, heart failure (HF), and on renal replacement therapy; monitor serum electrolytes periodically. Caution in patients with hepatic impairment (eg, biliary obstructive disorders); reduced clearance may be expected. Oliguria and/or progressive azotemia and (rarely) acute renal failure and/or death may occur in patients whose renal function is dependent on the RAS (eg, severe congestive heart failure [CHF]). Changes in renal function may occur in susceptible patients and with the dual blockade of the RAS (eg, adding an ACE inhibitor); monitor renal function. May increase SrCr/BUN in patients with renal artery stenosis.

ADVERSE REACTIONS: Upper respiratory tract infection, back pain, sinusitis, diarrhea, intermittent claudication, skin ulcer.

INTERACTIONS: See Contraindications. Avoid with aliskiren in patients with renal impairment (GFR <60 mL/min). Avoid with an ACE inhibitor. Increased exposure to ramipril and ramiprilat; concomitant use is not recommended. Hyperkalemia may occur with K+ supplements, K+-sparing diuretics, K+-containing salt substitutes, or other drugs that increase K+ levels. May increase digoxin levels; monitor digoxin levels upon initiating, adjusting, and discontinuing therapy. May increase serum lithium levels/toxicity; monitor lithium levels during concomitant use. NSAIDs, including selective COX-2, may deteriorate renal function; monitor renal function periodically. Antihypertensive effect may be attenuated by NSAIDs.

PREGNANCY: Category D, not for use in nursing.

MECHANISM OF ACTION: Angiotensin II receptor antagonist; blocks the vasoconstrictor and aldosterone-secreting effects of angiotensin II by selectively blocking the binding of angiotensin II to the AT_1 receptor in many tissues, such as vascular smooth muscle and adrenal gland.

PHARMACOKINETICS: Absorption: Absolute bioavailability: 40mg (42%), 160mg (58%); T_{max}=0.5-1 hr. **Distribution:** V_d=500L; plasma protein binding (>99.5%). **Metabolism:** Conjugation. **Elimination:** Feces (>97%, unchanged), urine (0.49%); $T_{1/2}$=24 hrs.

NURSING CONSIDERATIONS

Assessment: Assess for known hypersensitivity (eg, anaphylaxis or angioedema), biliary obstructive disorders, HF/CHF, unilateral/bilateral renal artery stenosis, hepatic/renal impairment, volume/salt depletion, dialysis patients, pregnancy/nursing status, and possible drug interactions.

Monitoring: Monitor for symptomatic hypotension and other adverse reactions. Monitor BP, ECG, hepatic/renal function, serum electrolytes.

Patient Counseling: Inform women of childbearing age about the consequences of exposure to the medication during pregnancy. Discuss treatment options with women planning to become pregnant. Instruct to report pregnancies to the physician as soon as possible.

Administration: Oral route. **Storage:** 25°C (77°F); excursions permitted to 15-30°C (59-86°F).

MICARDIS HCT   RX
hydrochlorothiazide - telmisartan (Boehringer Ingelheim)

> D/C when pregnancy is detected. Drugs that act directly on the renin-angiotensin system (RAS) can cause injury/death to the developing fetus.

THERAPEUTIC CLASS: Angiotensin II receptor antagonist/thiazide diuretic

INDICATIONS: Treatment of HTN.

DOSAGE: *Adults:* Uncontrolled BP on 80mg Telmisartan/Controlled BP on 25mg/day of HCTZ but with Hypokalemia: Initial: 80mg-12.5mg tab qd. Uncontrolled BP on 25mg/day of HCTZ: Initial: 80mg-12.5mg qd or 80mg-25mg tab qd. Titrate/Max: Increase to 160mg-25mg if BP uncontrolled after 2-4 weeks. Biliary Obstruction/Hepatic Insufficiency: Initial: 40mg-12.5mg tab under qd. Replacement Therapy: May substitute combination for titrated components.

HOW SUPPLIED: Tab: (Telmisartan-HCTZ) 40mg-12.5mg, 80mg-12.5mg, 80mg-25mg

CONTRAINDICATIONS: Anuria, hypersensitivity to sulfonamide-derived drugs. Coadministration with aliskiren in patients with diabetes.

WARNINGS/PRECAUTIONS: Not for initial therapy. Hypotension may occur in patients with activated RAS, such as volume- or Na⁺-depleted (eg, vigorously treated with diuretics); correct these conditions prior to therapy and monitor closely. Not recommended with severe renal impairment (CrCl ≤30mL/min) and severe hepatic impairment. HCTZ: Caution with hepatic impairment or progressive liver disease; may precipitate hepatic coma. May cause hypersensitivity reactions, exacerbation or activation of systemic lupus erythematosus (SLE), hyperuricemia or precipitation of frank gout, hyperglycemia, hypomagnesemia, hypercalcemia, and latent diabetes mellitus (DM). May cause an idiosyncratic reaction, resulting in acute transient myopia and acute angle-closure glaucoma; d/c as rapidly as possible. Observe for clinical signs of fluid or electrolyte imbalance (hyponatremia, hypochloremic alkalosis, and hypokalemia). Hypokalemia may develop, especially with brisk diuresis, severe cirrhosis, or after prolonged therapy. Hypokalemia may cause cardiac arrhythmia and may sensitize/exaggerate the response of the heart to toxic effects of digitalis. D/C before testing for parathyroid function. Enhanced effects in postsympathectomy patients. Increased cholesterol and TG levels reported. Caution with severe renal disease; may precipitate azotemia with renal disease. Telmisartan: Oliguria and/or progressive azotemia and (rarely) acute renal failure and/or death may occur in patients whose renal function is dependent on the RAS (eg, severe congestive heart failure [CHF]). Changes in renal function may occur in susceptible patients and with the dual blockade of the RAS (eg, by adding an ACE inhibitor to an ARB); monitor renal function. May increase SrCr/BUN in patients with renal artery stenosis.

ADVERSE REACTIONS: Upper respiratory tract infection, dizziness, sinusitis, fatigue, diarrhea.

INTERACTIONS: See Contraindications. NSAIDs, including selective COX-2 inhibitors, may decrease effects of diuretics and ARBs and may further deteriorate renal function. May increase risk of lithium toxicity; avoid concurrent use. HCTZ: Alcohol, barbiturates, or narcotics may potentiate orthostatic hypotension. Dosage adjustment of antidiabetic drugs (eg, PO agents, insulin) may be required. Additive effect or potentiation with other antihypertensive drugs. Anionic exchange resins (eg, cholestyramine and colestipol resins) may impair absorption. Corticosteroids and adrenocorticotropic hormone may intensify electrolyte depletion, particularly hypokalemia. May decrease response to pressor amines (eg, norepinephrine). May increase responsiveness to nondepolarizing skeletal muscle relaxant (eg, tubocurarine). Telmisartan: Avoid with aliskiren in patients with renal impairment (GFR <60mL/min). May increase digoxin levels; monitor digoxin levels. May increase exposure to ramipril; concomitant use not recommended. May slightly decrease warfarin levels. Possible inhibition of drugs metabolized by CYP2C19.

PREGNANCY: Category D, not for use in nursing.

MECHANISM OF ACTION: Telmisartan: Angiotensin II receptor antagonist; blocks the vasoconstrictor and aldosterone-secreting effects of angiotensin II by selectively blocking the binding of angiotensin II to the AT₁ receptor in many tissues, such as vascular smooth muscle and adrenal gland. HCTZ: Thiazide diuretic; has not been established. Affects renal tubular mechanisms of electrolyte reabsorption, directly increasing excretion of Na⁺ salt and Cl⁻ in approximately equivalent amounts.

PHARMACOKINETICS: Absorption: Telmisartan: Absolute bioavailability: 40mg (42%), 160mg (58%); T_{max}=0.5-1 hr. **Distribution:** Telmisartan: V_d=500L; plasma protein binding (>99.5%). HCTZ: Crosses placenta; found in breast milk. **Metabolism:** Telmisartan: Conjugation. **Elimination:**

Telmisartan: Feces (>97%, unchanged), urine (0.49%); T$_{1/2}$=24 hrs. HCTZ: Urine (61%, unchanged); T$_{1/2}$=5.6-14.8 hrs.

NURSING CONSIDERATIONS

Assessment: Assess for hypersensitivity to drugs and their components, anuria, sulfonamide-derived hypersensitivity, history of penicillin allergy, volume/salt depletion, SLE, DM, CHF, hepatic/renal impairment, biliary obstructive disorder, renal artery stenosis, cirrhosis, postsympathectomy patients, pregnancy/nursing status, and possible drug interactions. Obtain baseline BP.

Monitoring: Monitor for exacerbation/activation of SLE, idiosyncratic reaction, latent DM manifestations, hyperglycemia, hypercalcemia, hyperuricemia or precipitation of gout, hypersensitivity reactions, and other adverse reactions. Monitor BP, serum electrolytes, and renal function periodically.

Patient Counseling: Inform women of childbearing age about the consequences of exposure to the medication during pregnancy. Discuss treatment options with women planning to become pregnant. Instruct to report pregnancies to the physician as soon as possible. Caution that lightheadedness may occur, especially during the 1st days of therapy and should be instructed to report to physician. Instruct to d/c therapy and consult physician if syncope occurs. Caution patients that inadequate fluid intake, excessive perspiration, diarrhea, or vomiting can lead to an excessive fall in BP, with the same consequences of lightheadedness and possible syncope. Advise patient not to use K$^+$ supplements or salt substitutes that contain K$^+$ without consulting physician.

Administration: Oral route. **Storage:** 25°C (77°F); excursions permitted to 15-30°C (59-86°F).

MICRO-K RX
potassium chloride (Ther-Rx)

THERAPEUTIC CLASS: K$^+$ supplement

INDICATIONS: (For those unable to tolerate liquid or effervescent potassium preparations). Treatment and prevention of hypokalemia with or without metabolic alkalosis. Treatment of digitalis intoxication and hypokalemic familial periodic paralysis.

DOSAGE: *Adults:* Prevention: 20mEq/day. Hypokalemia: 40-100mEq/day. Divide dose if >20mEq. Take with meal and full glass of water or liquid. May sprinkle on soft food; swallow without chewing.

HOW SUPPLIED: Cap, Extended-Release: 8mEq, 10mEq

CONTRAINDICATIONS: Hyperkalemia, esophageal ulceration, delay in GI passage (from structural, pathological, pharmacologic causes [eg, anticholinergic agents]), cardiac patients with esophageal compression due to enlarged left atrium.

WARNINGS/PRECAUTIONS: Potentially fatal hyperkalemia may occur. Extreme caution with acidosis, cardiac and renal disease; monitor ECG and electrolytes. Hypokalemia with metabolic acidosis should be treated with an alkalinizing potassium salt (eg, potassium bicarbonate, potassium citrate). May produce ulcerative or stenotic GI lesions.

ADVERSE REACTIONS: Hyperkalemia, GI effects (obstruction, bleeding, ulceration), N/V, abdominal pain, diarrhea.

INTERACTIONS: See Contraindications. Risk of hyperkalemia with ACE inhibitors (eg, captopril, enalapril), K$^+$-sparing diuretics, and K$^+$ supplements.

PREGNANCY: Category C, safe for use in nursing.

MECHANISM OF ACTION: K$^+$ supplement; helps in maintenance of intracellular tonicity, transmission of nerve impulses, contraction of cardiac, skeletal, and smooth muscle, and maintenance of normal renal function.

NURSING CONSIDERATIONS

Assessment: Assess for conditions that impair excretion of K$^+$, hyperkalemia, esophageal compression due to enlarged left atrium, conditions causing arrest or delay in passage through GI, renal insufficiency, diabetes mellitus, and possible drug interactions.

Monitoring: Monitor serum K$^+$ levels regularly; renal function, ECG, and acid-base balance. Monitor for GI ulceration/obstruction/perforation, hyperkalemia, renal dysfunction, and hypersensitivity reactions.

Patient Counseling: Instruct to take with meals; swallow with full glass of water or other suitable liquid. Instruct to not crush, chew, or suck. Instruct to seek medical attention if symptoms of GI ulceration, obstruction, perforation (vomiting, abdominal pain, distention, GI bleeding), hyperkalemia, or hypersensitivity reactions occur.

Administration: Oral route. **Storage:** 20-25°C (68-77°F).

MICROZIDE

hydrochlorothiazide (Watson)

RX

THERAPEUTIC CLASS: Thiazide diuretic

INDICATIONS: Management of HTN either alone or in combination with other antihypertensives.

DOSAGE: *Adults:* Initial: 12.5mg qd. Max: 50mg/day.

HOW SUPPLIED: Cap: 12.5mg

CONTRAINDICATIONS: Anuria, sulfonamide hypersensitivity.

WARNINGS/PRECAUTIONS: May cause idiosyncratic reaction, resulting in acute transient myopia and acute angle-closure glaucoma; d/c as rapidly as possible. May manifest latent diabetes mellitus (DM). May precipitate azotemia with renal impairment. Hypokalemia reported; monitor serum electrolytes and for sign/symptoms of fluid/electrolyte disturbances. Dilutional hyponatremia may occur in edematous patients in hot weather. Hyperuricemia or acute gout may be precipitated. Caution with hepatic impairment; hepatic coma may occur with severe liver disease. Decreased Ca^{2+} excretion and changes in parathyroid glands with hypercalcemia and hypophosphatemia reported during prolonged use. D/C prior to parathyroid test.

ADVERSE REACTIONS: Weakness, hypotension, pancreatitis, jaundice, diarrhea, vomiting, hematologic abnormalities, anaphylactic reactions, electrolyte imbalance, muscle spasm, vertigo, renal failure, erythema multiforme, transient blurred vision, impotence.

INTERACTIONS: Potentiation of orthostatic hypotension with alcohol, barbiturates, narcotics. Additive effect or potentiation with antihypertensive drugs. Dose adjustment of antidiabetic drugs (oral agents or insulin) may be required. Reduced absorption with cholestyramine or colestipol. Increased risk of electrolyte depletion (eg, hypokalemia) with corticosteroids and adrenocorticotropic hormone. May decrease response to pressor amines (eg, norepinephrine). May increase responsiveness to nondepolarizing skeletal muscle relaxants (eg, tubocurarine). Increased risk of lithium toxicity; avoid with lithium. NSAIDs may reduce diuretic, natriuretic, and antihypertensive effects. May cause hypokalemia, which can sensitize or exaggerate the response of the heart to the toxic effects of digitalis.

PREGNANCY: Category B, not for use in nursing.

MECHANISM OF ACTION: Thiazide diuretic; blocks reabsorption of Na^+ and Cl^- ions, thereby increasing the quantity of Na^+ traversing the distal tubule and the volume of water excreted. Also decreases the excretion of Ca^{2+} and uric acid, may increase the excretion of iodide and may reduce GFR.

PHARMACOKINETICS: Absorption: Well-absorbed; C_{max}=70-490ng/mL; T_{max}=1-5 hrs. **Distribution:** Plasma protein binding (40-68%); crosses placenta; found in breast milk. **Elimination:** Urine (55-77%, >95% unchanged); $T_{1/2}$=6-15 hrs.

NURSING CONSIDERATIONS

Assessment: Assess for anuria, known hypersensitivity to sulfonamide-derived drugs, history of penicillin allergy, DM, risk for developing hypokalemia, impaired renal/hepatic function, edema, pregnancy/nursing status, and for possible drug interactions. Obtain baseline serum electrolytes.

Monitoring: Monitor for signs/symptoms of decreased visual acuity, ocular pain, azotemia, hypokalemia, fluid/electrolyte disturbances, dilutional hyponatremia, hyperuricemia or acute gout, and hepatic coma. Periodically monitor serum electrolytes in patients with risk for developing hypokalemia.

Patient Counseling: Counsel about signs/symptoms of fluid and electrolyte imbalance and advise to seek prompt medical attention.

Administration: Oral route. **Storage:** 20-25°C (68-77°F). Protect from light, moisture, freezing, -20°C (-4°F). Keep container tightly closed.

MINIPRESS

prazosin HCl (Pfizer)

RX

THERAPEUTIC CLASS: Alpha₁-blocker (quinazoline)

INDICATIONS: Treatment of HTN either alone or in combination with other antihypertensive drugs (eg, diuretics, β-blockers).

DOSAGE: *Adults:* Individualize dose according to BP response. Initial: 1mg bid-tid. Titrate: May slowly increase to a total of 20mg/day in divided doses. Usual: 6-15mg/day in divided doses. Doses >20mg usually do not increase efficacy; however, some may benefit from further increases up to 40mg/day in divided doses. Concomitant Use with a Diuretic or Other Antihypertensive Agent: Reduce to 1-2mg tid, then retitrate. Concomitant Use with a PDE-5 Inhibitor: Initiate PDE-5 inhibitor at the lowest dose.

M

HOW SUPPLIED: Cap: 1mg, 2mg, 5mg

WARNINGS/PRECAUTIONS: May cause syncope with sudden loss of consciousness; minimize syncopal episodes by limiting initial dose to 1mg, by subsequently increasing the dose slowly, and introducing any additional antihypertensive with caution. Two and 5mg caps are not indicated for initial therapy; always start on 1mg cap. Intraoperative floppy iris syndrome observed during cataract surgery in some patients treated with α_1-blockers. False (+) results may occur in screening tests for pheochromocytoma. D/C with elevated urinary vanillylmandelic acid levels and retest after 1 month.

ADVERSE REACTIONS: Dizziness, headache, drowsiness, lack of energy, weakness, palpitations, N/V, edema, orthostatic hypotension, dyspnea, syncope, depression, urinary frequency, diarrhea.

INTERACTIONS: Additive hypotensive effects with diuretics, β-blockers (eg, propranolol), or other antihypertensives. Additive BP lowering effects and symptomatic hypotension with PDE-5 inhibitors.

PREGNANCY: Category C, caution in nursing.

MECHANISM OF ACTION: α_1-blocker, quinazoline derivative; has not been established. Causes a decrease in total peripheral resistance and thought to have a direct relaxant action on vascular smooth muscle.

PHARMACOKINETICS: Absorption: T_{max}=3 hrs. **Distribution:** Plasma protein binding (highly bound). Found in breast milk. **Metabolism:** Extensive. Primarily by demethylation and conjugation. **Elimination:** Bile and feces; $T_{1/2}$=2-3 hrs.

NURSING CONSIDERATIONS

Assessment: Assess for drug hypersensitivity, pregnancy/nursing status, and for possible drug interactions. Assess baseline BP level.

Monitoring: Monitor for signs/symptoms of hypotension, dizziness, lightheadedness, syncope, and other adverse reactions. Monitor BP levels.

Patient Counseling: Inform that dizziness or drowsiness may occur after 1st dose; avoid driving or performing hazardous tasks for first 24 hrs after taking the drug or when dose is increased. Advise that dizziness, lightheadedness, or fainting may occur, especially when rising from a lying or sitting position; inform that getting up slowly may lessen these problems. Inform that these problems may also occur if taking alcohol, standing for long periods of time, exercising, or during hot weather. Advise to be careful about the amount of alcohol ingesting and to use extra care during exercise or hot weather, or if standing for long periods.

Administration: Oral route. **Storage:** <30°C (86°F)

MiraLax   OTC

polyethylene glycol 3350 (MSD Consumer)

THERAPEUTIC CLASS: Osmotic laxative

INDICATIONS: Relieves occasional constipation (irregularity). Generally produces a bowel movement in 1-3 days.

DOSAGE: *Adults:* Stir and dissolve 17g in any 4-8 oz. of beverage (cold/hot/room temperature) then drink. Use qd. Use no more than 7 days. (Bottle) Fill to top of white section in cap that is marked to indicate the correct dose (17g).
Pediatrics: ≥17 Yrs: Stir and dissolve 17g in any 4-8 oz. of beverage (cold/hot/room temperature) then drink. Use qd. Use no more than 7 days. (Bottle) Fill to top of white section in cap that is marked to indicate the correct dose (17g).

HOW SUPPLIED: Sol (Powder): 17g/dose [7 dose, 14 dose, 30 dose, bottle; 10^s, pkt]

WARNINGS/PRECAUTIONS: Do not use with kidney disease unless directed. Caution with N/V, abdominal pain, sudden change in bowel habits that lasts >2 weeks, and irritable bowel syndrome (IBS). Loose, watery, more frequent stools may occur. D/C if rectal bleeding or diarrhea develops; if nausea, bloating, cramping, or abdominal pain worsens; or if patient needs to use a laxative for >1 week.

ADVERSE REACTIONS: Loose, watery, more frequent stools.

PREGNANCY: Safety not known in pregnancy/nursing.

MECHANISM OF ACTION: Osmotic laxative.

NURSING CONSIDERATIONS

Assessment: Assess for allergy to the drug, kidney disease, N/V, abdominal pain, sudden change in bowel habits that lasts >2 weeks, IBS, and pregnancy/nursing status.

Monitoring: Monitor for rectal bleeding, diarrhea, or worsening of nausea, bloating, cramping, or abdominal pain. Monitor if patient needs to use a laxative for >1 week.

Patient Counseling: Instruct not to take more than directed. Inform that loose, watery, more frequent stools may occur. Instruct to d/c use and consult physician if rectal bleeding or diarrhea develops; if nausea, bloating, cramping, or abdominal pain worsens; or if patient needs to use a laxative for >1 week. Advise to inform physician if taking a prescription drug, or if pregnant/nursing.

Administration: Oral route. **Storage:** 20-25°C (68-77°F)

MIRAPEX   RX
pramipexole dihydrochloride (Boehringer Ingelheim)

THERAPEUTIC CLASS: Non-ergot dopamine agonist

INDICATIONS: Treatment of signs and symptoms of idiopathic Parkinson's disease and moderate to severe primary restless legs syndrome (RLS).

DOSAGE: *Adults:* If a significant interruption in therapy occurs, retitration may be warranted. Parkinson's Disease: Initial: 0.125mg tid. Titrate: May increase gradually not more frequently than every 5-7 days (eg, Week 2: 0.25mg tid; Week 3: 0.5mg tid; Week 4: 0.75mg tid; Week 5: 1mg tid; Week 6: 1.25mg tid; Week 7: 1.5mg tid). Maint: 0.5-1.5mg tid in equally divided doses. Renal Impairment: Mild: CrCl >50mL/min: Initial: 0.125mg tid. Max: 1.5mg tid. Moderate: CrCl 30-50mL/min: Initial: 0.125mg bid. Max: 0.75mg tid. Severe: CrCl 15-<30mL/min: Initial: 0.125mg qd. Max: 1.5mg qd. Discontinuation: Taper off at a rate of 0.75mg/day until daily dose has been reduced to 0.75mg then reduce dose by 0.375mg/day. RLS: Administer 2-3 hrs before hs. Initial: 0.125mg qd. Titrate: May increase dose every 4-7 days up to 0.5mg/day, if needed. Titration Step 1: 0.125 mg qd. Titration Step 2: 0.25mg qd. Titration Step 3: 0.5 mg qd. Moderate/Severe Renal Impairment (CrCl 20-60mL/min): Increase duration between titration steps to 14 days.

HOW SUPPLIED: Tab: 0.125mg, 0.25mg*, 0.5mg*, 0.75mg, 1mg*, 1.5mg* *scored

WARNINGS/PRECAUTIONS: Falling asleep during activities of daily living and somnolence reported; continually reassess for drowsiness or sleepiness, and d/c if significant daytime sleepiness or episodes of falling asleep during activities that require active participation develops. May impair mental/physical abilities. May cause orthostatic hypotension; monitor for signs/symptoms, especially during dose escalation. May cause intense urges to gamble, increased sexual urges, intense urges to spend money uncontrollably, binge eating, and/or other intense urges, and the inability to control these urges while on therapy; consider dose reduction or discontinuation of therapy. Hallucinations reported; risk increases with age. May cause or exacerbate preexisting dyskinesia. Caution with renal impairment. Rhabdomyolysis and retinal deterioration reported. Symptom complex resembling the neuroleptic maglinant syndrome reported with rapid dose reduction, withdrawal of, or changes in antiparkinsonian therapy. May cause fibrotic complications (eg, retroperitoneal fibrosis, pulmonary infiltrates, pleural effusion, pleural thickening, pericarditis, cardiac valvulopathy). Monitor for melanomas frequently and regularly; perform periodic skin examinations. Rebound and augmentation in RLS reported.

ADVERSE REACTIONS: Nausea, dizziness, somnolence, insomnia, constipation, asthenia, hallucinations, anorexia, peripheral edema, amnesia, confusion, headache, diarrhea, dreaming abnormalities, fatigue.

INTERACTIONS: Sedating medications or alcohol, and medications that increase plasma levels of pramipexole (eg, cimetidine) may increase risk of drowsiness. Dopamine antagonists, such as neuroleptics (phenothiazines, butyrophenones, thioxanthenes) or metoclopramide may diminish effectiveness. May potentiate dopaminergic side effects of levodopa; consider a reduction of the levodopa dose. Drugs secreted by the cationic transport system (eg, cimetidine, ranitidine, diltiazem, triamterene, verapamil, quinidine, quinine), amantadine, and other known organic cation transport substrates and/or inhibitors (eg, cisplatin, procainamide) may decrease oral clearance.

PREGNANCY: Category C, not for use in nursing.

MECHANISM OF ACTION: Non-ergot dopamine agonist; not established. In Parkinson's disease, suspected to stimulate dopamine receptors in the striatum.

PHARMACOKINETICS: Absorption: Rapid. Absolute bioavailability (>90%); T_{max} =2 hrs. **Distribution:** V_d=500L; plasma protein binding (15%). **Elimination:** Urine (90% unchanged); $T_{1/2}$=8 hrs (healthy), 12 hrs (elderly).

NURSING CONSIDERATIONS

Assessment: Assess for preexisting dyskinesia, renal impairment, pregnancy/nursing status, and possible drug interactions.

Monitoring: Monitor signs/symptoms of rhabdomyolysis, orthostatic hypotension, melanomas, fibrotic complications, hallucinations, impulse control/compulsive behaviors, drowsiness or sleepiness, retinal deterioration, withdrawal symptoms, and other adverse events.

Patient Counseling: Instruct to take as prescribed. If a dose is missed, advise not to double the next dose. Advise that the occurrence of nausea may be reduced if taken with food. Instruct not to take both immediate-release pramipexole and extended-release pramipexole. Advise and alert about the potential sedating effects, including somnolence and the possibility of falling asleep while engaged in activities of daily living; instruct not to drive a car or engage in other potentially dangerous activities until the patient has gained sufficient experience with pramipexole tabs to gauge whether or not it affects the patient's mental and/or motor performance adversely. Advise to inform physician if taking alcohol or other sedating medications. Inform of the possibility to experience intense urges to spend money uncontrollably, intense urges to gamble, increased sexual urges, binge eating and/or other intense urges, the inability to control these urges. Inform that hallucinations may occur. Advise that postural (orthostatic) hypotension may develop with or without symptoms. Instruct to notify physician if pregnant/intend to be pregnant during therapy or breastfeeding/intend to breastfeed.

Administration: Oral route. Take with or without food. **Storage:** 25°C (77°F); excursions permitted to 15-30°C (59-86°F). Protect from light.

MIRCETTE   RX
ethinyl estradiol - desogestrel (Teva)

> Cigarette smoking increases the risk of serious cardiovascular (CV) side effects. Risk increases with age and with heavy smoking (≥15 cigarettes/day) and is quite marked in women >35 yrs. Women who use oral contraceptives should be strongly advised not to smoke.

OTHER BRAND NAMES: Kariva (Barr)

THERAPEUTIC CLASS: Estrogen/progestogen combination

INDICATIONS: Prevention of pregnancy.

DOSAGE: *Adults:* 1 tab qd for 28 days, then repeat. Start 1st Sunday after menses begins or 1st day of menses.
Pediatrics: Postpubertal: 1 tab qd for 28 days, then repeat. Start 1st Sunday after menses begins or 1st day of menses.

HOW SUPPLIED: Tab: (Ethinyl Estradiol-Desogestrel) 0.02mg-0.15mg, (Ethinyl Estradiol) 0.01mg

CONTRAINDICATIONS: Thrombophlebitis or past history of deep vein thrombophlebitis, thromboembolic disorders (current or past history), suspected/known pregnancy, cerebral vascular or coronary artery disease, undiagnosed abnormal genital bleeding, cholestatic jaundice of pregnancy or jaundice with prior pill use, known/suspected breast carcinoma, carcinoma of the endometrium or other known/suspected estrogen-dependent neoplasia, hepatic adenomas or carcinomas.

WARNINGS/PRECAUTIONS: Increased risk of myocardial infarction (MI), vascular disease, thromboembolism, stroke, hepatic neoplasia, and gallbladder disease. Increased risk of morbidity and mortality with HTN, hyperlipidemias, obesity, and diabetes mellitus (DM). D/C at least 4 weeks prior to and for 2 weeks after elective surgery associated with an increased risk of thromboembolism and during and following prolonged immobilization, if feasible. Start use no earlier than 4 weeks after delivery in women who elect not to breastfeed. Caution in women with CV disease risk factors. May develop visual changes or changes in lens tolerance in contact lens wearers. Retinal thrombosis reported; d/c if unexplained partial or complete loss of vision, onset of proptosis or diplopia, papilledema, or retinal vascular lesions develop. Should not be used to induce withdrawal bleeding as a test for pregnancy, or to treat threatened or habitual abortion during pregnancy. May decrease glucose tolerance; monitor prediabetic and diabetic patients. May elevate BP; monitor closely and d/c use if significant BP elevation occurs. New onset/exacerbation of migraine, or recurrent, persistent, severe headache may develop; d/c if these occur. Breakthrough bleeding and spotting reported; rule out malignancy or pregnancy. D/C if jaundice develops. May be poorly metabolized in patients with impaired liver function. May cause fluid retention; caution with conditions that aggravate fluid retention. Caution with history of depression; d/c if depression recurs to a serious degree. Does not protect against HIV infection (AIDS) and other sexually transmitted diseases (STDs). Perform annual history/physical exam; monitor women with history of breast cancer. Not for use before menarche. May affect certain endocrine, LFTs, and blood components in laboratory tests.

ADVERSE REACTIONS: N/V, breakthrough bleeding, spotting, amenorrhea, migraine, mental depression, vaginal candidiasis, edema, weight changes, abdominal cramps/bloating, menstrual flow changes, pulmonary embolism, MI, HTN.

INTERACTIONS: Reduced efficacy and increased breakthrough bleeding and menstrual irregularities with rifampin, barbiturates, phenylbutazone, phenytoin sodium, carbamazepine, and possibly with griseofulvin, ampicillin, and tetracyclines. May decrease lamotrigine levels; dosage adjustment of lamotrigine may be necessary.

PREGNANCY: Category X, not for use in nursing.

MECHANISM OF ACTION: Estrogen/progestogen combination; acts by suppressing gonadotropins, primarily inhibiting ovulation, and causing other alterations, including changes in cervical mucus (increases difficulty of sperm entry into uterus) and endometrium (reduces likelihood of implantation).

PHARMACOKINETICS: Absorption: Rapid and almost complete. Relative bioavailability 100% (Desogestrel), 93-99% (Ethinyl estradiol). Oral administration on various days during dosing led to altered parameters; refer to PI. **Distribution:** Found in breast milk. Etonogestrel: Plasma protein binding (99%), sex hormone-binding globulin (primary). Ethinyl estradiol: Plasma albumin binding (98.3%). **Metabolism:** Desogestrel: Etonogestrel (active metabolite). Liver and intestinal mucosa via hydroxylation, glucuronidation, and sulfate conjugation. Ethinyl estradiol: Conjugation. **Elimination:** Urine, bile, feces. Etonogestrel: $T_{1/2}$=27.8 hrs. Ethinyl estradiol: $T_{1/2}$=23.9 hrs (combination), 18.9 hrs (0.01mg).

NURSING CONSIDERATIONS

Assessment: Assess for current or history of thrombophlebitis or thromboembolic disorders, history of HTN, hyperlipidemia, DM, obesity, breast cancer, nursing status, or any other conditions where treatment is contraindicated/cautioned, and possible drug interactions.

Monitoring: Monitor for MI, thromboembolism, stroke, hepatic neoplasia, and other adverse effects. Monitor BP with history of HTN, serum glucose levels in diabetic or prediabetic patients, lipid levels with hyperlipidemia, and for signs of worsening depression with previous history. Refer contact lens wearer to ophthalmologist if ocular changes develop. Perform annual history and physical exam. Monitor women with strong family history of breast cancer or have breast nodules. Monitor LFTs, PT, thyroxine binding-globulin, T3 and T4, and serum folate levels.

Patient Counseling: Counsel about potential adverse effects, and to avoid smoking while on therapy. Inform that drug does not protect against HIV infection and other STDs. Inform about pregnancy risk if pills are missed. Instruct to take at the same time every day and intervals between doses should not exceed 24 hrs. Instruct that when initiating a Sunday start regimen, to use another method of contraception until after first 7 consecutive days of administration. Instruct if one "active" pill is missed to take as soon as remembered, and take next pill at regular time.

Administration: Oral route. **Storage:** 20-25°C (68-77°F).

M

MIRENA   RX
levonorgestrel (Bayer Healthcare)

THERAPEUTIC CLASS: Progestogen

INDICATIONS: Intrauterine contraception for up to 5 yrs. Treatment of heavy menstrual bleeding in women who choose to use intrauterine contraception as their method of contraception. Recommended for women who have had at least one child.

DOSAGE: *Adults:* Insert with the provided inserter into the uterine cavity within 7 days of onset of menstruation or immediately after a 1st trimester abortion. Replace after 5 yrs if continued use is desired.

HOW SUPPLIED: Intrauterine Insert: 52mg

CONTRAINDICATIONS: Pregnancy or suspicion of pregnancy, congenital or acquired uterine anomaly including fibroids if they distort the uterine cavity, acute or history of pelvic inflammatory disease (PID) unless there has been a subsequent intrauterine pregnancy, postpartum endometritis or infected abortion in the past 3 months, known/suspected uterine or cervical neoplasia or unresolved abnormal Pap smear, genital bleeding of unknown etiology, untreated acute cervicitis or vaginitis including bacterial vaginosis or other lower genital tract infections until infection is controlled, acute liver disease or liver tumor (benign or malignant), conditions associated with increased susceptibility to pelvic infections, previously inserted IUD that is not removed, known/suspected breast carcinoma.

WARNINGS/PRECAUTIONS: Should be inserted by a trained healthcare provider who is familiar with the insertion instructions. If pregnancy occurs while device is in place, evaluate for ectopic pregnancy and remove device; removal or manipulation may result in pregnancy loss. Increased risk of septic abortion, miscarriage, sepsis, premature delivery/labor, and congenital anomalies if intrauterine pregnancy occurs. Group A streptococcal sepsis (GAS) reported; aseptic technique during insertion of device is essential. Does not protect against sexually transmitted diseases (STDs). Associated with an increased risk of PID and actinomycosis; remove device and initiate antibiotic therapy. May alter bleeding pattern and result in spotting, irregular bleeding, heavy bleeding, oligomenorrhea, and amenorrhea; if bleeding irregularities develop during prolonged treatment, perform appropriate diagnostic measures to rule out endometrial pathology. Perforation or penetration of the uterine wall/cervix and embedment in myometrium may occur and may result in pregnancy; remove device when these occur. May increase risk of perforation in women with fixed retroverted uteri, during lactation, and postpartum; delay insertion a minimum of 6 weeks after delivery or until uterine involution is complete. If involution is substantially delayed, consider waiting until 12 weeks postpartum. Partial or complete expulsion may occur;

replace within 7 days of menstrual period after ruling out pregnancy. May cause enlarged ovarian follicles. Breast cancer reported. Caution in patients who have coagulopathy, migraine/headache, marked increase of BP, severe arterial disease (eg, stroke, myocardial infarction), increased risk of infective endocarditis, and in patients who require anticoagulants, chronic corticosteroid therapy or insulin. Syncope, bradycardia, or other neurovascular episodes may occur during insertion of device, especially in patients with a predisposition to these conditions or cervical stenosis. Remove device if patient has new onset menorrhagia and/or metrorrhagia producing anemia, STDs, pelvic infection, endometritis, intractable pelvic pain, severe dyspareunia, or endometrial or cervical malignancy. Consider removal of the system if migraine/headache, jaundice, marked BP increase, or severe arterial disease arise for the 1st time. Removal may be associated with some pain and/or bleeding or neurovascular episodes. May affect glucose tolerance; monitor blood glucose levels in diabetic patients. Not indicated for use before menarche.

ADVERSE REACTIONS: Uterine/vaginal bleeding alterations, amenorrhea, intermenstrual bleeding, spotting, abdominal/pelvic pain, ovarian cysts, headache/migraine, acne, depressed/altered mood, menorrhagia, breast tenderness/pain, vaginal discharge, IUD expulsion.

INTERACTIONS: Drugs or herbal products that induce enzymes, including CYP3A4 (eg, barbiturates, bosentan, carbamazepine, felbamate, griseofulvin, oxcarbazepine, phenytoin, rifampin, St. John's wort, topiramate) may decrease levels. HIV protease inhibitors or non-nucleoside reverse transcriptase inhibitors may significantly increase or decrease plasma levels.

PREGNANCY: Contraindicated in pregnancy, caution in nursing.

MECHANISM OF ACTION: Progestogen; has not been conclusively demonstrated. Thickens cervical mucus (preventing passage of sperm into uterus), inhibits sperm capacitation or survival, and alters endometrium.

PHARMACOKINETICS: Distribution: V_d=1.8L/kg; plasma protein binding (97.5-99%); found in breast milk. **Metabolism:** Conjugation; sulfate and glucuronide (lesser extent) conjugates (metabolites). **Elimination:** Urine (45%), feces (32%); (PO) $T_{1/2}$=17 hrs.

NURSING CONSIDERATIONS

Assessment: Assess for any conditions where treatment is contraindicated or cautioned, nursing status, and possible drug interactions. Perform complete medical/social history (including that of the partner) and physical exam, including a pelvic exam, Pap smear, breast exam, and appropriate tests for STDs. Prior to insertion, determine degree of patency of the endocervical canal and the internal os and the direction and depth of the uterine cavity.

Monitoring: Monitor for intrauterine/ectopic pregnancy, GAS, PID, migraine/headache, jaundice, marked BP increase, severe arterial disease, and other adverse reactions. Monitor blood glucose in diabetics. During insertion, monitor for decreased pulse, perspiration, or pallor. Reexamine/evaluate 4-12 weeks after insertion and once a year thereafter, or more frequently if clinically indicated. Check if thread is still visible and for length of thread.

Patient Counseling: Inform that drug does not protect against HIV infection (AIDS) and other STDs. Inform of risks/benefits of the device. Counsel that irregular/prolonged bleeding and spotting, and/or cramps may occur during 1st few weeks after insertion; instruct to contact physician if symptoms continue or become severe. Instruct to contact healthcare provider if experiencing stroke or heart attack, very severe or migraine headaches, unexplained fever, yellowing of skin or whites of the eyes, pelvic pain or pain during sex, unusual vaginal discharge, genital sores, severe or prolonged vaginal bleeding, or if patient suspects pregnancy, becomes HIV positive (including partner), is exposed to STDs, or cannot feel device's threads. Instruct how to check after menstrual period that threads still protrude from cervix and caution not to pull on the threads and displace device. Inform that no contraceptive protection exists if device is displaced or expelled.

Administration: Intrauterine route. Refer to PI for insertion, removal, and continuation of contraception after removal instructions. **Storage:** 25°C (77°F); excursions permitted to 15-30°C (59-86°F).

M-M-R II   RX
rubella vaccine live - measles vaccine live - mumps vaccine live (Merck)

THERAPEUTIC CLASS: Vaccine

INDICATIONS: Simultaneous vaccination against measles, mumps, and rubella in individuals ≥12 months of age. May be recommended in infants 6-12 months of age in outbreak situations. Refer to PI for other vaccination considerations.

DOSAGE: *Adults:* 0.5mL SQ into outer aspect of upper arm.
Pediatrics: 0.5mL SQ into outer aspect of upper arm (1st dose at 12-15 months of age). Administer 2nd dose at 4-6 yrs of age. Measles Outbreak: May give 1st dose at 6-12 months of age. Give 2nd dose at 12-15 months of age followed by revaccination at elementary school entry.

HOW SUPPLIED: Inj: 0.5mL

CONTRAINDICATIONS: Hypersensitivity to gelatin, pregnancy, anaphylactic/anaphylactoid reactions to neomycin, febrile respiratory illness or other active febrile infection, immunosuppressive therapy (except corticosteroids as replacement therapy), blood dyscrasias, leukemia, lymphomas of any type, malignant neoplasms affecting bone marrow or lymphatic systems, primary and acquired immunodeficiency states (including immunosuppression associated with AIDS or other clinical manifestations of HIV infection, cellular immune deficiencies, hypogammaglobulinemic and dysgammaglobulinemic states), family history of congenital or hereditary immunodeficiency.

WARNINGS/PRECAUTIONS: Caution with history of cerebral injury, individual or family histories of convulsions or any other condition in which stress due to fever should be avoided. Extreme caution with history of anaphylactic/anaphylactoid, or other immediate reactions (eg, hives, swelling of mouth and throat, difficulty breathing, hypotension, shock) subsequent to egg ingestion. Neomycin allergy often manifests as a contact dermatitis; a history of contact dermatitis to neomycin is not a contraindication. Have adequate treatment provisions, including epinephrine inj (1:1000), available for immediate use should an anaphylactic/anaphylactoid reaction occur. HIV infected children and young adults who are not immunosuppressed may be vaccinated but vaccine may be less effective than for uninfected persons; monitor closely for vaccine-preventable diseases. Severe thrombocytopenia may develop in individuals with current thrombocytopenia; individuals who experienced thrombocytopenia with 1st dose may also develop thrombocytopenia with repeat doses. Evaluate serologic status to determine need for additional doses. Ensure that inj does not enter a blood vessel. Excretion of small amounts of the live attenuated rubella virus from the nose or throat 7-28 days after vaccination reported. Avoid with active untreated tuberculosis (TB). May not result in protection in 100% of vaccinees. Persons vaccinated with inactivated vaccine followed within 3 months by live vaccine should be revaccinated with 2 doses of live vaccine. May result in temporary depression of tuberculin skin sensitivity if given individually; administer skin test either before or simultaneously.

ADVERSE REACTIONS: Panniculitis, atypical measles, fever, syncope, headache, dizziness, malaise, diarrhea, N/V, irritability, arthralgia, arthritis, pneumonia, sore throat, Stevens-Johnson syndrome.

INTERACTIONS: See Contraindications. Do not give with immune globulin (IG); may interfere with expected immune response. May be given 1 month before or after administration of other live viral vaccines. Defer vaccination for ≥3 months following administration of IG (human), or blood/plasma transfusions. Concurrent administration with diphtheria, tetanus, pertussis and/or oral poliovirus vaccines is not recommended.

PREGNANCY: Category C, caution in nursing.

MECHANISM OF ACTION: Vaccine; may induce antibodies that protect against measles, mumps, and rubella.

PHARMACOKINETICS: Distribution: Live Attenuated Rubella Vaccine: Found in breast milk.

NURSING CONSIDERATIONS

Assessment: Assess for hypersensitivity to any component of the vaccine, immune and current health/medical status, vaccination history, thrombocytopenia, active untreated TB, any other conditions where treatment is contraindicated or cautioned, pregnancy/nursing status, and possible drug interactions.

Monitoring: Monitor for anaphylactic/anaphylactoid reactions, thrombocytopenia, vaccine-preventable diseases in HIV patients, and other adverse reactions.

Patient Counseling: Inform of benefits/risks of vaccination. Instruct to report any serious adverse reactions. Instruct to avoid pregnancy for 3 months after vaccination and inform of the reasons for this precaution.

Administration: SQ route. Refer to PI for proper reconstitution and administration procedures.
Storage: Unreconstituted: -50 to 8°C (-58 to 46°F). Protect from light. Before Reconstitution: 2-8°C (36-46°F). May refrigerate diluent or store separately at room temperature; do not freeze diluent. Reconstituted: 2-8°C (36-46°F) in a dark place; discard if not used within 8 hrs.

MOBIC   RX
meloxicam (Boehringer Ingelheim)

> NSAIDs may cause an increased risk of serious CV thrombotic events, myocardial infarction, stroke, and serious GI adverse events, including bleeding, ulceration, and perforation of the stomach or intestines. Elderly patients at greater risk for serious GI events. Contraindicated for the treatment of perioperative pain in the setting of coronary artery bypass graft (CABG) surgery.

THERAPEUTIC CLASS: NSAID

INDICATIONS: Relief of signs and symptoms of osteoarthritis (OA) and rheumatoid arthritis (RA). Relief of signs and symptoms of pauciarticular/polyarticular course juvenile RA in patients ≥2 yrs.

DOSAGE: *Adults:* OA/RA: Initial/Maint: 7.5mg qd. Max: 15mg/day. Hemodialysis: Max: 7.5mg/day. *Pediatrics:* ≥2 Yrs: Juvenile RA: Individualize dose. Usual: 0.125mg/kg qd. Max: 7.5mg/day.

HOW SUPPLIED: Sus: 7.5mg/5mL; Tab: 7.5mg, 15mg

CONTRAINDICATIONS: Aspirin (ASA) or other NSAID allergy that precipitates asthma, urticaria, or allergic-type reactions. Treatment of perioperative pain in the setting of CABG surgery.

WARNINGS/PRECAUTIONS: Use lowest effective dose for the shortest duration possible. Extreme caution with history of ulcer disease or GI bleeding. May cause elevations of LFTs; d/c if liver disease develops, or if systemic manifestations occur. May lead to onset of new HTN, or worsening of preexisting HTN. Fluid retention and edema reported. Renal papillary necrosis, renal insufficiency, acute renal failure, and other renal injury reported after long-term use. Not recommended for use with severe renal impairment (CrCl <20mL/min). Caution in patients with considerable dehydration; rehydrate 1st, then start therapy. Caution in debilitated patients, with preexisting kidney disease, and asthma. Closely monitor patients with significant renal impairment. Avoid with ASA-triad/ASA-sensitive asthma. May cause anaphylactoid reactions and serious skin adverse events (eg, exfoliative dermatitis, Stevens-Johnson syndrome, toxic epidermal necrolysis); d/c at 1st appearance of rash or other signs of hypersensitivity. Avoid use starting at 30 weeks gestation; may cause premature closure of ductus arteriosus. Not a substitute for corticosteroids or for treatment of corticosteroid insufficiency. May mask signs of inflammation and fever. Anemia may occur; with long-term use, monitor Hgb/Hct if symptoms of anemia develop. May inhibit platelet aggregation and prolong bleeding time. May be associated with a reversible delay in ovulation; not recommended in women with difficulties conceiving, or who are undergoing investigation of infertility.

ADVERSE REACTIONS: Abdominal pain, diarrhea, dyspepsia, nausea, headache, anemia, arthralgia, insomnia, upper respiratory tract infection, urinary tract infection, dizziness, pain, pharyngitis, edema, influenza-like symptoms.

INTERACTIONS: Patients taking ACE inhibitors, thiazides, and loop diuretics (eg, furosemide) may have impaired response to these therapies. Risk of renal toxicity when coadministered with diuretics, ACE inhibitors, and angiotensin II receptor antagonists. Increased risk of GI bleeding with anticoagulants (eg, warfarin), smoking, alcohol, and oral corticosteroids. May diminish antihypertensive effect of ACE inhibitors. Not recommended with ASA; increased rate of GI ulceration or other complications with low-dose ASA. May elevate lithium plasma levels; observe for signs of lithium toxicity. May increase cyclosporine and methotrexate toxicities. (Sus) Not recommended with sodium polystyrene sulfonate (Kayexalate).

PREGNANCY: Category C (<30 weeks gestation) and D (≥30 weeks gestation), not for use in nursing.

MECHANISM OF ACTION: NSAIDs; has not been established. Suspected to inhibit prostaglandin synthetase, resulting in reduced formation of prostaglandins, thromboxanes, and prostacyclin.

PHARMACOKINETICS: Absorption: Administration of variable doses in different populations resulted in different parameters. Absolute bioavailability (89%). **Distribution:** V_d=10L, plasma protein binding (99.4%); crosses placenta. **Metabolism:** Liver (extensive); oxidation via CYP2C9 (major), CYP3A4 (minor). **Elimination:** Urine (0.2% unchanged), feces (1.6% unchanged); $T_{1/2}$=15-20 hrs.

NURSING CONSIDERATIONS

Assessment: Assess for cardiovascular disease (CVD), risk factors for CVD, ASA-triad, coagulation disorders, any other conditions where treatment is contraindicated or cautioned, renal/hepatic dysfunction, pregnancy/nursing status, and possible drug interactions. Assess use in elderly and debilitated patients.

Monitoring: Monitor for signs/symptoms of CV thrombotic events, HTN, GI events, fluid retention, edema, and anaphylactoid/skin reactions. Monitor BP, renal function, and LFTs. Perform periodic monitoring of CBC and chemistry profile with long-term use.

Patient Counseling: Advise to seek medical attention if symptoms of cardiovascular events (eg, chest pain, SOB, weakness, slurring of speech), GI ulceration and bleeding (eg, epigastric pain, dyspepsia, melena, hematemesis), hepatotoxicity (eg, nausea, fatigue, lethargy, pruritus, jaundice, right upper quadrant tenderness, flu-like symptoms), anaphylactoid reaction (eg, difficulty breathing, swelling of face/throat), skin rash, blisters, fever, hypersensitivity reaction (eg, itching), weight gain, or edema occur. Instruct to avoid use starting at 30 weeks gestation. Advise females of reproductive potential who desire pregnancy that drug may be associated with a reversible delay in ovulation.

Administration: Oral route. (Sus) Shake gently before using. **Storage:** 25°C (77°F); excursions permitted to 15-30°C (59-86°F). Keep tab in a dry place.

MONODOX   RX
doxycycline monohydrate (Aqua)

THERAPEUTIC CLASS: Tetracycline derivative

INDICATIONS: Treatment of the following infections caused by susceptible microorganisms: Rocky Mountain spotted fever, typhus fever and the typhus group, Q fever, rickettsialpox, tick fevers, respiratory tract infections, lymphogranuloma venereum, psittacosis (ornithosis), trachoma, inclusion conjunctivitis, uncomplicated urethral/endocervical/rectal infections (in adults), nongonococcal urethritis, relapsing fever, chancroid, plague, tularemia, cholera, *Campylobacter fetus* infections, brucellosis (in conjunction with streptomycin), bartonellosis, granuloma inguinale, urinary tract infections (UTIs), and anthrax (including inhalational anthrax [postexposure]). Treatment of infections caused by susceptible strains of *Escherichia coli*, *Enterobacter aerogenes*, *Shigella* species, and *Acinetobacter* species. When penicillin (PCN) is contraindicated, treatment of the following infections caused by susceptible microorganisms: uncomplicated gonorrhea, syphilis, yaws, listeriosis, Vincent's infection, actinomycosis, and infections caused by *Clostridium* species. Adjunctive therapy in acute intestinal amebiasis and severe acne.

DOSAGE: *Adults:* Initial: 100mg q12h or 50mg q6h on 1st day. Maint: 100mg qd or 50mg q12h. More Severe Infections (Chronic UTIs): 100mg q12h. Uncomplicated Gonococcal Infections (Except Anorectal Infections in Men): 100mg bid for 7 days or as an alternate single visit dose of 300mg stat followed in 1 hr by a second 300mg dose. Acute Epididymo-Orchitis: 100mg bid for at least 10 days. Primary/Secondary Syphilis: 300mg/day in divided doses for at least 10 days. Uncomplicated Urethral/Endocervical/Rectal Infection or Nongonococcal Urethritis: 100mg bid for at least 7 days. Inhalational Anthrax (Postexposure): 100mg bid for 60 days. Streptococcal Infections: Continue therapy for 10 days. Take with adequate amounts of fluid. *Pediatrics:* Inhalation Anthrax (Postexposure): ≥100 lbs: 100mg bid for 60 days. <100 lbs: 1mg/lb bid for 60 days. >8 Yrs: Infections: Usual: >100 lbs: Initial: 100mg q12h or 50mg q6h on 1st day. Maint: 100mg qd or 50mg q12h. More Severe Infections (Chronic UTIs): 100mg q12h. ≤100 lbs: 2mg/lb divided into 2 doses on 1st day, followed by 1mg/lb qd or as 2 divided doses, on subsequent days. More Severe Infections: Up to 2mg/lb. Streptococcal Infections: Continue therapy for 10 days. Take with adequate amounts of fluid.

HOW SUPPLIED: Cap: 50mg, 75mg, 100mg

WARNINGS/PRECAUTIONS: May cause permanent discoloration of the teeth (yellow-gray-brown) if used during tooth development (last half of pregnancy, infancy, and childhood to 8 yrs of age); do not use in this age group, except for anthrax. Enamel hypoplasia reported. *Clostridium difficile*-associated diarrhea (CDAD) reported; d/c if CDAD is suspected or confirmed. May decrease fibula growth rate in prematures. May cause an increase in BUN. Photosensitivity, manifested by an exaggerated sunburn reaction, reported; d/c at the 1st evidence of skin erythema. May result in bacterial resistance if used in the absence of proven or suspected bacterial infection, or a prophylactic indication; take appropriate measures if superinfection develops. Associated with intracranial HTN (pseudotumor cerebri); increased risk in women of childbearing age who are overweight or have a history of intracranial HTN. If visual disturbance occurs, prompt ophthalmologic evaluation is warranted. Intracranial pressure can remain elevated for weeks after drug cessation; monitor patients until they stabilize. Incision and drainage or other surgical procedures should be performed in conjunction with antibacterial therapy when indicated. False elevations of urinary catecholamine levels may occur due to interference with the fluorescence test.

ADVERSE REACTIONS: Diarrhea, hepatotoxicity, maculopapular/erythematous rash, Stevens-Johnson syndrome, toxic epidermal necrolysis, anorexia, N/V, urticaria, serum sickness, pericarditis, hemolytic anemia, thrombocytopenia, neutropenia, eosinophilia.

INTERACTIONS: Avoid concomitant use with isotretinoin; may increase risk of intracranial HTN. Depresses plasma prothrombin activity; may require downward adjustment of anticoagulant dose. May interfere with bactericidal action of PCN; avoid concurrent use. Impaired absorption with antacids containing aluminum, Ca^{2+}, or Mg^{2+}, and iron-containing preparations. Decreased $T_{1/2}$ with barbiturates, carbamazepine, and phenytoin. Fatal renal toxicity reported with methoxyflurane. May render oral contraceptives less effective.

PREGNANCY: Category D, not for use in nursing.

MECHANISM OF ACTION: Tetracycline; has bacteriostatic activity. Inhibits bacterial protein synthesis by binding to the 30S ribosomal subunit.

PHARMACOKINETICS: Absorption: Readily absorbed; virtually complete. (200mg, Normal adults) C_{max}=3.61mcg/mL; T_{max}=2.6 hrs. **Distribution:** Found in breast milk. **Elimination:** Urine (40%/72 hrs in CrCl 75mL/min, 1-5%/72 hrs in CrCl <10mL/min), feces; (200mg, Normal adults) $T_{1/2}$=16.33 hrs.

M

NURSING CONSIDERATIONS

Assessment: Assess for hypersensitivity to drug or any tetracyclines, risk for intracranial HTN, pregnancy/nursing status, and possible drug interactions. Perform culture and susceptibility tests. In venereal disease when coexistent syphilis is suspected, perform a dark-field examination and blood serology.

Monitoring: Monitor for CDAD, photosensitivity, skin erythema, superinfection, intracranial HTN, visual disturbance, and other adverse reactions. In long-term therapy, perform periodic laboratory evaluations of organ systems, including hematopoietic, renal, and hepatic studies. In venereal disease when coexistent syphilis is suspected, repeat blood serology monthly for at least 4 months.

Patient Counseling: Apprise of the potential hazard to fetus if used during pregnancy. Advise to avoid excessive sunlight or artificial UV light, and to d/c therapy if phototoxicity (eg, skin eruptions) occurs; advise to consider use of sunscreen or sunblock. Inform that absorption of drug is reduced when taken with bismuth subsalicylate, or with foods, especially those that contain Ca^{2+}. Inform that drug may increase incidence of vaginal candidiasis. Inform that diarrhea is a common problem caused by therapy, which usually ends when therapy is discontinued. Instruct to immediately contact physician if watery and bloody stools (with or without stomach cramps and fever) occur, even as late as ≥2 months after the last dose. Counsel that therapy should only be used to treat bacterial, not viral (eg, common cold), infections. Instruct to take exactly ud, even if patient feels better early in the course of therapy. Inform that skipping doses or not completing the full course of therapy may decrease effectiveness of treatment and increase bacterial resistance.

Administration: Oral route. Administer with adequate amounts of fluid. May be given with food if gastric irritation occurs. **Storage:** 20-25°C (68-77°F); excursions permitted to 15-30°C (59-86°F).

MORPHINE
morphine sulfate (Various)

CII

> Oral sol is available in 10mg/5mL, 20mg/5mL, and 100mg/5mL concentrations. The 100mg/5mL (20mg/mL) concentration is indicated for use in opioid-tolerant patients only. Use caution when prescribing and administering to avoid dosing errors due to confusion between different concentrations and between mg and mL, which could result in accidental overdose and death. Ensure the proper dose is communicated and dispensed. Keep out of reach of children. Seek emergency medical help immediately in case of accidental ingestion.

THERAPEUTIC CLASS: Opioid analgesic

INDICATIONS: Relief of moderate to severe acute and chronic pain where use of an opioid analgesic is appropriate. (Sol, 100mg/5mL) Relief of moderate to severe acute and chronic pain in opioid-tolerant patients.

DOSAGE: *Adults:* Individualize dose. Opioid-Naive Patients: Initial: 10-20mg (sol) or 15-30mg (tab) q4h PRN for pain. Titrate based upon the individual patient's response to the initial dose. Conversion from Parenteral to PO Formulation: Anywhere from 3-6mg PO dose may be required to provide pain relief equivalent to 1mg parenteral dose. Conversion from Parenteral PO Non-Morphine Opioids to PO Morphine: Close observation and dose adjustment is required. Refer to published relative potency information. Conversion from Controlled-Release PO Formulation to PO Formulation: Dose adjustment with close observation is necessary. Maint: Continue to re-evaluate with special attention to the maint of pain control and side effects. Periodically reassess the continued need for opioid analgesic use during chronic use especially for non-cancer-related pain (or pain associated with other terminal illness). Taper dose gradually. Elderly: Start at lower end of dosing range.

HOW SUPPLIED: Sol: 10mg/5mL [100mL, 500mL], 20mg/5mL [100mL, 500mL], 100mg/5mL [30mL, 120mL]; Tab: 15mg*, 30mg* *scored

CONTRAINDICATIONS: Respiratory depression in absence of resuscitative equipment, acute or severe bronchial asthma or hypercarbia, has or suspected of having paralytic ileus.

WARNINGS/PRECAUTIONS: Increased risk of respiratory depression in elderly or debilitated patients and in those with conditions accompanied by hypoxia, hypercapnia, or upper airway obstruction. Caution and consider alternative nonopioid analgesics with chronic obstructive pulmonary disease or cor pulmonale, substantially decreased respiratory reserve (eg, severe kyphoscoliosis), hypoxia, hypercapnia, or preexisting respiratory depression. Contains morphine sulfate, a Schedule II controlled substance, which has a high potential for abuse and is subject to misuse, abuse, or diversion. The possible respiratory depressant effects and the potential to elevate CSF pressure may be markedly exaggerated in the presence of head injury, intracranial lesions, or preexisting increase in intracranial pressure (ICP); may obscure neurologic signs of further increased ICP in patients with head injuries. May cause orthostatic hypotension and syncope in ambulatory patients. May cause severe hypotension when ability to maintain BP has been compromised by a depleted blood volume. Caution with circulatory shock. Avoid with GI obstruction, especially paralytic ileus; may obscure diagnosis or clinical course with acute abdominal conditions. Caution with biliary tract disease, including acute pancreatitis; may cause spasm of the sphincter of Oddi and diminish biliary and pancreatic secretions. Caution with and reduce dose in patients with severe renal or hepatic impairment, Addison's disease, hypothyroidism, prostatic hypertrophy, or urethral stricture, and in elderly or debilitated. Caution with CNS depression, toxic psychosis, acute alcoholism, and delirium tremens. May aggravate convulsions in patients with convulsive disorders and may induce seizures. May impair mental/physical abilities.

ADVERSE REACTIONS: Respiratory depression, apnea, circulatory depression, respiratory arrest, shock, cardiac arrest, lightheadedness, dizziness, constipation, somnolence, sedation, N/V, sweating.

INTERACTIONS: Caution with CNS depressants (eg, sedatives, hypnotics, general anesthetics, antiemetics, phenothiazines, tranquilizers, other opioids, illicit drugs, alcohol); may increase the risk of respiratory depression, hypotension, profound sedation, or coma. May enhance the neuromuscular-blocking action of skeletal muscle relaxants and produce an increased degree of respiratory depression. Avoid with mixed agonist/antagonist analgesics (eg, pentazocine, nalbuphine, butorphanol). Precipitated apnea, confusion, and muscle twitching reported with cimetidine. Potentiated action by MAOIs; allow at least 14 days after stopping MAOIs before initiating treatment. May result in increased risk of urinary retention and/or severe constipation, which may lead to paralytic ileus with anticholinergics or other medications with anticholinergic activity. Caution with P-glycoprotein inhibitors.

PREGNANCY: Category C, not for use in nursing.

MECHANISM OF ACTION: Opioid analgesic; precise mechanism unknown. Specific CNS opiate receptors and endogenous compounds with morphine-like activity have been identified throughout the brain and spinal cord and are likely to play a role in the expression and perception of analgesic effects. Causes respiratory depression, in part by a direct effect on the brainstem respiratory centers, and depresses cough reflex by direct effect on the cough center in the medulla.

PHARMACOKINETICS: Absorption: Bioavailability (<40%); C_{max}=78ng/mL (tab), 58ng/mL (sol). **Distribution:** V_d=1-6L/kg; plasma protein binding (20-35%); crosses placenta, found in breast milk. **Metabolism:** Liver via conjugation; 3- and 6-glucuronide (metabolites). **Elimination:** Urine (10% unchanged), feces (7-10%); $T_{1/2}$=2 hrs (IV).

NURSING CONSIDERATIONS

Assessment: Assess for degree of opioid tolerance, level of pain intensity, type of pain, patient's general condition and medical status, or any other conditions where treatment is contraindicated or cautioned, pregnancy/nursing status, and possible drug interactions.

Monitoring: Monitor for respiratory depression, CSF pressure elevation, orthostatic hypotension, syncope, hypotension, aggravation of convulsions/seizures, and other adverse reactions.

Patient Counseling: Advise to take only ud and not to adjust dose without consulting a physician. Inform physician if pregnant or plan to become pregnant prior to therapy. Counsel on the importance of safely tapering the dose. Inform of potential for severe constipation. Inform that therapy may produce physical or psychological dependence. Caution against performing hazardous tasks (eg, operating machinery/driving). Advise to avoid alcohol or CNS depressants except by the orders of the prescribing physician during therapy. Instruct to keep in a secure place out of reach of children, and when no longer needed, instruct to destroy the unused tabs by flushing down the toilet.

Administration: Oral route. (Sol, 100mg/5mL) Used only for patients who have already been titrated to a stable analgesic regimen using lower strengths and who can benefit from use of a smaller volume of sol; always use the enclosed calibrated PO syringe. **Storage:** 15-30°C (59-86°F). Protect from moisture.

MOXATAG   RX
amoxicillin (Middlebrook)

THERAPEUTIC CLASS: Semisynthetic ampicillin derivative

INDICATIONS: Treatment of tonsillitis and/or pharyngitis secondary to *Streptococcus pyogenes* in adults and pediatric patients ≥12 yrs of age.

DOSAGE: *Adults:* Take 775mg qd within 1 hr of finishing a meal for 10 days. Do not chew or crush. *Pediatrics:* ≥12 Yrs: Take 775mg qd within 1 hr of finishing a meal for 10 days. Do not chew or crush.

HOW SUPPLIED: Tab, Extended Release: 775mg

WARNINGS/PRECAUTIONS: Serious, fatal anaphylactic reactions may occur. *Clostridium difficile*-associated diarrhea (CDAD) reported. May result in bacterial resistance with prolonged use or use in the absence of a proven/suspected bacterial infection or a prophylactic indication; take appropriate measures if superinfection develops. Avoid use in patients with mononucleosis;

may cause erythematous skin rash. Not recommended for use in severe renal impairment (CrCl <30mL/min) or hemodialysis. Lab test interactions may occur.

ADVERSE REACTIONS: Vulvovaginal mycotic infection, diarrhea, N/V, abdominal pain, headache.

INTERACTIONS: Concurrent use with probenecid may increase and prolong blood levels; decreases renal tubular secretion of amoxicillin. Chloramphenicol, macrolides, sulfonamides, and tetracyclines may interfere with bactericidal effects. Lowers estrogen reabsorption and reduces efficacy of combined oral estrogen/progesterone contraceptives.

PREGNANCY: Category B, caution in nursing.

MECHANISM OF ACTION: Ampicillin analog; bactericidal action against susceptible organisms during the stage of multiplication; acts through inhibition of biosynthesis of cell wall mucopeptide.

PHARMACOKINETICS: Absorption: C_{max} =6.6 mcg/mL. T_{max} =3.1 hrs. **Distribution:** Plasma protein binding (20%). **Elimination:** Urine (unchanged); $T_{1/2}$=1.5 hrs.

NURSING CONSIDERATIONS

Assessment: Assess for history of allergic reaction to penicillins, cephalosporins, or other allergens, infectious mononucleosis, phenylketonuria, pregnancy/nursing status, and for possible drug interactions.

Monitoring: Monitor for serious anaphylactic reactions, erythematous skin rash, development of drug resistance or superinfection with mycotic or bacterial pathogen, signs/symptoms of CDAD (may range from mild diarrhea to fatal colitis). Monitor for false (+) reactions for urinary glucose test. Caution in dose selection in elderly; monitor renal function.

Patient Counseling: Instruct to not chew or crush. Inform drug treats bacterial, not viral, infections. Instruct to take exactly ud; skipping doses or not completing full course may decrease effectiveness and increase resistance. Inform about potential benefits/risks; notify physician if watery/bloody diarrhea (with/without stomach cramps and fever) is experienced, which may occur as late as 2 months after treatment. Notify physician of serious hypersensitivity reactions, pregnancy, or nursing.

Administration: Oral route. **Storage:** 25°C (77°F). Excursion permitted to 15-30°C (59-86°).

MOXEZA   RX
moxifloxacin HCl (Alcon)

THERAPEUTIC CLASS: Fluoroquinolone

INDICATIONS: Treatment of bacterial conjunctivitis caused by susceptible strains of organisms.

DOSAGE: *Adults:* 1 drop bid for 7 days in the affected eye(s).
Pediatrics: ≥4 Months: 1 drop bid for 7 days in the affected eye(s).

HOW SUPPLIED: Sol: 0.5% [3mL]

WARNINGS/PRECAUTIONS: For topical ophthalmic use only; should not be introduced directly into the anterior chamber of the eye. Serious and sometimes fatal hypersensitivity reactions reported with systemic use; d/c and institute appropriate therapy if allergic reaction occurs. Prolonged use may cause overgrowth of nonsusceptible organisms, including fungi. D/C use and consider alternative therapy if superinfection occurs. Avoid wearing contact lenses when signs/symptoms of bacterial conjunctivitis are present.

ADVERSE REACTIONS: Eye irritation, pyrexia, conjunctivitis.

PREGNANCY: Category C, caution in nursing.

MECHANISM OF ACTION: Fluoroquinolone antibiotic; inhibition of topoisomerase II (DNA gyrase) and topoisomerase IV. DNA gyrase is an essential enzyme involved in replication, transcription, and repair of bacterial DNA. Topoisomerase IV is an enzyme known to play a key role in partitioning of chromosomal DNA during bacterial cell division.

PHARMACOKINETICS: Absorption: AUC=8.17ng•hr/mL. **Distribution:** Presumed to be excreted in breast milk.

NURSING CONSIDERATIONS

Assessment: Assess severity of infection, symptoms, and pregnancy/nursing status.

Monitoring: Monitor for signs/symptoms of hypersensitivity/anaphylactic reactions and other adverse reactions. Monitor for superinfection; examine with magnification (eg, slit lamp biomicroscopy) and fluorescein staining, where appropriate.

Patient Counseling: Advise on proper use to prevent bacterial contamination. Instruct to d/c medication and contact physician if rash or allergic reaction occurs. Advise not to wear contact lenses if signs/symptoms of bacterial conjunctivitis are present.

Administration: Ocular route. Do not inject into eye. **Storage:** 2-25°C (36-77°F).

MS Contin

morphine sulfate (Purdue Pharma)

Contains morphine, an opioid agonist and Schedule II controlled substance with an abuse liability similar to other opioid agonists, legal or illicit; assess each patient's risk for opioid abuse or addiction prior to prescribing. Routinely monitor for signs of misuse, abuse, and addiction. Respiratory depression, including fatal cases, may occur even when used as recommended; proper dosing and titration are essential. Monitor for respiratory depression, especially during initiation or following a dose increase. Should only be prescribed by healthcare professionals who are knowledgeable in the use of potent opioids for the management of chronic pain. Accidental ingestion, especially in children, can result in fatal overdose. Swallow tab whole; crushing, dissolving, or chewing the tab can cause rapid release and absorption of a potentially fatal dose.

THERAPEUTIC CLASS: Opioid analgesic

INDICATIONS: Management of moderate to severe pain when a continuous, around-the-clock opioid analgesic is needed for an extended period of time.

DOSAGE: *Adults:* Individualize dose. The 100mg and 200mg tabs are for opioid-tolerant patients only. Refer to PI for the factors to consider when selecting an initial dose. First Opioid Analgesic: Initial: Begin treatment using immediate-release (IR) formulation. Conversion from Other PO Morphine: Give 1/2 of daily requirement q12h or give 1/3 of daily requirement q8h. Conversion from Parenteral Morphine: 2-6mg may be required to provide analgesia equivalent to 1mg of parenteral. Dose approximately 3X the daily parenteral requirement is typically sufficient. Conversion from Other Parenteral or PO Non-Morphine Opioids: Initial: Give 1/2 of estimated daily requirement. Supplement with IR morphine. May give 1st dose with the last dose of any IR opioid. Titrate and Maint: Individually titrate to a dose that provides adequate analgesia and minimizes adverse reactions. May adjust dose every 1-2 days. Breakthrough Pain: May require dose adjustment or rescue medication with appropriate dose of IR medication. If signs of excessive opioid-related adverse reactions observed, reduce next dose; adjust dose to obtain appropriate balance between pain management and opioid-related adverse reactions. Discontinuation: Use gradual downward titration; avoid abrupt discontinuation. Elderly: Start at the low end of dosing range.

HOW SUPPLIED: Tab, Controlled-Release: 15mg, 30mg, 60mg, 100mg, 200mg

CONTRAINDICATIONS: Significant respiratory depression, acute or severe bronchial asthma in an unmonitored setting or in the absence of resuscitative equipment, and known or suspected paralytic ileus.

WARNINGS/PRECAUTIONS: Not for use as PRN analgesic, for mild pain or acute pain, pain not expected to persist for an extended period of time, postoperative pain unless the patient is already receiving chronic opioid therapy prior to surgery or if postoperative pain is expected to be moderate to severe and persist for an extended period of time, and in the immediate postoperative period (first 24 hrs after surgery) for patients not previously taking the drug. Respiratory depression is more likely to occur in elderly, cachectic, or debilitated patients; monitor closely when initiating and titrating, and when given with drugs that depress respiration. Monitor for respiratory depression and consider alternative nonopioid analgesics in patients with significant chronic obstructive pulmonary disease (COPD) or cor pulmonale, patients having a substantially decreased respiratory reserve, hypoxia, hypercapnia, or preexisting respiratory depression. May cause severe hypotension, especially in patients with compromised ability to maintain BP. Avoid with circulatory shock, impaired consciousness, or coma. Monitor for signs of sedation and respiratory depression in patients susceptible to the intracranial effects of carbon dioxide retention (eg, those with increased intracranial pressure [ICP] or brain tumors). May obscure clinical course in patients with head injury. Avoid with GI obstruction. May cause spasm of sphincter of Oddi; monitor for worsening symptoms in patients with biliary tract disease (eg, acute pancreatitis). May aggravate convulsions in patients with convulsive disorders and may induce or aggravate seizures; monitor for worsened seizure control in patients with history of seizure disorders. May impair mental/physical abilities. Caution in elderly.

ADVERSE REACTIONS: Respiratory depression, constipation, dizziness, sedation, N/V, sweating, dysphoria, euphoric mood.

INTERACTIONS: CNS depressants (eg, sedatives or hypnotics, general anesthetics, phenothiazines, tranquilizers, alcohol, anxiolytics, neuroleptics, muscle relaxants, other opioids, and illicit drugs) may increase risk of respiratory depression, hypotension, profound sedation, or coma; reduce initial dose of 1 or both agents. Avoid use with mixed agonist/antagonist analgesics (eg, pentazocine, nalbuphine, butorphanol); may reduce analgesic effect or may precipitate withdrawal symptoms. May enhance neuromuscular-blocking action and produce increased respiratory depression with skeletal muscle relaxants. MAOIs have been reported to potentiate the effects of morphine anxiety, confusion, and significant depression of respiration or coma; avoid use or within 14 days of MAOI use. Confusion and severe respiratory depression in a patient undergoing hemodialysis reported when concurrently administered with cimetidine. May reduce efficacy of diuretics. Anticholinergics may increase risk of urinary retention and/or severe constipation, which may lead to paralytic ileus. May increase absorption/exposure with p-glycoprotein inhibitors (eg, quinidine) by about 2-fold.

PREGNANCY: Category C, not for use in nursing.

MECHANISM OF ACTION: Opioid analgesic; acts as a full agonist, binds with and activates opioid receptors at sites in the periaqueductal and periventricular grey matter, the ventromedial medulla and the spinal cord to produce analgesia.

PHARMACOKINETICS: Absorption: Oral bioavailability (20-40%). **Distribution:** V_d=3-4L/kg; plasma protein binding (30-35%); distributed to skeletal muscle, kidneys, liver, intestinal tract, lungs, spleen, and brain; crosses placental membranes; found in breast milk. **Metabolism:** Liver via glucuronidation and sulfation; (metabolites) morphine-3-glucuronide (M3G, about 50%), morphine-6-glucuronide (about 5-15%), morphine-3-etheral sulfate. **Elimination:** Urine (primary as M3G, 10% unchanged), bile (small); (IV) $T_{1/2}$=2-4 hrs.

NURSING CONSIDERATIONS

Assessment: Assess for personal/family history or risk factors for drug abuse or addiction, general condition and medical status, opioid experience/tolerance, pain severity/type, previous opioid daily dose, potency, and type of prior analgesics used, respiratory depression, COPD or other respiratory complications, GI obstruction, paralytic ileus, renal/hepatic impairment, pregnancy/nursing status, possible drug interactions, and any other conditions where treatment is contraindicated or cautioned.

Monitoring: Monitor for signs/symptoms of respiratory depression, orthostatic hypotension, syncope, symptoms of worsening biliary tract disease, aggravation/induction of seizures, tolerance, physical dependence, mental/physical impairment, and withdrawal syndrome. Monitor for signs of increased ICP. Routinely monitor for signs of misuse, abuse, and addiction. Periodically reassess the continued need of therapy.

Patient Counseling: Inform that drug has potential for abuse; instruct not to share drug with others and to take steps to protect from theft or misuse. Discuss risks of life-threatening respiratory depression, orthostatic hypotension, and syncope. Advise to store drug securely; accidental exposure, especially in children, can result in serious harm/death. Instruct to dispose unused drug by flushing down the toilet. Inform about risks of concomitant use of alcohol and other CNS depressants; advise not to use such drugs unless supervised by physician. Instruct on how to properly take the medication. Inform that therapy may impair physical/mental abilities; advise patients not to perform potentially hazardous activities (eg, driving a car, operating heavy machinery) until they know how they will react to the medication. Advise of the potential for severe constipation, including management instructions, and when to seek medical attention. Advise how to recognize anaphylaxis and when to seek medical attention. Inform females that drug can cause fetal harm; notify physician if pregnant/plan to become pregnant.

Administration: Oral route. Swallow whole. Do not crush, dissolve, or chew. **Storage:** 25°C (77°F); excursions permitted between 15-30°C (59-86°F).

MULTAQ   RX
dronedarone (Sanofi-Aventis)

> Doubles the risk of death in patients with symptomatic heart failure (HF), with recent decompensation, requiring hospitalization or NYHA Class IV HF; contraindicated in these patients. Doubles the risk of death, stroke, and hospitalization for HF in patients with permanent atrial fibrillation (A-fib); contraindicated in patients in A-fib who will not or cannot be cardioverted into normal sinus rhythm.

THERAPEUTIC CLASS: Class III antiarrhythmic

INDICATIONS: To reduce the risk of hospitalization for A-fib in patients in sinus rhythm with a history of paroxysmal or persistent A-fib.

DOSAGE: *Adults:* 400mg bid. Take as 1 tab with am meal and 1 tab with pm meal.

HOW SUPPLIED: Tab: 400mg

CONTRAINDICATIONS: Permanent A-fib, symptomatic HF with recent decompensation requiring hospitalization or NYHA Class IV symptoms, 2nd- or 3rd-degree atrioventricular block or sick sinus syndrome (except when used with a functioning pacemaker), bradycardia <50 bpm, liver or lung toxicity related to previous use of amiodarone, QTc Bazett interval ≥500 msec or PR interval >280 msec, severe hepatic impairment, women who are or may become pregnant, nursing mothers. Concomitant use of strong CYP3A inhibitors (eg, ketoconazole, clarithromycin, nefazodone), drugs or herbal products that prolong QT interval and might increase risk of torsades de pointes (eg, phenothiazine antipsychotics, TCAs, certain oral macrolide antibiotics, Class I and III antiarrhythmics).

WARNINGS/PRECAUTIONS: Monitor cardiac rhythm no less often than every 3 months. Cardiovert patients or d/c drug if patients are in A-fib. Only initiate in patients who are receiving appropriate antithrombotic therapy. New onset or worsening of HF reported; d/c if HF develops or worsens and requires hospitalization. Hepatocellular liver injury (including acute liver failure requiring transplant) reported; d/c if hepatic injury is suspected and test serum enzymes, AST, ALT, alkaline phosphatase, and serum bilirubin. Do not restart therapy without another explanation for observed liver injury. Interstitial lung disease (including pneumonitis and pulmonary fibrosis) reported. Onset of dyspnea or nonproductive cough may be related to pulmonary toxicity; evaluate patients carefully. D/C if pulmonary toxicity is confirmed. K^+ levels should be within normal range prior to and during therapy. May induce moderate QTc (Bazett) prolongation. Increase in SrCr, pre-renal azotemia, and acute renal failure often in the setting of HF or hypovolemia reported. Premenopausal women who have not undergone hysterectomy/oophorectomy must use effective contraception while on therapy.

ADVERSE REACTIONS: QT prolongation, SrCr increase, diarrhea, N/V, abdominal pain, asthenic conditions, bradycardia, rashes, pruritus, eczema, dermatitis, allergic dermatitis.

INTERACTIONS: See Contraindications. Hypokalemia/hypomagnesemia may occur with K^+-depleting diuretics. May increase exposure to digoxin. Digoxin may also potentiate electrophysiologic effects; consider discontinuing or halve the dose of digoxin and closely monitor serum levels and for toxicity if digoxin treatment is continued. Calcium channel blockers (CCBs) may potentiate effects on conduction and may increase exposure. Bradycardia more frequently observed with β-blockers. Give a low dose of CCB or β-blockers initially and increase only after ECG verification of good tolerability. Avoid grapefruit juice, rifampin, or other CYP3A inducers (eg, phenobarbital, carbamazepine, phenytoin, St. John's wort). May increase exposure of simvastatin/simvastatin acid, CCBs, dabigatran, P-glycoprotein substrates, and CYP2D6 substrates (eg, β-blockers, TCAs, SSRIs). Avoid doses >10mg qd of simvastatin. May increase plasma levels of tacrolimus, sirolimus, and other CYP3A substrates with a narrow therapeutic range; monitor concentrations and adjust dosage appropriately. Clinically significant INR elevations with oral anticoagulants and increased S-warfarin exposure reported; monitor INR after initiating therapy in patients taking warfarin.

PREGNANCY: Category X, not for use in nursing.

MECHANISM OF ACTION: Benzofuran derivative; has not been established. Has antiarrhythmic properties belonging to all 4 Vaughan-Williams classes.

PHARMACOKINETICS: Absorption: Absolute bioavailability (4% without food, 15% with high-fat meal); T_{max}=3-6 hrs (fed). **Distribution:** Plasma protein binding (>98%); (IV) V_d=1400L. **Metabolism:** Extensive via CYP3A; N-debutylation; N-debutyl metabolite (active). **Elimination:** Urine (6%, metabolites), feces (84%, metabolites); $T_{1/2}$=13-19 hrs.

NURSING CONSIDERATIONS

Assessment: Assess for recent HF decompensation, permanent A-fib, hepatic impairment, any other conditions where treatment is contraindicated/cautioned, pregnancy/nursing status, and possible drug interactions. Assess serum K^+ levels.

Monitoring: Monitor for signs/symptoms of new/worsening HF, hepatic injury, pulmonary toxicity, and QT interval prolongation. Monitor cardiac rhythm no less often than every 3 months, hepatic serum enzymes periodically, especially during first 6 months, and renal function periodically.

Patient Counseling: Instruct to take with meals and not to take with grapefruit juice. If a dose is missed, advise to take next dose at the regularly scheduled time and not to double the dose. Counsel to consult physician if signs/symptoms of HF or potential liver injury occur and before stopping the treatment. Advise to inform physician of any history of HF, rhythm disturbance other than A-fib or atrial flutter, or predisposing conditions, such as uncorrected hypokalemia. Advise to report any use of other prescription, nonprescription medication, or herbal products, particularly St. John's wort. Counsel patients of childbearing potential about appropriate contraceptive choices while on therapy.

Administration: Oral route. **Storage:** 25°C (77°F); excursions permitted to 15-30°C (59-86°F).

MYCAMINE   RX
micafungin sodium (Astellas)

THERAPEUTIC CLASS: Echinocandin

INDICATIONS: Treatment of candidemia, acute disseminated candidiasis, *Candida* peritonitis and abscesses, and esophageal candidiasis in adult and pediatric patients ≥4 months of age. Prophylaxis of *Candida* infections in adult and pediatric patients ≥4 months of age undergoing hematopoietic stem cell transplantation (HSCT).

M

DOSAGE: *Adults:* Candidemia/Acute Disseminated Candidiasis/*Candida* Peritonitis and Abscesses: 100mg IV qd (mean 15 days; range 10-47 days). Esophageal Candidiasis: 150mg IV qd (mean 15 days; range 10-30 days). *Candida* Infections Prophylaxis in HSCT: 50mg IV qd (mean 19 days; range 6-51 days).

Pediatrics: ≥4 Months: Candidemia/Acute Disseminated Candidiasis/*Candida* Peritonitis and Abscesses: 2mg/kg qd. Max: 100mg/day. Esophageal Candidiasis: >30kg: 2.5mg/kg qd. Max: 150mg/day. ≤30kg: 3mg/kg qd. *Candida* Infections Prophylaxis in HSCT: 1mg/kg qd. Max: 50mg/day.

HOW SUPPLIED: Inj: 50mg, 100mg

WARNINGS/PRECAUTIONS: Isolated cases of serious hypersensitivity reactions (eg, anaphylaxis, anaphylactoid reactions, shock) reported; d/c and administer appropriate treatment if these occur. Acute intravascular hemolysis, hemolytic anemia, and hemoglobinuria reported; monitor for worsening of hemolysis or hemolytic anemia and evaluate the risks/benefits of continuing therapy if evident. LFT abnormalities reported; monitor for worsening hepatic function and evaluate the risks/benefits of continuing therapy if evident. Hepatic abnormalities, hepatic impairment, hepatitis, and hepatic failure reported in patients taking multiple concomitant medications with serious underlying conditions. Elevations in BUN and creatinine reported, and isolated cases of significant renal impairment and acute renal failure reported; monitor for worsening of renal function in patients who develop abnormal renal function tests during therapy.

ADVERSE REACTIONS: Diarrhea, pyrexia, neutropenia, thrombocytopenia, anemia, rash, headache, insomnia, N/V, hypoglycemia, phlebitis, anxiety, tachycardia, abdominal pain, alanine aminotransferase increased.

INTERACTIONS: Monitor for sirolimus, nifedipine, or itraconazole toxicity; reduce dose of these drugs if necessary.

PREGNANCY: Category C, caution in nursing.

MECHANISM OF ACTION: Echinocandin; inhibits the synthesis of 1,3-β-D-glucan, an essential component of fungal cell walls.

PHARMACOKINETICS: Absorption: IV infusion of variable doses resulted in different parameters. **Distribution:** V_d=0.39L/kg (terminal phase); plasma protein binding (>99%). **Metabolism:** Metabolized to M-1 (catechol form) by arylsulfatase and further metabolized to M-2 (methoxy form) by catechol-O-methyltransferase. M-5 is formed (hydroxylation) catalyzed by CYP450 isoenzymes. **Elimination:** (25mg) Urine and feces (82.5%), feces (71%).

NURSING CONSIDERATIONS

Assessment: Assess for drug hypersensitivity, hematologic abnormalities, renal/hepatic impairment, pregnancy/nursing status, and possible drug interactions.

Monitoring: Monitor for hypersensitivity reactions, LFT abnormalities, worsening renal function, hematological effects, and other adverse reactions.

Patient Counseling: Counsel about the benefits/risks of treatment. Inform of the serious adverse effects (eg, hypersensitivity reactions, hematological effects, hepatic/renal effects). Instruct to inform healthcare provider if any unusual symptom develops, any known symptom persists or worsens, or if taking any other medications, including OTC medications.

Administration: IV route. Infuse over 1 hr. Do not mix or co-infuse with other medications. To minimize the risk of infusion reactions, concentrations >1.5mg/mL should be administered via central catheter in pediatric patients. Refer to PI for reconstitution, dilution, preparation, and administration techniques. **Storage:** Unopened Vials: 25°C (77°F); excursions permitted to 15-30°C (59-86°F). Reconstituted/Diluted Infusion: 25°C (77°F) for up to 24 hrs. Diluted Infusion: Protect from light.

MYFORTIC   RX
mycophenolic acid (Novartis)

Use during pregnancy is associated with increased risks of pregnancy loss and congenital malformations; counsel females of reproductive potential regarding pregnancy prevention and planning. Immunosuppression may lead to increased risk of lymphoma and other malignancies, particularly of the skin. Increased susceptibility to infections (bacterial, viral, fungal, protozoal, opportunistic). Only physicians experienced in immunosuppressive therapy and management of organ transplant patients should prescribe mycophenolic acid. Manage patients in facilities equipped and staffed with adequate laboratory and supportive medical resources. Physician responsible for maintenance therapy should have complete information requisite for patient follow-up.

THERAPEUTIC CLASS: Inosine monophosphate dehydrogenase inhibitor

INDICATIONS: Prophylaxis of organ rejection in adult patients receiving a kidney transplant and in pediatric patients ≥5 yrs of age who are at least 6 months post kidney transplant; use with cyclosporine and corticosteroids.

DOSAGE: *Adults:* Take on an empty stomach, 1 hr before or 2 hrs after food intake. Usual: 720mg bid (1440mg total daily dose).

Pediatrics: ≥5 Yrs: Take on an empty stomach, 1 hr before or 2 hrs after food intake. Usual: 400mg/m² bid. Max: 720mg bid. BSA >1.58m²: 1440mg daily dose (four 180mg tabs or two 360mg tabs bid). BSA 1.19-1.58m²: 1080mg daily dose (three 180mg tabs or one 180mg tab + one 360mg tab bid).

HOW SUPPLIED: Tab, Delayed-Release: 180mg, 360mg

WARNINGS/PRECAUTIONS: Should not be used interchangeably with mycophenolate mofetil (MMF) tabs and caps without medical supervision. Females of reproductive potential should have a serum or urine pregnancy test (sensitivity of at least 25 mIU/mL) immediately before starting therapy; repeat test after 8-10 days and during routine follow-up visits. Acceptable birth control must be used during therapy and for 6 weeks after discontinuation unless patient chooses abstinence. Consider alternative immunosuppressants with less potential for embryofetal toxicity in patients considering pregnancy. Limit exposure to sunlight and UV light in patients at increased risk for skin cancer. Polyomavirus-associated nephropathy (PVAN), JC virus associated progressive multifocal leukoencephalopathy (PML), cytomegalovirus (CMV) infections, reactivation of hepatitis B (HBV) or hepatitis C (HCV) reported; consider reduction in immunosuppression for patients who develop evidence of new or reactivated viral infections. PVAN, especially due to BK virus infection, may lead to deteriorating renal function and renal graft loss. Consider PML in differential diagnosis in patients reporting neurological symptoms and consider consultation with a neurologist as clinically indicated. Monitor HBV or HCV infected patients for clinical/lab signs of active HBV or HCV infection. Cases of pure red cell aplasia (PRCA) reported when used with other immunosuppressive agents. D/C or reduce dose if blood dyscrasias occur (neutropenia [absolute neutrophil count <1.3 x 10³/μL] or anemia). GI bleeding (requiring hospitalization), intestinal perforations, gastric ulcers, and duodenal ulcers reported; caution with active serious digestive system disease. Avoid with rare hereditary deficiency of hypoxanthine-guanine phosphoribosyl-transferase (HGPRT) (eg, Lesch-Nyhan and Kelley-Seegmiller syndromes). Caution in elderly.

ADVERSE REACTIONS: Lymphoma, skin malignancies, anemia, leukopenia, constipation, N/V, diarrhea, dyspepsia, infections, insomnia, postoperative pain.

INTERACTIONS: Mg^{2+}- and aluminum-containing antacids may decrease levels; do not administer simultaneously. Avoid concomitant use with azathioprine, MMF, and norfloxacin-metronidazole combination. Cholestyramine or other agents that may interfere with enterohepatic recirculation or drugs that may bind bile acids (eg, bile acid sequestrates or oral activated charcoal) may reduce efficacy; avoid concomitant use. Avoid live attenuated vaccines. Sevelamer may decrease levels; do not administer simultaneously with sevelamer and other Ca^{2+} free phosphate binders. Cyclosporine may decrease levels; caution when switching from cyclosporine to other immunosuppressive drugs or from other immunosuppressive drugs to cyclosporine. Decreased levels with rifampin; avoid concomitant use unless the benefit outweighs the risk. May decrease effects of hormonal contraceptives; coadminister with caution, and additional barrier contraceptive methods must be used. Drugs that undergo renal tubular secretion (eg, acyclovir/valacyclovir, ganciclovir/valganciclovir) may increase levels of both drugs; monitor blood cell counts. Drugs that alter the GI flora (eg, ciprofloxacin or amoxicillin plus clavulanic acid) may disrupt enterohepatic recirculation.

PREGNANCY: Category D, not for use in nursing.

MECHANISM OF ACTION: Inosine monophosphate dehydrogenase inhibitor; inhibits the de novo pathway of guanosine nucleotide synthesis without incorporation to deoxyribonucleic acid.

PHARMACOKINETICS: Absorption: Absolute bioavailability (72%); T_{max}=1.5-2.75 hrs (median). **Distribution:** V_d=54L; plasma protein binding (>98%), (82% mycophenolic acid glucuronide [MPAG]). **Metabolism:** Glucuronyl transferase; MPAG (major metabolite). **Elimination:** Urine (>60% MPAG, 3% unchanged), bile; $T_{1/2}$=8-16 hrs, 13-17 hrs (MPAG).

NURSING CONSIDERATIONS

Assessment: Assess for hypersensitivity to the drug, hepatic/renal impairment, hereditary deficiency of HGPRT (eg, Lesch-Nyhan and Kelley-Seegmiller syndromes), active digestive disease, pregnancy/nursing status, and for possible drug interactions.

Monitoring: Monitor for signs/symptoms of lymphomas, skin cancer and other malignancies, GI bleeding/perforation, infections, blood dyscrasias (eg, PRCA), and other adverse reactions. Monitor CBC weekly during the 1st month, twice monthly for the 2nd and 3rd month of therapy, and then monthly through 1st yr. Monitor pregnancy status by obtaining pregnancy test 8-10 days after initiation of therapy and repeatedly during follow-up visits.

Patient Counseling: Inform that use in pregnancy is associated with an increased risk of 1st trimester pregnancy loss and congenital malformation; discuss pregnancy testing, prevention (including acceptable contraception methods), and planning. Discuss appropriate alternative immunosuppressants with less potential for embryofetal toxicity in patients who are considering pregnancy. Advise not to breastfeed during therapy. Inform about increased risk of developing lymphomas and other malignancies; advise to limit exposure to sunlight and UV light by wearing protective clothing and using sunscreen with high protection factor. Inform about increased risk of developing a variety of infections, including opportunistic infections, due to immunosuppression. Inform about risk for developing blood dyscrasias and instruct to report if experiencing any symptoms of infection, unexpected bruising, bleeding, or any other manifestation of bone marrow suppression. Inform that therapy may cause GI tract complications, including bleeding, intestinal perforations, and gastric or duodenal ulcers; advise to contact healthcare provider if symptoms of GI bleeding or sudden onset or persistent abdominal pain occurs. Inform that therapy may interfere with the usual response to immunizations. Advise to report to physician the use of any other medications while on therapy. Encourage to enroll in the pregnancy registry if patient becomes pregnant while on therapy.

Administration: Oral route. Swallow whole; do not crush, chew, or cut. **Storage:** 25°C (77°F); excursions permitted to 15-30°C (59-86°F). Protect from moisture.

NABUMETONE RX
nabumetone (Various)

NSAIDs may increase risk of serious cardiovascular (CV) thrombotic events, myocardial infarction (MI), stroke and serious GI adverse events including bleeding, ulceration, and perforation of the stomach or intestines. Contraindicated for the treatment of perioperative pain in the setting of coronary artery bypass graft (CABG) surgery.

THERAPEUTIC CLASS: NSAID

INDICATIONS: Relief of signs and symptoms of osteoarthritis and rheumatoid arthritis.

DOSAGE: *Adults:* Initial: 1000mg qd with or without food. Titrate: May give 1500-2000mg depending on clinical response to initial therapy. Max: 2000mg/day given qd-bid. Renal impairment: Moderate: Initial: ≤750mg qd. Severe: Initial: ≤500mg qd.

HOW SUPPLIED: Tab: 500mg, 750mg

CONTRAINDICATIONS: History of asthma, urticaria, or allergic-type reactions after taking aspirin (ASA) or other NSAIDs. Treatment of perioperative pain in the setting of CABG surgery.

WARNINGS/PRECAUTIONS: Use lowest effective dose for shortest duration possible to minimize risk for CV events and adverse GI events. May lead to onset of new HTN or worsening of preexisting HTN; caution with HTN and monitor BP closely. Fluid retention and edema reported; caution with fluid retention or heart failure. Renal papillary necrosis and other renal injury reported after long-term use. Not recommended for use with advanced renal disease; if therapy must be initiated, monitor renal function closely. Anaphylactoid reactions may occur. Should not be given with ASA triad. May cause serious skin adverse events (eg, exfoliative dermatitis, Stevens-Johnson syndrome, and toxic epidermal necrolysis). Avoid in late pregnancy; may cause premature closure of ductus arteriosus. May cause elevations of LFTs; d/c if liver disease develops or systemic manifestations occur. Caution in elderly. Anemia may occur; monitor Hgb/Hct if signs or symptoms of anemia develop. May inhibit platelet aggregation and prolong bleeding time; monitor with coagulation disorders. Caution with asthma and avoid with ASA-sensitive asthma. May induce photosensitivity.

ADVERSE REACTIONS: Diarrhea, dyspepsia, abdominal pain, constipation, flatulence, N/V, positive stool guaiac, dizziness, headache, pruritus, rash, tinnitus, edema.

INTERACTIONS: Caution with warfarin and other protein-bound drugs. May decrease natriuretic effect of furosemide and thiazides; possible renal failure risk. May elevate lithium and methotrexate levels. May diminish antihypertensive effect of ACE inhibitors. Avoid concomitant ASA. May increase risk of GI bleeding with concomitant use of oral corticosteroids, anticoagulants or alcohol.

PREGNANCY: Category C, not for use in nursing.

MECHANISM OF ACTION: NSAID (naphthylalkanone derivative); suspected to inhibit prostaglandin synthesis, exerts anti-inflammatory, analgesic, and antipyretic actions.

PHARMACOKINETICS: Absorption: Well-absorbed (GIT). PO administration of variable doses resulted in different parameters. **Distribution:** Plasma protein binding (>99%). **Metabolism:** Liver (extensive biotransformation), 6-methoxy-2-naphthylacetic acid (active metabolite). **Elimination:** Urine (approximately 80%), feces (9%); $T_{1/2}$=24 hrs.

NURSING CONSIDERATIONS

Assessment: Assess LFTs, renal function, CBC, and coagulation profile. Assess for history of CABG surgery, asthma and allergic reactions to ASA or other NSAIDs, active ulceration or chronic inflammation of GI tract, CV disease, asthma, alcohol intake, pregnancy/nursing status. Note other diseases/conditions and drug therapies.

Monitoring: Monitor for hypersensitivity reactions, CV thrombotic events, MI, stroke, GI bleeding, asthma, and skin adverse effects. Monitor BP, LFTs, renal function, CBC with differential and platelet count, coagulation profile, ocular effects, and photosensitivity.

Patient Counseling: Counsel about potential side effects; seek medical attention if any develop, especially serious CV events or adverse GI events. Counsel about possible drug interactions and to take as prescribed. Advise women not to use in late pregnancy.

Administration: Oral route. **Storage:** 20-25°C (68-77°F). Dispense in tight, light-resistant container.

NAMENDA   RX
memantine HCl (Forest)

OTHER BRAND NAMES: Namenda XR (Forest)

THERAPEUTIC CLASS: NMDA receptor antagonist

INDICATIONS: Treatment of moderate to severe dementia of the Alzheimer's type.

DOSAGE: *Adults*: (Sol, Tab) Initial: 5mg qd. Titrate: Increase in 5mg increments to 10mg/day (5mg bid), 15mg/day (5mg and 10mg as separate doses), and 20mg/day (10mg bid) at ≥1 week intervals. Dosage shown to be effective in controlled clinical trials is 20mg/day. Severe Renal Impairment: (CrCl 5-29mL/min): Target Dose: 5mg bid. (Cap, Extended-Release [ER]) Initial: 7mg qd. Titrate: Increase in 7mg increments to 28mg qd at ≥1-week intervals. Max/Target Dose: 28mg qd. Severe Renal Impairment (CrCl 5-29mL/min): Target dose: 14mg/day. Switching from Tabs to Cap, ER: Switch from 10mg bid tabs to 28mg qd caps the day following last dose of 10mg tab. Severe Renal Impairment: Switch from 5mg bid tabs to 14mg qd caps the day following last dose of 5mg tab.

HOW SUPPLIED: Sol: 2mg/mL [360mL]; Tab: 5mg, 10mg; Titration-Pack: 5mg [28^s], 10mg [21^s]. Cap, ER: 7mg, 14mg, 21mg, 28mg; Titration Pack: 7mg [7^s], 14mg [7^s], 21mg [7^s], 28mg [7^s].

WARNINGS/PRECAUTIONS: Conditions that raise urine pH may decrease urinary elimination, resulting in increased plasma levels. Use not systematically evaluated with seizure disorders. Caution in patients with severe hepatic impairment.

ADVERSE REACTIONS: Dizziness, headache, constipation, confusion, HTN, coughing, somnolence, hallucination, vomiting, back pain, (Sol, Tab) pain, (Cap, ER) diarrhea, influenza, weight gain, depression.

INTERACTIONS: Caution with other N-methyl-D-aspartate (NMDA) antagonists (eg, amantadine, ketamine, dextromethorphan) and drugs that alter urine pH towards the alkaline condition (eg, carbonic anhydrase inhibitors, sodium bicarbonate). (Cap, ER) Coadministration with drugs eliminated via renal (cationic system) mechanism (eg, HCTZ, triamterene, metformin, cimetidine, ranitidine, quinidine, nicotine) may result in altered plasma levels of both agents.

PREGNANCY: Category B, caution in nursing.

MECHANISM OF ACTION: NMDA receptor antagonist; postulated to exert its therapeutic effect through its action as a low to moderate affinity uncompetitive (open-channel) NMDA receptor antagonist, which binds preferentially to the NMDA receptor-operated cation channels.

PHARMACOKINETICS: Absorption: (Sol, Tab) T_{max}=3-7 hrs. (Cap, ER, multiple dose) T_{max}=9-12 hrs. **Distribution**: V_d=9-11L/kg. Plasma protein binding (45%). **Metabolism**: Liver (partial); N-glucuronide conjugate, 6-hydroxy memantine, 1-nitroso-deaminated memantine (metabolites). **Elimination**: Urine (48%, unchanged); $T_{1/2}$=60-80 hrs.

NURSING CONSIDERATIONS

Assessment: Assess for hypersensitivity to drug, conditions that raise urine pH, seizure disorder, renal/hepatic impairment, pregnancy/nursing status, and possible drug interactions.

Monitoring: Monitor for hypersensitivity reactions and other adverse reactions. Monitor renal/hepatic function.

Patient Counseling: (Cap, ER; Sol; Tab) Instruct to take as prescribed. Inform about possible side effects and instruct to notify physician if any develop. (Sol, Tab) Instruct to follow dose titration schedule and not to resume dosing without consulting physician if there has been a failure to take the medication for several days. (Tab) Instruct not to use any damaged or tampered tabs. (Sol) Instruct on how to use the oral solution dosing device. Inform of the patient instruction sheet enclosed with the product and instruct to address any questions to physician or pharmacist.

Administration: Oral route. May take with or without food. (Sol, Tab) If a single dose is missed, take next dose as scheduled and do not double dose; if missed for several days, dosing may need to be resumed at lower doses and retitrated. (Sol) Do not mix with any other liquid. Administer with a dosing device (syringe, syringe adaptor cap, tubing, other supplies needed) that comes with the drug. Use syringe to withdraw correct volume of oral solution and squirt slowly into the corner of the mouth. (Cap, ER) Swallow cap whole; do not divide, chew or crush. May be opened, sprinkled on applesauce, and swallowed. **Storage**: 25°C (77°F); excursions permitted to 15-30°C (59-86°F).

NAPRELAN

RX

naproxen sodium (Shionogi)

NSAIDs may increase risk of serious cardiovascular thrombotic events, myocardial infarction (MI), and stroke; increased risk with duration of use and with cardiovascular disease (CVD) or risk factors for CVD. Increased risk of serious GI adverse events (eg, bleeding, ulceration, and stomach/intestinal perforation) that can be fatal and occur anytime during use without warning symptoms; elderly patients are at a greater risk. Contraindicated for treatment of perioperative pain in the setting of coronary artery bypass graft (CABG) surgery.

THERAPEUTIC CLASS: NSAID

INDICATIONS: Treatment of rheumatoid arthritis (RA), osteoarthritis (OA), ankylosing spondylitis (AS), tendinitis, bursitis, acute gout, and primary dysmenorrhea. Relief of mild to moderate pain.

DOSAGE: *Adults;* RA/OA/AS: Initial: 750mg or 1g qd. Titrate: Adjust dose/frequency up or down depending on clinical response; may increase to 1.5g qd for limited periods if patient can tolerate lower doses well. Pain/Primary Dysmenorrhea/Tendinitis/Bursitis: Initial: 1g qd (or 1.5g qd for a limited period). Max: 1g/day thereafter. Acute Gout: 1st Day: 1-1.5g qd. Succeeding Days: 1g qd until attack subsides. Elderly/Renal/Hepatic Impairment: Start at lower end of dosing range.

HOW SUPPLIED: Tab, Controlled-Release: 375mg, 500mg, 750mg

CONTRAINDICATIONS: History of asthma, urticaria, or allergic-type reactions with aspirin (ASA) or other NSAIDs. Treatment of perioperative pain in the setting of CABG surgery.

WARNINGS/PRECAUTIONS: Use lowest effective dose for the shortest duration possible. May cause HTN or worsen preexisting HTN; monitor BP closely. Fluid retention and edema reported; caution with fluid retention or heart failure (HF). Caution with history of ulcer disease, GI bleeding, or risk factors for GI bleeding; monitor for GI ulceration/bleeding, and d/c if serious GI event occurs. Renal injury reported with long-term use; increased risk with renal/hepatic impairment, heart failure, and elderly. Not recommended with advanced renal disease or moderate to severe renal impairment (CrCl <30mL/min); monitor renal function closely if therapy is initiated. Anaphylactoid reactions may occur. Caution with asthma and avoid with ASA-sensitive asthma and the ASA triad. May cause serious skin reactions (eg, exfoliative dermatitis, Stevens-Johnson syndrome, toxic epidermal necrolysis); d/c at 1st appearance of skin rash/hypersensitivity. Avoid in late pregnancy; may cause premature closure of ductus arteriosus. Not a substitute for corticosteroids nor treatment for corticosteroid insufficiency; may mask signs of inflammation and fever. May cause elevated LFTs or severe hepatic reactions; d/c if liver disease or systemic manifestations occur, and if abnormal LFTs persist/worsen. Anemia reported; monitor Hgb/Hct if anemia develops. May inhibit platelet aggregation and prolong bleeding time; monitor patients with coagulation disorders.

ADVERSE REACTIONS: Cardiovascular thrombotic events, MI, stroke, GI events, headache, dyspepsia, flu syndrome, pain, infection, nausea, diarrhea, constipation, rhinitis, sinusitis, urinary tract infection.

INTERACTIONS: Increased risk of GI bleeding with oral corticosteroids, anticoagulants, alcohol use, and smoking. Risk of renal toxicity with diuretics and ACE inhibitors. Monitor patients receiving anticoagulants. May diminish antihypertensive effect of ACE inhibitors. Not recommended with ASA. May reduce natriuretic effect of loop (eg, furosemide) or thiazide diuretics; monitor for signs of renal failure and diuretic efficacy. May increase lithium levels; monitor for lithium toxicity. May enhance methotrexate toxicity; caution with concomitant use. Synergistic effect on GI bleeding with warfarin.

PREGNANCY: Category C, not for use in nursing.

MECHANISM OF ACTION: NSAID; not established. Inhibition of prostaglandin synthesis thought to be involved in anti-inflammatory effect.

PHARMACOKINETICS: Absorption: Rapid and complete. Bioavailability (95%); (1g qd multiple dose) C_{max}=94mcg/mL, T_{max}=5 hrs, AUC=1448mcg•hr/mL. **Distribution:** V_d=0.16L/kg; plasma protein binding (>99%); found in breast milk. **Metabolism:** Extensive; 6-O-desmethyl naproxen metabolite. **Elimination:** Urine (<1% unchanged, <1% 6-O-desmethyl naproxen, 66-92% conjugates), feces (<5%); $T_{1/2}$=15 hrs.

NURSING CONSIDERATIONS

Assessment: Assess for history of asthma, urticaria, or allergic-type reactions with ASA or other NSAIDs, ASA triad, CVD, risk factors for CVD, HTN, fluid retention, heart failure, history of ulcer disease, history of/risk factors for GI bleeding, general health status, renal/hepatic function, coagulation disorders, pregnancy/nursing status, and possible drug interactions. Obtain baseline CBC and BP.

Monitoring: Monitor BP, CBC, bleeding time, LFTs, renal function, and chemistry profile periodically. Monitor for GI bleeding/ulceration/perforation, CV thrombotic events, MI, stroke, HTN, fluid retention, edema, and skin/allergic reactions.

Patient Counseling: Inform to seek medical advice if symptoms of CV events (eg, chest pain, SOB, weakness, slurred speech), GI ulceration/bleeding (eg, epigastric pain, dyspepsia, melena, hematemesis), skin/hypersensitivity reactions (eg, rash, blisters, fever, itching), unexplained weight gain or edema, hepatotoxicity (eg, nausea, fatigue, lethargy, pruritus, jaundice, right upper quadrant tenderness, flu-like symptoms), or anaphylactoid reactions (eg, face/throat swelling, difficulty breathing) occur. Instruct to avoid in late pregnancy.

Administration: Oral route. **Storage:** 20-25°C (68-77°F).

NAPROSYN   RX
naproxen (Genentech)

NSAIDs may increase risk of serious cardiovascular thrombotic events, myocardial infarction (MI), and stroke; increased risk with duration of use and with cardiovascular disease (CVD) or risk factors for CVD. Increased risk of serious GI adverse events (eg, bleeding, ulceration, and stomach/intestinal perforation) that can be fatal and occur anytime during use without warning symptoms; elderly patients are at a greater risk. Contraindicated for treatment of perioperative pain in the setting of coronary artery bypass graft (CABG) surgery.

OTHER BRAND NAMES: Anaprox DS (Genentech) - Anaprox (Genentech) - EC-Naprosyn (Genentech)

THERAPEUTIC CLASS: NSAID

INDICATIONS: Relief of signs and symptoms of rheumatoid arthritis (RA), osteoarthritis (OA), ankylosing spondylitis (AS), and juvenile arthritis (JA). (Naprosyn/Anaprox/Anaprox DS) Relief of signs and symptoms of tendonitis, bursitis, and acute gout, and management of pain and primary dysmenorrhea.

DOSAGE: *Adults:* RA/OA/AS: (Naprosyn) 250mg, 375mg, or 500mg bid. (EC-Naprosyn) 375mg or 500mg bid. (Anaprox) 275mg bid. (Anaprox DS) 550mg bid. Titrate: Adjust dose/frequency up or down depending on clinical response; may increase to 1500mg/day for ≤6 months if patient can tolerate lower doses well. Pain/Dysmenorrhea/Tendonitis/Bursitis: (Anaprox/Anaprox DS) Initial: 550mg, then 550mg q12h or 275mg q6-8h as required. Max: 1375mg/day initially, 1100mg/day thereafter. Acute Gout: (Naprosyn) Initial: 750mg, then 250mg q8h until attack subsides. (Anaprox) Initial: 825mg, then 275mg q8h until attack subsides. Elderly/Renal/Hepatic Impairment: Consider lower dose.
Pediatrics: ≥2 Yrs: JA: (Sus) Usual: 5mg/kg bid. Refer to PI for additional information. Renal/Hepatic Impairment: Consider lower dose.

HOW SUPPLIED: Sus: (Naprosyn) 125mg/5mL [473mL]; Tab: (Naprosyn) 250mg*, 375mg, 500mg*, (Anaprox [naproxen sodium]) 275mg, (Anaprox DS [naproxen sodium]) 550mg*; Tab, Delayed-Release: (EC-Naprosyn) 375mg, 500mg *scored

CONTRAINDICATIONS: History of asthma, urticaria, or other allergic-type reactions with aspirin (ASA) or other NSAIDs. Treatment of perioperative pain in the setting of CABG surgery.

WARNINGS/PRECAUTIONS: Use lowest effective dose for the shortest duration possible. May cause HTN or worsen preexisting HTN; monitor BP closely. Fluid retention and edema reported; caution with fluid retention, HTN, or heart failure (HF). Caution with prior history of ulcer disease, GI bleeding, and risk factors for GI bleeding; monitor for GI ulceration/bleeding and d/c if serious GI event occurs. May exacerbate inflammatory bowel disease. Renal injury reported with long-term use; increased risk with renal/hepatic impairment, hypovolemia, HF, salt depletion, and in elderly. Not recommended with advanced renal disease or moderate to severe renal impairment (CrCl <30mL/min); monitor renal function closely and hydrate adequately. D/C if signs and symptoms consistent with renal disease develop. Anaphylactoid reactions may occur. Caution with asthma and avoid with ASA-sensitive asthma and the ASA triad. May cause serious skin adverse events (eg, exfoliative dermatitis, Stevens-Johnson syndrome, toxic epidermal necrolysis); d/c at 1st appearance of skin rash/hypersensitivity. Avoid in late pregnancy; may cause premature closure of ductus arteriosus. Not a substitute for corticosteroids or for the treatment of corticosteroid insufficiency. May mask signs of inflammation and fever. Periodically monitor Hgb if initial Hgb ≤10g and receiving long-term therapy. Perform ophthalmic studies if visual changes/disturbances occur. May cause elevations of LFTs or severe hepatic reactions; d/c if liver disease or systemic manifestations occur, or if abnormal LFTs persist/worsen. Caution with chronic alcoholic liver disease and other diseases with decreased/abnormal plasma proteins if high doses are administered; dosage adjustment may be required. Anemia reported; monitor Hgb/Hct if anemia develops. May inhibit platelet aggregation and prolong bleeding time; monitor patients with coagulation disorders. Monitor CBC and chemistry profile periodically with long-term treatment. (Sus, Anaprox/Anaprox DS) Contains Na⁺; caution with severely restricted Na⁺ intake. (EC-Naprosyn) Not recommended for initial treatment of acute pain.

ADVERSE REACTIONS: Cardiovascular (CV) thrombotic events, MI, stroke, GI adverse events, edema, drowsiness, dizziness, constipation, heartburn, abdominal pain, nausea, headache, tinnitus, dyspnea, pruritus.

INTERACTIONS: Avoid with other naproxen products. Not recommended with ASA. Risk of renal toxicity with diuretics, ACE inhibitors, and ARBs. May reduce natriuretic effect of loop (eg, furosemide) or thiazide diuretics; monitor for signs of renal failure and diuretic efficacy. May diminish antihypertensive effect of ACE inhibitors, ARBs, or β-blockers (eg, propranolol); monitor changes in BP. May result in deterioration of renal function, including possible acute renal failure with ACE inhibitors or ARBs; monitor closely for signs of worsening renal function. May enhance methotrexate toxicity; caution with concomitant use. May increase lithium levels and reduce renal lithium clearance; monitor for lithium toxicity. Increased risk of GI bleeding with SSRIs, oral corticosteroids, anticoagulants, alcohol, and smoking; monitor carefully. Synergistic effect on GI bleeding with warfarin. Potential for interaction with other albumin-bound drugs (eg, coumarin-type anticoagulants, sulfonylureas, hydantoins, other NSAIDs, ASA); dose adjustment with hydantoin, sulfonamide, or sulfonylurea may be required. Probenecid significantly increases plasma levels and extends $T_{1/2}$. Antacids, sucralfate, and cholestyramine can delay absorption. (EC-Naprosyn) Not recommended with H_2-blockers, sucralfate, or intensive antacid therapy.

PREGNANCY: Category C, not for use in nursing.

MECHANISM OF ACTION: NSAID; not established. May be related to prostaglandin synthetase inhibition.

PHARMACOKINETICS: Absorption: Rapid and complete. Bioavailability (95%). Naprosyn: C_{max}=97.4mcg/mL, AUC=767mcg•hr/mL, T_{max}=2-4 hrs (tab), 1-4 hrs (sus). EC-Naprosyn: C_{max}=94.9mcg/mL, AUC=845mcg•hr/mL, T_{max}=4 hrs. Anaprox (naproxen sodium): T_{max}=1-2 hrs. **Distribution:** V_d=0.16L/kg; plasma protein binding (>99%); found in breast milk. **Metabolism:** Liver (extensive); 6-O-desmethyl naproxen (metabolite). **Elimination:** Urine (95%; <1% unchanged, <1% 6-O-desmethyl naproxen, 66-92% conjugates), feces (≤3%); $T_{1/2}$=12-17 hrs.

NURSING CONSIDERATIONS

Assessment: Assess for history of asthma, urticaria, or allergic-type reactions with ASA or other NSAIDs, ASA triad, CVD, risk factors for CVD, HTN, fluid retention, HF, salt restriction, history of ulcer disease, history of/risk factors for GI bleeding, general health status, history of IBD, renal/hepatic impairment, hypovolemia, decreased/abnormal plasma proteins, coagulation disorders, pregnancy/nursing status, and for possible drug interactions. Obtain baseline CBC and BP.

Monitoring: Monitor for GI bleeding/ulceration/perforation, CV thrombotic events, MI, stroke, HTN, fluid retention, edema, and skin/allergic reactions. Monitor BP, CBC, LFTs, renal function, and chemistry profile periodically.

Patient Counseling: Inform to seek medical advice if symptoms of CV events (eg, chest pain, SOB, weakness, slurring of speech), GI ulceration/bleeding (eg, epigastric pain, dyspepsia, melena, hematemesis), skin/hypersensitivity reactions (eg, rash, itching, blisters, fever), unexplained weight gain or edema, hepatotoxicity (eg, nausea, fatigue, lethargy, pruritus, jaundice, right upper quadrant tenderness, flu-like symptoms), or anaphylactoid reactions (eg, difficulty breathing, face/throat swelling) occur. Instruct to avoid use in late pregnancy. Instruct to use caution when performing activities that require alertness if drowsiness, dizziness, vertigo, or depression occurs.

Administration: Oral route. (EC-Naprosyn) Do not chew, crush, or break. **Storage:** 15-30°C (59-86°F). (Sus) Avoid excessive heat, >40°C (104°F). Shake gently before use.

NARDIL RX
phenelzine sulfate (Parke-Davis)

> Antidepressants increased the risk of suicidal thinking and behavior (suicidality) in children, adolescents, and young adults in short-term studies of major depressive disorder and other psychiatric disorders. Monitor and observe closely for clinical worsening, suicidality, or unusual changes in behavior in patients who are started on antidepressant therapy. Not approved for use in pediatric patients.

THERAPEUTIC CLASS: Monoamine oxidase inhibitor

INDICATIONS: Treatment of atypical, nonendogenous or neurotic depression not responsive to other antidepressants.

DOSAGE: *Adults:* Initial: 15mg tid. Titrate: Increase to 60-90mg/day at a fairly rapid pace consistent with patient tolerance until maximum benefit. Maint: Reduce slowly over several weeks to 15mg qd or qod.

HOW SUPPLIED: Tab: 15mg

CONTRAINDICATIONS: Pheochromocytoma, congestive heart failure (CHF), severe renal impairment or renal disease, history of liver disease, and abnormal LFTs. Concomitant use of meperidine, guanethidine, sympathomimetic drugs (eg, amphetamines, cocaine, methylphenidate, dopamine, epinephrine, norepinephrine), or related compounds (eg, methyldopa, L-dopa, L-tryptophan, L-tyrosine, phenylalanine), high tyramine- or dopamine-containing food, excessive caffeine and chocolate, dextromethorphan, CNS depressants (eg, alcohol, certain narcotics), local anesthesia containing sympathomimetic vasoconstrictors, and spinal anesthesia. Elective surgery requiring general anesthesia. ≥14 days should elapse between discontinuation of therapy and start of another antidepressant (including other MAOIs), buspirone HCl, bupropion HCl, and serotonin reuptake inhibitor (except fluoxetine). Allow ≥5 weeks between discontinuation of fluoxetine and initiation of therapy.

WARNINGS/PRECAUTIONS: Hypertensive crises and intracranial bleeding reported; monitor BP frequently and d/c use if palpitation or frequent headaches occur. Postural hypotension may occur. Caution with epilepsy, diabetes mellitus (DM), and patients on insulin or hypoglycemic agents. Hypomania and agitation reported following long-term use. May cause excessive stimulation in schizophrenics.

ADVERSE REACTIONS: Dizziness, headache, drowsiness, sleep disturbances, fatigue, weakness, tremors, constipation, dry mouth, GI disturbances, elevated serum transaminases, weight gain, postural hypotension, edema, sexual disturbances.

INTERACTIONS: See Contraindications. Avoid with sauerkraut, any spoiled or improperly refrigerated, handled, or stored protein-rich foods such as meats, fish, and dairy products, and OTC cold and cough preparations, nasal decongestants (tabs, drops, or spray), hay-fever/sinus/asthma inhalant medications, antiappetite medicines, weight-reducing preparations, and "pep" pills. Reduce dose of barbiturates. Caution with rauwolfia alkaloids. Exaggerated hypotensive effects with antihypertensives (eg, thiazides, β-blockers); use with caution. May potentiate hypoglycemic agents; requirements for insulin or oral hypoglycemic agents may be decreased.

PREGNANCY: Safety not known in pregnancy/nursing.

MECHANISM OF ACTION: MAOI; inhibits MAO activity.

PHARMACOKINETICS: Absorption: (30mg) C_{max}=19.8ng/mL, T_{max}=43 min. **Metabolism:** Extensive; oxidation via MAO; acetylation (minor). **Elimination:** Urine (73%); $T_{1/2}$=11.6 hrs (30mg).

NURSING CONSIDERATIONS

Assessment: Assess for pheochromocytoma, CHF, history of liver disease, bipolar disorder risk (detailed psychiatric history, family history of suicide, bipolar disorder, and depression), epilepsy, schizophrenia, manic-depressive state, DM, renal/hepatic impairment, drug hypersensitivity, pregnancy/nursing status, and possible drug interactions.

Monitoring: Monitor for clinical worsening, suicidality, unusual changes in behavior, hypertensive crisis, postural hypotension, hypomania, increased insulin sensitivity, increased psychosis, and activation of mania. Monitor BP frequently.

Patient Counseling: Inform patients, families, and caregivers about benefits/risks of therapy, including potential for clinical worsening and suicide risk. Instruct to notify physician if symptoms/adverse reactions occur during treatment or when adjusting the dose (eg, palpitations, tachycardia). Counsel to avoid concomitant intake of alcohol, foods with high tyramine content, certain OTC (eg, dextromethorphan) and prescription drugs, excessive quantities of caffeine and chocolate.

Administration: Oral route. **Storage:** 15-30°C (59-86°F).

NASONEX   RX
mometasone furoate monohydrate (Schering Corporation)

THERAPEUTIC CLASS: Corticosteroid

INDICATIONS: Treatment of nasal symptoms of seasonal and perennial allergic rhinitis and relief of nasal congestion associated with seasonal allergic rhinitis in patients ≥2 yrs of age. Prophylaxis of nasal symptoms of seasonal allergic rhinitis in patients ≥12 yrs of age. Treatment of nasal polyps in patients ≥18 yrs of age.

DOSAGE: *Adults:* Treatment (Seasonal/Perennial Allergic Rhinitis)/Prophylaxis and Treatment of Nasal Congestion (Seasonal Allergic Rhinitis): 2 sprays/nostril qd. Prophylaxis may start 2-4 weeks before pollen season. Nasal Polyps: 2 sprays/nostril qd-bid.
Pediatrics: ≥12 Yrs: Treatment (Seasonal/Perennial Allergic Rhinitis)/Prophylaxis and Treatment of Nasal Congestion (Seasonal Allergic Rhinitis): 2 sprays/nostril qd. Prophylaxis may start 2-4 weeks before pollen season. 2-11 Yrs: Treatment (Seasonal/Perennial Allergic Rhinitis)/Nasal Congestion (Seasonal Allergic Rhinitis): 1 spray/nostril qd.

HOW SUPPLIED: Spray: 50mcg/spray [17g]

WARNINGS/PRECAUTIONS: Local nasal effects (eg, epistaxis, *Candida* infections of nose and pharynx, nasal septum perforation, impaired wound healing) may occur; d/c when infection occurs. Glaucoma and/or cataracts may develop; monitor closely in patients with change in vision, history of increased intraocular pressure (IOP), glaucoma, and/or cataracts. D/C if hypersensitivity reactions, including instances of wheezing, occur. May increase susceptibility to infections; caution with active/quiescent tuberculosis (TB), ocular herpes simplex, or untreated bacterial, fungal, and systemic viral infections. Hypercorticism and adrenal suppression may appear when used at higher than recommended doses or in susceptible individuals at recommended doses; d/c slowly if such changes occur. May reduce growth velocity of pediatrics; monitor growth routinely.

ADVERSE REACTIONS: Headache, viral infection, pharyngitis, epistaxis/blood-tinged mucus, cough, upper respiratory tract infection, dysmenorrhea, musculoskeletal pain, sinusitis, N/V.

INTERACTIONS: May increase plasma concentrations with ketoconazole.

PREGNANCY: Category C, caution with nursing.

MECHANISM OF ACTION: Corticosteroid; not established. Demonstrates anti-inflammatory properties and is shown to have wide range of effects on multiple cell types (eg, mast cells, eosinophils, neutrophils, macrophages, lymphocytes) and mediators (eg, histamine, eicosanoids, leukotrienes, cytokines) involved in inflammation.

PHARMACOKINETICS: Absorption: Bioavailability (<1%). **Distribution:** Plasma protein binding (98-99%). **Metabolism:** Liver (extensive) via CYP3A4. **Elimination:** Bile (as metabolites); urine (limited extent); (IV) $T_{1/2}$=5.8 hrs.

NURSING CONSIDERATIONS

Assessment: Assess for previous hypersensitivity, active/quiescent TB, infections, ocular herpes simplex, change in vision, history of IOP, glaucoma or cataracts, recent nasal septum ulcers, nasal surgery/trauma, pregnancy/nursing status, and possible drug interactions.

Monitoring: Monitor for acute adrenal insufficiency, hypercorticism, nasal or pharyngeal *Candida* infections, suppression of growth velocity in children, hypersensitivity reactions, wheezing, nasal septum perforation, changes in vision, glaucoma, cataracts, increased IOP, epistaxis, wound healing, worsening of infections, and other adverse reactions.

Patient Counseling: Advise to take ud at regular intervals and not to increase prescribed dosage. Inform patients that treatment may be associated with adverse reactions (eg, epistaxis, nasal septum perforation, *Candida* infection). Inform that glaucoma and/or cataracts may develop. Counsel to avoid exposure to chickenpox or measles and to immediately consult a physician if exposed. Contact physician if symptoms worsen or do not improve. Supervise young children during administration. Advise patient to take missed dose as soon as remembered. Counsel on proper priming and administration techniques.

Administration: Intranasal route. Refer to PI for proper administration. **Storage:** 25°C (77°F); excursions permitted to 15-30°C (59-86°F). Protect from light.

NATACYN
natamycin (Alcon)

RX

THERAPEUTIC CLASS: Tetraene polyene antifungal

INDICATIONS: Treatment of fungal blepharitis, conjunctivitis, and keratitis caused by susceptible organisms. Effectiveness as a single agent in fungal endophthalmitis has not been established.

DOSAGE: *Adults:* Keratitis: 1 drop q1-2h for 3-4 days, then 1 drop 6-8 times daily for 14-21 days or until the resolution of infection. Reduce dose at 4-7 day intervals. Blepharitis/Conjunctivitis: 1 drop 4-6 times daily.

HOW SUPPLIED: Sus: 5% [15mL]

WARNINGS/PRECAUTIONS: For topical ophthalmic use only, not for injection. Failure of improvement of keratitis following 7-10 days of administration suggests that the infection may be caused by a microorganism not susceptible to natamycin. Continuation of therapy should be based on clinical reevaluation and additional lab tests. Adherence of sus to areas of epithelial ulceration or retention of the sus in the fornices occurs regularly.

ADVERSE REACTIONS: Allergic reaction, change in vision, chest pain, corneal opacity, dyspnea, eye discomfort, eye edema, eye hyperemia, eye irritation, eye pain, foreign body sensation, paresthesia, tearing.

PREGNANCY: Category C, caution in nursing.

MECHANISM OF ACTION: Tetraene polyene antifungal; binds to sterol moiety of the fungal cell membrane. Polyenesterol complex alters permeability of membrane to produce depletion of essential cellular constituents.

PHARMACOKINETICS: Absorption: GI (poor).

NURSING CONSIDERATIONS

Assessment: Assess proper diagnosis through clinical and lab evaluation (eg, smear and culture of corneal scrapings). Assess use in pregnant/nursing females.

Monitoring: Monitor for clinical response. In patients with keratitis, reassess therapy if no response within 7 to 10 days.

Patient Counseling: Advise not to touch dropper tip to any surface to avoid contamination of sus. Instruct not to wear contact lenses if have signs/symptoms of fungal blepharitis, conjunctivitis, and keratitis.

Administration: Ocular route. Shake well before use. **Storage:** 2-24°C (36-75°F). Do not freeze. Avoid exposure to light and excessive heat.

NATAZIA RX
estradiol valerate - dienogest (Bayer Healthcare)

Cigarette smoking increases risk of serious cardiovascular (CV) events from combination oral contraceptive (COC) use. Risk increases with age (>35 yrs) and with the number of cigarettes smoked. Should not be used by women who are >35 yrs and smoke.

THERAPEUTIC CLASS: Estrogen/progestogen combination

INDICATIONS: Prevention of pregnancy. Treatment of heavy menstrual bleeding in women without organic pathology who choose to use an oral contraceptive as their method of contraception.

DOSAGE: *Adults*: 1 tab qd at the same time for 28 days, then repeat. Take in the order directed on the blister pack. Start on Day 1 of menses or not earlier than 4 weeks postpartum for postpartum women who do not breastfeed or after 2nd trimester abortion. When starting therapy, use a nonhormonal back-up contraceptive method for first 9 days of therapy. If vomiting or diarrhea occurs within 3-4 hrs after taking a colored tab, consider it as a missed tab. Refer to PI when switching from combination hormonal method or progestin-only method.
Pediatrics: Postpubertal: 1 tab qd at the same time for 28 days, then repeat. Take in the order directed on the blister pack. Start on Day 1 of menses or not earlier than 4 weeks postpartum for postpartum women who do not breastfeed or after 2nd trimester abortion. When starting therapy, use a nonhormonal back-up contraceptive method for first 9 days of therapy. If vomiting/diarrhea occurs within 3-4 hrs after taking a colored tab, consider it a missed tab. Refer to PI when switching from combination hormonal method or progestin-only method.

HOW SUPPLIED: Tab: (Estradiol Valerate) 1mg, 3mg; Tab: (Estradiol Valerate-Dienogest) 2mg-2mg, 2mg-3mg

CONTRAINDICATIONS: High risk of arterial/venous thrombotic diseases (eg, smoking if >35 yrs, history/presence of deep vein thrombosis/pulmonary embolism, cerebrovascular disease, coronary artery disease, thrombogenic valvular or thrombogenic rhythm diseases of the heart [eg, subacute bacterial endocarditis with valvular disease, or atrial fibrillation], inherited/acquired hypercoagulopathies, uncontrolled HTN, diabetes mellitus [DM] with vascular disease, headaches with focal neurological symptoms or migraine with/without aura if >35 yrs), undiagnosed abnormal uterine bleeding, history/presence of breast or other estrogen-/progestin-sensitive cancer, benign/malignant liver tumors, liver disease, pregnancy.

WARNINGS/PRECAUTIONS: Increased risk of venous thromboembolism (VTE) and arterial thrombosis (eg, stroke, myocardial infarction [MI]); greatest risk of VTE during the first 6 months of COC use and is present after initially starting COC or restarting (after ≥4 weeks pill-free interval) the same or different COC. D/C if arterial/venous thrombotic event occurs. D/C at least 4 weeks before and through 2 weeks after major surgery or other surgeries known to have an elevated risk of thromboembolism. Start therapy no earlier than 4 weeks postpartum in women who do not breastfeed. Caution with CV disease risk factors. D/C if there is unexplained loss of vision, proptosis, diplopia, papilledema, or retinal vascular lesions; evaluate for retinal vein thrombosis immediately. May increase risk of breast or cervical cancer, intraepithelial neoplasia, gallbladder disease, hepatic adenomas, and hepatocellular carcinoma; d/c if jaundice develops. Cholestasis may occur with history of pregnancy-related cholestasis. Increased BP reported; d/c if BP rises significantly. May decrease glucose tolerance; monitor prediabetic and diabetic women. Consider alternative contraception with uncontrolled dyslipidemia. Increased risk of pancreatitis with hypertriglyceridemia or family history thereof. May increase frequency/severity of migraine; d/c if new headaches that are recurrent, persistent, or severe develop. May cause bleeding irregularities (eg, breakthrough bleeding, spotting, amenorrhea); rule out pregnancy or malignancies. Not for use as a test for pregnancy, or to treat threatened or habitual abortion during pregnancy. Caution with history of depression; d/c if depression recurs to serious degree. May change results of lab tests (eg, coagulation factors, lipids, glucose tolerance, binding proteins). May induce/exacerbate angioedema in patients with hereditary angioedema. Chloasma may occur; women with chloasma should avoid sun exposure or UV radiation. Not for use before menarche or evaluated in women with BMI >30kg/m².

ADVERSE REACTIONS: N/V, headache, migraine, menstrual disorders, breast pain/discomfort/tenderness, acne, increased weight, mood changes.

N

INTERACTIONS: Agents that induce certain enzymes, including CYP3A4 (eg, barbiturates, bosentan, felbamate, griseofulvin, oxcarbazepine, topiramate) may decrease COC efficacy and/ or increase breakthrough bleeding; consider alternative contraceptive or a back-up method when using moderate or weak inducers and continue back-up contraception for 28 days after discontinuation of the inducer. Avoid with strong CYP3A4 inducers (eg, carbamazepine, phenytoin, rifampicin, St. John's wort) and for at least 28 days after discontinuation of these inducers. Strong CYP3A4 inhibitors (eg, ketoconazole) and moderate CYP3A4 inhibitors (eg, erythromycin) may increase dienogest and estradiol levels. Other CYP3A4 inhibitors (eg, azole antifungals, cimetidine, verapamil, macrolides, diltiazem, antidepressants, grapefruit juice) may increase dienogest levels. Significant changes (increase/decrease) in plasma estrogen and progestin levels may occur with some HIV/hepatitis C virus protease inhibitors or with non-nucleoside reverse transcriptase inhibitors. Pregnancy reported with antibiotics. May decrease plasma concentrations of lamotrigine and reduce seizure control; may need dosage adjustment. Increases thyroid-binding globulin; may need to increase dose of thyroid hormone in patients on thyroid hormone replacement therapy.

PREGNANCY: Contraindicated in pregnancy, not for use in nursing.

MECHANISM OF ACTION: Estrogen/progestin COC; acts primarily by suppressing ovulation. Also causes cervical mucus changes that inhibit sperm penetration and endometrial changes that reduce the likelihood of implantation.

PHARMACOKINETICS: Absorption: Dienogest: Bioavailability (91%); C_{max}=91.7ng/mL, T_{max}=1 hr, $AUC_{(0-24\ hr)}$=964ng/mL; Estradiol: C_{max}=73.3pg/mL, T_{max}=6 hrs, $AUC_{(0-24\ hr)}$=1301pg•hr/mL. **Distribution:** Estradiol: V_d=1.2L/kg (IV); bound to sex hormone-binding globulin (38%) and albumin (60%); found in breast milk. Dienogest: V_d=46L (IV); bound to albumin (90%); found in breast milk. **Metabolism:** Estradiol: Extensive 1st pass effect; CYP3A; estrone and its sulfate or glucuronide conjugates (main metabolites); Dienogest: extensive (hydroxylation, conjugation), CYP3A4 (main). **Elimination:** Estradiol: Urine (main), feces (10%), $T_{1/2}$=14 hrs; Dienogest: Renal (main); $T_{1/2}$=11 hrs.

NURSING CONSIDERATIONS

Assessment: Assess for renal impairment, abnormal uterine bleeding, adrenal insufficiency, and known or suspected pregnancy and other conditions where treatment is cautioned or contraindicated. Assess use in women who are >35 yrs and smoke, have CV disease and arterial/venous thrombosis risk factors, predisposition to hyperkalemia, pregnancy-related cholestasis, HTN, DM, uncontrolled dyslipidemia, history of hypertriglyceridemia, history of depression, hereditary angioedema, and history of chloasma. Assess for possible drug interactions.

Monitoring: Monitor for bleeding irregularities, venous/arterial thrombotic and thromboembolic events, cervical cancer or intraepithelial neoplasia, retinal vein thrombosis or any other ophthalmic changes, jaundice, acute/chronic disturbances in liver function, new/worsening headaches or migraines, serious depression, cholestasis with history of pregnancy-related cholestasis, and pancreatitis. Monitor K^+ levels, thyroid function if receiving thyroid replacement therapy, glucose levels in DM or prediabetes, lipids with dyslipidemia, liver function, and check BP annually.

Patient Counseling: Counsel that cigarette smoking increases the risk of serious CV events from COC use and to avoid use in women who are >35 yrs of age and smoke. Inform that drug does not protect against HIV infection and other sexually transmitted diseases. Instruct to take at the same time every day, preferably pm pc or hs. Counsel on what to do if pills are missed or if vomiting occurs within 4 hrs after tablet-taking. Inform that amenorrhea may occur and pregnancy should be ruled out if amenorrhea occurs in ≥2 consecutive cycles. Advise to inform physician of preexisting medical conditions and/or drugs currently being taken. Counsel to use an additional method of contraception when enzyme inducers are used with COCs. Counsel any patient who starts medication postpartum, and who has not yet had a period, to use an additional method of contraception until have taken medication for 9 consecutive days. Instruct to d/c if pregnancy occurs during treatment.

Administration: Oral route. Do not skip a dose or delay intake by >12 hrs. **Storage:** 25°C (77°F); excursions permitted to 15-30°C (59-86°F).

NATRECOR   RX
nesiritide (Scios Inc.)

THERAPEUTIC CLASS: Human B-type natriuretic peptide

INDICATIONS: Treatment of acutely decompensated heart failure (HF) with dyspnea at rest or with minimal activity.

DOSAGE: *Adults:* 2mcg/kg IV bolus over 60 sec, then 0.01mcg/kg/min continuous IV infusion. Refer to PI for Weight-Adjusted Bolus Volume and Infusion Flow Rate. Reduce dose or d/c therapy if hypotension occurs. Once stabilized, may subsequently restart at a dose that is reduced by 30% (with no bolus administration). Do not up-titrate more frequently than q3h. Use central hemodynamic monitoring and do not exceed 0.03mcg/kg/min.

HOW SUPPLIED: Inj: 1.5mg

CONTRAINDICATIONS: Persistent systolic BP (SBP) <100mm Hg prior to therapy, cardiogenic shock.

WARNINGS/PRECAUTIONS: May cause hypotension; administer only in settings where BP can be monitored closely and hypotension aggressively treated. Avoid with low cardiac filling pressures. Avoid in patients for whom vasodilators are inappropriate (eg, significant valvular stenosis, restrictive or obstructive cardiomyopathy, constrictive pericarditis, pericardial tamponade, or other conditions in which cardiac output is dependent on venous return, or for patients suspected to have low cardiac filling pressures). May decrease renal function; monitor SrCr during and after therapy. Azotemia reported in patients with severe HF. Serious hypersensitivity/allergic reactions reported; some may require treatment with epinephrine, oxygen, IV fluids, antihistamines, corticosteroids, pressor amines and airway management, as clinically indicated. Determine previous hypersensitivity reaction to other recombinant peptides before therapy; d/c if allergic reaction occurs.

ADVERSE REACTIONS: Hypotension, back pain, nausea, headache, dizziness.

INTERACTIONS: Increased risk of hypotension with drugs affecting the renin-angiotensin system (eg, angiotensin receptor blockers and/or ACE inhibitors) or other afterload reducers.

PREGNANCY: Category C, caution in nursing.

MECHANISM OF ACTION: Human B-type natriuretic peptide; binds to the particulate guanylate cyclase receptor of vascular smooth muscle and endothelial cells, leading to increased intracellular concentrations of guanosine 3'5'-cyclic monophosphate and smooth muscle relaxation.

PHARMACOKINETICS: Distribution: V_d=0.19L/kg. **Elimination:** $T_{1/2}$=18 min.

NURSING CONSIDERATIONS

Assessment: Assess for known hypersensitivity to drug or any of its components, cardiogenic shock, persistent SBP <100mm Hg, low cardiac filling pressures, conditions where vasodilators are inappropriate, pregnancy/nursing status, and possible drug interactions.

Monitoring: Monitor for hypotension, hypersensitivity/allergic reactions, and other adverse reactions. Monitor BP and hemodynamic parameters. Monitor SrCr both during and after therapy has been completed.

Patient Counseling: Advise of the potential benefits and risks of therapy. Advise to notify physician or healthcare professional if symptoms of hypotension occur.

Administration: IV route. Refer to PI for preparation and administration instructions. **Storage:** <25°C (77°F). Do not freeze. Protect from light. Reconstituted Sol: 2-25°C (36-77°F) for up to 24 hrs.

N

NATROBA   RX
spinosad (ParaPRO/Pernix Therapeutics)

THERAPEUTIC CLASS: Pediculocide

INDICATIONS: Topical treatment of head lice infestation in patients ≥4 yrs of age.

DOSAGE: *Adults:* Apply up to 120mL to adequately cover dry scalp and hair. Leave on for 10 min, then thoroughly rinse off with warm water. Apply 2nd treatment if live lice seen 7 days after the 1st.
Pediatrics: ≥4 Yrs: Apply up to 120mL to adequately cover dry scalp and hair. Leave on for 10 min, then thoroughly rinse off with warm water. Apply 2nd treatment if live lice seen 7 days after the 1st.

HOW SUPPLIED: Sus: 0.9% [120mL]

WARNINGS/PRECAUTIONS: Not for PO, ophthalmic, or intravaginal use. Contains benzyl alcohol; avoid in neonates and infants <6 months of age. Should be used in the context of an overall lice management program (eg, washing of recently worn clothing and personal care items).

ADVERSE REACTIONS: Application-site erythema/irritation, ocular erythema.

PREGNANCY: Category B, caution in nursing.

MECHANISM OF ACTION: Pediculocide; causes neuronal excitation in insects; lice become paralyzed and die after periods of hyperexcitation.

NURSING CONSIDERATIONS

Assessment: Assess pregnancy/nursing status.

Monitoring: Monitor for presence of live lice after 7 days of 1st treatment.

Patient Counseling: Advise to use only on dry scalp and hair. Instruct not to swallow. Instruct to rinse thoroughly with water if medication gets in or near the eyes. Advise to wash hands after application. Inform to use on children only under direct supervision of an adult. Advise to consult physician if pregnant/breastfeeding.

Administration: Topical route. Shake well before use. Avoid contact with eyes. **Storage:** 25°C (77°F); excursions permitted between 15-30°C (59-86°F).

NAVANE   RX
thiothixene (Pfizer)

> Elderly patients with dementia-related psychosis treated with antipsychotic drugs are at an increased risk of death; most deaths appeared to be cardiovascular (CV) (eg, heart failure, sudden death) or infectious (eg, pneumonia) in nature. Navane is not approved for the treatment of patients with dementia-related psychosis.

THERAPEUTIC CLASS: Thioxanthene

INDICATIONS: Management of schizophrenia.

DOSAGE: *Adults:* Individualize dose. Mild Condition: Initial: 2mg tid. Titrate: May increase to 15mg/day. Severe Condition: Initial: 5mg bid. Usual: 20-30mg/day. Max: 60mg/day.
Pediatrics: ≥12 Yrs: Individualize dose. Mild Condition: Initial: 2mg tid. Titrate: May increase to 15mg/day. Severe Condition: Initial: 5mg bid. Usual: 20-30mg/day. Max: 60mg/day.

HOW SUPPLIED: Cap: 1mg, 2mg, 5mg, 10mg

CONTRAINDICATIONS: Circulatory collapse, comatose states, CNS depression, blood dyscrasias.

WARNINGS/PRECAUTIONS: May cause tardive dyskinesia (TD) and neuroleptic malignant syndrome (NMS); d/c if this develops. May impair mental/physical abilities. May mask signs of overdosage of toxic drugs and obscure conditions, such as intestinal obstruction and brain tumor. Caution with history of convulsive disorders or in a state of alcohol withdrawal; may lower convulsive threshold. Monitor for pigmentary retinopathy and lenticular pigmentation. Caution with CV disease, extreme heat exposure, activities requiring alertness. May elevate prolactin levels. May cause leukopenia, neutropenia, and agranulocytosis; consider discontinuing at 1st sign of significant decline in WBC in absence of other causes and when absolute neutrophil count is <1000/mm³. False positive pregnancy tests may occur. Risk for extrapyramidal symptoms (EPS) and/or withdrawal symptoms following delivery in neonates exposed during 3rd trimester of pregnancy.

ADVERSE REACTIONS: NMS, TD, tachycardia, hypotension, lightheadedness, syncope, drowsiness, restlessness, agitation, insomnia, EPS, cerebral edema, CSF abnormalities, allergic reactions, hematologic effects.

INTERACTIONS: Possible additive effects with hypotensive agents, CNS depressants, and alcohol. Increased clearance with hepatic microsomal enzyme inducers (eg, carbamazepine). Potentiates the actions of barbiturates. Caution with atropine or related drugs. Paradoxical effects (lowering of BP) with pressor agents (eg, epinephrine).

PREGNANCY: Safety is not known in pregnancy and nursing.

MECHANISM OF ACTION: Thioxanthene derivative; antipsychotic agent.

NURSING CONSIDERATIONS

Assessment: Assess for dementia-related psychosis in elderly, history of convulsive disorders, history of CV disorders, CNS depression, circulatory collapse, comatose state, blood dyscrasias, alcohol intake, infections, intestinal obstruction, brain tumor, possibility of extreme heat exposure, previous hypersensitivity to the drug, pregnancy/nursing status, and possible drug interactions. Obtain baseline vital signs, CBC, LFTs, prolactin levels.

Monitoring: Monitor for hypersensitivity reactions, TD, NMS, CV effects, visual disturbances, and EPS. Monitor LFTs, bilirubin, CBC, prolactin, and blood glucose.

Patient Counseling: Inform about the risks of treatment, particularly about the possibility of developing TD. Advise about risk of chronic use of drug. Warn to use caution when performing hazardous tasks (operating machinery/driving). Warn about possible additive effects (eg, hypotension) when drug is combined with hypotensive agents, CNS depressants and/or alcohol.

Administration: Oral route.

NEORAL   RX
cyclosporine (Novartis)

Should only be prescribed by physicians experienced in management of systemic immunosuppressive therapy for indicated diseases. Manage patients in facilities equipped and staffed with adequate laboratory and supportive medical resources. Increased susceptibility to infection and development of neoplasia (eg, lymphoma) may result from immuno-suppression. May be coadministered with other immunosuppressive agents in kidney, liver, and heart transplant patients. Not bioequivalent to Sandimmune and cannot be used interchangeably without physician supervision. Caution in switching from Sandimmune. Monitor cyclosporine blood concentrations in transplant and rheumatoid arthritis (RA) patients to avoid toxicity due to high concentrations. Dose adjustments should be made to minimize possible organ rejection due to low concentrations in transplant patients. Increased risk of developing skin malignancies in psoriasis patients previously treated with PUVA, methotrexate (MTX) or other immunosuppressive agents, UVB, coal tar, or radiation therapy. May cause systemic HTN and nephrotoxicity. Monitor for renal dysfunction including, structural kidney damage, during therapy.

THERAPEUTIC CLASS: Cyclic polypeptide immunosuppressant

INDICATIONS: Prophylaxis of organ rejection in kidney, liver, and heart allogeneic transplants. Treatment of severe, active RA where disease has not adequately responded to MTX. May be used in combination with MTX in RA not responding adequately to MTX alone. Treatment of nonimmunocompromised adults with severe (eg, extensive and/or disabling), recalcitrant, plaque psoriasis who failed to respond to at least one systemic therapy (eg, PUVA, retinoids, MTX) or in patients for whom other systemic therapies are contraindicated, or cannot be tolerated.

DOSAGE: *Adults:* Always give bid. Administer on a consistent schedule with regard to time of day and relation to meals. Newly Transplanted Patients: Initial: May give 4-12 hrs prior to transplant or postoperatively. Dose may vary depending on transplanted organ and other immunosuppressive agents included in protocol. Renal Transplant: 9±3mg/kg/day. Liver Transplant: 8±4mg/kg/day. Heart Transplant: 7±3mg/kg/day. Adjust subsequent dose to achieve a predefined blood concentration. Adjunct therapy with adrenal corticosteroid recommended initially; dose adjustments of adrenal corticosteroids must be made according to the clinical situation. Conversion from Sandimmune: Start with same daily dose as was previously used with Sandimmune, (1:1 dose conversion). Adjust subsequent dose to attain a pre-conversion blood trough concentration. Monitor blood levels every 4-7 days while adjusting to trough levels. Transplant Patients with Poor Sandimmune Absorption: Caution when converting patients at doses >10mg/kg/day. Titrate dose individually based on trough concentrations, tolerability, and clinical response. Measure blood trough concentration at least 2X a week until stabilized within desired range. Renal Impairment in Transplant Patients: Reduce dose if indicated. RA: Initial: 2.5mg/kg/day. Titrate: May be increased by 0.5-0.75mg/kg/day after 8 weeks and again after 12 weeks. Max: 4mg/kg/day. Combined with MTX (up to 15mg/week): ≤3mg/kg/day. D/C therapy if no benefit is seen by 16 weeks of treatment. Psoriasis: Initial: 2.5mg/kg/day for 4 weeks. If no significant clinical improvement occurs, may increase dosage at 2-week intervals. Titrate: May increase by approximately 0.5mg/kg/day based on clinical response. Max: 4mg/kg/day. D/C if satisfactory response cannot be achieved after 6 weeks at 4mg/kg/day or the patient's maximum tolerated dose. (RA/Psoriasis) Reduce dose by 25-50% if adverse events (eg, HTN) occur. D/C if reduction is not effective. Elderly: Start at lower end of dosing range. Severe Hepatic Impairment: Reduce dose.

HOW SUPPLIED: Cap: 25mg, 100mg; Sol: 100mg/mL [50mL]

CONTRAINDICATIONS: RA/Psoriasis: Abnormal renal function, uncontrolled HTN, malignancies. Psoriasis: Concomitant PUVA or UVB therapy, MTX, other immunosuppressants, coal tar, or radiation therapy.

WARNINGS/PRECAUTIONS: May cause hepatotoxicity and liver injury (eg, cholestasis, jaundice, hepatitis, liver failure). Elevations of SrCr and BUN may occur and reflect a reduction in GFR; closely monitor renal function and consider frequent dose adjustments. Elevations in SrCr and BUN levels do not necessarily indicate rejection; evaluate patient before initiating dose adjustment. Thrombocytopenia and microangiopathic hemolytic anemia, resulting in graft failure, significant hyperkalemia (sometimes associated with hyperchloremic metabolic acidosis) and hyperuricemia reported. Avoid excessive sun exposure. Oversuppression of the immune system resulting in increased risk of infection/malignancy may occur; caution with a multiple immunosuppressant regimen. Increased risk of developing bacterial, viral, fungal, protozoal, and opportunistic infections (eg, polyomavirus infections). JC virus-associated progressive multifocal leukoencephalopathy and polyomavirus-/BK virus-associated nephropathy reported; consider reduction in immunosuppression if develops. Convulsions, encephalopathy including posterior reversible encephalopathy syndrome, and rarely, optic disc edema reported. Evaluate before and during treatment for development of malignancies. In RA patients, monitor BP on 2 occasions and obtain 2 baseline SrCr levels before treatment, then monitor BP and SrCr every 2 weeks for the first 3 months of treatment, and then monthly if the patient is stable or more frequently during dose adjustments. In psoriasis patients, assess BP on 2 occasions and obtain baseline SrCr, BUN, CBC, Mg²⁺, K⁺, uric acid, and lipids before treatment, then monitor every 2 weeks for the first

3 months of therapy, and then monthly if the patient is stable or more frequently during dose adjustments. Monitor CBC and LFTs monthly with MTX. Monitor SrCr after initiation or increases in NSAID dose for RA. Consider the alcohol content of the drug when given to patients in whom alcohol intake should be avoided or minimized (eg, pregnant or breastfeeding women, patients presenting with liver disease or epilepsy, alcoholic patients, or pediatric patients). HTN may occur and persist, which may require antihypertensive therapy. Caution in elderly.

ADVERSE REACTIONS: Increased susceptibility to infection, lymphoma, renal dysfunction, HTN, hirsutism/hypertrichosis, tremor, headache, gum hyperplasia, diarrhea, N/V, paresthesia, hypertriglyceridemia, hyperesthesia.

INTERACTIONS: See Boxed Warning and Contraindications. Avoid with K^+-sparing diuretics, aliskiren, orlistat, grapefruit, and grapefruit juice. Vaccinations may be less effective; avoid live vaccines during therapy. Frequent gingival hyperplasia reported with nifedipine; avoid concomitant use with nifedipine in patients in whom gingival hyperplasia develops as a side effect of cyclosporine. Caution with rifabutin, nephrotoxic drugs, HIV protease inhibitors (eg, indinavir, nelfinavir, ritonavir, saquinavir), K^+-sparing drugs (eg, ACE inhibitors, angiotensin II receptor antagonists), K^+-containing drugs, and K^+-rich diet. Ciprofloxacin, gentamicin, tobramycin, vancomycin, trimethoprim with sulfamethoxazole, melphalan, amphotericin B, ketoconazole, azapropazon, colchicine, diclofenac, naproxen, sulindac, cimetidine, ranitidine, tacrolimus, fibric acid derivatives (eg, bezafibrate, fenofibrate), MTX, and NSAIDs may potentiate renal dysfunction. Diltiazem, nicardipine, verapamil, fluconazole, itraconazole, ketoconazole, voriconazole, azithromycin, clarithromycin, erythromycin, quinupristin/dalfopristin, methylprednisolone, allopurinol, amiodarone, bromocriptine, colchicine, danazol, imatinib, metoclopramide, nefazodone, oral contraceptives, grapefruit, grapefruit juice, HIV protease inhibitors, boceprevir, telaprevir may increase levels. Nafcillin, rifampin, carbamazepine, oxcarbazepine, phenobarbital, phenytoin, bosentan, octreotide, orlistat, sulfinpyrazone, terbinafine, ticlopidine, or St. John's wort may decrease levels. May increase levels of ambrisentan, bosentan, and CYP3A4 and/or P-glycoprotein (P-gp) substrates. CYP3A4 and/or P-gp inducers and inhibitors may alter levels; may require dose adjustments. May reduce clearance of digoxin, colchicine, prednisolone, HMG-CoA reductase inhibitors (statins), repaglinide, NSAIDs, sirolimus, and etoposide. Digitalis toxicity reported when used with digoxin; monitor digoxin levels. May increase levels and enhance toxic effects (eg, myopathy, neuropathy) of colchicine; may reduce colchicine dose. Myotoxicity cases seen with statins; temporarily withhold or d/c therapy if signs of myopathy develop or with risk factors predisposing to severe renal injury, including renal failure, secondary to rhabdomyolysis. May increase levels of repaglinide, thereby increasing the risk of hypoglycemia. High doses of cyclosporine may increase the exposure to anthracycline antibiotics (eg, doxorubicin, mitoxantrone, daunorubicin) in cancer patients. May double diclofenac blood levels. May increase MTX levels and decrease levels of active metabolite of MTX. May elevate SrCr and increase levels of sirolimus; give 4 hrs after cyclosporine administration. Convulsions reported with high-dose methylprednisolone. Calcium antagonists may interfere with cyclosporine metabolism.

PREGNANCY: Category C, not for use in nursing.

MECHANISM OF ACTION: Cyclic polypeptide immunosuppressant; results from specific and reversible inhibition of immunocompetent lymphocytes in the G_0- and G_1-phase of the cell cycle. T-lymphocytes are preferentially inhibited with T-helper cell as main target while also possibly suppressing T-suppressor cells. Also inhibits lymphokine production and release (eg, interleukin-2).

PHARMACOKINETICS: Absorption: Incomplete; T_{max}=1.5-2 hrs. Pharmacokinetic parameters varied with different indications (renal, liver, RA, and/or psoriasis). **Distribution:** V_d=3-5L/kg (IV); plasma protein binding (90%); found in breast milk. **Metabolism:** (Extensive) Liver via CYP3A, to a lesser extent GI tract and kidneys. M1, M9, and M4N (major metabolites); oxidation and demethylation pathways. **Elimination:** Bile (primary), urine (6%, 0.1% unchanged); $T_{1/2}$=8.4 hrs.

NURSING CONSIDERATIONS

Assessment: Assess for hypersensitivity to the drug, renal dysfunction, uncontrolled HTN, presence of malignancies, pregnancy/nursing status, and possible drug interactions. RA: Before initiating treatment, assess BP (on at least 2 occasions) and obtain 2 SrCr levels. Psoriasis: Prior to treatment, perform dermatological and physical examination, including measuring BP. Assess for presence of occult infections and for the presence of tumors. Assess for atypical skin lesions and biopsy them. Obtain baseline SrCr (at least twice), BUN, LFTs, bilirubin, CBC, Mg^{2+}, K^+, uric acid, and lipid levels.

Monitoring: Monitor for signs/symptoms of hepatotoxicity, liver injury, nephrotoxicity, thrombocytopenia, microangiopathic hemolytic anemia, HTN, hyperkalemia, lymphomas and other malignancies, serious/opportunistic/polyomavirus infections, convulsions and other neurotoxicities, and other adverse reactions. Monitor cyclosporine blood concentrations routinely in transplant patients and periodically in RA patients. RA: Monitor BP and SrCr every 2 weeks during the initial 3 months of treatment, then monthly if patient is stable. Monitor SrCr and BP after an increase of the dose of NSAIDs and after initiation of new NSAID therapy. If coadministered with MTX, monitor CBC and LFTs monthly. Psoriasis: Monitor for occult infections and tumors. Monitor SrCr,

BUN, BP, CBC, uric acid, K$^+$, lipids, and Mg^{2+} levels every 2 weeks during first 3 months of treatment, then monthly if stable.

Patient Counseling: Instruct to contact physician before changing formulations of cyclosporine, which may require dose changes. Inform that repeated lab tests are required while on therapy. Advise of the potential risks if used during pregnancy and inform of the increased risk of neoplasia, HTN, and renal dysfunction. Inform that vaccinations may be less effective and to avoid live vaccines during therapy. Advise to take the medication on a consistent schedule with regard to time and meals, and to avoid grapefruit and grapefruit juice. Inform to avoid excessive sun exposure.

Administration: Oral route. (Sol) Dilute oral sol with orange or apple juice that is at room temperature. Avoid diluting oral sol with grapefruit juice. Refer to PI for recommendations for administration. **Storage:** 20-25°C (68-77°F). (Sol) Use within 2 months upon opening. Do not refrigerate. At <20°C (68°F) may form gel; light flocculation, or formation of light sediment may occur; warm at 25°C (77°C) to reverse changes.

NESINA RX
alogliptin (Takeda)

THERAPEUTIC CLASS: Dipeptidyl peptidase-4 inhibitor

INDICATIONS: Adjunct to diet and exercise to improve glycemic control in adults with type 2 diabetes mellitus (DM).

DOSAGE: *Adults:* Usual: 25mg qd. Renal Impairment: Moderate (CrCl 30-<60mL/min): 12.5mg qd. Severe (CrCl 15-<30mL/min)/End-Stage Renal Disease (CrCl <15 mL/min or requiring hemodialysis): 6.25mg qd.

HOW SUPPLIED: Tab: 6.25mg, 12.5mg, 25mg

WARNINGS/PRECAUTIONS: Not for use in type 1 DM or for treatment of diabetic ketoacidosis. Acute pancreatitis reported; d/c if pancreatitis is suspected and initiate appropriate management. Serious hypersensitivity reactions reported; d/c if suspected, assess for other potential causes, and institute alternative treatment. Caution with history of angioedema with another dipeptidyl peptidase-4 (DPP-4) inhibitor. Fatal/nonfatal hepatic failure and serum ALT >3X ULN reported; initiate with caution in patients with abnormal LFTs. Interrupt treatment and investigate probable cause if clinically significant liver enzyme elevations and abnormal LFTs persist/worsen; do not restart without another explanation for abnormal LFTs. No conclusive evidence of macrovascular risk reduction.

ADVERSE REACTIONS: Hypoglycemia, nasopharyngitis, headache, upper respiratory infection.

INTERACTIONS: May require lower dose of insulin therapy or insulin secretagogue (eg, sulfonylurea) to reduce risk of hypoglycemia.

PREGNANCY: Category B, caution in nursing.

MECHANISM OF ACTION: DPP-4 inhibitor; slows inactivation of incretin hormones, thereby increasing their bloodstream concentrations and reducing fasting and postprandial glucose concentrations in a glucose-dependent manner.

PHARMACOKINETICS: Absorption: Absolute bioavailability (100%); T$_{max}$=1-2 hrs. **Distribution**: V$_d$=417L; plasma protein binding (20%). **Metabolism**: Via CYP2D6 and CYP3A4; N-demethylated alogliptin, M-I (active metabolite) and N-acetylated alogliptin, M-II. **Elimination**: Feces (13%), urine (76%, 60-71% unchanged); T$_{1/2}$= 21 hrs.

NURSING CONSIDERATIONS

Assessment: Assess renal/hepatic function, previous hypersensitivity to the drug, history of pancreatitis, type of DM, diabetic ketoacidosis, history of angioedema with another DPP-4 inhibitor, pregnancy/nursing status, and possible drug interactions. Obtain baseline FPG and HbA1c.

Monitoring: Monitor for pancreatitis and hypersensitivity reactions. Monitor FPG, HbA1c, renal/hepatic function periodically.

Patient Counseling: Inform of risks/benefits of therapy. Inform of signs/symptoms of pancreatitis (eg, severe/persistent abdominal pain, sometimes radiating to the back, vomiting); instruct to d/c promptly and contact physician if persistent severe abdominal pain occurs. Inform that allergic reactions (eg, skin rash, hives, face/lips/tongue/throat swelling, difficulty of breathing/swallowing) and liver injury have been reported; instruct to d/c and seek medical advice promptly if these occur. Inform that hypoglycemia can occur, particularly when therapy is used in combination with insulin or sulfonylurea; explain risks/symptoms/appropriate management of hypoglycemia. Instruct to take only ud; if a dose is missed, advise not to double next dose. Instruct to inform physician if unusual symptom develops or if a symptom persists/worsens.

Administration: Oral route. May be taken with or without food. May be administered without regard to timing of hemodialysis. **Storage:** 25°C (77°F); excursions permitted to 15-30°C (59-86°F).

NEULASTA   RX
pegfilgrastim (Amgen)

THERAPEUTIC CLASS: Granulocyte colony-stimulating factor

INDICATIONS: To decrease the incidence of infection, as manifested by febrile neutropenia, in patients with nonmyeloid malignancies receiving myelosuppressive anticancer drugs associated with a clinically significant incidence of febrile neutropenia.

DOSAGE: *Adults:* 6mg SQ once per chemotherapy cycle. Do not administer between 14 days before and 24 hrs after administration of cytotoxic chemotherapy.

HOW SUPPLIED: Inj: 6mg/0.6mL

WARNINGS/PRECAUTIONS: Splenic rupture, including fatal cases, may occur; evaluate for an enlarged spleen or splenic rupture if left upper abdominal or shoulder pain occurs. Acute respiratory distress syndrome (ARDS) may occur; evaluate for ARDS if fever and lung infiltrates or respiratory distress develops, and d/c if ARDS develops. Serious allergic reactions (eg, anaphylaxis) may occur; permanently d/c if serious allergic reactions occur. Severe and sometimes fatal sickle cell crises may occur in patients with sickle cell disorders. May act as a growth factor for any tumor type. Needle cover on prefilled syringe contains latex; do not administer to persons with latex allergies. Increased hematopoietic activity of the bone marrow in response to therapy may result in transiently positive bone imaging changes; consider this when interpreting bone-imaging results.

ADVERSE REACTIONS: Bone pain, pain in extremity.

PREGNANCY: Category C, caution in nursing.

MECHANISM OF ACTION: Granulocyte colony-stimulating factor; acts on hematopoietic cells by binding to specific cell surface receptors, thereby stimulating proliferation, differentiation, commitment, and end cell functional activation.

PHARMACOKINETICS: Elimination: $T_{1/2}$=15-80 hrs.

NURSING CONSIDERATIONS

Assessment: Assess for history of hypersensitivity to pegfilgrastim or filgrastim, latex allergy, sickle cell disorders, pregnancy/nursing status, and possible drug interactions.

Monitoring: Monitor for enlarged spleen/splenic rupture, ARDS, serious allergic reactions, sickle cell crises (in patients with sickle cell disorders), and other adverse reactions.

Patient Counseling: Advise of the risks of therapy (eg, splenic rupture, ARDS, serious allergic reactions, sickle cell crisis). Instruct to immediately contact physician if left upper quadrant or shoulder pain, SOB, signs/symptoms of sickle cell crisis or infection, flushing, dizziness, or rash develops. Encourage women who become pregnant during treatment to enroll in Amgen's Pregnancy Surveillance Program.

Administration: SQ route. **Storage:** 2-8°C (36-46°F). Protect from light. Do not shake. Discard syringes stored at room temperature for >48 hrs. Avoid freezing; if frozen, thaw in the refrigerator before administration. Discard syringe if frozen more than once.

NEUMEGA   RX
oprelvekin (Wyeth)

> Allergic or hypersensitivity reactions, including anaphylaxis, reported; permanently d/c if this develops.

THERAPEUTIC CLASS: Thrombopoietic agent

INDICATIONS: Prevention of severe thrombocytopenia and reduction of the need for platelet transfusions following myelosuppressive chemotherapy in adults with nonmyeloid malignancies who are at high risk of severe thrombocytopenia.

DOSAGE: *Adults:* 50mcg/kg SQ qd. Initiate 6-24 hrs after chemotherapy completion. Continue therapy until post-nadir platelet count is ≥50,000/μL. Max: 21 days/treatment course. D/C at least 2 days before starting the next chemotherapy cycle. May give for up to 6 cycles following chemotherapy. Severe Renal Impairment (CrCl <30mL/min): 25mcg/kg SQ.

HOW SUPPLIED: Inj: 5mg

WARNINGS/PRECAUTIONS: Not indicated following myeloablative chemotherapy. May cause serious fluid retention; caution in congestive heart failure (CHF) patients, patients who may be susceptible to developing CHF, patients receiving aggressive hydration, patients with history of heart failure who are well-compensated and receiving appropriate medical therapy, and patients who may develop fluid retention as a result of associated medical conditions or whose medical condition may be exacerbated by fluid retention. Monitor preexisting fluid collections; consider drainage if medically indicated. Moderate decreases in Hgb, Hct, and RBCs reported.

Cardiovascular events, including arrhythmias and pulmonary edema, reported. Caution in history of atrial arrhythmias. Papilledema reported; caution in patients with preexisting papilledema, or with tumors involving the CNS. Changes in visual acuity and/or visual field defects may occur in patients with papilledema. Obtain CBC before chemotherapy and at regular intervals during therapy. Monitor platelet counts during expected nadir time and until adequate recovery has occurred (post-nadir counts ≥50,000/µL).

ADVERSE REACTIONS: Edema, dyspnea, tachycardia, conjunctival injection, palpitations, atrial arrhythmias, pleural effusions, syncope, pneumonia, neutropenic fever, headache, N/V, mucositis, diarrhea.

INTERACTIONS: Perform close monitoring of fluid and electrolyte status in patients receiving chronic diuretic therapy.

PREGNANCY: Category C, not for use in nursing.

MECHANISM OF ACTION: Thrombopoietic agent; stimulates megakaryocytopoiesis and thrombopoiesis.

PHARMACOKINETICS: Absorption: Absolute bioavailability (>80%); C_{max}=17.4ng/mL; T_{max}=3.2 hrs. **Elimination:** Urine; $T_{1/2}$=6.9 hrs.

NURSING CONSIDERATIONS

Assessment: Assess for conditions where treatment is contraindicated or cautioned, pregnancy/nursing status, and possible drug interactions. Obtain baseline CBC prior to chemotherapy.

Monitoring: Monitor for signs/symptoms of hypersensitivity reactions, papilledema, fluid retention, pleural/pericardial effusion, atrial arrhythmias, and other adverse reactions. Periodically monitor CBC (including platelet counts), fluid balance, fluid and electrolyte status (chronic diuretic therapy).

Patient Counseling: Inform of pregnancy risks. Instruct on the proper dose, method for reconstituting and administering, and importance of proper disposal of the product when used outside of the hospital or office setting. Inform of the serious and most common adverse reactions associated with the product. Advise to immediately seek medical attention if any of the signs or symptoms of allergic or hypersensitivity reactions (edema, difficulty breathing, swallowing or talking, SOB, wheezing, chest pain, throat tightness, lightheadedness), worsening of dyspnea, or symptoms attributable to atrial arrhythmia occur.

Administration: SQ route. Administer in either the abdomen, thigh, or hip (upper arm if not self-injecting). Refer to PI for preparation of the product. **Storage:** 2-8°C (36-46°F). Protect powder from light. Do not freeze. Reconstituted: 2-8°C (36-46°F) or up to 25°C (77°F). Do not freeze or shake.

NEUPOGEN
filgrastim (Amgen)

RX

THERAPEUTIC CLASS: Granulocyte colony-stimulating factor

INDICATIONS: To decrease incidence of infection, as manifested by febrile neutropenia, in patients with nonmyeloid malignancies receiving myelosuppressive anticancer drugs associated with a significant incidence of severe neutropenia with fever. To reduce the time to neutrophil recovery and duration of fever, following induction or consolidation chemotherapy treatment of adults with acute myeloid leukemia (AML). To reduce the duration of neutropenia and neutropenia-related clinical sequelae in patients with nonmyeloid malignancies undergoing myeloablative chemotherapy followed by marrow transplantation. For mobilization of hematopoietic progenitor cells into the peripheral blood for collection by leukapheresis. For chronic administration to reduce incidence and duration of sequelae of neutropenia in symptomatic patients with congenital, cyclic, or idiopathic neutropenia.

DOSAGE: *Adults:* Receiving Myelosuppressive Chemotherapy: Initial: 5mcg/kg/day qd by SQ bolus inj, by short IV infusion (15-30 min), or by continuous SQ/IV infusion. Titrate: May increase in increments of 5mcg/kg for each chemotherapy cycle, according to duration and severity of absolute neutrophil count (ANC) nadir. Administer no earlier than 24 hrs after the administration of cytotoxic chemotherapy; do not administer in the period 24 hrs before the administration of chemotherapy. Administer daily for up to 2 weeks, until ANC has reached 10,000/mm³ following the expected chemotherapy-induced neutrophil nadir. D/C if ANC surpasses 10,000/mm³ after the expected chemotherapy-induced neutrophil nadir. Receiving Bone Marrow Transplant: 10mcg/kg/day by IV infusion of 4 or 24 hrs, or as continuous 24-hr SQ infusion. Administer 1st dose at least 24 hrs after cytotoxic chemotherapy and at least 24 hrs after bone marrow infusion. Refer to PI for dose adjustments against neutrophil response. Peripheral Blood Progenitor Cell Collection and Therapy: 10mcg/kg/day SQ, either as bolus or continuous infusion, for at least 4 days before the 1st leukapheresis procedure and continue until the last leukapheresis. Administration of therapy for 6-7 days with leukapheresis on Days 5, 6, and 7 was found to be safe and effective. Monitor neutrophil counts after 4 days of therapy, and consider dose modification if WBC >100,000/mm³ develops. Severe Chronic Neutropenia (SCN): Initial: 6mcg/kg SQ bid every day (congenital) or 5mcg/kg SQ qd every day (idiopathic/cyclic). Titrate: Adjust dose based on clinical course and ANC.

HOW SUPPLIED: Inj: 300mcg/mL, 480mcg/1.6mL [vial]; 300mcg/0.5mL, 480mcg/0.8mL [prefilled syringe]

CONTRAINDICATIONS: Hypersensitivity to *Escherichia coli*-derived proteins.

WARNINGS/PRECAUTIONS: Allergic-type reactions reported. Splenic rupture, including fatal cases, reported; evaluate for enlarged spleen or splenic rupture if left upper abdominal and/or shoulder tip pain occur. Acute respiratory distress syndrome (ARDS) reported; evaluate for ARDS if fever, lung infiltrates, or respiratory distress develops. If ARDS occurs, withhold therapy until resolved, or d/c. Severe sickle cell crises, in some cases resulting in death, reported in patients with sickle cell disorders; only physicians qualified in the treatment of patients with sickle cell disorders should prescribe therapy for such patients, and only after careful consideration of the potential risks and benefits. Cytogenetic abnormalities, transformation to myelodysplastic syndrome, and AML observed in patients treated for SCN; consider risks and benefits of continuing therapy if abnormal cytogenetics or myelodysplasia develops in patients with SCN. May act as a growth factor for any tumor type. Monitor CBC twice a week in patients receiving myelosuppressive chemotherapy to avoid potential complications of excessive leukocytosis. Premature discontinuation of therapy, prior to the time of recovery from the expected neutrophil nadir, is generally not recommended. Potential for immunogenicity. Cutaneous vasculitis reported. Thrombocytopenia reported; closely monitor platelet counts. Consider transient positive bone-imaging changes when interpreting bone-imaging results.

ADVERSE REACTIONS: N/V, skeletal pain, diarrhea, neutropenic fever, mucositis, fatigue, anorexia, dyspnea, headache, cough, splenomegaly, petechiae, stomatitis, hemorrhagic events, alopecia.

INTERACTIONS: Avoid simultaneous use with chemotherapy and radiation therapy. Caution with drugs that may potentiate the release of neutrophils (eg, lithium).

PREGNANCY: Category C, caution in nursing.

MECHANISM OF ACTION: Granulocyte colony-stimulating factor; acts on hematopoietic cells by binding to specific cell surface receptors and stimulating proliferation, differentiation commitment, and some end-cell functional activation.

PHARMACOKINETICS: Absorption: (SQ) C_{max}=4ng/mL (3.45mcg/kg), 49ng/mL (11.5mcg/kg); T_{max}=2-8 hrs. **Distribution:** V_d=150mL/kg. **Elimination:** $T_{1/2}$=3.5 hrs, 231 min (34.5mcg/kg IV), 210 min (3.45mcg/kg SQ).

NURSING CONSIDERATIONS

Assessment: Assess for hypersensitivity to the drug or to *E. coli*-derived proteins, sickle cell disorder, pregnancy/nursing status, and possible drug interactions. Obtain CBC and platelet counts prior to chemotherapy and at least 3X/week following marrow transplantation.

Monitoring: Monitor for allergic-type reactions, enlarged spleen/splenic rupture, ARDS, sickle cell crises (in patients with sickle cell disorders), cutaneous vasculitis, thrombocytopenia, and other adverse reactions. In patients receiving myelosuppressive chemotherapy, monitor CBC and platelet counts at regular intervals (twice per week). In patients with SCN, monitor CBC with differential and platelet counts twice weekly during the initial 4 weeks of therapy and during the 2 weeks following any dose adjustment, and, once patient is clinically stable, monthly during the 1st yr of treatment; thereafter, if clinically stable, routinely monitor with regular CBCs (as clinically indicated but at least quarterly). Perform annual bone marrow and cytogenetic evaluations throughout the duration of treatment in patients with congenital neutropenia.

Patient Counseling: Inform of the risks and benefits of therapy and instruct to report any adverse reactions (eg, left upper abdominal and/or shoulder tip pain). Encourage women who become pregnant or are nursing during treatment to enroll in Amgen's Pregnancy or Lactation Surveillance Program. Inform that the needle cover of the prefilled syringe contains dry natural rubber (a derivative of latex).

Administration: SQ/IV route. Refer to PI for dilution and administration instructions. **Storage:** 2-8°C (36-46°F). Avoid shaking. Prior to inj, may be allowed to reach room temperature for a max of 24 hrs; discard any vial or prefilled syringe left at room temperature for >24 hrs.

NEURONTIN   RX
gabapentin (Parke-Davis)

THERAPEUTIC CLASS: GABA analog

INDICATIONS: Adjunctive therapy in the treatment of partial seizures with and without secondary generalization in patients >12 yrs of age with epilepsy. Adjunctive therapy in the treatment of partial seizures in pediatric patients 3-12 yrs of age. Management of postherpetic neuralgia (PHN) in adults.

DOSAGE: *Adults:* Epilepsy: Initial: 300mg tid. Titrate: If necessary, may increase up to 1800mg/day given in 3 divided doses. Max: 3600mg/day. The max time between doses should not exceed 12 hrs. PHN: Initial: 300mg single dose on Day 1, then 300mg bid on Day 2, and 300mg tid on Day 3. Titrate: Increase PRN for pain relief to 600mg tid. Refer to PI for dosage in renal impairment. Dose Reduction/Substitution/Discontinuation: Should be done gradually over a minimum of 1 week. Elderly: Start at lower end of dosing range.
Pediatrics: Epilepsy: >12 Yrs: Initial: 300mg tid. Titrate: If necessary, may increase up to 1800mg/day given in 3 divided doses. Max: 3600mg/day. Refer to PI for dosage in renal impairment. 3-12 Yrs: Initial: 10-15mg/kg/day given in 3 divided doses. Titrate: Increase to effective dose over a period of 3 days. Usual: ≥5 Yrs: 25-35mg/kg/day given in 3 divided doses. 3-4 Yrs: 40mg/kg/day given in 3 divided doses. Max: 50mg/kg/day. The max time between doses should not exceed 12 hrs. Dose Reduction/Substitution/Discontinuation: Should be done gradually over a minimum of 1 week.

HOW SUPPLIED: Cap: 100mg, 300mg, 400mg; Sol: 250mg/5mL [470mL]; Tab: 600mg*, 800mg* *scored

WARNINGS/PRECAUTIONS: Increases the risk of suicidal thoughts or behavior; monitor for the emergence or worsening of depression, suicidal thoughts or behavior, and/or any unusual changes in mood or behavior. Use in pediatric patients 3-12 yrs of age is associated with CNS-related adverse events. Do not abruptly d/c; may increase seizure frequency. May have tumorigenic potential. Sudden and unexplained deaths reported in patients with epilepsy. Drug reaction with eosinophilia and systemic symptoms (DRESS)/multiorgan hypersensitivity reported; evaluate immediately if signs/symptoms (eg, fever, lymphadenopathy) are present and d/c if an alternative etiology cannot be established. Lab test interactions may occur. Caution in elderly.

ADVERSE REACTIONS: Dizziness, somnolence, fatigue, peripheral edema, hostility, diarrhea, asthenia, infection, dry mouth, nystagmus, constipation, N/V, headache, ataxia, fever.

INTERACTIONS: Decreased bioavailability with Maalox; take gabapentin at least 2 hrs following Maalox administration. Increased levels with naproxen sodium. Decreases levels of hydrocodone in a dose-dependent manner. Increased exposure with hydrocodone or controlled-release morphine cap.

PREGNANCY: Category C, caution in nursing.

MECHANISM OF ACTION: Gamma-aminobutyric acid analog; not established. Suspected to bind to areas of the brain, including neocortex and hippocampus (animals). Analgesic Effects: Prevents allodynia and hyperalgesia (animals).

PHARMACOKINETICS: Absorption: Administration of variable doses resulted in different parameters. **Distribution:** Plasma protein binding (<3%); found in breast milk; (150mg IV) V_d=58L. **Elimination:** Renal (unchanged); $T_{1/2}$=5-7 hrs.

NURSING CONSIDERATIONS

Assessment: Assess for renal impairment, previous hypersensitivity to the drug, depression, preexisting tumors, history of drug abuse, pregnancy/nursing status, and possible drug interactions.

Monitoring: Monitor for emergence or worsening of depression, suicidal thoughts or behavior, unusual changes in mood/behavior, development/worsening of tumors, DRESS, hypersensitivity, withdrawal precipitated seizures, signs/symptoms of misuse or abuse, and other adverse reactions.

Patient Counseling: Instruct to take drug only as prescribed. Counsel that treatment may increase the risk of suicidal thoughts and behavior; advise to report to physician any behaviors of concern. Inform that therapy may cause dizziness, somnolence, and other signs/symptoms of CNS depression; advise not to drive or operate complex machinery until effects on mental and/or motor performance are known. Encourage to enroll in North American Antiepileptic Drug Pregnancy Registry if patient becomes pregnant. Advise to immediately report to physician any rash or other signs/symptoms of hypersensitivity (eg, fever, lymphadenopathy). Inform that scored tabs can be broken in order to administer a half-tab; advise to take the unused half-tab as the next dose and to discard if not used within several days of breaking.

Administration: Oral route. Take with or without food. **Storage:** (Cap/Tab) 25°C (77°F); excursions permitted to 15-30°C (59-86°F). (Sol) 2-8°C (36-46°F).

NEVANAC   RX
nepafenac (Alcon)

THERAPEUTIC CLASS: NSAID
INDICATIONS: Treatment of pain and inflammation associated with cataract surgery.

DOSAGE: *Adults:* 1 drop to affected eye tid beginning 1 day prior to cataract surgery. Continue on day of surgery and throughout first 2 weeks of postoperative period.
Pediatrics: ≥10 Yrs: 1 drop to affected eye tid beginning 1 day prior to cataract surgery. Continue on day of surgery and throughout first 2 weeks of postoperative period.

HOW SUPPLIED: Sus: 0.1% [3mL]

WARNINGS/PRECAUTIONS: Potential for increased bleeding time due to interference with thrombocyte aggregation. Increased bleeding of ocular tissue (eg, hyphemas); caution with known bleeding tendencies that may prolong bleeding time. May slow or delay healing, or result in keratitis. Continued use may be sight threatening due to epithelial breakdown, corneal thinning, erosion, ulceration, or perforation; d/c if corneal epithelial breakdown occurs. Caution with complicated ocular surgeries, corneal denervation, corneal epithelial defects, diabetes mellitus (DM), ocular surface diseases (eg, dry eye syndrome), rheumatoid arthritis (RA), or repeat ocular surgeries within a short period of time. Increased risk for occurrence and severity of corneal adverse events if used >1 day prior to surgery or use beyond 14 days postsurgery. Avoid use with contact lenses and during late pregnancy.

ADVERSE REACTIONS: Capsular opacity, decreased visual acuity, foreign body sensation, increased intraocular pressure, sticky sensation, conjunctival edema, corneal edema, dry eye, lid margin crusting, ocular discomfort, ocular hyperemia/pain/pruritus, photophobia, tearing.

INTERACTIONS: Increased potential for healing problems with topical steroids. Caution with agents that may prolong bleeding time.

PREGNANCY: Category C, caution in nursing.

MECHANISM OF ACTION: NSAID; inhibits prostaglandin biosynthesis.

PHARMACOKINETICS: Absorption: C_{max}=0.310ng/mL (nepafenac), 0.422ng/mL (amfenac, metabolite). **Metabolism:** Hydrolysis via ocular tissue hydrolases to amfenac.

NURSING CONSIDERATIONS

Assessment: Assess for drug hypersensitivity, bleeding tendencies, complicated or repeated ocular surgeries, corneal denervation, corneal epithelial defects, DM, ocular surface diseases, RA, if using contact lenses, pregnancy/nursing status, and possible drug interactions.

Monitoring: Monitor for hypersensitivity reactions, wound healing problems, keratitis, bleeding time, bleeding of ocular tissues in conjunction with ocular surgery, and evidence of epithelial corneal breakdown.

Patient Counseling: Inform of possibility that slow or delayed healing may occur. Advise on proper use to prevent bacterial contamination, and shake bottle well before use. Instruct if using >1 ophthalmic medication, separate by 5 min, and not use while wearing contact lenses. Instruct to immediately notify physician if intercurrent ocular condition (eg, trauma or infection) occurs or undergoing ocular surgery to assess continuation of therapy.

Administration: Intraocular route. Administer 5 min apart if using >1 topical medication. **Storage:** 2-25°C (36-77°F).

NEXAVAR   RX
sorafenib (Bayer Healthcare)

THERAPEUTIC CLASS: Multikinase inhibitor

INDICATIONS: Treatment of unresectable hepatocellular carcinoma and advanced renal cell carcinoma. Treatment of locally recurrent or metastatic, progressive, differentiated thyroid carcinoma (DTC) that is refractory to radioactive iodine treatment.

DOSAGE: *Adults:* Usual: 400mg bid without food (at least 1 hr ac or 2 hrs pc). Continue until patient is no longer clinically benefiting from therapy or until unacceptable toxicity occurs. Refer to PI for dose modifications for suspected adverse drug reactions.

HOW SUPPLIED: Tab: 200mg

CONTRAINDICATIONS: Concomitant use with carboplatin and paclitaxel in patients with squamous cell lung cancer.

WARNINGS/PRECAUTIONS: HTN, cardiac ischemia, and/or infarction reported; temporary or permanent discontinuation should be considered. Increased risk of bleeding may occur; consider permanent discontinuation if bleeding necessitates medical intervention. Hand-foot skin reaction and rash reported; may require topical treatment, temporary interruption, and/or dose modification, or permanent discontinuation in severe or persistent cases. Severe dermatologic toxicities, including Stevens-Johnson syndrome (SJS) and toxic epidermal necrolysis (TEN) reported; d/c if SJS or TEN are suspected. D/C if GI perforation occurs. Temporarily interrupt therapy when undergoing major surgical procedures. May prolong QT/QTc interval; avoid in patients with congenital long QT syndrome. Monitor electrolytes and ECG in patients with congestive heart failure (CHF), bradyarrhythmias, and in patients taking drugs known to prolong QT interval (eg, Class

Ia and III antiarrhythmics). Correct electrolyte abnormalities (Mg^{2+}, K^+, Ca^{2+}). Interrupt treatment if QTc interval is >500 msec or for an increase from baseline ≥60 msec. Drug-induced hepatitis, and increased bilirubin and INR may occur; d/c in case of significantly increased transaminases without alternative explanation (eg, viral hepatitis or progressing underlying malignancy). May impair exogenous thyroid suppression; monitor TSH levels monthly and adjust thyroid replacement medication as needed in patients with DTC. May cause fetal harm.

ADVERSE REACTIONS: HTN, fatigue, weight loss, rash, hand-foot skin reaction, alopecia, pruritus, diarrhea, N/V, abdominal pain, anorexia, constipation, hemorrhage, infection, decreased appetite.

INTERACTIONS: See Contraindications. Avoid with gemcitabine/cisplatin in squamous cell lung cancer patients. Avoid with strong CYP3A4 inducers (eg, carbamazepine, dexamethasone, phenobarbital, phenytoin, rifampin, rifabutin, St. John's wort). Infrequent bleeding or increased INR with warfarin; monitor for changes in PT, INR, or bleeding episodes. Decreased exposure with oral neomycin.

PREGNANCY: Category D, not for use in nursing.

MECHANISM OF ACTION: Multikinase inhibitor; inhibits multiple intracellular (c-CRAF, BRAF and mutant BRAF) and cell surface kinases (KIT, FLT-3, RET, RET/PTC, VEGFR-1, VEGFR-2, VEGFR-3, and PDGFR-β) thought to be involved in tumor cell signaling, angiogenesis, and apoptosis.

PHARMACOKINETICS: Absorption: T_{max}=3 hrs. **Distribution:** Plasma protein binding (99.5%). **Metabolism:** Liver via oxidation and glucuronidation; CYP3A4, UGT1A9; pyridine N-oxide (metabolite). **Elimination:** (100mg Sol) Feces (77%, 51% unchanged), urine (19% glucuronidated metabolites). $T_{1/2}$=25-48 hrs.

NURSING CONSIDERATIONS

Assessment: Assess for bleeding disorders, upcoming major surgical procedures, CHF, bradyarrhythmias, electrolyte abnormalities, drug hypersensitivity, pregnancy/nursing status, and possible drug interactions.

Monitoring: Monitor BP weekly during the first 6 weeks and periodically thereafter. Monitor for cardiac ischemia/infarction, hemorrhage, HTN, dermatologic toxicities, GI perforation, QT/QTc prolongation, and other adverse reactions. Monitor electrolytes (eg, Mg^{2+}, Ca^{2+}, K^+) and ECG in patients with CHF, bradyarrhythmias, and in patients taking drugs known to prolong QT interval. Monitor LFTs regularly, and TSH levels monthly. Monitor patients taking concomitant warfarin for changes in PT, INR, or clinical bleeding episodes.

Patient Counseling: Counsel about possible side effects and to report any episodes of bleeding, chest pain, or other symptoms of cardiac ischemia. Inform that HTN may develop, especially during the first 6 weeks; and that BP should be monitored regularly during therapy. Inform of possible occurrence of hand-foot skin reaction and rash during therapy and appropriate countermeasures. Advise that GI perforation and drug-induced hepatitis may occur and to report signs/symptoms of hepatitis. Inform that temporary interruption is recommended in patients undergoing major surgical procedures. Counsel patients with history of prolonged QT interval that treatment can worsen the condition. Inform that the drug may cause birth defects or fetal loss during pregnancy; both males and females should use effective birth control during treatment and for at least 2 weeks after stopping therapy. Instruct to notify physician if patient becomes pregnant while on therapy. Advise against breastfeeding.

Administration: Oral route. **Storage:** 25°C (77°F); excursions permitted to 15-30°C (59-86°F). Store in a dry place.

NEXIUM IV   RX
esomeprazole sodium (AstraZeneca)

THERAPEUTIC CLASS: Proton pump inhibitor

INDICATIONS: Short-term treatment of gastroesophageal reflux disease with erosive esophagitis in adults and pediatrics 1 month to 17 yrs, when PO therapy is not possible or appropriate.

DOSAGE: *Adults:* 20mg or 40mg qd IV inj (no less than 3 min) or infusion (10-30 min) for up to 10 days. Severe Liver Impairment (Child-Pugh Class C): Max: 20mg/day. D/C and switch to PO as soon as possible/appropriate.
Pediatrics: IV infusion over 10-30 min. 1-17 yrs: ≥55kg: 20mg qd. <55kg: 10mg qd. 1 month-<1 yr: 0.5mg/kg qd. Severe Liver Impairment (Child-Pugh Class C): Max: 20mg/day. D/C and switch to PO as soon as possible/appropriate.

HOW SUPPLIED: Inj: 20mg, 40mg

WARNINGS/PRECAUTIONS: Symptomatic response does not preclude the presence of gastric malignancy. Atrophic gastritis reported with long-term use. May increase risk of *Clostridium difficile*-associated diarrhea (CDAD), especially in hospitalized patients. May increase risk of osteoporosis-related fractures of the hip, wrist, or spine, especially with high-dose and long-term therapy. Use lowest dose and shortest duration possible. Hypomagnesemia reported and may require magnesium replacement and d/c of therapy; consider monitoring of magnesium levels prior to and periodically during therapy with prolonged treatment. Drug-induced decrease in gastric acidity results in enterochromaffin-like cell hyperplasia and increased chromogranin A levels; may interfere with investigations for neuroendocrine tumors.

ADVERSE REACTIONS: Headache, flatulence, nausea, abdominal pain, diarrhea, dry mouth.

INTERACTIONS: CYP2C19 or 3A4 inducers may decrease levels; avoid concomitant use of St. John's wort or rifampin. Reduced pharmacological activity of clopidogrel; avoid concomitant use. May reduce atazanavir and nelfinavir levels; concomitant use not recommended. May change absorption or levels of antiretrovirals. May increase levels of saquinavir, cilostazol, and tacrolimus; consider saquinavir and cilostazol dose reduction. Monitor for increases in INR and PT with warfarin. Decreased clearance of diazepam. Increased levels with combined inhibitors of CYP2C19 and 3A4 (eg, voriconazole). May interfere with absorption of drugs where gastric pH is an important determinant of bioavailability (eg, decreased absorption of ketoconazole, atazanavir, iron salts, and erlotinib). Increased absorption and exposure of digoxin; monitor levels. May inhibit metabolism of CYP2C19 substrates. Caution with digoxin or other drugs that may cause hypomagnesemia (eg, diuretics). May elevate and prolong levels of methotrexate (MTX) and/or its metabolite, possibly leading to toxicities; consider temporary withdrawal of therapy with high-dose MTX.

PREGNANCY: Category B, not for use in nursing.

MECHANISM OF ACTION: Proton pump inhibitor; suppresses gastric acid secretion by specific inhibition of the H^+/K^+-ATPase in the gastric parietal cell. Blocks the final step of acid production.

PHARMACOKINETICS: Absorption: C_{max}=3.86µmol/L (20mg), 7.51µmol/L (40mg). AUC=5.11µmol•hr/L (20mg), 16.21µmol•hr/L (40mg). **Distribution:** V_d=16L; plasma protein binding (97%). **Metabolism:** Liver (extensive) via CYP2C19 (major) into hydroxyl and desmethyl metabolites, and via CYP3A4 into sulphone metabolite. **Elimination:** Urine (primary, <1% unchanged), feces. $T_{1/2}$=1.05 hrs (20mg), 1.41 hrs (40mg).

NURSING CONSIDERATIONS

Assessment: Assess for hypersensitivity to the drug or substituted benzimidazoles, hepatic function, risk for osteoporosis-related fractures, pregnancy/nursing status, and possible drug interactions. Obtain baseline magnesium levels.

Monitoring: Monitor for signs/symptoms of atrophic gastritis, bone fractures, hypomagnesemia, hypersensitivity reactions, CDAD, and other adverse reactions. Monitor magnesium levels periodically. Monitor LFTs.

Patient Counseling: Advise to notify physician if taking other medications. Inform that antacids may be used while on therapy. Advise to report and seek care for diarrhea that does not improve or if cardiovascular/neurological symptoms occur (eg, palpitations, dizziness, seizures, and tetany).

Administration: IV route. Refer to PI for preparation and administration instructions. Should not be administered concomitantly with any other medications through same IV site and/or tubing. Always flush IV line both prior to and after administration. **Storage:** 25°C (77°F); excursions permitted to 15-30°C (59-86°F). Protect from light. Reconstituted Sol: up to 30°C (86°F); use within 12 hrs after reconstitution.

NEXIUM ORAL   RX
esomeprazole magnesium (AstraZeneca)

THERAPEUTIC CLASS: Proton pump inhibitor

INDICATIONS: Short-term treatment (4-8 weeks) and maintenance (up to 6 months) in the healing and symptomatic resolution of erosive esophagitis. Short-term treatment (up to 6 weeks) of erosive esophagitis due to acid-mediated gastroesophageal reflux disease (GERD) in infants 1 month to <1 yr of age. Short-term treatment (4-8 weeks) of heartburn and other symptoms associated with GERD in adults and children ≥1 yr of age. Reduction in occurrence of gastric ulcers associated with continuous NSAID therapy in patients at risk for developing gastric ulcers. Long-term treatment of pathological hypersecretory conditions (eg, Zollinger-Ellison syndrome). In combination with amoxicillin and clarithromycin for the treatment of *Helicobacter pylori* infection and duodenal ulcer (DU) disease (active or history of within the past 5 yrs) for *H. pylori* eradication to reduce the risk of DU recurrence.

DOSAGE: *Adults:* Take at least 1 hr ac. Erosive Esophagitis: Healing: 20mg or 40mg qd for 4-8 weeks; may extend treatment for additional 4-8 weeks if not healed. Maint of Healing: 20mg qd for up to 6 months. Symptomatic GERD: 20mg qd for 4 weeks; may extend treatment for additional 4 weeks if symptoms do not resolve completely. Risk Reduction of NSAID-Associated Gastric Ulcer: 20mg or 40mg qd for up to 6 months. *H. pylori* Eradication: Triple Therapy:

40mg qd + amoxicillin 1000mg bid + clarithromycin 500mg bid, all for 10 days. Pathological Hypersecretory Conditions: 40mg bid; adjust dose to individual patient needs. Doses up to 240mg qd have been administered. Severe Liver Impairment (Child-Pugh Class C): Max: 20mg/day.

Pediatrics: Take at least 1 hr ac. 12-17 Yrs: Healing of Erosive Esophagitis: 20mg or 40mg qd for 4-8 weeks. Symptomatic GERD: 20mg qd for 4 weeks. 1-11 Yrs: Symptomatic GERD: 10mg qd for up to 8 weeks. Max: 1mg/kg/day. Healing of Erosive Esophagitis: ≥20kg: 10mg or 20mg qd for 8 weeks. Max: 1mg/kg/day. <20kg: 10mg qd for 8 weeks. Max: 1mg/kg/day. Erosive Esophagitis due to Acid-Mediated GERD: 1 Month-<1 Yr: >7.5-12kg: 10mg qd for up to 6 weeks. >5-7.5kg: 5mg qd for up to 6 weeks. 3-5kg: 2.5mg qd for up to 6 weeks. Severe Liver Impairment (Child-Pugh Class C): Max: 20mg/day.

HOW SUPPLIED: Cap, Delayed-Release: 20mg, 40mg; Sus, Delayed-Release: 2.5mg, 5mg, 10mg, 20mg, 40mg (granules/pkt)

WARNINGS/PRECAUTIONS: Symptomatic response does not preclude the presence of gastric malignancy. Atrophic gastritis reported with long-term use. May increase risk of *Clostridium difficile*-associated diarrhea (CDAD), especially in hospitalized patients. May increase risk for osteoporosis-related fractures of the hip, wrist, or spine, especially with high-dose and long-term therapy. Use lowest dose and shortest duration possible. Hypomagnesemia reported and may require Mg^{2+} replacement and discontinuation of therapy; consider monitoring of Mg^{2+} levels prior to and periodically during therapy with prolonged treatment. Drug-induced decrease in gastric acidity results in enterochromaffin-like cell hyperplasia and increased chromogranin A levels; may interfere with investigations for neuroendocrine tumors.

ADVERSE REACTIONS: Headache, diarrhea, abdominal pain.

INTERACTIONS: CYP2C19 or 3A4 inducers may decrease levels; avoid concomitant use of St. John's wort or rifampin. Reduced pharmacological activity of clopidogrel; avoid concomitant use. May reduce atazanavir and nelfinavir levels; concomitant use not recommended. May change absorption or levels of antiretrovirals. May increase levels of saquinavir, cilostazol, and tacrolimus; consider saquinavir and cilostazol dose reduction. May interfere with absorption of drugs where gastric pH is an important determinant of bioavailability; ketoconazole, atazanavir, iron salts, and erlotinib absorption can decrease while digoxin absorption can increase. Monitor for increases in INR and PT with warfarin. Decreased clearance of diazepam. Increased levels with combined inhibitors of CYP2C19 and 3A4 (eg, voriconazole). Increased levels of esomeprazole and 14-hydroxyclarithromycin with amoxicillin and clarithromycin. May inhibit metabolism of CYP2C19 substrates. Caution with digoxin or other drugs that may cause hypomagnesemia (eg, diuretics). May elevate and prolong levels of methotrexate (MTX) and/or its metabolite, possibly leading to toxicities; consider temporary withdrawal of therapy with high-dose MTX.

PREGNANCY: Category B, not for use in nursing.

MECHANISM OF ACTION: Proton pump inhibitor (PPI); suppresses gastric acid secretion by specific inhibition of the H^+/K^+-ATPase in the gastric parietal cell. Blocks the final step of acid production.

PHARMACOKINETICS: Absorption: C_{max}=2.1μmol/L (20mg), 4.7μmol/L (40mg); T_{max}=1.6 hrs; AUC=4.2μmol•hr/L (20mg), 12.6μmol•hr/L (40mg). Refer to PI for pharmacokinetic parameters in pediatrics. **Distribution:** V_d=16L; plasma protein binding (97%). **Metabolism:** Liver (extensive) via CYP2C19 (major) into hydroxy and desmethyl metabolites, and via CYP3A4 into sulphone metabolites. **Elimination:** Urine (80% metabolites, <1% unchanged), feces; $T_{1/2}$=1.2 hrs (20mg), 1.5 hrs (40mg).

NURSING CONSIDERATIONS

Assessment: Assess for hypersensitivity to PPIs, hepatic dysfunction, risk for osteoporosis-related fractures, pregnancy/nursing status, and possible drug interactions. Obtain baseline Mg^{2+} levels.

Monitoring: Monitor for signs/symptoms of atrophic gastritis, bone fractures, hypomagnesemia, hypersensitivity reactions, CDAD, and other adverse reactions. Monitor Mg^{2+} levels periodically. Monitor LFTs. Monitor for increases in INR and PT with warfarin.

Patient Counseling: Advise to notify physician if taking other medications. Inform that antacids may be used while on therapy. Instruct not to chew or crush cap; if opening cap to mix granules with food, mix with applesauce only. Inform about proper technique for administration of opened cap or oral sus. Counsel regarding the correct amount of water to use when mixing dose of oral sus. Advise to immediately report and seek care for diarrhea that does not improve or if cardio-vascular/neurological symptoms occur (eg, palpitations, dizziness, seizures, tetany).

Administration: Oral route. Take at least 1 hr ac. May be given via gastric/NG route. Refer to PI for preparation and administration instructions. **Storage:** 25°C (77°F); excursions permitted to 15-30°C (59-86°F).

NEXTERONE   RX
amiodarone HCl (Baxter)

OTHER BRAND NAMES: Amiodarone (Hospira)

THERAPEUTIC CLASS: Class III antiarrhythmic

INDICATIONS: Initiation of treatment and prophylaxis of frequently recurring ventricular fibrillation (VF) and hemodynamically unstable ventricular tachycardia (VT) refractory to other therapy. Treatment of patients with VT/VF for whom PO amiodarone is indicated, but who are unable to take PO medication.

DOSAGE: *Adults:* May individualize first 24-hr dose. Max Initial Infusion Rate: 30mg/min. LD: 150mg IV over first 10 min (15mg/min), then 360mg IV over next 6 hrs (1mg/min). Maint: 540mg IV over remaining 18 hrs (0.5mg/min). After first 24 hrs, continue maint infusion rate of 720mg/24 hrs (0.5mg/min); may increase rate to achieve arrhythmia suppression. Maint infusion of up to 0.5mg/min can be continued for 2-3 weeks. Max Concentration (Infusions >1 hr): 2mg/mL (unless a central venous catheter is used). Breakthrough Episodes of VF/Hemodynamically Unstable VT: use 150mg supplemental infusions over 10 min. Switching to PO Amiodarone (assuming a 720mg/day IV infusion): <1 week of IV Infusion: Initial: 800-1600mg/day; 1-3 weeks of IV Infusion: Initial: 600-800mg/day; >3 weeks of IV Infusion: Initial: 400mg/day. Elderly: Start at lower end of dosing range.

HOW SUPPLIED: Inj: 1.5mg/mL [100mL], 1.8mg/mL [200mL]

CONTRAINDICATIONS: Cardiogenic shock, marked sinus bradycardia, 2nd- or 3rd-degree atrioventricular (AV) block unless a functioning pacemaker is available.

WARNINGS/PRECAUTIONS: Hypotension reported; treat initially by slowing the infusion. Bradycardia reported; slow infusion rate or d/c treatment. Ensure availability of temporary pacemaker in patients with known predisposition to bradycardia or AV block. Elevations of hepatic enzymes reported; potential risk for hepatic injury. Acute centrolobular confluent hepatocellular necrosis leading to hepatic coma, acute renal failure, and death may occur at a much higher LD concentration and much faster rate of infusion than recommended. Consider d/c or reducing rate of administration with evidence of progressive hepatic injury. May worsen or precipitate a new arrhythmia; monitor for QTc prolongation. Early-onset pulmonary toxicity, pulmonary fibrosis and adult respiratory distress syndrome (ARDS) reported. Optic neuropathy/neuritis may occur; perform ophthalmic examination if symptoms of visual impairment appear. Not intended for long-term maint use. May cause thyroid dysfunction, which may lead to potentially fatal breakthrough or exacerbated arrhythmias. Hypo- and hyperthyroidism, thyroid nodules/cancer/dysfunction reported; evaluate thyroid function prior to treatment and periodically thereafter. Hyperthyroidism may result in thyrotoxicosis and arrhythmia breakthrough or aggravation. May cause fetal harm. Corneal refractive laser surgery devices may be contraindicated. Correct hypokalemia or hypomagnesemia prior to initiation of therapy. Caution in elderly.

ADVERSE REACTIONS: Hypotension, asystole, cardiac arrest, pulseless electrical activity, cardiogenic shock, congestive heart failure, bradycardia, liver function test abnormalities, nausea, VT, AV block.

INTERACTIONS: Potential for drug interactions may persist after d/c due to long half-life. Inhibitors of CYP3A (eg, protease inhibitors, cimetidine) and CYP2C8 may increase levels. Do not take grapefruit juice during treatment. QT prolongation and torsades de pointes with concomitant loratadine and trazodone reported. May increase levels of CYP1A2/CYP2C9/CYP2D6/CYP3A and P-glycoprotein substrates. May elevate plasma levels of cyclosporine, digoxin, quinidine, procainamide, phenytoin, flecainide. D/C or reduce digitalis dose by 50%. Reduce quinidine and procainamide doses by 1/3. Myopathy/rhabdomyolysis reported with HMG-CoA reductase inhibitors that are CYP3A4 substrates; limit simvastatin dose to 20mg/day, lovastatin to 40mg/day, and lower the initial and maint doses of other CYP3A4 substrates (eg, atorvastatin). May potentiate bradycardia, sinus arrest, and AV block with β-receptor blocking agents (eg, propranolol) or calcium channel antagonists (eg, verapamil, diltiazem); use with caution. May increase PT with warfarin-type anticoagulant; reduce anticoagulant dose by 1/3 to 1/2. Concomitant use with clopidogrel may result in ineffective inhibition of platelet aggregation. CYP3A inducers (eg, rifampin, St. John's wort) may decrease levels. May cause hypotension, bradycardia, and decreased cardiac output with fentanyl. Seizures and sinus bradycardia reported with lidocaine. May inhibit metabolism of dextromethorphan. Cholestyramine may decrease levels and half-life. QTc prolongation with disopyramide, fluoroquinolones, macrolides, and azoles. Use with propranolol, diltiazem, verapamil may result in hemodynamic and electrophysiologic interactions. May be more sensitive to myocardial depressant and conduction defects of halogenated inhalational anesthetics. May impair metabolism of phenytoin, dextromethorphan, and methotrexate. Action of antithyroid drugs may be delayed in amiodarone-induced thyrotoxicosis. Radioactive iodine therapy is contraindicated with amiodarone-induced hyperthyroidism. Monitor electrolyte and acid-base balance with concomitant diuretics. Initiate any added antiarrhythmic drug at a lower than usual dose.

PREGNANCY: Category D, not for use in nursing.

MECHANISM OF ACTION: Class III antiarrhythmic; blocks sodium, calcium, and potassium channels; exerts noncompetitive antisympathetic action, and negative chronotropic and dromotropic effects; lengthens cardiac action potential, decreases cardiac workload and myocardial oxygen consumption.

PHARMACOKINETICS: Absorption: C_{max}=7-26mg/L (150mg IV). **Distribution:** Plasma protein binding (>96%); crosses the placenta, found in breast milk. **Metabolism:** CYP3A, 2C8; N-desethylamiodarone (major active metabolite). **Elimination:** Urine, bile; $T_{1/2}$=9-36 days (amiodarone); 9-30 days (N-desethylamiodarone).

NURSING CONSIDERATIONS

Assessment: Assess for cardiogenic shock, marked sinus bradycardia, 2nd- or 3rd-degree AV block, functioning pacemaker, thyroid dysfunction, hypersensitivity, pregnancy/nursing status, and possible drug interactions. Prior to initiation, correct hypokalemia and hypomagnesemia.

Monitoring: Monitor for hypotension, bradycardia, AV block, acute centrolobular hepatocellular necrosis, hepatic coma, acute renal failure, hepatic injury, worsening of existing or precipitation of new arrhythmia, ARDS, pulmonary toxicity, pulmonary fibrosis, optic neuropathy/neuritis, hypo/hyperthyroidism, thyroid nodules, thyroid cancer, QTc prolongation. Monitor LFTs and thyroid function. Perform perioperative monitoring for patients undergoing general anesthesia. Perform regular ophthalmic examination (eg, fundoscopy and slit-lamp exams) during administration.

Patient Counseling: Inform about benefits and risks of therapy. Instruct to d/c nursing while on therapy. Inform that corneal refractive laser surgery may be contraindicated. Counsel not to take with grapefruit juice, over-the-counter cough medicine (that commonly contains dextromethorphan), and St. John's wort during therapy. Discuss symptoms of hypo- and hyperthyroidism, particularly if transitioned to PO therapy.

Administration: IV route. Refer to PI for instructions on administration and preparation. **Storage:** 20-25°C (68-77°F); excursions permitted to 15-30°C (59-86°F). Protect from light and excessive heat. Protect from freezing.

NIASPAN
niacin (AbbVie)

RX N

THERAPEUTIC CLASS: Nicotinic acid

INDICATIONS: To reduce elevated total cholesterol (total-C), LDL-C, apolipoprotein B, and TG levels, and to increase HDL-C in primary hyperlipidemia and mixed dyslipidemia. In combination with simvastatin or lovastatin, for the treatment of primary hyperlipidemia and mixed dyslipidemia when treatment with monotherapy is inadequate. To reduce the risk of recurrent nonfatal myocardial infarction (MI) in patients with history of MI and hyperlipidemia. In combination with a bile acid binding resin, to slow progression or promote regression of atherosclerotic disease in patients with history of coronary artery disease and hyperlipidemia, and to reduce elevated total-C and LDL-C levels in adults with primary hyperlipidemia. Adjunctive therapy for treatment of adults with severe hypertriglyceridemia who present a risk of pancreatitis and who do not respond adequately to diet.

DOSAGE: *Adults:* >16 Yrs: Take at hs after a low-fat snack. Individualize dose. Initial: 500mg. Titrate: Increase by 500mg every 4 weeks. After Week 8, titrate to patient response and tolerance. If response to 1000mg qd is inadequate, increase to 1500mg qd; may subsequently increase to 2000mg qd. Do not increase daily dose by >500mg in any 4-week period. Maint: 1000-2000mg qhs. Max: 2000mg/day. Women may respond at lower doses than men. Do not interchange three 500mg tabs with two 750mg tabs. May take aspirin (ASA) (up to 325mg) 30 min prior to treatment to reduce flushing. If therapy is discontinued for an extended period, reinstitution should include a titration phase. Refer to PI for concomitant therapy with lovastatin/simvastatin.

HOW SUPPLIED: Tab, Extended-Release: 500mg, 750mg, 1000mg

CONTRAINDICATIONS: Active liver disease or unexplained persistent elevations in hepatic transaminases, active peptic ulcer disease (PUD), arterial bleeding.

WARNINGS/PRECAUTIONS: At doses of 1500-2000mg/day, in combination with simvastatin, did not reduce the incidence of cardiovascular (CV) events more than simvastatin in patients with CV disease and mean baseline LDL-C levels of 74mg/dL. Do not substitute for equivalent doses of sustained-release (modified-release, timed-release) niacin or immediate-release (IR) (crystalline) niacin; severe hepatic toxicity, including fulminant hepatic necrosis, may occur. If switching from IR niacin, initiate with low doses (500mg at hs) and titrate to desired therapeutic response. Caution in patients with unstable angina or in the acute phase of MI, particularly if also receiving vasoactive drugs (eg, nitrates, calcium channel blockers, adrenergic blocking agents).

Caution in patients with renal impairment, or who consume substantial quantities of alcohol, and/ or have history of liver disease. Closely observe patients with history of jaundice, hepatobiliary disease, or peptic ulcer. Associated with abnormal LFTs; monitor LFTs (eg, AST, ALT) before treatment, every 6-12 weeks for the 1st yr, and periodically thereafter (eg, 6-month intervals). If elevated serum transaminase levels develop, measurements should be repeated promptly and then performed more frequently. D/C if transaminase levels progress, particularly if they rise to 3X ULN and are persistent, or if associated with nausea, fever, and/or malaise. May increase FPG; closely monitor diabetic/potentially diabetic patients (particularly during 1st few months of therapy or dose adjustment), and adjust diet and/or hypoglycemic therapy if necessary. Associated with dose-related reductions in platelet count and phosphorus (P) levels; periodically monitor P levels in patients at risk for hypophosphatemia. Associated with increases in PT; carefully evaluate patients undergoing surgery. Elevated uric acid levels reported; caution in patients predisposed to gout. Lab test interactions may occur.

ADVERSE REACTIONS: Flushing (warmth, redness, itching, and/or tingling), diarrhea, N/V, increased cough, pruritus, rash.

INTERACTIONS: Avoid ingestion of alcohol, hot drinks, or spicy foods around the time of administration; may increase flushing and pruritus. Use caution when prescribing niacin (≥1g/day) with statins; may increase risk of myopathy and rhabdomyolysis. Separate dosing from bile acid-binding resins by at least 4-6 hrs. ASA may decrease the metabolic clearance of nicotinic acid. May potentiate the effects of ganglionic blocking agents and vasoactive drugs, resulting in postural hypotension. Vitamins or other nutritional supplements containing large doses of niacin or related compounds (eg, nicotinamide) may potentiate adverse effects. Use caution with anticoagulants; monitor platelet counts and PT.

PREGNANCY: Category C, not for use in nursing.

MECHANISM OF ACTION: Nicotinic acid; not established. May partially inhibit release of free fatty acids from adipose tissue, and increase lipoprotein lipase activity, which may increase the rate of chylomicron TG removal from plasma. Decreases the rate of hepatic synthesis of VLDL and LDL, and does not appear to affect fecal excretion of fats, sterols, or bile acids.

PHARMACOKINETICS: Absorption: T_{max} =5 hrs. **Distribution:** Found in breast milk. **Metabolism:** Liver (rapid; extensive and saturable 1st-pass); nicotinuric acid (via conjugation), nicotinamide adenine dinucleotide (metabolites). **Elimination:** Urine (60-76%; up to 12% unchanged).

NURSING CONSIDERATIONS

Assessment: Assess for history of/active liver disease or PUD, unexplained persistent hepatic transaminase elevations, arterial bleeding, history of jaundice or hepatobiliary disease, renal impairment, predisposing factors for myopathy/rhabdomyolysis, risk for hypophosphatemia, drug hypersensitivity, any other conditions where treatment is contraindicated or cautioned, pregnancy/nursing status, and possible drug interactions. Obtain baseline LFTs and lipid levels.

Monitoring: Monitor for signs/symptoms of rhabdomyolysis, liver dysfunction, decreases in platelet counts and P levels, increases in PT and uric acid levels, and other adverse reactions. Monitor LFTs every 6-12 weeks for the 1st yr and periodically thereafter, and lipid levels. Frequently monitor blood glucose. Periodically monitor P levels in patients at risk for hypophosphatemia. Monitor PT and platelet counts with anticoagulants.

Patient Counseling: Advise to adhere to the National Cholesterol Education Program-recommended diet, a regular exercise program, and periodic testing of a fasting lipid panel. Instruct to contact physician before restarting therapy if dosing is interrupted for any length of time. Instruct to notify physician of any unexplained muscle pain, tenderness or weakness, dizziness, changes in blood glucose if diabetic, and all medications being taken (eg, vitamins or other nutritional supplements containing niacin or nicotinamide). Inform that flushing may occur and may subside after several weeks of consistent use of therapy. Instruct that if awakened by flushing at night, to get up slowly, especially if feeling dizzy or faint, or taking BP medications. Advise of the symptoms of flushing and how they differ from the symptoms of MI. Instruct to avoid ingestion of alcohol, hot beverages, and spicy foods around the time of administration to minimize flushing. Advise to d/c use and contact physician if pregnant.

Administration: Oral route. Take at hs after a low-fat snack. Swallow tab whole; do not break, crush, or chew. Avoid administration on an empty stomach to reduce flushing, pruritus, and GI distress. **Storage:** 20-25°C (68-77°F).

NIFEDIPINE   RX
nifedipine (Various)

OTHER BRAND NAMES: Procardia (Pfizer)

THERAPEUTIC CLASS: Calcium channel blocker (dihydropyridine)

INDICATIONS: Management of vasospastic angina and chronic stable angina without evidence of vasospasm in patients who remain symptomatic despite adequate doses of β-blockers and/or organic nitrates, or who cannot tolerate those agents.

DOSAGE: *Adults:* Initial: 10mg tid. Usual: 10-20mg tid or 20-30mg tid-qid with evidence of coronary artery spasm. Titrate over a 7- to 14-day period. If symptoms warrant (eg, activity level, attack frequency, SL nitroglycerin consumption) dose may be increased from 10mg tid to 20mg tid, then 30mg tid over a 3-day period. Ischemic hospitalized patients may increase in 10mg increments over 4- to 6-hr periods; single dose should rarely exceed 30mg. Max: 180mg/day. Elderly: Start at the low end of the dosing range.

HOW SUPPLIED: Cap: 10mg (Procardia), 20mg

WARNINGS/PRECAUTIONS: May cause hypotension; monitor BP initially and with titration. Not for acute reduction of BP or control of essential HTN. May increase frequency, duration and/or severity of angina or acute myocardial infarction (MI), particularly with severe obstructive coronary artery disease (CAD). Avoid with acute coronary syndrome and within 1 or 2 weeks after MI. May develop congestive heart failure (CHF), especially with aortic stenosis. Peripheral edema associated with vasodilation may occur; patients with angina complicated by CHF, rule out peripheral edema caused by left ventricular dysfunction. Transient elevations of enzymes (eg, alkaline phosphatase, CPK, LDH, SGOT, SGPT), cholestasis with/without jaundice, and allergic hepatitis reported. May decrease platelet aggregation and increase bleeding time. Positive direct Coombs test with/without hemolytic anemia reported. Reversible elevation in BUN and SrCr reported rarely in patients with chronic renal insufficiency. Caution in elderly. Taper dose upon discontinuation.

ADVERSE REACTIONS: Dizziness, lightheadedness, giddiness, flushing, heat sensation, heartburn, muscle cramps, tremor, headache, weakness, nausea, peripheral edema, nervousness/mood changes, palpitation.

INTERACTIONS: β-blockers may increase risk of CHF, severe hypotension, or angina exacerbation; avoid abrupt β-blocker withdrawal. Severe hypotension and/or increased fluid volume reported together with β-blockers and fentanyl or other narcotic analgesics. May increase digoxin levels; monitor when initiating, adjusting, and discontinuing therapy to avoid over- or under-digitalization. May decrease plasma levels of quinidine. May increase PT with coumarin anticoagulants. Cimetidine and grapefruit juice may increase levels. Monitor with other medications known to lower BP.

PREGNANCY: Category C, safety not known in nursing.

MECHANISM OF ACTION: Calcium channel blocker; inhibits Ca^{2+} ion influx into cardiac muscle and smooth muscle. Angina: Has not been established; believed to act by relaxation and prevention of coronary artery spasm and reduction of oxygen utilization.

PHARMACOKINETICS: Absorption: Rapid and fully absorbed; T_{max}=30 min. **Distribution:** Plasma protein binding (92-98%). **Metabolism:** Liver, extensive. **Elimination:** Urine (80%); $T_{1/2}$=2 hrs.

NURSING CONSIDERATIONS

Assessment: Assess for CHF, severe obstructive CAD, aortic stenosis, hepatic/renal impairment, essential HTN, recent MI, recent β-blocker withdrawal, pregnancy/nursing status, and possible drug interactions.

Monitoring: Monitor for excessive hypotension, increased frequency, duration and/or severity of angina and/or acute MI (especially during initiation and dose titration), CHF, peripheral edema (determine cause), cholestasis with or without jaundice and allergic hepatitis. Monitor BP, LFTs, BUN, SrCr, for decreased platelet aggregation, and increased bleeding time.

Patient Counseling: Inform about potential risks/benefits of drug. Advise to swallow cap whole.

Administration: Oral route. Swallow cap whole. **Storage:** 15-25°C (59-77°F). Protect from light and moisture.

NILANDRON   RX
nilutamide (Sanofi-Aventis)

> Interstitial pneumonitis reported. Reports of interstitial changes, including pulmonary fibrosis that led to hospitalization and death, reported rarely. Symptoms included exertional dyspnea, cough, chest pain, and fever. X-rays showed interstitial or alveolo-interstitial changes, and pulmonary function tests revealed a restrictive pattern with decreased DLco. Perform routine chest x-ray prior to initiating treatment; consider baseline pulmonary function tests. Instruct patients to report any new or worsening SOB during treatment. If symptoms occur, d/c immediately until it can be determined if symptoms are drug related.

THERAPEUTIC CLASS: Nonsteroidal antiandrogen

INDICATIONS: In combination with surgical castration for the treatment of metastatic prostate cancer (Stage D_2).

DOSAGE: *Adults:* Usual: 300mg qd for 30 days, followed thereafter by 150mg qd.

HOW SUPPLIED: Tab: 150mg

CONTRAINDICATIONS: Severe hepatic impairment, severe respiratory insufficiency.

WARNINGS/PRECAUTIONS: For max benefit, begin treatment on the same day as or on the day after surgical castration. Hepatotoxicity reported; measure serum transaminase levels prior to initiation, at regular intervals for first 4 months of treatment, and periodically thereafter. Obtain LFTs at 1st sign/symptom suggestive of liver dysfunction; d/c immediately if jaundice develops or ALT >2X ULN and closely monitor LFTs until resolution. Not for use in women, particularly for non-serious or non-life-threatening conditions. Isolated cases of aplastic anemia reported. Patients whose disease progresses while on therapy may experience clinical improvement with discontinuation.

ADVERSE REACTIONS: Interstitial pneumonitis, hot flushes, impaired adaptation to dark, nausea, urinary tract infection, increased AST/ALT, dizziness, constipation, abnormal vision, dyspnea, HTN.

INTERACTIONS: May reduce metabolism of CYP450 substrates in vitro; may increase serum $T_{1/2}$ of drugs with a low therapeutic margin (eg, vitamin K antagonists, phenytoin, theophylline), leading to a toxic level; dosage of these drugs or others with similar metabolism may need to be modified. Monitor PT and reduce dose of vitamin K antagonists if necessary.

PREGNANCY: Category C, safety not known in nursing.

MECHANISM OF ACTION: Nonsteroidal antiandrogen; blocks effects of testosterone at the androgen receptor level in vitro and interacts with the androgen receptor and prevents the normal androgenic response in vivo.

PHARMACOKINETICS: Absorption: Rapid and complete. **Metabolism:** Extensive, via oxidation. **Elimination:** Urine (62%, <2% unchanged), feces (1.4%-7%); $T_{1/2}$=38-59.1 hrs (100-300mg single dose).

NURSING CONSIDERATIONS

Assessment: Assess for severe hepatic impairment, severe respiratory insufficiency, hypersensitivity to drug or any of its component, and possible drug interactions. Perform routine chest x-ray, and obtain baseline pulmonary function tests and hepatic enzymes.

Monitoring: Monitor for signs/symptoms of interstitial pneumonitis, hepatotoxicity, and disease progression. Measure serum transaminase levels at regular intervals for first 4 months of treatment, and periodically thereafter. Obtain LFTs at first sign/symptom suggestive of liver dysfunction.

Patient Counseling: Inform that therapy should be started on the day of, or on the day after, surgical castration; advise not to interrupt or d/c dosing without consulting physician. Instruct to report any new or worsening dyspnea. Advise to consult physician should N/V, abdominal pain, or jaundice occur. Instruct to avoid intake of alcoholic beverages if experiencing alcohol intolerance. Counsel to wear tinted glasses to alleviate the delayed adaptation to dark; caution about driving at night and through tunnels.

Administration: Oral route. **Storage:** 25°C (77°F); excursions permitted between 15-30°C (59-86°F). Protect from light.

NIRAVAM
alprazolam (Azur)

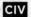

THERAPEUTIC CLASS: Benzodiazepine

INDICATIONS: Treatment of generalized anxiety disorder and panic disorder, with or without agoraphobia.

DOSAGE: *Adults:* Individualize dose. Anxiety: Initial: 0.25-0.5mg tid. Titrate: May increase every 3-4 days. Max: 4mg/day in divided doses. Panic Disorder: Initial: 0.5mg tid. Titrate: May increase by no more than 1mg/day every 3-4 days depending on response; slower titration to doses >4mg/day. Usual: 1-10mg/day. Daily Dose Reduction/Discontinuation: Decrease dose gradually (no more than 0.5mg/day every 3 days). Elderly/Advanced Liver Disease/Debilitating Disease: Initial: 0.25mg bid-tid. Titrate: Increase gradually PRN and as tolerated.

HOW SUPPLIED: Tab, Disintegrating: 0.25mg*, 0.5mg*, 1mg*, 2mg* *scored

CONTRAINDICATIONS: Acute narrow-angle glaucoma, coadministration with potent CYP3A4 inhibitors (eg, ketoconazole, itraconazole).

WARNINGS/PRECAUTIONS: Seizures, including status epilepticus reported with dose reduction or abrupt discontinuation. Use may lead to physical and psychological dependence; prescribe for short periods and periodically reassess the need for continued treatment. Increased risk of dependence with doses >4mg/day, treatment for >12 weeks, and in panic disorder patients. May cause fetal harm. Avoid use during 1st trimester of pregnancy; may increase risk of congenital anomalies. May impair mental/physical abilities. Hypomania and mania reported in patients with depression. Early morning anxiety and emergence of anxiety symptoms between doses reported; give same total daily dose divided as more frequent administrations. Withdrawal reactions may occur; reduce dose or d/c therapy gradually. Has a weak uricosuric effect. Decreased systemic elimination rate with alcoholic liver disease and obesity. Caution with severe depression, suicidal ideation/plans, impaired renal/hepatic/pulmonary function, elderly, and debilitated. Slow disintegration or dissolution, resulting in slowed or decreased absorption with diseases that cause dry mouth or raise stomach pH.

ADVERSE REACTIONS: Sedation, fatigue/tiredness, impaired coordination, irritability, memory impairment, increased/decreased appetite, cognitive disorder, weight gain/loss, constipation, dysarthria, lightheadedness, dry mouth, decreased/increased libido.

INTERACTIONS: See Contraindications. Avoid with other azole-type antifungals. Caution with alcohol, other CNS depressants, propoxyphene, diltiazem, isoniazid, macrolide antibiotics (eg, erythromycin, clarithromycin), grapefruit juice, sertraline, paroxetine, ergotamine, cyclosporine, amiodarone, nicardipine, nifedipine, and other CYP3A inhibitors. Increased plasma levels of imipramine and desipramine. Additive CNS depressant effects with psychotropics, anticonvulsants, antihistaminics, alcohol, and other drugs that produce CNS depression. Slow disintegration or dissolution, resulting in slowed or decreased absorption with drugs that cause dry mouth or raise stomach pH. Increased concentration with nefazodone, fluvoxamine, and cimetidine; consider dose reduction of alprazolam. Increased concentration with fluoxetine and oral contraceptives; use with caution. Decreased levels with CYP3A inducers, propoxyphene, carbamazepine, and smoking.

PREGNANCY: Category D, not for use in nursing.

MECHANISM OF ACTION: Benzodiazepine; not established. Binds to gamma-aminobutyric acid (GABA) receptors in the brain and enhances GABA-mediated synaptic inhibition; such actions may be responsible for the efficacy in anxiety disorder and panic disorder.

PHARMACOKINETICS: Absorption: Readily absorbed; C_{max}=8-37ng/mL (0.5-3mg); T_{max}=1.5-2 hrs. **Distribution:** Plasma protein binding (80%); crosses placenta; found in breast milk. **Metabolism:** Extensive. Liver via CYP3A4; 4-hydroxyalprazolam and α-hydroxyalprazolam (major metabolites). **Elimination:** Urine, $T_{1/2}$=12.5 hrs.

NURSING CONSIDERATIONS

Assessment: Assess for known sensitivity to drug, acute narrow-angle glaucoma, depression, suicidal ideation, renal/hepatic/pulmonary impairment, debilitation, obesity, diseases that cause dry mouth or raise stomach pH, history of alcohol/substance abuse, history of seizures/epilepsy, pregnancy/nursing status, and possible drug interactions. Assess for risk of dependence among panic disorder patients.

Monitoring: Monitor for dependence, rebound/withdrawal symptoms (eg, seizures), early morning anxiety and emergence of anxiety symptoms, CNS depression, hypomania, mania, suicidality, and other treatment-emergent symptoms. Reassess usefulness of therapy periodically.

Patient Counseling: Instruct not to remove tab from the bottle until just prior to dosing and inform of proper administration. Advise to inform physician about any alcohol consumption and medicine taken; alcohol should generally be avoided while taking this medication. Instruct to inform physician of pregnancy/nursing status. Advise not to drive or operate dangerous machinery until they are familiar with the effects of this medication. Advise not to increase/decrease dose or abruptly d/c therapy without consulting physician; instruct to follow gradual dosage tapering schedule. Inform of risks associated with doses >4mg/day.

Administration: Oral route. Remove tab from bottle with dry hands and immediately place tab on top of the tongue. Refer to PI for additional handling/administration instructions. **Storage:** 20-25°C (68-77°F); excursions permitted to 15-30°C (59-86°F). Protect from moisture.

NITRO-DUR   RX
nitroglycerin (Merck)

OTHER BRAND NAMES: Minitran (Medicis)

THERAPEUTIC CLASS: Nitrate vasodilator

INDICATIONS: Prevention of angina pectoris due to coronary artery disease.

DOSAGE: *Adults:* Initial: 0.2-0.4mg/hr patch for 12-14 hrs/day. Remove patch for 10-12 hrs/day. (Nitro-Dur) Elderly: Start at low end of dosing range.

HOW SUPPLIED: Patch: (Minitran) 0.1mg/hr, 0.2mg/hr, 0.4mg/hr, 0.6mg/hr [30s]; (Nitro-Dur) 0.1mg/hr, 0.2mg/hr, 0.3mg/hr, 0.4mg/hr, 0.6mg/hr, 0.8mg/hr [30s]

WARNINGS/PRECAUTIONS: Not useful in aborting an acute angina attack. Benefits of use with acute myocardial infarction (MI) or congestive heart failure (CHF) have not been established; perform careful clinical or hemodynamic monitoring to avoid hazards of hypotension and tachycardia if electing to use in these conditions. Do not discharge defibrillator/cardioverter through a paddle electrode that overlies the patch; may cause damage to paddles and burns to patient. Severe hypotension may occur; caution with volume depletion, hypotension, in the elderly, and in patients on multiple medications. Nitroglycerin-induced hypotension may be accompanied by paradoxal bradycardia and increased angina pectoris. May aggravate angina caused by hypertrophic cardiomyopathy. Tolerance and physical dependence observed; chest pain, acute MI, and death reported during temporary withdrawal.

ADVERSE REACTIONS: Headache, lightheadedness, hypotension, syncope, increased angina.

INTERACTIONS: Phosphodiesterase inhibitors (eg, sildenafil) amplify vasodilatory effects, which can result in severe hypotension. Vasodilating effects may be additive with those of other vasodilators (eg, alcohol). (Minitran) Marked symptomatic orthostatic hypotension reported with calcium channel blockers; dose adjustments of either class of agents may be necessary.

PREGNANCY: Category C, caution in nursing.

MECHANISM OF ACTION: Nitrate vasodilator; relaxes vascular smooth muscle producing dilatation of peripheral arteries and veins, especially the latter. Dilatation of veins leads to reduced left ventricular end-diastolic pressure and pulmonary capillary wedge pressure (preload). Arteriolar relaxation reduces systemic vascular resistance, systolic arterial pressure, and mean arterial pressure (afterload). Also dilates the coronary arteries.

PHARMACOKINETICS: Distribution: V_d=3L/kg. **Metabolism:** Extrahepatic metabolism (RBC and vascular walls); inorganic nitrate and the 1,2- and 1,3-dinitroglycerols (metabolites). **Elimination:** $T_{1/2}$=3 min.

NURSING CONSIDERATIONS

Assessment: Assess for previous drug hypersensitivity, acute MI, CHF, severe hypotension or volume depletion, angina caused by hypertrophic cardiomyopathy, pregnancy/nursing status, and possible drug interactions.

Monitoring: Monitor for hypotension, paradoxical bradycardia, increased angina pectoris, tolerance, physical dependence, and methemoglobinemia. In patients with acute MI and CHF, perform careful clinical or hemodynamic monitoring for hypotension and tachycardia.

Patient Counseling: Advise that daily headaches may accompany treatment; instruct to avoid altering schedule of treatment as the headaches are a marker of the activity of the medication and loss of headache may be associated with loss of antianginal efficacy. Counsel to carefully follow dosing regimen, including a 10-12 hrs nitrate-free period. Inform that treatment may be associated with lightheadedness on standing, especially just after rising from recumbent or seated position; inform that this effect may be more frequent if also consuming alcohol. Instruct to appropriately discard patch after use.

Administration: Transdermal route. **Storage:** (Minitran) 15-30°C (59-86°F). Avoid extreme temperatures and/or humidity. (Nitro-Dur) 25°C (77°F); excursions permitted to 15-30°C (59-86°F). Do not refrigerate.

NITROLINGUAL   RX
nitroglycerin (Arbor)

THERAPEUTIC CLASS: Nitrate vasodilator

INDICATIONS: Acute relief of an attack or prophylaxis of angina pectoris due to coronary artery disease.

DOSAGE: *Adults:* Acute Relief: 1 or 2 sprays at the onset of attack onto or under the tongue. Max: 3 sprays/15 min. If chest pain persists, prompt medical attention is recommended. Prophylaxis: May be used 5-10 min prior to engaging in activities that might precipitate an acute attack.

HOW SUPPLIED: Spray: 400mcg/spray

CONTRAINDICATIONS: Concomitant use with certain drugs for erectile dysfunction (phosphodiesterase inhibitors).

WARNINGS/PRECAUTIONS: Use during the early days of acute myocardial infarction (AMI) requires particular attention to hemodynamic monitoring and clinical status. Severe hypotension may occur; caution with volume depletion from diuretic therapy or in patients with low systolic BP (eg, <90mmHg). Paradoxical bradycardia and increased angina pectoris may accompany nitroglycerin-induced hypotension. May aggravate angina caused by hypertrophic cardiomyopathy. Tolerance and cross-tolerance to other nitrates and nitrites may occur.

ADVERSE REACTIONS: Headache, dizziness, paresthesia.

INTERACTIONS: See Contraindications. Alcohol may enhance hypotensive effects. Decreased or increased effect of other agents that depend on vascular smooth muscle as the final common path. Marked symptomatic orthostatic hypotension reported with concomitant use of calcium channel blockers and oral controlled-release nitroglycerin; dose adjustment of either class may be necessary.

PREGNANCY: Category C, caution in nursing.

MECHANISM OF ACTION: Nitrate vasodilator; relaxation of vascular smooth muscle, producing a vasodilator effect on both peripheral arteries and veins, with more prominent effects on the latter.

PHARMACOKINETICS: Absorption: (Healthy) C_{max}=1041pg/mL•min, T_{max}=7.5 min, AUC=12,769pg/mL•min. **Metabolism:** Liver (rapid) via reductase enzyme to glycerol nitrate metabolites and inorganic nitrates; hydrolysis to 1,2- and 1,3-dinitroglycerols (active metabolites).

NURSING CONSIDERATIONS

Assessment: Assess for volume-depletion, systolic BP, hypertrophic cardiomyopathy, drug hypersensitivity, pregnancy/nursing status, and possible drug interactions.

Monitoring: Monitor for hypotension, paradoxical bradycardia, increased angina pectoris, tolerance, and other adverse reactions. Perform clinical or hemodynamic monitoring with use during the early days of AMI.

Patient Counseling: Inform about the risks and benefits of therapy. Instruct to use ud and not to use with certain medications for erectile dysfunction (PDE5 inhibitors) because of the risk of hypotension. Instruct to familiarize with the position of the spray orifice to facilitate orientation for administration at night.

Administration: Sublingual route. Do not inhale. Do not shake. Do not expectorate medication or rinse mouth for 5-10 min after administration. Refer to PI for further administration instructions. **Storage:** 25°C (77°F); excursions permitted to 15-30°C (59-85°F). Do not forcefully open, burn container after use, or spray toward flames.

NITROSTAT

RX

nitroglycerin (Parke-Davis)

THERAPEUTIC CLASS: Nitrate vasodilator

INDICATIONS: Acute relief of an attack or acute prophylaxis of angina pectoris due to coronary artery disease.

DOSAGE: *Adults:* Treatment: 1 tab SL or in buccal pouch at 1st sign of acute attack. May repeat every 5 min until relief is obtained. If pain persists after a total of 3 tabs in 15 min, or if pain is different than typically experienced, prompt medical attention is recommended. Prophylaxis: Take 5-10 min prior to engaging in activities that may cause acute attack. Elderly: Start at lower end of dosing range.

HOW SUPPLIED: Tab, SL: 0.3mg, 0.4mg, 0.6mg

CONTRAINDICATIONS: Early myocardial infarction (MI), severe anemia, increased intracranial pressure (ICP), patients who are using a PDE-5 inhibitor (eg, sildenafil citrate, tadalafil, vardenafil hydrochloride).

WARNINGS/PRECAUTIONS: Use smallest dose required for effective relief of acute attack; excessive use may lead to tolerance. Severe hypotension, particularly with upright posture, may occur with small doses; caution with volume-depletion or hypotension. Nitroglycerin-induced hypotension may be accompanied by paradoxical bradycardia and increased angina pectoris. May aggravate angina caused by hypertrophic cardiomyopathy. As tolerance to other forms of nitroglycerin develops, effect on exercise tolerance is blunted. Physical dependence may occur. D/C if blurred vision or dry mouth occurs. Excessive dosage may produce severe headaches. SL nitroglycerin may cause nitrate tolerance in patients who maintain high continuous nitrate levels for more than 10-12 hrs daily. Caution in elderly.

ADVERSE REACTIONS: Headache, vertigo, dizziness, weakness, palpitation, syncope, flushing, drug rash, exfoliative dermatitis.

INTERACTIONS: See Contraindications. Antihypertensive drugs, β-adrenergic blockers, or phenothiazines may cause additive hypotensive effects. Calcium channel blockers may cause marked orthostatic hypotension. Alcohol may cause hypotension. Aspirin may enhance vasodilatory and hemodynamic effects. Caution with alteplase therapy. IV nitroglycerin reduces anticoagulant effect of heparin; monitor activated PTT during concomitant use. TCAs (eg, amitriptyline, desipramine, doxepin) and anticholinergics may make SL tab dissolution difficult. Avoid ergotamine and related drugs or monitor for ergotism symptoms if unavoidable. Long-acting nitrates may decrease therapeutic effect.

PREGNANCY: Category C, caution in nursing.

MECHANISM OF ACTION: Nitrate vasodilator; forms free radical nitric oxide that activates guanylate cyclase, resulting in an increase of guanosine 3'5' monophosphate in smooth muscle and other tissues leading to dephosphorylation of myosin light chains, which regulate contractile state in smooth muscle, resulting in vasodilatation. **PHARMACOKINETICS: Absorption:** (SL) Rapid. Absolute bioavailability (40%). (0.3mg x 2 doses) C_{max}=2.3ng/mL, T_{max}=6.4 min, AUC=14.9ng•mL/min; (0.6mg x 1 dose) C_{max}=2.1ng/mL, T_{max}=7.2 min, AUC=14.9ng•mL/min. **Distribution:** (IV) V_d=3.3L/kg; plasma protein binding (60%). **Metabolism:** Liver via reductase enzyme to glycerol nitrate metabolites to glycerol and organic nitrate; 1,2- and 1,3-dinitroglycerin (major metabolites). **Elimination:** $T_{1/2}$=2.8 min (0.3mg x 2 doses), 2.6 min (0.6mg x 1 dose).

NURSING CONSIDERATIONS

Assessment: Assess for early MI, severe anemia, increased ICP, hypotension, volume depletion, angina caused by hypertrophic cardiomyopathy, known hypersensitivity to the drug, pregnancy/nursing status, and possible drug interactions.

Monitoring: Monitor for hypotension, paradoxical bradycardia, increased/aggravated angina pectoris, tolerance, physical dependence, blurring of vision, drying of mouth, headache, and other adverse reactions. In patients with an acute MI or congestive heart failure, perform careful clinical or hemodynamic monitoring for hypotension and tachycardia.

Patient Counseling: Counsel on the proper dosage and administration of the drug. Instruct to take tab sublingually; do not chew, crush, or swallow. Advise to sit down when taking the drug and to use caution when returning to standing position. Inform about side effects of the drug (eg, headaches, lightheadedness upon standing, burning or tingling sensation when administered SL). Counsel that lightheadedness may be more frequent in patients who have consumed alcohol. Instruct to keep in original glass container and to tightly cap after each use.

Administration: SL route. Do not swallow tabs; intended for SL or buccal administration. Administer in sitting position. **Storage:** 20-25°C (68-77°F).

NIZATIDINE RX

nizatidine (Sandoz)

OTHER BRAND NAMES: Axid (Braintree)

THERAPEUTIC CLASS: H_2-blocker

INDICATIONS: Treatment of active duodenal ulcer (DU) and benign gastric ulcer (GU) for up to 8 weeks. Maintenance therapy for DU after healing of an active DU. Treatment of endoscopically diagnosed esophagitis, including erosive and ulcerative esophagitis, and heartburn due to gastroesophageal reflux disease (GERD) for up to 12 weeks. (Sol) Treatment of endoscopically diagnosed esophagitis, including erosive and ulcerative esophagitis, and heartburn due to GERD for up to 8 weeks in pediatrics ≥12 yrs of age.

DOSAGE: *Adults:* Active DU/Active Benign GU: Usual: 300mg qhs or 150mg bid up to 8 weeks. Maint of Healed Active DU: 150mg qhs up to 1 yr. GERD: 150mg bid up to 12 weeks. Renal Impairment: CrCl 20-50mL/min: 150mg/day. Maint: 150mg qod. CrCl <20mL/min: 150mg qod. Maint: 150mg every 3 days.
Pediatrics: ≥12 Yrs: (Sol) Erosive Esophagitis/GERD: 150mg bid up to 8 weeks. Max: 300mg/day. Renal Impairment: CrCl 20-50mL/min: 150mg/day. Maint: 150mg qod. CrCl <20mL/min: 150mg qod. Maint: 150mg every 3 days.

HOW SUPPLIED: Cap: 150mg, 300mg; Sol: (Axid) 15mg/mL [480mL]

WARNINGS/PRECAUTIONS: Caution with moderate to severe renal insufficiency; reduce dose. Symptomatic response does not preclude the presence of gastric malignancy. False positive tests for urobilinogen with Multistix may occur. Caution in elderly.

ADVERSE REACTIONS: Headache, abdominal pain, pain, asthenia, diarrhea, N/V, flatulence, dyspepsia, rhinitis, pharyngitis, dizziness, cough, fever, irritability.

INTERACTIONS: May elevate serum salicylate levels with high dose (3900mg/day) aspirin. Inhibits gastric acid secretion stimulated by caffeine, betazole, and pentagastrin. May decrease absorption with antacids consisting of aluminum and magnesium hydroxides with simethicone. Fatal thrombocytopenia reported with concomitant use of another H_2-receptor antagonist.

PREGNANCY: Category B, not for use in nursing.

MECHANISM OF ACTION: H_2-receptor antagonist; competitive, reversible inhibitor of histamine at the histamine H_2-receptors, particularly those in the gastric parietal cells.

PHARMACOKINETICS: Absorption: Absolute bioavailability (>70%); C_{max}=700-1800mcg/L (150mg dose), 1400-3600mcg/L (300mg dose); T_{max}=0.5-3 hrs. **Distribution:** V_d=0.8-1.5L/kg; plasma protein binding (35%); found in breast milk. **Metabolism:** N2-monodesmethylnizatidine (principal metabolite). **Elimination:** Urine (>90%, 60% unchanged); feces (<6%); $T_{1/2}$=1-2 hrs, 3.5-11 hrs.

NURSING CONSIDERATIONS

Assessment: Assess for hypersensitivity to other H$_2$-receptor antagonists, renal dysfunction, presence of gastric malignancy, pregnancy/nursing status, and possible drug interactions.

Monitoring: Monitor for hypersensitivity, other adverse reactions, and signs of clinical improvement.

Patient Counseling: Inform of the risks/benefits of therapy. Advise to take medication exactly as prescribed. Instruct to contact physician if signs/symptoms of hypersensitivity or other adverse reaction develops. Counsel pregnant/nursing females about risks of use.

Administration: Oral route. **Storage:** Cap: 20-25°C (68-77°F). Sol: 25°C (77°F); excursions permitted to 15-30°C (59-86°F).

NORCO
hydrocodone bitartrate - acetaminophen (Watson)

CIII

> Associated with cases of acute liver failure, at times resulting in liver transplant and death. Most cases of liver injury are associated with acetaminophen (APAP) use at doses >4000mg/day, and often involve >1 APAP-containing product.

THERAPEUTIC CLASS: Opioid analgesic

INDICATIONS: Relief of moderate to moderately severe pain.

DOSAGE: *Adults:* Adjust dose according to severity of pain and response. (5mg-325mg) Usual: 1 or 2 tabs q4-6h PRN. Max: 8 tabs/day. (7.5mg-325mg, 10mg-325mg) Usual: 1 tab q4-6h PRN. Max: 6 tabs/day. Elderly: Start at lower end of dosing range.

HOW SUPPLIED: Tab: (Hydrocodone-APAP) 5mg-325mg*, 7.5mg-325mg*, 10mg-325mg* *scored

WARNINGS/PRECAUTIONS: Increased risk of acute liver failure in patients with underlying liver disease. Hypersensitivity and anaphylaxis reported; d/c if signs/symptoms occur. May produce dose-related respiratory depression at high doses or in sensitive patients, and irregular and periodic breathing. Respiratory depressant effects and capacity for elevating CSF pressure may be markedly exaggerated in the presence of head injury, other intracranial lesions, or a preexisting increase in intracranial pressure. May obscure diagnosis or clinical course of head injuries and acute abdominal conditions. Caution with severe hepatic/renal impairment, hypothyroidism, Addison's disease, prostatic hypertrophy, urethral stricture, and in elderly or debilitated patients. Suppresses the cough reflex; caution in postoperative use and in patients with pulmonary disease. May impair mental/physical abilities. Lab test interactions may occur. Physical dependence and tolerance may develop.

ADVERSE REACTIONS: Acute liver failure, lightheadedness, dizziness, sedation, N/V.

INTERACTIONS: Increased risk of acute liver failure with alcohol ingestion. Additive CNS depression with narcotics, antihistamines, antipsychotics, antianxiety agents, or other CNS depressants (eg, alcohol); avoid concurrent use, or use in reduced dosages. Concomitant use with MAOIs or TCAs may increase the effect of either the antidepressant or hydrocodone.

PREGNANCY: Category C, not for use in nursing.

MECHANISM OF ACTION: Hydrocodone: Opioid analgesic; has not been established. Believed to relate to the existence of opiate receptors in the CNS. APAP: Nonopiate, nonsalicylate analgesic, and antipyretic; has not been established. Involves peripheral influences. Antipyretic activity is mediated through hypothalamic heat-regulating centers. Inhibits prostaglandin synthetase.

PHARMACOKINETICS: Absorption: Hydrocodone: (10mg) C_{max}=23.6ng/mL; T_{max}=1.3 hrs. APAP: Rapid. **Distribution:** APAP: Found in breast milk. **Metabolism:** Hydrocodone: O-demethylation, N-demethylation, and 6-ketoreduction. APAP: Liver via conjugation. **Elimination:** Hydrocodone: (10mg) $T_{1/2}$=3.8 hrs. APAP: Urine (85%); $T_{1/2}$=1.25-3 hrs.

NURSING CONSIDERATIONS

Assessment: Assess for level of pain intensity, type of pain, patient's general condition and medical status, or any other conditions where treatment is contraindicated or cautioned. Assess for history of drug hypersensitivity, renal/hepatic/pulmonary impairment, pregnancy/nursing status, and possible drug interactions.

Monitoring: Monitor for acute liver failure, hypersensitivity reactions, anaphylaxis, respiratory depression, elevation in CSF pressure, physical dependence, tolerance, and other adverse reactions. Monitor effects of therapy with serial LFTs and/or renal function tests in patients with severe hepatic/renal disease.

Patient Counseling: Instruct to d/c therapy and contact physician immediately if signs of allergy (eg, rash, difficulty breathing) develop. Instruct to look for APAP on package labels and not to use >1 APAP-containing product. Instruct to seek medical attention immediately upon ingestion of >4000mg/day of APAP, even if patient is feeling well. Inform that drug may impair mental/physical abilities required for the performance of potentially hazardous tasks (eg, operating machinery/driving). Instruct to avoid alcohol and other CNS depressants. Inform that drug may be habit-forming; instruct to take ud.

Administration: Oral route. **Storage:** (5mg-325mg) 15-30°C (59-86°F). (7.5mg-325mg, 10mg-325mg) 20-25°C (68-77°F).

NORDITROPIN   RX
somatropin rdna origin (Novo Nordisk)

THERAPEUTIC CLASS: Recombinant human growth hormone

INDICATIONS: Treatment of pediatric patients with growth failure due to inadequate secretion of endogenous growth hormone (GH). Treatment of pediatric patients with short stature associated with Noonan syndrome, Turner syndrome (TS), and those who were born small for gestational age (SGA) with no catch-up growth by 2-4 yrs of age. Replacement of endogenous GH in adults with adult-onset or childhood-onset GH deficiency (GHD).

DOSAGE: *Adults:* GHD: Weight-Based: Initial: ≤0.004mg/kg/day SQ. Titrate: May increase to ≤0.016mg/kg/day after 6 weeks according to individual requirements. Non-Weight Based: Initial: 0.2mg/day SQ (range, 0.15-0.30mg/day). Titrate: May increase gradually every 1-2 months by increments of 0.1-0.2mg/day based on response and serum insulin-like growth factor-I (IGF-I) concentrations. Decrease dose as necessary based on adverse events and/or serum IGF-I concentrations above the age- and gender-specific normal range. Maint: Individualize dose. Elderly: Start at lower end of dosing range and consider smaller dose increments. Estrogen-replete women may need higher doses than men.
Pediatrics: Individualize dose. GHD: 0.024-0.034mg/kg/day SQ 6-7X/week. Noonan Syndrome: Up to 0.066mg/kg/day SQ. TS/SGA: Up to 0.067mg/kg/day SQ. Refer to PI for further details.

HOW SUPPLIED: Inj: (FlexPro) 5mg/1.5mL, 10mg/1.5mL, 15mg/1.5mL; (NordiFlex) 30mg/3mL

CONTRAINDICATIONS: Acute critical illness due to complications following open heart surgery, abdominal surgery, multiple accidental trauma, or with acute respiratory failure. Pediatric patients with Prader-Willi syndrome (PWS) who are severely obese, with history of upper airway obstruction or sleep apnea, or have severe respiratory impairment. Pediatric patients with growth failure due to genetically confirmed PWS. Active malignancy, or progression or recurrence of underlying intracranial tumor. Active proliferative or severe nonproliferative diabetic retinopathy. Growth promotion in pediatric patients with closed epiphyses.

WARNINGS/PRECAUTIONS: Reevaluate adults with epiphyseal closure previously treated with replacement therapy in childhood. Treatment for short stature should be discontinued when epiphyses are fused. Implement effective weight control in patients with PWS and treat respiratory infections aggressively. Monitor for malignant transformation of skin lesions. Undiagnosed impaired glucose tolerance and overt diabetes mellitus (DM) may be unmasked, and new-onset type 2 DM reported. Intracranial HTN with papilledema, visual changes, headache, N/V reported; d/c therapy if papilledema occurs. Fluid retention in adults may occur. Hypothyroidism may become evident or worsen, and undiagnosed/untreated hypothyroidism may prevent optimal response. Monitor other hormonal replacement treatments in patients with hypopituitarism. Slipped capital femoral epiphysis and progression of scoliosis may occur in pediatric patients. Increased risk of ear/hearing disorders and cardiovascular (CV) disorders in TS patients. Tissue atrophy may occur; rotate inj site. Allergic reactions may occur. Serum levels of inorganic phosphorus, alkaline phosphatase, parathyroid hormone, and IGF-I may increase. Pancreatitis rarely reported. Caution in elderly.

ADVERSE REACTIONS: Gastroenteritis, ear infection, influenza, inj-site reaction, peripheral/leg edema, arthralgia, headache, increased sweating, myalgia, bronchitis, flu-like symptoms, HTN, paresthesia, skeletal pain, laryngitis.

INTERACTIONS: Use with glucocorticoid therapy may attenuate growth-promoting effects in children; carefully adjust glucocorticoid replacement dosing. Inhibits 11β-hydroxysteroid dehydrogenase type 1, resulting in reduced serum cortisol concentrations; may need glucocorticoid replacement/dose adjustments in glucocorticoid therapy (eg, cortisone acetate, prednisone). May alter clearance of compounds metabolized by CYP450 liver enzymes (eg, corticosteroids, anticonvulsants, cyclosporine); monitor carefully. May increase clearance of antipyrine. May require greater dose with oral estrogen replacement. May need to adjust dose of antihyperglycemics and thyroid hormone replacement therapy.

PREGNANCY: Category C, caution in nursing.

MECHANISM OF ACTION: Recombinant human GH; binds to dimeric GH receptor in cell membrane of target cells, resulting in intracellular signal transduction.

PHARMACOKINETICS: Absorption: T_{max}=4-5 hrs; C_{max}=13.8ng/mL (4mg), 17.1ng/mL (8mg). **Elimination:** $T_{1/2}$=7-10 hrs.

NURSING CONSIDERATIONS

Assessment: Assess for PWS, preexisting DM or impaired glucose tolerance, diabetic retinopathy, active malignancy, history of scoliosis, hypothyroidism, hypopituitarism, any other conditions where treatment is contraindicated or cautioned, pregnancy/nursing status, and possible drug interactions. Perform funduscopic exam.

Monitoring: Monitor for growth, clinical response, compliance, malignant transformation of skin lesions, fluid retention, intracranial HTN, allergic reactions, pancreatitis, and slipped capital femoral epiphysis and progression of scoliosis in pediatric patients (eg, onset of limp, hip or knee pain). Perform periodic thyroid function tests, funduscopic exam, and monitor glucose levels. In patients with PWS, monitor weight as well as signs of respiratory infections, sleep apnea, and upper airway obstruction. In patients with preexisting tumors or GHD secondary to intracranial lesion, monitor for progression/recurrence of underlying disease process. In patients with TS, monitor for ear/hearing/CV disorders.

Patient Counseling: Inform about potential benefits and risks of therapy, proper administration, usage and disposal, and caution against any reuse of needles and syringes.

Administration: SQ route. Refer to PI for preparation and administration instructions. **Storage:** Unused: 2-8°C (36-46°F). Do not freeze. Avoid direct light. In-use: 2-8°C (36-46°F) and use within 4 weeks or store at ≤25°C (77°F) for up to 3 weeks. Discard unused portions.

NORINYL 1/50   RX
norethindrone - mestranol (Watson)

> Cigarette smoking increases the risk of serious CV side effects. Risk increases with age (>35 yrs) and with heavy smoking (≥15 cigarettes/day). Women who use oral contraceptives should be strongly advised not to smoke.

OTHER BRAND NAMES: Necon 1/50 (Watson)

THERAPEUTIC CLASS: Estrogen/progestogen combination

INDICATIONS: Prevention of pregnancy.

DOSAGE: *Adults:* 1 tab qd for 28 days, then repeat. Start 1st Sunday after menses begin or 1st day of menses.
Pediatrics: Postpubertal Adolescents: 1 tab qd for 28 days, then repeat. Start 1st Sunday after menses begin or 1st day of menses.

HOW SUPPLIED: Tab: (Mestranol-Norethindrone) 0.05mg-1mg

CONTRAINDICATIONS: Thrombophlebitis, thromboembolic disorders, history of deep vein thrombophlebitis (DVT), cerebral vascular or coronary artery disease, carcinoma of the endometrium or other known or suspected estrogen-dependent neoplasia, undiagnosed abnormal genital bleeding, cholestatic jaundice of pregnancy or jaundice with prior pill use, hepatic adenomas or carcinomas, known or suspected carcinoma of the breast, and pregnancy. (Norinyl 1/50) Benign liver tumors.

WARNINGS/PRECAUTIONS: Increased risk of myocardial infarction, vascular disease, thromboembolism, stroke, gallbladder disease, and hepatic neoplasia. Increased risk of morbidity and mortality in patients with HTN, hyperlipidemias, obesity, and diabetes. May increase risk of breast cancer and cancer of the reproductive organs. Retinal thrombosis reported; d/c if unexplained partial or complete loss of vision occurs, onset of proptosis or diplopia, papilledema, or retinal vascular lesions develop. May cause glucose intolerance; monitor prediabetic and diabetic patients. May cause fluid retention and increase BP; monitor closely and d/c if significant elevation of BP occurs. Breakthrough bleeding and spotting reported; rule out malignancy or pregnancy. May cause onset or exacerbation of a migraine or development of a headache. May develop visual changes with contact lenses. May elevate LDL levels or cause other lipid effects. D/C if jaundice develops. Caution with history of depression; d/c if depression recurs to serious degree. Not indicated for use before menarche. Does not protect against HIV infection (AIDS) and other sexually transmitted diseases (STDs). May affect certain endocrine, LFTs, and blood components in laboratory tests. Ectopic and intrauterine pregnancies may occur with contraceptive failures. Should not be used to induce withdrawal bleeding as a test for pregnancy, or to treat threatened or habitual abortion during pregnancy.

ADVERSE REACTIONS: N/V, breakthrough bleeding, spotting, amenorrhea, migraine, mental depression, vaginal candidiasis, edema, weight changes, abdominal cramps/bloating, menstrual flow changes, melasma.

INTERACTIONS: Reduced effects, increased breakthrough bleeding, and menstrual irregularities with rifampin, barbiturates, phenylbutazone, phenytoin Na⁺, and possibly with griseofulvin, ampicillin, tetracyclines, and (Necon 1/50) carbamazepine.

PREGNANCY: Category X, not for use in nursing.

MECHANISM OF ACTION: Estrogen/progestogen oral contraceptive; suppresses gonadotropins. Primarily inhibits ovulation. Also causes changes in cervical mucus (increases difficulty of sperm entry into uterus) and endometrium (reduces likelihood of implantation).

PHARMACOKINETICS: Distribution: Found in breast milk.

NURSING CONSIDERATIONS

Assessment: Assess for thrombophlebitis, thromboembolic disorders, history of DVT or thromboembolic disorders, any other conditions where treatment is contraindicated or cautioned. Assess for pregnancy/nursing status, and for possible drug interactions. Assess use in patients with hyperlipidemia, HTN, obesity, diabetes, history of depression, and in patients >35 yrs of age who smoke ≥15 cigarettes/day. (Norinyl 1/50) Assess for benign liver tumors.

Monitoring: Monitor for MI, thromboembolism, stroke, and other adverse effects. Monitor glucose levels in diabetic or prediabetic patients, BP with history of HTN, and lipid levels with history of hyperlipidemia. Monitor for signs of liver dysfunction (eg, jaundice), and signs of worsening depression with previous history. Refer patients with contact lenses to ophthalmologist if ocular changes develop. Perform annual physical exam while on therapy.

Patient Counseling: Inform that therapy does not protect against HIV infection and other STDs. Inform of potential risks/benefits of oral contraceptives. When initiating treatment, instruct to use additional form of contraception until after 7 days on therapy. Instruct to take 1 pill at same time daily at intervals not exceeding 24 hrs. Inform that if dose is missed, to take as soon as possible; instruct to take next dose at regularly scheduled time. Instruct to continue medication if spotting or breakthrough bleeding occurs; instruct to notify physician if symptoms persist. Inform that missing a pill can cause spotting or light bleeding. Advise not to smoke while on therapy.

Administration: Oral route. **Storage:** 15-25°C (59-77°F) (Norinyl 1/50); 20-25°C (68-77°F) (Necon 1/50).

NOROXIN   RX
norfloxacin (Merck)

> Fluoroquinolones are associated with an increased risk of tendinitis and tendon rupture in all ages. Risk is further increased in patients >60 yrs, patients taking corticosteroids, and with kidney, heart, or lung transplants. May exacerbate muscle weakness with myasthenia gravis; avoid in patients with known history of myasthenia gravis.

THERAPEUTIC CLASS: Fluoroquinolone

INDICATIONS: Treatment of complicated and uncomplicated urinary tract infections (UTIs) (including cystitis), uncomplicated urethral and cervical gonorrhea, and prostatitis caused by susceptible strains of designated microorganisms in adults.

DOSAGE: *Adults:* Uncomplicated Gonorrhea: 800mg single dose. Acute/Chronic Prostatitis: 400mg q12h for 28 days. Uncomplicated UTIs: 400mg q12h for 3 days (*Escherichia coli, Klebsiella pneumoniae,* or *Proteus mirabilis*) or 7-10 days (other organisms). Complicated UTIs: 400mg q12h for 10-21 days. Renal Impairment (CrCl ≤30mL/min/1.73m^2): 400mg qd.

HOW SUPPLIED: Tab: 400mg

CONTRAINDICATIONS: History of tendinitis or tendon rupture associated with use of quinolones.

WARNINGS/PRECAUTIONS: D/C if pain, swelling, inflammation, or rupture of a tendon occurs. Convulsions reported. Increased intracranial pressure (ICP) (including pseudotumor cerebri), toxic psychoses, and CNS stimulation may occur; d/c and institute appropriate measures if CNS events occur. Caution with known or suspected CNS disorders (eg, severe cerebral arteriosclerosis, epilepsy) or other factors that predispose to seizures. Serious and occasionally fatal hypersensitivity (anaphylactic) reactions reported; d/c immediately at the 1st appearance of a skin rash, jaundice, or any other sign of hypersensitivity and institute supportive measures. *Clostridium difficile*-associated diarrhea (CDAD) reported; d/c if CDAD is suspected or confirmed. Rare cases of sensory or sensorimotor axonal polyneuropathy, resulting in paresthesias, hypoesthesias, dysesthesias, and weakness reported; d/c if symptoms of neuropathy occur. Not shown to be effective in the treatment of syphilis. May mask or delay symptoms of incubating syphilis if used in high doses for short periods of time to treat gonorrhea; perform serologic test for syphilis at the time of gonorrhea diagnosis and repeat after 3 months of therapy. Maintain adequate hydration. May cause photosensitivity/phototoxicity reactions; d/c if phototoxicity occurs. Avoid excessive exposure to sun/UV light. Hemolytic reactions reported with G6PD deficiency. May result in bacterial resistance if used in the absence of a proven/suspected bacterial infection or a prophylactic indication. Caution with risk factors for torsades de pointes (eg, known QT prolongation, uncorrected hypokalemia). Caution in elderly and in patients with renal impairment.

ADVERSE REACTIONS: Tendinitis, tendon rupture, dizziness, nausea, headache, abdominal cramping, asthenia, rash.

INTERACTIONS: See Boxed Warning. Concomitant use with drugs metabolized by CYP1A2 (eg, caffeine, clozapine, ropinirole, tacrine, theophylline, tizanidine) may result in increased substrate drug concentrations when given in usual doses. May increase theophylline and cyclosporine levels; monitor levels and adjust dose of theophylline and cyclosporine as required. May enhance effects of oral anticoagulants, including warfarin or its derivatives; closely monitor PT or other suitable coagulation tests. On rare occasions, may result in severe hypoglycemia if coadministered with glyburide (a sulfonylurea agent); monitor blood glucose levels. Diminished urinary excretion with probenecid. Avoid with nitrofurantoin; may antagonize antibacterial effect in the urinary tract. Multivitamins or other products containing iron or zinc, antacids or sucralfate, and didanosine (chewable/buffered tabs, pediatric oral sol) may interfere with absorption; space dose by 2 hrs. May reduce clearance of caffeine. Caution with NSAIDs; may increase the risk of CNS stimulation and convulsive seizures. Caution with drugs that can result in prolongation of the QT interval (eg, Class IA or Class III antiarrhythmics).

PREGNANCY: Category C, not for use in nursing.

MECHANISM OF ACTION: Fluoroquinolone; inhibits bacterial DNA synthesis, inhibits ATP-dependent DNA supercoiling reaction catalyzed by DNA gyrase, inhibits relaxation of supercoiled DNA, and promotes double-stranded DNA breakage.

PHARMACOKINETICS: Absorption: Rapid; C_{max}=0.8mcg/mL (200mg), 1.5mcg/mL (400mg), 2.4mcg/mL (800mg); T_{max}=1 hr. Refer to PI for different pharmacokinetic parameters of different age groups. **Distribution:** Plasma protein binding (10-15%). **Elimination:** Urine (26-32% unchanged, 5-8% active metabolites); feces (30%); $T_{1/2}$=3-4 hrs.

NURSING CONSIDERATIONS

Assessment: Assess for risk factors for developing tendinitis and tendon rupture, history of myasthenia gravis, drug hypersensitivity, CNS disorders or factors that may predispose to seizures, QT interval prolongation, uncorrected hypokalemia, G6PD deficiency, renal impairment, pregnancy/nursing status, and possible drug interactions. Obtain culture and susceptibility tests. Perform serologic test for syphilis in patients with gonorrhea.

Monitoring: Monitor for tendinitis, tendon rupture, convulsions, increased ICP, toxic psychoses, CNS stimulation, CDAD, peripheral neuropathy, photosensitivity/phototoxicity reactions, hypersensitivity reactions, and other adverse reactions. Monitor for muscle weakness in patients with myasthenia gravis. Periodically repeat culture and susceptibility testing during therapy. Perform follow-up serologic test for syphilis after 3 months in patients with gonorrhea.

Patient Counseling: Inform that drug only treats bacterial, not viral (eg, common cold), infections. Instruct to take exactly ud; advise that skipping doses or not completing full course may decrease effectiveness and increase resistance. Instruct to notify physician if symptoms of pain, swelling, or inflammation of a tendon, or weakness or inability to move joints occur; advise to rest and refrain from exercise and to d/c therapy. Instruct to inform physician of any history of QT prolongation, proarrhythmic conditions, or convulsions. Inform to d/c and notify physician if an allergic reaction, skin rash, or symptoms of peripheral neuropathy develop. Instruct to notify physician if patient experiences worsening muscle weakness or breathing problems, sunburn-like reaction or skin eruption, or if watery and bloody stools (even ≥2 months after last dose) develop. Inform that drug may cause dizziness and lightheadedness; caution with activities requiring mental alertness and coordination. Advise to minimize or avoid exposure to natural or artificial sunlight (eg, tanning beds or UVA/B treatment). Instruct to notify physician of all medications currently being used.

Administration: Oral route. Take at least 1 hr ac or at least 2 hrs pc or ingestion of milk and/or other dairy products. Take with a glass of water. Space dose by 2 hrs from multivitamins or other products containing iron or zinc, antacids, or Videx (didanosine) chewable/buffered tabs or the pediatric powder for oral sol. **Storage:** 25°C (77°F); excursions permitted to 15-30°C (59-86°F).

NORPACE   RX
disopyramide phosphate (Pharmacia & Upjohn)

> In a long-term clinical study in patients with asymptomatic non-life-threatening ventricular arrhythmias who had a myocardial infarction, an excessive mortality or non-fatal cardiac arrest rate was seen in patients treated with encainide or flecainide compared to placebo. Considering the known proarrhythmic properties of Norpace or Norpace CR and the lack of evidence of improved survival, its use should be reserved for patients with life-threatening ventricular arrhythmias.

OTHER BRAND NAMES: Norpace CR (Pharmacia & Upjohn)

THERAPEUTIC CLASS: Class I antiarrhythmic

INDICATIONS: Treatment of documented life-threatening ventricular arrhythmias.

DOSAGE: *Adults:* Usual: 400-800mg/day in divided dose. Recommended: 150mg q6h immediate-release (IR) or 300mg q12h extended-release (CR). Adjust dose with anticholinergic effects. Weight <110 lbs/Moderate Hepatic or Renal Insufficiency (CrCl >40mL/min): 100mg q6h IR or

200mg q12h CR. Severe Renal Insufficiency (with or without initial 150mg LD): CrCl 30-40mL/min: 100mg q8h IR. CrCl 15-30mL/min: 100mg q12h IR. CrCl <15mL/min: 100mg q24h IR. Rapid Control of Ventricular Arrhythmia: LD: 300mg IR (200mg if <110 lbs). Follow with maint dose. Cardiomyopathy/Cardiac Decompensation: Initial: 100mg q6-8h IR. Adjust gradually. See PI if no response or toxicity occurs. Elderly: Start at low end of dosing range.
Pediatrics: 12-18 Yrs: 6-15mg/kg/day. 4-12 Yrs: 10-15mg/kg/day. 1-4 Yrs: 10-20mg/kg/day. <1 Yr: 10-30mg/kg/day. Give in equally divided doses q6h. Hospitalize patient during initial therapy. Start dose titration at lower end of range.

HOW SUPPLIED: Cap: (Norpace) 100mg, 150mg; Cap, Extended-Release: (Norpace CR) 100mg, 150mg

CONTRAINDICATIONS: Cardiogenic shock, 2nd- or 3rd-degree atrioventricular block (if no pacemaker present), congenital QT prolongation.

WARNINGS/PRECAUTIONS: May cause or worsen congestive heart failure (CHF) and produce hypotension due to negative inotropic properties. Reduce dose if 1st-degree heart block occurs. Avoid with urinary retention, glaucoma, and myasthenia gravis unless adequate overriding measures taken. Atrial flutter/fibrillation; digitalize 1st. Monitor closely or withdraw if QT prolongation >25% occurs and ectopy continues. D/C if QRS widening >25% occurs. Avoid LD with cardiomyopathy or cardiac decompensation. Correct K^+ abnormalities before therapy. Reduce dose with renal/hepatic dysfunction; monitor ECG. Avoid CR formulation with CrCl ≤40mL/min. Caution with sick sinus syndrome, Wolff-Parkinson-White syndrome, bundle branch block, or elderly. May significantly lower blood glucose.

ADVERSE REACTIONS: Dry mouth, urinary retention/frequency/urgency, constipation, blurred vision, GI effects, dizziness, fatigue, headache.

INTERACTIONS: Avoid type IA and IC antiarrhythmics, and propranolol except in unresponsive, life-threatening arrhythmias. Hepatic enzyme inducers may lower levels. Avoid within 48 hrs before or 24 hrs after verapamil. Possible fatal interactions with CYP3A4 inhibitors. Monitor blood glucose with β-blockers, alcohol.

PREGNANCY: Category C, not for use in nursing.

MECHANISM OF ACTION: Type I antiarrhythmic; decreases rate of diastolic depolarization in cells with augmented automaticity, decreases upstroke velocity, and increases action potential duration of normal cardiac cells. Decreases disparity in refractoriness between infracted and adjacent normally perfused myocardium and has no effect on α- or β-adrenergic receptors.

PHARMACOKINETICS: Absorption: Rapid and complete; C_{max} =2.22mcg/mL, T_{max} =4.5 hrs. **Distribution:** Plasma protein binding (50-65%). **Metabolism:** Liver. **Elimination:** Urine (50% unchanged), (20% mono-N-dealkylated metabolite), (10% other metabolite); $T_{1/2}$ =11.65 hrs.

NURSING CONSIDERATIONS

Assessment: Prior to therapy, patients with atrial flutter/fibrillation should be digitalized and K^+ abnormalities should be corrected. Assess for cardiogenic shock, preexisting 2nd- or 3rd-degree heart block, presence of functioning pacemaker, sick sinus syndrome (bradycardia/tachycardia syndrome), Wolff-Parkinson-White syndrome, bundle branch block, congenital QT prolongation, myocardial infarction, life-threatening arrhythmia, CHF, cardiomyopathy or myocarditis, chronic malnutrition, hepatic/renal impairment, alcohol intake, glaucoma, myasthenia gravis, urinary retention or BPH, pregnancy/nursing status, and possible drug interactions.

Monitoring: Monitor for hypotension, HF, PR interval prolongation, widening of QRS, hypoglycemia, heart block, urinary retention, and myasthenia crisis.

Patient Counseling: Inform about risks/benefits; report adverse reactions. Instruct to notify physician if pregnant/nursing.

Administration: Oral route. **Storage:** 25°C (77°F); excursions permitted to 15-30°C (59-86°F).

NORVASC   RX
amlodipine besylate (Pfizer)

THERAPEUTIC CLASS: Calcium channel blocker (dihydropyridine)

INDICATIONS: Treatment of HTN or coronary artery disease (CAD), including chronic stable or vasospastic (Prinzmetal's/variant) angina, alone or in combination with other antihypertensives or antianginals, respectively. To reduce risks of hospitalization due to angina and to reduce the risk of coronary revascularization procedure in patients with recently documented CAD by angiography and without heart failure or ejection fraction <40%.

DOSAGE: *Adults:* HTN: Initial: 5mg qd. Adjust according to BP goals; wait 7-14 days between titration steps. If clinically warranted, titrate more rapidly and assess patient frequently. Max: 10mg qd. Small/Fragile/Elderly/Hepatic Insufficiency/Concomitant Antihypertensives: 2.5mg qd. Chronic Stable/Vasospastic Angina: Usual: 5-10mg qd. Elderly/Hepatic Insufficiency: Give lower

dose. CAD: Usual: 5-10mg qd. Elderly: Start at lower end of dosing range.
Pediatrics: 6-17 Yrs: HTN: Usual: 2.5-5mg qd. Max: 5mg qd.

HOW SUPPLIED: Tab: 2.5mg, 5mg, 10mg

WARNINGS/PRECAUTIONS: May cause symptomatic hypotension, particularly in patients with severe aortic stenosis. Worsening angina and acute myocardial infarction (MI) may develop after starting or increasing the dose, particularly with severe obstructive CAD. Titrate slowly in patients with severe hepatic impairment, and caution in elderly.

ADVERSE REACTIONS: Edema, palpitations, dizziness, fatigue, flushing.

INTERACTIONS: Diltiazem increased systemic exposure in elderly hypertensive patients. Strong inhibitors of CYP3A4 (eg, ketoconazole, itraconazole, ritonavir) may increase plasma concentrations to greater extent; monitor for symptoms of hypotension and edema with CYP3A4 inhibitors. Monitor BP if coadministered with CYP3A4 inducers. May increase simvastatin exposure; limit dose of simvastatin to 20mg daily. Increased cyclosporine trough levels reported in renal transplant patients.

PREGNANCY: Category C, not for use in nursing.

MECHANISM OF ACTION: Calcium channel blocker (dihydropyridine); inhibits the transmembrane influx of Ca^{2+} ions into vascular smooth muscle and cardiac muscle. Acts directly on vascular smooth muscle to cause a reduction in peripheral vascular resistance and reduction in BP.

PHARMACOKINETICS: Absorption: Absolute bioavailability (64-90%); T_{max}=6-12 hrs. **Distribution:** Plasma protein binding (93%). **Metabolism:** Hepatic. **Elimination:** Urine (10% parent compound; 60% metabolites), $T_{1/2}$=30-50 hrs.

NURSING CONSIDERATIONS

Assessment: Assess for hypersensitivity to the drug, severe aortic stenosis, hepatic function, pregnancy/nursing status, and possible drug interactions. Obtain baseline BP.

Monitoring: Monitor for worsening of angina, MI, and other adverse reactions. Monitor BP.

Patient Counseling: Inform of the risks/benefits of therapy. Counsel about potential adverse effects; advise to seek medical attention if any develop. Instruct to take as prescribed.

Administration: Oral route. **Storage:** 15-30°C (59-86°F).

NORVIR
RX
ritonavir (AbbVie)

Coadministration with several classes of drugs, including sedative hypnotics, antiarrhythmics, or ergot alkaloid preparations may result in potentially serious and/or life-threatening adverse events due to possible effects of ritonavir (RTV) on the hepatic metabolism of certain drugs. Review medications taken by patients prior to prescribing RTV or when prescribing other medications to patients already taking RTV.

THERAPEUTIC CLASS: Protease inhibitor

INDICATIONS: Treatment of HIV-1 infection in combination with other antiretrovirals.

DOSAGE: *Adults:* Initial: 300mg bid. Titrate: Increase at 2- to 3-day intervals by 100mg bid. Maint/Max: 600mg bid. Elderly: Start at lower end of dosing range. Take with meals. Refer to PI for general dosing guidelines.
Pediatrics: >1 Month: Initial: 250mg/m² bid. Titrate: Increase at 2- to 3-day intervals by 50mg/m² bid. Maint: 350-400mg/m² bid or highest tolerated dose. Max: 600mg bid. Take with meals. Refer to PI for pediatric dosage guidelines.

HOW SUPPLIED: Cap: 100mg; Sol: 80mg/mL [240mL]; Tab: 100mg

CONTRAINDICATIONS: Coadministration with voriconazole or St. John's wort. Coadministration of RTV with several classes of drugs (including sedative hypnotics, antiarrhythmics, or ergot alkaloid preparations) is contraindicated and may result in potentially serious and/or life-threatening adverse events due to possible effects of RTV on the hepatic metabolism of these drugs (eg, alfuzosin HCl, amiodarone, flecainide, propafenone, quinidine, dihydroergotamine, ergonovine, ergotamine, methylergonovine, cisapride, lovastatin, simvastatin, pimozide, sildenafil when used for treatment of pulmonary arterial HTN, triazolam, oral midazolam).

WARNINGS/PRECAUTIONS: Hepatic transaminase elevations >5X ULN, clinical hepatitis, and jaundice reported; increased risk with underlying hepatitis B or C. Caution with preexisting liver diseases, liver enzyme abnormalities, or hepatitis; consider increased AST/ALT monitoring, especially during first 3 months of therapy. Not recommended in severe hepatic impairment. Pancreatitis reported; d/c if diagnosed. Allergic reactions, anaphylaxis, Stevens-Johnson syndrome, and toxic epidermal necrolysis reported; d/c if severe reactions develop. Prolonged PR interval and 2nd- or 3rd-degree atrioventricular (AV) block may occur; caution with underlying structural heart disease, preexisting conduction system abnormalities, ischemic heart disease, and cardiomyopathies. May elevate TG and total cholesterol levels. New onset or exacerbation of diabetes mellitus (DM), hyperglycemia, diabetic ketoacidosis, immune reconstitution syndrome, autoimmune disorders (eg, Graves' disease, polymyositis, Guillain-Barre syndrome) in the setting of immune reconstitution, and redistribution/accumulation of body fat reported. Increased bleeding in patients with hemophilia type A and B reported. Various degrees of cross-resistance observed. Caution in elderly. (Sol) Contains alcohol and propylene glycol; do not administer to preterm neonates in the immediate postnatal period because of possible toxicities; if benefit outweighs potential risk, monitor infants closely for increases in serum osmolality and SrCr, and for drug-related toxicity.

ADVERSE REACTIONS: Diarrhea, N/V, abdominal pain, dizziness, dysgeusia, paresthesia, peripheral neuropathy, rash, fatigue/asthenia, arthralgia, back pain, coughing, oropharyngeal pain, pruritus, flushing.

INTERACTIONS: See Boxed Warning and Contraindications. Coadministration with CYP3A substrates for which elevated plasma concentrations are associated with serious and/or life-threatening reactions is contraindicated. Not recommended with fluticasone, other glucocorticoids that are metabolized by CYP3A, salmeterol, and high doses of itraconazole or ketoconazole. Avoid with colchicine in patients with renal/hepatic impairment, saquinavir/rifampin/RTV combination, avanafil, and rivaroxaban. Delavirdine may increase levels and rifampin may decrease levels. May increase levels of CYP3A or 2D6 substrates, atazanavir, darunavir, amprenavir, saquinavir, tipranavir, maraviroc, normeperidine, vincristine, vinblastine, dasatinib, nilotinib, antiarrhythmics, rivaroxaban, carbamazepine, clonazepam, ethosuximide, nefazodone, SSRIs, TCAs, desipramine, trazodone, dronabinol, ketoconazole, itraconazole, salmeterol, fluticasone, colchicine, clarithromycin, rifabutin, quinine, β-blockers, avanafil, vardenafil, sildenafil, tadalafil, calcium channel blockers, digoxin, bosentan, atorvastatin, rosuvastatin, immunosuppressants, neuroleptics, sedative/hypnotics, parenteral midazolam, glucocorticoids, methamphetamine, and fentanyl. May decrease levels of voriconazole, raltegravir, meperidine, theophylline, divalproex, lamotrigine, phenytoin, bupropion, atovaquone, methadone, and ethinyl estradiol. Caution with other drugs that prolong the PR interval, particularly with those drugs metabolized by CYP3A. May alter concentrations of warfarin (monitor INR) and indinavir. May need dose decrease of tramadol, and propoxyphene. Refer to PI for dosing modifications when used with certain concomitant therapies. (Cap/Sol) Contains alcohol; may produce disulfiram-like reactions with disulfiram or metronidazole.

PREGNANCY: Category B, not for use in nursing.

MECHANISM OF ACTION: HIV protease inhibitor; renders enzyme incapable of processing *gag-pol* polyprotein precursor, which leads to production of noninfectious immature HIV-1 particles.

PHARMACOKINETICS: Absorption: (Sol) T_{max}=2 hrs (fasting), 4 hrs (fed); (Cap) AUC=121.7, (Sol) AUC=129mg•hr/mL. **Distribution:** Plasma protein binding (98-99%). **Metabolism:** CYP3A, CYP2D6 (oxidation); isopropylthiazole (major metabolite). **Elimination:** (Sol) Urine (11.3%, 3.5% unchanged), feces (86.4%, 33.8% unchanged); $T_{1/2}$=3-5 hrs.

NURSING CONSIDERATIONS

Assessment: Assess for previous hypersensitivity to the drug, preexisting liver diseases, hepatitis, DM, hemophilia type A or B, underlying cardiac problems, lipid disorders, pregnancy/nursing status, and possible drug interactions. Obtain baseline ECG, AST, ALT, gamma-glutamyl transferase (GGT), CPK, uric acid, TG, and cholesterol levels.

Monitoring: Monitor for signs/symptoms of anaphylaxis or allergic reactions, hepatitis, jaundice, hepatic dysfunction, new onset or exacerbation of DM, hyperglycemia, diabetic ketoacidosis, pancreatitis, AV block, cardiac conduction abnormalities, immune reconstitution syndrome, autoimmune disorders, fat redistribution or accumulation, and for other adverse reactions. Monitor for bleeding in patients with hemophilia type A or B. Monitor ECG, LFTs, GGT, CPK, uric acid, TG, and cholesterol levels. Frequently monitor INR during coadministration with warfarin.

Patient Counseling: Counsel to take prescribed dose ud. Instruct to inform physician if weight changes in children occur. Inform that therapy is not a cure for HIV-1 infection and illnesses associated with HIV-1 infection may still be experienced. Advise to practice safe sex, use latex or polyurethane condoms, not to share personal items (eg, toothbrush, razor blades), needles, or other inj equipment, and not to breastfeed. Advise to notify physician of any use of Rx, OTC, or herbal products, particularly St. John's wort. Advise to use additional or alternative contraceptive measures if receiving estrogen-based hormonal contraceptives. Inform that use with certain drugs may increase risk of hypotension, visual changes, and priapism; instruct to contact physician if any of these symptoms occur. Counsel about potential adverse effects; instruct to report symptoms such as dizziness, lightheadedness, abnormal heart rhythm, or loss of consciousness.

Administration: Oral route. Take with meals. Tab: Swallow whole; do not crush, break, or chew. Sol: Shake well before use. May mix with chocolate milk, Ensure, or Advera within 1 hr of dosing. **Storage:** Cap: 2-8°C (36-46°F). May not require refrigeration if used within 30 days and stored below 25°C (77°F). Protect from light. Avoid exposure to excessive heat. Sol: 20-25°C (68-77°F). Do not refrigerate. Avoid exposure to excessive heat. Tab: ≤30°C (86°F). Exposure up to 50°C (122°F) for 7 days permitted. Dispense in original container or USP equivalent tight container (≤60mL). Exposure to high humidity outside the original or USP equivalent tight container (≤60mL) for >2 weeks is not recommended.

NOVOLIN 70/30   OTC
insulin human, rdna origin - insulin, human (isophane/regular) (Novo Nordisk)

THERAPEUTIC CLASS: Insulin

INDICATIONS: To control hyperglycemia in diabetes.

DOSAGE: *Adults:* Individualize dose.
Pediatrics: Individualize dose.

HOW SUPPLIED: Inj: (Isophane-Regular) 70 U-30 U/mL [10mL]

WARNINGS/PRECAUTIONS: Avoid in patients with hypoglycemia. Any change of insulin should be made cautiously and only under medical supervision. Hyperglycemia may occur if dosage is not taken. Hyperglycemia may lead to diabetic ketoacidosis if not treated; may cause loss of consciousness, coma, or death. May need to change dosage with illness, stress, diet change, physical activity/exercise, other medicines or surgery. May impair physical and mental abililities. Hypoglycemia may occur; monitor for symptoms of hypoglycemia (eg, sweating, dizziness, hunger, blurred vision, headache). Serious allergic reaction, inj-site reaction, hand/feet swelling, vision changes, and hypokalemia may occur. May cause lipodystrophy; rotate inj site.

ADVERSE REACTIONS: Hypoglycemia, allergic reaction, inj-site reaction, lipodystrophy, hand/feet swelling, vision changes, hypokalemia.

INTERACTIONS: Avoid with alcohol (eg, beer, wine); may affect blood glucose.

PREGNANCY: Safety not known in pregnancy/nursing.

MECHANISM OF ACTION: Insulin; structurally identical to insulin produced by the human pancreas that is used to control high blood glucose in patients with diabetes mellitus.

NURSING CONSIDERATIONS

Assessment: Assess for medical conditions, hypoglycemia, alcohol consumption, hypersensitivity, pregnancy/nursing status, and for possible drug interactions. Obtain baseline blood glucose levels.

Monitoring: Monitor for signs of hypoglycemia, hypokalemia, vision changes, lipodystrophy, inj-site reaction, hand/feet swelling, and allergic reactions. Monitor blood glucose levels.

Patient Counseling: Inform about potential risks and benefits of taking insulin and possible adverse reactions. Counsel on proper administration techniques, lifestyle management, regular blood glucose monitoring, signs and symptoms of hypoglycemia/hyperglycemia, management of hypoglycemia/hyperglycemia, and proper storage of insulin. Advise to consult physician during periods of stress, illness, diet/physical activity changes, or surgery for possible changes in insulin dosage. Instruct to exercise caution when driving or operating machinery. Instruct to always check carefully for correct type of insulin before administering. Instruct to notify physician of all medicines that are being taken.

Administration: SQ route. Inject in abdomen, upper arms, buttocks, or upper legs. Rotate inj site. Do not mix with any insulins. Refer to labeling for administration techniques. **Storage:** (Unopened) 2-8°C (36-46°F) or if refrigeration not possible, ≤25°C (77°F) for ≤6 weeks. Do not freeze. Protect from light. (Opened) <25°C (77°F) for ≤6 weeks; discard unused portion after 6 weeks. Keep away from direct heat/light.

NOVOLIN R   OTC
insulin, human regular (rdna origin) (Novo Nordisk)

THERAPEUTIC CLASS: Insulin

INDICATIONS: To improve glycemic control in adults and children with diabetes mellitus.

DOSAGE: *Adults:* Individualize dose. Usual: 0.5-1 U/kg/day. (SQ) Inject approximately 30 min prior to the start of a meal. Use with intermediate- or long-acting insulin. (IV) 0.05-1 U/mL in infusion systems with 0.9% NaCl, D5W, or D10W with 40 mmol/L of potassium chloride. Renal/Hepatic Impairment: May need to reduce dose.
Pediatrics: Individualize dose. Usual: 0.5-1 U/kg/day. (SQ) Inject approximately 30 min prior to the start of a meal. Use with intermediate- or long-acting insulin. (IV) 0.05-1 U/mL in infusion systems with 0.9% NaCl, D5W, or D10W with 40 mmol/L of potassium chloride. Renal/Hepatic Impairment: May need to reduce dose.

HOW SUPPLIED: Inj: 100 U/mL [10mL]

CONTRAINDICATIONS: Episodes of hypoglycemia.

WARNINGS/PRECAUTIONS: Any change of insulin dose should be made cautiously and only under medical supervision. Changing from one insulin product to another or changing the strength may result in the need for a change in dosage. The time course of therapy's action may vary in different individuals or at different times in the same individual and is dependent on dose, site of inj, local blood supply, temperature, and physical activity. May require dose adjustments in patients who change their level of physical activity or meal plan. Stress, illness, or emotional disturbance may alter insulin requirements. Hypoglycemia may occur; caution in patients with hypoglycemia unawareness and those predisposed to hypoglycemia (eg, those who fast or have erratic food intake, pediatrics, elderly). Hypoglycemia may impair mental/physical abilities. Hypokalemia may occur; caution in patients who may be at risk. Hyperglycemia, diabetic ketoacidosis, or hyperosmolar hyperglycemic non-ketotic syndrome may develop if taken less than needed. Redness, swelling, or itching at inj site may occur. Contains metacresol as excipient; localized reactions and generalized myalgias reported. Severe, life-threatening, generalized allergy (eg, anaphylaxis) may occur. Insulin mixtures should not be administered IV. Increases in titers of anti-insulin antibodies reported. May be administered IV under medical supervision; close monitoring of blood glucose and K$^+$ is required. Use in insulin pumps not recommended. Has not been studied in patients <2 yrs or pediatric patients with type 2 diabetes.

ADVERSE REACTIONS: Hypoglycemia, inj-site reaction, lipodystrophy, weight gain, peripheral edema, transitory reversible ophthalmologic refraction disorder, diabetic retinopathy worsening, peripheral neuropathy.

INTERACTIONS: May require dose adjustment and close monitoring with drugs that may increase blood glucose-lowering effect and susceptibility to hypoglycemia (oral antidiabetic drugs, pramlintide acetate, ACE inhibitors, disopyramide, fibrates, fluoxetine, MAOIs, propoxyphene, salicylates, somatostatin analogs [eg, octreotide], sulfonamide antibiotics), drugs that may reduce blood glucose-lowering effect leading to worsening of glycemic control (corticosteroids, niacin, danazol, diuretics, sympathomimetic agents [eg, epinephrine, salbutamol, terbutaline], isoniazid, phenothiazine derivatives, somatropin, thyroid hormones, estrogens, progestogens, atypical antipsychotics), or drugs that may either potentiate or weaken blood glucose-lowering effect (β-blockers, clonidine, lithium salts). Alcohol may increase susceptibility to hypoglycemia. Pentamidine may cause hypoglycemia, sometimes followed by hyperglycemia. Hypoglycemic signs may be reduced or absent with sympatholytics (eg, β-blockers, clonidine, guanethidine, reserpine). Caution with K$^+$-lowering drugs or drugs sensitive to serum K$^+$ concentrations.

PREGNANCY: Category B, caution in nursing.

MECHANISM OF ACTION: Insulin; regulates glucose metabolism. Binds to insulin receptors on muscle and adipocytes and lowers blood glucose by facilitating the cellular uptake of glucose and simultaneously inhibiting the output of glucose from the liver.

PHARMACOKINETICS: Absorption: T$_{max}$=1.5-2.5 hrs (0.1 U/kg SQ).

NURSING CONSIDERATIONS

Assessment: Assess for predisposal to hypoglycemia, risk of hypokalemia, hypersensitivity, renal/hepatic impairment, pregnancy/nursing status, and possible drug interactions. Obtain baseline blood glucose and HbA1c levels.

Monitoring: Monitor for signs and symptoms of hypoglycemia, lipodystrophy, allergic reactions, and other adverse effects. Monitor blood glucose, HbA1c, and K$^+$ concentrations (frequently during IV).

Patient Counseling: Inform about potential risks and benefits of therapy, including possible adverse reactions. Counsel on inj technique, lifestyle management, regular glucose monitoring, periodic HbA1c testing, recognition and management of hypo- and hyperglycemia, adherence to meal planning, complications of therapy, timing of dose, instruction in the use of inj devices, and proper storage. Instruct to exercise caution when driving or operating machinery. Instruct to inform physician if pregnant/breastfeeding or intend to become pregnant. Instruct to always carefully check that they are administering the correct insulin to avoid medication errors.

Administration: SQ/IV route. Inject SQ in abdomen, buttocks, thigh, or upper arm. Rotate inj sites within same region. **Storage:** Unopened: 2-8°C (36-46°F) or, if carried as a spare or if refrigeration not possible, <25°C (77°F) for 42 days. Do not freeze. Protect from light. Do not expose to heat/light. Opened: <25°C (77°F) for 42 days, away from heat/light. Do not refrigerate after 1st use.

NOVOLOG   RX
insulin aspart, rdna origin (Novo Nordisk)

THERAPEUTIC CLASS: Insulin

INDICATIONS: To improve glycemic control in adults and children with diabetes mellitus.

DOSAGE: *Adults:* Individualize dose. Total Daily Insulin Requirement: Usual: 0.5-1 U/kg/day. (SQ) Give immediately within 5-10 min ac. Use with an intermediate- or long-acting insulin. When used in a meal-related SQ inj treatment regimen, 50% to 70% of total requirement may be provided by insulin aspart and the remainder provided by an intermediate- or long-acting insulin. Continuous

SQ Insulin Infusion (CSII) by External Pump: Infuse premeal boluses immediately (within 5-10 min) ac. Initial: Based on the total daily insulin dose of the previous regimen. Usual: 50% of total dose given as meal-related boluses and the remainder given as basal infusion. (IV) Use at concentrations from 0.05-1 U/mL in infusion systems using polypropylene infusion bags. Renal/Hepatic Impairment: May need to reduce dose.

Pediatrics: ≥2 Yrs: Individualize dose. Total Daily Insulin Requirement: Usual: 0.5-1 U/kg/day. (SQ) Give immediately within 5-10 min ac. Use with an intermediate or long-acting insulin. When used in a meal-related SQ inj treatment regimen, 50% to 70% of total requirement may be provided by insulin aspart and the remainder provided by an intermediate- or long-acting insulin. CSII by External Pump: Infuse premeal boluses immediately (within 5-10 min) ac. Initial: Based on the total daily insulin dose of the previous regimen. Usual: 50% of total dose given as meal-related boluses and the remainder given as basal infusion. Renal/Hepatic Impairment: May need to reduce dose.

HOW SUPPLIED: Inj: 100 U/mL [3mL, FlexPen, FlexTouch, PenFill cartridges; 10mL, vial]

CONTRAINDICATIONS: During episodes of hypoglycemia.

WARNINGS/PRECAUTIONS: Any change of insulin dose should be made cautiously and under medical supervision. Changing from one insulin product to another or changing the insulin strength may result in the need for a change in dosage. Illness, emotional disturbances, or other stresses may alter insulin requirements. Do not share needles, FlexPen, or FlexTouch. Hypoglycemia may occur; caution in patients with hypoglycemia unawareness and in patients predisposed to hypoglycemia. Hypoglycemia may impair ability to concentrate and react. Hypokalemia may occur; caution in patients who may be at risk. Careful glucose monitoring and dose adjustments may be necessary with renal/hepatic impairment. Redness, swelling, or itching at the inj site may occur. Localized reactions and generalized myalgias reported with injected metacresol, an excipient in NovoLog. Severe, life-threatening, generalized allergy, including anaphylaxis, may occur. Increases in anti-insulin antibodies observed. Malfunction of the insulin pump or infusion set, or insulin degradation can lead to a rapid onset of hyperglycemia and ketosis; prompt identification and correction of the cause is necessary. Train patients using continuous SQ infusion pump therapy how to administer by inj and to have alternate insulin therapy available in case of pump failure. IV administration should be under medical supervision with close monitoring of blood glucose and K⁺ levels.

ADVERSE REACTIONS: Hypoglycemia, headache, hyporeflexia, onychomycosis, sensory disturbance, urinary tract infection, nausea, diarrhea, chest pain, abdominal pain, skin disorder, sinusitis, weight gain, peripheral edema, lipodystrophy.

INTERACTIONS: May require insulin dose adjustment and close monitoring with drugs that may increase blood glucose-lowering effect and susceptibility to hypoglycemia (eg, oral antidiabetic products, pramlintide, ACE inhibitors, disopyramide, fibrates, fluoxetine, MAOIs, propoxyphene, salicylates, somatostatin analogs [eg, octreotide], sulfonamide antibiotics), drugs that may reduce blood glucose-lowering effect (eg, corticosteroids, niacin, danazol, diuretics, sympathomimetic agents [eg, epinephrine, salbutamol, terbutaline], isoniazid, phenothiazine derivatives, somatropin, thyroid hormones, estrogens, progestogens [eg, in oral contraceptives], atypical antipsychotics), or drugs that may potentiate or weaken blood glucose-lowering effect (β-blockers, clonidine, lithium salts, alcohol). Pentamidine may cause hypoglycemia, sometimes followed by hyperglycemia. Signs of hyperglycemia may be reduced or absent with sympatholytics (eg, β-blockers, clonidine, guanethidine, reserpine). Caution with K⁺-lowering drugs or drugs sensitive to serum K⁺ levels. Observe for signs/symptoms of heart failure (HF) if treated concomitantly with a peroxisome proliferator-activated receptor (PPAR)-gamma agonist (eg, thiazolidinedione); consider discontinuation or dose reduction of the PPAR-gamma agonist if HF develops.

PREGNANCY: Category B, caution in nursing.

MECHANISM OF ACTION: Insulin aspart (rDNA origin); regulates glucose metabolism. Binds to the insulin receptors on muscle and fat cells and lowers blood glucose by facilitating the cellular uptake of glucose and simultaneously inhibiting the output of glucose from the liver.

PHARMACOKINETICS: Absorption: C_{max}=82mU/L; T_{max}=40-50 min (median). **Distribution:** Plasma protein binding (<10%). **Elimination:** $T_{1/2}$=81 min.

NURSING CONSIDERATIONS

Assessment: Assess for predisposition to hypoglycemia, risk of hypokalemia, hypersensitivity, renal/hepatic impairment, pregnancy/nursing status, and possible drug interactions. Obtain baseline blood glucose and HbA1c levels.

Monitoring: Monitor for signs/symptoms of hypoglycemia, hypokalemia, allergic reactions, and other adverse effects. Monitor blood glucose, HbA1c, K⁺ levels, and renal/hepatic function.

Patient Counseling: Inform about potential side effects (eg, hypoglycemia, allergic reactions, weight gain, allergic reactions). Inform that the ability to concentrate and react may be impaired as a result of hypoglycemia; advise to use caution when driving or operating machinery. Counsel on proper administration techniques, lifestyle management, adherence to meal planning, regular glucose monitoring, periodic HbA1c testing, recognition and management of hypo- and hyperglycemia, complications of insulin therapy, timing of dose, instruction in the use of inj or SQ insulin infusion pump, and proper storage of insulin. Instruct to always carefully check that appropriate insulin is administered to avoid medication errors.

Administration: SQ/IV route. Inject SQ in the abdominal region, buttocks, thigh, or upper arm, or give by continuous SQ infusion by an external insulin pump; rotate inj sites within the same region. If mixed with NPH human insulin, draw NovoLog into syringe 1st, and inject mixture immediately after mixing. Do not mix with any other insulin or diluent when used in an external SQ infusion pump. Do not administer insulin mixtures intravenously. Refer to PI for further instructions on preparation, handling, and administration. **Storage:** Refer to PI for storage conditions for vial, PenFill cartridges, FlexPen, and FlexTouch. Pump: Discard insulin in reservoir after at least every 6 days of use. Discard insulin if exposed to >37°C (98.6°F). Change infusion set and infusion set insertion site at least every 3 days. Diluted Novolog: <30°C (86°F) for 28 days. Storage in Infusion Fluids: Room temperature for 24 hrs.

NOVOLOG MIX 70/30 RX

insulin aspart, rdna origin - insulin aspart protamine, rdna origin (Novo Nordisk)

THERAPEUTIC CLASS: Insulin

INDICATIONS: To improve glycemic control in patients with diabetes mellitus (DM).

DOSAGE: *Adults:* Individualize dose. Type 1 DM: Inject SQ bid within 15 min ac. Type 2 DM: Inject SQ bid within 15 min ac or pc. Hepatic/Renal Impairment: May need to reduce dose. Elderly: Start at lower end of dosing range.

HOW SUPPLIED: Inj: (Insulin Aspart Protamine-Insulin Aspart) 70 U-30 U/mL [3mL, FlexPen; 10mL, vial]

CONTRAINDICATIONS: During episodes of hypoglycemia.

WARNINGS/PRECAUTIONS: Any change of insulin should be made cautiously and under medical supervision. Changing from one insulin product to another, changing the insulin strength, illness, emotional stress, and other physiologic stress in addition to changes in meals and exercise may result in the need for a change in dosage. Do not share needles or FlexPen. Hypoglycemia may occur; caution in patients with hypoglycemia unawareness and in patients predisposed to hypoglycemia. Hypokalemia may occur; caution in patients who may be at risk. Caution with renal/hepatic impairment. Inj-site reactions (eg, erythema, edema, pruritus) may occur. Localized reactions and generalized myalgias reported with the use of cresol, a component in NovoLog 70/30. Severe, life-threatening, generalized allergic reactions, including anaphylactic reactions, may occur. Changes in cross-reactive antibodies reported. Caution in elderly.

ADVERSE REACTIONS: Hypoglycemia, headache, influenza-like symptoms, dyspepsia, back pain, diarrhea, pharyngitis, rhinitis, skeletal pain, upper respiratory tract infection, neuropathy, abdominal pain, weight gain, peripheral edema, lipodystrophy.

INTERACTIONS: May require insulin dose adjustment and close monitoring with drugs that may increase blood glucose-lowering effect and susceptibility to hypoglycemia (eg, oral antidiabetic products, pramlintide, ACE inhibitors, disopyramide, fibrates, fluoxetine, MAOIs, propoxyphene, salicylates, somatostatin analogs [eg, octreotide], sulfonamide antibiotics), drugs that may reduce blood glucose-lowering effect (eg, corticosteroids, niacin, danazol, diuretics, sympathomimetic agents [eg, epinephrine, salbutamol, terbutaline], isoniazid, phenothiazine derivatives, somatropin, thyroid hormones, estrogens, progestogens [eg, in oral contraceptives], atypical antipsychotics), or drugs that may potentiate or weaken blood glucose-lowering effect (β-blockers, clonidine, lithium salts, alcohol). Pentamidine may cause hypoglycemia, sometimes followed by hyperglycemia. Signs of hypoglycemia may be reduced or absent with sympatholytics (eg, β-blockers, clonidine, guanethidine, reserpine). Caution with K^+-lowering drugs or drugs sensitive to serum K^+ levels. Observe for signs/symptoms of heart failure (HF) if treated concomitantly with a peroxisome proliferator-activated receptor (PPAR)-gamma agonist (eg, thiazolidinedione); consider discontinuation or dose reduction of the PPAR-gamma agonist if HF develops.

PREGNANCY: Category B, caution in nursing.

MECHANISM OF ACTION: Insulin; regulates glucose metabolism. Binds to the insulin receptors on muscle, liver, and fat cells and lowers blood glucose by facilitating the cellular uptake of glucose and simultaneously inhibiting the output of glucose from the liver.

PHARMACOKINETICS: Absorption: Rapid; (0.2 U/kg) C_{max}=23.4mU/L, T_{max}=60 min; (0.3 U/kg) C_{max}=61.3mU/L, T_{max}=85 min. **Distribution:** Plasma protein binding (0-9%). **Elimination:** $T_{1/2}$=8-9 hrs.

NURSING CONSIDERATIONS

Assessment: Assess for predisposition to hypoglycemia, risk of hypokalemia, renal/hepatic impairment, hypersensitivity, pregnancy/nursing status, and possible drug interactions. Obtain baseline blood glucose and HbA1c levels.

Monitoring: Monitor for signs and symptoms of hypoglycemia, hypokalemia, allergic reactions, and other adverse effects. Monitor blood glucose, HbA1c, and K⁺ levels. Monitor renal/hepatic function.

Patient Counseling: Inform about potential risks and benefits of therapy. Counsel on proper administration techniques, lifestyle management, regular glucose monitoring, periodic HbA1c testing, recognition and management of hypo- and hyperglycemia, adherence to meal planning, complications of insulin therapy, timing of dose, instruction in the use of inj devices, and proper storage of insulin. Inform that the ability to concentrate and react may be impaired as a result of hypoglycemia; advise to use caution when driving or operating machinery. Advise to always check carefully that appropriate insulin is administered to avoid medication errors.

Administration: SQ route. Inject SQ in the abdominal region, buttocks, thigh, or upper arm. Rotate inj sites. Do not mix with other insulins or use intravenously or in an insulin infusion pump. Refer to PI for resuspension instructions and further administration instructions. **Storage:** Refer to PI for storage conditions for vial and FlexPen.

NOXAFIL   RX
posaconazole (Merck)

THERAPEUTIC CLASS: Azole antifungal

INDICATIONS: Prophylaxis of invasive *Aspergillus* and *Candida* infections in patients (≥13 yrs of age [tab/sus], ≥18 yrs of age [inj]), who are at high risk of developing these infections due to being severely immunocompromised, such as hematopoietic stem cell transplant recipients with graft-versus-host disease or those with hematologic malignancies with prolonged neutropenia from chemotherapy. (Sus) Treatment of oropharyngeal candidiasis, including oropharyngeal candidiasis refractory to itraconazole and/or fluconazole.

DOSAGE: *Adults:* ≥18 Yrs: Prophylaxis of Invasive *Aspergillus* and *Candida* Infections: (Inj/Tab) LD: 300mg bid on the 1st day. Maint: 300mg qd, starting on the 2nd day. Duration of therapy is based on recovery from neutropenia or immunosuppression. (Sus) Usual: 200mg (5mL) tid. Duration of therapy is based on recovery from neutropenia or immunosuppression. Oropharyngeal Candidiasis: (Sus) LD: 100mg (2.5mL) bid on 1st day. Maint: 100mg qd for 13 days. Oropharyngeal Candidiasis Refractory to Itraconazole and/or Fluconazole: (Sus) 400mg (10mL) bid. Duration of therapy is based on severity of underlying disease and clinical response. *Pediatrics:* ≥13 Yrs: Prophylaxis of Invasive *Aspergillus* and *Candida* Infections: (Tab) LD: 300mg bid on the 1st day. Maint: 300mg qd, starting on the 2nd day. Duration of therapy is based on recovery from neutropenia or immunosuppression. (Sus) Usual: 200mg (5mL) tid. Duration of therapy is based on recovery from neutropenia or immunosuppression. Oropharyngeal Candidiasis: (Sus) LD: 100mg (2.5mL) bid on 1st day. Maint: 100mg qd for 13 days. Oropharyngeal Candidiasis Refractory to Itraconazole and/or Fluconazole: (Sus) 400mg (10mL) bid. Duration of therapy is based on severity of underlying disease and clinical response.

HOW SUPPLIED: Inj: 18mg/mL [16.7mL]; Sus: 40mg/mL [105mL]; Tab, Delayed Release: 100mg

CONTRAINDICATIONS: Coadministration with sirolimus, CYP3A4 substrates that prolong the QT interval (eg, pimozide, quinidine), HMG-CoA reductase inhibitors that are primarily metabolized through CYP3A4 (eg, atorvastatin, lovastatin, simvastatin), and ergot alkaloids (ergotamine, dihydroergotamine).

WARNINGS/PRECAUTIONS: Do not use tablet and sus interchangeably. Prolongation of the QT interval and cases of torsades de pointes reported; caution with potentially proarrhythmic conditions. Rigorous attempts to correct K⁺, Mg²⁺, and Ca²⁺ should be made before initiating treatment. Hepatic reactions (eg, mild to moderate elevations in ALT, AST, alkaline phosphatase, total bilirubin, and/or clinical hepatitis) reported. Cases of more severe hepatic reactions, including cholestasis or hepatic failure, reported in patients with serious underlying medical conditions (eg, hematologic malignancy). Evaluate LFTs at the start of and during the course of therapy; monitor for the development of more severe hepatic injury in patients who develop abnormal LFTs during therapy. Consider discontinuation if signs/symptoms of liver disease develop that may be attributable to therapy. Monitor closely for breakthrough fungal infections in patients weighing >120kg. (Inj) Avoid with moderate or severe renal impairment (estimated GFR <50 mL/min), unless an assessment of the benefit/risk justifies the use of inj. Monitor SrCr levels closely in patients with moderate or severe renal impairment; consider changing to oral therapy if increases occur. (Tab/Sus) Monitor closely for breakthrough fungal infections in patients with severe renal impairment and severe diarrhea or vomiting.

ADVERSE REACTIONS: Fever, headache, anemia, thrombocytopenia, diarrhea, N/V, abdominal pain, cough, rash, hypokalemia, constipation, HTN, edema peripheral, hypomagnesemia, epistaxis.

INTERACTIONS: See Contraindications. May increase whole blood trough concentrations of cyclosporine and tacrolimus; monitor tacrolimus or cyclosporine whole blood trough concentrations frequently during and at discontinuation of posaconazole treatment, and the dose of cyclosporine or tacrolimus should be adjusted accordingly. Avoid with phenytoin, rifabutin, and efavirenz, unless benefit outweighs risk. If phenytoin is required, closely monitor for break-through fungal infections closely and frequently monitor phenytoin concentrations closely; consider phenytoin dose reduction. If rifabutin is required, closely monitor for breakthrough fungal infections as well as frequent monitoring of CBC and adverse events due to increased rifabutin plasma concentrations (eg, uveitis, leukopenia). Fosamprenavir may decrease levels; monitor for breakthrough fungal infections. May increase levels of vinca alkaloids; consider dose adjustment of vinca alkaloid. May increase levels of midazolam and other benzodiazepines metabolized by CYP3A4 (eg, alprazolam, triazolam). May increase levels of calcium channel blockers (CCBs) metabolized by CYP3A4 (eg, verapamil, diltiazem, nifedipine, nicardipine, felodipine), and other drugs that are metabolized through CYP3A4 (eg, atazanavir, ritonavir); monitor for adverse effects and toxicity; dose reduction of CCBs may be needed. Increased digoxin levels reported; monitor digoxin plasma levels. Inhibitors or inducers of UDP glucuronosyltransferase or P-glycoprotein may affect posaconazole levels. Monitor glucose levels with glipizide. (Sus) Avoid with cimetidine and esomeprazole, unless benefit outweighs risks. Cimetidine, esomeprazole, and metoclopramide may decrease levels; monitor for breakthrough fungal infections.

PREGNANCY: Category C, not for use in nursing.

MECHANISM OF ACTION: Triazole antifungal agent; blocks synthesis of ergosterol, a key component of the fungal cell membrane, through inhibition of cytochrome P-450-dependent enzyme lanosterol 14α-demethylase, resulting in accumulation of methylated sterol precursors and depletion of ergosterol within the cell membrane, thus weakening the structure and function of the fungal cell membrane.

PHARMACOKINETICS: Absorption: Administration of variable doses resulted in different pharmacokinetic parameters. **Distribution:** V_d=261L (IV); plasma protein binding (>98%). **Metabolism:** Via UDP glucuronidation; glucuronide conjugates (metabolites). **Elimination:** (Sus) Feces (71%, 66% unchanged), urine (13%, <0.2% unchanged); $T_{1/2}$=27 hrs (inj), 26-31 hrs (tab), 35 hrs (sus).

NURSING CONSIDERATIONS

Assessment: Assess for hypersensitivity to any component of the drug or to other azole antifungals, proarrhythmic conditions, renal impairment, serious underlying medical conditions (eg, hematologic malignancy), pregnancy/nursing status, and for possible drug interactions. Obtain baseline LFTs.

Monitoring: Monitor for signs/symptoms of hypersensitivity reactions, hepatic reactions, QT prolongation, torsades de pointes, and other adverse reactions. Monitor LFTs during the course of therapy. Monitor closely for breakthrough fungal infections in patients weighing >120kg. (Tab/Sus) Monitor closely for breakthrough fungal infections in patients with severe renal impairment and severe diarrhea or vomiting.

Patient Counseling: Advise patients to inform physician of all medications being taken and if they have a heart condition or circulatory disease, liver disease, are pregnant or plan to become pregnant or breastfeed, or if have ever had an allergic reaction to other antifungal medications. Advise patients to inform physician if they develop severe diarrhea or vomiting, flu-like symptoms, itching, eyes/skin that turn yellow, swelling of a leg or SOB, notice a change in HR/heart rhythm, or if they feel more tired than usual. (Tab) Instruct that if a dose is missed, take as soon as remember; advise to skip the missed dose and go back to the regular schedule if do not remember until it is within 12 hrs of the next dose. Instruct not to double the next dose or take more than the prescribed dose.

Administration: Oral/IV route. (Inj) Administer via a central venous line, including a central venous catheter or peripherally inserted central catheter by slow IV infusion over 90 min. If central venous catheter is not available, inj may be administered through a peripheral venous catheter by slow IV infusion over 30 min as a single dose in advance of central venous line placement or to bridge the period during which a central venous line is replaced or is in use for other IV treatment. Refer to PI for further instructions for use. (Sus) Take during or immediately (eg, within 20 min) following a full meal. If a full meal cannot be eaten, take with a liquid nutritional supplement or an acidic carbonated beverage (eg, ginger ale). Shake well before use. Refer to PI for further administration instructions. (Tab) Take with food. Swallow whole; do not break, crush, dissolve, or chew tab before swallowing. **Storage:** (Inj) 2-8°C (36-46°F). (Sus) 25°C (77°F); excursions permitted to 15-30°C (59-86°F). Do not freeze. (Tab) 20-25°C (68-77°F); excursions permitted to 15-30°C (59-86°F).

Nplate
romiplostim (Amgen)

RX

THERAPEUTIC CLASS: Thrombopoietin receptor agonist

INDICATIONS: Treatment of thrombocytopenia in patients with chronic immune thrombocy-topenia (ITP) who have had an insufficient response to corticosteroids, immunoglobulins, or splenectomy.

DOSAGE: *Adults:* Administer as a weekly SQ inj. Initial: 1mcg/kg based on actual body weight. Titrate: Adjust weekly dose by increments of 1mcg/kg until platelet count is ≥50 x 10^9/L. Max: 10mcg/kg/week. Platelet Count <50 x 10^9/L: Increase dose by 1mcg/kg. Platelet Count >200 x 10^9/L for 2 Consecutive Weeks: Reduce dose by 1mcg/kg. Platelet Count >400 x 10^9/L: Do not dose; continue assessing platelet count weekly. After platelet count falls to <200 x 10^9/L, resume therapy at a dose reduced by 1mcg/kg. D/C if platelet count does not increase to a level suf-ficient to avoid clinically important bleeding after 4 weeks of therapy at the max weekly dose. Use with Concomitant Medical ITP Therapies (eg, Corticosteroids, Danazol, Azathioprine, IV Immunoglobulin, and Anti-D Immunoglobulin): May reduce or d/c medical ITP therapies if plate-let count is ≥50 x 10^9/L.

HOW SUPPLIED: Inj: 250mcg, 500mcg [vial]

WARNINGS/PRECAUTIONS: Not for the treatment of thrombocytopenia due to myelodysplastic syndrome (MDS) or any cause of thrombocytopenia other than chronic ITP; progression from MDS to acute myelogenous leukemia has been observed. Use only in patients with ITP whose de-gree of thrombocytopenia and clinical condition increases the risk for bleeding. Do not use in an attempt to normalize platelet counts. Use lowest dose to achieve and maintain a platelet count ≥50 x 10^9/L. Thrombotic/thromboembolic complications may occur. Portal vein thrombosis reported in patients with chronic liver disease. May increase risk for development or progression of reticulin fiber formation within the bone marrow; consider a bone marrow biopsy to include staining for fibrosis if new or worsening morphological abnormalities or cytopenias occur. Worsened thrombocytopenia reported after discontinuation; following discontinuation, obtain weekly CBCs, including platelet counts, for at least 2 weeks, and consider alternative treat-ments for worsening thrombocytopenia. If hyporesponsiveness or failure to maintain a platelet response occurs, search for causative factors (eg, neutralizing antibodies). Caution with renal/ hepatic impairment and in elderly.

ADVERSE REACTIONS: Headache, arthralgia, dizziness, insomnia, myalgia, pain in extremity, abdominal pain, shoulder pain, dyspepsia, development of antibodies, paresthesia.

PREGNANCY: Category C, not for use in nursing.

MECHANISM OF ACTION: Thrombopoietin (TPO) receptor agonist; increases platelet production through binding and activation of the TPO receptor.

PHARMACOKINETICS: Absorption: T_{max}=14 hrs (median). **Elimination:** $T_{1/2}$=3.5 days (median).

NURSING CONSIDERATIONS

Assessment: Assess for cause and degree of thrombocytopenia, hepatic/renal impairment, and pregnancy/nursing status.

Monitoring: Obtain CBCs, including platelet counts, weekly during dose adjustment phase, then monthly after establishment of a stable dose, and then weekly for at least 2 weeks after discon-tinuation. Monitor for thrombotic/thromboembolic complications, bone marrow reticulin fiber formation, new/worsening morphological abnormalities, cytopenias, hyporesponsiveness, and failure to maintain platelet response with therapy.

Patient Counseling: Inform of risks and benefits of therapy. Advise that the risks associated with long-term administration are unknown. Counsel to avoid situations or medications that may in-crease risk for bleeding. Inform pregnant women that they may enroll in the pregnancy registry.

Administration: SQ route. Refer to PI for preparation and administration instructions. **Storage:** 2-8°C (36-46°F). Do not freeze. Protect from light. Reconstituted: 25°C (77°F) or 2-8°C (36-46°F) for up to 24 hrs prior to administration. Protect from light. Discard unused portion.

NUCYNTA `CII`
tapentadol (Janssen)

THERAPEUTIC CLASS: Central acting analgesic

INDICATIONS: Management of moderate to severe acute pain in adults.

DOSAGE: *Adults:* Individualize dose. Refer to PI for the factors to consider when selecting an initial dose. Usual: 50mg, 75mg, or 100mg q4-6h depending upon pain intensity. Day 1: May give 2nd dose 1 hr after 1st dose if pain relief is inadequate, then 50mg, 75mg, or 100mg q4-6h. Adjust dose to maintain adequate analgesia with acceptable tolerability. Max: 700mg on Day 1, then 600mg/day thereafter. Periodically reassess continued need for use during chronic therapy, es-pecially for noncancer-related pain. Moderate Hepatic Impairment (Child-Pugh Score 7-9): Initial: 50mg no more frequently than once q8h. Max: 3 doses/24 hrs. Cessation of Therapy: Taper dose gradually. Elderly: Start at lower end of dosing range.

HOW SUPPLIED: Tab: 50mg, 75mg, 100mg

CONTRAINDICATIONS: Significant respiratory depression, acute or severe bronchial asthma or hypercarbia in an unmonitored setting or in the absence of resuscitative equipment, known or suspected paralytic ileus, and patients receiving MAOIs or who have taken them within the last 14 days.

WARNINGS/PRECAUTIONS: Abuse liability similar to other opioid agonists legal or illicit; assess each patient's risk for opioid abuse or addiction prior to prescribing. Routinely monitor all patients for signs of misuse, abuse, and addiction; misuse or abuse by crushing, chewing, snorting, or injecting will pose a significant risk that could result in overdose and death. Respiratory depression, if not immediately recognized and treated, may lead to respiratory arrest and death. Accidental ingestion, especially in children, can result in fatal overdose. Respiratory depression is more likely to occur in elderly, cachectic, or debilitated patients; monitor closely, particularly when given with drugs that depress respiration. Monitor for respiratory depression and consider use of alternative nonopioid analgesics in patients with significant chronic obstructive pulmonary disease (COPD) or cor pulmonale, and in patients with a substantially decreased respiratory reserve, hypoxia, hypercarbia, or preexisting respiratory depression. May cause severe hypotension. Monitor for signs of sedation and respiratory depression in patients susceptible to the intracranial effects of carbon dioxide retention (eg, those with evidence of increased intracranial pressure or brain tumors). May obscure clinical course in patients with a head injury. Avoid with circulatory shock, impaired consciousness, or coma. May aggravate convulsions in patients with convulsive disorders and may induce or aggravate seizures; monitor for worsened seizure control in patients with history of seizure disorders. May cause spasm of sphincter of Oddi; monitor for worsening symptoms in patients with biliary tract disease (eg, acute pancreatitis). Withdrawal symptoms may occur if discontinued abruptly. May impair mental/physical abilities. Monitor for respiratory/CNS depression with moderate hepatic impairment. Avoid use with severe renal/hepatic impairment. Not for use during and immediately prior to labor.

ADVERSE REACTIONS: N/V, dizziness, somnolence, constipation, pruritus, dry mouth, hyperhidrosis, fatigue.

INTERACTIONS: See Contraindications. Avoid use with alcoholic beverages or medications containing alcohol, other opioids, or drugs of abuse; may have additive effects. CNS depressants (eg, sedatives or hypnotics, general anesthetics, phenothiazines, tranquilizers, alcohol, anxiolytics, neuroleptics, muscle relaxants, other opioids, illicit drugs) may increase risk of respiratory depression, hypotension, profound sedation, or coma; start tapentadol at 1/3 to 1/2 of the usual dose and consider using a lower dose of concomitant CNS depressant. Serotonin syndrome may occur with serotonergic drugs (eg, SSRIs, SNRIs, TCAs, triptans, drugs that affect the serotonergic neurotransmitter system [eg, mirtazapine, trazodone, tramadol]), and drugs that may impair metabolism of serotonin (eg, MAOIs); use with caution. Avoid use with mixed agonist/antagonist analgesics (eg, butorphanol, nalbuphine, pentazocine), and partial agonists (eg, buprenorphine); may precipitate withdrawal symptoms. Anticholinergics may increase risk of urinary retention and/or severe constipation, which may lead to paralytic ileus.

PREGNANCY: Category C, not for use in nursing.

MECHANISM OF ACTION: Centrally acting synthetic analgesic; not established. Suspected to be due to μ-opioid agonist activity and the inhibition of norepinephrine reuptake.

PHARMACOKINETICS: Absorption: T_{max}=1.25 hrs; absolute bioavailability (32%). **Distribution:** (IV) V_d=540L; plasma protein binding (20%); crosses placenta. **Metabolism:** Conjugation; N-desmethyl tapentadol by CYP2C9 and CYP2C19; hydroxy tapentadol by CYP2D6. **Elimination:** Kidneys (99%); urine (3% unchanged, 70% conjugated); $T_{1/2}$=4 hrs.

NURSING CONSIDERATIONS

Assessment: Assess for personal/family history or risk factors for drug abuse or addiction, general condition and medical status, opioid experience/tolerance, pain type/severity, previous opioid daily dose, potency and type of prior analgesics used, respiratory depression, COPD or other respiratory complications, GI obstruction, paralytic ileus, renal/hepatic impairment, pregnancy/nursing status, possible drug interactions, and any other condition where treatment is contraindicated or cautioned.

Monitoring: Monitor for improvement of pain, signs/symptoms of respiratory depression, hypotension, symptoms of worsening biliary tract disease, aggravation/induction of seizure, tolerance, physical dependence, mental/physical impairment, serotonin syndrome, and other adverse reactions. Routinely monitor for signs of misuse, abuse, and addiction. Periodically reassess continued need for use during chronic therapy, especially for noncancer-related pain.

Patient Counseling: Instruct to take only as prescribed and not to d/c without first discussing the need for a tapering regimen with prescriber. Inform that drug has potential for abuse; instruct not to share drug with others and to take steps to protect from theft or misuse. Discuss the risks of respiratory depression, orthostatic hypotension, syncope, severe constipation, and anaphylaxis; counsel on how to recognize symptoms and when to seek medical attention. Inform that accidental exposure may result in serious harm or death; advise to dispose unused tabs by flushing them down the toilet. Inform about risks of concomitant use of alcohol, other CNS depressants, MAOIs, and serotonergic drugs; instruct to notify physician if taking/planning to take additional medications. Instruct to not consume alcoholic beverages, or take prescription and OTC products that contain alcohol, during treatment. Counsel that drug may cause seizures if at risk for seizures or if patient has epilepsy; advise to d/c therapy and seek medical attention if seizures occur during therapy. Inform that drug may impair the ability to perform potentially hazardous activities (eg, driving a car or operating heavy machinery); advise not to perform such tasks until patients know how they will react to the medication. Advise females that drug can cause fetal harm; instruct to notify physician if pregnant/planning to become pregnant.

Administration: Oral route. Take with or without food. **Storage:** ≤25°C (77°F); excursions permitted to 15-30°C (59-86°F). Protect from moisture.

NUCYNTA ER   `CII`
tapentadol (Janssen)

Exposes users to risks of addiction, abuse, and misuse, leading to overdose and death; assess each patient's risk prior to prescribing and monitor regularly for development of these behaviors/conditions. Serious, life-threatening, or fatal respiratory depression may occur; monitor during initiation or following a dose increase. Crushing, dissolving, or chewing tab can cause rapid release and absorption of potentially fatal dose; instruct patients to swallow tab whole. Accidental ingestion, especially by children, can result in a fatal overdose. Prolonged use during pregnancy can result in neonatal opioid withdrawal syndrome; advise pregnant women of the risk and ensure availability of appropriate treatment. Avoid use with alcoholic beverages or medications containing alcohol; may result in increased levels and potentially fatal overdose of tapentadol.

THERAPEUTIC CLASS: Central acting analgesic

INDICATIONS: Treatment of pain/neuropathic pain associated with diabetic peripheral neuropathy in adults severe enough to require daily, around-the-clock, long-term opioid treatment and for which alternative treatment options are inadequate.

DOSAGE: *Adults:* Individualize dose. Titrate to adequate analgesia with dose increases of 50mg no more than bid every 3 days. Max: 500mg/day. First Opioid Analgesic/Nonopioid Tolerant: Initial: 50mg bid (q12h). Conversion from Nucynta: Use the equivalent total daily dose of Nucynta, divided into 2 equal doses of Nucynta ER separated by approximately 12-hr intervals. Conversion from Other Opioids: D/C all other around-the-clock opioids when therapy is initiated. Give 1/2 of estimated daily tapentadol requirement as the initial dose; manage inadequate analgesia by supplementation with immediate-release rescue medication. Discontinuation: Gradual downward titration. Moderate Hepatic Impairment (Child-Pugh Score 7-9): Initial: 50mg, administer no more frequently than once q24h. Max: 100mg qd. Elderly: Start at lower end of dosing range. Refer to PI for further dosage information.

HOW SUPPLIED: Tab, Extended-Release: 50mg, 100mg, 150mg, 200mg, 250mg

CONTRAINDICATIONS: Significant respiratory depression, acute or severe bronchial asthma or hypercarbia in an unmonitored setting or in the absence of resuscitative equipment, known or suspected paralytic ileus, patients receiving MAOIs or who have taken them within the last 14 days.

WARNINGS/PRECAUTIONS: Reserve for use in patients for whom alternative treatment options are ineffective, not tolerated, or would be otherwise inadequate to provide sufficient management of pain. Should only be prescribed by healthcare professionals who are knowledgeable in the use of potent opioids for management of chronic pain. D/C all other tapentadol and tramadol products when initiating and during therapy. Life-threatening respiratory depression is more likely to occur in elderly, cachectic, or debilitated patients. Consider alternative nonopioid analgesics in patients with significant chronic obstructive pulmonary disease or cor pulmonale, and in patients having a substantially decreased respiratory reserve, hypoxia, hypercarbia, or preexisting respiratory depression. May cause severe hypotension; increased risk in patients whose ability to maintain BP is compromised by a reduced blood volume or concurrent administration of certain CNS depressants. Avoid with circulatory shock, impaired consciousness, or coma. Monitor patients who may be susceptible to intracranial effects of carbon dioxide retention for signs of sedation and respiratory depression when initiating therapy. May obscure clinical course in patients with head injury. May aggravate convulsions and induce/aggravate seizures. May cause spasm of sphincter of Oddi; monitor patients with biliary tract disease (eg, acute pancreatitis). May impair mental/physical abilities. Monitor for respiratory/CNS depression with moderate hepatic impairment. Not recommended with severe renal/hepatic impairment.

ADVERSE REACTIONS: Respiratory depression, N/V, dizziness, constipation, headache, somnolence, fatigue, dry mouth, hyperhidrosis, pruritus, insomnia, dyspepsia, diarrhea, decreased appetite, anxiety.

INTERACTIONS: See Boxed Warning and Contraindications. Hypotension, profound sedation, coma, and respiratory depression may occur with CNS depressants (eg, sedatives, anxiolytics, hypnotics); if coadministration is required, consider dose reduction of one or both agents. Serotonin syndrome may occur with serotonergic drugs (eg, SSRIs, SNRIs, TCAs, triptans, drugs that affect serotonergic neurotransmitter system) and drugs that may impair metabolism of serotonin (eg, MAOIs). Avoid use of mixed agonist/antagonist (eg, nalbuphine, pentazocine, butorphanol) and partial agonists (eg, buprenorphine) analgesics; may reduce analgesic effects and/or precipitate withdrawal symptoms. Enhanced neuromuscular blocking action and increased degree of respiratory depression with skeletal muscle relaxants. Anticholinergics may increase risk of urinary retention and/or severe constipation, which may lead to paralytic ileus.

PREGNANCY: Category C, not for use in nursing.

MECHANISM OF ACTION: Centrally acting synthetic analgesic; not established. Suspected to be due to μ-opioid receptor agonist activity and the inhibition of norepinephrine reuptake.

PHARMACOKINETICS: Absorption: T_{max}=3-6 hrs; absolute bioavailability (32%). **Distribution:** (IV) V_d=540L; plasma protein binding (20%); crosses placenta. **Metabolism:** Conjugation; N-desmethyl tapentadol by CYP2C9 and CYP2C19; hydroxy tapentadol by CYP2D6. **Elimination:** Kidneys (99%), urine (3% unchanged, 70% conjugated); $T_{1/2}$=5 hrs.

NURSING CONSIDERATIONS

Assessment: Assess for abuse/addiction risk, opioid experience/tolerance, pain type/severity, pregnancy/nursing status, possible drug interactions, and any other condition where treatment is contraindicated or cautioned.

Monitoring: Monitor for signs/symptoms of respiratory depression, hypotension, symptoms of worsening biliary tract disease, aggravation/induction of seizure, mental/physical impairment, serotonin syndrome, and other adverse reactions. Routinely monitor for signs of misuse, abuse, and addiction.

Patient Counseling: Inform that drug has potential for abuse and addiction; instruct not to share drug with others and to take steps to protect from theft or misuse. Inform about risk of accidental exposure and advise to store securely and to dispose unused tabs by flushing them down the toilet. Inform about the risks of life-threatening respiratory depression, orthostatic hypotension, and syncope. Inform about risks of concomitant use of alcohol, other CNS depressants, MAOIs, and serotonergic drugs; instruct to notify physician if taking/planning to take additional medications. Instruct to not consume alcoholic beverages or take prescription/OTC products that contain alcohol during treatment. Counsel on the risk for seizures and advise to d/c therapy and seek medical attention if seizures occur. Advise to use ud. Inform that drug may impair the ability to perform potentially hazardous activities; advise not to perform such tasks until patients know how they will react to medication. Advise of potential for severe constipation, including management instructions. Advise how to recognize anaphylaxis and when to seek medical attention. Advise females that drug can cause fetal harm; instruct to notify physician if pregnant/planning to become pregnant.

Administration: Oral route. Take 1 tab at a time, with enough water to ensure complete swallowing immediately after placing in the mouth. Swallow tab whole; do not cut, crush, dissolve, or chew. **Storage:** ≤25°C (77°F); excursions permitted to 15-30°C (59-86°F). Protect from moisture.

NUTROPIN   RX
somatropin rdna origin (Genentech)

OTHER BRAND NAMES: Nutropin AQ (Genentech)

THERAPEUTIC CLASS: Recombinant human growth hormone

INDICATIONS: Treatment of pediatric patients with growth failure due to inadequate endogenous growth hormone (GH) secretion or associated with chronic kidney disease (CKD) up to the time of renal transplantation, idiopathic short stature (ISS), or short stature associated with Turner syndrome (TS). Replacement of endogenous GH in adults with adult-onset or childhood-onset GH deficiency (GHD).

DOSAGE: *Adults:* GHD: Weight-Based: Initial: ≤0.006mg/kg qd SQ. Titrate: May increase based on individual requirements. Max: >35 Yrs: 0.0125mg/kg qd. ≤35 Yrs: 0.025mg/kg qd. Non-Weight Based: Initial: 0.2mg/day SQ (range, 0.15-0.30mg/day). Titrate: May increase gradually every 1-2 months by increments of 0.1-0.2mg/day based on clinical response and insulin-like growth factor-I (IGF-I) concentrations. Maint: Individualize dose. Elderly: Consider lower starting dose and smaller dose increments.
Pediatrics: Individualize dose. Divide weekly dose into daily SQ inj. GHD: Up to 0.3mg/kg/week. May use up to 0.7mg/kg/week in pubertal patients. CKD: Up to 0.35mg/kg/week. Hemodialysis: Give hs or at least 3-4 hrs after dialysis. Chronic Cycling Peritoneal Dialysis: Give in am after completion of dialysis. Chronic Ambulatory Peritoneal Dialysis: Give in pm during overnight exchange. ISS: Up to 0.3mg/kg/week. TS: Up to 0.375mg/kg/week divided into equal doses 3-7X/week SQ.

HOW SUPPLIED: Inj: 10mg; (AQ) 10mg/2mL [vial], 10mg/2mL, 20mg/2mL [pen cartridge], 5mg/2mL, 10mg/2mL, 20mg/2mL [NuSpin]

CONTRAINDICATIONS: Acute critical illness due to complications following open heart surgery, abdominal surgery, multiple accidental trauma, or with acute respiratory failure. Active malignancy, evidence of progression or recurrence of an underlying intracranial tumor, or active proliferative or severe nonproliferative diabetic retinopathy. Pediatric patients with Prader-Willi syndrome (PWS) who are severely obese, have a history of upper airway obstruction or sleep apnea, have severe respiratory impairment, or with closed epiphysis.

WARNINGS/PRECAUTIONS: Increased mortality reported in patients with acute critical illnesses. Fatalities reported in patients with PWS; evaluate for signs of upper airway obstruction and sleep apnea (eg, new/increased snoring) and interrupt therapy if these signs occur. Implement effective weight control in patients with PWS. Examine for progression/recurrence of underlying disease in patients with preexisting tumors or GHD secondary to an intracranial lesion. Monitor for malignant transformation of skin lesions. Undiagnosed impaired glucose tolerance and overt diabetes mellitus (DM) may be unmasked. New-onset type 2 DM reported; monitor glucose levels. Intracranial HTN with papilledema, visual changes, headache, N/V reported; perform funduscopic exam before and during therapy; d/c therapy if papilledema occurs. Fluid retention in adults may occur. Monitor other hormonal replacement treatments in patients with hypopituitarism. Undiagnosed/untreated hypothyroidism may prevent optimal response. Hypothyroidism may become evident or worsen; perform periodic thyroid function tests. Slipped capital femoral epiphysis (SCFE) and progression of scoliosis may occur in pediatric patients. Increased risk of ear/hearing disorders and cardiovascular (CV) disorders in TS patients. Periodically examine children with growth failure secondary to CKD for evidence of renal osteodystrophy progression. Tissue atrophy may occur when administered at the same site over a long period of time. Allergic reactions may occur. Serum levels of inorganic phosphorus, alkaline phosphatase, parathyroid hormone, and IGF-I may increase. Pancreatitis rarely reported; monitor for persistent severe abdominal pain. Diluent contains benzyl alcohol. Caution in elderly.

ADVERSE REACTIONS: Arthralgia, edema, joint disorders, ear disorders, glucose intolerance, inj-site reactions/rashes.

INTERACTIONS: May inhibit 11β-hydroxysteroid dehydrogenase type 1, resulting in reduced serum cortisol concentrations; may need glucocorticoid replacement or dose adjustments of glucocorticoid therapy (eg, cortisone acetate, prednisone). Glucocorticoid therapy may attenuate growth-promoting effects in children; carefully adjust glucocorticoid replacement therapy. May increase clearance of antipyrine. May alter clearance of compounds metabolized by CYP450 liver enzymes (eg, corticosteroids, sex steroids, anticonvulsants, cyclosporine); monitor carefully. Oral estrogen replacement may increase dose requirements. May need to adjust dose of insulin and/or oral/injectable hypoglycemic agents, and thyroid hormone replacement therapy.

PREGNANCY: Category C, caution in nursing.

MECHANISM OF ACTION: Recombinant human GH; binds to dimeric GH receptors in cell membranes of target tissue cells resulting in intracellular signal transduction.

PHARMACOKINETICS: Absorption: Absolute bioavailability (81%), C_{max}=71.1mcg/L, T_{max}=3.9 hrs, AUC=677mcg•hr/L. **Distribution:** V_d=50mL/kg. **Metabolism:** Liver and kidneys. **Elimination:** $T_{1/2}$=2.1 hrs.

NURSING CONSIDERATIONS

Assessment: Assess for preexisting DM or impaired glucose tolerance, hypothyroidism, hypopituitarism, history of scoliosis, any other conditions where treatment is contraindicated or cautioned, pregnancy/nursing status, and possible drug interactions. Perform funduscopic exam. Obtain x-rays of the hip in CKD patients. Assess for hypersensitivity to benzyl alcohol.

Monitoring: Monitor growth, clinical response, compliance, malignant transformation of skin lesions, fluid retention, weight control, respiratory status, intracranial HTN, allergic reactions, pancreatitis, and SCFE and progression of scoliosis in pediatric patients (eg, onset of limp, hip or knee pain). Perform periodic thyroid function tests, funduscopic exam, and monitor glucose levels. In patients with TS, monitor for ear disorders (eg, otitis media) and CV disorders. In patients with preexisting tumors or GHD secondary to an intracranial lesion, monitor for progression/recurrence of underlying disease process.

Patient Counseling: Inform about potential benefits and risks of therapy, proper administration, usage and disposal, and caution against reuse of needles and syringes. Instruct to notify physician if any adverse reactions develop.

Administration: SQ route. Refer to PI for preparation and administration instructions. **Storage:** 2-8°C (36-46°F). Avoid freezing. Reconstituted Sol: Stable for 14 days at 2-8°C (36-46°F). Avoid freezing. (AQ) Stable for 28 days after initial use at 2-8°C (36-46°F). Avoid freezing. Protect from light.

NUVARING   RX
etonogestrel - ethinyl estradiol (Merck)

> Cigarette smoking increases the risk of serious cardiovascular (CV) events. Risk increases with age and with number of cigarettes smoked. Not for use by women >35 yrs of age and smoke.

THERAPEUTIC CLASS: Estrogen/progestogen combination

INDICATIONS: Prevention of pregnancy.

DOSAGE: *Adults:* Insert ring vaginally. Ring is to remain in place continuously for 3 weeks. Remove for 1-week break, then insert a new ring on same day of week as the last ring was removed. No Hormonal Contraceptive Use in the Preceding Cycle: May insert ring on Days 1-5 of menstrual bleeding. If inserted on Days 2-5 of cycle, use an additional barrier method of contraception (eg, male condom with spermicide) for the first 7 days. Changing from a Combination Hormonal Contraceptive: May switch on any day, but at the latest on the day following the usual hormone-free interval. Changing from Progestin-Only Method (Progestin-Only Pill [POP], Implant, Inj, or Progestogen-Releasing Intrauterine System [IUS]): May switch on any day from the POP; start using on the day after taking last POP. May switch from an implant or IUS on the day of its removal and from an injectable on the day when the next inj is due. In all cases, additional barrier method (eg, male condom with spermicide) should be used for the first 7 days. Use After Abortion/Miscarriage: May start within 5 days following a complete 1st trimester abortion/miscarriage. No need to use an additional method of contraception. If not started within 5 days, follow instructions for "no hormonal contraceptive use in the preceding cycle." Following Childbirth or 2nd Trimester Abortion/Miscarriage: May be initiated no earlier than 4 weeks postpartum in women who elect not to breastfeed, or 4 weeks after a 2nd trimester abortion/miscarriage. If use is begun postpartum, use an additional method of contraception (eg, male condom with spermicide) for the first 7 days.

Pediatrics: Postpubertal: Insert ring vaginally. Ring is to remain in place continuously for 3 weeks. Remove for 1-week break, then insert a new ring on same day of week as the last ring was removed. No Hormonal Contraceptive Use in the Preceding Cycle: May insert ring on Days 1-5 of menstrual bleeding. If inserted on Days 2-5 of cycle, use an additional barrier method of contraception (eg, male condom with spermicide) for the first 7 days. Changing from a Combination Hormonal Contraceptive: May switch any day, but at the latest on the day following the usual hormone-free interval. Changing from Progestin-Only Method (POP, Implant, Inj, or IUS): May switch on any day from the POP; start using on the day after taking last POP. May switch from an implant or IUS on the day of its removal and from an injectable on the day when the next inj is due. In all cases, additional barrier method (eg, male condom with spermicide) should be used for the first 7 days. Use After Abortion/Miscarriage: May start within 5 days following a complete 1st trimester abortion/miscarriage. No need to use an additional method of contraception. If not started within 5 days, follow instructions for "no hormonal contraceptive use in the preceding cycle." Following Childbirth or 2nd Trimester Abortion/Miscarriage: May be initiated no earlier than 4 weeks postpartum in women who elect not to breastfeed, or 4 weeks after a 2nd trimester abortion/miscarriage. If use is begun postpartum, use an additional method of contraception (eg, male condom with spermicide) for the first 7 days.

HOW SUPPLIED: Vaginal ring: (Ethinyl Estradiol-Etonogestrel) 0.015mg-0.120mg/day

CONTRAINDICATIONS: A high risk of arterial or venous thrombotic diseases including women who are known to smoke, if >35 yrs of age; current or history of deep vein thrombosis or pulmonary embolism; cerebrovascular disease; coronary artery disease; thrombogenic valvular or thrombogenic rhythm diseases of the heart (eg, subacute bacterial endocarditis with valvular disease, or atrial fibrillation); inherited or acquired hypercoagulopathies; uncontrolled HTN; diabetes mellitus with vascular disease; headaches with focal neurological symptoms or migraine headaches with aura; >35 yrs of age with any migraine headaches. Benign or malignant liver tumors or liver disease; undiagnosed abnormal uterine bleeding; pregnancy; current or history of breast cancer or other estrogen- or progestin-sensitive cancer.

WARNINGS/PRECAUTIONS: For vaginal use only. Consider possibility of ovulation and conception prior to 1st use. Increased risk of a venous thromboembolic event (VTE) and arterial thromboses. D/C if unexplained loss of vision, proptosis, diplopia, papilledema, or retinal vascular lesions develop; evaluate for retinal vein thrombosis immediately. D/C at least 4 weeks prior to and 2 weeks after major surgery associated with an elevated risk of thromboembolism and during and following prolonged immobilization, if feasible. Start use no earlier than 4 weeks after delivery in women who elect not to breastfeed. Caution in women with CV disease risk factors. If patient exhibits signs/symptoms of toxic shock syndrome (TSS), consider possibility of this diagnosis and initiate appropriate medical evaluation and treatment. Acute or chronic disturbances of liver function may necessitate discontinuation until LFTs return to normal and combined hormonal contraceptive causation has been excluded. D/C if jaundice develops. Increased risk of cervical cancer or intraepithelial neoplasia, hepatic adenoma, hepatocellular carcinoma, and gallbladder disease. Increase in BP reported; increase is more likely in older women and with extended duration of use. Monitor BP in women with well-controlled HTN; d/c if BP rises significantly. May decrease glucose tolerance; monitor prediabetic and diabetic women. Consider alternative contraception with uncontrolled dyslipidemia. May increase risk of pancreatitis with hypertriglyceridemia or a family history thereof. D/C if indicated and evaluate cause if new headaches that are recurrent, persistent, or severe develop. Consider discontinuation in case of increased frequency or severity of migraine during use. Unscheduled (breakthrough or intracyclic) bleeding and spotting reported, especially during the first 3 months of use; check for causes (eg, pregnancy, malignancy) if bleeding persists or occurs after previously regular cycles. Consider possibility of pregnancy and take appropriate diagnostic measures if scheduled (withdrawal) bleeding does not occur and patient has not adhered to prescribed dosing schedule or patient has adhered to prescribed regimen and misses 2 consecutive periods. Caution with history of depression; d/c if it recurs to a serious degree. May induce or exacerbate angioedema in patients with hereditary angioedema. Chloasma may occur; avoid exposure to sun or UV radiation in women with a tendency to chloasma. May not be suitable for women with conditions that make the vagina more susceptible to vaginal irritation or ulceration. Vaginal/cervical erosion or ulceration and inadvertent insertion into urinary bladder reported; assess for ring insertion into urinary bladder with persistent urinary symptoms and if unable to locate ring. May be expelled while removing tampon, during intercourse, or with straining during a bowel movement. Cases of disconnection of the ring at the weld joint reported; discard the ring and replace it with a new ring if ring has disconnected. May interfere with correct placement and position of a diaphragm. May influence results of certain laboratory tests.

ADVERSE REACTIONS: Vaginitis, headache, mood changes, device-related events, vaginal discharge, increased weight, N/V, vaginal discomfort, breast pain, dysmenorrhea, abdominal pain.

INTERACTIONS: May decrease plasma concentrations and potentially diminish effectiveness or increase breakthrough bleeding when used concomitantly with drugs or herbal products that induce CYP3A4 (eg, phenytoin, barbiturates, carbamazepine, bosentan, felbamate, griseofulvin, oxcarbazepine, rifampicin, topiramate, rifabutin, rufinamide, aprepitant, products containing St. John's wort); use an alternative method of contraception or a back-up method when used concomitantly with enzyme inducers, and continue back-up contraception for 28 days after discontinuing enzyme inducers. Atorvastatin, ascorbic acid, acetaminophen, CYP3A4 inhibitors (eg, itraconazole, voriconazole, fluconazole, grapefruit juice, ketoconazole), and vaginal miconazole nitrate may increase plasma hormone levels. HIV protease inhibitors (eg, nelfinavir, ritonavir, [fos]amprenavir/ritonavir, indinavir, atazanavir/ritonavir), hepatitis C virus protease inhibitors (eg, boceprevir, telaprevir), and non-nucleoside reverse transcriptase inhibitors (eg, nevirapine, etravirine) may cause significant changes in plasma levels. May inhibit the metabolism of other compounds (eg, cyclosporine, prednisolone, theophylline, tizanidine, voriconazole) and increase their plasma concentrations. May decrease levels of acetaminophen, clofibric acid, morphine, salicylic acid, and temazepam. May decrease levels of lamotrigine and reduce seizure control; dosage adjustments of lamotrigine may be necessary. May raise serum concentrations of thyroxine-binding globulin and cortisol-binding globulin; may need to increase dose of replacement thyroid hormone or cortisol therapy.

PREGNANCY: Contraindicated in pregnancy, not for use in nursing.

MECHANISM OF ACTION: Estrogen/progestogen combination; acts by suppression of gonadotropins. Primarily inhibits ovulation. Also produces other alterations, including changes in the cervical mucus (increasing difficulty of sperm entry into the uterus) and the endometrium (reducing likelihood of implantation).

PHARMACOKINETICS: Absorption: Etonogestrel: Rapid; bioavailability (100%); C_{max}=1716pg/mL; T_{max}=200.3 hrs. Ethinyl estradiol: Rapid; bioavailability (56%); C_{max}=34.7pg/mL; T_{max}=59.3 hrs. **Distribution:** Found in breast milk. Etonogestrel: Serum albumin binding (66%), sex hormone-binding globulin (32%). Ethinyl estradiol: Serum albumin binding (98.5%). **Metabolism:** Hepatic via CYP3A4. Ethinyl estradiol: aromatic hydroxylation. **Elimination:** Urine, bile, feces; Etonogestrel: $T_{1/2}$=29.3 hrs; Ethinyl estradiol: $T_{1/2}$=44.7 hrs.

NURSING CONSIDERATIONS

Assessment: Assess for high risk of arterial or venous thrombotic diseases; benign or malignant liver tumors; liver disease; undiagnosed, abnormal uterine bleeding; presence or history of breast cancer or other estrogen- or progestin-sensitive cancer; pregnancy; and any other conditions where treatment is contraindicated/cautioned. Assess nursing status and for possible drug interactions.

Monitoring: Monitor for arterial thrombotic or venous thromboembolic events, TSS, hepatic adenomas, hepatocellular carcinoma, gallbladder disease, and other adverse effects. Monitor lipid levels with hyperlipidemia, BP with history of HTN, serum glucose levels in diabetic or prediabetic patients, and for signs of worsening depression with previous history. Have a yearly visit with patient for a BP check and for other indicated healthcare.

Patient Counseling: Inform of risks and benefits of therapy. Inform that cigarette smoking increases risk of serious CV events. Inform of increased risk of VTE. Counsel that therapy does not protect against HIV infection (AIDS) or other sexually transmitted diseases. Instruct not to use during pregnancy and to d/c if pregnancy is planned or occurs during use. Instruct to use a barrier method of contraception when ring is out for >3 continuous hrs until ring has been used continuously for at least 7 days. Counsel to use a back-up or alternative method of contraception when enzyme inducers are concomitantly used. Inform that breast milk production may be reduced with use. Instruct postpartum women who have not yet had a normal period, to use an additional non-hormonal method of contraception for the first 7 days. Instruct on proper usage and what to do if non compliant with timing of insertion and removal. Inform that amenorrhea may occur. Advise that pregnancy should be ruled out in the event of amenorrhea, if ring has been out of the vagina for >3 consecutive hrs, if ring-free interval was extended >1 week, if a period was missed for ≥2 consecutive cycles, or if ring has been retained for >4 weeks.

Administration: Intravaginal route. Refer to PI for further administration instructions. **Storage:** 2-8°C (36-46°F). After dispensing, store up to 4 months at 25°C (77°F); excursions permitted to 15-30°C (59-86°F). Avoid direct sunlight or above 30°C (86°F).

NUVIGIL
armodafinil (Cephalon)

CIV

THERAPEUTIC CLASS: Wakefulness-promoting agent

INDICATIONS: To improve wakefulness in adults with excessive sleepiness associated with obstructive sleep apnea (OSA), narcolepsy, or shift work disorder (SWD).

DOSAGE: *Adults:* OSA/Narcolepsy: 150-250mg qam. SWD: 150mg qd approximately 1 hr prior to work shift. Severe Hepatic Impairment with/without Cirrhosis: Reduce dose. Elderly: Consider lower doses.

HOW SUPPLIED: Tab: 50mg, 150mg, 200mg, 250mg

WARNINGS/PRECAUTIONS: Use only in patients who have had a complete evaluation of excessive sleepiness, and in whom a diagnosis of narcolepsy, OSA, or SWD has been made in accordance with International Classification of Sleep Disorders (ICSD) or Diagnostic and Statistical Manual of Mental Disorders (DSM) diagnostic criteria. Not indicated as treatment for underlying obstruction in OSA; if continuous positive airway pressure (CPAP) is the treatment of choice, treat with CPAP for an adequate period of time prior to initiation of therapy. Rare cases of serious or life-threatening rash, including Stevens-Johnson syndrome (SJS), toxic epidermal necrolysis (TEN), and drug rash with eosinophilia and systemic symptoms (DRESS) reported; d/c treatment at 1st sign of rash, unless rash is clearly not drug-related. Angioedema, anaphylactoid reactions, multiorgan hypersensitivity reactions, and psychiatric adverse experiences reported; d/c treatment if symptoms develop. Caution with cardiovascular disease (CVD) (eg, recent history of myocardial infarction, unstable angina). Avoid in patients with history of left ventricular hypertrophy or with mitral valve prolapse who have experienced mitral valve prolapse syndrome (eg, ischemic ECG changes, chest pain, arrhythmia) with CNS stimulants. May impair mental/physical abilities. Level of wakefulness may not return to normal in patients with abnormal levels of sleepiness. Potential for abuse. Caution in elderly.

ADVERSE REACTIONS: Headache, nausea, dizziness, insomnia, diarrhea, dry mouth, anxiety, depression, rash.

INTERACTIONS: Reduced exposure of CYP3A4/5 substrates (eg, cyclosporine, midazolam, triazolam); consider dose adjustment of these drugs. Effectiveness of steroidal contraceptives may be reduced during and for 1 month after discontinuation of therapy; alternative or concomitant methods of contraception are recommended. Cyclosporine levels may be reduced; monitor levels and consider dosage adjustment. Increased exposure of CYP2C19 substrates (eg, omeprazole, diazepam, phenytoin); dosage reduction of these drugs may be required. Frequently monitor PT/INR with warfarin.

PREGNANCY: Category C, caution in nursing.

MECHANISM OF ACTION: Wakefulness-promoting agent; not established. Binds to the dopamine transporter and inhibits dopamine reuptake.

PHARMACOKINETICS: Absorption: Readily absorbed. T_{max}=2 hrs (fasted). **Distribution:** V_d=42L. (Modafinil) Plasma protein binding (60%). **Metabolism:** Liver via hydrolytic deamidation, S-oxidation, aromatic ring hydroxylation, and glucuronide conjugation; CYP3A4/5. **Elimination:** (Modafinil) Feces (1%), urine (80%, <10% parent compound). $T_{1/2}$=15 hrs.

NURSING CONSIDERATIONS

Assessment: Assess for hypersensitivity to modafinil or to drug, hepatic impairment, psychosis, depression, mania, left ventricular hypertrophy, mitral valve prolapse, other CVD, pregnancy/nursing status, and possible drug interactions. Perform a complete evaluation of excessive sleepiness and confirm diagnosis of narcolepsy, OSA, and/or SWD in accordance with ICSD or DSM diagnostic criteria.

Monitoring: Monitor for serious rash, SJS, TEN, DRESS, angioedema, anaphylaxis, hypersensitivity reactions, multiorgan hypersensitivity reactions, psychiatric adverse symptoms, and other adverse reactions. Monitor for signs of misuse or abuse. Monitor HR and BP. If used adjunctively with CPAP, monitor for CPAP compliance periodically. Frequently reassess degree of sleepiness; reevaluate long-term usefulness periodically if prescribed for an extended time. Consider close monitoring in elderly. Monitor PT/INR frequently with warfarin.

Patient Counseling: Inform that drug is not a replacement for sleep. Inform that therapy may improve but not eliminate the abnormal tendency to fall asleep; instruct not to alter previous behavior with regard to potentially dangerous activities or other activities requiring appropriate levels of wakefulness, until and unless treatment has shown to produce levels of wakefulness that permit such activities. Inform of importance of continuing previously prescribed treatments. Advise to avoid alcohol during therapy. Advise to notify physician if pregnant, intending to become pregnant, or nursing. Caution about increased risk of pregnancy when using steroidal contraceptives and for 1 month after discontinuation of therapy. Instruct to inform physician if taking/planning to take any prescribed or OTC drugs. Instruct to d/c and notify physician if rash, hives, mouth sores, blisters, peeling skin, trouble swallowing or breathing or related allergic phenomenon, depression, anxiety, or signs of psychosis or mania develop.

Administration: Oral route. **Storage:** 20-25°C (68-77°F).

NYSTATIN ORAL   RX
nystatin (Various)

THERAPEUTIC CLASS: Polyene antifungal

INDICATIONS: (Sus) Treatment of oral candidiasis. (Tab) Treatment of non-esophageal mucus membrane GI candidiasis.

DOSAGE: *Adults:* (Sus) Oral Candidiasis: 4-6mL qid (1/2 of dose in each side of mouth). Retain in mouth as long as possible before swallowing. Continue treatment for at least 48 hrs after perioral symptoms disappear and cultures demonstrate eradication of *Candida albicans*. (Tab) Non-Esophageal GI Candidiasis: 1-2 tab tid. Continue treatment for at least 48 hrs after clinical cure. *Pediatrics:* (Sus) Oral Candidiasis: 4-6mL qid (1/2 of dose in each side of mouth). Retain in mouth as long as possible before swallowing. Infants: 2mL qid. Premature/Low Birth Weight Infants: 1mL qid. Continue treatment for at least 48 hrs after perioral symptoms disappear and cultures demonstrate eradication of *C. albicans*.

HOW SUPPLIED: Sus: 100,000 U/mL [60mL, 473mL]; Tab: 500,000 U

WARNINGS/PRECAUTIONS: Not for use in treatment of systemic mycoses. D/C if sensitization/irritation occurs.

ADVERSE REACTIONS: Oral irritation/sensitization, diarrhea, N/V, GI upset/disturbances.

PREGNANCY: Category C, caution in nursing.

MECHANISM OF ACTION: Polyene antifungal; binds to sterols in the cell membrane of susceptible *Candida* species with a resultant change in membrane permeability, allowing leakage of intracellular components.

PHARMACOKINETICS: Elimination: Feces (unchanged).

NURSING CONSIDERATIONS

Assessment: Assess for history of hypersensitivity to the drug or any of its components, and pregnancy/nursing status. Confirm diagnosis of candidiasis.

Monitoring: Monitor for oral irritation/sensitization, and other adverse reactions.

Patient Counseling: Advise to notify physician if any adverse reactions (eg, sensitization, irritation) occur. Instruct to inform physician if pregnant, planning to become pregnant, or breastfeeding.

Administration: Oral route. (Sus) Shake well before using. In infants and young children, use dropper to place 1/2 of dose in each side of mouth; avoid feeding for 5-10 min. **Storage:** 20-25°C (68-77°F). (Sus) Avoid freezing.

N

OFIRMEV
acetaminophen (Cadence)

RX

> Caution when prescribing, preparing, and administering therapy to avoid dosing errors that could result in accidental overdose and death. Ensure that the dose in mg and mL is not confused, the dosing is based on weight for patients <50kg, infusion pumps are properly programmed, and the total daily dose of acetaminophen (APAP) from all sources does not exceed max daily limits. Associated with cases of acute liver failure, at times resulting in liver transplant and death. Most cases of liver injury are associated with APAP use at doses that exceed the max daily limits, and often involve >1 APAP-containing product.

THERAPEUTIC CLASS: Analgesic

INDICATIONS: Management of mild to moderate pain, management of moderate to severe pain with adjunctive opioid analgesics, and for reduction of fever.

DOSAGE: *Adults:* ≥50kg: Usual: 1000mg q6h or 650mg q4h. Max: 1000mg/dose; 4000mg/day. <50kg: Usual: 15mg/kg q6h or 12.5mg/kg q4h. Max: 15mg/kg/dose (up to 750mg); 75mg/kg/day (up to 3750mg). Hepatic Impairment/Active Liver Disease: May reduce total daily dose. Severe Renal Impairment (CrCl ≤30mL/min): May extend dosing intervals and reduce total daily dose. *Pediatrics:* ≥13 Yrs: ≥50kg: Usual: 1000mg q6h or 650mg q4h. Max: 1000mg/dose; 4000mg/day. <50kg: Usual: 15mg/kg q6h or 12.5mg/kg q4h. Max: 15mg/kg/dose (up to 750mg); 75mg/kg/day (up to 3750mg). 2-12 Yrs: Usual: 15mg/kg q6h or 12.5mg/kg q4h. Max: 15mg/kg/dose (up to 750mg); 75mg/kg/day (up to 3750mg). Hepatic Impairment/Active Liver Disease: May reduce total daily dose. Severe Renal Impairment (CrCl ≤30mL/min): May extend dosing intervals and a reduce total daily dose.

HOW SUPPLIED: Inj: 10mg/mL [100mL]

CONTRAINDICATIONS: Severe hepatic impairment or severe active liver disease.

WARNINGS/PRECAUTIONS: Caution with hepatic impairment or active hepatic disease, alcoholism, chronic malnutrition, severe hypovolemia (eg, due to dehydration or blood loss), or severe renal impairment (CrCl ≤30mL/min). May cause serious skin reactions (eg, acute generalized exanthematous pustulosis, Stevens-Johnson syndrome, toxic epidermal necrolysis); d/c at the 1st appearance of skin rash or any other sign of hypersensitivity. Hypersensitivity and anaphylaxis reported; d/c immediately if symptoms occur. Do not use with APAP allergy.

ADVERSE REACTIONS: Liver failure, N/V, headache, insomnia, constipation, pruritus, agitation, atelectasis.

INTERACTIONS: Substances that induce or regulate CYP2E1 may alter the metabolism and increase hepatotoxic potential. Excessive alcohol use may induce hepatic cytochromes, but ethanol may also inhibit metabolism. Increased INR in some patients stabilized on sodium warfarin; more frequent assessment of INR may be appropriate.

PREGNANCY: Category C, caution in nursing.

MECHANISM OF ACTION: Nonopiate, nonsalicylate analgesic and antipyretic; not established. Thought to primarily involve central actions.

PHARMACOKINETICS: Absorption: Administration of variable doses to different age groups resulted in different pharmacokinetic parameters. **Distribution:** Plasma protein binding (10-25%); widely distributed throughout most body tissues except fat; (PO) found in breast milk. **Metabolism:** Liver; glucuronide and sulfate conjugation, and oxidation via CYP2E1; N-acetyl-p-benzoquinone imine (intermediate metabolite). **Elimination:** Urine (>90% within 24 hrs, <5% unconjugated).

NURSING CONSIDERATIONS

Assessment: Assess for previous hypersensitivity, alcoholism, chronic malnutrition, severe hypovolemia, hepatic/renal impairment, pregnancy/nursing status, and possible drug interactions.

Monitoring: Monitor for signs/symptoms of hypersensitivity and anaphylaxis, acute liver failure, serious skin reactions, and other adverse reactions. Monitor the end of infusion to prevent the possibility of air embolism, especially in cases where therapy is the primary infusion. Monitor INR frequently in patients stabilized on sodium warfarin.

Patient Counseling: Inform about the risks and benefits of therapy. Instruct not to exceed the recommended dose. Instruct to notify physician if any adverse reactions occur or if pregnant/nursing or planning to become pregnant. Counsel about possible drug interactions.

Administration: IV route. Administer by IV infusion. Do not add other medications to the vial or infusion device; physically incompatible with diazepam and chlorpromazine HCl. Refer to PI for further administration instructions. **Storage:** 20-25°C (68-77°F). Use within 6 hrs after opening. Do not refrigerate or freeze.

OFLOXACIN

RX

ofloxacin (Various)

> Fluoroquinolones are associated with an increased risk of tendinitis and tendon rupture in all ages. Risk is further increased in patients >60 yrs of age, taking corticosteroids, and with kidney, heart, or lung transplants. May exacerbate muscle weakness with myasthenia gravis; avoid with known history of myasthenia gravis.

THERAPEUTIC CLASS: Fluoroquinolone

INDICATIONS: Treatment of acute bacterial exacerbation of chronic bronchitis (ABECB), community-acquired pneumonia (CAP), uncomplicated skin and skin structure infections (SSSIs), acute uncomplicated urethral and cervical gonorrhea, nongonococcal urethritis and cervicitis, mixed infections of urethra and cervix, acute pelvic inflammatory disease (PID), uncomplicated cystitis, complicated urinary tract infections (UTIs), and prostatitis.

DOSAGE: *Adults:* ABECB/CAP/SSSI: 400mg q12h for 10 days. Cervicitis/Urethritis/Mixed Infection of Urethra and Cervix: 300mg q12h for 7 days. Gonorrhea: 400mg single dose. PID: 400mg q12h for 10-14 days. Cystitis: 200mg q12h for 3 days (*Escherichia coli* or *Klebsiella pneumoniae*) or 7 days (other approved pathogens). UTI: 200mg q12h for 10 days. Prostatitis: 300mg q12h for 6 weeks. Renal Impairment: CrCl 20-50mL/min: After normal initial dose, adjust dose as usual recommended unit dose q24h. CrCl <20mL/min: After normal initial dose, adjust dose as 50% of the usual recommended unit dose q24h. Severe Hepatic Impairment: Max: 400mg/day.

HOW SUPPLIED: Tab: 200mg, 300mg, 400mg

WARNINGS/PRECAUTIONS: D/C if pain, swelling, inflammation, or rupture of a tendon occurs. Convulsions, increased intracranial pressure (including pseudotumor cerebri), and toxic psychosis reported. CNS stimulation may occur; d/c and institute appropriate measures if reactions occur. Caution with CNS disorder or risk factors that may predispose to seizures or lower seizure threshold. Serious and occasionally fatal hypersensitivity and/or anaphylactic reactions reported; d/c immediately at the 1st appearance of skin rash, jaundice, or any other sign of hypersensitivity and institute supportive measures. Rare cases of sensory or sensorimotor axonal polyneuropathy resulting in paresthesias, hypoesthesias, dysesthesias, and weakness reported; d/c if symptoms occur. *Clostridium difficile*-associated diarrhea (CDAD) reported; d/c if CDAD suspected or confirmed. May result in bacterial resistance when use in the absence of a proven/strongly suspected bacterial infection or a prophylactic indication. Not shown to be effective in the treatment of syphilis. Maintain adequate hydration to prevent formation of highly concentrated urine. D/C therapy if photosensitivity/phototoxicity occurs. Prolongation of the QT interval on ECG, arrhythmia, and torsades de pointes reported; avoid with known QT interval prolongation or uncorrected hypokalemia. Caution in the presence of renal or hepatic insufficiency/impairment and in elderly, especially those on corticosteroids. Lab test interactions may occur.

ADVERSE REACTIONS: Tendinitis, tendon rupture, N/V, insomnia, headache, dizziness, diarrhea, external genital pruritus in women, vaginitis, abdominal pain/cramps, chest pain, decreased appetite, dry mouth, dysgeusia, fatigue.

INTERACTIONS: See Boxed Warning. Caution with drugs that may lower the seizure threshold. May prolong QT interval; avoid with Class IA (eg, quinidine, procainamide) or Class III (eg, amiodarone, sotalol) antiarrhythmics. Administration with antacids containing Ca^{2+}, Mg^{2+}, or aluminum, with sucralfate, with divalent or trivalent cations (eg, iron), or with multivitamins containing zinc or with didanosine, chewable/buffered tab or pediatric powder for oral solution may result in lower systemic levels; do not take within the 2-hr period before or after ofloxacin administration. Cimetidine may interfere with elimination. May elevate cyclosporine levels. May prolong $T_{1/2}$ of drugs metabolized by CYP450 (eg, cyclosporine, methylxanthines). NSAIDs may increase risk of CNS stimulation and convulsive seizures. Probenecid may affect renal tubular secretion. May increase theophylline levels and increase risk of theophylline-related adverse reactions; monitor theophylline levels closely and adjust theophylline dose, if appropriate. May enhance effects of warfarin or its derivatives; monitor PT or other suitable coagulation test. Disturbances of blood glucose with antidiabetic agents reported; monitor blood glucose levels and d/c if hypoglycemia occurs.

PREGNANCY: Category C, not for use in nursing.

MECHANISM OF ACTION: Fluoroquinolone; inhibits bacterial topoisomerase IV and DNA gyrase, enzymes required for DNA replication, transcription, repair, and recombination.

PHARMACOKINETICS: Absorption: Bioavailability (98%); T_{max}=1-2 hrs. Oral administration of variable doses resulted in different parameters. **Distribution:** Plasma protein binding (32%); found in breast milk. **Elimination:** Urine (65-80% unchanged, <5% desmethyl and N-oxide metabolites), feces (4-8%); (Biphasic) $T_{1/2}$=4-5 hrs and 20-25 hrs (multiple doses).

NURSING CONSIDERATIONS

Assessment: Assess for risk factors for developing tendinitis and tendon rupture, history of myasthenia gravis, drug hypersensitivity, epilepsy, CNS disorders, risk factors that may predispose to seizures or lower seizure threshold, QT interval prolongation, uncorrected hypokalemia, renal/hepatic dysfunction, pregnancy/nursing status, and possible drug interactions. Obtain baseline culture and susceptibility tests. Perform serologic test for syphilis in patients with gonorrhea.

Monitoring: Monitor for tendinitis or tendon rupture, CNS effects, signs/symptoms of hypersensitivity reactions, CDAD, peripheral neuropathy, photosensitivity/phototoxicity reactions, ECG changes, and other adverse reactions. Monitor renal/hepatic/hematopoietic function with prolonged use. Perform periodic culture and susceptibility testing. Perform follow-up serologic test for syphilis after 3 months. Monitor PT or other coagulation tests with warfarin or its derivatives.

Patient Counseling: Advise to notify physician if pain, swelling, or inflammation of a tendon, or weakness or inability to move joints develops; instruct to d/c therapy and rest/refrain from exercise. Instruct to notify physician if experiencing worsening muscle weakness or breathing problems, sunburn-like reaction or skin eruption, and of all medications and supplements currently being taken. Inform that drug treats only bacterial, not viral (eg, common cold), infections. Counsel to take exactly ud; inform that skipping doses or not completing full course of therapy may decrease effectiveness and increase bacterial resistance. Advise to drink fluids liberally. Instruct to d/c and notify physician if signs/symptoms of hypersensitivity reactions/allergic reactions or peripheral neuropathy develop. Inform that drug may cause dizziness and lightheadedness; advise to assess reaction to therapy before engaging in activities that require mental alertness or coordination. Counsel to minimize or avoid exposure to natural/artificial sunlight. Advise diabetic patients being treated with insulin or oral hypoglycemic drug to d/c therapy immediately if hypoglycemic reaction occurs and consult a physician. Instruct to notify physician of any history of convulsions. Advise to contact physician as soon as possible if watery and bloody stools (with or without stomach cramps and fever) develop. Instruct to notify physician if any symptoms of QT prolongation, including prolonged heart palpitations, or loss of consciousness occur. Advise not to take mineral supplements, vitamins with iron or minerals, antacids containing Ca^{2+}, Mg^{2+} or aluminum, sucralfate, didanosine, chewable/buffered tab or pediatric powder for oral solution within the 2-hr period before or after taking ofloxacin.

Administration: Oral route. Take without regard to meals. **Storage:** 20-25°C (68-77°F).

OFLOXACIN OTIC   RX
ofloxacin (Various)

THERAPEUTIC CLASS: Fluoroquinolone

INDICATIONS: Treatment of otitis externa in patients ≥6 months of age, chronic suppurative otitis media in patients ≥12 yrs of age with perforated tympanic membranes, and acute otitis media in patients ≥1 yr of age with tympanostomy tubes.

DOSAGE: *Adults:* Otitis Externa: 10 drops (0.5mL) into affected ear qd for 7 days. Chronic Suppurative Otitis Media with Perforated Tympanic Membrane: 10 drops (0.5mL) bid into affected ear for 14 days. Pump tragus 4 times by pushing inward to facilitate penetration into the middle ear.
Pediatrics: Otitis Externa: ≥13 Yrs: 10 drops (0.5mL) into affected ear qd for 7 days. 6 months-13 Yrs: 5 drops (0.25mL) into affected ear qd for 7 days. Chronic Suppurative Otitis Media with Perforated Tympanic Membrane: ≥12 Yrs: 10 drops (0.5mL) bid into affected ear for 14 days. Pump tragus 4 times by pushing inward to facilitate penetration into the middle ear. Acute Otitis Media with Tympanostomy Tubes: 1-12 Yrs: 5 drops (0.25mL) bid into affected ear for 10 days. Pump tragus 4 times by pushing inward to facilitate penetration into the middle ear.

HOW SUPPLIED: Sol: 0.3% [5mL, 10mL]

WARNINGS/PRECAUTIONS: D/C if hypersensitivity reaction occurs. Prolonged use may result in overgrowth of nonsusceptible organisms; reevaluate if no improvement after one week. If otorrhea persists after a full course, or if two or more episodes occur within 6 months, further evaluation is recommended. Not for injection or ophthalmic use.

ADVERSE REACTIONS: Pruritus, application-site reaction, taste perversion.

PREGNANCY: Category C, not for use in nursing.

MECHANISM OF ACTION: Fluoroquinolone; exerts antibacterial activity by inhibiting DNA gyrase, an enzyme required for DNA replication, repair, deactivation, and transcription.

PHARMACOKINETICS: Absorption: (Perforated tympanic membrane) C_{max}=10ng/mL.

NURSING CONSIDERATIONS

Assessment: Assess for drug hypersensitivity, preexisting cholesteatoma, foreign body or tumor, pregnancy/nursing status.

Monitoring: Monitor for anaphylactic reactions, cardiovascular collapse, loss of consciousness, angioedema, airway obstruction, dyspnea, urticaria and itching, overgrowth of nonsusceptible organisms, for improvement/persistence of otorrhea.

Patient Counseling: Counsel to avoid touching applicator tip to fingers or other surfaces to avoid contamination. D/C and instruct to contact physician if signs of allergy occur. Instruct patients to warm bottle by holding for 1-2 min, to avoid dizziness that may result from instillation of a cold solution. Instruct to lie with affected ear upward, before instilling the drops; maintain position for 5 min. Instruct to repeat if necessary, for opposite ear.

Administration: Otic route. **Storage:** 20-25°C (68-77°F). Protect from light.

OLEPTRO   RX
trazodone HCl (Angelini Pharma)

> Antidepressants increased the risk of suicidal thinking and behavior (suicidality) in children, adolescents and young adults in short-term studies of major depressive disorder (MDD) and other psychiatric disorders. Monitor and observe closely for clinical worsening, suicidality, or unusual changes in behavior. Not approved for use in pediatric patients.

THERAPEUTIC CLASS: Triazolopyridine derivative

INDICATIONS: Treatment of MDD.

DOSAGE: *Adults:* Initial: 150mg qd preferably at hs on an empty stomach. Titrate: May increase by 75mg/day every 3 days. Max: 375mg qd. Once adequate response is achieved, reduce dose gradually, with subsequent adjustment depending on therapeutic response. Maint: Generally recommended to continue treatment for several months after an initial response. Maintain on the lowest effective dose and periodically reassess to determine the continued need for maintenance treatment. Switching to or from MAOIs Intended to Treat Psychiatric Disorders: Allow at least 14 days to elapse between discontinuation of an MAOI and initiation of therapy, and vice versa. Refer to PI for instructions if using with other MAOIs (eg, linezolid, methylene blue).

HOW SUPPLIED: Tab, Extended Release: 150mg*, 300mg* *scored

CONTRAINDICATIONS: Concomitant use with an MAOI intended to treat psychiatric disorders or use within 14 days of stopping an MAOI, and vice versa. Starting treatment in patients being treated with MAOIs, such as linezolid or IV methylene blue.

WARNINGS/PRECAUTIONS: Not approved for treatment of bipolar depression. Monitor for withdrawal symptoms when treatment is discontinued; reduce dose gradually whenever possible. Serotonin syndrome reported; d/c immediately and initiate supportive symptomatic treatment. May increase the likelihood of precipitation of a mixed/manic episode in patients at risk for bipolar disorder. May cause QT/QTc interval prolongation and torsades de pointes. Not recommended for use during the initial recovery phase of myocardial infarction (MI). May cause cardiac arrhythmias and hypotension, including orthostatic hypotension and syncope. May increase risk of bleeding events. Priapism rarely reported; caution in men with conditions that may predispose to priapism (eg, sickle cell anemia, multiple myeloma, leukemia) or with penile anatomical deformation (eg, angulation, cavernosal fibrosis, Peyronie's disease); d/c with erection lasting >6 hrs (painful or not). Hyponatremia may occur; d/c and institute appropriate medical intervention. May cause somnolence or sedation and may impair mental/physical abilities. Caution with hepatic/renal impairment and elderly.

ADVERSE REACTIONS: Somnolence, sedation, headache, dry mouth, dizziness, nausea, fatigue, diarrhea, constipation, back pain, blurred vision, sexual dysfunction.

INTERACTIONS: See Contraindications. May cause serotonin syndrome with other serotonergic drugs (eg, triptans, fentanyl, buspirone, St. John's wort) and with drugs that impair serotonin metabolism; d/c immediately if this occurs. May enhance response to alcohol, barbiturates and other CNS depressants. Increased risk of cardiac arrhythmia with drugs that prolong QT interval or CYP3A4 inhibitors. CYP3A4 inhibitors (eg, ritonavir, ketoconazole, indinavir) may increase levels with the potential for adverse effects. Potent CYP3A4 inhibitors may increase risk of cardiac arrhythmia; consider lower dose of trazodone. Carbamazepine may decrease levels; monitor to determine if a dose increase is required. Increased serum digoxin or phenytoin levels reported; monitor serum levels and adjust dose PRN. Concomitant use with an antihypertensive may require reduction in the dose of the antihypertensive drug. Monitor and use caution with NSAIDs, aspirin, and other drugs that affect coagulation or bleeding. Increased risk of hyponatremia with diuretics. May alter PT in patients on warfarin.

PREGNANCY: Category C, caution in nursing.

MECHANISM OF ACTION: Triazolopyridine derivative; mechanism not established. Suspected to be related to its potentiation of serotonergic activity in the CNS. Preclinical studies show selective inhibition of neuronal reuptake of serotonin and activity as an antagonist at 5-HT-2A/2C serotonin receptors.

PHARMACOKINETICS: Absorption: Well-absorbed; (300mg qd dose) AUC=29131ng•h/mL, C_{max}=1812ng/mL; (Single dose 300mg, fasted) C_{max}=1188ng/mL, T_{max}=9 hrs. **Distribution:** Plasma protein binding (89-95%). **Metabolism:** Liver (extensive); CYP3A4 via oxidative cleavage; m-chlorophenylpiperazine (active metabolite). **Elimination:** Urine (70-75%, <1% unchanged); $T_{1/2}$=10 hrs.

NURSING CONSIDERATIONS

Assessment: Assess for psychiatric history including family history of suicide, bipolar disorder, and depression, for cardiac disease (eg, MI), conditions that may predispose to priapism, penile anatomical deformation, arrhythmias, hepatic/renal impairment, pregnancy/nursing status, and possible drug interactions.

Monitoring: Monitor for signs/symptoms of clinical worsening, suicidality, unusual changes in behavior, serotonin syndrome, QT/QTc interval prolongation, cardiac arrhythmias, orthostatic hypotension, syncope, bleeding events, priapism, hyponatremia, hepatic/renal impairment, and for other adverse reactions.

Patient Counseling: Advise about the benefits and risks of therapy. Instruct patients and caregivers to notify physician if signs of clinical worsening, changes in behavior, or suicidality occur. Instruct men to immediately d/c use and contact physician if erection lasts >6 hrs, whether painful or not. Inform that withdrawal symptoms may occur. Caution against performing potentially hazardous tasks. Inform that therapy may enhance response to alcohol, barbiturates, and other CNS depressants. Instruct to notify physician if pregnant, plan to become pregnant, or nursing.

Administration: Oral route. Do not chew or crush. Take at the same time every day, preferably at hs, on empty stomach. **Storage:** 15-30°C (59-86°F). Keep in tight, light-resistant containers.

Oʟᴜx-E   RX
clobetasol propionate (Stiefel)

THERAPEUTIC CLASS: Corticosteroid

INDICATIONS: Treatment of inflammatory and pruritic manifestations of corticosteroid-responsive dermatoses in patients ≥12 yrs of age.

DOSAGE: *Adults:* Apply a thin layer to affected area(s) bid (am and pm), for up to 2 consecutive weeks. Max: 50g/week or 21 capfuls/week.
Pediatrics: ≥12 Yrs: Apply a thin layer to affected area(s) bid (am and pm), for up to 2 consecutive weeks. Max: 50g/week or 21 capfuls/week.

HOW SUPPLIED: Foam: 0.05% [50g, 100g]

WARNINGS/PRECAUTIONS: May cause reversible hypothalamic pituitary adrenal (HPA) axis suppression with the potential for glucocorticosteroid insufficiency, Cushing's syndrome, hyperglycemia, and unmasking of latent diabetes mellitus; withdraw, reduce frequency, or substitute a less potent steroid if HPA-axis suppression occurs. Manifestations of adrenal insufficiency may require systemic corticosteroids. Pediatric patients may be more susceptible to systemic toxicity. Local adverse reactions are more likely to occur with occlusive use, prolonged use, or use of higher potency corticosteroids. D/C if irritation occurs. Use appropriate antimicrobial agent with skin infections; d/c until infection is treated. Avoid application to eyes, face, groin, axillae, and area of skin atrophy. Flammable; avoid fire, flame, or smoking during and immediately following application. Do not apply on the chest if used during lactation. D/C if control is achieved.

ADVERSE REACTIONS: Application-site reaction, application-site atrophy, folliculitis, acneiform eruptions, hypopigmentation, perioral dermatitis, allergic contact dermatitis, secondary infection, irritation, striae, miliaria.

INTERACTIONS: Use of >1 corticosteroid-containing product may increase the total systemic corticosteroid exposure.

PREGNANCY: Category C, caution in nursing.

MECHANISM OF ACTION: Corticosteroid; not established. Plays a role in cellular signaling, immune function, inflammation, and protein regulation.

PHARMACOKINETICS: Absorption: Percutaneous. C_{max}=59pg/mL, T_{max}=5 hrs (post-dose on Day 8). **Distribution:** Found in breast milk (systemically administered). **Metabolism:** Liver. **Elimination:** Kidneys, bile.

NURSING CONSIDERATIONS

Assessment: Assess for presence of concomitant skin infections, severity of dermatoses, factors that predispose to HPA-axis suppression, pregnancy/nursing status, and possible drug interactions.

Monitoring: Monitor for signs/symptoms of HPA-axis suppression, Cushing's syndrome, hyperglycemia, irritation, allergic contact dermatitis (eg, failure to heal), and skin infections. Monitor for systemic toxicity, linear growth retardation, delayed weight gain, and intracranial HTN in pediatric patients. Monitor response to therapy.

Patient Counseling: Counsel to use externally and exactly ud; avoid use on face, skin folds (eg, underarms, groin), eyes, or other mucous membranes. Advise to wash hands after use. Advise not to bandage or wrap treatment area, unless directed by physician. Counsel to contact physician if any local or systemic adverse reactions occur, if no improvement is seen after 2 weeks, or if surgery is contemplated. Advise that foam is flammable; avoid fire, flame, or smoking during application. Advise to d/c when control is achieved.

Administration: Topical route. Shake can, hold upside down, and depress the actuator. Dispense small amount (about a capful) and gently massage into the affected area(s) until foam is absorbed. **Storage:** 20-25°C (68-77°F); excursions permitted between 15-30°C (59-86°F). Do not puncture or incinerate container. Do not expose to heat or store above 49°C (120°F).

OMNARIS   RX
ciclesonide (Sunovion)

THERAPEUTIC CLASS: Non-halogenated glucocorticoid

INDICATIONS: Treatment of nasal symptoms associated with seasonal allergic rhinitis in adults/ children ≥6 yrs of age and with perennial allergic rhinitis in adults/adolescents ≥12 yrs of age.

DOSAGE: *Adults:* Seasonal/Perennial Allergic Rhinitis: 2 sprays/nostril qd. Max: 2 sprays/nostril/ day (200mcg/day). Elderly: Start at low end of dosing range.
Pediatrics: Perennial Allergic Rhinitis: ≥12 Yrs: 2 sprays/nostril qd. Max: 2 sprays/nostril/day (200mcg/day). Seasonal Allergic Rhinitis: ≥6 Yrs: 2 sprays/nostril qd. Max: 2 sprays/nostril/day (200mcg/day).

HOW SUPPLIED: Spray: 50mcg/spray [12.5g]

WARNINGS/PRECAUTIONS: Epistaxis reported. *Candida albicans* infections of the nose or pharynx may occur; examine periodically and treat accordingly. Nasal septal perforation may occur; avoid spraying directly onto nasal septum. May impair wound healing; avoid with recent nasal septal ulcers, nasal surgery, or nasal trauma until healing has occurred. Glaucoma and/or cataracts may develop. Risk for more severe/fatal course of infections (eg, chickenpox, measles); avoid exposure in patients who have not had these diseases or have not been properly immunized. May increase susceptibility to infections; caution with active or quiescent tuberculosis (TB), untreated local or systemic fungal/bacterial infections, systemic viral or parasitic infections, or ocular herpes simplex. D/C slowly if hypercorticism and adrenal suppression occur. Risk of adrenal insufficiency and withdrawal symptoms when replacing systemic corticosteroids with topical corticosteroids. May exacerbate symptoms of asthma and other conditions requiring long-term systemic corticosteroid use with rapid dose decrease. May reduce growth velocity in pediatric patients. Caution in elderly.

ADVERSE REACTIONS: Headache, epistaxis, nasopharyngitis, back pain, pharyngolaryngeal pain, sinusitis, influenza, nasal discomfort, bronchitis, urinary tract infection, cough.

INTERACTIONS: Ketoconazole may increase exposure of the active metabolite des-ciclesonide.

PREGNANCY: Category C, caution in nursing.

MECHANISM OF ACTION: Non-halogenated glucocorticoid; not established. Shown to have a wide range of effects on multiple cell types and mediators involved in allergic inflammation.

PHARMACOKINETICS: Absorption: Des-ciclesonide: C_{max}=<30pg/mL. **Distribution:** (IV) V_d=2.9L/kg (Ciclesonide), 12.1L/kg (des-ciclesonide); plasma protein binding (≥99%). **Metabolism:** Hydrolysis by esterases to des-ciclesonide (active metabolite); further metabolism in liver, via CYP3A4, CYP2D6. **Elimination:** (IV) Feces (66%), urine (≤20%).

NURSING CONSIDERATIONS

Assessment: Assess for drug hypersensitivity, TB, any infections, ocular herpes simplex, history of increased IOP, glaucoma, cataracts, recent nasal septal ulcers, nasal surgery/trauma, use of other inhaled or systemic corticosteroids, pregnancy/nursing status, and possible drug interactions. Assess if patients have not been immunized or exposed to infections, such as measles or chickenpox.

Monitoring: Monitor for hypercorticism, adrenal suppression, TB, infections, ocular herpes simplex, chickenpox, and measles. Monitor for epistaxis, nasal septal perforation, growth velocity in children, wound healing, visual changes, hypoadrenalism in infants born to mothers receiving corticosteroids during pregnancy, and hypersensitivity reactions. Monitor for adrenal insufficiency and withdrawal symptoms when replacing systemic with topical corticosteroids.

Patient Counseling: Counsel on appropriate priming and administration of spray; avoid spraying in eyes or directly onto nasal septum. Instruct to take ud at regular intervals; not to exceed prescribed dosage. Instruct to contact physician if symptoms do not improve by a reasonable time (over 1-2 weeks in seasonal allergic rhinitis and 5 weeks in perennial allergic rhinitis) or if condition worsens. Counsel about risks of epistaxis, nasal ulceration, *Candida* infections, and other adverse reactions. Instruct to avoid exposure to chickenpox or measles and to consult physician if exposed to chickenpox or measles. Inform that worsening of existing TB infections, fungal/bacterial/viral/parasitic infections, or ocular herpes simplex may occur. Instruct to inform physician if change in vision occurs.

Administration: Intranasal route. Shake bottle gently and prime pump by actuating 8X before initial use. Reprime with 1 spray or until fine mist appears if not used for 4 consecutive days. **Storage:** 25°C (77°F); excursions permitted to 15-30°C (59-86°F). Do not freeze. Discard after 4 months after removal from pouch or after 120 actuations following initial priming, whichever comes 1st.

OMNITROPE   RX
somatropin rdna origin (Sandoz)

THERAPEUTIC CLASS: Recombinant human growth hormone

INDICATIONS: Treatment of pediatrics with growth failure due to inadequate secretion of endogenous growth hormone (GH), Prader-Willi syndrome (PWS), and Turner syndrome (TS). Treatment of growth failure in pediatrics born small for gestational age (SGA) who fail to manifest catch-up growth by 2 yrs of age, and idiopathic short stature (ISS) in pediatrics whose epiphyses are not closed. Replacement of endogenous GH in adults with adult-onset or childhood-onset GH deficiency (GHD).

DOSAGE: *Adults:* Divide weekly dose over 6 or 7 days of SQ inj (preferably in pm). GHD: Weight-Based: Initial: Not more than 0.04mg/kg/week given as daily SQ inj. Titrate: May increase at 4- to 8-week intervals. Max: 0.08mg/kg/week. Non Weight-Based: Initial: 0.2mg/day (range, 0.15-0.30mg/day). Titrate: May increase gradually every 1-2 months by increments of 0.1-0.2mg/day based on clinical response and serum insulin-like growth factor-I (IGF-I) concentrations. Maint: Individualize dose. Elderly: Start at lower end of dosing range and consider smaller dose increments.
Pediatrics: Individualize dose. Divide weekly dose over 6 or 7 days of SQ inj (preferably in pm). GHD: 0.16-0.24mg/kg/week. PWS: 0.24mg/kg/week. SGA: Up to 0.48mg/kg/week. TS: 0.33mg/kg/week. ISS: Up to 0.47mg/kg/week.

HOW SUPPLIED: Inj: 5.8mg (vial); 5mg/1.5mL, 10mg/1.5mL (cartridge)

CONTRAINDICATIONS: Acute critical illness due to complications following open heart surgery, abdominal surgery, multiple accidental trauma, or with acute respiratory failure. Patients with PWS who are severely obese, with history of upper airway obstruction or sleep apnea, or with severe respiratory impairment. Active malignancy, or progression or recurrence of underlying intracranial tumor. Active proliferative or severe non-proliferative diabetic retinopathy, pediatric patients with closed epiphyses.

WARNINGS/PRECAUTIONS: Increased mortality reported in patients with acute critical illness. Fatalities reported in pediatric patients with PWS. Evaluate PWS patients for signs of upper airway obstruction and sleep apnea before treatment; d/c therapy if signs (eg, new/increased snoring) occur. Implement effective weight control in patients with PWS and treat respiratory infections aggressively. Examine for progression/recurrence of underlying disease process in those with preexisting tumors or GHD secondary to intracranial lesion. Monitor for malignant transformation of skin lesions. May decrease insulin sensitivity, as well as unmask undiagnosed impaired glucose tolerance and overt diabetes mellitus (DM). New-onset type 2 DM reported. Intracranial HTN with papilledema, visual changes, headache, N/V reported; perform funduscopic exam before and during therapy and d/c if papilledema occurs. Fluid retention in adults may occur. Monitor other hormonal replacement treatments in patients with hypopituitarism. Undiagnosed/untreated hypothyroidism may prevent optimal response. Hypothyroidism may become evident/worsen in patients with GHD. Slipped capital femoral epiphysis and progression of scoliosis may occur. Increased risk of ear/hearing and cardiovascular disorders reported in TS patients. Tissue atrophy may occur when administered at the same site over prolonged periods; can be avoided by rotating the inj site. Local/systemic allergic reactions may occur. Serum levels of inorganic phosphorus, alkaline phosphatase, parathyroid hormone, and IGF-I may increase. Pancreatitis rarely reported. Caution in elderly. (5mg/1.5mL cartridge, 5.8mg/vial) Contains benzyl alcohol.

ADVERSE REACTIONS: Elevated HbA1c, eosinophilia, hematoma.

INTERACTIONS: Use with glucocorticoid therapy may attenuate growth-promoting effects in children; carefully adjust glucocorticoid replacement dosing. May inhibit 11β-hydroxysteroid dehydrogenase type 1, resulting in reduced serum cortisol concentrations; may need glucocorticoid replacement/dose adjustments of glucocorticoid therapy (eg, cortisone acetate, prednisone). May increase clearance of antipyrine. May alter clearance of compounds metabolized by CYP450 liver enzymes (eg, corticosteroids, sex steroids, anticonvulsants, cyclosporine); monitor carefully. May require larger dose with oral estrogen replacement. May need to adjust dose of insulin and/or oral hypoglycemic agents in diabetic patients and thyroid hormone replacement therapy in patients with thyroid dysfunction.

PREGNANCY: Category B, caution in nursing.

MECHANISM OF ACTION: Recombinant human GH; binds to dimeric GH receptor in cell membrane of target cells resulting in intracellular signal transduction.

PHARMACOKINETICS: Absorption: C_{max}=72-74mcg/L; T_{max}=4 hrs. **Metabolism:** Liver and kidneys (proteolytic degradation). **Elimination:** $T_{1/2}$=2.5-2.8 hrs.

NURSING CONSIDERATIONS

Assessment: Assess for PWS, preexisting DM or impaired glucose tolerance, diabetic retinopathy, active malignancy, history of scoliosis, hypothyroidism, hypopituitarism, otitis media/other ear disorders in TS, pregnancy/nursing status, possible drug interactions, or any other conditions where treatment is contraindicated or cautioned. Perform funduscopic exam.

Monitoring: Monitor for growth, clinical response, compliance, malignant transformation of skin lesions, fluid retention, allergic reactions, pancreatitis, and slipped capital femoral epiphysis and progression of scoliosis in pediatric patients. Perform periodic thyroid function tests, funduscopic exam, and monitoring of glucose levels. In patients with PWS, monitor weight as well as signs of respiratory infections, sleep apnea, and upper airway obstruction. In patients with preexisting tumors or GHD secondary to intracranial lesion, monitor for progression/recurrence of underlying disease process. In patients with TS, monitor for ear/hearing/cardiovascular disorders.

Patient Counseling: Inform about potential benefits and risks of therapy, proper administration, usage and disposal, and caution against any reuse of needles and syringes.

Administration: SQ route. Refer to PI for preparation and administration instructions. **Storage:** 2-8°C (36-46°F). Keep in carton to protect from light. Do not freeze. (Cartridge) After 1st Use: Keep in pen at 2-8°C (36-46°F) for a max of 28 days. (Vial) Reconstituted: Use within 3 weeks. After First Use: Store in carton at 2-8°C (36-46°F).

ONGLYZA   RX
saxagliptin (Bristol-Myers Squibb/ AstraZeneca)

THERAPEUTIC CLASS: Dipeptidyl peptidase-4 inhibitor

INDICATIONS: Adjunct to diet and exercise to improve glycemic control in adults with type 2 diabetes mellitus (DM).

DOSAGE: *Adults:* Usual: 2.5mg or 5mg qd. Moderate or Severe Renal Impairment/End-Stage Renal Disease Requiring Hemodialysis (CrCl ≤50mL/min): 2.5mg qd. Administer following hemodialysis. With Strong CYP3A4/5 Inhibitors: 2.5mg qd. With Insulin Secretagogue (eg, Sulfonylurea)/Insulin: May require lower dose of insulin secretagogue or insulin.

HOW SUPPLIED: Tab: 2.5mg, 5mg

WARNINGS/PRECAUTIONS: Not for treatment of type 1 DM or diabetic ketoacidosis. Not studied in patients with a history of pancreatitis. Acute pancreatitis reported; d/c if pancreatitis is suspected. Serious hypersensitivity reactions reported; if suspected, d/c therapy, assess for other potential causes, and institute alternative treatment. Caution in patients with history of angioedema to another dipeptidyl peptidase-4 (DPP-4) inhibitor and in elderly. No conclusive evidence of macrovascular risk reduction.

ADVERSE REACTIONS: Upper respiratory tract infection, urinary tract infection, headache, peripheral edema.

INTERACTIONS: May require lower dose of insulin secretagogue (eg, sulfonylurea) or insulin to minimize risk of hypoglycemia. Ketoconazole or other strong CYP3A4/5 inhibitors (eg, atazanavir, clarithromycin, itraconazole, nefazodone) may increase plasma concentrations. Strong CYP3A4/5 inducers and inhibitors may alter pharmacokinetics of saxagliptin and its active metabolite.

PREGNANCY: Category B, caution in nursing.

MECHANISM OF ACTION: DPP-4 inhibitor; slows the inactivation of the incretin hormones, thereby increasing their bloodstream concentrations and reducing fasting and postprandial glucose concentrations in a glucose-dependent manner.

PHARMACOKINETICS: Absorption: C_{max}=24ng/mL, 47ng/mL (5-hydroxy saxagliptin); AUC=78ng•hr/mL, 214ng•hr/mL (5-hydroxy saxagliptin); T_{max}(median)=2 hrs, 4 hrs (5-hydroxy saxagliptin). **Metabolism:** CYP3A4/5; 5-hydroxy saxagliptin (active metabolite). **Elimination:** Feces (22%), urine (24% unchanged, 36% 5-hydroxy saxagliptin); $T_{1/2}$=2.5 hrs, 3.1 hrs (5-hydroxy saxagliptin).

NURSING CONSIDERATIONS

Assessment: Assess for previous hypersensitivity to the drug, history of pancreatitis, type of DM, diabetic ketoacidosis, history of angioedema to another DPP-4 inhibitor, pregnancy/nursing status, and possible drug interactions. Obtain baseline renal function, and FPG and HbA1c levels.

Monitoring: Monitor for pancreatitis, hypersensitivity reactions, and other adverse reactions. Monitor FPG, HbA1c, and renal function periodically. Measure lymphocyte count when clinically indicated (eg, settings of unusual or prolonged infection).

Patient Counseling: Inform of the potential risks, benefits, and alternative modes of therapy. Advise on the importance of adherence to dietary instructions, regular physical activity, periodic blood glucose monitoring and HbA1c testing, recognition and management of hypoglycemia and hyperglycemia, and assessment of diabetic complications. Instruct to seek medical advice promptly during periods of stress as medication requirements may change. Instruct to d/c use and notify physician if signs and symptoms of pancreatitis or allergic reactions occur. Counsel to inform physician if any unusual symptom develops, or if any existing symptom persists or worsens. Inform that if a dose was missed, to take the next dose as prescribed, unless otherwise instructed by physician; instruct not to take an extra dose the next day.

Administration: Oral route. Take regardless of meals. Do not split or cut tab. **Storage:** 20-25°C (68-77°F); excursions permitted to 15-30°C (59-86°F).

OPSUMIT   RX
macitentan (Actelion)

> Do not administer to a pregnant female; may cause fetal harm. Exclude pregnancy before the start of treatment, monthly during treatment, and 1 month after stopping treatment. Prevent pregnancy during and for 1 month after stopping treatment; use acceptable methods of contraception. For all female patients, available only through a restricted program called the OPSUMIT Risk Evaluation and Mitigation Strategy (REMS) Program.

THERAPEUTIC CLASS: Endothelin receptor antagonist

INDICATIONS: Treatment of pulmonary arterial HTN (World Health Organization Group 1) to delay disease progression.

DOSAGE: *Adults:* 10mg qd. Max: 10mg qd.

HOW SUPPLIED: Tab: 10mg

CONTRAINDICATIONS: Pregnancy.

WARNINGS/PRECAUTIONS: May cause elevations of aminotransferases, hepatotoxicity, and liver failure; obtain liver enzyme tests prior to initiation of treatment and repeat during treatment as clinically indicated. D/C therapy if clinically relevant aminotransferase elevations occur, or if elevations are accompanied by an increase in bilirubin >2X ULN, or by clinical symptoms of hepatotoxicity. Decreases in Hgb concentration and Hct reported; measure Hgb prior to initiation of treatment and repeat during treatment as clinically indicated. Not recommended in patients with severe anemia. If signs of pulmonary edema occur, consider the possibility of associated pulmonary veno-occlusive disease (PVOD); d/c if confirmed. May decrease sperm count.

ADVERSE REACTIONS: Anemia, nasopharyngitis/pharyngitis, bronchitis, headache, influenza, urinary tract infection.

INTERACTIONS: Strong CYP3A inducers (eg, rifampin) may significantly reduce exposure; avoid use. Strong CYP3A4 inhibitors (eg, ketoconazole, ritonavir) may approximately double exposure; avoid use.

PREGNANCY: Category X, not for use in nursing.

MECHANISM OF ACTION: Endothelin (ET) receptor antagonist; prevents the binding of ET-1 to both ET_A and ET_B receptors. Displays high affinity and sustained occupancy of the ET receptors in human pulmonary arterial smooth muscle cells.

PHARMACOKINETICS: Absorption: T_{max}=8 hrs. **Distribution:** V_d=50L, 40L (active metabolite); plasma protein binding (>99%). **Metabolism:** CYP3A4, CYP2C19 (minor); oxidative depropylation of the sulfamide (primary). **Elimination:** Urine (50%), feces (24%); $T_{1/2}$=16 hrs, 48 hrs (active metabolite).

NURSING CONSIDERATIONS

Assessment: Assess for pregnancy/nursing status, and possible drug interactions. Obtain baseline liver enzyme tests and Hgb levels.

Monitoring: Monitor for signs/symptoms of pulmonary edema, PVOD, hepatic impairment, and other adverse reactions. Obtain pregnancy tests monthly during treatment and 1 month after discontinuation of treatment. Monitor liver enzyme tests and Hgb levels as clinically indicated.

Patient Counseling: Counsel on the risk of fetal harm when used during pregnancy; instruct females of reproductive potential to use effective contraception during therapy and for 1 month after stopping treatment. Instruct to contact physician immediately if pregnancy is suspected. Inform female patients that they must enroll in the OPSUMIT REMS Program. Educate and counsel females of reproductive potential on the use of emergency contraception in the event of unprotected sex or contraceptive failure. Advise prepubertal females to immediately report to physician any reproductive status changes. Advise of the importance of Hgb testing. Educate patients on signs of hepatotoxicity.

Administration: Oral route. Do not split, crush, or chew tabs. May take with or without food. **Storage:** 20-25°C (68-77°F); excursions permitted from 15-30°C (59-86°F).

OPTIVAR   RX
azelastine HCl (Meda)

THERAPEUTIC CLASS: H₁-antagonist

INDICATIONS: Treatment of itching of the eye associated with allergic conjunctivitis.

DOSAGE: *Adults:* Usual: 1 drop into each affected eye bid.
Pediatrics: ≥3 Yrs: Usual: 1 drop into each affected eye bid.

HOW SUPPLIED: Sol: 0.05% [6mL]

WARNINGS/PRECAUTIONS: For ocular use only; not for inj or PO use.

ADVERSE REACTIONS: Eye burning/stinging, headaches, bitter taste, asthma, conjunctivitis, dyspnea, eye pain, fatigue, influenza-like symptoms, pharyngitis, pruritus, rhinitis, temporary blurring.

PREGNANCY: Category C, caution in nursing.

MECHANISM OF ACTION: Selective H₁ antagonist; inhibits release of histamine and other mediators from cells (eg, mast cells) involved in the allergic response and decreases chemotaxis and activation of eosinophils.

PHARMACOKINETICS: Absorption: Low. **Distribution:** V_d=14.5L/kg (IV/PO); plasma protein binding (88%). **Metabolism:** CYP450; N-desmethylazelastine (principal metabolite). **Elimination:** (PO) Feces (75%, <10% unchanged); $T_{1/2}$= 22 hrs (IV/PO).

NURSING CONSIDERATIONS

Assessment: Assess for drug hypersensitivity and pregnancy/nursing status.

Monitoring: Monitor for adverse events.

Patient Counseling: Advise not to touch dropper tip to any surface, to prevent contamination. Instruct to keep bottle tightly closed when not in use. Advise not to wear contact lenses if eye is red. Inform that drug is not used to treat contact lens-related irritation. Instruct patients who wear soft contact lenses and whose eyes are not red to wait at least 10 min after instillation before inserting contact lenses.

Administration: Ocular route. **Storage:** 2-25°C (36-77°F).

ORACEA   RX
doxycycline (Galderma)

THERAPEUTIC CLASS: Tetracycline derivative

INDICATIONS: Treatment of only the inflammatory lesions (papules and pustules) of rosacea in adults.

DOSAGE: *Adults:* 40mg qam. Take on an empty stomach, preferably at least 1 hr ac or 2 hrs pc. Elderly: Start at lower end of dosing range.

HOW SUPPLIED: Cap: 40mg

WARNINGS/PRECAUTIONS: Do not use for treating bacterial infections, providing antibacterial prophylaxis, or reducing the numbers of (or eliminating) microorganisms associated with any bacterial disease. May cause fetal harm. May cause permanent discoloration of the teeth (yellow-gray-brown) if used during tooth development (last half of pregnancy, infancy, childhood up to 8 yrs of age). Enamel hypoplasia reported. Do not use during tooth development unless other drugs are not likely to be effective or are contraindicated. May decrease fibula growth rate in premature infants. *Clostridium difficile*-associated diarrhea (CDAD) reported; d/c if CDAD is suspected or confirmed. May result in overgrowth of non-susceptible microorganisms, including fungi; d/c and institute appropriate therapy if superinfection occurs. Caution in patients with a history of or predisposition to *Candida* overgrowth. Bacterial resistance may develop; use only as indicated and do not exceed recommended dosage. Photosensitivity manifested by an exaggerated sunburn reaction reported. Development of autoimmune syndromes reported; d/c immediately and perform LFTs, antinuclear antibodies (ANA), CBC, and other appropriate tests in symptomatic patients. Tissue hyperpigmentation reported. May increase BUN. Caution in patients with renal impairment; may lead to excessive systemic accumulations and possible liver toxicity; lower than usual total dosages are indicated and if therapy is prolonged, serum drug level determinations may be advisable. Associated with pseudotumor cerebri (benign intracranial HTN) in adults and bulging fontanels in infants. Lab test interactions may occur. Caution in elderly.

ADVERSE REACTIONS: Nasopharyngitis, sinusitis, diarrhea, HTN.

INTERACTIONS: Depresses plasma prothrombin activity; may require downward adjustment of anticoagulant dosage. May interfere with bactericidal action of penicillin; avoid concurrent use. Fatal renal toxicity reported with methoxyflurane. Bismuth subsalicylate, proton pump inhibitors, antacids containing aluminum, Ca^{2+}, or Mg^{2+}, and iron-containing preparations may impair absorption. May interfere with the effectiveness of low dose oral contraceptives. Avoid concurrent use with oral retinoids (eg, isotretinoin, acitretin); pseudotumor cerebri reported. Barbiturates, carbamazepine, and phenytoin decrease the $T_{1/2}$ of doxycycline.

PREGNANCY: Category D, not for use in nursing.

MECHANISM OF ACTION: Tetracycline derivative; anti-inflammatory mechanism has not been established.

PHARMACOKINETICS: Absorption: (Healthy) Single dose: C_{max}=510ng/mL; T_{max}=3 hrs; AUC=9227ng•hr/mL. Steady-state: C_{max}=600ng/mL; T_{max}=2 hrs; AUC=7543ng•hr/mL. **Distribution:** Plasma protein binding (>90%); crosses the placenta, found in breast milk. **Elimination:** Urine (unchanged), feces (unchanged); $T_{1/2}$=21.2 hrs (single dose), 23.2 hrs (steady-state).

NURSING CONSIDERATIONS

Assessment: Assess for hypersensitivity to drug and other tetracyclines, renal impairment, history of or predisposition to *Candida* overgrowth, visual disturbances, pregnancy/nursing status, and possible drug interactions.

Monitoring: Monitor for signs/symptoms of CDAD, superinfection, photosensitivity, autoimmune syndromes, tissue hyperpigmentation, and other adverse reactions. Monitor serum drug levels in patients with renal impairment if therapy is prolonged. Routinely check for papilledema while on treatment. Perform periodic lab evaluations of organ systems, including hematopoietic, renal, and hepatic studies. If symptoms of autoimmune syndrome occur, perform LFTs, ANA, CBC, and other appropriate tests.

Patient Counseling: Inform that drug should not be used by pregnant or breastfeeding women nor by individuals of either gender who are attempting to conceive a child. Inform that drug may render oral contraceptives less effective; advise females to use a second form of contraception. Inform that pseudomembranous colitis and pseudotumor cerebri may occur; instruct to seek immediate medical attention if watery/bloody stools, or headache or blurred vision occur. Inform that photosensitivity, manifested by an exaggerated sunburn reaction, was observed; instruct to minimize/avoid exposure to natural or artificial sunlight and d/c at 1st evidence of sunburn, advise to wear loose-fitting clothes, and discuss other sun protection measures. Inform that medication may cause autoimmune syndromes; instruct to d/c and contact physician if arthralgia, fever, rash, or malaise develops. Inform that drug may cause discoloration of skin, scars, teeth, or gums. Instruct to take exactly ud. Inform that increasing doses beyond 40mg qam may increase likelihood that bacteria will develop resistance and will not be treatable by other antibacterial drugs in the future.

Administration: Oral route. Take on an empty stomach. Administer with adequate amounts of fluid to reduce the risk of esophageal irritation and ulceration. **Storage:** 15-30°C (59-86°F).

ORAVIG   RX
miconazole (Praelia)

THERAPEUTIC CLASS: Azole antifungal

INDICATIONS: Local treatment of oropharyngeal candidiasis in adults.

DOSAGE: *Adults:* ≥16 Yrs: Apply 1 tab to the upper gum region (canine fossa) qd for 14 consecutive days.

HOW SUPPLIED: Tab, Buccal: 50mg

CONTRAINDICATIONS: Hypersensitivity (eg, anaphylaxis) to milk protein concentrate.

WARNINGS/PRECAUTIONS: Allergic reactions, including anaphylactic reactions and hypersensitivity, reported; d/c immediately at the 1st sign of hypersensitivity. Caution with hepatic impairment.

ADVERSE REACTIONS: Diarrhea, N/V, headache, dysgeusia.

INTERACTIONS: May enhance anticoagulant effects of warfarin; closely monitor PT, INR, or other suitable anticoagulation tests, and for evidence of bleeding. May interact with drugs metabolized through CYP2C9 and CYP3A4 (eg, oral hypoglycemics, phenytoin, ergot alkaloids).

PREGNANCY: Category C, caution in nursing.

MECHANISM OF ACTION: Azole antifungal; inhibits the enzyme CYP450 14α-demethylase, leading to inhibition of ergosterol synthesis, an essential component of the fungal cell membrane. Affects the synthesis of TG and fatty acids and inhibits oxidative and peroxidative enzymes, increasing the amount of reactive oxygen species within the cell.

PHARMACOKINETICS: Absorption: Minimal systemic absorption (max salivary concentrations of 15mcg/mL at 7 hrs). **Metabolism:** Liver. **Elimination:** Urine (<1%, unchanged); $T_{1/2}$=24 hrs (healthy, systemic administration).

NURSING CONSIDERATIONS

Assessment: Assess for hypersensitivity to drug, milk protein concentrate, or any other component of the product, hepatic impairment, pregnancy/nursing status, and possible drug interactions.

Monitoring: Monitor for signs/symptoms of hypersensitivity and other adverse reactions. Closely monitor PT, INR, or other suitable anticoagulation tests, and for evidence of bleeding with warfarin.

Patient Counseling: Instruct on proper application of the tab. Inform that subsequent applications should be made to alternate sides of the gum. Advise that if tab does not stick or falls off within first 6 hrs, the same tab should be repositioned immediately; instruct to place a new tab if tab still does not adhere. Instruct to drink a glass of water and apply a new tab only once if tab is swallowed within first 6 hrs. Instruct to not apply a new tab until the next, regularly scheduled dose, if tab falls off or swallowed after it was in place for ≥6 hrs. Counsel to avoid situations that could interfere with the sticking of the tab (eg, touching/pressing tab after placement, wearing upper denture, chewing gum, hitting tab when brushing teeth, rinsing mouth too vigorously). Advise to d/c and contact physician if hives, skin rash, other symptoms of an allergic reaction, or application-site swelling/pain develops. Inform that patients may experience other adverse reactions, including diarrhea, headache, nausea, and change in taste.

Administration: Buccal route. Apply in the upper gum region qam, after brushing the teeth. Do not crush, chew, or swallow tab. Refer to PI for further administration instructions. **Storage:** 20-25°C (68-77°F); excursions between 15-30°C (59-86°F) permitted at room temperature. Protect from moisture.

ORENCIA   RX
abatacept (Bristol-Myers Squibb)

THERAPEUTIC CLASS: Selective costimulation modulator

INDICATIONS: To reduce signs and symptoms, induce major clinical response, inhibit progression of structural damage, and improve physical function in adults with moderate to severe active rheumatoid arthritis (RA); may be used as monotherapy or concomitantly with disease-modifying antirheumatic drugs other than TNF antagonists. To reduce signs and symptoms in pediatric patients ≥6 yrs of age with moderate to severe active polyarticular juvenile idiopathic arthritis (JIA); may be used as monotherapy or concomitantly with methotrexate.

DOSAGE: *Adults:* RA: IV Regimen: Give as an IV infusion over 30 min. Initial: >100kg: 1000mg. 60-100kg: 750mg. <60kg: 500mg. Maint: Give succeeding infusions at 2 and 4 weeks after the 1st infusion and every 4 weeks thereafter. SQ Regimen: 125mg SQ inj once weekly. May initiate with or without an IV LD. If initiating with an IV LD, initiate with a single IV infusion (as per body weight categories listed in the IV regimen), followed by the first 125mg SQ inj within a day of the IV infusion. Switching from IV to SQ Regimen: Give the 1st SQ dose instead of the next scheduled IV dose.
Pediatrics: 6-17 Yrs: JIA: Give as an IV infusion over 30 min. Initial: ≥75kg: Follow adult IV dosing regimen. Max: 1000mg. <75kg: 10mg/kg. Maint: Give succeeding infusions at 2 and 4 weeks after the 1st infusion and every 4 weeks thereafter.

HOW SUPPLIED: Inj: 125mg/mL [prefilled syringe], 250mg [vial]

WARNINGS/PRECAUTIONS: Anaphylaxis and anaphylactoid reactions may occur; permanently d/c and institute appropriate therapy if an anaphylactic or other serious allergic reaction occurs. Serious infections, including sepsis and pneumonia, reported; caution in patients with history of recurrent infections, underlying conditions that may predispose to infections, or chronic, latent, or localized infections. Immunosuppressive therapy may further predispose to infections; d/c if serious infection develops. Screen for latent tuberculosis (TB) infection and viral hepatitis prior to initiation of therapy; treat patients testing positive for TB prior to therapy. Hepatitis B reactivation reported with antirheumatic therapies. JIA patients should be brought up to date with all immunizations prior to initiation of therapy. Caution in patients with chronic obstructive pulmonary disease (COPD). May affect host defenses against infections and malignancies. Caution in elderly. (IV) Contains maltose that may react with glucose dehydrogenase pyrroloquinolinequinone based glucose monitoring and may result in falsely elevated blood glucose readings on the day of infusion; consider methods that do not react with maltose in patients requiring blood glucose monitoring.

ADVERSE REACTIONS: Headache, upper respiratory tract infection, nasopharyngitis, nausea, sinusitis, urinary tract infection, influenza, bronchitis, dizziness, cough, back pain, HTN, dyspepsia, rash, pain in extremities.

INTERACTIONS: May increase risk of serious infections with TNF antagonists; concomitant use is not recommended. Concomitant use with other biologic RA therapy (eg, anakinra) is not recommended. Do not use live vaccines concurrently with therapy or within 3 months of its discontinuation.

PREGNANCY: Category C, not for use in nursing.

MECHANISM OF ACTION: Selective costimulation modulator; inhibits T cell activation by binding to CD80 and CD86, thereby blocking interaction with CD28.

PHARMACOKINETICS: Absorption: (SQ) Bioavailability (78.6%). C_{max}=295mcg/mL (RA patients, IV), 48.1mcg/mL (RA patients, SQ), 217mcg/mL (JIA patients). **Distribution:** V_d=0.07L/kg (RA patients, IV), 0.11L/kg (RA patients, SQ). **Elimination:** $T_{1/2}$=13.1 days (RA patients, IV), 14.3 days (RA patients, SQ).

NURSING CONSIDERATIONS

Assessment: Assess for previous hypersensitivity to drug, history of recurrent infections, chronic/latent/localized infections, underlying conditions that may predispose to infection, COPD, pregnancy/nursing status, and possible drug interactions. Assess immunization history in pediatric patients. Screen for latent TB infection with a tuberculin skin test and for viral hepatitis.

Monitoring: Monitor for signs/symptoms of hypersensitivity, infection, hepatitis B reactivation, worsening of respiratory status, immunosuppression, malignancies, and other adverse reactions.

Patient Counseling: Instruct to immediately contact physician if an allergic reaction or infection occurs. Inform that patient may be tested for TB prior to therapy. Counsel not to receive live vaccines during therapy or within 3 months of its discontinuation. Inform caregivers that patients with JIA should be brought up to date with all immunizations prior to therapy and instruct to discuss with physician how to best handle future immunizations once therapy has been initiated. Instruct to inform physician if pregnant/nursing or planning to become pregnant. Inform that the formulation for IV administration contains maltose, which can give falsely elevated blood glucose readings on the day of administration with certain blood glucose monitors; advise to discuss with physician methods that do not react with maltose.

Administration: IV/SQ routes. Refer to PI for preparation and administration instructions. **Storage:** 2-8°C (36-46°F). Protect from light; store in original package until time of use. Do not allow prefilled syringe to freeze. Diluted Sol: Room temperature or 2-8°C (36-46°F); discard if not used within 24 hrs.

ORTHO EVRA   RX
ethinyl estradiol - norelgestromin (Janssen)

> Cigarette smoking increases risk of serious cardiovascular (CV) events, particularly in women >35 years of age, and with the number of cigarettes smoked. Should not be used by women who are >35 yrs of age and smoke. May increase risk of venous thromboembolism (VTE) among users of Ortho Evra compared to women who use certain oral contraceptives. Has higher steady state concentrations and a lower peak concentration than oral contraceptives.

THERAPEUTIC CLASS: Estrogen/progestogen combination

INDICATIONS: Prevention of pregnancy.

DOSAGE: *Adults:* Start during the first 24 hrs of menstrual period or on the 1st Sunday after menstrual period begins. Apply patch each week on the same day for 3 weeks. Week 4 is patch-free. There should not be more than a 7-day patch-free interval between dosing cycles. Only 1 patch should be worn at a time. Refer to PI for further dosing guidelines.
Pediatrics: Postpubertal: Start during the first 24 hrs of menstrual period or on the 1st Sunday after menstrual period begins. Apply patch each week on the same day for 3 weeks. Week 4 is patch-free. There should not be more than a 7-day patch-free interval between dosing cycles. Only 1 patch should be worn at a time. Refer to PI for further dosing guidelines.

HOW SUPPLIED: Patch: (Ethinyl Estradiol [EE]-Norelgestromin [NGMN]): 0.75mg-6mg [1ˢ, 3ˢ]

CONTRAINDICATIONS: High risk of arterial/venous thrombotic diseases (eg, smoking if >35 yrs of age, history/presence of deep vein thrombosis/pulmonary embolism, inherited or acquired hypercoagulopathies, cerebrovascular disease, coronary artery disease, thrombogenic valvular or thrombogenic rhythm diseases of the heart [eg, subacute bacterial endocarditis with valvular disease, or atrial fibrillation], uncontrolled HTN; diabetes mellitus with vascular disease, headaches with focal neurologic symptoms or migraine headaches with aura, >35 yrs of age with any migraine headaches), benign or malignant liver tumors or liver disease, undiagnosed abnormal uterine bleeding, pregnancy, current or history of breast cancer or other estrogen- or progestin-sensitive cancer.

WARNINGS/PRECAUTIONS: May be less effective in preventing pregnancy in women who weigh ≥198 lbs (90kg). Increased risk of arterial thromboses. D/C if an arterial or deep venous thrombotic event occurs. D/C if unexplained loss of vision, proptosis, diplopia, papilledema, or retinal vascular lesions develop; evaluate for retinal vein thrombosis immediately. D/C at least 4 weeks before and through 2 weeks after major surgery or other surgeries associated with an elevated risk of VTE and during prolonged immobilization, if feasible. Start use no earlier than 4 weeks after delivery in women who are not breastfeeding. Caution in women with cardiovascular disease risk factors. D/C if jaundice develops. Hepatic adenomas and increased risk of hepatocellular carcinoma reported. Increase in BP reported. Monitor BP in women with well-controlled HTN; d/c if BP rises significantly. Increased risk of cervical cancer or intraepithelial neoplasia, and gallbladder disease. May decrease glucose tolerance; monitor prediabetic and diabetic women. Consider alternative contraception with uncontrolled dyslipidemia. May increase risk of pancreatitis with hypertriglyceridemia or a family history thereof. D/C if indicated and evaluate cause if new headaches that are recurrent, persistent, or severe develop. Consider discontinuation in case of increased frequency or severity of migraine during use. Unscheduled bleeding and spotting reported. Consider non-hormonal causes and take adequate diagnostic measures to rule out malignancy, other pathology, or pregnancy in the event of unscheduled bleeding. Consider possibility of pregnancy in the event of amenorrhea. Amenorrhea or oligomenorrhea may occur after discontinuation of therapy. Caution with history of depression; d/c if depression recurs to a serious degree. May induce or exacerbate symptoms of angioedema in patients with hereditary angioedema. Chloasma may occur; avoid exposure to sun or UV radiation in women with a tendency to chloasma. May influence the results of certain laboratory tests.

ADVERSE REACTIONS: Breast symptoms (eg, breast discomfort, engorgement, pain); vaginal bleeding, menstrual disorders; dysmenorrhea; emotional lability; diarrhea; headache; application-site disorder; N/V; abdominal pain; dizziness; mood, affect and anxiety disorders; vaginal yeast infection.

INTERACTIONS: May decrease plasma concentrations and potentially diminish effectiveness or increase breakthrough bleeding when used concomitantly with drugs or herbal products that induce certain enzymes, including CYP3A4 (eg, phenytoin, barbiturates, carbamazepine, bosentan, felbamate, griseofulvin, oxcarbazepine, rifampicin, topiramate, rifabutin, rufinamide, aprepitant, products containing St. John's wort); use an alternative method of contraception or a back-up method when used concomitantly with enzyme inducers, and continue back-up contraception for 28 days after discontinuing the enzyme inducer. Atorvastatin or rosuvastatin may increase ethinyl estradiol exposure; ascorbic acid and acetaminophen (APAP) may increase ethinyl estradiol levels. CYP3A4 inhibitors (eg, itraconazole, voriconazole, fluconazole, grapefruit juice, ketoconazole) may increase plasma hormone levels. HIV protease inhibitors (eg, nelfinavir, ritonavir, darunavir/ritonavir, [fos] amprenavir/ritonavir, lopinavir/ritonavir, tipranavir/ritonavir, indinavir, atazanavir/ritonavir), hepatitis C virus protease inhibitors, or non-nucleoside reverse transcriptase inhibitors (eg, nevirapine, etravirine) may cause significant changes in plasma concentrations of estrogen and/or progestin. May inhibit the metabolism of other compounds (eg, cyclosporine, prednisolone, theophylline, tizanidine, voriconazole) and increase their plasma concentrations. May decrease concentrations of APAP, clofibric acid, morphine, salicylic acid, and temazepam. May decrease levels of lamotrigine and reduce seizure control; dosage adjustments of lamotrigine may be necessary. Increases serum concentration of thyroid-binding globulin; may need to increase dose of thyroid hormone replacement.

PREGNANCY: Contraindicated in pregnancy, caution in nursing.

MECHANISM OF ACTION: Estrogen/progestogen combination; acts by suppression of gonadotropins. Primarily inhibits ovulation. Also produces other alterations including changes in the cervical mucus (increases difficulty of sperm entry into the uterus) and endometrium (reduces likelihood of implantation).

PHARMACOKINETICS: Absorption: EE: AUC_{0-168}=12971pg•h/mL; C_{max}=97.4pg/mL. NGMN: AUC_{0-168}=145ng•h/mL; C_{max}=1.12ng/mL. Refer to PI for additional parameters. **Distribution:** Found in breast milk. EE: Serum albumin binding (extensive). NGMN: Serum protein binding (>97%). **Metabolism:** EE: Hydroxylated, glucuronide, and sulfate conjugates (metabolites). NGMN: Hepatic; hydroxylated and conjugated metabolites, norgestrel (metabolite). **Elimination:** Urine, feces (metabolites); $T_{1/2}$=17 hrs (EE), 28 hrs (NGMN).

NURSING CONSIDERATIONS

Assessment: Assess for risk of arterial or venous thrombotic diseases, benign or malignant liver tumors, liver disease, undiagnosed abnormal uterine bleeding, presence or history of breast cancer or other estrogen- or progestin-sensitive cancer, pregnancy, and any other conditions where treatment is contraindicated/cautioned. Assess for nursing status and possible drug interactions.

Monitoring: Monitor for arterial thrombotic or VTE events, hepatic adenomas, hepatocellular carcinoma, gallbladder disease, and other adverse effects. Monitor lipid levels with hyperlipidemia, BP with history of HTN, serum glucose levels in diabetic and prediabetic patients, thyroid function if receiving thyroid replacement therapy, and for signs of worsening depression with previous history. Schedule a yearly visit with patient for a BP check and for other indicated healthcare.

Patient Counseling: Inform of risks and benefits of therapy. Inform that cigarette smoking increases risk of serious CV events, and that women who are >35 yrs of age and smoke should not use combined hormonal contraceptives. Counsel that therapy does not protect against HIV infection (AIDS) and other sexually transmitted diseases. Instruct not to use during pregnancy and to d/c if pregnancy occurs during use. Instruct to apply a single patch on the same day every week (Weeks 1 through 3). Instruct patient on what to do in the event a patch is missed. Instruct to use a nonhormonal back up method of contraception for the first 7 days of the first cycle if started using therapy on the 1st Sunday after menses begin. Counsel to use a back-up or alternative method of contraception when enzyme inducers are concomitantly used. Inform that breast milk production may be reduced with use. Instruct postpartum women who have not yet had a normal period, to use an additional method of contraception for the 7 consecutive days. Inform that amenorrhea may occur. Advise that pregnancy should be ruled out in the event of amenorrhea in 2 or more consecutive cycles. Advise that insufficient drug delivery occurs when patch becomes partially or completely detached and remains detached.

Administration: Transdermal route. Apply immediately upon removal from protective pouch. Apply to clean and dry skin on upper outer arm, abdomen, buttock, or back in a place where it will not be rubbed by tight clothing. Do not cut, damage or alter patch in any way. Refer to PI for further administration instructions. **Storage:** 25°C (77°F); excursions permitted to 15-30°C (59-86°F). Store patches in their protective pouches. Do not store in the refrigerator or freezer.

ORTHO TRI-CYCLEN   RX
ethinyl estradiol - norgestimate (Janssen)

> Cigarette smoking increases risk of serious cardiovascular (CV) events. Risk increases with age (>35 yrs) and with the number of cigarettes smoked. Should not be used by women who are >35 yrs of age and smoke.

OTHER BRAND NAMES: Tri-Sprintec (Teva) - TriNessa (Watson) - Tri-Previfem (Qualitest)

THERAPEUTIC CLASS: Estrogen/progestogen combination

INDICATIONS: Prevention of pregnancy. Treatment of moderate acne vulgaris in females ≥15 yrs of age who have no known contraindication to oral contraceptive therapy, desire oral contraceptive for birth control, and have achieved menarche.

DOSAGE: *Adults:* Contraception/Acne: 1 tab qd for 28 days, then repeat. Start 1st Sunday after menses begins or 1st day of menses.
Pediatrics: Postpubertal: Contraception/Acne (≥15 Yrs): 1 tab qd for 28 days, then repeat. Start 1st Sunday after menses begins or 1st day of menses.

HOW SUPPLIED: Tab: (Ethinyl Estradiol [EE]-Norgestimate) 0.035mg-0.18mg, 0.035mg-0.215mg, 0.035mg-0.25mg

CONTRAINDICATIONS: Thrombophlebitis or thromboembolic disorders, past history of deep vein thrombophlebitis or thromboembolic disorders, cerebral vascular or coronary artery disease (current or past history), valvular heart disease with complications, diabetes with vascular involvement, headaches with focal neurological symptoms, major surgery with prolonged immobilization, known or suspected carcinoma of the breast or personal history of breast cancer, carcinoma of the endometrium or other known or suspected estrogen-dependent neoplasia, undiagnosed abnormal genital bleeding, cholestatic jaundice of pregnancy or jaundice with prior pill use, acute or chronic hepatocellular disease with abnormal liver function, hepatic adenomas or carcinomas, known or suspected pregnancy. (Ortho Tri-Cyclen, Tri-Previfem, TriNessa) Known thrombophilic conditions, persistent BP values of ≥160 mm Hg systolic or ≥100 mm Hg diastolic. (Tri-Sprintec) Severe HTN.

WARNINGS/PRECAUTIONS: For the first cycle of a Sunday Start regimen, use another method of contraception until after the first 7 consecutive days of administration. Not indicated for use in emergency contraception. Increased risk of myocardial infarction (MI), vascular disease, thromboembolism, stroke, hepatic neoplasia, and gallbladder disease. May increase risk of breast cancer and cancer of the reproductive organs. Increased risk of morbidity and mortality if other risk factors (eg, HTN, hyperlipidemia, obesity, diabetes mellitus [DM]) are present. D/C at least 4 weeks prior to and for 2 weeks after elective surgery of a type associated with an increased risk of thromboembolism, and during and following prolonged immobilization, if feasible. Caution in women with CV disease risk factors. Contact lens wearers who develop visual changes or changes in lens tolerance should be assessed by an ophthalmologist. Retinal thrombosis reported; d/c if unexplained partial or complete loss of vision occurs, onset of proptosis or diplopia, papilledema, or retinal vascular lesions develop. Should not be used to induce withdrawal bleeding as a test for pregnancy, or to treat threatened or habitual abortion during pregnancy. May cause glucose intolerance; monitor prediabetic and diabetic patients. May elevate LDL levels or cause other lipid abnormalities. D/C and evaluate the cause if new onset/exacerbation of migraine or recurrent, persistent, severe headache with a new pattern develops. May increase BP; monitor closely and d/c if significant elevation of BP occurs and cannot be adequately controlled. Breakthrough bleeding and spotting reported; rule out malignancies or pregnancy. Post-pill amenorrhea or oligomenorrhea may occur. D/C if jaundice develops. May cause fluid retention; caution and monitor patients with conditions that may be aggravated by fluid retention. Monitor closely with depression and d/c if depression recurs to a serious degree. Ectopic and intrauterine pregnancies may occur in contraceptive failures. May affect certain endocrine, LFTs, and blood components in laboratory tests. Perform annual history/physical exam; monitor closely women with a strong family history of breast cancer or who have breast nodules. Rule out pregnancy if two consecutive periods are missed; d/c if pregnancy is confirmed.

ADVERSE REACTIONS: N/V, breakthrough bleeding, GI symptoms (eg, abdominal cramps, bloating), spotting, menstrual flow changes, amenorrhea, migraine, depression, vaginal candidiasis, edema, weight changes, change in cervical erosion and secretion, melasma, cholestatic jaundice, change in corneal curvature.

INTERACTIONS: May decrease levels and potentially diminish effectiveness or increase breakthrough bleeding when used concomitantly with drugs or herbal products that induce certain enzymes, including CYP3A4 (eg, phenytoin, barbiturates, carbamazepine, bosentan, felbamate, griseofulvin, oxcarbazepine, rifampicin, topiramate, rifabutin, rufinamide, aprepitant, St. John's wort); use an alternative or back-up method of contraception and continue back-up contraception for 28 days after discontinuing the enzyme inducer. Atorvastatin or rosuvastatin may increase EE exposure; ascorbic acid and acetaminophen (APAP) may increase EE levels. May increase levels with CYP3A4 inhibitors (eg, itraconazole, voriconazole, fluconazole, grapefruit juice, ketoconazole). Significant level changes (increase or decrease) noted with HIV protease inhibitors (decreased [eg, nelfinavir, ritonavir, darunavir/ritonavir, (fos)amprenavir/ritonavir, lopinavir/ritonavir, tipranavir/ritonavir] or increased [eg, indinavir, atazanavir/ritonavir])/HCV protease inhibitors (decreased [eg, boceprevir, telaprevir]) or with non-nucleoside reverse transcriptase inhibitors (decreased [eg, nevirapine] or increased [eg, etravirine]). Colesevelam reported to significantly decrease EE exposure; decreased drug interaction reported when the two drug products are given 4 hrs apart. May inhibit metabolism and increase levels of other compounds (eg, cyclosporine, prednisolone, theophylline, tizanidine, voriconazole). May decrease levels of APAP, clofibric acid, morphine, salicylic acid, and temazepam. May significantly decrease levels of lamotrigine; dosage adjustment of lamotrigine may be needed. May increase serum levels of thyroid-binding globulins; increased dose of thyroid hormone may be needed in patients on thyroid hormone replacement therapy.

PREGNANCY: Category X, not for use in nursing.

MECHANISM OF ACTION: Estrogen/progestogen oral contraceptive; acts by suppression of gonadotropins to inhibit ovulation. Also causes changes in the cervical mucus (increasing the difficulty of sperm entry into the uterus) and the endometrium (reducing the likelihood of implantation).

PHARMACOKINETICS: Absorption: Rapid. Administration on various days of dosing cycle led to different parameters; refer to PI. **Distribution:** Found in breast milk. Norelgestromin and norgestrel: Serum protein binding (>97%; norelgestromin bound to albumin; norgestrel bound primarily to sex hormone-binding globulin). EE: Serum protein binding (>97% to albumin). **Metabolism:** Norgestimate: GI tract and/or liver (first-pass). Norelgestromin (primary, active metabolite): Liver; norgestrel (active metabolite), hydroxylated and conjugated metabolites. EE: Hydroxylated metabolites and their glucuronide and sulfate conjugates. **Elimination:** Urine and feces (EE and norgestimate metabolites) (Norgestimate metabolites: 47% urine and 37% feces).

NURSING CONSIDERATIONS

Assessment: Assess for thrombophlebitis or thromboembolic disorders, past history of deep vein thrombophlebitis or thromboembolic disorders, cerebral vascular or coronary artery disease (current or past history), valvular heart disease with complications, diabetes with vascular involvement, headaches with focal neurological symptoms, pregnancy, hypersensitivity, or any other conditions where treatment is contraindicated or cautioned. Assess nursing status and for possible drug interactions.

Monitoring: Monitor for signs/symptoms of MI, thromboembolism/thrombotic disease, stroke, and other adverse effects. Monitor BP with history of HTN, serum glucose levels in DM or prediabetic patients, lipid levels with history of hyperlipidemia, and for signs of worsening depression with previous history. Monitor liver function and for signs of jaundice. Refer contact lens wearers who develop visual changes or changes in lens tolerance to an ophthalmologist. Monitor serum folate levels in patients who become pregnant shortly after discontinuation. Perform annual history and physical exam.

Patient Counseling: Inform that drug does not protect against HIV infection (AIDS) and other sexually transmitted diseases. Advise to avoid smoking while on medication. Counsel about potential adverse effects. Instruct to take exactly ud, at intervals not exceeding 24 hrs. Instruct on what to do if doses are missed. Advise about risk of pregnancy if doses are missed. Instruct to d/c if pregnancy is confirmed/suspected. Counsel that efficacy may decrease if vomiting/diarrhea develops or if taking certain medicines; instruct to use a back-up method of contraception. Inform that spotting, light bleeding, or stomach sickness may occur during first 1-3 packs of pills; advise not to d/c medication and to notify physician if symptoms persist.

Administration: Oral route. **Storage:** (Ortho Tri-Cyclen, TriNessa) 25°C (77°F), excursions permitted to 15-30°C (59-86°F); (Tri-Previfem, Tri-Sprintec) 20-25°C (68-77°F). Protect from light.

ORTHO TRI-CYCLEN LO   RX

ethinyl estradiol - norgestimate (Ortho-McNeil)

> Cigarette smoking increases risk of serious cardiovascular (CV) side effects. Risk increases with age (>35 yrs) and with heavy smoking (≥15 cigarettes/day). Women who use oral contraceptives are strongly advised not to smoke.

THERAPEUTIC CLASS: Estrogen/progestogen combination

INDICATIONS: Prevention of pregnancy.

DOSAGE: *Adults:* 1 tab qd for 28 days, then repeat. Start 1st Sunday after menses begins or 1st day of menses.
Pediatrics: Postpubertal: 1 tab qd for 28 days, then repeat. Start 1st Sunday after menses begins or 1st day of menses.

HOW SUPPLIED: Tab: (Ethinyl Estradiol-Norgestimate) 0.025mg-0.18mg, 0.025mg-0.215mg, 0.025mg-0.25mg

CONTRAINDICATIONS: Thrombophlebitis or past history of deep vein thrombophlebitis, thromboembolic disorders (current or past history), cerebral vascular or coronary artery disease (current or past history), valvular heart disease with complications, severe HTN, diabetes mellitus (DM) with vascular involvement, headaches with focal neurological symptoms, major surgery with prolonged immobilization, breast cancer (current or past history), endometrial cancer, other known or suspected estrogen dependent neoplasia, undiagnosed abnormal genital bleeding, cholestatic jaundice of pregnancy or jaundice with prior pill use, hepatic adenomas or carcinomas, known or suspected pregnancy.

WARNINGS/PRECAUTIONS: Increased risk of myocardial infarction (MI), vascular disease, thromboembolism, stroke, hepatic neoplasia, and gallbladder disease. May increase risk of breast cancer and cancer of the reproductive organs. Increased risk of morbidity and mortality with HTN, hyperlipidemia, obesity, and DM. D/C at least 4 weeks prior to and 2 weeks post-elective surgery with increased risk of thromboembolism and during and following prolonged immobilization. Caution in women with CV disease risk factors. May develop visual changes with contact lenses. Retinal thrombosis reported; d/c if unexplained partial or complete loss of vision or other ophthalmic irregularities occur. May cause glucose intolerance, elevated LDL, other lipid abnormalities, or exacerbate migraine headaches. May cause increased BP and fluid retention; d/c if significant BP elevations occur. Breakthrough bleeding and spotting reported; rule out malignancies or pregnancy. Not indicated for use before menarche. May affect certain endocrine, LFTs, and blood components in laboratory tests. Perform annual history/physical exam; monitor women with history of breast cancer.

ADVERSE REACTIONS: N/V, breakthrough bleeding, spotting, amenorrhea, migraine, depression, vaginal candidiasis, edema, weight changes, melasma, breast changes, changes in cervical erosion and secretion, allergic rash.

INTERACTIONS: Reduced effects resulting in pregnancy or breakthrough bleeding with antibiotics, anticonvulsants, and other drugs that increase the metabolism of contraceptive steroids (eg, rifampin, phenytoin, carbamazepine). Anti-HIV protease inhibitors may increase or decrease plasma levels. Atorvastatin, ascorbic acid, acetaminophen (APAP), and CYP3A4 inhibitors (eg, itraconazole, ketoconazole) may increase plasma ethinyl estradiol levels. Increased plasma levels of cyclosporine, prednisolone, and theophylline have been reported. Decreased plasma concentration of APAP and increased the clearance of temazepam, salicylic acid, morphine, and clofibric acid. May significantly decrease plasma levels of lamotrigine; dosage adjustment of lamotrigine may be necessary.

PREGNANCY: Category X, not for use in nursing.

MECHANISM OF ACTION: Estrogen/progestogen oral contraceptive; acts by suppression of gonadotropins and inhibits ovulation. Also increases difficulty of sperm entry into the uterus and reduces the likelihood of implantation.

PHARMACOKINETICS: Absorption: Rapid. **Distribution:** Found in breast milk. Norgestimate/Ethinyl estradiol: Serum protein binding (>97%). **Metabolism:** Norgestimate: GI tract and/or liver, 1st pass mechanism. Norelgestromin (active major metabolite): Hepatic, norgestrel (active metabolite). Ethinyl estradiol: Hydroxylated, glucuronide, and sulfate conjugates. **Elimination:** Urine, feces; $T_{1/2}$=28.1 hrs (norelgestromin), 36.4 hrs (norgestrel), 17.7 hrs (ethinyl estradiol).

NURSING CONSIDERATIONS

Assessment: Assess for current or history of thrombophlebitis or thromboembolic disorders, history of HTN, hyperlipidemia, DM, obesity, breast cancer, and any other conditions where treatment is contraindicated or cautioned. Assess use in women >35 yrs of age, smokers (≥15 cigarettes/day). Assess pregnancy/nursing status and for possible drug interactions.

Monitoring: Monitor for signs/symptoms of MI, thromboembolism, stroke, hepatic neoplasia, and other adverse effects. Monitor BP with history of HTN, serum glucose levels in DM or prediabetic patients, lipid levels with history of hyperlipidemia, and for signs of worsening depression with previous history. Monitor liver function and for signs of liver toxicity. Refer to an ophthalmologist if ocular changes develop.

Patient Counseling: Inform that the drug does not protect against HIV infection (AIDS) and other sexually transmitted diseases. Counsel about potential adverse effects. Advise to avoid smoking. Instruct to take exactly ud at intervals not exceeding 24 hrs. Advise about risks of pregnancy if dose is missed. Inform that if one dose is missed, take as soon as possible and take next pill at regular scheduled time. Inform that patient may experience spotting, light bleeding, or nausea during the first 1-3 packs of pills; advise not to d/c medication and if symptoms persist, notify physician. Instruct to d/c if pregnancy is confirmed/suspected.

Administration: Oral route. **Storage:** 25°C (77°F); excursions permitted to 15-30°C (59-86°F). Protect from light.

ORTHO-CYCLEN RX
ethinyl estradiol - norgestimate (Janssen)

> Cigarette smoking increases risk of serious cardiovascular (CV) events. Risk increases with age (>35 yrs) and with the number of cigarettes smoked. Should not be used by women who are >35 yrs of age and smoke.

OTHER BRAND NAMES: Sprintec (Teva) - MonoNessa (Watson) - Previfem (Qualitest)

THERAPEUTIC CLASS: Estrogen/progestogen combination

INDICATIONS: Prevention of pregnancy.

DOSAGE: *Adults:* 1 tab qd for 28 days, then repeat. Start 1st Sunday after menses begins or 1st day of menses.
Pediatrics: Postpubertal: 1 tab qd for 28 days, then repeat. Start 1st Sunday after menses begins or 1st day of menses.

HOW SUPPLIED: Tab: (Ethinyl Estradiol [EE]-Norgestimate) 0.035mg-0.25mg

CONTRAINDICATIONS: Thrombophlebitis or thromboembolic disorders, past history of deep vein thrombophlebitis or thromboembolic disorders, cerebral vascular or coronary artery disease (current or past history), valvular heart disease with complications, diabetes with vascular involvement, headaches with focal neurological symptoms, major surgery with prolonged immobilization, known or suspected carcinoma of the breast or personal history of breast cancer, carcinoma of the endometrium or other known or suspected estrogen-dependent neoplasia, undiagnosed abnormal genital bleeding, cholestatic jaundice of pregnancy or jaundice with prior pill use, acute or chronic hepatocellular disease with abnormal liver function, hepatic adenomas or carcinomas, known or suspected pregnancy. (Ortho-Cyclen, Previfem) Known thrombophilic conditions, persistent BP values of ≥160 mm Hg systolic or ≥100 mm Hg diastolic. (MonoNessa, Sprintec) Severe HTN.

WARNINGS/PRECAUTIONS: For the first cycle of a Sunday Start regimen, use another method of contraception until after the first 7 consecutive days of administration. Not indicated for use in emergency contraception. Increased risk of myocardial infarction (MI), vascular disease, thromboembolism, stroke, hepatic neoplasia, and gallbladder disease. May increase risk of breast cancer and cancer of the reproductive organs. Increased risk of morbidity and mortality if other risk factors (eg, HTN, hyperlipidemia, obesity, diabetes mellitus [DM]) are present. D/C at least 4 weeks prior to and for 2 weeks after elective surgery of a type associated with an increased risk of thromboembolism, and during and following prolonged immobilization, if feasible. Contact lens wearers who develop visual changes or changes in lens tolerance should be assessed by an ophthalmologist. Retinal thrombosis reported; d/c if unexplained partial or complete loss of vision occurs, onset of proptosis or diplopia, papilledema, or retinal vascular lesions develop. Should not be used to induce withdrawal bleeding as a test for pregnancy, or to treat threatened or habitual abortion during pregnancy. May cause glucose intolerance; monitor prediabetic and diabetic patients. May elevate LDL levels or cause other lipid abnormalities. D/C and evaluate the cause if new onset/exacerbation of migraine or recurrent, persistent, severe headache with a new pattern develops. May increase BP; monitor closely and d/c if significant elevation of BP occurs and cannot be adequately controlled. Breakthrough bleeding and spotting reported; rule out malignancies or pregnancy. Post-pill amenorrhea or oligomenorrhea may occur. D/C if jaundice develops. May cause fluid retention. Monitor closely with depression and d/c if depression recurs to a serious degree. Ectopic and intrauterine pregnancies may occur in contraceptive failures. May affect certain endocrine, LFTs, and blood components in laboratory tests. Rule out pregnancy if two consecutive periods are missed.

ADVERSE REACTIONS: N/V, breakthrough bleeding, GI symptoms (eg, abdominal cramps, bloating), spotting, menstrual flow changes, amenorrhea, migraine, depression, vaginal candidiasis, edema, weight changes, change in cervical erosion and secretion, melasma, cholestatic jaundice, change in corneal curvature.

INTERACTIONS: May decrease levels and potentially diminish effectiveness or increase breakthrough bleeding when used concomitantly with drugs or herbal products that induce certain enzymes, including CYP3A4 (eg, phenytoin, barbiturates, carbamazepine); use an alternative or back-up method of contraception and continue back-up contraception for 28 days after discontinuing the enzyme inducer. Atorvastatin or rosuvastatin may increase EE exposure; ascorbic acid and acetaminophen (APAP) may increase EE levels. Increased levels with CYP3A4 inhibitors (eg, itraconazole, voriconazole, fluconazole). Significant level changes (decreased/increased) noted with HIV protease inhibitors (decreased [eg, nelfinavir, darunavir/ritonavir, (fos)amprenavir/ritonavir] or increased [eg, indinavir, atazanavir/ritonavir])/HCV protease inhibitors (decreased [eg, boceprevir, telaprevir]) or with non-nucleoside reverse transcriptase inhibitors (decreased [eg, nevirapine] or increased [eg, etravirine]). Colesevelam reported to significantly decrease EE exposure; decreased drug interaction reported when the two drug products are given 4 hrs apart. May inhibit metabolism and increase levels of other compounds (eg, cyclosporine, prednisolone, theophylline). May decrease levels of APAP, clofibric acid, morphine, salicylic acid, and temazepam. May significantly decrease levels of lamotrigine; dosage adjustment of lamotrigine may be needed. May increase serum levels of thyroid-binding globulins; increased dose of thyroid hormone may be needed in patients on thyroid hormone replacement therapy.

PREGNANCY: Category X, not for use in nursing.

MECHANISM OF ACTION: Estrogen/progestogen oral contraceptive; acts by suppression of gonadotropins to inhibit ovulation. Also causes changes in the cervical mucus (increasing the difficulty of sperm entry into the uterus) and the endometrium (reducing the likelihood of implantation).

PHARMACOKINETICS: Absorption: Rapid. Administration on various days of dosing cycle led to different parameters; refer to PI. **Distribution:** Found in breast milk. Norelgestromin and norgestrel: Serum protein binding (>97%; norelgestromin bound to albumin; norgestrel bound primarily to sex hormone-binding globulin). EE: Serum protein binding (>97% to albumin). **Metabolism:** Norgestimate: GI tract and/or liver (first-pass). Norelgestromin (primary, active metabolite): Liver; norgestrel (active metabolite), hydroxylated and conjugated metabolites. EE: Hydroxylated metabolites and their glucuronide and sulfate conjugates. **Elimination:** Urine and feces (EE and norgestimate metabolites) (Norgestimate metabolites: 47% urine and 37% feces).

NURSING CONSIDERATIONS

Assessment: Assess for thrombophlebitis or thromboembolic disorders, past history of deep vein thrombophlebitis or thromboembolic disorders, cerebral vascular or coronary artery disease (current or past history), valvular heart disease with complications, diabetes with vascular involvement, headaches with focal neurological symptoms, pregnancy/nursing status, hypersensitivity, and for any other conditions where treatment is contraindicated or cautioned. Assess for possible drug interactions.

Monitoring: Monitor for signs/symptoms of MI, thromboembolism/thrombotic disease, stroke, and other adverse effects. Monitor BP with history of HTN, serum glucose levels in DM or prediabetic patients, lipid levels with history of hyperlipidemia, and for signs of worsening depression with previous history. Monitor liver function and for signs of jaundice. Refer contact lens wearers who develop visual changes or changes in lens tolerance to an ophthalmologist. Monitor serum folate levels in patients who become pregnant shortly after discontinuation. Perform annual history and physical exam.

Patient Counseling: Inform that drug does not protect against HIV infection (AIDS) and other sexually transmitted diseases. Advise to avoid smoking while on medication. Counsel about potential adverse effects. Instruct to take exactly ud, at intervals not exceeding 24 hrs. Instruct on what to do if doses are missed. Advise about risk of pregnancy if doses are missed. Instruct to d/c if pregnancy is confirmed/suspected. Counsel that efficacy may decrease if vomiting/diarrhea develops or if taking certain medicines; instruct to use a back-up method of contraception. Inform that spotting, light bleeding, or stomach sickness may occur during first 1-3 packs of pills; advise not to d/c medication and to notify physician if symptoms persist.

Administration: Oral route. **Storage:** (Ortho-Cyclen, MonoNessa) 25°C (77°F); excursions permitted to 15-30°C (59-86°F). (Previfem, Sprintec) 20-25°C (68-77°F). Protect from light.

OSENI   RX
pioglitazone - alogliptin (Takeda)

> Thiazolidinediones, including pioglitazone, cause or exacerbate congestive heart failure (CHF) in some patients. After initiation and dose increases, monitor carefully for signs and symptoms of heart failure (HF); manage accordingly and consider discontinuation or dose reduction if HF develops. Not recommended with symptomatic HF. Contraindicated with established NYHA Class III or IV HF.

THERAPEUTIC CLASS: Dipeptidyl peptidase-4 inhibitor/thiazolidinedione

INDICATIONS: Adjunct to diet and exercise to improve glycemic control in adults with type 2 diabetes mellitus (DM) in multiple clinical settings when treatment with both alogliptin and pioglitazone is appropriate.

DOSAGE: *Adults:* Initial: Inadequately Controlled on Diet and Exercise/Inadequately Controlled on Metformin Monotherapy/On Alogliptin who Require Additional Glycemic Control: 25mg-15mg or 25mg-30mg qd. On Pioglitazone who Require Additional Glycemic Control: 25mg-15mg, 25mg-30mg, or 25mg-45mg qd as appropriate based upon current therapy. Switching from Alogliptin Coadministered with Pioglitazone: Dose of alogliptin and pioglitazone based upon current therapy. With CHF (NYHA Class I or II): 25mg-15mg qd. Titrate: Adjust based on glycemic response as determined by HbA1c. Max: 25mg-45mg qd. Moderate Renal Impairment (CrCl ≥30-<60mL/min): 12.5mg-15mg, 12.5mg-30mg, or 12.5mg-45mg qd. Coadministration with Strong CYP2C8 Inhibitors (eg, gemfibrozil): Max: 25mg-15mg qd.

HOW SUPPLIED: Tab: (Alogliptin-Pioglitazone) 12.5mg-15mg, 12.5mg-30mg, 12.5mg-45mg, 25mg-15mg, 25mg-30mg, 25mg-45mg

CONTRAINDICATIONS: NYHA Class III or IV HF.

WARNINGS/PRECAUTIONS: Not for use with type 1 DM or for treatment of diabetic ketoacidosis. Not recommended with severe renal impairment or end-stage renal disease. No conclusive evidence of macrovascular risk reduction. Fatal and nonfatal hepatic events reported; obtain baseline LFTs, and initiate with caution in patients with abnormal LFTs. Measure LFTs promptly in patients who report symptoms that may indicate liver injury. If abnormal LFTs (ALT >3X ULN) are reported, interrupt treatment and investigate for the probable cause, and do not restart therapy without another explanation for the LFT abnormalities. Alogliptin: Acute pancreatitis reported; d/c if suspected and initiate appropriate management. Serious hypersensitivity reactions reported; d/c if suspected, assess for other potential causes, and institute alternative treatment for diabetes. Caution with history of angioedema to another dipeptidyl peptidase-4 (DPP-4) inhibitor. Pioglitazone: Dose-related edema reported. Increased incidence of bone fractures reported in females. Not for use in patients with active bladder cancer; consider benefits versus risks in patients with a prior history of bladder cancer. Macular edema reported; promptly refer to an ophthalmologist if visual symptoms occur. May result in ovulation in some premenopausal anovulatory women, which may increase risk for pregnancy; adequate contraception is recommended.

ADVERSE REACTIONS: Nasopharyngitis, back pain, upper respiratory tract infection, influenza, hypoglycemia, CHF.

INTERACTIONS: May require lower dose of insulin or insulin secretagogue to minimize risk of hypoglycemia. Pioglitazone: Increased exposure and $T_{1/2}$ with strong CYP2C8 inhibitors (eg, gemfibrozil). CYP2C8 inducers (eg, rifampin) may decrease exposure; if a CYP2C8 inducer is started or stopped during treatment, dose may need to be adjusted based on clinical response. May cause dose-related fluid retention when used with other antidiabetic medications, most commonly with insulin.

PREGNANCY: Category C, not for use in nursing.

MECHANISM OF ACTION: Alogliptin: DPP-4 inhibitor; slows inactivation of incretin hormones, thereby increasing their bloodstream concentrations and reducing fasting and postprandial glucose concentrations in a glucose-dependent manner. Pioglitazone: Thiazolidinedione; improves insulin sensitivity in muscle and adipose tissue while inhibiting hepatic gluconeogenesis.

PHARMACOKINETICS: Absorption: Alogliptin: Absolute bioavailability (100%). Pioglitazone: T_{max}=within 2 hrs, 3-4 hrs (with food). **Distribution:** Alogliptin: V_d=417L (IV); plasma protein binding (20%). Pioglitazone: V_d=0.63L/kg; plasma protein binding (>99%). **Metabolism:** Alogliptin: via CYP2D6 and CYP3A4, N-demethylated alogliptin, M-I (active metabolite), and N-acetylated alogliptin, M-II. Pioglitazone: Hydroxylation and oxidation (extensive), CYP2C8, CYP3A4; M-III [keto derivative] and M-IV [hydroxyl derivative] (active metabolites). **Elimination:** Alogliptin: Urine (76%, 60-71% unchanged), feces (13%). Pioglitazone: Urine (15-30%), feces; $T_{1/2}$=3-7 hrs (pioglitazone), 16-24 hrs (metabolites).

NURSING CONSIDERATIONS

Assessment: Assess for HF or risk of HF, edema, renal/hepatic function, bone health, history of pancreatitis, diabetic ketoacidosis, active/history of bladder cancer, history of angioedema to another DPP-4 inhibitor, pregnancy/nursing status, and possible drug interactions. Obtain FPG and HbA1c.

Monitoring: Monitor for signs/symptoms of CHF, pancreatitis, hypersensitivity reactions, fractures, visual symptoms, and other adverse reactions. Monitor LFTs, FPG, and HbA1c. Monitor renal function periodically.

Patient Counseling: Inform of the potential risks and benefits of therapy. Instruct to immediately report to physician any symptoms that may indicate HF. Inform that pancreatitis may occur; instruct to promptly d/c use and contact physician if persistent severe abdominal pain occurs. Instruct to d/c use and seek medical advice promptly if signs/symptoms of allergic reactions, liver injury, or bladder cancer occur. Inform that hypoglycemia can occur; explain the risks, symptoms, and appropriate management. Counsel premenopausal women to use adequate contraception during treatment. Advise not to double the next dose if a dose is missed. Instruct to inform physician if an unusual symptom develops or if a symptom persists or worsens.

Administration: Oral route. May be taken with or without food. Do not split before swallowing.
Storage: 25°C (77°F); excursions permitted to 15-30°C (59-86°F). Protect from moisture and humidity.

OSMOPREP   RX
monobasic sodium phosphate monohydrate - dibasic sodium phosphate (Salix)

> Rare, but serious, acute phosphate nephropathy reported; some cases resulted in permanent renal impairment and some patients required long-term dialysis. Patients at increased risk may include those with increased age, hypovolemia, increased bowel transit time (eg, bowel obstruction), active colitis, or baseline kidney disease, and those using medicines that affect renal perfusion or function (eg, diuretics, ACE inhibitors, ARBs, and possibly NSAIDs). Use the dose and dosing regimen as recommended (pm/am split dose).

THERAPEUTIC CLASS: Bowel cleanser

INDICATIONS: For cleansing of the colon as a preparation for colonoscopy in adults ≥18 yrs of age.

DOSAGE: *Adults:* ≥18 Yrs: Evening Before Colonoscopy: Take 4 tabs with 8 oz. of clear liquids every 15 min for a total of 20 tabs. Day of Colonoscopy: Starting 3-5 hrs before procedure, take 4 tabs with 8 oz. of clear liquids every 15 min for a total of 12 tabs.

HOW SUPPLIED: Tab: (Sodium Phosphate Monobasic Monohydrate-Sodium Phosphate Dibasic Anhydrous) 1.102g-0.398g

CONTRAINDICATIONS: Biopsy-proven acute phosphate nephropathy, GI obstruction, gastric bypass or stapling surgery, bowel perforation, toxic colitis, toxic megacolon.

WARNINGS/PRECAUTIONS: Do not use within 7 days of previous administration. Rare, but serious, renal failure and nephrocalcinosis reported. Caution with renal impairment (CrCl <30mL/min), history of acute phosphate nephropathy, known or suspected electrolyte disturbances (eg, dehydration), or with conditions that increase the risk for fluid and electrolyte disturbances or increase the risk of seizure (eg, hyponatremia). Adequately hydrate before, during, and after use. If significant vomiting or signs of dehydration develop, consider performing postcolonoscopy lab tests (electrolytes, SrCr, and BUN). Correct electrolyte abnormalities before treatment. Do not administer additional laxative or purgative agents, particularly additional sodium phosphate-based purgative or enema products. Serious arrhythmias rarely reported; consider predose and postcolonoscopy ECGs in patients at increased risk of serious cardiac arrhythmias. Generalized tonic-clonic seizures and/or loss of consciousness rarely reported; caution with history of seizures. May induce colonic mucosal aphthous ulcerations; consider this in patients with known or suspected inflammatory bowel disease (IBD). Caution with acute exacerbation of chronic IBD, impaired gag reflex, in patients prone to regurgitation or aspiration, and in elderly.

ADVERSE REACTIONS: Acute phosphate nephropathy, abdominal bloating, abdominal pain, N/V, dizziness, headache, hyperphosphatemia, hypokalemia.

INTERACTIONS: See Boxed Warning. PO medication administered within 1 hr of the start of each dose may be flushed from GI tract and may not be absorbed properly. Caution with drugs that may affect electrolyte levels (eg, diuretics), increase the risk of arrhythmias, prolong QT interval, and lower the seizure threshold (eg, TCAs). Caution in patients withdrawing from alcohol or benzodiazepines.

PREGNANCY: Category C, caution in nursing.

MECHANISM OF ACTION: Osmotic laxative; thought to be through the osmotic effect of Na^+, causing large amounts of water to be drawn into the colon, promoting evacuation.

NURSING CONSIDERATIONS

Assessment: Assess for biopsy-proven acute phosphate nephropathy, GI obstruction, gastric bypass or stapling surgery, bowel perforation, toxic colitis, toxic megacolon, risk of acute phosphate nephropathy, electrolyte abnormalities, or any other conditions where treatment is cautioned. Assess for hypersensitivity, pregnancy/nursing status, and possible drug interactions. Consider performing baseline lab tests (electrolytes, SrCr, and BUN). Consider predose ECGs in patients at increased risk of serious cardiac arrhythmias.

Monitoring: Monitor for acute phosphate nephropathy, arrhythmias, generalized tonic-clonic seizures, loss of consciousness, colonic mucosal aphthous ulcerations, and other adverse reactions. Consider performing postcolonoscopy lab tests. Consider postcolonoscopy ECGs in patients at increased risk of serious cardiac arrhythmias.

Patient Counseling: Instruct to notify physician if patient has a history of renal disease or takes medication for BP, or cardiac/renal disease. Explain the importance of taking the recommended fluid regimen and advise to hydrate adequately before, during, and after use. Instruct to contact physician if experiencing symptoms of dehydration, or worsening of bloating, abdominal pain, N/V, or headache. Counsel not to take with other laxatives or enemas made with sodium phosphate.

Administration: Oral route. Do not drink any liquids colored purple or red. **Storage:** 25°C (77°F); excursions permitted to 15-30°C (59-86°F).

OVCON-35   RX
ethinyl estradiol - norethindrone (Warner Chilcott)

> Cigarette smoking increases the risk of serious cardiovascular (CV) side effects. Risk increases with age (>35 yrs) and with heavy smoking (≥15 cigarettes/day). Women who use oral contraceptives should be strongly advised not to smoke.

OTHER BRAND NAMES: Balziva (Barr)

THERAPEUTIC CLASS: Estrogen/progestogen combination

INDICATIONS: Prevention of pregnancy.

DOSAGE: *Adults:* 1 tab qd for 28 days, then repeat regimen on the next day after the last tab. Start on the 1st day of menses or 1st Sunday after menses begin. For the 1st cycle of a Sunday start regimen, use back-up method if having intercourse before taking the seven pills. *Pediatrics:* Postpubertal Adolescents: 1 tab qd for 28 days, then repeat regimen on the next day after the last tab. Start on the 1st day of menses or 1st Sunday after menses begin. For the 1st cycle of a Sunday start regimen, use back-up method if having intercourse before taking the seven pills.

HOW SUPPLIED: Tab: (Ethinyl Estradiol-Norethindrone) (Ovcon-35, Balziva) 0.035mg-0.4mg

CONTRAINDICATIONS: Thrombophlebitis, current or history of thromboembolic disorders, past history of deep vein thrombophlebitis, cerebrovascular or coronary artery disease (CAD), known or suspected carcinoma of the breast, endometrial carcinoma or other known or suspected estrogen-dependent neoplasia, undiagnosed abnormal genital bleeding, cholestatic jaundice of pregnancy or jaundice with prior pill use, hepatic adenomas or carcinomas, known or suspected pregnancy.

WARNINGS/PRECAUTIONS: Increased risk of myocardial infarction (MI), thromboembolism, cerebrovascular events, gallbladder disease, and hepatic neoplasia. May increase risk of breast cancer and cervical intraepithelial neoplasia. May cause benign hepatic adenomas. Retinal thrombosis reported; d/c if unexplained partial or complete loss of vision, onset of proptosis or diplopia, papilledema, or retinal vascular lesions develop. Increased risk of gallbladder surgery reported. May cause glucose intolerance. May cause fluid retention and increase BP; d/c if significant elevation of BP occurs. May cause migraine or development of headaches; d/c and evaluate the cause. Breakthrough bleeding and spotting reported; rule out malignancy or pregnancy. D/C if jaundice develops. Monitor closely with depression and d/c if depression recurs to serious degree. May develop visual changes or changes in contact lens tolerance. Use back-up method of contraception with significant GI disturbance.

ADVERSE REACTIONS: N/V, breakthrough bleeding, GI symptoms, spotting, menstrual flow changes, amenorrhea, migraine, depression, vaginal candidiasis, edema, weight changes, cervical ectropion and secretion changes.

INTERACTIONS: Reduced effects, increased breakthrough bleeding, and menstrual irregularities with rifampin, barbiturates, phenylbutazone, phenytoin sodium, and possibly with griseofulvin, ampicillin, and tetracyclines.

PREGNANCY: Category X, not for use in nursing.

MECHANISM OF ACTION: Estrogen/progestogen combination oral contraceptive; acts by suppressing gonadotropins. Primarily inhibits ovulation, but also increases difficulty of sperm entry into the uterus and reduces the likelihood of implantation.

PHARMACOKINETICS: Distribution: Found in breast milk.

NURSING CONSIDERATIONS

Assessment: Assess for pregnancy/nursing status, possible drug interactions, and conditions where treatment is contraindicated or cautioned. Assess use in patients >35 yrs of age who smoke ≥15 cigarettes/day, and with HTN, hyperlipidemia, obesity, and diabetes mellitus.

Monitoring: Monitor for signs/symptoms of thromboembolism, stroke, MI, and other adverse effects. Monitor BP in patients with a history of HTN, HTN-related disease, or renal disease. Monitor for signs of depression in patients with a history of depression. Perform annual history and physical exam. Monitor serum glucose levels in prediabetic and diabetic patients. Monitor lipid levels in patients with a history of hyperlipidemia.

Patient Counseling: Inform that medication does not protect against HIV (AIDS) and other STDs. Counsel about possible serious side effects. Advise to avoid smoking while on therapy. If dose is missed, refer to PI for instructions. Inform that if spotting, light bleeding, or nausea occurs during first 1-3 packs of pills, to not d/c medication and if symptoms persist, to notify physician. Inform if vomiting or diarrhea occurs or if taking other medications, efficacy may decrease; instruct to use backup method of contraception. Refer patients with contact lenses to an ophthalmologist if changes in vision or lens tolerance develop.

Administration: Oral route. **Storage:** (Ovcon 35, Balziva) 20-25°C (68-77°F).

OXTELLAR XR   RX
oxcarbazepine (Supernus)

THERAPEUTIC CLASS: Dibenzazepine

INDICATIONS: Adjunctive therapy of partial seizures in adults and in children 6-17 yrs of age.

DOSAGE: *Adults:* Administer on an empty stomach (at least 1 hr ac or at least 2 hrs pc). Initial: 600mg qd for 1 week. Titrate: May increase at weekly intervals in 600mg/day increments. Usual: 1200-2400mg qd. Renal Impairment (CrCl <30mL/min): Initial: 1/2 the usual initial dose (300mg qd). Titrate: May increase at weekly intervals in 300-450mg/day increments to achieve desired clinical response. Geriatrics: Initial: Consider starting at 300-450mg qd. Titrate: May increase at weekly intervals in 300-450mg/day increments to achieve desired clinical effect. Concomitant Enzyme Inducing Antiepileptic Drugs (AEDs) (eg, carbamazepine, phenobarbital, phenytoin): Dose increases may be necessary. Initial: Consider 900mg qd. Conversion From Immediate-Release (IR) to Extended-Release (ER): Higher doses may be necessary.
Pediatrics: Administer on an empty stomach (at least 1 hr ac or at least 2 hrs pc). 6-17 yrs: Initial: 8-10mg/kg (up to 600mg) qd for 1 week. Titrate: May increase at weekly intervals in 8-10mg/kg increments (up to 600mg) qd. Target Maint Dose (Achieved Over 2-3 Weeks): >39kg: 1800mg qd. 29.1-39kg: 1200mg qd. 20-29kg: 900mg qd. Renal Impairment (CrCl <30mL/min): Initial: 1/2 the usual initial dose. Titrate: May increase at weekly intervals in 300-450mg/day increments to achieve desired clinical response. Concomitant AEDs (eg, carbamazepine/phenobarbital/phenytoin): Dose increases may be necessary. Conversion From IR to ER: Higher doses may be necessary.

HOW SUPPLIED: Tab, Extended-Release: 150mg, 300mg, 600mg

WARNINGS/PRECAUTIONS: Clinically significant hyponatremia may develop; measure serum Na levels during treatment if symptoms of hyponatremia develop, and particularly if receiving concomitant medications known to decrease serum Na levels (eg, drugs associated with inappropriate antidiuretic hormone secretion). Anaphylaxis and angioedema involving the larynx, glottis, lips, and eyelids reported with immediate-release oxcarbazepine; d/c if any of these reactions develop, do not rechallenge and initiate alternative treatment. Treat patients with history of hypersensitivity reactions to carbamazepine only if potential benefit justifies potential risk; d/c immediately if signs/symptoms of hypersensitivity develop. Serious dermatological reactions (eg, Stevens-Johnson syndrome, toxic epidermal necrolysis) reported with immediate-release oxcarbazepine; consider d/c and prescribing another AED if a skin reaction develops. Increased risk of suicidal thoughts or behavior; monitor for emergence or worsening of depression, suicidal thoughts or behavior, and/or any unusual changes in mood or behavior. Withdraw gradually to minimize potential of increased seizure frequency. Multiorgan hypersensitivity reactions reported with IR oxcarbazepine; d/c and initiate an alternative treatment if suspected. Pancytopenia, agranulocytosis, and leukopenia reported; consider d/c if any evidence of these hematologic events develop. Levels may decrease during pregnancy; monitor during pregnancy and through the postpartum period. Immediate-release oxcarbazepine associated with decreases in T4, without changes in T3 or TSH. Caution with severe renal impairment and in the elderly. Not recommended with severe hepatic impairment.

ADVERSE REACTIONS: Dizziness, somnolence, headache, balance disorder, tremor, vomiting, diplopia, asthenia, fatigue, ataxia, nystagmus, blurred vision, visual impairment, dyspepsia, sinusitis.

INTERACTIONS: AEDs that are CYP450 inducers (eg, carbamazepine, phenobarbital, phenytoin), valproic acid, and verapamil may decrease 10-monohydroxy derivative (MHD) levels. May inhibit CYP2C19 and induce CYP3A4/5 with potentially important effects on levels of other drugs. May decrease levels of dihydropyridine calcium antagonists (eg, felodipine), oral contraceptives (eg, ethinyl estradiol, levonorgestrel), and cyclosporine.

PREGNANCY: Category C, not for use in nursing.

MECHANISM OF ACTION: Dibenzazepine; not established. Oxcarbazepine and MHD suspected to exert antiseizure effects through blockade of voltage-sensitive Na^+ channels, resulting in stabilization of hyperexcited neural membranes, inhibition of repetitive neuronal firing, and diminution of propagation of synaptic impulses. Also, increased K^+ conductance and modulation of high-voltage activated calcium channels may contribute to the anticonvulsant effects.

PHARMACOKINETICS: Absorption: (1200mg qd) T_{max}=7 hrs (MHD). **Distribution:** Found in breast milk. (MHD) V_d=49L; plasma protein binding (40%). **Metabolism:** Liver; reduction by cytosolic enzymes to MHD (active metabolite). (MHD) Conjugation with glucuronic acid. **Elimination:** (Immediate-Release Formulation) Urine (>95%, <1% unchanged), feces (<4%). $T_{1/2}$=7-11 hrs (oxcarbazepine), 9-11 hrs (MHD).

NURSING CONSIDERATIONS

Assessment: Assess for hypersensitivity to drug or history of hypersensitivity to carbamazepine, depression, renal/hepatic impairment, pregnancy/nursing status, and for possible drug interactions.

Monitoring: Monitor for signs/symptoms of hyponatremia, anaphylaxis, angioedema, dermatological/hematologic reactions, emergence/worsening of depression, suicidal thoughts or behavior and/or any unusual changes in mood or behavior, multiorgan hypersensitivity reactions, and other adverse reactions. Monitor patients during pregnancy and through the postpartum period.

Patient Counseling: Advise to report symptoms of low Na and fever associated with other organ system involvement (eg, rash, lymphadenopathy). Instruct to report immediately signs/symptoms suggesting angioedema and to d/c therapy until consulting with physician. Instruct to contact physician immediately if a hypersensitivity reaction, symptoms suggestive of blood disorders, or if a skin reaction occurs. Inform female patients of childbearing age that concurrent use with hormonal contraceptives may render this method of contraception less effective; advise to use additional nonhormonal forms of contraception. Counsel that therapy may increase risk of suicidal thoughts or behavior and to be alert for emergence/worsening of symptoms of depression, any unusual changes in mood/behavior, or emergence of suicidal thoughts, behavior, or thoughts about self-harm; instruct to immediately report behaviors of concern to healthcare providers. Advise to use caution if taking alcohol while on therapy, due to possible additive sedative effect. Inform that therapy may cause dizziness and somnolence; advise not to drive/operate machinery until effects have been determined. Encourage to enroll in the North American Antiepileptic Drug Pregnancy Registry if become pregnant.

Administration: Oral route. Take tab whole with water or other liquid; do not cut, crush, or chew. **Storage:** 25°C (77°F); excursions permitted to 15-30°C (59-86°F). Protect from light and moisture.

OXYBUTYNIN   RX
oxybutynin chloride (Various)

THERAPEUTIC CLASS: Anticholinergic

INDICATIONS: Relief of symptoms of bladder instability associated with voiding in patients with uninhibited neurogenic or reflex neurogenic bladder (eg, urgency, frequency, urinary leakage, urge incontinence, dysuria).

DOSAGE: *Adults:* Usual: 5mg bid-tid. Max: 5mg qid. Frail Elderly: Initial: 2.5mg bid-tid. Elderly: Start at lower end of doing range.
Pediatrics: ≥5 Yrs: Usual: 5mg bid. Max: 5mg tid.

HOW SUPPLIED: Syrup: 5mg/5mL [118mL, 473mL]; Tab: 5mg* *scored

CONTRAINDICATIONS: Urinary retention, gastric retention and other severe decreased GI motility conditions, uncontrolled narrow-angle glaucoma, and in patients at risk for these conditions.

WARNINGS/PRECAUTIONS: Angioedema of the face, lips, tongue and/or larynx reported; d/c if involvement of the tongue, hypopharynx, or larynx occurs. Variety of CNS anticholinergic effects reported; consider dose reduction or discontinuation. May aggravate symptoms of hyperthyroidism, coronary heart disease (CHD), congestive heart failure (CHF), cardiac arrhythmias, hiatal hernia, tachycardia, HTN, myasthenia gravis, and prostatic hypertrophy. Caution with preexisting dementia treated with cholinesterase inhibitors; hepatic/renal impairment, myasthenia gravis, clinically significant bladder outflow obstruction, GI obstructive disorders, ulcerative colitis, intestinal atony, gastroesophageal reflux disorder (GERD), and in frail elderly.

ADVERSE REACTIONS: Dry mouth, dizziness, constipation, somnolence, nausea, blurred vision, urinary hesitation, headache, urinary tract infection, nervousness, dyspepsia, urinary retention, insomnia.

INTERACTIONS: May increase frequency and/or severity of adverse effects with other anticholinergics or with other agents which produce dry mouth, constipation, somnolence, and/or other anticholinergic effects. May alter GI absorption of other drugs due to GI motility effects; caution with drugs with narrow therapeutic index. Increased levels with ketoconazole. CYP3A4 inhibitors (eg, antimycotics, macrolides) may alter mean pharmacokinetic parameters; caution when coadministered. Caution with drugs that can cause or exacerbate esophagitis (eg, bisphosphonates).

PREGNANCY: Category B, caution in nursing.

MECHANISM OF ACTION: Antispasmodic/anticholinergic agent; inhibits muscarinic action of acetylcholine on smooth muscle exerting direct antispasmodic effect; relaxes smooth muscle of bladder.

PHARMACOKINETICS: Absorption: Rapid. Absolute bioavailability (6%); T_{max}=1 hr. Refer to PI for pediatric, isomer, and metabolite parameters. **Distribution:** (IV) V_d=193L; plasma protein binding (>99%, >97% desethyloxybutynin). **Metabolism:** Liver via CYP3A4; desethyloxybutynin (active metabolite). **Elimination:** Urine (<0.1%, unchanged; <0.1%, desethyloxybutynin); $T_{1/2}$=2-3 hrs.

NURSING CONSIDERATIONS

Assessment: Assess for urinary and gastric retention, and other severe decreased GI motility conditions, uncontrolled narrow-angle glaucoma, preexisting dementia, hepatic/renal impairment, myasthenia gravis, hyperthyroidism, CHD, CHF, hypersensitivity to the drug, and other conditions where treatment is contraindicated or cautioned, pregnancy/nursing status, and possible drug interactions.

Monitoring: Monitor for aggravation of myasthenia gravis, hyperthyroidism, CHD, CHF, cardiac arrhythmias, hiatal hernia, tachycardia, HTN, and prostatic hypertrophy symptoms. Monitor for signs of anticholinergic CNS effects, hypersensitivity reactions, and other adverse reactions.

Patient Counseling: Inform that angioedema may occur and could result in life-threatening airway obstruction; advise to promptly d/c therapy and seek medical attention if tongue/laryngopharynx edema or difficulty breathing occurs. Inform that heat prostration may occur when administered in high environmental temperature. Inform that drug may produce drowsiness or blurred vision; advise to exercise caution. Inform that alcohol may enhance drowsiness.

Administration: Oral route. **Storage:** (Tab) 20-25°C (68-77°F). (Syrup) 15°-30°C (59-86°F).

OXYCODONE TABLETS $\qquad$ CII
oxycodone HCl (Various)

OTHER BRAND NAMES: Roxicodone (Mallinckrodt)

THERAPEUTIC CLASS: Opioid analgesic

INDICATIONS: Management of moderate to severe pain.

DOSAGE: *Adults:* Opioid-Naive: Initial: 5-15mg q4-6h PRN. Titrate: Adjust dose based upon response. For chronic pain, give on an around-the-clock basis. For severe chronic pain, give q4-6h at the lowest effective dose. Cessation: D/C gradually; decrease by 25-50% per day. Raise dose to previous level and titrate down more slowly if withdrawal symptoms occur. Hepatic/Renal Impairment: Initial: Dose conservatively. Titrate: Adjust according to clinical situation. Refer to PI for conversion from fixed-ratio opioid/acetaminophen, opioid/aspirin, or opioid/nonsteroidal combination drugs.

HOW SUPPLIED: Tab: 10mg*, 20mg*; (Roxicodone) 5mg*, 15mg*, 30mg* *scored

CONTRAINDICATIONS: Significant respiratory depression (in unmonitored settings or the absence of resuscitative equipment), paralytic ileus, acute or severe bronchial asthma or hypercarbia.

WARNINGS/PRECAUTIONS: Respiratory depression may occur; extreme caution with significant chronic obstructive pulmonary disease or cor pulmonale, substantially decreased respiratory reserve, hypoxia, hypercapnia, preexisting respiratory depression, and in the elderly/debilitated. May cause severe hypotension; caution with circulatory shock. May produce orthostatic hypotension in ambulatory patients. Respiratory depressant effects and capacity to elevate CSF pressure may be markedly exaggerated in the presence of head injury, other intracranial lesions, or preexisting increased intracranial pressure. May obscure the clinical course of patients with head injuries. Caution with acute alcoholism, adrenocortical insufficiency (eg, Addison's disease), convulsive disorders, CNS depression or coma, delirium tremens, kyphoscoliosis associated with respiratory depression, myxedema or hypothyroidism, prostatic hypertrophy or urethral stricture, severe hepatic/renal/pulmonary impairment, and toxic psychosis. May obscure diagnosis or clinical course in patients with acute abdominal conditions. May aggravate convulsions with convulsive disorders and may induce or aggravate seizures in some clinical settings. Potential for tolerance and physical dependence. May cause spasm of the sphincter of Oddi; caution with biliary tract disease, including acute pancreatitis. May cause increases in serum amylase levels. Not recommended for use during or immediately prior to labor. May impair mental/physical abilities. Abuse liability similar to other opioids.

ADVERSE REACTIONS: Respiratory depression/arrest, circulatory depression, cardiac arrest, hypotension, shock, N/V, constipation, headache, pruritus, insomnia, dizziness, asthenia, somnolence.

INTERACTIONS: CYP2D6 inhibitors may block the partial metabolism to oxymorphone. May enhance neuromuscular blocking action of skeletal muscle relaxants and increase respiratory depression. Additive CNS depression with other CNS depressants (eg, narcotics, general anesthetics, tranquilizers, alcohol); when combination is contemplated, reduce dose of one or both agents. Mixed agonist/antagonist analgesics (eg, pentazocine, nalbuphine, buprenorphine) may reduce analgesic effect and/or precipitate withdrawal symptoms. Not recommended with MAOIs or within 14 days of stopping such treatment. May cause severe hypotension with phenothiazines or other agents that compromise vasomotor tone.

PREGNANCY: Category B, not for use in nursing.

MECHANISM OF ACTION: Opioid analgesic; pure opioid agonist. Has not been established. Specific CNS opioid receptors for endogenous compounds with opioid-like activity have been identified throughout the brain and spinal cord and play a role in analgesic effects.

PHARMACOKINETICS: Absorption: Absolute bioavailability (60-87%). Administration of multiple doses resulted in different parameters. **Distribution:** V_d=2.6L/kg (IV); plasma protein binding (45%); found in breast milk. **Metabolism:** Extensively metabolized to noroxycodone (major metabolite), oxymorphone (via CYP2D6), and their glucuronides. **Elimination:** Urine; $T_{1/2}$=3.5-4 hrs.

NURSING CONSIDERATIONS

Assessment: Assess for level of pain intensity, type of pain, patient's general condition and medical status, or any other conditions where treatment is contraindicated or cautioned. Assess for drug hypersensitivity, renal/hepatic/pulmonary impairment, pregnancy/nursing status, and possible drug interactions.

Monitoring: Monitor for signs/symptoms of respiratory depression, hypotension, convulsions/seizures, spasm of the sphincter of Oddi, increases in serum amylase levels, tolerance, physical dependence, and other adverse reactions. Reassess the continued need for therapy.

Patient Counseling: Advise to report episodes of breakthrough pain and adverse experiences occurring during therapy. Instruct to not adjust the dose without consulting physician. Inform that drug may impair mental/physical abilities required for the performance of potentially hazardous tasks. Counsel to avoid alcohol or other CNS depressants, except by the order of physician. Advise to consult physician regarding effects when used during pregnancy. Inform that drug has potential for abuse and should be protected from theft and never be given to anyone other than for whom it was prescribed. Counsel that if taking medication for more than a few weeks and need to d/c therapy, to avoid abrupt withdrawal, as dosing will need to be tapered.

Administration: Oral route. **Storage:** 25°C (77°F); excursions permitted to 15-30°C (59-86°F). Protect from moisture.

OXYCONTIN CII
oxycodone HCl (Purdue Pharma)

> Exposes users to risks of addiction, abuse, and misuse, leading to overdose and death; assess each patient's risk prior to prescribing and monitor regularly for development of these behaviors/conditions. Serious, life-threatening, or fatal respiratory depression may occur; monitor during initiation or following a dose increase. Crushing, dissolving, or chewing tab can cause rapid release and absorption of potentially fatal dose; instruct patients to swallow tab whole. Accidental ingestion, especially by children, can result in a fatal overdose. Prolonged use during pregnancy can result in neonatal opioid withdrawal syndrome; advise pregnant women of the risk and ensure availability of appropriate treatment. Concomitant use of CYP3A4 inhibitors or discontinuation of CYP3A4 inducers can result in oxycodone overdose; monitor patients receiving concomitant CYP3A4 inhibitors/inducers.

THERAPEUTIC CLASS: Opioid analgesic

INDICATIONS: Management of severe pain that requires daily, around-the-clock, long-term opioid treatment and for which alternative treatment options are inadequate.

DOSAGE: *Adults:* Initial: First Opioid Analgesic/Nonopioid Tolerant: 10mg q12h. Conversion from Other Oral Oxycodone Formulations: 1/2 of total daily dose q12h. Conversion from Other Opioids: D/C all other around-the-clock opioids when therapy is initiated. Initial: 10mg q12h. Conversion from Transdermal Fentanyl: 10mg q12h for each 25mcg/hr fentanyl transdermal patch; administer dose 18 hrs following removal of patch. Titrate: Individualize dose. May increase total daily dose by 25-50% of current dose every 1-2 days. Hepatic Impairment: Initial: 1/3 to 1/2 the usual starting dose followed by careful dose titration. Renal Impairment: Follow conservative dose initiation and adjust accordingly. Discontinuation: Use gradual downward titration. Elderly: Reduce starting dose to 1/3 to 1/2 the usual dose in debilitated, nonopioid tolerant patients. Refer to PI for further dosage information.

HOW SUPPLIED: Tab, Extended-Release: 10mg, 15mg, 20mg, 30mg, 40mg, 60mg, 80mg

CONTRAINDICATIONS: Significant respiratory depression, acute or severe bronchial asthma in unmonitored settings or in the absence of resuscitative equipment, known or suspected paralytic ileus and GI obstruction.

WARNINGS/PRECAUTIONS: Reserve use in patients for whom alternative treatment options are ineffective, not tolerated, or would be otherwise inadequate to provide sufficient management of pain. Should only be prescribed by healthcare professionals who are knowledgeable in the use of potent opioids for management of chronic pain. 60mg and 80mg tabs, a single dose >40mg, or a total daily dose >80mg are only for use in opioid-tolerant patients. Life-threatening respiratory depression is more likely to occur in elderly, cachectic, or debilitated patients. Consider alternative nonopioid analgesics in patients with significant chronic obstructive pulmonary disease (COPD) or cor pulmonale, and in patients having a substantially decreased respiratory reserve,

O

hypoxia, hypercapnia, or preexisting respiratory depression. May cause severe hypotension, orthostatic hypotension, and syncope; increased risk in patients whose ability to maintain BP has already been compromised by a reduced blood volume or concurrent administration of certain CNS depressants. Avoid with circulatory shock. Monitor patients who may be susceptible to intracranial effects of carbon dioxide retention for signs of sedation and respiratory depression when initiating therapy. Therapy may obscure clinical course in patient with head injury. Avoid with impaired consciousness or coma. Difficulty in swallowing tab, intestinal obstruction, and exacerbation of diverticulitis reported; consider alternative analgesic in patients who have difficulty swallowing or have underlying GI disorders that may predispose them to obstruction. May cause spasm of sphincter of Oddi and increase in serum amylase; monitor patients with biliary tract disease. May aggravate convulsions and induce/aggravate seizures. May impair mental or physical abilities. Urine drug test may not detect oxycodone reliably. Not recommended for use immediately prior to labor.

ADVERSE REACTIONS: Respiratory depression, constipation, N/V, somnolence, dizziness, pruritus, headache, dry mouth, asthenia, sweating, apnea, respiratory arrest, circulatory depression, hypotension.

INTERACTIONS: See Boxed Warning. Respiratory depression, hypotension, and profound sedation or coma may occur with CNS depressants (eg, sedatives, anxiolytics, neuroleptics); if coadministration is required, consider dose reduction of one or both agents. Monitor use in elderly, cachectic, and debilitated patients when coadministered with other drugs that depress respiration. May enhance neuromuscular blocking action of true skeletal muscle relaxants and increase respiratory depression. CYP3A4 inhibitors (eg, erythromycin, ketoconazole, ritonavir) may increase levels of oxycodone and prolong opioid effects; these effects could be more pronounced with concomitant use of CYP2D6 and 3A4 inhibitors. CYP3A4 inducers (eg, rifampin, carbamazepine, phenytoin) may decrease levels and cause lack of efficacy, or development of abstinence syndrome. If coadministration is necessary, use with caution when initiating oxycodone treatment in patients currently taking, or discontinuing CYP3A4 inhibitors/inducers. Mixed agonist/antagonists (eg, pentazocine, nalbuphine, butorphanol) or partial agonist (buprenorphine) may reduce analgesic effect or precipitate withdrawal symptoms; avoid coadministration. May reduce efficacy of diuretics and lead to acute urinary retention. Anticholinergics or other medications with anticholinergic activity may increase risk of urinary retention and/or severe constipation and lead to paralytic ileus.

PREGNANCY: Category C, not for use in nursing.

MECHANISM OF ACTION: Full opioid agonist; not established. Specific CNS opioid receptors have been identified throughout the brain and spinal cord and are thought to play a role in analgesic effect.

PHARMACOKINETICS: Absorption: Oral bioavailability (60-87%). Administration of variable doses resulted in different parameters. **Distribution:** V_d=2.6L/kg (IV); plasma protein binding (45%); crosses placenta; found in breast milk. **Metabolism:** Extensive; via CYP3A mediated N-demethylation to noroxycodone and CYP2D6 mediated O-demethylation to oxymorphone; noroxycodone and noroxymorphone (major metabolites). **Elimination:** Urine; $T_{1/2}$=4.5 hrs.

NURSING CONSIDERATIONS

Assessment: Assess for abuse/addiction risk, pain intensity, prior opioid therapy, opioid tolerance, respiratory depression, drug hypersensitivity, pregnancy/nursing status, possible drug interactions, or any other conditions where treatment is contraindicated or cautioned.

Monitoring: Monitor for respiratory depression (especially within first 24-72 hrs of initiation), hypotension, seizures/convulsions, and other adverse reactions. Monitor BP and serum amylase levels. Routinely monitor for signs of misuse, abuse, and addiction. Periodically reassess the continued need for therapy.

Patient Counseling: Inform that use of drug can result in addiction, abuse, and misuse; instruct not to share with others and to take steps to protect from theft or misuse. Inform patients about risk of respiratory depression. Advise to store securely and dispose unused tabs by flushing down the toilet. Inform female patients of reproductive potential that prolonged use during pregnancy may result in neonatal opioid withdrawal syndrome and instruct to inform physician if pregnant or planning to become pregnant. Inform that potentially serious additive effects may occur when used with CNS depressants, and not to use such drugs unless supervised by healthcare provider. Instruct about proper administration instructions. Inform that drug may cause orthostatic hypotension, syncope, impair the ability to perform potentially hazardous activities; advise to not perform such tasks until they know how they will react to medication. Advise of potential for severe constipation, including management instructions. Advise how to recognize anaphylaxis and when to seek medical attention.

Administration: Oral route. Swallow tab whole; do not crush, dissolve, or chew. Do not pre-soak, lick, or wet tab prior to placing in mouth. Take 1 tab at a time with enough water. **Storage:** 25°C (77°F); excursions permitted to 15-30°C (59-86°F).

OXYTROL   RX
oxybutynin (Watson)

THERAPEUTIC CLASS: Muscarinic antagonist

INDICATIONS: Treatment of overactive bladder with symptoms of urge urinary incontinence, urgency, and frequency.

DOSAGE: *Adults:* Apply one 3.9mg/day system to dry, intact skin on the abdomen, hip, or buttock twice weekly (every 3 or 4 days). Select a new application site with each new system to avoid reapplication to the same site within 7 days.

HOW SUPPLIED: Patch: 3.9mg/day [8s]

CONTRAINDICATIONS: Urinary retention, gastric retention, uncontrolled narrow-angle glaucoma.

WARNINGS/PRECAUTIONS: Caution with bladder outflow obstruction, GI obstructive disorders, gastroesophageal reflux disease (GERD), and myasthenia gravis. May decrease GI motility; caution with ulcerative colitis (UC) or intestinal atony. CNS anticholinergic effects reported; consider discontinuation if these occur. May impair mental/physical abilities. Angioedema may occur; d/c and provide appropriate therapy if this occurs. D/C if skin hypersensitivity develops.

ADVERSE REACTIONS: Application-site reactions (pruritus, erythema, vesicles, rash), dry mouth, diarrhea, constipation.

INTERACTIONS: Concomitant use with other anticholinergic drugs may increase the frequency and/or severity of dry mouth, constipation, somnolence, and/or other anticholinergic-like effects. May alter the absorption of other drugs due to anticholinergic effects on GI motility. Caution with drugs that can cause or exacerbate esophagitis (eg, bisphosphonates).

PREGNANCY: Category B, caution in nursing.

MECHANISM OF ACTION: Muscarinic antagonist; acts as a competitive antagonist of acetylcholine at postganglionic muscarinic receptors, resulting in relaxation of bladder smooth muscle.

PHARMACOKINETICS: Absorption: Administration of variable doses resulted in different parameters. **Distribution:** (IV) V_d=193L. **Metabolism:** Liver (extensive) via CYP3A4; N-desethyloxybutynin (active metabolite). **Elimination:** Urine (<0.1% unchanged, <0.1% N-desethyloxybutynin); $T_{1/2}$=7-8 hrs following patch removal.

NURSING CONSIDERATIONS

Assessment: Assess for urinary/gastric retention, uncontrolled narrow-angle glaucoma, bladder outflow obstruction, GI obstructive disorders, UC, intestinal atony, GERD, myasthenia gravis, pregnancy/nursing status, and possible drug interactions.

Monitoring: Monitor for urinary retention, gastric retention, anticholinergic CNS effects (particularly after beginning treatment), angioedema, skin hypersensitivity, exacerbation of symptoms of myasthenia gravis, and other adverse reactions.

Patient Counseling: Instruct to discard used patch in household trash in a manner that prevents accidental application or ingestion by children, pets, or others. Inform that drug may produce adverse reactions related to anticholinergic activity (eg, urinary retention, constipation, dizziness, blurred vision). Advise that heat prostration may occur when the drug is used in a hot environment. Instruct to avoid driving or operating heavy machinery until effects have been determined. Inform that drowsiness may be worsened by alcohol. Advise to promptly d/c therapy and seek immediate medical attention if symptoms consistent with angioedema occur.

Administration: Transdermal route. Apply immediately after removal from the protective pouch. **Storage:** 20-25°C (68-77°F). Protect from moisture and humidity. Do not store outside the sealed pouch.

PACLITAXEL   RX
paclitaxel (Various)

> Should be administered under supervision of a physician experienced in the use of cancer chemotherapeutic agents. Anaphylaxis and severe hypersensitivity reactions reported; pretreat with corticosteroids, diphenhydramine, and H_2 antagonists. Fatal reactions have occurred despite premedication. Do not rechallenge if severe hypersensitivity reaction occurs. Should not be given to patients with solid tumors having baseline neutrophil counts of <1500 cells/mm³ and with AIDS-related Kaposi's sarcoma having baseline neutrophil count of <1000 cells/mm³. Perform peripheral blood cell counts frequently to monitor occurrence of bone marrow suppression, primarily neutropenia.

THERAPEUTIC CLASS: Antimicrotubule agent

INDICATIONS: First-line (in combination with cisplatin) and subsequent therapy for the treatment of advanced ovarian carcinoma. Adjuvant treatment of node-positive breast cancer administered sequentially to standard doxorubicin-containing combination chemotherapy. Treatment of breast cancer after failure of combination chemotherapy for metastatic disease or relapse within 6 months of adjuvant chemotherapy. Second-line treatment of AIDS-related Kaposi's sarcoma. First-line treatment of non-small cell lung cancer (NSCLC) in combination with cisplatin in patients who are not candidates for potentially curative surgery and/or radiation therapy.

DOSAGE: *Adults:* Premedicate with dexamethasone (20mg PO 12 and 6 hrs before inj), diphehy-dramine or its equivalent (50mg IV 30-60 min prior to inj), and cimetidine (300mg) or ranitidine (50mg) IV 30-60 min before inj. Ovarian Carcinoma: Previously Untreated: 175mg/m^2 IV over 3 hrs or 135mg/m^2 IV over 24 hrs every 3 weeks followed by cisplatin 75mg/m^2. Previously Treated: Usual: 135mg/m^2 IV or 175mg/m^2 IV over 3 hrs every 3 weeks. Breast Cancer: Adjuvant Therapy: Usual: 175mg/m^2 IV over 3 hrs every 3 weeks for 4 courses given sequentially to doxorubicin-containing combination chemotherapy. Failure of Initial Chemotherapy for Metastatic Disease or Relapse within 6 Months of Chemotherapy: 175mg/m^2 IV over 3 hrs every 3 weeks. NSCLC: Usual: 135mg/m^2 IV over 24 hrs every 3 weeks followed by cisplatin 75mg/m^2. Kaposi's Sarcoma: Usual: 135mg/m^2 IV over 3 hrs every 3 weeks or 100mg/m^2 IV over 3 hrs every 2 weeks. Reduce dose by 20% for subsequent courses of paclitaxel inj in patients who experience severe neutropenia (neutrophils <500 cells/mm^3 for a week or longer) or severe peripheral neuropathy. Refer to PI for dosing in patients with hepatic impairment and modifications in patients with advanced HIV disease.

HOW SUPPLIED: Inj: 30mg/5mL, 100mg/16.7mL, 150mg/25mL, 300mg/50mL

CONTRAINDICATIONS: Hypersensitivity to drugs formulated in polyoxyl 35 castor oil, NF; solid tumor patients with baseline neutrophils <1500 cells/mm^3, or AIDS-related Kaposi's sarcoma patients with baseline neutrophils <1000 cells/mm^3.

WARNINGS/PRECAUTIONS: Severe conduction abnormalities reported; administer appropriate therapy and perform continuous cardiac monitoring during subsequent therapy. May cause fetal harm during pregnancy. Hypotension, bradycardia, and HTN reported. Contains dehydrated alcohol; CNS and other alcohol effects may occur. Caution in patients with bilirubin >2X ULN and in elderly. Inj-site reactions and peripheral neuropathy reported.

ADVERSE REACTIONS: Anaphylaxis, bone marrow suppression, neutropenia, infections, bleeding, abnormal ECG, hypotension, peripheral neuropathy, myalgia/arthralgia, N/V, diarrhea, alopecia, inj-site reactions.

INTERACTIONS: Myelosuppression more profound when given after cisplatin than with the alternate sequence. Caution with CYP3A4 substrates (eg, midazolam, buspirone, felodipine), inducers (eg, rifampicin, carbamazepine), and inhibitors (eg, atazanavir, clarithromycin, ketoconazole). Caution with CYP2C8 substrates (eg, repaglinide, rosiglitazone), inhibitors (eg, gemfibrozil), and inducers (eg, rifampin). May increase doxorubicin levels.

PREGNANCY: Category D, not for use in nursing.

MECHANISM OF ACTION: Antimicrotubule agent; promotes assembly of microtubules from tubulin dimers and stabilizes microtubules by preventing depolymerization and induces abnormal arrays or bundles of microtubules throughout the cell cycle and multiple asters of microtubules during mitosis.

PHARMACOKINETICS: Absorption: IV administration of multiple doses resulted in different parameters. **Distribution:** V_d=227-688L/m^2; plasma protein binding (89-98%). **Metabolism:** Liver via CYP2C8 (major), CYP3A4 (minor). 6α-hydroxypaclitaxel (major metabolite); 3'-*p*-hydroxy-paclitaxel and 6α, 3'-*p*-dihydroxypaclitaxel (minor metabolites). **Elimination:** Urine (1.3-12.6% unchanged), feces (71%, 5% unchanged).

NURSING CONSIDERATIONS

Assessment: Assess for hypersensitivity (polyoxyl 35 castor oil, NF), hepatic impairment, bilirubin levels, pregnancy/nursing status, and possible drug interactions. Assess for baseline neutrophil count in patients with solid tumors or with Kaposi's sarcoma.

Monitoring: Monitor for signs/symptoms of anaphylaxis/hypersensitivity reactions, inj-site reactions, myelosuppression, toxicity, and other adverse reactions. Monitor blood count frequently and vital signs frequently during 1st hr of infusion. Monitor cardiac function in patients with serious conduction abnormalities and when used in combination with doxorubicin.

Patient Counseling: Inform about risks and benefits of therapy. Advise that drug may cause fetal harm; advise women of childbearing potential to avoid becoming pregnant. Advise to report to healthcare provider for any signs of an allergic reaction or signs of infection. Advise to inform physician of liver/heart problems and breastfeeding status or plans to breastfeed.

Administration: IV route. Refer to PI for preparation and administration procedures. **Storage:** Undiluted: 20-25°C (68-77°F). Retain in the original package to protect from light. Diluted Sol: Ambient temperature approximately 25°C (77°F) and room lighting conditions for up to 27 hrs.

PAMELOR

RX

nortriptyline HCl (Mallinckrodt)

Antidepressants increased the risk of suicidal thinking and behavior (suicidality) in short-term studies in children, adolescents, and young adults with major depressive disorder (MDD) and other psychiatric disorders. Monitor and observe closely for clinical worsening, suicidality, or unusual changes in behavior in patients who are started on antidepressant therapy. Nortriptyline is not approved for use in pediatric patients.

THERAPEUTIC CLASS: Tricyclic antidepressant

INDICATIONS: Relief of symptoms of depression.

DOSAGE: *Adults:* 25mg tid-qid. Max: 150mg/day. Total daily dose may be given once a day. Monitor serum levels if dose >100mg/day. Elderly/Adolescents: 30-50mg/day in single or divided doses.

HOW SUPPLIED: Cap: 10mg, 25mg, 50mg, 75mg; Sol: 10mg/5mL

CONTRAINDICATIONS: MAOI use within 14 days, acute recovery period following myocardial infarction (MI).

WARNINGS/PRECAUTIONS: MI, arrhythmia, and strokes have occurred. Caution with cardiovascular disease (CVD), glaucoma, history of urinary retention, and hyperthyroidism. May lower seizure threshold, exacerbate psychosis or activate schizophrenia, cause symptoms of mania in bipolar disease, or alter glucose levels. D/C several days prior to elective surgery.

ADVERSE REACTIONS: Arrhythmias, hypotension, HTN, tachycardia, MI, heart block, stroke, confusion, hallucination, insomnia, tremors, ataxia, dry mouth, blurred vision, skin rash.

INTERACTIONS: See Contraindications. May block guanethidine effects. Arrhythmia risk with thyroid agents. Alcohol may potentiate effects. "Stimulating" effect with reserpine. Monitor with anticholinergic and sympathomimetic drugs. Increased plasma levels with cimetidine. Hypoglycemia reported with chlorpropamide. SSRIs, antidepressants, phenothiazines, propafenone, flecainide, and CYP2D6 inhibitors (eg, quinidine) may potentiate effects. Decreased clearance with quinidine.

PREGNANCY: Safety during pregnancy and nursing not known.

MECHANISM OF ACTION: Tricyclic antidepressant; inhibits activity of histamine, 5-hydroxytryptamine, and acetylcholine; increases pressor effect of norepinephrine, blocks pressor response of phenethylamine, and interferes with transport, release, and storage of catecholamine.

NURSING CONSIDERATIONS

Assessment: Assess for acute recovery period after MI, bipolar disorder risk, history of mania, unrecognized/history of schizophrenia, possible drug interactions, history of seizures, CVD, hyperthyroidism, diabetes mellitus, glaucoma, urinary retention, history of agitation or overactivity, and pregnancy/nursing status.

Monitoring: Periodically monitor blood glucose. Monitor for signs/symptoms of clinical worsening, mania, cardiovascular events, increasing psychosis, increasing anxiety/agitation, mydriasis, hypo/hyperglycemia, seizures, cognitive/motor impairment.

Patient Counseling: Advise to avoid alcohol. Instruct to seek medical attention for symptoms of activation of mania, seizures, clinical worsening, cardiovascular events, increasing psychosis, increasing anxiety/agitation, mydriasis, and hypo- or hyperglycemia. Inform that physical/mental abilities may be impaired.

Administration: Oral route. **Storage:** 20-25°C (68-77°F).

PANCREAZE

RX

pancrelipase (Janssen)

THERAPEUTIC CLASS: Pancreatic enzyme supplement

INDICATIONS: Treatment of exocrine pancreatic insufficiency due to cystic fibrosis or other conditions.

DOSAGE: *Adults:* Individualize dose based on clinical symptoms, degree of steatorrhea present, and fat content of diet. Start at the lowest recommended dose and increase gradually. Initial: 500 lipase U/kg/meal. Max: 2500 lipase U/kg/meal (or ≤10,000 lipase U/kg/day) or <4000 lipase U/g fat ingested/day. Half of the dose used for meals should be given with each snack. Reduce dose in older patients. Refer to PI for the dosing limitations.

Pediatrics: Individualize dose based on clinical symptoms, degree of steatorrhea present, and fat content of diet. Start at the lowest recommended dose and increase gradually. ≥4 Yrs: Initial: 500 lipase U/kg/meal. Max: 2500 lipase U/kg/meal (or ≤10,000 lipase U/kg/day) or <4000 lipase U/g fat ingested/day. Half of the dose used for meals should be given with each snack. >12 Months-<4 Yrs: Initial: 1000 lipase U/kg/meal. Max: 2500 lipase U/kg/meal (or ≤10,000 lipase U/kg/day) or <4000 lipase U/g fat ingested/day. ≤12 Months: May give 2000-4000 lipase U/120mL of formula or per breastfeeding. Refer to PI for the dosing limitations.

HOW SUPPLIED: Cap, Delayed-Release: (Lipase-Protease-Amylase) 4200 U-10,000 U-17,500 U; 10,500 U-25,000 U-43,750 U; 16,800 U-40,000 U-70,000 U; 21,000 U-37,000 U-61,000 U

WARNINGS/PRECAUTIONS: Not interchangeable with other pancrelipase products. Fibrosing colonopathy reported; monitor closely for progression to stricture formation. Caution with doses >2500 lipase U/kg/meal (or >10,000 lipase U/kg/day); use only if these doses are documented to be effective by 3-day fecal fat measures indicating significant improvement. Examine patients receiving >6000 lipase U/kg/meal; immediately decrease dose or titrate dose downward to a lower range. Ensure that no drug is retained in the mouth. If mixed with soft food, swallow mixture immediately and follow with water or juice to ensure complete ingestion. Do not crush or chew or mix in foods with pH >4.5; may disrupt enteric coating of cap, resulting in early release of enzymes, irritation of oral mucosa, and/or loss of enzyme activity. Caution in patients with gout, renal impairment, or hyperuricemia; may increase blood uric acid levels. Risk for transmission of viral diseases. Caution with known allergy to proteins of porcine origin; severe allergic reactions reported.

ADVERSE REACTIONS: Abdominal pain, flatulence, diarrhea.

PREGNANCY: Category C, caution in nursing.

MECHANISM OF ACTION: Pancreatic enzyme supplement; catalyzes the hydrolysis of fats to monoglyceride, glycerol, and free fatty acids, proteins into peptides and amino acids, and starches into dextrins and short chain sugars (eg, maltose, maltriose) in the duodenum and proximal small intestine, thereby acting like digestive enzymes physiologically secreted by the pancreas.

NURSING CONSIDERATIONS

Assessment: Assess for known allergy to porcine proteins, gout, renal impairment, hyperuricemia, and pregnancy/nursing status.

Monitoring: Monitor for fibrosing colonopathy, stricture formation, oral mucosa irritation, viral diseases, allergic reactions, and other adverse reactions. Monitor serum uric acid levels.

Patient Counseling: Instruct to take ud with food and sufficient fluids. Inform that if a dose is missed, take the next dose with the next meal/snack ud; instruct not to double dose. Inform that cap contents can be sprinkled on soft acidic foods (eg, applesauce), if necessary. Instruct to notify physician if pregnant/breastfeeding or planning to become pregnant/breastfeed during therapy. Inform that doses >6000 lipase U/kg/meal have been associated with colonic strictures in children <12 yrs of age. Advise to contact physician immediately if allergic reactions develop.

Administration: Oral route. Take during meals or snacks, with sufficient fluid. Swallow whole; do not crush or chew caps/cap contents. Do not retain in mouth. Do not mix directly into formula or breastmilk. Refer to PI for proper administration instructions. **Storage:** ≤25°C (77°F). Avoid heat. Protect from moisture. Store in original container.

PARCOPA   RX
levodopa - carbidopa (Jazz)

THERAPEUTIC CLASS: Dopa-decarboxylase inhibitor/dopamine precursor

INDICATIONS: Treatment of symptoms of idiopathic Parkinson's disease (paralysis agitans), postencephalitic parkinsonism, and symptomatic parkinsonism.

DOSAGE: *Adults:* Individualize dose. Determine dose by careful titration. Available in a 1:4 ratio of carbidopa to levodopa (25/100) and a 1:10 ratio (25/250, 10/100); tabs of the 2 ratios may be given separately or combined PRN to provide optimum dosage. (25mg-100mg) Initial: 1 tab tid. Titrate: May increase by 1 tab qd or qod, as necessary, until 8 tabs/day is reached. (10mg-100mg) Initial: 1 tab tid-qid. Titrate: May increase by 1 tab qd or qod until 8 tabs/day (2 tabs qid) is reached. Transfer from Levodopa: D/C at least 12 hrs before starting therapy. Daily dosage should be chosen that will provide approximately 25% of previous levodopa dosage. Previously Taking <1500mg/day of Levodopa: Initial: 1 tab (25mg-100mg) tid or qid. Previously Taking >1500mg/day of Levodopa: Initial: 1 tab (25mg-250mg) tid or qid. Maint: 70-100mg/day of carbidopa should be provided. May substitute 1 tab of 25mg-100mg for each 10mg-100mg when greater proportion of carbidopa is required. When more levodopa is required, substitute 25mg-250mg for 25mg-100mg or 10mg-100mg. May increase dosage of 25mg-250mg by 1/2 or 1 tab qd or qod to a max of 8 tabs/day if necessary. Max: 200mg/day of carbidopa. Refer to PI for information on the addition of other antiparkinsonian medications and interruption of therapy.

HOW SUPPLIED: Tab, Disintegrating: (Carbidopa-Levodopa) 10mg-100mg*, 25mg-100mg*, 25mg-250mg* *scored

CONTRAINDICATIONS: During or within 2 weeks of using nonselective MAOIs; narrow-angle glaucoma; suspicious, undiagnosed skin lesions, or history of melanoma.

WARNINGS/PRECAUTIONS: Dyskinesias may occur; may require dose reduction. May cause mental disturbances; monitor for depression with concomitant suicidal tendencies. Caution with past or current psychoses, severe cardiovascular (CV) or pulmonary disease, bronchial asthma, renal/hepatic/endocrine disease, or chronic wide-angle glaucoma. Caution with history of myocardial infarction (MI) with residual atrial, nodal, or ventricular arrhythmias; monitor cardiac function with particular care during the period of initial dosage adjustment, in a facility with provisions for intensive cardiac care. May increase possibility of upper GI hemorrhage in patients with a history of peptic ulcer. Sporadic cases of a symptom complex resembling neuroleptic malignant syndrome (NMS) reported during dose reduction or withdrawal. Periodically evaluate hepatic, hematopoietic, CV, and renal function if on extended therapy. May be associated with somnolence and very rarely episodes of sudden onset of sleep; may impair physical/mental abilities. Monitor for melanomas frequently and on a regular basis. Abnormalities in lab tests may include elevations of LFTs (eg, alkaline phosphatase, AST, ALT, lactic dehydrogenase, bilirubin) and abnormalities in BUN and positive Coombs test, reported. May cause lab test interactions. Cases of falsely diagnosed pheochromocytoma reported very rarely; caution when interpreting the plasma and urine levels of catecholamines and their metabolites.

ADVERSE REACTIONS: Dyskinesias (eg, choreiform, dystonic, other involuntary movements), nausea.

INTERACTIONS: See Contraindications. Symptomatic postural hypotension reported with concomitant use of antihypertensives drugs; dosage adjustment of the antihypertensive drug may be required. Use with selegiline may cause severe orthostatic hypotension. HTN and dyskinesia may occur with TCAs. May reduce effects of levodopa when use concomitantly with dopamine D_2 receptor antagonists (eg, phenothiazines, butyrophenones, risperidone), and isoniazid. Beneficial effects of levodopa in Parkinson's disease reported to be reversed by phenytoin and papaverine; monitor for loss of therapeutic response. Iron salts may reduce the bioavailability of levodopa and carbidopa. Metoclopramide may increase the bioavailability of levodopa and may also adversely affect disease control.

PREGNANCY: Category C, caution in nursing.

MECHANISM OF ACTION: Dopa-decarboxylase inhibitor/dopamine precursor. Carbidopa: Inhibits decarboxylation of peripheral levodopa. Levodopa: Crosses blood-brain barrier and presumably converted to dopamine in the brain.

PHARMACOKINETICS: Absorption: Carbidopa: Bioavailability (99%). **Elimination:** Urine.

NURSING CONSIDERATIONS

Assessment: Assess for narrow-angle/chronic wide-angle glaucoma; suspicious/undiagnosed skin lesions or history of melanoma; presence of or history of psychoses; history of peptic ulcer; severe CV or pulmonary disease; bronchial asthma; hepatic, renal, or endocrine disease; history of MI with residual atrial, nodal, or ventricular arrhythmias; pregnancy/nursing status; and possible drug interactions.

Monitoring: Monitor for dyskinesias, mental disturbances, depression with suicidal tendencies, somnolence, NMS, upper GI hemorrhage in patients with a history of peptic ulcer, and other adverse reactions. Monitor cardiac function in patients with a history of MI who have residual atrial, nodal, or ventricular arrhythmias. Monitor for LFT elevations and BUN abnormalities. For patients on extended therapy, perform periodic evaluation of hepatic, hematopoetic, CV, and renal function. Monitor for melanomas frequently and on a regular basis. Monitor for changes in intraocular pressure in patients with chronic wide-angle glaucoma. Monitor closely during the dose adjustment period.

Patient Counseling: Inform phenylketonuric patients that drug contains phenylalanine. Instruct not to remove tabs from the bottle until just prior to dosing. Instruct to gently remove the tab from the bottle with dry hands and to immediately place the tab on top of the tongue to dissolve and be swallowed with saliva. Inform that therapy is an immediate-release formulation designed to begin release of ingredients within 30 min. Advise to take at regular intervals according to the schedule outlined by the physician. Instruct to cautioned not to change the prescribed dosage regimen and not to add any additional antiparkinson medications, including other carbidopa and levodopa preparations, without consulting the physician. Advise that sometimes a "wearing-off" effect may occur at the end of the dosing interval; notify physician if such response poses a problem to lifestyle. Advise that occasionally, dark color (red, brown, or black) may appear in saliva, urine, or sweat after ingestion of therapy. Inform that high protein diet, excessive acidity, and iron salts may reduce clinical effectiveness. Advise to exercise caution while driving or operating machinery; instruct to refrain from these activities if have experienced somnolence and/or sudden sleep onset. Instruct to inform physician if new or increase gambling urges, or sexual or other intense urges develop.

Administration: Oral route. Refer to PI for use/handling instructions. **Storage:** 20-25°C (68-77°F); excursions permitted to 15-30°C (59-86°F). Protect from moisture and light.

PARLODEL   RX
bromocriptine mesylate (Validus)

THERAPEUTIC CLASS: Dopamine receptor agonist

INDICATIONS: Treatment of dysfunctions associated with hyperprolactinemia, including amenorrhea with or without galactorrhea, infertility, or hypogonadism. Treatment of prolactin-secreting adenomas, acromegaly, and signs and symptoms of idiopathic or postencephalitic Parkinson's disease.

DOSAGE: *Adults:* Take with food. Hyperprolactinemia: Initial: 1/2-1 tab qd. Titrate: May add 1 tab (2.5mg) every 2-7 days. Usual: 2.5-15mg/day. Acromegaly: Initial: 1/2-1 tab before hs for 3 days. Titrate: May add 1/2-1 tab every 3-7 days. Reevaluate monthly and adjust dose based on reductions of growth hormone or clinical response. Usual: 20-30mg/day. Max: 100mg/day. Withdraw for 4-8 weeks on a yearly basis if being treated with pituitary irradiation. Parkinson's Disease: Maintain levodopa dose during introductory period, if possible. Initial: 1/2 tab bid. Titrate: May increase every 14-28 days by 2.5mg/day. If levodopa dose has to be reduced because of adverse reactions, increase the daily dose of bromocriptine gradually in small (2.5mg) increments. Max: 100mg/day. Elderly: Start at lower end of dosing range.
Pediatrics: Take with food. Prolactin-Secreting Adenoma: ≥16 Yrs: Initial: 1/2-1 tab qd. Titrate: May add 1 tab (2.5mg) every 2-7 days. Usual: 2.5-15mg/day. 11-15 Yrs: Initial: 1/2-1 tab qd. Titrate: May be increased as tolerated. Usual: 2.5-10mg/day.

HOW SUPPLIED: Cap: 5mg; Tab: 2.5mg* *scored

CONTRAINDICATIONS: Uncontrolled HTN, postpartum period in women with history of coronary artery disease (CAD) and other severe cardiovascular (CV) conditions unless withdrawal is medically contraindicated, pregnancy if treating hyperprolactinemia. Hypertensive disorders of pregnancy (eg, eclampsia, preeclampsia, or pregnancy-induced HTN) if used to treat acromegaly, prolactinoma, or Parkinson's disease, unless withdrawal is medically contraindicated.

WARNINGS/PRECAUTIONS: Perform complete evaluation of the pituitary before treatment. Safety during pregnancy not established; use contraceptive measures, other than oral contraceptives, during treatment. D/C treatment if patient becomes pregnant. Somnolence and episodes of sudden sleep onset may occur, particularly to patients with Parkinson's disease; consider dose reduction or termination of therapy. May impair physical/mental abilities. Symptomatic hypotension may occur. HTN, myocardial infarction (MI), seizures, and stroke reported (rare) in postpartum women; not recommended for prevention of physiological lactation. D/C and evaluate promptly if HTN, severe, progressive or unremitting headache (with or without visual disturbance), or evidence of CNS toxicity develops. Pleural and pericardial effusions, pleural and pulmonary fibrosis, constrictive pericarditis, and retroperitoneal fibrosis reported, particularly on long-term and high-dose treatment; consider discontinuation of therapy. Caution with history of psychosis or CV disease. Avoid with hereditary problems of galactose intolerance, severe lactase deficiency, or glucose-galactose malabsorption. Visual field deterioration may develop; consider dose reduction in patients with macroprolactinoma. CSF rhinorrhea reported in patients with prolactin-secreting adenomas. Cold-sensitive digital vasospasm and possible tumor expansion reported in acromegalic patients; d/c therapy and consider alternative procedures if tumor expansion develops. Severe GI bleeding in patients with peptic ulcers reported. Safety during long-term use (>2 yrs) for Parkinson's disease not established. May cause confusion and mental disturbances with high doses; caution with mild degrees of dementia. May cause hallucinations (visual or auditory) with or without concomitant levodopa; dosage reduction or discontinuation of therapy may be required. May cause intense urges to gamble, increased sexual urges, intense urges to spend money uncontrollably, and other intense urges; consider dose reduction or d/c therapy. Caution with history of MI with residual atrial, nodal, or ventricular arrhythmia. Regularly monitor for melanomas. Symptom complex resembling the neuroleptic malignant syndrome (NMS) reported with rapid dose reduction, withdrawal of, or changes in antiparkinsonian therapy. Caution with renal/liver impairment and in elderly.

ADVERSE REACTIONS: Confusion, hallucinations, headache, drowsiness, visual disturbance, hypotension, nasal congestion, N/V, dizziness, constipation, anorexia, dry mouth, indigestion/dyspepsia, fatigue, lightheadedness.

INTERACTIONS: Not recommended with other ergot alkaloids. May potentiate side effects with alcohol. May interact with dopamine antagonists, butyrophenones, and certain other agents. May decrease efficacy with phenothiazines, haloperidol, metoclopramide, and pimozide. Caution with strong CYP3A4 inhibitors (eg, azole antimycotics, HIV protease inhibitors). Increased plasma levels with macrolide antibiotics (eg, erythromycin) and octreotide. Caution in patients recently treated or on concomitant therapy with drugs that can alter BP; concomitant use in puerperium is not recommended.

PREGNANCY: Category B, not for use in nursing.

MECHANISM OF ACTION: Dopamine receptor agonist; activates postsynaptic dopamine receptors and modulates the secretion of prolactin from the anterior pituitary by secreting a prolactin inhibitory factor.

PHARMACOKINETICS: Absorption: (Healthy) C_{max} =465pg/mL (fasted, 2 x 2.5mg), 628pg/mL (5mg bid); AUC=2377pg•hr/mL; T_{max}=2.5 hrs. **Distribution:** Plasma protein binding (90-96%). **Metabolism:** Liver (extensive); via CYP3A and hydroxylation. **Elimination:** Feces (82%), urine (5.6%); $T_{1/2}$=4.85 hrs.

NURSING CONSIDERATIONS

Assessment: Assess for previous hypersensitivity to ergot alkaloids, uncontrolled HTN, history of CAD or other severe CV conditions, pituitary tumors, dementia, history of psychosis, unexplained pleuropulmonary disorders, history of peptic ulcer or GI bleeding, hereditary problems of galactose intolerance, severe lactase deficiency or glucose-galactose malabsorption, macroadenomas, renal/hepatic disease, pregnancy/nursing status, and possible drug interactions. Perform complete pituitary evaluation.

Monitoring: Monitor for GI bleeding, somnolence, episodes of sudden sleep onset, seizures, stroke, MI, pleural and pericardial effusions, pleural and pulmonary fibrosis, constrictive pericarditis, retroperitoneal fibrosis, cold sensitive digital vasospasm, peptic ulcers, enlargement of a previously undetected or existing prolactin-secreting tumor, symptom complex resembling NMS, confusion and mental disturbances, and other adverse reactions. Monitor prolactin levels. Monitor visual fields in patients with macroprolactinoma; rapidly progressive visual field loss should be evaluated by a neurosurgeon. Periodically evaluate hepatic, hematopoietic, CV, and renal function. Periodic monitoring of BP, particularly during 1st weeks of therapy is prudent. Perform pregnancy test at least every 4 weeks during amenorrhea, and for every missed menstrual period once menses are reinitiated. Periodic skin exam should be performed by qualified individuals (eg, dermatologist).

Patient Counseling: Inform that dizziness, drowsiness, faintness, fainting, and syncope may occur during treatment. Advise that somnolence and episodes of sudden sleep onset may occur and instruct not to engage in activities requiring rapid and precise responses. Instruct patients with hyperprolactinemic states associated with macroadenoma or those who have had previous transsphenoidal surgery to report any persistent watery nasal discharge. Inform patients with macroadenoma that discontinuation of therapy may be associated with rapid regrowth of tumor and recurrence of their original symptoms. Advise of the possibility that patients may experience intense urges to spend money uncontrollably, intense urges to gamble, increased sexual urges, and the inability to control these urges while on therapy. Inform that hypotensive reactions may occasionally occur and result in reduced alertness.

Administration: Oral route. Take with food. **Storage:** <25°C (77°F).

PATANOL
olopatadine HCl (Alcon)

RX

THERAPEUTIC CLASS: H_1-antagonist and mast cell stabilizer

INDICATIONS: Allergic conjunctivitis.

DOSAGE: *Adults:* 1 drop bid, q6-8h.
Pediatrics: ≥3 Yrs: 1 drop bid, q6-8h.

HOW SUPPLIED: Sol: 0.1% [5mL]

WARNINGS/PRECAUTIONS: May reinsert contact lens 10 min after dosing if eye is not red. Not for injection or oral use.

ADVERSE REACTIONS: Headache, asthenia, blurred vision, burning, stinging, cold syndrome, dry eye, foreign body sensation, hyperemia, hypersensitivity, keratitis, lid edema, nausea, pharyngitis, pruritus, rhinitis.

PREGNANCY: Category C, caution in nursing.

MECHANISM OF ACTION: Antihistaminic drug; relatively selective histamine H_1-antagonist; inhibits the type 1 immediate hypersensitivity reaction, including inhibition of histamine induced effects on human conjunctival epithelial cells.

PHARMACOKINETICS: Absorption: C_{max}=0.5-1.3ng/mL; T_{max}=2 hrs. **Metabolism:** Metabolites: Mono-desmethyl and N-oxide. **Elimination:** Urine (60-70% parent drug).

NURSING CONSIDERATIONS

Assessment: Assess for drug hypersensitivity.

Monitoring: Monitor for headache and other adverse reactions.

Patient Counseling: Counsel not to wear contact lenses if eye is red; wait at least 10 min after instillation to wear contact lenses. Instruct to avoid touching tip of container to eye or any other surface to avoid contamination.

Administration: Ocular route. **Storage:** 4-25°C (39-77°F). Keep bottle tightly closed.

PAXIL   RX
paroxetine HCl (GlaxoSmithKline)

> Antidepressants increased the risk of suicidal thinking and behavior (suicidality) in short-term studies in children, adolescents, and young adults with major depressive disorder (MDD) and other psychiatric disorders. Monitor and observe closely for clinical worsening, suicidality, or unusual changes in behavior in patients who are started on antidepressant therapy. Not approved for use in pediatric patients.

THERAPEUTIC CLASS: Selective serotonin reuptake inhibitor

INDICATIONS: Treatment of MDD, panic disorder with or without agoraphobia, obsessive compulsive disorder (OCD), social anxiety disorder (SAD), generalized anxiety disorder (GAD), and post-traumatic stress disorder (PTSD).

DOSAGE: *Adults:* Give qd, usually in the am. To titrate, may increase in 10mg/day increments at intervals of ≥1 week. Maintain on lowest effective dose. MDD: Initial: 20mg/day. Max: 50mg/day. Maint: Efficacy is maintained for periods of up to 1 year with doses that averaged about 30mg. OCD: Initial: 20mg/day. Usual: 40mg qd. Max: 60mg/day. Panic Disorder: Initial: 10mg/day. Usual: 40mg/day. Max: 60mg/day. GAD: Initial/Usual: 20mg/day. Dose Range: 20-50mg/day. SAD: Initial/Usual: 20mg/day. Dose Range: 20-60mg/day; no additional benefiit for doses >20mg/day. PTSD: Initial: 20mg/day. Dose Range: 20-50mg/day. Elderly/Debilitated/Severe Renal/Hepatic Impairment: Initial: 10mg/day. Max: 40mg/day. 3rd Trimester Pregnancy: Taper dose. Allow ≥14-day interval between discontinuation of an MAOI and start of paroxetine and vice versa. Use with Reversible MAOIs (eg, linezolid, methylene blue) and Discontinuation of Treatment: Refer to PI.

HOW SUPPLIED: Sus: 10mg/5mL [250mL]; Tab: 10mg*, 20mg*, 30mg, 40mg *scored

CONTRAINDICATIONS: Use with MAOIs intended to treat depression with, or within 14 days of treatment. Do not start treatment in patients being treated with a reversible MAOI (eg, linezolid, methylene blue). Concomitant use with thioridazine or pimozide.

WARNINGS/PRECAUTIONS: Not approved for treatment of bipolar depression. Serotonin syndrome or neuroleptic malignant syndrome (NMS)-like reactions reported. Increased risk of congenital malformations reported in 1st trimester of pregnancy. Neonatal complications requiring prolonged hospitalization, respiratory support, and tube feeding may develop in neonates exposed in the late 3rd trimester. Activation of mania/hypomania reported. Caution with history of seizures; d/c if seizures occur. Adverse reactions (eg, dysphoric mood, irritability) upon discontinuation reported; avoid abrupt withdrawal. Akathisia may develop. Hyponatremia reported; caution in elderly and volume-depleted patients. May increase risk of bleeding events. Bone fracture risk reported; consider pathological fracture in patients with unexplained bone pain, point tenderness, swelling, or bruising. Caution with disease/conditions that could affect metabolism or hemodynamic responses, narrow-angle glaucoma, severe renal/hepatic impairment, and in elderly and debilitated patients. May impair mental/physical abilities.

ADVERSE REACTIONS: Suicidality, somnolence, headache, insomnia, nausea, asthenia, abnormal ejaculation, dry mouth, constipation, dizziness, diarrhea, decreased libido, sweating, decreased appetite, tremor.

INTERACTIONS: See Contraindications. Serotonin syndrome or NMS-like reactions reported when used alone and in combination with serotonergic drugs (eg, triptans, fentanyl, St. John's wort), drugs that impair serotonin metabolism, antipsychotics, and dopamine antagonists. Use with other SSRIs, SNRIs, or tryptophan is not recommended. Avoid alcohol. Concomitant use with aspirin (ASA), NSAIDs, warfarin, and other anticoagulants may increase risk of bleeding events. Use with diuretics may increase risk of developing hyponatremia. Metabolism and pharmacokinetics of paroxetine may be affected by induction or inhibition of drug-metabolizing enzymes. Increased levels with cimetidine. Reduced levels with phenobarbital, phenytoin, and fosamprenavir/ritonavir. Increased phenytoin level after 4 weeks of coadministration. Caution with drugs that are metabolized by CYP2D6 (eg, phenothiazines, risperidone, type 1C antiarrhythmics) and with drugs that inhibit CYP2D6 (eg, quinidine). May increase levels of desipramine, risperidone, and atomoxetine. May reduce efficacy of tamoxifen. May inhibit metabolism of TCAs. May displace other highly protein-bound drugs. Decreased levels of digoxin seen. May increase procyclidine levels; reduce dose if anticholinergic effects are seen. Severe hypotension reported when added to chronic metoprolol treatment. May elevate theophylline levels. Caution with lithium. May decrease phenytoin levels.

PREGNANCY: Category D, caution in nursing.

MECHANISM OF ACTION: SSRI; inhibits CNS neuronal reuptake of serotonin.

PHARMACOKINETICS: Absorption: Complete; Tab (30mg): C_{max}=61.7ng/mL; T_{max}=5.2 hrs. **Distribution:** Plasma protein binding (93-95%); found in breast milk. **Metabolism:** Extensive; oxidation and methylation via CYP2D6. **Elimination:** Sol (30 mg): Urine (62%, metabolites; 2%, parent compound); feces (36%, metabolites; <1%, parent compound); Tab (30 mg): $T_{1/2}$=21 hrs.

NURSING CONSIDERATIONS

Assessment: Assess for history of seizures or mania, volume depletion, diseases/conditions that alter metabolism or hemodynamic responses, hepatic/renal impairment, narrow-angle glaucoma, previous hypersensitivity, pregnancy/nursing status, and for possible drug interactions. Assess use in the elderly or debilitated patients. Screen for bipolar disorder.

Monitoring: Monitor for signs/symptoms of clinical worsening, serotonin syndrome or NMS-like reactions, seizures, manic episodes, akathisia, bone fracture, hyponatremia especially in the elderly, and abnormal bleeding. Upon discontinuation, monitor for symptoms. Periodically reassess need for continued therapy. Regularly monitor weight and growth of children and adolescents.

Patient Counseling: Instruct to swallow whole, not to chew or crush, and to avoid alcohol. Instruct to notify physician of all prescription or OTC drugs currently taking or planning to take. Caution on risk of serotonin syndrome with concomitant use of triptans, tramadol, or other serotonergic agents. Instruct patient, families, and caregivers to report emergence of anxiety, agitation, panic attacks, insomnia, irritability, hostility, aggressiveness, impulsivity, akathisia, hypomania, mania, unusual changes in behavior, worsening of depression, and suicidal ideation, especially during drug initiation or dose adjustment. Caution against hazardous tasks. Inform that improvement may be noticed in 1-4 weeks; instruct to continue therapy ud. Instruct to notify physician if pregnant/intend to become pregnant, or breastfeeding. Caution about concomitant use with NSAIDs, ASA, warfarin, or other drugs that affect coagulation.

Administration: Oral route. (Sus) Shake well before use. **Storage:** (Tab): 15-30°C (59-86°F). (Sus): ≤25°C (77°F).

PAXIL CR

RX

paroxetine HCl (GlaxoSmithKline)

> Antidepressants increased the risk of suicidal thinking and behavior (suicidality) in short-term studies in children, adolescents, and young adults with major depressive disorder (MDD) and other psychiatric disorders. Monitor and observe closely for clinical worsening, suicidality, or unusual changes in behavior in patients who are started on antidepressant therapy. Not approved for use in pediatric patients.

THERAPEUTIC CLASS: Selective serotonin reuptake inhibitor

INDICATIONS: Treatment of MDD, panic disorder with or without agoraphobia, social anxiety disorder (SAD), and premenstrual dysphoric disorder (PMDD).

DOSAGE: *Adults:* Give qd, usually in the am with/without food. MDD: Initial: 25mg/day. Titrate: May increase by 12.5mg/day at intervals of ≥1 week. Max: 62.5mg/day. Panic Disorder: Initial: 12.5mg/day. Titrate: May increase by 12.5mg/day at intervals of ≥1 week. Max: 75mg/day. SAD: Initial: 12.5mg/day. Titrate: May increase by 12.5mg/day at intervals of ≥1 week. Max: 37.5mg/day. PMDD: Initial: 12.5mg/day. Give either qd throughout menstrual cycle or limit to luteal phase. 25mg/day also shown to be effective. Titrate: Changes should occur at intervals of ≥1 week. Elderly/Debilitated/Severe Renal/Hepatic Impairment: Initial: 12.5mg/day. Max: 50mg/day. 3rd Trimester Pregnancy: Taper dose. Allow ≥14-day interval between discontinuation of an MAOI and start of paroxetine and vice versa. Use with Reversible MAOIs (eg, linezolid, methylene blue) and Discontinuation of Treatment: Refer to PI.

HOW SUPPLIED: Tab, Controlled-Release: 12.5mg, 25mg, 37.5mg

CONTRAINDICATIONS: Use with MAOIs intended to treat depression with, or within 14 days of treatment. Do not start treatment in patients being treated with a reversible MAOI (eg, linezolid, methylene blue). Concomitant use with thioridazine or pimozide.

WARNINGS/PRECAUTIONS: Not approved for treatment of bipolar depression. Serotonin syndrome or neuroleptic malignant syndrome (NMS)-like reactions reported. Increased risk of congenital malformations reported in 1st trimester of pregnancy. Neonatal complications requiring prolonged hospitalization, respiratory support, and tube feeding may develop in neonates exposed in the late 3rd trimester. Activation of mania/hypomania reported. Caution with history of seizures; d/c if seizures occur. Adverse reactions upon discontinuation (eg, dysphoric mood, irritability) reported; avoid abrupt withdrawal. Akathisia may develop. Hyponatremia reported; caution in elderly and volume-depleted patients. May increase risk of bleeding events. Bone fracture risk reported; consider pathological fracture in patients with unexplained bone pain, point tenderness, swelling, or bruising. Caution with disease/conditions that could affect metabolism or hemodynamic responses, narrow-angle glaucoma, severe renal/hepatic impairment, and in elderly and debilitated patients. May impair mental/physical abilities.

P

ADVERSE REACTIONS: Suicidality, somnolence, insomnia, nausea, asthenia, abnormal ejaculation, dry mouth, constipation, dizziness, diarrhea, decreased libido, sweating, abnormal vision, headache, tremor.

INTERACTIONS: See Contraindications. Serotonin syndrome or NMS-like reactions reported when used alone and in combination with serotonergic drugs (eg, triptans, fentanyl, St. John's wort), drugs that impair serotonin metabolism, antipsychotics, and dopamine antagonists. Use with other SSRIs, SNRIs, or tryptophan is not recommended. Avoid alcohol. Concomitant use with aspirin (ASA), NSAIDs, warfarin, and other drugs that may affect coagulation may increase risk of bleeding events. Use with diuretics may increase risk of developing hyponatremia. Metabolism and pharmacokinetics may be affected by induction or inhibition of drug-metabolizing enzymes. Increased levels with cimetidine. Reduced levels with phenobarbital, phenytoin, and fosamprenavir/ritonavir. Increased phenytoin level after 4 weeks of coadministration reported. Caution with drugs that are metabolized by CYP2D6 (eg, phenothiazines, risperidone, type 1C antiarrhythmics) and with drugs that inhibit CYP2D6 (eg, quinidine). May increase levels of desipramine, risperidone, atomoxetine. May reduce efficacy of tamoxifen. May inhibit metabolism of TCAs. May displace or be displaced by other highly protein-bound drugs. Decreased levels of digoxin seen. May increase procyclidine levels; reduce dose if anticholinergic effects are seen. Severe hypotension may occur when added to chronic metoprolol treatment. May elevate theophylline levels. Caution with lithium. May decrease phenytoin levels.

PREGNANCY: Category D, caution in nursing.

MECHANISM OF ACTION: SSRI; inhibits CNS neuronal reuptake of serotonin.

PHARMACOKINETICS: Absorption: Complete; administration of variable doses resulted in different parameters; T_{max}=6-10 hrs. **Distribution:** Plasma protein binding (93-95%); found in breast milk. **Metabolism:** Extensive; oxidation and methylation via CYP2D6. **Elimination:** Sol: Urine (62%, metabolites; 2%, parent); feces (36%, metabolites; <1%, parent). $T_{1/2}$=15-20 hrs.

NURSING CONSIDERATIONS

Assessment: Assess for history of seizures or mania, volume depletion, diseases/conditions that affect metabolism or hemodynamic response, hepatic/renal impairment, narrow-angle glaucoma, previous hypersensitivity, pregnancy/nursing status, and for possible drug interactions. Assess use in the elderly or debilitated patients. Screen for bipolar disorder.

Monitoring: Monitor for signs/symptoms of clinical worsening, serotonin syndrome or NMS-like reactions, seizures, mania, akathisia, bone fracture, hyponatremia especially in the elderly, and abnormal bleeding. Upon discontinuation, monitor for symptoms. Periodically reassess need for continued therapy. Regularly monitor weight and growth of children and adolescents.

Patient Counseling: Inform patient to swallow whole, not to chew or crush, and to avoid alcohol use. Instruct to notify physician of all prescription or OTC drugs currently taking or planning to take. Caution on risk of serotonin syndrome with concomitant use of triptans, tramadol, or other serotonergic agents. Instruct patient, families, and caregivers to report emergence of anxiety, agitation, panic attacks, insomnia, irritability, hostility, aggressiveness, impulsivity, akathisia, hypomania, mania, unusual changes in behavior, worsening of depression, and suicidal ideation, especially during drug initiation or dose adjustment. Caution against hazardous tasks. Inform that improvement may be noticed in 1-4 weeks; instruct to continue therapy ud. Instruct to notify physician if pregnant/intend to become pregnant, or breastfeeding. Caution on concomitant use with NSAIDs, ASA, warfarin, or other drugs that affect coagulation.

Administration: Oral route. **Storage:** ≤25°C (77°F). (Generic) 20-25°C (68-77°F).

PEDIAPRED   RX
prednisolone sodium phosphate (Royal)

THERAPEUTIC CLASS: Glucocorticoid

INDICATIONS: Steroid-responsive dermatoses.

DOSAGE: *Adults:* Initial: 5-60mg/day depending on disease and response. Maint: Decrease dose by small amounts to lowest effective dose. MS Exacerbations: 200mg qd for 1 week, then 80mg qod for 1 month.
Pediatrics: Initial: 0.14-2mg/kg/day given tid-qid. Nephrotic Syndrome: 20mg/m² tid for 4 weeks, then 40mg/m² qod for 4 weeks. Uncontrolled Asthma: 1-2mg/kg/day in single or divided doses until peak expiratory rate of 80% is achieved (usually 3-10 days).

HOW SUPPLIED: Sol: 5mg/5mL [120mL]

CONTRAINDICATIONS: Systemic fungal infections.

WARNINGS/PRECAUTIONS: May produce reversible hypothalamic-pituitary-adrenal axis suppression. Adjust dose during stress or change in thyroid status. May mask signs of infection or cause new infections. May activate latent amebiasis. Avoid with cerebral malaria. Avoid exposure to chickenpox or measles. Not for treatment of optic neuritis or active ocular herpes simplex. May cause elevation of BP or intraocular pressure (IOP), cataracts, glaucoma, optic nerve damage, Kaposi's sarcoma, psychic derangements, salt/water retention, increased excretion of K$^+$ and/or Ca^{2+}, osteoporosis, growth suppression in children, or secondary ocular infections. Caution with strongyloides, chronic heart failure, diverticulitis, HTN, renal insufficiency, fresh intestinal anastomoses, active or latent peptic ulcer, and ulcerative colitis. Enhanced effect in hypothyroidism or cirrhosis. Avoid abrupt withdrawal. Caution in elderly due to increased risk of corticosteroid-induced side effects; start at low end of dosing range and monitor bone mineral density.

ADVERSE REACTIONS: Edema, fluid/electrolyte disturbances, osteoporosis, muscle weakness, pancreatitis, peptic ulcer, impaired wound healing, increased intracranial pressure, cushingoid state, hirsutism, menstrual irregularities, growth suppression in children, glaucoma, nausea, weight gain.

INTERACTIONS: Enhanced metabolism with barbiturates, phenytoin, ephedrine, and rifampin. Use with cyclosporine may increase activity of both drugs; convulsions reported with concomitant use. Decreased metabolism with estrogens or ketoconazole. May inhibit response to warfarin. Increased risk of GI side effects with aspirin or other NSAIDs. May increase clearance of salicylates. High doses or concurrent neuromuscular drugs may cause acute myopathy. Enhanced possibility of hypokalemia when given with K$^+$-depleting agents. May produce severe weakness in myasthenia gravis patients on anticholinesterase agents. Avoid live vaccines with immunosuppressive doses. Possible diminished response with killed or inactivated vaccines. May increase blood glucose; adjust antidiabetic agents. May suppress reactions to skin tests.

PREGNANCY: Category C, caution in nursing.

MECHANISM OF ACTION: Synthetic adrenocorticoid steroid; promotes gluconeogenesis, increases deposition of glycogen in the liver, inhibits glucose utilization, and increases catabolism of protein, lipolysis, and glomerular filtration that leads to increased urinary excretion of urate and Ca^{2+}.

PHARMACOKINETICS: Absorption: Rapidly absorbed from GI tract. **Distribution:** Plasma protein binding (70-90%); found in breast milk. **Metabolism:** Liver. **Elimination:** Urine (as sulfate and glucuronide congugates); T$_{1/2}$=2-4 hrs.

NURSING CONSIDERATIONS

Assessment: Assess for systemic fungal/other infections, active tuberculosis, vaccination history, HTN, congestive heart failure, renal insufficiency, ophthalmic disease, osteoporosis, thyroid status, hepatic impairment, nonspecific ulcerative colitis, ulcers, pregnancy/nursing status, and possible drug interactions.

Monitoring: Monitor for adrenocortical insufficiency, occurrence of infections, psychic derangement, cataracts, acute myopathy, Kaposi's sarcoma, fluid retention, and measurement of serum electrolytes, TSH, LFTs, glucose, IOP, and BP.

Patient Counseling: Advise not to d/c therapy abruptly or without medical supervision. Instruct to avoid exposure to chickenpox or measles; report immediately if exposed. Advise to implement dietary salt restriction and K$^+$ supplementation.

Administration: Oral route. **Storage:** 4-25°C (39-77°F).

PEDIARIX   RX
acellular pertussis - hepatitis B (recombinant) - inactivated poliovirus - diphtheria toxoid - tetanus toxoid (GlaxoSmithKline)

THERAPEUTIC CLASS: Toxoid/vaccine combination

INDICATIONS: Active immunization against diphtheria, tetanus, pertussis, infection caused by all known subtypes of hepatitis B virus (HBV), and poliomyelitis in infants born of hepatitis B surface antigen (HBsAg)-negative mothers, beginning as early as 6 weeks of age through 6 yrs of age (prior to 7th birthday).

DOSAGE: *Pediatrics:* 6 Weeks to 6 Yrs: 3 doses of 0.5mL IM at 2, 4, and 6 months (at intervals of 6-8 weeks, preferably 8 weeks). May be used to complete the first 3 doses of DTaP series in children who have received 1 or 2 doses of Infanrix and are also scheduled to receive other vaccine components of Pediarix. May be used to complete the HBV vaccination series following 1 or 2 doses of another HBV vaccine, including vaccines from other manufacturers, in children born of HBsAg-negative mothers who are also scheduled to receive the other components of Pediarix. May be used to complete the first 3 doses of the inactivated poliovirus vaccine (IPV) series in children who have received 1 or 2 doses of IPV from other manufacturers and are scheduled to receive other components of Pediarix. May use Infanrix and Kinrix to complete DTaP and IPV series; refer to prescribing information for further details.

HOW SUPPLIED: Inj: 0.5mL [prefilled syringe]

P

CONTRAINDICATIONS: Encephalopathy (eg, coma, decreased level of consciousness, prolonged seizures) within 7 days of administration of a previous pertussis-containing vaccine that is not attributable to another identifiable cause, progressive neurologic disorder (including infantile spasms, uncontrolled epilepsy, or progressive encephalopathy). Severe allergic reaction (eg, anaphylaxis) to yeast, neomycin, or polymyxin B.

WARNINGS/PRECAUTIONS: Use in infants is associated with higher risk of fever relative to separately administered vaccines. Evaluate potential benefits and risks of vaccine administration if Guillain-Barre syndrome occurs within 6 weeks of receipt of a prior tetanus toxoid-containing vaccine. Tip caps of prefilled syringes may contain natural rubber latex; may cause allergic reactions in latex-sensitive individuals. Syncope may occur and can be accompanied by transient neurological signs. Evaluate the potential benefits and risks of vaccine administration if any of the following events occur in temporal relation to receipt of a pertussis-containing vaccine: temperature ≥40.5°C (105°F) within 48 hrs not due to another identifiable cause; collapse or shock-like state occurring within 48 hrs; persistent, inconsolable crying lasting ≥3 hrs, occurring within 48 hrs; or seizures with or without fever occurring within 3 days. May administer an antipyretic at the time of vaccination and for the ensuing 24 hrs in children at higher risk for seizures. Apnea following IM administration observed in premature infants; consider infant's medical status, and the potential benefits and possible risks of vaccination. Review immunization history for possible vaccine sensitivity; appropriate treatment should be available for possible allergic reactions.

ADVERSE REACTIONS: Local inj-site reactions (pain, redness, swelling), fever, irritability/fussiness, drowsiness, loss of appetite.

INTERACTIONS: Immunosuppressive therapies, including irradiation, antimetabolites, alkylating agents, cytotoxic drugs, and corticosteroids (used in greater than physiologic doses), may reduce immune response to vaccine.

PREGNANCY: Category C, safety not known in nursing.

MECHANISM OF ACTION: Toxoid/vaccine combination; provides active immunization by producing antibodies against diphtheria toxin, tetanus toxin, pertussis, hepatitis B, and poliovirus infections.

NURSING CONSIDERATIONS

Assessment: Assess for history of encephalopathy, development of Guillain-Barre syndrome following a prior tetanus toxoid-containing vaccine, progressive neurologic disorder, immunosuppression, risk for seizures, possible drug interactions, and hypersensitivity to latex, yeast, neomycin, or polymyxin B. Review immunization history for possible vaccine sensitivity and previous vaccination-related adverse reactions. Assess use in premature infants.

Monitoring: Monitor for signs/symptoms of Guillain-Barre syndrome, allergic reactions, syncope, neurological signs, apnea in premature infants, and other adverse reactions.

Patient Counseling: Inform parents/guardians about potential benefits/risks of immunization, and of the importance of completing the immunization series. Counsel parents/guardians about potential adverse reactions; instruct to report any adverse events to physician.

Administration: IM route. Do not administer IV, intradermally, or SQ. Do not mix with any other vaccine in the same syringe or vial. Administer other vaccines separately, at different inj site. Refer to PI for preparation and administration instructions. **Storage:** 2-8°C (36-46°F). Do not freeze. Discard if frozen.

PEGASYS
peginterferon alfa-2a (Genentech)

RX

> May cause or aggravate fatal or life-threatening neuropsychiatric, autoimmune, ischemic, and infectious disorders. Monitor closely with periodic clinical and lab evaluations. D/C with severe or worsening signs or symptoms of these conditions. Use with ribavirin may cause birth defects, fetal death, and hemolytic anemia. Refer to the individual PI for more information on ribavirin.

THERAPEUTIC CLASS: Pegylated virus proliferation inhibitor

INDICATIONS: Treatment of chronic hepatitis C (CHC) virus infection, alone or in combination with Copegus, in patients ≥5 yrs of age with compensated liver disease and not previously treated with interferon-alfa. Treatment of HBeAg-positive and HBeAg-negative chronic hepatitis B (CHB) in adults with compensated liver disease, evidence of viral replication, and liver inflammation.

DOSAGE: *Adults:* CHC: 180mcg SQ once weekly for 48 weeks. With Copegus: 180mcg SQ once weekly. Genotype 2 and 3: Treat for 24 weeks. Genotype 1 and 4: Treat for 48 weeks. CHC w/ HIV Coinfection: 180mcg SQ once weekly for 48 weeks. With Copegus: 180mcg SQ once weekly for 48 weeks, regardless of genotype. CHB: 180mcg SQ once weekly for 48 weeks. Renal Impairment: CrCl 30-50mL/min: 180mcg once weekly. Hemodialysis/CrCl <30mL/min: 135mcg once weekly. Refer to PI for Copegus dosage, dose modification, and discontinuation of therapy.

Pediatrics: ≥5 Yrs: CHC: With Copegus: 180mcg/1.73m^2 x BSA SQ once weekly. Max: 180mcg SQ once weekly. Genotype 2 and 3: Treat for 24 weeks. For Other Genotypes: Treat for 48 weeks. Refer to PI for Copegus dosage, dose modification, and discontinuation of therapy.

HOW SUPPLIED: Inj: 180mcg/0.5mL [prefilled syringe]; 180mcg/0.5mL, 135mcg/0.5mL [ProClick autoinjector]; 180mcg/mL [vial]

CONTRAINDICATIONS: Autoimmune hepatitis, hepatic decompensation (Child-Pugh score >6 [Class B and C]) in cirrhotic patients before treatment, hepatic decompensation with Child-Pugh score ≥6 in cirrhotic CHC patients coinfected with HIV before treatment, neonates, and infants (contains benzyl alcohol). When used with Copegus, refer to PI for additional contraindications.

WARNINGS/PRECAUTIONS: Life-threatening neuropsychiatric reactions may occur; extreme caution with history of depression; d/c immediately in severe cases and institute psychiatric intervention. Caution with preexisting cardiac disease and autoimmune disorders. May cause bone marrow suppression and severe cytopenias; d/c if severe decrease in neutrophil or platelet count develops. May cause or aggravate hypo/hyperthyroidism, and pulmonary disorders. Hypo/hyperglycemia, diabetes mellitus, ischemic and hemorrhagic cerebrovascular events, autoimmune/ophthalmologic disorders reported. CHC patients with cirrhosis may be at risk for hepatic decompensation and death. Exacerbation of hepatitis B reported; d/c immediately if hepatic decompensation with increase in ALT occurs. Serious infections, severe acute hypersensitivity reactions, ulcerative or hemorrhagic/ischemic colitis, and pancreatitis reported; d/c if any of these develop. D/C with new or worsening ophthalmologic disorders, pulmonary infiltrates or pulmonary function impairment, and pancytopenia. Peripheral neuropathy reported in combination with telbivudine. May delay growth in pediatrics. May impair fertility in women. Caution with CrCl <50mL/min and in elderly.

ADVERSE REACTIONS: Inj-site reactions, fatigue/asthenia, diarrhea, pyrexia, rigors, N/V, anorexia, neutropenia, myalgia, headache, irritability/anxiety/nervousness, insomnia, depression, alopecia, dizziness.

INTERACTIONS: May inhibit CYP1A2 and increase AUC levels of theophylline; monitor theophylline serum levels and consider dose adjustments. May increase levels of methadone; monitor for toxicity. Hepatic decompensation can occur with concomitant use of nucleoside reverse transcriptase inhibitors (NRTIs) and peginterferon alfa-2a/ribavirin; refer to PI for respective NRTIs for guidance regarding toxicity management. Concomitant use of peginterferon alfa-2a/ribavirin with zidovudine may cause severe neutropenia and severe anemia; reduce dose or d/c if worsening toxicities occur.

PREGNANCY: Category C, Category X (with ribavirin); not for use in nursing.

MECHANISM OF ACTION: Interferon alfa-2a; binds to human type 1 interferon receptor leading to receptor dimerization, which activates multiple intracellular signal transduction pathways initially mediated by the JAK/STAT pathway. Expected to have pleiotropic biological effects in the body.

PHARMACOKINETICS: Absorption: T_{max}=72-96 hrs. **Elimination:** $T_{1/2}$=160 hrs (CHC).

NURSING CONSIDERATIONS

Assessment: Assess for neuropsychiatric, autoimmune, ischemic or infectious disorders, hepatic/renal impairment, risk of severe anemia, known hypersensitivity reactions, pregnancy/nursing status, possible drug interactions, or any other conditions where treatment is contraindicated or cautioned. Obtain baseline CBC, TSH, CD4$^+$ (HIV), and eye exam. Perform ECG for preexisting cardiac diseases prior to therapy. Obtain pregnancy test in women of childbearing potential.

Monitoring: Monitor for neuropsychiatric, autoimmune, ischemic, infectious disorders, bone marrow toxicities, cardiovascular disorders, cerebrovascular disorders, or other adverse reactions. Monitor hematological (Weeks 2 and 4), biochemical tests (Week 4), LFTs, TSH (every 12 weeks). Perform periodic eye exams in patients with preexisting ophthalmologic disorders. Perform monthly pregnancy tests if on combination therapy with Copegus and for 6 months after discontinuation. Monitor CBC, clinical status, and hepatic/renal function.

Patient Counseling: Counsel on benefits and risks of therapy. Advise not to use drug in combination with Copegus for pregnant women or men whose female partners are pregnant; perform monthly pregnancy tests. Inform of the teratogenic/embryocidal risks; use two forms of effective contraception during and for 6 months post-therapy. Inform that drug is not known to prevent transmission of HCV/HBV infection to others; lab evaluation is required prior to therapy, and periodically thereafter. Counsel to avoid alcohol, and avoid driving or operating machinery if dizziness, confusion, somnolence, or fatigue occurs. Instruct to remain well hydrated, and not to switch to other brand of interferon without consulting physician. Instruct on the proper preparation, administration, and disposal techniques; do not reuse any needles and syringes.

Administration: SQ route. Administer in abdomen or thigh. **Storage:** 2-8°C (36-46°F). Do not leave out of the refrigerator for ≥24 hrs. Do not freeze or shake. Protect from light.

P

PegIntron

RX

peginterferon alfa-2b (Merck)

> May cause or aggravate fatal or life-threatening neuropsychiatric, autoimmune, ischemic, and infectious disorders. Closely monitor patients with periodic clinical and laboratory evaluations. D/C with persistently severe or worsening signs/symptoms of these conditions. When used with ribavirin, refer to the individual monograph.

THERAPEUTIC CLASS: Pegylated virus proliferation inhibitor

INDICATIONS: Treatment of chronic hepatitis C (CHC) in patients with compensated liver disease in combination with Rebetol (ribavirin) and an approved hepatitis C virus (HCV) NS3/4A protease inhibitor in adult patients with HCV genotype 1 infection. Treatment of CHC in patients with compensated liver disease in combination with Rebetol in patients with genotypes other than 1, pediatric patients (3-17 yrs of age), or in patients with genotype 1 infection where use of another HCV NS3/4A protease inhibitor is not warranted based on tolerability, contraindications, or other clinical factors. Treatment of CHC as monotherapy in patients with compensated liver disease if there are contraindications to or significant intolerance of Rebetol and for use only in previously untreated adult patients.

DOSAGE: *Adults:* Monotherapy: 1mcg/kg/week SQ for 1 yr administered on the same day of the week. Moderate Renal Dysfunction (CrCl 30-50mL/min): Reduce dose by 25%. Severe Renal Dysfunction (CrCl 10-29mL/min)/Hemodialysis: Reduce dose by 50%. Combination Therapy: 1.5mcg/kg/week SQ with 800-1400mg Rebetol PO based on body weight; refer to PI of the specific HCV NS3/4A protease inhibitor for dosing regimen. Take Rebetol with food. Treatment with PegIntron/Rebetol of Interferon Alfa-Naive Patients: Genotype 1: Treat for 48 weeks. Genotype 2 and 3: Treat for 24 weeks. Retreatment with PegIntron/Rebetol of Prior Treatment Failures: Retreat for 48 weeks, regardless of HCV genotype. Refer to PI for volume of PegIntron to be injected, dose modifications, and discontinuation.
Pediatrics: 3-17 Yrs: Combination Therapy: 60mcg/m²/week SQ with 15mg/kg/day Rebetol PO in 2 divided doses. Take Rebetol with food. Remain on pediatric dosing regimen if 18th birthday was reached while receiving therapy. Genotype 1: Treat for 48 weeks. Genotype 2 and 3: Treat for 24 weeks. Refer to PI for volume of PegIntron to be injected, dose modifications, and discontinuation.

HOW SUPPLIED: Inj: 50mcg/0.5mL, 80mcg/0.5mL, 120mcg/0.5mL, 150mcg/0.5mL [vial, Redipen, Selectdose]

CONTRAINDICATIONS: Autoimmune hepatitis, hepatic decompensation (Child-Pugh score >6 [class B and C]) in cirrhotic CHC patients before or during treatment. When used with ribavirin, refer to the individual monograph.

WARNINGS/PRECAUTIONS: Caution with history of psychiatric disorders. Monitor during treatment and in the 6-month follow-up period if psychiatric problems develop; d/c if symptoms persist or worsen, or if suicidal ideation or aggressive behavior is identified. Cases of encephalopathy reported with higher doses. Cardiovascular (CV) events reported; caution with CV disease (CVD) (eg, myocardial infarction [MI], arrhythmia). Hyperglycemia, diabetes mellitus, and new/worsening hypothyroidism and hyperthyroidism reported; do not begin/continue therapy in patients with these conditions who cannot be controlled with medication. Ophthalmologic disorders may be induced or aggravated; conduct baseline eye exam and periodically monitor patients with preexisting ophthalmologic disorders. D/C if new or worsening ophthalmologic disorders occur. Ischemic and hemorrhagic cerebrovascular events reported. Suppresses bone marrow function; d/c if severe decreases in neutrophil or platelet counts develop. May rarely be associated with aplastic anemia. Autoimmune/pulmonary/dental/periodontal disorders, pancreatitis, ulcerative or hemorrhagic/ischemic colitis, increases in SrCr/ALT/TG levels, and hypersensitivity reactions have been observed. Caution with autoimmune disorders, debilitating medical conditions (eg, history of pulmonary disease), and in elderly. Suspend combination treatment if pulmonary infiltrates or pulmonary function impairment develops. D/C if signs/symptoms of pancreatitis, colitis, or hypersensitivity reactions occur. CHC patients with cirrhosis may be at risk for hepatic decompensation and death. Monitor patients with renal impairment for toxicity; adjust dose or d/c therapy. Use monotherapy with caution and avoid combination therapy with ribavirin in patients with CrCl <50mL/min. Weight loss and growth inhibition (including long-term growth inhibition) reported in pediatric patients during combination therapy with Rebetol.

ADVERSE REACTIONS: Neuropsychiatric/autoimmune/ischemic/infectious disorders, headache, fatigue/asthenia, rigors, N/V, abdominal pain, anorexia, emotional lability/irritability, myalgia, fever, inj-site inflammation/erythema.

INTERACTIONS: May decrease therapeutic effects of CYP2C8/9 (eg, warfarin, phenytoin) or CYP2D6 (eg, flecainide) substrates. May increase methadone concentrations; monitor for signs/symptoms of increased narcotic effect. Closely monitor for toxicities, especially hepatic decompensation and anemia, with nucleoside reverse transcriptase inhibitors (NRTIs); consider dose reduction or discontinuation of interferon, ribavirin, or both, or discontinuation of NRTIs if worsening clinical toxicities occur. Concomitant use of peginterferon alpha and ribavirin with zidovudine may cause severe neutropenia and severe anemia. Peripheral neuropathy reported when used in combination with telbivudine.

PREGNANCY: Category C, Category X (with ribavirin); not for use in nursing.

MECHANISM OF ACTION: Pegylated virus proliferation inhibitor; binds to and activates the human type 1 interferon receptor. Upon binding, the receptor subunits dimerize and activate multiple intracellular signal transduction pathways.

PHARMACOKINETICS: Absorption: T_{max}=15-44 hrs. **Elimination:** $T_{1/2}$=40 hrs (HCV-infected).

NURSING CONSIDERATIONS

Assessment: Assess for history of MI, arrhythmia, and psychiatric disorders; presence of CVD, endocrine, autoimmune, and ophthalmologic disorders; hepatic/renal impairment; drug hypersensitivity; any other conditions where treatment is contraindicated or cautioned; pregnancy/nursing status; and possible drug interactions. Obtain baseline CBC, blood chemistry, and eye exam. Perform ECG in patients with preexisting cardiac abnormalities.

Monitoring: Monitor CBC, blood chemistry, renal function, TG levels, HCV-RNA, and complete eye and dental exams periodically. Monitor for signs/symptoms of autoimmune, cerebrovascular, infectious, endocrine, and pulmonary disorders; CV and neuropsychiatric events; bone marrow toxicity; hepatic decompensation; colitis; pancreatitis; hypersensitivity reactions; and other adverse reactions.

Patient Counseling: Inform of benefits and risks of therapy. Advise to report immediately any symptoms of depression or suicidal ideation to physician. Instruct to use at least 2 forms of contraception and to avoid pregnancy during treatment with combination therapy and for 6 months post-therapy. Instruct to brush teeth thoroughly bid and to have regular dental examinations when used in combination with Rebetol; if vomiting occurs, advise to rinse out mouth afterwards. Counsel that flu-like symptoms associated with treatment may be minimized by hs administration of the drug or by using antipyretics. Inform that chest x-ray or other tests may be needed if fever, cough, SOB, or other symptoms of a lung problem develop. Advise to remain well-hydrated. Instruct self-administering patients on the importance of site selection, rotating inj sites, and proper disposal of needles, syringes, and Redipen/Selectdose; caution against reuse.

Administration: SQ route. Refer to PI for preparation and administration instructions. **Storage:** (Redipen/Selectdose) 2-8°C (36-46°F). (Vial) 25°C (77°F); excursions permitted to 15-30°C (59-86°F). (Redipen/Selectdose/Vial) Reconstituted Sol: Use immediately, but may store for up to 24 hrs at 2-8°C (36-46°F). Do not freeze. Keep away from heat.

PENICILLIN VK   RX

penicillin V potassium (Various)

THERAPEUTIC CLASS: Penicillin

INDICATIONS: Treatment of mild to moderately severe bacterial infections due to penicillin (PCN) G-sensitive microorganisms (eg, infections of the respiratory tract, oropharynx, skin and soft tissue), and infections such as scarlet fever or mild erysipelas. Prevention of recurrence following rheumatic fever and/or chorea. May be useful as prophylaxis against bacterial endocarditis in patients with congenital heart disease or rheumatic or other acquired valvular heart disease who are undergoing dental procedures and surgical procedures of the upper respiratory tract.

DOSAGE: *Adults:* Determine dose according to the sensitivity of the causative organism and severity of infection, and adjust based on clinical response. Usual: Streptococcal Infections (Scarlet Fever/Erysipelas/Upper Respiratory Tract): 125-250mg q6-8h for 10 days. Pneumococcal Infections (Otitis Media/Respiratory Tract): 250-500mg q6h until afebrile for at least 2 days. Staphylococcus Infections (Skin/Soft Tissue)/Fusospirochetosis (Oropharynx): 250-500mg q6-8h. Rheumatic Fever/Chorea Prevention: 125-250mg bid on a continuous basis. Bacterial Endocarditis Prophylaxis: 2g one hr before procedure and then 1g after 6 hrs.
Pediatrics: ≥12 Yrs: Determine dose according to the sensitivity of the causative organism and severity of infection, and adjust based on clinical response. Usual: Streptococcal Infections (Scarlet Fever/Erysipelas/Upper Respiratory Tract): 125-250mg q6-8h for 10 days. Pneumococcal Infections (Otitis Media/Respiratory Tract): 250-500mg q6h until afebrile for at least 2 days. Staphylococcus Infections (Skin/Soft Tissue)/Fusospirochetosis (Oropharynx): 250-500mg q6-8h. Rheumatic Fever/Chorea Prevention: 125-250mg bid on a continuous basis. Bacterial Endocarditis Prophylaxis: 2g or 1g (<60 lbs) one hr before procedure and then 1g or 500mg (<60 lbs) after 6 hrs.

HOW SUPPLIED: Sol: 125mg/5mL [100mL, 200mL], 250mg/5mL [100mL, 200mL]; Tab: 250mg, 500mg

WARNINGS/PRECAUTIONS: Not for treatment of severe pneumonia, empyema, bacteremia, pericarditis, meningitis, and arthritis during the acute stage. Necessary dental care should be accomplished in infections involving the gum tissue. Oral PCN should not be used in patients at particularly high risk for endocarditis (eg, those with prosthetic heart valves or surgically constructed systemic pulmonary shunts). Should not be used as adjunctive prophylaxis for genitourinary instrumentation/surgery, lower intestinal tract surgery, sigmoidoscopy, and childbirth. Serious and fatal anaphylactic reactions reported; caution with a history of hypersensitivity to PCN, cephalosporins, and/or multiple allergens. Caution with history of significant allergies and/or asthma. D/C if an allergic reaction occurs and institute appropriate therapy. *Clostridium difficile*-associated diarrhea (CDAD) reported; d/c therapy if CDAD is suspected/confirmed. Use in the absence of a proven/strongly suspected bacterial infection or a prophylactic indication is unlikely to provide benefit and increases the risk of drug-resistant bacteria. Prolonged use may promote overgrowth of nonsusceptible organisms; take appropriate measures if superinfection develops. Oral route of administration should not be relied upon with severe illness, N/V, gastric dilatation, cardiospasm, or intestinal hypermotility. Obtain cultures following completion of treatment for streptococcal infections.

ADVERSE REACTIONS: Epigastric distress, N/V, diarrhea, black hairy tongue, hypersensitivity reactions (skin eruptions, urticaria, other serum-sickness like reactions, laryngeal edema, anaphylaxis), fever, eosinophilia.

PREGNANCY: Safety in pregnancy/nursing not known.

MECHANISM OF ACTION: PCN; exerts a bactericidal action against PCN-sensitive microorganisms during the stage of active multiplication. Acts through inhibition of biosynthesis of cell-wall mucopeptide.

PHARMACOKINETICS: Distribution: Plasma protein binding (80%). **Elimination:** Urine.

NURSING CONSIDERATIONS

Assessment: Assess for previous hypersensitivity reactions to PCNs/cephalosporins or other allergens, history of asthma, N/V, gastric dilatation, severe illness, cardiospasm, intestinal hypermotility, and pregnancy/nursing status. Obtain cultures and sensitivity tests, especially in suspected staphylococcal infections.

Monitoring: Monitor for signs/symptoms of hypersensitivity reactions, CDAD, superinfections, and other adverse reactions. Obtain cultures following completion of treatment of streptococcal infections.

Patient Counseling: Counsel that therapy only treats bacterial, not viral (eg, common cold), infections. Instruct to take ud; inform that skipping doses or not completing the full course of therapy may decrease effectiveness and increase resistance. Inform that diarrhea may occur. Instruct to seek medical attention if watery and bloody stools (with or without stomach cramps and fever) occur even after ≥2 months of discontinuing therapy.

Administration: Oral route. Refer to PI for directions for mixing solution. **Storage:** 20-25°C (68-77°F). (Reconstituted Sol) Store in a refrigerator. Discard any unused portion after 14 days.

PENLAC   RX
ciclopirox (Valeant)

THERAPEUTIC CLASS: Broad-spectrum antifungal

INDICATIONS: Mild to moderate onychomycosis of fingernails or toenails without lunula involvement due to *Trichophyton rubrum* in immunocompetent patients.

DOSAGE: *Adults:* Apply evenly over the entire plate qd (preferably at hs or 8 hrs before washing) to nail bed, hyponychium, and the under surface of nail plate when it is free of nail bed (eg, onycholysis). Apply daily over previous coat and remove with alcohol every 7 days. Repeat regimen for up to 48 weeks.
Pediatrics: ≥12 Yrs: Apply evenly over the entire plate qd (preferably at hs or 8 hrs before washing) to nail bed, hyponychium, and the under surface of nail plate when it is free of nail bed (eg, onycholysis). Apply daily over previous coat and remove with alcohol every 7 days. Repeat regimen for up to 48 weeks.

HOW SUPPLIED: Sol: 8% [6.6mL]

WARNINGS/PRECAUTIONS: Not for ophthalmic, oral, or intravaginal use; for use on nails and immediately adjacent skin only. Should be used as a component of a comprehensive management program for onychomycosis and should be used only under medical supervision by a healthcare professional who has special competence in the diagnosis and treatment of nail disorders, including minor nail procedures. D/C and treat appropriately if sensitivity reaction or chemical irritation occurs. Caution with removal of infected nail in patients with a history of insulin-dependent diabetes mellitus (DM) or diabetic neuropathy.

ADVERSE REACTIONS: Periungual erythema, erythema of the proximal nail fold, nail shape change, nail irritation, ingrown toenail, nail discoloration.

INTERACTIONS: Avoid with systemic antifungal agents for onychomycosis.

PREGNANCY: Category B, caution in nursing.

MECHANISM OF ACTION: Broad spectrum antifungal; not established. Suggested to act by chelation of polyvalent cations, resulting in the inhibition of the metal-dependent enzymes responsible for degradation of peroxides within fungal cell.

PHARMACOKINETICS: Absorption: (PO) Rapid. **Metabolism:** Glucuronidation. **Elimination:** Urine (<5% of applied topical dose).

NURSING CONSIDERATIONS

Assessment: Assess for insulin-dependent DM, diabetic neuropathy, drug hypersensitivity, pregnancy/nursing status, and possible drug interactions.

Monitoring: Monitor for sensitivity reactions, chemical irritation, and other adverse reactions. Perform frequent (eg, monthly) removal of unattached infected nails, trimming of onycholytic nail, and filing of any excess horny material.

Patient Counseling: Advise to avoid contact with the eyes and mucous membranes. Instruct to apply medication evenly over entire nail plate and 5mm of surrounding skin. Advise that if possible, the medication should be applied to the nail bed, hyponychium, and the under surface of the nail plate when it is free of the nail bed (eg, onycholysis). Instruct to notify physician if signs of increased irritation at the application site develop. Instruct to inform physician if patient has diabetes or problems with numbness in toes or fingers for consideration of appropriate nail management program. Instruct to file away (with emery board) loose nail material and trim nails as required or ud. Advise to not use nail polish or other nail cosmetic products on the treated nails. Instruct not to use medication near open flame. Inform that it may take up to 48 weeks of daily application of the medication (including monthly professional removal of unattached infected nails) to achieve a clear or almost clear nail.

Administration: Topical route. Refer to PI for further administration instructions. **Storage:** 15-30°C (59-86°F). Flammable; keep away from heat and flame. Protect from light.

PENNSAID   RX
diclofenac sodium (Mallinckrodt)

> NSAIDs may increase risk of serious cardiovascular (CV) thrombotic events, myocardial infarction, and stroke; increased risk with duration of use and with CV disease (CVD) or risk factors for CVD. Contraindicated in the perioperative setting of coronary artery bypass graft (CABG) surgery. May increase risk of serious GI adverse events (eg, bleeding, ulceration, stomach/intestinal perforation), which can be fatal and may occur at any time during use without warning symptoms; elderly patients are at greater risk.

THERAPEUTIC CLASS: NSAID

INDICATIONS: Treatment of signs and symptoms of osteoarthritis of the knee(s).

DOSAGE: *Adults:* Apply to clean, dry skin. (1.5%) 40 drops/knee qid. (2%) 40mg (2 pump actuations) on each painful knee bid.

HOW SUPPLIED: Sol: 1.5% [150mL], 2% [112g]

CONTRAINDICATIONS: Patients who have experienced asthma, urticaria, or allergic-type reactions after taking aspirin (ASA) or other NSAIDs. Perioperative setting of CABG surgery.

WARNINGS/PRECAUTIONS: Use the lowest effective dose for the shortest duration possible. Extreme caution with history of ulcer disease or GI bleeding, or risk factors for GI bleeding (eg, longer duration of NSAID therapy, older age, poor general health status); monitor for signs/symptoms of GI ulcer/bleeding. May cause elevation of LFTs, hepatotoxicity, severe hepatic reactions, or liver injury; measure LFTs periodically with long-term therapy (monitor within 4-8 weeks after initiation). D/C therapy immediately if abnormal LFTs persist/worsen, liver disease develops, or systemic manifestations occur. May lead to new onset or worsening of preexisting HTN; caution with HTN, and monitor BP closely. Fluid retention and edema reported; caution with fluid retention or heart failure (HF). Use caution when initiating treatment in patients with considerable dehydration. Consider correcting fluid status prior to initiation of treatment. Renal papillary necrosis and other renal injury reported with long-term use. Renal toxicity reported in patients in whom renal prostaglandins have a compensatory role in the maintenance of renal perfusion; increased risk with renal/hepatic impairment, HF, and in elderly. Not recommended with advanced renal disease; if therapy must be initiated, closely monitor renal function. D/C if abnormal renal tests persist/worsen. Anaphylactoid reactions may occur; do not prescribe to patients with ASA-triad. Do not apply to open skin wounds, infections, inflammations, or exfoliative dermatitis; may affect absorption and tolerability of the drug. May cause serious skin adverse events; d/c at 1st appearance of skin rash or any other signs of hypersensitivity. Avoid in pregnant/nursing women or those intending to become pregnant. Caution with preexisting asthma and avoid with ASA-sensitive asthma. Avoid exposing treated knee(s) to natural or artificial sunlight. Avoid contact with eyes and mucosa. Not a substitute for corticosteroids or for the treatment of corticosteroid insufficiency. May mask signs of inflammation and fever. Anemia may occur; check Hgb/Hct if signs/symptoms of anemia or blood loss develop. May inhibit platelet aggregation and prolong bleeding time; monitor patients with coagulation disorders. Caution in elderly/debilitated.

ADVERSE REACTIONS: Application-site skin reactions (dry skin, pruritus, contact dermatitis, exfoliation, erythema), dyspepsia, pharyngitis, abdominal pain, infection, flatulence, diarrhea, nausea, constipation, edema, rash.

INTERACTIONS: Not recommended with ASA; potential for increased adverse effects. Increased risk of GI bleeding with oral corticosteroids or anticoagulants (eg, warfarin), smoking, and alcohol. Caution with drugs that are potentially hepatotoxic (eg, acetaminophen [APAP], certain antibiotics, antiepileptics). May diminish the antihypertensive effect of ACE inhibitors. May reduce the natriuretic effect of thiazide and loop (eg, furosemide) diuretics. Increased risk of renal toxicity with diuretics and ACE inhibitors; monitor renal function. May elevate lithium levels; observe for signs of lithium toxicity. May enhance methotrexate toxicity; use caution when coadministered. May increase cyclosporine's nephrotoxicity; use caution when coadministered. Concomitant use with oral NSAIDs resulted in a higher rate of rectal hemorrhage and more frequent abnormal SrCr, urea, and Hgb; avoid combination unless benefit outweighs risk and conduct periodic lab tests. Wait until the treated area is completely dry before applying sunscreen, insect repellant, lotion, moisturizer, cosmetics, or other topical medication to the same skin surface of the treated knee(s). Monitor patients receiving anticoagulants.

PREGNANCY: Category C (<30 weeks gestation) and D (≥30 weeks gestation), not for use in nursing.

MECHANISM OF ACTION: NSAID; inhibits the enzyme, cyclooxygenase, an early component of the arachidonic acid cascade, resulting in the reduced formation of prostaglandins, thromboxanes, and prostacylin.

PHARMACOKINETICS: Absorption: Administration of multiple doses resulted in different parameters. **Distribution:** Plasma protein binding (>99%). **Metabolism:** 4'-hydroxy-diclofenac (major metabolite) via CYP2C9; glucuronidation or sulfation, and acylglucuronidation (via UGT2B7) and oxidation (via CPY2C8). **Elimination:** Bile and urine. (1.5%) $T_{1/2}$=36.7 hrs (single dose), 79 hrs (multiple dose).

NURSING CONSIDERATIONS

Assessment: Assess for history of asthma, urticaria, or allergic-type reactions with ASA or other NSAIDs, ASA-triad, CVD, risk factors for CVD, history of ulcer disease or GI bleeding, risk factors for GI bleeding, coagulation disorders, renal/hepatic impairment, any other conditions where treatment is contraindicated or cautioned, fluid status, pregnancy/nursing status, and possible drug interactions. Assess application site for open wounds, infections, inflammations, and exfoliative dermatitis.

Monitoring: Monitor for CV/GI events, anaphylactoid/skin/hypersensitivity reactions, hematological effects, and other adverse reactions. Monitor BP, LFTs, renal function, CBC, and chemistry profile.

Patient Counseling: Instruct to seek medical advice if signs and symptoms of CV events, GI ulceration/bleeding, hepatotoxicity, skin/hypersensitivity reactions, unexplained weight gain or edema, and anaphylactoid reactions occur. Advise to d/c therapy immediately and contact physician if any type of generalized rash develops. Advise to contact physician as soon as possible if any type of localized application-site rash develops. Instruct not to apply to open skin wounds, infections, inflammations, or exfoliative dermatitis. Instruct to wait until the area treated with drug is completely dry before applying sunscreen, insect repellant, lotion, moisturizer, cosmetics, or other topical medication. Instruct to minimize or avoid exposure of treated knee(s) to natural or artificial sunlight. Instruct women who are pregnant or intending to become pregnant not to use the product. Instruct to avoid contact with the eyes and mucosa; advise that if eye contact occurs, to immediately wash out the eye with water or saline and consult physician if irritation persists for >1 hr. Caution to avoid taking unprescribed APAP while using the drug. Advise to avoid showering/bathing for at least 30 min after application, to wash and dry hands after use, to avoid wearing clothing over the treated knee(s) until the treated knee(s) is dry, and not to apply external heat and/or occlusive dressings to treated knee(s). (1.5%) Advise to avoid skin-to-skin contact between other people and the knee(s) to which drug was applied until the knee(s) is completely dry.

Administration: Topical route. Refer to PI for administration instructions. (2%) Prime pump before 1st use. Refer to PI for priming instructions. **Storage:** 25°C (77°F); excursions permitted to 15-30°C (59-86°F).

Pᴇɴᴛᴀsᴀ   RX
mesalamine (Shire)

THERAPEUTIC CLASS: 5-aminosalicylic acid derivative

INDICATIONS: Induction of remission and treatment of mildly to moderately active ulcerative colitis.

DOSAGE: *Adults:* Usual: 1g (4 caps of 250mg or 2 caps of 500mg) qid. May be given up to 8 weeks.

HOW SUPPLIED: Cap, Controlled-Release: 250mg, 500mg

WARNINGS/PRECAUTIONS: Caution with impaired hepatic and renal function. Has been associated with an acute intolerance syndrome (eg, acute abdominal pain, cramping, bloody diarrhea) that may be difficult to distinguish from a flare of inflammatory bowel disease; d/c if suspected. If a rechallenge is performed later in order to validate the hypersensitivity, it should be carried out under close medical supervision at reduced dose and only if clearly needed. Nephrotic syndrome and interstitial nephritis reported; monitor patients with preexisting renal disease, increased BUN or SrCr, or proteinuria especially during the initial phase of therapy. Nephrotoxicity should be suspected in patients developing renal dysfunction during treatment. May interfere with lab tests.

ADVERSE REACTIONS: Diarrhea, nausea.

PREGNANCY: Category B, caution in nursing.

MECHANISM OF ACTION: 5-aminosalicylic acid derivative; not established. Suspected to diminish inflammation by blocking cyclooxygenase and inhibiting prostaglandin production in the colon.

PHARMACOKINETICS: Absorption: (1g dose) C_{max}=1mcg/mL, T_{max}=3 hrs. (N-acetylmesalamine) C_{max}=1.8mcg/mL, T_{max}=3 hrs. **Distribution:** Crosses the placenta; found in breast milk. **Metabolism:** N-acetylmesalamine (major metabolite). **Elimination:** Feces, urine (19-30%, N-acetylmesalamine); (IV) $T_{1/2}$=42 min.

NURSING CONSIDERATIONS

Assessment: Assess for hypersensitivity to the drug or salicylates, hepatic/renal impairment, and pregnancy/nursing status.

Monitoring: Monitor for acute intolerance syndrome, hypersensitivity reaction, and other adverse reactions. Monitor renal function. Monitor patients with preexisting renal disease, increased BUN or SrCr, or proteinuria especially during the initial phase of therapy.

Patient Counseling: Inform of the risks/benefits of therapy. Advise to take ud. Advise to seek medical attention if symptoms of acute intolerance syndrome and hypersensitivity reactions occur.

Administration: Oral route. **Storage:** 25°C (77°F); excursions permitted to 15-30°C (59-86°F).

PERCOCET `CII`
oxycodone HCl - acetaminophen (Endo)

> Associated with cases of acute liver failure, at times resulting in liver transplant and death. Most cases of liver injury are associated with acetaminophen (APAP) use at doses >4000mg/day, and often involve >1 APAP-containing product.

OTHER BRAND NAMES: Endocet (Qualitest)

THERAPEUTIC CLASS: Opioid analgesic

INDICATIONS: Relief of moderate to moderately severe pain.

DOSAGE: *Adults:* (2.5mg-325mg) Usual: 1 or 2 tabs q6h PRN. Max: 12 tabs/day. (5mg-325mg) Usual: 1 tab q6h PRN. Max: 12 tabs/day. (7.5mg-325mg) Usual: 1 tab q6h PRN. Max: 8 tabs/day. (10mg-325mg) Usual: 1 tab q6h PRN. Max: 6 tabs/day. If pain is constant, give at regular intervals on an around-the-clock schedule. Do not exceed 4g/day of APAP. Cessation: Taper dose gradually.

HOW SUPPLIED: Tab: (Oxycodone-APAP) 2.5mg-325mg, 5mg-325mg*, 7.5mg-325mg, 10mg-325mg *scored

CONTRAINDICATIONS: Oxycodone: Significant respiratory depression (in unmonitored settings or absence of resuscitative equipment), acute or severe bronchial asthma or hypercarbia, suspected/known paralytic ileus.

WARNINGS/PRECAUTIONS: May be abused in a manner similar to other opioid agonists. Respiratory depression may occur; use extreme caution and consider alternative nonopioid analgesics in patients with acute asthma, chronic obstructive pulmonary disorder, cor pulmonale, preexisting respiratory impairment, or in the elderly or debilitated. Respiratory depressant effects may be markedly exaggerated in the presence of head injury, other intracranial lesions or preexisting increase in intracranial pressure. Produces effects on pupillary response and consciousness that may obscure neurologic signs of worsening in patients with head injuries. May cause severe hypotension; caution with circulatory shock. May produce orthostatic hypotension in ambulatory patients. Increased risk of acute liver failure in patients with underlying liver disease. May cause serious skin reactions (eg, acute generalized exanthematous pustulosis, Stevens-Johnson syndrome, toxic epidermal necrolysis), which can be fatal; d/c at the 1st appearance of skin rash or any other sign of hypersensitivity. Hypersensitivity and anaphylaxis reported; d/c immediately if signs/symptoms occur. May obscure diagnosis or clinical course in patients with acute abdominal conditions. Caution with CNS depression, hypothyroidism, Addison's disease, prostatic hypertrophy, urethral stricture, acute alcoholism, delirium tremens, kyphoscoliosis with respiratory depression, myxedema, toxic psychosis, hepatic/renal/pulmonary impairment, and in elderly/debilitated. May aggravate convulsions with convulsive disorders and may induce or aggravate seizures in some clinical settings. Monitor for decreased bowel motility in postoperative patients. May cause spasm of the sphincter of Oddi; caution with biliary tract disease, including acute pancreatitis. May cause increases in serum amylase level. Physical dependence and tolerance may occur. Do not abruptly d/c. Lab test interactions may occur. Not recommended for use during and immediately prior to labor and delivery.

ADVERSE REACTIONS: Lightheadedness, dizziness, drowsiness/sedation, N/V, respiratory depression, apnea, respiratory arrest, circulatory depression, hypotension, shock.

INTERACTIONS: Oxycodone: May cause severe hypotension after coadministration with drugs that compromise vasomotor tone (eg, phenothiazines). May enhance neuromuscular-blocking action of skeletal muscle relaxants and increase respiratory depression. Additive CNS depression with CNS depressants (eg, general anesthetics, phenothiazines, tranquilizers, alcohol); use in reduced dosages. Coadministration with anticholinergics may produce paralytic ileus. Agonist/antagonist analgesics (eg, pentazocine, nalbuphine, naltrexone, butorphanol) may reduce the analgesic effect or precipitate withdrawal symptoms; use with caution. APAP: Increased risk of acute liver failure with alcohol; hepatotoxicity reported in chronic alcoholics. Increase in glucuronidation resulting in increased plasma clearance and decreased $T_{1/2}$ with oral contraceptives. Propranolol and probenecid may increase pharmacologic/therapeutic effects. May decrease effects of loop diuretics, lamotrigine, and zidovudine.

PREGNANCY: Category C, not for use in nursing.

MECHANISM OF ACTION: Oxycodone: Opioid analgesic; semisynthetic pure opioid agonist whose principal therapeutic action is analgesia. Effects are mediated by receptors (eg, μ and kappa) in the CNS for endogenous opioid-like compounds (eg, endorphins, enkephalins). APAP: Nonopiate, nonsalicylate analgesic and antipyretic; site and mechanism for the analgesic effect not established. Antipyretic effect is accomplished through inhibition of endogenous pyrogen action on the hypothalamic heat-regulating centers.

PHARMACOKINETICS: Absorption: Oxycodone: Absolute bioavailability (87%). APAP: Rapid and almost complete from GI tract. **Distribution:** Oxycodone: Found in breast milk. Oxycodone: Plasma protein binding (45%); V_d=211.9L (IV); crosses the placenta. **Metabolism:** Oxycodone: N-dealkylation to noroxycodone (1st-pass); O-demethylation via CYP2D6 to oxymorphone. APAP: Liver via CYP450; conjugation with glucuronic acid and (lesser extent) sulfuric acid and cysteine; N acetyl-p-benzoquinoneimine (toxic metabolite). **Elimination:** Oxycodone: Urine (8-14% unchanged); $T_{1/2}$=3.51 hrs. APAP: Urine (90-100%).

NURSING CONSIDERATIONS

Assessment: Assess for level of pain intensity, type of pain, patient's general condition and medical status, or any other conditions where treatment is contraindicated or cautioned. Assess for drug hypersensitivity, renal/hepatic/pulmonary impairment, pregnancy/nursing status, and possible drug interactions.

Monitoring: Monitor for acute liver failure, respiratory depression, hypotension, skin/hypersensitivity/anaphylactic reactions, convulsions/seizures, decreased bowel motility in postoperative patients, spasm of sphincter of Oddi, increases in serum amylase levels, physical dependence, tolerance, and other adverse reactions.

Patient Counseling: Advise to d/c use and contact physician immediately if signs of allergy develop. Instruct to look for APAP on package labels and not to use >1 APAP-containing product. Instruct to seek medical attention immediately upon ingestion of >4000mg/day of APAP, even if patient is feeling well. Inform about the signs of serious skin reactions. Advise to destroy unused tabs by flushing down the toilet. Inform that drug may impair mental/physical abilities required to perform hazardous tasks. Instruct to avoid alcohol or other CNS depressants. Advise not to adjust dose without consulting physician and not to abruptly d/c if on treatment for more than a few weeks. Inform that drug has potential for abuse and should be protected from theft. Instruct to consult physician if pregnant, planning to become pregnant, or breastfeeding.

Administration: Oral route. **Storage:** 20-25°C (68-77°F).

PERCODAN CII

oxycodone HCl - aspirin (Endo)

OTHER BRAND NAMES: Endodan (Endo)

THERAPEUTIC CLASS: Opioid analgesic

INDICATIONS: Management of moderate to moderately severe pain.

DOSAGE: *Adults:* Usual: 1 tab q6h PRN for pain. Titrate: Adjust according to severity of pain and response. Max: (aspirin [ASA]) 4g/day or 12 tabs/day. Cessation of Therapy: Taper dose gradually.

HOW SUPPLIED: Tab: (ASA-Oxycodone HCl) 325mg-4.8355mg* *scored

CONTRAINDICATIONS: ASA: Hemophilia, children/teenagers with viral infections, NSAID allergy, and syndrome of asthma, rhinitis, and nasal polyps. Oxycodone: Significant respiratory depression (in unmonitored settings or absence of resuscitative equipment), acute/severe bronchial asthma or hypercarbia, and known/suspected paralytic ileus.

WARNINGS/PRECAUTIONS: Oxycodone: May be abused in a manner similar to other opioid agonists. May cause respiratory depression; extreme caution with acute asthma, chronic obstructive pulmonary disorder, cor pulmonale, or preexisting respiratory impairment. Respiratory depressant effects may be markedly exaggerated in the presence of head injury, other intracranial lesions, or preexisting increased intracranial pressure. Produces effects on pupillary response and consciousness, which may obscure neurologic signs of worsening in patients with head injuries. May cause severe hypotension; caution in circulatory shock. May produce orthostatic hypotension in ambulatory patients. Caution with CNS depression, hypothyroidism, Addison's disease, prostatic hypertrophy, urethral stricture, acute alcoholism, delirium tremens, kyphoscoliosis with respiratory depression, myxedema, toxic psychosis, severe hepatic/pulmonary/renal impairment, and in elderly/debilitated. May obscure diagnosis or clinical course of acute abdominal conditions. May induce or aggravate convulsions/seizures. Monitor for decreased bowel motility in postoperative patients. May cause spasm of the sphincter of Oddi; caution with biliary tract disease, including acute pancreatitis. Physical dependence and tolerance may occur. ASA: May inhibit platelet function. GI side effects reported; monitor for signs of ulceration and bleeding. May cause gastric mucosal irritation and bleeding; avoid with history of active peptic ulcer disease. May cause elevated hepatic enzymes, BUN, SrCr, and amylase, hyperkalemia, proteinuria, and prolonged bleeding time. May cause fetal harm; avoid use during pregnancy, especially in the 3rd trimester. Avoid with severe renal failure (GFR <10mL/min), or with severe hepatic insufficiency. May increase protein-bound iodine result. Avoid use 1 week prior to and during labor and delivery.

ADVERSE REACTIONS: Respiratory depression, apnea, respiratory arrest, circulatory depression, hypotension, shock, lightheadedness, dizziness, drowsiness, sedation, N/V.

INTERACTIONS: ASA: May increase concentrations of acetazolamide, leading to toxicity. May diminish effects of ACE inhibitors, β-blockers, and diuretics. Bleeding risk increased with anticoagulants (eg, warfarin, heparin) and chronic, heavy alcohol use. May decrease total concentration of phenytoin and increase serum valproic acid levels. May enhance serious side effects and toxicity of methotrexate and ketorolac. Avoid with NSAIDs; may increase bleeding or lead to decreased renal function. May increase serum glucose-lowering action of insulin and sulfonylureas, leading to hypoglycemia. Antagonizes uricosuric action of probenecid or sulfinpyrazone. Oxycodone: May enhance neuromuscular-blocking action of skeletal muscle relaxants and increase respiratory depression. Additive CNS depression with opioid analgesics, general anesthetics, centrally acting antiemetics, phenothiazines, tranquilizers, sedative-hypnotics, or other CNS depressants (eg, alcohol); reduce dose of one or both agents. May cause severe hypotension with drugs that compromise vasomotor tone (eg, phenothiazines). Mixed agonist/antagonist analgesics (eg, pentazocine, nalbuphine, naltrexone, butorphanol) may reduce analgesic effect and/or may precipitate withdrawal symptoms. Increased concentrations with CYP3A4 inhibitors (eg, macrolides, azole antifungals, protease inhibitors). Decreased concentrations with CYP450 inducers (eg, rifampin, carbamazepine, phenytoin).

PREGNANCY: Category B (oxycodone) and D (ASA), not for use in nursing.

MECHANISM OF ACTION: ASA: NSAID; inhibits prostaglandin production, including those involved in inflammation. In CNS, works on hypothalamus heat-regulating center to reduce fever. Oxycodone: Opioid analgesic; pure opioid agonist. Principal therapeutic action is analgesia. Effects are mediated by receptors (notably μ and kappa) in the CNS for endogenous opioid-like compounds (eg, endorphins, enkephalins).

PHARMACOKINETICS: Absorption: ASA: Rapid from the stomach. Oxycodone: Absolute bioavailability (87%). **Distribution:** Found in breast milk; crosses placenta. Oxycodone: V_d=211.9L (IV); plasma protein binding (45%). **Metabolism:** ASA: Liver by microsomal enzymes; hydrolysis to salicylate. Oxycodone: Extensive by CYP3A4-mediated N-demethylation to noroxycodone (major); further oxidation to noroxymorphone (active). **Elimination:** ASA: Urine (80-100%; 10%, unchanged salicylate); $T_{1/2}$=15 min (ASA), 2-3 hrs (salicylate). Oxycodone: Urine (8-14%, unchanged); $T_{1/2}$=3.51 hrs.

NURSING CONSIDERATIONS

Assessment: Assess for degree of opioid tolerance, level of pain intensity, type of pain, patient's general condition and medical status, any other conditions where treatment is contraindicated or cautioned, renal/hepatic function, pregnancy/nursing status, and possible drug interactions.

Monitoring: Monitor for signs/symptoms of respiratory depression, elevations in CSF pressure, hypotension, seizures/convulsions, decreased bowel motility in postoperative patients, spasm of sphincter of Oddi, GI ulceration and/or bleeding, physical dependence, tolerance, abuse/addiction, and other adverse reactions. Monitor platelet/renal/hepatic function.

Patient Counseling: Instruct to dispose of unused tabs by flushing down the toilet. Instruct not to adjust dose without consulting physician. Advise that drug may impair mental and/or physical abilities. Instruct to avoid alcohol or other CNS depressants. Advise to consult physician if pregnant, planning to become pregnant, or nursing. Inform that if taking medication for more than a few weeks, to avoid abrupt withdrawal; advise that dosing will need to be tapered. Inform that drug has potential for abuse, to protect it from theft, and not to give to anyone. Advise that drug may cause or worsen constipation; instruct to notify physician for any past history of constipation.

Administration: Oral route. **Storage:** 25°C (77°F); excursions permitted to 15-30°C (59-86°F).

PERFOROMIST   RX
formoterol fumarate (Mylan Specialty)

Long-acting β₂-adrenergic agonists (LABA) may increase risk of asthma-related death. Contraindicated in asthma without use of a long-term asthma control medication.

THERAPEUTIC CLASS: Beta$_2$-agonist

INDICATIONS: Long-term maintenance treatment of bronchoconstriction in patients with chronic obstructive pulmonary disease (COPD), including chronic bronchitis and emphysema.

DOSAGE: *Adults:* 20mcg bid (am and pm) by nebulization. Max: 40mcg/day.

HOW SUPPLIED: Sol, Inhalation: 20mcg/2mL

CONTRAINDICATIONS: Asthma without use of a long-term asthma control medication.

WARNINGS/PRECAUTIONS: Not for acutely deteriorating COPD, or relief of acute symptoms. Cardiovascular (CV) effects and fatalities reported with excessive use; do not use excessively or with other LABA. D/C if paradoxical bronchospasm or CV effects occur. ECG changes reported. Caution with CV disorders, convulsive disorders, thyrotoxicosis, and in patients unusually responsive to sympathomimetic amines. Hypokalemia, hyperglycemia, and immediate hypersensitivity reactions may occur.

ADVERSE REACTIONS: Diarrhea, nausea, CV events, COPD exacerbation, nasopharyngitis, dry mouth.

INTERACTIONS: Adrenergic drugs may potentiate sympathetic effects; use with caution. Xanthine derivatives, steroids, or diuretics may potentiate any hypokalemic effect. ECG changes and/or hypokalemia that may result from non-K⁺ sparing diuretics (eg, loop/thiazide diuretics) can be acutely worsened; use with caution. MAOIs, TCAs, and drugs known to prolong QTc interval may potentiate effect on CV system; use with extreme caution. β-blockers may block effects and produce severe bronchospasm in COPD patients; if needed, consider cardioselective β-blocker with caution.

PREGNANCY: Category C, caution in nursing.

MECHANISM OF ACTION: LABA (β$_2$-agonist); acts as bronchodilator, stimulates intracellular adenyl cyclase, the enzyme that catalyzes the conversion of ATP to cAMP.

PHARMACOKINETICS: Distribution: Plasma protein binding (61-64%). **Metabolism:** Direct glucuronidation via UGT1A1, 1A8, 1A9, 2B7, 2B15; O-demethylation via CYP2D6, 2C19, 2C9, 2A6. **Elimination:** Urine (1.1-1.7%, unchanged).

NURSING CONSIDERATIONS

Assessment: Assess for acute COPD deteriorations, asthma, use of control medication, CV disorders, convulsive disorders, thyrotoxicosis, diabetes mellitus (DM), pregnancy/nursing status, and possible drug interactions. Assess use in patients unusually responsive to sympathomimetic amines.

Monitoring: Monitor for signs of COPD destabilization, serious asthma exacerbations, paradoxical bronchospasm, CV effects, hypokalemia, hyperglycemia, aggravation of DM and ketoacidosis, and immediate hypersensitivity reactions. Monitor pulse rate, BP, ECG changes, serum K⁺, and blood glucose levels.

Patient Counseling: Inform of the risks and benefits of therapy. Instruct to seek medical attention if symptoms worsen despite recommended doses, if treatment becomes less effective, or if short-acting β₂-agonist (eg, albuterol) is needed more than usual. Advise not to ingest inhalation sol, and not to exceed prescribed dose or d/c unless directed by physician. Instruct to d/c regular use of short-acting β₂-agonists and use only for symptomatic relief of acute symptoms. Counsel not to use with other inhalers containing LABA or mix with other drugs. Inform of the common adverse reactions (eg, palpitations, chest pain, rapid HR).

Administration: Oral inhalation route. Administer only via standard jet nebulizer (PARI-LC Plus) connected to an air compressor (Proneb) with adequate airflow and equipped with a facemask or mouthpiece. Remove from foil pouch only immediately before use. **Storage:** Prior to Dispensing: 2-8°C (36-46°F). After Dispensing: 2-25°C (36-77°F) for ≤3 months. Protect from heat.

PERJETA   RX
pertuzumab (Genentech)

> May result in subclinical and clinical cardiac failure; evaluate left ventricular function prior to and during treatment. D/C treatment for a confirmed clinically significant decrease in left ventricular function. Exposure during pregnancy may result in embryo-fetal death and birth defects; advise patients of these risks and the need for effective contraception.

THERAPEUTIC CLASS: Monoclonal antibody/HER2-blocker

INDICATIONS: In combination with trastuzumab and docetaxel, for the treatment of patients with human epidermal growth factor receptor 2 (HER2)-positive metastatic breast cancer who have not received prior anti-HER2 therapy or chemotherapy for metastatic disease, and for the neoadjuvant treatment of patients with HER2-positive, locally advanced, inflammatory, or early stage breast cancer (either >2cm in diameter or node positive) as part of a complete treatment regimen for early breast cancer.

DOSAGE: *Adults:* Initial: 840mg IV infusion over 60 min, followed every 3 weeks by a dose of 420mg IV infusion over 30-60 min. Administer pertuzumab, trastuzumab, and docetaxel sequentially; may give pertuzumab and trastuzumab in any order, then administer docetaxel after pertuzumab and trastuzumab. Observe for 30-60 min after each pertuzumab infusion and before commencement of any subsequent infusion of trastuzumab or docetaxel. Neoadjuvant Treatment of Breast Cancer: Administer preoperatively every 3 weeks for 3-6 cycles; see PI. Refer to PI for trastuzumab and docetaxel dosing and for dose modifications.

HOW SUPPLIED: Inj: 420mg/14mL

WARNINGS/PRECAUTIONS: Monitor for oligohydramnios if pregnancy occurs during therapy; if this occurs, perform fetal testing appropriate for gestational age. Infusion-related reactions reported; observe closely for 60 min after the 1st infusion and for 30 min after subsequent infusions. Consider permanent discontinuation in patients with severe infusion reactions. Hypersensitivity/anaphylaxis reactions reported; medications/emergency equipment should be available for immediate use. Detection of HER2 protein overexpression is necessary for appropriate patient selection. Patients who have received prior anthracyclines or prior radiotherapy to the chest area may be at higher risk of decreased left ventricular ejection fraction (LVEF).

ADVERSE REACTIONS: Cardiac failure, diarrhea, alopecia, neutropenia, N/V, fatigue, rash, peripheral neuropathy, leukopenia, mucosal inflammation, anemia, myalgia, decreased appetite, headache, dyspepsia.

PREGNANCY: Category D, not for use in nursing.

MECHANISM OF ACTION: Monoclonal antibody/HER2 blocker; inhibits ligand-initiated intracellular signaling pathways, which can result in cell growth arrest and apoptosis. Also mediates antibody-dependent cell-mediated cytotoxicity.

PHARMACOKINETICS: Elimination: $T_{1/2}$=18 days (median).

NURSING CONSIDERATIONS

Assessment: Assess for hypersensitivity to drug and pregnancy/nursing status. Assess LVEF prior to initiation of therapy. Assess HER2 status; should be performed by laboratories with demonstrated proficiency in the specific technology being utilized.

Monitoring: Monitor for infusion-related reactions, hypersensitivity/anaphylaxis reactions, and other adverse reactions. Monitor LVEF at regular intervals (eg, every 3 months in the metastatic setting and every 6 weeks in the neoadjuvant setting).

Patient Counseling: Inform that exposure to drug may result in fetal harm, including embryo-fetal death or birth defects; advise females of reproductive potential to use effective contraception while on therapy and for 6 months following the last dose. Instruct to contact physician immediately if pregnancy is suspected. Encourage women exposed to pertuzumab during pregnancy to enroll in the MotHER Pregnancy Registry. Advise not to breastfeed during therapy.

Administration: IV route. Administer as an IV infusion only; do not administer as an IV push or bolus. Do not mix with other drugs. Refer to PI for preparation for administration. **Storage:** 2-8°C

(36-46°F) until time of use. Protect from light. Do not freeze or shake. Diluted Sol: 2-8°C (36-46°F) for up to 24 hrs.

PHENERGAN INJECTION RX
promethazine HCl (Teva)

> Do not use in pediatric patients <2 yrs because of potential for fatal respiratory depression. Caution when used in pediatric patients ≥2 yrs. Injection may cause severe chemical irritation and damage to tissue regardless of the route of administration. Irritation and damage may result from perivascular extravasation, unintentional intra-arterial injection, or intraneuronal/perineuronal infiltration; surgical intervention may be required. Preferred route of administration is deep IM injection.

OTHER BRAND NAMES: Promethazine Injection (Teva)

THERAPEUTIC CLASS: Phenothiazine derivative

INDICATIONS: Amelioration of allergic reactions to blood or plasma. In anaphylaxis as an adjunct to epinephrine and other standard measures after acute symptoms have been controlled. For other uncomplicated allergic conditions of the immediate type when oral therapy is not possible or contraindicated. For sedation and relief of apprehension to produce light sleep. Active treatment of motion sickness. Prevention and control of N/V associated with certain types of anesthesia and surgery. Adjunct to analgesics for the control of postoperative pain. Preoperative, postoperative, and obstetric (during labor) sedation. IV in special surgical situations such as repeated bronchoscopy, ophthalmic surgery, and poor-risk patients, with reduced amounts of meperidine or other narcotic analgesic as adjunct to anesthesia and analgesia.

DOSAGE: *Adults:* (IM/IV) IM route is preferred. Allergy: Initial: 25mg, may repeat within 2 hrs. Adjust to the smallest adequate amount to relieve symptoms. For continued therapy, oral route preferred. Sedation: 25-50mg qhs in hospitalized patients. N/V: Usual: 12.5-25mg, not to be repeated more frequently than q4h. Preoperative/Postoperative Adjunct: 25-50mg. May be combined with appropriately reduced doses of analgesics and atropine-like drugs. Obstetrics: 50mg in early stages of labor, 25-75mg in established labor may be given with an appropriately reduced dose of any desired narcotic; may repeat once or twice q4h in normal labor. Max: 100mg/24 hrs of labor. Do not give IV administration >25mg/mL and rate should not exceed 25mg/min. Elderly: Start at lower end of dosing range.
Pediatrics: ≥2 yrs: Dose should not exceed half of suggested adult dose. Premedication Adjunct: Usual: 1.1 mg/kg body weight in combination with an appropriately reduced dose of narcotic or barbiturate and appropriate dose of an atropine-like drug. Do not give IV administration >25mg/mL and rate should not exceed 25mg/min.

HOW SUPPLIED: Inj: 25mg/mL, 50mg/mL

CONTRAINDICATIONS: Children <2 yrs, comatose states, intra-arterial or SQ injection.

WARNINGS/PRECAUTIONS: Not recommended for uncomplicated vomiting in pediatrics. May impair physical/mental ability. Fatal respiratory depression reported; avoid with compromised respiratory function or patients at risk of respiratory failure (eg, chronic obstructive pulmonary disease [COPD], sleep apnea). May lower seizure threshold. Caution with bone marrow depression; leukopenia and agranulocytosis reported. Neuroleptic malignant syndrome (NMS) reported. Sulfite sensitivity may occur; caution especially in asthmatics. Avoid in pediatrics with Reye's syndrome or other hepatic diseases. Hallucinations and convulsions may occur in pediatrics. Increased susceptibility to dystonias in acutely ill pediatric patients with dehydration. May inhibit platelet aggregation in the newborn when used in pregnant women within 2 weeks of delivery. Caution with narrow-angle glaucoma, prostatic hypertrophy, stenosing peptic ulcer, bladder-neck or pyloroduodenal obstruction, cardiovascular (CV) disease, hepatic dysfunction. Cholestatic jaundice reported. May cause false interpretations of diagnostic pregnancy tests and may increase blood glucose. Caution in the elderly.

ADVERSE REACTIONS: Respiratory depression, severe tissue injury, drowsiness, dizziness, tinnitus, blurred vision, dry mouth, increased or decreased BP, urticaria, N/V, blood dyscrasia, gangrene.

INTERACTIONS: Concomitant use with respiratory depressants in pediatric patients may result in death. May increase, prolong, or intensify sedation when used concomitantly with CNS depressants (eg, alcohol, sedative/hypnotics [including barbiturates], general anesthetics, narcotics, TCAs, tranquilizers); avoid concomitant use or reduce dose. Reduce dose of barbiturates by at least 50% if given concomitantly. Reduce dose of narcotics by 25-50% if given concomitantly. Caution with drugs that alter seizure threshold (eg, narcotics, local anesthetics). Leukopenia and agranulocytosis reported when used with other known marrow-toxic agents. Do not use epinephrine for promethazine injection overdose. Caution with anticholinergics. Possible adverse reactions with MAOIs. NMS reported alone and in combination with antipsychotics.

PREGNANCY: Category C, not for use in nursing.

MECHANISM OF ACTION: Phenothiazine derivative/H₁ receptor antagonist; possesses antihistamine (does not block release of histamine), sedative, anti-motion sickness, antiemetic, and anticholinergic effects.

PHARMACOKINETICS: Metabolism: Liver; sulfoxides, N-desmethylpromethazine (metabolites). **Elimination:** Urine; $T_{1/2}$=9-16 hrs (IV), 9.8 hrs (IM).

NURSING CONSIDERATIONS

Assessment: Assess for history of seizure disorder, compromised respiratory function or risk of respiratory failure (eg, COPD, sleep apnea), bone marrow depression, sulfite hypersensitivity, asthma, narrow-angle glaucoma, prostatic hypertrophy, stenosing peptic ulcer, pyloroduodenal obstruction, bladder-neck obstruction, CV disease, hepatic impairment, pregnancy/nursing status, and for possible drug interactions. Assess age of patient and presence of a comatose state. In pediatrics, assess for Reye's syndrome or presence of acute illness with dehydration.

Monitoring: Monitor for signs/symptoms of respiratory depression, seizures, leukopenia, agranulocytosis, NMS, cholestatic jaundice, injection-site reactions, and for hypersensitivity reactions. Monitor for hallucinations, convulsions, extrapyramidal symptoms and dystonia in pediatrics. In newborns, monitor platelet count, when used in pregnant women within 2 weeks of delivery.

Patient Counseling: Advise regarding risk of respiratory depression and risk of tissue injury. May impair physical/mental abilities. Seek medical attention if symptoms of respiratory depression, seizures, infections, NMS (hyperpyrexia, muscle rigidity, autonomic instability), injection-site reactions (burning, pain, erythema), or hypersensitivity reactions occur. Avoid alcohol, certain other medications with possible interactions, and prolonged sun exposure.

Administration: IV, IM route. If pain occurs during IV injection, stop immediately and evaluate for possible arterial injection or perivascular extravasation. Inspect before use and discard if either color or particulate is observed. **Storage:** 20-25°C (68-77°F). Protect from light.

PHENOBARBITAL
phenobarbital (Various)

CIV

THERAPEUTIC CLASS: Barbiturate

INDICATIONS: As an anticonvulsant for treatment of generalized/partial seizures and as a sedative.

DOSAGE: *Adults:* (Elixir/16.2mg, 32.4mg, 64.8mg, 97.2mg Tab) Individualize dose. Consider age, weight, and condition. Daytime Sedation: 30-120mg in 2-3 divided doses. Max: 400mg/24 hrs. Hypnotic: 100-200mg. Anticonvulsant: 60-200mg/day. Elderly/Debilitated/Renal Impairment or Hepatic Disease: Reduce dose. (15mg, 30mg, 60mg, 100mg Tab) Sedation: 30-120mg/day in 2 or 3 divided doses. Hypnotic: 100-320mg. Anticonvulsant: 50-100mg bid or tid.
Pediatrics: (Elixir/16.2mg, 32.4mg, 64.8mg, 97.2mg Tab) Individualize dose. Consider age, weight, and condition. Anticonvulsant: 3-6mg/kg/day. Debilitated/Renal Impairment or Hepatic Disease: Reduce dose. (15mg, 30mg, 60mg, 100mg Tab) Sedation: 6mg/kg/day in 3 divided doses. Anticonvulsant: 15-50mg bid or tid.

HOW SUPPLIED: Elixir: 20mg/5mL [473mL]; Tab: 15mg, 16.2mg*, 30mg*, 32.4mg*, 60mg, 64.8mg*, 97.2mg*, 100mg* *scored

CONTRAINDICATIONS: Marked impairment of liver function or respiratory disease in which dyspnea or obstruction is evident. (Elixir/16.2mg, 32.4mg, 64.8mg, 97.2mg Tab) History of manifest/latent porphyria. (15mg, 30mg, 60mg, 100mg Tab) Personal or familial history of acute intermittent porphyria, known previous addiction to sedative/hypnotic group.

WARNINGS/PRECAUTIONS: Caution with borderline hypoadrenal function and history of drug abuse or dependence. Caution in patients who are mentally depressed or with suicidal tendencies. Caution when prescribing large amounts to patients with a history of emotional disturbances. Elderly or debilitated patients may react with marked excitement, depression, or confusion. (15mg, 30mg, 60mg, 100mg Tab) May increase reaction to painful stimuli in small doses; cannot be relied upon to relieve pain or even produce sedation or sleep in the presence of severe pain if taken alone. Caution with decreased liver function. (Elixir/16.2mg, 32.4mg, 64.8mg, 97.2mg Tab) Caution with acute or chronic pain; may induce paradoxical excitement or mask important symptoms. Some persons, especially children, may repeatedly produce excitement rather than depression. Caution in patients with hepatic damage; initiate therapy in reduced doses. Avoid in patients showing premonitory signs of hepatic coma. May cause fetal damage. Use during labor may result in respiratory depression in the newborn. Cognitive deficits reported in children taking drug for complicated febrile seizures. May be habit-forming; limit prescription and dispensing to amount required for the interval until the next appointment. Withdraw gradually in patients taking excessive doses over long periods of time.

ADVERSE REACTIONS: Respiratory/CNS depression, apnea, circulatory collapse, hypersensitivity reactions, N/V, headache, somnolence.

INTERACTIONS: May produce additive depressant effects with other CNS depressants (eg, other sedatives/hypnotics, antihistamines, tranquilizers, alcohol). May diminish systemic effects of exogenous corticosteroids (eg, hydrocortisone). Decreased anticoagulant response of oral anticoagulants (eg, warfarin, acenocoumarol, dicumarol, phenprocoumon); determine PT frequently. Dose adjustments of anticoagulants may be required if barbiturates are added to or withdrawn from the dosage regimen. (Elixir/16.2mg, 32.4mg, 64.8mg, 97.2mg Tab) Dose adjustments of corticosteroids may be required if barbiturates are added to or withdrawn from the dosage regimen. May decrease griseofulvin levels; avoid concomitant use. May shorten $T_{1/2}$ of doxycycline for as long as 2 weeks after barbiturate therapy is discontinued; monitor response to doxycycline closely if given concurrently. Monitor phenytoin and barbiturate blood levels frequently when given concurrently. Increased levels with sodium valproate and valproic acid; closely monitor barbiturate blood levels and adjust dose as indicated. MAOIs may prolong effects. May decrease effect of estradiol with pretreatment or with concurrent use. Pregnancy reported with oral contraceptives; may suggest use of alternative contraceptive method.

PREGNANCY: Category B (15mg, 30mg, 60mg, 100mg Tab) and D (Elixir/16.2mg, 32.4mg, 64.8mg, 97.2mg Tab), caution in nursing.

MECHANISM OF ACTION: Barbiturate; CNS depressant. Depresses sensory cortex, decreases motor activity, alters cerebellar function, and produces drowsiness, sedation, and hypnosis.

PHARMACOKINETICS: Distribution: Crosses the placenta; found in breast milk. **Metabolism:** Hepatic. **Elimination:** Urine (25-50% unchanged), feces; $T_{1/2}$=53-118 hrs (adults), 60-180 hrs (children and newborns <48 hrs old).

NURSING CONSIDERATIONS

Assessment: Assess for known barbiturate hypersensitivity, history of porphyria, respiratory disease with evident dyspnea or obstruction, hypoadrenal function, suicidal tendencies, history of drug abuse or dependence, mental depression, hepatic impairment, debilitation, pain, pregnancy/nursing status, and possible drug interactions. (Elixir/16.2mg, 32.4mg, 64.8mg, 97.2mg Tab) Assess for renal impairment.

Monitoring: Monitor for marked excitement, depression, and confusion in elderly and debilitated patients. Monitor for tolerance, psychological and physical dependence, and withdrawal symptoms. Monitor PT frequently if used with coumarin anticoagulants. (Elixir/16.2mg, 32.4mg, 64.8mg, 97.2mg Tab) Monitor for paradoxical excitement and for masking of symptoms in patients with acute/chronic pain. Monitor for cognitive deficits in children with complicated febrile seizures. Perform periodic laboratory evaluation of hematopoietic, renal, and hepatic systems during prolonged therapy.

Patient Counseling: Inform that medication may impair mental/physical abilities required for the performance of potentially hazardous tasks (eg, driving/operating machinery); advise to use caution. (Elixir/16.2mg, 32.4mg, 64.8mg, 97.2mg Tab) Inform of the risk of psychological and/or physical dependence; instruct not to increase dose without consulting physician. Instruct to avoid alcohol while on therapy; inform that use of other CNS depressants (eg, alcohol, narcotics, tranquilizers, antihistamines) may result in additional CNS depressant effects.

Administration: Oral route. **Storage:** 20-25°C (68-77°F). (15mg, 30mg, 60mg, 100mg Tab) Protect from light and moisture.

PHENYTEK   RX
phenytoin sodium (Mylan)

THERAPEUTIC CLASS: Hydantoin

INDICATIONS: Control of generalized tonic-clonic (grand mal) and complex partial (psychomotor, temporal lobe) seizures. Prevention and treatment of seizures during or following neurosurgery.

DOSAGE: *Adults:* Individualize dose. Do not change dose at intervals <7-10 days. Divided Daily Dosing: No Previous Treatment: Initial: 100mg tid. Maint: 100mg tid-qid. Titrate: May increase up to 200mg tid, if necessary. QD Dosing: May consider 300mg qd if seizure is controlled on divided doses of three 100mg caps daily. LD (Clinic/Hospital): Initial: 1g in 3 divided doses (400mg, 300mg, 300mg) at 2-hr intervals. Maint: Start maintenance dose 24 hrs after LD. Do not give oral loading regimen in patients with history of renal/liver disease. Elderly: May require lower or less frequent dosing.
Pediatrics: Individualize dose. Do not change dose at intervals <7-10 days. Initial: 5mg/kg/day in 2 or 3 equally divided doses. Maint: 4-8mg/kg/day. Max: 300mg/day. >6 Yrs: May require the minimum adult dose (300mg/day).

HOW SUPPLIED: Cap, Extended-Release (ER): 200mg, 300mg

CONTRAINDICATIONS: Coadministration with delavirdine.

WARNINGS/PRECAUTIONS: Caution in the interpretation of total phenytoin plasma levels with renal/hepatic disease, or in those with hypoalbuminemia. Avoid abrupt withdrawal; may precipitate status epilepticus. May increase risk of suicidal thoughts/behavior; monitor for emergence/worsening of depression, suicidal thoughts/behavior, and/or any unusual changes in mood/behavior. Serious and sometimes fatal dermatologic reactions, including toxic epidermal necrolysis (TEN) and Stevens-Johnson syndrome (SJS) reported; d/c at 1st sign of rash, unless the rash is clearly not drug-related. Do not resume therapy and consider alternative therapy if signs/symptoms suggest SJS/TEN. Consider avoiding use as an alternative for carbamazepine in patients positive for HLA-B*1502. Drug reaction with eosinophilia and systemic symptoms (DRESS)/multiorgan hypersensitivity reported; evaluate immediately if signs/symptoms (eg, rash, fever, lymphadenopathy) are present and d/c if an alternative etiology cannot be established. Caution with history/immediate family history of hypersensitivity to structurally similar drugs (eg, carboxamides, barbiturates, succinimides, oxazolidinediones); consider alternatives to therapy. Acute hepatotoxicity (eg, acute hepatic failure) reported; d/c immediately and do not readminister. Hematopoietic complications and lymphadenopathy reported; follow-up observation for an extended period is indicated and every effort should be made to achieve seizure control using alternative antiepileptic drugs in all cases of lymphadenopathy. Decreased bone mineral density and bone fractures reported during chronic use; consider screening and initiating treatment as appropriate. Caution with porphyria, hepatic impairment, and in elderly, or gravely ill patients. Increase in seizure frequency may occur during pregnancy. Bleeding disorder in newborns may occur; give vitamin K to mother before delivery and to neonate after birth. Check plasma levels immediately if early signs of dose-related CNS toxicity develop. Hyperglycemia reported; may increase serum glucose levels in diabetics. Not indicated for seizures due to hypoglycemia or other metabolic causes. Not effective for absence (petit mal) seizures; if tonic-clonic (grand mal) and absence (petit mal) seizures are present, combined drug therapy is needed. May produce confusional states at levels sustained above optimal range; reduce dose if plasma levels are excessive, or d/c if symptoms persist. Lab test interactions may occur.

ADVERSE REACTIONS: Rash, nystagmus, ataxia, slurred speech, decreased coordination, somnolence, mental confusion, dizziness, insomnia, transient nervousness, motor twitching, N/V, headache, altered taste sensation, Peyronie's disease.

INTERACTIONS: See Contraindications. Acute alcohol intake, amiodarone, antiepileptic agents (eg, felbamate, oxcarbazepine, topiramate), azoles (eg, fluconazole, ketoconazole, itraconazole), chloramphenicol, chlordiazepoxide, cimetidine, diazepam, disulfiram, estrogens, ethosuximide, fluorouracil, fluoxetine, fluvoxamine, H_2-antagonists, halothane, isoniazid, methylphenidate, phenothiazines, omeprazole, salicylates, sertraline, succinamides, sulfonamides, ticlopidine, tolbutamide, trazodone, and warfarin may increase levels. Carbamazepine, chronic alcohol abuse, nelfinavir, reserpine, ritonavir, and sucralfate may decrease levels. Ingestion times of phenytoin and antacid preparations containing Ca^{2+} should be staggered in patients with low serum phenytoin levels to prevent absorption problems. Phenobarbital, sodium valproate, and valproic acid may increase or decrease levels. May impair efficacy of azoles, corticosteroids, doxycycline, estrogens, furosemide, irinotecan, oral contraceptives, paclitaxel, paroxetine, quinidine, rifampin, sertraline, teniposide, theophylline, vitamin D, and warfarin. Increased and decreased PT/INR responses reported with warfarin. May decrease levels of certain HIV antivirals (eg, amprenavir, efavirenz, lopinavir/ritonavir) and anti-epileptic agents. Avoid with enteral feeding preparations and/or nutritional supplements.

PREGNANCY: Category D, not for use in nursing.

MECHANISM OF ACTION: Hydantoin; inhibits seizure activity by promoting Na^+ efflux from neurons and stabilizing the threshold against hyperexcitability caused by excessive stimulation or environmental changes capable of reducing membrane Na^+ gradient. Reduces the maximal activity of the brain stem centers responsible for the tonic phase of tonic-clonic (grand mal) seizures.

PHARMACOKINETICS: Absorption: T_{max}=4-12 hrs. **Distribution:** Plasma protein binding (high); found in breast milk. **Metabolism:** Liver (hydroxylation). **Elimination:** Bile (mostly inactive metabolites), urine; $T_{1/2}$=22 hrs.

NURSING CONSIDERATIONS

Assessment: Assess for history of hypersensitivity to the drug, its inactive ingredients, or other hydantoins, alcohol use, hepatic/renal impairment, grave illness, porphyria, seizures due to hypoglycemic or other metabolic causes, absence seizures, any other conditions where treatment is cautioned, pregnancy/nursing status, and possible drug interactions.

Monitoring: Monitor for signs/symptoms of hypersensitivity reactions, dermatologic reactions, DRESS/multiorgan hypersensitivity, hepatotoxicity, hematopoietic complications, lymphadenopathy, decreased bone mineral density, bone fractures, exacerbation of porphyria, hyperglycemia, and other adverse reactions. Monitor for emergence/worsening of depression, suicidal thoughts/behavior, and/or any unusual changes in mood/behavior. Monitor serum levels; monitor when switching from a product formulated with the free acid to a another with the Na^+ salt and vice versa.

Patient Counseling: Instruct to take only as prescribed. Advise of the importance of adhering strictly to the prescribed dosage regimen, and of informing physician of any clinical condition in which it is not possible to take the drug orally as prescribed (eg, surgery). Counsel about the early toxic signs/symptoms of potential hematologic, dermatologic, hypersensitivity, or hepatic reactions; instruct to immediately report any occurrence to physician even if mild or when occurring after extended use. Caution on the use of other drugs or alcoholic beverages without first seeking physician's advice. Stress the importance of good dental hygiene to minimize development of gingival hyperplasia and its complications. Advise to notify physician immediately if depression, suicidal thoughts, behavior, or thoughts about self-harm emerge. Encourage patients to enroll in the North American Antiepileptic Drug Pregnancy Registry.

Administration: Oral route. **Storage:** 20-25°C (68-77°F). Protect from light and moisture.

PHOSLYRA   RX
calcium acetate (Fresenius)

THERAPEUTIC CLASS: Phosphate binder

INDICATIONS: To reduce serum phosphorus in end-stage renal disease patients.

DOSAGE: *Adults:* Initial: 10mL with each meal. Titrate: Every 2-3 weeks until acceptable serum phosphorus level is reached. Increase dose gradually to lower serum phosphate levels to the target range, as long as hypercalcemia does not develop. Maint: 15-20mL with each meal.

HOW SUPPLIED: Sol: 667mg/5mL [473mL]

CONTRAINDICATIONS: Hypercalcemia.

WARNINGS/PRECAUTIONS: May develop hypercalcemia. Monitor serum Ca^{2+} twice weekly during early dose adjustment period. If hypercalcemia develops, reduce dose or d/c immediately depending on severity. Chronic hypercalcemia may lead to vascular calcification and other soft-tissue calcification; radiographic evaluation of suspected anatomical region may be helpful in early detection of soft-tissue calcification. Maintain serum calcium-phosphorus (Ca^{2+} x P) product <$55mg^2/dL^2$. Caution in elderly.

ADVERSE REACTIONS: Diarrhea, dizziness, edema, weakness.

INTERACTIONS: Avoid with other Ca^{2+} supplements, including Ca^{2+}-based nonprescription antacids. Hypercalcemia may aggravate digitalis toxicity. May induce laxative effect with other products containing maltitol. May decrease bioavailability of tetracyclines or fluoroquinolones (eg, ciprofloxacin). Administer oral medication where a reduction in the bioavailability of that medication would have a clinically significant effect on its safety/efficacy 1 hr before or 3 hrs after therapy. Monitor blood levels of concomitant drugs that have a narrow therapeutic range.

PREGNANCY: Category C, caution in nursing.

MECHANISM OF ACTION: Phosphate binder; combines with dietary phosphate to form insoluble Ca^{2+}-phosphate complex, resulting in decreased serum phosphorus (P) concentrations.

PHARMACOKINETICS: Distribution: Found in breast milk.

NURSING CONSIDERATIONS

Assessment: Assess for hypercalcemia, pregnancy/nursing status, and for possible drug interactions.

Monitoring: Monitor for hypercalcemia, confusion, delirium, stupor, coma, anorexia, N/V, vascular and other soft-tissue calcification. Monitor serum Ca^{2+} twice weekly early in treatment, during dose adjustment, and periodically thereafter. Monitor for serum P levels periodically.

Patient Counseling: Instruct to take with meals, adhere to prescribed diets, and to avoid use of nonprescription antacids. Inform about symptoms of hypercalcemia. Advise patients who are taking oral medication to take the drug 1 hr before or 3 hrs after calcium acetate.

Administration: Oral route. **Storage:** 25°C (77°F); excursions permitted to 15-30°C (59-86°F).

PLAQUENIL   RX
hydroxychloroquine sulfate (Sanofi-Aventis)

Before prescribing, physicians should be completely familiar with the complete prescribing information.

THERAPEUTIC CLASS: Quinine derivative

INDICATIONS: Suppression and treatment of acute attacks of malaria due to *Plasmodium vivax*, *P. malariae*, *P. ovale* and susceptible strains of *P. falciparum*. Treatment of lupus erythematosus (chronic discoid and systemic) and acute or chronic rheumatoid arthritis (RA).

DOSAGE: *Adults:* Malaria: Suppression: 400mg on exactly the same day of each week. Begin 2 weeks prior to exposure if circumstances permit. If failing this, may give 800mg initial double (loading) dose in 2 divided doses, 6 hrs apart. Continue therapy for 8 weeks after leaving the endemic area. Acute Attack: 800mg, followed by 400mg 6-8 hrs later, then 400mg on each of 2 consecutive days. May also give 800mg single dose as alternative. Lupus Erythematosus: Initial: 400mg qd-bid for several weeks or months depending on response. Prolonged Maint: 200-400mg/day. RA: Initial: 400-600mg qd with meal or milk. May require temporary reduction of the initial dose in some patients with troublesome side effects. Later (5-10 days), may gradually increase dose to optimum response level. Maint: After 4-12 weeks, 200-400mg qd with food or milk. May resume therapy or continue on an intermittent schedule if relapse occurs after drug withdrawal.

Pediatrics: Malaria: Suppression: 5mg/kg (calculated as base/kg) weekly. Max: 400mg/dose. Begin 2 weeks prior to exposure if circumstances permit. If failing this, may give 10mg base/kg in 2 divided doses, 6 hrs apart. Continue therapy for 8 weeks after leaving the endemic area. Acute Attack: 1st Dose: 10mg base/kg. Max: 620mg base single dose. 2nd Dose: 5mg base/kg 6 hrs after 1st dose. Max: 310mg base single dose. 3rd Dose: 5mg base/kg 18 hrs after 2nd dose. 4th Dose: 5mg base/kg 24 hrs after 3rd dose.

HOW SUPPLIED: Tab: 200mg (200mg tab=155mg base)

CONTRAINDICATIONS: Long-term therapy in children or in the presence of retinal/visual field changes attributable to any 4-aminoquinoline compound.

WARNINGS/PRECAUTIONS: Not effective against chloroquine-resistant strains of *P. falciparum*. Carefully examine for visual acuity, central visual field and color vision including fundoscopy prior to long-term therapy; repeat exam at least annually. Irreversible retinal damage reported with long-term or high dosage of 4-aminoquinoline therapy. Perform baseline and periodic (every 3 months) ophthalmologic exams with prolonged therapy. Increased risk of retinal toxicity if recommended daily dose is exceeded sharply. D/C therapy immediately if any visual disturbance occurs and closely observe for possible progression of the abnormality. Retinal and visual disturbances may progress even after discontinuation of therapy. Suicidal behavior reported. May precipitate a severe attack of psoriasis and may exacerbate porphyria; avoid use in these conditions unless benefits outweigh possible hazard. Avoid in pregnancy except in the suppression/treatment of malaria if benefit outweighs the risk. Caution with hepatic disease, alcoholism, and G6PD deficiency. Perform periodic blood cell counts with prolonged therapy; d/c therapy if any severe blood disorder appears which is not attributable to the disease under treatment. (Lupus erythematosus/RA) Examine all patients periodically including testing of knee and ankle reflexes; d/c treatment if muscular weakness occurs. Dermatologic reactions may occur with a significant tendency to produce dermatitis. Caution with impaired renal function and/or metabolic acidosis. In treatment of RA, d/c if no improvement occurs after 6 months.

ADVERSE REACTIONS: Dizziness, headache, convulsions, diarrhea, nervousness, emotional lability, psychosis, suicidal behavior, retinopathy with changes in pigmentation, visual field defects, erythema multiforme, Stevens-Johnson syndrome, toxic epidermal necrolysis, photosensitivity, exfoliative dermatitis.

INTERACTIONS: Caution with hepatotoxic drugs.

PREGNANCY: Safety in pregnancy and nursing not known.

MECHANISM OF ACTION: Quinine derivative; has not been established. Possesses antimalarial action.

NURSING CONSIDERATIONS

Assessment: Assess for retinal or visual field defects, psoriasis, porphyria, hepatic/renal disease, alcoholism, G6PD deficiency, chloroquine-resistant strains of *P. falciparum*, or any other conditions where treatment is contraindicated or cautioned, pregnancy/nursing status, and possible drug interactions. Perform baseline ophthalmologic exams with prolonged therapy.

Monitoring: Monitor for retinal/visual disturbances, severe psoriasis attack, exacerbation of porphyria, dermatologic reactions, and other adverse reactions. Perform periodic (every 3 months) ophthalmologic exams with prolonged therapy and monitor CBC with differential and platelet count. Periodically test for knee and ankle reflexes in RA patients.

Patient Counseling: Counsel about adverse effects and to d/c drug and seek medical attention if any signs/symptoms develop. Advise about need for periodic follow-up.

Administration: Oral route. (RA) Take with meal or glass of milk. **Storage:** Room temperature up to 30°C (86°F).

PLAVIX   RX

clopidogrel bisulfate (Bristol-Myers Squibb/Sanofi-Aventis)

> Effectiveness is dependent on activation to an active metabolite via CYP2C19. Poor metabolizers of CYP2C19 with acute coronary syndrome (ACS) or undergoing percutaneous coronary intervention treated with clopidogrel at recommended doses exhibit higher cardiovascular (CV) event rates than patients with normal CYP2C19 function. Tests are available to identify a patient's CYP2C19 genotype; these tests can be used as an aid in determining therapeutic strategy. Consider alternative treatment or treatment strategies in patients identified as CYP2C19 poor metabolizers.

THERAPEUTIC CLASS: Platelet aggregation inhibitor

INDICATIONS: To decrease the rate of combined endpoint of CV death, myocardial infarction (MI), stroke, or refractory ischemia in patients with non-ST-segment elevation ACS (unstable angina [UA]/non-ST-elevation MI [NSTEMI]), including patients who are to be managed medically and those who are to be managed with coronary revascularization. To reduce the rate of death from any cause and the rate of combined endpoint of death, reinfarction, or stroke in patients with ST-elevation MI (STEMI). To reduce the rate of combined endpoint of new ischemic stroke, new MI, and other vascular death in patients with history of recent MI, recent stroke, or established peripheral arterial disease.

DOSAGE: *Adults:* UA/NSTEMI: LD: 300mg. Maint: 75mg qd. Initiate aspirin (ASA) (75-325mg qd) and continue in combination with clopidogrel. STEMI: 75mg qd with ASA (75-325mg qd), with or without thrombolytics. May initiate with or without a LD. Recent MI/Recent Stroke/Peripheral Arterial Disease: 75mg qd.

HOW SUPPLIED: Tab: 75mg, 300mg

CONTRAINDICATIONS: Active pathological bleeding (eg, peptic ulcer, intracranial hemorrhage).

WARNINGS/PRECAUTIONS: Increases the risk of bleeding; d/c 5 days prior to surgery if an antiplatelet effect is not desired. Avoid lapses in therapy; if therapy must be temporarily discontinued, restart as soon as possible. Premature discontinuation may increase risk of CV events. Thrombotic thrombocytopenic purpura (TTP) reported. Hypersensitivity (eg, rash, angioedema, hematologic reaction) reported, including in patients with a history of hypersensitivity or hematologic reaction to other thienopyridines.

ADVERSE REACTIONS: Bleeding.

INTERACTIONS: Reduced antiplatelet activity with omeprazole or esomeprazole; avoid concomitant use, or consider using another acid-reducing agent with minimal or no CYP2C19 inhibitory effect on the formation of clopidogrel active metabolite when coadministration of a proton pump inhibitor is required. Certain CYP2C19 inhibitors may reduce platelet inhibition. NSAIDs, warfarin, SSRIs, SNRIs, and ASA may increase risk of bleeding.

PREGNANCY: Category B, not for use in nursing.

MECHANISM OF ACTION: Platelet activation and aggregation inhibitor; irreversibly and selectively inhibits the binding of adenosine diphosphate (ADP) to its platelet $P2Y_{12}$ receptor and the subsequent ADP-mediated activation of the glycoprotein GPIIb/IIIa complex.

PHARMACOKINETICS: Absorption: Rapid. T_{max}=30-60 min (active thiol metabolite). **Metabolism:** Extensive via esterases (leading to hydrolysis) and via multiple CYP450 enzymes; active thiol metabolite (principally by CYP2C19). **Elimination:** Urine (50%), feces (46%); $T_{1/2}$=6 hrs, 30 min (active thiol metabolite).

NURSING CONSIDERATIONS

Assessment: Assess for active pathological bleeding, hypersensitivity to drug or another thienopyridine, CYP2C19 genotype, pregnancy/nursing status, and possible drug interactions. Assess use in patients at risk for increased bleeding (eg, undergoing surgery).

Monitoring: Monitor for bleeding, TTP, hypersensitivity, and other adverse reactions.

Patient Counseling: Inform about the benefits and risks of treatment. Instruct to take exactly as prescribed and not to d/c without consulting the prescribing physician. Inform that they will bruise and bleed more easily and that bleeding will take longer than usual to stop. Advise to report any unanticipated, prolonged, or excessive bleeding, or blood in stool or urine. Instruct to seek prompt medical attention if unexplained fever, weakness, extreme skin paleness, purple skin patches, yellowing of the skin or eyes, or neurological changes occur. Instruct to notify physician or dentist about therapy before scheduling any invasive procedure. Advise to inform physician of all medications they are taking or planning to take.

Administration: Oral route. May be administered with or without food. **Storage:** 25°C (77°F); excursions permitted to 15-30°C (59-86°F).

PLETAL

RX

cilostazol (Otsuka America)

Contraindicated with congestive heart failure (CHF) of any severity due to possible decrease in survival.

THERAPEUTIC CLASS: Phosphodiesterase III inhibitor

INDICATIONS: Reduction of symptoms of intermittent claudication.

DOSAGE: *Adults:* Usual: 100mg bid, at least 1/2 hr before or 2 hrs after breakfast and dinner. Concomitant CYP3A4/CYP2C19 Inhibitors: Consider 50mg bid.

HOW SUPPLIED: Tab: 50mg, 100mg

CONTRAINDICATIONS: CHF of any severity. Hemostatic disorders or active pathologic bleeding (eg, peptic ulcer, intracranial bleeding).

WARNINGS/PRECAUTIONS: Thrombocytopenia/leukopenia progressing to agranulocytosis rarely reported. Special caution with moderate/severe hepatic impairment, severe renal impairment (CrCl <25mL/min). Caution with thrombocytopenia and in patients at risk of bleeding from surgery or pathologic processes.

ADVERSE REACTIONS: Headache, palpitation, tachycardia, abnormal stools, diarrhea, peripheral edema, dizziness, infection, rhinitis, pharyngitis, nausea, back pain, dyspepsia.

INTERACTIONS: May increase levels with CYP3A4 inhibitors (eg, ketoconazole, fluvoxamine, erythromycin, grapefruit juice) or CYP2C19 inhibitors (eg, omeprazole); consider reducing dose. Caution with clopidogrel and other antiplatelet agents. Smoking may decrease levels.

PREGNANCY: Category C, not for use in nursing.

MECHANISM OF ACTION: Phosphodiesterase III inhibitor; not established. Suspected to inhibit phosphodiesterase activity and suppress cAMP degradation resulting in an increase of cAMP in platelets and blood vessels, leading to inhibition of platelet aggregation and vasodilation.

PHARMACOKINETICS: Distribution: Plasma protein binding (95-98%). **Metabolism:** Liver (extensive) via CYP450 3A4 (primary), 2C19; 3,4-dehydro-cilostazol, 4'-trans-hydroxy-cilostazol (major active metabolites). **Elimination:** Urine (74%), feces (20%); $T_{1/2}$=11-13 hrs.

NURSING CONSIDERATIONS

Assessment: Assess for CHF, hemostatic disorders, active pathologic bleeding, renal/hepatic function, hypersensitivity to drug, pregnancy/nursing status, and possible drug interactions.

Monitoring: Monitor for signs/symptoms of thrombocytopenia, leukopenia, agranulocytosis, and other adverse reactions.

Patient Counseling: Advise to take at least 30 min before or 2 hrs after food. Inform that benefits of medication may not be immediate; treatment may be required for up to 12 weeks before beneficial effect is experienced.

Administration: Oral route. **Storage:** 25°C (77°F); excursions permitted to 15-30°C (59-86°F).

PNEUMOVAX 23

RX

pneumococcal vaccine polyvalent (Merck)

THERAPEUTIC CLASS: Vaccine

INDICATIONS: Active immunization for the prevention of pneumococcal disease caused by the 23 serotypes contained in the vaccine in persons ≥50 yrs of age and persons aged ≥2 yrs who are at increased risk for pneumococcal disease.

DOSAGE: *Adults:* Single 0.5mL dose SQ/IM into the deltoid muscle or lateral mid-thigh. *Pediatrics:* ≥2 Yrs: Single 0.5mL dose SQ/IM into the deltoid muscle or lateral mid-thigh.

HOW SUPPLIED: Inj: 0.5mL [single-dose, 5-dose vial]

WARNINGS/PRECAUTIONS: Do not inject intravascularly or intradermally. Defer vaccination in patients with moderate or severe acute illness. Caution with severely compromised cardiovascular (CV) and/or pulmonary function in those whom a systemic reaction would pose a significant risk. Does not replace the need for antibiotic prophylaxis (eg, penicillin) against pneumococcal infection; do not d/c use of antibiotic prophylaxis after vaccination in patients who require antibiotic prophylaxis. Response to vaccine may be diminished in immunocompromised individuals. May not prevent pneumococcal meningitis in patients with chronic CSF leakage resulting from congenital lesions, skull fractures, or neurosurgical procedures. Will not prevent disease caused by capsular types of pneumococcus other than those contained in the vaccine. Advisory Committee on Immunization Practices has recommendations for revaccination for persons at high risk who were previously vaccinated with Pneumovax 23; routine revaccination of immunocompetent patients previously vaccinated with a 23-valent vaccine is not recommended.

P

ADVERSE REACTIONS: Local inj-site reactions (eg, pain, soreness, tenderness, swelling, induration, erythema), asthenia, fatigue, myalgia, headache.

INTERACTIONS: Persons receiving immunosuppressive therapies may have a diminished immune response to the vaccine. Reduced immune response to zoster vaccine live with concurrent administration; separate vaccinations by at least 4 weeks.

PREGNANCY: Category C, caution in nursing.

MECHANISM OF ACTION: Vaccine; induces antibodies that enhance opsonization, phagocytosis, and killing of pneumococci by leukocytes and other phagocytic cells.

NURSING CONSIDERATIONS

Assessment: Assess for history of hypersensitivity to any component of the vaccine, health/immune status, vaccination history, compromised CV/pulmonary function, chronic CSF leakage, moderate or severe acute illness, pregnancy/nursing status, and possible drug interactions.

Monitoring: Monitor patients with compromised CV and/or pulmonary function. Monitor for hypersensitivity reactions and for other possible adverse reactions.

Patient Counseling: Inform of potential benefits/risks of vaccination. Inform that the vaccine may not offer 100% protection from pneumococcal infection. With each immunization, provide the patient or parent/guardian with the vaccine information statements required by the National Childhood Vaccine Injury Act of 1986. Instruct to inform physician of any adverse reactions.

Administration: IM or SQ route. Inject into the deltoid muscle or lateral mid-thigh. Do not mix with other vaccines in the same syringe or vial. **Storage:** 2-8°C (36-46°F).

POTABA   RX
aminobenzoate potassium (Glenwood)

THERAPEUTIC CLASS: Vitamin B complex

INDICATIONS: Possibly effective in the treatment of scleroderma, dermatomyositis, morphea, linear scleroderma, pemphigus, and Peyronie's disease.

DOSAGE: *Adults:* 12g/day, given in 4-6 divided doses. Take with meals and at hs with snack. *Pediatrics:* 1g/day, given in divided doses for each 10 lbs of body weight. Take with meals and at hs with snack.

HOW SUPPLIED: Cap: 0.5g

CONTRAINDICATIONS: Concomitant use with sulfonamides.

WARNINGS/PRECAUTIONS: If anorexia or nausea occurs, interrupt therapy until the patient is eating normally again. Caution with renal disease. D/C if hypersensitivity reaction occurs.

ADVERSE REACTIONS: Anorexia, nausea, fever, rash.

INTERACTIONS: See Contraindications.

PREGNANCY: Safety not known in pregnancy/nursing.

MECHANISM OF ACTION: Vitamin B complex; it is suggested that the antifibrosis action is due to its mediation of increased oxygen uptake at the tissue level, which enhances MAO activity and prevents or brings about regression of fibrosis.

NURSING CONSIDERATIONS

Assessment: Assess for renal disease, pregnancy/nursing status, and possible drug interactions.

Monitoring: Monitor for anorexia, nausea, hypersensitivity reactions, and other adverse reactions.

Patient Counseling: Inform of the possible adverse reactions (eg, anorexia, nausea, fever, rash). Advise to d/c if hypersensitivity reaction should occur.

Administration: Oral route. Take with meals and at hs with snack.

PRADAXA   RX
dabigatran etexilate mesylate (Boehringer Ingelheim)

Discontinuing therapy places patients at an increased risk of thrombotic events. If therapy must be discontinued for a reason other than pathological bleeding, consider coverage with another anticoagulant.

THERAPEUTIC CLASS: Direct thrombin inhibitor

INDICATIONS: To reduce the risk of stroke and systemic embolism in patients with nonvalvular atrial fibrillation (A-fib).

DOSAGE: *Adults:* CrCl >30mL/min: Usual: 150mg bid. CrCl 15-30mL/min: Usual: 75mg bid. Concomitant Dronedarone/Systemic Ketoconazole with CrCl 30-50mL/min: Consider reducing dabigatran dose to 75mg bid. Conversion from Warfarin: D/C warfarin and start therapy when INR <2.0. Conversion to Warfarin: Start warfarin 3 days (CrCl ≥50mL/min), 2 days (CrCl 30-50mL/min), or 1 day (CrCl 15-30mL/min) before discontinuing therapy. Conversion from Parenteral Anticoagulants: Start 0-2 hrs before the time that the next dose of parenteral drug was to have been administered, or at time of discontinuation of a continuously administered parenteral drug (eg, IV unfractionated heparin). Conversion to Parenteral Anticoagulant: Wait 12 hrs (CrCl ≥30mL/min) or 24 hrs (CrCl <30mL/min) after last dose before initiating parenteral drug. Surgery and Interventions: D/C 1-2 days (CrCl ≥50mL/min) or 3-5 days (CrCl <50mL/min) before invasive or surgical procedures, if possible. Consider longer times for patients undergoing major surgery, spinal puncture, or placement of a spinal or epidural catheter or port, in whom complete hemostasis may be required.

HOW SUPPLIED: Cap: 75mg, 150mg

CONTRAINDICATIONS: Active pathological bleeding and in patients with mechanical prosthetic heart valve.

WARNINGS/PRECAUTIONS: Periodically monitor renal function as clinically indicated; adjust therapy accordingly. D/C therapy in patients who develop acute renal failure and consider alternative anticoagulant therapy. Increases risk of bleeding and may cause significant and, sometimes, fatal bleeding; promptly evaluate for any signs/symptoms of blood loss. D/C therapy in patients with active pathological bleeding. Renal impairment may increase anticoagulant activity and $T_{1/2}$. Consider administration of platelet concentrates in cases where thrombocytopenia is present or long-acting antiplatelet drugs have been used. Use for the prophylaxis of thromboembolic events in patients with A-fib in the setting of other forms of valvular heart disease (including the presence of a bioprosthetic heart valve) is not recommended.

ADVERSE REACTIONS: GI reactions, bleeding.

INTERACTIONS: Risk factors for bleeding include the concomitant use of other drugs that increase the risk of bleeding (eg, antiplatelet agents, heparin, fibrinolytics, chronic use of NSAIDs). P-glycoprotein (P-gp) inducers (eg, rifampin) may reduce exposure; avoid concomitant use. Concomitant use of P-gp inhibitors (eg, dronedarone, systemic ketoconazole) in patients with renal impairment may increase exposure; consider reducing dose of dabigatran in moderate renal impairment (CrCl 30-50mL/min) and avoid combination in patients with severe renal impairment (CrCl 15-30mL/min). Quinidine, clopidogrel, verapamil, and amiodarone may increase levels.

PREGNANCY: Category C, caution in nursing.

MECHANISM OF ACTION: Direct thrombin inhibitor; prevents the development of a thrombus. Both free and clot-bound thrombin and thrombin-induced platelet aggregation are inhibited by the active moieties.

PHARMACOKINETICS: Absorption: Absolute bioavailability (3-7%); T_{max}=1 hr (fasted, healthy). **Distribution:** Plasma protein binding (35%); V_d=50-70L. **Metabolism:** Esterase-catalyzed hydrolysis, conjugation; acyl glucuronides (active metabolites). **Elimination:** Urine (7%), feces (86%); $T_{1/2}$=12-17 hrs (healthy). Refer to PI for pharmacokinetic parameters in renally impaired patients.

NURSING CONSIDERATIONS

Assessment: Assess for active pathological bleeding, mechanical prosthetic heart valve, history of serious hypersensitivity reaction to drug, A-fib in the setting of other forms of valvular heart disease, risk factors for bleeding, pregnancy/nursing status, and possible drug interactions. Assess renal function.

Monitoring: Monitor for bleeding, GI adverse reactions, hypersensitivity reactions, and other adverse events. Periodically monitor renal function as clinically indicated. When necessary, monitor anticoagulant activity by using activated PTT or ecarin clotting time, and not INR.

Patient Counseling: Instruct to take exactly as prescribed and not to d/c without talking to physician. Instruct to keep drug in original bottle to protect from moisture and not to put it in pill boxes/organizers. When >1 bottle is dispensed, instruct to open only 1 bottle at a time. Instruct to remove only 1 cap from the opened bottle at the time of use and to immediately and tightly close bottle. Inform that bleeding may be longer and occur more easily. Instruct to call physician if any signs/symptoms of bleeding, dyspepsia, or gastritis occur. Instruct to inform physician of intake of dabigatran before any invasive procedure (including dental procedures) is scheduled. Advise patients to list all prescription/OTC medications or dietary supplements they may be taking or planning to take. Instruct to inform physician if patient will have or have had surgery to place a prosthetic heart valve. Instruct that if a dose is missed, to take that dose as soon as possible on the same day or skip it if cannot be taken at least 6 hrs before the next scheduled dose. Instruct not to double dose.

Administration: Oral route. Take with a full glass of water. Swallow cap whole; do not break, chew, or empty the contents. **Storage:** 25°C (77°F); excursions permitted to 15-30°C (59-86°F). Store in original package to protect from moisture. Once bottle is opened, use within 4 months; keep tightly closed.

PRANDIMET   RX
metformin HCl - repaglinide (Novo Nordisk)

> Lactic acidosis may occur due to metformin accumulation; risk increases with conditions such as sepsis, dehydration, excess alcohol intake, hepatic impairment, renal impairment, and acute congestive heart failure (CHF). If acidosis is suspected, d/c and hospitalize patient immediately.

THERAPEUTIC CLASS: Biguanide/meglitinide

INDICATIONS: Adjunct to diet and exercise to improve glycemic control in adults with type 2 diabetes mellitus (DM) who are already treated with a meglitinide and metformin, or who have inadequate glycemic control on a meglitinide alone or metformin alone.

DOSAGE: *Adults:* Individualize dose. Administer bid-tid up to 4mg-1000mg/meal. Take dose within 15-30 min ac. Inadequately Controlled with Metformin Monotherapy: Initial: 1mg-500mg bid. Titrate: Gradually escalate dose (based on glycemic response) to reduce risk of hypoglycemia. Inadequately Controlled with Meglitinide Monotherapy: Initial: 500mg of metformin component bid. Titrate: Gradually escalate dose (based on glycemic response) to reduce GI side effects. Refer to PI if switching from current repaglinide/metformin combination. Max: 10mg-2500mg/day.

HOW SUPPLIED: Tab: (Repaglinide-Metformin) 1mg-500mg, 2mg-500mg

CONTRAINDICATIONS: Renal impairment (eg, SrCr ≥1.5mg/dL [males], ≥1.4mg/dL [females], or abnormal CrCl), acute or chronic metabolic acidosis, including diabetic ketoacidosis, concomitant gemfibrozil.

WARNINGS/PRECAUTIONS: Do not initiate in patients ≥80 yrs of age unless renal function is normal. Temporarily d/c at the time of or prior to intravascular contrast studies with iodinated materials, and withhold for 48 hrs subsequent to the procedure and reinstitute only if renal function is normal. Avoid with hepatic impairment. May cause hypoglycemia; risk increased in elderly, debilitated, or malnourished patients, or with adrenal or pituitary insufficiency. May decrease vitamin B12 levels; measure hematologic parameters annually. Suspend temporarily for any surgical procedure (except minor procedures not associated with restricted food and fluid intake); restart when oral intake is resumed and renal function is normal. Temporary loss of glycemic control may occur when exposed to stress; may need to withhold therapy and temporarily administer insulin. D/C promptly in hypoxic states (eg, acute CHF, shock, acute myocardial infarction). Evaluate promptly for evidence of ketoacidosis or lactic acidosis if laboratory abnormalities or clinical illness develops; d/c immediately if acidosis occurs.

ADVERSE REACTIONS: Lactic acidosis, GI system disorder, symptomatic hypoglycemia, headache, diarrhea, nausea, upper respiratory tract infection.

INTERACTIONS: See Contraindications. May increase C_{max} of fenofibrate. Metformin: Alcohol potentiates effect of metformin on lactate metabolism. Caution with drugs that may affect renal function or result in significant hemodynamic change or may interfere with the disposition of metformin, such as cationic drugs eliminated by renal tubular secretion (eg, amiloride, digoxin, morphine). Cimetidine, furosemide, nifedipine, and ibuprofen may increase levels. Propranolol may decrease levels. May decrease levels of furosemide. Repaglinide: Not for use in combination with NPH-insulin. Risk of hypoglycemia increased with alcohol. Hypoglycemia may be difficult to recognize with β-adrenergic blocking drugs. CYP2C8 inhibitors, CYP3A4 inhibitors, or CYP2C8/3A4 inducers may alter pharmacokinetics and pharmacodynamics. Clarithromycin, deferasirox, fenofibrate, gemfibrozil, itraconazole, ketoconazole, simvastatin, trimethoprim, and OATP1B1 inhibitors (eg, cyclosporine) may increase levels. Levonorgestrel/ethinyl estradiol combination may decrease area under the curve and increase C_{max}. Nifedipine and rifampin may decrease levels. May increase levels of ethinyl estradiol.

PREGNANCY: Category C, not for use in nursing.

MECHANISM OF ACTION: Metformin: Biguanide; decreases hepatic glucose production, decreases intestinal absorption of glucose, and improves insulin sensitivity by increasing peripheral glucose uptake and utilization. Repaglinide: Meglitinide; lowers blood glucose levels by stimulating the release of insulin from the pancreas.

PHARMACOKINETICS: Absorption: Administration of variable doses resulted in different pharmacokinetic parameters. Metformin: Absolute bioavailability (50-60%) (fasted). Repaglinide: Absolute bioavailability (56%); T_{max}=1 hr. **Distribution:** Metformin: V_d=654L. Repaglinide: (IV) V_d=31L; plasma protein binding (>98%). **Metabolism:** Repaglinide: Complete. CYP2C8, 3A4; oxidation, and direct conjugation with glucuronic acid; oxidized dicarboxylic acid (M2), aromatic amine (M1), acyl glucuronide (M7) (major metabolites). **Elimination:** Metformin: Urine (90%); $T_{1/2}$=6.2 hrs (plasma), 17.6 hrs (blood). Repaglinide: Feces (90%, <2% unchanged), urine (8%, 0.1% unchanged); $T_{1/2}$=1 hr.

NURSING CONSIDERATIONS

Assessment: Assess for metabolic acidosis, diabetic ketoacidosis, type of DM, renal/hepatic function, risk factors for lactic acidosis, susceptibility to hypoglycemia, drug hypersensitivity, pregnancy/nursing status, and possible drug interactions. Assess if patient is planning to undergo any surgical procedure or is under any form of stress. Obtain baseline FPG and HbA1c.

Monitoring: Monitor for lactic acidosis, clinical illness, hypoxic states, and other adverse reactions. Monitor renal function, especially in elderly patients, at least annually. Monitor vitamin B12 levels in patients predisposed to develop subnormal vitamin B12 levels. Monitor FPG, HbA1c, and hematologic parameters periodically.

Patient Counseling: Inform of potential risks/advantages of therapy, alternative modes of therapy, the importance of adherence to dietary instructions, regular exercise program, and regular testing of blood glucose, HbA1c, renal function, and hematologic parameters. Inform about risks of hypoglycemia and lactic acidosis, their symptoms and treatment, and predisposing conditions. Instruct to seek medical advice during periods of stress as medication needs may change. Advise to d/c drug immediately and notify physician if unexplained hyperventilation, myalgia, malaise, unusual somnolence, or other nonspecific symptoms occur. Instruct to take drug with meals; if a meal is skipped, instruct to skip the dose for that meal. Counsel against excessive alcohol intake.

Administration: Oral route. **Storage:** ≤25°C (77°F). Protect from moisture.

PRANDIN   RX
repaglinide (Novo Nordisk)

THERAPEUTIC CLASS: Meglitinide

INDICATIONS: Adjunct to diet and exercise to improve glycemic control in adults with type 2 diabetes mellitus (DM).

DOSAGE: *Adults:* Administer dose within 15-30 min ac, bid-qid in response to changes in meal pattern. Initial: Not Previously Treated or HbA1c <8%: 0.5mg. Previously Treated or HbA1c ≥8%: 1mg or 2mg. Titrate: May double preprandial dose up to 4mg at no less than 1-week intervals. Usual Range: 0.5-4mg. Max: 16mg/day. Severe Renal Impairment (CrCl 20-40mL/min): Initial: 0.5mg ac; titrate carefully. Hepatic Impairment: Utilize longer intervals between dose adjustments to fully assess response.

HOW SUPPLIED: Tab: 0.5mg, 1mg, 2mg

CONTRAINDICATIONS: Diabetic ketoacidosis with or without coma, type 1 DM, concomitant gemfibrozil.

WARNINGS/PRECAUTIONS: May cause hypoglycemia; risk increased in elderly, debilitated or malnourished patients, or with adrenal, pituitary, hepatic, or severe renal insufficiency. Loss of glycemic control may occur when exposed to stress; may need to d/c therapy and administer insulin. Secondary failure may occur; assess adequate dose adjustment and adherence to diet before classifying a patient as a secondary failure. Caution with hepatic impairment.

ADVERSE REACTIONS: Hypoglycemia, upper respiratory infection, headache, rhinitis, sinusitis, bronchitis, arthralgia, back pain, N/V, diarrhea, dyspepsia, constipation, paresthesia, chest pain.

INTERACTIONS: See Contraindications. Not for use in combination with NPH-insulin. CYP3A4 and/or CYP2C8 inducers (eg, barbiturates, carbamazepine), CYP3A4 inhibitors (eg, erythromycin), and CYP2C8 inhibitors (eg, montelukast) may alter metabolism; use with caution. OATP1B1 inhibitors (eg, cyclosporine), itraconazole, ketoconazole, clarithromycin, trimethoprim, and deferasirox may increase levels. Rifampin may decrease levels. NSAIDs, highly protein-bound drugs, salicylates, sulfonamides, cyclosporine, chloramphenicol, coumarins, probenecid, MAOIs, β-blockers, alcohol, and >1 glucose-lowering drug may potentiate hypoglycemic action. Thiazides and other diuretics, corticosteroids, phenothiazines, thyroid products, estrogens, oral contraceptives, phenytoin, nicotinic acid, sympathomimetics, calcium channel blockers, and isoniazid tend to produce hyperglycemia and may lead to loss of glycemic control. β-blockers may mask hypoglycemia. May increase ethinyl estradiol levels and levonorgestrel C_{max}. Levonorgestrel/ethinyl estradiol combination and simvastatin may increase C_{max}.

PREGNANCY: Category C, not for use in nursing.

MECHANISM OF ACTION: Meglitinide; lowers blood glucose levels by stimulating the release of insulin from the pancreas.

PHARMACOKINETICS: Absorption: Rapid and complete. Absolute bioavailability (56%); T_{max}=1 hr. See PI for parameters of different doses. **Distribution:** (IV) V_d=31L; plasma protein binding (>98%). **Metabolism:** CYP2C8, 3A4; oxidation, and direct conjugation with glucuronic acid; oxidized dicarboxylic acid (M2), aromatic amine (M1), acyl glucuronide (M7) (major metabolites). **Elimination:** Feces (90%, <2% unchanged), urine (8%, 0.1% unchanged); $T_{1/2}$=1-1.4 hrs.

NURSING CONSIDERATIONS

Assessment: Assess for diabetic ketoacidosis, type 1 DM, adrenal/pituitary/hepatic/severe renal insufficiency, drug hypersensitivity, pregnancy/nursing status, and possible drug interactions. Assess FPG, postprandial glucose (PPG), and HbA1c.

Monitoring: Monitor for hypo/hyperglycemia, secondary failure, and other adverse events. Monitor FPG, PPG, HbA1c, and renal/hepatic function.

Patient Counseling: Inform of potential risks/benefits of therapy, alternative modes of therapy, the importance of adherence to dietary instructions, regular exercise program, and regular blood glucose and HbA1c testing. Inform about risks of hypoglycemia, its symptoms and treatment, and predisposing conditions. Instruct to take drug ac (bid-qid preprandially); if a meal is skipped (or an extra meal is added), instruct to skip (or add) a dose for that meal.

Administration: Oral route. **Storage:** ≤25°C (77°F). Protect from moisture.

PRAVACHOL   RX
pravastatin sodium (Bristol-Myers Squibb)

THERAPEUTIC CLASS: HMG-CoA reductase inhibitor

INDICATIONS: Adjunct to diet to decrease total cholesterol, LDL, apolipoprotein B, and TG levels, and to increase HDL levels in primary hypercholesterolemia and mixed dyslipidemia, elevated serum TG levels, heterozygous familial hypercholesterolemia (≥8 years of age), and in prevention of coronary and cardiovascular disease.

DOSAGE: *Adults:* Initial: 40mg qd. Titrate: May increase to 80mg qd if 40mg qd does not achieve desired cholesterol levels. Significant Renal Impairment: Initial: 10mg qd. Concomitant Lipid-Altering Therapy: Give either 1 hr or more before or at least 4 hrs following the resin. Concomitant Immunosuppressive: Initial: 10mg qhs. Titrate: Increase dose cautiously. Usual Max: 20mg/day. Concomitant Cyclosporine: Limit to 20mg qd. Concomitant Clarithromycin: Limit to 40mg qd.
Pediatrics: 14-18 Yrs: Initial: 40mg qd. Max: 40mg. 8-13 Yrs: Usual: 20mg qd. Max: 20mg. Concomitant Lipid-Altering Therapy: Give either 1 hr or more before or at least 4 hrs following the resin. Concomitant Immunosuppressive: Initial: 10mg qhs. Titrate: Increase dose cautiously. Usual Max: 20mg/day. Concomitant Cyclosporine: Limit to 20mg qd. Concomitant Clarithromycin: Limit to 40mg qd.

HOW SUPPLIED: Tab: 10mg, 20mg, 40mg, 80mg

CONTRAINDICATIONS: Active liver disease or unexplained, persistent elevations of serum transaminases, women who are pregnant or may become pregnant, and nursing mothers.

WARNINGS/PRECAUTIONS: Has not been studied in conditions where the major lipoprotein abnormality is elevation of chylomicrons (Fredrickson Types I and V). Rare cases of rhabdomyolysis with acute renal failure secondary to myoglobinuria reported. Increased risk of rhabdomyolysis in patients with history of renal impairment. Uncomplicated myalgia and myopathy (including immune-mediated necrotizing myopathy [IMNM]) reported; d/c if markedly elevated CPK levels occur or myopathy is diagnosed/suspected. Temporarily withhold if experiencing an acute or serious condition predisposing to development of renal failure secondary to rhabdomyolysis. May cause biochemical liver function abnormalities; perform LFTs prior to initiation of therapy and when clinically indicated. Caution with recent (<6 months) history of liver disease, signs that may suggest liver disease, in heavy alcohol users, and elderly. Fatal and nonfatal hepatic failure reported (rare); promptly interrupt therapy if serious liver injury with clinical symptoms and/or hyperbilirubinemia or jaundice occurs; do not restart if alternate etiology is not found. May blunt adrenal or gonadal steroid hormone production. Evaluate patients who display clinical evidence of endocrine dysfunction.

ADVERSE REACTIONS: N/V, diarrhea, sinus abnormality, rash, fatigue, musculoskeletal pain and trauma, cough, muscle cramps, dizziness, headache, upper respiratory tract infection, influenza, chest pain.

INTERACTIONS: Increased risk of myopathy with cyclosporine, fibrates, niacin (nicotinic acid), erythromycin, clarithromycin, colchicine, and gemfibrozil; caution with colchicine and fibrates, and avoid with gemfibrozil. Niacin may enhance risk of skeletal muscle effects; consider dose reduction. Caution with drugs that may diminish levels or activity of steroid hormones (eg, ketoconazole, spironolactone, cimetidine).

PREGNANCY: Category X, not for use in nursing.

MECHANISM OF ACTION: HMG-CoA reductase inhibitor; inhibits the conversion of HMG-CoA to mevalonate, an early and rate-limiting step in the biosynthetic pathway for cholesterol. Reduces VLDL and TG and increases HDL.

PHARMACOKINETICS: Absorption: Absolute bioavailability (17%); T_{max}=1-1.5 hrs; (fasted) C_{max}=26.5ng/mL, AUC=59.8ng•hr/mL. **Distribution:** Plasma protein binding (50%); found in breast milk. **Metabolism:** Liver (extensive) via isomerization and enzymatic ring hydroxylation; 3α-hydroxyisomeric metabolite (active). **Elimination:** Feces (70%), urine (20%); $T_{1/2}$=1.8 hrs.

NURSING CONSIDERATIONS

Assessment: Assess for active liver disease or unexplained, persistent elevations of serum transaminases, hypersensitivity to the drug, predisposing factors for myopathy, alcohol intake, pregnancy/nursing status, and possible drug interactions. Obtain baseline LFTs.

Monitoring: Monitor for signs/symptoms of rhabdomyolysis and myopathy (including IMNM), endocrine dysfunction, and other adverse reactions. Monitor lipid profile and CPK levels. Perform LFTs when clinically indicated.

Patient Counseling: Advise to report promptly unexplained muscle pain, tenderness, or weakness, particularly if accompanied by malaise or fever or if these muscle signs or symptoms persist after discontinuing. Advise to immediately report any symptoms of liver injury, including fatigue, anorexia, right upper abdominal discomfort, dark urine, or jaundice. Counsel females of childbearing potential on appropriate contraceptive methods while on therapy.

Administration: Oral route. Take with or without food. **Storage:** 25°C (77°F); excursions permitted to 15-30°C (59-86°F). Protect from light.

PRECEDEX   RX
dexmedetomidine HCl (Hospira)

THERAPEUTIC CLASS: Alpha$_2$-agonist

INDICATIONS: For sedation of initially intubated and mechanically ventilated patients during treatment in an intensive care setting. For sedation of non-intubated patients prior to and/or during surgical and other procedures.

DOSAGE: *Adults:* Individualize dose. Administer by continuous infusion (using a controlled infusion device) not to exceed 24 hrs. Intensive Care Unit Sedation: LD: 1mcg/kg IV infusion over 10 min. May not be required for patients being converted from alternate sedative therapy. Maint: 0.2-0.7mcg/kg/hr. Adjust infusion rate to achieve desired level of sedation. Elderly (>65 Yrs)/ Hepatic Impairment: Consider dose reduction. Procedural Sedation: LD: 1mcg/kg (0.5mcg/kg for less invasive procedures [eg, ophthalmic surgery]) IV infusion over 10 min. Maint: Initial: 0.6mcg/kg/hr. Titrate: Adjust to achieve desired clinical effect. Range: 0.2-1mcg/kg/hr. Adjust infusion rate to achieve targeted level of sedation. Awake Fiberoptic Intubation Patients: LD: 1mcg/kg IV infusion over 10 min. Maint: 0.7mcg/kg/hr until endotracheal tube is secured. Elderly (>65 Yrs): LD: 0.5mcg/kg IV infusion over 10 min. Maint: Consider dose reduction. Hepatic Impairment: Consider dose reduction. Concomitant Anesthetics, Sedatives, Hypnotics, or Opioids: May require dose reduction of dexmedetomidine or the concomitant drug.

HOW SUPPLIED: Inj: 100mcg/mL [2mL, vial], 4mcg/mL [50mL, 100mL, bottle]

WARNINGS/PRECAUTIONS: Should be administered only by persons skilled in the management of patients in the intensive care or operating room setting. Monitor patients continuously during administration. Hypotension, bradycardia, and sinus arrest reported; treat appropriately. Hypotension and/or bradycardia may be more pronounced in patients with hypovolemia, diabetes mellitus (DM), chronic HTN, and in elderly. Caution with advanced heart block and/or severe ventricular dysfunction. Transient HTN observed primarily during the LD; reduction of loading infusion rate may be desirable. Arousability and alertness reported in some patients upon stimulation. Withdrawal events reported with intensive care unit sedation; if tachycardia and/or HTN occurs after discontinuation, supportive therapy is indicated. Use beyond 24 hrs has been associated with tolerance, tachyphylaxis, and a dose-related increase in adverse reactions.

ADVERSE REACTIONS: Hypotension, HTN, bradycardia, dry mouth, tachycardia, N/V, atrial fibrillation, fever, anemia, hypovolemia, hypoxia, atelectasis, agitation, respiratory depression/failure.

INTERACTIONS: Coadministration with anesthetics, sedatives, hypnotics, and opioids (eg, sevoflurane, isoflurane, propofol, alfentanil, midazolam) may lead to enhancement of effects; may require dose reduction of dexmedetomidine or the concomitant drug. Caution with vasodilators or negative chronotropic agents.

PREGNANCY: Category C, caution in nursing.

MECHANISM OF ACTION: Selective α$_2$-adrenergic agonist; possesses sedative properties.

PHARMACOKINETICS: Distribution: V_d=118L; plasma protein binding (94%). **Metabolism:** Direct N-glucuronidation, aliphatic hydroxylation (via CYP2A6), and N-methylation. **Elimination:** Urine (95%), feces (4%); $T_{1/2}$=2 hrs.

NURSING CONSIDERATIONS

Assessment: Assess for advanced heart block, severe ventricular dysfunction, hepatic impairment, hypovolemia, DM, chronic HTN, pregnancy/nursing status, and possible drug interactions.

Monitoring: Monitor for hypotension, bradycardia, sinus arrest, transient HTN, withdrawal events, and other adverse reactions.

Patient Counseling: When infused for >6 hrs, instruct to report nervousness, agitation, and headaches that may occur for up to 48 hrs. Instruct to report symptoms that occur within 48 hrs after administration (eg, weakness, confusion, excessive sweating, weight loss, abdominal pain, salt cravings, diarrhea, constipation, dizziness, lightheadedness).

Administration: IV route. Do not coadminister through the same IV catheter with blood or plasma. Refer to PI for preparation and administration instructions and compatibility information.
Storage: 25°C (77°F); excursions allowed from 15-30°C (59-86°F).

PRECOSE RX
acarbose (Bayer Healthcare)

THERAPEUTIC CLASS: Alpha-glucosidase inhibitor

INDICATIONS: Adjunct to diet and exercise to improve glycemic control in adults with type 2 diabetes mellitus.

DOSAGE: *Adults:* Initial: 25mg tid with 1st bite of each main meal. May also initiate at 25mg qd to minimize GI side effects then increase gradually to 25mg tid. Titrate: After reaching 25mg tid, may increase to 50mg tid at 4- to 8-week intervals, then further to 100mg tid PRN. Maint Range: 50-100mg tid. Max: >60kg: 100mg tid. ≤60kg: 50mg tid. If no further reduction in postprandial glucose or HbA1c observed with 100mg tid, consider reducing dose.

HOW SUPPLIED: Tab: 25mg, 50mg, 100mg

CONTRAINDICATIONS: Diabetic ketoacidosis, cirrhosis, inflammatory bowel disease, colonic ulceration, partial intestinal obstruction or predisposition to it, chronic intestinal diseases with marked disorders of digestion or absorption, and conditions that may deteriorate from increased intestinal gas formation.

WARNINGS/PRECAUTIONS: Not recommended with significant renal dysfunction (SrCr >2mg/dL). Elevated serum transaminase levels, fulminant hepatitis, and hyperbilirubinemia reported; monitor serum transaminase levels every 3 months for 1st year, then periodically. Reduce dose or d/c if elevated serum transaminases persist. Loss of control of blood glucose may occur when exposed to stress; temporary insulin therapy may be necessary. Pneumatosis cystoides intestinalis reported; d/c and perform appropriate diagnostic imaging if this is suspected. Reduce dose temporarily or permanently if strongly distressing symptoms develop in spite of adherence to the diabetic diet. Inhibits hydrolysis of sucrose to glucose and fructose; use oral glucose (dextrose) instead of sucrose (cane sugar) in treatment of mild to moderate hypoglycemia.

ADVERSE REACTIONS: Flatulence, diarrhea, abdominal pain.

INTERACTIONS: Closely observe for loss of blood glucose control with thiazides and other diuretics, corticosteroids, phenothiazines, thyroid products, estrogens, oral contraceptives, phenytoin, nicotinic acid, sympathomimetics, calcium channel blockers, and isoniazid. Intestinal adsorbents (eg, charcoal) and digestive enzyme preparations containing carbohydrate-splitting enzymes (eg, amylase, pancreatin) may reduce effect; avoid concomitant use. May affect digoxin bioavailability; may require dose adjustment of digoxin. May reduce peak plasma level of metformin. Increased potential for hypoglycemia with insulin or sulfonylureas; adjust dose if hypoglycemia occurs.

PREGNANCY: Category B, not for use in nursing.

MECHANISM OF ACTION: α-glucosidase inhibitor; competitively and reversibly inhibits pancreatic α-amylase and membrane-bound intestinal α-glucoside hydrolase enzymes.

PHARMACOKINETICS: Absorption: Active Drug: Bioavailability (<2%); T_{max}=1 hr. **Metabolism:** GI tract by intestinal bacteria and digestive enzymes; 4-methylpyrogallol derivatives (major metabolites). **Elimination:** Urine (<2%), feces (51%, unabsorbed); $T_{1/2}$=2 hrs.

NURSING CONSIDERATIONS

Assessment: Assess for renal dysfunction, diabetic ketoacidosis, cirrhosis, inflammatory bowel disease, colonic ulceration, partial intestinal obstruction or predisposition to it, chronic intestinal diseases with marked disorders of digestion or absorption, conditions that may deteriorate from increased intestinal gas formation, previous hypersensitivity to the drug, pregnancy/nursing status, and possible drug interactions.

Monitoring: Monitor FPG, HbA1c, LFTs, and renal function. Monitor serum transaminases every 3 months for 1st year, then periodically. Monitor for signs/symptoms of hypoglycemia and pneumatosis cystoides intestinalis.

Patient Counseling: Instruct to take tid at the start of each main meal. Inform about importance of adhering to dietary instructions, a regular exercise program, and regular testing of urine and blood glucose. Counsel about risks, signs/symptoms, treatment of hypoglycemia, and conditions that predispose to its development. Instruct to have readily available source of glucose (dextrose, D-glucose) to treat symptoms of low blood sugar. Inform that side effects (GI effects such as flatulence, diarrhea, abdominal discomfort) usually develop during the 1st few weeks of therapy and generally diminish in frequency and intensity with time.

Administration: Oral route. **Storage:** ≤25°C (≤77°F). Protect from moisture.

PRED FORTE   RX
prednisolone acetate (Allergan)

THERAPEUTIC CLASS: Corticosteroid

INDICATIONS: Treatment of steroid-responsive inflammation of the palpebral and bulbar conjunctiva, cornea, and anterior segment of the globe.

DOSAGE: *Adults:* Instill 1-2 drops into the conjunctival sac bid-qid. May increase dosing frequency if necessary during the initial 24-48 hrs. Reevaluate if signs/symptoms fail to improve after 2 days.

HOW SUPPLIED: Sus: 1% [1mL, 5mL, 10mL, 15mL]

CONTRAINDICATIONS: Most viral diseases of the cornea and conjunctiva (eg, epithelial herpes simplex keratitis [dendritic keratitis], vaccinia, varicella), mycobacterial infection of the eye, and fungal diseases of ocular structures.

WARNINGS/PRECAUTIONS: Prolonged use may result in glaucoma with damage to the optic nerve, defects in visual acuity and fields of vision, and in posterior subcapsular cataract formation; caution with glaucoma. Prolonged use may suppress the host immune response and increase the hazard of secondary ocular infections. Use of topical corticosteroids in the presence of thin corneal or scleral tissue, which may be caused by various ocular diseases or long-term use of topical corticosteroids, may lead to perforation. Acute purulent infections of the eye may be masked or activity enhanced. Routinely monitor intraocular pressure (IOP) if used for ≥10 days. May delay healing and increase incidence of bleb formation after cataract surgery. May prolong the course and may exacerbate the severity of many viral infections of the eye (including herpes simplex). Caution with history of herpes simplex; frequent slit lamp microscopy is recommended. Contains sodium bisulfite; allergic-type reactions, including anaphylactic symptoms and life-threatening or less severe asthmatic episodes in certain susceptible patients, may occur. Initial prescription and renewal of the medication order beyond 20mL of sus should be made only after examination of the patient with the aid of magnification (eg, slit lamp biomicroscopy) and, where appropriate, fluorescein staining. Fungal infections of the cornea may develop coincidentally with long-term use; suspect fungal invasion in any persistent corneal ulceration and take fungal cultures when appropriate. Caution not to d/c therapy prematurely. Not effective in mustard gas keratitis and Sjogren's keratoconjunctivitis.

ADVERSE REACTIONS: Elevation of IOP, glaucoma, optic nerve damage, posterior subcapsular cataract formation, delayed wound healing, acute anterior uveitis, perforation of globe, burning/stinging upon instillation, ocular irritation, secondary ocular infection, visual disturbance, foreign body sensation.

PREGNANCY: Category C, not for use in nursing.

MECHANISM OF ACTION: Glucocorticoid; inhibits the edema, fibrin deposition, capillary dilation, and phagocytic migration of the acute inflammatory response, as well as capillary proliferation, deposition of collagen, and scar formation.

PHARMACOKINETICS: Distribution: Found in breast milk (systemically administered).

NURSING CONSIDERATIONS

Assessment: Assess for previous drug hypersensitivity, viral diseases of the cornea and conjunctiva, mycobacterial infection of the eye, fungal diseases of ocular structures, glaucoma, thinning of the cornea/sclera, history of herpes simplex, and pregnancy/nursing status. Perform examination of patient with the aid of magnification (eg, slit lamp biomicroscopy, fluorescein staining). Assess use in patients who have undergone recent cataract surgery.

Monitoring: Monitor for glaucoma with damage to the optic nerve, defects in visual acuity and fields of vision, posterior subcapsular cataract formation, perforation of the cornea/sclera, secondary ocular infections, fungal infections, masking of existing infections, and other adverse reactions. Reevaluate if signs/symptoms fail to improve after 2 days. Monitor IOP during prolonged use (≥10 days). Perform examination of patient with the aid of magnification (eg, slit lamp biomicroscopy, fluorescein staining) before renewal of medication order beyond 20mL.

Patient Counseling: Advise to d/c use and consult physician if inflammation or pain persists >48 hrs or becomes aggravated. Instruct to use caution to avoid touching the bottle tip to eyelids or to any other surface to prevent contamination. Inform that the use of the bottle by >1 person may spread infection. Instruct to keep the bottle tightly closed when not in use.

Administration: Ocular route. Shake well before use. **Storage:** ≤25°C (77°F) in an upright position. Protect from freezing.

Pᴿᴇᴅɴɪꜱᴏɴᴇ   RX
prednisone (Roxane)

THERAPEUTIC CLASS: Glucocorticoid

INDICATIONS: Steroid-responsive disorders.

DOSAGE: *Adults:* Individualize dose. Initial: 5-60mg/day depending on disease and response. Maint: Decrease dose by small amounts to lowest effective dose. Withdraw gradually after long-term therapy. Acute Exacerbations of Multiple Sclerosis (MS): 200mg/day for 1 week followed by 80mg qod for 1 month. Alternate Day Therapy (ADT): Twice the usual daily dose administered every other am. Refer to PI for detailed information for ADT. Elderly: Start at lower end of dosing range.
Pediatrics: Individualize dose. Initial: 5-60mg/day depending on disease and response. Maint: Decrease dose by small amounts to lowest effective dose. Withdraw gradually after long-term therapy. Acute Exacerbations of MS: 200mg/day for 1 week followed by 80mg qod for 1 month. ADT: Twice the usual daily dose administered every other am. Refer to PI for detailed information for ADT.

HOW SUPPLIED: Sol: 5mg/mL [30mL], 5mg/5mL [120mL, 500mL]; Tab: 1mg*, 2.5mg*, 5mg*, 10mg*, 20mg*, 50mg* *scored

CONTRAINDICATIONS: Systemic fungal infections.

WARNINGS/PRECAUTIONS: Rare instances of anaphylactoid reactions reported. May need to increase dose before, during, and after stressful situations. May cause BP elevation, salt/water retention, increased K⁺ excretion. Caution in patients with left ventricular free wall rupture after a recent myocardial infarction. May produce reversible hypothalamic-pituitary-adrenal axis suppression with the potential for glucocorticosteroid insufficiency after withdrawal. Changes in thyroid status may necessitate dose adjustment. May increase susceptibility to infections, mask signs of current infection, activate latent disease, or exacerbate intercurrent infections. May exacerbate systemic fungal infections; avoid use unless needed to control drug reactions. Rule out latent or active amebiasis before initiating therapy. Caution with known or suspected *Strongyloides* infestation, active/latent tuberculosis (TB) or tuberculin reactivity, active/latent peptic ulcers, diverticulitis, fresh intestinal anastomoses, and nonspecific ulcerative colitis. Not for use in cerebral malaria and active ocular herpes simplex. More serious/fatal course of chickenpox and measles reported. May produce posterior subcapsular cataracts, glaucoma with possible optic nerve damage, and enhance establishment of secondary ocular infections. Not recommended in optic neuritis treatment. Avoid abrupt withdrawal. Drug-induced secondary adrenocortical insufficiency may be minimized by gradual dose reduction. Enhanced effect in patients with cirrhosis. May decrease bone formation and increase bone resorption, and may lead to inhibition of bone growth in pediatric patients and development of osteoporosis at any age. Acute myopathy reported with use of high doses. Creatinine kinase elevation, psychiatric derangements, and aggravation of emotional instability or psychotic tendencies may occur. May elevate intraocular pressure (IOP); monitor IOP if used for >6 weeks. May suppress reactions to skin tests.

ADVERSE REACTIONS: Anaphylactoid reactions, HTN, osteoporosis, muscle weakness, menstrual irregularities, insomnia, impaired wound healing, ulcerative esophagitis, increased sweating, decreased carbohydrate tolerance, glaucoma, weight gain, nausea, malaise, anemia.

INTERACTIONS: Live or live, attenuated vaccines are contraindicated with immunosuppressive doses. May diminish response to toxoids and live or inactivated vaccines. Hypokalemia may develop with K⁺-depleting agents (eg, amphotericin B, diuretics). Cardiac enlargement and congestive heart failure (CHF) may occur with concomitant use of amphotericin B. Macrolide antibiotics may decrease clearance. May produce severe weakness in myasthenia gravis patients with anticholinesterase agents (eg, neostigmine, pyridostigmine); d/c anticholinesterase agents at least 24 hrs before start of therapy and monitor for possible respiratory support if concomitant therapy must occur. Monitor coagulation indices frequently with warfarin. Dose adjustment of antidiabetic agents may be required. May decrease serum concentration of isoniazid. Caution with bupropion; employ low initial dosing and small gradual increase. Cholestyramine may increase clearance. Convulsions and increased activity of both drugs reported with cyclosporine. Digitalis glycosides may increase risk of arrhythmias due to hypokalemia. Estrogens may decrease hepatic metabolism, thereby increasing their effect. Increased risk of tendon rupture in elderly with concomitant fluoroquinolones. CYP3A4 inducers (eg, barbiturates, phenytoin, carbamazepine, rifampin) may enhance metabolism and may require increase in corticosteroid dose. CYP3A4 inhibitors (eg, ketoconazole, ritonavir, erythromycin) may increase plasma concentrations. Other drugs that are metabolized by CYP3A4 (eg, indinavir, erythromycin) may increase their clearance, resulting in decreased plasma concentration. Increased risk of corticosteroid side effects with ketoconazole. Aspirin (ASA) or other NSAIDs may increase risk of GI side effects. Caution with ASA in hypoprothrombinemia patients. May increase clearance of salicylates. Decreased therapeutic effect with phenytoin. Increased doses of quetiapine may be required to maintain control of schizophrenia symptoms. Caution with thalidomide; toxic epidermal necrolysis reported. Acute myopathy reported with neuromuscular blocking drugs (eg, pancuronium).

PREGNANCY: Category C, not for use in nursing.

MECHANISM OF ACTION: Anti-inflammatory glucocorticoid; causes profound and varied metabolic effects and modifies the body's immune responses to diverse stimuli.

PHARMACOKINETICS: Absorption: Readily absorbed (GI tract). **Distribution:** Found in breast milk (systemically administered).

NURSING CONSIDERATIONS

Assessment: Assess for vaccination history, unusual stress, CHF, HTN, renal impairment, systemic fungal/other current infections, active TB, thyroid status, risk of osteoporosis, emotional instability or psychotic tendencies, any other condition where treatment is cautioned, pregnancy/nursing status, and possible drug interactions.

Monitoring: Monitor for adrenocortical insufficiency, salt/water retention, new infections, change in thyroid status, posterior subcapsular cataracts, glaucoma, optic nerve damage, secondary ocular infections, Kaposi's sarcoma, psychiatric derangements, emotional instability or aggravation of psychotic tendencies, and other adverse reactions. Monitor IOP, BP, serum K^+ and Ca^{2+} levels. Monitor growth and development of infants/children on prolonged therapy (including bone growth) and for hypoadrenalism in infants born to mothers who received substantial doses.

Patient Counseling: Instruct not to d/c therapy abruptly or without medical supervision. Advise to avoid exposure to chickenpox or measles; instruct to report immediately if exposed. Advise regarding dietary salt restriction and K^+ supplementation.

Administration: Oral route. Refer to PI for further administration instructions. **Storage:** 25°C (77°F); excursions permitted to 15-30°C (59-86°F). (Tab) Protect from moisture.

PREMARIN TABLETS   RX
conjugated estrogens (Wyeth)

> Estrogens increase the risk of endometrial cancer. Perform adequate diagnostic measures, including endometrial sampling, to rule out malignancy with undiagnosed persistent or recurring abnormal genital bleeding. Should not be used for the prevention of cardiovascular disease or dementia. Increased risks of myocardial infarction (MI), stroke, invasive breast cancer, pulmonary embolism (PE), and deep vein thrombosis (DVT) in postmenopausal women (50-79 yrs of age) reported. Increased risk of developing probable dementia in postmenopausal women ≥65 yrs of age reported. Should be prescribed at the lowest effective dose for the shortest duration consistent with treatment goals and risks.

THERAPEUTIC CLASS: Estrogen

INDICATIONS: Treatment of moderate to severe vasomotor symptoms and/or vulvar/vaginal atrophy due to menopause. Treatment of hypoestrogenism due to hypogonadism, castration, or primary ovarian failure. Palliative treatment of breast cancer in patients with metastatic disease. Palliative treatment of advanced androgen-dependent carcinoma of the prostate. Prevention of postmenopausal osteoporosis.

DOSAGE: *Adults:* Vasomotor Symptoms/Vulvar and Vaginal Atrophy/Prevention of Osteoporosis: Initial: 0.3mg qd continuously or cyclically (eg, 25 days on, 5 days off). Adjust subsequent dose based on response [including bone mineral density [BMD] response for osteoporosis]. Female Hypogonadism: 0.3 or 0.625mg qd cyclically (eg, 3 weeks on and 1 week off). Adjust dose based on severity of symptoms and response of the endometrium. Female Castration/Primary Ovarian Failure: 1.25mg qd cyclically. Adjust dose based on severity of symptoms and response. Breast Cancer: 10mg tid for minimum 3 months. Prostate Cancer: 1.25-2.5mg (two 1.25mg) tid. Use lowest effective dose and for the shortest duration consistent with treatment goals and risk. Reevaluate at 3- to 6-month intervals.

HOW SUPPLIED: Tab: 0.3mg, 0.45mg, 0.625mg, 0.9mg, 1.25mg

CONTRAINDICATIONS: Undiagnosed abnormal genital bleeding, known/suspected/history of breast cancer unless being treated for metastatic disease, known/suspected estrogen-dependent neoplasia, active/history of DVT/PE, active/history of arterial thromboembolic disease (eg, stroke, MI), liver dysfunction/disease, thrombophilic disorders (eg, protein C, protein S, or antithrombin deficiency), known/suspected pregnancy.

WARNINGS/PRECAUTIONS: Increased risk of stroke, DVT, PE, and MI reported; d/c immediately if any of these events occur or are suspected. Caution in patients with risk factors for arterial vascular disease and/or venous thromboembolism. If feasible, d/c at least 4-6 weeks before surgery of the type associated with an increased risk of thromboembolism, or during periods of prolonged immobilization. May increase risk of breast/endometrial/ovarian cancer, and gallbladder disease. Consider addition of progestin for women with a uterus or with residual endometriosis post-hysterectomy. May lead to severe hypercalcemia in patients with breast cancer and bone metastases; d/c and take appropriate measures if hypercalcemia occurs. Retinal vascular thrombosis reported; if visual abnormalities or migraine occurs, d/c pending examination. If examination reveals papilledema or retinal vascular lesions, d/c permanently. Anaphylaxis and angioedema involving tongue, larynx, face, hands, and feet requiring medical intervention reported; d/c if anaphylactic reaction with or without angioedema occurs. May induce or exacerbate symptoms of angioedema, particularly in women with hereditary angioedema. May elevate BP and thyroid-binding globulin levels. May elevate plasma TG; consider discontinuation if pancreatitis occurs. Caution with history of cholestatic jaundice associated with past estrogen use or with pregnancy; d/c in case of recurrence. May cause fluid retention. Caution with hypoparathyroidism; hypocalcemia may occur. May exacerbate endometriosis, asthma, diabetes mellitus (DM), epilepsy, migraine, porphyria, systemic lupus erythematosus (SLE), and hepatic hemangiomas. May affect certain endocrine and blood components in laboratory tests.

ADVERSE REACTIONS: Abdominal pain, asthenia, back pain, headache, infection, pain, arthralgia, leg cramps, breast pain, vaginal hemorrhage, vaginitis, flatulence, flu syndrome, diarrhea, nausea.

INTERACTIONS: CYP3A4 inducers (eg, St. John's wort, phenobarbital, carbamazepine, rifampin) may decrease levels, which may decrease therapeutic effects and/or change uterine bleeding profile. CYP3A4 inhibitors (eg, erythromycin, ketoconazole, ritonavir, grapefruit juice) may increase levels. Women concomitantly receiving thyroid hormone replacement therapy and estrogens may require increased doses of their thyroid replacement therapy.

PREGNANCY: Contraindicated in pregnancy, not for use in nursing.

MECHANISM OF ACTION: Estrogen; binds to nuclear receptors in estrogen-responsive tissues. Reduces elevated levels of gonadotropins, luteinizing hormone, and follicle-stimulating hormone in postmenopausal women.

PHARMACOKINETICS: Absorption: Well-absorbed; PO administration of variable doses resulted in different parameters; refer to PI. **Distribution:** Largely bound to sex hormone-binding globulin and albumin; found in breast milk. **Metabolism:** Liver to estrone (metabolite), estriol (major urinary metabolite); sulfate and glucuronide conjugation (liver); gut hydrolysis; CYP3A4 (partial metabolism). **Elimination:** Urine (parent drug and metabolites).

NURSING CONSIDERATIONS

Assessment: Assess for undiagnosed abnormal genital bleeding, estrogen-dependent neoplasia, presence or history of breast cancer, arterial thromboembolic disease, DVT/PE, thrombophilic disorders, previous hypersensitivity, or any other conditions where treatment is contraindicated or cautioned. Assess for cardiac or renal dysfunction, pregnancy/nursing status, need for progestin therapy, and possible drug interactions.

Monitoring: Monitor for signs/symptoms of cardiovascular events, malignant neoplasms, dementia, gallbladder disease, hypercalcemia, visual abnormalities, pancreatitis, hypertriglyceridemia, elevated BP, cholestatic jaundice, hypothyroidism, fluid retention, exacerbation of endometriosis and other conditions. Perform annual breast exam; schedule mammography based on age, risk factors, and prior mammogram results. Periodically evaluate (3- to 6-month intervals), including BMD, to determine need for therapy. Monitor thyroid function in women on thyroid replacement therapy. If undiagnosed persistent or recurring genital bleeding occurs; perform adequate diagnostic measures (eg, endometrial sampling) to rule out malignancies.

Patient Counseling: Inform that drug increases risk for uterine cancer, heart attack, stroke, breast cancer, blood clots, and dementia. Instruct to report any breast lumps, unusual vaginal bleeding, dizziness and faintness, changes in speech, severe headaches, chest pain, SOB, leg pains, changes in vision, or vomiting. Advise to notify physician if planning surgery or bed rest. Instruct to take medication at same time daily and to perform monthly self-breast exams. Instruct to take exactly ud.

Administration: Oral route. **Storage:** 20-25°C (68-77°F); excursions permitted to 15-30°C (59-86°F).

PREMARIN VAGINAL   RX
conjugated estrogens (Wyeth)

Estrogens increase the risk of endometrial cancer. Perform adequate diagnostic measures, including endometrial sampling, to rule out malignancy with undiagnosed persistent or recurring abnormal genital bleeding. Should not be used for the prevention of cardiovascular disease (CVD) or dementia. Increased risks of myocardial infarction (MI), stroke, invasive breast cancer, pulmonary embolism (PE), and deep vein thrombosis (DVT) in postmenopausal women (50-79 yrs of age) reported. Increased risk of developing probable dementia in postmenopausal women ≥65 yrs of age reported. Should be prescribed at the lowest effective dose for the shortest duration consistent with treatment goals and risks.

THERAPEUTIC CLASS: Estrogen

INDICATIONS: Treatment of atrophic vaginitis and kraurosis vulvae, and moderate to severe dyspareunia, a symptom of vulvar and vaginal atrophy due to menopause.

DOSAGE: *Adults:* Atrophic Vaginitis/Kraurosis Vulvae: Initial: 0.5g intravaginally cyclically (21 days on, then 7 days off). Titrate: May increase to 0.5-2g based on individual response. Moderate to Severe Dyspareunia: 0.5g intravaginally 2X/week (eg, Monday and Thursday) continuously or cyclically (21 days on, then 7 days off).

HOW SUPPLIED: Cre: 0.625mg/g [30g, 42.5g]

CONTRAINDICATIONS: Undiagnosed abnormal genital bleeding, known/suspected/history of breast cancer, known/suspected estrogen-dependent neoplasia, active/history of DVT/PE, active/history of arterial thromboembolic disease (eg, stroke, MI), liver dysfunction/disease, thrombophilic disorders (eg, protein C, protein S, or antithrombin deficiency), or known/suspected pregnancy.

WARNINGS/PRECAUTIONS: D/C therapy immediately if stroke, DVT, PE, or MI occurs or are suspected. Caution in patients with risk factors for arterial vascular disease and/or venous thromboembolism (VTE). If feasible, d/c at least 4-6 weeks before surgery of the type associated with an increased risk of thromboembolism, or during periods of prolonged immobilization. May increase risk of gallbladder disease requiring surgery and ovarian cancer. Consider addition of progestin for women with a uterus or with residual endometriosis post-hysterectomy. May lead to severe hypercalcemia in patients with breast cancer and bone metastases; d/c and take appropriate measures if hypercalcemia occurs. Retinal vascular thrombosis reported; if visual abnormalities or migraine occurs, d/c pending examination. If examination reveals papilledema or retinal vascular lesions, d/c permanently. May elevate BP, thyroid-binding globulin levels, and plasma TG. Consider discontinuation if pancreatitis occurs. Caution with history of cholestatic jaundice associated with past estrogen use or pregnancy; d/c in case of recurrence. May cause fluid retention. Caution with hypoparathyroidism; hypocalcemia may occur. Anaphylaxis and angioedema reported with PO treatment. May induce or exacerbate symptoms of angioedema in women with hereditary angioedema. May exacerbate endometriosis, asthma, diabetes mellitus (DM), epilepsy, migraine, porphyria, systemic lupus erythematosus (SLE), and hepatic hemangiomas. May weaken and contribute to the failure of condoms, diaphragms, or cervical caps made of latex or rubber. May affect certain endocrine and blood components in laboratory tests.

ADVERSE REACTIONS: Breast pain, headache.

INTERACTIONS: CYP3A4 inducers (eg, St. John's wort, phenobarbital, carbamazepine, rifampin) may decrease levels, which may decrease therapeutic effects and/or change uterine bleeding profile. CYP3A4 inhibitors (eg, erythromycin, ketoconazole, ritonavir, grapefruit juice) may increase levels. Women concomitantly receiving thyroid hormone replacement therapy and estrogens may require increased doses of thyroid replacement therapy.

PREGNANCY: Contraindicated in pregnancy, not for use in nursing.

MECHANISM OF ACTION: Estrogen; binds to nuclear receptors in estrogen-responsive tissues. Reduces elevated levels of gonadotropins, luteinizing hormone, and follicle-stimulating hormone in postmenopausal women.

PHARMACOKINETICS: Absorption: Well-absorbed through the skin and mucus membranes; refer to PI for parameters. **Distribution:** Largely bound to sex hormone-binding globulin and albumin; found in breast milk. **Metabolism:** Liver to estrone (metabolite), estriol (major urinary metabolite); sulfate and glucuronide conjugation (liver); gut hydrolysis; CYP3A4 (partial metabolism). **Elimination:** Urine (parent compound and metabolites).

NURSING CONSIDERATIONS

Assessment: Assess for abnormal genital bleeding, estrogen-dependent neoplasia, presence/history of breast cancer, arterial thromboembolic disease, DVT/PE, hereditary angioedema, previous hypersensitivity, thrombophilic disorders, or any other conditions where treatment is contraindicated or cautioned. Assess use in women ≥65 yrs of age, those with DM, asthma, epilepsy, migraines or porphyria, SLE, and hepatic hemangiomas. Assess for cardiac or renal dysfunction, pregnancy/nursing status, need for progestin therapy, and possible drug interactions.

Monitoring: Monitor for signs/symptoms of cardiovascular events, malignant neoplasms, dementia, gallbladder disease, hypercalcemia, visual abnormalities, pancreatitis, hypertriglyceridemia, cholestatic jaundice, hypothyroidism, fluid retention, exacerbation of endometriosis and other conditions. Perform annual breast exam; schedule mammography based on age, risk factors, and prior mammogram results. Regularly monitor BP, thyroid function in women on thyroid replacement therapy, and periodically evaluate to determine need for treatment. Perform adequate diagnostic measures (eg, endometrial sampling) to rule out malignancies if undiagnosed persistent or recurring genital bleeding occurs.

Patient Counseling: Advise to notify physician if signs/symptoms of unusual vaginal bleeding occur. Inform about possible serious adverse reactions (eg, CVD, malignant neoplasms, and probable dementia) and possible less serious but common adverse reactions (eg, headache, breast pain/tenderness, N/V). Instruct on how to use the applicator. Instruct to perform monthly breast self-examination. Inform that medication may weaken barrier contraceptives (eg, latex or rubber condoms, diaphragms, cervical caps).

Administration: Intravaginal route. Refer to PI for instructions on use of applicator. **Storage:** 20-25°C (68-77°F); excursions permitted to 15-30°C (59-86°F).

PREMPHASE   RX
medroxyprogesterone acetate - conjugated estrogens (Wyeth)

> Estrogens increase the risk of endometrial cancer. Perform adequate diagnostic measures, including endometrial sampling, to rule out malignancy in postmenopausal women with undiagnosed persistent or recurring abnormal genital bleeding. Should not be used for the prevention of cardiovascular disease (CVD) or dementia. Increased risk of myocardial infarction (MI), stroke, invasive breast cancer, pulmonary embolism (PE), and deep vein thrombosis (DVT) in postmenopausal women (50-79 yrs of age) reported. Increased risk of developing probable dementia in postmenopausal women ≥65 yrs of age reported. Should be prescribed at the lowest effective dose and for the shortest duration consistent with treatment goals and risks.

OTHER BRAND NAMES: Prempro (Wyeth)

THERAPEUTIC CLASS: Estrogen/progestogen combination

INDICATIONS: Treatment of moderate to severe vasomotor symptoms and/or vulvar and vaginal atrophy due to menopause, and prevention of postmenopausal osteoporosis.

DOSAGE: *Adults:* (Premphase) One 0.625mg tab qd on Days 1-14 and one 0.625mg-5mg tab qd on Days 15-28. (Prempro) 1 tab qd. Reevaluate treatment need periodically.

HOW SUPPLIED: Tab: (Premphase) (Conjugated Estrogens [CE]) 0.625mg, (CE-Medroxyprogesterone) 0.625mg-5mg; (Prempro) (CE-Medroxyprogesterone) 0.3mg-1.5mg, 0.45mg-1.5mg, 0.625mg-2.5mg, 0.625mg-5mg

CONTRAINDICATIONS: Undiagnosed abnormal genital bleeding, known/suspected/history of breast cancer, known/suspected estrogen-dependent neoplasia, active or history of DVT/PE/ arterial thromboembolic disease (eg, stroke, MI), known liver dysfunction/disease, known protein C/protein S/antithrombin deficiency, or other known thrombophilic disorders, known/suspected pregnancy.

WARNINGS/PRECAUTIONS: D/C immediately if PE, DVT, stroke, or MI occurs or is suspected. Caution in patients with risk factors for arterial vascular disease and/or venous thrombo-embolism (VTE). If feasible, d/c at least 4-6 weeks before surgery of the type associated with an increased risk of thromboembolism, or during periods of prolonged immobilization. May increase risk of gallbladder disease requiring surgery. May lead to severe hypercalcemia in patients with breast cancer and bone metastases; d/c and take appropriate measures if hypercalcemia occurs. Retinal vascular thrombosis reported; d/c pending examination if sudden partial/complete loss of vision or sudden onset of proptosis, diplopia, or migraine occurs. D/C permanently if examination reveals papilledema or retinal vascular lesions. May increase BP and thyroid-binding globulin levels. May be associated with elevations of plasma TG; consider discontinuation if pancreatitis occurs. Caution with history of cholestatic jaundice associated with past estrogen use or with pregnancy; d/c in case of recurrence. May cause fluid retention. Caution with hypoparathyroid-ism; hypocalcemia may occur. Anaphylaxis and angioedema reported. May exacerbate symptoms of angioedema in women with hereditary angioedema. May exacerbate endometriosis, asthma, DM, epilepsy, migraine, porphyria, SLE, and hepatic hemangiomas. May affect certain endocrine and blood components in laboratory tests.

ADVERSE REACTIONS: MI, stroke, invasive breast cancer, PE, DVT, probable dementia, breast pain, headache, abdominal pain, dysmenorrhea, nausea, depression, leukorrhea, flatulence, asthenia.

INTERACTIONS: CYP3A4 inducers (eg, St. John's wort, phenobarbital, carbamazepine, rifampin) may decrease levels, which may decrease therapeutic effects and/or change uterine bleed-ing profile. CYP3A4 inhibitors (eg, erythromycin, ketoconazole, ritonavir, grapefruit juice) may increase levels. Aminoglutethimide may significantly depress bioavailability of medroxyproges-terone acetate (MPA). Patients concomitantly receiving thyroid hormone replacement therapy and estrogens may require increased doses of their thyroid replacement therapy; monitor thyroid function.

PREGNANCY: Contraindicated in pregnancy, not for use in nursing.

MECHANISM OF ACTION: CE: Estrogen; binds to nuclear receptors in estrogen-responsive tis-sues. Reduces elevated levels of gonadotropins, luteinizing hormone, and follicle-stimulating hor-mone in postmenopausal women. MPA: Progesterone derivative; parenterally administered MPA inhibits gonadotropin production, which prevents follicular maturation and ovulation.

PHARMACOKINETICS: Absorption: Well-absorbed. Administration of variable doses resulted in different parameters. **Distribution:** Found in breast milk. CE: Largely bound to sex hormone-binding globulin and albumin. MPA: Plasma protein binding (90%). **Metabolism:** CE: Liver to estrone (metabolite) and estriol (major urinary metabolite); enterohepatic recirculation via sulfate and glucuronide conjugation in the liver; biliary secretion of conjugates into the intestine; hydrolysis in the intestine; reabsorption. MPA: Liver via hydroxylation, with subsequent conjugation. **Elimination:** CE: Urine (parent compound and metabolites). MPA: Urine (metabolites).

NURSING CONSIDERATIONS

Assessment: Assess for abnormal genital bleeding, presence/history of breast cancer, estrogen-dependent neoplasia, active or history of DVT/PE/arterial thromboembolic disease, liver dysfunction/disease, thrombophilic disorders, known anaphylactic reaction or angioedema to the drug, cardiac or renal dysfunction, other conditions where treatment is contraindicated or cautioned, pregnancy/nursing status, and possible drug interactions.

Monitoring: Monitor for signs/symptoms of CVD, malignant neoplasms, dementia, gallbladder disease, hypercalcemia, visual abnormalities, BP and plasma TG elevations, pancreatitis, cholestatic jaundice, hypothyroidism, fluid retention, anaphylaxis, angioedema, and exacerbation of endometriosis and other conditions. Perform annual breast examinations; schedule mammography based on patient age, risk factors, and prior mammogram results. Perform adequate diagnostic measures (eg, endometrial sampling) in patients with undiagnosed persistent or recurring genital bleeding. Perform periodic evaluation to determine treatment need.

Patient Counseling: Inform of the importance of reporting abnormal vaginal bleeding to physician as soon as possible. Advise of possible serious adverse reactions of therapy (eg, CVD, malignant neoplasms, probable dementia) and of possible less serious but common adverse reactions (eg, headache, breast pain and tenderness, N/V). Instruct to have yearly breast examinations by a healthcare provider and perform monthly breast self-examinations.

Administration: Oral route. **Storage:** 20-25°C (68-77°F); excursions permitted to 15-30°C (59-86°F).

PREPOPIK   RX
sodium picosulfate - magnesium oxide - anhydrous citric acid (Ferring)

THERAPEUTIC CLASS: Bowel cleanser

INDICATIONS: Cleansing of the colon as a preparation for colonoscopy in adults.

DOSAGE: *Adults:* Split-Dose Regimen: Take 1st dose during pm before the colonoscopy (eg, 5-9 pm), followed by five 8-oz. drinks of clear liquids before bed (consume within 5 hrs). Take 2nd dose next day, 5 hrs before the colonoscopy, followed by at least three 8-oz. drinks of clear liquids before the colonoscopy (consume within 5 hrs up until 2 hrs before the time of colonoscopy). Day-Before Regimen: Take 1st dose in afternoon or early pm (eg, 4-6 pm) before the colonoscopy followed by five 8 oz. drinks of clear liquids before next dose (consume within 5 hrs). Take 2nd dose 6 hrs later in the late pm (eg, 10 pm-12 am) the night before the colonoscopy followed by three 8 oz. drinks before bed (consume within 5 hrs). If severe bloating, distention, or abdominal pain occurs following the 1st dose, delay the 2nd dose until symptoms resolve.

HOW SUPPLIED: Sol (powder): (Na Picosulfate-Magnesium Oxide-Anhydrous Citric Acid) 10mg-3.5g-12g [16.1g]

CONTRAINDICATIONS: Severely reduced renal function (CrCl <30mL/min), GI obstruction or ileus, bowel perforation, toxic colitis or toxic megacolon, gastric retention.

WARNINGS/PRECAUTIONS: May cause fluid/electrolyte disturbances, arrhythmias, and generalized tonic-clonic seizures; correct fluid and electrolyte abnormalities prior to treatment. Caution with congestive heart failure (CHF) when replacing fluids. If vomiting or signs of dehydration (including signs of orthostatic hypotension) develops after treatment, perform postcolonoscopy lab tests (eg, electrolytes, SrCr, BUN) and treat accordingly. Caution with impaired renal function and severe ulcerative colitis. May produce colonic mucosal aphthous ulceration. Serious cases of ischemic colitis reported. Caution in patients prone to regurgitation/aspiration or with impaired gag reflex. Direct ingestion of undissolved powder may increase risk of N/V, dehydration, and electrolyte disturbance. Rule out GI obstruction/perforation before administration.

ADVERSE REACTIONS: Orthostatic changes, electrolyte abnormalities, headache, N/V, abdominal distention/pain/cramping.

INTERACTIONS: Increased risk of colonic mucosal aphthous ulceration with stimulant laxatives. Caution with drugs that increase the risk of fluid and electrolyte abnormalities, affect renal function (eg, diuretics, ACE inhibitors, angiotensin receptor blockers, NSAIDs), drugs associated with hypokalemia (eg, corticosteroid, cardiac glycosides) or hyponatremia, drugs that lower seizure threshold (eg, TCAs), drugs known to induce antidiuretic hormone secretion (eg, SSRIs, antipsychotics, carbamazepine), and in patients withdrawing from alcohol or benzodiazepines. Caution with drugs that increase the risk for arrhythmias and prolonged QT in the setting of fluid and electrolyte abnormalities. Oral medications given within 1 hr of administration may be flushed from GI tract and may not be absorbed. Take tetracycline and fluoroquinolone antibiot-

P

ics, iron, digoxin, chlorpromazine, and penicillamine at least 2 hrs before and not <6 hrs after administration. Reduced efficacy with antibiotics.

PREGNANCY: Category B, caution in nursing.

MECHANISM OF ACTION: Bowel cleanser: Stimulant and osmotic laxative; produces a purgative effect which produces watery diarrhea.

PHARMACOKINETICS: Absorption: Na Picosulfate: C_{max}=3.2ng/mL, T_{max}=7 hrs. Magnesium: (Post initial pkt) C_{max}=1.9mEq/L, T_{max}=10 hrs. **Metabolism:** Na Picosulfate: intestinal bacteria to bis-(p-hydroxy-phenyl)-pyridyl-2-methane (active metabolite). **Elimination:** Na Picosulfate: Urine (0.19% unchanged), $T_{1/2}$=7.4 hrs.

NURSING CONSIDERATIONS

Assessment: Assess for previous hypersensitivity to any of the components, electrolyte abnormalities, risk for arrhythmias, CHF, seizures, renal impairment, ileus, GI obstruction/perforation, gastric retention, toxic colitis/megacolon, ulcerative colitis, impaired gag reflex, regurgitation or aspiration tendencies, pregnancy/nursing status, and possible drug interactions. Perform predose lab tests (eg, electrolytes, SrCr, BUN) and ECG.

Monitoring: Monitor for fluid/electrolyte disturbances, arrhythmias, seizures, GI ulceration, colitis, bloating, abdominal distention/pain, and other adverse reactions. Perform postcolonoscopy lab tests and ECG.

Patient Counseling: Advise to adequately hydrate before, during, and after use. Instruct not to take other laxatives during therapy. Inform that if they experience severe bloating, distention or abdominal pain, delay the 2nd administration until the symptoms resolve. Instruct to contact their healthcare provider if they develop signs/symptoms of dehydration, have trouble swallowing, or are prone to regurgitation or aspiration. Inform that product is not for direct ingestion.

Administration: Oral route. Refer to PI reconstitution instruction. **Storage:** 25°C (77°F); excursions permitted to 15-30°C (59-86°F).

PREVACID   RX
lansoprazole (Takeda)

OTHER BRAND NAMES: Prevacid SoluTab (Takeda)

THERAPEUTIC CLASS: Proton pump inhibitor

INDICATIONS: Short-term treatment of active duodenal ulcer (DU), active benign gastric ulcer (GU), and erosive esophagitis (EE). Maint of healing of DU and EE. Treatment and risk reduction of NSAID-associated GU. Treatment of heartburn and other symptoms associated with gastroesophageal reflux disease (GERD). Long-term treatment of pathological hypersecretory conditions (eg, Zollinger-Ellison syndrome). Combination therapy with amoxicillin +/- clarithromycin for *Helicobacter pylori* eradication to reduce the risk of DU recurrence.

DOSAGE: *Adults:* Take before eating. DU: Short-Term Treatment: 15mg qd for 4 weeks. Maint of Healing of DU: 15mg qd. Short-Term Treatment of Benign GU: 30mg qd for up to 8 weeks. NSAID-associated GU: Healing: 30mg qd for 8 weeks. Risk Reduction: 15mg qd for up to 12 weeks. GERD: Short-Term Treatment of Symptomatic GERD: 15mg qd for up to 8 weeks. Short-Term Treatment of EE: 30mg qd for up to 8 weeks. May give for 8 more weeks if healing does not occur. If there is recurrence of EE, an additional 8-week course may be considered. Maint of Healing of EE: 15mg qd. Pathological Hypersecretory Conditions: Initial: 60mg qd. Titrate: Individualize dose. Max: 90mg bid. Divide dose if >120mg/day. *H. pylori* Eradication to Reduce Risk of DU Recurrence: Triple Therapy: 30mg + amoxicillin 1000mg + clarithromycin 500mg, all bid (q12h) for 10 or 14 days. Dual Therapy: 30mg + amoxicillin 1000mg, both tid (q8h) for 14 days. Severe Hepatic Impairment: Consider dose adjustment.
Pediatrics: Take before eating. 12-17 Yrs: Short-Term Treatment of Symptomatic GERD: Nonerosive GERD: 15mg qd for up to 8 weeks. EE: 30mg qd for up to 8 weeks. 1-11 Yrs: Short-Term Treatment of Symptomatic GERD/EE: >30kg: 30mg qd for up to 12 weeks; may increase up to 30mg bid after ≥2 weeks if symptomatic. ≤30kg: 15mg qd for up to 12 weeks; may increase up to 30mg bid after ≥2 weeks if symptomatic. Severe Hepatic Impairment: Consider dose adjustment.

HOW SUPPLIED: Cap, Delayed-Release: 15mg, 30mg; Tab, Disintegrating (SoluTab): 15mg, 30mg

WARNINGS/PRECAUTIONS: Symptomatic response does not preclude the presence of gastric malignancy. May increase risk for *Clostridium difficile*-associated diarrhea (CDAD), especially in hospitalized patients. May increase risk for osteoporosis-related fractures of the hip, wrist, or spine, especially with high-dose and long-term therapy. Use lowest dose and shortest duration appropriate to the condition being treated. Hypomagnesemia reported; Mg^{2+} replacement and discontinuation of therapy may be required. (Tab, Disintegrating) Contains phenylalanine.

ADVERSE REACTIONS: Abdominal pain, constipation, diarrhea, nausea, dizziness, headache.

INTERACTIONS: Substantially decreases atazanavir concentrations; concomitant use is not recommended. May alter absorption of other drugs where gastric pH is an important determinant of oral bioavailability (eg, ampicillin esters, digoxin, iron salts, ketoconazole). Delayed absorption and reduced bioavailability with sucralfate; give at least 30 min prior to sucralfate. May increase theophylline clearance; may require theophylline dose titration when lansoprazole is started or stopped. Monitor for increases in INR and PT with warfarin. May increase tacrolimus levels. May elevate and prolong levels of methotrexate leading to toxicities; consider temporary withdrawal of therapy with high-dose methotrexate. Caution with digoxin or other drugs that may cause hypomagnesemia (eg, diuretics).

PREGNANCY: Category B, not for use in nursing.

MECHANISM OF ACTION: Proton pump inhibitor; suppresses gastric acid secretion by specific inhibition of the (H^+/K^+)-ATPase enzyme system at the secretory surface of the gastric parietal cell.

PHARMACOKINETICS: Absorption: Rapid; absolute bioavailability (>80%); T_{max}=1.7 hrs. **Distribution:** Plasma protein binding (97%). **Metabolism:** Liver (extensive). **Elimination:** Urine (1/3), feces (2/3); $T_{1/2}$=<2 hrs.

NURSING CONSIDERATIONS

Assessment: Assess for hepatic insufficiency, risk for osteoporosis, phenylketonuria, previous hypersensitivity to the drug, pregnancy/nursing status, and possible drug interactions. Obtain baseline Mg^{2+} levels.

Monitoring: Monitor for signs/symptoms of bone fractures, CDAD, hypersensitivity reactions, and other adverse reactions. Monitor Mg^{2+} levels periodically.

Patient Counseling: Advise to seek immediate medical attention if diarrhea does not improve or cardiovascular/neurological symptoms (eg, palpitations, dizziness, seizures, tetany) develop. Instruct to take exactly ud. Inform of alternative methods of administration if patient has swallowing difficulties.

Administration: Oral route. Take before eating. May also be administered via NG tube. Do not crush, break, cut, or chew. Swallow caps whole. Allow tab to disintegrate on tongue until particles can be swallowed. Refer to PI for additional administration instructions. **Storage:** 25°C (77°F); excursions permitted to 15-30°C (59-86°F).

PREVPAC

RX

clarithromycin - lansoprazole - amoxicillin (Takeda)

P

THERAPEUTIC CLASS: *H. pylori* treatment combination

INDICATIONS: Treatment of *H. pylori* infection associated with active duodenal ulcer and to reduce the risk of duodenal ulcer recurrence.

DOSAGE: *Adults:* 1g amoxicillin, 500mg clarithromycin and 30mg lansoprazole, all bid (am and pm) ac for 10 or 14 days. Swallow each pill whole. Renal Impairment (with or without hepatic impairment): Decrease clarithromycin dose or prolong intervals.

HOW SUPPLIED: Cap: (Amoxicillin) 500mg, Tab: (Clarithromycin) 500mg, Cap, Delayed-Release: (Lansoprazole) 30mg

CONTRAINDICATIONS: Concomitant use with cisapride, pimozide, astemizole, terfenadine, ergotamine, or dihydroergotamine.

WARNINGS/PRECAUTIONS: Serious and occasional fatal hypersensitivity reactions reported in patients on penicillin (PCN) therapy. Avoid if CrCl <30mL/min. Caution with cephalosporin/PCN allergy; anaphylactic reactions have been reported. Pseudomembranous colitis reported. D/C if superinfections occur. Caution in elderly. Do not use clarithromycin during pregnancy. Symptomatic response to lansoprazole does not preclude the presence of gastric malignancy. *Clostridium difficile*-associated diarrhea (CDAD) reported. D/C if confirmed. Exacerbation of symptoms with myasthenia gravis and new onset of myasthenic syndrome reported with clarithromycin.

ADVERSE REACTIONS: Diarrhea, taste perversion, headache, abdominal pain, dark stools, myalgia, confusion, respiratory disorders, skin reactions, vaginitis.

INTERACTIONS: See Contraindications. Lansoprazole: May interfere with absorption of drugs dependent on gastric pH for bioavailability (eg, ketoconazole, ampicillin esters, iron salts, digoxin). Monitor increase in INR and PT with concomitant use of warfarin. Amoxicillin: May decrease renal tubular secretion when coadministered with probenecid. May interfere with bactericidal effects of PCN with chloramphenicol, macrolides, sulfonamides, and tetracycline. Clarithromycin: May increase theophylline and carbamazepine levels. Simultaneous administration with zidovudine resulted in decreased steady-state zidovudine levels in HIV-infected patients. Elevated digoxin levels in patients receiving concomitant digoxin. May lead to increased exposure to colchicine when coadministered; monitor for toxicity. May increase or prolong both therapeutic and adverse effects with erythromycin. Torsades de pointes may occur with quinidine or disopyramide. May increase systemic exposure of sildenafil; consider dose reduction.

PREGNANCY: Category C, not for use in nursing.

MECHANISM OF ACTION: Lansoprazole: Substituted benzimidazole; inhibits gastric acid secretion. Amoxicillin: Semi-synthetic antibiotic; has broad spectrum of bactericidal activity against many gram-positive and gram-negative microorganisms. Clarithromycin: Semi-synthetic macrolide antibiotic.

PHARMACOKINETICS: Absorption: Lansoprazole: Rapidly absorbed; absolute bioavailability (80%); T_{max}=1.7 hrs. Amoxicillin: Rapidly absorbed. Clarithromycin: Rapidly absorbed; absolute bioavailability (50%); T_{max}=2-2.5 hrs. **Distribution:** Lansoprazole: Plasma protein binding (97%); found in breast milk. Amoxicillin: Plasma protein binding (approximately 20%). Clarithromycin: Found in breast milk. **Metabolism:** Lansoprazole: Liver (extensive). Clarithromycin: 14-OH clarithromycin (active metabolite). **Elimination:** Lansoprazole: Urine, feces; $T_{1/2}$=<2 hrs. Amoxicillin: Urine (60%); $T_{1/2}$=61.3 min. Clarithromycin: Urine (30%); $T_{1/2}$=5-7 hrs; (metabolite) $T_{1/2}$=7-9 hrs.

NURSING CONSIDERATIONS

Assessment: Assess for hypersensitivity to other macrolides, PCNs, or cephalosporins. Assess for proper diagnosis of susceptible bacteria (eg, cultures), pregnancy/nursing status, renal impairment, gastric malignancy, presence of bacterial infection, and possible drug interactions.

Monitoring: Monitor for signs/symptoms of drug interactions, hypersensitivity reactions, pseudomembranous colitis and CDAD, and development of superinfections.

Patient Counseling: Instruct to take each dose twice per day before eating; swallow pill whole. Instruct to notify physician of all medications currently being taken. Inform that drug treats bacterial, not viral, infections. Instruct to take exactly ud; skipping doses may decrease effectiveness and increase antibiotic resistance. Instruct to avoid pregnancy/nursing during therapy and contact physician if diarrhea occurs.

Administration: Oral route. **Storage:** 20-25°C (68-77°F). Protect from light and moisture.

PREZISTA   RX
darunavir (Janssen)

THERAPEUTIC CLASS: Protease inhibitor

INDICATIONS: Treatment of HIV-1 infection in adult and pediatric (≥3 yrs of age) patients in combination with ritonavir (RTV) and other antiretroviral agents.

DOSAGE: *Adults:* Treatment-Naive/Treatment-Experienced with No Darunavir Resistance Associated Substitutions: 800mg (one 800mg tab, two 400mg tabs, or two 4mL sus administrations) with RTV 100mg qd. Treatment-Experienced with At Least 1 Darunavir Resistance Associated Substitution or with No Feasible Genotypic Testing: 600mg (one 600mg tab or 6mL sus) with RTV 100mg bid. Take with food. Refer to PI for dose modifications when used with certain concomitant therapies.
Pediatrics: 3-<18 Yrs: Refer to PI for appropriate dose based on body weight (kg). Do not exceed recommended adult dose. Take with food. Refer to PI for dose modifications when used with certain concomitant therapies.

HOW SUPPLIED: Sus: 100mg/mL [200mL]; Tab: 75mg, 150mg, 400mg, 600mg, 800mg

CONTRAINDICATIONS: Concomitant use with drugs that are highly dependent on CYP3A for clearance and for which elevated plasma concentrations are associated with serious and/or life-threatening events, and with certain other drugs that may lead to reduced efficacy of darunavir (eg, alfuzosin, dihydroergotamine, ergonovine, ergotamine, methylergonovine, cisapride, pimozide, oral midazolam, triazolam, St. John's wort, lovastatin, simvastatin, rifampin, sildenafil [when used to treat pulmonary arterial HTN]).

WARNINGS/PRECAUTIONS: Must be coadministered with RTV and food to achieve desired effect. Drug-induced hepatitis and liver injury reported; perform appropriate laboratory testing prior to therapy and monitor during treatment; consider performing increased AST/ALT monitoring in patients with underlying chronic hepatitis, cirrhosis, or those with pretreatment transaminase elevations. Consider interruption or discontinuation of therapy if evidence of new/worsening liver dysfunction occurs. Increased risk for liver function abnormalities in patients with preexisting liver dysfunction, including chronic active hepatitis B or C. Avoid in patients with severe hepatic impairment. Severe skin reactions sometimes accompanied by fever and/or transaminase elevations, Stevens-Johnson syndrome (SJS), toxic epidermal necrolysis (TEN), and acute generalized exanthematous pustulosis, reported; d/c if severe skin reactions develop. Caution in patients with a known sulfonamide allergy. New onset diabetes mellitus (DM), exacerbation of preexisting DM, hyperglycemia, and diabetic ketoacidosis reported. Immune reconstitution syndrome, autoimmune disorders (eg, Graves' disease, polymyositis, Guillain-Barre syndrome) in the setting of immune reconstitution, redistribution/accumulation of body fat, and increased bleeding in hemophilia type A and B reported. Caution in elderly patients.

ADVERSE REACTIONS: Diarrhea, N/V, headache, abdominal pain, rash, asthenia, anorexia, pruritus, fatigue, decreased appetite.

INTERACTIONS: See Contraindications. Avoid with colchicine in patients with renal/hepatic impairment. Not recommended with lopinavir/RTV, saquinavir, boceprevir, telaprevir, salmeterol, and other protease inhibitors (except atazanavir and indinavir). Avoid with voriconazole unless an assessment of the benefit/risk ratio justifies use of voriconazole. May increase levels of CYP3A and CYP2D6 substrates, indinavir, maraviroc, antiarrhythmics, digoxin, carbamazepine, trazodone, desipramine, clarithromycin, ketoconazole, itraconazole, colchicine, rifabutin, β-blockers, parenteral midazolam, calcium channel blockers, inhaled fluticasone, bosentan, pravastatin, atorvastatin, rosuvastatin, immunosuppressants, salmeterol, norbuprenorphine, neuroleptics, sildenafil for erectile dysfunction, vardenafil, and tadalafil. May decrease levels of phenytoin, phenobarbital, voriconazole, warfarin (monitor INR), methadone, boceprevir, telaprevir, ethinyl estradiol, norethindrone, sertraline, and paroxetine. CYP3A inhibitors, ketoconazole, itraconazole, indinavir, and rifabutin may increase levels. CYP3A inducers, systemic dexamethasone, lopinavir/RTV, saquinavir, boceprevir, and telaprevir may decrease levels. Give didanosine 1 hr before or 2 hrs after administration. Increased lumefantrine exposure may increase the risk of QT prolongation; caution with artemether/lumefantrine. May require initiation or dose adjustments of insulin or oral hypoglycemics for treatment of DM.

PREGNANCY: Category C, not for use in nursing.

MECHANISM OF ACTION: Protease inhibitor; selectively inhibits the cleavage of HIV-1 encoded Gag-Pol polyproteins in infected cells, thereby preventing the formation of mature virus particles.

PHARMACOKINETICS: Absorption: Absolute oral bioavailability (37%) darunavir, (82%) darunavir/RTV; T_{max}=2.5-4 hrs. **Distribution:** Plasma protein binding (95%). **Metabolism:** Hepatic (extensive); oxidation via CYP3A. **Elimination:** Darunavir/RTV: Feces (79.5%, 41.2%, unchanged), urine (13.9%, 7.7%, unchanged); $T_{1/2}$=15 hrs.

NURSING CONSIDERATIONS

Assessment: Assess for sulfonamide allergy, liver dysfunction, hemophilia, preexisting DM, pregnancy/nursing status, and possible drug interactions. Assess ability to swallow tab in children ≥15kg. In treatment-experienced patients, assess treatment history and perform phenotypic or genotypic testing.

Monitoring: Monitor for signs/symptoms of hepatotoxicity, severe skin reactions (eg, SJS, TEN, acute generalized exanthematous pustulosis), new onset/exacerbation of DM, diabetic ketoacidosis, fat redistribution/accumulation, immune reconstitution syndrome, autoimmune disorders, and other adverse reactions. In patients with hemophilia, monitor for bleeding events. Consider performing increased AST/ALT monitoring in patients with underlying chronic hepatitis, cirrhosis, or those with pretreatment transaminase elevations. Monitor INR during coadministration with warfarin.

Patient Counseling: Inform that therapy is not a cure for HIV and that illnesses associated with HIV may continue. Advise to avoid doing things that can spread HIV infection to others. Advise to take with food and to swallow tab whole with a drink; instruct not to alter dose or d/c without consulting physician. Counsel to take drug immediately for missed dose <6 hrs and <12 hrs, for bid and qd dosing respectively, and take the next dose at regular scheduled time. Instruct that if a dose is missed by >6 hrs or >12 hrs, for bid and qd dosing respectively, take the next dose as scheduled; instruct not to double the dose. Advise about the signs/symptoms of liver problems. Inform that mild to severe skin reactions may develop; advise to d/c immediately if signs/symptoms of severe skin reactions develop. Instruct to notify physician if taking any other prescription, OTC, or herbal medication. Instruct to use alternative contraceptive measures if on estrogen-based contraceptive during therapy. Inform that redistribution and accumulation of body fat may occur.

Administration: Oral route. Take with food. (Sus) May use if swallowing tab is difficult. Shake well before each use. **Storage:** 25°C (77°F); excursions permitted to 15-30°C (59-86°F). (Sus) Do not refrigerate or freeze. Avoid exposure to excessive heat.

PRILOSEC   RX
omeprazole (AstraZeneca)

THERAPEUTIC CLASS: Proton pump inhibitor

INDICATIONS: Short-term treatment of active duodenal ulcer (DU) and active benign gastric ulcer (GU) in adults. Treatment of heartburn and other symptoms associated with gastroesophageal reflux disease (GERD) in adults and pediatric patients. Short-term treatment and maintenance of healing of erosive esophagitis (EE) in adults and pediatric patients. Long-term treatment of pathological hypersecretory conditions (eg, Zollinger-Ellison syndrome, multiple endocrine adenomas, systemic mastocytosis) in adults. Combination therapy with clarithromycin +/- amoxicillin in *Helicobacter pylori* infection and DU disease for *H. pylori* eradication in adults.

DOSAGE: *Adults:* Take ac. Active DU: 20mg qd for 4-8 weeks. GERD: Without Esophageal Lesions: 20mg qd for up to 4 weeks. With EE and Accompanying Symptoms: 20mg qd for 4-8 weeks. Maint of Healing of EE: 20mg qd. GU: 40mg qd for 4-8 weeks. Hypersecretory Conditions: Initial: 60mg qd. Titrate: Adjust to individual needs and continue for as long as clinically indicated. Doses up to 120mg tid have been administered. Give >80mg/day in divided doses. *H. pylori* Eradication: Triple Therapy: 20mg + clarithromycin 500mg + amoxicillin 1000mg, each given bid for 10 days. Give additional 18 days of omeprazole 20mg qd if ulcer is present at the time of initiation of therapy. Dual Therapy: 40mg qd + clarithromycin 500mg tid for 14 days. Give additional 14 days of omeprazole 20mg qd if ulcer is present at the time of initiation of therapy. Hepatic Impairment/Asian Population: Consider dose reduction, particularly for mainte-nance of healing of EE.
Pediatrics: 1-16 Yrs: Take ac. GERD/Maint of Healing of EE: ≥20kg: 20mg/day. 10-<20kg: 10mg/day. 5-<10kg: 5mg/day. Hepatic Impairment/Asian Population: Consider dose reduction, particularly for maintenance of healing of EE.

HOW SUPPLIED: Cap, Delayed-Release: 10mg, 20mg, 40mg; Sus, Delayed-Release: (Magnesium) 2.5mg, 10mg (granules/pkt)

WARNINGS/PRECAUTIONS: Symptomatic response does not preclude the presence of gastric malignancy. Atrophic gastritis reported with long-term use. May increase risk of *Clostridium difficile*-associated diarrhea (CDAD), especially in hospitalized patients. May increase risk for osteoporosis-related fractures of the hip, wrist, or spine, especially with high-dose and long-term therapy. Use lowest dose and shortest duration appropriate to the condition being treated. Hypomagnesemia reported and may require Mg^{2+} replacement and discontinuation of therapy; consider monitoring Mg^{2+} levels prior to and periodically during therapy with prolonged treat-ment. Drug-induced decrease in gastric acidity results in enterochromaffin-like cell hyperplasia and increased chromogranin A (CgA) levels, which may interfere with investigations for neuroen-docrine tumors; temporarily d/c treatment before assessing CgA levels.

ADVERSE REACTIONS: Headache, diarrhea, abdominal pain, N/V, flatulence.

INTERACTIONS: May reduce atazanavir and nelfinavir levels; concomitant use not recommend-ed. May change absorption or levels of antiretrovirals. May interfere with absorption of drugs where gastric pH is an important determinant of bioavailability (eg, ketoconazole, ampicillin esters, iron salts, erlotinib, digoxin). May prolong elimination of drugs metabolized by oxidation in the liver (eg, diazepam, warfarin, phenytoin). Monitor patients taking drugs metabolized by CYP450 (eg, cyclosporine, disulfiram, benzodiazepines). Monitor for increases in INR and PT with warfarin. Voriconazole (a combined inhibitor of CYP2C19 and CYP3A4) may increase levels. Decreased levels with CYP2C19 or CYP3A4 inducers; avoid with St. John's wort or rifampin. Reduces pharmacological activity of clopidogrel; avoid concomitant use. May increase levels of saquinavir, cilostazol, and tacrolimus; consider saquinavir and cilostazol dose reduction. Caution with digoxin or other drugs that may cause hypomagnesemia (eg, diuretics). May elevate and prolong levels of methotrexate (MTX) and/or its metabolite, possibly leading to toxicities; con-sider temporary withdrawal of therapy with high-dose MTX.

PREGNANCY: Category C, caution in nursing.

MECHANISM OF ACTION: Proton pump inhibitor; substituted benzimidazole that suppresses gastric acid secretion by specific inhibition of the H^+/K^+ ATPase enzyme system at the secretory surface of the gastric parietal cell.

PHARMACOKINETICS: Absorption: Rapid. Absolute bioavailability (30-40%); T_{max}=0.5-3.5 hrs. **Distribution:** Plasma protein binding (95%); found in breast milk. **Metabolism:** Extensive via CYP450. **Elimination:** Urine (77%, metabolites), feces; $T_{1/2}$=0.5-1 hr.

NURSING CONSIDERATIONS

Assessment: Assess for hypersensitivity to the drug, risk for osteoporosis-related fractures, hepatic impairment, pregnancy/nursing status, and possible drug interactions.

Monitoring: Monitor for signs/symptoms of atrophic gastritis, bone fractures, hypersensitivity reactions, CDAD, and other adverse reactions. Monitor INR and PT when given with warfarin.

Patient Counseling: Advise to immediately report and seek care for diarrhea that does not improve and for any cardiovascular/neurological symptoms (eg, palpitations, dizziness, seizures, tetany). Inform of alternative administration options if patient has difficulty swallowing.

Administration: Oral route. Take ac. (Cap) Swallow whole or, alternatively, open cap and sprinkle all pellets on 1 tbsp of applesauce, then swallow immediately with a glass of cool water; do not chew or crush the pellets. (Sus) May be given via gastric/NG tube. Refer to PI for administra-tion instructions. **Storage:** (Cap) 15-30°C (59-86°F). Protect from light and moisture. (Sus) 25°C (77°F); excursions permitted to 15-30°C (59-86°F).

PRINIVIL
lisinopril (Merck)

> D/C when pregnancy is detected. Drugs that act directly on the renin-angiotensin system can cause injury and death to the developing fetus.

THERAPEUTIC CLASS: ACE inhibitor

INDICATIONS: Treatment of HTN alone as initial therapy or concomitantly with other classes of antihypertensive agents. Adjunctive therapy in the management of heart failure (HF) if inadequately responding to diuretics and digitalis. Treatment of hemodynamically stable patients within 24 hrs of acute myocardial infarction (AMI), to improve survival.

DOSAGE: *Adults:* HTN: Not Receiving Diuretics: Initial: 10mg qd. Titrate: Adjust dose according to BP response. Usual: 20-40mg qd. Max: 80mg. May add a low-dose diuretic if BP is not controlled. Receiving Diuretics: D/C diuretic 2-3 days prior to therapy. Adjust dose according to BP response. If diuretic cannot be discontinued, give initial lisinopril dose of 5mg under medical supervision for at least 2 hrs and until BP has stabilized for at least an additional 1 hr. CrCl 10-30mL/min: Initial: 5mg qd. CrCl <10mL/min: Initial: 2.5mg qd. Titrate: May increase until BP is controlled. Max: 40mg/day. HF: Initial: 5mg qd. Usual: 5-20mg qd. HF with Hyponatremia or CrCl ≤30mL/min or SrCr >3mg/dL: Initial: 2.5mg qd under close medical supervision. AMI: 5mg within 24 hrs, followed by 5mg after 24 hrs, 10mg after 48 hrs, and then 10mg qd for 6 weeks. Patients with Systolic BP (SBP) ≤120mmHg when Treatment is Started or During First 3 Days After the Infarct: 2.5mg. Maint: 5mg/day with temporary reductions to 2.5mg if needed if SBP ≤100mmHg occurs. D/C if SBP <90mmHg for >1 hr occurs. Elderly: Start at lower end of dosing range.
Pediatrics: ≥6 Yrs: HTN: Initial: 0.07mg/kg qd (up to 5mg total). Titrate: Adjust dose according to BP response. Max: 0.61mg/kg (or 40mg).

HOW SUPPLIED: Tab: 5mg*, 10mg*, 20mg* *scored

CONTRAINDICATIONS: Hereditary or idiopathic angioedema, history of ACE inhibitor-associated angioedema. Coadministration with aliskiren in patients with diabetes.

WARNINGS/PRECAUTIONS: Not recommended in pediatric patients with GFR <30mL/min/1.73m². Head/neck angioedema reported; d/c and administer appropriate therapy. Intestinal angioedema reported; monitor for abdominal pain. More reports of angioedema in blacks than nonblacks. Anaphylactoid reactions reported during desensitization with hymenoptera venom, dialysis with high-flux membranes, and LDL apheresis with dextran sulfate absorption. Caution when initiating therapy in AMI patients with renal impairment (SrCr >2mg/dL) and in HF patients. Excessive hypotension, sometimes associated with oliguria and/or progressive azotemia, and rarely with acute renal failure and/or death may occur; monitor closely. If symptomatic hypotension develops, dose reduction or discontinuation of therapy or concomitant diuretic may be necessary. Rare cases of leukopenia/neutropenia and bone marrow depression reported; consider monitoring of WBCs in patients with collagen vascular disease and renal disease. Rarely, syndrome that starts with cholestatic jaundice or hepatitis progressing to fulminant hepatic necrosis and (sometimes) death reported; d/c if jaundice or marked hepatic enzyme elevations occur. Caution with left ventricular outflow obstruction. May cause changes in renal function. May increase BUN and SrCr in patients with renal artery stenosis or with no preexisting renal vascular disease. Hyperkalemia and persistent nonproductive cough reported. Hypotension may occur with major surgery or during anesthesia. Caution in elderly.

ADVERSE REACTIONS: Hypotension, dizziness, headache, diarrhea, cough, chest pain, hyperkalemia.

INTERACTIONS: See Contraindications. Hypotension risk and increased BUN and SrCr with diuretics. Increased hypoglycemic risk with insulin or oral hypoglycemics. NSAIDs, including selective COX-2 inhibitors, may diminish effect and may cause further deterioration of renal function. Dual blockade of the renin-angiotensin-aldosterone system (RAAS) is associated with increased risks of hypotension, syncope, hyperkalemia, and changes in renal function (including acute renal failure); closely monitor BP, renal function, and electrolytes with concomitant agents that affect the RAAS. Avoid with aliskiren in patients with renal impairment (GFR <60mL/min). Increased risk of hyperkalemia with K⁺-sparing diuretics, K⁺ supplements, or K⁺-containing salt substitutes; use with caution and frequently monitor serum K⁺. Concomitant K⁺-sparing agents should generally not be used with HF. Lithium toxicity reported; frequently monitor serum lithium levels. Nitritoid reactions reported with injectable gold.

PREGNANCY: Category D, not for use in nursing.

MECHANISM OF ACTION: ACE inhibitor; decreases plasma angiotensin II, which leads to decreased vasopressor activity and decreased aldosterone secretion.

PHARMACOKINETICS: Absorption: T_{max}=7 hrs (adults), 6 hrs (pediatric patients). **Distribution:** Crosses placenta. **Elimination:** Urine (unchanged); $T_{1/2}$=12 hrs.

P

NURSING CONSIDERATIONS

Assessment: Assess for hereditary or idiopathic angioedema, collagen vascular disease, left ventricular outflow obstruction, renal artery stenosis, risk factors for hyperkalemia, risk of excessive hypotension, history of ACE inhibitor-associated angioedema, renal function, hypersensitivity to the drug, pregnancy/nursing status, and possible drug interactions.

Monitoring: Monitor for angioedema, anaphylactoid reactions, hyperkalemia, and other adverse reactions. Monitor WBCs in patients with collagen vascular disease and renal disease. Monitor BP, LFTs, and renal function.

Patient Counseling: Instruct to d/c therapy and to immediately report signs/symptoms of angioedema. Instruct to report lightheadedness, especially during 1st few days of therapy; advise to d/c and consult with a physician if actual syncope occurs. Advise that excessive perspiration, dehydration, diarrhea, or vomiting may lead to fall in BP; instruct to consult with a physician. Advise not to use salt substitutes containing K⁺ without consulting physician. Advise diabetic patients to monitor for hypoglycemia. Instruct to report any indication of infection (eg, sore throat, fever) that may be a sign of leukopenia/neutropenia. Inform about fetal risks if taken during pregnancy and discuss treatment options in women planning to become pregnant; instruct to report pregnancy to physician as soon as possible.

Administration: Oral route. Refer to PI for instruction for preparation of sus. Shake sus before each use. **Storage:** (Tab) 15-30°C (59-86°F). Protect from moisture. (Sus) ≤25°C (77°F) for up to 4 weeks.

PRISTIQ RX
desvenlafaxine (Wyeth)

> Antidepressants increased the risk of suicidal thoughts and behavior in children, adolescents, and young adults in short-term studies. Monitor and observe closely for worsening, and emergence of suicidal thoughts and behaviors. Not approved for use in pediatric patients.

THERAPEUTIC CLASS: Serotonin and norepinephrine reuptake inhibitor

INDICATIONS: Treatment of major depressive disorder.

DOSAGE: *Adults:* Usual: 50mg qd. Doses up to 400mg were effective but with no additional benefit; more frequent adverse reactions at higher doses reported. Moderate Renal Impairment (CrCl 30-50mL/min): Max: 50mg/day. Severe Renal Impairment (CrCl <30mL/min) or End-Stage Renal Disease: Max: 50mg qod. Do not give supplemental doses after dialysis. Moderate-Severe Hepatic Impairment: Usual: 50mg/day. Max: 100mg/day. Periodically reassess the need for continued treatment. Discontinuation of Treatment: Consider resuming previously prescribed dose if intolerable symptoms occur following a decrease in dose or upon discontinuation of treatment. May continue decreasing the dose subsequently but at a more gradual rate. Switching from Other Antidepressants: Tapering of the initial antidepressant may be necessary to minimize discontinuation symptoms. Switching to/from an MAOI for Psychiatric Disorders: Allow at least 14 days between discontinuation of an MAOI and initiation of treatment, and allow at least 7 days between discontinuation of treatment and initiation of an MAOI. Use with Other MAOIs (eg, Linezolid, IV Methylene Blue): Refer to PI.

HOW SUPPLIED: Tab, Extended-Release: 50mg, 100mg

CONTRAINDICATIONS: Use of an MAOI intended to treat psychiatric disorders either concomitantly or within 7 days of stopping treatment. Treatment within 14 days of stopping an MAOI to treat psychiatric disorders. Starting treatment in patients being treated with other MAOIs (eg, linezolid, IV methylene blue).

WARNINGS/PRECAUTIONS: Not approved for the treatment of bipolar depression. Serotonin syndrome reported; d/c immediately if symptoms occur and initiate supportive symptomatic treatment. Caution with preexisting HTN, cardiovascular (CV) or cerebrovascular conditions that might be compromised by increases in BP. Consider dose reduction or discontinuation of therapy if sustained increases in BP occur. May increase risk of bleeding events. Mydriasis reported; monitor patients with increased intraocular pressure (IOP) or those at risk of acute narrow-angle glaucoma. Activation of mania/hypomania reported; caution with history or family history of mania/hypomania. Discontinuation symptoms reported. Avoid abrupt discontinuation; gradually reduce dose whenever possible. Seizures reported; caution with seizure disorder. Hyponatremia may occur; caution in elderly and volume-depleted patients. Consider discontinuation in patients with symptomatic hyponatremia and institute appropriate medical intervention. Consider discontinuation of therapy if interstitial lung disease and eosinophilic pneumonia occur. False (+) urine immunoassay screening tests for phencyclidine and amphetamines reported.

ADVERSE REACTIONS: N/V, dry mouth, dizziness, insomnia, somnolence, hyperhidrosis, constipation, anxiety, decreased appetite, tremor, mydriasis, erectile dysfunction, anorgasmia, fatigue, vision blurred.

INTERACTIONS: See Contraindications. Avoid with other desvenlafaxine-containing products or venlafaxine products; may increase levels and increase dose-related adverse reactions. Avoid alcohol consumption. May cause serotonin syndrome with other serotonergic drugs (eg, triptans, TCAs, fentanyl, lithium, tramadol, tryptophan, buspirone, St. John's wort) and with drugs that impair metabolism of serotonin; d/c immediately if serotonin syndrome occurs. Caution with NSAIDs, aspirin (ASA), warfarin, and other drugs that affect coagulation or bleeding due to increased risk of bleeding. May increase risk of hyponatremia with diuretics. Potent CYP3A4 inhibitors (eg, ketoconazole) may increase levels. CYP2D6 substrates (eg, desipramine, atomoxetine, dextromethorphan, metoprolol, nebivolol, perphenazine, tolterodine) should be dosed at the original level when coadministered with 100mg desvenlafaxine or lower, or when desvenlafaxine is discontinued; reduce the dose of these substrates by up to 1/2 if coadministered with 400mg of desvenlafaxine.

PREGNANCY: Category C, not for use in nursing.

MECHANISM OF ACTION: SNRI; has not been established. Thought to be related to the potentiation of serotonin and norepinephrine in the CNS through inhibition of their reuptake.

PHARMACOKINETICS: Absorption: Absolute bioavailability (80%). **Distribution:** Plasma protein binding (30%); V_d=3.4L/kg (IV); found in breast milk. **Metabolism:** Conjugation via UGT isoforms (primary) and N-demethylation via CYP3A4 (minor). **Elimination:** Urine (45% unchanged, 19% glucuronide metabolite, <5% oxidative metabolite). $T_{1/2}$=10-11.1 hrs.

NURSING CONSIDERATIONS

Assessment: Assess for risk for bipolar disorder, history of mania/hypomania, history of seizures, seizure disorders, HTN, CV/cerebrovascular conditions, increased IOP, risk factors for acute narrow-angle glaucoma, volume depletion, hypersensitivity to the drug, hepatic/renal impairment, pregnancy/nursing status, and possible drug interactions.

Monitoring: Monitor for signs/symptoms of clinical worsening (eg, suicidality, unusual changes in behavior), serotonin syndrome, abnormal bleeding, mydriasis, activation of mania/hypomania, seizures, hyponatremia, interstitial lung disease, eosinophilic pneumonia, and other adverse reactions. Monitor BP, LFTs, and renal function. Monitor for discontinuation symptoms (eg, dysphoric mood, irritability, agitation) when discontinuing therapy. Monitor carefully in patients receiving warfarin therapy when treatment is initiated or discontinued. Periodically reassess to determine the need for continued treatment.

Patient Counseling: Advise patients, families and caregivers about the benefits and risks of treatment and counsel on its appropriate use. Counsel patients, families, and caregivers to look for the emergence of suicidality, especially early during treatment and when the dose is adjusted up or down. Caution about the risk of serotonin syndrome, particularly with the concomitant use with other serotonergic agents. Inform that concomitant use with ASA, NSAIDs, warfarin, or other drugs that affect coagulation may increase the risk of bleeding. Advise to monitor BP regularly, to observe for signs/symptoms of activation of mania/hypomania, to avoid alcohol, and not to d/c therapy without notifying physician. Caution against operating hazardous machinery (including automobiles) until reasonably certain that therapy does not adversely affect ability to engage in such activities. Advise to notify physician if allergic phenomena (eg, rash, hives, swelling, difficulty breathing) develop, if pregnant, intend to become pregnant, or if breastfeeding. Inform that an inert matrix tab may pass in the stool or via colostomy.

Administration: Oral route. Take at the same time each day, with or without food. Swallow tab whole with fluid; do not divide, crush, chew, or dissolve. **Storage:** 20-25°C (68-77°F); excursions permitted to 15-30°C (59-86°F).

PROAIR HFA   RX
albuterol sulfate (Teva)

THERAPEUTIC CLASS: Beta$_2$-agonist

INDICATIONS: Treatment or prevention of bronchospasm with reversible obstructive airway disease and prevention of exercise-induced bronchospasm (EIB) in patients ≥4 yrs of age.

DOSAGE: *Adults*: Treatment/Prevention of Bronchospasm: 2 inh q4-6h; 1 inh q4h may be sufficient in some patients. EIB Prevention: 2 inh 15-30 min prior to exercise. Elderly: Start at lower end of dosing range.
Pediatrics: ≥4 Yrs: Treatment/Prevention of Bronchospasm: 2 inh q4-6h; 1 inh q4h may be sufficient in some patients. EIB Prevention: 2 inh 15-30 min prior to exercise.

HOW SUPPLIED: MDI: 90mcg/inh [200 actuations]

WARNINGS/PRECAUTIONS: If more doses than usual are needed, this may be a marker of destabilization of asthma and may require reevaluation of the patient and treatment regimen; antiinflammatory treatment (eg, corticosteroids) may be needed. May produce paradoxical bronchospasm; d/c immediately and institute alternative therapy if this occurs. D/C if cardiovascular

(CV) effects occur. ECG changes and immediate hypersensitivity reactions may occur. Fatalities reported with excessive use; do not exceed recommended dose. Caution with CV disorders, convulsive disorders, hyperthyroidism, diabetes mellitus (DM), and in patients unusually responsive to sympathomimetic amines. May produce significant hypokalemia and BP changes. Aggravation of preexisting DM and ketoacidosis reported with large doses of IV albuterol. Caution in elderly and when administering high doses in patients with renal impairment.

ADVERSE REACTIONS: Pharyngitis, headache, rhinitis, dizziness, musculoskeletal pain, tachycardia.

INTERACTIONS: Avoid with other short-acting sympathomimetic aerosol bronchodilators; caution with additional adrenergic drugs administered by any route. Use with β-blockers may block pulmonary effect and produce severe bronchospasm in asthmatic patients; avoid concomitant use. If needed, consider cardioselective β-blockers. ECG changes and/or hypokalemia caused by non-K⁺-sparing diuretics (eg, loop, thiazide) may be worsened; consider monitoring K⁺ levels. May decrease digoxin levels; monitor serum digoxin levels. Use extreme caution with MAOIs and TCAs, or within 2 weeks of discontinuation of such agents; consider alternative therapy in patients taking MAOIs or TCAs.

PREGNANCY: Category C, not for use in nursing.

MECHANISM OF ACTION: β_2-agonist; activates β_2-adrenergic receptors on airway smooth muscle leading to activation of adenylcyclase and to an increase in cAMP.

PHARMACOKINETICS: Absorption: C_{max}=4100pg/mL; AUC=28,426pg/mL•hr. **Metabolism:** GI tract via SULTIA3 (sulfotransferase). **Elimination:** Urine (80-100%), feces (<20%); $T_{1/2}$=6 hrs.

NURSING CONSIDERATIONS

Assessment: Assess for history of hypersensitivity to drug, CV disorders, convulsive disorders, hyperthyroidism, DM, renal impairment, pregnancy/nursing status, and possible drug interactions. Assess use in patients unusually responsive to sympathomimetic amines.

Monitoring: Monitor for paradoxical bronchospasm, deterioration of asthma, CV effects, ECG changes, hypokalemia, immediate hypersensitivity reactions, and other adverse reactions. Monitor BP, HR, and ECG changes. Monitor renal function in elderly.

Patient Counseling: Counsel not to increase dose/frequency of doses without consulting physician. Advise to seek immediate medical attention if treatment becomes less effective for symptomatic relief, symptoms become worse, and/or there is a need to use product more frequently than usual. Inform that drug may cause paradoxical bronchospasm; instruct to d/c if this occurs. Instruct to take concurrent inhaled drugs and other asthma medications only ud. Inform of the common adverse effects of treatment (eg, palpitations, chest pain, rapid HR, tremor, nervousness). Instruct to notify physician if pregnant/nursing.

Administration: Oral inhalation route. Shake well before use. Prime inhaler before use for the 1st time or if inhaler has not been used for >2 weeks by releasing 3 sprays into the air, away from face. Avoid spraying in eyes. Refer to PI for further administration instructions. **Storage:** 15-25°C (59-77°F). Protect from freezing and direct sunlight. Contents under pressure; do not puncture or incinerate. Exposure to temperatures >49°C (120°F) may cause bursting.

PROBENECID/COLCHICINE   RX
colchicine - probenecid (Various)

THERAPEUTIC CLASS: Uricosuric

INDICATIONS: Chronic gouty arthritis complicated by frequent, recurrent acute gout attacks.

DOSAGE: *Adults:* Initial: 1 tab qd for 1 week, then 1 tab bid. Maint: Continue dosage that will maintain normal serum urate levels. May reduce dose by 1 tab every 6 months if acute attacks are absent ≥6 months and serum urate levels remain normal. Renal Impairment: 2 tabs/day. Titrate: May increase dose by 1 tab every 4 weeks if symptoms not controlled or 24 hr uric acid excretion is not >700mg. Max: 4 tabs/day. Decrease dose if gastric intolerance occurs.

HOW SUPPLIED: Tab: (Probenecid-Colchicine) 500mg-0.5mg

CONTRAINDICATIONS: Blood dyscrasias, uric acid kidney stones, children <2 yrs of age, pregnancy, initiating therapy before acute gout attack subsides, coadministration with salicylates.

WARNINGS/PRECAUTIONS: Exacerbation of gout may occur. Severe allergic reactions and anaphylaxis reported rarely; d/c if hypersensitivity occurs. Caution with history of peptic ulcer. Hematuria, renal colic, costovertebral pain, and formation of uric acid stones reported; maintain liberal fluid intake and alkalization of urine. May not be effective in chronic renal insufficiency (GFR ≤30mL/min). Reversible azoospermia reported. Colchicine is an established mutagen; may be carcinogenic.

ADVERSE REACTIONS: Headache, dizziness, fever, pruritus, acute gouty arthritis, purpura, leukopenia, peripheral neuritis, muscular weakness, N/V, urticaria, anemia, dermatitis, alopecia.

INTERACTIONS: See Contraindications. Salicylates and pyrazinamide antagonize uricosuric effects; use acetaminophen (APAP) if mild analgesic is needed. Probenecid increases plasma levels of penicillin and other β-lactams; psychic disturbances reported. Methotrexate levels increased with coadministration; reduce dose and monitor levels. May prolong/enhance effects of sulfonylureas; increased risk of hypoglycemia. Increased $T_{1/2}$ and levels of indomethacin, naproxen, ketoprofen, meclofenamate, lorazepam, APAP, and rifampin. Increased levels of sulindac and sulfonamides; monitor sulfonamide levels with prolonged use. Inhibits renal transport of amino hippuric acid, aminosalicylic acid, indomethacin, sodium iodomethamate and related iodinated organic acids, 17-ketosteroids, pantothenic acid, phenolsulfonphthalein, sulfonamides, and sulfonylureas. Possible falsely high plasma levels of theophylline. Decreases hepatic/renal excretion of sulfobromophthalein. May require significantly less thiopental for induction of anesthesia.

PREGNANCY: Contraindicated in pregnancy; safety not known in nursing.

MECHANISM OF ACTION: Probenecid: Uricosuric/renal tubular blocking agent; increases urinary excretion of uric acid and decreases serum urate levels. Colchicine: Colchicum alkaloid; not established. Has prophylactic, suppressive effect helping to reduce incidence of acute attacks and to relieve residual pain and mild discomfort.

NURSING CONSIDERATIONS

Assessment: Assess for known blood dyscrasias, uric acid kidney stones, acute/chronic gout attack, history of peptic ulcer, renal function, hypersensitivity to drug, pregnancy/nursing status, and possible drug interactions.

Monitoring: Monitor for signs/symptoms of gout exacerbation, allergic reactions, hematuria, renal colic, costovertebral pain, and uric acid stone formation. Monitor serum uric acid levels.

Patient Counseling: Inform about the risks and benefits of therapy and importance of liberal fluid intake. Advise to seek medical attention if symptoms of allergic reaction, hematuria, renal colic, or costovertebral pain occur.

Administration: Oral route. **Storage:** 20-25°C (68-77°F). Protect from light.

PROCARDIA XL
nifedipine (Pfizer)

RX

OTHER BRAND NAMES: Nifedical XL (Teva)

THERAPEUTIC CLASS: Calcium channel blocker (dihydropyridine)

INDICATIONS: Management of vasospastic angina and chronic stable angina without evidence of vasospasm in patients who remain symptomatic despite adequate doses of β-blockers and/or organic nitrates or who cannot tolerate those agents. Treatment of HTN alone or with other antihypertensive agents.

DOSAGE: *Adults:* Angina/HTN: Initial: 30 or 60mg qd. Titrate over a 7- to 14-day period (usual) but may proceed more rapidly if symptoms warrant. Max: 120mg/day. Caution with doses >90mg for angina. Switching from Nifedipine Cap Alone or with Other Antianginal Agents: Use nearest equivalent daily dose. Titrate as clinically warranted.

HOW SUPPLIED: Tab, Extended-Release: 30mg, 60mg, 90mg; (Nifedical XL) 30mg, 60mg

WARNINGS/PRECAUTIONS: May cause hypotension; monitor BP initially and with titration. May increase frequency, duration, and/or severity of angina or acute myocardial infarction, particularly with severe obstructive coronary artery disease. May develop congestive heart failure (CHF), especially with tight aortic stenosis. GI obstruction and bezoars reported; caution with altered GI anatomy and hypomotility disorders. Peripheral edema associated with vasodilation may occur; rule out peripheral edema caused by left ventricular dysfunction in patients with angina or HTN complicated by CHF. Transient elevations of enzymes (eg, alkaline phosphatase, CPK, LDH, SGOT, SGPT), cholestasis with/without jaundice, and allergic hepatitis reported rarely. May decrease platelet aggregation and increase bleeding time. Positive direct Coombs test with or without hemolytic anemia reported. Reversible elevation in BUN and SrCr reported rarely in patients with chronic renal insufficiency. (Procardia XL) Tablet adherence to GI wall with ulceration reported.

ADVERSE REACTIONS: Dizziness, headache, nausea, fatigue, constipation, edema.

INTERACTIONS: β-blockers may increase risk of CHF, severe hypotension, or angina exacerbation; avoid abrupt β-blocker withdrawal. Severe hypotension and/or increased fluid volume reported together with β-blockers and fentanyl or other narcotic analgesics. May increase digoxin levels; monitor digoxin levels when initiating, adjusting, and discontinuing therapy to avoid over- or under-digitalization. May increase PT with coumarin anticoagulants. Cimetidine may increase levels. Decreased serum K+ levels with diuretics. Monitor with other medications known to lower BP. Increased risk of GI obstruction with H_2-histamine blockers, NSAIDs, laxatives, anticholinergic agents, levothyroxine, (Procardia XL) opiates, and neuromuscular blocking agents.

PREGNANCY: Category C, safety not known in nursing.

MECHANISM OF ACTION: Calcium channel blocker; inhibits Ca^{2+} ion influx into cardiac muscle and smooth muscle. Angina: not established; believed to act by relaxation and prevention of coronary artery spasm and reduction of oxygen utilization. HTN: Peripheral arterial vasodilation resulting in reduction in peripheral vascular resistance.

PHARMACOKINETICS: Absorption: Complete. Bioavailability (86%). **Distribution:** Plasma protein binding (92-98%, Procardia XL) (90-98%, Nifedical XL). **Metabolism:** Liver, extensive. **Elimination:** Urine (60-80%, metabolites; <0.1%, unchanged), feces (metabolites); $T_{1/2}$=2 hrs.

NURSING CONSIDERATIONS

Assessment: Assess for CHF, severe obstructive CAD, aortic stenosis, hepatic/renal impairment, altered GI anatomy (eg, severe GI narrowing, colon cancer, small bowel obstruction, bowel resection, gastric bypass, vertical banded gastroplasty, colostomy, diverticulitis, diverticulosis, inflammatory bowel disease), hypomotility disorders (eg, constipation, gastroesophageal reflux disease, ileus, obesity, hypothyroidism, diabetes), recent β-blocker withdrawal, pregnancy/nursing status, and possible drug interactions.

Monitoring: Monitor for excessive hypotension, increased frequency, duration and/or severity of angina and/or acute MI (especially during initiation and dose titration), CHF, signs/symptoms of GI obstruction, peripheral edema (determine cause), cholestasis with/without jaundice, and allergic hepatitis. Monitor BP, LFTs, BUN, SrCr, for decreased platelet aggregation, and increased bleeding time.

Patient Counseling: Advise to take exactly as prescribed. Instruct to swallow tablet whole; not to chew, divide, or crush. Counsel about adverse effects; advise to report any. (Procardia XL) Inform that it is normal to occasionally observe a tablet-like material in the stool.

Administration: Oral route. **Storage:** Protect from moisture and humidity. (Procardia XL) <30°C (86°F). (Nifedical XL) 25°C (77°F); excursions permitted to 15-30°C (59-86°F).

PROCENTRA `CII`
dextroamphetamine sulfate (FSC Laboratories)

> High potential for abuse. Prolonged use may lead to drug dependence and must be avoided. Misuse may cause sudden death and serious cardiovascular adverse events.

THERAPEUTIC CLASS: Sympathomimetic amine

INDICATIONS: Treatment of narcolepsy and attention-deficit hyperactivity disorder (ADHD).

DOSAGE: *Adults:* Narcolepsy: Initial: 10mg/day. Titrate: May increase in increments of 10mg at weekly intervals. Usual: 5-60mg/day in divided doses. Give 1st dose on awakening; additional doses (1 or 2) at intervals of 4-6 hrs. Avoid late pm doses.
Pediatrics: Give 1st dose on awakening; additional doses (1 or 2) at intervals of 4-6 hrs. Avoid late pm doses. Narcolepsy: ≥12 Yrs: Initial: 10mg/day. Titrate: May increase in increments of 10mg at weekly intervals. 6-12 Yrs: Initial: 5mg/day. Titrate: May increase in increments of 5mg at weekly intervals. Usual: 5-60mg/day in divided doses. ADHD: ≥6 Yrs: Initial: 5mg qd or bid. Titrate: May increase in increments of 5mg at weekly intervals. Only in rare cases will it be necessary to exceed a total of 40mg/day. 3-5 Yrs: Initial: 2.5mg/day. Titrate: May increase in increments of 2.5mg at weekly intervals.

HOW SUPPLIED: Sol: 5mg/5mL (473mL)

CONTRAINDICATIONS: Advanced arteriosclerosis, symptomatic cardiovascular disease (CVD), moderate to severe HTN, hyperthyroidism, glaucoma, agitated states, and history of drug abuse. During or within 14 days following MAOI use.

WARNINGS/PRECAUTIONS: Sudden death reported in children and adolescents with structural cardiac abnormalities or other serious heart problems. Sudden death, stroke, and myocardial infarction (MI) reported in adults. Avoid with known serious structural cardiac abnormalities, cardiomyopathy, serious heart rhythm abnormalities, coronary artery disease, or other serious cardiac problems. May cause a modest increase in average BP and HR. Prior to treatment, obtain medical history and perform physical exam to assess for presence of cardiac disease. Promptly perform cardiac evaluation if symptoms of cardiac disease develop during treatment. May exacerbate symptoms of behavior disturbance and thought disorder in patients with preexisting psychotic disorder. May induce mixed/manic episodes in patients with comorbid bipolar disorder. May cause treatment-emergent psychotic or manic symptoms in children and adolescents without a prior history of psychotic illness or mania; consider discontinuation if such symptoms occur. Aggressive behavior or hostility reported in children and adolescents with ADHD. May cause long-term suppression of growth in children; monitor growth, and may need to interrupt treatment in patients not growing or gaining height or weight as expected. May lower convulsive threshold; d/c if seizures occur. Difficulties with accommodation and blurring of vision reported. May exacerbate motor and phonic tics, and Tourette's syndrome. May elevate plasma corticosteroid levels and interfere with urinary steroid determinations.

ADVERSE REACTIONS: Palpitations, tachycardia, BP elevation, dizziness, insomnia, euphoria, dyskinesia, tremor, headache, dryness of mouth, diarrhea, constipation, urticaria, impotence, changes in libido.

INTERACTIONS: See Contraindications. GI acidifying agents (eg, guanethidine, reserpine, glutamic acid, ascorbic acid, fruit juices) and urinary acidifying agents (eg, ammonium chloride, sodium acid phosphate) lower blood levels and efficacy. Inhibits adrenergic blockers. GI alkalizing agents (eg, sodium bicarbonate) and urinary alkalinizing agents (eg, acetazolamide, some thiazides) increase blood levels and therefore potentiate actions. May enhance activity of TCAs or sympathomimetic agents. Desipramine or protriptyline and possibly other TCAs cause striking and sustained increases in the concentration of d-amphetamine in the brain; cardiovascular effects can be potentiated. May counteract sedative effects of antihistamines. May antagonize effect of antihypertensives. Chlorpromazine and haloperidol block dopamine and norepinephrine reuptake, thus inhibiting central stimulant effects. May delay intestinal absorption of ethosuximide, phenobarbital, and phenytoin; coadministration with phenobarbital or phenytoin may produce a synergistic anticonvulsant action. Lithium carbonate may inhibit stimulatory effects. Potentiates analgesic effect of meperidine. Acidifying agents used in methenamine therapy increase urinary excretion and reduce efficacy. Enhances adrenergic effect of norepinephrine. In cases of propoxyphene overdosage, CNS stimulation is potentiated and fatal convulsions can occur. Inhibits hypotensive effect of veratrum alkaloids.

PREGNANCY: Category C, not for use in nursing.

MECHANISM OF ACTION: Sympathomimetic amine; not established. Has CNS stimulant activity.

PHARMACOKINETICS: Absorption: (Healthy) C_{max}=33.2ng/mL. **Distribution:** Found in breast milk. **Elimination:** (Healthy) Urine (38%); $T_{1/2}$=11.75 hrs.

NURSING CONSIDERATIONS

Assessment: Assess for hypersensitivity/idiosyncrasy to sympathomimetic amines, advanced arteriosclerosis, symptomatic CVD, moderate to severe HTN, hyperthyroidism, glaucoma, agitated states, history of drug abuse, tics, Tourette's syndrome, preexisting psychotic disorder, risk for/comorbid bipolar disorder, cardiac disease, medical conditions that might be compromised by increases in BP or HR, any other conditions where treatment is cautioned, pregnancy/nursing status, and possible drug interactions.

Monitoring: Monitor for changes in HR and BP, signs/symptoms of cardiac disease, exacerbation of behavioral disturbance and thought disorder, psychosis, mania, appearance of or worsening of aggressive behavior or hostility, seizures, visual disturbances, exacerbation of motor and phonic tics or Tourette's syndrome, and other adverse reactions. In pediatric patients, monitor growth.

Patient Counseling: Inform about benefits and risks of treatment. Counsel that drug has high potential for abuse. Caution against engaging in potentially hazardous activities.

Administration: Oral route. Avoid late pm doses. **Storage:** 20-25°C (68-77°F).

P

PROCHLORPERAZINE   RX
prochlorperazine (Various)

> Elderly patients with dementia-related psychosis treated with antipsychotic drugs are at an increased risk of death; most deaths appeared to be cardiovascular (CV) (eg, heart failure, sudden death) or infectious (eg, pneumonia) in nature. Treatment with conventional antipsychotic drugs may similarly increase mortality. Not approved for the treatment of patients with dementia-related psychosis.

THERAPEUTIC CLASS: Phenothiazine derivative

INDICATIONS: Control of severe N/V. Treatment of schizophrenia. (Tab) Short-term treatment of generalized nonpsychotic anxiety.

DOSAGE: *Adults:* N/V: (Tab) Usual: 5mg or 10mg PO tid-qid. Daily dose >40mg should only be used in resistant cases. (IM) Initial: 5-10mg IM q3-4h PRN. Max: 40mg/day. (IV) 2.5-10mg slow IV inj or infusion at rate ≤5mg/min. Max: 10mg single dose and 40mg/day. N/V with Surgery: (IM) 5-10mg IM 1-2 hrs before induction of anesthesia (repeat once in 30 min if necessary). (IV) 5-10mg as slow IV inj or infusion 15-30 min before induction of anesthesia. To control acute symptoms during or after surgery, repeat once if necessary. Max: 40mg/day. Nonpsychotic Anxiety: (Tab) Usual: 5mg tid-qid. Max: 20mg/day, not longer than 12 weeks. Psychotic Disorders (Schizophrenia): (Tab) Mild/Outpatient: 5-10mg tid-qid. Moderate-Severe/Hospitalized: Initial: 10mg tid-qid. May increase dose gradually in small increments every 2-3 days. Severe: (Tab) 100-150mg/day. (IM) Initial: 10-20mg, may repeat q2-4h if neccessary (or, in resistant cases, every hr). Switch to PO after obtaining control at the same dosage level or higher. Prolonged Parenteral Therapy: 10-20mg IM q4-6h. Debilitated or Emaciated Adults: Increase more gradually. Elderly: Start at lower end of dosing range and increase more gradually. *Pediatrics:* N/V: ≥2 Yrs, ≥20 lbs: (Tab) 40-85 lbs: 2.5mg tid or 5mg bid. Max: 15mg/day. 30-39 lbs: 2.5mg bid-tid. Max: 10mg/day. 20-29 lbs: Usual: 2.5mg qd-bid. Max: 7.5mg/day. Severe N/V: (IM)

0.06mg/lb. Control is usually obtained with 1 dose. Psychotic Disorders (Schizophrenia): (Tab) 2-12 Yrs: Initial: 2.5mg bid-tid. Do not give >10mg on the 1st day. Increase dose based on patient's response. 6-12 Yrs: Max: 25mg/day. 2-5 Yrs: Max: 20mg/day. (IM) <12 Yrs: 0.06mg/lb. Control is usually obtained with 1 dose. Switch to PO after obtaining control at the same dosage level or higher.

HOW SUPPLIED: Inj: (Edisylate) 5mg/mL [2mL, 10mL]; Tab: (Maleate) 5mg, 10mg

CONTRAINDICATIONS: Comatose states, concomitant large doses of CNS depressants (eg, alcohol, barbiturates, narcotics), pediatric surgery, pediatrics <2 yrs of age or <20 lbs.

WARNINGS/PRECAUTIONS: Secondary extrapyramidal symptoms can occur. Tardive dyskinesia (TD) may develop, especially in elderly and during long-term use. Neuroleptic malignant syndrome (NMS) reported; d/c if it occurs and institute appropriate treatment. Caution during reintroduction of therapy as NMS recurrence reported. Avoid in patients with bone marrow depression, previous hypersensitivity reaction, and in pregnant women. May impair mental and/or physical abilities, especially during the 1st few days of therapy. May mask symptoms of overdose of other drugs, and obscure diagnosis of intestinal obstruction, brain tumor, and Reye's syndrome; avoid in children/adolescents whose signs and symptoms suggest Reye's syndrome. May cause hypotension; caution with large doses and parenteral administration in patients with impaired CV system. May interfere with thermoregulation; caution in patients exposed to extreme heat. Evaluate therapy periodically with prolonged use. Leukopenia/neutropenia/agranulocytosis reported; monitor during 1st few months of therapy, and d/c at 1st sign of leukopenia or if severe neutropenia (absolute neutrophil count <1000/mm^3) occurs. Caution with glaucoma, in children with dehydration or acute illness, and in elderly. May produce α-adrenergic blockade, lower seizure threshold, or elevate prolactin levels. D/C 48 hrs before myelography; may resume after 24 hrs postprocedure.

ADVERSE REACTIONS: NMS, cholestatic jaundice, leukopenia, agranulocytosis, drowsiness, dizziness, amenorrhea, blurred vision, skin reactions, hypotension, motor restlessness, extrapyramidal symptoms, TD, dystonia, pseudoparkinsonism.

INTERACTIONS: See Contraindications. May intensify and prolong action of CNS depressants (eg, alcohol, anesthetics, narcotics), atropine, and organophosphorus insecticides. May decrease oral anticoagulant effects. Thiazide diuretics accentuate orthostatic hypotension. Increased levels of both drugs with propranolol. Anticonvulsants may need dosage adjustment; may lower convulsive threshold. May interfere with metabolism of phenytoin and precipitate toxicity. Risk of encephalopathic syndrome occurs with lithium. May antagonize antihypertensive effects of guanethidine and related compounds. Avoid use prior to myelography with metrizamide; vomiting as a sign of toxicity of cancer chemotherapeutic drugs may be obscured by the antiemetic effect. May reverse effect of epinephrine. May cause paradoxical further lowering of BP with epinephrine and other pressor agents (excluding norepinephrine bitartrate and phenylephrine HCl).

PREGNANCY: Safety is not known in pregnancy; caution in nursing.

MECHANISM OF ACTION: Phenothiazine derivative; antiemetic and antipsychotic.

PHARMACOKINETICS: Distribution: Excreted in breast milk.

NURSING CONSIDERATIONS

Assessment: Assess for Reye's syndrome, TD, pregnancy/nursing status, possible drug interactions, impaired CV system, breast cancer, glaucoma, bone marrow depression, preexisting low WBC count, history of drug-induced leukopenia/neutropenia, history of psychosis, and seizure disorder. Assess use in children with acute illness or dehydration, elderly, debilitated, or emaciated patients.

Monitoring: Monitor for extrapyramidal symptoms, signs/symptoms of TD, NMS, hypotension, fever, sore throat, infection, jaundice, motor restlessness, dystonia, pseudoparkinsonism, and hypersensitivity reactions. Monitor CBC, WBC, and prolactin levels. Conduct liver studies if fever with grippe-like symptoms occur.

Patient Counseling: Inform about the risks and benefits of therapy. Instruct to avoid engaging in hazardous activities and exposure to extreme heat. Counsel to seek medical attention if symptoms of TD, NMS, hypotension, mydriasis, encephalopathic syndrome, sore throat, infection, deep sleep, or hypersensitivity reactions occur.

Administration: IV, IM, Oral route. (Inj) Inspect visually for particulate matter and discoloration. Discard if marked discoloration noted. Inject deeply into upper, outer quadrant of the buttock. SQ is not advisable because of local irritation. May be administered either undiluted or diluted in isotonic solution. When given IV, do not use bolus injection. Do not mix with other agents in the syringe. Avoid getting injection solution on hands or clothing because of potential contact dermatitis. **Storage:** Tab, Inj: 20-25°C (68-77°F). Protect from light. (Inj) Do not freeze.

PROCRIT   RX
epoetin alfa (Janssen)

Increased risk of death, myocardial infarction, stroke, venous thromboembolism, thrombosis of vascular access, and tumor progression or recurrence. Use the lowest dose sufficient to reduce/avoid the need for RBC transfusions. Chronic kidney disease (CKD): Greater risks for death, serious adverse cardiovascular (CV) reactions, and stroke when administered to target Hgb level >11g/dL. Cancer: Shortened overall survival and/or increased risk of tumor progression or recurrence in patients with breast, non-small-cell lung, head and neck, lymphoid, and cervical cancers. Must enroll in and comply with the ESA APPRISE Oncology Program to prescribe and/or dispense drug to patients. Use only for anemia from myelosuppressive chemotherapy. Not indicated for patients receiving myelosuppressive chemotherapy when anticipated outcome is cure. D/C following completion of chemotherapy course. Perisurgery: Due to increased risk of deep venous thrombosis (DVT), DVT prophylaxis is recommended.

THERAPEUTIC CLASS: Erythropoiesis stimulator

INDICATIONS: Treatment of anemia due to CKD, including patients on and not on dialysis; anemia due to zidovudine administered at ≤4200mg/week in HIV-infected patients with endogenous serum erythropoietin levels of ≤500 mU/mL; anemic patients with nonmyeloid malignancies where anemia is due to the effect of concomitant myelosuppressive chemotherapy, and, upon initiation, there is a minimum of 2 additional months of planned chemotherapy. To reduce the need for allogeneic RBC transfusions in patients with perioperative Hgb >10 to ≤13g/dL who are at high risk for perioperative blood loss from elective, noncardiac, nonvascular surgery.

DOSAGE: *Adults:* Initiate when Hgb is <10g/dL (see PI for additional parameters). CKD on Dialysis/Not on Dialysis: Initial: 50-100 U/kg IV/SQ 3X weekly. IV route is recommended for patients on dialysis. Titrate: Adjust dose based on Hgb levels; see PI. Zidovudine-Treated HIV-Infected Patients: Initial: 100 U/kg IV/SQ 3X weekly. Titrate: Adjust dose based on Hgb levels; see PI. Patients on Chemotherapy: Initial: 150 U/kg SQ 3X weekly or 40,000 U SQ weekly until completion of a chemotherapy course. Titrate: Adjust dose based on Hgb levels; see PI. Surgery Patients: Usual: 300 U/kg/day SQ qd for 10 days before, on the day of, and for 4 days after surgery; or 600 U/kg SQ in 4 doses administered 21, 14, and 7 days before surgery and on the day of surgery. DVT prophylaxis is recommended. Individualize dose selection and adjustment for the elderly to achieve/maintain target Hgb.
Pediatrics: Initiate when Hgb is <10g/dL (see PI for additional parameters). 5-18 Yrs: Patients on Chemotherapy: Initial: 600 U/kg IV weekly until completion of a chemotherapy course. Titrate: Adjust dose based on Hgb levels; see PI. Max: 60,000 U weekly. 1 Month-16 Yrs: CKD on Dialysis: Initial: 50 U/kg IV/SQ 3X weekly. IV route is recommended for patients on dialysis. Titrate: Adjust dose based on Hgb levels; see PI.

HOW SUPPLIED: Inj: 2000 U/mL, 3000 U/mL, 4000 U/mL, 10,000 U/mL, 40,000 U/mL [Single-dose]; 10,000 U/mL, 20,000 U/mL [Multidose]

CONTRAINDICATIONS: Uncontrolled HTN, pure red cell aplasia (PRCA) that begins after treatment with epoetin alfa or other erythropoietin drugs. Multidose: Neonates, infants, pregnant women, and nursing mothers.

WARNINGS/PRECAUTIONS: Not indicated for use in patients with cancer who are receiving hormonal agents, biologic products, or radiotherapy, unless also receiving concomitant myelosuppressive chemotherapy; in patients scheduled for surgery who are willing to donate autologous blood; in patients undergoing cardiac/vascular surgery, or as a substitute for RBC transfusions in patients requiring immediate correction of anemia. Evaluate transferrin saturation and serum ferritin prior to and during treatment; administer supplemental iron when serum ferritin is <100mcg/L or serum transferrin saturation is <20%. Correct/exclude other causes of anemia (eg, vitamin deficiency, metabolic/chronic inflammatory conditions, bleeding) before initiating therapy. Hypertensive encephalopathy and seizures reported with CKD. Appropriately control HTN prior to initiation of and during treatment; reduce/withhold therapy if BP becomes difficult to control. PRCA and severe anemia, with or without other cytopenias that arise following development of neutralizing antibodies to erythropoietin reported. Withhold and evaluate for neutralizing antibodies to erythropoietin if severe anemia and low reticulocyte count develop; d/c permanently if PRCA develops, and do not switch to other erythropoiesis-stimulating agents. Immediately and permanently d/c if a serious allergic or anaphylactic reaction occurs. Contains albumin; may carry an extremely remote risk for transmission of viral diseases or Creutzfeldt-Jakob disease. May require adjustment in dialysis prescriptions and increased anticoagulation with heparin to prevent clotting of extracorporeal circuit during hemodialysis. Multidose vial contains benzyl alcohol; benzyl alcohol associated with serious adverse events and death, particularly in pediatric patients.

ADVERSE REACTIONS: CV/thromboembolic reactions, tumor progression/recurrence, pyrexia, N/V, HTN, cough, arthralgia, myalgia, pruritus, rash, headache, injection-site pain, stomatitis, dizziness.

PREGNANCY: Category C, caution in nursing.

MECHANISM OF ACTION: Erythropoiesis-stimulating glycoprotein; stimulates erythropoiesis by the same mechanism as endogenous erythropoietin.

PHARMACOKINETICS: Absorption: Adults and Pediatrics with CKD: (SQ) T_{max}=5-24 hrs. Anemic Cancer Patients: (SQ) T_{max}=13.3 hrs (150 U/kg), 38 hrs (40,000 U). **Elimination:** Adults and Pediatrics with CKD: (IV) $T_{1/2}$=4-13 hrs. Anemic Cancer Patients: (SQ) $T_{1/2}$=16-67 hrs.

NURSING CONSIDERATIONS

Assessment: Assess for uncontrolled HTN, previous hypersensitivity to the drug, causes of anemia, pregnancy/nursing status, and other conditions where treatment is cautioned/contraindicated. Obtain baseline Hgb levels, transferrin saturation, and serum ferritin.

Monitoring: Monitor for signs/symptoms of an allergic reaction, CV/thromboembolic events, stroke, premonitory neurologic symptoms, PRCA, severe anemia, and progression/recurrence of tumor. Monitor Hgb (weekly until stable), BP, transferrin saturation, and serum ferritin.

Patient Counseling: Inform about risks/benefits of therapy, increased risks of mortality, serious CV reactions, thromboembolic reactions, stroke, and tumor progression/recurrence, need to have regular laboratory tests for Hgb, and for cancer patients to sign the patient-physician acknowledgment form prior to therapy. Instruct to undergo regular BP monitoring, adhere to prescribed antihypertensive regimen, and follow recommended dietary restrictions. Advise to contact physician if new onset neurologic symptoms or changes in seizure frequency occur, or if any other adverse reactions develop. Inform that risks are associated with benzyl alcohol in neonates, infants, pregnant women, and nursing mothers. Instruct regarding proper disposal and caution against the reuse of needles, syringes, or unused portions of single-dose vials.

Administration: IV/SQ route. IV route recommended in hemodialysis patients. Do not dilute. Do not mix with other drug sol; refer to PI for admixing exceptions. **Storage:** 2-8°C (36-46°F). Do not freeze or shake. Protect from light. Discard unused portions of multidose vials 21 days after initial entry.

PROGRAF   RX
tacrolimus (Astellas)

> Immunosuppression may lead to increased risk of lymphoma and other malignancies, particularly of the skin. Increased susceptibility to infections (bacterial, viral, fungal, protozoal, opportunistic). Should only be prescribed by physicians experienced in immunosuppressive therapy and management of organ transplant patients.

THERAPEUTIC CLASS: Macrolide immunosuppressant

INDICATIONS: Prophylaxis of organ rejection in patients receiving allogeneic kidney, liver, and heart transplants with concomitant adrenal corticosteroids. In heart and kidney transplant patients, azathioprine or mycophenolate mofetil (MMF) coadministration is recommended.

DOSAGE: *Adults:* Initial: Administer no sooner than 6 hrs after liver/heart transplant. May administer within 24 hrs of kidney transplant, but should be delayed until renal function has recovered. Adjunct therapy with adrenal corticosteroids is recommended early post-transplant. (PO) Administer daily dose as 2 divided doses, q12h. Kidney Transplant: 0.2mg/kg/day in combination with azathioprine or 0.1mg/kg/day in combination with MMF/Interleukin-2 receptor antagonist. Liver Transplant: 0.10-0.15mg/kg/day. Heart Transplant: 0.075mg/kg/day. Titrate based on clinical assessments of rejection and tolerability. Maint: Lower dosage may be sufficient. Black patients may require higher doses. If receiving IV infusion, give 1st PO dose 8-12 hrs after d/c of IV infusion. (Inj) Give as continuous IV infusion if patient cannot tolerate PO. D/C as soon as patient can tolerate PO, usually within 2-3 days. Initial: Kidney/Liver Transplant: 0.03-0.05mg/kg/day. Heart Transplant: 0.01mg/kg/day. Adult patients should receive doses at the lower end of the dosing range. Refer to PI for dose adjustments in renal/hepatic impairment. Elderly: Start at lower end of dosing range.
Pediatrics: Liver Transplant: Initial: (PO) 0.15-0.2mg/kg/day as 2 divided doses, q12h. (Inj) 0.03-0.05mg/kg/day IV if necessary. Refer to PI for dose adjustments in renal/hepatic impairment.

HOW SUPPLIED: Cap: 0.5mg, 1mg, 5mg; Inj: 5mg/mL [1mL]

CONTRAINDICATIONS: (Inj) Hypersensitivity to polyoxyl 60 hydrogenated castor oil (HCO-60).

WARNINGS/PRECAUTIONS: Limit exposure to sunlight and UV light in patients at increased risk for skin cancer. Increased risk for polyoma virus infections, cytomegalovirus (CMV) viremia, and CMV disease. Polyoma virus-associated nephropathy reported; may lead to renal dysfunction and kidney graft loss. Progressive multifocal leukoencephalopathy (PML) reported; consider PML in differential diagnosis in patients reporting neurological symptoms and consider consultation with a neurologist. May cause new onset diabetes mellitus; closely monitor blood glucose concentrations. May cause acute/chronic nephrotoxicity; closely monitor patients with renal dysfunction. Consider changing to another immunosuppressive therapy in patients with persistent SrCr elevations unresponsive to dose adjustments. May cause neurotoxicity (eg, posterior reversible encephalopathy syndrome [PRES], delirium, coma); if PRES is suspected or diagnosed, maintain BP control and immediately reduce immunosuppression. Hyperkalemia and HTN reported. Myocardial hypertrophy reported; consider dose reduction or d/c if diagnosed. Pure red cell aplasia (PRCA) reported; consider d/c if diagnosed. Caution in elderly. (Inj) Anaphylactic reactions may occur; should be reserved for patients unable to take cap orally. Patients should be under continuous observation for at least the 1st 30 min following the start of infusion and at frequent intervals thereafter; stop infusion if signs/symptoms of anaphylaxis occur.

ADVERSE REACTIONS: Lymphoma, malignancies, infection, tremor, HTN, abnormal renal function, headache, insomnia, hyperglycemia, hyperkalemia, hypomagnesemia, diarrhea, N/V, paresthesia.

INTERACTIONS: Do not use with cyclosporine; d/c tacrolimus or cyclosporine at least 24 hrs before initiating the other. Not recommended with sirolimus in liver and heart transplant. Safety and efficacy with sirolimus not established in kidney transplant. Increased levels with CYP3A inhibitors (eg, lansoprazole, omeprazole, cimetidine). Decreased levels with CYP3A inducers. May increase mycophenolic acid (MPA) exposure after crossover from cyclosporine to tacrolimus in patients concomitantly receiving MPA-containing products. Avoid grapefruit or grapefruit juice and consider avoiding nelfinavir. Monitor whole blood concentrations and adjust dose with concomitant protease inhibitors (eg, ritonavir, telaprevir, boceprevir), calcium channel blockers (CCBs) (eg, verapamil, diltiazem, nifedipine, nicardipine), erythromycin, clarithromycin, troleandomycin, chloramphenicol, rifampin, rifabutin, phenytoin, carbamazepine, phenobarbital, St. John's wort, magnesium and aluminum hydroxide antacids, bromocriptine, nefazodone, metoclopramide, danazol, ethinyl estradiol, amiodarone, or methylprednisolone, or when concomitant use of antifungal drugs (eg, azoles, caspofungin) with tacrolimus is initiated or d/c. May increase levels of phenytoin; monitor phenytoin levels and adjust phenytoin dose PRN. Caution with CYP3A4 inhibitors (eg, antifungals, CCBs, macrolide antibiotics). Additive/synergistic impairment of renal function with drugs that may be associated with renal dysfunction (eg, aminoglycosides, ganciclovir, amphotericin B, cisplatin, nucleotide reverse transcriptase inhibitors, protease inhibitors). Caution prior to use of other agents or antihypertensive agents associated with hyperkalemia (eg, K⁺-sparing diuretics, ACE inhibitors, ARBs). Strong CYP3A4 inhibitors/inducers not recommended without tacrolimus dose adjustments and subsequent close monitoring of tacrolimus whole blood trough concentrations and tacrolimus-associated adverse reactions. Reduce tacrolimus dose, closely monitor tacrolimus whole blood concentrations, and monitor for QT prolongation when coadministered with CYP3A4 substrates and/or inhibitors that also have the potential to prolong the QT interval. Amiodarone may increase whole blood concentrations with or without concurrent QT prolongation. Avoid live vaccines.

PREGNANCY: Category C, not for use in nursing.

MECHANISM OF ACTION: Macrolide immunosuppressant; not established. Suspected to inhibit T-lymphocyte activation. Binds to intracellular protein, FKBP-12, forming a complex of tacrolimus-FKBP-12, calcium, calmodulin, and calcineurin, inhibiting phosphatase activity of calcineurin. Effect may prevent dephosphorylation and translocation of nuclear factor of activated T-cells, a nuclear component thought to initiate gene transcription for the formation of lymphokines.

PHARMACOKINETICS: Absorption: (PO) Incomplete and variable. Refer to PI for parameters in different populations. **Distribution:** Plasma protein binding (99%), crosses placenta, found in breast milk. **Metabolism:** Liver, via CYP3A (demethylation and hydroxylation); 13-demethyl tacrolimus (major metabolite); 31-demethyl (active metabolite). **Elimination:** (PO) Feces (92.6%), urine (2.3%). (IV) Feces (92.4%); urine (<1% unchanged). Refer to PI for $T_{1/2}$ values in different populations.

NURSING CONSIDERATIONS

Assessment: Assess for renal/hepatic impairment, hypersensitivity to the drug, Epstein Barr virus/CMV seronegativity, pregnancy/nursing status, and possible drug interactions. (Inj) Assess for hypersensitivity to HCO-60 (polyoxyl 60 hydrogenated castor oil).

Monitoring: Monitor tacrolimus blood concentrations in conjunction with other laboratory and clinical parameters (hepatic/renal dysfunction, addition or d/c of potential interacting drugs, post-transplant time). Monitor for signs/symptoms of neurotoxicity, lymphomas and other malignancies, HTN, myocardial hypertrophy, PRCA, and various infections. Monitor serum K⁺ and glucose concentrations. (Inj) Monitor for anaphylactic reactions.

Patient Counseling: Advise to take medicine at the same 12-hr interval every day and not to eat grapefruit or drink grapefruit juice in combination with the drug. Advise to limit exposure to sunlight and UV light by wearing protective clothing and to use sunscreen with high protection factor. Instruct to contact physician if frequent urination, increased thirst or hunger, vision changes, deliriums, tremors, or any symptoms of infection develop. Advise to attend all visits and complete all blood tests ordered by their medical team. Instruct to inform physician if patient plans to become pregnant or breastfeed or when they start or stop taking any medication (prescription and nonprescription, natural/herbal, nutritional supplements, vitamins).

Administration: Oral/IV route. (Cap) Take consistently with or without food. (Inj) Refer to PI for preparation and administration instructions. **Storage:** Cap: 25°C (77°F); excursions permitted to

15-30°C (59-86°F). Inj: 5-25°C (41-77°F). Diluted Sol: store in glass or polyethylene containers and discard after 24 hrs.

PROLIA   RX
denosumab (Amgen)

THERAPEUTIC CLASS: IgG$_2$ monoclonal antibody

INDICATIONS: Treatment of postmenopausal women with osteoporosis or to increase bone mass in men with osteoporosis at high risk for fracture (eg, history of osteoporotic fracture, multiple risk factors for fracture) or patients who have failed or are intolerant to other available osteoporosis therapy. As treatment to increase bone mass in women at high risk for fracture receiving adjuvant aromatase inhibitor therapy for breast cancer. As treatment to increase bone mass in men at high risk for fracture receiving androgen deprivation therapy for nonmetastatic prostate cancer.

DOSAGE: *Adults:* 60mg as a single SQ inj once every 6 months. If a dose is missed, administer as soon as patient is available and schedule inj every 6 months from date of last inj. All patients should receive Ca^{2+} 1000mg daily and at least 400 IU vitamin D daily.

HOW SUPPLIED: Inj: 60mg/mL [prefilled syringe, vial]

CONTRAINDICATIONS: Hypocalcemia, pregnancy.

WARNINGS/PRECAUTIONS: Should be administered by a healthcare professional. Do not give with other drugs that contain the same active ingredient (eg, Xgeva). Hypersensitivity, including anaphylaxis, reported; d/c further use and initiate appropriate therapy if anaphylactic/allergic reaction occurs. Hypocalcemia may be exacerbated; correct preexisting hypocalcemia prior to initiating therapy. Monitor Ca^{2+} and mineral levels (phosphorus [P] and Mg^{2+}) in patients predisposed to hypocalcemia and disturbances of mineral metabolism (eg, history of hypoparathyroidism, thyroid/parathyroid surgery, malabsorption syndromes, excision of the small intestine, severe renal impairment [CrCl <30mL/min] or receiving dialysis). Endocarditis and serious skin, abdomen, urinary tract, and ear infections leading to hospitalization reported. Increased risk for serious infections in patients with an impaired immune system. Epidermal and dermal adverse events may occur; consider discontinuing therapy if severe symptoms develop. Osteonecrosis of the jaw (ONJ) may occur; routine oral exam should be performed prior to initiation of treatment. Consider a dental examination with appropriate preventive dentistry prior to treatment in patients with risk factors for ONJ (eg, invasive dental procedures, diagnosis of cancer, concomitant therapies [eg, chemotherapy, corticosteroids], poor oral hygiene, comorbid disorders [eg, periodontal and/or other preexisting dental disease, anemia, coagulopathy, infection, ill-fitting dentures]). Atypical low-energy or low-trauma fractures of the femoral shaft reported; consider interruption of therapy. Significant suppression of bone remodeling as evidenced by markers of bone turnover and bone histomorphometry reported. Potential for fetal exposure to denosumab when a man treated with denosumab has unprotected sexual intercourse with a pregnant partner.

ADVERSE REACTIONS: Back pain, anemia, vertigo, upper abdominal pain, peripheral edema, cystitis, upper respiratory tract infection, pneumonia, hypercholesterolemia, pain in extremity, musculoskeletal pain, bone pain, sciatica, arthralgia, nasopharyngitis.

INTERACTIONS: Immunosuppressant agents may increase the risk of serious infections.

PREGNANCY: Category X, not for use in nursing.

MECHANISM OF ACTION: IgG$_2$ monoclonal antibody; binds to receptor activator of nuclear factor kappa-B ligand (RANKL) and prevents RANKL from activating its receptor, RANK, on the surface of osteoclasts and their precursors, thereby decreasing bone resorption and increasing bone mass and strength in both cortical and trabecular bone.

PHARMACOKINETICS: Absorption: (60mg SQ, after fasting) C_{max}=6.75mcg/mL, T_{max}=10 days, $AUC_{0-16\ weeks}$=316mcg•day/mL. **Elimination:** $T_{1/2}$=25.4 days.

NURSING CONSIDERATIONS

Assessment: Assess for drug hypersensitivity, preexisting hypocalcemia, history of hypoparathyroidism, thyroid/parathyroid surgery, malabsorption syndromes, excision of the small intestine, renal impairment, impairment of the immune system, risk factors for ONJ, pregnancy/nursing status, and possible drug interactions. Consider performing a dental examination with appropriate preventive dentistry in patients with risk factors for ONJ.

Monitoring: Monitor for signs/symptoms of hypocalcemia, infections (eg, cellulitis), hypersensitivity, dermatological reactions, ONJ, atypical fractures, delayed fracture healing, and other adverse reactions. Monitor Ca^{2+} and mineral levels (P and Mg^{2+}).

Patient Counseling: Counsel not to take with other drugs with the same active ingredient. Inform about the signs/symptoms of hypocalcemia and the importance of maintaining Ca^{2+} levels with adequate Ca^{2+} and vitamin D supplementation. Advise to seek prompt medical attention if signs/

symptoms of hypocalcemia, infections, dermatological reactions, and hypersensitivity reactions develop. Advise to maintain good oral hygiene during treatment and to inform dentist prior to dental procedures of current treatment. Instruct to inform physician or dentist if patient experiences persistent pain and/or slow healing of the mouth or jaw after dental surgery. Advise to report new or unusual thigh, hip, or groin pain. Counsel of the potential fetal exposure when a man treated with therapy has unprotected sexual intercourse with a pregnant partner. Inform that therapy should not be used if pregnant or nursing. Counsel to adhere to proper schedule of administration.

Administration: SQ route. Administer in the upper arm/thigh, or abdomen. Refer to PI for preparation and administration instructions. **Storage:** 2-8°C (36-46°F). Do not freeze. Prior to administration, may allow to reach room temperature (≤25°C [77°F]). Use within 14 days. Protect from direct light and heat. Avoid vigorous shaking.

PROMACTA   RX
eltrombopag (GlaxoSmithKline)

> May increase risk of hepatic decompensation in patients with chronic hepatitis C when given in combination with interferon and ribavirin.

THERAPEUTIC CLASS: Thrombopoietin-receptor agonist

INDICATIONS: Treatment of thrombocytopenia in patients with chronic immune (idiopathic) thrombocytopenia purpura (ITP) who have had an insufficient response to corticosteroids, immunoglobulins, or splenectomy. Treatment of thrombocytopenia in patients with chronic hepatitis C to allow the initiation and maintenance of interferon-based therapy.

DOSAGE: *Adults:* Chronic ITP: Initial: 50mg qd. East Asian Ancestry/Mild to Severe Hepatic Impairment (Child-Pugh Class A, B, C): Initial: 25mg qd. East Asian Ancestry with Hepatic Impairment (Child-Pugh Class A, B, C): Initial: 12.5mg qd. Titrate: Adjust the dose to achieve and maintain platelet count ≥50 x 10^9/L. Max: 75mg/day. Refer to PI for monitoring and dose adjustments. Hepatic Impairment (Child-Pugh A, B, C): After initiating therapy or after any subsequent dosing increase, wait 3 weeks before increasing the dose. Modify dosage regimen of concomitant ITP medications; do not administer >1 dose of eltrombopag within any 24-hr period. D/C if platelet count does not increase to a sufficient level after 4 weeks of therapy at max daily dose of 75mg. Chronic Hepatitis C-Associated Thrombocytopenia: Initial: 25mg qd. Titrate: Adjust dose in 25mg increments every 2 weeks as necessary to achieve the target platelet count required to initiate antiviral therapy. During antiviral therapy, adjust dose to avoid dose reductions of peginterferon. Max: 100mg/day. Refer to PI for monitoring and dose adjustments. D/C therapy when antiviral therapy is discontinued.

HOW SUPPLIED: Tab: 12.5mg, 25mg, 50mg, 75mg, 100mg

WARNINGS/PRECAUTIONS: Should not be used to normalize platelet counts. Should only be used in patients with ITP whose degree of thrombocytopenia and clinical condition increase the risk for bleeding. Use lowest dose to achieve and maintain a platelet count ≥50 x 10^9/L as necessary to reduce the risk for bleeding. Liver enzyme elevations and indirect hyperbilirubinemia may occur; if bilirubin is elevated, perform fractionation. D/C if ALT levels increase to ≥3X ULN in patients with normal liver function or ≥3X baseline in patients with pretreatment elevations in transaminases, and are progressively increasing or persistent for ≥4 weeks, or accompanied by increased direct bilirubin, or accompanied by clinical symptoms of liver injury or evidence for hepatic decompensation. Hepatotoxicity may reoccur with reinitiation; caution with reintroduction of therapy and measure LFTs weekly. If liver test abnormalities persist, worsen or reoccur, then permanently d/c therapy. Thrombotic/thromboembolic complications may result from increase in platelet counts; caution in patients with known risk factors for thromboembolism (eg, factor V Leiden, antithrombin III deficiency, antiphospholipid syndrome, chronic liver disease). Development or worsening of cataracts reported. Closely monitor patients with renal impairment.

ADVERSE REACTIONS: Headache, N/V, diarrhea, upper respiratory tract infection, hyperbilirubinemia, cataract, increased ALT/AST, myalgia, urinary tract infection, oropharyngeal pain, pharyngitis, back pain, influenza, anemia, pyrexia, fatigue.

INTERACTIONS: See Boxed Warning. Do not take within 4 hrs of any medications or products containing polyvalent cations, such as antacids, dairy products, and mineral supplements. Caution with substrates of organic anion transporting polypeptide 1B1 (eg, atorvastatin, bosentan, glyburide) or breast cancer resistant protein (eg, imatinib, irinotecan, methotrexate); monitor for signs/symptoms of excessive exposure and consider dose reduction of these drugs. Lopinavir/ritonavir may decrease plasma exposure.

PREGNANCY: Category C, not for use in nursing.

P

MECHANISM OF ACTION: Thrombopoietin (TPO)-receptor agonist; interacts with the transmembrane domain of the human TPO receptor and initiates signaling cascades that induce proliferation and differentiation of megakaryocytes from bone marrow progenitor cells.

PHARMACOKINETICS: Absorption: T_{max}=2-6 hrs. **Distribution:** Plasma protein binding (>99%). **Metabolism:** Extensive; cleavage, oxidation (via CYP1A2, CYP2C8), and conjugation with glucuronic acid (via UGT1A1, UGT1A3), glutathione, or cysteine. **Elimination:** Urine (31%), feces (59%, 20% unchanged); $T_{1/2}$=26-35 hrs (ITP).

NURSING CONSIDERATIONS

Assessment: Assess for degree of thrombocytopenia, risk factors for thromboembolism, renal/hepatic impairment, pregnancy/nursing status, and for possible drug interactions. Obtain baseline CBCs with differentials, including platelet counts, and LFTs. Perform a baseline ocular exam.

Monitoring: Monitor for thrombotic/thromboembolic complications, hepatotoxicity, hepatic decompensation in patients with chronic hepatitis C, cataracts, and other adverse reactions. Closely monitor patients with renal impairment. Monitor LFTs every 2 weeks during dose adjustment phase, then monthly following establishment of a stable dose. If abnormal LFT levels are detected, repeat tests within 3-5 days. If the abnormalities are confirmed, monitor serum LFT tests weekly until resolved or stabilized. Perform regular ocular exam. Monitor platelet counts every week prior to starting antiviral therapy in patients with chronic hepatitis C. Monitor CBCs with differentials, including platelets counts, weekly during therapy until a stable platelet count is achieved. Obtain CBCs with differentials, including platelet counts, monthly thereafter and then weekly for at least 4 weeks after discontinuation.

Patient Counseling: Inform about the risks and benefits of therapy. Inform that therapy may be associated with hepatobiliary lab abnormalities. Advise patients with chronic hepatitis C and cirrhosis that hepatic decompensation may occur when receiving alfa interferon therapy. Advise to avoid situations or medications that may increase risk for bleeding and to report to physician any signs/symptoms of liver problems immediately. Inform that thrombocytopenia and risk of bleeding may reoccur upon discontinuation, particularly if therapy is discontinued while on anticoagulants/antiplatelet agents. Inform that excessive dose may result in excessive platelet counts and risk for thrombotic/thromboembolic complications. Advise to have a baseline ocular exam prior to administration of therapy and be monitored for signs/symptoms of cataracts during therapy.

Administration: Oral route. Take on empty stomach (1 hr ac or 2 hrs pc). Allow at least a 4-hr interval between therapy and other medications (eg, antacids), Ca^{2+}-rich foods (eg, dairy products and Ca^{2+} fortified juices), or supplements containing polyvalent cations, such as iron, Ca^{2+}, aluminum, Mg^{2+}, selenium, and zinc. **Storage:** 20-25°C (68-77°F); excursions permitted to 15-30°C (59-86°F).

PROMETHAZINE   RX
promethazine HCl (Various)

> Promethazine HCl should not be used in patients <2 yrs of age; potential for fatal respiratory depression. Caution when administering to patients ≥2 yrs of age; use lowest effective dose and avoid concomitant administration of respiratory depressants.

OTHER BRAND NAMES: Phenadoz (Various) - Promethegan (G & W Labs)

THERAPEUTIC CLASS: Phenothiazine derivative

INDICATIONS: Allergic and vasomotor rhinitis, allergic conjunctivitis, allergic reactions to blood or plasma, dermographism, mild allergic skin manifestation of urticaria and angioedema. Preoperative, postoperative, or obstetric sedation. Adjunct in anaphylactic reactions. Prevention and control of N/V with certain types of anesthesia and surgery. Active and prophylactic treatment of motion sickness. Sedation, relief of apprehension, production of light sleep. Adjunct with meperidine or other analgesics for postoperative pain. Antiemetic in postoperative patients.

DOSAGE: *Adults:* Allergy: Usual: 25mg qhs or 12.5mg ac and hs; may give 6.25-12.5mg tid. Adjust to lowest effective dose after initiation. Motion Sickness: Initial: 25mg 30-60 min before travel, repeat after 8-12 hrs if necessary. Maint: 25mg bid, on arising and before pm meal. Prevention/Control of N/V: Prevention: Usual: 25mg, may repeat q4-6h as necessary. Control: Usual: 25mg, then 12.5-25mg q4-6h as necessary. Sedation: 25-50mg qhs. Preoperative: Usual: 50mg. Postoperative/Adjunctive with analgesics: 25-50mg.
Pediatrics: ≥2 yrs: Allergy: Usual: 25mg qhs or 12.5mg ac and hs; may give 6.25-12.5mg tid. Adjust to lowest effective dose after initiation. Motion Sickness: 12.5-25mg bid. Prevention/Control of N/V: Prevention: Usual: 25mg, may repeat q4-6h as necessary. Control: Usual: 0.5mg/lb. Adjust dose based on patient age/weight and severity of condition. Sedation: 12.5-25mg hs. Preoperative: Usual: 0.5mg/lb. Postoperative/Adjunctive with analgesics: 12.5-25mg.

HOW SUPPLIED: Sup: (Phenadoz, Promethazine) 12.5mg, 25mg, (Promethegan) 50mg; Syrup: (Promethazine): 6.25mg/5mL [118mL, 237mL, 473mL] Tab: (Promethazine) 12.5mg*, 25mg*, 50mg *scored

CONTRAINDICATIONS: Treatment of lower respiratory tract symptoms, including asthma. Comatose states, pediatric patients <2 yrs.

WARNINGS/PRECAUTIONS: Avoid in pediatric patients whose signs and symptoms may suggest Reye's syndrome or other hepatic diseases. May impair mental/physical abilities. May lower seizure threshold; caution with seizure disorders. May lead to potentially fatal respiratory depression; avoid with compromised respiratory function (eg, chronic obstructive pulmonary disease, sleep apnea). Caution with bone marrow depression; leukopenia and agranulocytosis reported. Neuroleptic malignant syndrome (NMS) reported; d/c immediately. Hallucinations and convulsions may occur in pediatric patients. Acutely ill pediatric patients who are dehydrated may have increased susceptibility to dystonias. Not recommended for uncomplicated vomiting in pediatric patients; should be limited to prolonged vomiting of known etiology. Caution with narrow-angle glaucoma, prostatic hypertrophy, stenosing peptic ulcer, bladder-neck or pyloroduodenal obstruction, cardiovascular (CV) disease, hepatic impairment. Cholestatic jaundice reported. Caution in elderly patients.

ADVERSE REACTIONS: Drowsiness, sedation, blurred vision, dizziness, increased or decreased BP, urticaria, dry mouth, N/V, respiratory depression, hallucination, leukopenia, apnea, NMS.

INTERACTIONS: See Boxed Warning. May increase rates of extrapyramidal effects with concomitant MAOI use. May increase, prolong, or intensify the sedative action of other CNS depressants, such as alcohol, sedatives/hypnotics (including barbiturates), narcotics, narcotic analgesics, general anesthetics, TCAs, tranquilizers; avoid such agents or reduce dosages. Reduce barbiturate dose by at least one-half and narcotic analgesics by one-quarter to one-half. May reverse vasopressor effect of epinephrine. Caution with medications that may affect seizure threshold (eg, narcotics, local anesthetics). Caution with anticholinergics. Leukopenia and agranulocytosis reported, usually with marrow-toxic agents. NMS reported in combination with antipsychotics.

PREGNANCY: Category C, not for use in nursing.

MECHANISM OF ACTION: Phenothiazine derivative; H_1 receptor-blocking agent (antihistaminic action) and provides sedative and antiemetic effects.

PHARMACOKINETICS: Absorption: Well-absorbed from GI tract. **Metabolism:** Liver; sulfoxides, N-demethylpromethazine (metabolites). **Elimination:** Urine.

NURSING CONSIDERATIONS

Assessment: Assess for drug hypersensitivity or prior idiosyncratic reaction to phenothiazines, or any other conditions where treatment is contraindicated or cautioned. Assess for pregnancy/nursing status and for possible drug interaction. Assess for signs/symptoms of Reye's syndrome, hepatic diseases, or encephalopathy in pediatrics.

Monitoring: Monitor for signs/symptoms of CNS/respiratory depression, NMS, seizures, cholestatic jaundice, leukopenia, agranulocytosis. Monitor for hallucinations, convulsions, extrapyramidal symptoms, respiratory depression, dystonias in pediatric patients. Monitor for false positive and false negative pregnancy tests, blood glucose levels, and BP. Monitor platelet count in newborns when used in pregnant women within 2 weeks of delivery.

Patient Counseling: Inform that drowsiness or impairment of mental and/or physical abilities may occur. Counsel to report involuntary muscle movements. Instruct to avoid alcohol use, prolonged sun exposure, and concomitant use of other CNS depressants.

Administration: Oral and rectal route. **Storage:** (Tab) 20-25°C (68-77°F). Protect from light. (Sup) 2-8°C (36-46°F).

PROMETHAZINE VC/CODEINE — CV
phenylephrine HCl - promethazine HCl - codeine phosphate (Qualitest)

> Contraindicated in pediatric patients <6 yrs of age. Concomitant administration of promethazine products with other respiratory depressants is associated with respiratory depression, and sometimes death, in pediatric patients. Respiratory depression, including fatalities, have been reported with use of promethazine HCl in patients <2 yrs of age.

THERAPEUTIC CLASS: Antitussive/phenothiazine derivative/sympathomimetic

INDICATIONS: Temporary relief of coughs and upper respiratory symptoms (eg, nasal congestion) associated with allergy or the common cold.

DOSAGE: *Adults:* 5mL q4-6h. Max: 30mL/24hr. Elderly: Start at lower end of dosing range. *Pediatrics:* ≥12 Yrs: 5mL q4-6h. Max: 30mL/24hr. 6-<12 Yrs: 2.5-5mL q4-6h. Max: 30mL/24hr.

HOW SUPPLIED: Syrup: (Codeine Phosphate-Promethazine HCl-Phenylephrine HCl) 10mg-6.25mg-5mg/5mL [118mL, 237mL, 473mL]

CONTRAINDICATIONS: Concomitant use with MAOIs, comatose states, treatment of lower respiratory tract symptoms (eg, asthma), HTN, peripheral vascular insufficiency, pediatric patients <6 yrs of age.

WARNINGS/PRECAUTIONS: Should only be given to a pregnant woman if clearly needed. Caution in elderly. Codeine: Do not increase dose if cough fails to respond to treatment. May cause/aggravate constipation. Caution in atopic children. Capacity to elevate CSF pressure and respiratory depressant effects may be markedly exaggerated in head injury, intracranial lesions, or with preexisting increase in intracranial pressure. May obscure clinical course in patients with head injuries. Avoid with acute febrile illness with productive cough or in chronic respiratory disease. May produce orthostatic hypotension in ambulatory patients. Give with caution and reduce initial dose with acute abdominal conditions, convulsive disorders, significant hepatic/renal impairment, fever, hypothyroidism, Addison's disease, ulcerative colitis, prostatic hypertrophy, recent GI or urinary tract surgery, and in the very young, elderly, or debilitated. Use lowest effective dose for the shortest period of time. Potential for abuse and dependence. Promethazine: May impair mental/physical abilities. May lead to potentially fatal respiratory depression; avoid with compromised respiratory function (eg, chronic obstructive pulmonary disease, sleep apnea). May lower seizure threshold. Leukopenia and agranulocytosis reported, especially when given with other marrow-toxic agents. Neuroleptic malignant syndrome (NMS) reported; d/c immediately if NMS occurs. Hallucinations and convulsions may occur in pediatric patients. Acutely ill pediatric patients who are dehydrated may have increased susceptibility to dystonias. Cholestatic jaundice reported. Caution with narrow-angle glaucoma, prostatic hypertrophy, stenosing peptic ulcer, pyloroduodenal/bladder-neck obstruction, cardiovascular disease, or with impaired liver function. May increase blood glucose. Phenylephrine: Caution with diabetes mellitus, thyroid, and heart diseases. May cause urinary retention in men with symptomatic BPH. May decrease cardiac output; use extreme caution with arteriosclerosis, the elderly, and/or patients with initially poor cerebral or coronary circulation.

ADVERSE REACTIONS: Drowsiness, dizziness, anxiety, sedation, tremor, blurred vision, dry mouth, increased or decreased BP, N/V, respiratory depression, urinary retention, NMS, constipation.

INTERACTIONS: See Boxed Warning and Contraindications. Promethazine: May increase, prolong, or intensify the sedative action of other CNS depressants (eg, alcohol, narcotics, general anesthetics, tranquilizers); avoid such agents or administer in reduced doses. Reduce dose of barbiturate by at least one-half and narcotic analgesics by one-quarter to one-half. May reverse vasopressor effect of epinephrine. Caution with other agents with anticholinergic properties and drugs that also affect seizure threshold (eg, narcotics, local anesthetics). Phenylephrine: Pressor response increased with TCAs and decreased with prior administration of phentolamine or other α-adrenergic blockers. Ergot alkaloids may cause excessive rise in BP. Tachycardia or other arrhythmias may occur with bronchodilator sympathomimetics, epinephrine, or other sympathomimetics. Reflex bradycardia blocked and pressor response enhanced with atropine sulfate. Cardiostimulating effects blocked with prior administration of propranolol or other β-adrenergic blockers. Synergistic adrenergic response with diet preparations (eg, amphetamines, phenylpropanolamine).

PREGNANCY: Category C, caution in nursing.

MECHANISM OF ACTION: Codeine: Narcotic analgesic/antitussive; primary effects are on CNS and GI tract. Promethazine: Phenothiazine derivative; blocks H_1 receptor and provides sedative and antiemetic effects. Phenylephrine: Sympathomimetic amine; potent postsynaptic-α-receptor agonist with little effect on β-receptors of heart. Causes vasoconstriction and has a mild central stimulant effect.

PHARMACOKINETICS: Absorption: Codeine/Promethazine: Well-absorbed. Phenylephrine: Irregularly absorbed. **Distribution:** Codeine: Crosses placenta; found in breast milk. **Metabolism:** Codeine: Liver via O-demethylation, N-demethylation, and partial conjugation with glucuronic acid. Promethazine: Liver; sulfoxides and N-demethylpromethazine (metabolites). Phenylephrine: Liver and intestine via monoamine oxidase. **Elimination:** Codeine: Urine (primary; inactive metabolites and free/conjugated morphine), feces (negligible amount; parent compound and metabolites). Promethazine: Urine (metabolites).

NURSING CONSIDERATIONS

Assessment: Assess for drug hypersensitivity or idiosyncrasy, history of drug abuse/dependence, or any other conditions where treatment is contraindicated or cautioned. Assess BP, pregnancy/nursing status, and for possible drug interactions.

Monitoring: Monitor for signs/symptoms of CNS and respiratory depression, constipation, leukopenia, agranulocytosis, cholestatic jaundice, seizures, NMS, and orthostatic hypotension. Monitor for urinary retention in men with BPH. Monitor pediatric patients for hallucinations, convulsions, and dystonias. Monitor glucose levels. Reevaluate 5 days or sooner if cough is unresponsive to treatment.

Patient Counseling: Instruct to measure medication with an accurate measuring device. Inform that therapy may cause marked drowsiness and may impair mental and/or physical abilities required for performing hazardous tasks; advise to avoid such activities until it is known that they do not become drowsy or dizzy with the therapy. Counsel to avoid the use of alcohol and other CNS depressants while on therapy, report any involuntary muscle movements, and avoid prolonged sun exposure. Inform that therapy may produce orthostatic hypotension. Inform about risks and the signs of morphine overdose. Instruct nursing mothers to notify pediatrician immediately, or get emergency medical attention, if signs of morphine toxicity (eg, increased sleepiness, difficulty breastfeeding, breathing difficulties, limpness) are noticed in their infants.

Administration: Oral route. **Storage:** 20-25°C (68-77°F).

PROMETHAZINE W/CODEINE CV
promethazine HCl - codeine phosphate (Various)

> Contraindicated in pediatric patients <6 yrs of age. Concomitant administration of promethazine products with other respiratory depressants is associated with respiratory depression, and sometimes death, in pediatric patients. Respiratory depression, including fatalities, have been reported with use of promethazine in pediatric patients <2 yrs of age.

OTHER BRAND NAMES: Prometh w/ Codeine (Actavis)

THERAPEUTIC CLASS: Antitussive/phenothiazine derivative

INDICATIONS: Temporary relief of cough and upper respiratory symptoms associated with allergy or the common cold.

DOSAGE: *Adults:* 5mL q4-6h. Max: 30mL/24hr. Elderly: Start at lower end of dosing range. *Pediatrics:* ≥12 Yrs: 5mL q4-6h. Max: 30mL/24hr. 6-<12 Yrs: 2.5-5mL q4-6h. Max: 30mL/24hr.

HOW SUPPLIED: Syrup: (Codeine Phosphate-Promethazine HCl) 10mg-6.25mg/5mL [118mL, 273mL, 473mL]

CONTRAINDICATIONS: Comatose states, treatment of lower respiratory tract symptoms (eg, asthma), pediatric patients <6 yrs of age.

WARNINGS/PRECAUTIONS: Should only be given to a pregnant woman if clearly needed. Caution in elderly. Codeine: Do not increase dose if cough fails to respond to treatment. May cause/aggravate constipation. Caution in atopic children. Capacity to elevate CSF pressure and respiratory depressant effects may be markedly exaggerated in head injury, intracranial lesions, or with preexisting increase in intracranial pressure. May obscure clinical course in patients with head injuries. Avoid with acute febrile illness with productive cough or in chronic respiratory disease. May produce orthostatic hypotension in ambulatory patients. Give with caution and reduce initial dose with acute abdominal conditions, convulsive disorders, significant hepatic/renal impairment, fever, hypothyroidism, Addison's disease, ulcerative colitis, prostatic hypertrophy, recent GI or urinary tract surgery, and in the very young, elderly, or debilitated. Use lowest effective dose for the shortest period of time. Potential for abuse and dependence. Promethazine: May impair mental/physical abilities. May lead to potentially fatal respiratory depression; avoid with compromised respiratory function (eg, chronic obstructive pulmonary disease, sleep apnea). May lower seizure threshold. Leukopenia and agranulocytosis reported, especially when given with other marrow-toxic agents. Neuroleptic malignant syndrome (NMS) reported; d/c immediately if NMS occurs. Hallucinations and convulsions may occur in pediatric patients. Acutely ill pediatric patients who are dehydrated may have increased susceptibility to dystonias. Cholestatic jaundice reported. Caution with narrow-angle glaucoma, prostatic hypertrophy, stenosing peptic ulcer, pyloroduodenal/bladder-neck obstruction, cardiovascular disease, or with impaired liver function. May increase blood glucose.

ADVERSE REACTIONS: Drowsiness, dizziness, sedation, blurred vision, dry mouth, increased or decreased BP, N/V, constipation, urinary retention, leukopenia, agranulocytosis, respiratory depression, NMS.

INTERACTIONS: See Boxed Warning. Possible interaction with MAOIs (eg, increased incidence of extrapyramidal effects); consider initial small test dose. Promethazine: May increase, prolong, or intensify the sedative action of other CNS depressants (eg, alcohol, narcotics, general anesthetics, tranquilizers); avoid such agents or administer in reduced doses. Reduce dose of barbiturate by at least one-half and narcotic analgesic by one-quarter to one-half. May reverse vasopressor effect of epinephrine. Caution with other agents with anticholinergic properties and drugs that also affect seizure threshold (eg, narcotics, local anesthetics).

PREGNANCY: Category C, caution in nursing.

MECHANISM OF ACTION: Codeine: Narcotic analgesic/antitussive; primary effects are on CNS and GI tract. Promethazine: Phenothiazine derivative; blocks H_1 receptor and provides sedative and antiemetic effects.

PHARMACOKINETICS: Absorption: Well-absorbed. **Distribution:** Codeine: Crosses placenta; found in breast milk. **Metabolism:** Codeine: Liver via O-demethylation, N-demethylation, and partial conjugation with glucuronic acid. Promethazine: Liver; sulfoxides and N-demethylpromethazine (metabolites). **Elimination:** Codeine: Urine (primary; inactive me-

P

tabolites and free/conjugated morphine), feces (negligible amount; parent compound and metabolites). Promethazine: Urine (metabolites).

NURSING CONSIDERATIONS

Assessment: Assess for drug hypersensitivity or idiosyncrasy, history of drug abuse/dependence, or any other conditions where treatment is contraindicated or cautioned. Assess BP, pregnancy/nursing status, and for possible drug interactions.

Monitoring: Monitor for signs/symptoms of CNS and respiratory depression, constipation, leukopenia, agranulocytosis, cholestatic jaundice, seizures, NMS, orthostatic hypotension, and abuse and dependence. Monitor pediatric patients for hallucinations, convulsions, and dystonias. Monitor glucose levels. Reevaluate 5 days or sooner if cough is unresponsive to treatment.

Patient Counseling: Instruct to measure medication with an accurate measuring device. Inform that therapy may cause drowsiness and may impair mental and/or physical abilities required for performing potentially hazardous tasks; advise to avoid such activities until it is known that they do not become drowsy or dizzy with the therapy. Instruct to avoid the use of alcohol and other CNS depressants while on therapy. Instruct to report any involuntary muscle movements. Instruct to avoid prolonged sun exposure. Inform that therapy may produce orthostatic hypotension. Inform about risks and the signs of morphine overdose. Instruct nursing mothers to notify pediatrician immediately, or get emergency medical attention, if signs of morphine toxicity (eg, increased sleepiness, difficulty breastfeeding, breathing difficulties, limpness) are noticed in their infants.

Administration: Oral route. **Storage:** 20-25°C (68-77°F).

PROPECIA RX
finasteride (Merck)

THERAPEUTIC CLASS: Type II 5 alpha-reductase inhibitor

INDICATIONS: Treatment of male pattern hair loss (androgenetic alopecia) in men only.

DOSAGE: *Adults:* Usual: 1 tab (1mg) qd for ≥3 months. Continued use is recommended to sustain benefit; reevaluate periodically.

HOW SUPPLIED: Tab: 1mg

CONTRAINDICATIONS: Pregnancy, women of child bearing potential.

WARNINGS/PRECAUTIONS: Withdrawal of treatment may lead to reversal of effect within 12 months. Potential risk to male fetus; broken or crushed tabs should not be handled by pregnant women or women who may potentially be pregnant. May decrease serum prostate specific antigen (PSA) levels during therapy or in the presence of prostate cancer; any confirmed increase from lowest PSA value during treatment may signal presence of prostate cancer and should be evaluated. May increase risk of high-grade prostate cancer. Caution with liver dysfunction.

ADVERSE REACTIONS: Decreased libido, erectile dysfunction, ejaculation disorder.

PREGNANCY: Category X, not for use in nursing.

MECHANISM OF ACTION: Type II 5α-reductase inhibitor; blocks peripheral conversion of testosterone to 5α-dihydrotestosterone (DHT), resulting in significant decreases in serum and tissue DHT concentrations.

PHARMACOKINETICS: Absorption: Absolute bioavailability (65%); C_{max}=9.2ng/mL; T_{max}=1-2 hrs; $AUC_{(0-24\ hr)}$=53ng•hr/mL. **Distribution:** V_d=76L; plasma protein binding (90%). **Metabolism:** Liver (extensive) via CYP3A4; t-butyl side chain monohydroxylated and monocarboxylic acid (metabolites). **Elimination:** Urine (39%, metabolites), feces (57%); $T_{1/2}$=5-6 hrs (18-60 yrs of age), 8 hrs (>70 yrs of age).

NURSING CONSIDERATIONS

Assessment: Assess for liver dysfunction and previous hypersensitivity to the drug and its components. Obtain baseline PSA levels.

Monitoring: Monitor for hypersensitivity reactions or other adverse reactions. Monitor PSA levels.

Patient Counseling: Instruct pregnant or potentially pregnant women not to handle crushed or broken tabs due to possible absorption and potential risk to male fetus; advise to immediately wash contact area with soap and water if contact occurs. Inform that there was an increase in high-grade prostate cancer in men treated with 5α-reductase inhibitors indicated for BPH treatment. Instruct to promptly report any changes in breasts (eg, lumps, pain, nipple discharge) to physician.

Administration: Oral route. Take with or without meals. **Storage:** 15-30°C (59-86°F). Protect from moisture.

PROPRANOLOL

RX

propranolol HCl (Various)

THERAPEUTIC CLASS: Nonselective beta-blocker

INDICATIONS: (PO) Management of HTN (alone or in combination with other antihypertensives), atrial fibrillation (A-fib), familial or hereditary essential tremor, hypertrophic subaortic stenosis, and angina pectoris due to coronary atherosclerosis. Reduction of cardiovascular mortality post-myocardial infarction (MI). Adjunct to control BP and reduce symptoms of pheochromocytoma. Common migraine headache prophylaxis. (Inj) For life-threatening arrhythmias or those occurring under anesthesia (supraventricular/ventricular tachycardia, tachyarrhythmia of digitalis intoxication, resistant tachyarrhythmia due to excessive catecholamine action during anesthesia).

DOSAGE: *Adults:* (PO) Individualize dose. HTN: Initial: 40mg bid. Titrate: May increase gradually until adequate BP control is achieved. Usual Maint: 120-240mg/day. In some instances, 640mg/day may be required. If control is not adequate with bid dosing, a larger dose, or tid therapy may achieve a better control. Angina: 80-320mg/day given bid-qid. A-Fib: 10-30mg tid or qid ac and at hs. MI: Initial: 40mg tid. Titrate: Increase to 60-80mg tid after 1 month as tolerated. Usual: 180-240mg/day in divided doses (either bid or tid). Max: 240mg/day. Migraine: Initial: 80mg/day in divided doses. Usual: 160-240mg/day. Titrate: May increase gradually for optimum prophylaxis. D/C gradually if a satisfactory response is not obtained within 4-6 weeks after reaching max dose. Tremor: Initial: 40mg bid. Usual/Maint: 120mg/day. Occasional: 240-320mg/day PRN. Hypertrophic Subaortic Stenosis: Usual: 20-40mg tid or qid ac and at hs. Pheochromocytoma: Usual: 60mg/day in divided doses for 3 days before surgery with α-adrenergic blocker. Inoperable Tumor: Usual: 30mg/day in divided doses with α-adrenergic blocker. (Inj) Usual: 1-3mg IV at ≤1mg/min. May give a 2nd dose if necessary after 2 min then do not give additional drug in <4 hrs. Do not give additional dose when desired alteration in rate/rhythm is achieved. Transfer to PO therapy as soon as possible. Hepatic Insufficiency: Consider lower dose. (Inj/PO) Elderly: Start at lower end of dosing range.

HOW SUPPLIED: Inj: 1mg/mL; Sol: 20mg/5mL, 40mg/5mL [500mL]; Tab: 10mg*, 20mg*, 40mg*, 60mg*, 80mg* *scored

CONTRAINDICATIONS: Cardiogenic shock, sinus bradycardia and >1st-degree block, bronchial asthma.

WARNINGS/PRECAUTIONS: Exacerbation of angina and MI following abrupt discontinuation reported; when discontinuation is planned, reduce dose gradually over at least a few weeks. Reinstitute therapy if exacerbation of angina occurs upon interruption and take other measures for management of angina pectoris; follow same procedure in patients at risk of occult atherosclerotic heart disease who are given propranolol for other indication since coronary artery disease may be unrecognized. May precipitate more severe failure in patients with congestive heart failure (CHF); avoid with overt CHF and caution in patients with history of heart failure (HF) who are well-compensated and are receiving additional therapies. Caution with bronchospastic lung disease, hepatic/renal impairment, Wolff-Parkinson-White (WPW) syndrome, and tachycardia. Chronically administered therapy should not be routinely withdrawn prior to major surgery; however, may augment risks of general anesthesia and surgical procedures. May mask acute hypoglycemia and hyperthyroidism signs/symptoms. May be more difficult to adjust insulin dose in labile insulin-dependent diabetics. Abrupt withdrawal may be followed by an exacerbation of symptoms of hyperthyroidism, including thyroid storm. May reduce intraocular pressure (IOP). Hypersensitivity/anaphylactic/cutaneous reactions reported. Patients with history of severe anaphylactic reaction to a variety of allergens may be more reactive to repeated accidental/diagnostic/therapeutic challenge; may be unresponsive to usual doses of epinephrine. Elevated serum K+, transaminases, and alkaline phosphatase levels reported. Increases in BUN reported in patients with severe HF. Not for treatment of hypertensive emergencies. Caution in elderly. (PO) Not indicated for migraine attack that has started and tremor associated with parkinsonism. Continued use in patients without history of HF may lead to cardiac failure.

ADVERSE REACTIONS: Bradycardia, CHF, hypotension, lightheadedness, mental depression, N/V, agranulocytosis, respiratory distress.

INTERACTIONS: Administration with CYP450 (2D6, 1A2, 2C19) substrates, inducers, and inhibitors may lead to clinically relevant drug interactions. Increased levels and/or toxicity with substrates/inhibitors of CYP2D6 (eg, amiodarone, cimetidine, fluoxetine, ritonavir), CYP1A2 (eg, imipramine, ciprofloxacin, isoniazid, theophylline), and CYP2C19 (eg, fluconazole, teniposide, tolbutamide). Decreased blood levels with hepatic enzyme inducers (eg, rifampin, ethanol, phenytoin, phenobarbital). May increase levels of propafenone, lidocaine, nifedipine, zolmitriptan, rizatriptan, diazepam and its metabolites. Increased levels with nisoldipine, nicardipine, and chlorpromazine. May decrease theophylline clearance. Increased thioridazine plasma and metabolite (mesoridazine) concentrations with doses ≥160mg/day. Decreased levels with aluminum hydroxide gel, cholestyramine, and colestipol. May decrease levels of lovastatin and pravastatin. Increased warfarin levels and PT; monitor PT. Additive effect with propafenone and amiodarone. Caution with drugs that slow atrioventricular (AV) nodal conduction (eg, digitalis, lidocaine,

795

calcium channel blockers); increased risk of bradycardia with digitalis. Significant bradycardia, HF, and cardiovascular collapse reported with concomitant verapamil. Bradycardia, hypotension, high-degree heart block, and HF reported with concomitant diltiazem. Concomitant ACE inhibitors may cause hypotension. May antagonize effects of clonidine; administer cautiously to patients withdrawing from clonidine. Prolongation of 1st dose hypotension may occur with concomitant prazosin. Postural hypotension reported with concomitant terazosin or doxazosin. Monitor for excessive reduction of resting sympathetic nervous activity with catecholamine-depleting drugs (eg, reserpine). Patients on long-term therapy may experience uncontrolled HTN with concomitant epinephrine. β-receptor agonists (eg, dobutamine, isoproterenol) may reverse effects. NSAIDs (eg, indomethacin) may blunt the antihypertensive effect. Coadministration with methoxyflurane and trichloroethylene may depress myocardial contractility. Hypotension and cardiac arrest reported with concomitant haloperidol. Thyroxine may result in a lower than expected T3 concentration when coadministered with propranolol. May exacerbate hypotensive effects of MAOIs or TCAs. (Inj) Severe bradycardia, asystole, and HF reported with concomitant disopyramide. Increased bronchial hyperreactivity with ACE inhibitors. (PO) Increased levels with alcohol.

PREGNANCY: Category C, caution in nursing.

MECHANISM OF ACTION: Nonselective β-adrenergic receptor blocker. (PO) HTN: Not established; proposed to decrease cardiac output, inhibit renin release, and lessen tonic sympathetic nerve outflow from vasomotor centers in the brain. Angina: Reduces the oxygen requirement of the heart at any given level of effort by blocking the catecholamine-induced increases in the HR, systolic BP, and the velocity and extent of myocardial contraction. Migraine: Not established; β-adrenergic receptors have been demonstrated in the pial vessels of the brain. Tremor: Not established; $β_2$ receptors may be involved and a central effect is also possible. (Inj) Arrhythmia: Decreases the activity of both normal and ectopic pacemaker cells and AV nodal conduction velocity.

PHARMACOKINETICS: Absorption: (PO) Almost complete. Bioavailability (25%); T_{max}=1-4 hrs. **Distribution:** V_d=4-5L/kg; plasma protein binding (90%); found in breast milk, (PO) crosses placenta. **Metabolism:** Liver (extensive); hydroxylation (CYP2D6), N-dealkylation, oxidation (CYP1A2, 2D6), and glucuronidation. Propranolol glucuronide, naphthyloxylactic acid, glucuronic acid, and sulfate conjugates of 4-hydroxy propranolol (major metabolites). **Elimination:** Urine; $T_{1/2}$=3-6 hrs (PO), 2-5.5 hrs (Inj).

NURSING CONSIDERATIONS

Assessment: Assess for cardiogenic shock, sinus bradycardia, AV heart block, bronchial asthma, CHF, bronchospastic lung disease, hyperthyroidism, diabetes, WPW syndrome, tachycardia, hepatic/renal impairment, history/presence of HF, risk for occult atherosclerotic heart disease, hypersensitivity to drug, pregnancy/nursing status, and possible drug interactions.

Monitoring: Monitor for signs/symptoms of cardiac failure, hypoglycemia, decreased IOP, hyperthyroidism, withdrawal symptoms, hypersensitivity reactions, and other adverse reactions. (Inj) Monitor ECG and central venous pressure. (PO) For HTN (bid dosing), measure BP near the end of dosing interval to determine satisfactory BP control.

Patient Counseling: Instruct not to interrupt or d/c therapy without physician's advise. Inform that therapy may interfere with glaucoma screening test.

Administration: Oral/IV route. **Storage:** 20-25°C (68-77°F); (Sol) excursions permitted to 15-30°C (59-86°F). (Inj) Protect from freezing and excessive heat. (Tab) Protect from light.

PROPYLTHIOURACIL   RX
propylthiouracil (Various)

> Severe liver injury and acute liver failure reported; some cases have been fatal or required liver transplantation. Reserve use only for those who cannot tolerate methimazole and in whom radioactive iodine therapy or surgery are not appropriate for the management of hyperthyroidism. Treatment of choice during or just prior to the 1st trimester of pregnancy due to risk of fetal abnormalities associated with methimazole.

THERAPEUTIC CLASS: Thiourea-derivative antithyroid agent

INDICATIONS: Patients with Graves' disease with hyperthyroidism or toxic multinodular goiter who are intolerant of methimazole and for whom surgery or radioactive iodine therapy is not an appropriate treatment option. To ameliorate symptoms of hyperthyroidism in preparation for thyroidectomy or radioactive iodine therapy in patients who are intolerant of methimazole.

DOSAGE: *Adults:* Initial: 300mg/day. Severe Hyperthyroidism/Very Large Goiters: Initial: 400mg/day; occasionally may require 600-900mg/day. Maint: 100-150mg/day. Give daily dose in 3 equal doses, q8h. Elderly: Start at lower end of dosing range.
Pediatrics: ≥6 Yrs: Initial: 50mg/day in 3 equal doses, q8h. Titrate: Carefully increase based on clinical response and evaluation of TSH and free T4 levels.

HOW SUPPLIED: Tab: 50mg* *scored

WARNINGS/PRECAUTIONS: Not recommended for pediatric patients except when methimazole is not well-tolerated and surgery or radioactive iodine therapy are not appropriate. D/C if hepatic dysfunction, agranulocytosis, aplastic anemia, pancytopenia, anti-neutrophilic cytoplasmic antibodies (ANCA)-positive vasculitis, hepatitis, interstitial pneumonitis, fever, or exfoliative dermatitis develops. May cause hypothyroidism; adjust dose to maintain euthyroid state. Fetal goiter and cretinism may occur when given during pregnancy. May cause hypoprothrombinemia and bleeding; monitor PT, especially before surgery. Monitor thyroid function tests periodically.

ADVERSE REACTIONS: Agranulocytosis, liver injury, liver failure, thrombocytopenia, aplastic anemia, hepatitis, periarteritis, hypoprothrombinemia, skin rash, urticaria, N/V, epigastric distress, arthralgia, paresthesias.

INTERACTIONS: May increase activity of oral anticoagulants (eg, warfarin); consider additional monitoring of PT/INR. Hyperthyroidism may increase clearance of β-blockers; may need reduced β-blocker dose when patient becomes euthyroid. Digitalis glycoside levels may be increased when patient becomes euthyroid; may need to reduce digitalis dose. Theophylline clearance may decrease when patient becomes euthyroid; may need reduced theophylline dose. Caution with other drugs that cause agranulocytosis.

PREGNANCY: Category D, safety not known in nursing.

MECHANISM OF ACTION: Thiourea-derivate antithyroid agent; inhibits the synthesis of thyroid hormones and the conversion of thyroxine to triiodothyronine in peripheral tissues.

PHARMACOKINETICS: Absorption: Readily absorbed. **Distribution:** Found in breast milk, crosses placenta. **Metabolism:** Extensive. **Elimination:** Urine (35%).

NURSING CONSIDERATIONS

Assessment: Assess for previous hypersensitivity to the drug, hepatic impairment, pregnancy/nursing status, and possible drug interactions.

Monitoring: Monitor for signs/symptoms of hepatic dysfunction, agranulocytosis, leukopenia, thrombocytopenia, aplastic anemia, pancytopenia, ANCA-positive vasculitis, interstitial pneumonitis, fever, exfoliative dermatitis, and hypothyroidism. Monitor CBC with differential, PT, TSH, free T4 levels, AST, ALT, bilirubin, and alkaline phosphatase.

Patient Counseling: Instruct to inform physician if pregnant/nursing or planning to become pregnant. Advise to report signs/symptoms of illness (eg, fever, sore throat, skin eruptions, headache, general malaise) and hepatic dysfunction. Inform about the risk of liver failure.

Administration: Oral route. **Storage:** 15-30°C (59-86°F).

PROSCAR
finasteride (Merck)

RX

THERAPEUTIC CLASS: Type II 5 alpha-reductase inhibitor

INDICATIONS: Treatment of symptomatic BPH in men with an enlarged prostate. To reduce risk of symptomatic progression of BPH (a confirmed ≥4 point increase in American Urological Association symptom score) in combination with doxazosin.

DOSAGE: *Adults:* Monotherapy/Combination with Doxazosin: 5mg qd.

HOW SUPPLIED: Tab: 5mg

CONTRAINDICATIONS: Women who are or may potentially be pregnant.

WARNINGS/PRECAUTIONS: Not approved for the prevention of prostate cancer. May decrease serum prostate specific antigen (PSA) concentration during therapy or in the presence of prostate cancer; establish a new baseline PSA at least 6 months after starting treatment and monitor PSA periodically thereafter. Any confirmed increase from lowest PSA value during treatment may signal presence of prostate cancer. May increase risk of high-grade prostate cancer. Potential risk to male fetus; broken or crushed tabs should not be handled by pregnant women or women who may potentially be pregnant. May decrease ejaculate volume and total sperm per ejaculate. Prior to treatment initiation, consider other urological conditions that may cause similar symptoms; BPH and prostate cancer may coexist. Monitor for obstructive uropathy in patients with large residual urinary volume and/or severely diminished urinary flow; such patients may not be candidates for therapy. Caution with liver dysfunction.

ADVERSE REACTIONS: Impotence, decreased libido, decreased ejaculate volume, asthenia, postural hypotension, dizziness, abnormal ejaculation.

PREGNANCY: Category X, not for use in nursing.

MECHANISM OF ACTION: Type II 5α-reductase inhibitor; competitively and specifically inhibits type II 5α-reductase with which it forms a stable enzyme complex, inhibiting metabolism of testosterone to 5α-dihydrotestosterone.

PHARMACOKINETICS: Absorption: Absolute bioavailability (63%); C_{max}=37ng/mL; T_{max}=1-2 hrs. Refer to PI for different pharmacokinetic parameters of different age groups. **Distribution:** V_d=76L; plasma protein binding (90%). **Metabolism:** Liver (extensive) via CYP3A4; t-butyl side chain monohydroxylated and monocarboxylic acid (metabolites). **Elimination:** Urine (39% as metabolites), feces (57%); $T_{1/2}$=6 hrs (45-60 yrs of age), 8 hrs (≥70 yrs of age).

NURSING CONSIDERATIONS

Assessment: Assess for liver dysfunction, previous hypersensitivity to the drug, other urological conditions that may cause similar symptoms, residual urinary volume, and diminished urinary flow.

Monitoring: Monitor for obstructive uropathy in patients with large residual urinary volume and/or severely diminished urinary flow. Monitor for signs/symptoms of prostate cancer, hypersensitivity reactions, and other adverse reactions. Obtain baseline PSA levels at least 6 months after starting treatment and monitor PSA periodically thereafter.

Patient Counseling: Inform that therapy may increase risk of high-grade prostate cancer. Instruct pregnant or potentially pregnant females not to handle crushed or broken tabs due to possible absorption and potential risk to male fetus; advise to immediately wash contact area with soap and water if contact occurs. Advise that the volume of ejaculate may be decreased and impotence/decreased libido may occur. Instruct to promptly report to physician any changes in breasts (eg, lumps, pain, nipple discharge).

Administration: Oral route. Take with or without meals. **Storage:** Room temperature <30°C (86°F). Protect from light.

PROTAMINE SULFATE   RX
protamine sulfate (Various)

> May cause severe hypotension, cardiovascular (CV) collapse, noncardiogenic pulmonary edema, catastrophic pulmonary vasoconstriction, and pulmonary HTN; risk factors include high dose/overdose, rapid/previous administration, repeated doses, and current/previous use of protamine-containing drugs. Risk to benefit of administration should be carefully considered with presence of any risk factors. Should not be given when bleeding occurs without prior heparin use.

THERAPEUTIC CLASS: Heparin antagonist

INDICATIONS: Management of heparin overdose.

DOSAGE: *Adults:* Administer as very slow IV infusion over 10 min in doses not to exceed 50mg. Determine dose by blood coagulation studies. Each mg neutralizes not less than 100 USP heparin units.

HOW SUPPLIED: Inj: 10mg/mL [5mL, 25mL]

WARNINGS/PRECAUTIONS: May cause allergic reactions with fish hypersensitivity. Rapid administration may cause severe hypotensive and anaphylactoid-like reactions. Caution in cardiac surgeries; hyperheparinemia or bleeding reported. Previous exposure to protamine/protamine-containing insulin may induce humoral immune response; severe hypersensitivity reaction, including life-threatening anaphylaxis reported. Increased risk of antiprotamine antibodies in infertile or vasectomized men.

ADVERSE REACTIONS: Hypotension, bradycardia, transitory flushing/feeling of warmth, lassitude, dyspnea, N/V, back pain, anaphylaxis that causes severe respiratory distress, circulatory collapse, noncardiogenic pulmonary edema, acute pulmonary HTN.

INTERACTIONS: Incompatible with certain antibiotics, such as cephalosporins and penicillins. Concomitant or previous use of protamine-containing drugs (eg, NPH insulin, protamine zinc insulin, certain beta-blockers) is risk factor for severe adverse events; see Boxed Warning.

PREGNANCY: Category C, caution in nursing.

MECHANISM OF ACTION: Heparin antagonist; has anticoagulant effects when administered alone, however, when given in presence of heparin, a stable salt is formed and anticoagulant activity of both drugs is lost.

NURSING CONSIDERATIONS

Assessment: Assess for fish allergy, previous vasectomy, previous exposure, severe left ventricular dysfunction, abnormal preoperative pulmonary hemodynamics, and possible drug interactions. Assess blood coagulation studies for appropriate dosage.

Monitoring: Monitor for hypersensitivity/allergic reactions, hypotension, CV collapse, pulmonary edema, and pulmonary HTN. Monitor blood coagulation studies.

Administration: Slow IV infusion. Large-size 25mL vials are designed for antiheparin treatment only when large doses of heparin have been given during surgery. **Storage:** 20-25°C (68-77°F). Do not freeze.

PROTONIX   RX
pantoprazole sodium (Wyeth)

OTHER BRAND NAMES: Protonix IV (Wyeth)

THERAPEUTIC CLASS: Proton pump inhibitor

INDICATIONS: (Tab/Sus) Short-term treatment (up to 8 weeks) in the healing and symptomatic relief of erosive esophagitis (EE) associated with gastroesophageal reflux disease (GERD) in adults and pediatric patients ≥5 yrs of age. Maintenance of healing of EE and reduction in relapse rates of daytime and nighttime heartburn symptoms in adults with GERD. Long-term treatment of pathological hypersecretory conditions, including Zollinger-Ellison syndrome. (IV) Short-term treatment (7-10 days) of adults with GERD and a history of EE. Treatment of pathological hypersecretory conditions, including Zollinger-Ellison syndrome, in adults.

DOSAGE: *Adults:* (Tab/Sus) Treatment of EE Associated with GERD: 40mg qd for up to 8 weeks. May consider additional 8-week course if not healed after 8 weeks of treatment. Maintenance of Healing of EE: 40mg qd; controlled studies did not extend beyond 12 months. Pathological Hypersecretory Conditions: Usual: 40mg bid. Titrate: Adjust to individual needs and continue for as long as clinically indicated. Doses up to 240mg/day have been administered. If unable to swallow 40mg tab, may give two 20mg tabs. (IV) GERD Associated with History of EE: 40mg qd by IV infusion for 7-10 days. D/C as soon as the patient is able to receive treatment with tab/sus. Pathological Hypersecretory Conditions: Usual: 80mg IV q12h. Titrate: Adjust frequency based on acid output; may increase to 80mg q8h if higher dosage is needed. Doses >240mg/day and duration >6 days not studied.
Pediatrics: ≥5 Yrs: (Tab/Sus) Treatment of EE Associated with GERD: ≥40kg: 40mg qd for up to 8 weeks. ≥15kg to <40kg: 20mg qd for up to 8 weeks. If unable to swallow 40mg tab, may give two 20mg tabs. Do not divide the 40mg pkt to create a 20mg dosage for pediatric patients unable to take tab.

HOW SUPPLIED: Inj: 40mg; Sus, Delayed-Release: 40mg (granules/pkt); Tab, Delayed-Release: 20mg, 40mg

WARNINGS/PRECAUTIONS: Symptomatic response does not preclude the presence of gastric malignancy. May increase risk of *Clostridium difficile*-associated diarrhea (CDAD), especially in hospitalized patients. May increase risk for osteoporosis-related fractures of the hip, wrist, or spine, especially with high-dose and long-term therapy. Use lowest dose and shortest duration appropriate to the condition being treated. Hypomagnesemia reported and may require Mg^{2+} replacement and discontinuation of therapy; consider monitoring Mg^{2+} levels prior to and periodically during therapy with prolonged treatment. Anaphylaxis and other serious reactions (eg, erythema multiforme, Stevens-Johnson syndrome, toxic epidermal necrolysis) reported. Lab test interactions may occur. (Tab/Sus) Atrophic gastritis noted with long-term therapy, particularly in patients who were *Helicobacter pylori* positive. Vitamin B12 deficiency caused by hypo- or achlorhydria may occur with long-term use (eg, >3 yrs). (IV) Thrombophlebitis reported. Contains edetate disodium (EDTA), a chelator of metal ions including zinc; consider zinc supplementation in patients prone to zinc deficiency. Mild, transient transaminase elevations observed in clinical studies.

ADVERSE REACTIONS: Headache, diarrhea, N/V, abdominal pain, flatulence, dizziness, rash, fever, upper respiratory infection, arthralgia.

INTERACTIONS: Concomitant use with atazanavir or nelfinavir is not recommended; may substantially decrease atazanavir or nelfinavir concentrations. Monitor for increases in INR and PT with warfarin. May interfere with absorption of drugs where gastric pH is an important determinant of bioavailability (eg, ketoconazole, ampicillin esters, iron salts, digoxin). Caution with digoxin or other drugs that may cause hypomagnesemia (eg, diuretics). May elevate and prolong levels of methotrexate (MTX) and/or its metabolite, possibly leading to toxicities; consider temporary withdrawal of therapy with high-dose MTX. (IV) Use caution when other EDTA-containing products are also coadministered IV.

PREGNANCY: Category B, not for use in nursing.

MECHANISM OF ACTION: Proton pump inhibitor; suppresses the final step in gastric acid production by covalently binding to the (H^+/K^+)-ATPase enzyme system at the secretory surface of the gastric parietal cell.

PHARMACOKINETICS: Absorption: Tab: Absolute bioavailability (77%). (40mg) C_{max}=2.5mcg/mL; T_{max}=2.5 hrs; AUC=4.8mcg•hr/mL. IV: (40mg) C_{max}=5.52mcg/mL; AUC=5.4mcg•hr/mL. Sus: Refer to PI. **Distribution:** V_d=11-23.6L; plasma protein binding (98%); (PO) found in breast milk. **Metabolism:** Liver (extensive) via demethylation, by CYP2C19, with subsequent sulfation; oxidation by CYP3A4. **Elimination:** (Healthy) Urine (71%), feces (18%); $T_{1/2}$=1 hr.

P

NURSING CONSIDERATIONS

Assessment: Assess for hypersensitivity to the drug, risk for osteoporosis-related fractures, pregnancy/nursing status, and possible drug interactions. Obtain baseline Mg^{2+} levels. (IV) Assess if prone to zinc deficiency.

Monitoring: Monitor for signs/symptoms of CDAD, bone fractures, hypersensitivity reactions, and other adverse reactions. Monitor Mg^{2+} levels periodically. (Tab/Sus) Monitor INR and PT when given with warfarin. (Tab/Sus) Monitor for signs/symptoms of atrophic gastritis and vitamin B12 deficiency. (IV) Monitor for thrombophlebitis, zinc deficiency, and transaminase elevations.

Patient Counseling: Inform of the most frequently occurring adverse reactions. Instruct to inform physician if any unusual symptom develops, or if any known symptom persists or worsens; advise to immediately report and seek care for any cardiovascular or neurological symptoms (eg, palpitation, dizziness, seizures, tetany) and for diarrhea that does not improve. Instruct to inform physician of all medications currently being taken, including OTC medications, as well as allergies to any medications. Inform that concomitant administration of antacids does not affect the absorption of the tabs. Advise that oral sus pkt is a fixed dose and cannot be divided to make smaller dose.

Administration: Oral/IV route. (Tab/Sus) Do not split, crush, or chew. (Tab) Swallow whole, with or without food. (Sus) Administer in 1 tsp of applesauce or apple juice approximately 30 min ac. May be administered via NG/gastrostomy tube. Refer to PI for preparation and administration instructions. (IV) Flush IV line before and after administration. Refer to PI for further preparation and administration instructions. **Storage:** 20-25°C (68-77°F); excursions permitted to 15-30°C (59-86°F). (IV) Protect from light. Refer to PI for reconstituted and admixed solution storage information.

PROTOPIC   RX
tacrolimus (Astellas)

> Rare cases of malignancy (eg, skin and lymphoma) reported with topical calcineurin inhibitors, including tacrolimus oint, although causal relationship has not been established. Avoid long-term use, and application should be limited to areas of involvement with atopic dermatitis. Not indicated for children <2 yrs of age; only 0.03% oint is indicated for children 2-15 yrs of age.

THERAPEUTIC CLASS: Macrolide immunosuppressant

INDICATIONS: Second-line therapy for short-term and noncontinuous chronic treatment of moderate to severe atopic dermatitis in nonimmunocompromised adults and children who have failed to respond adequately to other topical prescription treatments for atopic dermatitis, or when those treatments are not advisable.

DOSAGE: *Adults:* (0.03% or 0.1%) Apply thin layer to the affected skin bid until signs and symptoms resolve. Reexamine patient if signs and symptoms do not improve within 6 weeks. *Pediatrics:* 2-15 Yrs: (0.03%) Apply thin layer to the affected skin bid until signs and symptoms resolve. Reexamine patient if signs and symptoms do not improve within 6 weeks.

HOW SUPPLIED: Oint: 0.03%, 0.1% [30g, 60g, 100g]

WARNINGS/PRECAUTIONS: Long-term safety, beyond 1 yr of noncontinuous use, has not been established. Avoid with premalignant and malignant skin conditions. Not recommended for oral application, or in patients having skin conditions with a skin barrier defect where there is potential for increased systemic absorption (eg, Netherton's syndrome, lamellar ichthyosis, generalized erythroderma, cutaneous graft-versus-host disease). May cause local symptoms, such as skin burning or pruritus and may improve as the lesions of atopic dermatitis resolve. Resolve bacterial or viral infections at treatment sites before starting treatment. Increased risk of varicella zoster and herpes simplex virus (HSV) infection, or eczema herpeticum. Lymphadenopathy reported; d/c if etiology of lymphadenopathy is unknown, or in the presence of acute infectious mononucleosis. Minimize or avoid natural or artificial sunlight exposure during treatment. Rare cases of acute renal failure reported. Not for ophthalmic use. Do not use with occlusive dressings.

ADVERSE REACTIONS: Skin burning, pruritus, flu-like symptoms, allergic reaction, skin erythema, headache, skin infection, fever, herpes simplex, rhinitis, increased cough, asthma, pharyngitis, pustular rash, folliculitis.

INTERACTIONS: Caution with CYP3A4 inhibitors (eg, erythromycin, ketoconazole, calcium channel blockers, cimetidine) in patients with widespread and/or erythrodermic disease.

PREGNANCY: Category C, not for use in nursing.

MECHANISM OF ACTION: Macrolide immunosuppressant; not established in atopic dermatitis. Inhibits T-lymphocyte activation by 1st binding to an intracellular protein, FKBP-12. A complex of tacrolimus-FKBP-12, Ca^{2+}, calmodulin, and calcineurin is then formed and the phosphatase activity of calcineurin is inhibited. This has been shown to prevent the dephosphorylation and translocation of nuclear factor of activated T-cells (NF-AT), a nuclear component thought to initiate gene transcription for the formation of lymphokines.

PHARMACOKINETICS: Absorption: Absolute bioavailability (0.5%), C_{max}=<2ng/mL. **Distribution:** Plasma protein binding (99%); crosses placenta; found in breast milk. **Metabolism:** Extensive via CYP3A; demethylation and hydroxylation; 13-demethyl tacrolimus (major metabolite).

NURSING CONSIDERATIONS

Assessment: Assess for history of hypersensitivity to drug, premalignant/malignant skin conditions, conditions where there is potential for increased systemic absorption, bacterial or viral infections at treatment sites, renal impairment, pregnancy/nursing status, and possible drug interactions.

Monitoring: Monitor for skin malignancy, lymphoma, infections, local symptoms, lymphadenopathy, and acute renal failure. Monitor improvement of signs/symptoms of atopic dermatitis within 6 weeks.

Patient Counseling: Instruct to use drug exactly as prescribed, only on areas of skin that have eczema, and not to use continuously for a prolonged period. Advise to d/c medication when signs/symptoms of eczema subside. Instruct to consult physician if symptoms get worse, a skin infection develops, or if symptoms do not improve after 6 weeks. Advise caregivers applying the oint, or patients not treating their hands, to wash hands with soap and water after application. Counsel to not bathe, shower, or swim right after application. Advise to avoid getting oint in the eyes or mouth. Instruct to avoid artificial sunlight exposure during treatment, limit sun exposure, wear loose-fitting clothing that protects treated area from the sun, and not cover treated skin with bandages, dressings, or wraps.

Administration: Topical route. Rub in the minimum amount of oint gently and completely.
Storage: 25°C (77°F); excursions permitted to 15-30°C (59-86°F).

PROVENGE

RX

sipuleucel-T (Dendreon)

THERAPEUTIC CLASS: Immunomodulatory agent

INDICATIONS: Treatment of asymptomatic or minimally symptomatic metastatic castrate resistant (hormone refractory) prostate cancer.

DOSAGE: *Adults*: Usual: 3 complete doses (250mL each) given at approximately 2-week intervals via IV infusion over 60 min. If unable to give scheduled infusion, additional leukapheresis is needed. Premedication: PO acetaminophen and antihistamine (eg, diphenhydramine) 30 min prior to administration.

HOW SUPPLIED: Sus: 250mL

WARNINGS/PRECAUTIONS: For autologous use only. Acute infusion reactions reported; infusion rate may be decreased or stopped depending on severity of reaction; administer appropriate medical therapy PRN. Monitor closely with cardiac or pulmonary conditions. May transmit infectious diseases to healthcare professionals handling the product; employ universal precautions. Do not infuse until confirmation of product release has been received.

ADVERSE REACTIONS: Chills, fatigue, fever, back pain, N/V, joint ache, headache, paresthesia, anemia, constipation, infusion reactions, citrate toxicity, pain, dizziness.

INTERACTIONS: Immunosuppressive agents may alter efficacy and/or safety; evaluate whether it is appropriate to reduce or d/c immunosuppressive agents prior to treatment.

PREGNANCY: Safety in pregnancy and nursing not known.

MECHANISM OF ACTION: Immunomodulatory agent (autologous cellular immunotherapy); not established. Induces an immune response targeted against prostatic acid phosphatase, an antigen expressed in most prostate cancer.

NURSING CONSIDERATIONS

Assessment: Assess for history of cardiac or pulmonary conditions and possible drug interactions.

Monitoring: Monitor for signs and symptoms of infusion reactions, especially with cardiac or pulmonary conditions. Monitor for infectious sequelae in patients with central venous catheters.

Patient Counseling: Counsel on adhering to preparation instructions for leukapheresis procedure, possible side effects, and postprocedure care. Advise to report signs and symptoms of acute infusion reactions (eg, fever, chills, fatigue, breathing problems, dizziness, high BP, N/V, headache, muscle aches) and symptoms suggestive of cardiac arrhythmia. Instruct to notify physician if taking immunosuppressive agents. Inform of the need for a central venous catheter placement if peripheral venous access is not adequate, and counsel on the importance of catheter care; advise to inform physician if fever or any swelling or redness around the catheter site occurs. Inform of the need to undergo an additional leukapheresis if a scheduled dose is missed.

Administration: IV route. Begin infusion prior to expiration date and time; do not infuse expired product. Do not use a cell filter. Infuse IV over 60 min; observe patient for at least 30 min after each infusion. Refer to PI for modification for infusion reactions and preparation instructions.
Storage: Infusion bag must remain within the insulated polyurethane container until the time of administration; stable for ≤3 hrs at room temperature once removed. Do not remove from the outer cardboard shipping box. Refer to PI for complete handling instructions.

PROVERA   RX
medroxyprogesterone acetate (Pharmacia & Upjohn)

> Should not be used for the prevention of cardiovascular disease (CVD) or dementia. Increased risks of myocardial infarction (MI), stroke, invasive breast cancer, pulmonary embolism (PE), and deep vein thrombosis (DVT) in postmenopausal women (50-79 yrs of age) reported. Increased risk of developing probable dementia in postmenopausal women ≥65 yrs of age reported. Should be prescribed at the lowest effective dose and for the shortest duration consistent with treatment goals and risks.

THERAPEUTIC CLASS: Progestogen

INDICATIONS: Treatment of secondary amenorrhea and abnormal uterine bleeding due to hormonal imbalance in the absence of organic pathology, such as fibroids or uterine cancer. Reduce incidence of endometrial hyperplasia in non-hysterectomized postmenopausal women receiving daily oral 0.625mg conjugated estrogen.

DOSAGE: *Adults:* Secondary Amenorrhea: 5 or 10mg/day for 5-10 days; 10mg/day for 10 days, beginning at anytime, is used to induce optimum secretory transformation of primed endometrium. Abnormal Uterine Bleeding: 5 or 10mg/day for 5-10 days beginning on Day 16 or 21 of cycle; 10mg/day for 10 days, beginning on Day 16 of the cycle is recommended to produce an optimum secretory transformation of primed endometrium. Endometrial Hyperplasia: 5 or 10mg/day for 12-14 consecutive days/month beginning on Day 1 or 16 of cycle.

HOW SUPPLIED: Tab: 2.5mg*, 5mg*, 10mg* *scored

CONTRAINDICATIONS: Undiagnosed abnormal genital bleeding, known/suspected/history of breast cancer, known/suspected estrogen- or progesterone-dependent neoplasia, active or history of DVT/PE, active or recent arterial thromboembolic disease (eg, stroke, MI), known liver dysfunction or disease, missed abortion, known/suspected pregnancy, as a diagnostic test for pregnancy.

WARNINGS/PRECAUTIONS: Increased risk of cardiovascular events. Caution in patients with risk factors for arterial vascular disease and/or venous thromboembolism. Unopposed estrogen in women with a uterus has been associated with increased risk of endometrial cancer. May increase risk of ovarian cancer. Consider addition of a progestin for women with a uterus. If visual abnormalities or migraine occurs, d/c pending examination. If examination reveals papilledema or retinal vascular lesions, d/c permanently. In cases of undiagnosed abnormal vaginal bleeding, perform adequate diagnostic measures. Withdrawal bleeding may occur within 3-7 days after discontinuing therapy. May elevate BP. May increase plasma TG, leading to pancreatitis and other complications with preexisting hypertriglyceridemia. Caution with history of cholestatic jaundice; d/c in case of recurrence. May cause fluid retention. Caution with severe hypocalcemia. May exacerbate asthma, diabetes mellitus, epilepsy, migraine, porphyria, systemic lupus erythematosus, and hepatic hemangiomas. May affect certain endocrine, LFTs, and blood components in lab tests.

ADVERSE REACTIONS: Abnormal uterine bleeding, breast tenderness, galactorrhea, urticaria, pruritus, edema, rash, menstrual changes, change in weight, mental depression, insomnia, somnolence, dizziness, headache, nausea.

INTERACTIONS: Patients on thyroid replacement therapy may require higher doses of thyroid hormone.

PREGNANCY: Category X, not for use in nursing.

MECHANISM OF ACTION: Progestogen; transforms proliferative endometrium into secretory endometrium.

PHARMACOKINETICS: Absorption: Rapid. Administration of different doses resulted in different pharmacokinetic parameters; refer to PI. **Distribution:** Plasma protein binding (90%); found in breast milk. **Metabolism:** Extensive (hepatic) via hydroxylation with subsequent conjugation. **Elimination:** Urine.

NURSING CONSIDERATIONS

Assessment: Assess for abnormal genital bleeding, cardiac or renal dysfunction, presence or history of breast cancer, estrogen-progesterone-dependent neoplasias, DVT, PE, active or recent (within past yr) arterial thromboembolic disease, any other conditions where treatment is contraindicated or cautioned, need for progestin therapy, and for possible drug interactions.

Monitoring: Monitor for signs/symptoms of CVD, malignant neoplasms, visual abnormalities, hypertriglyceridemia, fluid retention, exacerbation of asthma, hypersensitivity reactions, and other conditions. Perform annual breast exam; schedule mammography based on age, risk factors, and prior mammogram results. Regularly monitor BP, thyroid function in patients on thyroid replacement therapy, and periodically evaluate (every 3-6 months) need for therapy. In cases of undiagnosed, persistent, or recurrent vaginal bleeding in women with uterus, perform adequate diagnostic measures (eg, endometrial sampling) to rule out malignancies.

Patient Counseling: Counsel about risk of birth defects if exposed to drug. Inform that drug may increase risk for breast cancer, uterine cancer, stroke, heart attack, blood clots, and dementia. Instruct to report breast lumps, unusual vaginal bleeding, dizziness/faintness, changes in speech, severe headaches, chest pain, SOB, leg pain, visual changes, or vomiting. Instruct to have an annual pelvic exam, breast exam, and mammogram. Advise to perform monthly self breast exams.

Administration: Oral route. **Storage:** 20-25°C (68-77°F).

PROVIGIL
modafinil (Cephalon)

THERAPEUTIC CLASS: Wakefulness-promoting agent

INDICATIONS: To improve wakefulness in patients with excessive sleepiness associated with narcolepsy, obstructive sleep apnea (OSA), shift work disorder (SWD). As adjunct to standard treatment for underlying obstruction in OSA.

DOSAGE: *Adults:* ≥17 Yrs: 200mg qd. Max: 400mg/day as single dose. Narcolepsy/OSA: Take as single dose in am. SWD: Take 1 hr prior to start of work shift. Severe Hepatic Impairment: 100mg qd. Elderly: Consider dose reduction.

HOW SUPPLIED: Tab: 100mg, 200mg* *scored

WARNINGS/PRECAUTIONS: Rare cases of severe or life-threatening rash (eg, Stevens-Johnson syndrome [SJS], toxic epidermal necrolysis [TEN], drug rash with eosinophilia and systemic symptoms [DRESS]) reported; d/c treatment at first sign. Angioedema, anaphylactoid reactions, multiorgan hypersensitivity and psychiatric adverse experiences reported; d/c treatment if symptoms develop. Caution with a history of psychosis, depression or mania. Caution with recent myocardial infarction (MI) or unstable angina. Avoid in patients with history of left ventricular hypertrophy or with mitral valve prolapse who have experienced mitral valve prolapse syndrome (eg, ischemic ECG changes, chest pain, arrhythmia) with CNS stimulants. May impair mental/physical abilities. Reduce dose with severe hepatic impairment. Use low dose in elderly. Doses up to 400mg/day have been well-tolerated, but there is no evidence that this dose confers additional benefit.

ADVERSE REACTIONS: Headache, nausea, nervousness, anxiety, insomnia, rhinitis, diarrhea, back pain, dizziness, dyspepsia, flu syndrome, dry mouth, anorexia, pharyngitis.

INTERACTIONS: Methylphenidate and dextroamphetamine may delay absorption. May reduce efficacy of steroidal contraceptives up to 1 month after discontinuation. Caution with MAOIs. CYP3A4 inducers (eg, carbamazepine, phenobarbital, rifampin) may decrease levels. CYP3A4 inhibitors (eg, ketoconazole, itraconazole) may increase levels. May increase levels of drugs metabolized by CYP2C19 (eg, diazepam, propranolol, phenytoin) or CYP2C9 (eg, warfarin). Monitor for toxicity with CYP2C19 substrates and PT/INR with warfarin. May increase levels of certain TCAs (eg, clomipramine, desipramine) and SSRIs in CYP2D6-deficient patients. May decrease levels of drugs metabolized by CYP3A4 (eg, cyclosporine, ethinyl estradiol, triazolam). May induce CYP1A2 and CYP2B6; caution with CYP1A2 and CYP2B6 substrates.

PREGNANCY: Category C, caution in nursing.

MECHANISM OF ACTION: Wakefulness-promoting agent; not established. Binds to dopamine transporter, inhibits dopamine reuptake, and results in increased extracellular dopamine levels in some brain regions.

PHARMACOKINETICS: Absorption: Rapid. T_{max}=2-4 hrs, delayed by 1 hr (fed). **Distribution:** V_d=0.9L/kg; plasma protein binding (60%). **Metabolism:** Liver via hydrolytic deamination, S-oxidation, aromatic ring hydroxylation, and glucuronide conjugation; CYP3A4. **Elimination:** Feces (1%), urine (80%, <10% parent compound); $T_{1/2}$=15 hrs.

NURSING CONSIDERATIONS

Assessment: Assess for hypersensitivity, hepatic impairment, pregnancy/nursing status, possible drug interactions, and a history of psychosis, depression, mania, left ventricular hypertrophy, or mitral valve prolapse. Assess for a recent history of MI or unstable angina. Use only in patients who have had complete evaluation of their excessive sleepiness, and in whom a diagnosis of either narcolepsy, OSA, and/or SWD has been made.

Monitoring: Monitor for serious rash, SJS, TEN, DRESS, angioedema, hypersensitivity, multiorgan hypersensitivity reactions, psychiatric adverse symptoms, and other adverse reactions. Monitor

BP. If used adjunctively with continuous positive airway pressure (CPAP), monitor for CPAP compliance. Periodically reevaluate long-term usefulness if prescribed for an extended time.

Patient Counseling: Advise that this is not a replacement for sleep. Inform that drug may improve but does not eliminate sleepiness. Instruct to avoid taking alcohol during therapy. Caution against hazardous tasks or performing other activities that require mental alertness. Instruct to notify physician if pregnant or intend to become pregnant, or if nursing during therapy. Caution about increased risk of pregnancy when using steroidal contraceptives and for 1 month after discontinuing therapy. Instruct to inform physician if taking or planning to take any prescribed or OTC drugs. Instruct to contact physician if chest pain, rash, depression, anxiety, or signs of psychosis or mania develop. Inform of importance of continuing previously prescribed treatments. Instruct to d/c and notify physician if rash, hives, mouth sores, blisters, peeling skin, trouble swallowing or breathing, or other allergic reactions develop.

Administration: Oral route. **Storage:** 20-25°C (68-77°F).

PROZAC
fluoxetine HCl (Lilly)

RX

Antidepressants increased the risk of suicidal thoughts and behavior in children, adolescents, and young adults in short-term studies. Monitor closely for worsening and for emergence of suicidal thoughts and behaviors in patients who are started on antidepressant therapy. Not approved for use in children <7 yrs of age.

THERAPEUTIC CLASS: Selective serotonin reuptake inhibitor

INDICATIONS: Acute and maintenance treatment of major depressive disorder (MDD) in patients ≥8 yrs of age and obsessive compulsive disorder (OCD) in patients ≥7 yrs of age. Acute and maintenance treatment of binge-eating and vomiting behaviors in adults with moderate to severe bulimia nervosa. Acute treatment of panic disorder, with or without agoraphobia in adults. Acute treatment of depressive episodes associated with bipolar I disorder and treatment-resistant depression (MDD in adults who failed to respond to 2 separate trials of different antidepressants) in combination with olanzapine.

DOSAGE: *Adults:* MDD: Initial: 20mg/day qam. Titrate: May consider dose increase after several weeks if improvement is insufficient. Doses >20mg/day may be given qd (am) or bid (am and noon). Max: 80mg/day. Prozac Weekly: Start 7 days after last daily dose of 20mg cap. Consider reestablishing a daily dosing regimen if satisfactory response is not maintained. Switching to a TCA: May need to reduce TCA dose and monitor TCA concentrations with coadministration or when therapy is discontinued. OCD: Initial: 20mg/day qam. Titrate: May consider dose increase after several weeks if improvement is insufficient. Doses >20mg/day may be given qd (am) or bid (am and noon). Usual: 20-60mg/day. Max: 80mg/day. Bulimia Nervosa: Usual: 60mg/day qam. May titrate up to this target dose over several days. Max: 60mg/day. Panic Disorder: Initial: 10mg/day. Titrate: Increase to 20mg/day after 1 week. May consider additional dose increase after several weeks if no clinical improvement observed. Max: 60mg/day. Depressive Episodes Associated with Bipolar I Disorder/Treatment-Resistant Depression: Initial: 20mg + 5mg olanzapine qpm. Titrate: Adjust dose based on efficacy and tolerability within dose range of 20-50mg + 5-12.5mg olanzapine (depressive episodes associated with bipolar I disorder) or 5-20mg olanzapine (treatment-resistant depression). Max: 75mg + 18mg olanzapine. Predisposition to Hypotension/Hepatic Impairment/Slow Metabolizers/Olanzapine-Sensitive: Initial: 20mg + 2.5-5mg olanzapine. Titrate: Increase cautiously. Periodically reassess the need for continued treatment. Concomitant Illness: May require dose adjustments. Hepatic Impairment (Cirrhosis)/Elderly: Use lower or less frequent dosage. Switching to/from an MAOI for Psychiatric Disorders: Allow at least 14 days between discontinuation of an MAOI and initiation of treatment, and allow at least 5 weeks between discontinuation of treatment and initiation of an MAOI. Use with Other MAOIs (eg, Linezolid, IV Methylene Blue): Refer to PI.
Pediatrics: MDD: ≥8 Yrs: Initial: 10 or 20mg/day. Titrate: Increase to 20mg/day after 1 week at 10mg/day. Lower Weight Children: Initial/Target: 10mg/day. Titrate: May consider dose increase to 20mg/day after several weeks if improvement is insufficient. Switching to a TCA: May need to reduce TCA dose and monitor TCA concentrations with coadministration or when therapy is discontinued. OCD: ≥7 Yrs: Adolescents and Higher Weight Children: Initial: 10mg/day. Titrate: Increase to 20mg/day after 2 weeks. May consider additional dose increases after several more weeks if improvement is insufficient. Usual: 20-60mg/day. Lower Weight Children: Initial: 10mg/day. Titrate: May consider additional dose increases after several weeks if improvement is insufficient. Usual: 20-30mg/day. Max: 60mg/day. Depressive Episodes Associated with Bipolar I Disorder: 10-17 Yrs: Initial: 20mg + 2.5mg olanzapine qpm. Titrate: Adjust dose based on efficacy and tolerability. Max: 50mg + 12mg olanzapine. Periodically reassess the need for continued treatment. Concomitant Illness: May require dose adjustments. Hepatic Impairment (Cirrhosis): Use lower or less frequent dosage. Switching to/from an MAOI for Psychiatric Disorders: Allow at least 14 days between discontinuation of an MAOI and initiation of treatment, and allow at least 5 weeks between discontinuation of treatment and initiation of an MAOI. Use with Other MAOIs (eg, Linezolid, IV Methylene Blue): Refer to PI.

HOW SUPPLIED: Cap: 10mg, 20mg, 40mg; Cap, Delayed-Release (Prozac Weekly): 90mg

CONTRAINDICATIONS: Use of an MAOI for psychiatric disorders either concomitantly or within 5 weeks of stopping treatment. Treatment within 14 days of stopping an MAOI for psychiatric disorders. Starting treatment in patients being treated with other MAOIs (eg, linezolid, IV methylene blue). Concomitant use with pimozide or thioridazine.

WARNINGS/PRECAUTIONS: Serotonin syndrome reported; d/c immediately and initiate supportive symptomatic treatment. Anaphylactoid and pulmonary reactions reported; d/c if unexplained allergic reaction or rash occurs. May precipitate mixed/manic episode in patients at risk for bipolar disorder; screen for risk of bipolar disorder prior to initiating treatment. Convulsions reported; caution in patients with history of seizures. Weight loss and anorexia reported; monitor weight change during therapy. May increase risk of bleeding reactions. Hyponatremia may occur; caution in elderly and volume-depleted patients. Consider discontinuation of treatment in patients with symptomatic hyponatremia and institute appropriate medical intervention. Mania/hypomania, anxiety, insomnia, and nervousness reported. QT interval prolongation and ventricular arrhythmia including torsades de pointes reported. Caution in patients with congenital long QT syndrome, previous history of QT prolongation, family history of long QT syndrome or sudden cardiac death, and other conditions that predispose to QT prolongation and ventricular arrhythmia; consider ECG assessment and periodic ECG monitoring when initiating treatment. Consider discontinuing treatment and obtaining cardiac evaluation if signs or symptoms of ventricular arrhythmia develop. May alter glycemic control in patients with diabetes. Mydriasis reported; caution with increased intraocular pressure (IOP) or those at risk for acute narrow-angle glaucoma. Caution in patients with diseases/conditions that could affect hemodynamic responses or metabolism. May impair mental/physical abilities. Long elimination $T_{1/2}$; changes in dose may not be fully reflected in plasma for several weeks. Adverse reactions reported upon discontinuation; avoid abrupt withdrawal.

ADVERSE REACTIONS: Somnolence, anorexia, anxiety, asthenia, diarrhea, dry mouth, dyspepsia, headache, insomnia, tremor, pharyngitis, flu syndrome, dizziness, nausea, nervousness.

INTERACTIONS: See Contraindications. Do not use thioridazine within 5 weeks of discontinuing therapy. Caution with CNS active drugs. Avoid with other drugs that cause QT prolongation (eg, specific antipsychotics [eg, ziprasidone, iloperidone, chlorpromazine, mesoridazine, droperidol], specific antibiotics [eg, erythromycin, gatifloxacin, moxifloxacin, sparfloxacin], Class 1A antiarrhythmics [eg, quinidine, procainamide], Class III antiarrhythmics [eg, amiodarone, sotalol], and others [eg, pentamidine, levomethadyl acetate, methadone, halofantrine, mefloquine, dolasetron mesylate, probucol, tacrolimus]). May cause serotonin syndrome with other serotonergic drugs (eg, triptans, TCAs, fentanyl, lithium, tramadol, tryptophan, buspirone, St. John's wort) and with drugs that impair metabolism of serotonin; d/c immediately if this occurs. Increased risk of bleeding with aspirin, NSAIDs, warfarin, and other anticoagulants. Rare reports of prolonged seizures with electroconvulsive therapy. Drugs that are tightly bound to plasma proteins (eg, warfarin, digitoxin) may cause a shift in plasma concentrations, resulting in an adverse effect. Caution with CYP2D6 substrates, including antidepressants (eg, TCAs), antipsychotics (eg, phenothiazines and most atypicals), and antiarrhythmics (eg, propafenone, flecainide). Consider decreasing dose of drugs metabolized by CYP2D6, especially drugs with narrow therapeutic index (eg, flecainide, propafenone, vinblastine, TCAs). May prolong $T_{1/2}$ of diazepam. May increase levels of phenytoin, carbamazepine, haloperidol, clozapine, imipramine, and desipramine. Coadministration with alprazolam resulted in increased alprazolam levels and further psychomotor performance decrement. Anticonvulsant toxicity reported with phenytoin and carbamazepine. Antidiabetic drugs (eg, insulin, oral hypoglycemics) may require dose adjustment. May cause lithium toxicity; monitor lithium levels. Increased risk of hyponatremia with diuretics. Increased levels with CYP2D6 inhibitors.

PREGNANCY: Category C, not for use in nursing.

MECHANISM OF ACTION: SSRI; has not been established. Presumed to be linked to its inhibition of CNS neuronal uptake of serotonin.

PHARMACOKINETICS: Absorption: (Single 40mg dose) C_{max}=15-55ng/mL, T_{max}=6-8 hrs. **Distribution:** Plasma protein binding (94.5%); crosses the placenta; found in breast milk. **Metabolism:** Liver (extensive) via CYP2D6; demethylation into norfluoxetine (active metabolite). **Elimination:** Kidney; $T_{1/2}$=1-3 days (acute administration), 4-6 days (chronic administration), 4-16 days (norfluoxetine, acute and chronic administration).

NURSING CONSIDERATIONS

Assessment: Assess for volume depletion, history of seizures, risk for/presence of bipolar disorder, disease/condition that affects metabolism or hemodynamic responses, diabetes, increased IOP, risk of acute narrow-angle glaucoma, congenital long QT syndrome, previous history of QT prolongation, family history of long QT syndrome or sudden cardiac death, other conditions that predispose to QT prolongation and ventricular arrhythmia, pregnancy/nursing status, and possible drug interactions. Consider ECG assessment if initiating treatment in patients with risk factors for QT prolongation and ventricular arrhythmia.

Monitoring: Monitor for clinical worsening, suicidality, unusual changes in behavior, allergic reactions, serotonin syndrome, bleeding reactions, altered appetite and weight, hyponatremia, seizures, activation of mania/hypomania, mydriasis, hypoglycemia, hyperglycemia, QT interval prolongation, ventricular arrhythmia, and other adverse reactions. Monitor height and weight periodically in children. Consider periodic ECG monitoring if initiating treatment in patients with risk factors for QT prolongation and ventricular arrhythmia. Periodically reassess need for continued treatment.

Patient Counseling: Inform of risks, benefits, and appropriate use of therapy. Counsel to be alert for the emergence of suicidality, unusual changes in behavior, or worsening of depression, especially early during treatment and when the dose is adjusted up or down. Inform about risk of serotonin syndrome with concomitant use with other serotonergic agents. Counsel to seek medical care immediately if rash/hives or unusual bruising/bleeding develop, or if experiencing signs/symptoms associated with serotonin syndrome or hyponatremia. Inform that QT interval prolongation and ventricular arrhythmia including torsades de pointes have been reported. Advise to avoid operating hazardous machinery or driving a car until effects of drug are known. Advise to inform physician if taking or planning to take any prescription or OTC drugs, if pregnant/intending to become pregnant, or if breastfeeding. Instruct to take ud, not to stop taking medication without consulting physician, and to consult physician if symptoms do not improve.

Administration: Oral route. Take with or without food. **Storage:** 15-30°C (59-86°F). (Cap) Protect from light.

Pᴜʟᴍɪᴄᴏʀᴛ   RX
budesonide (AstraZeneca)

OTHER BRAND NAMES: Pulmicort Respules (AstraZeneca) - Pulmicort Flexhaler (AstraZeneca)
THERAPEUTIC CLASS: Corticosteroid

INDICATIONS: (Flexhaler) Maintenance treatment of asthma as prophylactic therapy in patients ≥6 yrs of age. (Respules) Maintenance treatment of asthma and as prophylactic therapy in children 12 months to 8 yrs of age.

DOSAGE: *Adults:* ≥18 Yrs: (Flexhaler) Individualize dose. Initial: 180-360mcg bid. Max: 720mcg bid. Titrate to the lowest effective dose once asthma stability is achieved. Elderly: Start at lower end of dosing range.
Pediatrics: ≥6 Yrs: (Flexhaler) Individualize dose. Initial: 180-360mcg bid. Max: 360mcg bid. 1-8 Yrs: (Respules) Previous Bronchodilators Alone: Initial: 0.5mg qd or 0.25mg bid. Max: 0.5mg/day. Previous Inhaled Corticosteroids: Initial: 0.5mg qd or 0.25mg bid up to 0.5mg bid. Max: 1mg/day. Previous Oral Corticosteroids: Initial: 1mg qd or 0.5mg bid. Max: 1mg/day. Not Responding to Non-steroidal Therapy: Initial: 0.25mg qd. Titrate to the lowest effective dose once asthma stability is achieved. After 1 week of budesonide, gradually reduce PO corticosteroid dose. If once-daily treatment does not provide adequate control, increase total daily dose and/or administer as a divided dose.

HOW SUPPLIED: Powder, Inhalation: (Flexhaler) 90mcg/dose, 180mcg/dose. Sus, Inhalation: (Respules) 0.25mg/2mL, 0.5mg/2mL, 1mg/2mL [2mL]

CONTRAINDICATIONS: Primary treatment of status asthmaticus or other acute episodes of asthma where intensive measures are required. (Flexhaler) Severe hypersensitivity to milk proteins.

WARNINGS/PRECAUTIONS: *Candida albicans* infections of mouth and pharynx reported; treat and/or d/c if needed. Not indicated for the rapid relief of bronchospasm or other acute episodes of asthma; may require oral corticosteroids. Increased susceptibility to infections (eg, chickenpox, measles), may lead to serious/fatal course; if exposed, consider prophylaxis/treatment. Caution with tuberculosis (TB), untreated systemic fungal, bacterial, viral or parasitic infections, and ocular herpes simplex. Deaths due to adrenal insufficiency reported with transfer from systemic to inhaled corticosteroids (ICS); if oral corticosteroids are required, wean slowly from systemic steroid use after transferring to ICS. Transfer from systemic to inhalation therapy may unmask allergic conditions (eg, rhinitis, conjunctivitis). Observe for systemic corticosteroid withdrawal effects. Hypercorticism and adrenal suppression may appear; reduce dose slowly. Decreases in bone mineral density (BMD) reported; caution with chronic use of drugs that can reduce bone mass (eg, anticonvulsants, corticosteroids). May cause reduction in growth velocity in pediatrics. Glaucoma, increased intraocular pressure, and cataracts reported. Bronchospasm, with immediate increase in wheezing, may occur; d/c immediately. Rare cases of systemic eosinophilic conditions and vasculitis consistent with Churg-Strauss syndrome reported. Hypersensitivity reactions reported; d/c if signs and symptoms occur. (Flexhaler) Caution in elderly.

ADVERSE REACTIONS: Respiratory infection. (Flexhaler) Nasopharyngitis, headache, fever, sinusitis, pain, N/V, insomnia, dry mouth, weight gain. (Respules) Rhinitis, otitis media, coughing, viral infection, ear infection, gastroenteritis.

INTERACTIONS: Oral ketoconazole increases plasma levels of oral budesonide. Inhibition of metabolism and increased exposure with CYP3A4 inhibitors. Caution with ketoconazole and other known strong CYP3A4 inhibitors (eg, ritonavir, clarithromycin, itraconazole, nefazodone).

PREGNANCY: Category B, caution in nursing.

MECHANISM OF ACTION: Corticosteroid; not established. Shown to have inhibitory activities against multiple cell types and mediators involved in inflammatory and asthmatic response.

PHARMACOKINETICS: Absorption: Flexhaler: (Adults) T_{max}=10 min; C_{max}=0.6nmol/L (180mcg qd), 1.6nmol/L (360mcg bid). (Peds) T_{max}=15-30 min; C_{max}=0.4nmol/L (180mcg qd), 1.5nmol/L (360mcg bid). Respules: (4-6 yrs of age) Absolute bioavailability (6%); C_{max}=2.6nmol/L; T_{max}=20 min. **Distribution:** V_d=3L/kg; plasma protein binding (85-90%); found in breast milk. **Metabolism:** Liver (extensive) via CYP450 and CYP3A4; 16α-hydroxyprednisolone and 6β-hydroxybudesonide (major metabolites). **Elimination:** Urine and feces (metabolites); (IV) Urine (60%). Flexhaler: $T_{1/2}$=2-3 hrs. Respules: $T_{1/2}$=2.3 hrs.

NURSING CONSIDERATIONS

Assessment: Assess for concomitant diseases (eg, status asthmaticus, acute bronchospasm, other acute episodes of asthma), infections, major risk factors for decreased bone mineral content, history of eye disorders, hypersensitivity, pregnancy/nursing status, and possible drug interactions. Obtain baseline cortisol production levels. Assess lung function in oral corticosteroids withdrawal. (Flexhaler) Assess for severe milk protein hypersensitivity and hepatic disease.

Monitoring: Monitor for localized oral infections with *C. albicans*, worsening or acutely deteriorating asthma, systemic corticosteroid effects, decreased BMD, height in children, vision change, bronchospasm, and hypersensitivity reactions. (Flexhaler) Monitor for hepatic disease.

Patient Counseling: Advise to use at regular intervals and rinse mouth after inhalation; effectiveness depends on regular use. Instruct to d/c if oral candidiasis or hypersensitivity reactions occur. Inform that medication is not meant to relieve acute asthma symptoms and extra doses should not be used for that purpose. Instruct not to d/c without physician's guidance; symptoms may recur after discontinuation. Warn to avoid exposure to chickenpox or measles; if exposed, consult physician. Counsel that maximum benefit may not be achieved for ≥1-2 weeks (Flexhaler) or ≥4-6 weeks (Respules); instruct to notify physician if symptoms worsen or do not improve in that time frame. (Flexhaler) Instruct not to repeat inhalation even if the patient did not feel medication when inhaling; discard whole device after labeled number of inhalations have been used. Advise to carry a warning card indicating need for supplemental systemic corticosteroid during periods of stress or severe asthma attack if chronic systemic corticosteroids have been reduced or withdrawn. Instruct to consult physician if pregnant/breastfeeding or intend to become pregnant.

Administration: Oral inhalation route. After use, rinse mouth with water without swallowing. (Flexhaler) Prime prior to initial use and inhale deeply and forcefully each time the device is used. (Respules) Administer via jet nebulizer connected to air compressor with adequate air flow, equipped with mouthpiece or suitable face mask. Refer to PI for proper administration. **Storage:** (Flexhaler): 20-25°C (68-77°F). Cover tightly. Store in a dry place. (Respules): 20-25°C (68-77°F). Protect from light. Do not freeze. After aluminum foil opened, unused ampules stable for 2 weeks. Once opened, use promptly.

PYLERA   RX
bismuth subcitrate potassium - tetracycline HCl - metronidazole (Aptalis)

THERAPEUTIC CLASS: *H. pylori* treatment combination

INDICATIONS: Treatment of *Helicobacter pylori* infection and duodenal ulcer disease (active or history of within the past 5 yrs) to eradicate *H. pylori*, in combination with omeprazole.

DOSAGE: *Adults:* Usual: 3 caps qid for 10 days, pc and at hs. Take with omeprazole 20mg bid for 10 days after am and pm meals.

HOW SUPPLIED: Cap: (Bismuth-Metronidazole-Tetracycline) 140mg-125mg-125mg

CONTRAINDICATIONS: Use of methoxyflurane concomitantly, disulfiram within the last 2 weeks, and alcoholic beverages or other products containing propylene glycol during therapy and for at least 3 days after therapy. Severe renal impairment.

WARNINGS/PRECAUTIONS: May result in bacterial resistance if used in the absence of a proven or strongly suspected bacterial infection or a prophylactic indication. Caution with hepatic impairment and in the elderly. Bismuth: Neurotoxicity associated with excessive doses reported. May cause temporary and harmless darkening of the tongue and/or black stool. May interfere with x-ray diagnostic procedures of the GI tract. Metronidazole: Encephalopathy, optic and peripheral neuropathy, convulsive seizures, and aseptic meningitis reported. Known or previously unrecognized candidiasis may present more prominent symptoms; treat with an antifungal agent. Caution with evidence of or history of blood dyscrasia. Mild leukopenia reported; obtain total and differential leukocyte counts prior to and after therapy. May interfere with certain types of determinations of serum chemistry values (eg, AST, ALT, LDH, TG, and hexokinase glucose). Tetracycline: May cause fetal harm. May cause permanent teeth discoloration during tooth development (last half of pregnancy, infancy, and childhood to the age of 8 yrs) and enamel hypoplasia; avoid use in this age group. Maternal hepatotoxicity may occur if given during pregnancy at high doses (>2g IV). Pseudotumor cerebri reported. May result in overgrowth of nonsusceptible organisms (eg, fungi); d/c if superinfection occurs. Photosensitivity reported; avoid exposure to the sun or sun lamps and d/c treatment at the 1st evidence of skin erythema. May increase BUN.

ADVERSE REACTIONS: Abnormal feces, nausea, diarrhea, abdominal pain, asthenia, headache, dysgeusia.

INTERACTIONS: See Contraindications. May alter anticoagulant effects of warfarin and other oral coumarin anticoagulants; monitor PT, INR, or other suitable anticoagulation tests and for evidence of bleeding. Metronidazole: Short-term use may cause elevation of serum lithium concentrations and signs of lithium toxicity with high doses of lithium. Drugs that inhibit microsomal liver enzymes (eg, cimetidine) may decrease plasma clearance and prolong $T_{1/2}$. Drugs that induce microsomal liver enzymes (eg, phenytoin, phenobarbital) may accelerate elimination and reduce plasma concentrations. Impaired clearance of phenytoin reported; monitor phenytoin concentrations. Tetracycline: Oral contraceptives may become less effective and may cause breakthrough bleeding if given concomitantly. Antacids containing aluminum, Ca^{2+}, or Mg^{2+}; preparations containing iron, zinc, or sodium bicarbonate; or milk and dairy products may reduce absorption; do not consume concomitantly. May interfere with bactericidal action of penicillin; avoid coadministration.

PREGNANCY: Category D, not for use in nursing.

MECHANISM OF ACTION: *H. pylori* treatment combination; antimicrobial agent. Bismuth: Antibacterial action not well understood. Metronidazole: Metabolized through reductive pathways into reactive intermediates that have cytotoxic action. Tetracycline: Interacts with 30S subunit of the bacterial ribosome and inhibits protein synthesis.

PHARMACOKINETICS: Absorption: Metronidazole: Well-absorbed. Tetracycline: 60-90% (stomach and upper small intestine). Administration of the individual drugs as separate cap formulations or as Pylera resulted in variable pharmacokinetic parameters. **Distribution:** Bismuth: Plasma protein binding (>90%). Metronidazole: Plasma protein binding (<20%); found in breast milk. Tetracycline: Plasma protein binding (varying degrees); crosses placenta, found in breast milk. **Metabolism:** Metronidazole: Side-chain oxidation and glucuronide conjugation. **Elimination:** Bismuth: Urinary, biliary; $T_{1/2}$=5 days (blood and urine). Metronidazole: Urine (60-80%, 20% unchanged), feces (6-15%); $T_{1/2}$=8 hrs (normal patients). Tetracycline: Urine, feces.

NURSING CONSIDERATIONS

Assessment: Assess for drug hypersensitivity, history of blood dyscrasia, known or previously unrecognized candidiasis, hepatic/renal impairment, pregnancy/nursing status, and possible drug interactions. Obtain total and differential leukocyte counts prior to therapy.

Monitoring: Monitor for encephalopathy, peripheral neuropathy, convulsive seizures, aseptic meningitis, leukopenia, enamel hypoplasia, pseudotumor cerebri, superinfections, photosensitivity reactions, skin erythema, and other adverse reactions. Monitor total and differential leukocyte counts and BUN levels. Monitor PT, INR, or other suitable anticoagulation tests and for evidence of bleeding with warfarin and other oral coumarin anticoagulants.

Patient Counseling: Advise pregnant women that therapy may cause fetal harm. Advise to avoid breastfeeding while on therapy; instruct to d/c feeding or pump and discard breast milk during treatment and for 24 hrs after the last dose. Inform that therapy may cause allergic reactions; instruct to d/c therapy at 1st sign of urticaria, erythematous rash, flushing, fever or other symptoms of an allergic reaction. Inform of the risk of central and peripheral nervous system effects; inform to d/c and notify physician immediately if any neurologic symptoms occur. Instruct to avoid exposure to sun or sun lamps. Advise patients to notify physician of the use of any other medications while on therapy. Inform that temporary and harmless darkening of tongue, and/or black stool may occur. Inform of proper dosing information and instruct to take exactly ud; inform that skipping doses or not completing the full course of therapy may decrease effectiveness and increase likelihood of bacterial resistance. Advise not to take double doses; if a dose is missed, advise to continue normal dosing schedule until medication is gone. Instruct to inform physician if >4 doses are missed. Counsel that therapy should only be used to treat bacterial, not viral (eg, common cold), infections.

Administration: Oral route. Swallow cap whole with a full glass of water (8 oz.). **Storage:** 20-25°C (68-77°F).

QSYMIA

phentermine - topiramate (Vivus)

THERAPEUTIC CLASS: Anorectic sympathomimetic amine/sulfamate-substituted monosaccharide

INDICATIONS: Adjunct to a reduced-calorie diet and increased physical activity for chronic weight management in adults with an initial BMI of ≥30kg/m² (obese), or ≥27kg/m² (overweight) in the presence of at least 1 weight-related comorbidity (eg, HTN, type 2 diabetes mellitus [DM], or dyslipidemia).

DOSAGE: *Adults:* Determine BMI; refer to PI for BMI conversion chart. Avoid pm dose. Initial: 3.75mg-23mg qam for 14 days. Titrate: May increase to 7.5mg-46mg qam. Evaluate weight loss after 12 weeks of therapy with 7.5mg-46mg; d/c or escalate dose if patient has not lost at least 3% of baseline weight. Dose Escalation: Increase to 11.25mg-69mg qam for 14 days, followed by 15mg-92mg qam. Evaluate weight loss after an additional 12 weeks with 15mg-92mg; d/c if patient has not lost at least 5% of baseline weight. Use 3.75mg-23mg and 11.25mg-69mg strengths for titration purposes only. Discontinuation: D/C 15mg-92mg gradually by taking a dose qod for at least 1 week prior to stopping treatment. Moderate (CrCl ≥30-<50mL/min)/Severe (CrCl <30mL/min) Renal Impairment/Moderate Hepatic Impairment (Child-Pugh 7-9): Adjust dose. Max: 7.5mg-46mg qam. Elderly: Start at lower end of dosing range.

HOW SUPPLIED: Cap, Extended-Release: (Phentermine-Topiramate) 3.75mg-23mg, 7.5mg-46mg, 11.25mg-69mg, 15mg-92mg

CONTRAINDICATIONS: Pregnancy, glaucoma, hyperthyroidism, during or within 14 days of administration of MAOIs.

WARNINGS/PRECAUTIONS: May cause fetal harm; use effective contraception to prevent pregnancy. Available through a limited program under the Risk Evaluation and Mitigation Strategy. May increase resting HR; monitor resting HR regularly in all patients, especially those with cardiac or cerebrovascular disease or when initiating or increasing dose. Reduce dose or d/c if sustained increase in resting HR or persistent SrCr elevations occur. Increased risk of suicidal thoughts/behavior; monitor for emergence/worsening of depression, suicidal thoughts/behavior, and/or any unusual changes in mood or behavior, and d/c if these occur. Avoid with history of suicidal attempts or active suicidal ideation. Acute myopia associated with secondary angle closure glaucoma reported; d/c immediately to reverse symptoms. Mood/sleep disorders, including anxiety and insomnia, may occur; consider dose reduction or withdrawal for clinically significant or persistent symptoms. May impair physical/mental abilities; consider dose reduction or withdrawal if cognitive dysfunction persists. Hyperchloremic, non-anion gap, metabolic acidosis reported. Conditions that predispose to acidosis (eg, renal disease, severe respiratory disorders, status epilepticus, diarrhea, surgery, ketogenic diet) may be additive to the bicarbonate lowering effects of topiramate. Weight loss may increase risk of hypoglycemia in patients with type 2 DM treated with insulin and/or insulin secretagogues (eg, sulfonylureas), and risk of hypotension in those treated with antihypertensives; appropriate changes should be made to antidiabetic or antihypertensive therapy if hypoglycemia or hypotension develops. Seizures associated with abrupt withdrawal in individuals without history of seizures or epilepsy; taper dose gradually if using 15mg-92mg and monitor for seizures in situations where immediate termination of therapy is required. Avoid with end-stage renal disease on dialysis or severe hepatic impairment (Child-Pugh 10-15). Associated with kidney stone formation; increase fluid intake to increase urine output. Oligohidrosis reported; monitor for decreased sweating and increased body temperature during physical activity, especially in hot weather. May increase risk of hypokalemia. Potential for abuse. Lab test interactions may occur. Caution in elderly.

ADVERSE REACTIONS: Paresthesia, dry mouth, constipation, upper respiratory tract infection, headache, dysgeusia, insomnia, nasopharyngitis, dizziness, sinusitis, bronchitis, nausea, back pain, diarrhea, blurred vision.

INTERACTIONS: See Contraindications. May decrease exposure of ethinyl estradiol and increase exposure of norethindrone with single dose of oral contraceptive. Alcohol or CNS depressants (eg, barbiturates, benzodiazepines, sleep medications) may potentiate CNS depression. May potentiate the K⁺ wasting action of non-K⁺-sparing diuretics; monitor for hypokalemia. Avoid with other drugs that inhibit carbonic anhydrase (eg, zonisamide, acetazolamide, methazolamide, dichlorphenamide); may increase severity of metabolic acidosis and kidney stone formation. Caution with other drugs that predispose patients to heat-related disorders (eg, other carbonic anhydrase inhibitors, drugs with anticholinergic activity). Phenytoin or carbamazepine may decrease plasma levels. Concurrent administration of valproic acid has been associated with hyperammonemia with or without encephalopathy, and hypothermia.

PREGNANCY: Category X, not for use in nursing.

MECHANISM OF ACTION: Phentermine: Anorectic sympathomimetic amine; has not been established. Releases catecholamines in the hypothalamus, resulting in reduced appetite and decreased food consumption. Topiramate: Sulfamate-substituted monosaccharide; has not been established. Effect may be due to its effects on both appetite suppression and satiety enhancement, induced by combination of pharmacologic effects including augmenting the activity of the neurotransmitter gamma-aminobutyrate, modulation of voltage-gated ion channels, inhibition of AMPA/kainite excitatory glutamate receptors, or inhibition of carbonic anhydrase.

PHARMACOKINETICS: Absorption: (15mg-92mg Single Dose) Phentermine: C_{max}=49.1ng/mL, T_{max}=6 hrs, AUC_{0-t}=1990ng•hr/mL, AUC_{0-inf}=2000ng•hr/mL. Topiramate: C_{max}=1020ng/mL, T_{max}=9 hrs, AUC_{0-t}=61,600ng•hr/mL, AUC_{0-inf}=68,000ng•hr/mL. **Distribution:** Found in breast milk; Phentermine: V_d=348L; plasma protein binding (17.5%). Topiramate: Plasma protein binding (15-41%). **Metabolism:** Phentermine: CYP3A4 by p-hydroxylation and N-oxidation. Topiramate: Hydroxylation, hydrolysis, glucuronidation. **Elimination:** Phentermine: Urine (70-80% unchanged); $T_{1/2}$=20 hrs. Topiramate: Urine (70% unchanged); $T_{1/2}$=65 hrs.

NURSING CONSIDERATIONS

Assessment: Assess for known hypersensitivity or idiosyncrasy to sympathomimetic amines, glaucoma, hyperthyroidism, cardiac and cerebrovascular disease; history of behavioral/mood disorders, history of seizures, renal/hepatic dysfunction, or any other conditions where treatment is contraindicated or cautioned, pregnancy/nursing status, possible drug interactions. Obtain baseline HR and blood chemistry profile (eg, bicarbonate, creatinine, K^+, glucose).

Monitoring: Monitor for acute myopia, secondary angle-closure glaucoma, emergence/worsening of depression, suicidal thoughts or behavior, mood/sleep disorders, cognitive dysfunction, hyperchloremic metabolic acidosis, seizures, kidney stone formation, oligohidrosis, and hyperthermia. Monitor for HR regularly and blood chemistry profile (eg, bicarbonate, creatinine, K^+, glucose) periodically. Assess pregnancy status monthly during therapy.

Patient Counseling: Inform that therapy is for chronic weight management in conjunction with a reduced-calorie diet and increased physical activity. Inform that drug is only available through certified pharmacies. Instruct to inform physician about all medications, nutritional supplements, and vitamins (including any weight loss products) taken while on therapy. Instruct on how to properly take the medication. Instruct to avoid pregnancy/breastfeeding while on therapy and to notify physician immediately if patient becomes pregnant during treatment. Advise to report symptoms of sustained periods of heart pounding or racing while at rest, suicidal behavior/ideation, mood changes, depression, severe/persistent eye pain or significant visual changes, any changes in attention/concentration/memory, and/or difficulty finding words. Advise not to drive/operate machinery until they know how they will react to the medication. Instruct to notify physician about any factors that can increase the risk of acidosis (eg, prolonged diarrhea, surgery, high protein/low carbohydrate diet, and/or concomitant medications such as other carbonic anhydrase inhibitors) and to avoid alcohol while on therapy. Instruct diabetic patients to monitor blood glucose levels and to report symptoms of hypoglycemia to physician. Advise not to abruptly d/c therapy without notifying physician. Advise to increase fluid intake and report symptoms of severe side or back pain, and/or blood in urine to physician. Advise to monitor for decreased sweating and increased body temperature during physical activity, especially in hot weather.

Administration: Oral route. Take with or without food. **Storage:** 15-25°C (59-77°F). Protect from moisture.

QUILLIVANT XR
methylphenidate HCl (NextWave)

> High potential for abuse and dependence. Assess the risk of abuse prior to prescribing, and monitor for signs of abuse and dependence while on therapy.

THERAPEUTIC CLASS: Sympathomimetic amine

INDICATIONS: Treatment of attention-deficit hyperactivity disorder.

DOSAGE: *Adults:* Individualize dose. Initial: 20mg qam. Titrate: May be titrated weekly in increments of 10mg to 20mg. Max: 60mg/day. Maint/Extended Treatment: Periodically reevaluate long-term usefulness with trials off medication to assess functioning without pharmacotherapy. Reduce dose or d/c if necessary, if paradoxical aggravation of symptoms or other adverse events occur. D/C if no improvement observed after appropriate dosage adjustments over 1 month. *Pediatrics:* ≥6 Yrs: Individualize dose. Initial: 20mg qam. Titrate: May be titrated weekly in increments of 10mg to 20mg. Max: 60mg/day. Maint/Extended Treatment: Periodically reevaluate long-term usefulness with trials off medication to assess functioning without pharmacotherapy. Reduce dose or d/c if necessary, if paradoxical aggravation of symptoms or other adverse events occur. D/C if no improvement observed after appropriate dosage adjustments over 1 month.

HOW SUPPLIED: Sus, Extended-Release: 5mg/mL [60mL, 120mL, 150mL, 180mL]

CONTRAINDICATIONS: Treatment with or within 14 days following discontinuation of treatment with an MAOI.

WARNINGS/PRECAUTIONS: Sudden death reported in children and adolescents with structural cardiac abnormalities and other serious cardiac problems. Sudden death, stroke, and myocardial infarction (MI) reported in adults. Avoid with known structural cardiac abnormalities, cardiomyopathy, serious cardiac arrhythmias, coronary artery disease, or other serious cardiac problems. May increase BP and HR. May exacerbate symptoms of behavior disturbance and thought disorder in patients with a preexisting psychotic disorder. May induce a manic or mixed episode in patients with bipolar disorder. May cause psychotic or manic symptoms in patients without a prior history of psychotic illness or mania at recommended doses; consider discontinuation if such symptoms occur. Priapism reported; seek immediate medical attention if abnormally sustained or frequent and painful erections develop. Associated with peripheral vasculopathy, including Raynaud's phenomenon; monitor for digital changes. May cause long-term suppression of growth in pediatric patients; may need to interrupt treatment in patients not growing or gaining height or weight as expected.

ADVERSE REACTIONS: Affect lability, excoriation, initial insomnia, tic, decreased appetite, vomiting, motion sickness, eye pain, rash.

INTERACTIONS: See Contraindications.

PREGNANCY: Category C, not for use in nursing.

MECHANISM OF ACTION: Sympathomimetic amine; CNS stimulant. Thought to block the reuptake of norepinephrine and dopamine into the presynaptic neuron and increase the release of these monoamines into the extraneuronal space.

PHARMACOKINETICS: Absorption: d-methylphenidate: C_{max}=34.4ng/mL (children), 21.1ng/mL (adolescents), 17ng/mL (adults); T_{max}=4.05 hrs (median, children), 2 hrs (median, adolescents), 4 hrs (median, adults); AUC_{inf}=378hr•ng/mL (children), 178hr•ng/mL (adolescents), 163.2hr•ng/mL (adults). **Distribution:** Found in breast milk. **Metabolism:** Deesterification to α-phenyl-piperidine acetic acid [PPAA] (metabolite). **Elimination:** Urine (90%, 80% PPAA); (d-methylphenidate) $T_{1/2}$=5.2 hrs (adults/children), 5 hrs (adolescents).

NURSING CONSIDERATIONS

Assessment: Assess for drug hypersensitivity, cardiac problems, psychotic disorders, bipolar disorder, pregnancy/nursing status, and for possible drug interactions. Obtain baseline height/weight in children. Screen patients for risk factors for developing a manic episode and the risk of abuse before starting therapy.

Monitoring: Monitor for stroke, MI, HTN, tachycardia, exacerbations of behavior disturbances and thought disorders, psychotic or manic symptoms, digital changes, priapism, and other adverse reactions. Monitor growth in children. Monitor for signs of abuse and dependence. Periodically reevaluate long-term usefulness.

Patient Counseling: Inform about risks, benefits, and appropriate use of treatment. Counsel that drug has potential for abuse or dependence; instruct to keep medication in a safe place to prevent abuse. Advise of the potential for serious cardiovascular risks, including sudden death, MI, and stroke; instruct to contact physician immediately if symptoms, such as exertional chest pain, unexplained syncope, or other symptoms suggestive of cardiac disease develop. Advise that the drug can elevate BP and HR, can cause psychotic or manic symptoms even in patients without a prior history of psychotic symptoms or mania, and in pediatric patients can cause slowing of growth and weight loss. Advise of the possibility of priapism; instruct to seek immediate medical attention in the event of priapism. Inform about the risk of peripheral vasculopathy, including Raynaud's phenomenon; instruct to report to the physician any numbness, pain, skin color change, sensitivity to temperature in fingers or toes, and any signs of unexplained wounds appearing on fingers or toes. Instruct to inform physician if pregnant or intend to become pregnant during therapy. Advise of the potential fetal effects from use during pregnancy.

Administration: Oral route. Take with or without food. Vigorously shake bottle for at least 10 sec before each dose to ensure that the proper dose is administered. Use only with the oral dosing dispenser provided. Refer to PI for further administration and reconstitution instructions. **Storage:** 25°C (77°F); excursions permitted from 15-30°C (59-86°F). Stable for up to 4 months after reconstitution.

QUINIDINE GLUCONATE INJECTION   RX
quinidine gluconate (Various)

THERAPEUTIC CLASS: Class IA antiarrhythmic/schizonticide antimalarial

INDICATIONS: Treatment of life-threatening *Plasmodium falciparum* malaria. Conversion of atrial fibrillation/flutter (A-Fib/Flutter) to normal sinus rhythm. Treatment of ventricular arrhythmias.

DOSAGE: *Adults:* Malaria: LD: 15mg/kg base (24mg/kg gluconate) IV over 4 hrs. Maint: After 8 hrs, 7.5mg/kg (12mg/kg gluconate) IV q8h for 7 days. Alternate: Initial: 6.25mg/kg base (10mg/kg gluconate) IV over 1-2 hrs. Maint: 12.5mcg/kg/min base (20mcg/kg/min gluconate) IV

for 72 hrs. A-Fib/Flutter: 0.25mg/kg/min IV. Max: 5-10mg/kg IV. Consider alternate therapy if conversion to sinus rhythm not achieved. Ventricular Arrhythmia: Dosing regimens not adequately studied. Generally similar to A-Fib/Flutter. Renal/Hepatic Impairment or congestive heart failure (CHF): Reduce dose. Elderly: Start at low end of dosing range.
Pediatrics: Malaria: LD: 15mg/kg base (24mg/kg gluconate) IV over 4 hrs. Maint: After 8 hrs, 7.5mg/kg (12mg/kg gluconate) IV q8h for 7 days. Alternate: Initial: 6.25mg/kg base (10mg/kg gluconate) IV over 1-2 hrs. Maint: 12.5mcg/kg/min base (20mcg/kg/min gluconate) IV for 72 hrs.

HOW SUPPLIED: Inj: 80mg/mL [10mL]

CONTRAINDICATIONS: In the absence of a functional artificial pacemaker any cardiac rhythm dependent upon a junctional or idioventricular pacemaker (including with complete atrioventricular [AV] block), thrombocytopenic purpura with previous treatment, patients adversely affected by anticholinergics (eg, myasthenia gravis).

WARNINGS/PRECAUTIONS: Rapid infusion can cause peripheral vascular collapse and severe hypotension. May prolong QTc interval and may lead to torsades de pointes. Paradoxical increase in ventricular rate in A-Fib/Flutter. Caution in those at risk of complete AV block without implanted pacemakers, renal/hepatic dysfunction, elderly, and CHF. Physical/pharmacologic maneuvers to terminate paroxysmal supraventricular tachycardia may be ineffective. Exacerbated bradycardia in sick sinus syndrome.

ADVERSE REACTIONS: Upper GI distress, lightheadedness, fatigue, palpitations, weakness, visual problems, N/V, diarrhea, changes in sleeping habits, rash, headache, diarrhea, angina-like pain.

INTERACTIONS: Urine alkalinizers (eg, carbonic anhydrase inhibitors, sodium bicarbonate, thiazide diuretics) reduce renal elimination. CYP3A4 inducers (eg, phenobarbital, phenytoin, rifampin) may accelerate elimination. Verapamil and diltiazem decrease clearance. Caution with drugs metabolized by CYP2D6 (eg, mexiletine, phenothiazines, codeine) or by CYP3A4 (eg, nifedipine, felodipine, nicardipine). β-blockers may decrease clearance. May slow metabolism of nifedipine. Increases levels of digoxin, digitoxin, procainamide, and haloperidol. Increased levels with ketoconazole, amiodarone, and cimetidine. Potentiates warfarin and depolarizing and nondepolarizing neuromuscular blockers. Additive effects with anticholinergics, vasodilators, and negative inotropes. Antagonistic effects with cholinergics, vasoconstrictors, and positive inotropes.

PREGNANCY: Category C, not for use in nursing.

MECHANISM OF ACTION: Antimalarial schizonticide and antiarrhythmic agent with class 1a activity. Slows phase-0 depolarization by depressing the inward depolarizing Na^+ current, which slows conduction, prolongs effective refractory period, and reduces automaticity in the heart. Also has anticholinergic activity, negative ionotropic activity, and acts peripherally as an α-adrenergic antagonist.

PHARMACOKINETICS: Absorption: T_{max}=<2 hrs. **Distribution:** V_d=2-3L/kg; plasma protein binding (80-88%) in adults and older children, (50-70%) in pregnant women, infants, and neonates; found in breast milk. **Metabolism:** Liver, via CYP3A4 pathway. 3-hydroxy-quinidine (3HQ); major metabolite. **Elimination:** Urine (20% unchanged); $T_{1/2}$=6-8 hrs (adults), 3-4 hrs (pediatrics), and 12 hrs (3HQ).

NURSING CONSIDERATIONS

Assessment: Assess for structural heart disease, preexisting long-QT syndrome, implanted pacemaker, history of torsades de pointes, other conduction defects, thrombocytopenic purpura, CHF, renal/hepatic dysfunction, myasthenia gravis, pregnancy/nursing status, and possible drug/diet interactions.

Monitoring: Monitor for exacerbated bradycardia, paradoxical increase in ventricular rate in A-Fib/Flutter, torsades de pointes, life-threatening ventricular arrhythmia, hypotension, ventricular extrasystoles/tachycardia/flutter, and ventricular fibrillation. Continuously/carefully monitor ECG and BP.

Patient Counseling: Inform about risks/benefits of drug and report any adverse reactions. Instruct to notify physician if pregnant/nursing. Instruct to avoid grapefruit juice.

Administration: IV route. **Storage:** 25°C (77°F); excursions permitted to 15-30°C (59-86°F).

QUIXIN   RX
levofloxacin (Vistakon)

THERAPEUTIC CLASS: Fluoroquinolone

INDICATIONS: Treatment of bacterial conjunctivitis caused by susceptible strains of organisms.

DOSAGE: *Adults:* Days 1-2: 1-2 drops in affected eye(s) q2h while awake, up to 8X/day. Days 3-7: 1-2 drops in affected eye(s) q4h while awake, up to qid.
Pediatrics: ≥1 Yr: Days 1-2: 1-2 drops in affected eye(s) q2h while awake, up to 8X/day. Days 3-7: 1-2 drops in affected eye(s) q4h while awake, up to qid.

HOW SUPPLIED: Sol: 0.5% [5mL]

WARNINGS/PRECAUTIONS: Should not be injected subconjunctivally nor introduced directly to anterior chamber of the eye. D/C if allergic reaction or superinfection occurs; prolonged use may cause overgrowth of nonsusceptible organisms. Avoid wearing contact lenses if signs/symptoms of conjunctivitis present.

ADVERSE REACTIONS: Transient ocular burning, transient decreased vision, fever, foreign body sensation, headache, ocular pain/discomfort, pharyngitis, photophobia.

INTERACTIONS: Systemic quinolone therapy may increase theophylline levels, interfere with caffeine metabolism, enhance warfarin effects, and elevate SrCr with cyclosporine.

PREGNANCY: Category C, caution in nursing.

MECHANISM OF ACTION: Fluoroquinolone; inhibits bacterial topoisomerase IV and DNA gyrase, which are enzymes required for DNA replication, transcription, repair, and recombination.

PHARMACOKINETICS: Absorption: C_{max}=0.94ng/mL (single dose), 2.15ng/mL (multiple doses). **Distribution:** Presumed to be excreted in breast milk.

NURSING CONSIDERATIONS

Assessment: Assess for hypersensitivity to the drug or to other quinolones, use of contact lenses, pregnancy/nursing status, possible drug interactions, or any other conditions where treatment is contraindicated or cautioned.

Monitoring: Monitor for signs/symptoms of hypersensitivity or anaphylactic reaction, and overgrowth of nonsusceptible organisms. Perform eye exam using magnification (eg, slit-lamp biomicroscopy, fluorescein staining) if necessary.

Patient Counseling: Instruct to avoid contaminating applicator tip with material from eye, fingers, or other sources. Advise to not wear contact lenses if there are signs/symptoms of bacterial conjunctivitis. Instruct to d/c medication and contact physician if signs of hypersensitivity reaction (eg, rash) develop.

Administration: Ocular route. Do not inject subconjunctivally or introduce directly into anterior chamber of eye. **Storage:** 15-25°C (59-77°F).

QUTENZA   RX
capsaicin (Acorda)

THERAPEUTIC CLASS: Analgesic

INDICATIONS: Management of neuropathic pain associated with postherpetic neuralgia.

DOSAGE: *Adults:* A single 60-min application of up to 4 patches. May repeat every 3 months or as warranted by the return of pain (not more frequently than every 3 months). Apply to dry, intact skin.

HOW SUPPLIED: Patch: 179mg [8%]

WARNINGS/PRECAUTIONS: Do not apply to the face, scalp, or broken skin. Do not use near eyes or mucous membranes. Aerosolization may occur upon rapid removal; remove gently and slowly by rolling the adhesive side inward. If irritation of eyes or airways occur, flush with cool water. Inhalation can result in coughing or sneezing; provide supportive medical care if SOB develops. If skin not intended to be treated comes into contact with patch, apply cleansing gel for 1 min, then wipe off with dry gauze and wash with soap and water. May experience substantial procedural pain; treat with local cooling (eg, ice pack) and/or analgesic medication, such as opioids. HTN reported; monitor periodically. Increased risk of cardiovascular (CV) effects with unstable/poorly controlled HTN and history of CV/cerebrovascular events.

ADVERSE REACTIONS: Application-site erythema, pain, pruritus, papules, edema, nasopharyngitis, N/V.

PREGNANCY: Category B, safety not known in nursing.

MECHANISM OF ACTION: Analgesic; TRPV1 channel agonist. Causes an initial enhanced stimulation of the TRPV1-expressing cutaneous nociceptors that may be associated with painful sensations followed by pain relief thought to be mediated by a reduction in TRPV1-expressing nociceptive nerve endings.

PHARMACOKINETICS: Absorption: C_{max}=4.6ng/mL.

NURSING CONSIDERATIONS

Assessment: Assess application site, unstable/poorly controlled HTN, history of CV/cerebrovascular events, and pregnancy/nursing status.

Monitoring: Monitor for any hypersensitivity reactions and monitor BP periodically during treatment and for any possible side effects.

Patient Counseling: Inform that exposure of the skin to the patch may result in transient erythema and burning sensation. Instruct not to touch patch; may produce burning and/or stinging sensation. Instruct to inform physician if pregnant/breastfeeding, side effects becomes severe, or if eye/airway irritation occurs. Inform that treated area may be heat-sensitive (eg, hot showers/bath, direct sunlight, vigorous exercise) for a few days after treatment. Inform patients that they may be given medications such as opioids that may impair mental/physical abilities. Inform that a small transient increase in BP may occur during and shortly after treatment. Instruct to inform physician of any recent CV events.

Administration: Topical route. May cut patch to match size/shape of treatment area. Refer to PI for instructions for use. **Storage:** 20-25°C (68-77°F); excursions permitted between 15-30°C (59-86°F). Keep in sealed pouch immediately before use.

QVAR   RX
beclomethasone dipropionate (Teva)

THERAPEUTIC CLASS: Corticosteroid

INDICATIONS: Maintenance treatment of asthma as prophylactic therapy in patients ≥5 yrs of age. To reduce or eliminate the need for systemic corticosteroids in asthma patients requiring systemic corticosteroid administration.

DOSAGE: *Adults:* Previously on Bronchodilators Alone: Initial: 40-80mcg bid. Max: 320mcg bid. Previously on Inhaled Corticosteroids: Initial: 40-160mcg bid. Max: 320mcg bid. Taper to the lowest effective dose once desired effect is achieved. Maintained on Systemic Corticosteroids: Initial: Should be used concurrently with the usual maint dose of systemic corticosteroids. May attempt gradual reduction of systemic corticosteroid dose after 1 week on inhaled therapy by reducing the daily or alternate daily dose. Reductions may be made after an interval of 1 or 2 weeks, depending on the response. Elderly: Start at lower end of dosing range.
Pediatrics: ≥12 Yrs: Previously on Bronchodilators Alone: Initial: 40-80mcg bid. Max: 320mcg bid. Previously on Inhaled Corticosteroids: Initial: 40-160mcg bid. Max: 320mcg bid. 5-11 Yrs: Previously on Bronchodilators Alone/Inhaled Corticosteroids: Initial: 40mcg bid. Max: 80mcg bid. Taper to the lowest effective dose once desired effect is achieved. Maintained on Systemic Corticosteroids: Initial: Should be used concurrently with the usual maint dose of systemic corticosteroids. May attempt gradual reduction of systemic corticosteroid dose after 1 week on inhaled therapy by reducing the daily or alternate daily dose. Reductions may be made after an interval of 1 or 2 weeks, depending on the response.

HOW SUPPLIED: MDI: 40mcg/inh [7.3g, 8.7g], 80mcg/inh [4.2g, 7.3g, 8.7g]

CONTRAINDICATIONS: Primary treatment of status asthmaticus or other acute episodes of asthma where intensive measures are required.

WARNINGS/PRECAUTIONS: Deaths due to adrenal insufficiency have occurred during and after transfer from systemic corticosteroids to inhaled corticosteroids; monitor carefully. Resume oral corticosteroids (in large doses) immediately during stress or severe asthmatic attack. Transfer from systemic to inhalation therapy may unmask allergic conditions (eg, rhinitis, conjunctivitis, eczema). Risk for more severe/fatal course of infections (eg, chickenpox, measles); avoid exposure in patients who have not had these diseases or been properly immunized. If exposed, consider prophylaxis/treatment. Not a bronchodilator and is not indicated for rapid relief of bronchospasm. D/C, treat, and institute alternative therapy if bronchospasm occurs after dosing. Observe for systemic corticosteroid effects (eg, hypercorticism, adrenal suppression); if such changes appear, reduce dose slowly. Potential for reduced growth velocity in pediatric patients. Caution with active or quiescent tuberculosis (TB) infection, untreated systemic fungal, bacterial, parasitic, or viral infections, or ocular herpes simplex. Rare instances of glaucoma, increased intraocular pressure (IOP), and cataracts reported. Caution in elderly.

ADVERSE REACTIONS: Headache, pharyngitis, upper respiratory tract infection, rhinitis, increased asthma symptoms, oral symptoms (inhalation route), sinusitis, dysphonia, dysmenorrhea, coughing.

PREGNANCY: Category C, not for use in nursing.

MECHANISM OF ACTION: Corticosteroid; has multiple anti-inflammatory effects, inhibiting both inflammatory cells and release of inflammatory mediators.

PHARMACOKINETICS: Absorption: (Beclomethasone) C_{max}=88pg/mL, T_{max}= 0.5 hr; (Beclomethasone-17-monopropionate [17-BMP]) C_{max}=1419pg/mL, T_{max}=0.7 hr. **Distribution:** Found in breast milk; plasma protein binding (94-96%, 17-BMP) (in vitro). **Metabolism:** Liver (biotransformation) via CYP3A; 17-BMP, 21-BMP, beclomethasone (major metabolites). **Elimination:** Feces, urine (<10%); $T_{1/2}$= 2.8 hrs (17-BMP).

NURSING CONSIDERATIONS

Assessment: Assess for status asthmaticus, active or quiescent TB infections, untreated systemic fungal, bacterial, parasitic or viral infections, ocular herpes simplex, exposure to chickenpox or measles, and pregnancy/nursing status.

Monitoring: Monitor for bronchospasm, growth velocity in children, glaucoma, increased IOP, cataracts, hypercorticism, adrenal suppression/insufficiency, hypersensitivity reactions, and other adverse effects.

Patient Counseling: Inform about the risks and benefits of therapy. Advise to avoid exposure to chickenpox or measles; consult physician if exposed. Instruct to use drug at regular intervals ud and should not be stopped abruptly. Inform that drug is not intended for treatment of acute asthma. Counsel about the proper priming/use of inhaler and advise to rinse mouth after use. Advise to seek medical attention if worsening of existing TB, infections, or ocular herpes simplex occur, if symptoms do not improve or worsen, or during periods of stress or severe asthmatic attack.

Administration: Oral inhalation route. Prime prior to initial use or if not used for over 10 days. Refer to PI for directions for use. Should only be used with product's actuator and should not be used with any other inhalation drug product. **Storage:** 25°C (77°F); excursions permitted to 15-30°C (59-86°F). For optimal results, canister should be at room temperature when used.

RANEXA   RX
ranolazine (Gilead Sciences)

THERAPEUTIC CLASS: Miscellaneous antianginal

INDICATIONS: Treatment of chronic angina; may be used with β-blockers, nitrates, calcium channel blockers, antiplatelet therapy, lipid-lowering therapy, ACE inhibitors, and ARBs.

DOSAGE: *Adults:* Initial: 500mg bid. Titrate: May increase to 1000mg bid, PRN, based on clinical symptoms. Max: 1000mg bid. Concurrent Use with Moderate CYP3A Inhibitors (eg, Diltiazem, Verapamil, Erythromycin, Fluconazole, Grapefruit Juice or Grapefruit-Containing Products): Max: 500mg bid. Concurrent Use with P-glycoprotein (P-gp) Inhibitors (eg, Cyclosporine): Titrate dose based on clinical response. Elderly: Start at lower end of dosing range.

HOW SUPPLIED: Tab, Extended-Release: 500mg, 1000mg

CONTRAINDICATIONS: Liver cirrhosis, concomitant use with CYP3A inducers (eg, rifampin, rifabutin, rifapentine, phenobarbital, phenytoin, carbamazepine, St. John's wort) or strong CYP3A inhibitors (eg, ketoconazole, itraconazole, clarithromycin, nefazodone, nelfinavir, ritonavir, indinavir, saquinavir).

WARNINGS/PRECAUTIONS: May prolong QTc interval in a dose-related manner. Acute renal failure reported in patients with severe renal impairment (CrCl <30mL/min); d/c and treat appropriately if acute renal failure develops. Monitor renal function after initiation and periodically in patients with moderate to severe renal impairment (CrCl <60mL/min) for increases in SrCr accompanied by an increase in BUN. Caution in elderly.

ADVERSE REACTIONS: Dizziness, headache, constipation, N/V, abdominal pain, dyspepsia, anorexia, asthenia, peripheral edema, bradycardia, palpitations, confusion, dyspnea, hematuria, hyperhidrosis.

INTERACTIONS: See Contraindications and Dosage. P-gp inhibitors (eg, cyclosporine) may increase concentrations. May increase levels of simvastatin; limit simvastatin dose to 20mg qd. May increase concentrations of other sensitive CYP3A substrates (eg, lovastatin) and CYP3A substrates with a narrow therapeutic range (eg, cyclosporine, tacrolimus, sirolimus); may require dose adjustment of these drugs. May increase exposure to digoxin and CYP2D6 substrates (eg, TCAs, antipsychotics); may require digoxin dose adjustment and lower doses of CYP2D6 substrates. May increase levels of metformin; do not exceed 1700mg/day of metformin if coadministered with ranolazine 1000mg bid and monitor blood glucose levels and risks associated with high metformin exposure.

PREGNANCY: Category C, not for use in nursing.

MECHANISM OF ACTION: Antianginal; has not been established. Can inhibit the cardiac late Na$^+$ current.

PHARMACOKINETICS: Absorption: Highly variable. C_{max}=2600ng/mL (1000mg bid), T_{max}=2-5 hrs. **Distribution:** Plasma protein binding (62%). **Metabolism:** Intestine and liver (rapid and extensive) by CYP3A (major) and CYP2D6 (minor). **Elimination:** (Sol) Urine (75%), feces (25%); urine and feces (<5% unchanged); $T_{1/2}$=7 hrs, 6-22 hrs (metabolites).

NURSING CONSIDERATIONS

Assessment: Assess for liver cirrhosis, QT interval prolongation, renal impairment, pregnancy/nursing status, and possible drug interactions.

R

Monitoring: Monitor for ECG changes (eg, QT interval prolongation) and other adverse reactions. Monitor renal function (eg, SrCr, BUN) after initiation and periodically in patients with moderate to severe renal impairment.

Patient Counseling: Inform that drug will not abate an acute angina episode. Advise to inform physician of any other concurrent medications, including OTC drugs, and of any history of QTc prolongation, congenital long QT syndrome, or renal impairment. Inform about the risk of renal failure in patients with severe renal impairment. Instruct to limit grapefruit juice/products. Instruct to contact physician if fainting spells occur. Advise that therapy may cause dizziness and lightheadedness; instruct patients to know how they react to the drug before engaging in activities requiring mental alertness or coordination (eg, operating machinery, driving).

Administration: Oral route. Take with or without meals. Swallow tab whole; do not crush, break, or chew. **Storage:** 25°C (77°F); excursions permitted to 15-30°C (59-86°F).

RANITIDINE

RX

ranitidine HCl (Various)

OTHER BRAND NAMES: Zantac Oral (GlaxoSmithKline) - Zantac Injection (Covis)

THERAPEUTIC CLASS: H_2-blocker

INDICATIONS: (PO) Short-term treatment of active duodenal ulcer (DU) and benign gastric ulcer (GU). Maintenance therapy for DU and GU. Treatment of pathological hypersecretory conditions (eg, Zollinger-Ellison syndrome and systemic mastocytosis) and gastroesophageal reflux disease (GERD). Treatment and maintenance of healing of erosive esophagitis (EE). (Inj) For hospitalized patients with pathological hypersecretory conditions or intractable DU. As an alternative to oral therapy for short-term use in patients who are unable to take oral medication.

DOSAGE: *Adults:* (PO) Active DU: Usual: 150mg bid or 300mg qd after pm meal or at hs. Maint: 150mg at hs. Pathological Hypersecretory Conditions: 150mg bid. Adjust dose according to patient needs and continue as long as clinically indicated. Doses up to 6g/day have been employed with severe disease. Benign GU: Usual: 150mg bid. Maint: 150mg at hs. GERD: 150mg bid. EE: Usual: 150mg qid. Maint: 150mg bid. (Inj) Usual: 50mg IV/IM q6-8h or 6.25mg/hr continuous IV infusion. Intermittent IV Bolus: Inject at a rate ≤4mL/min (5 min). Intermittent IV Infusion: Infuse at a rate ≤5-7mL/min (15-20 min). Max: 400mg/day. Zollinger-Ellison Syndrome: Initial: 1mg/kg/hr. Titrate: May increase after 4 hrs by 0.5mg/kg/hr increments if gastric acid output is >10 mEq/hr or patient becomes symptomatic. Max: 2.5mg/kg/hr dose and 220mg/hr infusion rate. (PO/Inj) Renal Impairment: CrCl <50mL/min: 150mg PO q24h or 50mg IV/IM q18-24h. May increase dosing frequency to q12h or even further, with caution. Hemodialysis: Give dose at the end of treatment.
Pediatrics: 1 Month-16 Yrs: (PO) DU/GU: Usual: 2-4mg/kg bid. Max: 300mg/day. Maint of DU/GU: 2-4mg/kg qd. Max: 150mg/day. GERD/EE: 5-10mg/kg/day given as 2 divided doses. (Inj) DU: 2-4mg/kg/day IV given q6-8h. Max: 50mg IV q6-8h. (PO/Inj) Renal Impairment: CrCl <50mL/min: 150mg PO q24h or 50mg IV/IM q18-24h. May increase dosing frequency to q12h or even further, with caution. <1 Month: Neonatal Patients on Extracorporeal Membrane Oxygenation: 2mg/kg IV q12-24h or as continuous infusion.

HOW SUPPLIED: Cap: 150mg, 300mg; (Zantac) Inj: 25mg/mL [2mL, 6mL]; Syrup: 15mg/mL [16 fl. oz.]; Tab: 150mg, 300mg

WARNINGS/PRECAUTIONS: Symptomatic response does not preclude the presence of gastric malignancy. Caution with hepatic/renal dysfunction. May precipitate acute porphyric attacks in patients with acute porphyria; avoid with history of acute porphyria. False (+) tests for urine protein with Multistix may occur. Caution in elderly. D/C immediately if hepatocellular, cholestatic, or mixed hepatitis occurs. (Inj) Do not exceed recommended infusion rates; bradycardia reported with rapid infusion. ALT elevations reported; monitor if on IV therapy for ≥5 days at doses ≥100mg qid.

ADVERSE REACTIONS: Headache, constipation, diarrhea, N/V, abdominal discomfort/pain, rash.

INTERACTIONS: Procainamide plasma levels increased with high doses; monitor for procainamide toxicity on PO doses >300mg/day. Altered PT with warfarin; monitor PT closely. May impair absorption of atazanavir and delavirdine. Use with caution with atazanavir. Chronic use with delavirdine is not recommended. May increase exposure of triazolam, midazolam, and glipizide; monitor for excessive/prolonged sedation with oral midazolam and triazolam. May decrease exposure of ketoconazole and gefitinib.

PREGNANCY: Category B, caution in nursing.

MECHANISM OF ACTION: H_2-blocker; competitive, reversible inhibitor of histamine at histamine H_2-receptors, including receptors found on gastric cells.

PHARMACOKINETICS: Absorption: (PO, 150mg) Absolute bioavailability (50%); C_{max}=440-545ng/mL, T_{max}=2-3 hrs. (IM, 50mg) Rapid. Absolute bioavailability (90-100%); C_{max}=576ng/mL, T_{max}=≤15 min. Refer to PI for pediatric parameters. **Distribution:** V_d=1.4L/kg; serum protein binding (15%); found in breast milk. **Metabolism:** Liver, N-oxide (principal metabolite). **Elimination:** Feces, urine ([PO] 30% unchanged, [IV] 70% unchanged); $T_{1/2}$=(PO) 2.5-3 hrs, (IV) 2-2.5 hrs.

NURSING CONSIDERATIONS

Assessment: Assess for hypersensitivity to the drug, renal/hepatic function, history of acute porphyria, pregnancy/nursing status, and possible drug interactions.

Monitoring: Monitor for signs/symptoms of hepatic effects (eg, hepatitis, elevations in ALT values), hypersensitivity reactions, and other adverse reactions. Monitor PT in patients receiving warfarin.

Patient Counseling: Inform that antacids may be taken PRN for relief of pain. Instruct to notify physician if any adverse events develop.

Administration: Oral/IM/IV routes. **Storage:** Protect from light. Cap: 20-25°C (68-77°F) in a dry place. Tab: 15-30°C (59-86°F) in a dry place. Syrup: 4-25°C (39-77°F). Inj: 4-25°C (39-77°F); excursions permitted to 30°C (86°F). Stable for 48 hrs at room temperature when added or diluted with IV sol. Avoid excessive heat; brief exposure up to 40°C (104°F) does not adversely affect the product. Protect from freezing.

RAPAFLO   RX
silodosin (Watson)

THERAPEUTIC CLASS: Alpha$_1$-antagonist

INDICATIONS: Treatment of signs and symptoms of BPH.

DOSAGE: *Adults:* 8mg qd with a meal. Moderate Renal Impairment (CrCl 30-50mL/min): 4mg qd with a meal.

HOW SUPPLIED: Cap: 4mg, 8mg

CONTRAINDICATIONS: Severe renal impairment (CrCl <30mL/min), severe hepatic impairment (Child-Pugh score ≥10), and concomitant administration with strong CYP3A4 inhibitors (eg, ketoconazole, clarithromycin, itraconazole, ritonavir).

WARNINGS/PRECAUTIONS: Not for treatment of HTN. Postural hypotension and syncope may occur; may impair mental/physical abilities. Caution in patients with moderate renal impairment. Examine patients prior to therapy to rule out prostate cancer. Intraoperative floppy iris syndrome (IFIS) observed during cataract surgery in some patients on α$_1$-blockers or previously treated with α$_1$-blockers.

ADVERSE REACTIONS: Retrograde ejaculation, dizziness, diarrhea, orthostatic hypotension, headache, nasopharyngitis, nasal congestion.

INTERACTIONS: See Contraindications. Avoid with other α-blockers and strong P-glycoprotein (P-gp) inhibitors (eg, cyclosporine). Caution with antihypertensives. Coadministration with PDE-5 inhibitors may cause symptomatic hypotension; caution with use. Increased concentrations with P-gp inhibitors and moderate CYP3A4 inhibitors (eg, diltiazem, erythromycin, verapamil). UGT2B7 inhibitors (eg, probenecid, valproic acid, fluconazole) may potentially increase exposure.

PREGNANCY: Category B, safety not known in nursing.

MECHANISM OF ACTION: α$_1$-antagonist; blocks α$_1$-adrenoreceptors, causing smooth muscle relaxation in the bladder neck/base and prostate, resulting in improved urine flow and reduction in BPH symptoms.

PHARMACOKINETICS: Absorption: Absolute bioavailability (32%), C_{max}=61.6ng/mL, T_{max}=2.6 hrs, AUC_{ss}=373.4ng•hr/mL. **Distribution:** V_d=49.5L; plasma protein binding (97%). **Metabolism:** Glucuronidation, alcohol and aldehyde dehydrogenase, CYP3A4; KMD-3213G (main metabolite), KMD-3293 (2nd major metabolite). **Elimination:** Urine (33.5%), feces (54.9%); $T_{1/2}$=13.3 hrs.

NURSING CONSIDERATIONS

Assessment: Assess for drug hypersensitivity, renal/hepatic impairment, prostate cancer, and possible drug interactions.

Monitoring: Monitor for signs/symptoms of postural hypotension, syncope, IFIS during cataract surgery, and other adverse reactions.

Patient Counseling: Counsel about possible occurrence of symptoms related to postural hypotension (eg, dizziness); advise to use caution when driving, operating machinery, or performing hazardous tasks, particularly in patients with low BP or taking antihypertensives. Inform that most common side effect seen is an orgasm with reduced or no semen; inform that this side effect does not pose a safety concern and is reversible when drug is discontinued. Advise to notify ophthalmologist about the use of the drug before cataract surgery or other eye procedures, even if no longer taking silodosin.

R

Administration: Oral route. Take with a meal. Patients who have difficulty swallowing caps may sprinkle the cap powder on a tbsp of applesauce (should not be hot); swallow immediately (within 5 min) without chewing and follow with 8 oz. of cool water. Do not subdivide the contents of cap or store any powder/applesauce mixture for future use. **Storage:** 25°C (77°F); excursions permitted to 15-30°C (59-86°F). Protect from light and moisture.

RAPAMUNE RX
sirolimus (Wyeth)

> Increased susceptibility to infection and possible development of lymphoma and other malignancies may result from immunosuppression. Only physicians experienced in immunosuppressive therapy and management of renal transplant patients should use sirolimus. Use not recommended in liver or lung transplant patients. Excess mortality and graft loss in combination with tacrolimus reported in liver transplant patients. Increased hepatic artery thrombosis with cyclosporine or tacrolimus in liver transplant patients. Cases of bronchial anastomotic dehiscence, most fatal, reported in lung transplant patients.

THERAPEUTIC CLASS: Macrocyclic lactone immunosuppressant

INDICATIONS: Prophylaxis of organ rejection in patients ≥13 yrs of age receiving renal transplants.

DOSAGE: *Adults:* Give initial dose as soon as possible after transplantation. Give 4 hrs after cyclosporine. Maintain on a dose for at least 7-14 days before further dose adjustment. Refer to full PI for maintenance dose adjustments. Max: 40mg/day. If estimated dose is >40mg/day due to addition of LD, LD should be administered over 2 days. Monitor trough concentration at least 3-4 days after LD(s). Low-Moderate Immunologic Risk: Initial: Give with cyclosporine and corticosteroids. Give LD equivalent to 3X the maint dose. Progressively d/c cyclosporine over 4-8 weeks at 2-4 months following transplantation. Adjust dose to maintain blood trough concentration within target range. High-Immunologic Risk: Give with cyclosporine and corticosteroids for the first 12 months. LD: Up to 15mg on Day 1 post-transplantation. Maint: 5mg/day beginning on Day 2. Obtain trough level between Days 5 and 7 and adjust daily dose thereafter. Mild or Moderate Hepatic Impairment: Reduce maintenance dose by 1/3. Severe Hepatic Impairment: Reduce maintenance by 1/2. Low Body Weight (<40kg): Adjust initial dose based on BSA to 1mg/m²/day with a LD of 3mg/m². Elderly: Start at lower end of dosing range.
Pediatrics: ≥13 Yrs: Give initial dose as soon as possible after transplantation. Give 4 hrs after cyclosporine. Maintain on a dose for at least 7-14 days before further dose adjustment. Refer to full PI for maintenance dose adjustments. Max: 40mg/day. If estimated dose is >40mg/day due to addition of LD, LD should be administered over 2 days. Monitor trough concentration at least 3-4 days after LD(s). Low-Moderate Immunologic Risk: Initial: Give with cyclosporine and corticosteroids. Give LD equivalent to 3X the maint dose. Progressively d/c cyclosporine over 4-8 weeks at 2-4 months following transplantation. Adjust dose to maintain blood trough concentration within target range. Mild or Moderate Hepatic Impairment: Reduce maintenance dose by 1/3. Severe Hepatic Impairment: Reduce maintenance by 1/2. Low Body Weight (<40kg): Adjust initial dose based on BSA to 1mg/m²/day with a LD of 3mg/m².

HOW SUPPLIED: Sol: 1mg/mL [60mL]; Tab: 0.5mg, 1mg, 2mg

WARNINGS/PRECAUTIONS: Safety and efficacy of use in combination with cyclosporine and corticosteroids has not been studied beyond one year. Hypersensitivity reactions reported. Associated with the development of angioedema. Impaired wound healing, lymphocele, wound dehiscence, and fluid accumulation (eg, peripheral edema, lymphedema, pleural effusion, ascites, pericardial effusions) reported. May increase serum cholesterol and TG that may require treatment. May delay recovery of renal function in patients with delayed graft function. Proteinuria commonly observed. Increased risk for opportunistic infections, including activation of latent viral infections (eg, BK virus-associated nephropathy). Progressive multifocal leukoencephalopathy (PML) reported. Consider reduction in immunosuppression if BK virus nephropathy is suspected or if PML develops. Interstitial lung disease (eg, pneumonitis, bronchiolitis obliterans organizing pneumonia, pulmonary fibrosis) reported. Safety and efficacy of de novo use without cyclosporine is not established in renal transplant patients. Provide 1 yr prophylaxis for *Pneumocystis carinii* pneumonia and 3 months for cytomegalovirus after transplant. Patient sample concentration values from different assays may not be interchangeable. Increased risk of skin cancer; limit exposure to sunlight and UV light. Caution in elderly.

ADVERSE REACTIONS: Infection, lymphoma, malignancy, graft loss, peripheral edema, hypertriglyceridemia, HTN, constipation, hypercholesterolemia, increased creatinine, abdominal pain, diarrhea, headache.

INTERACTIONS: See Boxed Warning. CYP3A4 and P-glycoprotein (P-gp) inducers may decrease concentrations. CYP3A4 and P-gp inhibitors may increase concentrations. Avoid with strong inhibitors (eg, ketoconazole, erythromycin, clarithromycin) and strong inducers (eg, rifampin, rifabutin) of CYP3A4 and P-gp. May increase levels with cyclosporine, bromocriptine, cimetidine, cisapride, clotrimazole, danazol, diltiazem, fluconazole, protease inhibitors, metoclopramide, nicardipine, troleandomycin, and verapamil. May decrease levels with carbamazepine, phenobarbital, phenytoin, rifapentine, and St. John's wort. May increase verapamil concentration. Vaccines may be less effective; avoid live vaccines. Increases risk of angioedema with ACE inhibitors. Increased risk of calcineurin inhibitor-induced hemolytic uremic syndrome/thrombotic thrombocytopenic purpura/thrombotic microangiography with calcineurin inhibitor. Do not dilute or take with grapefruit juice. Caution with other nephrotoxic drugs (eg, aminoglycosides, amphotericin B). Monitor for possible development of rhabdomyolysis with HMG-CoA inhibitors and/or fibrates.

PREGNANCY: Category C, not for use in nursing.

MECHANISM OF ACTION: Immunosuppressant; inhibits T-lymphocyte activation and proliferation that occurs in response to antigenic and cytokine (interleukin [IL]-2, IL-4, and IL-15) stimulation by a mechanism distinct from that of other immunosuppressants. Also inhibits antibody production.

PHARMACOKINETICS: Absorption: (Sol) AUC=194ng•hr/mL, C_{max}=14.4ng/mL, T_{max}=2.1 hrs. (Tab) AUC=230ng•hr/mL, C_{max}=15ng/mL, T_{max}=3.5 hrs. Different pharmacokinetic data resulted from concentration-controlled trials of pediatric renal transplants. **Distribution:** V_d=12L/kg; plasma protein binding (92%). **Metabolism:** Intestinal wall and liver (extensive) via O-demethylation and/or hydroxylation; hydroxy, demethyl, and hydroxydemethyl (major metabolites). **Elimination:** Feces (91%), urine (2.2%); $T_{1/2}$=62 hrs.

NURSING CONSIDERATIONS

Assessment: Assess for drug hypersensitivity, immunologic risk, hepatic impairment, body weight/BMI, hyperlipidemia, infections, pregnancy/nursing status, and possible drug interactions.

Monitoring: Monitor for infections including opportunistic infections and activation of latent infections, development of PML, lymphoma/lymphoproliferative disease, other malignancies (particularly of the skin), signs and symptoms of graft loss, hypersensitivity reactions, interstitial lung disease, and hyperlipidemia. Monitor trough concentrations, especially in patients with altered drug metabolism, who weigh <40kg, and with hepatic impairment, and when a change is made during concurrent administration of strong CYP3A4 inducers or inhibitors. Monitor urinary protein excretion, renal/hepatic functions, cholesterol, TG, and BP.

Patient Counseling: Instruct patients to limit sunlight and UV light exposure by wearing protective clothing and using a sunscreen with a high protection. Inform patients about the potential risks during pregnancy and instruct to use effective contraception prior to, during therapy, and 12 weeks after therapy has been stopped.

Administration: Oral route. Give consistently with or without food. (Tab) Do not crush, chew, or split. (Sol) Refer to PI for proper dilution and administration. **Storage:** (Sol) 2-8°C (36-46°F), should be used within 1 month once opened. May store up to 25°C (77°F) for a short period (eg, not >15 days). (Tab) 20-25°C (68-77°F). Protect from light.

RAZADYNE ER

galantamine HBr (Janssen)

RX **R**

OTHER BRAND NAMES: Razadyne (Janssen)

THERAPEUTIC CLASS: Acetylcholinesterase inhibitor

INDICATIONS: Treatment of mild to moderate dementia of the Alzheimer's type.

DOSAGE: *Adults:* Usual: 16-24mg/day. Max: 24mg/day. Moderate Renal/Hepatic Impairment (Child-Pugh 7-9): Max: 16mg/day. (Sol, Tab) Initial: 4mg bid (8mg/day) with am and pm meals. Titrate: Increase to initial maint dose of 8mg bid (16mg/day) after a minimum of 4 weeks, then increase to 12mg bid (24mg/day) after a minimum of 4 weeks, if tolerated. Restart at the lowest dose and increase to current dose if therapy is interrupted for several days or longer. (Cap, Extended-Release [ER]) Initial: 8mg qd with am meal. Titrate: Increase to initial maint dose of 16mg qd after a minimum of 4 weeks, then increase to 24mg qd after a minimum of 4 weeks, if tolerated. Converting from Immediate-Release (IR) Tab: Take the last dose of IR tab in pm and start ER cap qd the next am. Converting from IR to ER should occur at the same total daily dose.

HOW SUPPLIED: Cap, ER: 8mg, 16mg, 24mg; Sol: 4mg/mL [100mL]; Tab: 4mg, 8mg, 12mg

WARNINGS/PRECAUTIONS: May lead to bradycardia and atrioventricular (AV) block due to vagotonic effects on sinoatrial and AV nodes; caution with supraventricular cardiac conduction disorders. Increased gastric acid secretion; monitor closely for symptoms of active/occult GI bleeding, especially in those with an increased risk for developing ulcers. May produce N/V, diarrhea, anorexia, and weight loss. May cause bladder outflow obstruction and generalized convulsions. Caution in patients with history of severe asthma or obstructive pulmonary disease. Deaths reported with mild cognitive impairment. Caution during dose titration in patients with moderate renal/hepatic impairment. Not recommended for severe hepatic/renal impairment.

ADVERSE REACTIONS: N/V, dizziness, anorexia, diarrhea, headache, urinary tract infection, weight decrease, depression, abdominal pain, dyspepsia, insomnia, fatigue, somnolence.

INTERACTIONS: Potential to interfere with anticholinergics. Synergistic effect with succinyl-choline, other cholinesterase inhibitors, similar neuromuscular blockers, or cholinergic agonists (eg, bethanechol). Increased levels with cimetidine, ketoconazole, erythromycin, and paroxetine. Caution with drugs that slow HR due to vagotonic effects. Monitor closely for symptoms of active/occult GI bleeding with concurrent NSAIDs.

PREGNANCY: Category B, not for use in nursing.

MECHANISM OF ACTION: Acetylcholinesterase inhibitor; not established. Exerts therapeutic effect by enhancing cholinergic function; increases concentration of acetylcholine through reversible inhibition of its hydrolysis by cholinesterase.

PHARMACOKINETICS: Absorption: Rapid and complete; absolute bioavailability (90%), T_{max} =1 hr. **Distribution:** V_d=175L; plasma protein binding (18%). **Metabolism:** CYP450 (2D6, 3A4); glucuronidation. **Elimination:** Urine (unchanged); $T_{1/2}$=7 hrs.

NURSING CONSIDERATIONS

Assessment: Assess for cardiovascular conditions, history of ulcer disease, severe asthma or obstructive pulmonary diseases, mild cognitive impairment, renal/hepatic function, pregnancy/nursing status, and possible drug interactions.

Monitoring: Monitor closely for symptoms of active or occult GI bleeding, cardiac conduction abnormalities, bladder outflow obstruction, convulsions, and other adverse reactions.

Patient Counseling: Instruct to take ud; advise that the most frequent adverse events associated with the use of the drug can be minimized by following the recommended dosage and administration. Advise to take the tab/sol preferably with am and pm meals; ER cap should be taken qam with food. Advise to ensure adequate fluid intake during treatment. Inform caregivers about the Instruction Sheet describing how the sol should be given; urge to read prior to administering the oral sol.

Administration: Oral route. **Storage:** 25°C (77°F); excursions permitted to 15-30°C (59-86°F). (Sol) Do not freeze.

REBETOL   RX
ribavirin (Merck)

Not for monotherapy treatment of chronic hepatitis C (CHC) virus infection. Primary toxicity is hemolytic anemia. Anemia associated with therapy may result in worsening of cardiac disease and lead to fatal and nonfatal myocardial infarctions. Avoid with history of significant/unstable cardiac disease. Contraindicated in women who are pregnant and in male partners of pregnant women. Extreme care must be taken to avoid pregnancy during therapy and for 6 months after completion of therapy. Use at least 2 reliable forms of effective contraception during treatment and for 6 months after discontinuation.

THERAPEUTIC CLASS: Nucleoside analogue

INDICATIONS: In combination with interferon alfa-2b (pegylated and nonpegylated) for treatment of CHC in patients ≥3 yrs of age with compensated liver disease.

DOSAGE: *Adults:* Take with food. Combination Therapy with PegIntron: 800-1400mg/day PO based on body weight (Refer to PI). Treat with PegIntron 1.5mcg/kg/week SQ. Interferon Alfa-Naive: Genotype 1: Treat for 48 weeks. Genotype 2 and 3: Treat for 24 weeks. Retreatment: Treat for 48 weeks, regardless of hepatitis C virus (HCV) genotype. Combination Therapy with Intron A: >75kg: 600mg qam and 600mg qpm. ≤75kg: 400mg qam and 600mg qpm. Treat with Intron A 3 million IU 3X weekly SQ. Interferon Alfa-Naive: Treat for 24-48 weeks. Individualize duration of treatment depending on baseline disease characteristics, response to therapy, and tolerability of regimen. Retreatment: Treat for 24 weeks. Elderly: Start at lower end of dosing range. Refer to PI for dose modifications and discontinuation.
Pediatrics: ≥3 Yrs: Take with food. Combination Therapy with PegIntron/Intron A: >73kg: 600mg qam and 600mg qpm. 60-73kg: 400mg qam and 600mg qpm. 47-59kg: 400mg qam and 400mg qpm. <47kg: (Sol) 15mg/kg/day divided into two doses. May use solution regardless of body weight. Treat with Intron A 3 million IU/m² 3X weekly SQ for 25-61kg (refer to adult dosing for >61kg) or PegIntron 60mcg/m²/week SQ. Genotype 1: Treat for 48 weeks. Genotype 2 or 3: Treat for 24 weeks. Remain on pediatric dosing while receiving therapy in combination with PegIntron when 18th birthday is reached. Refer to PI for dose modifications and discontinuation.

HOW SUPPLIED: Cap: 200mg; Sol: 40mg/mL [100mL]

CONTRAINDICATIONS: Women who are or may become pregnant, men whose female partners are pregnant, autoimmune hepatitis, hemoglobinopathies (eg, thalassemia major, sickle cell anemia), CrCl <50mL/min, coadministration with didanosine.

WARNINGS/PRECAUTIONS: Do not start therapy unless a negative pregnancy test has been obtained immediately prior to therapy. Suspend therapy in patients with signs and symptoms of pancreatitis; d/c therapy with confirmed pancreatitis. Pulmonary symptoms (eg, dyspnea, pulmonary infiltrates, pneumonitis, pulmonary HTN, pneumonia, sarcoidosis or exacerbation of sarcoidosis) reported; closely monitor and, if appropriate, d/c if pulmonary infiltrates or pulmonary function impairment develops. Alfa interferons may induce or aggravate ophthalmologic disorders (eg, decrease or loss of vision, retinopathy); perform eye exam in all patients prior to therapy, periodically with preexisting ophthalmologic disorders (eg, diabetic or hypertensive retinopathy), and if ocular symptoms develop during therapy. D/C if new or worsening ophthalmologic disorders develop. Severe decreases in neutrophil and platelet counts, and hematologic, endocrine (eg, TSH), and hepatic abnormalities may occur in combination with PegIntron; perform hematology and blood chemistry testing prior to therapy and periodically thereafter. Dental/periodontal disorders reported. Weight changes and growth inhibition (including long-term growth inhibition) reported in pediatric patients. Associated with significant adverse reactions (eg, severe depression and suicidal ideation, suppression of bone marrow function, autoimmune and infectious disorders, diabetes). Caution with preexisting cardiac disease; d/c if cardiovascular (CV) status deteriorates. Caution in the elderly. (Cap) Not for treatment of HIV infection, adenovirus, respiratory syncytial virus, parainfluenza, or influenza infections.

ADVERSE REACTIONS: Hemolytic anemia, inj-site reactions, headache, fatigue, rigors, fever, N/V, anorexia, myalgia, arthralgia, insomnia, irritability, depression, neutropenia, alopecia.

INTERACTIONS: See Contraindications. Closely monitor for toxicities, especially hepatic decompensation and anemia, with nucleoside reverse transcriptase inhibitors (NRTIs); consider dose reduction or discontinuation of interferon, ribavirin, or both, or discontinuation of NRTI if worsening clinical toxicities occur. May inhibit phosphorylation of lamivudine, stavudine, and zidovudine. Severe pancytopenia, bone marrow suppression, and myelotoxicity reported with azathioprine.

PREGNANCY: Category X, not for use in nursing.

MECHANISM OF ACTION: Nucleoside analogue; has not been established. Has direct antiviral activity in tissue culture against many RNA viruses; increases mutation frequency in the genomes of several viruses and ribavirin triphosphate inhibits HCV polymerase in a biochemical reaction.

PHARMACOKINETICS: Absorption: Rapid and extensive. (Cap) (Adults) Single-Dose: C_{max}=782ng/mL, T_{max}=1.7 hrs, AUC=13,400ng•hr/mL, absolute bioavailability (64%). Multiple-Dose: C_{max}=3680ng/mL, T_{max}=3 hrs, AUC=228,000ng•hr/mL. (Pediatrics) Multiple-Dose: C_{max}=3275ng/mL, T_{max}=1.9 hrs, AUC=29,774ng•hr/mL. (Adults) (Sol) Single-Dose: C_{max}=872ng/mL, T_{max}=1 hr, AUC=14,098ng•hr/mL. **Distribution:** (Adults) (Cap) Single-Dose: V_{d}=2825L. **Metabolism:** Nucleated cells (phosphorylation); deribosylation and amide hydrolysis. **Elimination:** Urine (61%), feces (12%). (Adults) (Cap) Single-Dose: $T_{1/2}$=43.6 hrs. Multiple Dose: $T_{1/2}$=298 hrs.

NURSING CONSIDERATIONS

Assessment: Assess for autoimmune hepatitis, hemoglobinopathies, depression, preexisting ophthalmologic disorders, history of or preexisting cardiac disease, hypersensitivity, and possible drug interactions. Assess nursing status and hepatic/renal/pulmonary function. Conduct pregnancy test (including female partners of male patients), standard hematologic tests, blood chemistries, ECG in patients with preexisting cardiac disease, and eye examination.

Monitoring: Monitor for anemia, worsening of cardiac disease, pancreatitis, renal/hepatic dysfunction, CV deterioration, pulmonary function impairment, new/worsening ophthalmologic disorders, and other adverse reactions. Monitor height and weight in pediatric patients. Perform standard hematologic tests, blood chemistries (eg, TSH), ECG, and HCV-RNA periodically. Obtain Hct and Hgb (Week 2 and 4 of therapy, and as clinically appropriate). Perform pregnancy test monthly during therapy and for 6 months after discontinuation of therapy (including female partners of male patients). Schedule regular dental exams.

Patient Counseling: Counsel on risk/benefits associated with treatment. Inform that anemia may develop. Advise that lab evaluations are required prior to starting therapy and periodically thereafter. Advise to be well-hydrated, especially during the initial stages of treatment. Inform of pregnancy risks. Instruct to use at least 2 forms of contraception and perform a monthly pregnancy test during therapy and for 6 months post-therapy (including female partners of male patients); advise to notify physician in the event of a pregnancy. Inform that appropriate precautions to prevent HCV transmission should be taken. Instruct to take missed doses as soon as possible during the same day and not to double next dose. Instruct to brush teeth bid and have regular dental exams; if vomiting occurs, advise to rinse out mouth afterwards.

Administration: Oral route. Take with food. (Cap) Do not open, crush, or break. **Storage:** (Cap) 25°C (77°F); excursions permitted to 15-30°C (59-86°F). (Sol) 2-8°C (36-46°F) or at 25°C (77°F); excursions permitted to 15-30°C (59-86°F).

REBIF   RX
interferon beta-1a (EMD Serono)

THERAPEUTIC CLASS: Biological response modifier

INDICATIONS: Treatment of patients with relapsing forms of multiple sclerosis to decrease the frequency of clinical exacerbations and delay the accumulation of physical disability.

DOSAGE: *Adults:* Initial: 20% of prescribed dose 3X/week. Titrate: Increase over a 4-week period. Target: 22mcg or 44mcg SQ 3X/week. Administer at the same time (preferably late afternoon or pm) on the same 3 days at least 48 hrs apart each week. Refer to PI for full titration schedule. Leukopenia/Elevated LFTs: May need to reduce dose or d/c administration until toxicity is resolved. Concurrent use of analgesics and/or antipyretics may help ameliorate flu-like symptoms on treatment days. Elderly: Start at lower end of dosing range.

HOW SUPPLIED: Inj: 22mcg/0.5mL, 44mcg/0.5mL [prefilled syringe, Rebidose autoinjector]; (Titration Pack) 8.8mcg/0.2mL, 22mcg/0.5mL [prefilled syringe, Rebidose autoinjector]

CONTRAINDICATIONS: History of hypersensitivity to human albumin.

WARNINGS/PRECAUTIONS: Depression, suicidal ideation, and suicide attempts reported; consider cessation of treatment if depression develops. Severe liver injury reported rarely; d/c immediately if jaundice or other symptoms of liver dysfunction appear. Asymptomatic elevation of hepatic transaminases (particularly ALT) may occur; caution with active liver disease, alcohol abuse, increased serum ALT (>2.5X ULN), or history of significant liver disease. Consider dose reduction if ALT rises >5X ULN; may gradually re-escalate dose when enzyme levels have normalized. Anaphylaxis (rare) and other allergic reactions (eg, skin rash, urticaria) reported. Contains albumin; carries an extremely remote risk for transmission of viral diseases or Creutzfeldt-Jakob disease. Seizures, leukopenia, and new or worsening thyroid abnormalities reported; regularly monitor for these conditions. Caution with preexisting seizure disorders and in elderly.

ADVERSE REACTIONS: Inj-site disorders, headache, fatigue, fever, rigors, chest pain, back pain, myalgia, abdominal pain, depression, elevation of liver enzymes, hematologic abnormalities.

INTERACTIONS: Due to the risk of neutropenia and lymphopenia, monitor with myelosuppressive agents. Consider the potential for hepatic injury when used in combination with other hepatotoxic products, or when new agents are added to the regimen.

PREGNANCY: Category C, caution in nursing.

MECHANISM OF ACTION: Biological response modifier; not established. Binding of interferon β to its receptors initiates a complex cascade of intracellular events that leads to the expression of numerous interferon-induced gene products and markers, including 2', 5'-oligoadenylate synthetase, β_2-microglobulin and neopterin, which may mediate some of the biological activities.

PHARMACOKINETICS: Absorption: C_{max}=5.1 IU/mL, T_{max}=16 hrs (median), AUC_{0-96}=294 IU•hr/mL. **Elimination:** $T_{1/2}$=69 hrs.

NURSING CONSIDERATIONS

Assessment: Assess for depression, history of or active liver disease, alcohol abuse, preexisting seizure disorder, thyroid dysfunction, myelosuppression, history of hypersensitivity to drug or to human albumin, pregnancy/nursing status, and possible drug interactions.

Monitoring: Monitor for depression, suicidal ideation, jaundice, allergic reactions, seizures, and other adverse reactions. Perform CBC and LFTs at regular intervals (1, 3, and 6 months) following initiation and then periodically thereafter in the absence of clinical symptoms; patients with myelosuppression may require more intensive monitoring of CBC, with differential and platelet counts. Perform thyroid function tests every 6 months in patients with a history of thyroid dysfunction, or as clinically indicated.

Patient Counseling: Instruct not to change the dose or the schedule of administration without consulting physician. Inform of the most common and the most severe adverse reactions associated with therapy; advise of the symptoms associated with these conditions and to report them to physician. Caution female patients about the abortifacient potential of the drug. Advise on how to properly administer the drug. Instruct in the use of aseptic technique when self-administering the drug and on the importance of rotating inj sites. Explain the importance of proper disposal of prefilled syringes and autoinjectors, and caution against reuse of these items.

Administration: SQ route. **Storage:** 2-8°C (36-46°F). Do not freeze. If refrigerator is not available, may store at 2-25°C (36-77°F) for up to 30 days and away from heat and light.

RECLAST   RX
zoledronic acid (Novartis)

THERAPEUTIC CLASS: Bisphosphonate

INDICATIONS: Treatment and prevention of osteoporosis in postmenopausal women, and glucocorticoid-induced osteoporosis in men and women who are either initiating or continuing systemic glucocorticoids in a daily dosage equivalent to 7.5mg or greater of prednisone and who are expected to remain on glucocorticoids for at least 12 months. Treatment to increase bone mass in men with osteoporosis and of Paget's disease of bone in men and women.

DOSAGE: *Adults:* Infuse IV over no less than 15 min at a constant rate. Treatment of Osteoporosis and Treatment/Prevention of Glucocorticoid-Induced Osteoporosis: 5mg once a yr. Prevention of Osteoporosis: 5mg once every 2 yrs. Paget's Disease: 5mg. May consider retreatment in patients who have relapsed (based on increases in serum alkaline phosphatase), who failed to achieve normalization of serum alkaline phosphatase, or with symptoms. Recommended Intake of Ca^{2+} in Osteoporosis: At least 1200mg/day. Recommended Intake of Vitamin D in Osteoporosis: 800-1000 IU/day. Recommended Intake of Ca^{2+} in Paget's Disease: 1500mg/day in divided doses (750mg bid or 500mg tid), particularly in the 2 weeks following administration. Recommended Intake of Vitamin D in Paget's Disease: 800 IU/day, particularly in the 2 weeks following administration. May give acetaminophen following administration to reduce incidence of acute-phase reaction symptoms. Reevaluate the need for continued therapy on a periodic basis.

HOW SUPPLIED: Inj: 5mg/100mL [bottle]

CONTRAINDICATIONS: Hypocalcemia, CrCl <35mL/min, acute renal impairment.

WARNINGS/PRECAUTIONS: Consider discontinuation after 3-5 yrs of use in patients at low-risk for fracture; periodically reevaluate risk for fracture in patients who d/c therapy. Hydrate prior to administration. Contains same active ingredient as Zometa; do not treat with Reclast if on concomitant therapy with Zometa. Treat preexisting hypocalcemia and disturbances of mineral metabolism prior to treatment; clinical monitoring of Ca^{2+} and mineral levels is highly recommended for these patients. Risk of hypocalcemia in Paget's disease. Withhold therapy until normovolemic status has been achieved if history or physical signs suggest dehydration. Caution with chronic renal impairment. Acute renal impairment, including renal failure, reported, especially in patients with preexisting renal compromise, advanced age, concomitant nephrotoxic medications or diuretic therapy, or severe dehydration. Obtain SrCr and calculate CrCl based on actual body weight before each dose. Assess fluid status in patients at increased risk of acute renal failure. Osteonecrosis of the jaw (ONJ) reported; perform routine oral exam prior to treatment. Avoid invasive dental procedures while on treatment in patients with concomitant risk factors (eg, cancer, chemotherapy, radiotherapy, corticosteroids, poor oral hygiene, preexisting dental disease or infection, anemia, coagulopathy) if possible. Atypical, low-energy, or low-trauma fractures of the femoral shaft reported; evaluate any patient with a history of bisphosphonate exposure who presents with thigh/groin pain to rule out an incomplete femur fracture, and consider interruption of therapy. Avoid pregnancy; may cause fetal harm. Severe and occasionally incapacitating bone, joint, and/or muscle pain reported; consider withholding future treatment if severe symptoms develop. Caution with aspirin (ASA) sensitivity; bronchoconstriction reported.

ADVERSE REACTIONS: Pain, chills, dizziness, osteoarthritis, fatigue, dyspnea, headache, HTN, influenza-like illness, myalgia, arthralgia, pyrexia, N/V, acute phase reaction.

INTERACTIONS: Caution with aminoglycosides; may have an additive effect to lower serum Ca^{2+} levels for prolonged periods. Caution with loop diuretics; may increase risk of hypocalcemia. Caution with other potentially nephrotoxic drugs (eg, NSAIDs). Renal impairment reported; in patients with renal impairment, exposure to concomitant medications that are primarily renally excreted (eg, digoxin) may increase.

PREGNANCY: Category D, not for use in nursing.

MECHANISM OF ACTION: Bisphosphonate; acts primarily on bone. Inhibits osteoclast-mediated bone resorption.

PHARMACOKINETICS: Distribution: Plasma protein binding (28% at 200ng/mL, 53% at 50ng/mL). **Elimination:** Urine (39%); $T_{1/2}$=146 hrs.

NURSING CONSIDERATIONS

Assessment: Assess for hypocalcemia, disturbances of mineral metabolism, risk factors for developing renal impairment and ONJ, ASA sensitivity, previous hypersensitivity to the drug, pregnancy/nursing status, and possible drug interactions. Obtain SrCr and calculate CrCl based on actual body weight before each dose. Assess fluid status in patients at increased risk of acute renal failure. Perform routine oral exam, and consider appropriate preventive dentistry in patients with a history of risk factors for ONJ.

Monitoring: Monitor for ONJ, atypical femur fracture, musculoskeletal pain, bronchoconstriction, and other adverse events. Monitor renal function and serum Ca^{2+}/mineral levels. Reevaluate the need for continued therapy on a periodic basis.

Patient Counseling: Inform about benefits/risks of therapy, and the importance of Ca^{2+} and vitamin D supplementation. Instruct to notify physician if patient has kidney problems, had surgery to remove some or all of parathyroid glands, had sections of intestine removed, takes any other medications, is unable to take Ca^{2+} supplements, is sensitive to ASA, is pregnant, planning to become pregnant, or breastfeeding. Advise to avoid becoming pregnant. Advise to eat and drink normally (at least 2 glasses of fluid, such as water, within a few hrs prior to infusion) on the day of treatment, before receiving the drug. Inform of the most commonly associated side effects of therapy and to consult physician if these symptoms persist. Instruct to inform physician or dentist if experiencing persistent pain and/or nonhealing sore of the mouth or jaw.

R

Administration: IV route. IV infusion should be followed by a 10mL normal saline flush of the IV line. Do not allow sol to come in contact with any Ca^{2+} or other divalent cation-containing sol. Administer as a single IV sol through a separate vented infusion line. **Storage:** 25°C (77°F); excursions permitted to 15-30°C (59-86°F). Stable for 24 hrs at 2-8°C (36-46°F) after opening. If refrigerated, allow to reach room temperature before administration.

RECOMBIVAX HB   RX
hepatitis B (recombinant) (Merck)

THERAPEUTIC CLASS: Vaccine

INDICATIONS: Vaccination against infection caused by all known subtypes of hepatitis B virus (HBV).

DOSAGE: *Adults:* ≥20 Yrs: Give IM into deltoid muscle. May be given SQ if at risk of hemorrhage. 3-Dose Regimen: 10mcg at 0, 1, 6 months. Predialysis/Dialysis (Dialysis Formulation): 40mcg at 0, 1, 6 months; consider booster/revaccination if anti-hepatitis B surface (HBs) level <10 mIU/mL 1-2 months after 3rd dose. Known/Presumed Exposure to Hepatitis B Surface Antigen (HBsAg): Follow 3-Dose Regimen giving 1st dose within 7 days of exposure. Give 0.06mL/kg IM hepatitis B immune globulin (HBIG) immediately after exposure and within 24 hrs if possible, at a separate site.
Pediatrics: Give IM into anterolateral thigh in infants/young children. May be given SQ if at risk of hemorrhage. 0-19 Yrs: 3-Dose Regimen (Pediatric/Adolescent Formulation): 5mcg at 0, 1, 6 months. 11-15 Yrs: 2-Dose Regimen (Adult Formulation): 10mcg at 0 and 4-6 months. Infants Born to HBsAg Positive/Unknown Status Mothers: Follow 3-Dose Regimen above. Give 0.5mL HBIG immediately in the opposite anterolateral thigh if the mother is determined to be HBsAg positive within 7 days of delivery. Known/Presumed Exposure to HBsAg: Follow 3-Dose Regimen giving 1st dose within 7 days of exposure. Give 0.06mL/kg IM HBIG immediately after exposure and within 24 hrs if possible, at a separate site.

HOW SUPPLIED: Inj: (Pediatric/Adolescent) 5mcg/0.5mL [vial, syringe]; (Adult) 10mcg/mL [vial, syringe]; (Dialysis) 40mcg/mL [vial]

CONTRAINDICATIONS: Hypersensitivity to yeast.

WARNINGS/PRECAUTIONS: Do not continue therapy if hypersensitivity occurs after inj. May not prevent hepatitis B with unrecognized infection at time of vaccination. Anaphylactoid reaction may occur; have epinephrine (1:1000) immediately available. Tip cap, vial stopper, and syringe plunger stopper contain dry natural latex rubber, which may cause allergic reactions in latex-sensitive individuals; use with caution. Delay vaccination with serious active infection (eg, febrile illness) unless withholding the vaccine entails a greater risk. Caution with severely compromised cardiopulmonary status or in whom a febrile or systemic reaction could pose a significant risk. Review vaccination history for previous vaccination-related adverse reactions.

ADVERSE REACTIONS: Irritability, fever, diarrhea, fatigue/weakness, diminished appetite, rhinitis, inj-site reactions.

PREGNANCY: Category C, caution in nursing.

MECHANISM OF ACTION: Vaccine; may produce immune response for protection against infection caused by all known subtypes of HBV.

NURSING CONSIDERATIONS

Assessment: Assess current health status, hypersensitivity to yeast or any component of the vaccine, and pregnancy/nursing status. Review vaccination history for possible vaccine sensitivity and previous vaccination-related adverse reactions.

Monitoring: Monitor for signs/symptoms of hypersensitivity reactions, inj-site reactions, immune response, and for systemic reactions. Perform annual antibody testing in hemodialysis patients to assess the need for booster doses.

Patient Counseling: Inform of potential benefits/risks of vaccination and the importance of completing the immunization series. Instruct to report inj-site reactions or any serious adverse reactions to physician.

Administration: IM route. Do not inject intradermally or IV. Avoid injection of a blood vessel. May be given SQ if at risk of hemorrhage following IM inj. Shake well before use. Should be used as supplied; no dilution or reconstitution is necessary. Refer to PI for further administration instructions. **Storage:** 2-8°C (36-46°F). Do not freeze.

REFLUDAN   RX
lepirudin (Bayer Healthcare)

THERAPEUTIC CLASS: Thrombin inhibitor

INDICATIONS: Anticoagulant for heparin-induced thrombocytopenia (HIT) and associated thromboembolic disease.

DOSAGE: *Adults:* LD: 0.4mg/kg (max 44mg) IV over 15-20 seconds. Initial: 0.15mg/kg/hr (max 16.5mg/hr) continuous infusion for 2-10 days. Adjust dose based on aPTT. If aPTT is above target range, stop infusion for 2 hrs and restart at 50% of previous rate. Check aPTT 4 hrs later. If aPTT is below target range, increase rate in steps of 20% and check aPTT 4 hrs later. Do not exceed 0.21mg/kg/hr. Renal Impairment: LD: 0.2mg/kg. Initial: CrCl 45-60mL/min: 0.075mg/kg/hr. CrCl 30-44mL/min: 0.045mg/kg/hr. CrCl 15-29 mL/min: 0.0225mg/kg/hr. CrCl <15mL/min: Hemodialysis: Avoid or stop infusion. Concomitant Thrombolytic Therapy: LD: 0.2mg/kg. Initial: 0.1mg/kg/hr.

HOW SUPPLIED: Inj: 50mg

WARNINGS/PRECAUTIONS: Risk of bleeding. Weigh risks/benefits with recent puncture of large vessels or organ biopsy, anomaly of vessels or organs, recent cerebrovascular accident (CVA), stroke, intracerebral surgery or other neuraxial procedures, severe uncontrolled HTN, bacterial endocarditis, advanced renal impairment, hemorrhagic diathesis, recent major surgery or bleeding. Avoid with baseline aPTT ratio of ≥2.5. Monitor aPTT 4 hrs after initiating infusion and at least qd. Liver injury may enhance anticoagulant effects. Antihirudin antibodies reported; may increase anticoagulant effects.

ADVERSE REACTIONS: Hemorrhagic events (eg, bleeding, anemia, hematoma, hematuria, epistaxis, hemothorax), fever, liver dysfunction, pneumonia, sepsis, allergic skin reactions, multiorgan failure.

INTERACTIONS: Thrombolytics increase risk of life-threatening intracranial bleeding or other bleeding complications and may enhance the effect on aPTT prolongation. Increased risk of bleeding with coumarin derivatives and other drugs that affect platelet function.

PREGNANCY: Category B, not for use in nursing.

MECHANISM OF ACTION: Thrombin inhibitor; binds to thrombin and thereby blocks its thrombogenic activity.

PHARMACOKINETICS: Absorption: C_{max}=1500ng/mL. **Distribution:** V_d=12.2L. **Metabolism:** Catabolic hydrolysis. **Elimination:** Urine (48%); $T_{1/2}$=1.3 hrs.

NURSING CONSIDERATIONS

Assessment: Assess for bleeding risk (eg, recent puncture of large vessels, recent cerebrovascular accident, severe uncontrolled HTN, bacterial endocarditis, hemorrhagic diathesis), presence of hepatic/renal dysfunction, nursing status, and drug interactions. Obtain baseline aPTT ratio.

Monitoring: Monitor for signs/symptoms of bleeding complications (eg, intracranial bleeding) and allergic reactions (eg, anaphylactic reactions). Monitor aPTT ratio 4 hrs after start of infusion and perform qd thereafter during treatment.

Patient Counseling: Instruct to notify physician immediately if any type of allergic reaction (eg, anaphylaxis) develops. Advise about increased risk of bleeding during therapy. Inform that laboratory monitoring is needed during therapy.

Administration: IV route. Do not mix with other drugs. Reconstitute: 1) Use Sterile Water for Inj, USP; or 0.9% for NaCl Inj, USP. 2) For rapid, complete reconstitution, inject 1mL of diluent into the vial and shake it gently. 3) Further dilute to final concentration of 5mg/mL. Dilute using 0.9% NaCl Inj USP, or 5% Dextrose Inj USP. 4) Warm to room temperature prior to administration. **Storage:** Unopened vials: 2-25°C (35.6-77°F). Reconstituted: Use immediately; will remain stable for 24 hrs at room temperature.

RELENZA   RX
zanamivir (GlaxoSmithKline)

THERAPEUTIC CLASS: Neuraminidase inhibitor

INDICATIONS: Treatment of uncomplicated acute illness due to influenza A and B virus in adults and pediatric patients ≥7 yrs of age who have been symptomatic for no more than 2 days. Prophylaxis of influenza in adults and pediatric patients ≥5 yrs of age.

DOSAGE: *Adults:* Treatment: 2 inh (10mg) q12h for 5 days. Take 2 doses on 1st day at least 2 hrs apart, then 12 hrs apart (eg, am and pm) at approximately the same time each day on subsequent days. Prophylaxis: Administer at same time each day. Household Setting: 2 inh (10mg) qd for 10 days. Community Outbreaks: 2 inh (10mg) qd for 28 days.
Pediatrics: Treatment: ≥7 Yrs: 2 inh (10mg) q12h for 5 days. Take 2 doses on 1st day at least 2 hrs apart, then 12 hrs apart (eg, am and pm) at approximately the same time each day on subsequent days. Prophylaxis: Administer at same time each day. ≥5 Yrs: Household Setting: 2 inh (10mg) qd for 10 days. Adolescents: Community Outbreaks: 2 inh (10mg) qd for 28 days.

HOW SUPPLIED: Powder, Inhalation: 5mg/inh [4 blisters/disk]

CONTRAINDICATIONS: History of allergic reaction to milk proteins.

WARNINGS/PRECAUTIONS: Not a substitute for early influenza vaccination on an annual basis. Emergence of resistance mutations can decrease drug effectiveness; consider available information on influenza drug susceptibility patterns and treatment effects when deciding whether to use therapy. Not recommended for treatment or prophylaxis of influenza in individuals with underlying airways disease (eg, asthma, chronic obstructive pulmonary disease) due to risk of bronchospasm. Serious cases of bronchospasm reported; d/c if bronchospasm or decline in respiratory function develops. Allergic-like reactions (eg, oropharyngeal edema, serious skin rashes, anaphylaxis) reported; d/c and institute appropriate treatment if an allergic reaction occurs or is suspected. Delirium and abnormal behavior leading to injury, primarily in pediatric patients, reported; monitor for abnormal behavior and evaluate risks and benefits of continuing treatment if neuropsychiatric symptoms occur. Serious bacterial infections may begin with influenza-like symptoms or may coexist with or occur during the course of influenza; treatment does not prevent these complications. Must not be made into an extemporaneous solution for administration by nebulization or mechanical ventilation. Administer only using provided device. Carefully evaluate the ability of young children to use the delivery system if therapy is considered.

ADVERSE REACTIONS: Diarrhea, nausea, sinusitis, ear/nose/throat infections, viral respiratory infections, cough, headaches, nasal signs/symptoms, throat/tonsil discomfort and pain.

INTERACTIONS: Avoid administration of live attenuated influenza vaccines within 2 weeks before or 48 hrs after zanamivir, unless medically indicated.

PREGNANCY: Category C, caution in nursing.

MECHANISM OF ACTION: Neuraminidase inhibitor; inhibits influenza virus neuraminidase, affecting release of viral particles.

PHARMACOKINETICS: Absorption: C_{max}=17-142ng/mL, 43ng/mL (median, pediatric patients); T_{max}=1-2 hrs; AUC=111-1364ng•hr/mL, 167ng•hr/mL (median, pediatric patients). **Distribution:** Plasma protein binding (<10%). **Elimination:** Urine (unchanged), feces (unabsorbed); $T_{1/2}$=2.5-5.1 hrs.

NURSING CONSIDERATIONS

Assessment: Assess for history of allergic reaction to milk proteins, airways disease, underlying medical conditions, pregnancy/nursing status, and for possible drug interactions.

Monitoring: Monitor for signs/symptoms of bronchospasm, allergic reactions, neuropsychiatric events (eg, delirium, abnormal behavior, seizures, hallucinations), and other adverse reactions.

Patient Counseling: Inform of the risk of bronchospasm; advise to stop and contact physician if increased respiratory symptoms (eg, worsening wheezing, SOB, or other signs/symptoms of bronchospasm) are experienced. If taking inhaled bronchodilators, counsel to use bronchodilators before taking the medication. Advise of the risk of neuropsychiatric events and to contact physician if experiencing signs of unusual behavior during treatment. Instruct patients in use of the delivery system; if prescribed for children, instruct parents or caregivers on proper administration and supervision. Inform that this medication does not reduce the risk of transmission of influenza to others.

Administration: Oral inhalational route. Do not puncture any blister until taking a dose using the Diskhaler. Refer to PI for further administration instructions. **Storage:** 25°C (77°F); excursions permitted to 15-30°C (59-86°F).

RELISTOR
methylnaltrexone bromide (Salix)

RX

THERAPEUTIC CLASS: Opioid antagonist

INDICATIONS: Treatment of opioid-induced constipation in patients with advanced illness who are receiving palliative care, when response to laxative therapy has not been sufficient.

DOSAGE: *Adults:* Usual Schedule: 1 dose qod PRN. Max: 1 dose/24 hrs. 62-114kg: 12mg SQ. 38-<62kg: 8mg SQ. <38kg or >114kg: 0.15mg/kg; calculate inj volume by multiplying weight in kg by 0.0075 and round up the volume to the nearest 0.1mL. Severe Renal Impairment (CrCl <30mL/min): Reduce dose by 1/2; prescribe single-use vials to ensure correct dosing. Do not prescribe prefilled syringes to patients requiring dosing calculated on a mg/kg basis; prescribe only in patients requiring an 8mg or 12mg dose.

HOW SUPPLIED: Inj: 12mg/0.6mL [vial, prefilled syringe], 8mg/0.4mL [prefilled syringe]

CONTRAINDICATIONS: Known/suspected mechanical GI obstruction.

WARNINGS/PRECAUTIONS: Cases of GI perforation (eg, stomach, duodenum, colon) reported in patients with conditions that may be associated with localized or diffuse reduction of structural integrity in the wall of GI tract (eg, cancer, peptic ulcer, Ogilvie's syndrome). Caution with known/suspected lesions of the GI tract. D/C therapy if severe/persistent/worsening abdominal symptoms develop or if severe/persistent diarrhea occurs.

ADVERSE REACTIONS: Abdominal pain, flatulence, nausea, dizziness, hyperhidrosis, diarrhea.

PREGNANCY: Category B, caution in nursing.

MECHANISM OF ACTION: Opioid antagonist; peripherally acting μ-opioid receptor antagonist in tissues such as GI tract. Decreases constipating effects of opioids without impacting opioid-mediated analgesic effects on the CNS.

PHARMACOKINETICS: Absorption: Administration of variable doses resulted in different pharmacokinetic parameters. **Distribution:** V_d=1.1L/kg; plasma protein binding (11-15.3%). **Metabolism:** Conjugated by sulfotransferase SULT1E1 and SULT2A1 isoforms to methylnaltrexone sulfate (weak metabolite); aldo-keto reductase 1C enzymes to methyl-6-naltrexol isomers (active metabolites). **Elimination:** (IV) Urine (53.6%), feces (17.3%); $T_{1/2}$=8 hrs.

NURSING CONSIDERATIONS

Assessment: Assess for mechanical GI obstruction, renal impairment, GI tract lesions, conditions associated with localized or diffuse reduction of structural integrity of the GI tract wall, and pregnancy/nursing status.

Monitoring: Monitor for signs/symptoms of GI perforation, severe/persistent/worsening abdominal symptoms, severe/persistent diarrhea, and other adverse reactions.

Patient Counseling: Instruct to take ud and inform of proper SQ technique. Instruct to d/c therapy and promptly notify physician if experiencing severe/persistent/worsening abdominal symptoms or severe/persistent diarrhea. Inform that common side effects include abdominal pain, flatulence, nausea, dizziness, and diarrhea. Advise to be within close proximity to toilet facilities once administered. Instruct to d/c therapy if opioid pain medication is stopped.

Administration: SQ route. Inject in the upper arm, abdomen, or thigh; rotate inj sites. **Storage:** 20-25°C (68-77°F); excursions permitted to 15-30°C (59-86°F). Do not freeze. Protect from light. (Vial) Once drawn into syringe, store at ambient room temperature and administer within 24 hrs if immediate administration is not possible. (Prefilled Syringe) Do not remove from the tray until ready to administer.

RELPAX   RX
eletriptan hydrobromide (Pfizer)

THERAPEUTIC CLASS: 5-HT$_{1B/1D}$ agonist

INDICATIONS: Acute treatment of migraine with or without aura.

DOSAGE: *Adults:* Individualize dose. Initial: 20 or 40mg at onset of headache. May repeat after 2 hrs if headache recurs after initial relief. Max: 40mg/dose or 80mg/day.

HOW SUPPLIED: Tab: 20mg, 40mg

CONTRAINDICATIONS: Ischemic heart disease (eg, angina pectoris, history of myocardial infarction [MI], or documented silent ischemia) or symptoms/findings consistent with ischemic heart disease, coronary artery vasospasm (eg, Prinzmetal's variant angina), or other significant underlying cardiovascular (CV) disease, cerebrovascular syndromes (eg, stroke, transient ischemic attacks), peripheral vascular disease (eg, ischemic bowel disease), uncontrolled HTN, hemiplegic/basilar migraine, use of other 5-HT$_1$ agonists or ergotamine-containing/ergot-type agents (eg, dihydroergotamine, methysergide) within 24 hrs, severe hepatic impairment.

WARNINGS/PRECAUTIONS: Has potential to cause coronary artery vasospasm; do not give with documented ischemic/vasospastic coronary artery disease (CAD). Not for patients in whom unrecognized CAD is predicted by presence of risk factors unless with a satisfactory CV evaluation; administer 1st dose under medical supervision and obtain ECG during interval immediately after administration to assess for cardiac ischemia. Monitor CV function with long-term intermittent use. Serious adverse cardiac events, cerebrovascular events, and vasospastic reactions (eg, coronary artery vasospasm, peripheral vascular ischemia, colonic ischemia) reported. Serotonin syndrome may occur. HTN and hypertensive crisis reported rarely. Caution with hepatic dysfunction. Possible long-term ophthalmologic effects. Avoid in elderly.

ADVERSE REACTIONS: Asthenia, dizziness, drowsiness, nausea, headache, paresthesia, dry mouth, flushing/feeling of warmth, chest tightness/pain/pressure, abdominal pain/cramps, dyspepsia, dysphagia.

INTERACTIONS: See Contraindications. Avoid use within 72 hrs of potent CYP3A4 inhibitors (eg, ketoconazole, clarithromycin, ritonavir). May cause additive prolonged vasospastic reaction with ergot-containing drugs. Serotonin syndrome reported with SSRIs or SNRIs. Propranolol, erythromycin, verapamil, and fluconazole may increase levels.

PREGNANCY: Category C, caution in nursing.

R

REMERON

MECHANISM OF ACTION: Selective 5-HT$_{1B/1D}$ agonist; binds with high affinity to 5-HT$_{1B/1D/1F}$ receptors. Suspected to perform its action by (1) activation of 5-HT$_{1B/1D}$ receptors located on intracranial blood vessels, including those on arteriovenous anastomoses, which leads to vasoconstriction and is correlated with relief of migraine headache, or (2) activation of 5-HT$_{1B/1D}$ receptors in trigeminal system, which results in inhibition of proinflammatory neuropeptide release.

PHARMACOKINETICS: Absorption: Well-absorbed; absolute bioavailability (50%); T$_{max}$=1.5 hrs. **Distribution:** V$_d$=138L; plasma protein binding (85%). **Metabolism:** via CYP3A4; N-demethylated metabolite (active). **Elimination:** Urine. T$_{1/2}$=4 hrs (parent drug), 13 hrs (metabolite).

NURSING CONSIDERATIONS

Assessment: Confirm diagnosis of migraine before therapy. Assess for ischemic heart disease (eg, angina pectoris, Prinzmetal's variant angina, MI or documented silent MI), ECG changes, or any other conditions where treatment is contraindicated or cautioned. Assess for hepatic/renal impairment, pregnancy/nursing status, and possible drug interactions.

Monitoring: Monitor for signs/symptoms of cardiac events, cerebrovascular events, peripheral vascular ischemia, colonic ischemia, serotonin syndrome, hypersensitivity reactions, ophthalmologic changes, and other adverse reactions. Monitor ECG during interval immediately after administration in patients with CAD risk factors. For patients on long-term intermittent therapy or with CAD risk factors, periodically monitor CV function. Monitor BP, weight, and LFTs.

Patient Counseling: Inform about potential risks of therapy (eg, serotonin syndrome) and possible drug interactions. Advise to take exactly as prescribed. Instruct to notify physician if any adverse reactions occur, or if pregnant/nursing or plan to become pregnant.

Administration: Oral route. **Storage:** 25°C (77°F); excursions permitted to 15-30°C (59-86°F).

REMERON
mirtazapine (Merck)

RX

Antidepressants increased the risk of suicidal thinking and behavior (suicidality) in children, adolescents, and young adults in short-term studies of major depressive disorder (MDD) and other psychiatric disorders. Monitor and observe closely for clinical worsening, suicidality, or unusual changes in behavior in patients who are started on antidepressant therapy. Not approved for use in pediatric patients.

OTHER BRAND NAMES: RemeronSolTab (Merck)

THERAPEUTIC CLASS: Piperazino-azepine

INDICATIONS: Treatment of MDD.

DOSAGE: *Adults:* Initial: 15mg qhs. Titrate: Dose changes should not be made at intervals of less than 1-2 weeks. Range: 15-45mg/day. Max: 45mg/day. Reassess periodically to determine the need for maintenance treatment and the appropriate dose. Switching to/from an MAOI for Psychiatric Disorders: Allow at least 14 days between discontinuation of an MAOI and initiation of treatment, and allow at least 14 days between discontinuation of treatment and initiation of an MAOI. Use with Other MAOIs (eg, Linezolid, IV Methylene Blue): Refer to PI.

HOW SUPPLIED: Tab: 15mg*, 30mg*, 45mg; Tab, Disintegrating: 15mg, 30mg, 45mg *scored

CONTRAINDICATIONS: Use of an MAOI for psychiatric disorders either concomitantly or within 14 days of stopping treatment. Treatment within 14 days of stopping an MAOI for psychiatric disorders. Starting treatment in a patient being treated with other MAOIs (eg, linezolid, IV methylene blue).

WARNINGS/PRECAUTIONS: Not approved for treatment of bipolar depression. May precipitate mixed/manic episode in patients at risk for bipolar disorder. Agranulocytosis and severe neutropenia reported; d/c if sore throat, fever, stomatitis, or other signs of infection develop, along with low WBC counts. Serotonin syndrome reported; d/c immediately and initiate supportive symptomatic treatment. Avoid abrupt discontinuation; gradual dose reduction is recommended. Akathisia/psychomotor restlessness reported; increasing the dose may be detrimental in patients who develop these symptoms. Hyponatremia reported. May impair mental/physical abilities. Somnolence, dizziness, increased appetite, weight gain, and elevation in cholesterol/TG/ALT levels reported. Mania/hypomania and seizures reported. Caution with hepatic/renal impairment, diseases/conditions affecting metabolism or hemodynamic responses, and in the elderly. May cause orthostatic hypotension; caution with cardiovascular (CV) or cerebrovascular disease that could be exacerbated by hypotension and conditions that predispose to hypotension.

ADVERSE REACTIONS: Somnolence, increased appetite, weight gain, dizziness, dry mouth, constipation, asthenia, flu syndrome, abnormal dreams, abnormal thinking.

INTERACTIONS: See Contraindications. May cause serotonin syndrome with other serotonergic drugs (eg, triptans, fentanyl, tramadol, St. John's wort) and with drugs that impair metabolism of serotonin. Caution with antihypertensives and drugs known to cause hyponatremia. Phenytoin, carbamazepine, and other hepatic metabolism inducers (eg, rifampicin) may decrease levels; may need to increase mirtazapine dose. Cimetidine and ketoconazole may increase levels; may need to decrease mirtazapine dose with cimetidine. Avoid with alcohol and diazepam or drugs similar to diazepam. Caution with potent CYP3A4 inhibitors, HIV protease inhibitors, azole antifungals, erythromycin, or nefazodone. Increased INR with warfarin; monitor INR.

PREGNANCY: Category C, caution in nursing.

MECHANISM OF ACTION: Piperazino-azepine; not established. Acts as an antagonist at central presynaptic α_2-adrenergic inhibitory autoreceptors and heteroreceptors, an action that is postulated to result in an increase in central noradrenergic and serotonergic activity.

PHARMACOKINETICS: Absorption: Rapid and complete; absolute bioavailability (50%); T_{max}=2 hrs. **Distribution:** Plasma protein binding (85%). **Metabolism:** Extensive; demethylation and hydroxylation via CYP2D6, CYP1A2, and CYP3A followed by glucuronide conjugation. **Elimination:** Urine (75%), feces (15%); $T_{1/2}$=20-40 hrs.

NURSING CONSIDERATIONS

Assessment: Assess for risk of bipolar disorder, hyponatremia, CV or cerebrovascular diseases, history of mania/hypomania, seizure, conditions that predispose to hypotension, renal/hepatic impairment, diseases/conditions affecting metabolism or hemodynamic response, pregnancy/nursing status, and possible drug interactions.

Monitoring: Monitor for signs/symptoms of clinical worsening, serotonin syndrome, akathisia, signs of infection (eg, sore throat, fever, stomatitis), somnolence, dizziness, increased appetite, weight gain, elevation in cholesterol/TG/ALT levels, hyponatremia, seizures, and other adverse reactions.

Patient Counseling: Inform about the benefits and risks of therapy. Advise families and caregivers of the need for close observation for signs of clinical worsening and suicidal risks and to report such signs to physician. Warn about risk of developing agranulocytosis and instruct to contact physician if signs of infection (eg, fever, chills, sore throat, mucous membrane ulceration) develop. Advise to use caution when engaging in hazardous activities. Advise that improvement may be noticed in 1-4 weeks of therapy, but to continue therapy ud. Advise to inform physician if taking or intend to take any prescription or OTC drugs. Instruct to avoid alcohol while on therapy. Instruct to inform physician if pregnant/nursing, become pregnant, or intend to become pregnant during therapy. (Tab, Disintegrating) Inform phenylketonuric patients that the tab contains phenylalanine.

Administration: Oral route. (Tab, Disintegrating) Use immediately after removal from blister. Place tab on the tongue; disintegrated tab can be swallowed with saliva. Do not split the tab. **Storage:** 25°C (77°F); excursions permitted to 15-30°C (59-86°F). Protect from light and moisture.

REMICADE   RX
infliximab (Janssen)

Increased risk for developing serious infections (eg, active tuberculosis [TB], latent TB reactivation, invasive fungal infections, bacterial/viral infections, opportunistic infections) leading to hospitalization or death, mostly with concomitant use with immunosuppressants (eg, methotrexate [MTX], corticosteroids). D/C if serious infection or sepsis develops. Active/latent reactivation TB may present with disseminated or extrapulmonary disease; test for latent TB before and during therapy and initiate treatment for latent TB prior to infliximab use. Invasive fungal infections reported; consider empiric antifungal therapy in patients at risk who develop severe systemic illness. Consider risks and benefits prior to therapy in patients with chronic or recurrent infection. Monitor patients for development of infection during and after treatment, including development of TB in patients who tested negative for latent TB infection prior to therapy. Lymphoma and other malignancies, some fatal, reported in children and adolescents. Postmarketing cases of aggressive and fatal hepatosplenic T-cell lymphoma (HSTCL) reported in patients with Crohn's disease (CD) or ulcerative colitis (UC) and the majority were in adolescent and young adult males; all of these patients were treated concomitantly with azathioprine or 6-mercaptopurine.

THERAPEUTIC CLASS: Monoclonal antibody/TNF-blocker

INDICATIONS: Reduce signs/symptoms, induce and maintain clinical remission in adults and pediatric patients ≥6 yrs of age with moderately to severely active CD when response to conventional therapy is inadequate. Reduce the number of draining enterocutaneous and rectovaginal fistulas and maintain fistula closure in adults with fistulizing CD. Reduce signs/symptoms, induce and maintain clinical remission in adults and pediatric patients ≥6 yrs of age, induce and maintain mucosal healing, and eliminate corticosteroid use in adults with moderately to severely active UC when response to conventional therapy is inadequate. Reduce signs/symptoms, inhibit progression of structural damage, and improve physical function with moderately to severely active rheumatoid arthritis (RA) (in combination with MTX) and psoriatic arthritis. Reduce signs/symptoms with active ankylosing spondylitis (AS). Treatment of adults with chronic, severe (eg, extensive and/or disabling) plaque psoriasis who are candidates for systemic therapy and when other systemic therapies are medically less appropriate.

DOSAGE: *Adults:* CD/Fistulizing CD: Induction Regimen: 5mg/kg IV at 0, 2, and 6 weeks. Maint: 5mg/kg every 8 weeks. Patients Who Respond and Then Lose Their Response: May increase to 10mg/kg. Consider discontinuation if no response by Week 14. UC/Psoriatic Arthritis (with or without MTX)/Plaque Psoriasis: Induction Regimen: 5mg/kg IV at 0, 2, and 6 weeks. Maint: 5mg/kg every 8 weeks. RA (with MTX): Induction Regimen: 3mg/kg IV at 0, 2, and 6 weeks. Maint: 3mg/kg every 8 weeks. Incomplete Response: May increase up to 10mg/kg or give as often as every 4 weeks. AS: Induction Regimen: 5mg/kg IV at 0, 2, and 6 weeks. Maint: 5mg/kg every 6 weeks.
Pediatrics: ≥6 Yrs: CD/UC: Induction Regimen: 5mg/kg IV at 0, 2, and 6 weeks. Maint: 5mg/kg every 8 weeks.

HOW SUPPLIED: Inj: 100mg

CONTRAINDICATIONS: Hypersensitivity to murine proteins. Moderate to severe heart failure (HF) (NYHA Class III/IV) with doses >5mg/kg.

WARNINGS/PRECAUTIONS: Do not initiate with an active infection. Increased risk of infection in patients >65 yrs of age and in patients with comorbid conditions; consider the risks prior to therapy for those who have resided or traveled in areas of endemic TB or mycoses, and with any underlying conditions predisposing to infection. Cases of acute/chronic leukemia, melanoma, and Merkel cell carcinoma reported. Caution in patients with moderate to severe chronic obstructive pulmonary disease (COPD), history of malignancy, or in continuing treatment in patients who develop malignancy during therapy. Hepatitis B virus (HBV) reactivation reported; if reactivation occurs, d/c and initiate antiviral therapy with appropriate supportive treatment. Severe hepatic reactions (eg, acute liver failure, jaundice, hepatitis, cholestasis) reported; d/c if jaundice or marked elevations of liver enzymes (eg, ≥5X ULN) develop. New onset (rare) HF and worsening of HF reported; d/c if new or worsening symptoms of HF occur. Leukopenia, neutropenia, thrombocytopenia, and pancytopenia reported; consider discontinuation of therapy if significant hematologic abnormalities occur. Caution in patients who have ongoing or history of significant hematologic abnormalities. Hypersensitivity reactions reported; d/c for severe hypersensitivity reactions. CNS manifestation of systemic vasculitis, seizures, and new onset/exacerbation of CNS demyelinating disorders reported (rare); caution in patients with these neurologic disorders and consider discontinuation if these disorders develop. Caution when switching from one biologic disease-modifying antirheumatic drug to another; overlapping biological activity may further increase risk of infection. May cause autoantibody formation and, rarely, may develop lupus-like syndrome; d/c if lupus-like syndrome develops. Caution in administration of live vaccines to infants born to female patients treated with infliximab during pregnancy. All pediatric patients should be up to date with all vaccinations prior to therapy. Caution in elderly.

ADVERSE REACTIONS: Serious infections, malignancies, infusion reactions, nausea, upper respiratory tract infection, anemia, rash, headache, sinusitis, pharyngitis, coughing, abdominal pain, diarrhea, bronchitis, leukopenia.

INTERACTIONS: See Boxed Warning. Avoid with live vaccines or therapeutic infectious agents. Avoid use with tocilizumab; possible increased immunosuppression and increased risk of infection. Not recommended with anakinra or abatacept; may increase risk of serious infections. Not recommended with other biological therapeutics used to treat the same conditions. MTX may decrease the incidence of anti-infliximab antibody production and increase infliximab concentrations. Upon initiation or discontinuation of infliximab in patients being treated with CYP450 substrates with a narrow therapeutic index, monitor therapeutic effect (eg, warfarin) or drug concentration (eg, cyclosporine, theophylline) and adjust individual dose of the drug product as needed.

PREGNANCY: Category B, not for use in nursing.

MECHANISM OF ACTION: Monoclonal antibody/TNF-α receptor blocker; neutralizes biological activity of TNF-α by binding with high affinity to the soluble and transmembrane forms of TNF-α and inhibits binding of TNF-α with its receptors.

PHARMACOKINETICS: Distribution: Crosses placenta. **Elimination:** $T_{1/2}$=7.7-9.5 days (median).

NURSING CONSIDERATIONS

Assessment: Assess for active/chronic/recurrent infection (eg, TB, HBV), history of an opportunistic infection, recent travel to areas of endemic TB or endemic mycoses, underlying conditions that may predispose to infection, HF, history of malignancy, moderate to severe COPD, inflammatory bowel disease, presence or history of significant hematologic abnormalities, neurologic disorders, previous hypersensitivity to drug or to murine proteins, risk factors for skin cancer, pregnancy/nursing status, and for possible drug interactions. Assess vaccination history in pediatric patients. Perform test for latent TB infection.

Monitoring: Monitor for sepsis, TB (active, reactivation, or latent), invasive fungal infections, or bacterial, viral, and other infections caused by opportunistic pathogens during and after therapy. Monitor for development of lymphoma, HSTCL, or other malignancies. Monitor for NMSCs in psoriasis patients, melanoma and Merkel cell carcinoma, new or worsening symptoms of HF, active HBV infection, hepatotoxicity, hematological events, hypersensitivity reactions,

CNS demyelinating disorders, lupus-like syndrome, and other adverse reactions. Monitor LFTs. Perform periodic skin examination, particularly in patients with risk factors for skin cancer.

Patient Counseling: Advise of potential risks and benefits of therapy. Inform that therapy may lower the ability of immune system to fight infections; instruct to immediately contact physician if any signs/symptoms of an infection develop, including TB and HBV reactivation. Counsel about the risks of lymphoma and other malignancies while on therapy. Advise to report to physician signs of new or worsening medical conditions (eg, heart disease, neurological disease, autoimmune disorders) and symptoms of cytopenia (eg, bruising, bleeding, persistent fever).

Administration: IV route. Refer to PI for administration and preparation instructions. **Storage:** 2-8°C (36-46°F).

RENAGEL   RX
sevelamer HCl (Genzyme)

THERAPEUTIC CLASS: Phosphate binder

INDICATIONS: Control of serum phosphorus (P) in patients with chronic kidney disease on dialysis.

DOSAGE: *Adults:* Take with meals. Not Taking Phosphate Binder: Initial: Serum P >5.5 and <7.5mg/dL: 800mg tid. Serum P ≥7.5 and <9mg/dL: 1200-1600mg tid. Serum P ≥9mg/dL: 1600mg tid. Switching from Calcium Acetate (667mg tab): Initial: Calcium acetate 1 tab/meal: 800mg/meal. Calcium acetate 2 tabs/meal: 1200-1600mg/meal. Calcium acetate 3 tabs/meal: 2000mg-2400mg/meal. Titrate: All Patients: Adjust based on serum P concentrations. Serum P >5.5mg/dL: Increase by 1 tab/meal at 2-week interval PRN. Serum P 3.5-5.5mg/dL: Maintain current dose. Serum P <3.5mg.dL: Decrease by 1 tab/meal at 2-week interval PRN. Elderly: Start at lower end of dosing range.

HOW SUPPLIED: Tab: 400mg, 800mg

CONTRAINDICATIONS: Bowel obstruction.

WARNINGS/PRECAUTIONS: Dysphagia and esophageal tablet retention reported with use of tab formulations; consider use of sus formulations in patients with history of swallowing disorder. Bowel obstruction and perforation reported. Monitor bicarbonate and Cl⁻ levels, and for reduced vitamin D, E, and K (clotting factors), and folic acid levels. Caution in elderly.

ADVERSE REACTIONS: N/V, abdominal pain, constipation, diarrhea, flatulence, dyspepsia, peritonitis.

INTERACTIONS: May decrease ciprofloxacin bioavailability by 50%. Very rare cases of increased TSH levels reported with levothyroxine; monitor TSH levels. When giving oral medication where reduction in bioavailability would have a clinically significant effect on its safety or efficacy, administer the drug ≥1 hr before or 3 hrs after sevelamer HCl and monitor blood levels of the drug. Caution with antiarrhythmic or antiseizure medications.

PREGNANCY: Category C, safety not known in nursing.

MECHANISM OF ACTION: Phosphate binder; contains multiple amines that exist in a protonated form in the intestine, and bind phosphate molecules through ionic and hydrogen bonding and decrease absorption, hence lowering phosphate concentration in the serum.

NURSING CONSIDERATIONS

Assessment: Assess for presence of bowel obstruction and other GI disorders (eg, dysphagia, swallowing disorders, GI motility disorders, GI tract surgery), pregnancy/nursing status, and possible drug interactions.

Monitoring: Monitor for bowel obstruction and perforation, dysphagia, esophageal tablet retention, and other adverse reactions. Monitor bicarbonate, Cl⁻, and folic acid levels, and for reduced vitamins D, E, and K (clotting factors).

Patient Counseling: Inform to take with meals and adhere to prescribed diets. Instruct to take other concomitant medication doses apart from sevelamer hydrochloride. Advise to report new onset or worsening of existing constipation to physician.

Administration: Oral route. **Storage:** 25°C (77°F); excursions permitted to 15-30°C (59-86°F). Protect from moisture.

RENVELA   RX
sevelamer carbonate (Genzyme)

THERAPEUTIC CLASS: Phosphate binder

INDICATIONS: Control of serum phosphorus (P) in patients with chronic kidney disease on dialysis.

ReoPro

DOSAGE: *Adults:* Take with meals. Not Taking Phosphate Binder: Initial: Serum P >5.5 and <7.5mg/dL: 0.8g tid. Serum P ≥7.5mg/dL: 1.6g tid. Switching from Sevelamer HCl/Switching Between Sevelamer Carbonate Tab and Powder: Use same dose in grams. Further titration may be necessary to achieve desired P levels. Switching from Calcium Acetate (667mg tab): Initial: 0.8g/meal if previously taking 1 tab calcium acetate/meal. 1.6g/meal if previously taking 2 tabs calcium acetate/meal. 2.4g/meal if previously taking 3 tabs calcium acetate/meal. Titrate: All Patients: May increase dose by 0.8g tid with meals at 2-week intervals PRN. Elderly: Start at low end of dosing range.

HOW SUPPLIED: Tab: 800mg; Powder: 0.8g/pkt, 2.4g/pkt

CONTRAINDICATIONS: Bowel obstruction.

WARNINGS/PRECAUTIONS: Dysphagia and esophageal tablet retention reported with use of tab formulation; consider use of sus in patient with history of swallowing disorder. Bowel obstruction and perforation reported. Safety not established in patients with dysphagia, swallowing disorders, severe GI motility disorders (eg, severe constipation, major GI tract surgery). Monitor bicarbonate and chloride levels, and for reduced vitamins D, E, and K (clotting factors), and folic acid levels. Caution in elderly.

ADVERSE REACTIONS: N/V, diarrhea, dyspepsia, abdominal pain, flatulence, constipation.

INTERACTIONS: May decrease ciprofloxacin bioavailability by 50%; consider dosing ≥1 hr before or 3 hrs after and monitor. Rare cases of increased TSH levels reported with levothyroxine; monitor TSH levels and for signs of hypothyroidism when used concomitantly.

PREGNANCY: Category C, safety not known in nursing.

MECHANISM OF ACTION: Phosphate binder; contains multiple amines that exist in a protonated form in the intestine, and bind phosphate molecules through ionic and hydrogen bonding and decrease absorption, hence lowering phosphate concentration in the serum.

NURSING CONSIDERATIONS

Assessment: Assess for presence of bowel obstruction and other GI disorders (eg, dysphagia, swallowing disorders, GI motility disorders, GI tract surgery), pregnancy/nursing status, and possible drug interactions.

Monitoring: Monitor for bowel obstruction and perforation, dysphagia, esophageal tablet retention, bicarbonate and Cl⁻ levels, and for reduced vitamins D, E, and K (clotting factors), and folic acid levels.

Patient Counseling: Inform to take with meals and adhere to prescribed diets. If taking an oral medication where reduced bioavailability would produce a clinically significant effect on safety or efficacy, advise to take medication ≥1 hr before or 3 hrs after dosing. Advise to report new onset or worsening of existing constipation to physician.

Administration: Oral route. Powder Preparation: Empty contents of pkt in cup and mix thoroughly with appropriate amount of water. Minimum Amount of Water: 0.8g: 1 oz./30mL/6 tsp/2 tbsp. 2.4g: 2 oz./60mL/4 tbsp. Vigorously stir just before drinking. Drink within 30 min. **Storage:** 25°C (77°F); excursions permitted to 15-30°C (59-86°F). Protect from moisture.

ReoPro   RX
abciximab (Lilly)

THERAPEUTIC CLASS: Glycoprotein IIb/IIIa inhibitor

INDICATIONS: Adjunct to percutaneous coronary intervention (PCI) for prevention of cardiac ischemic complications in patients undergoing PCI or with unstable angina unresponsive to conventional therapy when PCI is planned within 24 hrs. Intended for use with aspirin and heparin.

DOSAGE: *Adults:* PCI: 0.25mg/kg IV bolus given 10-60 min before start of PCI, followed by 0.125mcg/kg/min IV infusion (Max: 10mcg/min) for 12 hrs. Unstable Angina: 0.25mg/kg IV bolus followed by 10mcg/min infusion for 18-24 hrs, concluding 1 hr after PCI.

HOW SUPPLIED: Inj: 2mg/mL

CONTRAINDICATIONS: Active internal bleeding, recent (within 6 weeks) significant GI or genitourinary (GU) bleeding, cerebrovascular accident (CVA) within 2 yrs, CVA with significant residual neurological deficit, bleeding diathesis, oral anticoagulants within 7 days (unless PT ≤1.2x control), thrombocytopenia, recent (within 6 weeks) major surgery or trauma, intracranial neoplasm, arteriovenous malformation, aneurysm, severe uncontrolled HTN, history of vasculitis, IV dextran use before PCI or during an intervention. Hypersensitivity to murine proteins.

WARNINGS/PRECAUTIONS: Increased risk of bleeding. Monitor all potential bleeding sites (eg, catheter insertion sites, arterial and venous puncture sites, cutdown sites). Arterial/venous punctures, intramuscular injections, and use of urinary catheters, nasotracheal intubation, NG tubes, and automatic BP cuffs should be minimized. When obtaining IV access, noncompressible sites (eg, subclavian or jugular veins) should be avoided. Minimize vascular and other trauma. D/C if serious, uncontrollable bleeding, thrombocytopenia, or emergency surgery occurs. Anaphylaxis may occur. Antibody (HACA) formation may occur; risk of hypersensitivity, thrombocytopenia, decreased benefit with readministration. Monitor platelets, PT, APTT, and ACT before infusion.

ADVERSE REACTIONS: Bleeding, thrombocytopenia, hypotension, bradycardia, N/V, back/chest pain, headache.

INTERACTIONS: Caution with other drugs that affect hemostasis (eg, thrombolytics, heparin, oral anticoagulants, NSAIDs, dipyridamole, ticlopidine). Increased risk of bleeding with anticoagulants, thrombolytics, and antiplatelets. Possible allergic reactions with monoclonal antibody agents may occur in patients with HACA titers.

PREGNANCY: Category C, caution in nursing.

MECHANISM OF ACTION: Glycoprotein IIb/IIIa inhibitor; binds to the GPIIb/IIIa receptor and inhibits platelet aggregation by preventing the binding of fibrinogen, von Willebrand factor, and other adhesive molecules to GPIIb/IIIa receptor sites on activated platelets. Also binds to vitronectin receptor, which mediates the procoagulant properties of platelets and the proliferative properties of vascular endothelial and smooth muscle cells.

PHARMACOKINETICS: Elimination: $T_{1/2}$=30 min.

NURSING CONSIDERATIONS

Assessment: Assess for active internal bleeding, recent GI or GU bleeding, history of CVA, bleeding diathesis, thrombocytopenia, recent major surgery or trauma, intracranial neoplasm, arteriovenous malformation, aneurysm, severe uncontrolled HTN, presence or history of vasculitis, pregnancy/nursing status, and drug interactions. Obtain baseline PT, ACT, APTT, and platelet counts.

Monitoring: Monitor for signs/symptoms of bleeding; document and monitor vascular puncture sites. If hematoma develops, monitor for enlargement. Monitor for allergic reactions (eg, anaphylaxis) and thrombocytopenia. Check aPTT or ACT prior to arterial sheath removal; should not be removed unless aPTT ≤50 seconds or ACT ≤175 seconds. Monitor platelet counts 2-4 hrs following a bolus dose and 24 hrs prior to discharge.

Patient Counseling: Counsel to contact physician if hypersensitivity reactions (eg, anaphylaxis) develop. Inform patients that they will bleed and bruise more easily and take longer to stop bleeding. Instruct to report any unusual bleeding to physician.

Administration: IV infusion. In case of hypersensitivity reaction, epinephrine, dopamine, theophylline, antihistamines, and corticosteroids should be available for immediate use. Refer to PI for administration and preparation instructions. **Storage:** Store at 2-8°C (36-46°F). Do not freeze. Do not shake. Discard any unused portion left in vial.

REQUIP   RX
ropinirole (GlaxoSmithKline)

OTHER BRAND NAMES: Requip XL (GlaxoSmithKline)

THERAPEUTIC CLASS: Non-ergoline dopamine agonist

INDICATIONS: Treatment of signs and symptoms of idiopathic Parkinson's disease. (Tab) Treatment of moderate to severe primary restless legs syndrome (RLS).

DOSAGE: *Adults:* Parkinson's Disease: (Tab) Initial: 0.25mg tid. Titrate: May increase in weekly increments by 0.25mg tid. After Week 4, if necessary, may increase daily dose by 1.5mg/day on a weekly basis up to 9mg/day, then by up to 3mg/day weekly to a total dose of 24mg/day. Max: 24mg/day. Discontinuation: D/C gradually over a 7-day period; decrease frequency from tid to bid for 4 days, then qd for the remaining 3 days. (Tab, XL) Initial: 2mg qd for 1-2 weeks. Titrate: May increase by 2mg/day at ≥1-week intervals as appropriate, depending on therapeutic response and tolerability. Max: 24mg/day. Discontinuation: D/C gradually over a 7-day period. Switching from Immediate-Release (IR) to XL: Initial dose should match the total daily dose of IR formulation. Refer to PI for conversion from IR to XL. (Tab) RLS: Initial: 0.25mg qd, 1-3 hrs before hs. Titrate: May increase to 0.5mg qd on Days 3-7, 1mg qd on Week 2, then increase by 0.5mg weekly up to Week 6, and increase to 4mg on Week 7. Max: 4mg qd.

HOW SUPPLIED: Tab: 0.25mg, 0.5mg, 1mg, 2mg, 3mg, 4mg, 5mg; Tab, Extended-Release (XL): 2mg, 4mg, 6mg, 8mg, 12mg

WARNINGS/PRECAUTIONS: Falling asleep during activities of daily living reported; d/c if significant daytime sleepiness or episodes of falling asleep develop during activities that require active participation. May impair mental/physical abilities. Syncope, bradycardia, postural hypotension, hallucinations, fibrotic complications (eg, retroperitoneal fibrosis, pulmonary infiltrates, pleural effusion, pleural thickening, pericarditis, cardiac valvulopathy), and melanoma reported. Titrate with caution in patients with hepatic impairment. Symptom complex similar to neuroleptic malignant syndrome (NMS) reported in association with rapid dose reduction, withdrawal of, or changes in dopaminergic therapy. Caution with cardiovascular disease (CVD). (Tab, XL) May cause elevation of BP and changes in HR. Patients with major psychotic disorder should ordinarily not be treated because of risk of exacerbation of psychosis.

ADVERSE REACTIONS: N/V, somnolence, abdominal pain, dizziness, headache, constipation, orthostatic symptoms, syncope, hallucination. (Tab) Viral infection, pain, leg edema, fatigue, dyspepsia, confusion.

INTERACTIONS: May require adjustment of ropinirole dose if estrogen or a potent CYP1A2 inducer/inhibitor is stopped or started during treatment. Increased plasma levels with ciprofloxacin. Dopamine antagonists, such as neuroleptics (eg, phenothiazines, butyrophenones, thioxanthenes) or metoclopramide may diminish effectiveness. Increased clearance with smoking. May potentiate dopaminergic side effects of L-dopa and may cause and/or exacerbate preexisting dyskinesia in patients treated with L-dopa for Parkinson's disease. May increase risk of drowsiness with concomitant sedating medications and concomitant medications that increase ropinirole plasma levels.

PREGNANCY: Category C, not for use in nursing.

MECHANISM OF ACTION: Non-ergoline dopamine agonist; has not been established. Believed to stimulate postsynaptic dopamine D_2-type receptors within the caudate-putamen in the brain.

PHARMACOKINETICS: Absorption: Rapid. Absolute bioavailability (45-55%), T_{max}=1-2 hrs (IR), 6-10 hrs (XL). **Distribution:** V_d=7.5L/kg, plasma protein binding (40%). **Metabolism:** Liver via CYP1A2 (extensive); N-despropylation and hydroxylation. **Elimination:** Urine (<10% unchanged), $T_{1/2}$=6 hrs.

NURSING CONSIDERATIONS

Assessment: Assess for presence of sleep disorder, CVD, dyskinesia, major psychotic disorder, hepatic impairment, pregnancy/nursing status, and possible drug interactions.

Monitoring: Monitor symptom complex resembling NMS, syncope, bradycardia, postural hypotension, hallucinations, fibrotic complications, melanomas, daytime sleepiness/episodes of falling asleep, BP elevation, HR changes, and other adverse reactions. Perform dermatological screening periodically.

Patient Counseling: Instruct to take ud. Advise not to double the next dose if a dose is missed. Advise that postural (orthostatic) hypotension with/without symptoms (eg, dizziness, nausea, syncope, sweating) may develop; caution against rising rapidly after sitting or lying down for prolonged periods, especially at treatment initiation. Advise not to drive or participate in potentially dangerous activities, if increased somnolence or episodes of falling asleep during activities of daily living are experienced at any time during treatment. Caution patients taking other sedating medications, alcohol, or other CNS depressants concomitantly, or taking concomitant medications that increase plasma levels of ropinirole, because of possible additive effects. Inform that patients may experience hallucinations. Advise to report new or increased gambling urges, increased sexual urges, or if other intense urges occur. Instruct to inform physician if pregnant/intending to become pregnant or if breastfeeding/intending to breastfeed during therapy. (Tab, XL) Alert of the possibility of increase in BP and that significant increases/decreases in HR may be experienced during treatment.

Administration: Oral route. May be taken with or without food. (Tab, XL) Swallow whole; do not chew, crush, or divide. **Storage:** (Tab) 20-25°C (68-77°F). Protect from light and moisture. (Tab, XL) 25°C (77°F); excursions permitted to 15-30°C (59-86°F).

RESCRIPTOR   RX
delavirdine mesylate (ViiV Healthcare)

THERAPEUTIC CLASS: Non-nucleoside reverse transcriptase inhibitor

INDICATIONS: Treatment of HIV-1 infection in combination with at least 2 other active antiretroviral agents.

DOSAGE: *Adults:* Usual: 400mg (four 100mg or two 200mg tabs) tid. Take with acidic beverage (eg, orange or cranberry juice) if achlorhydric.
Pediatrics: ≥16 Yrs: Usual: 400mg (four 100mg or two 200mg tabs) tid. Take with acidic beverage (eg, orange or cranberry juice) if achlorhydric.

HOW SUPPLIED: Tab: 100mg, 200mg

CONTRAINDICATIONS: Coadminstration with CYP3A substrates that are associated with serious and/or life-threatening events at elevated plasma concentrations (eg, astemizole, terfenadine, dihydroergotamine, ergonovine, ergotamine, methylergonovine, cisapride, pimozide, alprazolam, midazolam, triazolam).

WARNINGS/PRECAUTIONS: Immune reconstitution syndrome reported. Autoimmune disorders (eg, Graves' disease, polymyositis, Guillain-Barre syndrome) have been reported to occur in the setting of immune reconstitution. Redistribution/accumulation of body fat reported. May confer cross-resistance to the other non-nucleoside reverse transcriptase inhibitors (NNRTIs). Severe rash (eg, erythema multiforme, Stevens-Johnson syndrome) reported; d/c use if this occurs. Caution with hepatic impairment and in elderly.

ADVERSE REACTIONS: Headache, fatigue, N/V, diarrhea, increased ALT/AST, rash, maculo-papular rash, pruritus, erythema, insomnia, upper respiratory infection, depressive symptoms, generalized abdominal pain.

INTERACTIONS: See Contraindications. Avoid with another NNRTI. Not recommended with lovastatin, simvastatin, St. John's wort, phenytoin, phenobarbital, carbamazepine, rifabutin, rifampin, or chronic use of H_2-receptor antagonists or PPIs. Increased risk of myopathy with HMG-CoA reductase inhibitors metabolized by CYP3A4 (eg, atorvastatin, cerivastatin). May increase levels of nelfinavir, lopinavir, ritonavir, amphetamines, trazodone, antiarrhythmics, war-farin (monitor INR), calcium channel blockers, atorvastatin, cerivastatin, fluvastatin, immunosup-pressants, CYP3A substrates, fluticasone, methadone, and ethinyl estradiol. May increase levels of maraviroc; maraviroc dose should be reduced. May increase levels of indinavir; consider dose reduction of indinavir. May increase levels of saquinavir; consider dose reduction of saquinavir (soft gelatin cap). May decrease levels of didanosine. Ketoconazole, fluoxetine, and CYP3A inhibi-tors may increase levels. Nelfinavir, didanosine, antacids, CYP3A inducers, H_2-receptor antago-nists, PPIs, and dexamethasone may decrease levels. May increase levels of clarithromycin; adjust clarithromycin dose in patients with impaired renal function. May increase levels of sildenafil; do not exceed a max single sildenafil dose of 25mg in a 48-hr period. Doses of an antacid and didanosine (buffered tabs) should be separated by at least 1 hr.

PREGNANCY: Category C, not for use in nursing.

MECHANISM OF ACTION: NNRTI; binds directly to reverse transcriptase and blocks RNA-dependent and DNA-dependent DNA polymerase activities.

PHARMACOKINETICS: Absorption: Rapid. (400mg tid) C_{max}=35µM, AUC=180µM•hr; T_{max}=1 hr. **Distribution:** Plasma protein binding (98%). **Metabolism:** Hepatic (N-desalkylation, pyridine hydroxylation) via CYP3A (major), 2D6. **Elimination:** (300mg tid multiple dose) Urine (51%, <5% unchanged), feces (44%); (400mg tid) $T_{1/2}$=5.8 hrs.

NURSING CONSIDERATIONS

Assessment: Assess for hypersensitivity, achlorhydria, hepatic impairment, pregnancy/nursing status, and possible drug interactions.

Monitoring: Monitor for severe rash or rash accompanied by symptoms (eg, fever, blistering, oral lesions, conjunctivitis, swelling, muscle joint aches), immune reconstitution syndrome, cross-resistance to other NNRTIs, fat redistribution, and other adverse reactions.

Patient Counseling: Inform patient that drug is not a cure for HIV-1 infection and that they may continue to experience illnesses associated with HIV-1 infection. Advise to avoid doing things that can spread HIV-1 infection to others. Inform to take as prescribed and to not alter the dose without consulting the physician. Advise patients with achlorhydria to take with acidic beverage (eg, orange or cranberry juice). Inform to take at least 1 hr apart if taking antacids. Advise to d/c and seek medical attention if severe rash or rash with symptoms such as fever, blistering, oral lesions, conjunctivitis, swelling, muscle or joint aches occur. Counsel that fat redistribution may occur. Advise to report use of any prescription or nonprescription medication or herbal products, particularly St. John's wort. Inform patients receiving sildenafil about increased risk of sildenafil-associated adverse events (eg, hypotension, visual changes, prolonged penile erection), and in-struct to promptly report any symptoms to the physician. Counsel to notify physician if pregnant or breastfeeding.

Administration: Oral route. Take with or without food. May disperse 100mg tabs in water prior to consumption. 200mg tabs should be taken as intact tabs. Refer to PI on how to prepare disper-sion. **Storage:** 20-25°C (68-77°F). Protect from high humidity.

R

RESTASIS   RX
cyclosporine (Allergan)

THERAPEUTIC CLASS: Topical immunomodulator

INDICATIONS: To increase tear production in patients whose tear production is presumed to be suppressed due to ocular inflammation associated with keratoconjunctivitis sicca.

DOSAGE: *Adults:* Instill 1 drop in ou q12h. With Artificial Tears: Allow 15-min interval between products.
Pediatrics: ≥16 Yrs: Instill 1 drop in ou q12h. With Artificial Tears: Allow 15-min interval between products.

HOW SUPPLIED: Emulsion: 0.05% [0.4mL]

WARNINGS/PRECAUTIONS: Increased tear production not seen in patients currently taking topical anti-inflammatory drugs or using punctal plugs. Do not touch vial tip to the eye or other surfaces to avoid the potential for eye injury and contamination. Do not administer in patients wearing contact lenses. Remove contact lenses prior to administration; may reinsert 15 min after administration.

ADVERSE REACTIONS: Ocular burning, conjunctival hyperemia, discharge, epiphora, eye pain, foreign body sensation, pruritus, stinging, visual disturbance (eg, blurring).

PREGNANCY: Category C, caution in nursing.

MECHANISM OF ACTION: Topical immunomodulator; not established. Thought to act as a partial immunomodulator.

PHARMACOKINETICS: Distribution: Found in breast milk (systemic administration).

NURSING CONSIDERATIONS

Assessment: Assess for hypersensitivity, contact lens use, and pregnancy/nursing status.

Monitoring: Monitor for signs/symptoms of ocular burning and other adverse reactions.

Patient Counseling: Instruct not to allow the vial tip to touch the eye or any surface. Advise to remove contact lenses before administration; inform that lenses may be reinserted 15 min following administration. Advise to use single-use vial immediately after opening and to discard the remaining contents immediately after administration.

Administration: Ocular route. Invert unit dose vial a few times to obtain uniform, white, opaque emulsion before using. **Storage:** 15-25°C (59-77°F).

RESTORIL   CIV
temazepam (Mallinckrodt)

THERAPEUTIC CLASS: Benzodiazepine

INDICATIONS: Short-term treatment of insomnia (7-10 days).

DOSAGE: *Adults:* Administer hs. Usual: 15mg. Range: 7.5-30mg. Transient Insomnia: 7.5mg may be sufficient. Elderly/Debilitated: Initiate with 7.5mg.

HOW SUPPLIED: Cap: 7.5mg, 15mg, 22.5mg, 30mg

CONTRAINDICATIONS: Women who are or may become pregnant.

WARNINGS/PRECAUTIONS: Initiate only after careful evaluation; failure of insomnia to remit after 7-10 days of treatment may indicate primary psychiatric and/or medical illness. Worsening of insomnia and emergence of thinking or behavior abnormalities may occur especially in elderly; use lowest possible effective dose. Behavioral changes (eg, decreased inhibition, bizarre behavior, agitation, hallucinations, depersonalization) and complex behavior (eg, sleep-driving) reported; strongly consider discontinuation if sleep-driving episode occurs. Amnesia and other neuropsychiatric symptoms may occur unpredictably. Worsening of depression, including suicidal thinking, reported. Withdrawal symptoms may occur after abrupt discontinuation. Rare cases of angioedema and anaphylaxis reported; do not rechallenge. Oversedation, confusion, and/or ataxia may develop with large doses in elderly and debilitated patients. Caution with hepatic/renal impairment, chronic pulmonary insufficiency, debilitated, severe or latent depression, and in elderly. Abnormal LFTs, renal function tests, and blood dyscrasias reported.

ADVERSE REACTIONS: Drowsiness, headache, fatigue, nervousness, lethargy, dizziness, nausea.

INTERACTIONS: Increased risk of complex behaviors with alcohol and CNS depressants. Potential additive effects with hypnotics and CNS depressants. Possible synergistic effect with diphenhydramine.

PREGNANCY: Category X, caution in nursing.

MECHANISM OF ACTION: Benzodiazepine hypnotic agent.

PHARMACOKINETICS: Absorption: Well-absorbed; C_{max}=865ng/mL; T_{max}=1.5 hrs. **Distribution:** Plasma protein binding (96% unchanged); crosses placenta. **Metabolism:** Complete; conjugation. **Elimination:** Urine (80-90%); $T_{1/2}$=3.5-18.4 hrs.

NURSING CONSIDERATIONS

Assessment: Assess for physical and/or psychiatric disorder, medical illness, severe or latent depression, renal/hepatic dysfunction, chronic pulmonary insufficiency, pregnancy/nursing status, alcohol use, and possible drug interactions.

Monitoring: Monitor for signs/symptoms of withdrawal, tolerance, abuse, dependence, abnormal thinking, behavioral changes, agitation, depersonalization, hallucinations, complex behaviors, amnesia, anxiety, neuropsychiatric symptoms, worsening of depression, suicidal thoughts and actions, angioedema, driving/psychomotor impairment, worsening of insomnia, thinking or behavioral abnormalities, and possible abuse/dependence.

Patient Counseling: Inform about the benefits and risks of treatment. Instruct patient to take as prescribed. Inform about the risks and possibility of physical/psychological dependence, memory problems, and complex behaviors (eg, sleep-driving). Caution against hazardous tasks (eg, operating machinery/driving). Advise not to drink alcohol. Instruct to notify physician if pregnant/planning to become pregnant.

Administration: Oral route. **Storage:** 20-25°C (68-77°F).

RETAVASE
reteplase (EKR)

RX

THERAPEUTIC CLASS: Thrombolytic agent

INDICATIONS: Management of acute myocardial infarction (AMI) in adults for the improvement of ventricular function following AMI, reduction of the incidence of congestive heart failure (CHF), and the reduction of mortality associated with AMI.

DOSAGE: *Adults:* Administer two 10 U bolus injections. Administer each bolus as IV inj over 2 min. Give 2nd bolus 30 min after 1st bolus inj. Do not administer other medications simultaneously via the same IV line.

HOW SUPPLIED: Inj: 10.4 U (18.1mg)

CONTRAINDICATIONS: Active internal bleeding; history of cerebrovascular accident (CVA); recent intracranial or intraspinal surgery or trauma; intracranial neoplasm; arteriovenous malformation or aneurysm; known bleeding diathesis; severe uncontrolled HTN.

WARNINGS/PRECAUTIONS: Bleeding is the most common complication during therapy; careful attention to all potential bleeding sites is required. If arterial puncture is necessary during administration, use an upper extremity vessel that is accessible to manual compression. Avoid IM inj and nonessential handling of patients. Perform venipuncture carefully and only if required. Weigh benefits/risks of therapy with recent major surgery, previous puncture of noncompressible vessels, cerebrovascular disease, recent GI or genitourinary (GU) bleeding, recent trauma, HTN, high likelihood of left heart thrombus, acute pericarditis, subacute bacterial endocarditis, hemostatic defects, severe hepatic or renal dysfunction, pregnancy, diabetic hemorrhagic retinopathy or other hemorrhagic ophthalmic conditions, septic thrombophlebitis or occluded AV cannula at a seriously infected site, advanced age, or any other condition in which bleeding would constitute a significant hazard or be difficult to manage. Cholesterol embolism reported. Coronary thrombolysis may result in arrhythmias associated with reperfusion. Do not administer 2nd bolus if an anaphylactoid reaction occurs. May affect results of coagulation tests and/or measurements of fibrinolytic activity.

ADVERSE REACTIONS: Bleeding, allergic reactions.

INTERACTIONS: Increased risk of bleeding with heparin, vitamin K antagonists, and drugs that alter platelet function (eg, ASA, dipyridamole, abciximab) if administered before, during, or after therapy. Concomitant use of anticoagulant therapy should be terminated if serious bleeding occurs.

PREGNANCY: Category C, caution in nursing.

MECHANISM OF ACTION: Thrombolytic agent; recombinant plasminogen activator that catalyzes the cleavage of endogenous plasminogen to generate plasmin. Plasmin in turn degrades the fibrin matrix of the thrombus, thereby exerting its thrombolytic action.

PHARMACOKINETICS: Metabolism: Hepatic. **Elimination:** Renal; $T_{1/2}$=13-16 min.

NURSING CONSIDERATIONS

Assessment: Assess for active internal bleeding, history of CVA, or any other conditions where treatment is contraindicated or cautioned. Assess for age, renal/hepatic function, pregnancy/nursing status, and possible drug interactions.

Monitoring: Monitor for signs/symptoms of bleeding, internal and superficial bleeding sites, bleeding at recent puncture sites, cholesterol embolism (eg, livedo reticularis, "purple toe" syndrome, MI, cerebral infarction, HTN, gangrenous digits), and arrhythmias. Monitor renal/hepatic function.

Patient Counseling: Inform the patient about the risks and benefits of the therapy. Instruct to contact physician if any unusual bleeding occurs or if any other adverse reaction develops. Advise to avoid IM injections while on therapy.

Administration: IV route. Refer to the PI for administration and reconstitution instructions. **Storage:** Unused vial: 2-25°C (36-77°F). Box should remain sealed until use to protect the lyophilisate from exposure to light. Reconstituted: 2-30°C (36-86°F); use within 4 hrs.

RETIN-A
tretinoin (Ortho Neutrogena)

RX

OTHER BRAND NAMES: Retin-A Micro (Ortho Neutrogena)

THERAPEUTIC CLASS: Retinoid

INDICATIONS: Topical treatment of acne vulgaris.

DOSAGE: *Adults:* Apply qpm/before retiring, to the skin where acne lesions appear, using enough to cover the entire effected area lightly. If the degree of local irritation warrants, d/c use temporarily, or d/c use altogether.
Pediatrics: ≥12 Yrs: (Retin-A Micro) Apply qpm, to the skin where acne lesions appear, using enough to cover the entire effected area lightly. If the degree of local irritation warrants, d/c use temporarily, or d/c use altogether.

HOW SUPPLIED: (Retin-A) Cre: 0.025%, 0.05%, 0.1% [20g, 45g]; Gel: 0.01%, 0.025% [15g, 45g]; (Retin-A Micro) Gel: 0.04%, 0.1% [20g, 45g, 50g]

WARNINGS/PRECAUTIONS: D/C therapy if a reaction suggesting sensitivity or chemical irritation occurs. Minimize exposure to sunlight, including sunlamps; avoid use with sunburn until fully recovered. Caution in patients who may be required to have considerable sun exposure and those with inherent sensitivity to sun. Use of sunscreen products and protective clothing over treated areas is recommended when exposure cannot be avoided. Extreme weather (eg, cold, wind) may irritate skin. Avoid eyes, lips, paranasal creases/angles of the nose, and mucous membranes. May cause transitory feeling of warmth or slight stinging; temporarily d/c use or reduce the frequency of application. Caution with severe irritation on eczematous skin. An apparent exacerbation of inflammatory lesions may occur during early weeks of therapy. (Retin-A) May induce severe skin local erythema and peeling at application site. Gels are flammable. (Retin-A Micro) Excessive dryness may be experienced; use an appropriate emollient during the day may be helpful.

ADVERSE REACTIONS: Red/edematous/blistered/crusted skin, hyper-/hypopigmentation.

INTERACTIONS: Caution with topical medications, medicated/abrasive soaps and cleansers, products with strong drying effect, products with high concentrations of alcohol, astringents, spices, or lime (Retin-A). Caution with preparations containing sulfur, resorcinol, or salicylic acid; allow effects of these agents to subside before initiation of treatment. (Retin-A Micro) Avoid contact with peel of limes. Caution with concomitant topical OTC acne preparations containing benzoyl peroxide.

PREGNANCY: Category C, caution in nursing.

MECHANISM OF ACTION: Retinoic acid derivative; not established. Responsible for decreasing cohesiveness of follicular epithelial cells with decreased microcomedo formation. Also, stimulates mitotic activity and increases turnover rate of follicular epithelial cells, causing extrusion of comedones.

NURSING CONSIDERATIONS

Assessment: Assess for drug hypersensitivity, sun exposure, sensitivity to sun, sunburn, eczematous skin, pregnancy/nursing status, and possible drug interactions.

Monitoring: Monitor for sensitivity reactions, irritation, local erythema or peeling at application site, and other adverse reactions. Closely monitor alterations of vehicle, drug concentration, or dose frequency by carefully observing therapeutic response and skin tolerance.

Patient Counseling: Instruct to d/c use and consult physician if irritation occurs. Advise to minimize exposure to sunlight, including sunlamps, or use sunscreen products and protective clothing over treated areas when exposure to sun cannot be avoided. Inform that weather extremes (eg, wind, cold) may be irritating to treated skin. Instruct to use ud, and to keep away from eyes, mouth, angles of the nose, and mucous membranes. Advise to inform physician of other topical medication or preparations being used, and if pregnant or breastfeeding. Inform that during the early weeks of therapy, an apparent exacerbation of inflammatory lesions may occur, which should not be considered a reason for discontinuation.

Administration: Topical route. If using cosmetics, thoroughly clean the areas to be treated before applying the medication. Refer to PI for further administration instructions. **Storage:** (Retin-A) Gel: <30°C (86°F). Cre: <27°C (80°F). (Retin-A Micro) Gel: 15-25°C (59-77°F).

RETROVIR

RX

zidovudine (ViiV Healthcare)

> Associated with hematologic toxicity (eg, neutropenia, severe anemia), particularly with advanced HIV-1 disease. Symptomatic myopathy associated with prolonged use. Lactic acidosis and severe hepatomegaly with steatosis, including fatal cases, reported with nucleoside analogues; suspend treatment if lactic acidosis or pronounced hepatotoxicity occurs.

THERAPEUTIC CLASS: Nucleoside reverse transcriptase inhibitor

INDICATIONS: Treatment of HIV-1 infection in combination with other antiretrovirals. Prevention of maternal-fetal HIV-1 transmission.

DOSAGE: *Adults:* HIV-1 Infection: (PO) 600mg/day in divided doses. (Inj) 1mg/kg IV over 1 hr 5-6X/day. Use only until PO therapy can be administered. Maternal-Fetal HIV Transmission: >14 Weeks of Pregnancy: Maternal Dosing: 100mg PO 5X/day until start of labor. During Labor and Delivery: 2mg/kg IV over 1 hr followed by continuous IV infusion of 1mg/kg/hr until clamping of umbilical cord. End-Stage Renal Disease (ESRD) on Dialysis: 100mg PO q6-8h or 1mg/kg IV q6-8h. Significant Anemia/Neutropenia: May require dose interruption and may resume therapy with adjunctive epoetin alfa therapy if marrow recovery occurs.
Pediatrics: HIV-1 Infection: 4 Weeks-<18 Yrs: (PO) BSA Based: 480mg/m²/day in divided doses (240mg/m² bid or 160mg/m² tid). Weight Based: ≥30kg: 300mg bid or 200mg tid. ≥9-<30kg: 9mg/kg bid or 6mg/kg tid. 4-<9kg: 12mg/kg bid or 8mg/kg tid. Maternal-Fetal HIV Transmission: Neonates: 2mg/kg PO q6h or 1.5mg/kg IV over 30 min q6h, starting within 12 hrs after birth and continuing through 6 weeks of age. ESRD on Dialysis: 100mg PO q6-8h or 1mg/kg IV q6-8h. Significant Anemia/Neutropenia: May require dose interruption and may resume therapy with adjunctive epoetin alfa therapy if marrow recovery occurs.

HOW SUPPLIED: Cap: 100mg; Inj: 10mg/mL [20mL]; Syrup: 10mg/mL [240mL]; Tab: 300mg

WARNINGS/PRECAUTIONS: Caution with granulocyte count <1000 cells/mm³ or Hgb <9.5g/dL; monitor blood counts frequently in patients with poor bone marrow reserve, particularly with advanced HIV-1 disease and periodically with other HIV-infected patients and with asymptomatic/early HIV-1 disease. If anemia or neutropenia develops, dosage adjustment/interruption may be necessary. Obesity and prolonged nucleoside exposure may be risk factors for lactic acidosis and severe hepatomegaly with steatosis. Caution with any known risk factors for liver disease and in elderly. Pancytopenia and immune reconstitution syndrome reported. Autoimmune disorders (eg, Graves' disease, polymyositis, Guillain-Barre syndrome) reported to occur in the setting of immune reconstitution and can occur many months after initiation of treatment. Reduce dose in severe renal impairment (CrCl <15mL/min). (PO) May cause redistribution/accumulation of body fat.

ADVERSE REACTIONS: Hematologic toxicity, myopathy, lactic acidosis, severe hepatomegaly with steatosis, headache, N/V, malaise, anorexia, asthenia, constipation, abdominal pain/cramps, arthralgia, chills.

INTERACTIONS: Avoid with stavudine, nucleoside analogues affecting DNA replication (eg, ribavirin), doxorubicin, and other combination products containing zidovudine. Hepatic decompensation may occur in HIV/hepatitis C virus (HCV) coinfected patients receiving interferon alfa with or without ribavirin; closely monitor for treatment-associated toxicities. May increase risk of hematologic toxicities with ganciclovir, interferon alfa, ribavirin, and other bone marrow suppressive or cytotoxic agents.

PREGNANCY: Category C, not for use in nursing.

MECHANISM OF ACTION: Synthetic nucleoside analogue; inhibits reverse transcriptase via DNA chain termination after incorporation of the nucleotide analogue.

PHARMACOKINETICS: Absorption: (PO) Rapid. Bioavailability (64%); T_{max}=0.5-1.5 hrs. (IV) C_{max}=1.06mcg/mL. **Distribution:** V_d=1.6L/kg; plasma protein binding (<38%); crosses the placenta; found in breast milk. **Metabolism:** Hepatic. 3'-azido-3'-deoxy-5'-O-β-D-glucopyranuronosylthymidine (major metabolite). **Elimination:** (PO) Urine (14% unchanged, 74% metabolite); $T_{1/2}$=0.5-3 hrs. (IV) Urine (18% unchanged, 60% metabolite); $T_{1/2}$=1.1 hrs. Refer to PI for pediatric patients and patients with renal impairment pharmacokinetic parameters.

NURSING CONSIDERATIONS

Assessment: Assess for hypersensitivity reactions, advanced HIV disease, risk factors for lactic acidosis, risk factors for liver disease, bone marrow compromise, renal/hepatic impairment, pregnancy/nursing status, and possible drug interactions. (PO) Assess ability to swallow cap or tab in children.

Monitoring: Monitor for signs/symptoms of hematologic toxicity, lactic acidosis, hepatomegaly with steatosis, myopathy, immune reconstitution syndrome, autoimmune disorders, fat redistribution/accumulation, and other adverse reactions. Monitor blood counts/hematologic indices periodically and the need for dosage adjustment.

Patient Counseling: Inform about risk for hematologic toxicities and advise on importance of close blood count monitoring while on therapy. Counsel about the possible occurrence of myopathy and myositis with pathological changes during prolonged use and that therapy may cause a rare but serious condition called lactic acidosis with liver enlargement (hepatomegaly). Inform that hepatic decompensation has occurred in HIV-1/HCV coinfected patients receiving combination antiretroviral therapy and interferon alfa with or without ribavirin. Instruct to avoid use with combination products that contain zidovudine. Inform that redistribution/accumulation of body fat may occur. Inform that the drug may cause headache, malaise, N/V, and anorexia in adults and fever, cough, and digestive disorders in pediatric patients. Advise to consult a physician if muscle weakness, SOB, symptoms of hepatitis or pancreatitis, or any other unexpected adverse events occur. Counsel that use of other medications may exacerbate toxicity. Inform pregnant women that HIV transmission may still occur in some cases despite therapy; instruct not to

R

breastfeed to prevent postnatal transmission. Inform that drug is not a cure for HIV-1 infection and that illness associated with HIV-1 may still be experienced. Advise to avoid doing things that can spread HIV-1 infection to others (eg, sharing of needles/inj equipment/personal items that can have blood or body fluids on them, having sex without protection, breastfeeding). Inform patients to take all HIV medications exactly as prescribed.

Administration: IV/Oral route. (PO) Take with or without food. (IV) Avoid rapid infusion and bolus inj; do not give IM. Refer to PI for method of preparation. **Storage:** (IV) 15-25°C (59-77°F). Protect from light. Diluted Sol: Stable for 24 hrs at room temperature and for 48 hrs if refrigerated at 2-8°C (36-46°F). Administer within 8 hrs if stored at 25°C (77°F) or 24 hrs if refrigerated at 2-8°C (36-46°F) to minimize contamination. (PO) 15-25°C (59-77°F). Protect caps from moisture.

REVATIO   RX
sildenafil (Pfizer)

THERAPEUTIC CLASS: Phosphodiesterase type 5 inhibitor

INDICATIONS: Treatment of pulmonary arterial HTN (PAH) (WHO Group I) in adults to improve exercise ability and delay clinical worsening.

DOSAGE: *Adults:* PO: 5mg or 20mg tid, 4-6 hrs apart. Max: 20mg tid. IV: 2.5mg or 10mg IV bolus tid.

HOW SUPPLIED: Inj: 10mg [12.5mL]; Sus: 10mg/mL [112mL]; Tab: 20mg

CONTRAINDICATIONS: Organic nitrates in any form, either regularly/intermittently.

WARNINGS/PRECAUTIONS: Adding sildenafil to bosentan therapy does not result in any beneficial effect on exercise capacity. Not recommended in children. Vasodilatory effects may adversely affect patients with resting hypotension (BP <90/50), fluid depletion, severe left ventricular outflow obstruction, or autonomic dysfunction. Not recommended with pulmonary veno-occlusive disease (PVOD); consider possibility of associated PVOD if signs of pulmonary edema occur. Non-arteritic anterior ischemic optic neuropathy (NAION) reported; seek immediate medical attention if sudden loss of vision in 1 or both eyes occurs. Caution with previous NAION in 1 eye and with retinitis pigmentosa. Cases of sudden decrease or loss of hearing, which may be accompanied by tinnitus and dizziness, reported. Caution in patients with anatomical penile deformation (eg, angulation, cavernosal fibrosis, Peyronie's disease) or with predisposition to priapism (eg, sickle-cell anemia, multiple myeloma, leukemia). Penile tissue damage and permanent loss of potency may result if priapism is not immediately treated. Vaso-occlusive crises requiring hospitalization reported in patients with pulmonary HTN secondary to sickle-cell disease. Caution in elderly. (Inj) Used as continued treatment in patients currently taking tab/sus and who are temporarily unable to take PO medication.

ADVERSE REACTIONS: Headache, dyspepsia, edema, epistaxis, pain in extremities, flushing, diarrhea, insomnia, dyspnea exacerbation, myalgia, nausea, nasal congestion, erythema, pyrexia, rhinitis.

INTERACTIONS: See Contraindications. Vasodilatory effects may adversely affect patients on antihypertensive therapy; monitor BP when given with antihypertensives. Reports of epistaxis with oral vitamin K antagonists. Retinal and eye hemorrhage reported with anticoagulants. Avoid with other PDE-5 inhibitors. Not recommended with ritonavir and other potent CYP3A inhibitors. Symptomatic postural hypotension with doxazosin reported. Additional reduction of supine BP with oral amlodipine reported.

PREGNANCY: Category B, caution in nursing.

MECHANISM OF ACTION: PDE-5 inhibitor; increases cGMP within pulmonary vascular smooth muscle cells, resulting in relaxation and vasodilation of pulmonary vascular bed and systemic circulation.

PHARMACOKINETICS: Absorption: (PO) Rapid; absolute bioavailability (41%); T_{max}=60 min (median) (fasted state). **Distribution:** V_d=105L; plasma protein binding (96%). **Metabolism:** CYP3A (major route) and CYP2C9 (minor route); N-desmethyl metabolite (active metabolite). **Elimination:** Feces (80% metabolites), urine (13% metabolites); $T_{1/2}$=4 hrs.

NURSING CONSIDERATIONS

Assessment: Assess for hypotension, fluid depletion, left ventricular outflow obstruction, autonomic dysfunction, PVOD, "crowded disc", age >50, diabetes, HTN, coronary artery disease, hyperlipidemia, smoking, previous NAION in one eye, retinitis pigmentosa, anatomical deformities of the penis, conditions predisposing to priapism, pulmonary HTN secondary to sickle-cell disease, hypersensitivity to drug, nursing/pregnancy status, and possible drug interactions. Obtain baseline BP.

Monitoring: Monitor for signs of pulmonary edema, decreased/sudden loss of vision or hearing, tinnitus, dizziness, epistaxis, priapism, vaso-occlusive crises, and hypersensitivity reactions. Monitor BP.

Patient Counseling: Counsel about risks and benefits of the drug. Inform that drug is also marketed as Viagra for male erectile dysfunction. Advise not to take Viagra or other PDE-5 inhibitors and organic nitrates during therapy. Advise to notify physician if sudden decrease/loss of vision or hearing occurs. Instruct to seek immediate medical attention if an erection persists >4 hrs.

Administration: Oral, IV route. Refer to PI for reconstitution of the powder for oral sus. **Storage:** (Tab, IV) 20-25°C (68-77°F); excursions permitted to 15-30°C (59-86°F). (Sus) <30°C (86°F). Protect from moisture. Constituted: <30°C (86°F) or 2-8°C (36-46°F). Do not freeze. Shelf-life: 60 days.

REVLIMID

lenalidomide (Celgene)

RX

Do not use during pregnancy; may cause birth defects or embryo-fetal death. Females of reproductive potential should have 2 negative pregnancy tests prior to treatment and must use 2 forms of contraception or continuously abstain from heterosexual sex during and for 4 weeks after treatment. Available only through a restricted distribution program, the Revlimid REMS program. May cause significant neutropenia and thrombocytopenia. Patients on therapy for del 5q myelodysplastic syndromes (MDS) should have their CBC monitored weekly for the first 8 weeks of therapy and at least monthly thereafter; may require dose interruption and/or reduction and use of blood product support and/or growth factors. Increased risk of deep vein thrombosis (DVT) and pulmonary embolism (PE) reported in patients with multiple myeloma treated with lenalidomide and dexamethasone; observe for signs/symptoms of thromboembolism. Instruct patients to seek medical care if symptoms such as SOB, chest pain, or arm or leg swelling develop. Consider taking prophylactic measures for venous thromboembolism based on assessment of individual's underlying risk factors.

THERAPEUTIC CLASS: Thalidomide analog

INDICATIONS: Treatment of transfusion-dependent anemia due to low- or intermediate-1-risk MDS associated with a deletion 5q cytogenetic abnormality with or without additional cytogenetic abnormalities. In combination with dexamethasone, for the treatment of multiple myeloma (MM) in patients who have received at least 1 prior therapy. Treatment of patients with mantle cell lymphoma (MCL) whose disease has relapsed or progressed after 2 prior therapies, 1 of which included bortezomib.

DOSAGE: *Adults:* MDS-Associated Anemia: Initial: 10mg/day. MM: Initial: 25mg qd on Days 1-21 of repeated 28-day cycles. Give dexamethasone 40mg qd on Days 1-4, 9-12, and 17-20 of each 28-day cycle for the first 4 cycles, then on Days 1-4 every 28 days. MCL: Initial: 25mg/day on Days 1-21 of repeated 28-day cycles for relapsed or refractory MCL. Continue treatment until disease progression or unacceptable toxicity. Renal Impairment: MDS-Associated Anemia: Moderate (CrCl 30-60mL/min): 5mg q24h. Severe (CrCl <30mL/min Not Requiring Dialysis): 2.5mg q24h. End-Stage Renal Disease (ESRD) (CrCl <30mL/min Requiring Dialysis): 2.5mg qd; on dialysis days, administer dose following dialysis. MM/MCL: Moderate (CrCl 30-60mL/min): 10mg q24h. Severe (CrCl <30mL/min Not Requiring Dialysis): 15mg q48h. ESRD (CrCl <30mL/min Requiring Dialysis): 5mg qd; on dialysis days, administer dose following dialysis. Refer to PI for dose adjustments based on platelet and/or absolute neutrophil counts.

HOW SUPPLIED: Cap: 2.5mg, 5mg, 10mg, 15mg, 20mg, 25mg

CONTRAINDICATIONS: Pregnancy.

WARNINGS/PRECAUTIONS: Not indicated and not recommended for the treatment of patients with chronic lymphocytic leukemia outside of controlled clinical trials; increased risk of death and serious adverse cardiovascular (CV) reactions reported. Avoid pregnancy for at least 4 weeks before beginning therapy, during therapy, during dose interruptions, and for at least 4 weeks after completing therapy; perform appropriate pregnancy tests prior to and during therapy. Male patients (including those who had a vasectomy) must always use a latex/synthetic condom during any sexual contact with females of reproductive potential during therapy and for up to 28 days after discontinuing therapy. Avoid sperm donation during therapy. Avoid blood donation during treatment and for 1 month following discontinuation. Patients on therapy for MM should have their CBC monitored every 2 weeks for the first 12 weeks of therapy and then monthly thereafter. Patients on therapy for MCL should have their CBC monitored weekly for the 1st cycle (28 days), every 2 weeks during cycles 2-4, and then monthly thereafter. Higher incidence of 2nd primary malignancies (particularly acute myelogenous leukemia and Hodgkin lymphoma) reported in patients with MM. Hepatic failure, including fatal cases, reported in combination with dexamethasone. D/C treatment upon elevation of liver enzymes and consider treatment at a lower dose after values return to baseline. Angioedema and serious dermatologic reactions reported; d/c if angioedema, Stevens-Johnson syndrome (SJS), toxic epidermal necrolysis (TEN), Grade 4 rash, or exfoliative or bullous rash is suspected and do not resume for these reactions. Consider treatment interruption or discontinuation for Grade 2-3 skin rash. Avoid with a prior history of Grade 4 rash associated with thalidomide treatment. Contains lactose. Tumor lysis syndrome reported; caution in patients with high tumor burden prior to treatment and monitor closely. Tumor flare reaction (TFR) reported in patients with MCL; withhold treatment in patients with Grade 3 or 4 TFR until TFR resolves to ≤Grade 1. Caution with renal impairment and in the elderly.

R

ADVERSE REACTIONS: Thrombocytopenia, neutropenia, PE, pruritus, rash, diarrhea, constipation, nausea, anemia, arthralgia, cough, pyrexia, peripheral edema, dizziness.

INTERACTIONS: May increase levels of digoxin; monitor digoxin levels periodically. Closely monitor PT and INR with warfarin in MM patients. Caution with erythropoietic agents or other agents that may increase risk of thrombosis (eg, estrogen-containing therapies) in MM patients.

PREGNANCY: Category X, not for use in nursing.

MECHANISM OF ACTION: Thalidomide analog; with immunomodulatory, antiangiogenic, and antineoplastic properties. Inhibits proliferation and induces apoptosis of certain hematopoietic tumor cells. Immunomodulatory properties include activation of T cells and natural killer (NK) cells, increased numbers of NKT cells, and inhibition of proinflammatory cytokines (eg, TNF-α and IL-6) by monocytes.

PHARMACOKINETICS: Absorption: Rapid. (Single/Multiple Dose) T_{max}=0.5-6 hrs. **Distribution:** Plasma protein binding (30%). **Metabolism:** Hydroxy-lenalidomide and N-acetyl-lenalidomide (metabolites). **Elimination:** Urine (90%, 82% unchanged), feces (4%); $T_{1/2}$=3-5 hrs.

NURSING CONSIDERATIONS

Assessment: Assess for renal/hepatic impairment, history of Grade 4 rash, risk factors for venous thromboembolism, high tumor burden, lactose intolerance, hypersensitivity to the drug, pregnancy/nursing status, and possible drug interactions. Perform pregnancy test 10-14 days before and 24 hrs prior to therapy. Obtain baseline CBC.

Monitoring: Monitor for signs/symptoms of venous thromboembolism, neutropenia, thrombocytopenia, angioedema, SJS, TEN, tumor lysis syndrome, TFR, 2nd primary malignancies, serious adverse CV reactions, and other adverse reactions. Perform pregnancy test weekly during 1st month, then repeat monthly (regular menstrual cycle) or every 2 weeks (irregular menstrual cycle) and perform pregnancy test if period is missed or if there is any abnormality with the patient's menstrual bleeding. Monitor CBC weekly for the first 8 weeks of therapy and monthly thereafter (MDS); every 2 weeks for the first 12 weeks and monthly thereafter (MM); weekly for the 1st cycle (28 days), every 2 weeks during cycles 2-4, and monthly thereafter (MCL). Monitor renal/hepatic function. Closely monitor PT and INR with warfarin in MM patients.

Patient Counseling: Instruct females of reproductive potential to avoid pregnancy, have monthly pregnancy tests, and to use 2 different forms of contraception, including at least 1 highly effective form simultaneously during therapy, during dose interruption, and for 4 weeks after completing therapy. Instruct to immediately d/c and contact physician if patient becomes pregnant, misses her menstrual period, experiences unusual menstrual bleeding, or if she stops taking birth control. Instruct males (including those who had a vasectomy) to always use a latex/synthetic condom during any sexual contact with females of reproductive potential during therapy and for up to 28 days after discontinuing therapy. Advise males not to donate sperm. Instruct not to donate blood during therapy, during dose interruptions, and for 1 month following discontinuation. Inform of the other risks associated with therapy. Instruct that if a dose is missed, may still take dose up to 12 hrs after the time dose is normally taken. Advise that if >12 hrs have elapsed, the dose for that day should be skipped; the dose for the next day should be taken at the usual time.

Administration: Oral route. Take at about the same time each day, with or without food. Swallow cap whole with water; do not open, crush, break, or chew. Wash the skin immediately and thoroughly with soap and water if powder from cap gets in contact with the skin. If drug contacts the mucous membranes, flush thoroughly with water. **Storage:** 20-25°C (68-77°F); excursions permitted to 15-30°C (59-86°F).

REYATAZ

RX

atazanavir sulfate (Bristol-Myers Squibb)

THERAPEUTIC CLASS: Protease inhibitor

INDICATIONS: Treatment of HIV-1 infection in combination with other antiretrovirals.

DOSAGE: *Adults:* Take with food. Therapy-Naive: 300mg with ritonavir (RTV) 100mg qd. If intolerant to RTV, give atazanavir (ATV) 400mg qd. End-Stage Renal Disease (ESRD) with Hemodialysis: 300mg with RTV 100mg. Therapy-Experienced: 300mg with RTV 100mg qd. 2nd/3rd Trimester Pregnancy with H_2-Receptor Antagonist or Tenofovir: 400mg with RTV 100mg qd. Moderate Hepatic Impairment (Child-Pugh Class B) Without Prior Virologic Failure: Consider 300mg qd.
Pediatrics: Take with food. 6-<18 Yrs: ≥40kg: 300mg with RTV 100mg qd. 20-<40kg: 200mg with RTV 100mg qd. 15-<20kg: 150mg with RTV 100mg qd. Therapy-Naive: ≥13 Yrs and ≥40kg: If intolerant to RTV, give ATV 400mg (without RTV) qd. Do not exceed recommended adult dose.

HOW SUPPLIED: Cap: 150mg, 200mg, 300mg

CONTRAINDICATIONS: Coadministration with CYP3A or UGT1A1 substrates, and drugs for which elevated plasma concentrations are associated with serious and/or life-threatening events, and

R

other drugs (eg, alfuzosin, rifampin, irinotecan, triazolam, oral midazolam, dihydroergotamine, ergotamine, ergonovine, methylergonovine, cisapride, St. John's wort, lovastatin, simvastatin, pimozide, sildenafil when used for pulmonary arterial HTN, indinavir).

WARNINGS/PRECAUTIONS: Not recommended without RTV for treatment-experienced adults/ pediatric patients with prior virologic failure and during pregnancy or postpartum period. Should not be administered to HIV treatment-experienced patients with ESRD managed with hemo-dialysis. Caution with mild to moderate hepatic impairment. Avoid with severe hepatic impairment. ATV/RTV is not recommended with hepatic impairment. May prolong PR interval; caution with preexisting conduction system diseases or with drugs that prolong PR interval. Rash and cases of Stevens-Johnson syndrome, erythema multiforme, and toxic skin eruptions, including drug rash with eosinophilia and systemic symptoms (DRESS) syndrome, reported; d/c if severe rash develops. May cause hyperbilirubinemia; dose reduction is not recommended and alternative antiretroviral therapy may be considered with jaundice or scleral icterus. Increased risk for further transaminase elevations or hepatic decompensation in patients with underlying hepatitis B or C infections or marked transaminase elevations; conduct LFTs prior to and during treatment. Nephrolithiasis and/or cholelithiasis reported; consider temporary interruption or discontinuation of therapy if signs/symptoms occur. New onset or exacerbation of diabetes mellitus (DM), hyperglycemia, diabetic ketoacidosis, immune reconstitution syndrome, autoimmune disorders (eg, Graves' disease, polymyositis, Guillain-Barre syndrome) in the setting of immune reconstitution, redistribution/accumulation of body fat, and increased bleeding with hemophilia A and B reported. Various degrees of cross-resistance observed. Caution in elderly.

ADVERSE REACTIONS: N/V, jaundice/scleral icterus, rash, myalgia, headache, abdominal pain, insomnia, peripheral neurologic symptoms, diarrhea, fever, AST/ALT elevations, neutropenia, hypoglycemia, extremity pain.

INTERACTIONS: See Contraindications. Not recommended with nevirapine, salmeterol, or (without RTV) tenofovir, carbamazepine, phenytoin, phenobarbital, bosentan, and buprenorphine. ATV/RTV is not recommended with other protease inhibitors, voriconazole, fluticasone propionate, and boceprevir. Avoid with efavirenz or PPIs in treatment-experienced patients. Avoid with colchicine in patients with renal/hepatic impairment. Caution with CYP2C8 substrates with narrow therapeutic indices (eg, paclitaxel, repaglinide) and oral contraceptives. CYP3A4 inducers, tenofovir, nevirapine, carbamazepine, boceprevir, phenytoin, phenobarbital, bosentan, efavirenz, PPIs, antacids, buffered medications, and H_2-receptor antagonists may decrease levels. Telaprevir, RTV, and clarithromycin may increase levels. Administer at least 2 hrs before or 1 hr after buffered formulations (eg, didanosine buffered or enteric-coated formulations) and antacids, and 12 hrs after PPIs. May increase levels of CYP3A or UGT1A1 substrates, tenofovir, nevirapine, saquinavir, amiodarone, bepridil, lidocaine (systemic), quinidine, TCAs, trazodone, itraconazole, ketoconazole, colchicine, rifabutin, parenteral midazolam, warfarin (monitor INR), diltiazem and other calcium channel blockers, bosentan, atorvastatin, rosuvastatin, norgestimate, norethindrone, fluticasone propionate, clarithromycin, buprenorphine, norbuprenorphine, immunosuppressants, and PDE-5 inhibitors. ATV/RTV may increase levels of carbamazepine. Rosuvastatin dose should not exceed 10mg/day. May decrease levels of didanosine, 14-OH clarithromycin (clarithromycin active metabolite), and telaprevir. ATV/RTV may decrease levels of phenytoin, phenobarbital, and lamotrigine. Voriconazole may alter levels. May alter levels of ethinyl estradiol.

PREGNANCY: Category B, not for use in nursing.

MECHANISM OF ACTION: HIV-1 protease inhibitor; selectively inhibits virus-specific processing of viral Gag and Gag-Pol polyproteins in HIV-1 infected cells, preventing formation of mature virions.

PHARMACOKINETICS: Absorption: Rapid. C_{max}=3152ng/mL, T_{max}=2.5 hrs, AUC=22262ng•hr/mL. **Distribution:** Plasma protein binding (86%). **Metabolism:** Liver (extensive); mono- and dioxygenation via CYP3A. **Elimination:** Urine (13%, 7% unchanged), feces (79%, 20% unchanged); $T_{1/2}$=7 hrs.

NURSING CONSIDERATIONS

Assessment: Assess renal/liver function, treatment history, known hypersensitivity, DM, hemophilia, conduction system disease, pregnancy/nursing status, and possible drug interactions. Obtain baseline LFTs in patients with underlying hepatitis B or C infections or marked transaminase elevations.

Monitoring: Monitor for cardiac conduction abnormalities, PR interval prolongation, rash, DRESS, hyperbilirubinemia, nephrolithiasis, cholelithiasis, new onset or exacerbation of DM, hyperglycemia, diabetic ketoacidosis, autoimmune disorders, immune reconstitution syndrome, fat redistribution/accumulation, cross-resistance among protease inhibitors, and other adverse reactions. Monitor LFTs in patients with underlying hepatitis B or C infections or marked transaminase elevations. Monitor for bleeding in patients with hemophilia. Closely monitor for adverse events during the first 2 months postpartum.

Patient Counseling: Inform that therapy is not a cure for HIV-1 infection, and patients may continue to experience illnesses associated with HIV-1 infections (eg, opportunistic infections).

R

Advise to avoid doing things that can spread HIV-1 infection to others. Advise to take ud and to take with food. Instruct to report use of any other medications or herbal products. Inform that mild rashes without other symptoms, redistribution or accumulation of body fat, or yellowing of the skin or whites of the eyes may occur. Inform that kidney stones and/or gallstones have been reported. Advise to consult physician if dizziness or lightheadedness occurs. Advise to d/c and seek medical evaluation immediately if signs or symptoms of severe skin reactions or hypersensitivity reactions develop.

Administration: Oral route. Take with food. Do not open cap. **Storage:** 25°C (77°F); excursions permitted to 15-30°C (59-86°F).

RHINOCORT AQUA RX
budesonide (AstraZeneca)

THERAPEUTIC CLASS: Corticosteroid

INDICATIONS: Treatment of nasal symptoms of seasonal or perennial allergic rhinitis in adults and children ≥6 yrs of age.

DOSAGE: *Adults:* Initial: 1 spray/nostril qd. Max: 4 sprays/nostril qd.
Pediatrics: ≥12 Yrs: Initial: 1 spray/nostril qd. Max: 4 sprays/nostril qd. 6-<12 Yrs: Initial: 1 spray/nostril qd. Max: 2 sprays/nostril qd.

HOW SUPPLIED: Spray: 32mcg/spray [8.6g]

WARNINGS/PRECAUTIONS: Local nasal effects (eg, epistaxis, *Candida* infections of the nose and pharynx, nasal septal perforation, impaired wound healing) may occur. May need to d/c treatment when *Candida* infection develops. Avoid in patients with recent nasal surgery, trauma, or septal ulcers until healing has occurred. Hypersensitivity reactions may occur. May cause immunosuppression; caution with active or quiescent tuberculosis (TB), untreated local or bacterial, systemic viral, or parasitic infections; or ocular herpes simplex. Hypercorticism and adrenal suppression may appear with higher than recommended dose or in susceptible individuals at recommended dose; d/c slowly. Adrenal insufficiency and withdrawal symptoms may occur when replacing a systemic with a topical corticosteroid. May reduce growth velocity in pediatric patients. Glaucoma, increased intraocular pressure (IOP), and cataracts reported. Caution with hepatic dysfunction.

ADVERSE REACTIONS: Pharyngitis, epistaxis, cough, bronchospasm, nasal irritation.

INTERACTIONS: Oral ketoconazole and other known strong CYP3A4 inhibitors (eg, ritonavir, clarithromycin, itraconazole, nefazodone) may increase plasma levels.

PREGNANCY: Category B, caution in nursing.

MECHANISM OF ACTION: Corticosteroid; not established. Possesses a wide range of inhibitory activities against multiple cell types and mediators involved in allergic-mediated inflammation.

PHARMACOKINETICS: Absorption: Absolute bioavailability (34%); C_{max}=0.3nmol/L; T_{max}=0.5 hr. **Distribution:** V_d=2-3L/kg, plasma protein binding (85-90%), found in breast milk. **Metabolism:** Liver (rapid, extensive) via CYP3A4; 16α-hydroxyprednisolone and 6β-hydroxybudesonide (major metabolites). **Elimination:** Urine (2/3 metabolites), feces; $T_{1/2}$=2-3 hrs.

NURSING CONSIDERATIONS

Assessment: Assess for history of hypersensitivity, increased IOP, glaucoma, and/or cataracts. Assess for recent nasal ulcers, surgery/trauma, active or quiescent TB, untreated local or systemic fungal or bacterial infections, systemic viral or parasitic infections, ocular herpes simplex, suppressed immune system, asthma or other conditions requiring chronic systemic corticosteroid therapy, pregnancy/nursing status, and possible drug interactions.

Monitoring: Monitor for acute adrenal insufficiency and withdrawal symptoms when replacing systemic corticosteroid with topical corticosteroid. Monitor for hypercorticism and/or HPA-axis suppression, disseminated infections (eg, chickenpox, measles), nasal or pharyngeal *Candida* infections, suppression of growth velocity in children, nasal septal perforation, epistaxis, change in vision, glaucoma, increased IOP, and cataracts.

Patient Counseling: Inform about the benefits and risks of the treatment. Take ud at regular intervals. Avoid exposure to chickenpox or measles. Instruct to consult physician immediately if exposed to chickenpox or measles, if existing infection worsens, or if episodes of epistaxis or nasal discomfort occur. Inform physician if a change in vision occurs.

Administration: Intranasal route. Shake gently before use. Refer to PI for further administration instructions. **Storage:** 20-25°C (68-77°F) with the valve up. Do not freeze. Protect from light.

RIASTAP
fibrinogen concentrate (human) (CSL Behring)

THERAPEUTIC CLASS: Plasma glycoprotein

INDICATIONS: Treatment of acute bleeding episodes in patients with congenital fibrinogen deficiency, including afibrinogenemia and hypofibrinogenemia.

DOSAGE: *Adults:* Individualize dose. Known Baseline Fibrinogen Level: Target plasma fibrinogen level based on bleeding type, actual measured plasma fibrinogen level, and body weight. Dose calculated as [target level (mg/dL)-measured level (mg/dL)]/1.7 (mg/dL per mg/kg body weight). Unknown Baseline Fibrinogen Level: Usual: 70mg/kg IV. Monitor fibrinogen level during treatment. A target fibrinogen level of 100mg/dL should be maintained until hemostasis is obtained.

HOW SUPPLIED: Inj: 900mg-1300mg

WARNINGS/PRECAUTIONS: For IV use only. Administer under medical supervision. Not indicated for dysfibrinogenemia. Allergic reactions may occur; d/c if symptoms of allergic or early signs of hypersensitivity reactions occur. Thromboembolic events reported; monitor for signs and symptoms of thrombosis. Made from human plasma; may contain infectious agents (eg, viruses) and theoretically, the Creutzfeldt-Jakob (CJD) agent that can cause disease. All infections thought to have been transmitted by product should be reported to manufacturer.

ADVERSE REACTIONS: Allergic reactions, chills, fever, headache, N/V, thromboembolic episodes.

PREGNANCY: Category C, safety not known in nursing.

MECHANISM OF ACTION: Plasma glycoprotein; physiological substrate of thrombin, factor XIIIa, and plasmin. Replaces the missing or low coagulation factor.

PHARMACOKINETICS: Absorption: C_{max}=140mg/dL, AUC=124.3mg•hr/mL (70mg/kg dose). **Distribution:** V_d=52.7mL/kg. **Elimination:** $T_{1/2}$=78.7 hrs.

NURSING CONSIDERATIONS

Assessment: Assess for drug hypersensitivity, dysfibrinogenemia, and pregnancy/nursing status. Assess fibrinogen levels.

Monitoring: Monitor for signs/symptoms of allergic/hypersensitivity reactions, thrombosis, and infection (eg, viruses). Monitor fibrinogen levels.

Patient Counseling: Inform of the signs of allergic/hypersensitivity reactions (eg, hives, chest tightness, wheezing, hypotension, anaphylaxis) and thrombotic events (eg, unexplained pleuritic, chest and/or leg pain or edema, hemoptysis, dyspnea, tachypnea, neurologic symptoms) and advise to report to physician if any of these occur. Inform of risks/benefits of therapy.

Administration: IV route. Refer to PI for preparation, reconstitution, and administration instructions. **Storage:** 2-25°C (36-77°F) up to 30 months. Protect from light. Do not freeze. Reconstituted: 20-25°C for 8 hrs. Do not freeze.

R

RIFAMATE
rifampin - isoniazid (Sanofi-Aventis)

> Severe and sometimes fatal hepatitis associated with isoniazid (INH) therapy may occur and may develop even after many months of treatment. The risk of developing hepatitis is age-related and increased with daily alcohol consumption. Monitor LFTs monthly. D/C promptly if signs of hepatic damage are detected. Give appropriate alternative treatment in patients with tuberculosis (TB). If INH must be reinstituted, do so only after symptoms and lab abnormalities have cleared. Restart in very small and gradually increasing doses and withdraw immediately if there is any indication of recurrent liver involvement. Defer treatment in persons with acute hepatic diseases.

THERAPEUTIC CLASS: Isonicotinic acid hydrazide/rifamycin derivative

INDICATIONS: Treatment of pulmonary TB in which organisms are susceptible and when patient has been titrated on the individual components and that this fixed dosage has been established to be therapeutically effective.

DOSAGE: *Adults:* 2 caps qd 1 hr ac or 2 hrs pc for at least 4 months. Treatment should be continued for longer if sputum/culture positive, if resistant organisms are present, or if HIV positive. *Pediatrics:* ≥15 Yrs: 2 caps qd 1 hr ac or 2 hrs pc for at least 4 months. Treatment should be continued for longer if sputum/culture positive, if resistant organisms are present, or if HIV positive.

HOW SUPPLIED: Cap: (INH-Rifampin) 150mg-300mg

CONTRAINDICATIONS: INH: Severe hepatic damage, severe adverse reactions to INH (eg, drug fever, chills, arthritis), acute liver disease, acute gout. Rifampin: Concomitant administration of atazanavir, darunavir, fosamprenavir, saquinavir, tipranavir, and ritonavir-boosted saquinavir.

WARNINGS/PRECAUTIONS: Not recommended for initial therapy of TB or preventive therapy. Not indicated for the treatment of meningococcal infections or asymptomatic carriers of *Neisseria meningitidis* to eliminate meningococci from the nasopharynx. Associated with liver dysfunction. Caution with impaired liver function; d/c if signs of hepatocellular damage occur. Caution with history of diabetes mellitus (DM) and in elderly. Concomitant administration of pyridoxine is recommended in the malnourished, in those predisposed to neuropathy (eg, alcoholics, diabetics), and in adolescents. Lab test interactions may occur. Rifampin: Hyperbilirubinemia may occur in the early days of treatment; assess need for treatment interruption. Porphyria exacerbation reported (isolated). Doses of >600mg qd or 2X weekly resulted in higher incidence of adverse reactions (flu syndrome, hematopoietic/cutaneous/GI/hepatic reactions, SOB, shock, anaphylaxis, renal failure). Not recommended for intermittent therapy; caution against intentional or accidental interruption of treatment since renal hypersensitivity reactions (rare) reported when therapy is resumed. May enhance metabolism of endogenous substrates (eg, adrenal/thyroid hormones, vitamin D). INH: D/C all drugs and evaluate patient at 1st sign of a hypersensitivity reaction. Carefully monitor patients with current chronic liver disease or severe renal dysfunction.

ADVERSE REACTIONS: Hepatitis, thrombocytopenia, hemolytic anemia, abnormal LFTs, fever, vasculitis, epigastric distress, anaphylactic reactions, peripheral neuropathy, N/V, BUN/serum uric acid elevations, eosinophilia, jaundice, pyridoxine deficiency, pellagra.

INTERACTIONS: See Contraindications. Avoid with halothane. Caution with other hepatotoxic drugs. Rifampin: Induces certain CYP450 enzymes; dosages of drugs metabolized by these enzymes may require adjustment when starting/stopping concomitant rifampin. May accelerate metabolism of anticonvulsants, digitoxin, antiarrhythmics, oral anticoagulants, antifungals, barbiturates, β-blockers, calcium channel blockers, chloramphenicol, clarithromycin, fluoroquinolones, corticosteroids, cyclosporine, cardiac glycosides, clofibrate, oral/systemic hormonal contraceptives, dapsone, diazepam, doxycycline, haloperidol, oral hypoglycemics, levothyroxine, methadone, narcotic analgesics, TCAs, progestins, quinine, tacrolimus, theophylline, and zidovudine; dosage adjustment of these drugs may be necessary. Decreased concentration of atovaquone, ketoconazole, enalaprilat, or sulfapyridine; adjust ketoconazole or enalapril dose if indicated. Decreased concentration with ketoconazole. Increased blood levels with atovaquone, probenecid, or cotrimoxazole. Antacids may reduce absorption; give daily doses at least 1 hr before antacids. Increases requirements for anticoagulant drugs of the coumarin type; perform PT daily or as frequently as necessary to establish and maintain required anticoagulant dose. Monitor for hepatotoxicity with INH. INH: Higher incidence of hepatitis with daily alcohol ingestion. Monitor renal function with enflurane. Inhibits certain CYP450 enzymes; dosages of drugs metabolized by these enzymes may require adjustment when starting/stopping therapy. Inhibits metabolism of anticonvulsants (eg, carbamazepine, phenytoin), benzodiazepines, haloperidol, ketoconazole, theophylline, and warfarin; dose adjustments of these drugs may be necessary. Decreased levels with corticosteroids (eg, prednisolone). Para-aminosalicylic acid may increase levels and $T_{1/2}$. Monitor for hepatotoxicity with rifampin. Exaggerates CNS effects of meperidine, cycloserine, and disulfiram. Levodopa may produce symptoms of excess catecholamine stimulation or lack of levodopa effect. May produce hyperglycemia and lead to loss of glucose control with oral hypoglycemics. Avoid foods containing tyramine (eg, cheese, red wine) or histamine (eg, skipjack, tuna, other tropical fish).

PREGNANCY: Category C, not for use in nursing.

MECHANISM OF ACTION: INH: Isonicotinic acid hydrazide; Inhibits the biosynthesis of mycolic acids, which are major components of the cell wall of *Mycobacterium tuberculosis*. Rifampin: Rifamycin derivative; inhibits DNA-dependent RNA polymerase activity in susceptible *M. tuberculosis* cells; interacts with bacterial RNA polymerase but does not inhibit the mammalian enzyme.

PHARMACOKINETICS: Absorption: Readily absorbed from GI tract. (INH) T_{max}=1-2 hrs. (Rifampin) C_{max}=10mcg/mL, T_{max}=1.5-3 hrs. **Distribution:** Crosses placenta; found in breast milk. (Rifampin) Plasma protein binding (80%). **Metabolism:** (INH) Liver via acetylation and dehydrazination. (Rifampin) Via deacetylation. **Elimination:** (INH) Urine (50-70% metabolites); $T_{1/2}$=1-4 hrs. (Rifampin) Bile, urine (≤30%, 50% unchanged); refer to PI for $T_{1/2}$.

NURSING CONSIDERATIONS

Assessment: Assess for history of hypersensitivity to any components of the drug, severe adverse reactions to INH, severe hepatic damage, acute liver disease, acute gout, DM, pregnancy/nursing status, and possible drug interactions. Perform bacteriologic smears or cultures and susceptibility tests to confirm diagnosis. Obtain baseline LFTs, bilirubin, SrCr, CBC, platelet count, and blood uric acid. Perform ophthalmologic exam.

Monitoring: Monitor for liver dysfunction, hyperbilirubinemia, hypersensitivity reactions, porphyria exacerbation, and other adverse reactions. Monitor LFTs every 2-4 weeks with impaired liver function. Perform periodic ophthalmologic exams, even without occurrence of visual symptoms. Repeat bacteriologic smears or cultures and susceptibility tests throughout therapy to monitor response to treatment. Monitor patients at least monthly.

Patient Counseling: Instruct to avoid foods containing tyramine (eg, cheese, red wine) and histamine (eg, skipjack, tuna, other tropical fish). Inform that drug may produce reddish discoloration of urine, sweat, sputum, and tears, and may permanently stain soft contact lenses. Inform that reliability of oral or other systemic contraceptives may be affected; advise to change to nonhormonal methods of birth control during therapy. Instruct to notify physician if fever, loss of appetite, malaise, N/V, darkened urine, yellowish discoloration of the skin and eyes, or pain/swelling of joints occurs. Advise to comply with the full course of therapy; inform of the importance of not missing any doses.

Administration: Oral route. Take 1 hr ac or 2 hrs pc with a full glass of water. **Storage:** 25°C (77°F); excursions permitted to 15-30°C (59-86°F). Protect from excessive humidity.

RIFATER   RX
pyrazinamide - rifampin - isoniazid (Sanofi-Aventis)

> Severe and sometimes fatal hepatitis associated with isoniazid (INH) therapy may occur even after many months of treatment. The risk of developing hepatitis is age-related and increased with daily alcohol consumption. Monitor LFTs at monthly intervals. D/C promptly if symptoms appear or signs of hepatic damage occur and give appropriate alternative treatment. If INH must be reinstituted, do so only after symptoms and lab abnormalities have cleared. Restart in very small and gradually increasing doses and withdraw immediately if there is any indication of recurrent liver involvement. Defer treatment in patients with acute hepatic diseases.

THERAPEUTIC CLASS: Isonicotinic acid hydrazide/nicotinamide analogue/rifamycin derivative

INDICATIONS: For initial phase of the short-course treatment of pulmonary tuberculosis.

DOSAGE: *Adults:* Administer as single daily dose 1 hr ac or 2 hrs pc with a full glass of water for 2 months. ≥55kg: 6 tabs qd. 45-54kg: 5 tabs qd. ≤44kg: 4 tabs qd.
Pediatrics: Administer as single daily dose 1 hr ac or 2 hrs pc with a full glass of water for 2 months. ≥15 Yrs: ≥55kg: 6 tabs qd. 45-54kg: 5 tabs qd. ≤44kg: 4 tabs qd.

HOW SUPPLIED: Tab: (INH-Pyrazinamide-Rifampin) 50mg-300mg-120mg

CONTRAINDICATIONS: INH: Severe hepatic damage, adverse reactions to INH (eg, drug fever, chills, arthritis), acute liver disease, and acute gout. Rifampin: Concomitant administration of atazanavir, darunavir, fosamprenavir, saquinavir, tipranavir, and ritonavir-boosted saquinavir.

WARNINGS/PRECAUTIONS: Associated with liver dysfunction. Caution in patients with impaired liver function; d/c if signs of hepatocellular damage occur. Caution with history of diabetes mellitus (DM) and in elderly. Concomitant administration of pyridoxine is recommended in the malnourished, in those predisposed to neuropathy (eg, alcoholics, diabetics), and in adolescents. Lab test interactions may occur. Rifampin: Hyperbilirubinemia may occur in the early days of treatment. A decision to interrupt treatment should be made after repeating tests, noting trends in levels, and considering clinical condition. Porphyria exacerbation reported (isolated). Doses of >600mg qd or 2X weekly resulted in higher incidence of adverse reactions (eg, flu syndrome, hematopoietic/cutaneous/GI/hepatic reactions, SOB, shock, anaphylaxis, renal failure). Not recommended for intermittent therapy; caution against intentional or accidental interruption of treatment since renal hypersensitivity reactions (rare) reported when therapy is resumed. May enhance metabolism of endogenous substrates (eg, adrenal/thyroid hormones, vitamin D). INH: Perform periodic ophthalmologic exams before and periodically thereafter. D/C all drugs and evaluate patient at the 1st sign of a hypersensitivity reaction. Carefully monitor patients with current chronic liver disease or severe renal dysfunction. Pyrazinamide: D/C and do not resume treatment if signs of hepatocellular damage or hyperuricemia accompanied by acute gouty arthritis appear; transfer to a regimen not containing pyrazinamide if acute gouty arthritis occurs without liver dysfunction.

ADVERSE REACTIONS: Hepatitis, N/V, digestive pain, diarrhea, sweating, headache, insomnia, rash, arthralgia, tightness in chest, coughing, angina, palpitation, hemoptysis, total pneumothorax, phlebitis.

INTERACTIONS: See Contraindications. Rifampin: Induces certain CYP450 enzymes; dosages of drugs metabolized by these enzymes may require adjustment when starting/stopping concomitant rifampin. May accelerate metabolism of anticonvulsants, digitoxin, antiarrhythmics (eg, disopyramide, mexiletine, quinidine, tocainide), oral anticoagulants, antifungals (eg, fluconazole, itraconazole, ketoconazole), barbiturates, β-blockers, calcium channel blockers (eg, diltiazem, nifedipine, verapamil), chloramphenicol, clarithromycin, fluoroquinolones (eg, ciprofloxacin), corticosteroids, cyclosporine, cardiac glycosides, clofibrate, oral or systemic hormonal contraceptives, dapsone, diazepam, doxycycline, haloperidol, oral hypoglycemics (eg, sulfonylureas), levothyroxine, methadone, narcotic analgesics, TCAs (eg, amitriptyline, nortriptyline), progestins, quinine, tacrolimus, theophylline, and zidovudine; dosage adjustment of these drugs may be necessary. Decreased concentration of atovaquone, ketoconazole, enalaprilat (active metabolite of enalapril), or sulfapyridine; adjust ketoconazole or enalapril dose if indicated. Decreased concentration with ketoconazole. Increased concentration with atovaquone, probenecid, or cotrimoxazole. Antacids may reduce absorption; give daily doses at least 1 hr before antacids. Increased

R

requirements for anticoagulant drugs of the coumarin type; perform PT daily or as frequently as necessary to establish and maintain required anticoagulant dose. Avoid with halothane. Monitor for hepatotoxicity with INH. INH: Higher incidence of hepatitis with daily alcohol ingestion. Monitor renal function with enflurane. Inhibits certain CYP450 enzymes; dosages of drugs metabolized by these enzymes may require adjustment when starting/stopping therapy. Inhibits metabolism of anticonvulsants (eg, carbamazepine, phenytoin, primidone, valproic acid), benzodiazepines (eg, diazepam), haloperidol, ketoconazole, theophylline, and warfarin; dose adjustments of these drugs may be necessary. Antacids and food may reduce absorption; take therapy on an empty stomach at least 1 hr before antacids/food. Decreased levels with corticosteroids (eg, prednisolone). Para-aminosalicylic acid may increase levels and $T_{1/2}$. Monitor for hepatotoxicity with rifampin. Exaggerates CNS effects of meperidine, cycloserine, and disulfiram. Levodopa may produce symptoms of excess catecholamine stimulation or lack of levodopa effect. May produce hyperglycemia and lead to loss of glucose control with oral hypoglycemics. Avoid foods containing tyramine (eg, cheese, red wine) or histamine (eg, skipjack, tuna, other tropical fish).

PREGNANCY: Category C, not for use in nursing.

MECHANISM OF ACTION: INH: Isonicotinic acid hydrazide; inhibits the biosynthesis of mycolic acids, which are major components of the cell wall of *Mycobacterium tuberculosis*. Pyrazinamide: Nicotinamide analogue; has not been established. Rifampin: Rifamycin derivative; inhibits DNA-dependent RNA polymerase activity in susceptible *M. tuberculosis* organisms. Interacts with bacterial RNA polymerase, but does not inhibit the mammalian enzyme.

PHARMACOKINETICS: Absorption: (5 tabs single dose) INH: Readily absorbed. Bioavailability (100.6%), C_{max}=3.09mcg/mL, T_{max}=1-2 hrs. Pyrazinamide: Well-absorbed. Bioavailability (96.8%), C_{max}=28.02mcg/mL, T_{max}=2 hrs. Rifampin: Readily absorbed. Bioavailability (88.8%), C_{max}=11.04mcg/mL. **Distribution:** Found in breast milk. INH: Crosses placenta. Pyrazinamide: Plasma protein binding (10%). Rifampin: Protein binding (80%). **Metabolism:** INH: Acetylation and dehydrazination. Pyrazinamide: Liver, via hydroxylation; pyrazinoic acid (major active metabolite). Rifampin: Via deacetylation. **Elimination:** INH: Urine (50-70% mostly metabolites); $T_{1/2}$=1-4 hrs. Pyrazinamide: Urine (70%, 4-14% unchanged); $T_{1/2}$=9-10 hrs. Rifampin: Urine (≤30%, 50% unchanged), bile. Refer to PI for $T_{1/2}$.

NURSING CONSIDERATIONS

Assessment: Assess for history of hypersensitivity to any components of the drug, severe adverse reactions to INH, severe hepatic damage, renal/hepatic impairment, acute gout, DM, pregnancy/nursing status, and possible drug interactions. Perform bacteriologic smears or cultures and susceptibility tests to confirm diagnosis. Obtain baseline LFTs, bilirubin, SrCr, CBC and platelet count, and blood uric acid. Perform ophthalmologic exam.

Monitoring: Monitor for liver dysfunction, hyperbilirubinemia, hyperuricemia, hypersensitivity reactions, acute gouty arthritis, porphyria exacerbation, and other adverse reactions. Monitor LFTs every 2-4 weeks with impaired liver function. Perform ophthalmologic exam periodically, even without occurrence of visual symptoms. Repeat bacteriologic smears or cultures and susceptibility tests throughout therapy to monitor response to treatment. Monitor PT daily or as frequently as necessary if used with anticoagulants. Monitor patients at least monthly; those with lab abnormalities should have follow-up lab testing if necessary.

Patient Counseling: Instruct to avoid foods containing tyramine and histamine. Inform that medication may produce reddish coloration of urine, sweat, sputum, and tears, and may permanently stain soft contact lenses. Inform that reliability of oral or other systemic contraceptives may be affected; advise to change to nonhormonal methods of birth control during therapy. Instruct to notify physician if fever, loss of appetite, malaise, N/V, darkened urine, yellowish discoloration of the skin and eyes, pain or swelling of joints occur. Advise to comply with the full course of therapy; inform of the importance of not missing any doses.

Administration: Oral route. Take 1 hr ac or 2 hrs pc with a full glass of water. **Storage:** 25°C (77°F); excursions permitted to 15-30°C (59-86°F). Protect from excessive humidity.

RILUTEK   RX
riluzole (Covis)

THERAPEUTIC CLASS: Benzothiazole

INDICATIONS: Treatment of amyotrophic lateral sclerosis (ALS). Extends survival and/or time to tracheostomy.

DOSAGE: *Adults:* 50mg q12h. Take 1 hr before or 2 hrs pc.

HOW SUPPLIED: Tab: 50mg

WARNINGS/PRECAUTIONS: Caution with hepatic impairment; monitor LFTs. D/C if ALT levels ≥5 x ULN or clinical jaundice develops. Clinical hepatitis reported. Neutropenia may occur; monitor

WBC count with febrile illness. Interstitial lung disease reported; perform chest radiography if respiratory symptoms develop. May impair mental/physical abilities. Caution in elderly.

ADVERSE REACTIONS: Asthenia, N/V, dizziness, decreased lung function, diarrhea, abdominal pain, vertigo, circumonal paresthesia, anorexia, somnolence, headache, anorexia, rhinitis, HTN.

INTERACTIONS: Caution with concomitant use with potentially hepatotoxic drugs (eg, allopurinol, methyldopa, sulfasalazine). CYP1A2 inhibitors may decrease elimination. CYP1A2 inducers may increase elimination.

PREGNANCY: Category C, not for use in nursing.

MECHANISM OF ACTION: Benzothiazole; mechanism not established. May inhibit the effect on glutamate release, inactivates voltage-dependent Na^{2+} channels, and interferes with intracellular events that follow transmitter binding at excitatory amino acid receptors.

PHARMACOKINETICS: Absorption: Well-absorbed; absolute bioavailability (60%). **Distribution:** Plasma protein binding (96%). **Metabolism:** Extensive; liver via CYP450 by hydroxylation and glucuronidation; N-hydroxyriluzole (major metabolite). **Elimination:** Urine (90% metabolites, 2% unchanged), feces (5%); $T_{1/2}$=12 hrs.

NURSING CONSIDERATIONS

Assessment: Assess for hepatic impairment, pregnancy/nursing status, alcohol intake, hypersensitivity, and possible drug interactions. Perform baseline LFTs.

Monitoring: Perform baseline LFTs before therapy, every month during first 3 months, every 3 months for the remainder of the 1st year, then periodically thereafter. Take WBC count and chest radiography if necessary. Monitor for signs/symptoms of febrile illness, liver toxicity, and hypersensitivity reactions.

Patient Counseling: Instruct to notify healthcare professional of any signs of febrile illness. Caution about hazardous tasks. Advise to notify healthcare professional if cough or SOB occur. Instruct to avoid use with excessive intake of alcohol. Instruct patient if a dose is missed, to take next tablet as originally planned.

Administration: Oral route. **Storage:** 20-25°C (68-77°F); protect from bright light.

RIOMET

metformin HCl (Ranbaxy)

RX

> Lactic acidosis may occur due to metformin accumulation; risk increases with the degree of renal dysfunction, patient's age, and in patients with unstable/acute congestive heart failure at risk of hypoperfusion and hypoxemia. Regularly monitor renal function and use minimum effective dose to decrease the risk. Do not initiate in patients ≥80 yrs of age unless, based on CrCl, renal function is not reduced. Withhold therapy in the presence of any condition associated with hypoxemia, dehydration, or sepsis. Avoid with clinical or laboratory evidence of hepatic disease. Caution against excessive alcohol intake since alcohol potentiates effects of metformin on lactate metabolism. Temporarily d/c therapy prior to any intravascular radiocontrast study and for any surgical procedure. D/C use and hospitalize patient if lactic acidosis occurs.

THERAPEUTIC CLASS: Biguanide

INDICATIONS: Adjunct to diet and exercise to improve glycemic control in adults and children with type 2 diabetes mellitus.

DOSAGE: *Adults:* Individualize dose. Take with meals. Initial: 500mg (5mL) bid or 850mg (8.5mL) qd. Titrate: Increase by 500mg weekly or 850mg every 2 weeks, up to a total of 2000mg/day (20mL/day) in divided doses, or may increase from 500mg bid to 850mg bid after 2 weeks. Max: 2550mg/day (25.5mL/day). Doses >2000mg may be better tolerated given tid. With Insulin: Initial: 500mg qd. Titrate: Increase by 500mg/week. Max: 2500mg/day (25mL/day). Decrease insulin dose by 10-25% when FPG concentrations decrease to <120mg/dL. Elderly/Debilitated/Malnourished: Dose conservatively; do not titrate to max.
Pediatrics: 10-16 Yrs: Individualize dose. Take with meals. Initial: 500mg (5mL) bid. Titrate: Increase by 500mg weekly. Max: 2000mg/day (20mL/day) in divided doses.

HOW SUPPLIED: Sol: 500mg/5mL [118mL, 473mL]

CONTRAINDICATIONS: Renal disease/dysfunction (eg, SrCr ≥1.5mg/dL [males], ≥1.4mg/dL [females], or abnormal CrCl). Acute/chronic metabolic acidosis, including diabetic ketoacidosis, with or without coma. Temporarily d/c if undergoing radiologic studies involving intravascular administration of iodinated contrast materials.

WARNINGS/PRECAUTIONS: Suspend temporarily for any surgical procedure (except minor procedures not associated with restricted intake of food and fluids); restart when oral intake is resumed and renal function is normal. May decrease vitamin B12 levels; monitor hematologic parameters annually. Evaluate for evidence of ketoacidosis or lactic acidosis if laboratory abnormalities or clinical illness develops; d/c if acidosis occurs. Temporary loss of glycemic control may occur when exposed to stress; may need to withhold therapy and temporarily administer insulin. May be combined with a sulfonylurea should secondary failure occur; may need to consider

R

therapeutic alternatives, including initiation of insulin, if secondary failure occurs with combination therapy. Caution in elderly. Not recommended for use during pregnancy.

ADVERSE REACTIONS: Lactic acidosis, diarrhea, N/V, flatulence, asthenia, abdominal discomfort, hypoglycemia, dyspnea, taste disorder, chest discomfort, flu syndrome, palpitations, indigestion, headache.

INTERACTIONS: See Boxed Warning and Contraindications. Furosemide, nifedipine, and oral cimetidine may increase levels. Cationic drugs that are eliminated by renal tubular secretion (eg, amiloride, morphine, quinidine, ranitidine, vancomycin) may potentially produce an interaction; adjust dose. Observe for loss of glycemic control with thiazides and other diuretics, corticosteroids, phenothiazines, thyroid products, estrogens, oral contraceptives, phenytoin, nicotinic acid, sympathomimetics, calcium channel blockers, and isoniazid. May decrease glyburide and furosemide levels. Caution with drugs that may affect renal function or result in significant hemodynamic change or may interfere with the disposition of metformin (eg, cationic drugs eliminated by renal tubular secretion). Hypoglycemia may occur during concomitant use with other glucose-lowering agents or ethanol. Hypoglycemia may be difficult to recognize with β-blockers.

PREGNANCY: Category B, not for use in nursing.

MECHANISM OF ACTION: Biguanide; decreases hepatic glucose production, decreases intestinal absorption of glucose, and improves insulin sensitivity by increasing peripheral glucose uptake and utilization.

PHARMACOKINETICS: Absorption: Administration under fed/fasting conditions resulted in various parameters. **Distribution:** V_d=654L (850mg). **Elimination:** Urine (90%); $T_{1/2}$=6.2 hrs (plasma), 17.6 hrs (blood).

NURSING CONSIDERATIONS

Assessment: Assess for metabolic acidosis, risk factors for lactic acidosis, renal/hepatic function, inadequate vitamin B12 or Ca^{2+} intake/absorption, hypersensitivity to the drug, pregnancy/nursing status, and possible drug interactions. Assess if patient is planning to undergo any surgical procedure or is under any form of stress. Obtain baseline FPG, HbA1c, and hematologic parameters.

Monitoring: Monitor for signs/symptoms of lactic acidosis, ketoacidosis, clinical illness, hypoxic states, and other adverse reactions. Perform routine serum vitamin B12 measurements at 2- to 3-yr intervals in patients predisposed to develop subnormal vitamin B12 levels. Monitor FPG, HbA1c, renal function, and hematologic parameters periodically.

Patient Counseling: Inform of risks, benefits, and alternative modes of therapy, and about the importance of adherence to dietary instructions, regular exercise program, and regular testing of blood glucose, HbA1c, renal function, and hematologic parameters. Advise of the risk of lactic acidosis and to d/c therapy immediately and notify physician if unexplained hyperventilation, myalgia, malaise, unusual somnolence, or other nonspecific symptoms occur. Counsel against excessive alcohol intake. Explain the risks, symptoms, and conditions that predispose to the development of hypoglycemia when initiating combination therapy with PO sulfonylureas and insulin.

Administration: Oral route. **Storage:** 15-30°C (59-86°F).

R

RISPERDAL   RX
risperidone (Janssen)

OTHER BRAND NAMES: Risperdal M-Tab (Janssen)

THERAPEUTIC CLASS: Benzisoxazole derivative

INDICATIONS: Treatment of schizophrenia in adults and adolescents (13-17 yrs of age). Treatment of acute manic or mixed episodes associated with bipolar I disorder as monotherapy in adults and pediatrics (10-17 yrs of age) or as adjunctive therapy with lithium or valproate in adults. Treatment of irritability associated with autistic disorder, including symptoms of aggression towards others, deliberate self-injuriousness, temper tantrums, and quickly changing moods, in children and adolescents (5-17 yrs of age).

DOSAGE: *Adults:* Schizophrenia: May be administered qd or bid. Initial: 2mg/day. Titrate: May increase at intervals of ≥24 hrs, by 1-2mg/day. Target: 4-8mg/day. Range: 4-16mg/day. Max: 16mg/day. Maint: 2-8mg/day. Bipolar Mania: Initial: 2-3mg/day. Titrate: May increase at intervals of ≥24 hrs, by 1mg/day. Target/Range: 1-6mg/day. Max: 6mg/day. If experiencing persistent somnolence, may divide daily dose bid. Severe Renal Impairment (CrCl <30mL/min) or Hepatic Impairment (10-15 points on Child Pugh System): Initial: 0.5mg bid. Titrate: May increase by ≤0.5mg bid. For doses >1.5mg bid, increase in intervals of ≥1 week. Refer to PI for dose adjustments with concomitant enzyme inducers, fluoxetine, or paroxetine. Elderly: Start at lower end of dosing range.

Pediatrics: Schizophrenia: 13-17 Yrs: Initial: 0.5mg qd in am or pm. Titrate: May increase at intervals of ≥24 hrs, by 0.5mg/day or 1mg/day. Target: 3mg/day. Range: 1-6mg/day. Max: 6mg/day. Bipolar Mania: 10-17 Yrs: Initial: 0.5mg qd in am or pm. Titrate: May increase at intervals of ≥24 hrs, by 0.5mg/day or 1mg/day. Target: 1-2.5mg/day. Range: 0.5-6mg/day. Max: 6mg/day. If experiencing persistent somnolence, may divide daily dose bid. Irritability Associated with Autistic Disorder: 5-17 Yrs: Total daily dose may be administered qd or divided bid. Initial: ≥20kg: 0.5mg/day. <20kg: 0.25mg/day. Titrate: May increase after a minimum of 4 days. Target: ≥20kg: 1mg/day. <20kg: 0.5mg/day. Maintain this dose for a minimum of 14 days. If not achieving sufficient response, may increase at intervals of ≥2 weeks, by 0.5mg/day (≥20kg) or 0.25mg/day (<20kg). Range: 0.5-3mg/day. Once sufficient response is achieved and maintained, consider gradually lowering the dose. If experiencing persistent somnolence, may give qd dose hs, divide daily dose bid, or reduce dose. Refer to PI for dose adjustments with concomitant enzyme inducers, fluoxetine, or paroxetine.

HOW SUPPLIED: Sol: 1mg/mL [30mL]; Tab: 0.25mg, 0.5mg, 1mg, 2mg, 3mg, 4mg; (M-Tab) Tab, Disintegrating: 0.5mg, 1mg, 2mg, 3mg, 4mg

WARNINGS/PRECAUTIONS: May cause neuroleptic malignant syndrome (NMS); d/c and treat immediately if this occurs. Tardive dyskinesia (TD) may develop; consider discontinuing if signs/symptoms appear. Associated with metabolic changes (eg, hyperglycemia, dyslipidemia, weight gain). Monitor regularly for worsening of glucose control in patients with diabetes mellitus (DM), and perform FPG testing at the beginning of treatment and periodically during treatment in patients with risk factors for DM. Elevates prolactin levels. May induce orthostatic hypotension. Leukopenia, neutropenia, and agranulocytosis reported; monitor CBC in patients with history of clinically significant low WBC counts or drug-induced leukopenia/neutropenia, and consider discontinuation at 1st sign of clinically significant decline in WBC counts without other causative factors. D/C and follow WBC counts until recovery in patients with severe neutropenia (absolute neutrophil count <1000/mm³). May impair mental/physical abilities. Seizures reported. Esophageal dysmotility and aspiration reported; caution in patients at risk for aspiration pneumonia. Priapism reported. May disrupt body temperature regulation; caution when prescribing for patients who will be exposed to temperature extremes. Patients with Parkinson's disease or dementia with Lewy bodies may experience increased sensitivity. Observe for drug misuse/abuse in patients with a history of drug abuse. Caution in elderly. (Tab, Disintegrating) Contains phenylalanine.

ADVERSE REACTIONS: Increased appetite, fatigue, N/V, constipation, parkinsonism, upper abdominal pain, anxiety, dizziness, tremor, sedation, akathisia, dystonia, blurred vision, stomach discomfort.

INTERACTIONS: CYP2D6 inhibitors (eg, fluoxetine, paroxetine, quinidine) interfere with conversion to 9-hydroxyrisperidone; adjust dose when used with CYP2D6 inhibitors. Enzyme inducers (eg, carbamazepine, phenytoin, rifampin, phenobarbital) may decrease concentrations; adjust dose when used with enzyme inducers. Increased valproate C_{max}. Caution with other centrally-acting drugs and alcohol. May enhance hypotensive effects of other therapeutic agents with this potential. May antagonize effects of levodopa and dopamine agonists. Decreased clearance with chronic use of clozapine.

PREGNANCY: Category C, not for use in nursing.

MECHANISM OF ACTION: Benzisoxazole derivative; not established. In schizophrenia, proposed to be mediated through a combination of dopamine type 2 (D_2) and serotonin type 2 ($5HT_2$) receptor antagonism.

PHARMACOKINETICS: Absorption: Well-absorbed. Absolute bioavailability (70%); T_{max}=1 hr, 3 hrs (9-hydroxyrisperidone, extensive metabolizers), 17 hrs (9-hydroxyrisperidone, poor metabolizers). **Distribution:** V_d=1-2L/kg; plasma protein binding (90%), (77%, 9-hydroxyrisperidone); found in breast milk. **Metabolism:** Liver (extensive); hydroxylation via CYP2D6 to 9-hydroxyrisperidone (major metabolite); N-dealkylation (minor pathway). **Elimination:** Urine (70%), feces (14%); $T_{1/2}$=3 hrs (extensive metabolizers), 20 hrs (poor metabolizers), 21 hrs (9-hydroxyrisperidone, extensive metabolizers), 30 hrs (9-hydroxyrisperidone, poor metabolizers).

NURSING CONSIDERATIONS

Assessment: Assess for dementia-related psychosis, DM, risk for hypotension, history of seizures, drug hypersensitivity or any other conditions where treatment is cautioned, hepatic/renal function, pregnancy/nursing status, and possible drug interactions. Obtain FPG in patients at risk for DM.

Monitoring: Monitor for NMS, TD, hyperglycemia, hyperprolactinemia, orthostatic hypotension, leukopenia, neutropenia, agranulocytosis, cognitive/motor impairment, seizures, esophageal dysmotility, aspiration, priapism, disruption of body temperature, and other adverse events. Monitor FPG in patients with DM or at risk for DM, lipid profile, and weight. Monitor CBC frequently during the 1st few months of therapy in patients with history of clinically significant low WBC or drug-induced leukopenia/neutropenia. In patients with clinically significant neutropenia, monitor for fever or other symptoms or signs of infection.

R

Patient Counseling: Advise about the risk of orthostatic hypotension, especially during the period of initial dose titration. Inform that therapy has the potential to impair judgment, thinking, or motor skills; advise to use caution when operating hazardous machinery. Instruct to notify physician if pregnant or planning to become pregnant, nursing, and if taking or planning to take any prescription or OTC drugs. Advise to avoid alcohol during treatment. Inform that orally disintegrating tab contains phenylalanine. Inform that treatment can be associated with hyperglycemia and DM, dyslipidemia, and weight gain. Inform about risk of TD.

Administration: Oral route. May be given with or without meals. (Sol/Tab, Disintegrating) Refer to PI for administration instructions/directions for use. **Storage:** 15-25°C (59-77°F). (Sol) Protect from light and freezing. (Tab) Protect from light and moisture.

RISPERDAL CONSTA   RX
risperidone (Ortho-McNeil/Janssen)

> Elderly patients with dementia-related psychosis treated with antipsychotic drugs are at an increased risk of death; most deaths appeared to be cardiovascular (CV) (eg, heart failure, sudden death) or infectious (eg, pneumonia) in nature. Not approved for the treatment of patients with dementia-related psychosis.

THERAPEUTIC CLASS: Benzisoxazole derivative

INDICATIONS: Treatment of schizophrenia. As monotherapy or adjunctive therapy to lithium or valproate for maintenance treatment of bipolar I disorder.

DOSAGE: *Adults:* Establish tolerability with oral formulation prior to treatment with inj in risperidone-naive patients. Give 1st inj with oral risperidone or other antipsychotic; continue for 3 weeks, then d/c oral therapy. Upward dose adjustment should not be made more frequently than every 4 weeks. Schizophrenia/Bipolar I Disorder: Usual: 25mg IM every 2 weeks. Titrate: May increase to 37.5mg or 50mg. Max: 50mg every 2 weeks. Hepatic/Renal Impairment: Prior to initiating IM therapy, administer 0.5mg PO bid during the 1st week. Titrate: May increase to 1mg PO bid or 2mg PO qd during the 2nd week. If total daily oral dose of ≥2mg is tolerated, start at 12.5mg or 25mg IM every 2 weeks. Elderly: 25mg IM every 2 weeks. Reinitiation: Supplement with oral risperidone or other antipsychotic. Switching from Other Antipsychotics: Continue previous antipsychotic for 3 weeks after 1st risperidone inj. Poor Tolerability: Initial: 12.5mg IM. Refer to PI for dose adjustments with concomitant enzyme inducers, fluoxetine, or paroxetine.

HOW SUPPLIED: Inj: 12.5mg, 25mg, 37.5mg, 50mg

WARNINGS/PRECAUTIONS: Neuroleptic malignant syndrome (NMS), tardive dyskinesia (TD), hyperprolactinemia reported. Associated with metabolic changes (eg, hyperglycemia, dyslipidemia, weight gain) that may increase CV/cerebrovascular risk. May induce orthostatic hypotension. Leukopenia, neutropenia, and agranulocytosis reported; d/c in cases of severe neutropenia (absolute neutrophil count <1000/mm^3). May impair mental/physical abilities. Seizures reported. Esophageal dysmotility and aspiration reported; caution in patients at risk for aspiration pneumonia. Priapism and thrombotic thrombocytopenic purpura (TTP) reported. May disrupt body temperature regulation; caution when exposed to extreme temperatures. May produce an antiemetic effect that may mask signs/symptoms of overdosage with certain drugs or conditions (eg, intestinal obstruction, Reye's syndrome, brain tumor). Closely supervise patients at high-risk of suicide. Increased sensitivity reported in patients with Parkinson's disease or dementia with Lewy bodies. Caution with diseases/conditions affecting metabolism or hemodynamic responses, renal/hepatic impairment, and in elderly. Intended for IM inj; avoid inadvertent inj into a blood vessel.

ADVERSE REACTIONS: Headache, dizziness, constipation, dyspepsia, akathisia, parkinsonism, weight increased, dry mouth, fatigue, pain in extremity, tremor, nausea, sedation, cough, pain.

INTERACTIONS: Caution with other centrally-acting drugs and alcohol. May enhance hypotensive effects of antihypertensive drugs. May antagonize effects of levodopa and dopamine agonists. Increases bioavailability of PO risperidone with cimetidine or ranitidine. Increased exposure with ranitidine. Decreased clearance with chronic use of clozapine. Increased valproate peak plasma concentrations with PO risperidone. Increased concentrations with fluoxetine, paroxetine, and other CYP2D6 inhibitors. Decreased concentrations with carbamazepine and other CYP3A4 enzyme inducers.

PREGNANCY: Category C, not for use in nursing.

MECHANISM OF ACTION: Benzisoxazole derivative; not established. In schizophrenia, proposed to be mediated through a combination of dopamine type 2 (D$_2$) and serotonin type 2 (5HT$_2$) receptor antagonism.

PHARMACOKINETICS: Distribution: Rapid; V$_d$=1-2L/kg; plasma protein binding (risperidone, 90%), (9-hydroxyrisperidone, 77%); found in breast milk. **Metabolism:** Liver (extensive) via CYP2D6; hydroxylation, N-dealkylation; 9-hydroxyrisperidone (major metabolite). **Elimination:** Urine (70%), feces (14%); T$_{1/2}$=3-6 days.

NURSING CONSIDERATIONS

Assessment: Assess for dementia-related psychosis, DM, risk for hypotension, history of seizures, or any other conditions where treatment is contraindicated or cautioned. Assess for hepatic/renal impairment, pregnancy/nursing status, and for possible drug interactions. Obtain baseline FPG in patients at risk for diabetes mellitus (DM).

Monitoring: Monitor for NMS, TD, hyperprolactinemia, orthostatic hypotension, cognitive and motor impairment, seizures, esophageal dysmotility, aspiration, priapism, TTP, metabolic changes, and disruption of body temperature. Monitor for signs of hyperglycemia; perform periodic monitoring of FPG levels in patients with DM or at risk for DM. Monitor for signs/symptoms of leukopenia, neutropenia (eg, fever, infection), and agranulocytosis; perform frequent monitoring of CBC in patients with history of clinically significant low WBC or drug-induced leukopenia/neutropenia. Monitor liver/renal function and weight.

Patient Counseling: Advise of risk of orthostatic hypotension and of nonpharmacologic interventions that will help reduce its occurrence. Inform that therapy has the potential to impair judgment, thinking, or motor skills; advise to use caution when operating hazardous machinery. Instruct to notify physician if pregnant or plan to become pregnant, and of all medications currently being taken. Instruct not to breastfeed while on therapy and for ≥12 weeks after last inj. Advise to avoid alcohol during treatment.

Administration: IM route. Deep IM into the gluteal or deltoid muscle every 2 weeks. Not for IV use. Refer to PI for complete instructions for use. **Storage**: 2-8°C (36-46°F). Protect from light. If refrigeration is unavailable, store at ≤25°C (77°F) for ≤7 days prior to administration.

RITALIN
methylphenidate HCl (Novartis)

CII

> Caution with history of drug dependence or alcoholism. Chronic abuse may lead to marked tolerance and psychological dependence with varying degrees of abnormal behavior. Frank psychotic episodes may occur, especially with parenteral abuse. Careful supervision is required during withdrawal from abusive use since severe depression may occur. Withdrawal following chronic use may unmask symptoms of underlying disorder that may require follow-up.

OTHER BRAND NAMES: Methylphenidate (Various) - Ritalin-SR (Novartis)

THERAPEUTIC CLASS: Sympathomimetic amine

INDICATIONS: Treatment of attention deficit disorders and narcolepsy.

DOSAGE: *Adults:* Individualize dose. (Tab) 10-60mg/day given in divided doses bid-tid 30-45 min ac. Take last dose before 6 pm if unable to sleep. (Tab, SR) May be used in place of methylphenidate tabs when the 8-hr dosage corresponds to the titrated 8-hr dosage of methylphenidate tabs.
Pediatrics: ≥6 Yrs: Individualize dose. Initiate in small doses, with gradual weekly increments. Max: 60mg/day. D/C if no improvement seen after appropriate dose adjustment over 1 month. (Tab) Initial: 5mg bid before breakfast and lunch. Titrate: Increase gradually by 5-10mg weekly. (Tab, SR) May be used in place of methylphenidate tabs when the 8-hr dosage corresponds to the titrated 8-hr dosage of methylphenidate tabs. Reduce dose or, if necessary, d/c if paradoxical aggravation of symptoms or other adverse effects occur. Periodically d/c to assess child's condition. Drug treatment should not and need not be indefinite and usually may be discontinued after puberty.

HOW SUPPLIED: Tab: (Ritalin) 5mg, 10mg*, 20mg*; Tab, Sustained-Release (SR): (Generic) 10mg, (Ritalin-SR) 20mg *scored

CONTRAINDICATIONS: Marked anxiety, tension, agitation, glaucoma, motor tics, or family history or diagnosis of Tourette's syndrome. Treatment with MAOIs or within a minimum of 14 days following discontinuation of an MAOI.

WARNINGS/PRECAUTIONS: Avoid with known serious structural cardiac abnormalities, cardiomyopathy, serious heart rhythm abnormalities, coronary artery disease, or other serious cardiac problems. Sudden death reported in children and adolescents with structural cardiac abnormalities or other serious heart problems. Sudden death, stroke, and myocardial infarction (MI) reported in adults. May increase BP and HR; caution with conditions that might be compromised by increases in BP/HR (eg, preexisting HTN, heart failure, recent MI, ventricular arrhythmia). Prior to treatment, obtain medical history (including assessment for family history of sudden death or ventricular arrhythmia) and perform physical exam to assess for presence of cardiac disease. Promptly perform cardiac evaluation if symptoms of cardiac disease develop. May exacerbate symptoms of behavior disturbance and thought disorder in patients with preexisting psychotic disorder. Caution in patients with comorbid bipolar disorder; may induce mixed/manic episode. May cause treatment-emergent psychotic or manic symptoms (eg, hallucinations, delusional thinking, mania) in children and adolescents without prior history of psychotic illness or mania; consider discontinuation if such symptoms occur. Aggressive behavior or hostility reported in children and adolescents. May cause long-term suppression of growth in children;

monitor growth, and may need to interrupt treatment in patients not growing or gaining height or weight as expected. May lower convulsive threshold; d/c if seizures occur. Associated with peripheral vasculopathy, including Raynaud's phenomenon; carefully observe for digital changes. Difficulties with accommodation and blurring of vision reported. Patients with an element of agitation may react adversely; d/c if necessary. (Ritalin/Ritalin-SR) Priapism, sometimes requiring surgical intervention, reported.

ADVERSE REACTIONS: Nervousness, insomnia, hypersensitivity reactions, anorexia, nausea, dizziness, palpitations, headache, dyskinesia, drowsiness, BP and pulse changes, tachycardia, angina, cardiac arrhythmia, abdominal pain.

INTERACTIONS: See Contraindications. Caution with pressor agents. May decrease effectiveness of drugs used to treat HTN. May inhibit metabolism of coumarin anticoagulants, anticonvulsants (eg, phenobarbital, phenytoin, primidone), and TCAs (eg, imipramine, clomipramine, desipramine); downward dose adjustment and monitoring of plasma drug concentration (or coagulation times for coumarin) of these drugs may be necessary when initiating or discontinuing methylphenidate.

PREGNANCY: Category C, caution in nursing.

MECHANISM OF ACTION: Sympathomimetic amine; mild CNS stimulant. Has not been established; thought to activate the brain stem arousal system and cortex to produce its stimulant effect.

PHARMACOKINETICS: Absorption: (Children) T_{max}=4.7 hrs (Tab, SR), 1.9 hrs (Tab). **Metabolism:** Deesterification to α-phenyl-2-piperidine acetic acid (ritalinic acid) (major metabolite). **Elimination:** Urine.

NURSING CONSIDERATIONS

Assessment: Assess for hypersensitivity to the drug, marked anxiety, tension, agitation, glaucoma, motor tics, family history or diagnosis of Tourette's syndrome, cardiovascular conditions, history of drug dependence or alcoholism, psychotic disorder, comorbid bipolar disorder, any other conditions where treatment is contraindicated or cautioned, pregnancy/nursing status, and possible drug interactions.

Monitoring: Monitor for changes in HR and BP, signs/symptoms of cardiac disease, exacerbation of behavior disturbance and thought disorder, psychosis, mania, appearance of or worsening of aggressive behavior or hostility, seizures, peripheral vasculopathy (including Raynaud's phenomenon), visual disturbances, and other adverse reactions. In pediatric patients, monitor growth. Perform periodic monitoring of CBC, differential, and platelet counts during prolonged therapy. (Ritalin/Ritalin-SR) Monitor for priapism.

Patient Counseling: Inform about the benefits and risks of therapy and counsel about appropriate use. Instruct to report to physician any new numbness, pain, skin color change, or sensitivity to temperature in fingers or toes, and to contact physician immediately if any signs of unexplained wounds appear on fingers or toes while taking the drug. (Ritalin/Ritalin-SR) Instruct to seek immediate medical attention in the event of priapism.

Administration: Oral route. (Tab, SR) Swallow tabs whole; do not crush or chew. **Storage:** (Ritalin/Ritalin-SR) 25°C (77°F); excursions permitted to 15-30°C (59-86°F). (Generic) 20-25°C (68-77°F). (Ritalin) Protect from light. (Tab, SR) Protect from moisture.

RITUXAN   RX
rituximab (Genentech)

> Serious, including fatal infusion reactions reported; deaths within 24 hrs of infusion have occurred. Monitor patients closely. D/C for severe reaction and treat for Grade 3/4 reactions. Severe, including fatal, mucocutaneous reactions may occur. Hepatitis B virus (HBV) reactivation can occur, in some cases resulting in fulminant hepatitis, hepatic failure, and death. Screen all patients for HBV infection before treatment initiation; monitor patients during and after treatment. D/C therapy and concomitant medications in the event of HBV reactivation. Fatal Progressive Multifocal Leukoencephalopathy (PML) may occur.

THERAPEUTIC CLASS: Monoclonal antibody/CD20-blocker

INDICATIONS: Treatment of non-Hodgkin's lymphoma (NHL) in patients with: relapsed or refractory, low-grade or follicular, CD20-positive, B-cell NHL as a single agent; previously untreated follicular, CD20-positive, B-cell NHL in combination with 1st-line chemotherapy, and in patients achieving a complete or partial response to rituximab in combination with chemotherapy, as single agent maintenance therapy; non-progressing (eg, stable disease), low-grade, CD20-positive, B-cell NHL, as a single agent, after 1st-line cyclophosphamide, vincristine, and prednisone (CVP) chemotherapy; previously untreated diffuse large B-cell, CD20-positive NHL in combination with cyclophosphamide, doxorubicin, vincristine, and prednisone (CHOP) or other anthracycline-based chemotherapy regimens. Treatment of previously untreated and previously treated CD20-positive chronic lymphocytic leukemia (CLL) in combination with fludarabine and cyclophosphamide (FC). Treatment of adult patients with moderately- to severely- active rheumatoid arthritis (RA) who had inadequate response to ≥1 TNF-antagonist therapies, in combination with methotrexate (MTX). Treatment of adult patients with granulomatosis with polyangiitis (GPA) (Wegener's granulomatosis) and microscopic polyangiitis (MPA), in combination with glucocorticoids.

DOSAGE: *Adults:* Premedicate before each infusion with acetaminophen and antihistamine. If administered according to the 90-min infusion rate, administer glucocorticoid component of chemotherapy regimen prior to infusion. Administer as IV infusion only. Relapsed/Refractory, Low-Grade/Follicular, CD20-Positive, B-Cell NHL: Usual: 375mg/m² once weekly for 4 or 8 doses. Retreatment: Usual: 375mg/m² once weekly for 4 doses. Previously Untreated, Follicular, CD20-Positive, B-Cell NHL: Usual: 375mg/m² on Day 1 of each chemotherapy cycle for up to 8 doses. Maint: In patients with complete or partial response, initiate 8 weeks after completion of rituximab in combination with chemotherapy. Give rituximab as single agent every 8 weeks for 12 doses. Non-progressing, Low-Grade, CD20-Positive, B-Cell NHL: Usual: 375mg/m² once weekly for 4 doses at 6-month intervals after completion of 6-8 CVP chemotherapy cycles. Max: 16 doses. Diffuse Large B-Cell NHL: Usual: 375mg/m² on Day 1 of each chemotherapy cycle for up to 8 infusions. CLL: Usual: 375mg/m² the day prior to initiation of FC chemotherapy, then 500mg/m² on Day 1 of cycles 2-6 (every 28 days). Refer to PI for dosing as a component of Zevalin. RA: Usual: Two-1000mg IV infusions separated by 2 weeks, in combination with MTX. Give methylprednisolone 100mg IV (or its equivalent) 30 min prior to each infusion. Give subsequent courses every 24 weeks or based on evaluation, but not sooner than every 16 weeks. GPA/MPA: Usual: 375mg/m² once weekly for 4 weeks. Give methylprednisolone 1000mg/day IV for 1-3 days followed by oral prednisone 1mg/kg/day (≤80mg/day and taper per clinical need) to treat severe vasculitis symptoms. Begin regimen within 14 days prior to or with initiation of rituximab therapy; may continue during and after the 4-week course of treatment.

HOW SUPPLIED: Inj: 100mg/10mL, 500mg/50mL

WARNINGS/PRECAUTIONS: Should only be administered by a healthcare professional with appropriate medical support to manage severe infusion reactions that can be fatal if they occur. Not recommended for use with severe, active infections. *Pneumocystis jiroveci* pneumonia (PCP) and antiherpetic viral prophylaxis is recommended for patients with CLL during treatment and for up to 12 months following treatment as appropriate. PCP prophylaxis is recommended for patients with GPA and MPA during treatment and for at least 6 months following last infusion. Potential for immunogenicity. Mucocutaneous reactions (eg, paraneoplastic pemphigus, Steven-Johnson syndrome, lichenoid dermatitis, vesiculobullous dermatitis, toxic epidermal necrolysis) reported. Acute renal failure, hyperkalemia, hypocalcemia, hyperuricemia, and/or hyperphosphatemia from tumor lysis may occur within 12-24 hrs after the 1st infusion. A high number of circulating malignant cells (≥25,000/mm³) or high tumor burden confers greater risk of tumor lysis syndrome (TLS); administer aggressive IV hydration and antihyperuricemic therapy in patients with high risk of TLS. Correct electrolyte abnormalities, monitor renal function, and fluid balance, and administer supportive care, including dialysis as indicated. Serious, including fatal, bacterial, fungal, and new/reactivated viral infections may occur during and following the completion of therapy; d/c before serious infections and institute anti-infective therapy. Infections reported in some patients with prolonged hypogammaglobulinemia (>11 months after rituximab exposure). D/C if serious/life-threatening cardiac arrhythmias occur. Perform cardiac monitoring during and after all infusions if arrhythmias develop or with history of arrhythmia/angina. Severe renal toxicity may occur in NHL; d/c if SrCr rises or oliguria occurs. Abdominal pain, bowel obstruction, and perforation may occur. Follow current immunization guidelines and administer non-live vaccines at least 4 weeks prior to therapy for RA patients. Obtain CBC and platelet count prior to each course in lymphoid malignancy patients, at weekly to monthly intervals (more frequently if cytopenia develops) during treatment with rituximab and chemotherapy, and at 2- to 4-month intervals during therapy in RA, GPA, or MPA patients. Not recommended in patients with RA who have not had prior inadequate response to one or more TNF antagonists.

ADVERSE REACTIONS: Infusion reactions, mucocutaneous reactions, Hepatitis B reactivation, PML, infections, fever, lymphopenia, chills, asthenia, neutropenia, headache, leukopenia, diarrhea, muscle spasms.

INTERACTIONS: Renal toxicity reported with cisplatin. Vaccination with live viral vaccines not recommended. Observe closely for signs of infection if biologic agents and/or disease modifying antirheumatic drugs are used concomitantly.

PREGNANCY: Category C, caution in nursing.

MECHANISM OF ACTION: Chimeric murine/human monoclonal IgG, kappa antibody/CD20 antigen blocker; binds to CD20 antigen on B-lymphocytes, and Fc domain recruits immune effector functions to mediate B-cell lysis, possibly by complement-dependent cytotoxicity and antibody-dependent cell-mediated cytotoxicity.

PHARMACOKINETICS: Absorption: RA: C_{max}=157mcg/mL (1st infusion), 183mcg/mL (2nd infusion), 318mcg/mL (2 x 500mg dose), 381mcg/mL (2 x 1000mg dose). **Distribution:** RA: V_d=3.1L. GPA/MPA: V_d=4.5L. **Elimination:** NHL: $T_{1/2}$=22 days, RA: $T_{1/2}$=18 days, CLL: $T_{1/2}$=32 days. GPA/MPA: $T_{1/2}$=23 days.

NURSING CONSIDERATIONS

Assessment: Assess for severe active infections, preexisting cardiac/pulmonary conditions, prior experience of cardiopulmonary adverse reactions, high number of circulating malignant cells (≥25,000/mm³), high tumor burden, electrolyte abnormalities, risk/preexisting HBV infection, hypogammaglobulinemia, history of arrhythmias or angina, or any other conditions where treatment is cautioned, pregnancy/nursing status, and possible drug interactions. Perform HBsAg and anti-HBc measurement before initiating treatment. Obtain CBC and platelet count.

Monitoring: Monitor fluid and electrolyte balance, cardiac/renal function, CBC, and platelet counts periodically. Monitor for signs/symptoms of infusion reactions, mucocutaneous reactions, hepatitis B reactivation, PML, new-onset neurologic manifestations, TLS, infections, arrhythmias, bowel obstruction/perforation, cytopenias, and other adverse reactions. Closely monitor for infusion reactions in patients with preexisting cardiac/pulmonary conditions, those who experienced prior cardiopulmonary adverse reactions, and those with high numbers of circulating malignant cells. Monitor patients with evidence of current or prior HBV infection for clinical and laboratory signs of hepatitis or HBV reactivation during and for several months following therapy.

Patient Counseling: Inform of risks of therapy and importance of assessing overall health status at each visit. Inform that drug is detectable in serum for up to 6 months following completion of therapy. Advise to use effective contraception during and for 12 months after therapy.

Administration: IV route. Do not administer as IV push/bolus; for IV infusion only. Refer to PI for infusion instructions and preparation for administration. **Storage:** 2-8°C (36-46°F). Protect from direct sunlight. Do not freeze or shake. Sol for Infusion: 2-8°C (36-46°F) for 24 hrs. Stable for additional 24 hrs at room temperature; however, store diluted solutions at 2-8°C (36-46°F).

ROBAXIN   RX
methocarbamol (Schwarz)

OTHER BRAND NAMES: Robaxin Injection (Baxter) - Robaxin-750 (Schwarz)

THERAPEUTIC CLASS: Muscular analgesic (central-acting)

INDICATIONS: Adjunct for relief of acute, painful musculoskeletal conditions.

DOSAGE: *Adults:* (PO) Initial: (500mg tab) 1500mg qid for 2-3 days. Maint: 1000mg qid. Initial: (750mg tab) 1500mg qid for 2-3 days. Maint: 750mg qid or 1500mg tid. Max: 6g/day for 2-3 days; 8g/day if severe. (Inj) Moderate Symptoms: 10mL IV/IM. IV Max Rate: 3mL undiluted drug/min. IM Max: 5mL into each gluteal region. Severe/Postop Condition: Max: 20-30mL/day up to 3 consecutive days. If feasible, continue with PO. Tetanus: 10-20mL up to 30mL. May repeat q6h until NG tube can be inserted. Continue with crushed tabs. Max: 24g/day PO.
Pediatrics: Tetanus: Initial: 15mg/kg or 500mg/m². Repeat q6h PRN. Max: 1.8g/m² for 3 consecutive days. Administer by injection into tubing or IV infusion.

HOW SUPPLIED: Inj: 100mg/mL [10mL]; Tab: 500mg, 750mg

CONTRAINDICATIONS: (Inj) Renal pathology with injection due to propylene glycol content.

WARNINGS/PRECAUTIONS: May impair mental/physical abilities. May cause color interference in certain screening tests for 5-hydroxy-indoleacetic acid (5-HIAA) and vanillylmandelic acid (VMA). Caution in epilepsy with the injection. Injection rate should not exceed 3mL/min. Avoid extravasation with injection. Avoid use of inj, particularly during early pregnancy.

ADVERSE REACTIONS: Lightheadedness, dizziness, drowsiness, nausea, urticaria, pruritus, rash, conjunctivitis, nasal congestion, blurred vision, headache, fever, seizures, syncope, flushing.

INTERACTIONS: Additive adverse effects with alcohol and other CNS depressants. May inhibit effect of pyridostigmine; caution in patients with myasthenia gravis receiving anticholinergics.

PREGNANCY: Category C, caution in nursing.

MECHANISM OF ACTION: Carbamate derivative of guaifenesin; not established, suspected to have CNS depressant with sedative and musculoskeletal relaxant properties.

PHARMACOKINETICS: Distribution: Plasma protein binding (46-50%). Found in breast milk. **Metabolism:** Via dealkylation, hydroxylation, and conjugation pathways. **Elimination:** Urine; $T_{1/2}$=1-2 hrs.

NURSING CONSIDERATIONS

Assessment: Assess for renal/hepatic impairment, myasthenia gravis, seizures, pregnancy/nursing status, alcohol intake, and drug interactions.

Monitoring: Monitor for congenital and fetal abnormalities if taken during pregnancy, for color interference in certain screening tests for 5-HIAA using nitrosonaphthol reagent and in screening tests for urinary VMA using Gitlow method.

Patient Counseling: Instruct to use caution while performing hazardous tasks. Warn to avoid alcohol or other CNS depressants. Instruct to notify physician if pregnant/nursing or if planning to become pregnant.

Administration: Oral route, IV infusion, and IM; careful supervision of dose and rate of injection.
Storage: 20-25°C (68-77°F), in tight container; excursions permitted to 15-30°C (59-86°F).

ROCALTROL   RX
calcitriol (Validus)

THERAPEUTIC CLASS: Vitamin D analog

INDICATIONS: Management of secondary hyperparathyroidism and resultant metabolic bone disease with moderate to severe chronic renal failure (CrCl 15-55mL/min) in patients not yet on dialysis. Management of hypocalcemia and resultant metabolic bone disease in patients undergoing chronic renal dialysis. Management of hypocalcemia and its clinical manifestations in patients with postsurgical hypoparathyroidism, idiopathic hypoparathyroidism, and pseudohypoparathyroidism.

DOSAGE: *Adults:* Hypoparathyroidism: Initial: 0.25mcg/day qam. Titrate: May increase at 2- to 4-week intervals. Usual: 0.5-2mcg/day qam. Predialysis: Initial: 0.25mcg/day. Titrate: May increase to 0.5mcg/day. Dialysis: Initial: 0.25mcg/day. Titrate: May increase by 0.25mcg/day at 4- to 8-week intervals. Patients with normal or slightly reduced Ca^{2+} levels may respond to 0.25mcg qod. Usual: 0.5-1mcg/day. D/C with hypercalcemia; when Ca^{2+} levels return to normal, continue therapy at a daily dose 0.25mcg lower than that previously used. Elderly: Start at lower end of dosing range.
Pediatrics: Hypoparathyroidism: ≥6 Yrs: Usual: 0.5-2mcg/day qam. 1-5 Yrs: Usual: 0.25-0.75mcg/day qam. Predialysis: ≥3 Yrs: Initial: 0.25mcg/day. Titrate: May increase to 0.5mcg/day. <3 Yrs: Initial: 10-15ng/kg/day. D/C with hypercalcemia; when Ca^{2+} levels return to normal, continue therapy at a daily dose 0.25mcg lower than that previously used.

HOW SUPPLIED: Cap: 0.25mcg, 0.5mcg; Sol: 1mcg/mL [15mL]

CONTRAINDICATIONS: Hypercalcemia or evidence of vitamin D toxicity.

WARNINGS/PRECAUTIONS: Administration in excess of daily requirements may cause hypercalcemia, hypercalciuria, and hyperphosphatemia. Chronic hypercalcemia may lead to generalized vascular calcification, nephrocalcinosis, and other soft tissue calcification. Serum Ca^{2+} times phosphate (Ca x P) product should not exceed 70 mg^2/dL^2. May increase serum inorganic phosphate levels, leading to ectopic calcification in patients with renal failure; use non-aluminum phosphate binders and low phosphate diet to control serum phosphate in dialysis patients. Caution in elderly and immobilized patients. If treatment switched from ergocalciferol, may take several months for ergocalciferol level in blood to return to baseline. In patients with normal renal function, chronic hypercalcemia may be associated with an increase in SrCr. Avoid dehydration in patients with normal renal function. When indicated, estimate daily dietary Ca^{2+} intake and adjust accordingly.

ADVERSE REACTIONS: Hypercalcemia, hypercalciuria, SrCr elevation, weakness, N/V, dry mouth, constipation, muscle and bone pain, metallic taste, polyuria, polydipsia, weight loss, hypersensitivity reactions.

INTERACTIONS: Avoid pharmacological doses of vitamin D products and derivatives during therapy. Avoid uncontrolled intake of additional Ca^{2+}-containing preparations. Avoid with Mg^{2+}-containing preparations (eg, antacids) in patients on chronic renal dialysis; use may lead to hypermagnesemia. May impair intestinal absorption with cholestyramine. Reduced blood levels with phenytoin or phenobarbital. Caution with thiazides; may cause hypercalcemia. Reduced serum endogenous concentrations with ketoconazole reported. Hypercalcemia may precipitate cardiac arrhythmias in patients on digitalis; use with caution. Functional antagonism with corticosteroids. Adjust dose of concomitant phosphate-binding agent.

PREGNANCY: Category C, not for use in nursing.

MECHANISM OF ACTION: Synthetic vitamin D analog; regulates absorption of Ca^{2+} from the GI tract and its utilization in the body.

PHARMACOKINETICS: Absorption: Rapid (intestine). T_{max}=3-6 hrs, 8-12 hrs (hemodialysis); C_{max}=116pmol/L (pediatrics). **Distribution:** Found in breast milk. **Metabolism:** Hydroxylation to 1α, $25R(OH)_2$-26, 23S-lactone D_3 (major metabolite). **Elimination:** Feces (primary), urine (10%, 1mcg dose); $T_{1/2}$=5-8 hrs (normal subjects), 16.2 hrs and 21.9 hrs (hemodialysis).

NURSING CONSIDERATIONS

Assessment: Assess for hypercalcemia, evidence of vitamin D toxicity, renal function, presence of immobilization, pregnancy/nursing status, and possible drug interactions. Obtain baseline levels of serum Ca^{2+}, phosphorus (P), alkaline phosphatase, creatinine, and intact parathyroid hormone (iPTH).

Monitoring: Monitor for hypercalcemia, hypercalciuria, and hyperphosphatemia. For dialysis patients, perform periodic monitoring of serum Ca^{2+}, P, Mg^{2+}, and alkaline phosphatase. For hypoparathyroid patients, perform periodic monitoring of serum Ca^{2+}, P, and 24-hr urinary Ca^{2+}.

R

For predialysis patients, perform monthly monitoring of serum Ca^{2+}, P, alkaline phosphatase, and creatinine for 6 months; then periodically, and periodic monitoring of iPTH every 3- to 4-months. Monitor serum Ca^{2+} levels ≥2X/week after all dosage changes and during titration periods.

Patient Counseling: Inform about compliance with dosage instructions, adherence to instructions about diet and Ca^{2+} supplementation, and avoidance of the use of unapproved nonprescription drugs. Carefully inform about symptoms of hypercalcemia. Advise to maintain adequate calcium intake at a minimum of 600mg/day.

Administration: Oral route. **Storage:** 15-30°C (59-86°F). Protect from light.

ROTATEQ   RX
rotavirus vaccine, live, pentavalent (Merck)

THERAPEUTIC CLASS: Vaccine

INDICATIONS: Prevention of rotavirus gastroenteritis caused by the serotypes G1, G2, G3, and G4 in infants between the ages of 6-32 weeks.

DOSAGE: *Pediatrics:* 6-32 Weeks: Administer series of 3 (2mL) doses PO starting at 6-12 weeks of age, with subsequent doses administered at 4- to 10-week intervals. Third dose should not be given after 32 weeks of age.

HOW SUPPLIED: Sol: 2mL

CONTRAINDICATIONS: Severe combined immunodeficiency disease (SCID) and history of intussusception.

WARNINGS/PRECAUTIONS: For PO use only. Appropriate treatment and supervision must be available to manage possible anaphylactic reactions following administration. Safety and efficacy data not available for administration to infants who are potentially immunocompromised. Caution in infants with a history of GI disorders (eg, active acute GI illness, chronic diarrhea, failure to thrive, history of congenital abdominal disorders, abdominal surgery). Intussusception reported. Shedding of vaccine virus in stool reported. Transmission of vaccine virus from vaccinees to unvaccinated contacts reported; caution when administering to individuals with immunodeficient close contacts. Consider delaying use with febrile illness. May not protect all vaccine recipients against rotavirus. Clinical data not available for postexposure prophylaxis or for level of protection provided with administration of an incomplete regimen. If an incomplete dose is administered (eg, infant spits or regurgitates vaccine), do not give replacement dose; continue to give any remaining doses in the recommended series.

ADVERSE REACTIONS: Irritability, fever, diarrhea, vomiting, nasopharyngitis, otitis media.

INTERACTIONS: Immunosuppressive therapies, including irradiation, antimetabolites, alkylating agents, cytotoxic drugs, and corticosteroids (used in greater than physiologic doses) may reduce immune response to vaccine.

PREGNANCY: Category C, safety not known in nursing.

MECHANISM OF ACTION: Vaccine; exact immunologic mechanism is unknown. Replicates in small intestine and induces immunity.

NURSING CONSIDERATIONS

Assessment: Assess for previous hypersensitivity to the vaccine, SCID, history of intussusception, immunization history, immunocompromised conditions, history of GI disorders, febrile illness, and possible drug interactions.

Monitoring: Monitor for hypersensitivity/anaphylactic reactions, intussusception, and other adverse events.

Patient Counseling: Inform parent/guardian of potential benefits/risks of vaccine. Instruct parent/guardian to inform physician of the current health status of patient and to report if patient has close contact with a family/household member who has a weak immune system. Advise to contact physician immediately if patient develops vomiting, diarrhea, severe stomach pain, or blood in the stool and advise to contact physician if any other adverse reactions develop.

Administration: Oral route. Gently squeeze liquid into infant's mouth toward the inner cheek until dosing tube is empty. Administer as soon as possible after being removed from refrigeration. Food or liquid consumption, including breast milk, before or after vaccination is not restricted. Do not mix with any other vaccines or sol. Do not reconstitute or dilute. Refer to PI for further information on instructions for use. **Storage:** 2-8°C (36-46°F). Protect from light.

ROXICET
oxycodone HCl - acetaminophen (Roxane)

> Associated with cases of acute liver failure, at times resulting in liver transplant and death. Most cases associated with acetaminophen (APAP) doses >4000mg/day and involved more than one APAP-containing product.

THERAPEUTIC CLASS: Analgesic combination

INDICATIONS: Relief of moderate to moderately severe pain.

DOSAGE: *Adults:* Usual: 5mL q6h PRN. Titrate: May need to exceed usual dose based on individual response, pain severity, and tolerance. Max: 60mL/day. Do not exceed 4g/day of APAP. Constant Pain: Give at regular intervals on an around-the-clock schedule.

HOW SUPPLIED: Sol: (Oxycodone-APAP) 5mg-325mg/5mL [5mL, 500mL]

CONTRAINDICATIONS: Oxycodone: Significant respiratory depression (in unmonitored settings or absence of resuscitative equipment), acute or severe bronchial asthma or hypercarbia, known/suspected paralytic ileus.

WARNINGS/PRECAUTIONS: Caution with CNS depression, elderly/debilitated patients, severe impairment of hepatic, pulmonary, or renal function, hypothyroidism, Addison's disease, prostatic hypertrophy, urethral stricture, acute alcoholism, delirium tremens, kyphoscoliosis with respiratory depression, myxedema, and toxic psychosis. Not recommended during and immediately prior to labor and delivery due to potential effects on respiratory function of the newborn. Oxycodone: May be abused in a manner similar to other opioid agonists. May cause respiratory depression; extreme caution with acute asthma, chronic obstructive pulmonary disorder, cor pulmonale, or preexisting respiratory impairment; consider nonopioid alternatives or use lowest effective dose and monitor carefully. Respiratory depressant effects may be markedly exaggerated in the presence of head injury, other intracranial lesions, or preexisting increased intracranial pressure. Produces effects on pupillary response and consciousness which may obscure neurologic signs of worsening in patients with head injuries. May cause severe hypotension; caution in patients with circulatory shock. May produce orthostatic hypotension in ambulatory patients. May obscure the diagnosis or clinical course of acute abdominal conditions. May induce or aggravate convulsions/seizures. Ileus may occur after intra-abdominal surgery; monitor for decreased bowel motility in postoperative patients. May cause spasm of the sphincter of Oddi and increase serum amylase; caution with biliary tract disease, including acute pancreatitis. Physical dependence and tolerance may occur. Anaphylaxis reported in patients with codeine hypersensitivity. Upon discontinuation, taper dose gradually if on therapy for more than a few weeks. Caution with hepatic/renal impairment. APAP: Hypersensitivity/anaphylaxis reported; d/c if symptoms occur. Increased risk of acute liver failure with underlying liver disease.

ADVERSE REACTIONS: Respiratory depression, apnea, respiratory arrest, circulatory depression, hypotension, shock, lightheadedness, dizziness, sedation, N/V, euphoria, dysphoria, constipation, pruritus.

INTERACTIONS: Oxycodone: May enhance neuromuscular-blocking action of skeletal muscle relaxants and increase respiratory depression. Additive CNS depression with opioid analgesics, general anesthetics, centrally acting antiemetics, phenothiazines, tranquilizers, sedative-hypnotics and other CNS depressants (eg, alcohol); reduce dose of one or both agents. May produce paralytic ileus with anticholinergics. Mixed agonist/antagonist analgesics (eg, pentazocine, nalbuphine, naltrexone, butorphanol) may reduce analgesic effect and/or precipitate withdrawal symptoms. May cause severe hypotension with drugs that compromise vasomotor tone (eg, phenothiazines). APAP: Increased risk of acute liver failure with alcohol ingestion; hepatotoxicity occurred in chronic alcoholics. Increase in glucuronidation and plasma clearance as well as decreased $T_{1/2}$ with oral contraceptives. Increased effects with propranolol and probenecid. May decrease effects of loop diuretics, lamotrigine, and zidovudine.

PREGNANCY: Category C, not for use in nursing.

MECHANISM OF ACTION: Oxycodone: Opioid analgesic; pure opioid agonist. Principal therapeutic effect is analgesia. Effects are mediated by receptors (notably µ and kappa) in the CNS for endogenous opioid-like compounds (eg, endorphins, enkephalins). APAP: Nonopiate, nonsalicylate analgesic and antipyretic; not established. Antipyretic effect occurs through inhibition of endogenous pyrogen action on the hypothalamic heat-regulating centers.

PHARMACOKINETICS: Absorption: Oxycodone: Absolute bioavailability (87%). APAP: Rapid and almost complete. **Distribution:** Oxycodone: Plasma protein binding (45%); (IV) V_d=211.9L; crosses placenta; found in breast milk. APAP: Plasma protein binding during acute intoxication (20-50%); found in breast milk. **Metabolism:** Oxycodone: N-dealkylation, O-demethylation via CYP2D6; noroxycodone, oxymorphone (metabolites). APAP: Liver via CYP450 (conjugation), N acetyl-p-benzoquinoneimine, N-acetylimidoquinone (toxic metabolite). **Elimination:** Oxycodone: Urine (8-14%, unchanged); $T_{1/2}$=3.51 hrs. APAP: Urine (90-100%).

NURSING CONSIDERATIONS

Assessment: Assess for drug hypersensitivity, severity and type of pain, respiratory depression, bronchial asthma, hypercarbia, paralytic ileus, level of consciousness, alcohol consumption, pregnancy/nursing status, renal/hepatic function, drug abuse potential, possible drug interactions, or any other conditions where treatment is contraindicated or cautioned.

Monitoring: Monitor for signs/symptoms of respiratory depression, elevations in CSF pressure, altered consciousness, hypotension, hepatotoxicity, convulsions, anaphylactic reactions, decreased bowel motility in postoperative patients, spasm of the sphincter of Oddi, serum amylase levels, physical dependence and tolerance, abuse or misuse of medication, hypersensitivity reactions, and withdrawal syndrome during discontinuation.

Patient Counseling: Instruct to keep out of reach of children. Advise to dispose of unused drug by flushing down the toilet. Advise to not adjust dosing without consulting physician. Inform that drug may impair mental/physical abilities required to perform hazardous tasks. Instruct to not combine with alcohol and other CNS depressants unless under recommendation and guidance of a physician. If on medication for more than a few weeks, instruct to consult physician for gradual discontinuation dose schedule. Inform that medication has potential for abuse; instruct to protect from theft. Advise to d/c and contact physician immediately if signs of allergy develop. Inform to not take >4000mg/day of APAP and to contact physician if the recommended dose is exceeded.

Administration: Oral route. **Storage:** 20-25°C (68-77°F).

ROZEREM   RX
 ramelteon (Takeda)

THERAPEUTIC CLASS: Melatonin receptor agonist

INDICATIONS: Treatment of insomnia characterized by difficulty with sleep onset.

DOSAGE: *Adults:* Usual: 8mg within 30 min of hs. Max: 8mg/day.

HOW SUPPLIED: Tab: 8mg

CONTRAINDICATIONS: Coadministration with fluvoxamine.

WARNINGS/PRECAUTIONS: Angioedema reported; do not rechallenge if angioedema develops. Sleep disturbances may manifest as a physical and/or psychiatric disorder; symptomatic treatment of insomnia should be initiated only after careful evaluation. Failure of insomnia to remit after 7-10 days of therapy may indicate presence of psychiatric and/or medical illness. Cognitive and behavior changes, hallucinations, amnesia, anxiety, other neuropsychiatric symptoms, and complex behaviors reported; d/c if complex sleep behavior occurs. Worsening of depression reported in primarily depressed patients. May impair physical/mental abilities. May affect reproductive hormones (eg, decreased testosterone levels, increased prolactin levels). Not recommended with severe sleep apnea. Do not use with severe hepatic impairment. Caution with moderate hepatic impairment.

ADVERSE REACTIONS: Dizziness, somnolence, fatigue, nausea, exacerbated insomnia.

INTERACTIONS: See Contraindications. Decreased efficacy with strong CYP inducers (eg, rifampin). Caution with less strong CYP1A2 inhibitors, strong CYP3A4 inhibitors (eg, ketoconazole), and strong CYP2C9 inhibitors (eg, fluconazole). Increased levels with donepezil and doxepin; monitor patients closely. Increased T_{max} of zolpidem; avoid use. Increased risk of complex behaviors with alcohol and other CNS depressants. Additive effect with alcohol; avoid alcohol use.

PREGNANCY: Category C, caution in nursing.

MECHANISM OF ACTION: Melatonin receptor agonist; activity at MT_1 and MT_2 receptors believed to contribute to sleep-promoting properties. These receptors, acted upon by endogenous melatonin, are thought to be involved in the maintenance of the circadian rhythm underlying the normal sleep-wake cycle.

PHARMACOKINETICS: Absorption: Rapid. Absolute bioavailability (1.8%); T_{max}=0.75 hr (fasted). **Distribution:** Plasma protein binding (82%). **Metabolism:** Oxidation via CYP1A2 (major), CYP2C, CYP3A4 (minor). M-II, M-IV, M-I, M-III (principal metabolites). **Elimination:** Urine and feces (<0.1% parent compound); $T_{1/2}$=1-2.6 hrs, 2-5 hrs (M-II). Refer to PI for PK parameters in elderly patients.

NURSING CONSIDERATIONS

Assessment: Assess for hepatic impairment, manifestations of physical and/or psychiatric disorder, depression, sleep apnea, other comorbid diagnoses, hypersensitivity, pregnancy/nursing status, and possible drug interactions.

Monitoring: Monitor for signs/symptoms of angioedema, exacerbations of insomnia, emergence of cognitive or behavioral abnormalities, worsening of depression, complex sleep behaviors, and anaphylactic/anaphylactoid reactions.

Patient Counseling: Inform patients, families, and caregivers about benefits and risks associated with treatment. Counsel for appropriate use and instruct to read Medication Guide. Inform that severe anaphylactic and anaphylactoid reactions may occur; advise to seek immediate medical attention. Instruct to report sleep-driving to doctor immediately. Instruct to consult healthcare provider if cessation of menses, galactorrhea in females, decreased libido, or fertility problems occur. Instruct to take within 30 min prior to hs and confine activities to those necessary to prepare for bed. Instruct to swallow tab whole; do not break.

Administration: Oral route. Do not take with or immediately after high-fat meal. **Storage:** 25°C (77°F); excursions permitted to 15-30°C (59-86°F). Protect from moisture and humidity.

RYTHMOL   RX
propafenone HCl (Qualitest)

> Increased rate of death or reversed cardiac arrest rate reported in patients treated with encainide or flecainide (Class 1C antiarrhythmics) in a study of patients with asymptomatic non-life-threatening ventricular arrhythmias who had a myocardial infarction (MI) >6 days but <2 yrs previously. Consider any 1C antiarrhythmic to have a significant proarrhythmic risk in patients with structural heart disease. Avoid in patients with non-life-threatening ventricular arrhythmias, even if experiencing unpleasant, but not life-threatening signs/symptoms.

OTHER BRAND NAMES: Propafenone (Qualitest)

THERAPEUTIC CLASS: Class IC antiarrhythmic

INDICATIONS: To prolong the time to recurrence of paroxysmal atrial fibrillation/flutter and paroxysmal supraventricular tachycardia associated with disabling symptoms in patients without structural heart disease. Treatment of life-threatening documented ventricular arrhythmias (eg, sustained ventricular tachycardia).

DOSAGE: *Adults:* Initial: 150mg q8h. Titrate: Individualize based on response and tolerance. May increase at a minimum of 3- to 4-day intervals to 225mg q8h. If additional therapeutic effect is needed, may increase to 300mg q8h. Max: 900mg/day. Elderly/Ventricular Arrhythmia with Marked Previous Myocardial Damage: Increase more gradually during initial phase. Hepatic Impairment/Significant QRS Widening/2nd- or 3rd-Degree Atrioventricular (AV) Block: Reduce dose. Elderly: Start at lower end of dosing range.

HOW SUPPLIED: Tab: 150mg*, 225mg* *scored

CONTRAINDICATIONS: Heart failure (HF), cardiogenic shock, known Brugada syndrome, bradycardia, marked hypotension, bronchospastic disorders or severe obstructive pulmonary disease, marked electrolyte imbalance, and sinoatrial, AV, and intraventricular disorders of impulse generation or conduction (eg, sick sinus node syndrome, AV block) in the absence of an artificial pacemaker.

WARNINGS/PRECAUTIONS: Do not use to control ventricular rate during atrial fibrillation. Concomitant treatment with drugs that increase the functional AV nodal refractory period is recommended. May cause new or worsened arrhythmias; evaluate ECG prior to and during therapy to determine if response supports continued treatment. Brugada syndrome may be unmasked after exposure to therapy; perform ECG after initiation of treatment and d/c if changes are suggestive of Brugada syndrome. May provoke overt HF. Conduction disturbances (eg, 1st to 3rd-degree AV block, bundle branch block, intraventricular conduction delay, bradycardia), agranulocytosis, positive antinuclear antibody (ANA) titers, and exacerbation of myasthenia gravis reported. D/C if persistent or worsening elevation of ANA titers detected. May alter pacing and sensing thresholds of implanted pacemakers and defibrillators; monitor and reprogram devices accordingly during and after therapy. Reversible, short-term drop (within normal range) in sperm count may occur. Treatment of ventricular arrhythmias should be initiated in the hospital. Caution in patients with renal/hepatic dysfunction and in elderly.

ADVERSE REACTIONS: Unusual taste, N/V, dizziness, constipation, headache, fatigue, blurred vision, weakness.

INTERACTIONS: Avoid with Class IA and III antiarrhythmics (eg, quinidine, amiodarone) and withhold these agents for at least 5 half-lives prior to therapy. Inhibitors of CYP2D6 (eg, desipramine, paroxetine, ritonavir, sertraline) and CYP3A4 (eg, ketoconazole, ritonavir, saquinavir, erythromycin, grapefruit juice) may increase levels; avoid simultaneous use with both a CYP2D6 and a CYP3A4 inhibitor. Amiodarone can affect conduction and repolarization; coadministration is not recommended. Fluoxetine may increase levels in extensive metabolizers. Rifampin may decrease levels and may increase norpropafenone (active metabolite) levels. May increase levels of digoxin, propranolol, metoprolol, and warfarin; monitor digoxin levels and INR. May result in severe adverse events (eg, convulsions, AV block, acute circulatory failure) with abrupt cessation of orlistat. May increase risk of CNS side effects of lidocaine. CYP1A2 inhibitors (eg, amiodarone, tobacco smoke) and cimetidine may increase levels.

PREGNANCY: Category C, not for use in nursing.

MECHANISM OF ACTION: Class 1C antiarrhythmic; has local anesthetic effects and direct stabilizing action on myocardial membranes. Reduces upstroke velocity (phase 0) of the monophasic action potential. Reduces the fast inward current carried by Na$^+$ ions in Purkinje fibers and myocardial fibers. Diastolic excitability threshold is increased and effective refractory period prolonged. Reduces spontaneous automaticity and depresses triggered activity.

PHARMACOKINETICS: Absorption: Complete; absolute bioavailability (3.4%, 150mg dose), (10.6%, 300mg dose); T_{max}=3.5 hrs. **Distribution:** (IV) V_d=252L; plasma protein binding (>95%); found in breast milk. **Metabolism:** Liver (rapid, extensive) via CYP3A4, 1A2, and 2D6; 5-hydroxypropafenone and N-depropylpropafenone (active metabolites). **Elimination:** $T_{1/2}$=2-10 hrs (>90% of patients), 10-32 hrs (<10% of patients).

NURSING CONSIDERATIONS

Assessment: Assess for HF, cardiogenic shock, sinoatrial/AV/intraventricular disorders, implanted pacemaker/defibrillator, bradycardia, marked hypotension, bronchospastic disorders or severe obstructive pulmonary disease, marked electrolyte imbalance, MI, renal/hepatic dysfunction, known Brugada syndrome, pregnancy/nursing status, and possible drug interactions. Evaluate ECG prior to therapy.

Monitoring: Monitor for proarrhythmic effects, signs/symptoms of conduction disturbances, agranulocytosis, HF, unmasking of Brugada syndrome, exacerbation of myasthenia gravis, and other adverse reactions. Monitor implanted pacemakers and defibrillators during and after therapy and reprogram accordingly. Evaluate ECG during therapy. Monitor ANA titers and renal/hepatic function. Monitor INR when given with warfarin.

Patient Counseling: Inform about risks/benefits of therapy. Advise to report symptoms that may be associated with electrolyte imbalance (eg, excessive/prolonged diarrhea, sweating, vomiting, loss of appetite, thirst) to physician. Inform to notify physician of all Rx, herbal/natural preparations, and OTC medications currently being taken or of any changes with these products. Instruct not to double the next dose if a dose is missed and to take next dose at the usual time.

Administration: Oral route. **Storage:** 25°C (77°F); excursions permitted to 15-30°C (59-86°F).

RYTHMOL SR   RX
propafenone HCl (GlaxoSmithKline)

> Increased rate of death or reversed cardiac arrest rate reported in patients treated with encainide or flecainide (Class 1C antiarrhythmics) in a study of patients with asymptomatic non-life-threatening ventricular arrhythmias who had a myocardial infarction (MI) >6 days but <2 yrs previously. Consider any 1C antiarrhythmics to have significant proarrhythmic risk in patients with structural heart disease. Avoid in patients with non-life-threatening ventricular arrhythmias, even if experiencing unpleasant, but not life-threatening signs/symptoms.

THERAPEUTIC CLASS: Class IC antiarrhythmic

INDICATIONS: To prolong the time to recurrence of symptomatic atrial fibrillation (A-fib) in patients with episodic (most likely paroxysmal or persistent) A-fib who do not have structural heart disease.

DOSAGE: *Adults:* Initial: 225mg q12h. Titrate: May increase at a minimum of 5-day intervals to 325mg q12h. If additional therapeutic effect is needed, may increase to 425mg q12h. Hepatic Impairment/Significant QRS Widening/2nd- or 3rd-degree Atrioventricular (AV) Block: Reduce dose.

HOW SUPPLIED: Cap, Extended-Release: 225mg, 325mg, 425mg

CONTRAINDICATIONS: Heart failure (HF), cardiogenic shock, known Brugada syndrome, bradycardia, marked hypotension, bronchospastic disorders or severe obstructive pulmonary disease, marked electrolyte imbalance, and sinoatrial, AV and intraventricular disorders of impulse generation or conduction (eg, sick sinus node syndrome, AV block) in the absence of an artificial pacemaker.

WARNINGS/PRECAUTIONS: Do not use to control ventricular rate during A-fib. Concomitant treatment with drugs that increase the functional AV nodal refractory period is recommended. May cause new or worsened arrhythmias; evaluate ECG prior to and during therapy. Brugada syndrome may be unmasked after exposure to therapy; perform ECG after initiation of treatment and d/c if changes are suggestive of Brugada syndrome. May provoke overt HF. Proarrhythmic effects more likely occur in patients with HF or severe MI. Conduction disturbances (eg, 1st-degree AV block), agranulocytosis, positive antinuclear antibody (ANA) titers, and exacerbation of myasthenia gravis reported. D/C if persistent or worsening elevation of ANA titers detected. May alter pacing and sensing thresholds of implanted pacemakers and defibrillators; monitor and reprogram devices accordingly during and after therapy. Reversible, short-term drop (within normal range) in sperm count may occur. Caution with renal/hepatic dysfunction.

ADVERSE REACTIONS: Dizziness, palpitations, chest pain, dyspnea, taste disturbance, nausea, fatigue, anxiety, constipation, upper respiratory tract infection, edema, influenza.

INTERACTIONS: Avoid with Class Ia and III antiarrhythmics (eg, quinidine, amiodarone) and withhold these agents for at least 5 half-lives prior to therapy. Inhibitors of CYP2D6 (eg, desipramine, paroxetine, ritonavir) and CYP3A4 (eg, ketoconazole, ritonavir, erythromycin, grapefruit juice) may increase levels; avoid simultaneous use with both a CYP2D6 and a CYP3A4 inhibitor. Amiodarone can affect conduction and repolarization; coadministration is not recommended. Fluoxetine may increase levels in extensive metabolizers. Rifampin may decrease levels and may increase norpropafenone (active metabolite) levels. May increase levels of digoxin, propranolol, metoprolol, and warfarin; monitor digoxin levels and INR. May result in severe adverse events (eg, convulsions, AV block, acute circulatory failure) with abrupt cessation of orlistat. May increase risk of CNS side effects of lidocaine. CYP1A2 inhibitors (eg, amiodarone, tobacco smoke) and cimetidine may increase levels.

PREGNANCY: Category C, not for use in nursing.

MECHANISM OF ACTION: Class 1C antiarrhythmic; has local anesthetic effects and direct stabilizing action on myocardial membranes. Reduces upstroke velocity (Phase 0) of the monophasic action potential. Reduces the fast inward current carried by Na$^+$ ions in Purkinje fibers and myocardial fibers. Diastolic excitability is increased and effective refractory period is prolonged. Reduces spontaneous automaticity and depresses triggered activity.

PHARMACOKINETICS: Absorption: T_{max}=3-8 hrs. **Distribution:** (IV) V_d=252L; plasma protein binding (>95%); found in breast milk. **Metabolism:** Liver (rapid, extensive) via CYP2D6, 3A4, and 1A2. 5-hydroxypropafenone and N-depropylpropafenone (active metabolites). **Elimination:** $T_{1/2}$=2-10 hrs (>90% of patients), $T_{1/2}$=10-32 hrs (<10% of patients).

NURSING CONSIDERATIONS

Assessment: Assess for HF, cardiogenic shock, sinoatrial/AV/intraventricular disorders, implanted pacemaker/defibrillator, bradycardia, marked hypotension, bronchospastic disorders or severe obstructive pulmonary disease, marked electrolyte imbalance, MI, renal/hepatic dysfunction, known Brugada syndrome, pregnancy/nursing status, and possible drug interactions. Evaluate ECG prior to therapy.

Monitoring: Monitor for proarrhythmic effects, signs/symptoms of conduction disturbances, agranulocytosis, HF, unmasking of Brugada syndrome, exacerbation of myasthenia gravis, and other adverse reactions. Monitor implanted pacemakers and defibrillators during and after therapy and reprogram accordingly. Evaluate ECG during therapy. Monitor ANA titers, LFTs, and renal/hepatic function.

Patient Counseling: Inform about risks/benefits of therapy. Advise to report symptoms that may be associated with electrolyte imbalance (eg, excessive/prolonged diarrhea, sweating, vomiting, loss of appetite, thirst). Inform to notify physician of all prescription, herbal/natural preparations, and OTC medications currently being taken or of any changes with these products. Instruct not to double the next dose if a dose is missed and to take next dose at the usual time.

Administration: Oral route. Take with or without food. Do not crush or further divide cap contents. **Storage:** 25°C (77°F); excursions permitted to 15-30°C (59-86°F).

SABRIL

RX

vigabatrin (Lundbeck)

> Causes permanent vision loss in infants, children, and adults; timing of onset is unpredictable. Causes permanent bilateral concentric visual field constriction in a high percentage of adult patients; in some cases may damage central retina and may decrease visual acuity. Risk of vision loss increases with increasing dose and cumulative exposure; use lowest dose and shortest exposure. D/C in patients who fail to show clinical benefit within 2-4 weeks (pediatric patients) or 3 months (adults) of initiation, or sooner if treatment failure is obvious. Vision loss may not be recognized until it is severe. Unless a patient is formally exempted from periodic ophthalmologic assessment, vision assessment is required at baseline (no later than 4 weeks after starting therapy), at least every 3 months during therapy and about 3-6 months after therapy is discontinued. Consider drug discontinuation, balancing benefit and risk, if visual loss is documented. Vision loss may worsen despite discontinuation of therapy. Unless benefit clearly outweighs the risk, avoid use with other drugs associated with serious adverse ophthalmic effects (eg, retinopathy, glaucoma) and in patients with, or at high risk of, other types of irreversible vision loss. Available only through restricted distribution program (SHARE).

THERAPEUTIC CLASS: GABA analog

INDICATIONS: (Sol) Monotherapy for pediatric patients (1 month-2 yrs of age) with infantile spasms (IS) for whom the potential benefits outweigh the potential risk of vision loss. (Tab) Adjunctive therapy for adults with refractory complex partial seizures (CPS) who have inadequately responded to several alternative treatments and for whom the potential benefits outweigh the risk of vision loss.

DOSAGE: *Adults:* (Tab) Refractory CPS: Initial: 500mg bid (1g/day). Titrate: May increase total daily dose in 500mg increments at weekly intervals. Usual: 1.5g bid (3g/day). Mild Renal Impairment (CrCl >50-80mL/min): Decrease dose by 25%. Moderate Renal Impairment (CrCl >30-50mL/min): Decrease dose by 50%. Severe Renal Impairment (CrCl >10-<30mL/min):

Decrease dose by 75%. Reduce dose gradually to d/c.
Pediatrics: 1 Month-2 Yrs: (Sol) IS: Initial: 50mg/kg/day in 2 divided doses. Titrate: May increase by 25-50mg/kg/day increments every 3 days. Max: 150mg/kg/day. Refer to PI for volume of individual doses. Reduce dose gradually to d/c.

HOW SUPPLIED: Sol: 500mg/pkt [50³]; Tab: 500mg* *scored

WARNINGS/PRECAUTIONS: Abnormal magnetic resonance imaging (MRI) signal changes involving the thalamus, basal ganglia, brain stem, and cerebellum observed in some infants. May increase risk of suicidal thoughts/behavior. May cause anemia, somnolence, fatigue, peripheral neuropathy, weight gain, and edema. Should be withdrawn gradually. May impair physical/mental abilities. May decrease ALT and AST plasma activity and may preclude the use of these markers, especially ALT, to detect hepatic injury. May increase amount of amino acids in the urine, possibly leading to false positive test for certain rare genetic metabolic diseases (eg, alpha aminoadipic aciduria). Caution with renal impairment and in elderly.

ADVERSE REACTIONS: Vision loss/visual field defects, vomiting, urinary tract infection, upper respiratory tract infection, lethargy, rash, somnolence, irritability, diarrhea, fever, constipation, sedation, influenza.

INTERACTIONS: See Boxed Warning. May decrease phenytoin plasma levels. May increase C_{max} and decrease T_{max} of clonazepam.

PREGNANCY: Category C, not for use in nursing.

MECHANISM OF ACTION: Gamma-aminobutyric acid (GABA) analog; has not been established. Believed to be the result of its action as an irreversible inhibitor of GABA transaminase, which results in increased levels of GABA in the CNS.

PHARMACOKINETICS: Absorption: Complete. T_{max}=1 hr (adults/children), 2.5 hrs (infants). **Distribution:** V_d=1.1L/kg; found in breast milk. **Elimination:** Urine (95%, 80% parent drug); $T_{1/2}$=7.5 hrs (adults), 5.7 hrs (infants).

NURSING CONSIDERATIONS

Assessment: Assess for renal impairment, underlying suicidal behavior/ideation, pregnancy/nursing status, and for drug interactions. Perform baseline vision assessment (no later than 4 weeks after starting therapy).

Monitoring: Monitor for worsening vision/visual field changes and vision loss, abnormal MRI signal changes, suicidal thoughts/behavior, emergence/worsening of depression, unusual changes in thoughts or behavior, anemia, somnolence, fatigue, peripheral neuropathy, weight gain, edema, and other adverse reactions. Monitor Hgb, Hct, and renal function. Perform vision assessment at least every 3 months during therapy and about 3-6 months after discontinuation of therapy. Monitor response to therapy and continued need for treatment periodically.

Patient Counseling: Inform of the risk of permanent vision loss, particularly loss of peripheral vision, and the need for vision monitoring. Instruct to notify physician if changes in vision occur. Advise that therapy may increase risk of suicidal thoughts and behavior; instruct to notify physician if any abnormal behaviors develop. Advise to not drive a car or operate other complex machinery until patients are familiar with the effects of therapy on their ability to perform such activities. Inform to notify physician if pregnant, plan to become pregnant, or if breastfeeding. Instruct to not abruptly d/c therapy. Inform of the possibility of developing abnormal MRI signal changes.

Administration: Oral route. Take with or without food. (Sol) Empty contents of pkt into an empty cup and dissolve with 10mL of cold/room temperature water per pkt using oral syringe. Final sol concentration should be 50mg/mL. Prepare each dose immediately prior to administration. Refer to PI for further preparation and administration instructions. **Storage:** 20-25°C (68-77°F).

SAMSCA   RX
tolvaptan (Otsuka America)

> Initiate and reinitiate therapy in patients only in a hospital where serum Na⁺ can be monitored closely. Osmotic demyelination resulting in dysarthria, mutism, dysphagia, lethargy, affective changes, spastic quadriparesis, seizures, coma, and death may occur due to rapid correction of hyponatremia (eg, >12mEq/L/24 hrs). Slower rates of correction may be advisable in susceptible patients (eg, with severe malnutrition, alcoholism, advanced liver disease).

THERAPEUTIC CLASS: Arginine vasopressin antagonist

INDICATIONS: Treatment of clinically significant hypervolemic and euvolemic hyponatremia (eg, serum Na⁺ <125mEq/L or less marked hyponatremia that is symptomatic and has resisted correction with fluid restriction), including patients with heart failure and syndrome of inappropriate antidiuretic hormone.

DOSAGE: *Adults:* Initial: 15mg qd. Titrate: Increase to 30mg qd, after at least 24 hrs. Max: 60mg qd, PRN to achieve desired level of serum Na⁺. Avoid fluid restriction during the first 24 hrs of therapy. Limit duration of therapy to 30 days to minimize the risk of liver injury.

HOW SUPPLIED: Tab: 15mg, 30mg

CONTRAINDICATIONS: Urgent need to raise serum Na⁺ acutely, inability to autoregulate fluid balance, hypovolemic hyponatremia, anuria, and concomitant use of strong CYP3A inhibitors (eg, clarithromycin, ketoconazole, itraconazole, ritonavir, indinavir, nelfinavir, saquinavir, nefazodone, telithromycin).

WARNINGS/PRECAUTIONS: Frequently monitor for changes in serum electrolytes and volume during initiation and titration. Allow to continue fluid ingestion in response to thirst. Resume fluid restriction and monitor for serum Na⁺ and volume status changes following discontinuation of therapy. D/C or interrupt therapy if patient develops elevation in serum Na⁺ too rapidly; consider hypotonic fluid administration. Serious and potentially fatal liver injury may occur; avoid use in patients with underlying liver disease, including cirrhosis, and d/c therapy in patients with symptoms that may indicate liver injury. May induce copious aquaresis. Dehydration and hypovolemia may occur, especially in potentially volume-depleted patients receiving diuretics or those who are fluid restricted; interrupt or d/c therapy and provide supportive care with careful management of vital signs, fluid balance, and electrolytes if signs/symptoms of hypovolemia develop. Concomitant use with hypertonic saline is not recommended. Increased serum K⁺ levels may occur; monitor serum K⁺ levels after initiation of therapy in patients with serum K⁺ >5mEq/L and those receiving drugs known to increase serum K⁺ levels. Not recommended for patients with CrCl <10mL/min.

ADVERSE REACTIONS: Osmotic demyelination, thirst, dry mouth, pollakiuria/polyuria, nausea, asthenia, constipation, hyperglycemia, pyrexia, anorexia.

INTERACTIONS: See Contraindications. Avoid with moderate CYP3A inhibitors (eg, erythromycin, fluconazole, aprepitant, diltiazem, verapamil). Avoid with CYP3A inducers (eg, rifampin, rifabutin, rifapentin, barbiturates, phenytoin, carbamazepine, St. John's wort); if coadministered, the dose of tolvaptan may need to be increased. Dose reduction of tolvaptan may be required when coadministered with P-glycoprotein inhibitors (eg, cyclosporine). Grapefruit juice may increase exposure. Increases exposure of digoxin. Higher incidence of hyperkalemia with ARBs, ACE inhibitors, and K⁺-sparing diuretics; monitor serum K⁺ levels. Not recommended with vasopressin V_2 agonist (eg, desmopressin).

PREGNANCY: Category C, not for use in nursing.

MECHANISM OF ACTION: Arginine vasopressin antagonist; antagonizes the effect of vasopressin and causes an increase in urine water excretion, resulting in an increase in free water clearance (aquaresis), a decrease in urine osmolality, and an increase in serum Na⁺ concentrations.

PHARMACOKINETICS: Absorption: T_{max}=2-4 hrs. **Distribution:** V_d=3L/kg; plasma protein binding (99%). **Metabolism:** Via CYP3A. **Elimination:** $T_{1/2}$=12 hrs.

NURSING CONSIDERATIONS

Assessment: Assess serum Na⁺ levels, neurologic status, ability to respond to thirst, renal/hepatic function, for hypersensitivity to drug, any other conditions where treatment is cautioned or contraindicated, pregnancy/nursing status, and possible drug interactions.

Monitoring: Monitor for osmotic demyelination, changes in serum Na⁺/electrolytes/volume, neurologic status, signs/symptoms of hypovolemia, liver injury, hypersensitivity reactions, and other adverse reactions. Monitor serum K⁺ levels in patients with serum K⁺ >5mEq/L and those receiving drugs known to increase serum K⁺ levels.

Patient Counseling: Advise to continue ingestion of fluid in response to thirst. Advise to resume fluid restriction following discontinuation of therapy. Instruct to inform physician if taking or plan to take any Rx or OTC drugs. Advise not to breastfeed during therapy.

Administration: Oral route. Take without regard to meals. **Storage:** 25°C (77°F); excursions permitted between 15-30°C (59-86°F).

SANCTURA XR   RX
trospium chloride (Allergan)

OTHER BRAND NAMES: Sanctura (Allergan)

THERAPEUTIC CLASS: Muscarinic antagonist

INDICATIONS: Treatment of overactive bladder with symptoms of urge urinary incontinence, urgency, and urinary frequency.

DOSAGE: *Adults:* (Tab) 20mg bid at least 1 hr ac or on an empty stomach. CrCl <30mL/min: 20mg qd at hs. Elderly (≥75 Yrs): May be titrated down to 20mg qd. (Cap) 60mg qam with water on an empty stomach, at least 1 hr ac.

S

HOW SUPPLIED: Cap, Extended-Release: 60mg; Tab: 20mg

CONTRAINDICATIONS: Urinary retention, gastric retention, uncontrolled narrow-angle glaucoma.

WARNINGS/PRECAUTIONS: Angioedema reported; d/c if the tongue, hypopharynx, or larynx is involved. Caution with clinically significant bladder outflow obstruction, GI obstructive disorders, moderate and severe hepatic impairment, and patients treated for controlled narrow-angle glaucoma. May decrease GI motility; caution with ulcerative colitis, intestinal atony, and myasthenia gravis. Associated with anticholinergic CNS effects; consider dose reduction or d/c if effects occur. (Cap) Not recommended with severe renal impairment (CrCl <30mL/min). Alcohol should not be consumed within 2 hrs of administration.

ADVERSE REACTIONS: Dry mouth, constipation, urinary tract infection. (Tab) Headache.

INTERACTIONS: May increase frequency and/or severity of dry mouth, constipation, and other anticholinergic pharmacologic effects with other antimuscarinic agents. May potentially alter the absorption of some concomitantly administered drugs due to effects on GI motility. May interact with other drugs that are eliminated by active tubular secretion (eg, procainamide, pancuronium, morphine, vancomycin, tenofovir). May enhance drowsiness with alcohol. Reduced levels with metformin. (Cap) Antacids containing aluminum hydroxide and magnesium carbonate may alter exposure.

PREGNANCY: Category C, caution in nursing.

MECHANISM OF ACTION: Muscarinic antagonist; reduces the tonus of smooth muscle in the bladder by antagonizing the effect of acetylcholine on muscarinic receptors.

PHARMACOKINETICS: Absorption: (Tab) Absolute bioavailability (9.6%); C_{max}=3.5ng/mL; T_{max}=5.3 hrs; AUC=36.4ng/mL•hr. (Cap) C_{max}=2ng/mL; T_{max}=5 hrs; AUC=18ng•hr/mL. **Distribution:** (Tab/Cap) Plasma protein binding (50-85%); V_d=395L (Tab), >600L (Cap). **Metabolism:** Ester hydrolysis with subsequent conjugation. **Elimination:** (Tab) Feces (85.2%), urine (5.8%, 60% unchanged); $T_{1/2}$=18.3 hrs (Tab), 35 hrs (Cap).

NURSING CONSIDERATIONS

Assessment: Assess for drug hypersensitivity, other conditions where treatment is contraindicated or cautioned, hepatic/renal impairment, pregnancy/nursing status, and for possible drug interactions.

Monitoring: Monitor for angioedema, anticholinergic CNS effects, urinary retention, gastric retention, and decreased GI motility. Monitor renal/hepatic function.

Patient Counseling: Inform that angioedema may occur and could result in life-threatening airway obstruction; instruct to d/c and seek medical attention if edema of the tongue/laryngopharynx or difficulty breathing occurs. Inform about the most common side effects (eg, dry mouth, constipation) and less common side effects (eg, trouble emptying the bladder, blurred vision, heat prostration). Advise not to drive or operate heavy machinery until patient knows how the drug affects him or her. Advise that alcohol may enhance drowsiness. (Cap) Advise that use of alcoholic beverages within 2 hrs of dosing is not recommended.

Administration: Oral route. **Storage:** 20-25°C (68-77°F); (Cap) excursions permitted between 15-30°C (59-86°F).

SANCUSO   RX
granisetron (Prostrakan)

THERAPEUTIC CLASS: 5-HT$_3$ receptor antagonist

INDICATIONS: Prevention of N/V in patients receiving moderately and/or highly emetogenic chemotherapy regimens of up to 5 consecutive days.

DOSAGE: *Adults:* Apply single patch to upper outer arm a minimum of 24 hrs before chemotherapy. May be applied up to a max of 48 hrs before chemotherapy as appropriate. Remove patch a minimum of 24 hrs after completion of chemotherapy. Can be worn for up to 7 days depending on duration of chemotherapy regimen.

HOW SUPPLIED: Patch: 3.1mg/24 hrs

WARNINGS/PRECAUTIONS: Avoid placing on red, irritated, or damaged skin. May mask progressive ileus and/or gastric distention caused by the underlying condition. Application-site reactions reported; remove patch if a generalized skin reaction or serious skin reactions occur. Avoid direct natural or artificial sunlight. Cover application site in case of risk of exposure to sunlight throughout the period of wear and for 10 days following removal. Caution in elderly.

ADVERSE REACTIONS: Constipation.

INTERACTIONS: Hepatic CYP450 enzyme (CYP1A1 and CYP3A4) inducers or inhibitors may alter clearance and $T_{1/2}$. In vitro inhibition of metabolism reported with ketoconazole. (IV) Increased total plasma clearance with phenobarbital.

PREGNANCY: Category B, caution in nursing.

MECHANISM OF ACTION: 5-HT$_3$ receptor antagonist; blocks serotonin stimulation and subsequent vomiting after emetogenic stimuli.

PHARMACOKINETICS: Absorption: T_{max}=48 hrs; C_{max}=5ng/mL; $AUC_{0-168hr}$=527ng•hr/mL. **Distribution:** Plasma protein binding (65%). **Metabolism:** N-demethylation and aromatic ring oxidation mediated by CYP450 3A. **Elimination:** (IV) Urine (12% unchanged, 49% metabolites), feces (34%).

NURSING CONSIDERATIONS

Assessment: Assess for drug hypersensitivity, GI history, pregnancy/nursing status, and possible drug interactions.

Monitoring: Monitor for hypersensitivity reactions, application-site or generalized skin reactions, and other adverse events.

Patient Counseling: Instruct to apply to clean, dry, intact healthy skin on upper outer arm and to not place on skin that is red, irritated, or damaged. Advise to inform physician if abdominal pain or swelling occurs. Advise to remove patch if severe or generalized skin reactions occur. Instruct to peel off gently. Advise to cover patch application site (eg, with clothing) if there is a risk of exposure to sunlight or sunlamps during the period of wear and for 10 days after removal.

Administration: Topical route. Refer to PI for proper application techniques. **Storage:** 20-25°C (68-77°F); excursions permitted between 15-30°C (59-86°F).

SANDOSTATIN LAR   RX
octreotide acetate (Novartis)

THERAPEUTIC CLASS: Somatostatin analog

INDICATIONS: Long-term maintenance therapy in acromegalic patients with inadequate response to surgery and/or radiotherapy or for whom surgery and/or radiotherapy is not an option. Long-term treatment of severe diarrhea and flushing episodes associated with metastatic carcinoid tumors, and profuse watery diarrhea associated with vasoactive intestinal peptide-secreting tumors (VIPomas).

DOSAGE: *Adults:* Administer IM in the gluteal region. Patients not currently receiving octreotide should begin therapy with Sandostatin inj; see PI for dosing. Acromegaly: Initial: 20mg at 4-week intervals for 3 months. Titrate: See PI for dose adjustment based on growth hormone (GH), insulin-like growth factor-1 (IGF-1) and/or clinical symptoms. Max: 40mg every 4 weeks. Withdraw yearly for 8 weeks to assess disease activity after pituitary irradiation. Resume therapy if GH or IGF-1 levels increase, and signs and symptoms recur. Carcinoid Tumors/VIPomas: Initial: 20mg at 4-week intervals for 2 months. Continue with Sandostatin injection SQ for at least 2 weeks before the switch. Titrate: If symptoms are not controlled, increase to 30mg every 4 weeks. If symptoms are controlled at 20mg, consider dose reduction to 10mg for a trial period. If symptoms recur increase dose to 20mg every 4 weeks. Max: 30mg every 4 weeks. For exacerbation of symptoms, give Sandostatin inj SQ for a few days at the dosage received prior to switching to depot. When symptoms are again controlled, the Sandostatin inj can be discontinued. Patients must be considered responders and tolerate the inj before switching to the depot. Renal Failure Requiring Dialysis/Cirrhotic Patients: Initial: 10mg every 4 weeks. Elderly: Start at lower end of dosing range.

HOW SUPPLIED: Inj, Depot: 10mg, 20mg, 30mg

WARNINGS/PRECAUTIONS: May inhibit gallbladder contractility and decrease bile secretion which may lead to gallbladder abnormalities or sludge. May alter balance between the counter-regulatory hormones, insulin, glucagon, and GH and lead to hypo- or hyperglycemia; monitor blood glucose levels when treatment is initiated or dose is altered and adjust antidiabetic treatment periodically. May result in hypothyroidism; monitor thyroid levels periodically. Cardiac conduction and other cardiovascular (CV) abnormalities may occur; caution in patients at risk. Depressed vitamin B12 levels and abnormal Schilling's test reported. Therapy may alter dietary fats absorption. Serum zinc may rise excessively when fluid loss is reversed for patients on TPN; monitor zinc levels. Caution in the elderly.

ADVERSE REACTIONS: Diarrhea, N/V, abdominal pain, flatulence, constipation, injection-site pain, upper respiratory infection, influenza-like symptoms, fatigue, dizziness, headache, cholelithiasis, back pain.

INTERACTIONS: May alter absorption of orally administered drugs. May decrease cyclosporine levels. May need dose adjustments of insulin, oral hypoglycemics, and bradycardia-inducing drugs (eg, β-blockers). Increased availability of bromocriptine. May decrease the metabolic clearance of drugs metabolized by CYP450; caution with other drugs metabolized by CYP3A4 with a low therapeutic index (eg, quinidine, terfenadine).

PREGNANCY: Category B, caution in nursing.

S

MECHANISM OF ACTION: Somatostatin analog; long acting. Exerts similar actions to natural hormone somatostatin, but is more potent in inhibiting GH, glucagon, and insulin. Like somatostatin, it also suppresses luteinizing hormone response to gonadotropin-releasing hormone, decreases splanchnic blood flow and inhibits release of serotonin, gastrin, vasoactive intestinal peptide, secretin, motilin, and pancreatic polypeptide.

PHARMACOKINETICS: Absorption: (SQ) Rapid, complete. C_{max}=5.2ng/mL; T_{max}=0.4 hrs; acromegaly: C_{max}=2.8ng/mL, T_{max}=0.7 hr. **Distribution:** V_d=13.6L; plasma protein binding (65%); acromegaly: V_d=21.6L, plasma protein binding (41.2%). **Elimination**: Urine (32%, unchanged); $T_{1/2}$=1.7-1.9 hrs.

NURSING CONSIDERATIONS

Assessment: Assess for renal/hepatic impairment, cardiac dysfunction, pregnancy/nursing status, and for possible drug interactions. Assess GH and IGF-1 levels and obtain baseline thyroid function tests (TSH, total and/or free T4).

Monitoring: Monitor for signs/symptoms of biliary tract abnormalities (eg, gallstones, biliary duct dilatation), hypo- and hyperglycemia, hypothyroidism, cardiac conduction abnormalities, and pancreatitis. Monitor zinc levels if receiving TPN. With acromegaly: Monitor GH and IGF-1 levels. With carcinoids: Monitor urinary 5-hydroxyindoleacetic acid, plasma serotonin levels, and plasma Substance P levels. With VIPoma: Monitor VIP levels. Monitor total and/or free T4 and vitamin B12 levels during chronic therapy.

Patient Counseling: Inform of risks and benefits of treatment. Advise patients with carcinoid tumors and VIPomas to adhere closely to scheduled return visits for reinjection to minimize exacerbation of symptoms. Advise patients with acromegaly to adhere to return visit schedule to help ensure steady control of GH and IGF-1 levels. Instruct to notify physician if any adverse reactions develop.

Administration: IM route. Avoid deltoid inj. Not for IV/SQ routes. Refer to PI for preparation and administration instructions. **Storage:** Refrigerate between 2-8°C (36-46°F). Protect from light until time of use.

SAPHRIS   RX
asenapine (Merck)

> Elderly patients with dementia-related psychosis treated with antipsychotic drugs are at an increased risk of death; most deaths appeared to be cardiovascular (CV) (eg, heart failure, sudden death) or infectious (eg, pneumonia) in nature. Not approved for treatment of dementia-related psychosis.

THERAPEUTIC CLASS: Dibenzapine derivative

INDICATIONS: Treatment of schizophrenia. As monotherapy or adjunctive therapy with either lithium or valproate for the acute treatment of manic or mixed episodes associated with bipolar I disorder.

DOSAGE: *Adults:* Schizophrenia: Acute Treatment: Initial/Usual: 5mg bid. Max: 10mg bid. Maint Treatment: Initial: 5mg bid. Titrate: May increase to 10mg bid after 1 week. Max: 10mg bid. Bipolar Disorder: Monotherapy: Initial/Max: 10mg bid. Titrate: May decrease to 5mg bid. Adjunctive Therapy (with Lithium/Valproate): Initial: 5mg bid. Titrate: May increase to 10mg bid. Max: 10mg bid. Continue treatment beyond acute response in responding patients. Switching from Other Antipsychotics: Minimize period of overlapping antipsychotics.

HOW SUPPLIED: Tab, SL: 5mg, 10mg

WARNINGS/PRECAUTIONS: Neuroleptic malignant syndrome (NMS) reported; d/c therapy and institute symptomatic treatment. May cause tardive dyskinesia (TD), especially in the elderly; d/c if this occurs. Hyperglycemia, in some cases extreme and associated with ketoacidosis or hyperosmolar coma or death, may occur; monitor glucose control regularly in patients with diabetes mellitus (DM) and FPG in patients at risk for DM. May cause weight gain. Hypersensitivity reactions reported usually after the 1st dose. May induce orthostatic hypotension and syncope; consider dose reduction if hypotension occurs. Caution with CV disease, cerebrovascular disease, or conditions that predispose to hypotension. Leukopenia, neutropenia, and agranulocytosis may occur; monitor CBC frequently during 1st few months in patients with preexisting low WBC or history of drug-induced leukopenia/neutropenia, and d/c at 1st sign of decline in WBC without causative factors. D/C therapy and follow WBC until recovery in patients with severe neutropenia (absolute neutrophil count <1000/mm³). May prolong QTc interval; avoid use with history of cardiac arrhythmias or in circumstances that may increase risk of torsades de pointes. May elevate prolactin levels. Seizures reported; caution with history of seizures or conditions that lower seizure threshold. Somnolence reported. May impair mental/physical abilities. May disrupt body's ability to reduce core body temperature. Caution with those at risk for suicide and in elderly patients. May cause esophageal dysmotility and aspiration; avoid in patients at risk for aspiration pneumonia. Not recommended in patients with severe hepatic impairment (Child-Pugh C).

ADVERSE REACTIONS: Somnolence, insomnia, headache, dizziness, extrapyramidal symptoms, akathisia, vomiting, oral hypoesthesia, constipation, weight increase, fatigue, increased appetite, anxiety, arthralgia, dyspepsia.

INTERACTIONS: Avoid use with other drugs known to prolong QTc, including Class 1A antiarrhythmics (eg, quinidine, procainamide), Class 3 antiarrhythmics (eg, amiodarone, sotalol), antipsychotics (eg, ziprasidone, chlorpromazine, thioridazine), and antibiotics (eg, gatifloxacin, moxifloxacin). Caution with other centrally acting drugs, alcohol, CYP2D6 substrates and inhibitors, drugs that can induce hypotension, bradycardia, respiratory or CNS depression, and drugs with anticholinergic activity. May enhance effects of antihypertensive agents. Fluvoxamine may increase levels. Imipramine may increase levels. Paroxetine, cimetidine, and carbamazepine may decrease levels.

PREGNANCY: Category C, not for use in nursing.

MECHANISM OF ACTION: Dibenzapine derivative; has not been established. Suggested that efficacy may be mediated through a combination of antagonist activity at dopamine type 2 and serotonin type 2A receptors.

PHARMACOKINETICS: Absorption: Rapid. (5mg) Absolute bioavailability (35%); C_{max}=4ng/mL; T_{max}=1 hr. **Distribution:** V_c=20-25L/kg; plasma protein binding (95%). **Metabolism:** Direct glucuronidation via UGT1A4 and oxidation via CYP1A2, and to a lesser extent 3A4 and 2D6. **Elimination:** Urine (50%), feces (40%); $T_{1/2}$=24 hrs.

NURSING CONSIDERATIONS

Assessment: Assess for dementia-related psychosis, history of cardiac arrhythmias, factors that may increase risk of torsades de pointes, risk for aspiration pneumonia, and conditions where treatment is cautioned. Assess for hepatic impairment, pregnancy/nursing status, known hypersensitivity to the drug, and possible drug interactions. Obtain baseline FPG in patients with DM or at risk for DM. Obtain baseline CBC if at risk for leukopenia/neutropenia.

Monitoring: Monitor for QT prolongation, NMS, TD, hyperglycemia, orthostatic hypotension, seizures, esophageal dysmotility, aspiration, suicidal ideation, hypersensitivity reactions, and other adverse effects. Monitor CBC frequently in patients with preexisting low WBC or history of drug-induced leukopenia/neutropenia. Monitor for fever or other signs/symptoms of infection in patients with neutropenia. Monitor weight regularly and hepatic function. Monitor FPG in patients with DM or at risk for DM. Reassess periodically to determine need for maintenance treatment.

Patient Counseling: Inform of the risks/benefits of therapy. Inform of the signs/symptoms of serious allergic reactions; instruct to seek immediate medical attention if serious allergic reaction develops. Inform that application-site reactions, including oral ulcers, blisters, peeling/sloughing, and inflammation, have been reported; instruct to monitor for these reactions. Inform about risk of developing NMS and counsel about its signs and symptoms. Inform of the need to monitor blood glucose in patients with DM or with risk factors for DM. Advise that weight gain may be experienced. Inform about risk of developing orthostatic hypotension. Advise patients with preexisting low WBC counts or history of drug-induced leukopenia/neutropenia to have their CBC monitored. Caution about performing activities requiring mental alertness. Instruct regarding appropriate care in avoiding overheating or dehydration. Advise to notify physician if taking/planning to take any prescription or OTC medications, or if pregnant/intend to become pregnant during therapy. Instruct to avoid breastfeeding and alcohol use while on therapy.

Administration: SL route. Place tab under tongue and allow to dissolve completely. Do not crush, chew, or swallow. Do not eat/drink for 10 min after administration. **Storage:** 15-30°C (59-86°F).

S

SAVELLA   RX
milnacipran HCl (Forest)

> Savella is a selective SNRI, similar to some drugs used for the treatment of depression and other psychiatric disorders. Antidepressants increased the risk of suicidal thinking and behavior (suicidality) in children, adolescents, and young adults in short-term studies of major depressive disorder (MDD) and other psychiatric disorders. Monitor appropriately and observe closely for clinical worsening, suicidality, or unusual behavioral changes in patients who are started on milnacipran. Not approved for use in the treatment of MDD and in pediatric patients.

THERAPEUTIC CLASS: Serotonin and norepinephrine reuptake inhibitor

INDICATIONS: Management of fibromyalgia.

DOSAGE: *Adults:* Day 1: 12.5mg qd. Days 2-3: 12.5mg bid. Days 4-7: 25mg bid. After Day 7/Usual: 50mg bid. May increase to 100mg bid based on individual response. Max: 100mg bid. Severe Renal Impairment (CrCl 5-29mL/min): Reduce maintenance dose by 50% to 25mg bid. May increase to 50mg bid based on individual response. Switching to/from an MAOI for Psychiatric Disorders: Allow at least 14 days between discontinuation of an MAOI and initiation of treatment, and allow at least 5 days between discontinuation of treatment and initiation of an MAOI. Use with Other MAOIs (eg, Linezolid, IV Methylene Blue): Refer to PI.

HOW SUPPLIED: Tab: 12.5mg, 25mg, 50mg, 100mg

CONTRAINDICATIONS: Use of an MAOI for psychiatric disorders either concomitantly or within 5 days of stopping treatment. Treatment within 14 days of stopping an MAOI for psychiatric disorders. Starting treatment in patients being treated with other MAOIs (eg, linezolid, IV methylene blue). Uncontrolled narrow-angle glaucoma.

WARNINGS/PRECAUTIONS: Serotonin syndrome reported; d/c immediately and initiate supportive symptomatic treatment. Associated with increase in BP and HR; treat preexisting HTN, preexisting tachyarrhythmias, and other cardiac diseases before starting therapy. Caution with significant HTN or cardiac disease. Consider dose reduction or discontinuation of therapy if sustained increase in BP or HR occurs. Increased liver enzymes and severe liver injury reported; d/c if jaundice or other evidence of liver dysfunction develops. Withdrawal symptoms and physical dependence reported; taper gradually and avoid abrupt discontinuation after extended use. Hyponatremia may occur; elderly and volume-depleted patients may be at greater risk. Consider discontinuation in patients with symptomatic hyponatremia. May increase risk of bleeding events. Caution with history of a seizure disorder or mania. May affect urethral resistance and micturition; caution with history of dysuria, notably in male patients with prostatic hypertrophy, prostatitis, and other lower urinary tract obstructive disorders. Male patients may experience testicular pain or ejaculation disorders. Mydriasis reported; caution with controlled narrow-angle glaucoma. May aggravate preexisting liver disease; avoid with substantial alcohol use or chronic liver disease. Caution with moderate renal impairment, severe hepatic impairment, and in the elderly. Not recommended with end-stage renal disease.

ADVERSE REACTIONS: N/V, headache, constipation, hot flush, insomnia, hyperhidrosis, palpitations, upper respiratory infection, increased HR, dry mouth, HTN, anxiety, dizziness, migraine, abdominal pain.

INTERACTIONS: See Contraindications. May cause serotonin syndrome with other serotonergic drugs (eg, triptans, TCAs, fentanyl, lithium, tramadol, tryptophan, buspirone, St. John's wort) and with drugs that impair metabolism of serotonin; d/c immediately if this occurs. If treatment with other serotonergic drugs is clinically warranted, patient should be made aware of potential risk for serotonin syndrome, particularly during dose initiation and dose increases. Paroxysmal HTN and possible arrhythmia may occur with epinephrine and norepinephrine. Increase in euphoria and postural hypotension observed in patients who switched from clomipramine; caution with other centrally acting drugs. Concomitant use with digoxin may potentiate adverse hemodynamic effects. Avoid with IV digoxin; postural hypotension and tachycardia reported. May inhibit antihypertensive effect of clonidine. Caution with NSAIDs, aspirin (ASA), warfarin, and other drugs that affect coagulation due to potential increased risk of bleeding. Caution with drugs that increase BP and HR. May increase risk of hyponatremia with diuretics.

PREGNANCY: Category C, caution in nursing.

MECHANISM OF ACTION: Selective SNRI; not established. May be associated with its potent inhibition of neuronal norepinephrine and serotonin reuptake without directly affecting uptake of dopamine or other neurotransmitters.

PHARMACOKINETICS: Absorption: Well-absorbed. Absolute bioavailability (85-90%); T_{max}=2-4 hrs. **Distribution:** Found in breast milk. (IV) V_d=400L; plasma protein binding (13%). **Metabolism:** l-milnacipran carbamoyl-O-glucuronide (major metabolite). **Elimination:** Urine (55% unchanged, 17% major metabolite); $T_{1/2}$=6-8 hrs.

NURSING CONSIDERATIONS

Assessment: Assess for narrow-angle glaucoma, HTN, tachyarrhythmias, cardiac diseases, depression, history of seizure disorder/mania/dysuria, prostatic hypertrophy, prostatitis, lower urinary tract obstructive disorders, volume depletion, renal/hepatic impairment, pregnancy/nursing status, and possible drug interactions. Assess alcohol use. Obtain baseline BP and HR.

Monitoring: Monitor for clinical worsening, suicidality, unusual changes in behavior, serotonin syndrome, hyponatremia, bleeding events, mydriasis, withdrawal symptoms, physical dependence, liver dysfunction, and other adverse reactions. Monitor for urethral resistance and micturition, testicular pain, and ejaculation disorders in male patients. Monitor BP and HR.

Patient Counseling: Inform about risks/benefits of therapy and counsel on its appropriate use. Advise to look for the emergence of suicidality, especially early during treatment and when the dose is adjusted up or down. Inform about the risk of serotonin syndrome, particularly with concomitant use with other serotonergic agents. Instruct to consult physician if symptoms of serotonin syndrome and emergence of suicidality occur. Advise to have BP and HR monitored regularly. Caution about the increased risk of abnormal bleeding with concomitant use of NSAIDs, ASA, and other drugs that affect coagulation. Inform that drug may impair mental/physical abilities; caution against operating machinery/driving motor vehicles until effects of drug are known. Instruct to discuss alcohol intake with physician prior to initiating therapy. Advise that withdrawal symptoms may occur with abrupt discontinuation. Advise that if a dose is missed, to skip the dose and take the next dose at the regular time. Instruct to notify physician if pregnant, intending to become pregnant, or if breastfeeding; encourage to enroll in the Savella Pregnancy Registry if patient becomes pregnant.

Administration: Oral route. Take with or without food. Taking with food may improve tolerability.
Storage: 25°C (77°F); excursions permitted to 15-30°C (59-86°F).

SEASONIQUE   RX
ethinyl estradiol - levonorgestrel (Teva)

> Cigarette smoking increases risk of serious cardiovascular (CV) events. Risk increases with age (>35 yrs of age) and with the number of cigarettes smoked. Should not be used by women who are >35 yrs of age and smoke.

OTHER BRAND NAMES: Camrese (Teva)

THERAPEUTIC CLASS: Estrogen/progestogen combination

INDICATIONS: Prevention of pregnancy.

DOSAGE: *Adults:* 1 tab qd at the same time every day for 91 days, then repeat. Start on the 1st Sunday after onset of menstruation. Use a nonhormonal back-up method of contraception (eg, condoms, spermicide) for the first 7 days of treatment. If patient does not immediately start the next pill pack, use a nonhormonal back-up method of contraception until patient has taken a light blue-green tab qd for 7 consecutive days.
Pediatrics: Postpubertal: 1 tab qd at the same time every day for 91 days, then repeat. Start on the 1st Sunday after onset of menstruation. Use a nonhormonal back-up method of contraception (eg, condoms, spermicide) for the first 7 days of treatment. If patient does not immediately start the next pill pack, use a nonhormonal back-up method of contraception until patient has taken a light blue-green tab qd for 7 consecutive days.

HOW SUPPLIED: Tab: (Levonorgestrel-Ethinyl Estradiol [EE]) 0.15mg-0.03mg; Tab: (EE) 0.01mg

CONTRAINDICATIONS: High risk of arterial/venous thrombotic diseases (eg, smoking if >35 yrs of age, history/presence of deep vein thrombosis/pulmonary embolism, cerebrovascular disease, coronary artery disease, thrombogenic valvular or thrombogenic rhythm diseases of the heart [eg, subacute bacterial endocarditis with valvular disease, or atrial fibrillation], inherited/acquired hypercoagulopathies, uncontrolled HTN, diabetes with vascular disease, headaches with focal neurological symptoms or migraine with/without aura if >35 yrs of age), undiagnosed abnormal genital bleeding, history/presence of breast or other estrogen-/progestin-sensitive cancer, benign/malignant liver tumors, liver disease, pregnancy.

WARNINGS/PRECAUTIONS: Increased risk of venous thromboembolism and arterial thrombosis (eg, stroke, myocardial infarction); d/c if an arterial/deep venous thrombotic event occurs. D/C at least 4 weeks before and through 2 weeks after major surgery or other surgeries known to have an elevated risk of thromboembolism. Start therapy no earlier than 4-6 weeks postpartum in women who do not breastfeed. Caution with CV disease risk factors. D/C if there is unexplained loss of vision, proptosis, diplopia, papilledema, or retinal vascular lesions; evaluate for retinal vein thrombosis immediately. May increase risk of cervical cancer, intraepithelial neoplasia, and gallbladder disease. D/C if jaundice develops. Hepatic adenoma and increased risk of hepatocellular carcinoma reported. Cholestasis may occur in women with a history of pregnancy-related cholestasis. Increase in BP reported. Monitor BP in women with well-controlled HTN; d/c if BP rises significantly. May decrease glucose tolerance; monitor prediabetic and diabetic women. Consider alternative contraception with uncontrolled dyslipidemias. May increase risk of pancreatitis with hypertriglyceridemia or family history thereof. Evaluate the cause and d/c if indicated if new headaches that are recurrent, persistent, or severe develop. Unscheduled bleeding and spotting may occur; rule out pregnancy or malignancies. Amenorrhea or oligomenorrhea may occur after discontinuing therapy. Caution with history of depression; d/c if depression recurs to a serious degree. May change results of laboratory tests (eg, coagulation factors, lipids, glucose tolerance, binding proteins). May induce/exacerbate angioedema in patients with hereditary angioedema. Chloasma may occur; women with chloasma should avoid sun exposure or UV radiation.

ADVERSE REACTIONS: Irregular and/or heavy uterine bleeding, weight gain, acne.

INTERACTIONS: Agents that induce certain enzymes, including CYP3A4 (eg, barbiturates, bosentan, carbamazepine, felbamate, griseofulvin, oxcarbazepine, phenytoin, rifampin, St. John's wort, topiramate), may decrease combination oral contraceptive (COC) efficacy or increase breakthrough bleeding; use additional or alternative contraceptive method. Significant changes (increase or decrease) in plasma estrogen and progestin levels reported with HIV protease inhibitors or non-nucleoside reverse transcriptase inhibitors. Pregnancy reported with antibiotics. Atorvastatin may increase ethinyl estradiol exposure; ascorbic acid and acetaminophen may increase ethinyl estradiol levels. CYP3A4 inhibitors (eg, itraconazole, ketoconazole) may increase plasma hormone levels. May decrease concentrations of lamotrigine and reduce seizure control; dosage adjustments of lamotrigine may be needed. Increases thyroid-binding globulin; may need to increase dose of thyroid hormone in patients on thyroid hormone replacement therapy.

S

PREGNANCY: Contraindicated in pregnancy, not for use in nursing.

MECHANISM OF ACTION: Estrogen/progestogen COC; acts primarily by suppressing ovulation. Also causes cervical mucus changes that inhibit sperm penetration and endometrial changes that reduce the likelihood of implantation.

PHARMACOKINETICS: Absorption: T_{max}=2 hrs. Levonorgestrel: Complete. Bioavailability (nearly 100%). EE: Bioavailability (43%). Administration on different days resulted in variable parameters; refer to PI. **Distribution:** Found in breast milk. Levonorgestrel: V_d=1.8L/kg; plasma protein binding (97.5-99%). EE: V_d=4.3L/kg; plasma protein binding (95-97%, albumin). **Metabolism:** Levonorgestrel: Sulfate and glucuronide conjugation. EE: 1st-pass (gut wall); liver by hydroxylation via CYP3A4; methylation and/or conjugation. **Elimination:** Levonorgestrel: Urine (45%) (levonorgestrel and metabolites), feces (32%)(mostly metabolites); $T_{1/2}$=34 hrs. EE: Urine, feces (metabolites); $T_{1/2}$=18 hrs.

NURSING CONSIDERATIONS

Assessment: Assess for high risk of arterial or venous thrombotic diseases; benign or malignant liver tumors; liver disease; undiagnosed abnormal genital bleeding; presence or history of breast cancer or other estrogen- or progestin-sensitive cancer; pregnancy; and any other conditions where treatment is contraindicated/cautioned. Assess nursing status and for possible drug interactions.

Monitoring: Monitor for arterial/deep venous thrombotic events, retinal vein thrombosis, cervical cancer or intraepithelial neoplasia, hepatic impairment, liver tumors, gallbladder disease, pancreatitis, new headaches or increased frequency or severity of migraines, bleeding irregularities, worsening depression with previous history, and other adverse reactions. Monitor BP with history of HTN, glucose levels in diabetic or prediabetic women, lipid levels with dyslipidemia, and thyroid function if receiving thyroid replacement therapy. Schedule a yearly visit with patient for a BP check and for other indicated health care.

Patient Counseling: Inform of benefits and risks of therapy. Counsel that cigarette smoking increases the risk of serious CV events, and that women who are >35 yrs of age and smoke should not use COCs. Inform that drug does not protect against HIV infection and other sexually transmitted diseases. Instruct on what to do if pills are missed. Inform that COCs may reduce breast milk production. Advise to inform physician of preexisting medical conditions and/or drugs currently being taken. Counsel women who start COCs postpartum, and who have not yet had a period, to use an additional method of contraception until after the first 7 consecutive days of administration. Inform that amenorrhea may occur and pregnancy should be ruled out if amenorrhea is associated with symptoms of pregnancy. Instruct to d/c if pregnancy occurs during treatment.

Administration: Oral route. Take at the same time every day. Refer to PI for further administration instructions. **Storage:** 20-25°C (68-77°F).

SECTRAL RX
acebutolol HCl (Promius Pharma)

THERAPEUTIC CLASS: Selective beta₁-blocker

INDICATIONS: Management of HTN alone or in combination with other antihypertensive agents (eg, thiazide-type diuretics) in adults. Management of ventricular premature beats.

DOSAGE: *Adults:* Mild-Moderate HTN: Initial: 400mg/day, given qd-bid. Usual: 200-800mg/day. Severe/Inadequate Control HTN: 1200mg/day, given bid. Ventricular Arrhythmia: Initial: 200mg bid. Maint: Increase gradually to 600-1200mg/day. Gradually reduce dose over a period of about 2 weeks to d/c. CrCl <50mL/min: Reduce daily dose by 50%. CrCl <25mL/min: Reduce daily dose by 75%. Elderly: Start at lower end of dosing range. Max: 800mg/day.

HOW SUPPLIED: Cap: 200mg, 400mg

CONTRAINDICATIONS: Persistently severe bradycardia, 2nd- and 3rd-degree heart block, overt cardiac failure, cardiogenic shock.

WARNINGS/PRECAUTIONS: Caution in patients with history of heart failure (HF) who are controlled with digitalis and/or diuretics. Cardiac failure may occur in patients with aortic or mitral valve disease or compromised left ventricular function; digitalize and/or give diuretic, and d/c acebutolol if cardiac failure continues. Exacerbation of ischemic heart disease and death reported with coronary artery disease (CAD); avoid abrupt withdrawal. Use low doses in patients with bronchospastic disease who do not respond to or cannot tolerate alternative treatment. Do not routinely withdraw prior to major surgery. Can precipitate/aggravate arterial insufficiency in patients with peripheral vascular disease (PVD). Caution with hepatic or renal dysfunction. May mask hypoglycemia in diabetics or hyperthyroidism symptoms (eg, tachycardia). Abrupt withdrawal may precipitate thyroid storm; thyrotoxicosis may occur. May be more reactive to repeated challenge with history of severe anaphylactic reaction to variety of allergens; may be unresponsive to usual doses of epinephrine. May develop antinuclear antibodies (ANA).

ADVERSE REACTIONS: Fatigue, dizziness, headache, constipation, diarrhea, dyspepsia, nausea, dyspnea, flatulence, micturition, insomnia.

INTERACTIONS: Possible additive effects with catecholamine-depleting drugs (eg, reserpine); monitor closely for hypotension and bradycardia. NSAIDs may reduce antihypertensive effects. Exaggerated hypertensive responses with α-adrenergic stimulants reported. May potentiate insulin-induced hypoglycemia. Digitalis glycosides may increase risk of bradycardia. May augment the risks of general anesthesia.

PREGNANCY: Category B, not for use in nursing.

MECHANISM OF ACTION: Cardioselective β-adrenoreceptor blocking agent; reduction in resting HR and decrease in exercise-induced tachycardia, reduction in cardiac output at rest and after exercise, reduction of systolic and diastolic BP at rest and post-exercise, and inhibition of isoproterenol-induced tachycardia.

PHARMACOKINETICS: Absorption: Well-absorbed; absolute bioavailability (40%); T_{max}=2.5 hrs; 3.5 hrs (diacetolol). **Distribution:** Plasma protein binding (26%); crosses placental barrier; found in breast milk. **Metabolism:** Diacetolol (major active metabolite). **Elimination:** Renal (30-40%), nonrenal (50-60%); $T_{1/2}$=3-4 hrs (acebutolol), 8-13 hrs (diacetolol).

NURSING CONSIDERATIONS

Assessment: Assess for bradycardia, cardiogenic shock, 2nd- and 3rd-degree heart block, overt cardiac failure, thyroid problems, hepatic/renal function, history of severe anaphylactic reaction, HF, CAD, bronchospastic disease, PVD, diabetes mellitus, pregnancy/nursing status, and possible drug interactions.

Monitoring: Monitor for cardiac failure, renal dysfunction, exacerbation of angina pectoris, and MI following abrupt withdrawal, thyrotoxicosis, ANA, and other adverse reactions.

Patient Counseling: Instruct to not interrupt or d/c therapy without consulting physician. Advise to consult physician if signs/symptoms of impending congestive heart failure or unexplained respiratory symptoms develop. Warn about possible hypertensive reactions from concomitant use of α-adrenergic stimulants, such as nasal decongestants used in OTC cold preparations.

Administration: Oral route. **Storage:** 20-25°C (68-77°F). Protect from light.

SELEGILINE   RX
selegiline HCl (Various)

OTHER BRAND NAMES: Eldepryl (Mylan)

THERAPEUTIC CLASS: Monoamine oxidase inhibitor (type B)

INDICATIONS: Adjunct in the management of parkinsonian patients being treated with levodopa/carbidopa who exhibit deterioration in the quality of their response to this therapy.

DOSAGE: *Adults:* 10mg/day as divided doses of 5mg each taken at breakfast and lunch. May attempt to reduce levodopa/carbidopa dose after 2-3 days of therapy. Further reductions of levodopa/carbidopa may be possible during continued selegiline therapy.

HOW SUPPLIED: Tab: 5mg; (Eldepryl) Cap: 5mg

CONTRAINDICATIONS: Concomitant use with meperidine or other opioids.

WARNINGS/PRECAUTIONS: Do not use at doses >10mg/day due to risks associated with non-selective inhibition of MAO. Exacerbation of levodopa-associated side effects may occur; may mitigate effects by reducing levodopa/carbidopa dose by 10-30%. Observe closely for atypical responses. Patients with Parkinson's disease have a higher risk of developing melanoma; monitor for melanomas frequently and on a regular basis.

ADVERSE REACTIONS: Nausea, dizziness/lightheadedness/fainting, abdominal pain, confusion, hallucinations, dry mouth.

INTERACTIONS: See Contraindications. Avoid with SSRIs (eg, fluoxetine, sertraline, paroxetine) and TCAs (eg, amitriptyline, protriptyline); severe toxicity reported. At least 14 days should elapse between discontinuation of selegiline and initiation of TCAs or SSRIs. At least 5 weeks (longer with chronic/high-dose fluoxetine) should elapse between discontinuation of fluoxetine and initiation of selegiline due to long $T_{1/2}$ of fluoxetine and its active metabolite. Hypertensive crises/reactions reported with ephedrine or tyramine-containing foods.

PREGNANCY: Category C, caution in nursing.

MECHANISM OF ACTION: MAOI (Type B); not established. Irreversibly inhibits MAO type B (selectivity is dose-dependent), blocking the catabolism of dopamine. May also act through other mechanisms to increase dopaminergic activity.

S

PHARMACOKINETICS: Absorption: C_{max}=1ng/mL. **Metabolism:** Extensive (presumably attributable to presystemic clearance in gut and liver); N-desmethylselegiline (active major metabolite), L-amphetamine and L-methamphetamine (major metabolites). **Elimination:** $T_{1/2}$=2 hrs (single dose), 10 hrs (steady state).

NURSING CONSIDERATIONS

Assessment: Assess for drug hypersensitivity, pregnancy/nursing status, and possible drug interactions.

Monitoring: Monitor for exacerbation of levodopa-associated side effects, atypical responses, and other adverse reactions. Monitor for melanomas frequently and on a regular basis.

Patient Counseling: Advise of the possible need to reduce levodopa dosage after initiation of therapy. Instruct not to exceed 10mg/day and explain the risk of using higher daily doses; provide a brief description of the 'cheese reaction.' Inform about the signs and symptoms associated with MAOI-induced hypertensive reactions; instruct to immediately report to physician any severe headache or other atypical/unusual symptoms not previously experienced. Instruct to inform physician if new or increased gambling urges, increased sexual urges, or other intense urges develop.

Administration: Oral route. Take at breakfast and at lunch. **Storage:** 20-25°C (68-77°F).

SELZENTRY

RX

maraviroc (ViiV Healthcare)

> Hepatotoxicity reported; may be preceded by severe rash or evidence of systemic allergic reaction (eg, fever, eosinophilia, elevated IgE). Immediately evaluate patients with signs or symptoms of hepatitis or allergic reaction.

THERAPEUTIC CLASS: CCR5 co-receptor antagonist

INDICATIONS: In combination with other antiretroviral agents for adults infected with only CCR5-tropic HIV-1.

DOSAGE: *Adults:* ≥18 Yrs: Concomitant Potent CYP3A Inhibitors (With/Without Potent CYP3A Inducer): 150mg bid. Other Concomitant Medications (eg, Tipranavir/Ritonavir, Nevirapine, Raltegravir, Nucleoside Reverse Transcriptase Inhibitors, Enfuvirtide): 300mg bid. Concomitant Potent CYP3A Inducers (Without Potent CYP3A Inhibitor): 600mg bid. Refer to PI for concomitant medications and dosing regimens based on renal function.

HOW SUPPLIED: Tab: 150mg, 300mg

CONTRAINDICATIONS: In patients with severe renal impairment or end-stage renal disease (ESRD) (CrCl <30mL/min) who are taking potent CYP3A inhibitors or inducers.

WARNINGS/PRECAUTIONS: Caution in patients with preexisting liver dysfunction or who are coinfected with viral hepatitis B or C. Consider discontinuation in patients with signs or symptoms of hepatitis, or with increased liver transaminases combined with rash or other systemic symptoms. Severe, potentially life-threatening skin and hypersensitivity reactions reported (eg, Stevens-Johnson syndrome, toxic epidermal necrolysis, drug rash with eosinophilia and systemic symptoms); d/c therapy and other suspected agents immediately if signs and symptoms develop. Cardiovascular (CV) events (eg, myocardial ischemia/infarction) and postural hypotension reported; caution in patients at increased risk for CV events and with history of or risk factors for postural hypotension or CV comorbidities. Increased risk of postural hypotension in patients with severe renal insufficiency or ESRD. Immune reconstitution syndrome reported. Autoimmune disorders (eg, Graves' disease, polymyositis, Guillain-Barre syndrome) reported in the setting of immune reconstitution and can occur many months after initiation of treatment. May increase risk of developing infections. May affect immune surveillance and lead to increased risk of malignancy. In treatment-naive patients, more subjects treated with maraviroc experienced virologic failure and developed lamivudine resistance compared with efavirenz. Caution in elderly.

ADVERSE REACTIONS: Hepatotoxicity, upper respiratory tract infections, cough, pyrexia, rash, dizziness.

INTERACTIONS: See Contraindications and dosage. Not recommended with St. John's wort or products containing St. John's wort; may substantially decrease levels and lead to loss of virologic response and possible resistance. Dose adjustment may be required with CYP3A inhibitors/inducers and P-glycoprotein inhibitors/inducers. Caution with medications known to lower BP.

PREGNANCY: Category B, not for use in nursing.

MECHANISM OF ACTION: CCR5 co-receptor antagonist; selectively binds to human chemokine receptor CCR5 present on cell membrane, preventing interaction of HIV-1 gp120 and CCR5 necessary for CCR5-tropic HIV-1 to enter cells.

PHARMACOKINETICS: Absorption: T_{max}=0.5-4 hrs (1-1200mg in uninfected volunteers); absolute bioavailability (23% [100mg], 33% [300mg]). Refer to PI for other pharmacokinetic parameters. **Distribution:** V_d=194L; plasma protein binding (76%). **Metabolism:** CYP3A (major); secondary amine (metabolite) via N-dealkylation. **Elimination:** Urine (20%, 8% unchanged), feces (76%, 25% unchanged); T$_{1/2}$=14-18 hrs.

NURSING CONSIDERATIONS

Assessment: Assess for renal and liver dysfunction, coinfection with hepatitis B or C, risk for CV events, history of or risk factors for postural hypotension and CV comorbidities, pregnancy/nursing status, and possible drug interactions. Conduct tropism testing to identify appropriate patients. Obtain baseline LFTs.

Monitoring: Monitor for signs/symptoms of hepatotoxicity, allergic reactions, skin/hypersensitivity reactions, immune reconstitution syndrome, CV events, postural hypotension, infections, malignancy, and other adverse reactions. Monitor LFTs as clinically indicated.

Patient Counseling: Inform that liver problems have been reported and advise to d/c therapy and seek medical attention if signs/symptoms of hepatitis or allergic reaction develop. Inform that therapy is not a cure for HIV-1 infection and patients may continue to experience illnesses associated with HIV-1 infection, including opportunistic infections. Instruct to avoid driving/operating machinery if dizziness occurs. Advise to remain under the care of a physician, to take all anti-HIV medicines as prescribed, and not to change dose or d/c therapy without consulting physician. Instruct to take missed dose as soon as possible; advise not to take missed dose if it is <6 hours before next scheduled dose and to take next dose at the regular time. Counsel to avoid doing things that can spread HIV-1 infection to others (eg, sharing of needles/inj equipment or personal items that can have blood/body fluids on them). Advise to always practice safe sex by using latex or polyurethane condoms. Instruct to avoid breastfeeding.

Administration: Oral route. Take with or without food. **Storage:** 25°C (77°F); excursions permitted between 15-30°C (59-86°F).

SENSIPAR
cinacalcet (Amgen)

RX

THERAPEUTIC CLASS: Calcimimetic agent

INDICATIONS: Treatment of secondary hyperparathyroidism (HPT) in patients with chronic kidney disease (CKD) on dialysis, of hypercalcemia in patients with parathyroid carcinoma, and of severe hypercalcemia in patients with primary HPT who are unable to undergo parathyroidectomy.

DOSAGE: *Adults:* Individualize dose. Secondary HPT with CKD on Dialysis: Initial: 30mg qd. Titrate: Increase no more frequently than every 2-4 weeks through sequential doses of 30mg, 60mg, 90mg, 120mg, and 180mg qd to target intact parathyroid hormone (iPTH) of 150-300pg/mL. Measure serum Ca^{2+} and phosphorus (P) within 1 week and iPTH between 1-4 weeks after initiation or dose adjustment. May be used alone or in combination with vitamin D sterols and/or phosphate binders. Hypercalcemia with Parathyroid Carcinoma/Primary HPT: Initial: 30mg bid. Titrate: Increase every 2-4 weeks through sequential doses of 30mg bid, 60mg bid, 90mg bid, and 90mg tid-qid PRN to normalize serum Ca^{2+} levels.

HOW SUPPLIED: Tab: 30mg, 60mg, 90mg

CONTRAINDICATIONS: Hypocalcemia.

WARNINGS/PRECAUTIONS: Lowers serum Ca^{2+}; monitor for hypocalcemia. If serum Ca^{2+} <8.4mg/dL but remains >7.5mg/dL, or if symptoms of hypocalcemia occur, Ca^{2+}-containing phosphate binders and/or vitamin D sterols can be used. If serum Ca^{2+} <7.5mg/dL, or if symptoms of hypocalcemia persist and dose of vitamin D cannot be increased, d/c therapy until Ca^{2+} levels reach 8mg/dL or symptoms resolve. Restart treatment using the next lowest dose. Avoid use in patients with CKD not on dialysis. Seizures reported; monitor serum Ca^{2+} particularly in patients with history of seizure disorder. Hypotension, worsening heart failure (HF), and/or arrhythmia reported in patients with impaired cardiac function. Adynamic bone disease may develop with iPTH levels <100pg/mL; reduce dose or d/c therapy if iPTH levels <150pg/mL. Monitor patients with moderate and severe hepatic impairment throughout treatment.

ADVERSE REACTIONS: N/V, diarrhea, myalgia, dizziness, asthenia, anorexia, paresthesia, fatigue, fracture, hypercalcemia, dehydration, anemia, arthralgia, depression.

INTERACTIONS: May require dose adjustment with CYP2D6 substrates (eg, desipramine, metoprolol, carvedilol) and particularly those with narrow therapeutic index (eg, flecainide, most TCAs). May require dose adjustment if a patient initiates or discontinues therapy with strong CYP3A4 inhibitors (eg, ketoconazole, itraconazole); closely monitor iPTH and serum Ca^{2+} levels. Increased area under the curve (AUC) and C$_{max}$ with ketoconazole. Decreased AUC with calcium carbonate and sevelamer HCl. Increased AUC and decreased C$_{max}$ with pantoprazole. May increase AUC and C$_{max}$ of desipramine, amitriptyline, and nortriptyline. May decrease AUC of warfarin. May increase AUC and decrease C$_{max}$ of midazolam.

PREGNANCY: Category C, not for use in nursing.

S

MECHANISM OF ACTION: Calcimimetic agent; lowers PTH levels by increasing the sensitivity of the Ca^{2+}-sensing receptor to extracellular Ca^{2+}.

PHARMACOKINETICS: Absorption: T_{max}=2-6 hrs. **Distribution:** V_d=1000L; plasma protein binding (93-97%). **Metabolism:** Via CYP3A4, 2D6, and 1A2; hydrocinnamic acid and glucuronidated dihydrodiols (major metabolites). **Elimination:** Urine (80%), feces (15%); $T_{1/2}$=30-40 hrs.

NURSING CONSIDERATIONS

Assessment: Assess for hypocalcemia, a history of seizure disorder, hepatic impairment, cardiac function, pregnancy/nursing status, and possible drug interactions. Assess serum Ca^{2+} levels prior to administration.

Monitoring: Monitor for seizures, signs/symptoms of hypocalcemia and adynamic bone disease. In patients with impaired cardiac function, monitor for hypotension, worsening HF, and/or arrhythmias. For patients with CKD on dialysis, monitor serum Ca^{2+} and P levels within 1 week and iPTH levels 1-4 weeks after initiation or dose adjustment. After maintenance dose is reached, measure serum Ca^{2+} and P levels monthly, and iPTH levels every 1-3 months. For patients with parathyroid carcinoma/primary HPT, measure serum Ca^{2+} levels within 1 week after drug initiation or dose adjustment; measure serum Ca^{2+} levels every 2 months after maintenance dose levels have been established. Monitor iPTH/Ca^{2+}/P levels with moderate and severe hepatic impairment.

Patient Counseling: Advise to take with food or shortly after a meal; instruct to take whole and not to divide. Inform of the importance of regular blood tests. Advise to report to physician if N/V and potential symptoms of hypocalcemia (eg, tingling/numbness of the skin, muscle pain/cramping) occur. Advise to report to their physician if taking medication to prevent seizures, have had seizures in the past, and experience any seizure episodes while on therapy.

Administration: Oral route. **Storage:** 25°C (77°F); excursions permitted to 15-30°C (59-86°F).

SEREVENT DISKUS   RX
salmeterol xinafoate (GlaxoSmithKline)

> Long-acting β_2-adrenergic agonists (LABA) may increase the risk of asthma-related death. Contraindicated in asthma without use of a long-term asthma control medication (eg, inhaled corticosteroid). Do not use for asthma adequately controlled on low or medium dose inhaled corticosteroids. LABA may increase risk of asthma-related hospitalization in pediatric and adolescent patients; ensure adherence with both long-term asthma control medication and LABA.

THERAPEUTIC CLASS: Beta$_2$-agonist

INDICATIONS: Treatment of asthma and prevention of bronchospasm only as concomitant therapy with a long-term asthma control medication (eg, inhaled corticosteroid) in patients ≥4 yrs of age with reversible obstructive airway disease, including patients with symptoms of nocturnal asthma. Prevention of exercise-induced bronchospasm (EIB) in patients ≥4 yrs of age. For the long-term, bid (am and pm) administration in the maintenance treatment of bronchospasm associated with chronic obstructive pulmonary disease (COPD) (eg, emphysema, chronic bronchitis).

DOSAGE: *Adults:* Asthma/COPD: 1 inh bid, am and pm (12 hrs apart). EIB: 1 inh ≥30 min before exercise (additional doses should not be used for 12 hrs after administration or if already on bid dose).
Pediatrics: ≥4 Yrs: Asthma: 1 inh bid, am and pm (12 hrs apart). EIB: 1 inh ≥30 min before exercise (additional doses should not be used for 12 hrs after administration or if already on bid dose).

HOW SUPPLIED: Disk, Inhalation: 50mcg/inh [28^s, 60^s]

CONTRAINDICATIONS: Treatment of asthma without concomitant use of long-term asthma control medication (eg, inhaled corticosteroid). Primary treatment of status asthmaticus or other acute episodes of asthma or COPD where intensive measures are required. Severe hypersensitivity to milk proteins.

WARNINGS/PRECAUTIONS: Should not be initiated during rapidly deteriorating or potentially life-threatening episodes of asthma or COPD. Increased use of inhaled, short-acting β_2-agonists (SABA) is a marker of deteriorating asthma; reevaluate and reassess treatment regimen. Should not be used for relief of acute symptoms; use SABA to relieve acute symptoms. At treatment initiation, regular use of an inhaled SABA should be discontinued. Not a substitute for oral/inhaled corticosteroids. Should not be used more often or at higher doses than recommended; cardiovascular (CV) effects and fatalities reported with excessive use. May produce paradoxical bronchospasm; d/c immediately, treat, and institute alternative therapy. Caution with cardiovascular disorders (CVDs) (eg, coronary insufficiency, cardiac arrhythmias, HTN), convulsive disorders, thyrotoxicosis, hepatic disease, diabetes mellitus (DM), those who are unusually responsive to sympathomimetic amines, and in the elderly. ECG changes (eg, flattening of T wave, QTc interval prolongation, ST segment depression) reported. Immediate hypersensitivity reactions, hypokalemia, and dose-related changes in blood glucose and/or serum K^+ may occur.

ADVERSE REACTIONS: Nasal/sinus congestion, pharyngitis, cough, viral respiratory infection, musculoskeletal pain, rhinitis, headache, tracheitis/bronchitis, influenza, throat irritation.

INTERACTIONS: Not recommended with strong CYP3A4 inhibitors (eg, ketoconazole, ritonavir, clarithromycin, nefazodone). Avoid with other medications containing LABA. Increased exposure with ketoconazole. Caution with non-K$^+$-sparing diuretics (eg, loop, thiazide). Use with β-blockers may produce severe bronchospasm; if needed, consider cardioselective β-blocker with caution. Extreme caution with MAOIs or TCAs, or within 2 weeks of discontinuation of these agents. Increased C$_{max}$ with erythromycin.

PREGNANCY: Category C, not for use in nursing.

MECHANISM OF ACTION: Selective LABA (β$_2$-agonist); stimulates intracellular adenyl cyclase, the enzyme that catalyzes the conversion of adenosine triphosphate to cAMP, producing relaxation of bronchial smooth muscles and inhibits the release of mediators of immediate hypersensitivity from mast cells.

PHARMACOKINETICS: Absorption: C$_{max}$=167pg/mL; T$_{max}$=20 min. **Distribution:** Plasma protein binding (96%). **Metabolism:** Liver (aliphatic oxidation) via CYP3A4; α-hydroxysalmeterol (metabolite). **Elimination:** Urine (25%), feces (60%); T$_{1/2}$=5.5 hrs.

NURSING CONSIDERATIONS

Assessment: Assess for asthma control, hypersensitivity to milk proteins, acute bronchospasm, rapidly deteriorating asthma or COPD, CVD, convulsive disorder, thyrotoxicosis, DM, hepatic disease, pregnancy/nursing status, and possible drug interactions. Obtain baseline lung function before therapy, serum K$^+$, and blood glucose levels.

Monitoring: Monitor lung function periodically. Monitor patients with hepatic disease. Monitor for paradoxical bronchospasm, CV effects, and hypersensitivity. Monitor asthma control, pulse rate, BP, ECG changes, serum K$^+$, and blood glucose levels.

Patient Counseling: Inform that drug may increase risk of asthma-related death. Inform that the medication should only be used as additional therapy when long-term asthma control medications do not adequately control asthma symptoms. Counsel that the medication is not meant to relieve acute asthma or exacerbations of COPD symptoms and extra doses should not be used for that purpose. Advise that therapy is not a substitute for oral or inhaled corticosteroids. Instruct to notify physician immediately if signs of seriously worsening asthma or COPD occur. Instruct not to change dosage or stop therapy unless directed by physician. Advise that additional LABA should not be used while on therapy. Inform of adverse effects (eg, palpitations, chest pain, rapid HR, tremor, nervousness). Inform patients treated for EIB that additional doses should not be used for 12 hrs and not to use additional doses.

Administration: Oral inhalation route. Refer to PI for proper administration and use. **Storage:** 20-25°C (68-77°F). Keep in dry place, away from direct heat or sunlight. Discard 6 weeks after removal from pouch or after all blisters have been used (when the dose indicator reads "0"), whichever comes 1st.

SEROQUEL   RX
quetiapine fumarate (AstraZeneca)

Elderly patients with dementia-related psychosis treated with antipsychotic drugs are at an increased risk of death. Not approved for the treatment of patients with dementia-related psychosis. Antidepressants increased the risk of suicidal thoughts and behavior in children, adolescents, and young adults in short-term studies. Monitor closely for worsening, and for emergence of suicidal thoughts and behaviors in patients who are started on antidepressant therapy. Not approved for use in pediatric patients <10 yrs of age.

THERAPEUTIC CLASS: Dibenzapine derivative

INDICATIONS: Treatment of schizophrenia in adults and adolescents (13-17 yrs of age). Acute treatment of manic episodes associated with bipolar I disorder, as monotherapy in adults and pediatric patients (10-17 yrs of age), and as an adjunct to lithium or divalproex in adults. Monotherapy for acute treatment of depressive episodes associated with bipolar disorder in adults. Maintenance treatment of bipolar I disorder as an adjunct to lithium or divalproex in adults.

DOSAGE: *Adults:* Schizophrenia: Initial: 25mg bid. Titrate: Increase in increments of 25-50mg divided 2 or 3 times on Days 2 and 3 to a range of 300-400mg by Day 4. Further adjustments can be made in increments of 25-50mg bid, in intervals of not <2 days. Usual: 150-750mg/day. Max: 750mg/day. Schizophrenia Maint: Usual: 400-800mg/day. Max: 800mg/day. Bipolar Mania: Monotherapy/Adjunct: Day 1: 100mg/day given bid. Day 2: 200mg/day given bid. Day 3: 300mg/day given bid. Day 4: 400mg/day given bid. Titrate: May further adjust to up to 800mg/day by Day 6 in increments of ≤200mg/day. Usual: 400-800mg/day. Max: 800mg/day. Bipolar Depression: Day 1: 50mg qhs. Day 2: 100mg qhs. Day 3: 200mg qhs. Day 4: 300mg qhs. Usual/Max: 300mg/day. Bipolar I Disorder Maint: Initial: 400-800mg/day given bid as adjunct to lithium or divalproex. Usual: 400-800mg/day. Max: 800mg/day. Elderly/Debilitated/Predisposed to Hypotension: Consider slower rate of titration and lower target dose. Elderly:

Initial: 50mg/day. Titrate: May increase in increments of 50mg/day. Hepatic Impairment: Initial: 25mg/day. Titrate: May increase in increments of 25-50mg/day. Refer to PI for dosing modifications when used with certain concomitant therapies, when reinitiating treatment, and if switching from other antipsychotics.

Pediatrics: Schizophrenia: 13-17 Yrs: Day 1: 25mg bid. Day 2: 100mg/day given bid. Day 3: 200mg/day given bid. Day 4: 300mg/day given bid. Day 5: 400mg/day given bid. Further adjustments should be made in increments ≤100mg/day. May administer tid based on response and tolerability. Usual: 400-800mg/day. Max: 800mg/day. Bipolar Mania: Monotherapy: 10-17 Yrs: Day 1: 25mg bid. Day 2: 100mg/day given bid. Day 3: 200mg/day given bid. Day 4: 300mg/day given bid. Day 5: 400mg/day given bid. Further adjustments should be made in increments ≤100mg/day. May administer tid based on response and tolerability. Usual: 400-600mg/day. Max: 600mg/day. Debilitated/Predisposition to Hypotension: Consider slower rate of titration and lower target dose. Hepatic Impairment: Initial: 25mg/day. Titrate: May be increased in increments of 25-50mg/day. Refer to PI for further information when reinitiating treatment, and if switching from other antipsychotics.

HOW SUPPLIED: Tab: 25mg, 50mg, 100mg, 200mg, 300mg, 400mg

WARNINGS/PRECAUTIONS: Initiate in pediatric patients only after a thorough diagnostic evaluation is conducted and careful consideration is given to the risks of therapy. Neuroleptic malignant syndrome (NMS) reported; d/c and institute symptomatic treatment. Hyperglycemia, in some cases extreme and associated with ketoacidosis or hyperosmolar coma or death, reported; monitor glucose regularly in patients with diabetes mellitus (DM) and FPG in patients at risk for DM. Alterations in lipids and weight gain observed. May cause tardive dyskinesia (TD), especially in the elderly; consider discontinuation if this occurs. May induce orthostatic hypotension. Leukopenia, neutropenia, and agranulocytosis reported; monitor CBC frequently during 1st few months in patients with preexisting low WBC count or history of drug-induced leukopenia/neutropenia, and d/c at 1st sign of decline in WBC count without causative factors. D/C therapy and follow WBC count until recovery in patients with severe neutropenia (absolute neutrophil count <1000/mm³). QT prolongation reported. Avoid in circumstances that may increase the risk of torsades de pointes and/or sudden death. Seizures reported; caution with conditions that lower seizure threshold. Decrease in thyroid hormone levels reported; measure TSH and free T4 at baseline and at follow-up in addition to clinical assessment. May elevate prolactin levels. May impair physical/mental abilities. May disrupt body's ability to reduce core body temperature. May cause esophageal dysmotility and aspiration; caution in patients at risk for aspiration pneumonia. Acute withdrawal symptoms (eg, N/V, insomnia) may occur after abrupt cessation; d/c gradually.

ADVERSE REACTIONS: Headache, somnolence, dizziness, dry mouth, constipation, dyspepsia, tachycardia, asthenia, agitation, pain, weight gain, ALT increased, abdominal pain, back pain, N/V.

INTERACTIONS: Caution with other centrally acting drugs and alcohol. Increased exposure with CYP3A4 inhibitors (eg, ketoconazole, ritonavir, nefazodone) and decreased exposure with CYP3A4 inducers (eg, phenytoin, carbamazepine, rifampin, St. John's wort); dose adjustment of quetiapine may be necessary. May enhance the effects of certain antihypertensives. May antagonize the effects of levodopa and dopamine agonists. QT prolongation reported with drugs known to cause electrolyte imbalance. Avoid with other drugs that are known to prolong QTc interval (eg, quinidine, amiodarone, ziprasidone, gatifloxacin, methadone). Caution with anticholinergic medications.

PREGNANCY: Category C, not for use in nursing.

MECHANISM OF ACTION: Dibenzothiazepine derivative; not established. Suspected to be mediated through a combination of dopamine type 2 (D_2) and serotonin type 2 ($5HT_2$) antagonism.

PHARMACOKINETICS: Absorption: Rapid. T_{max}=1.5 hrs. **Distribution:** V_d=10L/kg; plasma protein binding (83%); found in breast milk. **Metabolism:** Liver (extensive) via sulfoxidation and oxidation; CYP3A4; N-desalkyl quetiapine (active metabolite). **Elimination:** Urine (73%), feces (20%); $T_{1/2}$=6 hrs.

NURSING CONSIDERATIONS

Assessment: Assess for history of dementia-related psychosis, risk for hypotension, drug hypersensitivity, psychiatric disorders, hepatic impairment, other conditions where treatment is cautioned, pregnancy/nursing status, and possible drug interactions. Obtain baseline FPG in patients with DM or at risk for DM. Obtain baseline CBC if at risk for leukopenia/neutropenia. Obtain baseline TSH, and free T4. Obtain baseline BP in children and adolescents. Assess for cataracts by performing lens exam (eg, slit lamp exam).

Monitoring: Monitor for clinical worsening, suicidality, unusual changes in behavior, NMS, TD, hyperglycemia, orthostatic hypotension, hypothyroidism, seizures, aspiration, and other adverse effects. Monitor CBC frequently in patients with preexisting low WBC or history of drug-induced leukopenia/neutropenia. Monitor for fever or other signs/symptoms of infection in patients with neutropenia. Monitor weight regularly; monitor lipids, hepatic function, and FPG periodically. Monitor for cataract formation shortly after start of treatment, and at 6-month intervals

S

during chronic treatment. Monitor BP periodically during treatment in children and adolescents. Periodically reassess for continued need for maintenance treatment.

Patient Counseling: Inform of the risks and benefits of therapy. Instruct caregivers and patients to contact physician if signs of agitation, anxiety, panic attacks, insomnia, hostility, aggressiveness, impulsivity, akathisia, hypomania, mania, irritability, worsening of depression, changes in behavior, or suicidal ideation develop. Advise about signs/symptoms of NMS, symptoms of hyperglycemia and DM, weight gain, and risk of orthostatic hypotension. Instruct to avoid overheating and dehydration. Caution about performing activities requiring mental alertness. Instruct to notify physician if patient becomes pregnant or intends to become pregnant during therapy, and if patient is taking or plans to take any prescription or OTC drugs.

Administration: Oral route. Take with or without food. **Storage:** 25°C (77°F); excursions permitted to 15-30°C (59-86°F).

SEROQUEL XR

RX

quetiapine fumarate (AstraZeneca)

Elderly patients with dementia-related psychosis treated with antipsychotic drugs are at an increased risk of death. Not approved for the treatment of patients with dementia-related psychosis. Antidepressants increased the risk of suicidal thoughts and behavior in children, adolescents, and young adults in short-term studies. Monitor closely for worsening, and for emergence of suicidal thoughts and behaviors in patients who are started on antidepressant therapy. Not approved for use in pediatric patients <10 yrs of age.

THERAPEUTIC CLASS: Dibenzapine derivative

INDICATIONS: Treatment of schizophrenia in adults and adolescents (13-17 yrs of age). Acute treatment of manic or mixed episodes associated with bipolar I disorder, both as monotherapy and as an adjunct to lithium or divalproex in adults. Acute treatment of manic episodes associated with bipolar I disorder as monotherapy in pediatric patients (10-17 yrs of age). Acute treatment of depressive episodes associated with bipolar disorder, maintenance treatment of bipolar I disorder (adjunct to lithium or divalproex), and adjunctive therapy to antidepressants for the treatment of major depressive disorder (MDD) in adults.

DOSAGE: *Adults:* Administer qd in the pm. Schizophrenia: Initial: 300mg/day. Titrate: Dose increases may be made at intervals as short as 1 day and in increments of up to 300mg/day. Usual: 400-800mg/day. Max: 800mg/day. Schizophrenia Maint: Usual: 400-800mg/day. Max: 800mg/day. Bipolar I Disorder (Manic or Mixed): Monotherapy/Adjunct: Day 1: 300mg/day. Day 2: 600mg/day. Day 3: Between 400mg and 800mg/day. Usual: 400-800mg/day. Max: 800mg/day. Bipolar Disorder, Depressive Episodes: Day 1: 50mg/day. Day 2: 100mg/day. Day 3: 200mg/day. Day 4: 300mg/day. Usual/Max: 300mg/day. Bipolar I Disorder Maint (Adjunct to Lithium or Divalproex): Usual: 400-800mg/day. Max: 800mg/day. MDD (Adjunctive Therapy): Initial: Day 1: 50mg/day. Day 2: 50mg/day. Day 3: 150mg/day. Usual: 150-300mg/day. Max: 300mg/day. Elderly/Debilitated/Predisposition to Hypotension: Consider slower rate of titration and lower target dose. Elderly/Hepatic Impairment: Initial: 50mg/day. Titrate: May increase in increments of 50mg/day. Refer to PI for dose modifications when used concomitantly with other medications, when reinitiating treatment, if switching from Seroquel tabs to Seroquel XR tabs, and if switching from other antipsychotics.
Pediatrics: Administer qd in the pm. Schizophrenia: 13-17 Yrs: Day 1: 50mg/day. Day 2: 100mg/day. Day 3: 200mg/day. Day 4: 300mg/day. Day 5: 400mg/day. Usual: 400-800mg/day. Max: 800mg/day. Bipolar I Disorder (Manic): Monotherapy: 10-17 Yrs: Day 1: 50mg/day. Day 2: 100mg/day. Day 3: 200mg/day. Day 4: 300mg/day. Day 5: 400mg/day. Usual: 400-600mg/day. Max: 600mg/day. Debilitated/Predisposition to Hypotension: Consider slower rate of titration and lower target dose. Hepatic Impairment: Initial: 50mg/day. Titrate: May increase in increments of 50mg/day. Refer to PI for dose modifications when used concomitantly with other medications, when reinitiating treatment, if switching from Seroquel tabs to Seroquel XR tabs, and if switching from other antipsychotics.

HOW SUPPLIED: Tab, Extended-Release: 50mg, 150mg, 200mg, 300mg, 400mg

WARNINGS/PRECAUTIONS: Initiate in pediatric patients only after a thorough diagnostic evaluation is conducted and careful consideration is given to the risks of therapy. Neuroleptic malignant syndrome (NMS) reported; d/c and institute symptomatic treatment and monitor. Hyperglycemia, in some cases extreme and associated with ketoacidosis or hyperosmolar coma or death, reported; monitor glucose regularly in patients with diabetes mellitus (DM) and FPG in patients at risk for DM. Alterations in lipids and weight gain observed. May cause tardive dyskinesia (TD), especially in the elderly; consider discontinuation if this occurs. May induce orthostatic hypotension. Leukopenia, neutropenia, and agranulocytosis reported; monitor CBC frequently during 1st few months in patients with preexisting low WBC count or history of drug-induced leukopenia/neutropenia, and d/c at 1st sign of decline in WBC count without causative factors. D/C therapy and follow WBC count until recovery in patients with severe neutropenia (absolute neutrophil count <1000/mm³). QT prolongation reported. Avoid in circumstances that may increase the risk of torsades de pointes and/or sudden death. Seizures reported; caution with conditions that lower seizure threshold. Decrease in thyroid hormone levels reported; measure TSH and free T4 at baseline and at follow-up in addition to clinical assessment. May elevate prolactin levels. May impair physical/mental abilities. May disrupt body's ability to reduce core body temperature. May cause esophageal dysmotility and aspiration; caution in patients at risk for aspiration pneumonia. Acute withdrawal symptoms (eg, N/V, insomnia) may occur after abrupt cessation; d/c gradually.

ADVERSE REACTIONS: Dry mouth, constipation, dyspepsia, somnolence, dizziness, orthostatic hypotension, weight gain, fatigue, dysarthria, nasal congestion, extrapyramidal symptoms, increased appetite, back pain, abnormal dreams, irritability.

INTERACTIONS: Caution with other centrally acting drugs and alcohol. Increased exposure with CYP3A4 inhibitors (eg, ketoconazole, ritonavir, nefazodone) and decreased exposure with CYP3A4 inducers (eg, phenytoin, carbamazepine, rifampin, St. John's wort); dose adjustment of quetiapine may be necessary. May enhance the effects of certain antihypertensives. May antagonize the effects of levodopa and dopamine agonists. QT prolongation reported with drugs known to cause electrolyte imbalance. Avoid with other drugs that are known to prolong QTc interval (eg, quinidine, amiodarone, ziprasidone, gatifloxacin, methadone). Caution with anticholinergic medications.

PREGNANCY: Category C, not for use in nursing.

MECHANISM OF ACTION: Dibenzothiazepine derivative; not established. Suspected to be mediated through a combination of dopamine type 2 (D_2) and serotonin type 2A ($5HT_{2A}$) antagonism.

PHARMACOKINETICS: Absorption: T_{max}=6 hrs. **Distribution:** V_d=10L/kg; plasma protein binding (83%); found in breast milk. **Metabolism:** Liver (extensive) via sulfoxidation and oxidation; CYP3A4; norquetiapine (active metabolite). **Elimination:** Urine (73%), feces (20%); $T_{1/2}$=7 hrs (quetiapine), 12 hrs (norquetiapine).

NURSING CONSIDERATIONS

Assessment: Assess for history of dementia-related psychosis, risk for hypotension, drug hypersensitivity, psychiatric disorders, hepatic impairment, other conditions where treatment is cautioned, pregnancy/nursing status, and possible drug interactions. Obtain baseline FPG in patients with DM or at risk for DM. Obtain baseline CBC if at risk for leukopenia/neutropenia. Obtain baseline TSH, and free T4. Obtain baseline BP in children and adolescents. Assess for cataracts by performing lens exam (eg, slit lamp exam).

Monitoring: Monitor for clinical worsening, suicidality, unusual changes in behavior, NMS, TD, hyperglycemia, orthostatic hypotension, hypothyroidism, seizures, aspiration, and other adverse effects. Monitor CBC frequently in patients with preexisting low WBC or history of drug-induced leukopenia/neutropenia. Monitor for fever or other signs/symptoms of infection in patients with neutropenia. Monitor weight regularly, and lipids, hepatic function, and FPG periodically. Monitor for cataract formation at 6-month intervals during chronic treatment. Monitor BP periodically during treatment in children and adolescents. Periodically reassess for continued need for maintenance treatment.

Patient Counseling: Inform of the risks and benefits of therapy. Instruct caregivers and patients to contact physician if signs of agitation, anxiety, panic attacks, insomnia, hostility, aggressiveness, impulsivity, akathisia, hypomania, mania, irritability, worsening of depression, changes in behavior, or suicidal ideation develop. Advise about signs/symptoms of NMS, symptoms of hyperglycemia and DM, weight gain, or risk of orthostatic hypotension. Counsel to avoid overheating and dehydration. Caution about performing activities requiring mental alertness. Counsel to notify physician if patient becomes pregnant or intends to become pregnant during therapy, and if patient is taking or plans to take any prescription or OTC drugs.

Administration: Oral route. Swallow tab whole; do not split, crush, or chew. Take without food or with a light meal (approximately 300 calories). **Storage:** 25°C (77°F); excursions permitted to 15-30°C (59-86°F).

SF ROWASA   RX
mesalamine (Alaven)

OTHER BRAND NAMES: Rowasa (Alaven)

THERAPEUTIC CLASS: 5-aminosalicylic acid derivative

INDICATIONS: Treatment of active mild to moderate distal ulcerative colitis, proctosigmoiditis, or proctitis.

DOSAGE: *Adults:* Usual: 60mL units in one rectal instillation qhs for 3-6 weeks. Retain for 8 hrs.

HOW SUPPLIED: Sus: 4g/60mL

WARNINGS/PRECAUTIONS: Acute intolerance syndrome (eg, cramping, bloody diarrhea, abdominal pain, headache) may develop; d/c if signs and symptoms occur. Reevaluate history of sulfasalazine intolerance; if rechallenge is considered, perform under close supervision. Caution with sulfasalazine hypersensitivity; d/c if rash or fever occurs. Carefully monitor with preexisting renal disease; obtain baseline/periodic urinalysis, BUN, and creatinine. Worsening of colitis or symptoms of inflammatory bowel disease, including melena and hematochezia, may occur. Pancolitis, pericarditis (rare) reported. (Rowasa) Contains potassium metabisulfite; caution with sulfite sensitivity especially in asthmatics.

ADVERSE REACTIONS: Abdominal pain/cramps/discomfort, headache, flatulence, flu, fever, nausea, malaise/fatigue.

PREGNANCY: Category B, not for use in nursing.

MECHANISM OF ACTION: 5-aminosalicylic acid; has not been established. Suspected to diminish inflammation by blocking cyclo-oxygenase and inhibiting prostaglandin production in the colon.

PHARMACOKINETICS: Absorption: Colon: Poor. Extent dependent on retention time. **Metabolism:** Acetylation, N-acetyl-5-ASA (Metabolite). **Elimination:** Urine (10-30%), feces, $T_{1/2}$=0.5-1.5 hrs.

NURSING CONSIDERATIONS

Assessment: Assess for history of sulfasalazine intolerance, preexisting renal disease, hypersensitivity, pregnancy/nursing status, and possible drug interactions. Obtain baseline urinalysis, BUN, and creatinine. (Rowasa) Assess for history of asthma or atopic allergies.

Monitoring: Monitor urinalysis, BUN, and creatinine periodically. Monitor for signs/symptoms of acute intolerance syndrome, hypersensitivity, or allergic reaction.

Patient Counseling: Instruct on how to use. Advise that best results achieved if bowel emptied immediately before administration. Advise to seek medical attention if symptoms of acute intolerance syndrome, hypersensitivity, or allergic reactions occur. Instruct that if signs of rash or fever develop, to d/c therapy. Advise to choose a suitable location for administration.

Administration: Rectal route. Refer to PI for administration instructions. **Storage:** 20-25°C (68-77°F). Excursions permitted. Discard unwrapped bottles after 14 days and products with dark brown contents.

SILENOR   RX
doxepin (Somaxon)

THERAPEUTIC CLASS: H_1-antagonist

INDICATIONS: Treatment of insomnia characterized by difficulties with sleep maintenance.

DOSAGE: *Adults:* Individualize dose. Do not take within 3 hrs of a meal. Initial: 6mg qd within 30 min of hs. May decrease to 3mg. Max: 6mg/day. Elderly: ≥65 Yrs: Initial: 3mg qd. May increase to 6mg. Hepatic Impairment: Initial 3mg. Concomitant use with Cimetidine: Max: 3mg.

HOW SUPPLIED: Tab: 3mg, 6mg

CONTRAINDICATIONS: With or within 2 weeks of MAOIs. Untreated narrow-angle glaucoma, severe urinary retention.

WARNINGS/PRECAUTIONS: Evaluate comorbid diagnoses prior to initiation of treatment. Failure of remission after 7 to 10 days may indicate the presence of primary psychiatric and/or medical illness that should be evaluated. Complex behaviors (eg, sleep-driving), amnesia, anxiety and other neuropsychiatric symptoms reported; consider discontinuation if sleep-driving episode occurs. Worsening of depression reported. May impair physical/mental abilities. Caution in patients with compromised respiratory function. Avoid in patients with severe sleep apnea.

ADVERSE REACTIONS: Somnolence, sedation, upper respiratory tract infection, nasopharyngitis, HTN, gastroenteritis, dizziness, N/V.

INTERACTIONS: See Contraindications. Alcohol, CNS depressants, sedating antihistamines may potentiate sedative effects. Increased exposure with inhibitors of CYP2C19, CYP2D6, CYP1A2, and CYP2C9. Doubled exposure with cimetidine. Hypoglycemia reported when oral doxepin was added to tolazamide therapy. Increased blood concentration and decreased psychomotor function with sertraline.

PREGNANCY: Category C, caution in nursing.

MECHANISM OF ACTION: H_1-antagonist; mechanism unknown but is believed to exert its sleep maintenance effect by antagonizing the H_1 receptor.

PHARMACOKINETICS: Absorption: T_{max}=3.5 hrs; **Distribution:** V_d=11,930L; plasma protein binding (80%); found in breast milk. **Metabolism:** Extensive by oxidation and demethylation via CYP2C19, CYP2D6, CYP1A2, CYP2C9; N-desmethyldoxepin (nordoxepin) (primary metabolite). **Elimination:** Urine (<3%); $T_{1/2}$=15.3 hrs (doxepin), 31 hrs (nordoxepin).

NURSING CONSIDERATIONS

Assessment: Assess for untreated narrow-angle glaucoma, urinary retention, presence of a primary psychiatric and/or medical illness that may cause insomnia, depression, hepatic impairment, sleep apnea, pregnancy/nursing status, and possible drug interactions.

Monitoring: Monitor treatment response, sleep-driving, and worsening of depression such as suicidal ideation and actions.

Patient Counseling: Inform of benefits and risks associated with therapy. Counsel on appropriate use of medication. Instruct to contact physician if sleep-driving occurs or if patient performs other complex behaviors while not fully awake. Instruct to seek medical attention if symptoms of cognitive or behavioral abnormalities or if worsening of insomnia occurs. Inform that medication may cause sedation; caution against operating machinery (eg, automobiles) during therapy. Inform that use of alcohol, sedating antihistamines, or other CNS depressants may potentiate sedative effects of drug.

Administration: Oral route. Storage: 20°-25°C (68°-77°F). Protect from light.

SILVADENE   RX
silver sulfadiazine (Monarch Pharmaceuticals Inc.)

OTHER BRAND NAMES: SSD (Dr. Reddy's)

THERAPEUTIC CLASS: Sulfonamide

INDICATIONS: Adjunct for the prevention and treatment of wound sepsis in patients with 2nd- and 3rd-degree burns.

DOSAGE: *Adults:* Apply under sterile conditions qd-bid to a thickness of approximately 1/16 inch. Whenever necessary, reapply to any areas from which it has been removed due to patient activity. Reapply immediately after hydrotherapy. Continue treatment until satisfactory healing has occurred or until the burn site is ready for grafting.

HOW SUPPLIED: Cre: 1% [50g, 400g, 1000g (jar); 20g, 85g (tube)]; (SSD) 1% [50g, 400g (jar); 25g, 50g, 85g (tube)]; (SSD AF) 1% [50g, 400g]

CONTRAINDICATIONS: Pregnant women approaching or at term, premature infants, newborns during the first 2 months of life.

WARNINGS/PRECAUTIONS: Not for ophthalmic use. Potential cross-sensitivity with other sulfonamides; if allergic reactions attributable to treatment occur, weigh continuation of therapy against potential hazards of the particular allergic reaction. Fungal proliferation in and below the eschar may occur. Caution with G6PD deficiency; hemolysis may occur. Drug accumulation may occur if hepatic and renal functions become impaired and elimination of drug decreases; weigh discontinuation of therapy against the therapeutic benefit being achieved. In the treatment of burn wounds involving extensive areas of the body, serum sulfa concentrations may approach adult therapeutic levels (8-12mg%); monitor serum sulfa concentrations in these patients. Monitor renal function and check urine for sulfa crystals. Lab test interactions may occur. Adverse reactions associated with sulfonamides (eg, blood dyscrasias, dermatologic and allergic reactions, GI reactions, hepatitis and hepatocellular necrosis, CNS reactions, toxic nephrosis) may occur.

ADVERSE REACTIONS: Transient leukopenia, skin necrosis, erythema multiforme, skin discoloration, burning sensation, rash, interstitial nephritis.

INTERACTIONS: May inactivate topical proteolytic enzymes.

PREGNANCY: Category B, not for use in nursing.

MECHANISM OF ACTION: Sulfonamide; topical antibacterial. Bactericidal for many gram-negative and gram-positive bacteria as well as being effective against yeast; acts on cell membrane and cell wall to produce bactericidal effect.

NURSING CONSIDERATIONS

Assessment: Assess for hypersensitivity to drug, G6PD deficiency, renal/hepatic impairment, pregnancy/nursing status, and possible drug interactions.

Monitoring: Monitor for allergic reactions, fungal proliferation, renal/hepatic dysfunction, and other adverse effects. Check urine for sulfa crystals. Monitor serum sulfa concentrations in patients with wounds involving extensive areas of the body.

Patient Counseling: Inform of the risks and benefits of therapy. Instruct to use ud. Advise to notify physician if adverse reactions occur.

Administration: Topical route. Refer to PI for administration instructions. **Storage:** 15-30°C (59-86°F).

SIMBRINZA
brimonidine tartrate - brinzolamide (Alcon)

RX

THERAPEUTIC CLASS: Alpha$_2$-agonist/carbonic anhydrase inhibitor

INDICATIONS: Reduction of elevated intraocular pressure (IOP) in patients with open-angle glaucoma or ocular HTN.

DOSAGE: *Adults:* 1 drop in the affected eye(s) tid. Space dosing by at least 5 min if using >1 topical ophthalmic drug.
Pediatrics: ≥2 Yrs: 1 drop in the affected eye(s) tid. Space dosing by at least 5 min if using >1 topical ophthalmic drug.

HOW SUPPLIED: Sus: (Brinzolamide-Brimonidine) 1%-0.2% [8mL]

CONTRAINDICATIONS: Neonates and infants (<2 yrs of age).

WARNINGS/PRECAUTIONS: Systemically absorbed. Fatalities occurred due to severe reactions to sulfonamides, including Stevens-Johnson syndrome, toxic epidermal necrolysis, fulminant hepatic necrosis, agranulocytosis, aplastic anemia, and other blood dyscrasias. Sensitization may recur when a sulfonamide is readministered irrespective of route. D/C if signs of serious reactions or hypersensitivity occur. Caution with low endothelial cell counts; increased potential for corneal edema. Not recommended with severe renal impairment (CrCl <30mL/min). Contains benzalkonium chloride, which may be absorbed by soft contact lenses; contact lenses should be removed during instillation, but may be reinserted 15 min after instillation. Caution with severe cardiovascular disease (CVD), severe hepatic impairment, depression, cerebral or coronary insufficiency, Raynaud's phenomenon, orthostatic hypotension, or thromboangiitis obliterans. Bacterial keratitis reported with multidose containers.

ADVERSE REACTIONS: Blurred vision, eye irritation, dysgeusia, dry mouth, eye allergy.

INTERACTIONS: Potential additive systemic effects with oral carbonic anhydrase inhibitors; coadministration is not recommended. Acid-base alterations reported with high-dose salicylate therapy in patients treated with oral carbonic anhydrase inhibitors. Possible additive or potentiating effect with CNS depressants (eg, alcohol, opiates, barbiturates, sedatives, anesthetics). Caution with antihypertensives and/or cardiac glycosides. Caution with TCAs and MAOIs, which can affect the metabolism and uptake of circulating amines.

PREGNANCY: Category C, not for use in nursing.

MECHANISM OF ACTION: Brinzolamide: Carbonic anhydrase inhibitor; inhibits carbonic anhydrase in the ciliary processes of the eye to decrease aqueous humor secretion. Results in a reduction in elevated IOP. Brimonidine: α-$_2$ adrenergic receptor agonist; reduces aqueous humor production and increases uveoscleral outflow. Results in a reduction in IOP.

PHARMACOKINETICS: Absorption: Brinzolamide: Systemic. Brimonidine: T$_{max}$=1-4 hrs. **Distribution:** Brinzolamide: Plasma protein binding (60%). **Metabolism:** Brinzolamide: N-desethyl brinzolamide (metabolite). Brimonidine: Liver (extensive). **Elimination:** Brinzolamide: Urine (unchanged, metabolites); T$_{1/2}$=111 days (whole blood). Brimonidine: (PO) Urine (74%, unchanged and metabolites). T$_{1/2}$=3 hrs.

NURSING CONSIDERATIONS

S

Assessment: Assess for hypersensitivity to drug or to sulfonamides, low endothelial cell counts, renal/hepatic impairment, contact lens use, severe CVD, depression, cerebral or coronary insufficiency, Raynaud's phenomenon, orthostatic hypotension, thromboangiitis obliterans, pregnancy/nursing status, and possible drug interactions.

Monitoring: Monitor for sulfonamide hypersensitivity reactions, potentiation of syndromes associated with vascular insufficiency, bacterial keratitis, and other adverse reactions.

Patient Counseling: Advise to d/c use and consult physician if serious or unusual ocular or systemic reactions or signs of hypersensitivity occur. Inform that vision may be temporarily blurred following dosing and fatigue and/or drowsiness may be experienced; instruct to use caution in operating machinery, driving a motor vehicle, and engaging in other hazardous activities. Instruct that ocular sol, if handled improperly or if the tip of dispensing container contacts the eye or surrounding structures, can become contaminated by common bacteria known to cause ocular infections. Advise that contaminated sol may result in serious eye damage and subsequent loss of vision. Instruct to always replace cap after using. Advise not to use if sol changes color or becomes cloudy. Instruct to consult physician about the continued use of the present multidose container if having ocular surgery or if an intercurrent ocular condition (eg, trauma, infection) develops. If using >1 topical ophthalmic drug, instruct to administer the drugs at least 5 min apart. Advise that contact lenses should be removed during instillation, but may be reinserted 15 min after instillation.

Administration: Ocular route. Shake well before use. **Storage:** 2-25°C (36-77°F).

SIMCOR
niacin - simvastatin (AbbVie)

THERAPEUTIC CLASS: HMG-CoA reductase inhibitor/nicotinic acid

INDICATIONS: Adjunct to diet to reduce total cholesterol, LDL, apolipoprotein B, non-HDL, TG, or to increase HDL in primary hypercholesterolemia and mixed dyslipidemia, and to reduce TG in hypertriglyceridemia when treatment with simvastatin monotherapy or niacin extended-release (ER) monotherapy is considered inadequate.

DOSAGE: *Adults:* Take at hs with a low-fat snack. Not Currently on Niacin ER or Switching from Non-ER Niacin: Initial: 500mg-20mg qd. Additional Lipid Level Management Needed Despite Simvastatin 20-40mg: Initial: 500mg-40mg qd. Titrate: Niacin ER Component: Increase by no more than 500mg qd every 4 weeks. After Week 8, titrate to patient response and tolerance. Maint: 1000mg-20mg to 2000mg-40mg qd depending on tolerability and lipid levels. Max: 2000mg-40mg qd. If discontinued for >7 days, retitrate as tolerated. May take aspirin (ASA) (up to 325mg) 30 min prior to treatment to reduce flushing. Concomitant Amiodarone, Amlodipine, or Ranolazine: Max: 1000mg-20mg/day. Chinese Patients: Caution with doses >1000mg-20mg/day. Severe Renal Insufficiency: Do not start unless already tolerated ≥10mg simvastatin.

HOW SUPPLIED: Tab: (Niacin ER-Simvastatin) 500mg-20mg, 500mg-40mg, 750mg-20mg, 1000mg-20mg, 1000mg-40mg

CONTRAINDICATIONS: Active liver disease or unexplained persistent elevations in hepatic transaminase levels, active peptic ulcer disease (PUD), arterial bleeding, women who are or may become pregnant, and nursing mothers. Concomitant administration with strong CYP3A4 inhibitors (eg, itraconazole, ketoconazole, posaconazole, HIV protease inhibitors, boceprevir, telaprevir, erythromycin, clarithromycin, telithromycin, nefazodone), gemfibrozil, cyclosporine, danazol, verapamil, or diltiazem.

WARNINGS/PRECAUTIONS: No incremental benefit of Simcor on cardiovascular (CV) morbidity and mortality over and above that demonstrated for simvastatin monotherapy and niacin mono-therapy has been established. Niacin ER, at doses of 1500-2000mg/day, in combination with simvastatin, did not reduce the incidence of CV events more than simvastatin in patients with CV disease and mean baseline LDL levels of 74mg/dL. Should be substituted only for equivalent doses of niacin ER (Niaspan); do not substitute for equivalent doses of immediate-release (IR) (crystalline) niacin. Dose-related myopathy and/or rhabdomyolysis reported; predisposing factors include advanced age (≥65 yrs of age), female gender, uncontrolled hypothyroidism, and renal impairment. Immune-mediated necrotizing myopathy (IMNM) reported. D/C if markedly elevated CPK levels occur or myopathy is diagnosed/suspected, and temporarily withhold in any patient experiencing an acute or serious condition predisposing to development of renal failure secondary to rhabdomyolysis. Stop treatment for a few days before elective major surgery and when any major acute medical/surgical condition supervenes. Severe hepatic toxicity, including fulminant hepatic necrosis, reported when substituting sustained-release niacin for IR niacin at equivalent doses. Caution with substantial alcohol consumption and/or history of liver disease. May cause abnormal LFTs; obtain LFTs prior to initiation and repeat as clinically indicated. Fatal and nonfatal hepatic failure (rare) reported; promptly interrupt therapy if serious liver injury with clinical symptoms and/or hyperbilirubinemia or jaundice occurs and do not restart if no alternate etiology found. Increases in HbA1c and FPG levels reported; closely monitor diabetic/potentially diabetic patients (particularly during 1st few months of therapy), and adjust diet and/or hypoglycemic therapy or d/c Simcor if necessary. May reduce platelet count or phosphorus (P) levels, and increase PT or uric acid levels. Caution in patients predisposed to gout, with renal impairment, and in elderly.

ADVERSE REACTIONS: Flushing, headache, back pain, diarrhea, nausea, pruritus.

INTERACTIONS: See Contraindications. Avoid ingestion of alcohol, hot drinks, or spicy foods around the time of administration; may increase flushing and pruritus. Simvastatin: Due to the risk of myopathy, avoid with large quantities of grapefruit juice (>1 quart/day) and drugs that cause myopathy/rhabdomyolysis when given alone (eg, fibrates); caution with colchicine; do not exceed 1000mg-20mg/day with amiodarone, amlodipine, and ranolazine. Voriconazole may increase concentration; consider dose adjustment of Simcor to reduce risk of myopathy/rhabdomyolysis. Decreased C_{max} with propranolol. May increase digoxin concentrations; monitor patients taking digoxin when therapy is initiated. May potentiate effect of coumarin anticoagulants; determine PT before initiation and frequently during therapy. Niacin: ASA may decrease metabolic clearance. May potentiate effects of ganglionic blocking agents and vasoactive drugs, resulting in postural hypotension. Separate administration from bile acid-binding resins (eg, colestipol, cholestyramine) by at least 4-6 hrs. Nutritional supplements containing large doses of niacin or related compounds may potentiate adverse effects.

PREGNANCY: Category X, not for use in nursing.

MECHANISM OF ACTION: Niacin: Nicotinic acid; has not been established. May partially inhibit release of free fatty acids from adipose tissue, and increase lipoprotein lipase activity (which may increase rate of chylomicron TG removal from plasma). Decreases rate of hepatic synthesis of VLDL and LDL. Simvastatin: HMG-CoA reductase inhibitor; inhibits conversion of HMG-CoA to mevalonate. Reduces VLDL and TG, and increases HDL.

PHARMACOKINETICS: Absorption: Niacin: T_{max}=4.6-4.9 hrs. Simvastatin: T_{max}=1.9-2 hrs, 6.56 hrs (simvastatin acid); C_{max}=3.29ng/mL, $AUC_{(0-t)}$=30.81ng•hr/mL (simvastatin acid). **Distribution:** Niacin: Found in breast milk. **Metabolism:** Niacin: Liver (rapid and extensive 1st-pass); nicotinuric acid (via conjugation), nicotinamide adenine dinucleotide (metabolites). Simvastatin: Liver (rapid and extensive 1st-pass) via CYP3A4; β-hydroxyacid (simvastatin acid), 6'-hydroxy, 6'-hydroxymethyl, and 6'-exomethylene derivatives (major active metabolites). **Elimination:** Niacin: Urine (54%, 3.6% unchanged). Simvastatin: Feces (60%), urine (13%); $T_{1/2}$=4.2-4.9 hrs, 4.6-5 hrs (simvastatin acid).

NURSING CONSIDERATIONS

Assessment: Assess for history of/active liver disease, unexplained persistent hepatic transaminase elevations, active PUD, arterial bleeding, predisposing factors for myopathy, renal impairment, diabetes, any other conditions where treatment is contraindicated or cautioned, drug hypersensitivity, pregnancy/nursing status, and possible drug interactions. Assess lipid profile and LFTs.

Monitoring: Monitor for signs/symptoms of myopathy (including IMNM), rhabdomyolysis, liver/renal dysfunction, decreases in platelet counts and P levels, increases in PT and uric acid levels, and other adverse reactions. Monitor lipid profile, LFTs, blood glucose, and CPK levels. Check PT with coumarin anticoagulants.

Patient Counseling: Advise to adhere to their National Cholesterol Education Program-recommended diet, a regular exercise program, and periodic testing of a fasting lipid panel. Inform about substances that should be avoided during therapy, and advise to discuss all medications, both prescription and OTC, including vitamins or other nutritional supplements containing niacin or nicotinamide, with their physician. Instruct to report promptly any unexplained muscle pain, tenderness, or weakness, particularly if accompanied by malaise or fever or if these muscle signs or symptoms persist after discontinuation, any symptoms that may indicate liver injury, or if symptoms of dizziness occur. Advise to notify physician prior to restarting therapy if dosing is interrupted for any length of time, and of changes in blood glucose if diabetic. Inform that flushing may occur but may subside after several weeks of consistent use of therapy. If awakened by flushing at night, instruct to get up slowly, especially if feeling dizzy or faint, or taking BP medications. Instruct women to use an effective method of birth control to prevent pregnancy while on therapy, to d/c therapy and call physician if pregnant, and not to breastfeed while on therapy.

Administration: Oral route. Take at hs with a low-fat snack. Swallow whole; do not break, crush, or chew. Avoid administration on an empty stomach to reduce flushing, pruritus, and GI distress. **Storage:** 20-25°C (68-77°F).

SIMPONI RX
golimumab (Janssen)

S

Increased risk for developing serious infections (eg, active tuberculosis [TB], latent TB reactivation, invasive fungal infections, bacterial/viral infections, opportunistic infections) leading to hospitalization or death, mostly with concomitant use with immunosuppressants (eg, methotrexate [MTX] or corticosteroids). D/C if serious infection develops. Active TB/latent TB reactivation may present with disseminated or extrapulmonary disease; test for latent TB before and during therapy and initiate treatment for latent TB prior to therapy. Invasive fungal infections reported; consider empiric antifungal therapy in patients at risk who develop severe systemic illness. Consider risks and benefits prior to therapy in patients with chronic or recurrent infection. Monitor patients for development of infection during and after treatment, including development of TB in patients who tested (-) for latent TB infection prior to therapy. Lymphoma and other malignancies, some fatal, reported in children and adolescents.

THERAPEUTIC CLASS: Monoclonal antibody/TNF-blocker

INDICATIONS: Treatment of adults with moderately to severely active rheumatoid arthritis (RA) in combination with MTX, active psoriatic arthritis (PsA) alone or in combination with MTX, and active ankylosing spondylitis (AS). For inducing and maintaining clinical response, improving endoscopic appearance of the mucosa during induction, inducing clinical remission, and achieving and sustaining clinical remission in induction responders, in adults with moderately to severely active ulcerative colitis (UC) who have demonstrated corticosteroid dependence or who have had an inadequate response to or failed to tolerate oral aminosalicylates, oral corticosteroids, azathioprine, or 6-mercaptopurine.

DOSAGE: *Adults:* RA: 50mg SQ once a month in combination with MTX. May continue corticosteroids, nonbiologic disease-modifying antirheumatic drugs (DMARDs), and/or NSAIDs during treatment. PsA/AS: 50mg SQ once a month with or without MTX or other nonbiologic DMARDs. May continue corticosteroids, nonbiologic DMARDs, and/or NSAIDs during treatment.

UC: Induction: 200mg SQ at Week 0, followed by 100mg SQ at Week 2. Maint: 100mg SQ every 4 weeks.

HOW SUPPLIED: Inj: 50mg/0.5mL, 100mg/mL [prefilled SmartJect autoinjector, prefilled syringe]

WARNINGS/PRECAUTIONS: Do not initiate in patients with an active infection. Increased risk of infection in patients >65 yrs of age and in patients with comorbid conditions; consider the risks and benefits prior to therapy in patients who have resided or traveled in areas of endemic TB or endemic mycoses, and with any underlying conditions predisposing to infection. Hepatitis B virus (HBV) reactivation reported in chronic carriers; closely monitor for signs of active HBV infection during and for several months after therapy. D/C if reactivation occurs and initiate antiviral therapy with appropriate supportive treatment. Consider risks and benefits prior to initiating therapy in patients with a known malignancy other than a successfully treated nonmelanoma skin cancer or when considering continuing therapy in patients who develop a malignancy. All patients with UC who are at increased risk for dysplasia or colon carcinoma, or who had a prior history of dysplasia or colon carcinoma should be screened for dysplasia at regular intervals before therapy and throughout their disease course. Melanoma/Merkel cell carcinoma and worsening/new onset congestive heart failure (CHF) reported. Associated with rare cases of new onset or exacerbation of CNS (eg, multiple sclerosis) and peripheral (eg, Guillain-Barre syndrome) demyelinating disorders; consider discontinuation if these disorders develop. Caution when switching from one biological product to another biological product; overlapping biological activity may further increase risk of infection. Hematologic cytopenias (eg, neutropenia, aplastic anemia) reported. Serious systemic hypersensitivity reactions reported; d/c immediately if these reactions occur. Caution in elderly.

ADVERSE REACTIONS: Serious infection, malignancies, upper respiratory tract infection, nasopharyngitis, inj-site reactions, HTN, increased ALT/AST.

INTERACTIONS: See Boxed Warning. Not recommended with anakinra, abatacept, or biologics approved to treat RA, PsA, or AS; may increase risk of serious infections. Avoid with live vaccines and therapeutic infectious agents (eg, live attenuated bacteria [eg, BCG bladder instillation for the treatment of cancer]). Avoid administration of live vaccines to infants for 6 months following the mother's last golimumab injection during pregnancy. Upon initiation or discontinuation of therapy in patients being treated with CYP450 substrates with a narrow therapeutic index, monitor effect (eg, warfarin) or drug concentration (eg, cyclosporine, theophylline) and may adjust individual dose of the drug product as needed.

PREGNANCY: Category B, not for use in nursing.

MECHANISM OF ACTION: Monoclonal antibody/TNF-α receptor blocker; prevents the binding of TNF-α to its receptors, thereby inhibiting the biological activity of TNF-α.

PHARMACOKINETICS: Absorption: Absolute bioavailability (53%); C_{max}=3.2mcg/mL; T_{max}=2-6 days (median). **Distribution:** V_d=58-126mL/kg (IV); crosses the placenta. **Elimination:** (IV) $T_{1/2}$=2 weeks (median).

NURSING CONSIDERATIONS

Assessment: Assess for active/chronic/recurrent infection, history of an opportunistic infection, recent travel to areas of endemic TB or endemic mycoses, underlying conditions that may predispose to infection, malignancies, dysplasia (in UC patients), CHF, demyelinating disorders, significant cytopenias, latex sensitivity, risk factors for skin cancer, pregnancy/nursing status, and possible drug interactions. Test for latent TB infection and for HBV infection.

Monitoring: Monitor for development of infection during and after treatment. Monitor for HBV reactivation, malignancies, dysplasia, new or worsening CHF, demyelinating disorders, hematological events, hypersensitivity reactions, and other adverse reactions. Periodically evaluate for active TB and test for latent TB infection. Perform periodic skin examination, particularly in patients with risk factors for skin cancer.

Patient Counseling: Advise of the potential risks and benefits of therapy. Inform that therapy may lower the ability of immune system to fight infections; instruct to contact physician if any symptoms of infection develop. Counsel about the risk of lymphoma and other malignancies. Instruct patients sensitive to latex to not handle the needle cover on the prefilled syringe as well as the needle cover of the prefilled syringe within the autoinjector cap because it contains dry natural rubber (a derivative of latex). Advise to report any signs of new/worsening medical conditions (eg, CHF, demyelinating disorders, autoimmune diseases, liver disease, cytopenias, psoriasis).

Administration: SQ route. Refer to PI for administration instructions. **Storage:** 2-8°C (36-46°F). Protect from light. Do not freeze or shake.

SINEMET CR

RX

levodopa - carbidopa (Merck)

OTHER BRAND NAMES: Sinemet (Merck)

THERAPEUTIC CLASS: Dopa-decarboxylase inhibitor/dopamine precursor

INDICATIONS: Treatment of symptoms of idiopathic Parkinson's disease (paralysis agitans), postencephalitic parkinsonism, and symptomatic parkinsonism that may follow injury to the nervous system by carbon monoxide/manganese intoxication.

DOSAGE: *Adults:* Determine dose by careful titration. (Tab) Tabs with different ratios of carbidopa to levodopa may be given separately or combined PRN to provide optimum dosage. (25mg-100mg) Initial: 1 tab tid. Titrate: May increase by 1 tab qd or qod, as necessary, until 8 tabs/day is reached. (10mg-100mg) Initial: 1 tab tid-qid. Titrate: May increase by 1 tab qd or qod until 8 tabs/day (2 tabs qid) is reached. Transfer from Levodopa (d/c at least 12 hr before starting): Daily dosage should provide approximately 25% of previous levodopa dosage. <1500mg/day Levodopa: Initial: 1 tab (25mg-100mg) tid or qid. >1500mg/day Levodopa: Initial: 1 tab (25mg-250mg) tid or qid. Maint: 70-100mg/day of carbidopa should be provided. May substitute 1 tab of 25mg-100mg for each 10mg-100mg when greater proportion of carbidopa is required. When more levodopa is required, substitute 25mg-250mg for 25mg-100mg or 10mg-100mg. May increase dosage of 25mg-250mg by 1/2 or 1 tab qd or qod to a max of 8 tabs/day if necessary. Max: 200mg/day of carbidopa. (Tab, Extended-Release [ER]) Currently Treated with Levodopa without Decarboxylase Inhibitor: D/C levodopa at least 12 hr before starting. Substitute at a dosage that will provide approximately 25% of the previous levodopa dose. With Mild to Moderate Disease: Initial: 1 tab (50mg-200mg) bid. No Prior Levodopa Use: With Mild to Moderate Disease: Initial: 1 tab (50mg-200mg) bid at ≥6-hr intervals. Titration: May increase or decrease dose or interval depending upon therapeutic response following initiation of therapy. Most patients have been adequately treated with doses that provide 400-1600mg/day of levodopa given in divided doses at 4-8 hr intervals during the waking day. If given at intervals of <4 hrs and/or if the divided doses are not equal, give the smaller doses at the end of the day. An interval of at least 3 days between dosage adjustments is recommended. Refer to PI for Conversion to ER Tabs, Addition of Other Antiparkinson Medication, or Interruption of Therapy.

HOW SUPPLIED: (Carbidopa-Levodopa) Tab: 10mg-100mg, 25mg-100mg, 25mg-250mg; Tab, ER: 25mg-100mg, 50mg-200mg

CONTRAINDICATIONS: During or within 14 days of using nonselective MAOIs; narrow-angle glaucoma; suspicious, undiagnosed skin lesion, or history of melanoma.

WARNINGS/PRECAUTIONS: Dyskinesias may occur; may require dose reduction. May cause mental disturbances; monitor for depression with suicidal tendencies. Caution with past or current psychoses, severe cardiovascular (CV) or pulmonary disease, bronchial asthma, renal or hepatic disease, endocrine disease, chronic wide-angle glaucoma, or history of myocardial infarction (MI) with residual atrial, nodal, or ventricular arrhythmias. May increase the risk of upper GI hemorrhage; caution in history of peptic ulcer. Neuroleptic malignant syndrome (NMS) reported during dose reduction or withdrawal. Periodically evaluate hepatic, hematopoietic, CV, and renal function if on extended therapy. Somnolence and very rarely sudden onset of sleep reported; may impair physical/mental abilities. Monitor for melanomas frequently and on a regular basis. Abnormalities in laboratory tests, including elevations of LFTs and abnormalities in BUN, reported. Cases of falsely diagnosed pheochromocytoma reported very rarely; caution when interpreting the plasma and urine levels of catecholamines and their metabolites.

ADVERSE REACTIONS: Dyskinesias (eg, choreiform, dystonic, and other involuntary movements), nausea.

INTERACTIONS: See Contraindications. Symptomatic postural hypotension reported with concomitant use of antihypertensive drugs. Use with selegiline may cause severe orthostatic hypotension. HTN and dyskinesia may occur with TCAs. May reduce effects of levodopa when used concomitantly with dopamine D_2 receptor antagonists (eg, phenothiazines, butyrophenones, risperidone) and isoniazid. Caution with phenytoin, papaverine; therapeutic response may be reversed. Not recommended with dopamine-depleting agents (eg, reserpine, tetrabenazine) or other drugs known to deplete monoamine stores. Reduced bioavailability with iron salts. Metoclopramide may increase the bioavailability and may also adversely affect disease control.

PREGNANCY: Category C, caution in nursing.

MECHANISM OF ACTION: Dopa-decarboxylase inhibitor/dopamine precursor. Carbidopa: Inhibits decarboxylation of peripheral levodopa. Levodopa: Crosses blood-brain barrier and presumably converted to dopamine in the brain.

PHARMACOKINETICS: Absorption: Administration of variable doses resulted in different parameters. **Distribution:** Levodopa: Crosses the placenta; found in breast milk. **Elimination:** Levodopa: $T_{1/2}$=50 min, 1.5 hrs (in the presence of carbidopa).

S

NURSING CONSIDERATIONS

Assessment: Assess for narrow-angle/chronic wide-angle glaucoma, suspicious/undiagnosed skin lesions or history of melanoma, presence of or history of psychoses, history of peptic ulcer, severe CV or pulmonary disease, bronchial asthma, hepatic, renal, or endocrine disease, history of MI with residual atrial, nodal, or ventricular arrhythmias, pregnancy/nursing status, and for possible drug interactions.

Monitoring: Monitor for signs/symptoms of mental disturbances, depression with suicidal tendencies, somnolence, and NMS (eg, fever, muscle rigidity, involuntary movements). Monitor for signs/symptoms of upper GI hemorrhage in patients with a history of peptic ulcer. Monitor cardiac function in patients with a history of MI who have residual atrial, nodal, or ventricular arrhythmias. Monitor for LFT elevations and BUN abnormalities. For patients on extended therapy, perform periodic evaluation of hepatic, hematopoetic, CV, and renal function. Monitor for melanomas frequently and on a regular basis. Monitor IOP in chronic wide-angle glaucoma. Monitor closely during the dose adjustment period.

Patient Counseling: Instruct to take ud. Inform that discoloration of saliva, urine, or sweat may occur after ingestion. Inform that high protein diet, excessive acidity, or iron salts may reduce clinical effectiveness. Instruct to refrain from driving or operating machinery if somnolence and/or sudden sleep onset is experienced. Instruct to inform physician if new or increased gambling, sexual, or other intense urges develop. (Tab) Advise that "wearing-off" effect may occur at end of dosing interval; notify physician if such response poses a problem to lifestyle. (Tab, ER) Inform that onset of effect of the 1st morning dose may be delayed for up to 1 hr; instruct to notify physician if this poses a problem in treatment.

Administration: Oral route. (Tab, ER) Do not chew or crush. **Storage:** 25°C (77°F); excursions permitted to 15-30°C (59-86°F). Protect from light and moisture.

SINGULAIR   RX
montelukast sodium (Merck)

THERAPEUTIC CLASS: Leukotriene receptor antagonist

INDICATIONS: Prophylaxis and chronic treatment of asthma in adults and pediatric patients ≥12 months of age. Relief of symptoms of seasonal allergic rhinitis in patients ≥2 yrs of age and perennial allergic rhinitis in patients ≥6 months of age. Prevention of exercise-induced bronchoconstriction (EIB) in patients ≥6 yrs of age.

DOSAGE: *Adults:* Asthma: 10mg tab qpm. Seasonal/Perennial Allergic Rhinitis: 10mg tab qd. Patients with both asthma and allergic rhinitis should take 1 dose qpm. EIB: 10mg tab at least 2 hrs before exercise. Do not take an additional dose within 24 hrs of a previous dose.
Pediatrics: Asthma: ≥15 Yrs: 10mg tab qpm. 6-14 Yrs: 5mg chewable tab qpm. 2-5 Yrs: 4mg chewable tab or 4mg granules qpm. 12-23 Months: 4mg granules qpm. Seasonal/Perennial Allergic Rhinitis: ≥15 Yrs: 10mg tab qd. 6-14 Yrs: 5mg chewable tab qd. 2-5 Yrs: 4mg chewable tab or 4mg granules qd. Perennial Allergic Rhinitis: 6-23 Months: 4mg granules qd. Patients with both asthma and allergic rhinitis should take 1 dose qpm. EIB: ≥15 Yrs: 10mg tab at least 2 hrs before exercise. 6-14 Yrs: 5mg chewable tab at least 2 hrs before exercise. Do not take an additional dose within 24 hrs of a previous dose.

HOW SUPPLIED: Granules: 4mg/pkt; Tab, Chewable: 4mg, 5mg; Tab: 10mg

WARNINGS/PRECAUTIONS: Not for use in the reversal of bronchospasm in acute asthma attacks, including status asthmaticus; have appropriate rescue medication available. Therapy during acute exacerbations of asthma may be continued. Patients should have short-acting inhaled β-agonist available for rescue during exacerbations of asthma after exercise. Should not be abruptly substituted for inhaled or oral corticosteroids. Eosinophilic conditions reported. Neuropsychiatric events reported; evaluate risks and benefits of continuing treatment if such events occur. Chew tabs contain phenylalanine; caution with phenylketonuria. Avoid aspirin (ASA) and NSAIDs with known ASA sensitivity; has not been shown to truncate bronchoconstrictor response to ASA and other NSAIDs in ASA-sensitive asthmatic patients.

ADVERSE REACTIONS: Headache, pharyngitis, influenza, fever, sinusitis, diarrhea, upper respiratory tract infection, cough, abdominal pain, otitis media, rhinorrhea, otitis.

INTERACTIONS: Monitor with potent CYP450 inducers (eg, phenobarbital, rifampin).

PREGNANCY: Category B, caution in nursing.

MECHANISM OF ACTION: Leukotriene receptor antagonist; binds to cysteinyl leukotriene receptors found in the airway (including airway smooth muscle cells and airway macrophages) and on other proinflammatory cells (including eosinophils and certain myeloid stem cells). Inhibits physiologic actions of leukotrienes.

PHARMACOKINETICS: Absorption: Rapid. (10mg tab) T_{max}=3-4 hrs; oral bioavailability (64%). (5mg Chewable tab) T_{max}=2-2.5 hrs; oral bioavailability: fasted (73%), fed (63%). 2-5 yrs: (4mg Chewable tab) T_{max}=2 hrs (fasted). (4mg Granules) T_{max}=2.3 hrs (fasted), 6.4 hrs (fed).

Distribution: V$_d$=8-11L; plasma protein binding (>99%). **Metabolism:** Liver (extensive); CYP3A4, 2C8, and 2C9. **Elimination:** Biliary (major), feces (86%), urine (<0.2%); T$_{1/2}$=2.7-5.5 hrs.

NURSING CONSIDERATIONS

Assessment: Assess for drug hypersensitivity, phenylketonuria, asthma status, pregnancy/nursing status, and possible drug interactions.

Monitoring: Monitor for signs/symptoms of eosinophilia, vasculitic rash, worsening pulmonary symptoms, cardiac complications, neuropathy, neuropsychiatric events, hypersensitivity reactions, and other adverse reactions.

Patient Counseling: Advise to take daily as prescribed, even when asymptomatic, as well as during periods of worsening asthma; instruct to contact physician if asthma is not well controlled. Inform not to use for treatment of acute asthma attacks; inform that patient should have appropriate short-acting inhaled β-agonist medication available to treat asthma exacerbations. Advise to seek medical attention if short-acting inhaled bronchodilators are needed more than usual while on therapy or if more than the maximum number of inhalations of short-acting bronchodilator treatment prescribed for a 24-hour period are needed. Instruct not to decrease dose or d/c other anti-asthma medications unless instructed by physician. Advise to notify physician if symptoms of neuropsychiatric events occur. Advise patients with ASA sensitivity to continue avoiding ASA and NSAIDs while on therapy. Inform phenylketonuric patients that the 4mg and 5mg chewable tabs contain phenylalanine.

Administration: Oral route. Refer to PI for instructions for administration of granules. **Storage:** 25°C (77°F); excursions permitted to 15-30°C (59-86°F). Protect from light and moisture.

SKELAXIN   RX
metaxalone (King)

THERAPEUTIC CLASS: Muscular analgesic (central-acting)

INDICATIONS: Adjunct to rest, physical therapy, and other measures for the relief of discomforts associated with acute, painful musculoskeletal conditions.

DOSAGE: *Adults:* 800mg tid-qid.
Pediatrics: >12 Yrs: 800mg tid-qid.

HOW SUPPLIED: Tab: 800mg* *scored

CONTRAINDICATIONS: Known tendency to drug-induced, hemolytic, and other anemias. Significantly impaired renal/hepatic function.

WARNINGS/PRECAUTIONS: Caution with preexisting liver damage; perform serial LFTs. False-positive Benedict's tests reported; glucose-specific test will differentiate findings. Taking with food may enhance general CNS depression, especially in elderly patients.

ADVERSE REACTIONS: Drowsiness, dizziness, headache, nervousness, irritability, N/V, GI upset.

INTERACTIONS: Additive sedative effects with other CNS depressants (eg, alcohol, benzodiazepines, opioids, TCAs); use with caution if taking >1 CNS depressant simultaneously.

PREGNANCY: Not for use in pregnancy/nursing.

MECHANISM OF ACTION: Muscular analgesic (central-acting); has not been established. Activity may be due to general depression of CNS.

PHARMACOKINETICS: Absorption: (400mg) C$_{max}$=983ng/mL, T$_{max}$= 3.3 hrs; AUC=7479ng•hr/mL. (800mg) C$_{max}$=1816ng/mL, T$_{max}$=3 hrs; AUC=15,044ng•hr/mL. **Distribution:** V$_d$=800L. **Metabolism:** Liver; via CYP1A2, 2D6, 2E1, 3A4, and to a lesser extent CYP2C8, 2C9, C19. **Elimination:** Urine (metabolites); T$_{1/2}$=9 hrs (400mg), 8 hrs (800mg).

NURSING CONSIDERATIONS

Assessment: Assess for known tendency to drug-induced, hemolytic, or other anemias, significant renal/hepatic impairment, hypersensitivity to the drug, pregnancy/nursing status, and possible drug interactions.

Monitoring: Perform serial LFTs with preexisting liver damage. Monitor for signs/symptoms of CNS depression.

Patient Counseling: Inform that drug may impair mental and/or physical abilities required to perform hazardous tasks, especially when used with alcohol or other CNS depressants.

Administration: Oral route. Taking with food may enhance general CNS depression. **Storage:** 15-30°C (59-86°F).

S

SOLIRIS RX
eculizumab (Alexion)

Life-threatening and fatal meningococcal infections reported; may become rapidly life-threatening or fatal if not recognized and treated early. Comply with the most current Advisory Committee on Immunization Practices (ACIP) recommendations for meningococcal vaccination. Immunize patients with meningococcal vaccine at least 2 weeks prior to administering the 1st dose, unless risks of delaying therapy outweigh risk of meningococcal infection development. Monitor for early signs of meningococcal infections and evaluate immediately if infection suspected. Available only through a restricted program under a Risk Evaluation and Mitigation Strategy.

THERAPEUTIC CLASS: Monoclonal antibody/protein C5 blocker

INDICATIONS: Treatment of patients with paroxysmal nocturnal hemoglobinuria (PNH) to reduce hemolysis, and treatment of patients with atypical hemolytic uremic syndrome (aHUS) to inhibit complement-mediated thrombotic microangiopathy (TMA).

DOSAGE: *Adults:* ≥18 Yrs: PNH: Initial: 600mg weekly for the first 4 weeks. Maint: 900mg for the 5th dose 1 week later, then 900mg every 2 weeks thereafter. aHUS: Initial: 900mg weekly for the first 4 weeks. Maint: 1200mg for the 5th dose 1 week later, then 1200mg every 2 weeks thereafter. Refer to PI for supplemental dosing information after plasmapheresis/plasma exchange or fresh frozen plasma infusion.
Pediatrics: <18 Yrs: aHUS: ≥40kg: Induction: 900mg weekly x 4 doses. Maint: 1200mg at week 5, then 1200mg every 2 weeks. 30-<40kg: Induction: 600mg weekly x 2 doses. Maint: 900mg at week 3, then 900mg every 2 weeks. 20-<30kg: Induction: 600mg weekly x 2 doses. Maint: 600mg at week 3, then 600mg every 2 weeks. 10-<20kg: Induction: 600mg weekly x 1 dose. Maint: 300mg at week 2, then 300mg every 2 weeks. 5-<10kg: Induction: 300mg weekly x 1 dose. Maint: 300mg at week 2, then 300mg every 3 weeks. Refer to PI for supplemental dosing information after plasmapheresis/plasma exchange or fresh frozen plasma infusion.

HOW SUPPLIED: Inj: 10mg/mL [30mL]

CONTRAINDICATIONS: Patients with unresolved serious *Neisseria meningitidis* infection and patients not currently vaccinated against it.

WARNINGS/PRECAUTIONS: Not indicated for treatment of Shiga toxin *Escherichia coli*-related hemolytic uremic syndrome. May increase susceptibility to infections, especially with encapsulated bacteria; administer vaccinations for the prevention of *Streptococcus pneumoniae* and *Haemophilus influenza* type b (Hib) infections according to ACIP guidelines, and use caution with any systemic infection. Monitor PNH patients for at least 8 weeks after discontinuing therapy to detect hemolysis. Monitor aHUS patients for signs/symptoms of TMA complications during therapy and for at least 12 weeks after discontinuing therapy; consider reinstitution of therapy, plasma therapy, or appropriate organ-specific supportive measures if TMA complications occur after discontinuing therapy. May result in infusion reactions, including anaphylaxis or other hypersensitivity reactions; interrupt infusion and institute appropriate supportive measures if signs of cardiovascular instability or respiratory compromise occur.

ADVERSE REACTIONS: Meningococcal infections, headache, nasopharyngitis, back pain, N/V, urinary tract infection, HTN, upper respiratory tract infection, diarrhea, anemia, pyrexia, cough, nasal congestion, tachycardia.

PREGNANCY: Category C, caution in nursing.

MECHANISM OF ACTION: Monoclonal antibody/complement protein C5 blocker; specifically binds to complement protein C5 with high affinity, thereby inhibiting its cleavage to C5a and C5b and preventing the generation of the terminal complement complex C5b-9. Inhibits terminal complement-mediated intravascular hemolysis in PNH patients and complement-mediated TMA in patients with aHUS.

PHARMACOKINETICS: Absorption: C_{max}=194mcg/mL (PNH). **Distribution:** V_d=7.7L (PNH), 6.14L (aHUS); crosses the placenta; found in breast milk. **Elimination:** $T_{1/2}$=272 hrs (PNH), 291 hrs (aHUS).

NURSING CONSIDERATIONS

Assessment: Assess for unresolved serious *N. meningitidis* infection, meningococcal vaccination status, presence of a systemic infection, and pregnancy/nursing status. In patients with PNH, obtain baseline serum LDH levels. In patients with aHUS, obtain baseline serum LDH levels, platelet count, and SrCr levels.

Monitoring: Monitor for signs/symptoms of meningococcal infections, other infections, and infusion/hypersensitivity reactions. Monitor PNH patients after discontinuing therapy for at least 8 weeks to detect hemolysis; serum LDH levels may assist in monitoring effects. Monitor aHUS patients for signs of TMA by monitoring serial platelet counts, serum LDH levels, and SrCr levels during therapy and for at least 12 weeks after discontinuing therapy.

Patient Counseling: Counsel about risks/benefits of therapy, in particular, the risk of meningococcal infection, and the need to be monitored by a physician after discontinuing therapy.

Inform that patients are required to receive meningococcal vaccination at least 2 weeks prior to receiving the 1st dose of treatment, if not previously vaccinated, and that they are required to be revaccinated while on therapy. Inform about the signs/symptoms of a meningococcal infection, and advise to seek immediate medical attention if these signs/symptoms occur. Instruct patients to carry the Soliris Patient Safety Information Card with them at all times, until 3 months after the last dose. Inform parents/caregivers that their child being treated for aHUS should be vaccinated against *S. pneumoniae* and Hib.

Administration: IV route. Administer by IV infusion over 35 min; do not administer as an IV push or bolus inj. Refer to PI for preparation and administration instructions. **Storage:** 2-8°C (36-46°F). Protect from light. Do not freeze or shake. Admixed Sol: Stable for 24 hrs at 2-8°C (36-46°F) and at room temperature.

SOLU-CORTEF   RX
hydrocortisone sodium succinate (Pharmacia & Upjohn)

THERAPEUTIC CLASS: Glucocorticoid

INDICATIONS: Steroid-responsive disorders.

DOSAGE: *Adults:* Individualize dose. Initial: 100-500mg IV/IM, depending on disease being treated. May repeat dose at intervals of 2, 4, or 6 hrs. High-dose therapy should be continued only until patient is stabilized, usually not beyond 48-72 hrs. Maint: Decrease initial dosage in small decrements at appropriate time intervals until the lowest dosage that maintains an adequate clinical response is reached. Withdraw gradually after long-term therapy. Acute Exacerbations of Multiple Sclerosis: Usual: 800mg/day for 1 week followed by 320mg qod for 1 month. Liver Disease: May consider reducing dose. Elderly: Start at lower end of dosing range.
Pediatrics: Individualize dose. Initial: 0.56-8mg/kg/day IV/IM in 3 or 4 divided doses (20-240mg/m²bsa/day). Titrate: Adjust to the lowest effective dose.

HOW SUPPLIED: Inj: 100mg, 250mg, 500mg, 1000mg

CONTRAINDICATIONS: Systemic fungal infections, idiopathic thrombocytopenic purpura (IM corticosteroid preparations), intrathecal administration.

WARNINGS/PRECAUTIONS: May result in dermal and/or subdermal changes forming depressions in the skin at the inj site; exercise caution not to exceed recommended doses in injections. Anaphylactoid reactions (rare) may occur. May need to increase dose before, during, and after stressful situations. High doses should not be used for the treatment of traumatic brain injury. May cause elevation of BP, salt/water retention, and increased excretion of K^+ and Ca^{2+}. Associated with left ventricular free wall rupture after a recent myocardial infarction (MI); caution in these patients. Hypothalamic-pituitary-adrenal (HPA) axis suppression, Cushing's syndrome, and hyperglycemia reported; monitor chronic use. May produce reversible HPA-axis suppression with the potential for glucocorticosteroid insufficiency after withdrawal of treatment. Drug-induced secondary adrenocortical insufficiency may be minimized by gradual reduction of dosage. May cause decreased resistance and inability to localize infection. May mask some signs of current infection or cause new infections; do not use intra-articularly, intrabursally, or for intratendinous administration for local effect in the presence of acute local infection. May exacerbate systemic fungal infections; avoid use in the presence of such infections unless needed to control drug reactions. Rule out latent or active amebiasis before initiating therapy. Caution with Strongyloides infestation, active or latent tuberculosis (TB), congestive heart failure (CHF), HTN, renal insufficiency, osteoporosis, and ocular herpes simplex. Not for use in cerebral malaria or active ocular herpes simplex. More serious/fatal course of chickenpox and measles reported. Severe medical events associated with intrathecal route of administration. May produce posterior subcapsular cataracts, glaucoma with possible damage to the optic nerves, and may enhance the establishment of secondary ocular infections due to bacteria, fungi, or viruses. Kaposi's sarcoma reported. Caution with active or latent peptic ulcers, diverticulitis, fresh intestinal anastomoses and nonspecific ulcerative colitis; may increase risk of perforation. Enhanced effect in patients with cirrhosis. May decrease bone formation and increase bone resorption. Acute myopathy with high doses reported most often in patients with disorders of neuromuscular transmission (eg, myasthenia gravis) or concomitant neuromuscular blocking drugs (eg, pancuronium). Elevation of CK may occur. Changes in thyroid status may necessitate dose adjustment. Psychic derangements may appear and existing emotional instability or psychotic tendencies may be aggravated. May elevate intraocular pressure (IOP); monitor IOP if steroid therapy is >6 weeks. May suppress reactions to skin tests.

ADVERSE REACTIONS: Bradycardia, cardiac arrest, acne, allergic dermatitis, decreased carbohydrate and glucose tolerance, fluid retention, abdominal distention, bowel/bladder dysfunction, negative nitrogen balance, aseptic necrosis of femoral and humeral heads, convulsions, emotional instability, exophthalmoses, glaucoma, abnormal fat deposits.

INTERACTIONS: Aminoglutethimide may lead to a loss of corticosteroid-induced adrenal suppression. May develop hypokalemia with K^+-depleting agents (eg, amphotericin B, diuretics).

S

Reports of cardiac enlargement and CHF with amphotericin B. Macrolide antibiotics may cause a significant decrease in clearance. Concomitant use with anticholinesterase agents may produce severe weakness in patients with myasthenia gravis. May inhibit response to warfarin; frequently monitor coagulation indices. May increase blood glucose levels; may require dose adjustments of antidiabetic agents. May decrease serum levels of isoniazid. Cholestyramine may increase clearance. Increased activity of both drugs may occur with cyclosporine; convulsions reported with concurrent use. May increase risk of arrhythmias with digitalis glycosides. Estrogens, including oral contraceptives may decrease hepatic metabolism and enhance effect. Drugs that induce CYP3A4 (eg, barbiturates, phenytoin, carbamazepine, rifampin) may enhance metabolism and require corticosteroid dosage increase. Drugs that inhibit CYP3A4 (eg, ketoconazole, macrolide antibiotics such as erythromycin and troleandomycin) may increase plasma levels. Ketoconazole may increase risk of corticosteroid side effects. Aspirin or other NSAIDs may increase risk of GI side effects. Administration of live or live, attenuated vaccines is contraindicated in patients receiving immunosuppressive doses. Killed or inactivated vaccines may be administered, although response is unpredictable.

PREGNANCY: Category C, not for use in nursing.

MECHANISM OF ACTION: Glucocorticoid; causes profound and varied metabolic effects and modifies the body's immune responses to diverse stimuli.

PHARMACOKINETICS: Absorption: Readily absorbed from GI tract. **Distribution:** Found in breast milk (systemically administered).

NURSING CONSIDERATIONS

Assessment: Assess for hypersensitivity to drug, traumatic brain injury, CHF, renal insufficiency, systemic fungal infections, other current infections, active TB, vaccination status, unusual stress, ulcerative colitis, diverticulitis, HTN, recent MI, intestinal anastomoses, active or latent peptic ulcer, osteoporosis, myasthenia gravis, psychotic tendencies, cerebral malaria, active ocular herpes simplex, any other conditions where treatment is contraindicated or cautioned, pregnancy/nursing status, and possible drug interactions.

Monitoring: Monitor for anaphylactoid reactions, dermal and/or subdermal changes, growth/development (in pediatric patients), intestinal perforation and hemorrhage, infections, cataracts, glaucoma, osteoporosis, psychic derangements, Kaposi's sarcoma, acute myopathy, and other adverse reactions. Monitor for HPA-axis suppression, Cushing's syndrome, and hyperglycemia with chronic use. Monitor BP, HR, ECG, glucose, TSH, LFTs, CK, serum electrolytes, and IOP. Frequently monitor coagulation indices with warfarin.

Patient Counseling: Warn not to d/c abruptly or without medical supervision. Advise to inform any medical attendants that the patient is taking corticosteroids. Instruct to seek medical advice at once if fever or other signs of infection develop. Warn to avoid exposure to chickenpox or measles; advise to report immediately if exposed.

Administration: IM/IV routes. Avoid inj into deltoid muscle. Refer to PI for preparation and administration instructions. **Storage:** 20-25°C (68-77°F). Protect from light. Discard unused sol after 3 days.

SOLU-MEDROL   RX
methylprednisolone sodium succinate (Pharmacia & Upjohn)

THERAPEUTIC CLASS: Glucocorticoid

INDICATIONS: Steroid-responsive disorders when oral therapy is not feasible.

DOSAGE: *Adults:* Individualize dose. Initial: 10-40mg IV/IM inj or IV infusion, depending on disease. High-Dose Therapy: 30mg/kg IV over at least 30 min. May be repeated q4-6h for 48 hrs. High-dose therapy should continue only until patient is stabilized, usually not beyond 48-72 hrs. Maint: Decrease initial dosage in small decrements at appropriate time intervals until the lowest dosage that maintains an adequate clinical response is reached. Acute Exacerbations of Multiple Sclerosis: 160mg qd for a week followed by 64mg qod for 1 month. D/C if a period of spontaneous remission occurs in a chronic condition. Withdraw gradually after long-term therapy. Elderly: Start at lower end of dosing range.
Pediatrics: Individualize dose. Initial: 0.11-1.6mg/kg/day in 3 or 4 divided doses (3.2-48mg/m²/day); Uncontrolled Asthma: 1-2mg/kg/day in single or divided doses. Continue short-course ("burst") therapy until patient achieves a peak expiratory flow rate of 80% of personal best, or symptoms resolve (usually 3-10 days). Dose may be reduced and should be governed by severity of condition/response; should not be <0.5mg/kg/24 hr. D/C if a period of spontaneous remission occurs in a chronic condition. Withdraw gradually after long-term therapy.

HOW SUPPLIED: Inj: 40mg, 125mg, 500mg, 1g, 2g

CONTRAINDICATIONS: Systemic fungal infections, idiopathic thrombocytopenic purpura (IM preparations), intrathecal administration. Premature infants (formulations preserved with benzyl alcohol).

WARNINGS/PRECAUTIONS: Monitor for situations which may make dosage adjustments necessary (eg, change in clinical status secondary to remissions/exacerbations in the disease process, individual drug responsiveness, effect of patient exposure to stress). Formulations with preservative contain benzyl alcohol, which is potentially toxic to neural tissue. Exposure to excessive amounts of benzyl alcohol has been associated with toxicity, particularly in neonates. May result in dermal and/or subdermal changes forming depressions in the skin at the inj site; exercise caution not to exceed recommended doses. Anaphylactoid reactions (rare) may occur. May need to increase dose before, during, and after stressful situations. Do not use for the treatment of traumatic brain injury. May cause elevation of BP, salt/water retention, and increased excretion of K^+ and Ca^{2+}; dietary salt restriction and K^+ supplementation may be necessary. Caution in patients with recent myocardial infarction (MI). Monitor for hypothalamic-pituitary-adrenal (HPA) axis suppression, Cushing's syndrome, and hyperglycemia with chronic use. May produce reversible HPA-axis suppression with the potential for glucocorticosteroid insufficiency after withdrawal of treatment. Drug-induced secondary adrenocortical insufficiency may be minimized by gradual reduction of dosage. May mask signs of current infection or cause new infections; avoid use intra-articularly, intrabursally, or for intratendinous administration for local effect in the presence of acute local infection. May exacerbate systemic fungal infections. Rule out latent or active amebiasis before initiating therapy. Caution with *Strongyloides* infestation, active or latent tuberculosis (TB), HTN, congestive heart failure (CHF), renal insufficiency, osteoporosis, and ocular herpes simplex. Caution with active or latent peptic ulcers, diverticulitis, fresh intestinal anastomoses, and nonspecific ulcerative colitis; may increase risk of perforation. Signs of peritoneal irritation following GI perforation may be minimal/absent. Acute myopathy with high doses reported, most often in patients with disorders of neuromuscular transmission (eg, myasthenia gravis). More serious/fatal course of chickenpox and measles reported. Not for use in cerebral malaria or active ocular herpes simplex. Use of oral corticosteroids not recommended in the treatment of optic neuritis. May decrease bone formation and increase bone resorption, and may lead to inhibition of bone growth in pediatric patients and development of osteoporosis at any age; caution with increased risk of osteoporosis (eg, postmenopausal women). Psychic derangements may appear and existing emotional instability or psychotic tendencies may be aggravated. May elevate intraocular pressure (IOP); monitor IOP if used for >6 weeks. Severe medical events associated with intrathecal route of administration. May produce posterior subcapsular cataracts, glaucoma with possible damage to the optic nerves, and may enhance the establishment of secondary ocular infections due to bacteria, fungi, or viruses. Kaposi's sarcoma reported. Changes in thyroid status may necessitate dose adjustment. Elevation of creatine kinase (CK) may occur. May suppress reactions to skin tests. Avoid abrupt withdrawal. Avoid inj into deltoid muscle or into a previously infected site. Caution in elderly.

ADVERSE REACTIONS: Anaphylactoid reaction, HTN, osteoporosis, muscle weakness, menstrual irregularities, insomnia, impaired wound healing, manifestations of latent diabetes mellitus, ulcerative esophagitis, increased sweating, increased intracranial pressure, decreased carbohydrate/glucose tolerance, glaucoma, posterior subcapsular cataracts.

INTERACTIONS: Aminoglutethimide may lead to a loss of corticosteroid-induced adrenal suppression. May develop hypokalemia with K^+-depleting agents (eg, amphotericin B, diuretics). Reports of cardiac enlargement and CHF following concomitant use of amphotericin B and hydrocortisone. Macrolide antibiotics may cause a significant decrease in clearance. Concomitant use with anticholinesterase agents may produce severe weakness in patients with myasthenia gravis; d/c anticholinesterase agents at least 24 hrs before initiating therapy. May inhibit response to warfarin; frequently monitor coagulation indices. May increase blood glucose levels; dosage adjustments of antidiabetic agents may be required. May decrease serum levels of isoniazid. Cholestyramine may increase clearance. Increased activity of both drugs may occur with cyclosporine; convulsions reported with concurrent use. May increase risk of arrhythmias with digitalis glycosides. Estrogens, including oral contraceptives, may decrease hepatic metabolism and enhance effect. Drugs that induce CYP3A4 (eg, barbiturates, phenytoin, carbamazepine, rifampin) may enhance metabolism and require corticosteroid dosage increase. Drugs that inhibit CYP3A4 (eg, ketoconazole, macrolide antibiotics such as erythromycin and troleandomycin) may increase plasma levels. Ketoconazole may increase risk of corticosteroid side effects. Aspirin (ASA) or other NSAIDs may increase risk of GI side effects; caution with ASA in hypoprothrombinemia patients. May increase clearance of salicylates. Administration of live or live, attenuated vaccines is contraindicated in patients receiving immunosuppressive doses. Killed or inactivated vaccines may be administered, although response is unpredictable. Acute myopathy reported with neuromuscular blocking drugs (eg, pancuronium).

PREGNANCY: Category C, not for use in nursing.

MECHANISM OF ACTION: Glucocorticoid; causes profound and varied metabolic effects and modifies the body's immune responses to diverse stimuli.

PHARMACOKINETICS: Absorption: (IM) Rapid. **Distribution:** Found in breast milk.

S

NURSING CONSIDERATIONS

Assessment: Assess for hypersensitivity to drug, traumatic brain injury, CHF, renal insufficiency, systemic fungal infections, other current infections, active TB, vaccination status, unusual stress, ulcerative colitis, diverticulitis, HTN, recent MI, intestinal anastomoses, active or latent peptic ulcer, osteoporosis, myasthenia gravis, psychotic tendencies, cerebral malaria, active ocular herpes simplex, any other conditions where treatment is contraindicated or cautioned, pregnancy/nursing status, and possible drug interactions.

Monitoring: Monitor for anaphylactoid reactions, dermal and/or subdermal changes, growth/development (in pediatric patients), intestinal perforation, infections, cataracts, glaucoma, osteoporosis, psychic derangements, Kaposi's sarcoma, acute myopathy, and other adverse reactions. Monitor for HPA-axis suppression, Cushing's syndrome, and hyperglycemia with chronic use. Monitor BP, HR, ECG, glucose, TSH, LFTs, CK, serum electrolytes, IOP. Frequently monitor coagulation indices with warfarin.

Patient Counseling: Warn not to d/c abruptly or use without medical supervision. Instruct to seek medical advice at once if fever or other signs of infection develop. Warn to avoid exposure to chickenpox or measles; advise to report immediately if exposed.

Administration: IM/IV route. Do not dilute or mix with other solution. Refer to PI for preparation and administration instructions. **Storage:** 20-25°C (68-77°F). Protect from light. Use within 48 hrs after mixing.

SOMA   RX
carisoprodol (Meda)

THERAPEUTIC CLASS: Skeletal muscle relaxant (central-acting)

INDICATIONS: Relief of discomfort associated with acute, painful musculoskeletal conditions.

DOSAGE: *Adults:* ≥16 Yrs: 250-350mg tid and hs for up to 2-3 weeks.

HOW SUPPLIED: Tab: 250mg, 350mg

CONTRAINDICATIONS: History of acute intermittent porphyria.

WARNINGS/PRECAUTIONS: May impair mental/physical abilities. Drug abuse, dependence, and withdrawal reported with prolonged use. Withdrawal symptoms reported following abrupt cessation after prolonged use. Seizures reported in postmarketing surveillance. Caution with hepatic or renal dysfunction and in addiction-prone patients. Not studied in patients >65 yrs of age.

ADVERSE REACTIONS: Drowsiness, dizziness, headache.

INTERACTIONS: Additive sedative effects with other CNS depressants (eg, alcohol, benzodiazepines, opioids, TCAs); caution when coadministering. Concomitant use with meprobamate is not recommended. Increased exposure of carisoprodol and decreased exposure of meprobamate with CYP2C19 inhibitors (eg, omeprazole, fluvoxamine). Decreased exposure of carisoprodol and increased exposure of meprobamate with CYP2C19 inducers (eg, rifampin, St. John's wort). Induction effect on CYP2C19 seen with low-dose aspirin.

PREGNANCY: Category C, caution in nursing.

MECHANISM OF ACTION: Centrally acting muscle relaxant; not established. Suspected to be associated with altered interneuronal activity in the spinal cord and the descending reticular formation of the brain. Meprobamate, a metabolite, has anxiolytic and sedative properties.

PHARMACOKINETICS: Absorption: Carisoprodol: (250mg) C_{max}=1.2mcg/mL, T_{max}=1.5 hrs, AUC=4.5mcg•hr/mL; (350mg) C_{max}=1.8mcg/mL, T_{max}=1.7 hrs, AUC=7.0mcg•hr/mL. Meprobamate: (250mg) C_{max}=1.8mcg/mL, T_{max}= 3.6 hrs, AUC=32mcg•hr/mL; (350mg) C_{max}=2.5mcg/mL, T_{max}=4.5 hrs, AUC=46mcg•hr/mL. **Distribution:** Found in breast milk. **Metabolism:** Liver via CYP2C19. Meprobamate (metabolite). **Elimination:** Renal/Nonrenal route, Carisoprodol: $T_{1/2}$=1.7 hrs (250mg), 2.0 hrs (350mg). Meprobamate: $T_{1/2}$=9.7 hrs (250mg), 9.6 hrs (350mg).

NURSING CONSIDERATIONS

Assessment: Assess for acute intermittent porphyria, renal/hepatic impairment, seizures, history of addiction, use of alcohol/illegal drugs/drugs of abuse, pregnancy/nursing status, and possible drug interactions.

Monitoring: Monitor for signs/symptoms of CNS depression, drug abuse/dependence, and seizures.

Patient Counseling: Advise that drug may cause drowsiness and/or dizziness; instruct to avoid taking carisoprodol before engaging in hazardous tasks. Instruct to avoid alcohol, illegal drugs, drugs of abuse, or other CNS depressants. Inform that drug is limited to acute use. Instruct to notify physician if musculoskeletal symptoms persist. Inform of drug dependence/abuse potential.

Administration: Oral route. **Storage:** 20-25°C (68-77°F).

SOMAVERT   RX
pegvisomant (Pharmacia & Upjohn)

THERAPEUTIC CLASS: Growth hormone receptor antagonist

INDICATIONS: Treatment of acromegaly in patients who have had an inadequate response to surgery or radiation therapy, or for whom these therapies are not appropriate.

DOSAGE: *Adults:* LD: 40mg SQ. Maint: 10mg SQ qd. Titrate: Adjust dose by 5mg increments or decrements in 4- to 6-week intervals based on serum insulin-like growth factor-I (IGF-I) concentrations. Range: 10-30mg SQ qd. Max: 30mg SQ qd. Elderly: Start at lower end of dosing range. Refer to PI for recommendations based on LFTs.

HOW SUPPLIED: Inj: 10mg, 15mg, 20mg

WARNINGS/PRECAUTIONS: May improve glucose tolerance; carefully monitor patients with diabetes mellitus (DM). Transaminase elevations reported; obtain baseline LFTs, and monitor for development of LFT elevations or any other signs/symptoms of liver dysfunction during therapy. Cross-reactivity with growth hormone (GH) assays reported. Lipohypertrophy reported; rotate inj sites daily. Exercise caution and close monitoring when reinitiating therapy in patients with systemic hypersensitivity reactions. Administer LD under physician supervision. Caution in elderly.

ADVERSE REACTIONS: Infection, abnormal LFTs, pain, inj-site reaction, chest/back pain, diarrhea, nausea, flu syndrome, dizziness, paresthesia, HTN, sinusitis, peripheral edema.

INTERACTIONS: May need to reduce dose of insulin and/or oral hypoglycemics in DM patients. Higher doses may be needed to normalize IGF-I concentrations in patients taking opioids.

PREGNANCY: Category C, caution in nursing.

MECHANISM OF ACTION: GH receptor antagonist; selectively binds to GH receptors on cell surfaces, where it blocks binding of endogenous GH, and thus interferes with GH signal transduction. Inhibition of GH action results in decreased serum IGF-I concentrations, as well as other GH-responsive serum proteins.

PHARMACOKINETICS: Absorption: Absolute bioavailability (57%); T_{max}=33-77 hrs. **Distribution:** V_d=7L. **Elimination:** Urine (<1%); $T_{1/2}$=74-172 hrs.

NURSING CONSIDERATIONS

Assessment: Assess for DM, history of drug hypersensitivity, pregnancy/nursing status, and possible drug interactions. Obtain baseline LFTs.

Monitoring: Monitor for hypoglycemia (in patients with DM), signs/symptoms of liver dysfunction, hypersensitivity reactions, and other adverse reactions. Measure serum IGF-I concentrations every 4-6 weeks. Periodically monitor LFTs.

Patient Counseling: Inform that blood testing will be needed to check IGF-I levels and LFTs before/during treatment and that the dose may be changed based on the results of these tests. Instruct to notify physician if pregnant/breastfeeding. Advise of the most common reported adverse reactions (inj-site reaction, LFT elevations, pain, nausea, diarrhea). Instruct to immediately d/c therapy and contact physician if jaundice develops. Inform that GH-secreting tumors may enlarge in people with acromegaly and that these tumors need to be watched carefully and monitored by magnetic resonance imaging. Counsel that thickening under the skin may occur at the inj site that could lead to lumps and that switching sites may prevent or lessen this. Instruct on how to properly reconstitute and administer the drug.

Administration: SQ route. Refer to PI for reconstitution and administration instructions. **Storage:** 2-8°C (36-46°F). Do not freeze. Reconstituted Sol: Administer within 6 hrs. Do not shake.

SONATA   CIV
zaleplon (Pfizer)

THERAPEUTIC CLASS: Pyrazolopyrimidine (non-benzodiazepine)

INDICATIONS: Short-term treatment of insomnia.

DOSAGE: *Adults:* Individualize dose. Take immediately before hs or after going to bed and experiencing difficulty falling asleep. Insomnia: 10mg. Low Weight Patients: 5mg. Max: 20mg. Elderly/Debilitated: 5mg. Max: 10mg. Mild to Moderate Hepatic Impairment: 5mg. Concomitant Use with Cimetidine: Initial: 5mg.

HOW SUPPLIED: Cap: 5mg, 10mg

WARNINGS/PRECAUTIONS: Initiate only after careful evaluation; failure of insomnia to remit after 7-10 days of treatment may indicate presence of a primary psychiatric and/or medical illness. Use lowest effective dose, especially in elderly. Abnormal thinking and behavior changes reported. Complex behaviors (eg, sleep-driving) reported; consider discontinuation if sleep-driving occurs. Amnesia and other neuropsychiatric symptoms may occur unpredictably. Worsening of depression, including suicidal thoughts and actions, reported in primarily depressed patients; caution with signs/symptoms of depression. Withdrawal signs/symptoms reported following rapid dose decrease or abrupt discontinuation. May impair mental/physical abilities. Severe anaphylactic and anaphylactoid reactions reported; do not rechallenge if angioedema develops. May result in short-term memory impairment, hallucinations, impaired coordination, dizziness, and lightheadedness when taken while still up and about. Caution with diseases or conditions affecting metabolism or hemodynamic responses, or with compromised respiratory function. Carefully monitor patients with compromised respiration due to preexisting illness. Not recommended for use in patients with severe hepatic impairment or in women during pregnancy. Contains tartrazine, which may cause allergic-type reactions (including bronchial asthma) in certain susceptible persons. Has an abuse potential. Monitor patients at risk of habituation and dependence (eg, history of addiction to, or abuse of, drugs or alcohol).

ADVERSE REACTIONS: Headache, dizziness, nausea, asthenia, abdominal pain, somnolence, amnesia, eye pain, dysmenorrhea, paresthesia.

INTERACTIONS: Additive CNS depression with other psychotropic medications, anticonvulsants, antihistamines, narcotic analgesics, anesthetics, ethanol, and other CNS depressants; dosage adjustment may be necessary. Do not take with alcohol. Increased risk of complex behaviors with alcohol and other CNS depressants. Decreased C_{max} with promethazine. Decreased levels with rifampin (a potent CYP3A4 inducer); coadministration of a potent CYP3A4 inducer can lead to ineffectiveness of zaleplon. May consider alternative non-CYP3A4 substrate hypnotic agent in patients taking CYP3A4 inducers (eg, phenytoin, carbamazepine, phenobarbital). Strong selective CYP3A4 inhibitors (eg, erythromycin, ketoconazole) may increase levels. Increased levels with cimetidine; give an initial dose of 5mg.

PREGNANCY: Category C, not for use in nursing.

MECHANISM OF ACTION: Pyrazolopyrimidine (non-benzodiazepine) hypnotic agent; interacts with gamma-aminobutyric acid-benzodiazepine receptor complex.

PHARMACOKINETICS: Absorption: Rapid and almost complete. Absolute bioavailability (30%); T_{max}=1 hr. **Distribution:** Plasma protein binding (60%); found in breast milk. (IV) V_d=1.4L/kg. **Metabolism:** Liver (extensive) via aldehyde oxidation (primary), CYP3A4 (lesser extent). **Elimination:** Urine (<1% unchanged, 70% within 48 hrs, 71% within 6 days), feces (17% within 6 days); $T_{1/2}$=1 hr.

NURSING CONSIDERATIONS

Assessment: Assess for physical and/or psychiatric disorders, medical illness, depression, diseases/conditions affecting metabolism or hemodynamic responses, compromised respiratory function, hepatic impairment, risk of habituation and dependence, hypersensitivity, pregnancy/nursing status, and possible drug interactions.

Monitoring: Monitor for complex behaviors, emergence of any new behavioral signs/symptoms, anaphylactic/anaphylactoid reactions, angioedema, abuse, habituation, dependence, withdrawal symptoms, and other adverse reactions. Monitor elderly and/or debilitated patients closely.

Patient Counseling: Inform of the risks and benefits of therapy. Caution against engaging in hazardous occupations requiring complete mental alertness (eg, operating machinery, driving). Instruct to immediately report to physician if any adverse reactions (eg, sleep-driving or other complex behaviors) occur. Instruct to notify physician if pregnant/nursing or planning to become pregnant. Instruct not to take with alcohol. Inform that taking the drug with or immediately after a heavy, high-fat meal results in slower absorption and may reduce the effect of the drug on sleep latency.

Administration: Oral route. **Storage:** 20-25°C (68-77°F).

SORIATANE   RX
acitretin (Stiefel)

Avoid in pregnancy and avoid becoming pregnant during therapy and for at least 3 yrs after discontinuation of therapy; use 2 reliable forms of contraception simultaneously. Females should avoid ethanol during and for 2 months after discontinuation of therapy because it may increase the duration of teratogenic potential. Only use in females of reproductive potential with severe psoriasis unresponsive to or contraindicated with other therapies. Patient must have 2 negative urine/serum pregnancy tests with a sensitivity of at least 25 mIU/mL before receiving initial prescription. Contraception counseling should be done on a regular basis. It is not known whether residual acitretin in seminal fluid poses risk to a fetus while a male patient is taking the drug or after it is discontinued. Severe birth defects reported. Interferes with contraceptive effect of microdosed progestin "minipill" oral contraceptives. Caution not to self-medicate with herbal St. John's wort, because a possible interaction has been suggested with hormonal contraceptives, based on reports of breakthrough bleeding. Potential for hepatotoxicity; elevations of AST, ALT, gamma-glutamyl transpeptidase, or lactate dehydrogenase reported. D/C if hepatotoxicity is suspected.

THERAPEUTIC CLASS: Retinoid

INDICATIONS: Treatment of severe psoriasis in adults.

DOSAGE: *Adults:* Individualize dose. Initial: 25-50mg qd as single dose with main meal. Maint: 25-50mg qd may be given dependent upon response to initial treatment. May treat relapses as outlined for initial therapy. Concomitant Phototherapy: Decrease phototherapy dose, dependent on patient's individual response. Elderly: Start at lower end of dosing range.

HOW SUPPLIED: Cap: 10mg, 17.5mg, 25mg

CONTRAINDICATIONS: Pregnancy, severely impaired liver or kidney function, chronic abnormally elevated blood lipid values. Concomitant methotrexate and tetracyclines.

WARNINGS/PRECAUTIONS: Risk of hyperostosis, pancreatitis, and pseudotumor cerebri (benign intracranial HTN). D/C and undergo ophthalmologic evaluation if visual difficulties occur. Bone abnormalities of the vertebral column, knees, and ankles reported. Increased TG and cholesterol and decreased HDL reported; perform blood lipid determinations before therapy and again at 1- to 2-week intervals until lipid response to therapy is established, usually within 4-8 weeks. Caution in patients with an increased tendency to develop hypertriglyceridemia (eg, disturbances of lipid metabolism, diabetes mellitus [DM], obesity, increased alcohol intake, or familial history of these conditions). Blood sugar control problems and new cases of diabetes, including diabetic ketoacidosis, reported; monitor blood sugar levels very carefully in diabetics. Caution in elderly. Not indicated for treatment of acne.

ADVERSE REACTIONS: Hepatotoxicity, cheilitis, alopecia, skin peeling, rhinitis, dry skin, nail disorder, pruritus, rigors, xerophthalmia, dry mouth, epistaxis, arthralgia, spinal hyperostosis, erythematous rash.

INTERACTIONS: See Boxed Warning and Contraindications. Potentiates the blood glucose-lowering effect of glyburide; careful supervision of diabetic patients is recommended. Reduced protein binding effect of phenytoin. Avoid use with vitamin A and/or other oral retinoids; may increase risk of hypervitaminosis A.

PREGNANCY: Category X, not for use in nursing.

MECHANISM OF ACTION: Retinoid; has not been established.

PHARMACOKINETICS: Absorption: (Healthy, 50mg) C_{max}=416ng/mL, T_{max}=2.7 hrs. **Distribution:** Plasma protein binding (99.9%); found in breast milk. **Metabolism:** Extensive; via isomerization to cis-acitretin; both parent compound and isomer are further metabolized into chain-shortened breakdown products and conjugates. **Elimination:** Urine (16-53%, metabolites and conjugates); feces (34-54%, metabolites and conjugates); $T_{1/2}$=49 hrs (multiple dose), 63 hrs (cis-acitretin).

NURSING CONSIDERATIONS

Assessment: Assess for DM, obesity, alcohol intake, or familial history of these conditions, cardiovascular status, preexisting abnormalities of the spine or extremities, renal/hepatic function, pregnancy/nursing status, and possible drug interactions. Perform blood lipid determinations before initiating therapy.

Monitoring: Monitor for hepatotoxicity, hyperostosis, hypertriglyceridemia, myocardial infarction or other thromboembolic events, pancreatitis, pseudotumor cerebri, visual difficulties, and other adverse reactions. Perform appropriate examinations periodically in view of possible ossification abnormalities. Monitor blood sugar levels very carefully in diabetic patients. Repeat pregnancy test every month, during therapy, and every 3 months for at least 3 yrs after discontinuation of therapy. Monitor blood lipid determinations at 1- to 2-week intervals until lipid response to the drug is established during therapy.

Patient Counseling: Inform about the Pregnancy Prevention Actively Required During and After Treatment (*Do Your P.A.R.T.*) program and the risks of therapy. Advise to notify physician if pregnant or nursing. Advise to use 2 effective forms of contraception simultaneously at least 1 month prior to initiation of therapy. Advise against donating blood during or for at least 3 yrs following completion of therapy. Counsel to d/c therapy and notify physician immediately if psychiatric symptoms develop. Instruct not to ingest beverages or products containing ethanol while taking therapy and for 2 months after discontinuation of therapy. Warn to be cautious when driving or operating a vehicle at night, and not to give the drug to any other person. Inform to use caution when taking vitamin A supplements to avoid additive toxic effects. Instruct to avoid use of sun lamps and excessive exposure to sunlight.

Administration: Oral route. **Storage:** 15-25°C (59-77°F). Protect from light. Avoid exposure to high temperatures and humidity after the bottle is opened.

SORILUX

calcipotriene (Stiefel)

RX

THERAPEUTIC CLASS: Vitamin D3 derivative

S

INDICATIONS: Treatment of plaque psoriasis of the scalp and body in adults ≥18 yrs of age.

DOSAGE: *Adults:* ≥18 Yrs: Apply a thin layer bid to the affected areas and rub in gently and completely.

HOW SUPPLIED: Foam: 0.005% [60g, 120g]

CONTRAINDICATIONS: Hypercalcemia.

WARNINGS/PRECAUTIONS: Propellant in drug is flammable; avoid fire, flame, and smoking during and immediately following application. Hypercalcemia may occur; d/c treatment until normal Ca^{2+} levels are restored if elevation outside normal range occurs. Avoid excessive exposure of treated areas to natural or artificial sunlight. Limit or avoid use of phototherapy. Use not evaluated with erythrodermic, exfoliative, or pustular psoriasis. Avoid contact with the face and eyes.

ADVERSE REACTIONS: Application-site erythema/pain.

PREGNANCY: Category C, caution in nursing.

MECHANISM OF ACTION: Vitamin D3 analog; not established.

NURSING CONSIDERATIONS

Assessment: Assess for hypercalcemia and pregnancy/nursing status.

Monitoring: Monitor serum Ca^{2+} levels and for development of application-site erythema and/or pain.

Patient Counseling: Advise not to refrigerate or freeze the product. Instruct to avoid fire, flame, and smoking during and immediately following application and excessive exposure of the treated areas to natural or artificial sunlight (eg, tanning beds, sun lamps). If the foam gets on the face or in or near the eyes, advise to rinse thoroughly with water. Instruct to consult physician if there are no improvements after 8 weeks of treatment. Counsel to wash hands after application, unless treating the hands. Instruct to apply foam to the scalp when hair is dry.

Administration: Topical route. Not for PO, ophthalmic, or intravaginal use. **Storage:** 20-25°C (68-77°F); excursions permitted to 15-30°C (59-86°F). Do not puncture or incinerate. Do not expose to heat or to temperatures >49°C (120°F).

SOVALDI   RX
sofosbuvir (Gilead)

THERAPEUTIC CLASS: Nucleotide analogue inhibitor

INDICATIONS: Treatment of chronic hepatitis C infection as a component of a combination antiviral treatment regimen in patients with hepatitis C virus (HCV) genotype 1, 2, 3, or 4 infection, including those with hepatocellular carcinoma meeting Milan criteria (awaiting liver transplantation) and those with HCV/HIV-1 coinfection.

DOSAGE: *Adults:* Usual: 400mg qd. Genotype 1 or 4: Treat with sofosbuvir in combination with peginterferon alfa and ribavirin for 12 weeks; may consider sofosbuvir in combination with ribavirin for 24 weeks in patients with genotype 1 infection who are ineligible to receive an interferon-based regimen. Genotype 2: Treat with sofosbuvir in combination with ribavirin for 12 weeks. Genotype 3: Treat with sofosbuvir in combination with ribavirin for 24 weeks. Hepatocellular Carcinoma Awaiting Liver Transplantation: Treat with sofosbuvir in combination with ribavirin for up to 48 weeks or until time of transplant, whichever occurs 1st. Refer to PI for dose modification and discontinuation.

HOW SUPPLIED: Tab: 400mg

CONTRAINDICATIONS: Women who are pregnant or may become pregnant and men whose female partners are pregnant. Refer to the individual monographs for peginterferon alfa and ribavirin.

WARNINGS/PRECAUTIONS: Women of childbearing potential and their male partners must use 2 forms of effective contraception during treatment and for at least 6 months after discontinuation; perform routine monthly pregnancy tests during this time. Use 2 nonhormonal methods of contraception during treatment with concomitant ribavirin.

ADVERSE REACTIONS: Fatigue, headache, nausea, insomnia, anemia, pruritus, asthenia, rash, decreased appetite, chills, influenza-like illness, pyrexia, diarrhea, myalgia, irritability.

INTERACTIONS: Potent P-glycoprotein (P-gp) inducers in the intestine (eg, rifampin, St. John's wort) may significantly decrease concentrations and may lead to a reduced therapeutic effect; do not use with rifampin and St. John's wort. P-gp and/or breast cancer resistance protein inhibitors may increase concentration. Carbamazepine, phenytoin, phenobarbital, oxcarbazepine, rifabutin, rifapentine, and tipranavir/ritonavir may decrease concentrations, leading to reduced therapeutic effects; coadministration is not recommended.

PREGNANCY: Category B, Category X (with ribavirin or peginterferon alfa/ribavirin); not for use in nursing.

MECHANISM OF ACTION: Nucleotide analogue inhibitor; inhibits HCV NS5B RNA-dependent RNA polymerase, which is essential for viral replication.

PHARMACOKINETICS: Absorption: T_{max}=0.5-2 hrs, 2-4 hrs (GS-331007); (with ribavirin) AUC=828ng•hr/mL, 6790ng•hr/mL (GS-331007). **Distribution:** Plasma protein binding (61-65%). **Metabolism:** Liver (extensive) to GS-461203 (active); dephosphorylation to GS-331007 (major). **Elimination:** Urine (80%, 3.5% unchanged), feces (14%), expired air (2.5%); $T_{1/2}$ (median)=0.4 hr, 27 hrs (GS-331007).

NURSING CONSIDERATIONS

Assessment: Assess for pregnancy/nursing status and possible drug interactions.

Monitoring: Monitor for adverse reactions. Perform routine monthly pregnancy tests.

Patient Counseling: Advise women of childbearing potential and their male partners to use at least 2 forms of effective contraception (2 alternative nonhormonal methods) during therapy and for at least 6 months after treatment discontinuation. Instruct to notify physician immediately in the event of a pregnancy. Encourage patients who are HCV/HIV-1 coinfected and taking concomitant antiretrovirals to register in the Antiretroviral Pregnancy Registry. Inform that the effect of treatment of hepatitis C on transmission is unknown and that appropriate precautions to prevent HCV transmission during treatment or in the event of treatment failure should be taken. Advise to take ud, and not to reduce dose. Advise to take drug on a regular dosing schedule.

Administration: Oral route. Take with or without food. **Storage:** Room temperature <30°C (86°F).

SPIRIVA   RX
tiotropium bromide (Boehringer Ingelheim)

THERAPEUTIC CLASS: Anticholinergic bronchodilator

INDICATIONS: Long-term qd maint treatment of bronchospasm associated with chronic obstructive pulmonary disease (COPD), including chronic bronchitis and emphysema. Reduction of exacerbations in COPD patients.

DOSAGE: *Adults:* 2 inhalations of the powder contents of 1 cap (18mcg) qd with HandiHaler device.

HOW SUPPLIED: Cap, Inhalation: 18mcg

WARNINGS/PRECAUTIONS: Not for initial treatment of acute episodes of bronchospasm (eg, rescue therapy). D/C and consider alternative treatments if immediate hypersensitivity reactions (eg, angioedema, itching, rash) or paradoxical bronchospasm occurs. Caution with hypersensitivity to milk proteins or to atropine. Caution with narrow-angle glaucoma; observe for signs and symptoms of acute narrow-angle glaucoma. Caution with urinary retention; observe for signs and symptoms of prostatic hyperplasia or bladder-neck obstruction (eg, difficulty passing urine, painful urination). Monitor for anticholinergic effects in patients with moderate to severe renal impairment (CrCl ≤50mL/min).

ADVERSE REACTIONS: Dry mouth, sinusitis, constipation, abdominal pain, urinary tract infection, upper respiratory tract infection, chest pain, edema, vomiting, myalgia, moniliasis, rash, dyspepsia, pharyngitis, rhinitis.

INTERACTIONS: Avoid with other anticholinergic-containing drugs; may lead to an increase in anticholinergic adverse effects.

PREGNANCY: Category C, caution in nursing.

MECHANISM OF ACTION: Anticholinergic bronchodilator; inhibits M_3-receptors on smooth muscle leading to bronchodilation.

PHARMACOKINETICS: Absorption: Absolute bioavailability (19.5%); T_{max}=5 min. **Distribution:** V_d=32L/kg; plasma protein binding (72%). **Metabolism:** Liver (oxidation, conjugation) via CYP2D6, 3A4. **Elimination:** Urine (14%, inhalation), feces. $T_{1/2}$=5-6 days.

NURSING CONSIDERATIONS

Assessment: Assess for hypersensitivity to atropine or its derivatives, narrow-angle glaucoma, urinary retention, renal impairment, pregnancy/nursing status, and possible drug interactions.

Monitoring: Monitor for signs and symptoms of prostatic hyperplasia or bladder neck obstruction, worsening narrow-angle glaucoma, paradoxical bronchospasm, and hypersensitivity reactions.

Patient Counseling: Inform that contents of cap are for oral inhalation only and must not be swallowed. Advise to administer only via the HandiHaler device and that the device should not be used for other medications. Advise not to use as a rescue medication for immediate relief of breathing problems. Advise to seek medical attention if acute eye pain/discomfort, blurring of vision, visual halos or colored images, difficulty in passing urine or dysuria develop. Advise to use

S

caution when engaging in activities such as driving a vehicle or operating appliances/machinery. Inform that paradoxical bronchospasm may occur; d/c if this develops. Instruct not to allow the powder to enter into the eyes.

Administration: Oral inhalation route. Do not swallow caps. Use with HandiHaler device only. Refer to PI for illustrative and detailed administration procedures. **Storage:** 25°C (77°F); excursions permitted to 15-30°C (59-86°F). Do not expose to extreme temperatures or moisture. Do not store caps in the HandiHaler device.

SPORANOX RX
itraconazole (Janssen/Ortho Biotech)

Contraindicated with cisapride, oral midazolam, nisoldipine, felodipine, pimozide, quinidine, dofetilide, triazolam, levacetylmethadol (levomethadyl), lovastatin, simvastatin, ergot alkaloids (eg, dihydroergotamine, ergometrine [ergonovine], ergotamine, methylergometrine [methylergonovine]), or methadone. May increase plasma concentrations of drugs metabolized by potent CYP3A4 inhibitor pathway. Serious cardiovascular events (eg, QT prolongation, torsades de pointes, ventricular tachycardia, cardiac arrest, and/or sudden death) reported with cisapride, pimozide, methadone, levacetylmethadol, or quinidine. Reassess or d/c use if signs/symptoms of congestive heart failure (CHF) occur. (Cap) Do not use cap for onychomycosis with ventricular dysfunction (eg, CHF or history of CHF).

THERAPEUTIC CLASS: Azole antifungal

INDICATIONS: (Cap) Onychomycosis of the toenail and fingernail in nonimmunocompromised patients. Treatment of blastomycosis (pulmonary/extrapulmonary), and histoplasmosis (eg, chronic cavitary pulmonary disease and disseminated, nonmeningeal), and aspergillosis (pulmonary/extrapulmonary) if refractory to or intolerant of amphotericin B therapy. (Sol) Treatment of oropharyngeal and esophageal candidiasis.

DOSAGE: *Adults:* Cap: Take with full meal. If patient has achlorhydria or is taking gastric acid suppressors, give with cola beverage. Aspergillosis: 200-400mg/day. Blastomycosis/Histoplasmosis: 200mg qd. May increase in 100-mg increments if no improvement or if with evidence of progressive fungal disease. Max: 400mg/day. Give bid if dose >200mg/day. Life-Threatening Situations: LD: 200mg tid for first 3 days. Continue for minimum of 3 months and until infection subsides. Onychomycosis: Toenails: 200mg qd for 12 consecutive weeks. Fingernails: 200mg bid for 1 week, skip 3 weeks, then repeat. Sol: Take without food. Swish 10mL at a time for several seconds, then swallow. Candidiasis: Oropharyngeal: 200mg/day (20mL) for 1-2 weeks. If unresponsive/refractory to fluconazole tab, give 100mg (10mL) bid. Esophageal: 100mg/day (10mL) for minimum of 3 weeks. Continue for 2 weeks following resolution of symptoms. Max: 200mg/day (20mL) based on patient's response to therapy.

HOW SUPPLIED: Cap: 100mg [Pulsepak, 7 x 4 caps]; Sol: 10mg/mL [150mL]

CONTRAINDICATIONS: Concomitant use with cisapride, oral midazolam, nisoldipine, felodipine, pimozide, quinidine, dofetilide, triazolam, methadone, levacetylmethadol (levomethadyl), and HMG CoA-reductase inhibitors (eg, lovastatin, simvastatin) and ergot alkaloids (eg, dihydroergotamine, ergometrine, ergotamine, methylergometrine) metabolized by CYP3A4 . Evidence of ventricular dysfunction (eg, CHF/history of CHF) except for treatment of life-threatening or other serious infections. (Cap) Treatment of onychomycosis in pregnant patients or those contemplating pregnancy.

WARNINGS/PRECAUTIONS: Sol and caps should not be used interchangeably. Rare cases of hepatotoxicity reported. D/C if clinical signs/symptoms that are consistent with liver disease develop; perform LFTs. Use with elevated/abnormal liver enzymes, active liver disease, or in patients who experienced liver toxicity with other drugs is strongly discouraged. Caution with ischemic/valvular disease, pulmonary disease (eg, chronic obstructive pulmonary disease), renal/hepatic impairment, and other edematous disorders. CHF, peripheral edema, and pulmonary edema reported in patients treated for onychomycosis and/or systemic fungal infections. D/C if neuropathy occurs. Transient/permanent hearing loss reported that usually resolves upon discontinuation but can persist in some patients. Caution in elderly patients or when prescribed in patients with hypersensitivity to other azoles. (Sol) Consider alternative therapy if unresponsive in patients with cystic fibrosis. Not recommended for initiation of treatment in patients at immediate risk of systemic candidiasis.

ADVERSE REACTIONS: N/V, diarrhea, abdominal pain, chest pain, fever, cough, rash, dyspnea, increased sweating, headache, edema, myalgia, HTN, hepatic dysfunction, dyspepsia.

INTERACTIONS: See Boxed Warning and Contraindications. Not recommended with isoniazid, rifabutin, rifampin, and nevirapine. May increase levels of digoxin, disopyramide, coumarin-like drugs (eg, warfarin), carbamazepine, busulfan, docetaxel, vinca alkaloids, alprazolam, diazepam, calcium channel blockers (CCBs) (eg, dihydropyridines, verapamil), atorvastatin, cerivastatin, cyclosporine, tacrolimus, sirolimus, oral hypoglycemics, protease inhibitors (eg, indinavir, ritonavir, saquinavir), halofantrine, alfentanil, buspirone, certain glucocorticosteroids (eg, budesonide, dexamethasone, fluticasone, methylprednisolone), trimetrexate, cilostazol, eletriptan, and drugs metabolized by CYP3A4. Carbamazepine, phenobarbital, phenytoin, gastric acid suppressors/

neutralizers (eg, antacids, H$_2$-receptor antagonists, proton pump inhibitors), and CYP3A4 inducers may decrease levels. Erythromycin, clarithromycin, indinavir, ritonavir, and other CYP3A4 inhibitors may increase levels. Edema reported with dihydropyridine CCBs; adjust dose. Prolonged QT interval may occur with halofantrine. Fatal respiratory depression reported with fentanyl. May increase concentration of ergot alkaloids, causing ergotism. May reduce or inhibit the activity of polyenes (eg, amphotericin B). (Cap) Antacids or gastric secretion suppressors may impair absorption; administer antacid 1 hr before or 2 hrs after.

PREGNANCY: Category C, not for use in nursing.

MECHANISM OF ACTION: Azole antifungal agent; inhibits the CYP450-dependent synthesis of ergosterol, which is a vital component of fungal cell membranes.

PHARMACOKINETICS: Absorption: Absolute bioavailabilty (55%). PO administration of variable doses resulted in different parameters; refer to respective PIs for further details. **Metabolism:** Liver via CYP3A4; hydroxyitraconazole (major metabolite). **Distribution:** Plasma protein binding (99.8%, itraconazole), (99.5%, hydroxyitraconazole); found in breast milk. (IV) V$_d$=796L. **Elimination:** Urine (<0.03% parent drug, 40% inactive metabolites), feces (3-18%).

NURSING CONSIDERATIONS

Assessment: Assess for hypersensitivity to the drug or its excipients, proper diagnosis of fungal infection (eg, cultures, microscopic studies), ventricular dysfunction, ischemic/valvular disease, pulmonary disease, renal failure, hepatic impairment, edematous disorders, or any other conditions where treatment is cautioned or contraindicated. Assess pregnancy/nursing status and possible drug interactions.

Monitoring: Monitor for signs/symptoms of CHF, peripheral/pulmonary edema, hepatotoxicity, neuropathy, transient/permanent hearing loss, and other adverse reactions. Perform LFTs. Blood glucose concentrations should also be monitored when coadminstered with hypoglycemic agents. Monitor for prolongation of sedative effect if administered with parenteral midazolam.

Patient Counseling: Instruct to take cap with a full meal and oral sol in fasted state. Instruct not to interchange caps and oral sol. Counsel on signs/symptoms of CHF and liver dysfunction. Instruct to contact physician before taking any concomitant medications with the drug. Instruct to d/c therapy and inform physicians if hearing loss occurs. (Cap) Advise to avoid pregnancy while on medication and remain on contraceptives for 2 months following completion of therapy.

Administration: Oral route. **Storage:** (Cap): 15-25°C (59-77°F). Protect from light and moisture. (Sol): ≤25°C (77°F). Do not freeze.

SPRYCEL   RX
dasatinib (Bristol-Myers Squibb)

THERAPEUTIC CLASS: Kinase inhibitor

INDICATIONS: Treatment of adults with newly diagnosed Philadelphia chromosome-positive (Ph+) chronic myeloid leukemia (CML) in chronic phase. Treatment of adults with chronic, accelerated, or myeloid or lymphoid blast phase Ph+ CML with resistance or intolerance to prior therapy, including imatinib. Treatment of adults with Ph+ acute lymphoblastic leukemia (ALL) with resistance or intolerance to prior therapy.

DOSAGE: *Adults:* Chronic Phase CML: Initial: 100mg qd. Titrate: If no response, increase to 140mg qd. Accelerated Phase CML/Myeloid or Lymphoid Blast Phase CML/Ph+ ALL: Initial: 140mg qd. Titrate: If no response, increase to 180mg qd. Concomitant Strong CYP3A4 Inducers: Avoid use. If use is necessary, consider dose increase of dasatinib with careful monitoring for toxicity. Concomitant Strong CYP3A4 Inhibitors: Avoid use. If use is necessary, consider dose decrease of dasatinib to 20mg if taking 100mg qd, and to 40mg if taking 140mg qd, with careful monitoring for toxicity. If therapy is not tolerated after dose reduction, either d/c concomitant inhibitor and allow 1-week washout period before increasing dasatinib dose, or d/c dasatinib until end of treatment with inhibitor. Refer to PI for dose adjustment for adverse reactions.

HOW SUPPLIED: Tab: 20mg, 50mg, 70mg, 80mg, 100mg, 140mg

WARNINGS/PRECAUTIONS: Severe thrombocytopenia, neutropenia, and anemia reported; monitor CBCs weekly for first 2 months and monthly thereafter, or as clinically indicated. Manage myelosuppression by temporarily withholding therapy or by dose reduction. Severe CNS and GI hemorrhage, including fatalities and other cases of severe hemorrhage, reported. Severe fluid retention, ascites, pulmonary edema, and generalized edema reported; perform chest x-ray if symptoms suggestive of pleural effusion develop (eg, dyspnea, dry cough). QT prolongation reported; correct hypokalemia or hypomagnesemia prior to therapy. Cardiac adverse reactions reported; monitor for signs/symptoms consistent with cardiac dysfunction and treat appropriately. May increase risk of developing pulmonary arterial HTN (PAH); d/c permanently if PAH is confirmed. May cause fetal harm. Caution with hepatic impairment.

ADVERSE REACTIONS: Myelosuppression, fluid retention, diarrhea, N/V, headache, musculoskeletal pain, abdominal pain, hemorrhage, pneumonia, pyrexia, pleural effusion, dyspnea, skin rash, fatigue, myalgia.

INTERACTIONS: See Dosage. CYP3A4 inhibitors (eg, ketoconazole, clarithromycin, ritonavir) and grapefruit juice may increase levels. CYP3A4 inducers (eg, dexamethasone, phenytoin, carbamazepine) and St. John's wort may decrease levels. Avoid with antacids (eg, aluminum hydroxide/magnesium hydroxide); if use is necessary, administer antacid dose at least 2 hrs prior to or after dasatinib dose. H_2 antagonists (eg, famotidine) or proton pump inhibitors (eg, omeprazole) may reduce exposure; concomitant use is not recommended. May increase levels of simvastatin (a CYP3A4 substrate); caution with CYP3A4 substrates with narrow therapeutic index (eg, alfentanil, astemizole, ergotamine). Caution with anticoagulants or medications that inhibit platelet function. Antiarrhythmics or other QT-prolonging agents, and cumulative high-dose anthracycline therapy may increase risk of QT prolongation.

PREGNANCY: Category D, not for use in nursing.

MECHANISM OF ACTION: Kinase inhibitor; inhibits BCR-ABL, SRC family, c-KIT, EPHA2, and PDGFRβ kinases.

PHARMACOKINETICS: Absorption: T_{max}=0.5-6 hrs. **Distribution:** V_d=2505L; plasma protein binding (96% [parent], 93% [active metabolite]); crosses placenta. **Metabolism:** Extensive, primarily via CYP3A4. **Elimination:** Feces (85%, 19% unchanged), urine (4%, 0.1% unchanged); $T_{1/2}$=3-5 hrs.

NURSING CONSIDERATIONS

Assessment: Assess for signs/symptoms of underlying cardiopulmonary disease, hepatic impairment, presence or risk of QT prolongation, hypokalemia, hypomagnesemia, pregnancy/nursing status, and possible drug interactions.

Monitoring: Monitor for hemorrhage, cardiac dysfunction, myelosuppression, pleural effusion, fluid retention, QT prolongation, PAH, and other adverse reactions. Perform chest x-ray if symptoms of pleural effusion develop. Monitor CBCs weekly for first 2 months and monthly thereafter.

Patient Counseling: Inform of pregnancy risks; advise to avoid becoming pregnant during therapy and to contact physician if patient becomes pregnant, or if pregnancy is suspected. Instruct to seek medical attention if symptoms of hemorrhage, myelosuppression, fluid retention, significant N/V, diarrhea, headache, musculoskeletal pain, fatigue, or rash develop. Inform that product contains lactose.

Administration: Oral route. Swallow tab whole; do not crush or cut. Take with or without a meal, either in am or pm. **Storage:** 20-25°C (68-77°F); excursions permitted between 15-30°C (59-86°F).

STALEVO   RX
entacapone - levodopa - carbidopa (Novartis)

THERAPEUTIC CLASS: COMT inhibitor/dopa-decarboxylase inhibitor/dopamine precursor

INDICATIONS: Treatment of idiopathic Parkinson's disease; to substitute for equivalent doses of carbidopa/levodopa and entacapone previously administered as individual products, or to replace carbidopa/levodopa (without entacapone) for those experiencing signs and symptoms of end-of-dose "wearing off" (only for those taking ≤600mg/day levodopa without dyskinesias).

DOSAGE: *Adults:* ≤75 Yrs: Individualize dose. Titrate: Adjust according to desired therapeutic response. Currently Taking Carbidopa/Levodopa and Entacapone: May switch directly to corresponding strength of Stalevo with same amounts of carbidopa/levodopa. Currently Taking Carbidopa/Levodopa without Entacapone: Titrate individually with carbidopa/levodopa and entacapone, then transfer to corresponding dose once stabilized. Maint: Less Levodopa Required: Decrease strength of Stalevo at each administration or decrease frequency by extending time between doses. More Levodopa Required: Take next higher strength of Stalevo and/or increase frequency of doses. Max: 8 tabs/day (Stalevo 50, 75, 100, 125, 150); 6 tabs/day (Stalevo 200). Refer to PI for further dosing information when used concomitantly with other antiparkinsonian medications or general anesthesia.

HOW SUPPLIED: Tab: (Carbidopa-Levodopa-Entacapone): Stalevo 50: 12.5mg-50mg-200mg; Stalevo 75: 18.75mg-75mg-200mg; Stalevo 100: 25mg-100mg-200mg; Stalevo 125: 31.25mg-125mg-200mg; Stalevo 150: 37.5mg-150mg-200mg; Stalevo 200: 50mg-200mg-200mg

CONTRAINDICATIONS: Narrow-angle glaucoma; suspicious, undiagnosed skin lesions; history of melanoma. Nonselective MAOIs (eg, phenelzine, tranylcypromine); d/c nonselective MAOIs at least 2 weeks prior to therapy.

WARNINGS/PRECAUTIONS: CNS adverse effects may occur; may require dose reduction if dyskinesia or exacerbation of preexisting dyskinesia develop. Mental disturbances may occur; monitor for depression and suicidal tendencies. Caution with biliary obstruction, severe cardiovascular (CV)/pulmonary disease, bronchial asthma, renal/hepatic/endocrine disease, past or current psychoses, history of myocardial infarction with residual arrhythmias, and chronic wide-angle glaucoma. Caution with history of peptic ulcer; may increase the risk of upper GI hemorrhage. Symptom complex resembling neuroleptic malignant syndrome (NMS) reported in association with dose reduction or withdrawal; observe carefully if dose is reduced abruptly or discontinued, especially if receiving neuroleptics. Syncope, hypotension, hallucinations, rhabdomyolysis, hyperpyrexia, confusion, and fibrotic complications reported. Diarrhea and colitis reported with entacapone use; d/c if prolonged diarrhea develops and institute appropriate therapy. Melanomas may develop; perform periodic skin examination. Abnormalities in lab tests, including elevated LFTs, decreased BUN, creatinine and uric acid levels, positive Coombs test, false-positive reaction for urinary ketone bodies or false-negative glucose oxidase test may occur. Caution when interpreting plasma and urine levels of catecholamines and metabolites; falsely diagnosed pheochromocytoma reported. May decrease serum iron concentrations. May depress prolactin secretion and increase growth hormone levels.

ADVERSE REACTIONS: Dyskinesia, N/V, hyperkinesia, diarrhea, urine discoloration, hypokinesia, dizziness, abdominal pain, constipation, fatigue, back pain, dry mouth, dyspnea.

INTERACTIONS: See Contraindications. May result in increased HR, arrhythmias, and BP changes with drugs metabolized by catechol-O-methyltransferase (COMT) (eg, epinephrine, dopamine, α-methyldopa, isoetherine). Caution with drugs known to interfere with biliary excretion, glucuronidation, and intestinal β-glucuronidase (eg, probenecid, cholestyramine, erythromycin, ampicillin). Symptomatic postural hypotension reported when added with antihypertensives. Concomitant therapy with selegiline may be associated with severe orthostatic hypotension. HTN and dyskinesia may occur with TCAs. Reduced bioavailability with iron salts. Levodopa: Therapeutic response may be reversed by phenytoin and papaverine. Isoniazid and dopamine D_2 antagonists (eg, phenothiazines, butyrophenones, risperidone) may reduce therapeutic effects. Metoclopramide may increase the bioavailability and may also adversely affect disease control by its dopamine receptor antagonistic properties.

PREGNANCY: Category C, caution in nursing.

MECHANISM OF ACTION: Dopa-decarboxylase inhibitor/dopamine precursor/COMT inhibitor. Carbidopa: Inhibits the decarboxylation of peripheral levodopa, making more levodopa available for transport to the brain. Levodopa: Crosses blood-brain barrier and presumably converts to dopamine in brain. Entacapone: Sustains plasma levels of levodopa, resulting in more constant dopaminergic stimulation in brain.

PHARMACOKINETICS: Absorption: Levodopa: Rapid. (PO) Administration of variable doses resulted in different parameters. Entacapone: Rapid. C_{max}=1200-1500ng/mL; T_{max}=0.8-1.2 hrs; AUC=1250-1750ng•hr/mL. Carbidopa: Slower; C_{max}=40-225ng/mL; T_{max}=2.5-3.4 hrs; AUC=170-1200ng•hr/mL. **Distribution:** Plasma protein binding: Levodopa: (10-30%); Entacapone: (98%); Carbidopa: (36%). Levodopa: Crosses the placenta. **Metabolism:** Levodopa: Extensive decarboxylation by dopa decarboxylase and O-methylation by COMT. Entacapone: Isomerization; cis-isomer (active metabolite). Carbidopa: α-methyl-3-methoxy-4-hydroxyphenylpropionic acid, α-methyl-3,4-dihydroxyphenylpropionic acid (metabolites). **Elimination:** Levodopa: $T_{1/2}$=1.7 hrs. Entacapone: Feces (90%), urine (10%, 0.2% unchanged); $T_{1/2}$=0.8-1 hr. Carbidopa: Urine (30%, unchanged); $T_{1/2}$=1.6-2 hrs.

NURSING CONSIDERATIONS

Assessment: Assess for narrow-angle or chronic wide-angle glaucoma, preexisting dyskinesia, or any other conditions where treatment is contraindicated or cautioned. Assess for pregnancy/nursing status and possible drug interactions. Obtain intraocular pressure (IOP) in patients with chronic wide-angle glaucoma. Assess renal/hepatic function.

Monitoring: Monitor hematopoietic, CV/renal/hepatic function, and uric acid levels. Perform skin examination periodically. Monitor for signs/symptoms of mental disturbances, depression, suicidal tendencies, new/exacerbation of dyskinesia, NMS, rhabdomyolysis, diarrhea, colitis, upper GI hemorrhage, syncope, hypotension, melanomas, hallucinations, fibrotic complications, confusion, and hyperpyrexia. Monitor IOP in chronic wide-angle glaucoma.

Patient Counseling: Advise to take as prescribed. Inform that drug begins to release ingredients within 30 min after ingestion. Instruct to take at regular intervals, not to change dose regimen, and not to add any additional antiparkinsonian medications, including other carbidopa-levodopa preparations. Advise that "wearing-off" effect may occur at end of dosing interval; notify physician for possible treatment adjustments. Inform that discoloration of saliva, urine, or sweat may occur after ingestion. Counsel that high-protein diet, excessive acidity, and iron salts may reduce clinical effectiveness. Inform that hallucinations, postural hypotension, dizziness, nausea, syncope, sweating, diarrhea, and an increase in dyskinesia may occur. Take caution against rising rapidly after sitting or lying down, especially if in such position for prolonged periods. Instruct to avoid operating machinery/driving until sufficient experience is gained on therapy. Advise to take caution when taking other CNS depressants due to its additive sedative effects. Instruct to notify physician if pregnant, intend to become pregnant, or breastfeeding. Instruct to inform physician if new or increased gambling, sexual, or other intense urges develop.

Administration: Oral route. Do not fractionate tab. Administer only 1 tab at each dosing interval.
Storage: 25°C (77°F); excursions permitted to 15-30°C (59-86°F).

STARLIX   RX
nateglinide (Novartis)

THERAPEUTIC CLASS: Meglitinide

INDICATIONS: Adjunct to diet and exercise to improve glycemic control in adults with type 2 diabetes mellitus (DM).

DOSAGE: *Adults:* Monotherapy/Combination with Metformin or a Thiazolidinedione: Initial/Maint: 120mg tid, 1-30 min ac. May use 60mg dose tid in patients near goal HbA1c when treatment is initiated.

HOW SUPPLIED: Tab: 60mg, 120mg

CONTRAINDICATIONS: Type 1 DM, diabetic ketoacidosis.

WARNINGS/PRECAUTIONS: Risk of hypoglycemia increased with strenuous exercise, adrenal/pituitary insufficiency, severe renal impairment, and in elderly/malnourished patients. Autonomic neuropathy may mask hypoglycemia. Caution in moderate to severe hepatic impairment. Transient loss of glucose control may occur with fever, infection, trauma, or surgery; may need insulin therapy instead of nateglinide. Secondary failure (reduced effectiveness over a period of time) may occur.

ADVERSE REACTIONS: Upper respiratory infection (URI), flu symptoms, dizziness, arthropathy, diarrhea, hypoglycemia, back pain, jaundice, cholestatic hepatitis, elevated liver enzymes.

INTERACTIONS: Alcohol, NSAIDs, salicylates, MAOIs, nonselective β-blockers, guanethidine, and CYP2C9 inhibitors (eg, fluconazole, amiodarone, miconazole, oxandrolone) may potentiate hypoglycemia. Thiazides, corticosteroids, thyroid products, sympathomimetics, somatropin, rifampin, phenytoin, and dietary supplements (St. John's wort) may reduce hypoglycemic action of drug. Somatostatin analogues may potentiate/attenuate hypoglycemia. Reduced levels reported with liquid meals. β-blockers may mask hypoglycemic effects. Caution with highly protein-bound drugs.

PREGNANCY: Category C, not for use in nursing.

MECHANISM OF ACTION: Meglitinide; lowers blood glucose levels by stimulating insulin secretion from the pancreas.

PHARMACOKINETICS: Absorption: Rapidly absorbed. Absolute bioavailability (73%); T_{max}=1 hr. **Distribution:** V_d=10L (IV); plasma protein binding (98%). **Metabolism:** CYP2C9, 3A4; hydroxylation, glucuronide conjugation. **Elimination:** Urine (75%), feces; $T_{1/2}$=1.5 hrs.

NURSING CONSIDERATIONS

Assessment: Assess for diabetic ketoacidosis, type 1 DM, renal/hepatic impairment, adrenal/pituitary insufficiency, pregnancy/nursing status, other conditions where treatment is cautioned, and possible drug interactions. Assess FPG and HbA1c.

Monitoring: Monitor for hypo/hyperglycemia, diabetic ketoacidosis, secondary failure, URI, and other adverse reactions. Monitor FPG, HbA1c, renal function, and LFTs.

Patient Counseling: Inform of potential risks, benefits, alternate modes of therapy, and drug interactions. Instruct to take 1-30 min ac, but to skip scheduled dose if meal is skipped. Inform about importance of adherence to meal planning, regular physical activity, regular blood glucose monitoring, periodic HbA1c testing, recognition and management of hypo/hyperglycemia, and periodic assessment for diabetes complications. Advise to notify physician if any adverse events occur.

Administration: Oral route. **Storage:** 25°C (77°F); excursions permitted to 15-30°C (59-86°F).

STAVZOR

valproic acid (Noven)

Fatal hepatic failure reported, usually during first 6 months of treatment. Serious/fatal hepatotoxicity may be preceded by nonspecific symptoms (eg, malaise, weakness, lethargy, facial edema, anorexia, and vomiting) or loss of seizure control in patients with epilepsy; monitor closely. Monitor LFTs prior to therapy, and at frequent intervals thereafter, especially during first 6 months of treatment. Increased risk of developing fatal hepatotoxicity in children <2 yrs of age, especially if on multiple anticonvulsants, with congenital metabolic disorders, severe seizure disorders with mental retardation, and organic brain disease; use with extreme caution and as a sole agent. Increased risk of drug-induced acute liver failure and resultant deaths in patients with hereditary neurometabolic syndromes caused by DNA mutations of the mitochondrial DNA polymerase gamma (POLG) gene (eg, Alpers Huttenlocher syndrome). Contraindicated in patients known to have mitochondrial disorders caused by POLG mutations and children <2 yrs of age who are clinically suspected of having a mitochondrial disorder. In patients >2 yrs of age who are clinically suspected of having a hereditary mitochondrial disease, drug should only be used after other anticonvulsants have failed; closely monitor for the development of acute liver injury with regular clinical assessments and serum liver testing. May cause major congenital malformations, particularly neural tube defects (eg, spina bifida). May cause decreased IQ scores following in utero exposure. Contraindicated in pregnant women treated for prophylaxis of migraine; should only be used to treat pregnant women with epilepsy or bipolar disorder if other medications have failed to control their symptoms or are otherwise unacceptable. Do not administer to a woman of childbearing potential unless the drug is essential to the management of her medical condition; use effective contraception. Life-threatening pancreatitis reported; d/c if pancreatitis diagnosed and initiate appropriate treatment.

THERAPEUTIC CLASS: Carboxylic acid derivative

INDICATIONS: Treatment of manic episodes associated with bipolar disorder. In adults and children ≥10 yrs of age, monotherapy and adjunctive treatment of complex partial seizures that occur either in isolation or in association with other types of seizures. Sole and adjunctive therapy in treatment of simple/complex absence seizures, and adjunct for multiple seizure types that include absence seizures. Migraine headache prophylaxis.

DOSAGE: *Adults:* Mania: Initial: 750mg/day in divided doses. Titrate: Increase dose as rapidly as possible to achieve the lowest therapeutic dose that produces desired clinical effect or the desired range of plasma concentrations. Max: 60mg/kg/day. Complex Partial Seizures: Monotherapy/Conversion to Monotherapy/Adjunctive Therapy: Initial: 10-15mg/kg/day. Titrate: Increase by 5-10mg/kg/week until optimal response is achieved. Max: 60mg/kg/day. For adjunctive therapy, if total dose exceeds 250mg/day, give in 2-3 doses. When converting to monotherapy, reduce concomitant antiepilepsy drug by approximately 25% every 2 weeks, starting at initiation or delay by 1-2 weeks after start of therapy if there is concern that seizures are likely to occur with a reduction. Simple/Complex Absence Seizures: Initial: 15mg/kg/day. Titrate: Increase weekly by 5-10mg/kg/day until seizures are controlled or side effects preclude further increases. Max: 60mg/kg/day. If total dose exceeds 250mg/day, give in 2-3 doses. In epileptic patients previously receiving Depakene (valproic acid) therapy, initiate at the same daily dose and dosing schedule; a dosing schedule of bid or tid may be elected after the patient is stabilized. Migraine: Initial: 250mg bid. Some patients may benefit from doses up to 1000mg/day. Elderly: Reduce initial dose and titrate slowly. Consider decreasing the dose or discontinuing in patients with decreased food or fluid intake or excessive somnolence.
Pediatrics: ≥10 Yrs: Complex Partial Seizures: Monotherapy/Conversion to Monotherapy/Adjunctive Therapy: Initial: 10-15mg/kg/day. Titrate: Increase by 5-10mg/kg/week until optimal response is achieved. Max: 60mg/kg/day. For adjunctive therapy, if total dose exceeds 250mg/day, give in 2-3 doses. When converting to monotherapy, reduce concomitant antiepilepsy drug by approximately 25% every 2 weeks, starting at initiation, or delay by 1-2 weeks after start of therapy if there is concern that seizures are likely to occur with a reduction.

HOW SUPPLIED: Cap, Delayed-Release: 125mg, 250mg, 500mg

CONTRAINDICATIONS: Hepatic disease or significant hepatic dysfunction, known urea cycle disorders (UCD). Mitochondrial disorders caused by mutations in mitochondrial DNA POLG (eg, Alpers Huttenlocher syndrome) and children <2 yrs of age who are suspected of having a POLG-related disorder. Prophylaxis of migraine headaches in pregnant women.

WARNINGS/PRECAUTIONS: Caution in patients with a prior history of hepatic disease. D/C immediately if significant hepatic dysfunction (suspected or apparent) occurs. Hyperammonemic encephalopathy reported in UCD patients. D/C, initiate prompt treatment, and evaluate for underlying UCD, if symptoms of unexplained hyperammonemic encephalopathy develop. Prior to initiation of therapy, evaluate for UCD in high-risk patients (eg, those with a history of unexplained encephalopathy or coma, encephalopathy associated with a protein load, pregnancy-related or postpartum encephalopathy, unexplained mental retardation, or history of elevated plasma ammonia or glutamine). Increased risk of suicidal thoughts or behavior reported; monitor for the emergence/worsening of depression, suicidal thoughts or behavior, thoughts of self-harm, and/or any unusual changes in mood or behavior. Dose-related thrombocytopenia, inhibition of the secondary phase of platelet aggregation, and abnormal coagulation parameters (eg, low fibrinogen) reported; monitor platelet and coagulation parameters prior to therapy, periodically thereafter, and prior to planned surgery. Reduce dose or d/c if hemorrhage, bruising, or a disorder of hemostasis/coagulation occurs. Hyperammonemia reported and may be present

S

despite normal LFTs; consider hyperammonemic encephalopathy and measure ammonia levels if unexplained lethargy, vomiting, or mental status changes occur. Hypothermia reported both in conjunction with and in the absence of hyperammonemia. Multiorgan hypersensitivity reactions (rare) reported; d/c and initiate alternative treatment if this reaction is suspected. Caution in the elderly; monitor fluid/nutritional intake, and for dehydration, somnolence, and other adverse reactions. Altered thyroid function tests and urine ketone tests reported. Avoid abrupt discontinuation in patients in whom the drug is administered to prevent major seizures. May stimulate replication of HIV and cytomegalovirus.

ADVERSE REACTIONS: Hepatotoxicity, pancreatitis, tremor, N/V, somnolence, asthenia, dizziness, thrombocytopenia, alopecia, abdominal pain, diarrhea, infection, insomnia, diplopia, headache.

INTERACTIONS: Drugs that affect the level of expression of hepatic enzymes, particularly those that elevate levels of glucuronosyltransferases (eg, phenytoin, carbamazepine, phenobarbital, primidone) may increase valproate clearance. Increase monitoring of valproate and concomitant drug concentrations whenever enzyme-inducing drugs are introduced or withdrawn. Concomitant use with aspirin decreases protein binding and inhibits metabolism of valproate; use with caution. Carbapenem antibiotics (eg, ertapenem, imipenem, meropenem) may reduce serum concentrations to subtherapeutic levels, resulting in loss of seizure control; monitor serum valproic acid concentrations frequently after initiating carbapenem therapy. Rifampin increases valproate oral clearance and may require valproate dosage adjustment. Concomitant use with felbamate reported to increase valproate C_{max}; decrease in valproate dosage may be required. Reduces clearance of amitriptyline, nortriptyline, and lorazepam; consider monitoring amitriptyline levels and consider lowering the dose of amitriptyline/nortriptyline. Decreases serum levels of carbamazepine while increasing carbamazepine-10,11-epoxide serum levels. Inhibits metabolism of diazepam. Inhibits metabolism of ethosuximide; monitor serum concentrations of both drugs. Inhibits metabolism of phenobarbital and phenytoin; monitor drug serum concentrations and adjust dose appropriately. May inhibit metabolism of primidone. Breakthrough seizures reported with concomitant use with phenytoin. Use with clonazepam may induce absence status in patients with absence seizures. Increases $T_{1/2}$ of lamotrigine and serious skin reactions reported with concomitant use; reduce the dose of lamotrigine when coadministered. Concomitant use with topiramate associated with hypothermia and hyperammonemia with or without encephalopathy. Increased trough plasma levels reported with chlorpromazine. May displace protein-bound drugs (eg, phenytoin, carbamazepine, tolbutamide, warfarin); monitor coagulation tests when coadministered with warfarin. May decrease zidovudine clearance. Caution if taken with alcohol.

PREGNANCY: Category D (for epilepsy and for manic episodes associated with bipolar disorder), Category X (for prophylaxis of migraine headaches), not for use in nursing.

MECHANISM OF ACTION: Carboxylic acid derivative; has not been established. Activity in epilepsy is suggested to be related to increased gamma-aminobutyric acid concentrations in the brain.

PHARMACOKINETICS: Absorption: T_{max} =2 hrs (median) (fasted), 4.8 hrs (fed). **Distribution:** V_d=11L (total valproate), 92L (free valproate); found in breast milk. **Metabolism:** Liver via glucuronidation and mitochondrial β-oxidation (major); other oxidative mechanisms. **Elimination:** Urine (30-50% glucuronide conjugate, <3% unchanged); $T_{1/2}$=9-16 hrs (250-1000mg dose).

NURSING CONSIDERATIONS

Assessment: Assess for hepatic disease or significant hepatic dysfunction, history of hepatic disease, UCD, history of hypersensitivity to drug, mitochondrial disorders caused by mutations in mitochondrial POLG, any other conditions where treatment is contraindicated or cautioned, pregnancy/nursing status, or for possible drug interactions. Assess LFTs, CBC with platelet counts, and coagulation parameters.

Monitoring: Monitor for multiorgan hypersensitivity reactions, pancreatitis, hepatotoxicity, hyperammonemia, hypothermia, emergence/worsening of depression, suicidality or unusual changes in behavior, and other adverse reactions. Monitor LFTs frequently, especially during the first 6 months. Monitor ammonia levels, CBC with platelets, and coagulation parameters. Monitor fluid/nutritional intake and for dehydration and somnolence in elderly patients. Monitor coagulation tests when coadministered with warfarin.

Patient Counseling: Counsel about signs/symptoms of pancreatitis, hepatotoxicity, and hyperammonemic encephalopathy; advise to notify physician if any signs/symptoms occur. Inform pregnant women and women of childbearing potential about the risk in pregnancy (eg, birth defects, decreased IQ); advise to use effective contraception while on therapy and counsel about alternative therapeutic options. Advise to read medication guide. Instruct to notify physician if pregnant or intending to become pregnant. Encourage pregnant patients to enroll in the North American Antiepileptic Drug Pregnancy Registry. Advise to notify physician if depression, suicidal thoughts, behavior, or thoughts about self-harm emerge; instruct to report behaviors of concern to physician. Advise not to engage in hazardous activities (eg, driving, operating machinery) until the effects of the drug are known. Inform that a fever associated with other organ system involvement (eg, rash, lymphadenopathy) may be drug-related; instruct to report to physician immediately.

Administration: Oral route. Swallow cap whole. Take with food or slowly build up the dose from an initial low level if GI irritation occurs. **Storage:** 25°C (77°F); excursions permitted to 15-30°C (59-86°F).

STAXYN   RX
vardenafil HCl (GlaxoSmithKline)

THERAPEUTIC CLASS: Phosphodiesterase type 5 inhibitor

INDICATIONS: Treatment of erectile dysfunction (ED).

DOSAGE: *Adults:* 10mg PRN, 60 min before sexual activity. Max: 1 tab/day. Requires sexual stimulation for treatment response. Place on tongue to disintegrate. Take without liquid, and immediately upon removal from blister. Patients Stable on α-blocker Therapy: Initiate vardenafil at the lowest recommended dose. Use lower doses of vardenafil film-coated tab as initial therapy. Consider a time interval between dosing.

HOW SUPPLIED: Tab, Disintegrating: 10mg

CONTRAINDICATIONS: Concomitant use with nitrates (either regularly/intermittently) or nitric oxide donors.

WARNINGS/PRECAUTIONS: Not interchangeable with vardenafil 10mg film-coated tab (Levitra); prescribe film-coated tab if requiring a lower/higher dose. Increased sensitivity to vasodilatation effects with left ventricular outflow obstruction (eg, aortic stenosis, idiopathic hypertrophic subaortic stenosis). Has vasodilatory properties resulting in transient decreases in supine BP; prior to therapy, carefully consider if patients with cardiovascular (CV) disease may be affected by such vasodilatory effects. Prolonged erections >4 hrs and priapism reported; penile tissue damage and permanent loss of potency may result if priapism is not treated immediately. Avoid with moderate or severe hepatic impairment (Child-Pugh B or C), renal dialysis, hereditary degenerative retinal disorders (including retinitis pigmentosa), and congenital QT prolongation. Caution with bleeding disorders, active peptic ulcers, anatomical deformation of the penis (eg, angulation, cavernosal fibrosis, Peyronie's disease) or predisposition to priapism (eg, sickle cell anemia, multiple myeloma, leukemia). Rarely, non-arteritic anterior ischemic optic neuropathy (NAION) has been reported; d/c therapy if sudden loss of vision occurs. Increased risk of NAION in patients who had NAION in one eye. Sudden decrease or loss of hearing accompanied by tinnitus and dizziness reported; d/c therapy if this occurs. QT prolongation may occur; caution with known history of QT prolongation. Contains aspartame; may be harmful in phenylketonurics. Contains sorbitol; avoid with hereditary problems of fructose intolerance. Does not protect against sexually transmitted disease.

ADVERSE REACTIONS: Headache, flushing, nasal congestion.

INTERACTIONS: See Contraindications. Avoid use with Class IA (eg, quinidine, procainamide) or Class III (eg, amiodarone, sotalol) antiarrhythmics and other treatments for ED. Avoid with potent or moderate CYP3A4 inhibitors (eg, ketoconazole, itraconazole, ritonavir, indinavir, saquinavir, atazanavir, clarithromycin, erythromycin). Step-wise increase in α-blocker dose may be associated with further lowering of BP; caution when coadministering. Additive hypotensive effect with other antihypertensive agents. Caution with medications known to prolong QT interval.

PREGNANCY: Category B, not for use in nursing.

MECHANISM OF ACTION: Phosphodiesterase Type 5 inhibitor; enhances erectile function by increasing the amount of cyclic guanosine monophosphate, which triggers smooth muscle relaxations, allowing increased blood flow into the penis, resulting in erection.

PHARMACOKINETICS: Absorption: T_{max}=1.5 hrs (median). **Distribution:** V_{ss}=208L; plasma protein binding (95%). **Metabolism:** Via CYP3A4, CYP3A5, CYP2C. M1 (major metabolite). **Excretion:** Feces (91%-95%), urine (2%-6%); $T_{1/2}$=4-6 hrs (vardenafil), 3-5 hrs (M1).

NURSING CONSIDERATIONS

Assessment: Assess for left ventricular outflow obstruction, CV disease, congenital or history of QT prolongation, degenerative retinal disorders, retinitis pigmentosa, bleeding disorders, active peptic ulceration, anatomical deformation of the penis, conditions that may predispose to priapism, phenylketonuria, and renal/hepatic impairment. Assess potential underlying causes of erectile dysfunction, and for possible drug interactions.

Monitoring: Monitor for prolonged erection, priapism, vision changes (eg, NAION), hypersensitivity reactions, hearing impairment, and other adverse reactions. Monitor therapeutic effect when used in combination with other drugs. Monitor BP.

Patient Counseling: Discuss the risks and benefits of therapy. Instruct to take ud. Inform that it is not interchangeable with vardenafil film-coated tab (Levitra). Counsel that use of nitrates and α-blockers can cause hypotension resulting in dizziness, syncope, or even heart attack or stroke.

Instruct to contact the physician or healthcare provider if not satisfied with the quality of sexual performance or in case of unwanted effect. Inform that priapism may occur; if not treated immediately, penile tissue damage and permanent loss of potency may result. Instruct to stop the medication if sudden hearing loss, NAION, or loss of vision in one or both eyes occurs. Warn that therapy does not protect against sexually transmitted diseases. Advise to examine blisterpack before use and not to use if blisters are torn, broken, or missing.

Administration: Oral route. Place on tongue to disintegrate. Take without liquid and immediately upon removal from blister. Take without food. **Storage:** 25°C (77°F); excursions permitted to 15-30°C (59-86°F).

STELARA

ustekinumab (Janssen)

RX

THERAPEUTIC CLASS: Monoclonal antibody

INDICATIONS: Treatment of adults (≥18 yrs of age) with moderate to severe plaque psoriasis (Ps), who are candidates for phototherapy or systemic therapy. Treatment of adults (≥18 yrs of age) with active psoriatic arthritis (PsA) alone or in combination with methotrexate.

DOSAGE: *Adults:* ≥18 Yrs: Ps: >100kg: 90mg SQ initially and 4 weeks later, followed by 90mg SQ every 12 weeks. ≤100kg: 45mg SQ initially and 4 weeks later, followed by 45mg SQ every 12 weeks. PsA: 45mg SQ initially and 4 weeks later, followed by 45mg SQ every 12 weeks. With Coexistent Moderate to Severe Plaque Ps: >100kg: 90mg SQ initially and 4 weeks later, followed by 90mg SQ every 12 weeks.

HOW SUPPLIED: Inj: 45mg/0.5mL, 90mg/mL [prefilled syringe, vial]

WARNINGS/PRECAUTIONS: Serious bacterial, fungal, and viral infections reported. Should not be given to patients with any clinically important active infection, or until infection resolves or is adequately treated. Individuals genetically deficient in interleukin (IL)-12/IL-23 are particularly vulnerable to disseminated infections from mycobacteria (eg, nontuberculous, environmental mycobacteria), salmonella (eg, nontyphi strains), and Bacillus Calmette-Guerin (BCG) vaccinations; consider appropriate diagnostic testing (eg, tissue culture, stool culture) as dictated by clinical circumstances. Evaluate for tuberculosis (TB) infection prior to, during, and after treatment; do not administer to patients with active TB. Consider anti-TB therapy prior to initiation in patients with history of latent or active TB when an adequate course of treatment cannot be confirmed. Rapid appearance of multiple cutaneous squamous cell carcinomas reported in patients who had preexisting risk factors for developing non-melanoma skin cancer; closely monitor patients with history of prolonged immunosuppressant therapy, history of PUVA treatment, and patients >60 yrs of age. Hypersensitivity reactions (eg, anaphylaxis, angioedema) reported; institute appropriate therapy and d/c. Reversible posterior leukoencephalopathy syndrome (RPLS) reported; administer appropriate treatment and d/c if suspected. Prior to initiating therapy, patients should receive all immunizations appropriate for age as recommended by current immunization guidelines. Needle cover on prefilled syringe contains dry natural rubber and should not be handled by latex-sensitive individuals. Should only be given to patients who will be closely monitored and have regular follow-up visits with a physician.

ADVERSE REACTIONS: Infection, nasopharyngitis, upper respiratory tract infection, headache, fatigue, arthralgia, nausea.

INTERACTIONS: Do not give with live vaccines; caution when administering live vaccines to household contacts of patients receiving ustekinumab. BCG vaccines should not be given during treatment, for 1 yr prior to initiating treatment, or 1 yr following discontinuation of treatment. Non-live vaccinations received during course of therapy may not elicit an immune response sufficient to prevent disease. Consider monitoring for therapeutic effect (eg, for warfarin) or drug concentration (eg, for cyclosporine) with concomitant CYP450 substrates, particularly those with a narrow therapeutic index; adjust individual dose of the drug PRN. May decrease protective effect of allergen immunotherapy (decrease tolerance), which may increase the risk of an allergic reaction to a dose of allergen immunotherapy; caution in patients receiving or who have received allergen immunotherapy.

PREGNANCY: Category B, caution in nursing.

MECHANISM OF ACTION: Monoclonal antibody; binds with specificity to the shared p40 protein subunit used by both the IL-12 and IL-23 cytokines. In in vitro models, ustekinumab was shown to disrupt IL-12 and IL-23 mediated signaling and cytokine cascades by disrupting the interaction of these cytokines with a shared cell-surface receptor chain, IL-12Rβ1.

PHARMACOKINETICS: Absorption: (Psoriasis) T_{max}=13.5 days (median, 45mg), 7 days (median, 90mg). **Distribution:** (Psoriasis) V_d=161mL/kg (45mg), 179mL/kg (90mg); found in breast milk. **Elimination:** $T_{1/2}$=14.9-45.6 days (psoriasis).

NURSING CONSIDERATIONS

Assessment: Assess for drug hypersensitivity, active/chronic infection, history of recurrent infection, IL-12/IL-23 genetic deficiency, TB, immunization history, pregnancy/nursing status, and possible drug interactions.

Monitoring: Monitor for signs/symptoms of infection, appearance of non-melanoma skin cancer, TB during and after treatment, malignancies, hypersensitivity reactions, RPLS, and other adverse reactions.

Patient Counseling: Advise that therapy may lower the ability of the immune system to fight infections. Inform of the importance of communicating any history of infections to physician and to contact physician if any signs/symptoms of infection develop. Counsel about the risk of malignancies while on therapy. Advise to seek immediate medical attention if experiencing any symptoms of a serious allergic reaction. Inform of inj techniques and procedures. Advise not to reuse needles/syringes and instruct on proper disposal procedures.

Administration: SQ route. Refer to PI for general considerations and instructions for administration. **Storage:** 2-8°C (36-46°F). Store vials upright. Protect from light. Do not freeze or shake.

STENDRA RX
avanafil (Vivus)

THERAPEUTIC CLASS: Phosphodiesterase type 5 inhibitor

INDICATIONS: Treatment of erectile dysfunction (ED).

DOSAGE: *Adults:* Initial: 100mg PO PRN approximately 30 min before sexual activity. Titrate: May increase to a max dose of 200mg or decrease to 50mg. Max Frequency: Dose qd. Use the lowest dose that provides benefit. Sexual stimulation is required for response to treatment. With α-Blockers: Should be stable on α-blocker therapy prior to initiation of therapy. Initial: 50mg/day. With Moderate CYP3A4 Inhibitors: Max: 50mg, not to exceed once q24h.

HOW SUPPLIED: Tab: 50mg, 100mg, 200mg

CONTRAINDICATIONS: Organic nitrates, either taken regularly and/or intermittently, in any form.

WARNINGS/PRECAUTIONS: Potential for cardiac risk during sexual activity in patients with pre-existing cardiovascular disease (CVD); avoid in men for whom sexual activity is inadvisable due to underlying CV status. Patients with left ventricular outflow obstruction (eg, aortic stenosis, idiopathic hypertrophic subaortic stenosis) and severely impaired autonomic control of BP can be particularly sensitive to the actions of vasodilators (eg, avanafil). Not recommended in patients with myocardial infarction, stroke, life-threatening arrhythmia, coronary revascularization within the last 6 months, resting hypotension (BP <90/50 mmHg) or HTN (BP >170/100 mmHg), unstable angina, angina with sexual intercourse, NYHA Class 2 or greater congestive heart failure, and in patients with known hereditary degenerative retinal disorders (including retinitis pigmentosa). Prolonged erection (>4 hrs) and priapism (painful erections >6 hrs in duration) reported; caution with anatomical deformation of the penis (eg, angulation, cavernosal fibrosis, or Peyronie's disease), or conditions that may predispose to priapism (eg, sickle cell anemia, multiple myeloma, leukemia). Non-arteritic anterior ischemic optic neuropathy (NAION) rarely reported; d/c if sudden loss of vision is experienced in one or both eyes. Sudden decrease or loss of hearing, which may be accompanied by tinnitus or dizziness, reported; d/c if occurs. Does not protect against sexually transmitted diseases (eg, HIV). Avoid in patients with severe renal disease, on renal dialysis, or with severe hepatic disease.

ADVERSE REACTIONS: Headache, flushing, nasopharyngitis, nasal congestion, back pain, upper respiratory infection, ECG abnormal.

INTERACTIONS: See Contraindications. Not recommended with other PDE-5 inhibitors or ED therapy combinations. Not recommended with CYP inducers. Caution with α-blockers; may augment BP-lowering effect of α-blockers and other antihypertensives. May increase the risk of orthostatic signs/symptoms with substantial alcohol consumption. Avoid use with strong CYP3A4 inhibitors (eg, ketoconazole, ritonavir, clarithromycin, nefazodone). Increased levels with moderate CYP3A4 inhibitors (eg, erythromycin, amprenavir, diltiazem, fluconazole), other CYP3A4 inhibitors (eg, grapefruit juice). May increase levels of desipramine, omeprazole, and rosiglitazone. Amlodipine may increase levels. May potentiate the antiaggregatory effect of sodium nitroprusside.

PREGNANCY: Category C, safety not known in nursing.

MECHANISM OF ACTION: PDE-5 inhibitor; has no direct relaxant effect on isolated human corpus cavernosum, but enhances effect of nitric oxide by inhibiting PDE-5, which is responsible for degradation of cGMP in the corpus cavernosum.

PHARMACOKINETICS: Absorption: Rapid; (fasted) T_{max}=30-45 min. **Distribution:** Plasma protein binding (99%). **Metabolism:** Extensive; CYP3A4 (major), CYP2C isoform (minor); M4 and M16 (major circulating metabolites). **Elimination:** Feces (62% metabolites), urine (21% metabolites); $T_{1/2}$=5 hrs.

NURSING CONSIDERATIONS

Assessment: Assess for hypersensitivity to the drug, preexisting CVD, any other conditions where treatment is contraindicated/cautioned, and possible drug interactions. Assess to identify potential underlying causes of ED as well as treatment options.

Monitoring: Monitor for hypersensitivity reactions, NAION (eg, loss of vision), prolonged erection, priapism, cardiac risk, decrease or loss of hearing, and other adverse reactions.

Patient Counseling: Instruct to take as ud; discuss the appropriate use and its anticipated benefits. Instruct to seek medical assistance if prolonged erection persists >4 hrs. Inform of potential BP-lowering effect with α-blockers and other antihypertensive drugs. Inform of the potential cardiac risk of sexual activity in patients with preexisting CV risk factors. Inform that regular and/or intermittent use of organic nitrates is contraindicated. Advise to contact physician if new medications are prescribed by another healthcare provider. Advise to stop taking PDE-5 inhibitors and seek medical attention in the event of sudden loss of vision in one or both eyes or when sudden decrease or loss of hearing occurs. Inform patients that substantial consumption of alcohol (eg, >3 units) in combination with the medication may increase the potential for orthostatic signs/symptoms. Counsel patients about the protective measures necessary to guard against sexually transmitted diseases (eg, HIV).

Administration: Oral route. Take with or without food. **Storage:** 20-25°C (68-77°F); excursions permitted to 30°C (86°F). Protect from light.

STIVARGA   RX
regorafenib (Bayer Healthcare)

> Severe and sometimes fatal hepatotoxicity reported. Monitor hepatic function prior to and during treatment. Interrupt and then reduce or d/c treatment for hepatotoxicity as manifested by elevated LFTs or hepatocellular necrosis, depending upon severity and persistence.

THERAPEUTIC CLASS: Multikinase inhibitor

INDICATIONS: Treatment of metastatic colorectal cancer previously treated with fluoropyrimidine-, oxaliplatin- and irinotecan-based chemotherapy, an antivascular endothelial growth factor therapy, and, if KRAS wild type, an anti-epidermal growth factor receptor therapy. Treatment of locally advanced, unresectable or metastatic GI stromal tumor previously treated with imatinib mesylate and sunitinib malate.

DOSAGE: *Adults:* Usual: 160mg qd for the first 21 days of each 28-day cycle. Continue treatment until disease progression or unacceptable toxicity. Take at the same time each day with low-fat breakfast that contains <30% fat. Refer to PI for dose modifications.

HOW SUPPLIED: Tab: 40mg

WARNINGS/PRECAUTIONS: Increased incidence of hemorrhage reported; permanently d/c with severe or life-threatening hemorrhage. May increase incidence of adverse reactions involving the skin and SQ tissues (eg, hand-foot skin reaction [HFSR], toxic epidermal necrolysis, Stevens Johnson syndrome, severe rash); withhold, reduce dose, or permanently d/c treatment depending on severity and persistence of dermatologic toxicity. Increased incidence of HTN reported; temporarily or permanently withhold for severe or uncontrolled HTN; avoid initiation unless BP is adequately controlled. May increase incidence of myocardial ischemia and infarction; withhold if new or acute onset cardiac ischemia or infarction develops; resume only after resolution of acute cardiac ischemic events, if benefits outweigh risks of further cardiac ischemia. Reversible posterior leukoencephalopathy syndrome (RPLS) reported; perform evaluation for RPLS in any patient presenting with seizures, headache, visual disturbances, confusion, or altered mental function; d/c if RPLS develops. Permanently d/c if GI perforation or fistula develops. May impair wound healing; d/c at least 2 weeks prior to scheduled surgery. D/C in patients with wound dehiscence. May cause fetal harm; women and men should use effective contraception during treatment and up to 2 months after completion of therapy. Not recommended with severe hepatic impairment (Child-Pugh Class C).

ADVERSE REACTIONS: Hepatotoxicity, asthenia/fatigue, HFSR, diarrhea, decreased appetite/food intake, HTN, mucositis, dysphonia, infection, pain, decreased weight, GI/abdominal pain, rash, fever, nausea.

INTERACTIONS: Avoid concomitant use with strong CYP3A4 inducers (eg, rifampin, phenytoin, carbamazepine, phenobarbital, St. John's wort) and strong CYP3A4 inhibitors (eg, clarithromycin, grapefruit juice, itraconazole, ketoconazole, nefazodone, posaconazole, telithromycin, voriconazole). Monitor INR levels more frequently in patients receiving warfarin.

PREGNANCY: Category D, not for use in nursing.

MECHANISM OF ACTION: Multikinase inhibitor; inhibits multiple membrane-bound and intracellular kinases involved in normal cellular functions and in pathologic processes, such as oncogenesis, tumor angiogenesis, and maintenance of the tumor microenvironment.

PHARMACOKINETICS: Absorption: (Single 160mg dose) C_{max}=2.5mcg/mL, T_{max}=4 hrs (median), AUC=70.4mcg•h/mL. (Steady state) C_{max}=3.9mcg/mL, AUC=58.3mcg•h/mL. **Distribution:** Plasma protein binding (99.5%). **Metabolism:** CYP3A4, UGT1A9; M-2 (N-oxide) and M-5 (N-oxide and N-desmethyl) (active metabolites). **Elimination:** Urine (19%; 17% glucuronides), feces (71%; 47% parent compound, 24% metabolites); $T_{1/2}$=28 hrs (regorafenib), 25 hrs (M-2), 51 hrs (M-5).

NURSING CONSIDERATIONS

Assessment: Assess for scheduled/recent surgical procedures, hepatic dysfunction, HTN, pregnancy/nursing status, and possible drug interactions. Obtain baseline LFTs (ALT, AST, and bilirubin).

Monitoring: Monitor for hepatotoxicity, hemorrhage, dermatologic toxicity, HTN, myocardial ischemia or infarction, RPLS, wound dehiscence, GI perforation or fistula, and other adverse reactions. Monitor BP weekly for the first 6 weeks of treatment and then every cycle, or more frequently, as clinically indicated. Monitor LFTs at least every 2 weeks during the first 2 months of treatment, then monthly or more frequently as clinically indicated; monitor weekly in patients experiencing elevated LFTs until improvement to <3X ULN or baseline. Monitor INR levels more frequently in patients receiving warfarin.

Patient Counseling: Inform about the need to undergo monitoring for liver damage and instruct to immediately report to physician any signs or symptoms of severe liver damage. Advise to contact physician for any episode of bleeding, or if experiencing skin changes associated with redness, pain, blisters, bleeding, or swelling. Advise of the need for BP monitoring and to contact physician if BP is elevated, or if HTN symptoms occur. Instruct to seek immediate emergency help if experiencing chest pain, SOB, dizziness, or feeling like passing out. Advise to contact physician immediately if experiencing severe pain in the abdomen, persistent swelling of the abdomen, high fever, chills, N/V, severe diarrhea, or dehydration. Advise to inform physician if planning to undergo a surgical procedure or if had recent surgery. Advise women and men of the need for effective contraception during treatment and for up to 2 months after completion of treatment. Instruct women of reproductive potential to immediately contact physician if pregnancy is suspected or confirmed during or within 2 months of completing treatment. Advise nursing mothers that it is not known whether the drug is present in breast milk and discuss whether to d/c nursing or to d/c treatment. Inform to take any missed dose on the same day, as soon as they remember, and to not take 2 doses on the same day to make up for a dose missed on the previous day.

Administration: Oral route. Swallow tab whole with a low-fat breakfast that contains <30% fat. **Storage:** 25°C (77°F); excursions permitted to 15-30°C (59-86°F). Store tabs in original bottle and do not remove the desiccant. Keep the bottle tightly closed after 1st opening. Discard any unused tabs 7 weeks after opening the bottle.

STRATTERA RX
atomoxetine (Lilly)

S

> Increased risk of suicidal ideation in short-term studies in children or adolescents with attention-deficit hyperactivity disorder (ADHD); balance this risk with the clinical need. Closely monitor for suicidality (suicidal thinking and behavior), clinical worsening, or unusual changes in behavior. Not approved for major depressive disorder.

THERAPEUTIC CLASS: Selective norepinephrine reuptake inhibitor

INDICATIONS: Treatment of ADHD.

DOSAGE: *Adults:* Take as a single dose in the am or as evenly divided doses in the am and late afternoon/early pm. Initial: 40mg/day. Titrate: Increase after a minimum of 3 days to target dose of approximately 80mg/day; may increase after 2-4 additional weeks if optimal response is not achieved. Max: 100mg/day. Periodically reevaluate long-term usefulness. Refer to PI for dose adjustments for hepatic impairment, concomitant use with CYP2D6 inhibitors, and in patients known to be CYP2D6 poor metabolizers (PM).
Pediatrics: ≥6 Yrs: Take as a single dose in the am or as evenly divided doses in the am and late afternoon/early pm. >70kg: Initial: 40mg/day. Titrate: Increase after a minimum of 3 days to target dose of approximately 80mg/day; may increase after 2-4 additional weeks if optimal response is not achieved. Max: 100mg/day. ≤70kg: Initial: 0.5mg/kg/day. Titrate: Increase after a minimum of 3 days to target dose of approximately 1.2mg/kg/day. Max: 1.4mg/kg/day or 100mg/day, whichever is less. Periodically reevaluate long-term usefulness. Refer to PI for dose adjustments for hepatic impairment, concomitant use with CYP2D6 inhibitors, and in patients known to be CYP2D6 PM.

HOW SUPPLIED: Cap: 10mg, 18mg, 25mg, 40mg, 60mg, 80mg, 100mg

CONTRAINDICATIONS: Narrow-angle glaucoma, presence/history of pheochromocytoma, and severe cardiac/vascular disorders that would deteriorate with increases in BP/HR that would be clinically important (eg, 15-20mmHg in BP or 20 beats/min in HR). Concomitant use with an MAOI or within 2 weeks after discontinuation of an MAOI.

WARNINGS/PRECAUTIONS: May cause severe liver injury; d/c in patients with jaundice or laboratory evidence of liver injury, and do not restart therapy. Perform LFTs upon the 1st sign/symptom of liver dysfunction. Sudden death reported in children and adolescents with structural cardiac abnormalities or other serious heart problems. Sudden death, stroke, myocardial infarction reported in adults. Avoid in patients with known serious structural cardiac abnormalities, cardiomyopathy, serious heart rhythm abnormalities, coronary artery disease, or other serious cardiac problems. Promptly perform cardiac evaluation if symptoms suggestive of cardiac disease develop. May increase BP/HR; caution in patients whose underlying medical conditions could be worsened by increases in BP or HR. Orthostatic hypotension and syncope reported; caution with conditions predisposing to hypotension, or conditions associated with abrupt HR/BP changes. Caution in patients with comorbid bipolar disorder; may induce mixed/manic episode. May cause treatment-emergent psychotic or manic symptoms in children/adolescents without prior history of psychotic illness or mania; consider discontinuation if such symptoms occur. Monitor for appearance/worsening of aggressive behavior or hostility. Allergic reactions and priapism reported. May cause urinary retention/hesitation. Monitor growth in children.

ADVERSE REACTIONS: Abdominal pain, N/V, fatigue, decreased appetite, somnolence, headache, dry mouth, dizziness, insomnia, constipation, urinary hesitation, erectile dysfunction, irritability, weight decreased, hyperhidrosis.

INTERACTIONS: See Contraindications. Caution with systemically administered albuterol or other β_2 agonists; may potentiate CV effects of albuterol. Caution with antihypertensive drugs and pressor agents (eg, dopamine, dobutamine), or other drugs that increase BP. CYP2D6 inhibitors (eg, paroxetine, fluoxetine, quinidine) increase levels in extensive metabolizers (EM).

PREGNANCY: Category C, caution in nursing.

MECHANISM OF ACTION: Selective norepinephrine reuptake inhibitor; not established. May selectively inhibit the presynaptic norepinephrine transporter.

PHARMACOKINETICS: Absorption: Rapid; well-absorbed; absolute bioavailability (63% [EM], 94% [PM]); T_{max} =1-2 hrs. **Distribution:** V_d=0.85L/kg (IV); plasma protein binding (98%). **Metabolism:** Via CYP2D6; 4-hydroxyatomoxetine (major active metabolite), N-desmethylatomoxetine. **Elimination:** $T_{1/2}$=5 hrs. 4-hydroxyatomoxetine-O-glucuronide: Urine (>80%), feces (<17%).

NURSING CONSIDERATIONS

Assessment: Assess for hypersensitivity to drug, narrow-angle glaucoma, presence/history of pheochromocytoma, comorbid bipolar disorder, cardiovascular (CV) disorders, hepatic impairment, any other conditions where treatment is contraindicated or cautioned, pregnancy/nursing status, and possible drug interactions. Obtain baseline pulse and BP.

Monitoring: Monitor for signs/symptoms of CV events, liver injury, allergic reactions, emergence of psychosis/mania, suicidality, clinical worsening, aggressive or unusual changes in behavior, hostility, urinary retention/hesitation, priapism, and other adverse reactions. Monitor growth in children. Monitor pulse and BP following dose increases and periodically during therapy. Periodically reevaluate long-term usefulness.

Patient Counseling: Inform about risks, benefits, and appropriate use of therapy. Encourage patients, families, and caregivers to be alert for the emergence of agitation, irritability, and unusual changes in behavior, as well as the emergence of suicidality, especially early during treatment and when dose is adjusted; advise to report such symptoms to physician especially if severe, abrupt in onset, or not part of presenting symptoms. Advise to contact physician if symptoms of liver injury develop. Inform that priapism requires prompt medical attention. Inform that drug is an ocular irritant; if content of cap comes in contact with eye, instruct to immediately flush affected eye with water and obtain medical advice. Inform to notify physician if taking or planning to take any prescription or OTC medicines, dietary supplements, or herbal remedies. Instruct to notify physician if nursing, pregnant, or thinking of becoming pregnant. Caution when driving a car/operating hazardous machinery until reasonably certain that performance is not affected by therapy.

Administration: Oral route. Take whole with or without food; do not open cap. **Storage:** 25°C (77°F); excursions permitted to 15-30°C (59-86°F).

STRIANT   CIII
testosterone (Columbia Labs)

THERAPEUTIC CLASS: Androgen

INDICATIONS: Testosterone replacement therapy in males with primary or hypogonadotropic hypogonadism, congenital or acquired.

DOSAGE: *Adults:* 30mg q12h to gum region, just above the incisor tooth on either side of mouth. Rotate sites with each application. Hold system in place for 30 seconds. If buccal system falls off within the 12-hr dosing interval or falls out of position within 4 hrs prior to next dose, remove and apply new system. Do not chew or swallow.

HOW SUPPLIED: Tab, Buccal: 30mg [6 blister packs, 10 buccal systems/blister]

CONTRAINDICATIONS: Women. Carcinoma of the breast or known or suspected carcinoma of the prostate. Hypersensitivity to soy products.

WARNINGS/PRECAUTIONS: Caution in elderly; increased risk of prostatic hyperplasia/carcinoma. Risk of edema with preexisting cardiac, renal, or hepatic disease; d/c if edema occurs. May potentiate sleep apnea, especially with obesity or chronic lung diseases. Monitor Hgb, Hct, LFTs, prostate specific antigen (PSA), cholesterol, lipids, and serum testosterone. Gynecomastia frequently develops and occasionally persists.

ADVERSE REACTIONS: Gum/mouth irritation, bitter taste, gum pain/tenderness, headache, gynecomastia.

INTERACTIONS: May elevate oxyphenbutazone levels. May decrease blood glucose and, therefore, insulin requirements. Adrenocorticotropic hormone/corticosteroids may enhance edema formation; caution with cardiac or hepatic disease.

PREGNANCY: Category X, not for use in nursing.

MECHANISM OF ACTION: Androgen; responsible for normal growth and development of male sex organs and maintenance of secondary sex characteristics.

PHARMACOKINETICS: Absorption: T_{max}=10-12 hrs. **Distribution:** Sex hormone-binding globulin (40%), plasma protein binding. **Metabolism:** Estradiol, dihydrotestosterone (metabolites). **Elimination:** Urine, feces; $T_{1/2}$=10-100 min.

NURSING CONSIDERATIONS

Assessment: Assess for hypersensitivity to soy products, breast or prostate carcinoma, cardiac or renal/hepatic disease, obesity, chronic lung disease, diabetes mellitus, and possible drug interactions.

Monitoring: Periodically monitor Hgb, Hct, LFTs, PSA, cholesterol, and HDL. Obtain serum testosterone levels 4-12 weeks after initiation of therapy. Monitor for signs/symptoms of hypersensitivity reactions, edema with/without congestive heart failure, gynecomastia, prostatic hyperplasia/carcinoma in geriatrics, and potentiation of sleep apnea.

Patient Counseling: Instruct to apply against gums above incisors; if it fails to adhere, replace with new system. Explain that if system falls out 4 hrs prior to next dose, to replace with a new one until next scheduled dose. Advise to regularly inspect gums where applying system. Instruct to contact physician if abnormal findings on gums, too frequent or persistent erections, N/V, changes in skin color, ankle swelling, breathing disturbances, or hypersensitivity reactions occur.

Administration: Buccal route. Place rounded side surface of system against gum above incisor tooth and hold firmly in place with finger over lip and against product for 30 sec. To remove, slide gently downwards toward tooth to avoid scratching gums. **Storage:** 20-25°C (68-77°F). Protect from heat and moisture.

STRIBILD   RX
tenofovir disoproxil fumarate - emtricitabine - cobicistat - elvitegravir (Gilead)

Lactic acidosis and severe hepatomegaly with steatosis, including fatal cases, reported with the use of nucleoside analogues. Not approved for the treatment of chronic hepatitis B virus (HBV) infection. Severe acute exacerbations of hepatitis B reported in patients coinfected with HBV upon discontinuation of therapy; closely monitor hepatic function for at least several months. If appropriate, initiation of anti-hepatitis B therapy may be warranted.

THERAPEUTIC CLASS: HIV integrase strand transfer inhibitor/nucleoside analogue combination/pharmacokinetic enhancer

INDICATIONS: Complete regimen for the treatment of HIV-1 infection in antiretroviral treatment-naive adults.

DOSAGE: *Adults:* ≥18 Yrs: 1 tab qd with food.

HOW SUPPLIED: Tab: (Elvitegravir-Cobicistat-Emtricitabine-Tenofovir Disoproxil Fumarate [TDF]) 150mg-150mg-200mg-300mg

CONTRAINDICATIONS: Concomitant use with drugs that are highly dependent on CYP3A for clearance and for which elevated plasma concentrations are associated with serious and/or life-threatening reactions and with other drugs that may lead to reduced efficacy and possible resistance (eg, alfuzosin, rifampin, dihydroergotamine, ergotamine, methylergonovine, cisapride,

St. John's wort, lovastatin, simvastatin, pimozide, sildenafil [when used to treat pulmonary arterial HTN], triazolam, oral midazolam).

WARNINGS/PRECAUTIONS: Test for HBV infection and document estimated CrCl, urine glucose, and urine protein prior to initiation of therapy. Not recommended for use in patients with severe hepatic impairment. Renal impairment, including cases of acute renal failure and Fanconi syndrome, reported; d/c if estimated CrCl <50mL/min. Do not initiate therapy in patients with estimated CrCl <70mL/min. Immune reconstitution syndrome, autoimmune disorders (eg, Graves' disease, polymyositis, Guillain-Barre syndrome) in the setting of immune reconstitution, and redistribution/accumulation of body fat reported. Caution in elderly. Cobicistat: May cause modest increases in SrCr and modest declines in estimated CrCl without affecting renal glomerular function; closely monitor patients with confirmed increase in SrCr >0.4mg/dL from baseline for renal safety. TDF: Obesity and prolonged nucleoside exposure may be risk factors for lactic acidosis and severe hepatomegaly. Caution with known risk factors for liver disease. D/C if lactic acidosis or pronounced hepatotoxicity occurs. Decreased bone mineral density (BMD), increased biochemical markers of bone metabolism, and osteomalacia reported; consider assessment of BMD in patients with history of pathologic bone fracture or other risk factors for osteoporosis or bone loss. Arthralgias and muscle pain/weakness reported in cases of proximal renal tubulopathy. Consider hypophosphatemia and osteomalacia secondary to proximal renal tubulopathy in patients at risk of renal dysfunction who present with persistent or worsening bone or muscle symptoms.

ADVERSE REACTIONS: Lactic acidosis, severe hepatomegaly with steatosis, diarrhea, nausea, fatigue, headache, dizziness, insomnia, abnormal dreams, rash, creatine kinase/amylase elevation, hematuria.

INTERACTIONS: See Contraindications. Avoid with adefovir dipivoxil, rifabutin, rifapentine, salmeterol, emtricitabine or TDF, lamivudine, ritonavir, nephrotoxic agents (eg, high dose or multiple NSAIDs), or other antiretrovirals. Avoid with colchicine in patients with renal/hepatic impairment. Antacids (eg, aluminum and magnesium hydroxide) may lower elvitegravir levels; separate administration by at least 2 hrs. May increase levels of antiarrhythmics (eg, digoxin), clonazepam, ethosuximide, ketoconazole, itraconazole, voriconazole, β-blockers, calcium channel blockers, fluticasone (inhaled or nasal), bosentan, atorvastatin, immunosuppressants, neuroleptics, PDE-5 inhibitors, parenteral midazolam, and sedative/hypnotics (eg, benzodiazepines). May increase norgestimate and decrease ethinyl estradiol levels; caution with contraceptives containing norgestimate/ethinyl estradiol. May use alternative (nonhormonal) contraception if considering other hormonal contraceptives (eg, patch, vaginal ring, injectable) or oral contraceptives containing progestogens other than norgestimate. May increase levels of buprenorphine and norbuprenorphine and may decrease levels of naloxone. Monitor for sedation and cognitive effects upon coadministration with buprenorphine/naloxone. Monitor INR upon coadministration with warfarin. May increase levels of antidepressants (eg, SSRIs, TCAs, trazodone); carefully titrate antidepressant dose and monitor response. May increase levels of clarithromycin and/or cobicistat; reduce clarithromycin dose by 50% in patients with CrCl 50-60mL/min. May increase levels of telithromycin and/or cobicistat. May increase levels of substrates of CYP3A/2D6, P-glycoprotein, breast cancer resistance protein, or organic anion transporting polypeptides 1B1/1B3. CYP3A inhibitors may increase plasma levels of cobicistat. CYP3A inducers (eg, dexamethasone, carbamazepine, phenobarbital) may decrease elvitegravir and cobicistat levels and may result in loss of therapeutic effect and development of resistance. Drugs that reduce renal function or compete for active tubular secretion (eg, acyclovir, cidofovir, gentamicin) may increase levels of emtricitabine, tenofovir, and other renally eliminated drugs and may increase risk of adverse reactions. Elvitegravir may decrease levels of CYP2C9 substrates. Ketoconazole, itraconazole, or voriconazole may increase levels of elvitegravir and cobicistat. Cases of acute renal failure after initiation of high dose or multiple NSAIDs reported in patients with risk factors for renal dysfunction who appeared stable on TDF; consider alternatives to NSAIDs, if needed. Refer to PI for dosage adjustments with interacting drugs.

PREGNANCY: Category B, not for use in nursing.

MECHANISM OF ACTION: Elvitegravir: HIV-1 integrase strand inhibitor; inhibits the strand transfer activity of HIV-1 integrase, preventing the integration of HIV-1 deoxyribonucleic acid (DNA) into host genomic DNA, blocking the formation of HIV-1 provirus and propagation of the viral infection. Cobicistat: CYP3A inhibitor; inhibits CYP3A-mediated metabolism that leads to enhancement of systemic exposure of CYP3A substrates (eg, elvitegravir). Emtricitabine: Nucleoside analogue of cytidine; inhibits the activity of HIV-1 reverse transcriptase (RT) by competing with the natural substrate deoxycytidine 5'-triphosphate and by being incorporated into nascent viral DNA, resulting in chain termination. TDF: Acyclic nucleoside phosphonate diester analogue of adenosine monophosphate; inhibits the activity of HIV-1 RT by competing with the natural substrate deoxyadenosine 5'-triphosphate and, after incorporation into DNA, by DNA chain termination.

PHARMACOKINETICS: Absorption: Elvitegravir: C_{max}=1.7mcg/mL, AUC=23mcg•hr/mL, T_{max}=4 hrs. Cobicistat: C_{max}=1.1mcg/mL, AUC=8.3mcg•hr/mL, T_{max}=3 hrs. Emtricitabine: C_{max}=1.9mcg/mL, AUC=12.7mcg•hr/mL, T_{max}=3 hrs. TDF: C_{max}=0.45mcg/mL, AUC=4.4mcg•hr/mL, T_{max}=2 hrs.

Distribution: Elvitegravir: Plasma protein binding (98-99%). Cobicistat: Plasma protein binding (97-98%). Emtricitabine: Plasma protein binding (<4%); found in breast milk. TDF: Plasma protein binding (<0.7%); found in breast milk. **Metabolism:** Elvitegravir: CYP3A (major); glucuronidation via UGT1A1/3 enzymes. Cobicistat: CYP3A, CYP2D6 (minor). **Elimination:** Elvitegravir: Feces (94.8%), urine (6.7%); $T_{1/2}$=12.9 hrs (median). Cobicistat: Feces (86.2%), urine (8.2%); $T_{1/2}$=3.5 hrs (median). Emtricitabine/TDF: Urine.

NURSING CONSIDERATIONS

Assessment: Assess for obesity, prolonged nucleoside exposure, risk factors for liver disease, renal/hepatic impairment, pregnancy/nursing status, and possible drug interactions. Assess BMD in patients who have a history of pathological bone fracture or with other risk factors for osteoporosis or bone loss. Obtain baseline estimated CrCl, urine glucose, urine protein, and SrCr. Perform test for HBV infection prior to therapy.

Monitoring: Monitor for signs/symptoms of lactic acidosis, severe hepatomegaly with steatosis, new onset/worsening renal impairment, immune reconstitution syndrome, autoimmune disorders, fat redistribution/accumulation, decreased BMD, increased biochemical markers for bone metabolism, osteomalacia, and other adverse reactions. Monitor for exacerbations of hepatitis B in patients with coinfection for at least several months upon discontinuation of therapy. Monitor BMD, estimated CrCl, urine glucose, urine protein, and SrCr. Monitor serum phosphorus levels in patients at risk for renal impairment. Monitor INR upon coadministration with warfarin.

Patient Counseling: Advise patients to remain under care of a physician during therapy. Inform that therapy dose not cure HIV-1 infection and continuous therapy is necessary to control HIV-1 infection and decrease HIV-related illnesses. Advise to practice safe sex, to use latex or polyurethane condoms, not to share personal items (eg, toothbrush, razor blades), needles or other inj equipment, and not to breastfeed. Instruct to take on a regular dosing schedule with food and avoid missing doses. Instruct to contact physician if symptoms of lactic acidosis/pronounced hepatotoxicity (eg, N/V, unusual or unexpected stomach discomfort, weakness), or any symptoms of infection occur. Advise patients that fat redistribution/accumulation, renal impairment, and decreases in BMD may occur. Inform patients that hepatitis B testing is recommended prior to initiating therapy. Advise patients to report use of any prescription or nonprescription medication or herbal products, including St. John's wort.

Administration: Oral route. Take with food. **Storage:** 25°C (77°F); excursions permitted to 15-30°C (59-86°F).

SUBOXONE FILM   CIII
buprenorphine - naloxone (Reckitt Benckiser)

THERAPEUTIC CLASS: Partial opioid agonist/opioid antagonist

INDICATIONS: Maint treatment of opioid dependence and should be used as part of a complete treatment plan that includes counseling and psychosocial support.

DOSAGE: *Adults:* Administer SL as a single daily dose in patients initially inducted using Subutex (buprenorphine) SL tabs. Maint: Target Dose: 16mg-4mg/day. Titrate: Adjust dose progressively in increments/decrements of 2mg-0.5mg or 4mg-1mg to a level that maintains treatment and suppresses opioid withdrawal signs and symptoms. Range: 4mg-1mg to 24mg-6mg/day depending on the patient. Discontinuation of Therapy: Should be made as part of a comprehensive treatment plan. Switching Between SL Tab and SL Film: Start on the same dosage as the previously administered product, then adjust dose PRN. Hepatic Impairment: Adjust dose and observe for precipitated opioid withdrawal. Refer to PI for switching between SL film strengths. Elderly: Start at lower end of dosing range.

HOW SUPPLIED: Film, SL: (Buprenorphine-Naloxone) 2mg-0.5mg, 4mg-1mg, 8mg-2mg, 12mg-3mg

WARNINGS/PRECAUTIONS: Not appropriate as an analgesic. Hypersensitivity reactions and anaphylaxis reported. May precipitate opioid withdrawal signs and symptoms if administered before the agonist effects of the opioid have subsided. May impair mental/physical abilities. May produce orthostatic hypotension in ambulatory patients. Caution with myxedema, hypothyroidism, adrenal cortical insufficiency (eg, Addison's disease), CNS depression/coma, toxic psychoses, prostatic hypertrophy, urethral stricture, acute alcoholism, delirium tremens, hepatic impairment, kyphoscoliosis, and in elderly/debilitated patients. Buprenorphine: Potential for abuse. Significant respiratory depression reported. Reestablish adequate ventilation in case of overdose; may use higher doses and repeated administration of naloxone PRN to manage buprenorphine overdose. Accidental pediatric exposure can cause fatal respiratory depression. Chronic use produces physical dependence. Cytolytic hepatitis and hepatitis with jaundice reported; obtain LFTs prior to initiation and periodically thereafter. Neonatal withdrawal reported when used during pregnancy. May elevate CSF pressure; caution with head injuries, intracranial lesions, and other circumstances when CSF pressure may be increased. May produce miosis.

S

May increase intracholedochal pressure; caution with biliary tract dysfunction. May obscure the diagnosis or clinical course of patients with acute abdominal conditions.

ADVERSE REACTIONS: Oral hypoesthesia, constipation, glossodynia, oral mucosal erythema, vomiting, intoxication, disturbance in attention, palpitations, insomnia, withdrawal syndrome, hyperhidrosis, blurred vision.

INTERACTIONS: May cause respiratory depression, coma, and death with benzodiazepines or other CNS depressants (eg, alcohol). General anesthetics, opioid analgesics, benzodiazepines, phenothiazines, other tranquilizers, sedative/hypnotics, or other CNS depressants may increase CNS depression; consider dose reduction of 1 or both agents. Concomitant use with CYP3A4 inhibitors (eg, azole antifungals, macrolides, HIV protease inhibitors) may require dose reduction of 1 or both agents, and monitoring. Monitor for signs and symptoms of opioid withdrawal with CYP3A4 inducers (eg, efavirenz, phenobarbital, carbamazepine, phenytoin, rifampicin). Monitor dose if non-nucleoside reverse transcriptase inhibitors are added to treatment regimen. Some antiretroviral protease inhibitors with CYP3A4 inhibitory activity (eg, nelfinavir, lopinavir/ritonavir, ritonavir) have little effect on pharmacokinetics. Increased levels and sedation with atazanavir and atazanavir/ritonavir; consider dose reduction of buprenorphine. Concomitant use with potentially hepatotoxic drugs and ongoing injecting drug use may contribute to hepatic abnormalities. Caution with drugs that act on the CNS.

PREGNANCY: Category C, not for use in nursing.

MECHANISM OF ACTION: Buprenorphine: Partial agonist at the μ-opioid receptor and antagonist at the kappa-opioid receptor. Naloxone: Potent antagonist at the μ-opioid receptor.

PHARMACOKINETICS: Distribution: Plasma protein binding (96% buprenorphine; 45% naloxone); found in breast milk (buprenorphine). **Metabolism:** Buprenorphine: N-dealkylation via CYP3A4 and glucuronidation; norbuprenorphine (major metabolite). Naloxone: Glucuronidation, N-dealkylation, and reduction; naloxone-3-glucoronide (metabolite). **Elimination:** Buprenorphine: Urine (30%), feces (69%); $T_{1/2}$=24-42 hrs. Naloxone: $T_{1/2}$=2-12 hrs.

NURSING CONSIDERATIONS

Assessment: Assess for history of hypersensitivity to drug, debilitation, myxedema, hypothyroidism, acute alcoholism, adrenal cortical insufficiency (eg, Addison's disease), CNS depression or coma, toxic psychoses, prostatic hypertrophy, urethral stricture, delirium tremens, kyphoscoliosis, compromised respiratory function (eg, chronic obstructive pulmonary disease, cor pulmonale, decreased respiratory reserve, hypoxia, hypercapnia, preexisting respiratory depression), preexisting liver enzyme abnormalities, hepatitis B/hepatitis C virus infection, hepatic impairment, head injury, intracranial lesions and other circumstances in which cerebrospinal pressure may be increased, biliary tract dysfunction, acute abdominal conditions, pregnancy/nursing status, and possible drug interactions. Perform LFTs prior to therapy.

Monitoring: Monitor for hypersensitivity reactions, signs/symptoms of precipitated opioid withdrawal, impaired mental/physical ability, orthostatic hypotension, respiratory depression, drug abuse/dependence, cytolitic hepatitis, hepatitis with jaundice, elevation of CSF and intracholedochal pressure, miosis, changes in consciousness levels, and other adverse reactions. Monitor LFTs periodically. Monitor for symptoms related to over-dosing or under-dosing when switching between SL tab and SL film, or when switching between SL film strengths.

Patient Counseling: Warn about danger of self-administration of benzodiazepines and other CNS depressants, including alcohol, while on therapy. Advise that drug contains opioid that can be a target for abuse; keep film in a safe place, protected from theft and children. Instruct to seek medical attention immediately upon pediatric exposure to the drug and to never give the film to anyone else. Inform that drug may impair mental/physical abilities; caution especially during drug induction or dose adjustment and until certain that therapy does not adversely affect mental abilities. Advise to take film qd and to not change dose without consulting physician. Inform that treatment can cause dependence and that withdrawal syndrome may occur upon discontinuation. Counsel that drug may produce orthostatic hypotension in ambulatory individuals. Advise to report to physician all medications prescribed or currently being used. Advise women regarding possible effects during pregnancy and to not breastfeed. Advise to instruct family members that, in event of emergency, the treating physician or staff should be informed that patient is physically dependent on an opioid and that the patient is being treated with SL film.

Administration: SL route. Do not cut, chew, or swallow film. If an additional SL film is necessary, place it on the opposite side from the 1st film in a manner to minimize overlapping. Keep under the tongue until completely dissolved; should not be moved after placement. Refer to PI for information on clinical supervision and unstable patients. **Storage:** 25°C (77°F); excursions permitted to 15-30°C (59-86°F).

SUBSYS
fentanyl (Insys Therapeutics)

> Fatal respiratory depression may occur. Contraindicated in the management of acute or postoperative pain (eg, headache/migraine) and in opioid-nontolerant patients. Death reported upon accidental ingestion in children; keep out of reach of children. Concomitant use with CYP3A4 inhibitors may increase plasma levels, and may cause fatal respiratory depression. Do not convert patients on a mcg-per-mcg basis from any other fentanyl product to Subsys. Do not substitute for any other fentanyl products; may result in fatal overdose. Contains fentanyl with an abuse liability similar to other opioid analgesics. Available only through a restricted program called the Transmucosal Immediate-Release Fentanyl Risk Evaluation and Mitigation Strategy (TIRF REMS) Access program due to risk for misuse, abuse, addiction, and overdose. Outpatients, healthcare professionals who prescribe to outpatients, pharmacies, and distributors must enroll in the program.

THERAPEUTIC CLASS: Opioid analgesic

INDICATIONS: Management of breakthrough pain in adult cancer patients who are already receiving and are tolerant to around-the-clock opioid therapy for underlying persistent cancer pain.

DOSAGE: *Adults:* ≥18 Yrs: Initial: 100mcg. Switching from Actiq to Subsys: Refer to PI for initial dosing recommendations for patients on Actiq. Titrate: May take only 1 additional dose of the same strength for each breakthrough pain episode if pain is not relieved after 30 min. Max: 2 doses for any breakthrough pain episode; wait at least 4 hrs before treating another episode of breakthrough pain. Prescribe 200mcg units if there is a need to titrate to a 200mcg dose. Refer to PI for tabulated titration steps with corresponding dose strengths and units. Patient should have only 1 dose strength available at any time to reduce risk of overdose. Maint: Once titrated to an effective dose, use only 1 dose of the appropriate strength per breakthrough pain episode; limit consumption to ≤4 doses/day. Decrease subsequent doses if signs of excessive opioid effects appear. Only increase dose when single administration of current dose fails to adequately treat the breakthrough pain episode for several consecutive episodes. If >4 breakthrough pain episodes/day are experienced, reevaluate maintenance dose (around-the-clock) used for persistent pain.

HOW SUPPLIED: Spray: 100mcg/spray, 200mcg/spray, 400mcg/spray, 600mcg/spray, 800mcg/spray, 1200mcg/spray, 1600mcg/spray

CONTRAINDICATIONS: Opioid-nontolerant patients, management of acute or postoperative pain (eg, headache/migraine).

WARNINGS/PRECAUTIONS: Avoid use with ≥Grade 2 mucositis unless benefits outweigh potential risks. Increased risk of respiratory depression in patients with underlying respiratory disorders and in elderly/debilitated. May impair mental and/or physical abilities. Caution with chronic obstructive pulmonary disease or preexisting medical conditions predisposing to respiratory depression; may further decrease respiratory drive to the point of respiratory failure. Extreme caution in patients who may be susceptible to intracranial effects of carbon dioxide retention (eg, with evidence of increased intracranial pressure or impaired consciousness). May obscure clinical course of head injuries. Caution with bradyarrhythmias. Avoid use during labor and delivery. Caution with renal/hepatic impairment.

ADVERSE REACTIONS: Respiratory depression, circulatory depression, hypotension, shock, N/V, constipation, somnolence, dizziness, asthenia, dyspnea, anxiety.

INTERACTIONS: See Boxed Warning. Not recommended with an MAOI or within 14 days of discontinuation. Increased depressant effects with other CNS depressants (eg, other opioids, sedatives/hypnotics, general anesthetics, phenothiazines, tranquilizers, skeletal muscle relaxants, sedating antihistamines, alcoholic beverages); adjust dose of fentanyl if warranted. CYP3A4 inducers (eg, barbiturates, carbamazepine, efavirenz, glucocorticoids, modafinil, nevirapine, oxcarbazepine, phenobarbital, phenytoin, pioglitazone, rifabutin, rifampin, St. John's wort, troglitazone) may decrease levels. Respiratory depression may be more likely to occur when given in conjunction with other drugs that depress respiration.

PREGNANCY: Category C, not for use in nursing.

MECHANISM OF ACTION: Opioid analgesic; not established. Known to be μ-opioid receptor agonist; specific CNS opioid receptors for endogenous compounds with opioid-like activity have been identified throughout the brain and spinal cord and play a role in analgesic effects.

PHARMACOKINETICS: Absorption: Absolute bioavailability (76%). Administration of variable doses resulted in different parameters. **Distribution:** V_d=4L/kg; plasma protein binding (80-85%); crosses placenta; found in breast milk. **Metabolism:** Liver and intestinal mucosa via CYP3A4; norfentanyl (metabolite). **Elimination:** Urine (<7%, unchanged), feces (1%, unchanged); $T_{1/2}$=5-12 hrs.

NURSING CONSIDERATIONS

Assessment: Assess for degree of opioid tolerance, previous opioid dose, level of pain intensity, type of pain, patient's general condition and medical status, or any other conditions where treat-

S

ment is contraindicated or cautioned. Assess for intolerance or previous hypersensitivity, renal/hepatic function, pregnancy/nursing status, and possible drug interactions.

Monitoring: Monitor for signs/symptoms of respiratory depression, impairment of mental/physical abilities, bradycardia, drug abuse/addiction, and other adverse reactions. Closely monitor patients with Grade 1 mucositis or hepatic/renal impairment, and monitor elderly for respiratory depression and CNS effects.

Patient Counseling: Inform outpatients to enroll in the TIRF REMS Access program; instruct to sign a patient-prescriber agreement form to confirm understanding. Instruct to properly dispose of consumed units. Instruct not to take medication for acute or postoperative pain, pain from injuries, headache, migraine, or any other short-term pain. Advise to take drug as prescribed and avoid sharing it with anyone else. Instruct to notify physician if breakthrough pain is not alleviated or worsens after taking the medication. Inform that medication use may impair mental/physical abilities; caution against performing activities that require a high level of attention. Advise not to combine with alcohol, sleep aids, or tranquilizers, except if ordered by physician. Instruct to inform physician if pregnant or planning to become pregnant.

Administration: SL route. Refer to PI for proper administration and disposal. **Storage:** 20-25°C (68-77°F); excursions permitted between 15-30°C (59-86°F) until ready to use.

SULAR RX
nisoldipine (Shionogi)

THERAPEUTIC CLASS: Calcium channel blocker (dihydropyridine)

INDICATIONS: Treatment of HTN alone or in combination with other antihypertensive agents.

DOSAGE: *Adults:* Initial: 17mg qd. Titrate: May increase by 8.5mg/week or longer intervals. Maint: 17-34mg qd. Max: 34mg qd. Elderly/Hepatic Dysfunction: Initial: ≤8.5mg/day.

HOW SUPPLIED: Tab, Extended-Release: 8.5mg, 17mg, 25.5mg, 34mg

WARNINGS/PRECAUTIONS: May increase angina or acute myocardial infarction (MI) in patients with severe obstructive coronary artery disease (CAD). May cause hypotension; monitor BP initially or during titration. Caution with heart failure (HF) or compromised ventricular function, especially with concomitant β-blockers. Caution with severe hepatic dysfunction and in the elderly.

ADVERSE REACTIONS: Peripheral edema, headache, dizziness, pharyngitis, vasodilation, sinusitis, palpitations.

INTERACTIONS: Increased levels with cimetidine. Avoid with phenytoin, CYP3A4 inducers or inhibitors, and grapefruit juice. Decreased bioavailability with quinidine.

PREGNANCY: Category C, not for use in nursing.

MECHANISM OF ACTION: Calcium channel blocker (dihydropyridine); inhibits transmembrane influx of Ca^{2+} into vascular smooth muscle and cardiac muscle, resulting in dilation of arterioles and decreased peripheral vascular resistance.

PHARMACOKINETICS: Absorption: Well-absorbed. Absolute bioavailability (5%); T_{max}=9.2 hrs. C_{max} increases up to 245% with high fat meals. **Metabolism:** CYP3A4 via hydroxylation. **Distribution:** Plasma protein binding (>99%). **Elimination:** Urine (60-80%), feces; $T_{1/2}$=13.7 hrs.

NURSING CONSIDERATIONS

Assessment: Assess for CAD, HF, compromised ventricular function, pregnancy/nursing status, and possible drug interactions. Obtain baseline BP and LFTs.

Monitoring: Monitor for increased angina or MI in patients with severe obstructive CAD, and other adverse effects. Monitor BP and LFTs.

Patient Counseling: Instruct to swallow whole on an empty stomach; do not bite, divide, or crush. Instruct to avoid grapefruit juice pre/post dosing. Inform that drug contains tartrazine, which may cause allergic-type reactions, especially in those with aspirin hypersensitivity.

Administration: Oral route. Take on an empty stomach (1 hr ac or 2 hrs pc). Swallow whole; do not bite, divide, or crush. **Storage:** 20-25°C (68-77°F); excursions permitted to 15-30°C (59-86°F). Protect from light and moisture.

SULFAMETHOXAZOLE/TRIMETHOPRIM RX
sulfamethoxazole - trimethoprim (Various)

OTHER BRAND NAMES: Sulfatrim (STI) - Bactrim DS (AR Scientific) - Bactrim (AR Scientific)

THERAPEUTIC CLASS: Sulfonamide/tetrahydrofolic acid inhibitor

INDICATIONS: Treatment of *Pneumocystis jiroveci* pneumonia. Treatment of enteritis and urinary tract infections (UTIs) caused by susceptible strains of microorganisms. (Sus/Tab) Treatment of acute otitis media (pediatric patients), acute exacerbations of chronic bronchitis (AECB) (adults), and traveler's diarrhea (adults) caused by susceptible strains of microorganisms. Prophylaxis against *P. jiroveci* pneumonia in individuals who are immunosuppressed and considered to be at an increased risk of developing *P. jiroveci* pneumonia.

DOSAGE: *Adults:* (Inj) *P. jiroveci* Pneumonia: 15-20mg/kg/day (based on the trimethoprim [TMP] component) given in 3 or 4 equally divided doses q6-8h for up to 14 days. Severe UTIs/Shigellosis: 8-10mg/kg/day (based on the TMP component) given in equally divided doses q6h, q8h, or q12h for up to 14 days (severe UTIs) or 5 days (shigellosis). Max: 60mL/day. (Sus/Tab) UTIs/Shigellosis: Usual: One 800mg-160mg tab or two 400mg-80mg tabs or 4 tsp (20mL) sus q12h for 10-14 days (UTIs) or 5 days (shigellosis). AECB: Usual: One 800mg-160mg tab or two 400mg-80mg tabs or 4 tsp sus q12h for 14 days. *P. jiroveci* Pneumonia: Treatment: 75-100mg/kg sulfamethoxazole (SMX) and 15-20mg/kg TMP/24 hrs given in equally divided doses q6h for 14-21 days. Prophylaxis: One 800mg-160mg tab or 4 tsp sus daily. Traveler's Diarrhea: Usual: One 800mg-160mg tab or two 400mg-80mg tabs or 4 tsp sus q12h for 5 days. Refer to PI for dosing guidelines. (Inj/Sus/Tab) Renal Impairment: CrCl 15-30mL/min: 1/2 the usual regimen. CrCl <15mL/min: Use not recommended.
Pediatrics: ≥2 Months: (Inj) *P. jiroveci* Pneumonia: 15-20mg/kg/day (based on the TMP component) given in 3 or 4 equally divided doses q6-8h for up to 14 days. Severe UTIs/Shigellosis: 8-10mg/kg/day (based on the TMP component) given in equally divided doses q6h, q8h, or q12h for up to 14 days (severe UTIs) or 5 days (shigellosis). Max: 60mL/day. (Sus/Tab) UTIs/Shigellosis/Acute Otitis Media: 40mg/kg SMX and 8mg/kg TMP/24 hrs, given in 2 divided doses q12h for 10 days (UTIs/acute otitis media) or 5 days (shigellosis). *P. jiroveci* Pneumonia: Treatment: 75-100mg/kg SMX and 15-20mg/kg TMP/24 hrs given in equally divided doses q6h for 14-21 days. Prophylaxis: 750mg/m^2/day SMX with 150mg/m^2/day TMP given in equally divided doses bid, on 3 consecutive days/week. Max: 1600mg/day SMX and 320mg/day TMP. Refer to PI for dosing guidelines. (Inj/Sus/Tab) Renal Impairment: CrCl 15-30mL/min: 1/2 the usual regimen. CrCl <15mL/min: Use not recommended.

HOW SUPPLIED: (SMX-TMP) Inj: 80mg-16mg/mL [5mL, 10mL]; Sus: (Sulfatrim) 200mg-40mg/5mL [473mL]; Tab: (Bactrim) 400mg-80mg*, (Bactrim DS) 800mg-160mg* *scored

CONTRAINDICATIONS: Documented megaloblastic anemia due to folate deficiency, history of drug-induced immune thrombocytopenia with use of TMP and/or sulfonamides, and pediatrics <2 months of age. (Inj/Sus) Pregnant and nursing women. (Sus/Tab) Marked hepatic damage, and severe renal insufficiency when renal function status cannot be monitored.

WARNINGS/PRECAUTIONS: Fatalities, although rare, have occurred due to severe reactions, including Stevens-Johnson syndrome, toxic epidermal necrolysis, fulminant hepatic necrosis, agranulocytosis, aplastic anemia, thrombocytopenia, and other blood dyscrasias; d/c at the 1st appearance of skin rash or any sign of adverse reaction. Cough, SOB, and pulmonary infiltrates reported. Do not use for treatment of group A β-hemolytic streptococcal infections. *Clostridium difficile*-associated diarrhea (CDAD) reported; d/c if CDAD is suspected or confirmed. May result in bacterial resistance if used in the absence of proven or suspected bacterial infection or a prophylactic indication. Caution with hepatic/renal impairment, possible folate deficiency (eg, in the elderly, chronic alcoholics, those receiving anticonvulsant therapy, with malabsorption syndrome, and in malnutrition states), severe allergies or bronchial asthma, porphyria, and thyroid dysfunction. Hematological changes indicative of folic acid deficiency may occur in the elderly, or with preexisting folic acid deficiency or kidney failure; effects are reversible by folinic acid therapy. Hemolysis may occur in patients with G6PD deficiency. Cases of hypoglycemia in nondiabetic patients reported rarely. TMP may impair phenylalanine metabolism. AIDS patients may not tolerate or respond to therapy in the same manner as non-AIDS patients; increased incidence of side effects, particularly rash, fever, leukopenia, elevated transaminase values, and hyperkalemia, in AIDS patients being treated for *P. jiroveci* pneumonia; reevaluate therapy if skin rash or any sign of adverse reaction develops. May cause hyperkalemia in patients receiving high dosage of TMP, with underlying disorders of K$^+$ metabolism, with renal insufficiency, or when used concomitantly with drugs known to induce hyperkalemia; closely monitor serum K$^+$. Ensure adequate fluid intake and urinary output during treatment to prevent crystalluria. Slow acetylators may be more prone to idiosyncratic reactions to sulfonamides. D/C if a significant reduction in the count of any formed blood element is noted. Lab test interactions may occur. (Inj) Contains sodium metabisulfite, which may cause allergic-type reactions, including anaphylactic symptoms and life-threatening or less severe asthmatic episodes in certain susceptible people. Contains benzyl alcohol, which has been associated with an increased incidence of neurological and other complications (sometimes fatal) in newborns. Local irritation and inflammation due to extravascular infiltration of the infusion reported; d/c infusion and restart at another site if these occur. (Tab) Severe and symptomatic hyponatremia may occur, particularly in patients treated for *P. jiroveci* pneumonia; evaluation for hyponatremia and appropriate correction is necessary in symptomatic patients to prevent life-threatening complications. Use during pregnancy may be associated with an increased risk of congenital malformations.

ADVERSE REACTIONS: GI disturbances (N/V, anorexia), allergic skin reactions (eg, rash, urticaria).

S

INTERACTIONS: Increased incidence of thrombocytopenia with purpura reported in elderly concurrently receiving certain diuretics, primarily thiazides. May prolong PT with warfarin; caution with anticoagulants. May inhibit the hepatic metabolism of phenytoin; monitor for possible excessive phenytoin effect. May increase methotrexate concentrations. Marked but reversible nephrotoxicity reported with cyclosporine in renal transplant recipients. May increase digoxin levels, especially in the elderly; monitor digoxin levels. Increased SMX levels with indomethacin. Megaloblastic anemia may develop if used in patients receiving pyrimethamine as malaria prophylaxis in doses >25mg/week. May decrease efficacy of TCAs. Potentiates the effect of oral hypoglycemics. Toxic delirium reported with amantadine. Hyperkalemia in elderly patients reported after concomitant use with an ACE inhibitor. (Inj/Tab) Treatment failure and excess mortality reported when used concomitantly with leucovorin for the treatment of HIV positive patients with *P. jiroveci* pneumonia; avoid coadministration during treatment of *P. jiroveci* pneumonia. (Tab) Caution with drugs that are substrates of CYP2C8 (eg, pioglitazone, repaglinide, rosiglitazone), CYP2C9 (eg, glipizide, glyburide), or OCT2 (eg, memantine, metformin).

PREGNANCY: (Inj/Sus) Category C, not for use in nursing. (Tab) Category D, caution in nursing.

MECHANISM OF ACTION: SMX: Sulfonamide; inhibits bacterial synthesis of dihydrofolic acid by competing with para-aminobenzoic acid. TMP: Tetrahydrofolic acid inhibitor; blocks the production of tetrahydrofolic acid from dihydrofolic acid by binding to and reversibly inhibiting the required enzyme, dihydrofolate reductase. Thus, this combination blocks 2 consecutive steps in biosynthesis of nucleic acids and proteins essential to many bacteria.

PHARMACOKINETICS: Absorption: (PO) Rapid. T_{max}=1-4 hrs. (Inj) SMX: C_{max}=46.3mcg/mL. TMP: C_{max}=3.4mcg/mL. **Distribution:** Crosses placenta; found in breast milk. Plasma protein binding (70% [SMX], 44% [TMP]). **Metabolism:** SMX: N_4-acetylation. TMP: 1- and 3-oxides, 3'- and 4'-hydroxy derivatives (major metabolites). **Elimination:** (PO) Urine (84.5% total sulfonamide [30% as free SMX and remaining as N_4-acetylated metabolite], 66.8% free TMP). SMX: $T_{1/2}$=10 hrs. TMP: $T_{1/2}$=8-10 hrs. (Inj) Urine (7-12.7% free SMX, 17-42.4% free TMP, 36.7-56% total SMX). SMX: $T_{1/2}$=12.8 hrs. TMP: Refer to PI for $T_{1/2}$.

NURSING CONSIDERATIONS

Assessment: Assess for hypersensitivity to the drug, megaloblastic anemia, history of drug-induced immune thrombocytopenia, hepatic/renal impairment, folate deficiency, severe allergies, bronchial asthma, G6PD deficiency, porphyria, thyroid dysfunction, underlying disorders of K^+ metabolism, pregnancy/nursing status, and possible drug interactions.

Monitoring: Monitor for hypersensitivity and other fatal reactions, CDAD, folate deficiency, hypoglycemia, hyperkalemia, and other adverse reactions. Monitor hydration status. Perform CBC frequently, and urinalyses with careful microscopic exam and renal function tests. (Inj) Monitor for infusion reactions. (Tab) Monitor for hyponatremia.

Patient Counseling: Counsel that therapy should only be used to treat bacterial, not viral (eg, common cold), infections. Instruct to take exactly ud even if patient feels better early in the course of therapy. Inform that skipping doses or not completing the full course of therapy may decrease effectiveness of treatment and increase bacterial resistance. Instruct to maintain an adequate fluid intake. Inform that diarrhea is a common problem caused by therapy, which usually ends when therapy is discontinued. Instruct to immediately contact physician if watery and bloody stools (with or without stomach cramps and fever) occur, even as late as ≥2 months after having taken the last dose.

Administration: IV/Oral route. (Inj) Administer by IV infusion over 60-90 min; avoid rapid infusion or bolus inj. Dilute in D5W prior to administration. Do not mix with other drugs or solutions. Refer to PI for further preparation and administration instructions. (Sus) Shake well before using. **Storage:** 20-25°C (68-77°F). (Inj) Do not refrigerate. (Sus) Protect from light.

SUMAVEL DOSEPRO   RX
sumatriptan (Zogenix, Inc)

THERAPEUTIC CLASS: $5-HT_{1B/1D}$ agonist

INDICATIONS: Acute treatment of migraine, with or without aura, and acute treatment of cluster headache in adults.

DOSAGE: *Adults:* Administer only to the abdomen or thigh. Max Single Dose: 6mg SQ. Max Dose/24 Hrs: 12mg (doses separated by at least 1 hr). May be given at least 1 hr following a dose of another sumatriptan product. Consider a 2nd dose only if some response to 1st dose is observed. Migraine: May use a lower dose (4mg) if side effects are dose limiting. Elderly: Start at lower end of dosing range.

HOW SUPPLIED: Inj: 4mg/0.5mL, 6mg/0.5mL

CONTRAINDICATIONS: Ischemic coronary artery disease (CAD) (eg, angina pectoris, history of myocardial infarction [MI], documented silent ischemia), coronary artery vasospasm (eg,

Prinzmetal's variant angina), Wolff-Parkinson-White syndrome or arrhythmias associated with other cardiac accessory conduction pathway disorders, history of stroke or transient ischemic attack (TIA), history of hemiplegic/basilar migraine, peripheral vascular disease, ischemic bowel disease, uncontrolled HTN. Recent (eg, within 24 hrs) use of another 5-HT$_1$ agonist, or of ergot-amine-containing or ergot-type medication (eg, dihydroergotamine, methysergide). Concurrent administration or recent use (within 2 weeks) of an MAO-A inhibitor.

WARNINGS/PRECAUTIONS: May cause coronary artery vasospasm. Perform a cardiovascular (CV) evaluation in triptan-naive patients with multiple CV risk factors (eg, diabetes, HTN, smoking, obesity, strong family history of CAD, increased age) prior to therapy; if negative, consider administering 1st dose under medical supervision and obtain ECG immediately following administration. Perform periodic CV evaluation in these patients if on long-term intermittent use. Life-threatening cardiac rhythm disturbances (eg, ventricular tachycardia, ventricular fibrillation leading to death) reported; d/c if these occur. Sensations of tightness, pain, pressure, and heaviness in the precordium, throat, neck, and jaw may occur. Cerebral/subarachnoid hemorrhage, stroke, other cerebrovascular events, noncoronary vasospastic reactions (eg, peripheral vascular ischemia, GI vascular ischemia/infarction, Raynaud's syndrome, splenic infarction) reported. Rule out a vasospastic reaction in patients who experience symptoms/signs suggestive of noncoronary vasospasm reaction following any 5-HT$_1$ agonist use before receiving additional doses. Exclude other potentially serious neurologic conditions before treating headaches in patients not previously diagnosed as migraineurs, and in migraineurs who present with atypical symptoms. May cause transient and permanent blindness and significant partial vision loss. Overuse of acute migraine drugs may lead to exacerbation of headache; detoxification, including withdrawal of the overused drugs and treatment of withdrawal symptoms may be necessary. Serotonin syndrome may occur; d/c if serotonin syndrome is suspected. Significant elevation in BP, including hypertensive crisis, reported; monitor BP. Anaphylaxis, anaphylactoid, and hypersensitivity reactions may occur; caution with history of sensitivity to multiple allergens. Seizures reported; caution with history of epilepsy or conditions associated with a lowered seizure threshold. Reconsider the diagnosis of migraine before giving a 2nd dose if patient does not respond to the 1st dose of therapy. Not recommended for use in patients with severe hepatic impairment. Not indicated for prevention of migraine attacks. Use only if clear diagnosis of migraine or cluster headache has been established. Caution in elderly.

ADVERSE REACTIONS: Inj-site reaction, tingling, warm sensation, burning sensation, feeling of heaviness, pressure sensation, feeling of tightness, numbness, flushing, chest discomfort, weakness, dizziness, neck pain, paresthesia, N/V.

INTERACTIONS: See Contraindications. Serotonin syndrome reported with SSRIs, SNRIs, TCAs, or MAOIs.

PREGNANCY: Category C, not for use in nursing.

MECHANISM OF ACTION: 5-HT$_{1B/1D}$ agonist; thought to be due to the agonist effects at the 5-HT$_{1B/1D}$ receptors on intracranial blood vessels (including arteriovenous anastomoses) and sensory nerves of the trigeminal system, which result in cranial vessel constriction and inhibition of proinflammatory neuropeptide release.

PHARMACOKINETICS: Absorption: Bioavailability (97%); C$_{max}$=71.9ng/mL (thigh), 78.6ng/mL (abdomen); T$_{max}$=12 min. **Distribution:** (Healthy) Plasma protein binding (14-21%). **Elimination:** T$_{1/2}$=103 min (thigh), 102 min (abdomen).

NURSING CONSIDERATIONS

Assessment: Assess for CV disease, HTN, hemiplegic or basilar migraine, hypersensitivity to drug, hepatic impairment, any other conditions where treatment is contraindicated or cautioned, pregnancy/nursing status, and possible drug interactions. Perform CV evaluation with multiple CV risk factors. Confirm diagnosis of migraine or cluster headache and exclude other potentially serious neurological conditions prior to therapy.

Monitoring: Monitor for signs/symptoms of cardiac events (eg, coronary vasospasm, acute MI, arrhythmia, ECG changes), cerebrovascular events (eg, hemorrhage, stroke, TIA), noncoronary vasospastic reactions, blindness, vision loss, serotonin syndrome, anaphylactic/anaphylactoid/hypersensitivity reactions, HTN, seizures, and other adverse reactions. Perform periodic CV evaluation in patients on long-term intermittent use with risk factors for CAD. Reassess diagnosis if clinical response does not occur following 1st dose of therapy.

Patient Counseling: Inform that therapy may cause CV side effects and anaphylactic/anaphylactoid reactions. Instruct to seek medical attention if signs/symptoms of chest pain, SOB, irregular heartbeat, significant rise in BP, weakness, and slurring of speech occur. Inform that use of acute migraine drugs for ≥10 days/month may lead to an exacerbation of headache; encourage to record headache frequency and drug use (eg, by keeping a headache diary). Inform about the risk of serotonin syndrome, particularly during combined use with SSRIs, SNRIs, TCAs, and MAOIs. Inform that drug may cause somnolence and dizziness; instruct to evaluate ability to perform complex tasks during migraine attacks and after administration of drug. Inform that medication should not be used during pregnancy and instruct to notify physician if breastfeeding or plan to breastfeed. Instruct on proper use of product and to avoid IM or IV use. Instruct to use inj sites

S

on the abdomen (but not within 2 inches of the navel) or thigh with adequate SQ thickness to accommodate penetration of drug into the SQ space, and not on the arms or other areas of the body.

Administration: SQ route. Refer to PI for administration instructions. **Storage:** 20-25°C (68-77°F); excursions permitted between 15-30°C (59-86°F). Do not freeze. Protect from light.

SUPRAX   RX
cefixime (Lupin)

THERAPEUTIC CLASS: Cephalosporin (3rd generation)

INDICATIONS: Uncomplicated urinary tract infections, otitis media, pharyngitis, tonsillitis, acute exacerbation of chronic bronchitis, and uncomplicated gonorrhea (cervical/urethral) caused by susceptible isolates of microorganisms in adults and pediatrics ≥6 months of age.

DOSAGE: *Adults:* Usual: 400mg tab/cap qd or 1/2 tab q12h. Uncomplicated Gonorrhea: 400mg single dose. *Streptococcus pyogenes* Infections: Administer for at least 10 days. Renal Impairment: Refer to PI for dose adjustments.
Pediatrics: >12 Yrs or >45kg: Use adult dose. ≥6 Months: (Sus) 8mg/kg qd or 4mg/kg q12h. (Sus/Tab, Chewable) Refer to PI for Pediatric Dosage Chart. Otitis Media: Treat with chewable tab/sus. *S. pyogenes* Infections: Administer for at least 10 days.

HOW SUPPLIED: Cap: 400mg; Sus: 100mg/5mL [50mL, 75mL, 100mL], 200mg/5mL [25mL, 37.5mL, 50mL, 75mL, 100mL], 500mg/5mL [10mL, 20mL]; Tab, Chewable: 100mg, 150mg, 200mg; Tab: 400mg* *scored

WARNINGS/PRECAUTIONS: Do not substitute tab/cap for chewable tab or sus in the treatment of otitis media. Anaphylactic/anaphylactoid reactions reported. Cross hypersensitivity among β-lactam antibiotics reported; caution in patients with penicillin (PCN) sensitivity. D/C if an allergic reaction occurs. *Clostridium difficile*-associated diarrhea (CDAD) reported; d/c if CDAD suspected or confirmed. Carefully monitor patients on dialysis. May be associated with fall in prothrombin activity; caution in patients with renal/hepatic impairment, poor nutritional state, protracted course of antimicrobial therapy, and those previously stabilized on anticoagulant therapy. May result in bacterial resistance if used in the absence of proven/suspected bacterial infection. Lab test interactions may occur.

ADVERSE REACTIONS: Diarrhea, loose or frequent stools, abdominal pain, nausea, dyspepsia, flatulence.

INTERACTIONS: May increase levels of carbamazepine. Increased PT, with or without bleeding, with anticoagulants (eg, warfarin).

PREGNANCY: Category B, not for use in nursing.

MECHANISM OF ACTION: Cephalosporin (3rd generation); bactericidal, inhibits cell-wall synthesis.

PHARMACOKINETICS: Absorption: (Tab/Sus) 40-50%. C_{max}=2mcg/mL (200mg tab), 3.7mcg/mL (400mg tab), 3mcg/mL (200mg sus), 4.6mcg/mL (400mg sus); T_{max}=2-6 hrs (200mg tab, 400mg tab/sus), 2-5 hrs (200mg sus), 3-8 hrs (400mg cap). **Distribution:** Serum protein binding (65%). **Elimination:** Urine (50% unchanged); $T_{1/2}$=3-4 hrs but may range up to 9 hrs.

NURSING CONSIDERATIONS

Assessment: Assess for previous hypersensitivity to cephalosporins, PCNs, or other drugs. Assess renal/hepatic function, nutritional status, history of antimicrobial or anticoagulants use, pregnancy/nursing status, and for possible drug interactions.

Monitoring: Monitor for signs/symptoms of anaphylatic/anaphylactoid reactions and CDAD. Monitor PT and renal function.

Patient Counseling: Inform that therapy only treats bacterial, not viral (eg, common cold), infections. Instruct to take exactly ud; inform that skipping doses or not completing full course of therapy may decrease effectiveness and increase risk of bacterial resistance. Inform that diarrhea may be experienced as late as 2 or more months after last dose; instruct to contact physician if watery/bloody stools (with/without stomach cramps and fever) occur. Inform that chewable tabs contain phenylalanine.

Administration: Oral route. (Cap/Tab) Take with or without food. (Tab, Chewable) Chew or crush before swallowing. (Sus) Refer to PI for reconstitution directions. **Storage:** 20-25°C (68-77°F). (Sus) After reconstitution, store for 14 days either at room temperature, or under refrigeration; keep tightly closed. Shake well before use. Discard unused portion after 14 days.

Suprep   RX
potassium sulfate - magnesium sulfate - sodium sulfate (Braintree)

THERAPEUTIC CLASS: Bowel cleanser

INDICATIONS: Cleansing of colon as a preparation of colonoscopy in adults.

DOSAGE: *Adults:* Day Prior to Colonoscopy: May consume light breakfast or have only clear liquids. Early in evening prior to colonoscopy, dilute one bottle with 16 oz. of water and drink entire amount. Drink additional 32 oz. of water over the next hour. Day of Colonoscopy: Have only clear liquids until after colonoscopy. Morning of Colonoscopy (10-12 hrs after pm dose): Repeat steps taken on day prior with 2nd bottle. Complete Suprep Bowel Prep Kit and required water at least 1 hr prior to colonoscopy.

HOW SUPPLIED: Sol: (Sodium Sulfate-Potassium Sulfate-Magnesium Sulfate) 17.5g-3.13g-1.6g

CONTRAINDICATIONS: GI obstruction, bowel perforation, gastric retention, ileus, toxic colitis or toxic megaocolon.

WARNINGS/PRECAUTIONS: Hydrate adequately before, during, and after use. If significant vomiting or signs of dehydration occur, consider performing postcolonoscopy tests (eg, electrolytes, creatinine, BUN). Correct electrolyte abnormalities prior to use. Caution with conditions that may increase the risk of fluid/electrolyte disturbances and renal impairment. May increase uric acid levels. Serious arrhythmias reported rarely; caution in patients at increased risk of arrhythmias. Generalized tonic-clonic seizures and/or loss of consciousness reported; caution in patients at increased risk of seizures (eg, hyponatremia, alcohol or benzodiazepine withdrawal). May produce colonic mucosal aphthous ulcerations and ischemic colitis. If suspected, rule out GI obstruction or perforation prior to administration. Caution in patients with impaired gag reflex and patients prone to regurgitation or aspiration; observe during administration. Not for direct ingestion.

ADVERSE REACTIONS: Overall discomfort, abdominal distention, abdominal pain, N/V.

INTERACTIONS: Caution with concomitant use of medications that increase the risk for fluid and electrolyte disturbances or increase the risk of seizures (eg, TCAs), arrhythmias and prolonged QT. Caution with medications that may affect renal function (eg, diuretics, ACE inhibitors, angiotensin receptor blockers, NSAIDs). Concurrent use with stimulant laxatives may increase risk of colonic mucosal ulcerations and ischemic colitis. Absorption of oral medications may not occur if administered within an hr of the start of a Suprep dose.

PREGNANCY: Category C, caution in nursing.

MECHANISM OF ACTION: Bowel cleanser: sulfate salts provide sulfate anions that are poorly absorbed. The osmotic effect of the unabsorbed sulfate anions and the associated cations causes water to be retained within the GI tract.

PHARMACOKINETICS: Absorption: T_{max}=17 hrs (1st dose), 5 hrs (2nd dose). **Elimination:** Feces (primary), $T_{1/2}$=8.5 hrs.

NURSING CONSIDERATIONS

Assessment: Assess for GI obstruction, bowel perforation, or any other conditions where treatment is contraindicated or cautioned. Assess for pregnancy/nursing status, and for possible drug interactions. Obtain baseline electrolytes, creatinine, and BUN in patients with renal impairment. Perform baseline ECGs in patients at risk for arrhythmias.

Monitoring: Monitor for electrolyte abnormalities, cardiac arrhythmias, seizures, loss of consciousness, colonic mucosal ulcerations, ischemic colitis, and aspiration. Perform ECG in patients at increased risk of serious cardiac arrhythmias. Monitor electrolytes, creatinine, and BUN in patients with renal impairment.

Patient Counseling: Instruct to notify physician if patient has difficulty swallowing or is prone to regurgitation or aspiration. Instruct to dilute each bottle with water prior to ingestion and drink additional water ud by instructions. Advise that ingestion of undiluted solution may increase risk of N/V and dehydration. Inform that oral medications may not be absorbed properly if they are taken within 1 hr of starting each dose of Suprep Bowel Kit. Instruct not to take additional laxatives.

Administration: Oral Route. **Storage:** 20-25°C (68-77°F); excursions permitted between 15-30°C (59-86°F).

Sustiva   RX
efavirenz (Bristol-Myers Squibb)

THERAPEUTIC CLASS: Non-nucleoside reverse transcriptase inhibitor

INDICATIONS: In combination with other antiretroviral agents for the treatment of HIV-1 infection in adults and in pediatrics ≥3 months of age and weighing ≥3.5kg.

DOSAGE: *Adults:* Take on an empty stomach at hs. Usual: 600mg qd with a protease inhibitor and/or nucleoside analogue reverse transcriptase inhibitors. Concomitant Voriconazole: Reduce dose to 300mg qd using cap formulation; increase voriconazole maintenance dose to 400mg q12h. Concomitant Rifampin in Patients ≥50kg: Increase dose to 800mg qd. Refer to PI for further dosing modifications when used with certain concomitant therapies.
Pediatrics: ≥3 Months: Take on an empty stomach at hs. Usual: ≥40kg: 600mg qd. 32.5-<40kg: 400mg qd. 25-<32.5kg: 350mg qd. 20-<25kg: 300mg qd. 15-<20kg: 250mg qd. 7.5-<15kg: 200mg qd. 5-<7.5kg: 150mg qd. 3.5-<5kg: 100mg qd.

HOW SUPPLIED: Cap: 50mg, 200mg; Tab: 600mg

CONTRAINDICATIONS: Coadministration with CYP3A substrates for which elevated plasma concentrations are associated with serious and/or life-threatening reactions (eg, dihydroergotamine, ergonovine, ergotamine, methylergonovine, midazolam, triazolam, bepridil, cisapride, pimozide) or St. John's wort.

WARNINGS/PRECAUTIONS: Not for use as monotherapy or added on as a sole agent to a failing regimen. Not recommended with other efavirenz-containing products unless needed for dose adjustment. Serious psychiatric events reported; immediate medical evaluation is recommended if symptoms occur. CNS symptoms reported; dosing at hs may improve tolerability. May impair mental/physical abilities. Skin rash reported; d/c and administer appropriate treatment if severe rash associated with blistering, desquamation, mucosal involvement, or fever develops. Consider alternative therapy in patients who have had a life-threatening cutaneous reaction (eg, Stevens-Johnson syndrome). Consider prophylaxis with appropriate antihistamines before initiating therapy in pediatric patients. Avoid with moderate or severe hepatic impairment and use with caution with mild hepatic impairment and in the elderly. Hepatotoxicity reported; monitor liver enzymes before and during treatment with underlying hepatic disease, marked transaminase elevations, and with other medications associated with liver toxicity, and consider monitoring in patients without preexisting hepatic dysfunction/risk factors. Convulsions reported; caution with history of seizures. Lipid elevations, immune reconstitution syndrome, fat redistribution/accumulation, and autoimmune disorders (eg, Graves' disease, polymyositis, Guillain-Barre syndrome) in the setting of immune reconstitution reported. May cause fetal harm if administered during 1st trimester of pregnancy; avoid pregnancy during use. Use adequate contraceptive measures for 12 weeks after discontinuation.

ADVERSE REACTIONS: Rash, dizziness, N/V, headache, fatigue, insomnia, anxiety, diarrhea, depression, increased ALT/AST levels, hypercholesterolemia, CNS symptoms.

INTERACTIONS: See Contraindications. Avoid with other NNRTIs. Potential additive CNS effects with alcohol or psychoactive drugs. CYP3A substrates, inhibitors, or inducers may alter levels. May alter levels of warfarin and substrates of CYP2C9, 2C19, 3A4, or 2B6. Ritonavir and voriconazole may increase levels. CYP3A inducers (eg, phenobarbital, rifampin, rifabutin), telaprevir, carbamazepine, and anticonvulsants may decrease levels. May increase levels of ritonavir. May decrease levels of amprenavir, atazanavir (avoid combination in treatment-experienced patients), indinavir, lopinavir, saquinavir, maraviroc, raltegravir, boceprevir, telaprevir, carbamazepine, anticonvulsants (monitor levels), bupropion, sertraline, voriconazole, itraconazole, ketoconazole, clarithromycin, rifabutin, diltiazem or other calcium channel blockers, atorvastatin, pravastatin, simvastatin, norgestimate, norelgestromin, levonorgestrel, etonogestrel, immunosuppressants, and methadone. May decrease posaconazole levels; avoid concomitant use unless benefit outweighs risks.

PREGNANCY: Category D, not for use in nursing.

MECHANISM OF ACTION: NNRTI; mediated predominantly by noncompetitive inhibition of HIV-1 reverse transcriptase.

PHARMACOKINETICS: Absorption: T_{max}=3-5 hrs; (600mg qd) C_{max}=12.9µM, AUC=184µM•h.
Distribution: Plasma protein binding (99.5-99.75%). **Metabolism:** Via CYP3A and 2B6 (major) to hydroxylated metabolites with subsequent glucuronidation. **Elimination:** Urine (14-34%, <1% unchanged), feces (16-61%); $T_{1/2}$=40-55 hrs (multiple doses), 52-76 hrs (single dose).

NURSING CONSIDERATIONS

Assessment: Assess for underlying hepatic disease, history of inj drug use/seizures/cutaneous reaction, psychiatric history, hypersensitivity to the drug, pregnancy/nursing status, and possible drug interactions. Assess baseline LFTs and lipid profile (eg, cholesterol, TG).

Monitoring: Monitor for psychiatric events, CNS symptoms, skin rash, convulsions, immune reconstitution syndrome (eg, opportunistic infections), fat redistribution/accumulation, and other adverse reactions. Monitor LFTs during treatment with underlying hepatic disease, marked transaminase elevations, and with other medications associated with liver toxicity, and consider monitoring in patients without preexisting hepatic dysfunction/risk factors. Monitor lipid profile.

Patient Counseling: Inform that therapy is not a cure for HIV-1 infection and illnesses associated with HIV-1 infection may still be experienced. Advise to practice safe sex, use latex or polyurethane condoms, not to share personal items (eg, toothbrush, razor blades), needles or other inj equipment, and not to breastfeed. Advise to take medication every day as prescribed. Inform that CNS symptoms may occur during 1st weeks of therapy. Counsel that rash, psychiatric symptoms, and redistribution/accumulation of body fat may occur. Advise to avoid potentially hazardous tasks if experiencing CNS symptoms. Inform of the potential additive effects of the drug when used concomitantly with alcohol or psychoactive drugs. Instruct to seek medical attention if symptoms of rash and serious psychiatric events occur. Advise to inform physician of any history of mental illness or substance abuse. Counsel to avoid pregnancy while on therapy and to use adequate contraceptive measures for 12 weeks after discontinuation; instruct that barrier contraception must always be used in combination with other methods of contraception. Advise to report use of any prescription, OTC, or herbal products, particularly St. John's wort.

Administration: Oral route. Swallow cap/tab intact with liquid. (Cap) Sprinkle method is recommended for patients who cannot swallow cap/tab; see PI. **Storage:** 25°C (77°F); excursions permitted to 15-30°C (59-86°F).

SUTENT
sunitinib malate (Pfizer)

RX

Hepatotoxicity has been observed; may be severe, and deaths have been reported.

THERAPEUTIC CLASS: Multikinase inhibitor

INDICATIONS: Treatment of GI stromal tumor (GIST) after disease progression on or intolerance to imatinib mesylate, advanced renal cell carcinoma (RCC), and progressive, well-differentiated pancreatic neuroendocrine tumors (pNET) with unresectable locally advanced or metastatic disease.

DOSAGE: *Adults:* GIST/RCC: Usual: 50mg qd, on a schedule of 4 weeks on, followed by 2 weeks off. pNET: Usual: 37.5mg qd continuously without a scheduled-off treatment period. Dose interruption and/or dose modification in 12.5mg increments or decrements is recommended based on individual safety and tolerability. Max: 50mg/day (Phase 3 pNET Study). Concomitant Strong CYP3A4 Inhibitors: Consider dose reduction to a minimum of 37.5mg (GIST/RCC) or 25mg (pNET) qd. Concomitant CYP3A4 Inducers: Consider dose increase. Max: 87.5mg (GIST/RCC) or 62.5mg (pNET) qd.

HOW SUPPLIED: Cap: 12.5mg, 25mg, 50mg

WARNINGS/PRECAUTIONS: Interrupt therapy for Grade 3/4 hepatic adverse events; d/c if no resolution. Do not restart treatment if subsequently experiencing severe changes in LFTs or have other signs and symptoms of liver failure. May cause fetal harm; avoid pregnancy. Cardiovascular (CV) events, including decline in left ventricular ejection fraction (LVEF) to below lower limit of normal, reported; d/c in the presence of clinical manifestations of congestive heart failure, and interrupt and/or reduce dose with ejection fraction <50% and >20% below baseline. Dose-dependent QT interval prolongation and torsades de pointes observed; caution with history of QT interval prolongation, or preexisting cardiac disease, bradycardia, or electrolyte disturbances. Monitor for HTN and treat PRN; suspend temporarily in cases of severe HTN. Hemorrhagic events, including tumor-related hemorrhage, reported. Serious, sometimes fatal GI complications including GI perforation may occur rarely with intra-abdominal malignancies. Osteonecrosis of the jaw (ONJ) reported; exposure to risk factors (eg, dental disease) may increase the risk of ONJ. Tumor lysis syndrome (TLS) reported; closely monitor patients presenting with a high tumor burden prior to treatment and treat as clinically indicated. Observe closely for signs/symptoms of thyroid dysfunction, including hypo/hyperthyroidism and thyroiditis; monitor thyroid function and treat if signs/symptom/ occur. Cases of impaired wound healing reported; interrupt temporarily if patient will undergo major surgical procedures. Monitor for adrenal insufficiency in patients with stress, trauma, or severe infection.

ADVERSE REACTIONS: Hepatotoxicity, fatigue, fever, asthenia, diarrhea, N/V, mucositis/stomatitis, abdominal pain, HTN, rash, hand-foot syndrome, skin discoloration, altered taste, anorexia, bleeding.

INTERACTIONS: See Dosage. Caution with antiarrhythmics. Strong CYP3A4 inhibitors (eg, ketoconazole, nefazodone, ritonavir) and grapefruit may increase plasma concentrations; consider dose reduction. CYP3A4 inducers (eg, dexamethasone, phenytoin, rifampin) may decrease plasma concentrations; consider dose increase while monitoring for toxicity. Avoid with St. John's wort. Concomitant use with bisphosphonates may increase the risk of ONJ.

PREGNANCY: Category D, not for use in nursing.

MECHANISM OF ACTION: Multikinase inhibitor; inhibits multiple receptor tyrosine kinases, some of which are implicated in tumor growth, pathologic angiogenesis, and metastatic cancer progression.

PHARMACOKINETICS: Absorption: T_{max}=6-12 hrs. **Distribution:** V_d=2230L; plasma protein binding (95%), (90%, primary active metabolite). **Metabolism:** Liver via CYP3A4. **Elimination:** Feces (61%), urine (16%); (Healthy) $T_{1/2}$=40-60 hrs, 80-110 hrs (primary active metabolite).

NURSING CONSIDERATIONS

Assessment: Assess for cardiac events, electrolyte disturbances, dental disease, high tumor burden, pregnancy/nursing status, and possible drug interactions. Obtain baseline LFTs, LVEF, thyroid function, CBC with platelet count, serum chemistries (eg, phosphate), and urinalysis. Obtain a baseline evaluation of ejection fraction in patients without cardiac risk factors.

Monitoring: Monitor for signs/symptoms of CV events, HTN, hemorrhagic events, ONJ, TLS, adrenal insufficiency, seizures, reversible posterior leukoencephalopathy syndrome, pancreatitis, hepatotoxicity, muscle toxicity, thrombotic microangiopathy and proteinuria, and other adverse reactions. Monitor LFTs, LVEF, ECG, electrolytes (Mg^{+2}, K^+), thyroid function, CBC with platelet count, and serum chemistries (eg, phosphate).

Patient Counseling: Inform about the most commonly reported GI disorders and other adverse events that may occur. Advise that depigmentation of the hair or skin, and other possible dermatologic effects (eg, dryness, thickness or cracking of skin, blister or rash on the palms of the hands and soles of the feet) may occur during treatment. Advise patients to consider a dental examination and appropriate preventive dentistry prior to treatment. Advise to avoid invasive dental procedures if previously or concomitantly taking bisphosphonates. Advise to inform physician of all concomitant medications, including OTC medications and dietary supplements. Inform of pregnancy risks; advise women of childbearing potential to avoid becoming pregnant.

Administration: Oral route. Take with or without food. **Storage:** 25°C (77°F); excursions permitted to 15-30°C (59-86°F).

SYMBICORT   RX
formoterol fumarate dihydrate - budesonide (AstraZeneca)

> Long-acting β₂-adrenergic agonists (LABAs), such as formoterol, increase the risk of asthma-related death. LABAs may increase the risk of asthma-related hospitalization in pediatric patients and adolescents. Use only for patients not adequately controlled on a long-term asthma-control medication or whose disease severity clearly warrants initiation of treatment with both inhaled corticosteroids and LABA. Do not use if asthma is adequately controlled on low- or medium-dose inhaled corticosteroids.

THERAPEUTIC CLASS: Beta₂-agonist/corticosteroid

INDICATIONS: Treatment of asthma in patients ≥12 yrs of age. (160mcg-4.5mcg/inh) Maintenance treatment of airflow obstruction in patients with chronic obstructive pulmonary disease (COPD), including chronic bronchitis and emphysema.

DOSAGE: *Adults:* Asthma: 2 inh bid (am and pm, approximately q12h). Initial: Based on severity. Max: 160mcg-4.5mcg/inh bid. Not Responding After 1-2 Weeks of Therapy with 80mcg-4.5mcg/inh: Replace with 160mcg-4.5mcg/inh for better asthma control. COPD: 2 inh (160mcg-4.5mcg/inh) bid.
Pediatrics: ≥12 Yrs: Asthma: 2 inh bid (am and pm, approximately q12h). Initial: Based on severity. Max: 160mcg-4.5mcg/inh bid. Not Responding After 1-2 Weeks of Therapy with 80mcg-4.5mcg/inh: Replace with 160mcg-4.5mcg/inh for better asthma control.

HOW SUPPLIED: MDI: (Budesonide-Formoterol) 80mcg-4.5mcg/inh, 160mcg-4.5mcg/inh [60 inhalations, 120 inhalations]

CONTRAINDICATIONS: Primary treatment of status asthmaticus or other acute episodes of asthma or COPD where intensive measures are required.

WARNINGS/PRECAUTIONS: Not indicated for the relief of acute bronchospasm; take inhaled short-acting β₂-agonists (SABA) for immediate relief. Do not initiate during rapidly deteriorating/potentially life-threatening asthma or COPD. D/C regular use of oral/inhaled SABA when beginning treatment. Cardiovascular (CV) effects and fatalities reported with excessive use; do not use more often or at higher doses than recommended. *Candida albicans* infections of the mouth and pharynx reported; treat with appropriate local or systemic (eg, antifungal) therapy or, interrupt therapy if needed. Lower respiratory tract infections (eg, pneumonia) reported in patients with COPD. Increased susceptibility to infections. May lead to serious/fatal course of chickenpox or measles; avoid exposure and, if exposed, consider prophylaxis/treatment. Caution with active/quiescent tuberculosis (TB); untreated systemic fungal, bacterial, viral, or parasitic infections; or ocular herpes simplex. Deaths due to adrenal insufficiency reported with transfer from systemic to inhaled corticosteroids; if systemic corticosteroids are required, wean slowly from systemic steroid after transferring to therapy. Resume oral corticosteroids during periods of stress or a severe asthma attack if patient was previously withdrawn from systemic corticosteroid. Carefully monitor during withdrawal of oral corticosteroid. Transferring from systemic to inhalation therapy may unmask previously suppressed allergic conditions (eg, rhinitis, conjunctivitis, eczema, arthritis, eosinophilic conditions); monitor for systemic corticosteroid withdrawal effects. Observe carefully for any evidence of systemic corticosteroid effects; caution should be taken in observing patients postoperatively or during periods of stress for evidence of inadequate adrenal response. Reduce dose slowly if hypercorticism or adrenal suppression (including adrenal crisis) appears. May produce paradoxical bronchospasm; d/c immediately and institute alternative therapy. Immediate hypersensitivity reactions (eg, urticaria, angioedema, rash, bronchospasm) may occur. Caution with CV disorders (eg, coronary insufficiency, cardiac arrhythmias, HTN). Decreases in bone mineral density (BMD) reported; caution with major risk factors for decreased bone mineral content (eg, prolonged immobilization, family history of osteoporosis, postmenopausal status, tobacco use, advanced age, poor nutrition). May reduce growth velocity in pediatrics; use lowest effective dose. Glaucoma, increased intraocular pressure (IOP), cataracts, rare cases of systemic eosinophilic conditions, and vasculitis consistent with Churg-Strauss syndrome reported. Caution with convulsive disorders, thyrotoxicosis, diabetes mellitus (DM), ketoacidosis, hepatic impairment, and in patients unusually responsive to sympathomimetic amines. Clinically significant changes in blood glucose and/or serum K⁺ reported. Caution in elderly.

ADVERSE REACTIONS: Nasopharyngitis, headache, upper respiratory tract infection, pharyngolaryngeal pain, sinusitis, influenza, back pain, nasal congestion, stomach discomfort, oral candidiasis, bronchitis, vomiting.

INTERACTIONS: Do not use with other medications containing LABA (eg, salmeterol, formoterol fumarate, arformoterol tartrate); increased risk of CV effects. Caution with ketoconazole, other known strong CYP3A4 inhibitors (eg, ritonavir, nefazodone, telithromycin, itraconazole), and non-K⁺-sparing diuretics (eg, loop, thiazide). Caution with MAOIs or TCAs, or within 2 weeks of discontinuation of such agents. Concomitant use with β-blockers may produce severe bronchospasm in patients with asthma; consider cardioselective β-blockers and administer with caution. Caution with chronic use of drugs that can reduce bone mass (eg, anticonvulsants, oral corticosteroids).

PREGNANCY: Category C, not for use in nursing.

MECHANISM OF ACTION: Budesonide: Corticosteroid; shown to have inhibitory activities on multiple cell types and mediators involved in allergic and nonallergic mediated inflammation. Formoterol: LABA; attributable to stimulation of intracellular adenyl cyclase, that catalyzes the conversion of ATP to cAMP. Increased cAMP levels cause relaxation of bronchial smooth muscle and inhibition of release of mediators of immediate hypersensitivity from cells, especially mast cells.

PHARMACOKINETICS: Absorption: Rapid. Administration of various doses resulted in different pharmacokinetic parameters. **Distribution:** Budesonide: V_d=3L/kg; plasma protein binding (85-90%). Formoterol: Plasma protein binding (RR enantiomer, 46%), (SS enantiomer, 58%). **Metabolism:** Budesonide: Liver (rapid and extensive) via CYP3A4. Formoterol: Liver (direct glucuronidation and O-demethylation) via CYP2D6, CYP2C. **Elimination:** Budesonide: Urine (60%); feces. $T_{1/2}$=2-3 hrs. Formoterol: (Healthy) Urine (62%); feces (24%).

NURSING CONSIDERATIONS

Assessment: Assess use of long-term asthma control medication (eg, inhaled corticosteroids), status asthmaticus, acute asthma episodes, rapidly deteriorating asthma, bronchospasm, known hypersensitivity to any component of drug, risk factors for decreased bone mineral content, CV or convulsive disorders, other conditions where treatment is contraindicated or cautioned, pregnancy/nursing status, and possible drug interactions. Assess use in patients unusually responsive to sympathomimetic amines. Obtain baseline BMD, eye exam, and lung function.

Monitoring: Monitor for localized oral *C. albicans* infections, worsening or acutely deteriorating asthma, development of glaucoma, increased IOP, cataracts, CV/CNS effects, inhalation induced paradoxical bronchospasm, pneumonia, lower respiratory tract in patients with COPD, hypercorticism, adrenal suppression, hypersensitivity reactions, signs of increased drug exposure with hepatic impairment, and other adverse reactions. Monitor lung function, pulse rate, BP, ECG changes, blood glucose, and serum K⁺ levels. Monitor BMD periodically. Monitor growth in children.

Patient Counseling: Inform about increased risk of asthma-related death/hospitalization in pediatrics and adolescents. Instruct not to use to relieve acute asthma symptoms; treat acute symptoms with inhaled SABA for immediate relief. Instruct to notify physician immediately if experiencing decreased effectiveness of inhaled SABA, need for more inhalations of inhaled SABA than usual, or significant decrease in lung function. Instruct not to d/c without physician's guidance. Instruct not to use with other LABA for asthma and COPD. Advise that localized infections with *C. albicans* may occur in the mouth and pharynx. Instruct to contact physician if symptoms of pneumonia develop. Instruct to avoid exposure to chickenpox or measles and to consult physician without delay, if exposed. Inform of potential worsening of existing TB, fungal, bacterial, viral, or parasitic infections, or ocular herpes simplex. Inform about risks of hypercorticism and adrenal suppression, decreased BMD, cataracts or glaucoma, and reduced growth velocity in pediatric patients. Instruct to taper slowly from systemic corticosteroids if transferring to

S

budesonide-formoterol. Inform of adverse effects associated with β_2-agonists (eg, palpitations, chest pain, rapid HR, tremor, nervousness).

Administration: Oral inhalation route. After inhalation, rinse mouth with water without swallowing. Shake well for 5 sec before use. Refer to PI for proper priming and administration. **Storage:** 20-25°C (68-77°F). Store with mouthpiece down. Contents under pressure; do not puncture, incinerate, or store near heat or open flame. Discard when labeled number of inhalations have been used or within 3 months after removal from pouch.

SYMBYAX RX
fluoxetine HCl - olanzapine (Lilly)

> Antidepressants increased the risk of suicidal thinking and behavior (suicidality) in children, adolescents, and young adults in short-term studies of major depressive disorder (MDD) and other psychiatric disorders. Monitor and observe closely for clinical worsening, suicidality, or unusual changes in behavior in patients who are started on antidepressant therapy. Elderly patients with dementia-related psychosis treated with antipsychotic drugs are at an increased risk of death; most deaths appeared to be cardiovascular (eg, heart failure, sudden death) or infectious (eg, pneumonia) in nature. Not approved for use in pediatrics or for the treatment of patients with dementia-related psychosis.

THERAPEUTIC CLASS: Selective serotonin reuptake inhibitor/thienobenzodiazepine

INDICATIONS: Acute treatment of depressive episodes associated with bipolar I disorder and treatment-resistant depression (MDD patients who do not respond to 2 separate trials of different antidepressants of adequate dose and duration in the current episode) in adults.

DOSAGE: *Adults:* Depressive Episodes Associated with Bipolar I Disorder/Treatment-Resistant Depression: Initial: 6mg-25mg qpm. Dosing Range: Depressive Episodes Associated with Bipolar I Disorder: 6mg-12mg (olanzapine) and 25mg-50mg (fluoxetine). Treatment-Resistant Depression: 6mg-18mg (olanzapine) and 25mg-50mg (fluoxetine). Max: 18mg-75mg. Hypotension Risk/Hepatic Impairment/Slow Metabolizers/Olanzapine-Sensitive: Initial: 3mg-25mg to 6mg-25mg qpm. Titrate: Increase cautiously. Switching to/from an MAOI: Allow at least 14 days between discontinuation of an MAOI and initiation of treatment, and allow at least 5 weeks between discontinuation of treatment and initiation of an MAOI. Refer to PI for use with other MAOIs (eg, linezolid, methylene blue) and for elderly dosing.

HOW SUPPLIED: Cap: (Olanzapine-Fluoxetine): 3mg-25mg, 6mg-25mg, 6mg-50mg, 12mg-25mg, 12mg-50mg

CONTRAINDICATIONS: Use of an MAOI for psychiatric disorders either concomitantly or within 5 weeks of stopping treatment. Treatment within 14 days of stopping an MAOI for psychiatric disorders. Starting treatment in patients being treated with other MAOIs (eg, linezolid or IV methylene blue). Concomitant use with pimozide or thioridazine.

WARNINGS/PRECAUTIONS: Neuroleptic malignant syndrome (NMS) reported; d/c if symptoms occur and instill intensive symptomatic treatment and monitoring. May cause hyperglycemia; caution in patients with diabetes mellitus (DM) or borderline increased blood glucose levels. Hyperlipidemia, weight gain, and hyperprolactinemia reported. Serotonin syndrome reported; d/c immediately and initiate supportive symptomatic treatment. Anaphylactoid and pulmonary reactions reported; d/c if unexplained allergic reaction occurs. May increase precipitation of a manic episode. Tardive dyskinesia (TD) may develop; consider discontinuation if signs and symptoms appear. May induce orthostatic hypotension. Leukopenia, neutropenia, and agranulocytosis reported; d/c at 1st sign of clinically significant decline in WBC without causative factors or if severe neutropenia (absolute neutrophil count <1000/mm³) develops. May cause esophageal dysmotility and aspiration. Not approved for treatment of patients with Alzheimer's disease. Seizures reported; caution with conditions that potentially lower the seizure threshold. May increase risk of bleeding reactions. Hyponatremia reported; consider discontinuation in patients with symptomatic hyponatremia. May impair physical/mental abilities. May disrupt body's ability to reduce core body temperature; caution with conditions that may elevate core temperature (eg, strenuous exercise, extreme heat exposure, dehydration). Caution with clinically significant prostatic hypertrophy, narrow-angle glaucoma, history of paralytic ileus or related conditions, cardiac patients, diseases or conditions affecting hemodynamic responses, hepatic impairment, and in the elderly. Avoid abrupt withdrawal.

ADVERSE REACTIONS: Asthenia, somnolence, weight gain, increased appetite, disturbance in attention, peripheral edema, tremor, dry mouth, arthralgia, blurred vision, sedation, fatigue, flatulence, restlessness, hypersomnia.

INTERACTIONS: See Contraindications. Caution with CNS-active drugs, hepatotoxic drugs, and anticholinergic drugs. May enhance effects of certain antihypertensives. May potentiate orthostatic hypotension with diazepam and alcohol. May cause serotonin syndrome with other serotonergic drugs (eg, triptans, tramadol, St. John's wort) and with drugs that impair metabolism of serotonin; d/c immediately if this occurs. Increased risk of bleeding with aspirin, NSAIDs, warfarin, and other anticoagulants. Olanzapine: May antagonize effects of levodopa and dopamine agonists. Inducers of CYP1A2 or glucuronyl transferase (eg, carbamazepine, omeprazole, rifampin) may increase clearance. CYP1A2 inhibitors (eg, fluvoxamine, some fluoroquinolones) may decrease clearance. Fluoxetine: May increase levels of TCAs (eg, imipramine, desipramine). May cause lithium toxicity; monitor lithium levels. Increased risk of hyponatremia with diuretics. Caution with CYP2D6 substrates, including antidepressants (eg, TCAs), antipsychotics (eg, phenothiazines, most atypicals), vinblastine, and antiarrhythmics (eg, propafenone, flecainide). May increase levels of phenytoin, carbamazepine, haloperidol, clozapine, and alprazolam. May cause a shift in plasma concentration with drugs that are tightly bound to protein (eg, warfarin, digitoxin), resulting in an adverse effect. May prolong $T_{1/2}$ of diazepam. Rare reports of prolonged seizures with combined use of electroconvulsive therapy.

PREGNANCY: Category C, not for use in nursing.

MECHANISM OF ACTION: SSRI/Thienobenzodiazepine; unknown. Proposed that activation of serotonin, norepinephrine, and dopamine is responsible for its enhanced antidepressant effect. Fluoxetine: SSRI; inhibits serotonin transport; weak inhibitor of norepinephrine and dopamine transporters. Olanzapine: Thienobenzodiazepine; psychotropic agent with high affinity binding to $5HT_{2a/2c}$, $5HT_6$, D_{1-4}, H_1, and adrenergic $(\alpha)_1$-receptors.

PHARMACOKINETICS: Absorption: Fluoxetine: C_{max}=15-55ng/mL, T_{max}=6-8 hrs. Olanzapine: Well-absorbed; T_{max}=6 hrs. **Distribution:** Found in breast milk. Fluoxetine: Crosses placenta; plasma protein binding (94.5%). Olanzapine: V_d=1000L; plasma protein binding (93%). **Metabolism:** Fluoxetine: Liver (extensive) via CYP2D6; norfluoxetine (active metabolite). Olanzapine: Via direct glucuronidation and CYP450-mediated oxidation; 10-N-glucuronide and 4'-N-desmethyl olanzapine (major metabolites). **Elimination:** Fluoxetine: Kidneys; $T_{1/2}$=1-3 days (acute administration), 4-6 days (chronic administration). Olanzapine: Urine (57%, 7% unchanged), feces (30%); $T_{1/2}$=21-54 hrs.

NURSING CONSIDERATIONS

Assessment: Assess for DM, consequences of weight gain, MDD, mania, CVD, cerebrovascular disease, or any other conditions where treatment is contraindicated or cautioned. Assess for dementia-related psychosis, Alzheimer's disease in the elderly, pregnancy/nursing status, and possible drug interactions. Assess for predisposition to hypotension, hepatic impairment, slow metabolism, and pharmacodynamic sensitivity to olanzapine. Evaluate baseline CBC, FPG, lipid profile, and prolactin levels.

Monitoring: Monitor for signs/symptoms of NMS, serotonin syndrome, TD, clinical worsening, suicidality, unusual changes in behavior, worsening of glucose control, hyperglycemia, hyperlipidemia, weight gain, orthostatic hypotension, mania/hypomania, and other adverse effects. Perform periodic monitoring of FPG, lipid levels, and weight of patient. Perform frequent monitoring of CBC in patients with a history of clinically significant low WBC or drug-induced leukopenia/neutropenia. In patients with clinically significant neutropenia, monitor for fever or other signs/symptoms of infection.

Patient Counseling: Inform about risks and benefits of therapy. Advise patient, family, and caregivers to be alert for signs of behavior changes, worsening of depression, suicidal ideation, signs/symptoms of NMS, symptoms of hyperglycemia, hyponatremia, weight gain, and orthostatic hypotension; notify physician if these and other adverse reactions occur. Counsel to seek medical care immediately if rash, hives, or any increased or unusual bruising or bleeding develops. Counsel that drug may impair physical/mental abilities and to use caution when operating hazardous machinery, including automobiles. Advise regarding appropriate care in avoiding overheating and dehydration and to notify physician if they become severely ill or develop symptoms of dehydration. Instruct to notify physician if taking other drugs, pregnant, or planning to become pregnant. Instruct to avoid breastfeeding and alcohol intake. Counsel to take exactly as prescribed; instruct to continue even if symptoms improve.

Administration: Oral route. **Storage:** 25°C (77°F); excursions permitted to 15-30°C (59-86°F). Keep tightly closed; protect from moisture.

SYNERA   RX
tetracaine - lidocaine (Galen)

THERAPEUTIC CLASS: Local anesthetic

INDICATIONS: For use on intact skin to provide local dermal analgesia for superficial venous access and superficial dermatological procedures (eg, excision, electrodessication, shave biopsy of skin lesions).

DOSAGE: *Adults:* Venipuncture or IV Cannulation: Apply to intact skin for 20-30 min prior to procedure. Superficial Dermatological Procedures: Apply to intact skin for 30 min prior to procedure. Simultaneous or sequential application of multiple patches is not recommended; application of 1 additional patch at a new location to facilitate venous access is acceptable after a failed attempt.
Pediatrics: ≥3 Yrs: Venipuncture or IV Cannulation: Apply to intact skin for 20-30 min prior to

procedure. Superficial Dermatological Procedure: Apply to intact skin for 30 min prior to procedure. Simultaneous or sequential application of multiple (>2) patches is not recommended; application of 1 additional patch at a new location to facilitate venous access is acceptable after a failed attempt.

HOW SUPPLIED: Patch: (Lidocaine-Tetracaine) 70mg-70mg

CONTRAINDICATIONS: Known hypersensitivity to amide- or ester-type anesthetics or para-aminobenzoic acid (PABA).

WARNINGS/PRECAUTIONS: If irritation/burning sensation occurs during application, remove patch. Avoid contact with the eyes; if contact occurs, immediately wash out the eye with water or saline and protect the eye until sensation returns. Not recommended for use on mucous membranes or on areas with a compromised skin barrier. Application to broken or inflamed skin may result in toxic blood concentrations from increased absorption. Integrated heating component contains iron powder; remove patch before undergoing magnetic resonance imaging. Methemoglobinemia may occur; increased risk in patients with congenital or idiopathic methemoglobinemia, very young patients, or patients with G6PD deficiency. Allergic/anaphylactoid reactions may occur. Use with caution in patients who may be more sensitive to the systemic effects of lidocaine and tetracaine (eg, acutely ill, debilitated). Increased risk of toxicity in patients with severe hepatic disease or pseudocholinesterase deficiency.

ADVERSE REACTIONS: Local erythema/blanching/edema.

INTERACTIONS: Additive and potentially synergistic systemic toxic effects with Class I antiarrhythmics (eg, tocainide, mexiletine); use with caution. When used concomitantly with other products containing local anesthetic agents, consider the amount absorbed from all formulations due to additive and potentially synergistic systemic toxic effects. Increased risk for developing methemoglobinemia with drugs associated with drug-induced methemoglobinemia (eg, sulfonamides, acetaminophen, acetanilide, aniline dyes, benzocaine, chloroquine, dapsone, naphthalene, nitrates and nitrites, nitrofurantoin, nitroglycerin, nitroprusside, pamaquine, para-aminosalicylic acid, phenacetin, phenobarbital, phenytoin, primaquine, quinine).

PREGNANCY: Category B, caution in nursing.

MECHANISM OF ACTION: Lidocaine: Amide-type local anesthetic. Tetracaine: Ester-type local anesthetic. Both drugs block Na^+ channels required for the initiation and conduction of neuronal impulses, resulting in local anesthesia.

PHARMACOKINETICS: Absorption: Lidocaine: C_{max}=1.7ng/mL (adults), 63ng/mL (pediatrics); T_{max}=1.7 hrs (adults). Tetracaine: C_{max}<0.9ng/mL (adults), 65ng/mL (pediatrics). **Distribution:** Lidocaine: V_d=0.8-1.3L/kg (IV); plasma protein binding (75%); found in breast milk; crosses placenta. **Metabolism:** Lidocaine: Liver (rapid) by N-deethylation via CYP1A2 (primary) and CYP3A4 (minor); monoethylglycinexylidide, glycinexylidide (active metabolites). Tetracaine: Rapid hydrolysis by plasma esterases; PABA and diethylaminoethanol (primary metabolites). **Elimination:** Lidocaine: Urine (>98%; <10% unchanged [adults]); $T_{1/2}$=1.8 hrs (IV).

NURSING CONSIDERATIONS

Assessment: Assess for hypersensitivity to drug, local anesthetics of the amide- or ester-type, or PABA, congenital or idiopathic methemoglobinemia, G6PD deficiency, acute illness, debilitation, hepatic disease, pseudocholinesterase deficiency, pregnancy/nursing status, and possible drug interactions.

Monitoring: Monitor for methemoglobinemia, allergic/anaphylactoid reactions, toxicity, irritation, burning sensation, and other adverse reactions.

Patient Counseling: Instruct to avoid contact with the eyes. If contact occurs, instruct to immediately wash the eye with water or saline and to protect the eye until sensation returns. Advise that drug is not for use on mucous membranes or on areas with broken skin. Instruct to remove patch if skin irritation or a burning sensation occurs during application. Instruct to seek immediate emergency help if signs of an allergic/anaphylactoid reaction occur. Inform that use may lead to diminished or blocked sensation in the treated skin; instruct to avoid inadvertent trauma (rubbing, scratching, exposure to heat or cold) before complete sensation returns. Advise to contact physician if patient does not recall where to apply the patch.

Administration: Topical route. Use immediately after opening the pouch. Refer to PI for handling and disposal instructions. **Storage:** 25°C (77°F); excursions permitted to 15-30°C (59-86°F).

SYNERCID   RX
quinupristin - dalfopristin (Pfizer)

THERAPEUTIC CLASS: Streptogramin

INDICATIONS: Treatment of complicated skin and skin structure infections caused by *Staphylococcus aureus* (methicillin-susceptible) or *Streptococcus pyogenes*.

DOSAGE: *Adults:* Usual: 7.5mg/kg q12h for at least 7 days. Hepatic Cirrhosis (Child-Pugh A or B): May need dose reduction. Administer by IV infusion in D5W solution over a 60-min period. *Pediatrics:* ≥12 Yrs: Usual: 7.5mg/kg q12h for at least 7 days. Hepatic Cirrhosis (Child-Pugh A or B): May need dose reduction. Administer by IV infusion in D5W solution over a 60-min period.

HOW SUPPLIED: Inj: (Dalfopristin-Quinupristin) 350mg-150mg

WARNINGS/PRECAUTIONS: *Clostridium difficile*-associated diarrhea (CDAD) reported; d/c if CDAD is suspected or confirmed. Flush vein with D5W following completion of a peripheral infusion to minimize venous irritation; do not flush with saline or heparin. If moderate to severe venous irritation occurs after peripheral infusion of the drug diluted in 250mL of D5W, consider increasing infusion volume to 500 or 750mL, changing infusion site, or infusing by a peripherally inserted central catheter or central venous catheter. Arthralgia and myalgia, sometimes severe, reported. May promote the overgrowth of nonsusceptible organisms; take appropriate measures if superinfection occurs. Total bilirubin elevation >5X ULN observed.

ADVERSE REACTIONS: Infusion-site reactions (eg, inflammation, pain, edema), N/V, pain, rash, hyperbilirubinemia, arthralgia, myalgia.

INTERACTIONS: May increase plasma concentrations of drugs metabolized by CYP3A4 (eg, astemizole, terfenadine, delavirdine, nevirapine, indinavir, ritonavir, vinca alkaloids [eg, vinblastine], docetaxel, paclitaxel, midazolam, diazepam, dihydropyridines [eg, nifedipine], verapamil, diltiazem, HMG-CoA reductase inhibitors [eg, lovastatin], cisapride, cyclosporine, tacrolimus, methylprednisolone, carbamazepine, quinidine, lidocaine, disopyramide). Coadministration with CYP3A4 substrates that possess a narrow therapeutic window requires caution and monitoring of these drugs (eg, cyclosporine). Avoid with drugs metabolized by CYP3A4 that may prolong QTc interval. May inhibit gut metabolism of digoxin.

PREGNANCY: Category B, caution in nursing.

MECHANISM OF ACTION: Streptogramin antibiotic; components act synergistically on bacterial ribosome. Quinupristin: Inhibits the late phase of protein synthesis. Dalfopristin: Inhibits the early phase of protein synthesis.

PHARMACOKINETICS: Absorption: Quinupristin: C_{max}=3.2mcg/mL, AUC=7.2mcg•hr/mL; Dalfopristin: C_{max}=7.96mcg/mL, AUC=10.57mcg•hr/mL. **Distribution:** V_d=0.45L/kg (quinupristin); 0.24L/kg (dalfopristin). **Metabolism:** Quinupristin: 2 conjugated active metabolites (1 with glutathione; 1 with cysteine); Dalfopristin: 1 nonconjugated active metabolite, via hydrolysis. **Elimination:** Urine: 15% (quinupristin), 19% (dalfopristin), feces (75-77%); $T_{1/2}$=0.85 hrs (quinupristin), 0.70 hrs (dalfopristin).

NURSING CONSIDERATIONS

Assessment: Assess for known hypersensitivity to the drug or prior hypersensitivity to other streptogramins (eg, pristinamycin, virginiamycin), hepatic impairment, pregnancy/nursing status, and possible drug interactions.

Monitoring: Monitor for CDAD, venous irritation, arthralgia, myalgia, superinfection, and other adverse reactions. Monitor total bilirubin levels.

Patient Counseling: Inform about risks/benefits of therapy. Inform that diarrhea is a common problem caused by therapy that usually ends when therapy is discontinued; advise to contact physician immediately if watery and bloody stools (with or without stomach cramps and fever) develop, even as late as ≥2 months after the last dose.

Administration: IV route. Infuse over 60 min; flush only with D5W to minimize venous irritation. Refer to PI for preparation, administration, and compatibility information. **Storage:** 2-8°C (36-46°F). Dilute reconstituted solution within 30 min. Diluted Sol: Stable for 5 hrs at room temperature or for 54 hrs at 2-8°C (36-46°F). Do not freeze.

SYNTHROID   RX
levothyroxine sodium (AbbVie)

Do not use for the treatment of obesity or weight loss; doses within range of daily hormonal requirements are ineffective for weight reduction in euthyroid patients. Serious or life-threatening manifestations of toxicity may occur when given in larger doses, particularly when given in association with sympathomimetic amines.

THERAPEUTIC CLASS: Thyroid replacement hormone

INDICATIONS: Replacement or supplemental therapy in congenital or acquired hypothyroidism of any etiology, except transient hypothyroidism during the recovery phase of subacute thyroiditis. Treatment or prevention of various types of euthyroid goiters, including thyroid nodules, subacute or chronic lymphocytic thyroiditis, multinodular goiter and as an adjunct to surgery and radioiodine therapy for thyrotropin-dependent well-differentiated thyroid cancer.

DOSAGE: *Adults:* Individualize dose. Adjust dose based on periodic assessment of patient's clinical response and laboratory parameters. Give qd, preferably 30 min to 1 hr before breakfast. Take at least 4 hrs apart from drugs that are known to interfere with its absorption. Hypothyroidism: Usual: 1.7mcg/kg/day. >200mcg/day seldom required. >50 Yrs/<50 Yrs with Cardiac Disease: Initial: 25-50mcg/day. Titrate: Increase by 12.5-25mcg increments every 6-8 weeks, PRN until euthyroid. Elderly with Cardiac Disease: Initial: 12.5-25mcg/day. Titrate: Increase by 12.5-25mg increments every 4-6 weeks until euthyroid. Hypothyroidism: Initial: 12.5-25mcg/day. Titrate: Increase by 25mcg/day every 2-4 weeks until TSH level normalized. Secondary (Pituitary) or Tertiary (Hypothalamic) Hypothyroidism: Titrate: Increase until clinically euthyroid and the serum free-T4 level is restored to the upper half of the normal range. Pregnancy: May increase dose requirements. Subclinical Hypothyroidism: Lower doses may be adequate to normalize the serum TSH level (eg, 1mcg/kg/day). TSH Suppression in Well-Differentiated Thyroid Cancer and Thyroid Nodules: Individualize dose based on the specific disease and the patient being treated. Refer to PI for details.

Pediatrics: Individualize dose. Adjust dose based on periodic assessment of patient's clinical response and laboratory parameters. Give qd, preferably 30 min to 1 hr before breakfast. Take at least 4 hrs apart from drugs that are known to interfere with its absorption. Hypothyroidism: Growth/Puberty Complete: Usual: 1.7mcg/kg/day. >12 Yrs (Growth/Puberty Incomplete): 2-3mcg/kg/day. 6-12 Yrs: 4-5mcg/kg/day. 1-5 Yrs: 5-6mcg/kg/day. 6-12 months: 6-8mcg/kg/day. 3-6 months: 8-10mcg/kg/day. 0-3 months: 10-15mcg/kg/day. Infants at Risk for Cardiac Failure: Use lower starting dose (eg, 25mcg/day). Titrate: Increase dose in 4-6 weeks PRN. Infants with Serum T4 <5mcg/dL: Initial: 50mcg/day. Chronic/Severe Hypothyroidism: Children: Initial: 25mcg/day. Titrate: Increase by 25mcg increments every 2-4 weeks until desired effect is achieved. Minimize Hyperactivity in Older Children: Initial: Give 1/4 of full replacement dose. Titrate: Increase on a weekly basis by an amount equal to 1/4 the full recommended replacement dose until the full recommended replacement dose is reached. May crush tab and mix with 5-10mL of water.

HOW SUPPLIED: Tab: 25mcg*, 50mcg*, 75mcg*, 88mcg*, 100mcg*, 112mcg*, 125mcg*, 137mcg*, 150mcg*, 175mcg*, 200mcg*, 300mcg* *scored

CONTRAINDICATIONS: Untreated subclinical (suppressed serum TSH level with normal T3 level and T4 levels) or overt thyrotoxicosis of any etiology, acute myocardial infarction (MI), and uncorrected adrenal insufficiency.

WARNINGS/PRECAUTIONS: Should not be used in the treatment of male or female infertility unless associated with hypothyroidism. Contraindicated in patients with nontoxic diffuse goiter or nodular thyroid disease, particularly in the elderly or with underlying cardiovascular (CV) disease if serum TSH level is already suppressed; use with caution if TSH level is not suppressed and carefully monitor thyroid function. Has narrow therapeutic index; carefully titrate dose to avoid over- or under-treatment. May decrease bone mineral density (BMD) with long-term use; give minimum dose necessary to achieve desired clinical and biochemical response. Caution with CV disorders and the elderly. If cardiac symptoms develop or worsen, reduce or withhold dose for 1 week and then restart at lower dose. Overtreatment may produce CV effects (eg, increase in HR, increase in cardiac wall thickness, increase in cardiac contractility, precipitation of angina or arrhythmias). Monitor patients with coronary artery disease (CAD) closely during surgical procedures; may precipitate cardiac arrhythmias. Caution in patients with diabetes mellitus (DM). Patients with concomitant adrenal insufficiency should be treated with replacement glucocorticoids prior to therapy.

ADVERSE REACTIONS: Fatigue, increased appetite, weight loss, heat intolerance, headache, hyperactivity, irritability, insomnia, palpitations, arrhythmias, dyspnea, hair loss, menstrual irregularities, pseudotumor cerebri (children), slipped capital femoral epiphysis (children).

INTERACTIONS: Concurrent sympathomimetics may increase effects of sympathomimetics or thyroid hormone; may increase risk of coronary insufficiency with CAD. Upward dose adjustments may be needed for insulin and oral hypoglycemic agents. May decrease absorption with soybean flour, cottonseed meal, walnuts, and dietary fiber. May increase oral anticoagulant activity; adjust dose of anticoagulant and monitor PT. May decrease levels and effects of digitalis glycosides. Transient reduction in TSH secretion with dopamine/dopamine agonists, glucocorticoids, octreotide. Decreased thyroid hormone secretion with aminoglutethimide, amiodarone, iodide (including iodine-containing radiographic contrast agents), lithium, methimazole, propylthiouracil (PTU), sulfonamides, and tolbutamide. May increase thyroid hormone secretion with amiodarone and iodide. May decrease T4 absorption with antacids (aluminum and magnesium hydroxides), simethicone, bile acid sequestrants (cholestyramine, colestipol), calcium carbonate, cation exchange resins (kayexalate), ferrous sulfate, orlistat, and sucralfate; administer at least 4 hrs apart. May increase serum thyroxine-binding globulin (TBG) concentrations with clofibrate, estrogen-containing oral contraceptives, oral estrogens, heroin/methadone, 5-fluorouracil, mitotane, and tamoxifen. May decrease serum TBG concentrations with androgens/anabolic steroids, asparaginase, glucocorticoids, and slow-release nicotinic acid. May cause protein-binding site displacement with furosemide (>80mg IV), heparin, hydantoins, NSAIDs (fenamates, phenylbutazone), and salicylates (>2g/day). May alter T4 and T3 metabolism with carbamazepine, hydantoins, phenobarbital, and rifampin. May decrease T4 5'-deiodinase activity with amiodarone, β-adrenergic antagonists (eg, propranolol >160mg/day), glucocorticoids (eg, dexamethasone >4mg/day), and PTU. Concurrent use with tricyclic (eg, amitriptyline) and tetracyclic (eg, maprotiline) antidepressants may increase the therapeutic and toxic effects of both drugs. Coadministration with sertraline in patients stabilized on levothyroxine may result in increased levothyroxine requirements. Interferon-α may cause development of antithyroid microsomal antibodies and transient hypothyroidism, hyperthyroidism, or both. Interleukin-2 has been associated with transient painless thyroiditis. Excessive use with growth hormones (eg, somatropin, somatrem) may accelerate epiphyseal closure. Ketamine may produce marked HTN and tachycardia. May reduce uptake of radiographic agents. Decreased theophylline clearance may occur in hypothyroid patients. Altered levels of thyroid hormone and/or TSH levels with choral hydrate, diazepam, ethionamide, lovastatin, metoclopramide, 6-mercaptopurine, nitroprusside, para-aminosalicylate sodium, perphenazine, resorcinol (excessive topical use), and thiazide diuretics.

PREGNANCY: Category A, caution in nursing.

MECHANISM OF ACTION: Thyroid replacement hormone; mechanism not established. Suspected that principal effects are exerted through control of DNA transcription and protein synthesis.

PHARMACOKINETICS: Absorption: Majority absorbed from jejunum and upper ileum. **Distribution:** Plasma protein binding (>99%); found in breast milk. **Metabolism:** Sequential deiodination and conjugation in the liver (mainly), kidneys, and other tissues. **Elimination:** Urine; feces (approximately 20% unchanged). $T_{1/2}$=6-7 days (T4), ≤2 days (T3).

NURSING CONSIDERATIONS

Assessment: Assess for untreated subclinical or overt thyrotoxicosis, acute MI, uncorrected adrenal insufficiency, CAD, CV disorders, nontoxic diffuse goiter, nodular thyroid disease, DM, hypersensitivity, pregnancy/nursing status, and for possible drug interactions. In patients with secondary or tertiary hypothyroidism, assess for additional hypothalamic/pituitary hormone deficiencies. Assess TSH levels. In infants with congenital hypothyroidism, assess for other congenital anomalies.

Monitoring: Monitor for CV effects. In patients on long-term therapy, monitor for signs/symptoms of decreased BMD. In patients with nontoxic diffuse goiter or nodular thyroid disease, monitor for precipitation of thyrotoxicosis. In adults with primary hypothyroidism, perform periodic monitoring of serum TSH levels. In pediatric patients with congenital hypothyroidism, perform periodic monitoring of serum TSH levels and total or free T4 levels. In patients with secondary and tertiary hypothyroidism, perform periodic monitoring of serum free-T4 levels. Refer to PI for TSH and T4 monitoring parameters. Closely monitor PT if coadministered with an oral anticoagulant.

Patient Counseling: Instruct to notify physician if allergic to any foods or medicines, pregnant or plan to become pregnant, breastfeeding or taking any other drugs, including prescriptions and OTC preparations. Instruct to notify physician of any other medical conditions particularly heart disease, diabetes, clotting disorders, and adrenal or pituitary gland problems. Instruct not to stop or change dose unless directed by physician. Instruct to take on empty stomach, at least 1/2 to 1 hr before eating breakfast. Advise that partial hair loss may occur during the 1st few months of therapy, but is usually temporary. Instruct to notify physician or dentist prior to surgery about levothyroxine therapy. Inform that drug should not be used for weight control. Instruct to notify physician if rapid or irregular heartbeat, chest pain, SOB, leg cramps, headache, or any other unusual medical event occurs. Inform that dose may be increased during pregnancy. Inform that drug should not be administered within 4 hrs of agents such as iron/calcium supplements and antacids.

Administration: Oral route. **Storage:** 25°C (77°F); excursions permitted to 15-30°C (59-86°F). Protect from light and moisture.

TACHOSIL   RX
fibrin sealant (Baxter)

THERAPEUTIC CLASS: Fibrinogen/topical thrombin

INDICATIONS: For use with manual compression as adjunct to hemostasis for use in cardiovascular (CV) surgery when control of bleeding by standard surgical techniques (eg, suture, ligature, cautery) is ineffective or impractical.

DOSAGE: *Adults:* Apply the yellow, active side of the patch to the bleeding area. Determine the number of patches to be applied by the size of the bleeding area; refer to PI for max number of patches. Repeat application if not satisfied with placement of patch, or if bleeding still occurs during or after specified duration of compression.

HOW SUPPLIED: Patch: (Human fibrinogen-Human thrombin) 5.5mg-2.0 U/cm² [9.5cm x 4.8cm, 1ˢ; 4.8cm x 4.8cm, 2ˢ; 3.0cm x 2.5cm, 1ˢ, 5ˢ]

CONTRAINDICATIONS: Intravascular application, known anaphylactic or severe systemic reaction to horse proteins.

WARNINGS/PRECAUTIONS: Not for use in place of sutures or other form of mechanical ligation for the treatment of major arterial/venous bleeding. Thrombosis may occur if exposed intravascularly; for topical use on cardiac and vascular tissue only. Hypersensitivity reactions may occur with repetitive applications. Avoid application to contaminated or infected areas of the body, or in the presence of active infection. Contains collagen, which may adhere to bleeding surfaces. Avoid over-packing when placing into cavities or closed spaces; may cause compression of underlying tissue. Use the least amount of patches necessary to achieve hemostasis; do not pack. Excess patch material can become dislodged and migrate to other areas of the body. Remove unattached pieces of patch. Made from human plasma; may carry risk of transmitting infectious agents (eg, viruses, variant Creutzfeldt-Jakob disease [CJD] agent, CJD agent).

ADVERSE REACTIONS: Atrial fibrillation, pleural effusion, pyrexia.

PREGNANCY: Category C, caution in nursing.

MECHANISM OF ACTION: Fibrinogen/topical thrombin; fibrinogen-thrombin reaction initiates the last step in the cascade of biochemical reactions-conversion of fibrinogen into fibrin monomers that further polymerize to form the fibrin clot. Hemostasis is achieved when the formed fibrin clot adheres the collagen patch to the wound surface, thus providing a physical barrier to bleeding.

NURSING CONSIDERATIONS

Assessment: Assess for hypersensitivity reactions to human blood products or horse proteins, size of the bleeding area, and pregnancy/nursing status.

Monitoring: Monitor for signs/symptoms of thrombosis, hypersensitivity reactions, transmission of infectious agents (eg, viruses, CJD), and other adverse reactions.

Patient Counseling: Advise that drug is made from human blood, and may carry a risk of transmitting infectious agents (eg, viruses, CJD agent). Inform that patch may cause clot formation in blood vessels if exposed intravascularly; advise to consult physician if chest pain, SOB or difficulty speaking/swallowing, or leg tenderness/swelling develop. Instruct to consult physician if symptoms of B19 virus infection appear (fever, drowsiness, chills) followed about 2 weeks later by a rash and joint pain; inform that pregnant women (fetal infection), immunocompromised individuals, or those with increased erythropoiesis (eg, hemolytic anemia) are most seriously affected.

Administration: Transdermal route. Refer to PI for preparation and application of patch. **Storage:** 2-25°C (36-77°F). Does not require refrigeration. Do not freeze. Do not use if package is opened/damaged.

TAMIFLU   RX
oseltamivir phosphate (Genentech)

THERAPEUTIC CLASS: Neuraminidase inhibitor

INDICATIONS: Treatment of acute, uncomplicated illness due to influenza infection in patients ≥2 weeks of age who have been symptomatic for no more than 2 days. Prophylaxis of influenza in patients ≥1 yr of age.

DOSAGE: *Adults:* Treatment: Begin within 2 days of onset of symptoms or following close contact with infected individual, and treat for 5 days. Usual: 75mg bid. Renal Impairment (CrCl 10-30mL/min): 75mg qd. Prophylaxis: Begin after close contact with infected individual and give for at least 10 days. During community outbreak, treat up to 6 weeks (up to 12 weeks if immunocompromised). Usual: 75mg qd. Renal Impairment (CrCl 10-30mL/min): 75mg qod or 30mg qd. Refer to PI for treatment and prophylaxis dosing using oral sus in patients who cannot swallow cap. *Pediatrics:* Treatment: Begin within 2 days of onset of symptoms or following close contact with infected individual, and treat for 5 days. ≥13 Yrs: Usual: 75mg bid. 1-12 Yrs: Usual: ≥40.1kg: 75mg bid. 23.1-40kg: 60mg bid. 15.1-23kg: 45mg bid. ≤15kg: 30mg bid. 2 Weeks-<1 Yr: Usual: 3mg/kg bid. Renal Impairment (CrCl 10-30mL/min): 75mg qd. Prophylaxis: Begin after close contact with infected individual, and give for at least 10 days. During community outbreak, treat up to 6 weeks (up to 12 weeks if immunocompromised). ≥13 Yrs: Usual: 75mg qd. 1-12 Yrs: Usual: ≥40.1kg: 75mg qd. 23.1-40kg: 60mg qd. 15.1-23kg: 45mg qd. ≤15kg: 30mg qd. Renal Impairment (CrCl 10-30mL/min): 75mg qod or 30mg qd. Refer to PI for treatment and prophylaxis dosing using oral sus in patients who cannot swallow cap.

HOW SUPPLIED: Cap: 30mg, 45mg, 75mg; Sus: 6mg/mL [60mL]

WARNINGS/PRECAUTIONS: Not a substitute for early influenza vaccination on an annual basis. Emergence of resistance mutations can decrease drug effectiveness; consider available information on influenza drug susceptibility patterns and treatment effects when deciding whether to use treatment. Anaphylaxis and serious skin reactions (eg, toxic epidermal necrolysis, Stevens-Johnson syndrome, erythema multiforme) reported; d/c and institute appropriate treatment if an allergic-like reaction occurs or is suspected. Neuropsychiatric events (eg, hallucinations, delirium, abnormal behavior), in some cases resulting in fatal outcomes, reported; monitor for abnormal behavior and evaluate risks and benefits of continuing treatment if neuropsychiatric symptoms occur. Serious bacterial infections may begin with influenza-like symptoms or may coexist with or occur during the course of influenza; treatment does not prevent these complications.

ADVERSE REACTIONS: N/V, diarrhea, bronchitis, abdominal pain, dizziness, headache, cough, insomnia, vertigo, fatigue, otitis media, asthma, epistaxis, pneumonia, ear disorder.

INTERACTIONS: Avoid administration of live attenuated influenza vaccine within 2 weeks before or 48 hrs after oseltamivir, unless medically indicated. Probenecid may increase exposure.

PREGNANCY: Category C, caution in nursing.

MECHANISM OF ACTION: Neuraminidase inhibitor; inhibits influenza virus neuraminidase affecting release of viral particles.

PHARMACOKINETICS: Absorption: Readily absorbed from GI tract. Oseltamivir: C_{max}=65ng/mL; AUC_{0-12h}=112ng•hr/mL. Oseltamivir carboxylate: C_{max}=348ng/mL; AUC_{0-12h}=2719ng•hr/mL. **Distribution:** Oseltamivir: Plasma protein binding (42%). Oseltamivir carboxylate: Plasma protein binding (3%); (IV) V_d=23-26L. **Metabolism:** Extensive via hepatic esterases; oseltamivir carboxylate (active metabolite). **Elimination:** Oseltamivir: $T_{1/2}$=1-3 hrs. Oseltamivir carboxylate: Renal (>99%); $T_{1/2}$=6-10 hrs.

NURSING CONSIDERATIONS

Assessment: Assess for drug hypersensitivity, renal impairment, pregnancy/nursing status, and possible drug interactions.

Monitoring: Monitor for signs/symptoms of neuropsychiatric events, anaphylaxis/serious skin reactions, and other adverse reactions.

Patient Counseling: Advise of the risk of severe allergic reactions or serious skin reactions and to d/c and seek immediate medical attention if an allergic-like reaction occurs or is suspected. Advise of the risk of neuropsychiatric events and to contact physician if experiencing signs of abnormal behavior during treatment. Instruct to begin treatment as soon as possible from the 1st appearance of flu symptoms, and as soon as possible after exposure (for prevention). Instruct to take missed doses as soon as remembered, unless next scheduled dose is within 2 hrs, and then to continue at the usual times. Inform that the medication is not a substitute for flu vaccination. Inform that oral sus delivers 2g sorbitol/75mg dose; this is above the daily max limit of sorbitol for patients with hereditary fructose intolerance and may cause dyspepsia and diarrhea.

Administration: Oral route. May be taken with or without food. If oral sus is not available, may open caps and mix with sweetened liquids (eg, chocolate/corn syrup, caramel topping, or light brown sugar [dissolved in water]). Refer to PI for preparation of oral sus and emergency compounding of oral sus from caps. **Storage:** Cap/Dry Powder: 25°C (77°F); excursions permitted to 15-30°C (59-86°F). Constituted Sus: 2-8°C (36-46°F) for up to 17 days, or 25°C (77°F) for up to 10 days with excursions permitted to 15-30°C (59-86°F). Do not freeze.

TAMOXIFEN   RX
tamoxifen citrate (Various)

> Serious and life-threatening uterine malignancies (endometrial adenocarcinoma and uterine sarcoma), stroke, and pulmonary embolism (PE) reported in the risk-reduction setting; some of these events were fatal. Discuss the potential benefits versus the potential risks of these serious events with women at high-risk for breast cancer and women with ductal carcinoma in situ (DCIS) considering therapy for breast cancer risk reduction.

THERAPEUTIC CLASS: Antiestrogen

INDICATIONS: Treatment of metastatic breast cancer in women and men. Treatment of node-positive or axillary node-negative breast cancer in women following total or segmental mastectomy, axillary dissection, and breast irradiation. To reduce risk of invasive breast cancer in women with DCIS following breast surgery and radiation. To reduce incidence of breast cancer in high-risk women (those at least 35 yrs of age with a 5-yr predicted risk of breast cancer ≥1.67%, as calculated by the Gail Model).

DOSAGE: *Adults:* Breast Cancer Treatment: Usual: 20-40mg/day. Give dosages >20mg/day in divided doses (am and pm). Breast Cancer Incidence Reduction in High-Risk Women/DCIS: 20mg qd for 5 yrs.

HOW SUPPLIED: Tab: 10mg, 20mg

CONTRAINDICATIONS: (Breast Cancer Incidence Reduction in High-Risk Women/Women with DCIS) Women who require coumarin-type anticoagulant therapy or with history of deep vein thrombosis (DVT) or PE.

WARNINGS/PRECAUTIONS: Hypercalcemia reported in patients with bone metastases; take appropriate measures if hypercalcemia occurs, and, if severe, d/c therapy. Increased incidence of uterine malignancies reported; promptly evaluate any patient receiving or who has previously received therapy who reports abnormal vaginal bleeding. Perform annual gynecological examinations in patients receiving or who have previously received therapy. Increased incidence of endometrial changes, including hyperplasia and polyps, reported. Endometriosis, uterine fibroids, ovarian cysts (in premenopausal patients with advanced breast cancer), and menstrual irregularity or amenorrhea reported. Increased incidence of thromboembolic events (eg, DVT, PE) reported; for treatment of breast cancer, carefully consider risks and benefits of therapy with history of thromboembolic events. Malignant and nonmalignant (eg, changes in liver enzyme levels) effects on the liver, secondary primary tumors (non-uterine), ocular disturbances, increased incidence of cataracts and risk of having cataract surgery, thrombocytopenia, leukopenia, neutropenia, and pancytopenia reported. May cause fetal harm. Hyperlipidemias reported; may consider periodic monitoring of plasma TG and cholesterol in patients with preexisting hyperlipidemias.

ADVERSE REACTIONS: Uterine malignancies, stroke, PE, hot flashes, vaginal discharge, fatigue/asthenia, weight loss, flush, skin changes, N/V, irregular menses, fluid retention, pain.

INTERACTIONS: See Contraindications. For treatment of breast cancer, carefully monitor patient's PT with coumarin-type anticoagulants. Increased risk of thromboembolic events with cytotoxic agents or with chemotherapy. May reduce letrozole concentrations. Reduced concentrations with rifampin, aminoglutethimide, and phenobarbital. Medroxyprogesterone reduces concentrations of N-desmethyl tamoxifen (active metabolite). Increased levels with bromocriptine. May reduce anastrozole concentrations; avoid with anastrozole. Erythromycin, cyclosporine, nifedipine, and diltiazem may inhibit metabolism.

PREGNANCY: Category D, not for use in nursing.

MECHANISM OF ACTION: Nonsteroidal antiestrogen; competes with estrogen for binding sites in target tissues such as breast.

PHARMACOKINETICS: Absorption: C_{max}=40ng/mL, 15ng/mL (N-desmethyl tamoxifen); T_{max}=5 hrs. **Metabolism:** Extensive; N-desmethyl tamoxifen (active metabolite). **Elimination:** Feces; $T_{1/2}$=5-7 days.

NURSING CONSIDERATIONS

Assessment: Assess for history of thromboembolic events, preexisting hyperlipidemias, known hypersensitivity, pregnancy/nursing status, and possible drug interactions.

Monitoring: Monitor for signs/symptoms of uterine malignancies, stroke, thromboembolic events, hypercalcemia, ocular disturbances, and other adverse reactions. Periodically monitor plasma TG and cholesterol levels in patients with preexisting hyperlipidemias, and CBCs, including platelet counts and LFTs. Perform annual gynecological examinations.

Patient Counseling: Inform about potential risks and benefits of treatment. Advise premenopausal women not to become pregnant and to use nonhormonal contraception during therapy and for 2 months after discontinuation if sexually active. Instruct women to seek prompt medical attention if new breast lumps, vaginal bleeding, gynecologic symptoms (eg, menstrual irregularities, changes in vaginal discharge, pelvic pain/pressure), symptoms of leg swelling/tenderness, unexplained SOB, or changes in vision occur.

Administration: Oral route. **Storage:** 20-25°C (68-77°F).

TAPAZOLE   RX
methimazole (King)

THERAPEUTIC CLASS: Thyroid hormone synthesis inhibitor

INDICATIONS: Treatment of hyperthyroidism. To ameliorate hyperthyroidism prior to subtotal thyroidectomy or radioactive iodine therapy. Also indicated when thyroidectomy is contraindicated or not advisable.

DOSAGE: *Adults:* PO: Given in 3 equal doses at 8-hr intervals. Initial: Mild: 15mg/day. Moderately Severe: 30-40mg/day. Severe: 60mg/day. Maint: 5-15mg/day.
Pediatrics: PO: Given in 3 equal doses at 8-hr intervals. Initial: 0.4mg/kg/day. Maint: 1/2 of initial dose.

HOW SUPPLIED: Tab: 5mg*, 10mg* *scored

CONTRAINDICATIONS: Nursing mothers.

WARNINGS/PRECAUTIONS: Can cause fetal harm. Agranulocytosis, leukopenia, thrombocytopenia, and aplastic anemia (pancytopenia) may occur; monitor bone marrow function. D/C with agranulocytosis, aplastic anemia, hepatitis, or exfoliative dermatitis. Fulminant hepatitis, hepatic necrosis, and encephalopathy reported; d/c with liver abnormality, including transaminases >3X ULN. Monitor thyroid function periodically. May cause hypoprothrombinemia and bleeding; monitor PT.

ADVERSE REACTIONS: Agranulocytosis, granulocytopenia, thrombocytopenia, aplastic anemia, drug fever, lupus-like syndrome, insulin autoimmune syndrome, hepatitis, periarteritis, hypopro-thrombinemia, skin rash, urticaria, N/V, epigastric distress.

INTERACTIONS: May potentiate oral anticoagulants. β-blockers, digitalis, and theophylline may need dose reduction when patient becomes euthyroid. Caution with other drugs that cause agranulocytosis.

PREGNANCY: Category D, contraindicated in nursing.

MECHANISM OF ACTION: Inhibits synthesis of thyroid hormones.

PHARMACOKINETICS: Absorption: Readily absorbed (GI tract). **Distribution:** Crosses placenta and found in breast milk. **Elimination:** Urine.

NURSING CONSIDERATIONS

Assessment: Assess for drug hypersensitivity, pregnancy/nursing status, and possible drug interactions.

Monitoring: Monitor for signs of illness (eg, fever, sore throat, malaise, skin eruptions, headache), and hepatic dysfunction (eg, anorexia, upper quadrant pain). Monitor CBC, LFTs, PT, and bone marrow function. Monitor thyroid function periodically.

Patient Counseling: Instruct to inform physician if pregnant/nursing or planning to become pregnant. Instruct to report signs/symptoms of illness (eg, fever, general malaise, sore throat) to physician.

Administration: Oral route. **Storage:** 15-30°C (59-86°F).

TARCEVA   RX
erlotinib (Genentech)

THERAPEUTIC CLASS: Epidermal growth factor receptor tyrosine kinase inhibitor

INDICATIONS: First-line treatment of patients with metastatic non-small cell lung cancer (NSCLC) whose tumors have epidermal growth factor receptor (EGFR) exon 19 deletions or exon 21 (L858R) substitution mutations; treatment of locally advanced or metastatic NSCLC after failure of at least 1 prior chemotherapy regimen; maintenance treatment of locally advanced or metastatic NSCLC that has not progressed after 4 cycles of platinum-based 1st-line chemo-therapy. First-line treatment of locally advanced, unresectable, or metastatic pancreatic cancer in combination with gemcitabine.

DOSAGE: *Adults:* NSCLC: Usual: 150mg qd. Pancreatic Cancer: Usual: 100mg qd in combination with gemcitabine. Take on an empty stomach. Continue until disease progression or unaccept-able toxicity occurs. Refer to PI for dose modifications.

HOW SUPPLIED: Tab: 25mg, 100mg, 150mg

WARNINGS/PRECAUTIONS: Not recommended for use in combination with platinum-based chemotherapy. Serious interstitial lung disease (ILD) may occur; withhold for acute onset of new/progressive unexplained pulmonary symptoms. Renal failure; hepatotoxicity with or without hepatic impairment; hepatorenal syndrome; bullous, blistering, and exfoliative skin conditions; corneal perforation/ulceration and other ocular disorders (eg, abnormal eyelash growth, kera-toconjunctivitis sicca, keratitis); myocardial infarction (MI)/ischemia; cerebrovascular accidents (CVA); microangiopathic hemolytic anemia with thrombocytopenia; and fetal harm may occur. GI perforation may occur; increased risk in patients with prior history of peptic ulceration or diverticular disease.

ADVERSE REACTIONS: Rash, diarrhea, anorexia, fatigue, dyspnea, cough, N/V, infection, stoma-titis, pruritus, dry skin, conjunctivitis, keratoconjunctivitis sicca, back pain, chest pain.

INTERACTIONS: Concomitant use with antiangiogenic agents, corticosteroids, NSAIDs, and/or taxane-based chemotherapy may increase risk of GI perforation. Increased levels with potent CYP3A4 inhibitors (eg, ketoconazole), and with inhibitors of both CYP3A4 and CYP1A2 (eg, ciprofloxacin). Decreased levels with CYP3A4 inducers (eg, rifampicin). Cigarette smoking and drugs affecting gastric pH (eg, omeprazole, ranitidine) may decrease levels. INR elevations and bleeding events reported with coumarin-derived anticoagulants (eg, warfarin); monitor PT/INR regularly.

PREGNANCY: Category D, not for use in nursing.

MECHANISM OF ACTION: EGFR tyrosine kinase inhibitor; reversibly inhibits the kinase activity of EGFR, preventing autophosphorylation of tyrosine residues associated with the receptor and thereby inhibiting further downstream signaling.

PHARMACOKINETICS: Absorption: Bioavailability (60% without food, 100% with food); T_{max}=4 hrs. **Distribution:** V_d=232L; plasma protein binding (93%). **Metabolism:** CYP3A4 (major); 1A2, 1A1 (minor). **Elimination:** Feces (83%; 1% parent drug), urine (8%; 0.3% parent drug); $T_{1/2}$=36.2 hrs (median).

NURSING CONSIDERATIONS

Assessment: Assess for hepatic/renal impairment, dehydration, history of peptic ulceration or diverticular disease, pregnancy/nursing status, and possible drug interactions.

Monitoring: Monitor for signs and symptoms of ILD, hepatotoxicity, GI perforation, MI/ischemia, renal failure/insufficiency, CVA, microangiopathic hemolytic anemia with thrombocytopenia, ocular disorders, bullous and exfoliative skin disorders, and other adverse reactions. Monitor LFTs, renal function, and serum electrolytes. Regularly monitor PT/INR with coumarin-derived anticoagulants.

Patient Counseling: Inform of risks/benefits of therapy. Instruct to notify physician if onset or worsening of skin rash or development of bullous lesions or desquamation; severe/persistent diarrhea, N/V, anorexia; unexplained SOB or cough; or eye irritation occurs. Instruct to stop smoking and advise to contact physician for any changes in smoking status. Advise on the presentation of skin, hair and nail disorders. Instruct on initial management of rash or diarrhea. Counsel on pregnancy planning and prevention; advise females of reproductive potential to use highly effective contraception during treatment and for at least 2 weeks after the last dose. Advise to contact physician if pregnant or if pregnancy is suspected and to d/c nursing during treatment.

Administration: Oral route. Take on an empty stomach (at least 1 hr ac or 2 hrs pc). **Storage:** 25°C (77°F); excursions permitted to 15-30°C (59-86°F).

TARKA   RX
verapamil HCl - trandolapril (AbbVie)

> D/C when pregnancy is detected. Drugs that act directly on the renin-angiotensin system (RAS) can cause injury/death to the developing fetus.

THERAPEUTIC CLASS: ACE inhibitor/calcium channel blocker (nondihydropyridine)

INDICATIONS: Treatment of HTN.

DOSAGE: *Adults:* Begin therapy only after patient has either failed to achieve desired antihypertensive effect with monotherapy at max recommended dose and shortest dosing interval, or monotherapy dose cannot be increased further because of dose-limiting side effects. Replacement Therapy: Dose qd with food. Combination may be substituted for same component doses. Severe Liver Dysfunction: Give 30% of the normal verapamil dose.

HOW SUPPLIED: Tab, Extended-Release (ER): (Trandolapril-Verapamil ER) 2mg-180mg, 1mg-240mg, 2mg-240mg, 4mg-240mg

CONTRAINDICATIONS: Severe left ventricular dysfunction, hypotension (systolic BP <90mmHg), cardiogenic shock, sick sinus syndrome (except with functioning artificial ventricular pacemaker), 2nd- or 3rd-degree atrioventricular (AV) block (except with functioning artificial ventricular pacemaker), atrial fibrillation/atrial flutter (A-fib/A-flutter) and an accessory bypass tract (eg, Wolff-Parkinson-White, Lown-Ganong-Levine syndromes), and history of ACE inhibitor-associated angioedema. Coadministration with aliskiren in patients with diabetes.

WARNINGS/PRECAUTIONS: Not for initial therapy of HTN. Caution with impaired hepatic/renal function; monitor for abnormal PR interval prolongation. Trandolapril: Symptomatic hypotension may occur and is most likely in patients who are salt- or volume-depleted; correct the depletion prior to therapy. May cause excessive hypotension, which may be associated with oliguria or azotemia, and rarely, with acute renal failure and death in patients with congestive heart failure (CHF). May cause cholestatic jaundice, fulminant hepatic necrosis, and death; d/c if jaundice develops. Angioedema reported; d/c if laryngeal stridor or angioedema of the face, tongue, or glottis occurs and administer appropriate therapy. Anaphylactoid reactions reported during desensitization with hymenoptera venom, dialysis with high-flux membranes, and LDL apheresis with dextran sulfate absorption. Potential for agranulocytosis and neutropenia; monitor WBC in patients with collagen-vascular disease and/or renal disease. May increase BUN and SrCr with renal artery stenosis and without preexisting renal vascular disease; consider dose reduction and/or discontinuation. Hyperkalemia and persistent, nonproductive cough reported. Hypotension may occur with major surgery or during anesthesia. Verapamil: Has a negative inotropic effect; avoid with severe left ventricular dysfunction. May decrease BP, which may result in dizziness or symptomatic hypotension. Elevated transaminases with or without alkaline phosphatase/bilirubin elevation and hepatocellular injury reported. May lead to asymptomatic 1st-degree AV block and transient bradycardia. Reduce dose or d/c in marked 1st-degree block or progression to 2nd- or 3rd-degree AV block. Sinus bradycardia, 2nd-degree AV block, sinus arrest, and pulmonary edema/severe hypotension reported in patients with hypertrophic cardiomyopathy. May decrease neuromuscular transmission in patients with Duchenne's muscular dystrophy; reduce dose with attenuated neuromuscular transmission.

ADVERSE REACTIONS: 1st-degree AV block , constipation, cough, dizziness.

INTERACTIONS: See Contraindications. May cause additive hypotensive effects with diuretics, vasodilators, β-adrenergic blockers, and α-antagonists. Trandolapril: Avoid with aliskiren in patients with renal impairment (GFR <60mL/min). Dual blockade of the RAS is associated with increased risk of hypotension, hyperkalemia, and changes in renal function (including acute renal failure); closely monitor BP, renal function, and electrolytes with concomitant agents that also affect the RAS. Excessive BP reduction reported with diuretics. May increase risk of hyperkalemia with K⁺-sparing diuretics, K⁺ supplements, or K⁺-containing salt substitutes. May result in deterioration of renal function with NSAIDs, including selective COX-2 inhibitors. NSAIDs may also attenuate antihypertensive effect. May increase blood glucose-lowering effect of antidiabetic medications. Verapamil: Increased risk of lithium toxicity. Hypotension, bradyarrhythmias, and lactic acidosis were seen with clarithromycin and erythromycin. Not recommended with colchicine. Avoid disopyramide within 48 hrs before or 24 hrs after administration. Avoid concomitant quinidine use with hypertrophic cardiomyopathy; significant hypotension reported. Additive negative inotropic effect and prolongation of AV conduction with flecainide. Additive negative effects on HR, AV conduction, and/or cardiac contractility with β-adrenergic blockers. Inhalational anesthetics may depress cardiovascular activity. May potentiate activity of neuromuscular blocking agents (curare-like and depolarizing); reduce dose of either or both drugs. May increase levels of digoxin, prazosin, terazosin, simvastatin, lovastatin, atorvastatin, carbamazepine, cyclosporine, sirolimus, tacrolimus, theophylline, buspirone, midazolam, almotriptan, imipramine, doxorubicin, quinidine, metoprolol, propranolol, colchicine, and glyburide. CYP3A4 inhibitors (eg, erythromycin, telithromycin, ritonavir) may increase levels. CYP3A4 inducers (eg, rifampin, phenobarbital, sulfinpyrazone, St. John's wort) may decrease levels. Myopathy/rhabdomyolysis reported with HMG-CoA reductase inhibitors that are CYP3A4 substrates; limit simvastatin dose to 10mg/day, lovastatin dose to 40mg/day, and consider lower starting and maintenance doses for others.

PREGNANCY: Category D, not for use in nursing.

MECHANISM OF ACTION: Verapamil: Calcium channel blocker; modulates influx of ionic Ca^{2+} across the cell membrane of the arterial smooth muscle as well as in conductile and contractile myocardial cells. Decreases systemic vascular resistance, usually without orthostatic decreases in BP or reflex tachycardia. Trandolapril: ACE inhibitor; inhibition results in decreased plasma angiotensin II, which leads to decreased vasopressor activity and decreased aldosterone secretion.

PHARMACOKINETICS: Absorption: Verapamil: Absolute bioavailability (20-35%), T_{max}=4-15 hrs, 5-15 hrs (norverapamil). Trandolapril: Absolute bioavailability (10%, 70% trandolaprilat), T_{max}=0.5-2 hrs, 2-12 hrs (trandolaprilat). **Distribution:** Verapamil: Plasma protein binding (90%); found in breast milk. Trandolapril: Plasma protein binding (80%). **Metabolism:** Verapamil: Liver (extensive); norverapamil (active metabolite). Trandolapril: Trandolaprilat (active metabolite). **Elimination:** Verapamil: Urine (70% metabolite, 3-4% unchanged), feces (≥16% metabolite); $T_{1/2}$=6-11 hrs. Trandolapril: Urine (33%, <1% unchanged), feces (66%); $T_{1/2}$=6 hrs.

NURSING CONSIDERATIONS

Assessment: Assess for ventricular dysfunction, cardiogenic shock, sick sinus syndrome, AV block, A-fib/A-flutter and an accessory bypass tract, history of angioedema, diabetes, hepatic/renal impairment, CHF, hypertrophic cardiomyopathy, neuromuscular disorders, volume/salt depletion, collagen vascular disease, pregnancy/nursing status, and possible drug interactions.

Monitoring: Monitor for angioedema, cough, anaphylactoid reactions, hypotension, hepatic/renal impairment, cholestatic jaundice, fulminant hepatic necrosis, heart block, bradycardia, and agranulocytosis. Monitor BP and serum K⁺. Monitor WBC in patients with collagen vascular disease and/or renal disease.

Patient Counseling: Counsel regarding adverse effects (eg, angioedema, neutropenia, jaundice) and instruct to report any signs/symptoms. Inform of risks when taken during pregnancy; instruct to notify physician if patient is pregnant or becomes pregnant. Educate about need for periodic follow-ups and blood tests to rule out adverse effects and to monitor therapeutic effects.

Administration: Oral route. Take with food. **Storage:** 15-25°C (59-77°F).

TASIGNA   RX
nilotinib (Novartis)

> Prolongs QT interval. Prior to administration and periodically, monitor for hypokalemia or hypomagnesemia and correct deficiencies. Obtain ECGs to monitor QTc at baseline, 7 days after initiation, and periodically thereafter, and following any dose adjustments. Sudden deaths reported. Do not administer to patients with hypokalemia, hypomagnesemia, or long QT syndrome. Avoid with drugs known to prolong the QT interval and strong CYP3A4 inhibitors. Avoid food 2 hrs before and 1 hr after taking the dose.

THERAPEUTIC CLASS: Kinase inhibitor

INDICATIONS: Treatment of adults with newly diagnosed Philadelphia chromosome-positive chronic myeloid leukemia (Ph+ CML) in chronic phase (CP). Treatment of CP and accelerated phase (AP) Ph+ CML in adults resistant or intolerant to prior therapy that included imatinib.

DOSAGE: *Adults:* Newly Diagnosed Ph+ CML-CP: 300mg bid. Resistant or Intolerant Ph+ CML-CP and CML-AP: 400mg bid. Take at approximately 12-hr intervals and on an empty stomach. Refer to PI for dose adjustments or modifications based on hematologic and nonhematologic toxicities, QT prolongation, hepatic impairment, and drug interactions.

HOW SUPPLIED: Cap: 150mg, 200mg

CONTRAINDICATIONS: Hypokalemia, hypomagnesemia, long QT syndrome.

WARNINGS/PRECAUTIONS: Myelosuppression (eg, neutropenia, thrombocytopenia, anemia) may occur; perform CBC every 2 weeks for the first 2 months, then monthly thereafter, or as clinically indicated. Cardiovascular (CV) events, including arterial vascular occlusive events, reported; evaluate CV status and monitor and actively manage CV risk factors during therapy. May increase serum lipase; increased risk in patients with history of pancreatitis. Interrupt dosing and consider appropriate diagnostics to exclude pancreatitis if lipase elevations are accompanied by abdominal symptoms. May result in hepatotoxicity as measured by elevations in bilirubin, AST/ALT, and alkaline phosphatase. Monitor serum lipase levels and LFTs monthly or as clinically indicated. May cause hypophosphatemia, hypokalemia, hyperkalemia, hypocalcemia, and hyponatremia; correct electrolyte abnormalities prior to initiation and monitor periodically. Exposure is increased in patients with impaired hepatic function. Tumor lysis syndrome cases reported; maintain adequate hydration and correct uric acid levels prior to initiation. Reduced exposure in patients with total gastrectomy; perform more frequent monitoring and consider dose increase or alternative therapy. Contains lactose; not recommended with galactose intolerance, severe lactase deficiency with a severe degree of intolerance to lactose-containing products, or glucose-galactose malabsorption. May cause fetal harm. Caution with relevant cardiac disorders.

ADVERSE REACTIONS: QT prolongation, rash, pruritus, headache, nasopharyngitis, fatigue, N/V, alopecia, myalgia, arthralgia, abdominal pain, constipation, upper respiratory tract infection, diarrhea, cough.

INTERACTIONS: See Boxed Warning. Avoid with strong CYP3A4 inducers (eg, dexamethasone, phenytoin, carbamazepine, rifampin, rifabutin, rifapentine, phenobarbital), grapefruit products and other foods that inhibit CYP3A4, St. John's wort, and antiarrhythmic drugs. May increase concentrations of drugs eliminated by CYP3A4 (eg, midazolam), CYP2C8, CYP2C9, CYP2D6, and UGT1A1 enzymes and may decrease concentrations of drugs eliminated by CYP2B6, CYP2C8, and CYP2C9 enzymes; caution with substrates for these enzymes with narrow therapeutic index. May increase concentrations of P-glycoprotein (P-gp) substrates. Increased concentrations with P-gp inhibitors. Decreased solubility and reduced bioavailability with drugs that inhibit gastric acid secretion to elevate the gastric pH; concomitant use with PPIs is not recommended. Administer an H_2 blocker approximately 10 hrs before and 2 hrs after the dose of nilotinib. Administer an antacid approximately 2 hrs before or 2 hrs after the dose of nilotinib.

PREGNANCY: Category D, not for use in nursing.

MECHANISM OF ACTION: Kinase inhibitor; binds to and stabilizes the inactive conformation of the kinase domain of ABL protein.

PHARMACOKINETICS: Absorption: T_{max}=3 hrs. **Distribution:** Plasma protein binding (98%). **Metabolism:** Via oxidation and hydroxylation. **Elimination:** Feces (93%, 69% unchanged); $T_{1/2}$=17 hrs.

NURSING CONSIDERATIONS

Assessment: Assess for electrolyte abnormalities, history of pancreatitis, long QT syndrome, cardiac disorders, total gastrectomy, hepatic impairment, galactose intolerance, lactase deficiency, glucose-galactose malabsorption, pregnancy/nursing status, and possible drug interactions. Obtain baseline ECG, uric acid levels, and chemistry panels, including lipid profile and glucose.

Monitoring: Monitor for myelosuppression; perform CBC every 2 weeks for the first 2 months of therapy, then monthly thereafter or as clinically indicated. Periodically check chemistry panels, including electrolytes, lipid profile, and glucose. Monitor for signs/symptoms of QT prolongation; obtain ECG 7 days after initiation, periodically thereafter, and after any dose adjustments. Monitor for tumor lysis syndrome, hydration status, and CV status/risk factors. Monitor serum lipase levels and LFTs monthly or as clinically indicated.

Patient Counseling: Instruct to take ud. Advise to seek immediate medical attention with any symptoms suggestive of a CV event. Instruct not to consume grapefruit products at any time during treatment. Instruct to inform physician of other medicines being taken, including OTC drugs or herbal supplements (eg, St. John's wort). Advise women of childbearing potential to use highly effective contraceptives while on therapy. Instruct not to d/c or change dose without consulting physician.

Administration: Oral route. Take on an empty stomach; avoid food for at least 2 hrs before and 1 hr after taking the dose. Swallow caps whole, with water. May disperse contents of each cap in 1 tsp of applesauce if unable to swallow caps; take immediately (within 15 min) and do not store for future use. **Storage:** 25°C (77°F); excursions permitted between 15-30°C (59-86°F).

TASMAR   RX
tolcapone (Valeant)

Risk of potentially fatal, acute fulminant liver failure; should be used in patients with Parkinson's disease (PD) on levodopa/carbidopa who are experiencing symptom fluctuations and are not responding satisfactorily to or are not appropriate candidates for other adjunctive therapies. Withdraw treatment if patient fails to show benefit within 3 weeks of initiation. Do not initiate therapy if liver disease is clinically evident or if 2 ALT/AST values are >ULN. Caution with severe dyskinesia or dystonia. Monitor for evidence of emergent liver injury if used in face of the increased risk of liver injury. Do not consider retreatment in patients who develop evidence of hepatocellular injury while on therapy and are withdrawn from therapy for any reason. Determine ALT/AST at baseline/before increasing dose to 200mg tid and periodically (eg, every 2-4 weeks) for the first 6 months of therapy, then periodically thereafter. D/C if ALT/AST >2X ULN or if clinical signs/symptoms suggest the onset of hepatic dysfunction (eg, persistent nausea, fatigue, lethargy, anorexia, jaundice, dark urine, pruritus, right upper quadrant tenderness).

THERAPEUTIC CLASS: COMT inhibitor

INDICATIONS: Adjunct to levodopa/carbidopa for the treatment of signs and symptoms of idiopathic PD.

DOSAGE: *Adults:* Initial/Usual: 100mg tid. Titrate: Use 200mg tid only if anticipated clinical benefit is justified. D/C if patient fails to show the expected incremental benefit on 200mg dose after 3 weeks of treatment. May need to reduce daily levodopa dose to optimize response if daily levodopa dose is >600mg or if patient has moderate/severe dyskinesias prior to therapy. Take 1st dose of the day together with 1st dose of the day of levodopa/carbidopa; take subsequent doses 6 and 12 hrs later. May be combined with both the immediate and sustained release formulations of levodopa/carbidopa.

HOW SUPPLIED: Tab: 100mg

CONTRAINDICATIONS: Liver disease, patients withdrawn from therapy due to drug-induced hepatocellular injury, history of nontraumatic rhabdomyolysis or hyperpyrexia and confusion possibly related to medication.

WARNINGS/PRECAUTIONS: Falling asleep during activities of daily living and somnolence reported; continually reassess for drowsiness or sleepiness, and d/c if significant daytime sleepiness develops. May impair mental/physical abilities. Orthostatic hypotension, syncope, hallucinations, and hematuria reported. Incidence of hallucination may be increased in elderly >75 yrs of age. Diarrhea reported; appropriate work-up (including occult blood samples) is recommended in all cases of persistent diarrhea. May experience new or worsening mental status and behavioral changes, which may be severe, including psychotic-like behavior during treatment or after starting or increasing the dose. Avoid in patients with major psychotic disorder. May cause and/or exacerbate preexisting dyskinesia. May cause intense urges (eg, intense urges to gamble, increased sexual urges, intense urges to spend money, binge eating); consider dose reduction or discontinuation. Severe rhabdomyolysis and a symptom complex resembling neuroleptic malignant syndrome (NMS) (hyperpyrexia and confusion) reported. Caution with severe renal impairment. Retroperitoneal fibrosis, pulmonary infiltrates, pleural effusion, and pleural thickening reported with ergot derived dopaminergic agents; unknown if nonergot derived dopaminergic drugs cause these complications. May increase risk of developing melanoma; monitor for melanomas frequently and perform periodic skin exams. Withdrawal or abrupt dose reduction may lead to emergence of signs and symptoms of PD, or hyperpyrexia and confusion; if discontinuing treatment, closely monitor patient and adjust other dopaminergic treatments as needed.

ADVERSE REACTIONS: Fulminant liver failure, dyskinesia, dystonia, anorexia, muscle cramps, diarrhea, orthostatic complaints, hallucination, N/V, sleep disorder, somnolence, increased sweating, confusion, urine discoloration, dizziness.

INTERACTIONS: Consider dose reduction of drugs metabolized by catechol-O-methyltransferase (COMT), such as α-methyldopa, dobutamine, apomorphine, and isoproterenol, if coadministered. Avoid with nonselective MAOIs (eg, phenelzine, tranylcypromine). Symptom complex resembling NMS reported with concomitant administration of several medications affecting the CNS, such as monoaminergic (eg, MAOIs, TCAs, SSRIs) and anticholinergic agents. Caution with desipramine. Monitor coagulation parameters if coadministered with warfarin.

PREGNANCY: Category C, caution in nursing.

MECHANISM OF ACTION: COMT inhibitor; suspected to alter the plasma pharmacokinetics of levodopa, leading to more sustained plasma levels of levodopa when given in conjunction with levodopa/carbidopa.

PHARMACOKINETICS: Absorption: Rapid; absolute bioavailability (65%); C_{max}=3mcg/mL (100mg), 6mcg/mL (200mg); T_{max}=2 hrs. **Distribution:** V_d=9L; plasma protein binding (>99.9%). **Metabolism:** Liver; glucuronidation (main), methylation via COMT, oxidation via CYP3A4, CYP2A6. **Elimination:** Urine (60%, 0.5% unchanged), feces (40%); $T_{1/2}$=2-3 hrs.

T

NURSING CONSIDERATIONS

Assessment: Assess for hypersensitivity to the drug, liver disease, drug-induced hepatocellular injury, history of nontraumatic rhabdomyolysis or hyperpyrexia and confusion, renal impairment, dyskinesia, dystonia, major psychotic disorder, pregnancy/nursing status, other conditions where treatment is contraindicated or cautioned, and possible drug interactions. Obtain baseline LFTs.

Monitoring: Monitor for hypotension/syncope, diarrhea, dyskinesia, rhabdomyolysis, hematuria, fibrotic complications, melanomas, hallucinations, hyperpyrexia and confusion, mental/behavioral changes, impulse control/compulsive behaviors, drowsiness or sleepiness, and other adverse reactions. Perform LFTs and skin exams periodically.

Patient Counseling: Instruct to take ud. Inform of the benefits/risks of therapy. Advise that hallucinations, psychotic-like behavior, nausea, and possible increase in dyskinesia and/or dystonia may occur. Inform of the need for regular blood tests to monitor liver enzymes. Advise that orthostatic hypotension with/without symptoms may develop, especially at treatment initiation. Instruct to avoid driving a car or operating other complex machinery until sufficient experience is gained on therapy. Advise to use caution with CNS depressants because of possible additive sedative effects. Inform of signs/symptoms suggestive of hepatic injury; advise to contact physician immediately if these symptoms occur. Advise to inform physician if intense urges occur. Instruct to notify physician if pregnant/intending to become pregnant or if breastfeeding during therapy.

Administration: Oral route. Take with or without food. **Storage:** 20-25°C (68-77°F).

TAZICEF   RX
ceftazidime (Hospira)

THERAPEUTIC CLASS: Cephalosporin (3rd generation)

INDICATIONS: Treatment of lower respiratory tract (including pneumonia), bone and joint, gynecologic (including endometritis), intra-abdominal (including peritonitis), and CNS infections (including meningitis), bacterial septicemia, sepsis, skin and skin structure infections (SSSIs), and urinary tract infections (UTIs) caused by susceptible strains of microorganisms.

DOSAGE: *Adults:* Usual: 1g IV/IM q8-12h. Uncomplicated UTI: 250mg IM/IV q12h. Complicated UTI: 500mg IM/IV q8-12h. Bone and Joint Infections: 2g IV q12h. Uncomplicated Pneumonia/Mild SSSI: 500mg-1g IM/IV q8h. Serious Gynecologic/Intra-Abdominal/Meningitis/Severe Life-Threatening Infections: 2g IV q8h. Lung Infection Caused by Pseudomonas with Cystic Fibrosis (Normal Renal Function): 30-50mg/kg IV q8h. Max: 6g/day. Renal Impairment: May give initial LD of 1g. Maint: CrCl 31-50mL/min: 1g q12h. CrCl 16-30mL/min: 1g q24h. CrCl 6-15mL/min: 500mg q24h. CrCl <5mL/min: 500mg q48h. For severe infections (6g/day), renal impairment dose may be increased by 50% or the dosing frequency may be increased appropriately. Hemodialysis: Give 1g LD followed by 1g after each hemodialysis period. Intraperitoneal Dialysis/Continuous Ambulatory Peritoneal Dialysis: Give 1g LD followed by 500mg q24h, or add to fluid at 250mg/2L. Continue for 2 days after signs/symptoms of infection disappear; may require longer therapy with complicated infections.
Pediatrics: 1 Month-12 Yrs: 30-50mg/kg IV q8h. Max: 6g/day. Neonates (0-4 Weeks): 30mg/kg IV q12h. Higher doses should be reserved for immunocompromised patients with cystic fibrosis or meningitis. Continue for 2 days after signs/symptoms of infection disappear; may require longer therapy with complicated infections. Adjust dose in renal insufficiency; refer to PI.

HOW SUPPLIED: Inj: 1g, 2g. Also available as a Pharmacy Bulk Package. Refer to individual package insert for more information.

WARNINGS/PRECAUTIONS: Caution in penicillin (PCN)-sensitive patients; determine whether patient has had previous hypersensitivity reactions to cephalosporins, PCN, or other drugs. D/C if an allergic reaction occurs. *Clostridium difficile*-associated diarrhea (CDAD) reported; d/c if CDAD is suspected or confirmed. May result in overgrowth of nonsusceptible organisms with prolonged use or use in the absence of a proven or strongly suspected bacterial infection or prophylactic indication; take appropriate measures if superinfection develops. High and prolonged serum concentrations may occur in patients with transient or persistent reduction of urinary output. Elevated levels with renal insufficiency can lead to seizures, encephalopathy, coma, asterixis, neuromuscular excitability, and myoclonia. Risk of decreased prothrombin activity in patients with renal/hepatic impairment, poor nutritional state, and patients receiving a protracted course of therapy; monitor PT. Distal necrosis may occur after inadvertent intra-arterial administration. Lab test interactions may occur. Caution with impaired renal function, history of GI disease, particularly colitis, and in elderly.

ADVERSE REACTIONS: Phlebitis and inflammation at inj site, pruritus, rash, fever, diarrhea, N/V, abdominal pain, increased ALT/AST/GGT/LDH, eosinophilia.

INTERACTIONS: Nephrotoxicity reported with concomitant aminoglycosides or potent diuretics (eg, furosemide). Avoid with chloramphenicol; may antagonize effect of β-lactam antibiotics. May

T

affect the gut flora, leading to lower estrogen reabsorption and reduced efficacy of combined estrogen/progesterone oral contraceptives.

PREGNANCY: Category B, caution in nursing.

MECHANISM OF ACTION: Cephalosporin (3rd generation); bactericidal, exerting effect by inhibition of enzymes responsible for cell-wall synthesis.

PHARMACOKINETICS: Absorption: (IV/IM) Administration of variable doses resulted in different parameters. **Distribution:** Plasma protein binding (<10%); found in breast milk. **Elimination:** Urine (80-90% unchanged); $T_{1/2}$=1.9 hrs (IV), 2 hrs (IM).

NURSING CONSIDERATIONS

Assessment: Assess for previous hypersensitivity reaction to cephalosporins, PCNs or other drugs, renal/hepatic impairment, poor nutritional status, patients receiving protracted course of antibiotics, history of GI disease (eg, colitis), pregnancy/nursing status, and possible drug interactions.

Monitoring: Monitor for signs/symptoms of allergic reactions, CDAD, superinfection, and other adverse reactions. Monitor for seizures, encephalopathy, coma, asterixis, neuromuscular excitability, and myoclonia with renal impairment. Monitor renal function and PT. Perform periodic susceptibility testing.

Patient Counseling: Inform that drug only treats bacterial, not viral, infections. Instruct to take exactly ud; skipping doses or not completing full course of therapy may decrease effectiveness and increase the likelihood of bacterial resistance. Inform that diarrhea may occur and will usually end when therapy is discontinued. Instruct to contact physician as soon as possible if watery/bloody stools (with/without stomach cramps, fever) develop even as late as 2 months or more after having taken the last dose of therapy.

Administration: IV/IM routes. Refer to PI for administration procedures, direction for use of inj in ADD-Vantage vials, preparation of solutions, compatibility, and stability. **Storage:** (Dry state) 20-25°C (68-77°F). Protect from light.

TECFIDERA   RX
dimethyl fumarate (Biogen Idec)

THERAPEUTIC CLASS: Immunomodulatory agent

INDICATIONS: Treatment of patients with relapsing forms of multiple sclerosis.

DOSAGE: *Adults:* Initial: 120mg bid. Titrate: Increase to 240mg bid after 7 days.

HOW SUPPLIED: Cap, Delayed-Release: 120mg, 240mg

WARNINGS/PRECAUTIONS: May decrease lymphocyte counts; obtain a recent CBC (within 6 months) before initiating treatment, annually, and as clinically indicated. Consider withholding treatment in patients with serious infections until resolved. May cause flushing; administration with food may reduce the incidence.

ADVERSE REACTIONS: Flushing, abdominal pain, diarrhea, N/V, pruritus, rash, albuminuria, increased AST, dyspepsia, erythema.

PREGNANCY: Category C, caution in nursing.

MECHANISM OF ACTION: Immunomodulatory agent; not established. Dimethyl fumarate and the metabolite (monomethyl fumarate [MMF]) have been shown to activate the nuclear factor (erythroid-derived 2)-like 2 (Nrf2) pathway in vitro and in vivo. Nrf2 is involved in the cellular response to oxidative stress.

PHARMACOKINETICS: Absorption: MMF: C_{max}=1.87mg/L (with food), AUC=8.21mg•hr/L (with food), T_{max}=2-2.5 hrs. **Distribution:** MMF: V_d=53-73L; plasma protein binding (27%-45%). **Metabolism:** Extensive by rapid presystemic hydrolysis; MMF (active metabolite). **Elimination:** Primary Route: Exhalation of CO_2 (60%). Minor Route: Urine (16%), feces (1%); $T_{1/2}$=1 hr (MMF).

NURSING CONSIDERATIONS

Assessment: Assess for infection and pregnancy/nursing status. Obtain a recent CBC before initiating treatment.

Monitoring: Monitor for lymphopenia, flushing, and other adverse reactions. Monitor CBC annually and as clinically indicated.

Patient Counseling: Advise to contact physician if patient experiences persistent and/or severe flushing or GI reactions. Instruct to inform physician if patient is pregnant or plans to become pregnant while on therapy; encourage to enroll in the pregnancy registry if patient becomes pregnant while on therapy.

T

Administration: Oral route. Take with or without food. Swallow whole and intact; do not crush or chew. Cap content should not be sprinkled on food. **Storage:** 15-30°C (59-86°F). Protect from light. Once opened, discard bottle after 90 days.

TEFLARO
RX
ceftaroline fosamil (Forest)

THERAPEUTIC CLASS: Cephalosporin

INDICATIONS: Treatment of acute bacterial skin and skin structure infections (ABSSSIs) and community-acquired bacterial pneumonia (CABP).

DOSAGE: *Adults:* ≥18 Yrs: ABSSSI: 600mg q12h IV infusion over 1 hr for 5-14 days. CABP: 600mg q12h IV infusion over 1 hr for 5-7 days. Renal Impairment: Moderate (CrCl >30 to ≤50mL/min): 400mg IV (over 1 hr) q12h. Severe (CrCl ≥15 to ≤30mL/min): 300mg IV (over 1 hr) q12h. End-Stage Renal Disease (CrCl <15mL/min)/Hemodialysis: 200mg IV (over 1 hr) q12h. Elderly: Adjust dosage based on renal function.

HOW SUPPLIED: Inj: 400mg, 600mg

WARNINGS/PRECAUTIONS: Serious and occasionally fatal hypersensitivity and skin reactions reported; d/c if an allergic reaction occurs. Caution with penicillin (PCN) or other β-lactam allergy; cross-sensitivity may occur. *Clostridium difficile*-associated diarrhea (CDAD) reported; d/c if CDAD is suspected or confirmed. May result in bacterial resistance if used in the absence of a proven/suspected bacterial infection. Seroconversion from negative to a positive direct Coombs' test reported. If anemia develops, drug-induced hemolytic anemia should be considered. If drug-induced hemolytic anemia is suspected, consider discontinuation of therapy and administer supportive care if clinically indicated. Caution with renal impairment and in elderly.

ADVERSE REACTIONS: Diarrhea, nausea, rash.

PREGNANCY: Category B, caution in nursing.

MECHANISM OF ACTION: Cephalosporin; bactericidal action is mediated through binding to essential PCN-binding proteins.

PHARMACOKINETICS: Absorption: (Healthy) C_{max}=19mcg/mL (single 600mg dose), 21.3mcg/mL (multiple 600mg doses); T_{max}=1 hr (single 600mg dose), 0.92 hrs (multiple 600mg doses); AUC=56.8mcg•hr/mL (single 600mg dose), 56.3mcg•hr/mL (multiple 600mg doses). **Distribution:** (Healthy Males) V_d=20.3 L (median) (single 600mg dose); plasma protein binding (20%). **Metabolism:** Via phosphatase enzyme to ceftaroline; hydrolysis to ceftaroline M-1 (metabolite). **Elimination:** (Healthy Males) (single 600mg dose) Urine (88%, 64% ceftaroline, 2% metabolite), feces (6%); (Healthy) $T_{1/2}$=1.6 hrs (single 600mg dose), 2.66 hrs (multiple 600mg doses).

NURSING CONSIDERATIONS

Assessment: Assess for cephalosporin or other β-lactam allergy, drug hypersensitivity, renal impairment, pregnancy/nursing status, and possible drug interactions. Obtain appropriate specimens for microbiological examination to identify pathogen and determine susceptibility.

Monitoring: Monitor for signs/symptoms of hypersensitivity reactions, skin reactions, CDAD, drug-induced hemolytic anemia, and other adverse reactions. Monitor renal function, especially in elderly.

Patient Counseling: Advise that allergic reactions could occur and that serious reactions require immediate treatment. Advise to inform the physician about any previous hypersensitivity reactions to the drug, other β-lactams (including cephalosporins), or other allergens. Advise that antibacterial drugs should be used to treat only bacterial, not viral (eg, common cold), infections. Instruct to take ud; inform that skipping doses or not completing the full course may decrease effectiveness of treatment and increase bacterial resistance. Advise that diarrhea may occur; instruct to notify physician if severe watery or bloody diarrhea develops.

Administration: IV route. Refer to PI for information on preparation, administration, and stability. **Storage:** Unreconstituted: 25°C (77°F); excursions permitted to 15-30°C (59-86°F).

TEGRETOL
RX
carbamazepine (Novartis)

Serious and fatal dermatologic reactions, including toxic epidermal necrolysis (TEN) and Stevens-Johnson syndrome (SJS) reported; increased risk with presence of HLA-B*1502 allele. Screen patients with ancestry in genetically at risk populations for the presence of HLA-B*1502 prior to initiation of therapy. D/C at first sign of rash. Aplastic anemia and agranulocytosis reported; obtain complete baseline pretreatment hematological testing; consider discontinuing if evidence of bone marrow depression develops.

OTHER BRAND NAMES: Epitol (Teva) - Tegretol-XR (Novartis)

THERAPEUTIC CLASS: Carboxamide

INDICATIONS: Treatment of partial seizures with complex symptomatology (psychomotor, temporal lobe), generalized tonic-clonic seizures (grand mal), and mixed seizure patterns of these, or other partial or generalized seizures. Treatment of pain associated with true trigeminal or glossopharyngeal neuralgia.

DOSAGE: *Adults:* Epilepsy: Initial: (Tab/Tab, Extended Release [ER]) 200mg bid or (Sus) 1 tsp qid (400mg/day). Titrate: Increase at weekly intervals by adding up to 200mg/day bid (Tab, ER) or tid-qid (Tab/Sus/Tab, Chewable). Maint: 800-1200mg/day. Max: 1200mg/day but doses up to 1600mg/day have been used in rare instances. Combination Therapy: Add gradually while other anticonvulsants are maintained or gradually decreased (except phenytoin, which may have to be increased). Trigeminal Neuralgia: Initial (Day 1): (Tab/Tab, ER) 100mg bid or (Sus) 1/2 tsp qid (200mg/day). Titrate: May increase by up to 200mg/day using increments of 100mg q12h (Tab/Tab, ER) or 50mg (1/2 tsp) qid (Sus) PRN. Maint: 400-800mg/day. Max: 1200mg/day. Reevaluate every 3 months. Refer to PI for conversion from tab to sus or conversion from tab to tab, ER. Take with meals.
Pediatrics: Epilepsy: >12 Yrs: Initial: (Tab/Tab, ER) 200mg bid or (Sus) 1 tsp qid (400mg/day). Titrate: Increase at weekly intervals by adding up to 200mg/day given bid (Tab, ER) or tid-qid (Tab/Sus/Tab, Chewable). Maint: 800-1200mg/day. Max: >15 Yrs: 1200mg/day; 12-15 Yrs: 1000mg/day. 6-12 Yrs: Initial: (Tab/Tab, ER) 100mg bid or (Sus) 1/2 tsp qid (200mg/day). Titrate: Increase at weekly intervals by adding up to 100mg/day bid (Tab, ER) or tid-qid (Tab/Sus/Tab, Chewable). Maint: 400-800mg/day. Max: 1000mg/day. <6 Yrs: Initial: 10-20mg/kg/day bid-tid (Tab) or qid (Sus). Titrate: (Tab/Sus) Increase weekly to tid/qid. Maint: Optimal clinical response is achieved at daily doses <35mg/kg. Max: 35mg/kg/day. Combination Therapy: Add gradually while other anticonvulsants are maintained or gradually decreased (except phenytoin, which may have to be increased). Refer to PI for conversion from tab to sus or conversion from tab to tab, ER. Take with meals.

HOW SUPPLIED: Sus: (Tegretol) 100mg/5mL [450mL]; Tab: (Tegretol, Epitol) 200mg*; Tab, Chewable: (Tegretol) 100mg*; Tab, ER: (Tegretol-XR) 100mg, 200mg, 400mg *scored

CONTRAINDICATIONS: History of previous bone marrow depression, MAOI use within 14 days, hypersensitivity to tricyclic compounds (eg, amitriptyline, desipramine, imipramine, protriptyline, nortriptyline). Coadministration with nefazodone.

WARNINGS/PRECAUTIONS: Increased risk of suicidal thoughts or behavior reported. Avoid abrupt discontinuation when given to prevent major seizures; may precipitate status epilepticus with attendant hypoxia and threat to life. Avoid with history of hepatic porphyria (eg, acute intermittent porphyria, variegate porphyria, porphyria cutanea tarda); acute attacks reported. Withdraw gradually to minimize potential of increased seizure frequency. May cause fetal harm with pregnancy; neonatal seizures, respiratory depression, vomiting, and decreased feeding reported. Caution in patients with history of cardiac conduction disturbance, cardiac/hepatic/renal damage, adverse hematologic reactions to other drugs, previously interrupted course of carbamazepine, increased intraocular pressure (IOP), and mixed seizure disorder; atrioventricular heart block, hepatic effects, and increased frequency of generalized convulsions reported. Multiorgan hypersensitivity reactions reported; consider discontinuing if hypersensitivity develops. Caution with history of hypersensitivity reactions. Consider the possibility of activation of latent psychosis and, in the elderly, confusion or agitation. Avoid sus in patients with fructose intolerance. Not for relief of trivial aches or pains. Decrease in values of thyroid function tests, interference with some pregnancy tests, and hyponatremia reported.

ADVERSE REACTIONS: Dizziness, drowsiness, unsteadiness, N/V, bone marrow depression, multiorgan hypersensitivity, aplastic anemia, agranulocytosis, leukopenia, eosinophilia, SJS, TEN, liver dysfunction, cardiovascular complications.

INTERACTIONS: Occurrence of stool precipitate with other medicinal liquids or diluents. CYP3A4 inhibitors (eg, cimetidine, macrolides, azoles) may increase plasma levels. CYP3A4 inducers (eg, cisplatin, rifampin, theophylline) may decrease plasma levels. May increase plasma levels of clomipramine HCl, phenytoin, and primidone. May decrease levels of CYP3A4 substrates (eg, acetaminophen, alprazolam, warfarin); dose adjustments may be necessary. Insufficient plasma concentrations needed to achieve therapeutic effect with nefazodone; see Contraindications. May render hormonal contraceptives (eg, oral, levonorgestrel subdermal implant) less effective. Increased risk of neurotoxic side effects with lithium. Hypersensitivity reactions (oxcarbazepine, phenytoin, and phenobarbital) and alteration of thyroid function reported with other anticonvulsants. Higher prevalence of teratogenic effects with combination therapy in pregnant women. Increased isoniazid-induced hepatotoxicity with isoniazid. Symptomatic hyponatremia with some diuretics (eg, HCTZ, furosemide). Antagonizes effects of nondepolarizing muscle relaxants (eg, pancuronium). Consider the possible activation of latent psychosis, myocardial infarction, and confusion or agitation in the elderly when given with other tricyclic compounds.

PREGNANCY: Category D, not for use in nursing.

MECHANISM OF ACTION: Carboxamide; mechanism not established. Appears to act by reducing polysynaptic responses and blocking the post-tetanic potentiation. Depresses thalamic potential and bulbar and polysynaptic reflexes.

T

PHARMACOKINETICS: Absorption: T_{max}=1.5 hrs (Sus), 4-5 hrs (Tab), 3-12 hrs (Tab, ER). **Distribution:** Plasma protein binding (76%); crosses the placenta; found in breast milk. **Metabolism:** Liver via CYP3A4 to carbamazepine-10,11-epoxide (active metabolite). **Elimination:** Urine (72%; 3% unchanged), feces (28%); $T_{1/2}$=25-65 hrs (single dose); $T_{1/2}$=12-17 hrs (multiple doses).

NURSING CONSIDERATIONS

Assessment: Assess for history of hypersensitivity to carbamazepine and other anticonvulsants, conditions where treatment is contraindicated or cautioned, pregnancy/nursing status, and possible drug interactions. Perform detailed history and physical exam prior to treatment. Screen for HLA-B*1502 allele in suspected population. Obtain baseline CBC with platelet and reticulocyte counts, serum iron, LFTs, complete urinalysis, BUN determinations, lipid profile, and complete eye examination.

Monitoring: Monitor for hepatic failure, multiorgan hypersensitivity reactions, bone marrow depression, aplastic anemia, agranulocytosis, dermatological reactions (eg, SJS, TEN), new or worsening of seizure frequency, emergence or worsening of depression, suicidal thoughts/behavior, unusual changes in mood/behavior, latent psychosis, confusion or agitation in elderly patients, eye changes, and other adverse reactions. Periodically monitor WBC, platelet count, LFTs, complete urinalysis, BUN determinations, IOP, and serum drug levels. Include tests to detect defects during routine prenatal care in childbearing women.

Patient Counseling: Instruct to read Medication Guide before taking the drug. Instruct to report immediately if early toxic signs/symptoms of potential hematological problems, or if dermatological hypersensitivity or hepatic reactions occur. Instruct to notify physician if emergence or worsening of depression, unusual changes in mood or behavior, or suicidal thoughts/behavior, and thoughts about self-harm occur. Inform that drowsiness or dizziness may occur; caution against hazardous tasks. Advise to report the use of any other prescription, OTC, or herbal products. Instruct to exercise caution when taken with alcohol; may cause sedation. Instruct to notify physician if pregnant or intend to become pregnant. Encourage pregnant patients to enroll in North American Antiepileptic Drug (NAAED) Pregnancy Registry.

Administration: Oral route. (Sus) Shake well before using. (Tab, ER) Swallow whole; do not chew or crush. **Storage:** Sus: Do not store >30°C (86°F). Tab/Tab, Chewable: Do not store >30°C (86°F); Protect from light and moisture. Tab, ER: 15-30°C (59-86°F); (Epitol) 20-25°C (68-77°F). Protect from moisture.

TEKAMLO
aliskiren - amlodipine (Novartis)

RX

> D/C when pregnancy is detected. Drugs that act directly on the renin-angiotensin system can cause injury/death to the developing fetus.

THERAPEUTIC CLASS: Calcium channel blocker (dihydropyridine)/renin inhibitor

INDICATIONS: Treatment of HTN, alone or with other antihypertensive agents.

DOSAGE: *Adults:* Initial: 150mg-5mg qd. Titrate: Adjust dose PRN; increase up to 300mg-10mg qd if BP remains uncontrolled after 2-4 weeks. Max: 300mg-10mg qd. Add-On Therapy: Use if not adequately controlled with aliskiren alone or another dihydropyridine calcium channel blocker (CCB) alone. With dose-limiting adverse reactions to either component alone, switch to aliskiren-amlodipine containing a lower dose of that component. Replacement Therapy: Switch from separate tabs to a single tab of aliskiren-amlodipine containing the same doses. May increase dose of one or both components if BP control has not been satisfactory. Hepatic Impairment: Consider lower doses. Elderly: Consider lower initial doses.

HOW SUPPLIED: Tab: (Aliskiren-Amlodipine) 150mg-5mg, 150mg-10mg, 300mg-5mg, 300mg-10mg

CONTRAINDICATIONS: Concomitant use with ARBs or ACE inhibitors in patients with diabetes.

WARNINGS/PRECAUTIONS: Symptomatic hypotension may occur (eg, patients with marked volume/salt depletion, with severe aortic stenosis); correct volume/salt depletion prior to administration, or start treatment under close supervision. May cause changes in renal function; consider withholding or discontinuing therapy if significant decrease in renal function develops. Patients whose renal function may depend in part on the activity of the renin-angiotensin-aldosterone system (RAAS) (eg, renal artery stenosis, severe heart failure [HF], post-myocardial infarction [MI], volume depletion) may be at risk for developing acute renal failure. Aliskiren: Hypersensitivity/anaphylactic reactions and head/neck angioedema reported; d/c therapy immediately and do not readminister. May cause hyperkalemia; risk factors include renal insufficiency and diabetes. Amlodipine: May develop worsening of angina and acute MI after starting or increasing dose, particularly with severe obstructive coronary artery disease (CAD).

ADVERSE REACTIONS: Peripheral edema.

INTERACTIONS: See Contraindications. Avoid use with ARBs or ACE inhibitors in patients with moderate renal impairment (GFR <60mL/min). Aliskiren: Cyclosporine or itraconazole may increase levels; avoid concomitant use. NSAIDs, including selective COX-2 inhibitors, may deteriorate renal function and attenuate antihypertensive effect. Dual blockade of RAAS is associated with increased risks of hypotension, hyperkalemia, and changes in renal function (including acute renal failure); monitor BP, renal function, and electrolytes with concomitant agents that affect the RAAS. Oral coadministration with furosemide reduced exposure to furosemide; monitor diuretic effects. Risk of developing hyperkalemia with NSAIDs, K⁺ supplements, or K⁺-sparing diuretics. Amlodipine: May increase simvastatin exposure; limit simvastatin dose to 20mg/day. Increased systemic exposure with CYP3A inhibitors (moderate and strong) warranting dose reduction; monitor for symptoms of hypotension and edema to determine need for dose adjustment. Monitor BP when coadministered with CYP3A4 inducers.

PREGNANCY: Category D, not for use in nursing.

MECHANISM OF ACTION: Aliskiren: Direct renin inhibitor; decreases plasma renin activity and inhibits the conversion of angiotensinogen to angiotensin I. Amlodipine: Dihydropyridine CCB; inhibits the transmembrane influx of Ca^{2+} ions into vascular smooth muscle and cardiac muscle. Acts directly on vascular smooth muscle to cause a reduction in peripheral vascular resistance and reduction in BP.

PHARMACOKINETICS: Absorption: Aliskiren: Poor. Bioavailability (2.5%); T_{max}=1-3 hrs. Amlodipine: Absolute bioavailability (64-90%); T_{max}=6-12 hrs. **Distribution:** Amlodipine: Plasma protein binding (93%); V_d=21L/kg. **Metabolism:** Aliskiren: Via CYP3A4. Amlodipine: Hepatic (extensive). **Elimination:** Aliskiren: Urine (25% parent drug). Amlodipine: Urine (10% parent compound, 60% metabolites); $T_{1/2}$=30-50 hrs.

NURSING CONSIDERATIONS

Assessment: Assess for drug hypersensitivity, diabetes, volume/salt depletion, renal artery stenosis, HF, post-MI status, severe aortic stenosis, CAD, renal/hepatic impairment, pregnancy/nursing status, and possible drug interactions.

Monitoring: Monitor for signs/symptoms of hypotension, worsening of angina, acute MI, hyperkalemia, hypersensitivity/anaphylactic reactions, angioedema, airway obstruction, and other adverse reactions. Monitor BP and renal function periodically.

Patient Counseling: Inform women of childbearing age of the consequences of exposure during pregnancy and of the treatment options for women planning to become pregnant. Instruct to report pregnancy as soon as possible. Caution that lightheadedness may occur, especially during the 1st days of therapy; advise to contact physician if lightheadedness occurs. Advise to d/c and consult physician if syncope occurs. Caution that inadequate fluid intake, excessive perspiration, diarrhea, or vomiting can lead to an excessive fall in BP. Advise to d/c and immediately report any signs/symptoms of a severe allergic reaction or angioedema. Inform that angioedema (eg, laryngeal edema) may occur anytime during treatment. Instruct not to use K⁺ supplements or salt substitutes containing K⁺ without consulting physician.

Administration: Oral route. Establish a routine pattern for taking the drug with regard to meals; high-fat meals decrease absorption substantially. **Storage:** 25°C (77°F); excursions permitted to 15-30°C (59-86°F) in original container. Protect from heat and moisture.

TEKTURNA
aliskiren (Novartis)

RX

> D/C when pregnancy is detected. Drugs that act directly on the renin-angiotensin system can cause injury/death to the developing fetus.

THERAPEUTIC CLASS: Renin inhibitor

INDICATIONS: Treatment of HTN.

DOSAGE: *Adults:* Initial: 150mg qd. Titrate: May increase to 300mg qd if BP is not adequately controlled. Max: 300mg/day. May be administered with some other antihypertensive agents.

HOW SUPPLIED: Tab: 150mg, 300mg

CONTRAINDICATIONS: Coadministration with ARBs or ACE inhibitors in patients with diabetes.

WARNINGS/PRECAUTIONS: Hypersensitivity reactions (eg, anaphylactic reactions) and head/neck angioedema reported; d/c therapy immediately and do not readminister if anaphylactic reactions or angioedema develop. Symptomatic hypotension may occur in patients with marked volume depletion or with salt depletion; correct volume/salt depletion prior to administration, or start treatment under close medical supervision. May cause changes in renal function; consider withholding or discontinuing therapy if clinically significant decrease in renal function develops. Patients whose renal function may depend in part on the activity of the renin-angiotensin-aldosterone system (RAAS) (eg, renal artery stenosis, severe heart failure [HF], post-myocardial infarction [MI], volume depletion) may be at risk for developing acute renal failure. May cause hyperkalemia; risk factors include renal insufficiency and diabetes.

ADVERSE REACTIONS: Angioedema, diarrhea, cough, seizures, rash, elevated uric acid, gout, renal stones, increased BUN/SrCr.

INTERACTIONS: See Contraindications. Avoid with ARBs or ACE inhibitors in patients with moderate renal impairment (GFR <60mL/min). Cyclosporine or itraconazole may increase levels; avoid concomitant use. NSAIDs, including selective COX-2 inhibitors, may deteriorate renal function and may attenuate antihypertensive effect. Dual blockade of the RAAS is associated with increased risks of hypotension, hyperkalemia, and changes in renal function (including acute renal failure); monitor BP, renal function, and electrolytes with concomitant agents that affect the RAAS. Reduced furosemide exposure with concomitant use. Risk of developing hyperkalemia with NSAIDs, K⁺ supplements, or K⁺-sparing diuretics.

PREGNANCY: Category D, not for use in nursing.

MECHANISM OF ACTION: Direct renin inhibitor; decreases plasma renin activity and inhibits conversion of angiotensinogen to angiotensin I.

PHARMACOKINETICS: Absorption: Poor. Bioavailability (2.5%); T_{max}=1-3 hrs. **Metabolism:** Via CYP3A4. **Elimination:** Urine (25%, unchanged).

NURSING CONSIDERATIONS

Assessment: Assess for diabetes, volume/salt depletion, renal artery stenosis, HF, post-MI status, pregnancy/nursing status, and possible drug interactions.

Monitoring: Monitor for hypersensitivity/anaphylactic reactions, angioedema, and other adverse reactions. Monitor BP, renal function, and serum K⁺ periodically.

Patient Counseling: Inform women of childbearing age of the consequences of exposure during pregnancy and of the treatment options for women planning to become pregnant. Instruct to report pregnancy to physician as soon as possible. Advise to d/c therapy and to report immediately any signs/symptoms of a severe allergic reaction or angioedema. Caution that light-headedness may occur, especially during the 1st days of therapy; instruct to contact physician if lightheadedness occurs. Advise to d/c treatment and to consult physician if syncope occurs. Caution that inadequate fluid intake, excessive perspiration, diarrhea, or vomiting can lead to an excessive fall in BP. Instruct not to use K⁺ supplements or salt substitutes containing K⁺ without consulting physician.

Administration: Oral route. Establish a routine pattern for taking drug with regard to meals; high-fat meals decrease absorption substantially. **Storage:** 25°C (77°F); excursions permitted to 15-30°C (59-86°F). Protect from moisture.

TEKTURNA HCT   RX
aliskiren - hydrochlorothiazide (Novartis)

> D/C when pregnancy is detected. Drugs that act directly on the renin-angiotensin system can cause injury/death to the developing fetus.

THERAPEUTIC CLASS: Renin inhibitor/thiazide diuretic

INDICATIONS: Treatment of HTN. May be used in patients whose BP is not adequately controlled with aliskiren alone or HCTZ alone, patients whose BP is controlled with HCTZ alone but who experience hypokalemia, or patients who experience dose-limiting adverse reactions on either component alone. May be used as initial therapy in patients likely to need multiple drugs to achieve BP goals.

DOSAGE: *Adults:* Usual: Dose qd. May be administered with some other antihypertensive agents. Add-On/Initial Therapy: Initiate with 150mg-12.5mg qd PRN to control BP. Titrate: May increase if BP remains uncontrolled after 2-4 weeks. Max: 300mg-25mg qd. Replacement Therapy: May substitute for individually titrated components.

HOW SUPPLIED: Tab: (Aliskiren-HCTZ) 150mg-12.5mg, 150mg-25mg, 300mg-12.5mg, 300mg-25mg

CONTRAINDICATIONS: Coadministration with ARBs or ACE inhibitors in patients with diabetes. Anuria, sulfonamide-derived drug hypersensitivity.

WARNINGS/PRECAUTIONS: Not for initial therapy with intravascular volume depletion. Symptomatic hypotension may occur in patients with marked volume depletion or with salt depletion; correct volume/salt depletion prior to administration. Renal function changes may occur including acute renal failure; caution in patients whose renal function depend in part on the activity of the RAS (eg, renal artery stenosis, severe heart failure (HF), post-myocardial infarction (MI), or volume depletion). Consider withholding or discontinuing therapy if clinically significant decrease in renal function develops. May cause serum electrolyte abnormalities (eg, hyperkalemia, hypokalemia, hyponatremia, hypomagnesemia); correct hypokalemia and any coexisting hypomagnesemia prior to initiation. D/C if hypokalemia is accompanied by clinical signs (eg, muscular weakness, paresis, ECG alterations). Aliskiren: Hypersensitivity reactions (eg, anaphylactic reactions) and head/neck angioedema reported; d/c therapy immediately and do not readminister if anaphylactic reactions or angioedema develop. May cause hyperkalemia; risk factors include renal insufficiency and diabetes. HCTZ: May cause hypersensitivity reactions and exacerbation or activation of systemic lupus erythematosus (SLE). May cause idiosyncratic reaction, resulting in acute transient myopia and acute angle-closure glaucoma; d/c as rapidly as possible. May alter glucose tolerance and increase serum cholesterol and TG levels. May cause or exacerbate hyperuricemia and precipitate gout in susceptible patients. May cause hypercalcemia. Minor alterations of fluid and electrolyte balance may precipitate hepatic coma in patients with hepatic impairment or progressive liver disease.

ADVERSE REACTIONS: Dizziness, influenza, diarrhea, cough, vertigo, asthenia, arthralgia.

INTERACTIONS: See Contraindications. Avoid with ARBs or ACE inhibitors in patients with moderate renal impairment (GFR <60mL/min). Aliskiren: Cyclosporine or itraconazole may increase levels; avoid concomitant use. NSAIDs, including selective COX-2 inhibitors, may deteriorate renal function and may attenuate antihypertensive effect. Dual blockade of the renin-angiotensin-aldosterone system (RAAS) is associated with increased risks of hypotension, hyperkalemia, and changes in renal function (including acute renal failure); monitor BP, renal function, and electrolytes with concomitant agents that affect the RAAS. Reduced furosemide exposure with concomitant use. Risk of developing hyperkalemia with NSAIDs, K^+ supplements, or K^+-sparing diuretics. HCTZ: Dosage adjustment of antidiabetic drugs (oral agents and insulin) may be required. May increase risk of lithium toxicity; avoid concurrent use. Observe patients closely to determine if the desired effect of the diuretic is obtained when used concomitantly with NSAIDs. Administer at least 4 hrs before or 4-6 hrs after the administration of ion exchange resins (eg, cholestyramine, colestipol).

PREGNANCY: Category D, not for use in nursing.

MECHANISM OF ACTION: Aliskiren: Direct renin inhibitor; decreases plasma renin activity and inhibits conversion of angiotensinogen to angiotensin I. HCTZ: Thiazide diuretic; has not been established. Affects renal tubular mechanisms of electrolyte reabsorption, directly increasing excretion of Na^+ and Cl^- and indirectly reduces plasma volume.

PHARMACOKINETICS: Absorption: Aliskiren: Poor. Bioavailability (2.5%); T_{max}=1 hr (median). HCTZ: Absolute bioavailability (70%); T_{max}=2.5 hrs (median). **Distribution:** HCTZ: Plasma protein binding (40-70%, albumin); crosses placenta; found in breast milk. **Metabolism:** Aliskiren: Via CYP3A4. **Elimination:** Aliskiren: Urine (25%, unchanged). HCTZ: Urine (70%, unchanged); $T_{1/2}$=10 hrs.

NURSING CONSIDERATIONS

Assessment: Assess for diabetes, anuria, sulfonamide-derived drug hypersensitivity, history of penicillin allergy, volume/salt depletion, renal artery stenosis, HF, post-MI status, SLE, hypokalemia, hypomagnesemia, hepatic/renal impairment, pregnancy/nursing status, and possible drug interactions.

Monitoring: Monitor for signs/symptoms of electrolyte abnormalities, idiosyncratic reactions, hypersensitivity/anaphylactic reactions, angioedema, exacerbation/activation of SLE, hyperuricemia, precipitation of gout, and other adverse reactions. Monitor BP, renal function, and serum K^+ periodically. Monitor cholesterol, TG, and Ca^{2+} levels.

Patient Counseling: Instruct to inform physician if any unusual symptom develops, or if any known symptom persists or worsens. Inform women of childbearing age of the consequences of exposure during pregnancy and of the treatment options for women planning to become pregnant. Instruct to report pregnancy to physician as soon as possible. Caution that lightheadedness may occur, especially during the 1st days of therapy; instruct to contact physician if lightheadedness occurs. Advise to d/c treatment and to consult physician if syncope occurs. Caution that inadequate fluid intake, excessive perspiration, diarrhea, or vomiting can lead to an excessive fall in BP. Advise to d/c therapy and immediately report any signs/symptoms of a severe allergic reaction or angioedema. Instruct not to use K^+ supplements or salt substitutes containing K^+ without consulting physician.

Administration: Oral route. Establish a routine pattern for taking drug with regard to meals; high-fat meals decrease absorption substantially. **Storage:** 25°C (77°F); excursions permitted to 15-30°C (59-86°F). Protect from moisture.

TEMODAR   RX
temozolomide (Merck)

THERAPEUTIC CLASS: Alkylating agent (imidazotetrazine derivative)

INDICATIONS: Treatment of newly diagnosed glioblastoma multiforme (GBM) concomitantly with radiotherapy and then as maintenance treatment. Treatment of refractory anaplastic astrocytoma (eg, patients experiencing disease progression on a drug regimen containing nitrosourea and procarbazine).

DOSAGE: *Adults:* (IV/PO) Adjust according to nadir neutrophil and platelet counts of previous cycle and at time of initiating next cycle. Newly Diagnosed High Grade GBM: 75mg/m² daily for 42 days with focal radiotherapy. Maint: Cycle 1: 150mg/m² qd for 5 days followed by 23 days without treatment. Cycles 2-6: May increase to 200mg/m² at start of Cycle 2, if nonhematologic toxicity for Cycle 1 is Grade ≤2 (excluding alopecia, N/V), absolute neutrophil count (ANC) ≥1.5 x 10⁹/L, and platelet count ≥100 x 10⁹/L. Continue dose at 200 mg/m²/day for first 5 days of each subsequent cycle, unless toxicity occurs. Do not increase dose for subsequent cycles if dose was not increased at Cycle 2. Refer to PI for instructions on dose reduction or discontinuation during the maintenance phase. Refractory Anaplastic Astrocytoma: Initial: 150mg/m² qd for 5 consecutive days per 28-day cycle. May continue therapy until disease progression. Refer to PI for dose modifications for hematologic and nonhematologic toxicities.

HOW SUPPLIED: Cap: 5mg, 20mg, 100mg, 140mg, 180mg, 250mg; Inj: 100mg [vial]

CONTRAINDICATIONS: History of hypersensitivity to dacarbazine (DTIC).

WARNINGS/PRECAUTIONS: Myelosuppression may occur, including prolonged pancytopenia, which may result in aplastic anemia. Exposure to concomitant medications associated with aplastic anemia, including carbamazepine, phenytoin, sulfamethoxazole/trimethoprim, complicates assessment. Greater risk of myelosuppression in women and elderly patients. Cases of myelodysplastic syndrome and secondary malignancies, including myeloid leukemia, reported. *Pneumocystis carinii* pneumonia (PCP) prophylaxis is required in all patients with newly diagnosed GBM who are receiving concomitant radiotherapy for 42-day regimen; higher occurrence of PCP when administered during a longer dosing regimen. Monitor patients for the development of PCP, especially those receiving steroids. For the concomitant treatment phase with radiotherapy, obtain a CBC prior to initiation of treatment and weekly during treatment. For the 28-day treatment cycles, obtain a CBC prior to treatment on Day 1 and on Day 22 of each cycle. Perform weekly blood counts until recovery if the ANC <1.5 x 10⁹/L and platelet count <100 x 10⁹/L. May cause fetal harm if used during pregnancy. Caution with severe renal/hepatic impairment and in elderly. (Inj) Bioequivalence established only when inj is given over 90 min; infusion over a shorter or longer period may result in suboptimal dosing and may increase possibility of infusion related adverse reactions.

ADVERSE REACTIONS: Fatigue, alopecia, myelosuppression, N/V, anorexia, headache, constipation, fever, rash, convulsions, hemiparesis, diarrhea.

INTERACTIONS: Valproic acid may decrease oral clearance.

PREGNANCY: Category D, not for use in nursing.

MECHANISM OF ACTION: Alkylating agent (imidazotetrazine derivative); exerts action by alkylation of DNA. Alkylation (methylation) occurs mainly at the O^6 and N^7 positions of guanine.

PHARMACOKINETICS: Absorption: (PO) Rapid and complete, T_{max}=1 hr; C_{max}= 7.5mcg/mL, 282ng/mL 5-(3-methyltriazen-1-yl)-imidazole-4-carboxamide [MTIC]; AUC=23.4mcg•hr/mL, 864ng•hr/mL (MTIC). (IV) C_{max}=7.3mcg/mL, 276ng/mL (MTIC); AUC=24.6mcg•hr/mL, 891ng•hr/mL (MTIC). **Distribution:** V_d=0.4L/kg; plasma protein binding (15%). **Metabolism:** Via spontaneous hydrolysis; MTIC (major metabolite) to 5-amino-imidazole-4-carboxamide. **Elimination:** Urine (37.7%, 5.6% unchanged), feces (0.8%); $T_{1/2}$=1.8 hrs.

NURSING CONSIDERATIONS

Assessment: Assess for previous hypersensitivity to the drug, history of hypersensitivity to DTIC, myelosuppression, hepatic/renal impairment, pregnancy/nursing status, and possible drug interactions. Obtain baseline CBC and ANC.

Monitoring: Monitor for myelosuppression, PCP, myelodysplastic syndrome, secondary malignancies, and other adverse reactions. For the concomitant treatment phase with radiotherapy, obtain a CBC weekly during treatment. For the 28-day treatment cycles, obtain a CBC on Day 22. If ANC falls <1.5 x 10⁹/L and the platelet count falls <100 x 10⁹/L, obtain blood counts weekly until recovery. (Inj) Monitor for infusion-related reactions.

Patient Counseling: Instruct to take exactly as prescribed. Instruct to take rigorous precautions to avoid inhalation or contact with skin or mucous membranes if caps are accidentally opened or damaged. Inform about the most frequently occurring adverse effects (eg, N/V); instruct to seek medical attention if any of these develop.

Administration: Oral/IV route. Refer to PI for preparation and administration instructions. (Cap) Take on an empty stomach. Swallow whole with a glass of water; do not open or chew. May advise hs administration. Antiemetic therapy may be administered prior to and/or following administration. **Storage:** (Cap) 25°C (77°F); excursions permitted to 15-30°C (59-86°F). (Inj) 2-8°C (36-46°F). After reconstitution, store at 25°C (77°F); use within 14 hrs, including infusion time.

TENORETIC   RX
chlorthalidone - atenolol (AstraZeneca)

THERAPEUTIC CLASS: Monosulfamyl diuretic/selective beta$_1$-blocker

INDICATIONS: Treatment of HTN.

DOSAGE: *Adults:* Individualize dose. Initial: 50mg-25mg tab qd. May increase to 100mg-25mg tab qd. CrCl 15-35mL/min: Max: 50mg atenolol/day. CrCl <15mL/min: Max: 50mg atenolol qod. Elderly: Start at lower end of dosing range.

HOW SUPPLIED: Tab: (Atenolol-Chlorthalidone) 50mg-25mg*, 100mg-25mg *scored

CONTRAINDICATIONS: Sinus bradycardia, >1st-degree heart block, cardiogenic shock, overt cardiac failure, anuria, hypersensitivity to sulfonamide-derived drugs.

WARNINGS/PRECAUTIONS: Not for initial therapy. Avoid with untreated pheochromocytoma. May aggravate peripheral arterial circulatory disorders. Caution in elderly. Atenolol: May cause/precipitate heart failure (HF); d/c if cardiac failure continues despite adequate treatment. Caution in patients with impaired renal function. Avoid abrupt discontinuation; exacerbation of angina and myocardial infarction reported. Avoid with bronchospastic disease, but may use with caution if unresponsive/intolerant of other antihypertensive treatment. Chronically administered therapy should not be routinely withdrawn prior to major surgery; however, may augment risks of general anesthesia and surgical procedures. Caution in diabetic patients; may mask tachycardia occurring with hypoglycemia. May mask clinical signs of hyperthyroidism and precipitate thyroid storm with abrupt discontinuation. May cause fetal harm. Chlorthalidone: May precipitate azotemia with renal disease. If progressive renal impairment becomes evident, d/c therapy. Caution with impaired hepatic function or progressive liver disease; may precipitate hepatic coma. D/C prior to parathyroid function test. Decreased Ca^{2+} excretion observed. Altered parathyroid glands, with hypercalcemia and hypophosphatemia, seen with prolonged therapy. Hyperuricemia may occur, or acute gout may be precipitated. Fluid/electrolyte imbalance may develop. Sensitivity reactions may occur. Exacerbation/activation of systemic lupus erythematous (SLE) reported. May enhance effects in postsympathectomy patients.

ADVERSE REACTIONS: Bradycardia, dizziness, fatigue, nausea.

INTERACTIONS: May potentiate other antihypertensive agents. Observe for hypotension and/or marked bradycardia with catecholamine-depleting drugs (eg, reserpine). Additive effects with calcium channel blockers. Atenolol: Bradycardia, heart block, and rise of left ventricular end diastolic pressure may occur with verapamil or diltiazem. May cause severe bradycardia, asystole, and HF with disopyramide. Additive effects with amiodarone. Prostaglandin synthase inhibitors (eg, indomethacin) may decrease hypotensive effects. Exacerbates rebound HTN with clonidine withdrawal. May be unresponsive to usual doses of epinephrine. Digitalis glycosides may slow atrioventricular conduction and increase risk of bradycardia. Chlorthalidone: May alter insulin requirements in diabetic patients; latent diabetes mellitus (DM) may manifest. May develop hypokalemia with concomitant corticosteroids or adrenocorticotropic hormone. May decrease arterial response to norepinephrine. May increase responsiveness to tubocurarine. Avoid with lithium; risk of lithium toxicity.

PREGNANCY: Category D, caution in nursing.

MECHANISM OF ACTION: Atenolol: Cardioselective β-adrenoreceptor blocking agent; has not been established. Suspected to competitively antagonize catecholamines at peripheral adrenergic neuron sites, leading to decreased cardiac output; a central effect leading to reduced sympathetic outflow to the periphery and suppression of renin activity. Chlorthalidone: Monosulfamyl diuretic; acts on cortical diluting segment of ascending limb of Henle's loop and produces diuresis with increased excretion of Na^+ and Cl^-.

PHARMACOKINETICS: Absorption: Atenolol: Rapid, incomplete; T_{max}=2-4 hrs. **Distribution:** Crosses placenta. Atenolol: Plasma protein binding (6-16%); found in breast milk. **Elimination:** Atenolol: Renal excretion; feces (unchanged); $T_{1/2}$=6-7 hrs.

NURSING CONSIDERATIONS

Assessment: Assess for bradycardia, cardiogenic shock, >1st-degree heart block, overt cardiac failure, impaired renal/hepatic function, bronchospastic disease, peripheral vascular disease, DM, hyperthyroidism, pheochromocytoma, anuria, hypersensitivity to sulfonamide-derived drugs, serum electrolytes, parathyroid disease, pregnancy/nursing status, SLE, coronary artery disease, and possible drug interactions.

Monitoring: Monitor for cardiac failure, hepatic/renal function, withdrawal symptoms, hypersensitivity reactions, hyperuricemia or acute gout, and signs/symptoms of electrolyte imbalance. Monitor serum glucose, serum electrolytes, and BP.

Patient Counseling: Instruct not to interrupt or d/c therapy without consulting physician. Instruct to notify physician if signs/symptoms of impending congestive HF or unexplained respiratory symptoms develop. Counsel about signs/symptoms of electrolyte imbalance, and advise to seek prompt medical attention. Inform that drug may cause potential harm to fetus; instruct to inform physician if pregnant/planning to become pregnant.

Administration: Oral route. **Storage:** 20-25°C (68-77°F).

TENORMIN
atenolol (AstraZeneca)

RX

> Avoid abrupt discontinuation of therapy in patients with coronary artery disease (CAD). Severe exacerbation of angina and occurrence of myocardial infarction (MI) and ventricular arrhythmias reported in angina patients following abrupt discontinuation of β-blockers. If plan to d/c therapy, carefully observe and advise to limit physical activity. Promptly reinstitute therapy, at least temporarily, if angina worsens or acute coronary insufficiency develops. CAD may be unrecognized; may be prudent to avoid abrupt discontinuation in patients only treated for HTN.

THERAPEUTIC CLASS: Selective beta₁-blocker

INDICATIONS: Treatment of HTN alone or with other antihypertensives. Long-term management of angina pectoris. Management of hemodynamically stable patients with definite or suspected acute myocardial infarction (AMI) to reduce cardiovascular mortality.

DOSAGE: *Adults:* HTN: Initial: 50mg qd, either alone or with diuretic therapy. Titrate: May increase to 100mg qd after 1-2 weeks. Max: 100mg qd. Angina: Initial: 50mg qd. Titrate: May increase to 100mg qd after 1 week. Max: 200mg qd. AMI: Initial: 5mg IV over 5 min, repeat 10 min later. If tolerated, give 50mg PO 10 min after the last IV dose, followed by another 50mg PO 12 hrs later. Maint: 100mg qd or 50mg bid for 6-9 days or until discharge from the hospital. Renal Impairment/Elderly: HTN: Initial: 25mg qd. HTN/Angina/AMI: Max: CrCl 15-35mL/min: 50mg/day. CrCl <15mL/min: 25mg/day. Hemodialysis: 25-50mg after each dialysis.

HOW SUPPLIED: Tab: 25mg, 50mg*, 100mg *scored

CONTRAINDICATIONS: Sinus bradycardia, >1st-degree heart block, cardiogenic shock, overt cardiac failure.

WARNINGS/PRECAUTIONS: May cause/precipitate heart failure (HF); d/c if cardiac failure continues despite adequate treatment. Avoid with bronchospastic disease; may use with caution if unresponsive to/intolerant of other antihypertensive treatment. Chronically administered therapy should not be routinely withdrawn prior to major surgery; however, may augment risks of general anesthesia and surgical procedures. Caution in diabetic patients; may mask tachycardia occurring with hypoglycemia. May mask clinical signs of hyperthyroidism and may precipitate thyroid storm with abrupt discontinuation. Avoid with untreated pheochromocytoma. May cause fetal harm. May aggravate peripheral arterial circulatory disorders. Caution in elderly and those with renal impairment.

ADVERSE REACTIONS: Tiredness, dizziness, cold extremities, depression, fatigue, dyspnea, postural hypotension, bradycardia, leg pain, lightheadedness, lethargy, diarrhea, nausea, wheeziness.

INTERACTIONS: Additive effects with thiazide-type diuretics, catecholamine-depleting drugs (eg, reserpine), calcium channel blockers, and amiodarone. May cause severe bradycardia, asystole, and HF with disopyramide. Bradycardia and heart block can occur and left ventricular end diastolic pressure can rise with verapamil or diltiazem. Exacerbates rebound HTN with clonidine withdrawal. Prostaglandin synthase inhibitors (eg, indomethacin) may decrease hypotensive effects. May be unresponsive to usual doses of epinephrine. Concomitant use with digitalis glycosides may increase risk of bradycardia.

PREGNANCY: Category D, caution in nursing.

MECHANISM OF ACTION: Cardioselective β-adrenoreceptor-blocking agent; not established. Suspected to competitively antagonize catecholamines at peripheral (especially cardiac) adrenergic neuron sites, leading to decreased cardiac output; a central effect leading to reduced sympathetic outflow to the periphery and suppression of renin activity.

PHARMACOKINETICS: Absorption: Rapid, incomplete; T_{max}=2-4 hrs. **Distribution:** Plasma protein binding (6-16%); found in breast milk; crosses the placenta. **Elimination:** Urine (50%), feces (unchanged); $T_{1/2}$=6-7 hrs.

NURSING CONSIDERATIONS

Assessment: Assess for history of hypersensitivity, bradycardia, cardiogenic shock, >1st-degree heart block, overt cardiac failure, AMI, renal dysfunction, bronchospastic disease, conduction abnormalities, left ventricular dysfunction, peripheral arterial circulatory disorders, diabetes mellitus, hyperthyroidism, pheochromocytoma, pregnancy/nursing status, and for possible drug interactions.

Monitoring: Monitor for signs/symptoms of cardiac failure, and for masking of hyperthyroidism/hypoglycemia. Monitor renal function, pulse, and BP. Following abrupt discontinuation, monitor for thyroid storm and in patients with angina, monitor for severe exacerbation of angina, MI, and ventricular arrhythmias.

Patient Counseling: Instruct to take as prescribed. Advise not to interrupt or d/c therapy without first consulting physician. Counsel to notify physician if signs/symptoms of congestive HF or unexplained respiratory symptoms develop. Inform that drug may cause fetal harm; instruct to notify physician if pregnant or if considering becoming pregnant.

Administration: Oral route. **Storage:** 20-25°C (68-77°F).

TERAZOSIN   RX
terazosin HCl (Various)

THERAPEUTIC CLASS: Alpha$_1$-blocker (quinazoline)

INDICATIONS: Treatment of HTN and symptomatic BPH.

DOSAGE: *Adults:* If discontinued for several days or longer, restart using the initial dosing regimen. HTN: Initial: 1mg hs. Usual: 1-5mg qd. If response is substantially diminished at 24 hrs, may slowly increase dose or use bid regimen. Max: 40mg/day. BPH: Initial: 1mg qhs. Titrate: Increase stepwise to 2mg, 5mg, or 10mg qd. Usual: 10mg/day. Assess clinical response after 4-6 weeks. Max: 20mg/day.

HOW SUPPLIED: Cap: 1mg, 2mg, 5mg, 10mg

WARNINGS/PRECAUTIONS: May cause marked lowering of BP, especially postural hypotension and syncope with the 1st dose or 1st few days of therapy; similar effect may be anticipated if therapy is discontinued for several days and then restarted. May impair physical/mental abilities. Examine patients with BPH to rule out prostate cancer prior to initiation of therapy. Priapism reported. Intraoperative floppy iris syndrome observed during cataract surgery. Decreases in Hct, Hgb, WBCs, total protein and albumin reported.

ADVERSE REACTIONS: Asthenia, postural hypotension, headache, dizziness, dyspnea, nasal congestion, somnolence, palpitations, nausea, peripheral edema, pain in extremities.

INTERACTIONS: Caution with other antihypertensive agents; may need dose reduction or retitration of either agent. Increased levels with captopril. Hypotension reported with PDE-5 inhibitors.

PREGNANCY: Category C, caution in nursing.

MECHANISM OF ACTION: Alpha$_1$-blocker; (BPH) relaxes smooth muscle in bladder neck and prostate; (HTN) decreases total peripheral vascular resistance, causing decreased BP.

PHARMACOKINETICS: Absorption: Complete; T_{max}=1 hr. **Distribution:** Plasma protein binding (90-94%). **Elimination:** Feces (60%), urine (40%); $T_{1/2}$=12 hrs, 14 hrs (≥70 yrs), 11.4 hrs (20-39 yrs).

NURSING CONSIDERATIONS

Assessment: Assess BP, pregnancy/nursing status, and possible drug interactions. Rule out prostate cancer with BPH.

Monitoring: Monitor Hct, Hgb, WBCs, total protein/albumin, and BP periodically. Monitor for signs/symptoms of hypotension, priapism, and hypersensitivity reactions.

Patient Counseling: Inform of possibility of syncope and orthostatic symptoms, especially at initiation of therapy. Caution against driving or hazardous tasks for 12 hrs after 1st dose, dosage increase, or when resuming therapy after interruption. Avoid situations where injury could result, should syncope occur. Advise to sit or lie down when symptoms of low BP occur. Inform of possibility of priapism; advise to seek medical attention if it occurs and inform that it can lead to permanent erectile dysfunction if not brought to immediate medical attention.

Administration: Oral route. **Storage:** 20-25°C (68-77°F).

TESSALON   RX
benzonatate (Pfizer)

THERAPEUTIC CLASS: Non-narcotic antitussive

INDICATIONS: Symptomatic relief of cough.

DOSAGE: *Adults:* Usual: 100mg tid PRN. Max: 600mg/day in 3 divided doses. *Pediatrics:* >10 Yrs: Usual: 100mg tid PRN. Max: 600mg/day in 3 divided doses.

HOW SUPPLIED: Cap: 100mg

WARNINGS/PRECAUTIONS: Severe hypersensitivity reactions (eg, bronchospasm, laryngospasm, cardiovascular collapse) reported, possibly related to local anesthesia from sucking or chewing the cap instead of swallowing. Accidental ingestion resulting in death reported in children <10 yrs of age. May cause adverse CNS effects; caution with prior sensitivity to related agents, such as para-amino-benzoic acid based anesthetics (eg, procaine, tetracaine).

ADVERSE REACTIONS: Hypersensitivity reactions, sedation, headache, dizziness, constipation, nausea, GI upset, pruritus, skin eruptions, nasal congestion, numbness of the chest, sensation of burning in the eyes, vague "chilly" sensation.

INTERACTIONS: Bizarre behavior (eg, mental confusion, visual hallucinations) reported with other prescribed drugs. May cause adverse CNS effects with concomitant medications.

PREGNANCY: Category C, caution in nursing.

MECHANISM OF ACTION: Non-narcotic antitussive; acts peripherally by anesthetizing the stretch receptors located in the respiratory passages, lungs, and pleura by dampening their activity, thereby reducing cough reflex at its source.

NURSING CONSIDERATIONS

Assessment: Assess for hypersensitivity to the drug or related compounds, pregnancy/nursing status, and possible drug interactions.

Monitoring: Monitor for hypersensitivity reactions, CNS adverse effects, and other adverse reactions.

Patient Counseling: Inform to take ud. Instruct to refrain from oral ingestion of food or liquids if numbness or tingling of the tongue, mouth, throat, or face occurs until numbness resolves; advise to seek medical attention if symptoms worsen/persist. Inform that overdosage resulting to death may occur in adults.

Administration: Oral route. Swallow whole; do not break, chew, dissolve, cut, or crush. **Storage:** 25°C (77°F); excursions permitted to 15-30°C (59-86°F). Protect from light.

Teveten   RX
eprosartan mesylate (Abbott)

D/C when pregnancy is detected. Drugs that act directly on the renin-angiotensin system (RAS) can cause injury/death to the developing fetus.

THERAPEUTIC CLASS: Angiotensin II receptor antagonist

INDICATIONS: Treatment of HTN, alone or with other antihypertensives.

DOSAGE: *Adults:* Initial (Monotherapy and Not Volume-Depleted): 600mg qd. Usual: 400-800mg/day, given qd-bid. If antihypertensive effect is inadequate with qd regimen, give bid using same total daily dose or consider dose increase. Max: 800mg/day. Moderate and Severe Renal Impairment: Max: 600mg/day. Max BP reduction in most patients may take 2-3 weeks.

HOW SUPPLIED: Tab: 400mg, 600mg

CONTRAINDICATIONS: Coadminstration with aliskiren in patients with diabetes.

WARNINGS/PRECAUTIONS: In patients with an activated RAS (eg, volume- and/or salt-depleted patients receiving diuretics), symptomatic hypotension may occur; correct volume or salt depletion prior to therapy or monitor closely. Renal function changes reported. Oliguria and/or progressive azotemia may occur in patients whose renal function may depend on the renin-angiotensin-aldosterone system (eg, severe congestive heart failure [CHF]). Increases in SrCr or BUN reported in patients with renal artery stenosis. Dual blockade of the RAS is associated with increased risks of hypotension, hyperkalemia, and changes in renal function (including acute renal failure); closely monitor BP, renal function, and electrolytes with concomitant agents that also affect the RAS.

ADVERSE REACTIONS: Upper respiratory tract infection, rhinitis, pharyngitis, cough.

INTERACTIONS: See Contraindications. Avoid with aliskiren in patients with renal impairment (GFR <60mL/min). NSAIDs, including selective COX-2 inhibitors, may deteriorate renal function; monitor renal function periodically. Antihypertensive effect may be attenuated by NSAIDs.

PREGNANCY: Category D, not for use in nursing.

MECHANISM OF ACTION: Angiotensin II receptor antagonist; blocks vasoconstrictor and aldosterone-secreting effects of angiotensin II by selectively blocking binding of angiotensin II to AT_1 receptor found in many tissues.

PHARMACOKINETICS: Absorption: (300mg) Absolute bioavailability (13%); T_{max}=1-2 hrs (fasted). **Distribution:** V_d=308L; plasma protein binding (98%). **Elimination:** Feces (90%), urine (7%; 80%, unchanged); (multiple doses of 600mg) $T_{1/2}$=20 hrs.

NURSING CONSIDERATIONS

Assessment: Assess for volume or salt depletion, renal impairment, CHF, renal artery stenosis, diabetes, hypersensitivity to drug, pregnancy/nursing status, and possible drug interactions.

Monitoring: Monitor for signs/symptoms of hypotension, renal function changes, and other adverse reactions. Monitor BP.

Patient Counseling: Inform of pregnancy risks and instruct to contact physician immediately if patient becomes pregnant. Instruct to notify physician if any adverse reactions develop.

Administration: Oral route. Take with or without food. **Storage:** 20-25°C (68-77°F).

TEVETEN HCT   RX
eprosartan mesylate - hydrochlorothiazide (Abbott)

> D/C when pregnancy is detected. Drugs that act directly on the renin-angiotensin system (RAS) can cause injury/death to the developing fetus.

THERAPEUTIC CLASS: Angiotensin II receptor antagonist/thiazide diuretic

INDICATIONS: Treatment of HTN, alone or with other antihypertensives (eg, calcium channel blockers).

DOSAGE: *Adults:* Begin combination therapy only after failure to achieve desired effect with monotherapy. Refer to PI for monotherapy dosing. Replacement Therapy: May substitute for individual components. Usual (Not Volume-Depleted): 600mg-12.5mg qd. Titrate: May increase to 600mg-25mg qd. Max: 600mg-25mg qd. If additional BP control required, or to maintain bid dosing of monotherapy, 300mg eprosartan may be added qpm. Moderate and Severe Renal Impairment: Max: Eprosartan: 600mg qd. Max BP reduction in most patients may take 2-3 weeks.

HOW SUPPLIED: Tab: (Eprosartan-HCTZ) 600mg-12.5mg, 600mg-25mg

CONTRAINDICATIONS: Anuria, sulfonamide-derived drug hypersensitivity. Coadministration with aliskiren in patients with diabetes.

WARNINGS/PRECAUTIONS: Not for initial therapy of HTN. In patients with an activated RAS (eg, volume- and/or salt-depleted patients receiving diuretics), symptomatic hypotension may occur; correct volume or salt depletion prior to therapy or monitor closely. HCTZ: Caution with hepatic impairment or progressive liver disease; may precipitate hepatic coma. Hypersensitivity reactions may occur. May cause idiosyncratic reaction, resulting in acute transient myopia and acute angle-closure glaucoma; d/c as rapidly as possible. May exacerbate or activate systemic lupus erythematosus (SLE). Hyperuricemia may occur or frank gout may be precipitated. Hyperglycemia, hypomagnesemia, and hypercalcemia may occur. D/C prior to parathyroid test. May enhance effects in postsympathectomy patients. Observe for signs of fluid or electrolyte imbalance. May precipitate azotemia; caution with severe renal disease. Withhold or d/c with evident progressive renal impairment. Eprosartan: Renal function changes reported. Oliguria and/or progressive azotemia may occur in patients whose renal function may depend on the renin-angiotensin-aldosterone system (eg, severe congestive heart failure [CHF]). Increases in SrCr or BUN reported in patients with renal artery stenosis. Dual blockade of the RAS is associated with increased risks of hypotension, hyperkalemia, and changes in renal function (including acute renal failure); closely monitor BP, renal function, and electrolytes with concomitant agents that also affect the RAS.

ADVERSE REACTIONS: Dizziness, headache, back pain, fatigue, myalgia, upper respiratory tract infection.

INTERACTIONS: See Contraindications. NSAIDs, including selective COX-2 inhibitors, may decrease effects of diuretics and angiotensin II receptor antagonists and may further deteriorate renal function. Eprosartan: Avoid with aliskiren in patients with renal impairment (GFR <60mL/min). K^+-sparing diuretics (eg, spironolactone, triamterene, amiloride), K^+ supplements, or K^+-containing salt substitutes may increase serum K^+. HCTZ: Increased risk of lithium toxicity; avoid concurrent use. Alcohol, barbiturates, and narcotics may potentiate orthostatic hypotension. Dose adjustment of antidiabetic drugs (eg, PO agents, insulin) may be required. Additive effect or potentiation with other antihypertensives. Anionic exchange resins (eg, cholestyramine and colestipol resins) may impair absorption. Corticosteroids and adrenocorticotropic hormone may intensify electrolyte depletion, particularly hypokalemia. May decrease response to pressor amines (eg, norepinephrine). May increase responsiveness to nondepolarizing skeletal muscle relaxants (eg, tubocurarine).

PREGNANCY: Category D, not for use in nursing.

MECHANISM OF ACTION: Eprosartan: Angiotensin II receptor antagonist; blocks vasoconstrictor and aldosterone-secreting effects of angiotensin II by selectively blocking binding of angiotensin II to AT_1 receptor found in many tissues. HCTZ: Thiazide diuretic; has not been established. Affects the renal tubular mechanisms of electrolyte reabsorption, directly increasing excretion of Na^+ and Cl^- in approximately equivalent amounts.

PHARMACOKINETICS: Absorption: Eprosartan: (300mg) Absolute bioavailability (13%); T_{max}=1-2 hrs (fasted). **Distribution:** Eprosartan: V_d=308L; plasma protein binding (98%). HCTZ: Crosses placenta; found in breast milk. **Elimination:** Eprosartan: Feces (90%), urine (7%; 80%, unchanged); (multiple doses of 600mg) $T_{1/2}$=20 hrs. HCTZ: Urine (≥61%, unchanged); $T_{1/2}$=5.6-14.8 hrs.

NURSING CONSIDERATIONS

Assessment: Assess for anuria, sulfonamide-derived drug hypersensitivity, history of penicillin allergy, volume or salt depletion, renal/hepatic impairment, history of allergy or bronchial asthma, SLE, electrolyte imbalance, diabetes mellitus (DM), postsympathectomy status, CHF, renal artery stenosis, hypersensitivity to the drug, pregnancy/nursing status, and possible drug interactions.

Monitoring: Monitor for signs/symptoms of hypotension, hypersensitivity reactions, renal/hepatic impairment, idiosyncratic reaction, exacerbation/activation of SLE, hyperuricemia or precipitation of gout, latent DM, and other adverse effects. Monitor BP and serum electrolytes periodically.

Patient Counseling: Inform of pregnancy risks and instruct to contact physician immediately if patient becomes pregnant. Counsel that lightheadedness may occur, especially during 1st days of therapy; instruct to d/c therapy and consult physician if syncope occurs. Advise that inadequate fluid intake, excessive perspiration, diarrhea, or vomiting may lead to an excessive fall in BP, with the same consequences of lightheadedness and possible syncope. Instruct not to use K⁺ supplements or salt substitutes containing K⁺ without consulting physician.

Administration: Oral route. Take with or without food. **Storage:** 20-25°C (68-77°F).

THEOPHYLLINE ER   RX
theophylline (Various)

THERAPEUTIC CLASS: Methylxanthine

INDICATIONS: Treatment of the symptoms and reversible airflow obstruction associated with chronic asthma and other chronic lung disease (eg, emphysema, chronic bronchitis).

DOSAGE: *Adults:* 16-60 Yrs: Initial: 300-400mg qd (am or pm) for 3 days. Titrate: After 3 days, may increase to 400-600mg qd. After 3 more days, may increase dose >600mg according to blood levels. With Risk Factors for Impaired Clearance/Elderly (>60 yrs)/Not Feasible Serum Theophylline Concentrations: Max: 400mg/day. Conversion from Immediate-Release Theophylline: Give same daily dose as once daily. Refer to PI for other dosage instructions and dosage adjustment based on peak serum concentrations.
Pediatrics: 12-15 Yrs: >45kg: Initial: 300-400mg qd (am or pm) for 3 days. Titrate: After 3 days, may increase to 400-600mg qd. After 3 more days, may increase dose >600mg according to blood levels. <45kg: Initial: 12-14mg/kg/day up to a maximum of 300mg qd for 3 days. Titrate: After 3 days, may increase to 16mg/kg/day up to a maximum of 400mg qd. After 3 more days, may increase to 20mg/kg/day up to a maximum of 600mg qd. With Risk Factors for Impaired Clearance/Not Feasible Serum Theophylline Concentrations: Max: 16mg/kg/day up to a maximum of 400mg/day. Conversion from Immediate-Release Theophylline: Give same daily dose qd. Refer to PI for other dosage instructions and dosage adjustment based on peak serum concentrations.

HOW SUPPLIED: Tab, Extended-Release: 400mg*, 600mg* *scored

WARNINGS/PRECAUTIONS: Increased risk of exacerbation with active peptic ulcer disease, seizure disorders, and cardiac arrhythmias (not including bradyarrhythmias). Caution with risk factors for reduced clearance, such as in neonates, children <1 yr, and elderly (>60 yrs), acute pulmonary edema, congestive heart failure, fever (≥102°F for 24 hrs or lesser temperature for longer periods), cor pulmonale, hypothyroidism, liver disease, reduced renal function in infants <3 months of age, sepsis with multiorgan failure, and shock; risk for fatal toxicity if total daily dose is not appropriately reduced. Hyperthyroidism and cystic fibrosis are associated with increased clearance. If signs and symptoms of toxicity (eg, N/V, repetitive vomiting) occur, withhold therapy and monitor serum levels until they resolve. Avoid dose increase in response to acute exacerbation of symptoms of chronic lung disease. Measure peak steady-state serum theophylline concentration before increasing doses and limit dose increase to about 25% of the previous total daily dose to reduce risk of unintended excessive increase in serum levels.

ADVERSE REACTIONS: N/V, headache, insomnia, diarrhea, restlessness, tremors, hematemesis, hypokalemia, hyperglycemia, sinus tachycardia, hypotension/shock, nervousness, disorientation, arrhythmias, seizures.

INTERACTIONS: Blocks adenosine receptors. Alcohol, allopurinol, cimetidine, ciprofloxacin, clarithromycin, erythromycin, disulfiram, enoxacin, estrogen, fluvoxamine, interferon human recombinant α-A, methotrexate, mexiletine, pentoxifylline, propafenone, propranolol, tacrine, thiabendazole, ticlopidine, troleandomycin, and verapamil decreased theophylline clearance and increased its concentration. Aminoglutethimide, carbamazepine, isoproterenol (IV), moricizine, phenobarbital (after 2 weeks of phenobarbital use), phenytoin, rifampin, sulfinpyrazone increased theophylline clearance. May increase risk of ventricular arrhythmias with halothane. May lower theophylline seizure threshold with ketamine. May increase renal lithium clearance. Concomitant use with pancuronium may antagonize its nondepolarizing neuromuscular blocking effects; larger doses may be required. Diazepam, flurazepam, midazolam, and lorazepam may require larger doses to produce desired level of sedation. Increased frequency of nausea, nervousness, and insomnia with ephedrine. Decreased concentrations with St. John's wort. Phenytoin concentrations may be decreased.

PREGNANCY: Category C, caution in nursing.

MECHANISM OF ACTION: Methylxanthine; acts via smooth muscle relaxation and suppression of airway response to stimuli. Bronchodilatation suggested to be mediated by inhibiting two isozymes of phosphodiesterase. Also increases the force of contraction of diaphragmatic muscles due to enhancement of Ca^{2+} uptake through adenosine-mediated channel.

PHARMACOKINETICS: Absorption: Complete; bioavailability (59%, fasting). Administration of different doses resulted in different parameters. **Distribution:** V_d= 0.45L/kg; plasma protein binding (40%); crosses the placenta; found in breast milk. Metabolism: Liver (extensive); demethylation and hydroxylation via CYP1A2, 2E1, 3A3; caffeine and 3-methylxanthine (active metabolites). **Elimination:** Urine (10% unchanged), (50% unchanged in neonates). Elimination $T_{1/2}$ varied based on age and physiological states; refer to PI for details.

NURSING CONSIDERATIONS

Assessment: Assess use with any conditions where treatment is contraindicated or cautioned. Assess known hypersensitivity, renal/hepatic functions, pregnancy/nursing status, and possible drug interactions.

Monitoring: Carefully monitor serum drug levels (target unbound concentration: 6-12mcg/mL) for dose adjustments, drug toxicity, worsening of chronic illness, hepatic dysfunction. Monitor plasma glucose, uric acid, free fatty acids, cholesterol, HDL, LDL, LFTs, and urine-free cortisol excretion. When monitoring for signs and symptoms of toxicity (eg, nausea, repetitive vomiting), adjust dosage based on serum levels.

Patient Counseling: Instruct to seek medical attention if N/V, persistent headache, insomnia, or rapid heartbeat occur. Instruct to take once daily in morning or evening, consistently take with/without food, tablet may be split in half, and do not chew or crush. Counsel not to take St. John's wort concurrently but to consult physician before stopping St. John's wort. Inform physician if new illness (especially if accompanied with persistent fever) or worsening of chronic illness occurs, and if patient starts/stops smoking cigarettes or marijuana. Inform all physicians of theophylline use, especially if medication is being added or removed from treatment. Instruct not to alter the dose, timing of dose, or frequency of administration without consulting physician; instruct that if dose is missed, take next dose at the usual scheduled time and not to attempt to make up for the missed dose.

Administration: Oral route. **Storage:** 25°C (77°F); excursions permitted to 15-30°C (59-86°F).

Tiazac   RX
diltiazem HCl (Forest)

OTHER BRAND NAMES: Taztia XT (Watson)

THERAPEUTIC CLASS: Calcium channel blocker (nondihydropyridine)

INDICATIONS: Treatment of HTN alone or in combination with other antihypertensives. Treatment of chronic stable angina.

DOSAGE: *Adults:* Individualize dose. HTN: Initial (Monotherapy): 120-240mg qd. Titrate: Max effect usually observed by 14 days of therapy; schedule dose adjustments accordingly. Usual Range: 120-540mg qd. Max: 540mg qd. Angina: Initial: 120-180mg qd. Titrate: Carry out over 7-14 days, when necessary. Max: 540mg qd. Patients Treated with Other Diltiazem Formulations: May be switched to therapy at the nearest equivalent total daily dose. Refer to PI for information regarding concomitant use with other cardiovascular agents. Elderly: Start at lower end of dosing range.

HOW SUPPLIED: Cap, Extended-Release: 120mg, 180mg, 240mg, 300mg, 360mg, 420mg; (Taztia XT) 120mg, 180mg, 240mg, 300mg, 360mg

CONTRAINDICATIONS: Sick sinus syndrome and 2nd- or 3rd-degree atrioventricular (AV) block (except with a functioning ventricular pacemaker), severe hypotension (<90mmHg systolic), acute myocardial infarction (AMI) and pulmonary congestion documented by x-ray on admission.

WARNINGS/PRECAUTIONS: Prolongs AV node refractory periods without significantly prolonging sinus node recovery time, except in patients with sick sinus syndrome. Periods of asystole reported in a patient with Prinzmetal's angina. Worsening of congestive heart failure (CHF) reported in patients with preexisting ventricular dysfunction. Symptomatic hypotension may occur. Mild elevations of transaminases with and without concomitant alkaline phosphatase and bilirubin elevation reported. Significant elevations in enzymes (eg, alkaline phosphatase, LDH, AST, ALT) and other phenomena consistent with acute hepatic injury reported in rare instances. Monitor LFTs and renal function at regular intervals; caution with renal/hepatic dysfunction. Transient dermatological reactions and skin eruptions progressing to erythema multiforme and/

or exfoliative dermatitis have been reported; d/c if a dermatologic reaction persists. Caution in elderly.

ADVERSE REACTIONS: Peripheral edema, dizziness, headache, infection, pain, pharyngitis, dyspepsia, dyspnea, bronchitis, AV block, asthenia, vasodilation.

INTERACTIONS: Potential additive effects with other agents known to affect cardiac contractility and/or conduction; caution and careful titration are warranted. Additive effects in prolonging cardiac conduction with β-blockers or digitalis. CYP3A4 substrates, inhibitors, or inducers may have a significant impact on the efficacy and side effect profile of diltiazem; patients taking CYP3A4 substrates, especially patients with renal and/or hepatic impairment, may require dosage adjustment when starting or stopping concomitantly administered diltiazem. May potentiate depression of cardiac contractility, conductivity and automaticity, and vascular dilation associated with anesthetics; carefully titrate anesthetics and calcium channel blockers (CCBs) when used concomitantly. May increase levels of midazolam, triazolam, carbamazepine, quinidine, and lovastatin. May increase levels of propranolol; adjustment of the propranolol dose may be warranted. May increase levels of buspirone; dose adjustments may be necessary. Increased levels with cimetidine; adjustment of diltiazem dose may be warranted. Sinus bradycardia resulting in hospitalization and pacemaker insertion reported with clonidine; monitor HR. Monitor cyclosporine/digoxin concentrations, especially when diltiazem therapy is initiated, adjusted, or discontinued. Rifampin may decrease concentrations; avoid rifampin or any CYP3A4 inducer when possible, and consider alternative therapy. May increase simvastatin exposure; limit daily doses of simvastatin to 10mg and diltiazem to 240mg if coadministration is required. Risk of myopathy and rhabdomyolysis with statins metabolized by CYP3A4 may be increased. When possible, use a non-CYP3A4-metabolized statin; otherwise, consider dose adjustments for both agents and closely monitor for signs and symptoms of any statin-related adverse events. Additive antihypertensive effect when used with other antihypertensive agents; dosage of diltiazem or the concomitant antihypertensive may need to be adjusted.

PREGNANCY: Category C, not for use in nursing.

MECHANISM OF ACTION: CCB; inhibits cellular influx of Ca^{2+} during membrane depolarization of cardiac and vascular smooth muscle. HTN: Relaxes vascular smooth muscle, resulting in decreased peripheral vascular resistance. Angina: Produces increases in exercise tolerance, probably due to its ability to reduce myocardial oxygen demand; accomplished via reductions in HR and systemic BP at submaximal and maximal workloads.

PHARMACOKINETICS: Absorption: Well-absorbed from GI tract. (Immediate-Release) Absolute bioavailability (40%). **Distribution:** Plasma protein binding (70-80%); found in breast milk. **Metabolism:** Liver (extensive; substantial 1st-pass effect); desacetyldiltiazem (active), desmethyldiltiazem (primary metabolites). **Elimination:** Urine (2-4%, unchanged), bile; $T_{1/2}$=6.5 hrs.

NURSING CONSIDERATIONS

Assessment: Assess for sick sinus syndrome, 2nd- or 3rd-degree AV block, hypotension, AMI, pulmonary congestion, ventricular/renal/hepatic dysfunction, drug hypersensitivity, pregnancy/nursing status, and possible drug interactions.

Monitoring: Monitor for bradycardia, AV block, worsening of CHF, symptomatic hypotension, dermatological reactions, and other adverse reactions. Monitor LFTs and renal function at regular intervals. Monitor HR with clonidine.

Patient Counseling: Inform of risks and benefits of therapy. Instruct to take ud. Counsel to report any adverse reactions to physician. Inform that when administering with applesauce, it should not be hot and it should be soft enough to be swallowed without chewing.

Administration: Oral route. May sprinkle cap contents on a spoonful of applesauce. Swallow applesauce immediately without chewing and follow with a glass of cool water; do not store for future use. Subdividing contents of cap is not recommended. **Storage:** 25°C (77°F); excursions permitted to 15-30°C (59-86°F). Avoid excessive humidity. (Taztia XT) 20-25°C (68-77°F). Avoid excessive humidity.

TIGAN
RX
trimethobenzamide HCl (Various)

THERAPEUTIC CLASS: Emetic response modifier

INDICATIONS: Treatment of postoperative N/V, and nausea associated with gastroenteritis.

DOSAGE: *Adults:* Usual: (Cap) 300mg tid-qid. (Inj) 200mg IM tid-qid. Adjust according to indication, severity of symptoms, and response. Renal Impairment (CrCl ≤70mL/min/1.73m²): Reduce dose or increase dosing interval. Elderly: Start at lower end of dosing range.

HOW SUPPLIED: Cap: 300mg; Inj: 100mg/mL

CONTRAINDICATIONS: (Inj) Pediatric patients.

WARNINGS/PRECAUTIONS: May impair physical/mental abilities. Caution with acute febrile illness, encephalitides, gastroenteritis, dehydration, electrolyte imbalance, especially in children/elderly/debilitated; CNS reactions reported. Caution in the elderly and patients with renal impairment. May obscure diagnosis of appendicitis and signs of toxicity due to overdosage of other drugs. (Cap) Caution in children; may cause extrapyramidal symptoms (EPS), which may be confused with CNS signs of undiagnosed primary disease (eg, Reye's syndrome, other encephalopathy) and may unfavorably alter the course of Reye's syndrome due to hepatotoxic potential. Not recommended for uncomplicated vomiting in children.

ADVERSE REACTIONS: Parkinsonian-like symptoms, blood dyscrasias, blurred vision, coma, convulsions, mood depression, diarrhea, disorientation, dizziness, drowsiness, headache, jaundice, muscle cramps, opisthotonos.

INTERACTIONS: Caution with CNS-acting agents (phenothiazines, barbiturates, belladonna derivatives) in acute febrile illness, encephalitides, gastroenteritis, dehydration, and electrolyte imbalance due to potential CNS reactions. Adverse drug interaction reported with alcohol.

PREGNANCY: Safety in pregnancy and nursing not known.

MECHANISM OF ACTION: Not established; thought to involve chemoreceptor trigger zone, through which emetic impulses are conveyed to vomiting center (direct impulses to vomiting center apparently not similarly inhibited).

PHARMACOKINETICS: Absorption: T_{max}=30 min (IM 200mg), 45 min (cap 300mg). **Metabolism:** Oxidation, trimethobenzamide N-oxide (major metabolite). **Elimination:** Urine (30-50%, unchanged); $T_{1/2}$=7-9 hrs.

NURSING CONSIDERATIONS

Assessment: Assess for renal/hepatic impairment, Reye's syndrome in children, alcohol intake, acute febrile illness, encephalitides, gastroenteritis, dehydration, electrolyte imbalance, appendicitis, previous hypersensitivity to the drug, possible drug interactions, and any other conditions where treatment is contraindicated or cautioned.

Monitoring: Monitor renal function and for signs of hepatotoxicity, CNS reactions (eg, opisthotonos, convulsions, coma), EPS, hydration status, and electrolytes.

Patient Counseling: Advise that may cause drowsiness; caution against performing hazardous tasks (operating machinery/driving). Advise patients to not consume alcohol due to a potential drug interaction.

Administration: Oral and IM route. **Storage:** 25°C (77°F); excursions permitted to 15-30°C (59-86°F).

TIKOSYN   RX
dofetilide (Pfizer)

> To minimize risk of induced arrhythmia, for a minimum of 3 days, place patients initiated or reinitiated on therapy in a facility that can provide calculations of CrCl, continuous ECG monitoring, and cardiac resuscitation. Available only to hospitals and prescribers who have received appropriate dofetilide dosing and treatment initiation education.

THERAPEUTIC CLASS: Class III antiarrhythmic

INDICATIONS: Conversion of atrial fibrillation (A-fib)/atrial flutter (A-flutter) to normal sinus rhythm and maintenance of normal sinus rhythm in patients with highly symptomatic A-fib/A-flutter of >1 week duration who were converted to normal sinus rhythm.

DOSAGE: *Adults:* Individualize dose based on CrCl and QT interval (if HR <60bpm). Initial: CrCl >60mL/min: 500mcg bid. CrCl 40-60mL/min: 250mcg bid. CrCl 20-<40mL/min: 125mcg bid. Titrate: Check QTc 2-3 hrs after 1st dose and adjust dose if QTc >500 msec (550 msec in patients with ventricular conduction abnormalities) or increases by >15% from baseline. If initial dose is 500mcg bid, reduce dose to 250mcg bid. If initial dose is 250mcg bid, reduce dose to 125mcg bid. If initial dose is 125mcg bid, reduce dose to 125mcg qd. D/C therapy if at any time after the 2nd dose QTc >500 msec (550 msec in patients with ventricular conduction abnormalities). If renal function deteriorates, adjust dose following initial dosing. Max: CrCl >60mL/min: 500mcg bid. Refer to PI for complete dosing instructions.

HOW SUPPLIED: Cap: 125mcg, 250mcg, 500mcg

CONTRAINDICATIONS: Congenital or acquired long QT syndromes, baseline QT interval or QTc >440 msec (500 msec with ventricular conduction abnormalities), severe renal impairment (CrCl <20mL/min). Concomitant verapamil, HCTZ (alone/in combinations [eg, triamterene]), and inhibitors of renal cation transport system (eg, cimetidine, trimethoprim [alone/combination with sulfamethoxazole], ketoconazole, prochlorperazine, dolutegravir, megestrol).

WARNINGS/PRECAUTIONS: May cause serious ventricular arrhythmias, primarily torsades de pointes (TdP); risk of TdP can be reduced by controlling the plasma concentration through adjustment of the initial dofetilide dose according to CrCl and by monitoring the ECG. Calculate

CrCl before 1st dose. Caution in patients with severe hepatic impairment. Do not discharge patients within 12 hrs of conversion to normal sinus rhythm. Maintain normal K^+ levels prior to and during administration. Patients with A-Fib should be anticoagulated prior to cardioversion and may continue to use after cardioversion. Rehospitalize patient for 3 days anytime dose is increased. Consider electrical cardioversion if patient does not convert to normal sinus rhythm within 24 hrs of initiation of therapy. If dofetilide needs to be discontinued to allow dosing of other potentially interacting drug(s), a washout period of at least 2 days should be followed before starting the other drug(s). Caution in elderly.

ADVERSE REACTIONS: Headache, chest pain, dizziness, ventricular arrhythmia, ventricular tachycardia, TdP, respiratory tract infection, dyspnea, nausea, flu syndrome, insomnia, back pain, diarrhea, rash, abdominal pain.

INTERACTIONS: See Contraindications. Hypokalemia or hypomagnesemia may occur with K^+-depleting diuretics, increasing the potential for TdP. CYP3A4 inhibitors (eg, macrolides, protease inhibitors, serotonin reuptake inhibitors) and drugs actively secreted by cationic secretion (eg, triamterene, metformin, amiloride) may increase levels; caution when coadministered. Not recommended with drugs that prolong the QT interval (eg, phenothiazines, TCAs, certain oral macrolides). Withhold Class I and III antiarrhythmics for at least 3 half-lives prior to dosing with dofetilide. Do not initiate therapy until amiodarone levels are <0.3mcg/mL or until amiodarone has been withdrawn for at least 3 months. Higher occurrence of TdP with digoxin.

PREGNANCY: Category C, not for use in nursing.

MECHANISM OF ACTION: Class III antiarrhythmic; blocks cardiac ion channel carrying rapid component of delayed rectifier K^+ current, I_{Kr}.

PHARMACOKINETICS: Absorption: T_{max}=2-3 hrs (fasted). **Distribution:** V_d=3L/kg; plasma protein binding (60-70%). **Metabolism:** Liver via CYP3A4 through N-dealkylation and N-oxidation pathways. **Elimination:** Urine (80% unchanged, 20% metabolites); $T_{1/2}$=10 hrs.

NURSING CONSIDERATIONS

Assessment: Assess for previous hypersensitivity to drug, congenital or acquired long QT syndrome, renal/hepatic impairment, pregnancy/nursing status, and possible drug interactions. Correct K^+ levels prior to therapy. Obtain baseline ECG and CrCl prior to therapy.

Monitoring: Monitor serum K^+ levels and for development of ventricular arrhythmias (eg, TdP). After initiation or cardioversion, continuously monitor by ECG for a minimum of 3 days, or for a minimum of 12 hrs after electrical/pharmacological conversion to normal sinus rhythm, whichever is greater. Reevaluate renal function and QTc every 3 months, as medically warranted.

Patient Counseling: Inform about risks/benefits, need for compliance with prescribed dosing, potential drug interactions, and the need for periodic monitoring of QTc and renal function. Instruct to notify physician of any changes in medications and supplements or if hospitalized or prescribed a new medication for any condition. Counsel to report immediately any symptoms associated with electrolyte imbalance (eg, excessive/prolonged diarrhea, sweating, vomiting, loss of appetite, thirst). Instruct not to double the next dose if a dose is missed and take the next dose at the usual time.

Administration: Oral route. **Storage:** 15-30°C (59-86°F). Protect from humidity and moisture.

TIMENTIN   RX
ticarcillin disodium - clavulanate potassium (GlaxoSmithKline)

THERAPEUTIC CLASS: Beta-lactamase inhibitor/broad-spectrum penicillin

INDICATIONS: Treatment of lower respiratory, bone and joint, skin and skin structure, and urinary tract infections (UTIs); septicemia (including bacteremia); endometritis; and peritonitis.

DOSAGE: *Adults:* UTI/Systemic Infection: 3.1g (3g ticarcillin, 100mg clavulanate) IV q4-6h. Gynecologic Infections (Based on Ticarcillin Content): Moderate: 200mg/kg/day IV in divided doses q6h. Severe: 300mg/kg/day IV in divided doses q4h. <60kg (Based on Ticarcillin Content): 200-300mg/kg/day IV in divided doses q4-6h. Infuse over 30 min. Duration of therapy depends upon severity of infection, usually 10-14 days; may require more prolonged therapy in difficult and complicated infections. Renal Impairment: Refer to PI.
Pediatrics: ≥3 Months: ≥60kg: Mild to Moderate Infections: 3.1g (3g ticarcillin, 100mg clavulanate) IV q6h. Severe Infections: 3.1g IV q4h. <60kg (Based on Ticarcillin Content): Mild to Moderate Infections: 200mg/kg/day IV in divided doses q6h. Severe Infections: 300mg/kg/day IV in divided doses q4h. Infuse over 30 min. Duration of therapy depends upon severity of infection, usually 10-14 days; may require more prolonged therapy in difficult and complicated infections. Renal Impairment: Refer to PI.

HOW SUPPLIED: Inj: (Ticarcillin-Clavulanate) 3g-100mg [vial], 3g-100mg/100mL [Galaxy]. Also available as a Pharmacy Bulk Package.

WARNINGS/PRECAUTIONS: Serious and occasionally fatal hypersensitivity (anaphylactic) reactions reported; d/c and institute appropriate therapy if an allergic reaction occurs. *Clostridium difficile*-associated diarrhea (CDAD) reported; d/c if CDAD is suspected or confirmed. May cause convulsions when the recommended dose is exceeded, especially in the presence of renal impairment. Bleeding associated with abnormalities in coagulation tests may occur, especially in patients with renal impairment; d/c and institute appropriate therapy if bleeding manifestations appear. May result in bacterial resistance if used in the absence of proven or suspected bacterial infection; take appropriate measures if superinfection develops. Lab test interactions may occur. Hypokalemia reported; monitor serum K^+ in patients with fluid and electrolyte imbalance and in patients receiving prolonged therapy. Consider the Na^+ content of the drug (4.51mEq/g) in patients requiring restricted salt intake. Caution in elderly.

ADVERSE REACTIONS: Elevated eosinophils/AST/ALT, rash, nausea, diarrhea, phlebitis at inj site.

INTERACTIONS: Probenecid may increase serum concentrations and prolong $T_{1/2}$ of ticarcillin. May reduce efficacy of combined oral estrogen/progesterone contraceptives.

PREGNANCY: Category B, caution in nursing.

MECHANISM OF ACTION: Ticarcillin: Broad-spectrum penicillin (PCN); disrupts bacterial cell wall development by inhibiting peptidoglycan synthesis and/or by interacting with PCN-binding proteins. Clavulanic Acid: β-lactamase inhibitor; inactivates some β-lactamase enzymes commonly found in bacteria resistant to PCNs and cephalosporins.

PHARMACOKINETICS: **Absorption:** Ticarcillin: AUC=485mcg•hr/mL (adults), 339mcg•hr/mL (infants/children). Clavulanic Acid: AUC=8.2mcg•hr/mL (adults), 7mcg•hr/mL (infants/children). Refer to PI for C_{max} values. **Distribution:** Ticarcillin: Plasma protein binding (45%). Clavulanic Acid: Plasma protein binding (25%). **Elimination:** Ticarcillin: Urine (60-70%, unchanged); $T_{1/2}$=1.1 hrs (healthy adults), 4.4 hrs (neonates), 1 hr (infants/children). Clavulanic Acid: Urine (35-45%, unchanged); $T_{1/2}$=1.1 hrs (healthy adults), 1.9 hrs (neonates), 0.9 hr (infants/children).

NURSING CONSIDERATIONS

Assessment: Assess for previous hypersensitivity reactions to the drug, other β-lactam antibacterials (eg, PCNs, cephalosporins), or other allergens; renal/hepatic impairment; fluid/electrolyte imbalance; restricted salt intake; pregnancy/nursing status; and possible drug interactions.

Monitoring: Monitor for signs/symptoms of anaphylactic/allergic reactions, CDAD, convulsions, bleeding, superinfection, and other adverse reactions. Monitor serum K^+ in patients with fluid and electrolyte imbalance and in patients receiving prolonged therapy.

Patient Counseling: Counsel that drug should only be used to treat bacterial, not viral (eg, common cold), infections. Instruct to take exactly ud even if patient feels better early in the course of therapy. Inform that skipping doses or not completing the full course of therapy may decrease effectiveness of immediate treatment and increase bacterial resistance. Inform that diarrhea is a common problem caused by therapy, which usually ends when therapy is discontinued. Instruct to immediately contact physician if watery and bloody stools (with or without stomach cramps and fever) occur, even as late as ≥2 months after the last dose. Inform that drug contains a PCN that can cause allergic reactions in some individuals.

Administration: IV route. Administer by IV infusion over a 30-min period. When given with another antimicrobial (eg, aminoglycoside), administer each drug separately. Refer to PI for administration and directions for use. **Storage:** Vial/Pharmacy Bulk Package: ≤25°C (77°F). Galaxy: ≤-20°C (-4°F); Thawed Sol: 22°C (72°F) for 24 hrs or 4°C (39°F) for 7 days. Do not refreeze. Refer to PI for stability and handling instructions.

TIMOLOL   RX
timolol maleate (Various)

THERAPEUTIC CLASS: Nonselective beta-blocker

INDICATIONS: Treatment of HTN. To reduce cardiovascular mortality and risk of reinfarction with previous myocardial infarction (MI). Migraine prophylaxis.

DOSAGE: *Adults:* HTN: Initial: 10mg bid. Maint: 20-40mg/day. Wait at least 7 days between dose increases. Max: 60mg/day given bid. MI: 10mg bid. Migraine: Initial: 10mg bid. Maint: 20mg qd. Max: 30mg/day in divided doses. May decrease to 10mg qd. D/C if inadequate response after 6-8 weeks with max dose.

HOW SUPPLIED: Tab: 5mg, 10mg*, 20mg* *scored

CONTRAINDICATIONS: Active or history of bronchial asthma, severe chronic obstructive pulmonary disease (COPD), sinus bradycardia, 2nd- and 3rd-degree atrioventricular (AV) block, overt cardiac failure, cardiogenic shock.

WARNINGS/PRECAUTIONS: Caution with well-compensated cardiac failure, diabetes mellitus (DM), mild to moderate COPD, bronchospastic disease, dialysis, hepatic/renal impairment, or cerebrovascular insufficiency. Exacerbation of ischemic heart disease with abrupt cessation. May mask hyperthyroidism or hypoglycemia symptoms. Withdrawal before surgery is controversial. May potentiate weakness with myasthenia gravis. Can cause cardiac failure. Caution and consider monitoring renal function in elderly.

ADVERSE REACTIONS: Fatigue, headache, nausea, arrhythmia, pruritus, dizziness, dyspnea, asthenia, bradycardia.

INTERACTIONS: Possible additive effects and hypotension and/or marked bradycardia with catecholamine-depleting drugs. NSAIDs may reduce antihypertensive effects. Quinidine may potentiate β-blockade. AV conduction time prolonged with digitalis and either diltiazem or vera-pamil. Hypotension, AV conduction disturbances, and left ventricular failure reported with oral calcium antagonists; avoid with cardiac dysfunction. Caution with IV calcium antagonists, insulin, and oral hypoglycemics. May exacerbate rebound HTN following clonidine withdrawal. May block effects of epinephrine.

PREGNANCY: Category C, not for use in nursing.

MECHANISM OF ACTION: $β_1$- and $β_2$-adrenergic receptor blocking agent; reduces cardiac output and plasma renin activity.

PHARMACOKINETICS: Absorption: (PO) Completely absorbed (90%); T_{max}=2 hrs. **Metabolism:** Partially, by liver. **Excretion:** Kidneys; $T_{1/2}$=4 hrs.

NURSING CONSIDERATIONS

Assessment: Assess for bradycardia, cardiogenic shock, 2nd- and 3rd-degree heart block, overt cardiac failure, impaired hepatic/renal function, bronchospastic disease, peripheral vascular disease, DM, thyrotoxicosis, valvular heart disease, pregnancy/nursing status, and possible drug interactions.

Monitoring: Monitor for cardiac failure, HTN, renal function, exacerbation of ischemia following abrupt withdrawal, bronchospastic disease, anaphylactoid reactions, hypersensitivity reactions.

Patient Counseling: Counsel if signs suggest reduced cerebral blood flow; may need to d/c therapy. Instruct not to interrupt or d/c therapy without consulting physician. Counsel about signs/symptoms of congestive heart failure (CHF); instruct to notify physician if signs/symptoms of impending CHF or unexplained respiratory symptoms occur.

Administration: Oral route. **Storage:** 20-25°C (68-77°F); keep in a tight, light-resistant container.

Timoptic   RX
timolol maleate (Aton)

OTHER BRAND NAMES: Timoptic-XE (Aton) - Timoptic in Ocudose (Aton)

THERAPEUTIC CLASS: Nonselective beta-blocker

INDICATIONS: Treatment of elevated intraocular pressure (IOP) in patients with ocular HTN or open-angle glaucoma. (Ocudose) May be used when a patient is sensitive to the preservative in timolol maleate ophthalmic solution, benzalkonium chloride, or when use with a preservative free topical medication is advisable.

DOSAGE: *Adults:* (Sol/Ocudose) Initial: 1 drop (0.25%) in affected eye(s) bid. If clinical response is not adequate, may change to 1 drop (0.5%) in affected eye(s) bid. Maint: 1 drop (0.25-0.5%) in affected eye(s) qd. Max: 1 drop (0.5%) bid. (XE) Initial: 1 drop (0.25 or 0.5%) in the affected eye(s) qd. Max: 1 drop (0.5%) qd. Dose of other topically applied ophthalmic drugs should be adminis-tered at least 10 min prior to gel forming drops. (Sol/Ocudose/XE) Concomitant therapy can be instituted if IOP is still not at a satisfactory level. Evaluate IOP after 4 weeks.

HOW SUPPLIED: Sol: (Timoptic) 0.25% [5mL], 0.5% [5mL, 10mL]; Sol: (Timoptic Ocudose) 0.25%, 0.5% [0.2mL, 60^s]; Sol, Gel Forming: (Timoptic-XE) 0.25%, 0.5% [5mL]

CONTRAINDICATIONS: Bronchial asthma, history of bronchial asthma, severe chronic obstruc-tive pulmonary disease (COPD), sinus bradycardia, 2nd- or 3rd-degree atrioventricular (AV) block, overt cardiac failure, cardiogenic shock.

WARNINGS/PRECAUTIONS: Severe respiratory and cardiac reactions, including death, due to bronchospasm in patients with asthma and, rarely, death associated with cardiac failure report-ed. Caution with cardiac failure; d/c at 1st sign/symptom of cardiac failure. May mask the signs and symptoms of acute hypoglycemia; caution in patients subject to spontaneous hypoglycemia or diabetes mellitus (DM). May mask certain clinical signs (eg, tachycardia) of hyperthyroid-ism; carefully manage patients suspected of developing thyrotoxicosis. Avoid with COPD (eg, chronic bronchitis, emphysema), and history/known bronchospastic disease. Not for use alone in angle-closure glaucoma. May potentiate muscle weakness consistent with myasthenic symptoms (eg, diplopia, ptosis, generalized weakness); caution with myasthenia gravis or patients with myasthenic symptoms. Caution with cerebrovascular insufficiency; consider alternative therapy if signs/symptoms of reduced cerebral blood flow develop. Choroidal detachment after filtration procedures reported. May be more reactive to repeated challenge with history of atopy or severe anaphylactic reactions to variety of allergens; may be unresponsive to usual doses of epinephrine. (Sol/XE) Bacterial keratitis with the use of multiple-dose containers reported.

ADVERSE REACTIONS: Burning/stinging upon instillation. (XE) Ocular: blurred vision, pain, conjunctivitis, discharge, foreign-body sensation, itching, tearing. Systemic: headache, dizziness, upper respiratory infections.

INTERACTIONS: May potentially produce additive effects if used concomitantly with systemic β-blockers. Concomitant use of two topical β-adrenergic blocking agents is not recommended. Caution with oral/IV calcium antagonists because of possible AV conduction disturbances, left ventricular failure, or hypotension. Avoid oral/IV calcium antagonists with impaired cardiac function. Possible additive effects, production of hypotension and/or marked bradycardia may occur when used concomitantly with catecholamine-depleting drugs (eg, reserpine). Concomitant use with calcium antagonists and digitalis may cause additive effects in prolonging AV conduction time. Potentiated systemic β-blockade reported with concomitant use of CYP2D6 inhibitors (eg, quinidine, SSRIs). Mydriasis reported occasionally with epinephrine. May augment risks of general anesthesia in surgical procedures; protracted severe hypotension and difficulty in restarting and maintaining heartbeat reported; gradual withdrawal recommended. Caution with insulin or oral hypoglycemic agents.

PREGNANCY: Category C, not for use in nursing.

MECHANISM OF ACTION: Nonselective β-blocker; reduces elevated and normal IOP, whether or not accompanied by glaucoma. Ocular hypotensive action not clearly established; may be related to reduce aqueous formation and a slight increase in outflow capacity.

PHARMACOKINETICS: Absorption: (Sol/Ocudose) C_{max}=0.46ng/mL (am dose), 0.35ng/mL (afternoon dose); (XE) C_{max}=0.28ng/mL (am dose). **Distribution:** Found in breast milk.

NURSING CONSIDERATIONS

Assessment: Assess for presence or history of bronchial asthma, COPD (eg, bronchitis, emphysema), or any other conditions where treatment is contraindicated or cautioned. Assess for pregnancy/nursing status and possible drug interactions. Assess if planning to undergo major surgery. (Sol/XE) Assess for corneal disease or disruption of the ocular epithelial surface.

Monitoring: Monitor for signs/symptoms of cardiac failure, masking of signs/symptoms of hypoglycemia, masking of hyperthyroidism, thyrotoxicosis, reduced cerebral blood flow, choroidal detachment, anaphylaxis, keratitis and other adverse reactions. Evaluate IOP after 4 weeks of treatment.

Patient Counseling: Advise not to use product if patient has a presence or history of bronchial asthma, severe COPD, sinus bradycardia, 2nd- or 3rd-degree AV block, or cardiac failure. (Sol/XE) Instruct to avoid touching tip of container to eye or surrounding structures. Counsel to seek physician's advice on continued use of product if patient had prior ocular surgery or develops intercurrent ocular condition (eg, trauma or infection). Instruct to handle ocular solutions properly to avoid contamination; inform that using contaminated solution may result in serious eye damage. (Sol) Inform that drug contains benzalkonium chloride which may be absorbed by soft contact lenses. Instruct to remove contact lenses prior to administration and reinsert 15 min following administration. (Ocudose) Instruct about proper administration. Advise to use immediately after opening, and discard the individual unit and any remaining contents immediately after use. (XE) Instruct to invert the closed container and shake once before each use. Instruct to administer at least 10 min apart with other topical ophthalmic medications. Inform that ability to perform hazardous tasks (eg, operating machinery, driving motor vehicle) may be impaired.

Administration: Ocular route. **Storage:** 15-30°C (59-86°F). Avoid freezing. Protect from light. (Ocudose) Keep unit dose container in protective foil overwrap and use within 1 month after opening.

TINDAMAX   RX
tinidazole (Mission)

Carcinogenicity has been seen in mice and rats treated chronically with metronidazole. Although not reported for tinidazole, the two drugs are structurally related and have similar biologic effects. Use only for approved indications.

THERAPEUTIC CLASS: Antiprotozoal agent

INDICATIONS: Treatment of trichomoniasis caused by *Trichomonas vaginalis*, giardiasis caused by *Giardia duodenalis*, intestinal amebiasis and amebic liver abscess caused by *Entamoeba histolytica*, and bacterial vaginosis in nonpregnant women.

DOSAGE: *Adults:* Take with food. Trichomoniasis/Giardiasis: 2g single dose. For trichomoniasis, treat sexual partner with same dose and at same time. Amebiasis: Intestinal: 2g qd for 3 days. Amebic Liver Abscess: 2g qd for 3-5 days. Bacterial Vaginosis: 2g qd for 2 days or 1g qd for 5 days. Hemodialysis: If given on same day and prior to hemodialysis, give additional dose equivalent to one-half of recommended dose at the end of dialysis.

Pediatrics: >3 Yrs: Take with food. Giardiasis: 50mg/kg single dose. Amebiasis: Intestinal: 50mg/kg qd for 3 days. Amebic Liver Abscess: 50mg/kg qd for 3-5 days. Max (for all): 2g/day. May crush tabs in cherry syrup.

HOW SUPPLIED: Tab: 250mg*, 500mg* *scored

CONTRAINDICATIONS: Treatment during 1st trimester of pregnancy, nursing mothers during therapy and 3 days following last dose.

WARNINGS/PRECAUTIONS: Seizures, peripheral neuropathy reported. D/C if abnormal neurologic signs occur. Caution with hepatic impairment or blood dyscrasias. May develop vaginal candidiasis. May develop drug resistance if prescribed in absence of proven or strongly suspected bacterial infection. Caution in elderly.

ADVERSE REACTIONS: Metallic/bitter taste, N/V, vaginal fungal infection, anorexia, headache, dizziness, constipation, dyspepsia, cramps/epigastric discomfort, weakness, fatigue, malaise, convulsions, peripheral neuropathy.

INTERACTIONS: Avoid alcohol during therapy and for 3 days after use. Do not give if patient has taken disulfiram within the last 2 weeks. May potentiate oral anticoagulants. May prolong $T_{1/2}$ and reduce clearance of phenytoin (IV). May decrease clearance of fluorouracil, causing increased side effects; if concomitant use needed, monitor for toxicities. May increase levels of lithium, cyclosporine, and tacrolimus. Separate dosing with cholestyramine. Phenobarbital, rifampin, phenytoin, fosphenytoin, and other CYP3A4 inducers may decrease levels. Cimetidine, ketoconazole, and other CYP3A4 inhibitors may increase levels. Therapeutic effect antagonized by oxytetracycline.

PREGNANCY: Category C, not for use in nursing.

MECHANISM OF ACTION: Antiprotozoal, antibacterial agent; nitro group of tinidazole is reduced by cell extracts of *Trichomonas*. Free nitro radical generated as a result of this reduction may be responsible for antiprotozoal activity.

PHARMACOKINETICS: Absorption: Rapid, complete. (Fasted) C_{max}=47.7mcg/mL, T_{max}=1.6 hrs, AUC=901.6mcg.hr/mL at 72 hrs. **Distribution:** V_d=50L; plasma protein binding (12%); crosses blood-brain and placental barrier; found in breast milk. **Metabolism:** Mainly via oxidation, hydroxylation, conjugation; CYP3A4 mainly involved. **Elimination:** Urine (20-25% unchanged), feces (12%); $T_{1/2}$=12-14 hrs.

NURSING CONSIDERATIONS

Assessment: Assess for blood dyscrasias, seizures, pregnancy/nursing status, hypersensitivity and possible drug interactions. Assess for proven or strongly suspected bacterial infection to avoid drug resistance.

Monitoring: Monitor for convulsive seizures, peripheral neuropathy, vaginal candidiasis, drug resistance, hypersensitivity reactions (urticaria, pruritis, angioedema, erythema multiforme, Stevens-Johnson syndrome).

Patient Counseling: Advise to take with food to minimize epigastric discomfort and other GI side effects. Instruct to avoid alcohol and preparations containing ethanol and propylene glycol during therapy and for 3 days afterward to prevent abdominal cramps, N/V, headache, and flushing. Inform that therapy only treats bacterial, not viral (eg, common cold), infections. Instruct to take ud; skipping doses or not completing full course may decrease effectiveness and increase resistance.

Administration: Oral route. **Storage:** 20-25°C (68-77°F); excursions permitted to 15-30°C (59-86°F). Protect contents from light.

TIVICAY   RX
dolutegravir (ViiV Healthcare)

THERAPEUTIC CLASS: HIV-integrase strand transfer inhibitor

INDICATIONS: Treatment of HIV-1 infection in combination with other antiretroviral agents in adults and pediatric patients ≥12 yrs of age and weighing ≥40kg.

DOSAGE: *Adults:* Treatment-Naive/Treatment-Experienced Integrase Strand Transfer Inhibitor (INSTI)-Naive: 50mg qd. Coadministered with Efavirenz, Fosamprenavir/Ritonavir (RTV), Tipranavir/RTV, or Rifampin: 50mg bid. INSTI-Experienced with Certain INSTI-Associated Resistance Substitutions or Clinically Suspected INSTI Resistance: 50mg bid; alternative combinations that do not include metabolic inducers should be considered where possible. Max: 50mg bid.

Pediatrics: ≥12 Yrs (≥40kg): Treatment-Naive/Treatment-Experienced INSTI-Naive: 50mg qd. Coadministered with Efavirenz, Fosamprenavir/Ritonavir (RTV), Tipranavir/RTV, or Rifampin: 50mg bid.

HOW SUPPLIED: Tab: 50mg

CONTRAINDICATIONS: Coadministration with dofetilide.

WARNINGS/PRECAUTIONS: Hypersensitivity reactions reported; d/c therapy and other suspect agents immediately if signs/symptoms develop, monitor clinical status, including liver aminotransferases, and initiate appropriate therapy. Avoid with previous hypersensitivity to the product. Increased risk for worsening or development of transaminase elevations in patients with underlying hepatitis B or C; conduct appropriate lab testing prior to initiating therapy and monitor for hepatotoxicity during therapy. Redistribution/accumulation of body fat observed. Immune reconstitution syndrome reported. Autoimmune disorders (eg, Graves' disease, polymyositis, Guillain-Barre syndrome) reported in the setting of immune reconstitution and can occur many months after initiation of treatment. Caution in elderly. Not recommended with severe hepatic impairment. Caution in INSTI-experienced patients (with certain INSTI-associated resistance substitutions or clinically suspected INSTI resistance) with severe renal impairment.

ADVERSE REACTIONS: Insomnia, ALT/AST elevation, increased cholesterol/lipase, hyperglycemia.

INTERACTIONS: See Contraindications. Drugs that induce/inhibit UGT1A1, CYP3A, UGT1A3, UGT1A9, breast cancer resistance protein, and P-glycoprotein may decrease/increase levels, respectively. Decreased levels with etravirine; avoid etravirine use without coadministration of atazanavir/RTV, darunavir/RTV, or lopinavir/RTV. Decreased levels with nevirapine, oxcarbazepine, phenytoin, phenobarbital, carbamazepine, and St. John's wort; avoid coadministration. Administer 2 hrs before or 6 hrs after taking medications containing polyvalent cations (eg, cation-containing antacids/laxatives, sucralfate, oral iron/Ca^{2+} supplements, buffered medications). May increase levels of drugs eliminated via OCT2 (eg, metformin); close monitoring is recommended when initiating or discontinuing dolutegravir and metformin together and adjust metformin dose when necessary.

PREGNANCY: Category B, not for use in nursing.

MECHANISM OF ACTION: HIV-1 integrase strand transfer inhibitor; inhibits HIV integrase by binding to integrase active site and blocking the strand transfer step of retroviral deoxyribonucleic acid integration, which is essential for the HIV replication cycle.

PHARMACOKINETICS: Absorption: Adults: AUC=53.6mcg•hr/mL (50mg qd), 75.1mcg•hr/mL (50mg bid); C_{max}=3.67mcg/mL (50mg qd), 4.15mcg/mL (50mg bid); T_{max}=2-3 hrs. **Pediatrics:** C_{max}=3.49mcg/mL (50mg qd), AUC=46mcg•hr/mL (50mg qd). **Distribution:** Plasma protein binding (≥98.9%); V_d=17.4L (50mg qd). **Metabolism:** Via UGT1A1, CYP3A. **Elimination:** Urine (31%, <1% unchanged), feces (53% unchanged); $T_{1/2}$=14 hrs.

NURSING CONSIDERATIONS

Assessment: Assess for previous hypersensitivity to the drug, hepatitis B or C infection, renal/hepatic impairment, pregnancy/nursing status, and possible drug interactions.

Monitoring: Monitor for signs/symptoms of hypersensitivity reactions, redistribution/accumulation of body fat, immune reconstitution syndrome, autoimmune disorders, and other adverse reactions. If hypersensitivity reaction develops, monitor clinical status, including liver aminotransferases. Patients with underlying hepatic disease should be monitored for hepatotoxicity.

Patient Counseling: Instruct to d/c immediately and seek medical attention if rash develops and is associated with any of the following: fever, generally ill feeling, extreme tiredness, muscle or joint aches, blisters, oral lesions, eye inflammation, facial swelling, swelling of the eyes, lips, tongue, or mouth, breathing difficulty, and/or signs and symptoms of liver problems. Advise patients with underlying hepatitis B or C to have lab testing before and during therapy. Inform that fat redistribution/accumulation may occur. Advise to inform physician immediately of any symptoms of infection. Advise that therapy is not a cure for HIV or AIDS and patients may continue to experience illnesses associated with HIV. Instruct to take all HIV medications exactly as prescribed. Advise to avoid doing things that can spread HIV to others. Instruct to inform physician if unusual symptom develops, or if any known symptom persists or worsens. Instruct how to handle missed doses.

Administration: Oral route. Take with or without food. **Storage:** 25°C (77°F); excursions permitted to 15-30°C (59-86°F).

TNK<small>ASE</small>   RX
tenecteplase (Genentech)

THERAPEUTIC CLASS: Thrombolytic agent

INDICATIONS: To reduce mortality with acute myocardial infarction (AMI).

DOSAGE: *Adults:* Administer as single IV bolus over 5 sec. <60kg: 30mg. ≥60 to <70kg: 35mg. ≥70 to <80kg: 40mg. ≥80 to <90kg: 45mg. ≥90kg: 50mg. Max: 50mg/dose.

HOW SUPPLIED: Inj: 50mg

CONTRAINDICATIONS: Active internal bleeding, history of cerebrovascular accident (CVA), intracranial or intraspinal surgery or trauma within 2 months, intracranial neoplasm, arteriovenous (AV) malformation, aneurysm, bleeding diathesis, severe uncontrolled HTN.

WARNINGS/PRECAUTIONS: Weigh benefits/risks with recent major surgery, cerebrovascular disease, recent GI or genitourinary bleeding, recent trauma, HTN (systolic BP ≥180mmHg and/or diastolic BP ≥110mmHg), left heart thrombus, acute pericarditis, subacute bacterial endocarditis, hemostatic defects, severe hepatic dysfunction, pregnancy, diabetic hemorrhagic retinopathy or other hemorrhagic ophthalmic conditions, septic thrombophlebitis or occluded AV cannula at a seriously infected site, elderly, any other bleeding condition that is difficult to manage. Cholesterol embolism and internal/superficial bleeding reported. Arrhythmias may occur with reperfusion. Avoid IM injection, noncompressible arterial puncture, and internal jugular or subclavian venous puncture. Caution with readministration.

ADVERSE REACTIONS: Bleeding.

INTERACTIONS: Increased risk of bleeding with heparin, vitamin K antagonists, and drugs that alter platelet function (eg, aspirin, dipyridamole, GP IIb/IIIa inhibitors) before or after therapy. Weigh benefits/risks with oral anticoagulants, GP IIb/IIIa inhibitors.

PREGNANCY: Category C, caution in nursing.

MECHANISM OF ACTION: Thrombolytic agent; modified form of human tissue plasminogen activator (tPA) that binds to fibrin and converts plasminogen to plasmin.

PHARMACOKINETICS: Metabolism: Liver. **Elimination:** $T_{1/2}$=90-130 min.

NURSING CONSIDERATIONS

Assessment: Assess for active internal bleeding, history of CVA, or any other condition in which treatment is contraindicated or cautioned. Assess for hepatic function, pregnancy/nursing status, advanced age, and drug interactions.

Monitoring: Check for signs/symptoms of bleeding; if serious bleeding occurs, concomitant heparin or antiplatelet agents should be discontinued immediately. Monitor for cholesterol embolization (eg, livedo reticularis, "purple toe" syndrome, acute renal failure), arrhythmia, and hypersensitivity reactions (eg, anaphylaxis).

Patient Counseling: Counsel about increased risk of bleeding while on therapy. Instruct to contact physician if any type of unusual bleeding or hypersensitivity reactions develop.

Administration: IV route. Reconstitute just prior to use. 1) Inject 10mL of SWFI into vial. 2) Do not shake; gently swirl until contents completely dissolved. 3) May be administered as reconstituted solution (5mg/mL). **Storage:** Lyophilized vial: Store at controlled room temperature not exceeding 30°C (86°F), or under refrigeration 2-8°C (36-46°F). Reconstituted: 2-8°C (36-46°F); use within 8 hrs.

TobraDex   RX
dexamethasone - tobramycin (Alcon)

OTHER BRAND NAMES: TobraDex ST (Alcon)

THERAPEUTIC CLASS: Aminoglycoside/corticosteroid

INDICATIONS: Steroid-responsive inflammatory ocular condition and risk of/with superficial bacterial ocular infection caused by susceptible strains of microorganisms.

DOSAGE: *Adults:* (Sus) 1-2 drops into the conjunctival sac(s) q4-6h. Titrate: May increase to 1-2 drops q2h during the initial 24-48 hrs. (ST) 1 drop into conjunctival sac(s) q4-6h. Titrate: May increase to 1 drop q2h during the initial 24-48 hrs. (Sus/ST) Not more than 20mL should be initially prescribed. (Oint) Apply 1/2 inch ribbon in conjunctival sac(s) up to tid-qid. Not more than 8g should be initially prescribed.
Pediatrics: ≥2 Yrs: (Sus) 1-2 drops into the conjunctival sac(s) q4-6h. Titrate: May increase to 1-2 drops q2h during the initial 24-48 hrs. (ST) 1 drop into conjunctival sac(s) q4-6h. Titrate: May increase to 1 drop q2h during the initial 24-48 hrs. (Sus/ST) Not more than 20mL should be initially prescribed. (Oint) Apply 1/2 inch ribbon in conjunctival sac(s) up to tid-qid. Not more than 8g should be initially prescribed.

HOW SUPPLIED: Oint: (Tobramycin-Dexamethasone) 0.3%-0.1% [3.5g]; Sus: 0.3%-0.1% [2.5mL, 5mL, 10mL]; Sus (ST): 0.3%-0.05% [2.5mL, 5mL, 10mL]

CONTRAINDICATIONS: Viral diseases of the cornea and conjunctiva, epithelial herpes simplex keratitis (dendritic keratitis), vaccinia, varicella, mycobacterial infection, and fungal diseases of the eye.

WARNINGS/PRECAUTIONS: Prolonged use may result in glaucoma with optic nerve damage, visual acuity and field of vision defects, posterior subcapsular cataract formation, and may suppress host response and increase risk of secondary ocular infections. Perforations may occur with diseases causing thinning of the cornea or sclera. May mask/enhance existing infection in acute purulent conditions. Fungal infections of the cornea may occur; consider fungal invasion in any persistent corneal ulceration. (Oint/Sus) Not for injection into the eye. Routinely monitor intraocular pressure (IOP). D/C if sensitivity occurs. Cross-sensitivity to other aminoglycoside antibiotics may occur; d/c and institute appropriate therapy if hypersensitivity develops. May result in overgrowth of nonsusceptible organisms, including fungi; initiate appropriate therapy if superinfection occurs. (ST) Monitor IOP if to be used for ≥10 days. Reevaluate after 2 days if patient fails to improve. Use may prolong the course and may exacerbate the severity of many viral infections of the eye (including herpes simplex). May delay healing and increase the incidence of bleb formation after cataract surgery. (Oint) May retard corneal wound healing.

ADVERSE REACTIONS: Hypersensitivity, localized ocular toxicity, secondary infection, increased IOP, posterior subcapsular cataract formation, impaired wound healing.

INTERACTIONS: Monitor total serum concentrations if used concominantly with systemic aminoglycoside antibiotics.

PREGNANCY: Category C, caution in nursing.

MECHANISM OF ACTION: Tobramycin: Aminoglycoside antibiotic; provides action against susceptible organisms. Dexamethasone: Corticoid; suppresses inflammatory response and probably delays or slows healing.

NURSING CONSIDERATIONS

Assessment: Assess for epithelial herpes simplex keratitis (dendritic keratitis), vaccinia, varicella, other viral diseases of cornea or conjunctiva, mycobacterial infection and fungal diseases of eye, diseases that may cause thinning of cornea or sclera, other existing infections, pregnancy/nursing status, and for drug interactions. (ST) Assess for history of herpes simplex.

Monitoring: Monitor for signs/symptoms of hypersensitivity reactions, glaucoma, defects in visual acuity and fields of vision, posterior subcapsular cataracts, perforations, secondary infections, delayed wound healing. (ST) Monitor for IOP if used for ≥10 days, exacerbation of ocular viral infections, and bleb formation. (Oint/Sus) Routinely monitor IOP, and for development of superinfections.

Patient Counseling: Instruct not to touch dropper tip to any surface to avoid contaminating contents and not to wear contact lenses during therapy. (Sus/ST) Inform to shake well before use.

Administration: Ocular route. (Sus/ST) Shake well before use. (Oint) Tilt head back; place finger on cheek just under the eye and gently pull down until a "V" pocket is formed between eyeball and lower lid; apply recommended dose; avoid touching tip of tube to eye; look downward before closing eye. **Storage:** (Sus) 8-27°C (46-80°F); store upright. (Oint/ST): 2-25°C (36-77°F); protect ST from light.

TOFRANIL   RX
imipramine HCl (Mallinckrodt)

> Antidepressants increased the risk of suicidal thinking and behavior (suicidality) in short-term studies in children, adolescents, and young adults with major depressive disorder and other psychiatric disorders. Monitor and observe closely for clinical worsening, suicidality, or unusual changes in behavior in patients who are started on antidepressant therapy. Imipramine is not approved for use in pediatric patients except for use in patients with nocturnal enuresis.

THERAPEUTIC CLASS: Tricyclic antidepressant

INDICATIONS: Relief of symptoms of depression. Temporary adjunct in enuresis in children ≥6 yrs of age.

DOSAGE: *Adults:* Depression: Hospitalized Patients: Initial: 100mg/day in divided doses. Titrate: Increase gradually to 200mg/day; may increase to 250-300mg/day after 2 weeks. Outpatients: Initial: 75mg/day. Titrate: Increase to 150mg/day. Maint: 50-150mg/day. Max: 200mg/day. Elderly: Initial: 30-40mg/day. Max: 100mg/day.
Pediatrics: Depression: ≥12 Yrs: Initial: 30-40mg/day. Max: 100mg/day. Enuresis: ≥6 Yrs: Initial: 25mg/day 1 hr before hs. Titrate: 6-12 Yrs: If inadequate response in 1 week, increase to 50mg before hs. ≥12 Yrs: May increase to 75mg before hs after 1 week. Max: 2.5mg/kg/day. Taper dose gradually when discontinuing.

HOW SUPPLIED: Tab: 10mg, 25mg, 50mg

CONTRAINDICATIONS: Acute recovery period following myocardial infarction, MAOI coadministration or use within 14 days after stopping MAOI therapy.

WARNINGS/PRECAUTIONS: Not approved for use in treating bipolar depression. Extreme caution with cardiovascular (CV) disease, hyperthyroidism, urinary retention, narrow-angle glaucoma, increased intraocular pressure (IOP), and seizure disorders; cardiac surveillance required with CV disease. Caution with elderly, serious depression, renal and hepatic impairment. May alter glucose levels. May activate psychosis in schizophrenia. Manic or hypomanic episodes may occur; consider discontinuing until episode is relieved. May increase hazards with electroshock therapy. Photosensitivity reported. D/C prior to elective surgery. Monitor CBC with differential if fever and sore throat develops; d/c if neutropenia occurs. May impair mental/physical abilities.

ADVERSE REACTIONS: Suicidality, unusual changes in behavior, clinical worsening, sleep disorders, tiredness, mild GI disturbances, orthostatic hypotension, HTN, confusion, hallucinations, numbness, tremors, dry mouth, urticaria, N/V.

INTERACTIONS: See Contraindications. Metabolism may be inhibited by methylphenidate, CYP2D6 inhibitors (eg, quinidine, cimetidine, propafenone, flecainide); downward dosage adjustment may be required. Consider monitoring TCA plasma levels when coadministered with CYP2D6 inhibitors. Caution with SSRI coadministration and when switching between TCAs and SSRIs; wait sufficient time before starting therapy when switching from fluoxetine (eg, ≥5 weeks). Decreased levels with hepatic enzyme inducers (eg, barbiturates, phenytoin) and increased levels with hepatic enzyme inhibitors (eg, cimetidine, fluoxetine); dose adjustment of imipramine may be necessary. May block effects of clonidine, guanethidine, and similar agents. Additive effects with CNS depressants and alcohol. Extreme caution with drugs that lower BP and thyroid drugs. Additive effects (eg, paralytic ileus) with anticholinergics (including antiparkinsonism agents); monitor and adjust dosage carefully. Avoid use of preparations that contain a sympathomimetic amine (eg, epinephrine, norepinephrine); may potentiate catecholamine effects.

PREGNANCY: Not safe in pregnancy; not for use in nursing.

MECHANISM OF ACTION: Tricyclic antidepressant; mechanism unknown. Suspected to potentiate adrenergic synapses by blocking uptake of norepinephrine at nerve endings.

NURSING CONSIDERATIONS

Assessment: Assess for known hypersensitivity, renal/hepatic function, history of suicide, bipolar disorder, depression, urinary retention, narrow-angle glaucoma, hyperthyroidism, CV disease, seizures, pregnancy/nursing status, and possible drug interactions. Obtain baseline LFTs, ECG, IOP.

Monitoring: Monitor for clinical worsening, suicidality, or unusual changes in behavior, psychosis, seizures, CV disease, ECG, and blood sugar levels. Monitor CBC with differential if fever and sore throat develop.

Patient Counseling: Inform patients, families and caregivers about benefits/risks of therapy. Instruct to read and understand Medication Guide, and assist in understanding the contents. Instruct to notify the physician if clinical worsening, suicidality or unusual changes in behavior occur during treatment or when adjusting the dose. Inform that drug may impair mental/physical abilities required for performance of hazardous tasks.

Administration: Oral route. **Storage:** 20-25°C (68-77°F).

TOPAMAX   RX
topiramate (Janssen)

OTHER BRAND NAMES: Topamax Sprinkle (Janssen)

THERAPEUTIC CLASS: Sulfamate-substituted monosaccharide antiepileptic

INDICATIONS: Initial monotherapy in patients ≥2 yrs of age with partial onset or primary generalized tonic-clonic seizures. Adjunct therapy in patients ≥2 yrs of age with partial onset seizures or primary generalized tonic-clonic seizures and with seizures associated with Lennox-Gastaut syndrome. Migraine headache prophylaxis in adults.

DOSAGE: *Adults:* Monotherapy: Epilepsy: Initial: Week 1: 25mg bid. Titrate: Week 2: 50mg bid. Week 3: 75mg bid. Week 4: 100mg bid. Week 5: 150mg bid. Week 6: 200mg bid. Adjunct Therapy: Epilepsy/Lennox-Gastaut Syndrome: ≥17 Yrs: Initial: 25-50mg/day. Titrate: Increments of 25-50mg/day every week. Partial Onset: Usual: 200-400mg/day in 2 divided doses. Tonic-Clonic: Usual: 400mg/day in 2 divided doses. Migraine Prophylaxis: Initial: Week 1: 25mg qpm. Titrate: Week 2: 25mg bid. Week 3: 25mg qam and 50mg qpm. Week 4: 50mg bid. Usual: 100mg/day in 2 divided doses. CrCl <70mL/min: 50% of usual dose. Hemodialysis: May need supplemental dose.
Pediatrics: Monotherapy: Epilepsy: ≥10 Yrs: Initial: Week 1: 25mg bid. Titrate: Week 2: 50mg bid. Week 3: 75mg bid. Week 4: 100mg bid. Week 5: 150mg bid. Week 6: 200mg bid. 2-<10 Yrs: Based on weight. Initial: Week 1: 25mg/day qpm. Titrate: Week 2: Increase to 50mg/day (25mg bid) based on tolerability. May increase by 25-50mg/day each subsequent week as tolerated. Titrate to minimum maintenance dose over 5-7 weeks; may attempt max maintenance dose based upon tolerability and seizure control. Refer to PI for minimum/max maintenance dose recommendations. Adjunct Therapy: Epilepsy/Lennox-Gastaut Syndrome: 2-16 Yrs: Initial: Week 1: 25mg/day qpm (or <25mg/day, based on range of 1-3mg/kg/day). Titrate: Increase at 1- or 2-week intervals by 1-3mg/kg/day increments (in 2 divided doses) to achieve clinical response. Usual: 5-9mg/kg/day in 2 divided doses. CrCl <70mL/min: 50% of usual dose. Hemodialysis: May need supplemental dose.

HOW SUPPLIED: Cap: (Sprinkle) 15mg, 25mg; Tab: 25mg, 50mg, 100mg, 200mg

WARNINGS/PRECAUTIONS: Acute myopia associated with secondary angle-closure glaucoma reported; d/c immediately to reverse symptoms. Elevated intraocular pressure (IOP) of any etiology may lead to serious adverse events (eg, permanent loss of vision) if left untreated. Visual field defects reported in patients independent of elevated IOP; consider discontinuing therapy if visual problems occur. Oligohidrosis and hyperthermia reported, mostly in pediatrics; monitor for decreased sweating and increased body temperature. Hyperchloremic, non-anion gap, metabolic acidosis reported; d/c or reduce dose if metabolic acidosis develops/persists. If decision is to continue therapy, consider alkali treatment. Conditions or therapies that predispose to acidosis (eg, renal disease, severe respiratory disorders, status epilepticus, diarrhea, ketogenic diet, specific drugs) may be additive to the bicarbonate lowering effects. Increased risk of suicidal thoughts/behavior; monitor for the emergence/worsening of depression, suicidal thoughts/behavior, and/or any unusual changes in mood or behavior. Cognitive-related dysfunction, psychiatric/behavioral disturbances, and somnolence or fatigue reported. May cause cleft lip and/or palate in infants if used during pregnancy. D/C gradually to minimize the potential for seizure or increased seizure frequency; appropriate monitoring is recommended when rapid withdrawal is required. Sudden unexplained deaths in epilepsy reported. Patients with inborn errors of metabolism or reduced hepatic mitochondrial activity may be at an increased risk for hyperammonemia with or without encephalopathy; consider hyperammonemic encephalopathy and measure ammonia levels in patients who develop unexplained lethargy, vomiting, or changes in mental status associated with therapy. Kidney stone formation reported; hydration is recommended to reduce new stone formation. Paresthesia may occur. Lab test interactions may occur. Caution with renal/hepatic impairment and in elderly.

ADVERSE REACTIONS: Anorexia, anxiety, diarrhea, fatigue, fever, infection, weight decrease, cognitive problems, paresthesia, somnolence, taste perversion, mood problems, nausea, nervousness, confusion.

INTERACTIONS: Phenytoin or carbamazepine may decrease levels. Increase in systemic exposure of lithium observed following topiramate doses of ≤600mg/day; monitor lithium levels. May cause CNS depression and cognitive/neuropsychiatric adverse events with alcohol and other CNS depressants; use with extreme caution. May decrease contraceptive efficacy and increase breakthrough bleeding with combination oral contraceptives. Concurrent administration of valproic acid has been associated with hyperammonemia with or without encephalopathy, and hypothermia. Other carbonic anhydrase inhibitors (eg, zonisamide, acetazolamide, dichlorphenamide) may increase the severity of metabolic acidosis and may also increase the risk of kidney stone formation. Caution with agents that predispose patients to heat-related disorders (eg, carbonic anhydrase inhibitors, anticholinergics).

PREGNANCY: Category D, caution in nursing.

MECHANISM OF ACTION: Sulfamate-substituted monosaccharide; not established. Suspected to block voltage-dependent Na^+ channels, augment activity of the neurotransmitter gamma-aminobutyrate at some subtypes of the GABA-A receptor, antagonize the AMPA/kainate subtype of the glutamate receptor, and inhibit the carbonic anhydrase enzyme, particularly isoenzymes II and IV.

PHARMACOKINETICS: Absorption: Rapid. T_{max}=2 hrs (400mg). **Distribution:** Plasma protein binding (15-41%). **Metabolism:** Hydroxylation, hydrolysis, glucuronidation. **Elimination:** Urine (70% unchanged); $T_{1/2}$=21 hrs.

NURSING CONSIDERATIONS

Assessment: Assess for renal/hepatic dysfunction, predisposing factors for metabolic acidosis, inborn errors of metabolism, reduced hepatic mitochondrial activity, pregnancy/nursing status, and possible drug interactions. Obtain baseline serum bicarbonate and blood ammonia levels.

Monitoring: Monitor for signs/symptoms of acute myopia, secondary angle-closure glaucoma, visual field defects, oligohidrosis, hyperthermia, cognitive or neuropsychiatric adverse reactions, kidney stones, renal dysfunction, metabolic acidosis, paresthesia, hyperammonemia, and other adverse reactions. Monitor serum bicarbonate and blood ammonia levels.

Patient Counseling: Instruct to seek immediate medical attention if blurred vision, visual disturbances, periorbital pain, or suicidal thoughts/behavior occur and to closely monitor for decreased sweating or high/persistent fever. Warn about risk for metabolic acidosis. Advise to use caution when engaging in activities where loss of consciousness may result in serious danger (eg, swimming, driving, climbing in high places, operating machinery). Inform about risk for hyperammonemia with or without encephalopathy; instruct to contact physician if unexplained lethargy, vomiting, or mental status changes develop. Instruct to maintain adequate fluid intake to minimize risk of kidney stones. Inform of pregnancy risks. Encourage to enroll in the North American Antiepileptic Drug Pregnancy Registry if patient becomes pregnant.

Administration: Oral route. Take without regard to meals. (Cap) Swallow whole or sprinkle over soft food; swallow immediately; do not chew. (Tab) Do not break. **Storage:** Protect from moisture. (Tab) 15-30°C (59-86°F). (Cap) ≤25°C (77°F).

TOPROL-XL

RX

metoprolol succinate (AstraZeneca)

Exacerbation of angina and myocardial infarction (MI) reported following abrupt discontinuation. When discontinuing chronic therapy, particularly with ischemic heart disease, taper over 1-2 weeks with careful monitoring. If worsening of angina or acute coronary insufficiency develops, reinstate therapy promptly, at least temporarily, and take other appropriate measures. Caution patients against interruption or discontinuation of therapy without physician's advice.

THERAPEUTIC CLASS: Selective beta₁-blocker

INDICATIONS: Treatment of HTN alone or in combination with other antihypertensives. Long-term treatment of angina pectoris. Treatment of stable symptomatic (NYHA Class II or III) heart failure (HF) of ischemic, hypertensive, or cardiomyopathic origin.

DOSAGE: *Adults:* HTN: Initial: 25-100mg qd. Titrate: May increase at weekly (or longer) intervals. Max: 400mg/day. Angina: Initial: 100mg qd. Titrate: May gradually increase weekly. Max: 400mg/day. Reduce dose gradually over a period of 1-2 weeks if to be discontinued. HF: Initial: (NYHA Class II HF) 25mg qd or (Severe HF) 12.5mg qd for 2 weeks. Titrate: Double dose every 2 weeks to the highest dose level tolerated. Max: 200mg. Reduce dose if experiencing symptomatic bradycardia. Dose should not be increased until symptoms of worsening HF have been stabilized. Hepatic Impairment: May require lower initial dose; gradually increase dose to optimize therapy. Elderly: Start at low initial dose.
Pediatrics: ≥6 Yrs: HTN: Initial: 1mg/kg qd up to 50mg qd. Adjust dose according to BP response. Max: 2mg/kg (or up to 200mg) qd.

HOW SUPPLIED: Tab, Extended-Release: 25mg*, 50mg*, 100mg*, 200mg* *scored

CONTRAINDICATIONS: Severe bradycardia, 2nd- or 3rd-degree heart block, cardiogenic shock, decompensated cardiac failure, sick sinus syndrome (unless with a permanent pacemaker).

WARNINGS/PRECAUTIONS: Worsening cardiac failure may occur during up-titration; lower dose or temporarily d/c. Avoid with bronchospastic disease; may be used only with those who do not respond to or cannot tolerate other antihypertensive treatment. If used in the setting of pheochromocytoma, should be given in combination with an α-blocker, and only after α-blocker has been initiated; may cause a paradoxical increase in BP if administered alone. Avoid initiation of a high-dose regimen in patients undergoing noncardiac surgery. Chronically administered therapy should not be routinely withdrawn prior to major surgery; however, the impaired ability of the heart to respond to reflex adrenergic stimuli may augment the risks of general anesthesia and surgical procedures. May mask tachycardia occurring with hypoglycemia. May mask signs of hyperthyroidism, such as tachycardia; abrupt withdrawal may precipitate thyroid storm. Patients with a history of severe anaphylactic reaction to variety of allergens may be more reactive to repeated challenge and may be unresponsive to usual doses of epinephrine. May precipitate or aggravate symptoms of arterial insufficiency with peripheral vascular disease (PVD). Caution with hepatic impairment and in elderly.

ADVERSE REACTIONS: Tiredness, dizziness, depression, diarrhea, SOB, bradycardia, rash.

INTERACTIONS: Additive effects with catecholamine-depleting drugs (eg, reserpine, MAOIs). CYP2D6 inhibitors (eg, quinidine, fluoxetine, propafenone) may increase levels. Caution when used with verapamil and diltiazem. May increase the risk of bradycardia with digitalis glycosides, clonidine, diltiazem, and verapamil. When given concomitantly with clonidine, d/c several days before clonidine is gradually withdrawn; may exacerbate rebound HTN.

PREGNANCY: Category C, caution in nursing.

MECHANISM OF ACTION: β₁-selective adrenergic receptor blocker; not established. Proposed to decrease cardiac output, reduce sympathetic outflow to the periphery, and suppress renin activity.

PHARMACOKINETICS: Absorption: Rapid, complete. **Distribution:** Found in breast milk. **Metabolism:** Liver via CYP2D6. **Elimination:** Urine (<5% unchanged); $T_{1/2}$=3-7 hrs.

NURSING CONSIDERATIONS

Assessment: Assess for severe bradycardia, 2nd- or 3rd-degree heart block, cardiogenic shock, decompensated cardiac failure, sick sinus syndrome, presence of pacemaker, ischemic heart disease, bronchospastic disease, diabetes, hyperthyroidism, PVD, arterial insufficiency, hepatic impairment, pheochromocytoma, history of anaphylactic reactions, pregnancy/nursing status, and possible drug interactions.

Monitoring: Monitor for signs/symptoms of worsening cardiac failure during up-titration, hypoglycemia, precipitation of thyroid storm, precipitation/aggravation of arterial insufficiency in patients with PVD, anaphylactic reactions, and other adverse reactions. Monitor patients with ischemic heart disease.

Patient Counseling: Advise to take drug regularly and continuously, ud, preferably with or immediately following meals. Counsel that if dose is missed, take only the next scheduled dose (without doubling). Instruct not to interrupt or d/c therapy without consulting physician. Advise to avoid operating automobiles and machinery or engaging in other tasks requiring alertness. Instruct to contact physician if any difficulty in breathing occurs. Instruct to inform physician or dentist of medication use before any type of surgery. Advise HF patients to consult physician if experience signs/symptoms of worsening HF.

Administration: Oral route. Tab may be divided; do not crush or chew whole or half tab. **Storage:** 25°C (77°F); excursions permitted to 15-30°C (59-86°F).

TORISEL RX
temsirolimus (Wyeth)

THERAPEUTIC CLASS: mTOR inhibitor

INDICATIONS: Treatment of advanced renal cell carcinoma.

DOSAGE: *Adults:* 25mg IV over 30-60 min once a week. Premedication: Diphenhydramine IV (or similar antihistamine) 25-50mg 30 min before the start of each dose. Hold if absolute neutrophil count <1000/mm³, platelet count <75,000/mm³, or NCI CTCAE ≥Grade 3 adverse reactions. Once toxicities resolve to ≤Grade 2, restart with dose reduced by 5mg/week to a dose no lower than 15mg/week. Mild Hepatic Impairment: Reduce dose to 15mg/week. Concomitant Strong CYP3A4 Inhibitors: Consider dose reduction to 12.5mg/week. If strong inhibitor is discontinued, allow washout period of about 1 week before dose readjustment. Concomitant Strong CYP3A4 Inducers: Consider dose increase up to 50mg/week.

HOW SUPPLIED: Inj: 25mg/mL

CONTRAINDICATIONS: Patients with bilirubin >1.5X ULN.

WARNINGS/PRECAUTIONS: Hypersensitivity/infusion reactions observed; may occur very early in the 1st infusion. D/C infusion and observe for 30-60 min if hypersensitivity reaction develops. Caution with hypersensitivity to antihistamines (or patients who cannot receive an antihistamine for other medical reasons), polysorbate 80, or any other component. Give H_1 and/or H_2 receptor antagonist before restarting infusion. Caution with mild hepatic impairment; may need dose reduction. Hyperglycemia reported; may require initiation, or increase in the dose, of insulin and/or PO hypoglycemic agents. Monitor serum glucose before and during treatment. May cause immunosuppression; observe for infections. Interstitial lung disease (ILD) reported; withhold and consider empiric treatment with corticosteroids and/or antibiotics if clinically significant respiratory symptoms develop. Increases in serum TG and cholesterol reported; may require initiation, or increase in the dose, of lipid-lowering agents. Test serum TG and cholesterol before and during treatment. Bowel perforation may occur. Rapidly progressive and sometimes fatal acute renal failure not clearly related to disease progression reported. May cause abnormal wound healing; caution during perioperative period. Increased risk of intracerebral bleeding in patients with CNS tumors. Avoid use of live vaccines and close contact with those who have received live vaccines. May cause fetal harm; avoid pregnancy throughout treatment and for 3 months after discontinuation. Elderly may be more likely to experience certain adverse reactions (eg, diarrhea, edema, pneumonia). Monitor CBC weekly and chemistry panels every 2 weeks.

ADVERSE REACTIONS: Rash, asthenia, mucositis, N/V, edema, anorexia, dyspnea, cough, pain, pyrexia, diarrhea, abdominal pain, constipation, laboratory abnormalities.

INTERACTIONS: Avoid strong CYP3A4 inhibitors or strong CYP3A4/5 inducers; if unavoidable, adjust dose of temsirolimus accordingly. Do not take St. John's wort concomitantly. P-glycoprotein (P-gp) inhibitors may increase concentrations. May increase concentrations of P-gp substrates. Sunitinib may cause dose-limiting toxicity. ACE inhibitors may cause angioneurotic edema-type reactions. Anticoagulants increase risk of intracerebral bleeding. Interferon-α may increase incidence of multiple adverse reactions.

PREGNANCY: Category D, not for use in nursing.

MECHANISM OF ACTION: Mammalian target of rapamycin (mTOR) inhibitor; inhibits activity of mTOR that controls cell division, resulting in G1 growth arrest in treated tumor cells, inability to phosphorylate p70S6k and S6 ribosomal protein, and reduced levels of hypoxia-inducible factors HIF-1 and HIF-2α and the vascular endothelial growth factor.

PHARMACOKINETICS: Absorption: C_{max}=585ng/mL, AUC=1627ng•h/mL. **Distribution:** V_d=172L. **Metabolism:** Liver, via CYP3A4; sirolimus (active metabolite). **Elimination:** Urine (4.6%), feces (78%); $T_{1/2}$=17.3 hrs (temsirolimus), 54.6 hrs (sirolimus).

NURSING CONSIDERATIONS

Assessment: Assess for renal/hepatic impairment, CNS tumors, hypersensitivity, pregnancy/nursing status, and possible drug interactions. Obtain baseline bilirubin levels, lung radiograph, and serum glucose, cholesterol, and TG.

Monitoring: Monitor for hypersensitivity reactions, infections, ILD, clinical respiratory symptoms, bowel perforation, renal/hepatic impairment, intracerebral bleeding, wound healing complications, and other adverse events. Monitor CBCs, chemistry panels, and serum glucose, cholesterol, and TG levels.

Patient Counseling: Inform of possible serious allergic reactions despite premedication with antihistamines. Instruct women of childbearing potential and men with partners of childbearing potential to use reliable contraception throughout treatment and for 3 months after last dose. Advise that blood glucose, TG, and/or cholesterol levels may increase. Counsel on the risk of developing infections, ILD, bowel perforation, renal failure, abnormal wound healing, and intracerebral bleeding. Instruct to report to physician if any facial swelling, difficulty of breathing, excessive thirst or frequency of urination, new/worsening respiratory symptoms, new/worsening abdominal pain, or blood in their stools occurs. Instruct to avoid close contact with people who have received live vaccines.

Administration: IV route. Refer to PI for proper preparation and administration. **Storage:** 2-8°C (36-46°F). Concentrate-diluent mixture stable <25°C (77°F) up to 24 hrs. Protect from light.

TORSEMIDE   RX
torsemide (Various)

OTHER BRAND NAMES: Demadex (Meda)

THERAPEUTIC CLASS: Loop diuretic

INDICATIONS: Treatment of edema associated with congestive heart failure (CHF), renal disease, chronic renal failure (CRF), or hepatic disease. Treatment of HTN, alone or in combination with other antihypertensive agents. (Inj) Indicated when a rapid onset of diuresis is desired or when oral administration is impractical.

DOSAGE: *Adults:* PO/IV (as bolus over 2 min or continuous infusion): CHF: Initial: 10 or 20mg qd. Titrate: Double dose until desired response. Max: 200mg single dose. CRF: Initial: 20mg qd. Titrate: Double dose until desired response. Max: 200mg single dose. Hepatic Cirrhosis: Initial: 5 or 10mg qd with an aldosterone antagonist or K$^+$-sparing diuretic. Titrate: Double dose until desired response. Max: 40mg single dose. HTN: Initial: 5mg qd. Titrate: May increase to 10mg qd after 4-6 weeks, then may add additional antihypertensive agent if needed.

HOW SUPPLIED: Inj: 10mg/mL [2mL, 5mL]; Tab: (Demadex) 5mg*, 10mg*, 20mg*, 100mg* *scored

CONTRAINDICATIONS: Hypersensitivity to sulfonylureas, anuria.

WARNINGS/PRECAUTIONS: Caution in hepatic disease with cirrhosis and ascites; best to initiate therapy in a hospital. Tinnitus and hearing loss (usually reversible) reported. Excessive diuresis may cause dehydration, blood-volume reduction, and possible thrombosis and embolism, especially in elderly. Monitor for electrolyte imbalance, hypovolemia, or prerenal azotemia; if signs/symptoms occur, d/c until corrected and may be restarted at a lower dose. Increased risk of hypokalemia with liver cirrhosis, brisk diuresis, and inadequate oral intake of electrolytes. Diuretic-induced hypokalemia may produce arrhythmias in patients with cardiovascular disease (CVD). Hyperglycemia, hypokalemia, hypomagnesemia, hypercalcemia, and symptomatic gout reported. May increase BUN, SrCr, serum uric acid, total cholesterol, TG, and alkaline phosphatase. Decreased Hgb/Hct/erythrocyte count and increased WBC/platelet count reported.

ADVERSE REACTIONS: Headache, excessive urination, dizziness, hypotension, chest pain, atrial fibrillation, diarrhea, GI hemorrhage, rectal bleeding, rash, shunt thrombosis, syncope.

INTERACTIONS: Caution with aminoglycosides, ethacrynic acid, lithium, digitalis glycosides, and high-dose salicylates. Indomethacin partially inhibits natriuretic effect. Avoid simultaneous cholestyramine administration; may decrease oral drug absorption. Probenecid decreases diuretic activity. Reduces spironolactone clearance. Increased risk of hypokalemia with adrenocorticotropic hormone or corticosteroids. Possible renal dysfunction with NSAIDs (including aspirin). Increased exposure with digoxin.

PREGNANCY: Category B, caution in nursing.

MECHANISM OF ACTION: Loop diuretic; acts from within the lumen of the thick ascending limb of loop of Henle, inhibiting Na$^+$/K$^+$/2Cl$^-$-carrier system.

PHARMACOKINETICS: Absorption: (Tab) Bioavailability (80%); T$_{max}$=1 hr. **Distribution:** V$_d$=12-15L; plasma protein binding (>99%). **Metabolism:** Liver; Carboxylic acid derivative (major metabolite). **Elimination:** Urine (20%); T$_{1/2}$=3.5 hrs.

NURSING CONSIDERATIONS

Assessment: Assess for history of hypersensitivity to the drug or to sulfonylureas, anuria, CVD, renal/hepatic impairment, pregnancy/nursing status, and possible drug interactions.

Monitoring: Monitor for signs/symptoms of hypokalemia, electrolyte imbalance, hypovolemia, prerenal azotemia, arrhythmias, tinnitus, hearing loss, hypersensitivity reactions, renal/hepatic dysfunction and other adverse reactions. Monitor serum electrolytes, BUN, SrCr, uric acid, blood glucose, TG, total cholesterol, alkaline phosphatase, and CBC.

Patient Counseling: Inform of risks and benefits of therapy. Advise to seek medical attention if symptoms of hypokalemia, fluid/electrolyte imbalance, hypersensitivity, hearing loss or tinnitus occur.

Administration: IV/Oral route. (Inj) Flush IV line with normal saline before and after administration. Refer to PI for further administration instructions. **Storage:** (Inj) 20-25°C (68-77°F); do not freeze. (Tab) 15-30°C (59-86°F).

TOVIAZ   RX
fesoterodine fumarate (Pfizer)

THERAPEUTIC CLASS: Muscarinic antagonist

INDICATIONS: Treatment of overactive bladder with symptoms of urge urinary incontinence, urgency, and frequency.

DOSAGE: *Adults:* Initial: 4mg qd. Titrate: May increase to 8mg qd based on individual response and tolerability. Severe Renal Impairment (CrCl <30mL/min)/With Potent CYP3A4 Inhibitors (eg, ketoconazole, itraconazole, clarithromycin): Max: 4mg/day.

HOW SUPPLIED: Tab, Extended Release: 4mg, 8mg

CONTRAINDICATIONS: Urinary/gastric retention, uncontrolled narrow-angle glaucoma, hypersensitivity to tolterodine tartrate tab/extended-release cap.

WARNINGS/PRECAUTIONS: Not recommended with severe hepatic impairment (Child-Pugh C). Angioedema of the face, lips, tongue, and/or larynx reported; d/c and promptly provide appropriate therapy if angioedema occurs. Risk of urinary retention; caution with clinically significant bladder outlet obstruction. Caution with decreased GI motility (eg, severe constipation), controlled narrow-angle glaucoma, and myasthenia gravis. CNS anticholinergic effects (eg, headache, dizziness, and somnolence) reported; monitor for signs, particularly after beginning treatment or increasing the dose, and consider dose reduction or discontinuation if such effects occur.

ADVERSE REACTIONS: Dry mouth, constipation, urinary tract infection, dry eyes.

INTERACTIONS: May increase the frequency and/or severity of dry mouth, constipation, urinary retention, and other anticholinergic pharmacologic effects with other antimuscarinic agents that produce such effects. May potentially alter the absorption of some concomitantly administered drugs due to anticholinergic effects on GI motility. CYP3A4 inhibitors may increase levels; doses >4mg are not recommended in patients taking potent CYP3A4 inhibitors (eg, ketoconazole, itraconazole, clarithromycin). CYP2D6 inhibitors may increase levels. Rifampin or rifampicin may decrease levels.

PREGNANCY: Category C, caution in nursing.

MECHANISM OF ACTION: Muscarinic receptor antagonist; inhibits muscarinic receptors, which mediate contractions of urinary bladder smooth muscle and stimulation of salivary secretion.

PHARMACOKINETICS: Absorption: Well-absorbed. Bioavailability (52%, 5-hydroxymethyl tolterodine [5-HMT]); T_{max} =5 hrs (5-HMT). Variable doses resulted in different pharmacokinetic parameters in extensive and poor CYP2D6 metabolizers. **Distribution:** Plasma protein binding (50%, 5-HMT); V_d =169L (IV, 5-HMT). **Metabolism:** Rapid and extensive via hydrolysis; 5-HMT (active metabolite). 5-HMT further metabolized in liver via CYP2D6 and CYP3A4. **Elimination:** Urine (70%; 16%, 5-HMT), feces (7%); $T_{1/2}$ =7 hrs (5-HMT).

NURSING CONSIDERATIONS

Assessment: Assess for hypersensitivity to the drug or tolterodine tartrate, urinary/gastric retention, narrow-angle glaucoma, bladder outlet obstruction, decreased GI motility, severe constipation, myasthenia gravis, severe hepatic/renal impairment, pregnancy/nursing status, and possible drug interactions.

Monitoring: Monitor for angioedema, upper airway swelling, urinary retention, CNS anticholinergic effects, and other adverse reactions.

Patient Counseling: Inform that therapy may produce angioedema; instruct to promptly d/c therapy and seek immediate medical attention if edema of the tongue/laryngopharynx or difficulty in breathing occur. Counsel that therapy may produce clinically significant adverse effects (eg, constipation, urinary retention). Inform that blurred vision may occur; advise to exercise caution in decisions to engage in potentially dangerous activities until effects have been determined. Inform that heat prostration (due to decreased sweating) may occur when used in a hot environment. Inform that alcohol may enhance drowsiness caused by therapy.

T

Administration: Oral route. Take with or without food. Take tab with liquid and swallow whole; do not crush, chew, or divide. **Storage:** 20-25°C (68-77°F); excursions permitted between 15-30°C (59-86°F). Protect from moisture.

TRADJENTA RX
linagliptin (Boehringer Ingelheim)

THERAPEUTIC CLASS: Dipeptidyl peptidase-4 inhibitor

INDICATIONS: Adjunct to diet and exercise to improve glycemic control in adults with type 2 diabetes mellitus (DM).

DOSAGE: *Adults:* Usual: 5mg qd. With Insulin Secretagogue (eg, Sulfonylurea)/Insulin: May require lower dose of insulin secretagogue or insulin.

HOW SUPPLIED: Tab: 5mg

WARNINGS/PRECAUTIONS: Not for the treatment of type 1 DM or diabetic ketoacidosis. Acute pancreatitis reported; d/c if pancreatitis is suspected. No conclusive evidence of macrovascular risk reduction.

ADVERSE REACTIONS: Hypoglycemia, nasopharyngitis, diarrhea, back pain, arthralgia, upper respiratory tract infection, headache, cough, pain in extremity.

INTERACTIONS: Strong inducers of P-glycoprotein or CYP3A4 (eg, rifampin) may reduce efficacy; use of alternative treatments is strongly recommended. May require lower dose of insulin secretagogue (eg, sulfonylurea) or insulin to reduce risk of hypoglycemia.

PREGNANCY: Category B, caution in nursing.

MECHANISM OF ACTION: Dipeptidyl peptidase-4 inhibitor; degrades the incretin hormones glucagon-like peptide-1 and glucose-dependent insulinotropic polypeptide, thus increasing the concentrations of active incretin hormones, stimulating the release of insulin in a glucose-dependent manner, and decreasing glucagon levels in the circulation.

PHARMACOKINETICS: Absorption: Absolute bioavailability (30%); C_{max}=8.9nmol/L, T_{max}=1.5 hrs, AUC=139nmol•hr/L. **Distribution:** (IV) V_d=1110L; plasma protein binding (concentration-dependent). **Elimination:** Enterohepatic (80%), urine (5%); $T_{1/2}$=12 hrs.

NURSING CONSIDERATIONS

Assessment: Assess for history of hypersensitivity, type of DM, diabetic ketoacidosis, history of pancreatitis, pregnancy/nursing status, and possible drug interactions. Obtain baseline FPG and HbA1c levels.

Monitoring: Monitor for pancreatitis, hypersensitivity reactions, and other adverse reactions. Monitor blood glucose and HbA1c levels periodically.

Patient Counseling: Inform of the potential risks/benefits of therapy and alternative modes of therapy. Advise on the importance of adherence to dietary instructions, regular physical activity, periodic blood glucose monitoring and HbA1c testing, recognition/management of hypoglycemia/hyperglycemia, and assessment for diabetes complications. Instruct to promptly seek medical advice during periods of stress (eg, fever, trauma, infection, surgery) as medication requirements may change. Inform that acute pancreatitis has been reported; instruct to promptly d/c and contact physician if persistent severe abdominal pain occurs. Instruct to take as prescribed; advise not to double the next dose if missed. Counsel to inform physician or pharmacist if any unusual symptom develops or if any known symptom persists/worsens.

Administration: Oral route. May be taken with or without food. **Storage:** 25°C (77°F); excursions permitted to 15-30°C (59-86°F).

TRANSDERM SCOP RX
scopolamine (Novartis Consumer)

THERAPEUTIC CLASS: Anticholinergic

INDICATIONS: Prevention of N/V associated with motion sickness or recovery from anesthesia and/or opiate analgesia and surgery in adults.

DOSAGE: *Adults:* Motion Sickness N/V: 1 patch at least 4 hrs before the antiemetic effect is required. Replace patch after 3 days if therapy is required for >3 days. Postoperative N/V: 1 patch on the evening before surgery or 1 hr prior to cesarean section. Remove patch 24 hrs following surgery.

HOW SUPPLIED: Patch: 1.5mg [4^s]

CONTRAINDICATIONS: Angle closure glaucoma.

WARNINGS/PRECAUTIONS: May increase intraocular pressure (IOP) with open-angle glaucoma; monitor therapy and adjust during use. May cause temporary dilation of pupils and blurred vision if contact with eyes occurs. Caution with pyloric obstruction, urinary bladder neck obstruction, and intestinal obstruction. May aggravate seizures or psychosis. Idiosyncratic reactions may occur with ordinary therapeutic doses. Increased CNS effects may occur in elderly and with hepatic/renal impairment. May impair physical/mental abilities. Remove patch before undergoing a magnetic resonance imaging (MRI) scan; skin burns at the patch site reported. May interfere with gastric secretion test.

ADVERSE REACTIONS: Dry mouth, dizziness, somnolence, urinary retention, agitation, visual impairment, confusion, mydriasis, pharyngitis.

INTERACTIONS: May decrease absorption of oral medications due to decreased gastric motility and delayed gastric emptying. Caution with other drugs with CNS effects (eg, sedatives, tranquilizers, alcohol) and anticholinergic properties (eg, meclizine, TCAs, muscle relaxants).

PREGNANCY: Category C, caution in nursing.

MECHANISM OF ACTION: Anticholinergic agent; acts as competitive inhibitor at postganglionic muscarinic receptor sites of parasympathetic nervous system and on smooth muscles that respond to acetylcholine but lack cholinergic innervation. Acts in the CNS by blocking cholinergic transmission from vestibular nuclei to higher centers in the CNS and from reticular formation to the vomiting center.

PHARMACOKINETICS: Absorption: Well-absorbed. T_{max}=24 hrs. **Distribution:** Crosses placenta; found in breast milk. **Metabolism:** Extensive; conjugation. **Elimination:** Urine (<10%, <5% unchanged); $T_{1/2}$=9.5 hrs.

NURSING CONSIDERATIONS

Assessment: Assess for known hypersensitivity to the drug, glaucoma, pyloric obstruction, urinary bladder neck obstruction, intestinal obstruction, history of seizures or psychosis, hepatic/renal impairment, pregnancy/nursing status, and for possible drug interactions.

Monitoring: Monitor for aggravation of seizures or psychosis, idiosyncratic reactions (eg, agitation, hallucinations, paranoid behaviors, delusions), CNS effects, drowsiness, disorientation, confusion, withdrawal symptoms, and other adverse reactions. Monitor IOP in patients with open-angle glaucoma.

Patient Counseling: Inform elderly that patch may cause a greater likelihood of CNS effects and to seek medical care if patient becomes confused, disoriented, or dizzy while wearing the patch or after removing. Inform that patch may cause drowsiness, disorientation, and confusion; advise to use caution when engaging in activities that require mental alertness. Instruct to avoid alcohol. Instruct to seek medical care if withdrawal symptoms occur following abrupt discontinuation. Inform that patch may cause temporary dilation of pupils and blurred vision. Instruct to wash hands thoroughly with soap and water immediately after handling patch. Instruct to dispose the patch properly to avoid contact with children or pets. Advise to remove patch before undergoing an MRI to avoid skin burns. Instruct to use ud. Advise to remove the patch immediately and promptly contact physician if symptoms of acute angle closure glaucoma or difficulty in urinating is experienced.

Administration: Transdermal route. Apply only to skin in the postauricular area. After application, wash hands thoroughly with soap and water and dry. Wear only 1 patch at anytime. Do not cut patch. Discard patch if displaced and replace with a fresh patch. **Storage:** 20-25°C (68-77°F).

TRAVATAN Z   RX
travoprost (Alcon)

THERAPEUTIC CLASS: Prostaglandin analog

INDICATIONS: Reduction of elevated intraocular pressure (IOP) in patients with open-angle glaucoma or ocular HTN.

DOSAGE: *Adults:* 1 drop in affected eye(s) qd in pm. Space by at least 5 min if using >1 topical ophthalmic drug.
Pediatrics: ≥16 Yrs: 1 drop in affected eye(s) qd in pm. Space by at least 5 min if using >1 topical ophthalmic drug.

HOW SUPPLIED: Sol: 0.004% [2.5mL, 5mL]

WARNINGS/PRECAUTIONS: Changes to pigmented tissues, including increased pigmentation of iris (may be permanent), eyelid, and eyelashes (may be reversible) reported. Regularly examine patients with noticeably increased iris pigmentation. May cause changes to eyelashes and vellus hair in the treated eye. May exacerbate active intraocular inflammation (eg, uveitis). Macular edema, including cystoid macular edema, reported; caution with aphakic patients, pseudophakic patients with torn posterior lens capsule, or patients at risk of macular edema. Treatment of angle-closure, inflammatory, or neovascular glaucoma has not been evaluated. Bacterial keratitis reported with multidose container. Remove contact lenses prior to instillation; may reinsert 15 min after administration.

ADVERSE REACTIONS: Ocular hyperemia, foreign body sensation, decreased visual acuity, eye discomfort/pruritus/pain.

PREGNANCY: Category C, caution in nursing.

MECHANISM OF ACTION: Prostaglandin analog; not established. Selective FP prostanoid receptor agonist believed to reduce IOP by increasing uveoscleral outflow.

PHARMACOKINETICS: Absorption: C_{max}=0.018ng/mL; T_{max}=30 min. **Metabolism:** Cornea, via esterases to active free acid and systemically to inactive metabolites via β-oxidation and reduction. **Elimination:** Urine (<2%); $T_{1/2}$=45 min.

NURSING CONSIDERATIONS

Assessment: Assess for active intraocular inflammation (uveitis), active macular edema, aphakic/pseudophakic patients with torn posterior lens capsule, angle-closure, inflammatory, or neovascular glaucoma, and pregnancy/nursing status.

Monitoring: Monitor for increased pigmentation of the iris and periorbital tissue (eyelid); changes in eyelashes; macular edema; and bacterial keratitis.

Patient Counseling: Inform about risk of brown pigmentation of iris and darkening of eyelid skin. Inform about the possibility of eyelash and vellus hair changes. Advise to avoid touching tip of dispensing container to eye, surrounding structures, fingers, or any other surface, in order to avoid contamination of the sol. Advise to consult physician if having ocular surgery or if intercurrent ocular conditions (eg, trauma or infection) or ocular reactions develop. Instruct to remove contact lenses prior to instillation; reinsert 15 min after administration. Instruct to administer at least 5 min apart if using >1 topical ophthalmic drugs.

Administration: Ocular route. **Storage:** 2-25°C (36-77°F).

TRAZODONE   RX
trazodone HCl (Various)

Antidepressants increased the risk of suicidal thinking and behavior (suicidality) in children, adolescents and young adults in short-term studies of major depressive disorder (MDD) and other psychiatric disorders. Monitor and observe closely for clinical worsening, suicidality, or unusual changes in behavior. Not approved for use in pediatric patients.

THERAPEUTIC CLASS: Triazolopyridine derivative

INDICATIONS: Treatment of MDD.

DOSAGE: *Adults:* Initial: 150mg/day in divided doses after a meal or light snack. Titrate: May increase by 50mg/day every 3-4 days. Max: (Outpatient) 400mg/day in divided doses. (Inpatient) 600mg/day in divided doses. Once adequate response is achieved, reduce dose gradually, with subsequent adjustment, depending on therapeutic response. Maint: Generally recommended to continue treatment for several months after an initial response. Maintain on the lowest effective dose and periodically reassess to determine the continued need for maint treatment. Administer major portion of daily dose at hs or reduce dose if drowsiness occurs.

HOW SUPPLIED: Tab: 50mg*, 100mg*, 150mg*, 300mg* *scored

WARNINGS/PRECAUTIONS: May precipitate mixed/manic episodes in patients at risk for bipolar disorder. Not approved for treatment of bipolar depression. Monitor withdrawal symptoms while d/c treatment; gradually reduce dose whenever possible. Serotonin syndrome or neuroleptic malignant syndrome (NMS)-like reactions reported; d/c immediately and initiate supportive symptomatic treatment. May cause QT/QTc interval prolongation and torsades de pointes. Not for use during initial recovery phase of myocardial infarction (MI). Caution with cardiac disease; may cause cardiac arrhythmias. Hypotension, including orthostatic hypotension and syncope, reported. May increase risk of bleeding events. Rare cases of priapism reported; caution in men with conditions that may predispose to priapism (eg, sickle cell anemia, multiple myeloma, or leukemia) or with penile anatomical deformation (eg, angulation, cavernosal fibrosis, or Peyronie's disease); d/c with erection lasting >6 hrs (painful or not). Hyponatremia may occur; d/c and institute appropriate medical intervention. May cause somnolence or sedation and may impair physical/mental abilities. Withdrawal symptoms, including anxiety, agitation, and sleep disturbances, reported. Caution with hepatic/renal impairment and elderly.

ADVERSE REACTIONS: Drowsiness, dry mouth, headache, nervousness, N/V, blurred vision, abdominal/gastric disorder, nasal/sinus congestion, musculoskeletal aches/pains, tremors.

INTERACTIONS: May cause serotonin syndrome or NMS-like reactions with serotonergic drugs (eg, SSRIs, SNRIs, triptans), drugs which impair serotonin metabolism, antipsychotics, or other dopamine antagonists; d/c immediately and initiate therapy if these occur. Not recommended with serotonin precursors (eg, tryptophan). CYP3A4 inhibitors (eg, ritonavir, ketoconazole, indinavir, itraconazole) may increase levels with the potential for adverse effects. Potent

CYP3A4 inhibitors may increase risk of cardiac arrhythmia; consider lower dose of trazodone. Carbamazepine decreases levels; monitor to determine if a dose increase is required. Increased serum digoxin or phenytoin levels reported; monitor serum levels and adjust dose PRN. Do not use with MAOIs or within 14 days of d/c an MAOI. May enhance response to alcohol, barbiturates, and other CNS depressants. May alter PT in patients on warfarin. Concomitant use with an antihypertensive may require a dose reduction of the antihypertensive drug. Monitor and use caution with NSAIDs, aspirin, and other drugs that affect coagulation or bleeding. Increased risk of hyponatremia with diuretics. May increase risk of cardiac arrhythmia with drugs that prolong QT interval.

PREGNANCY: Category C, caution in nursing.

MECHANISM OF ACTION: Triazolopyridine derivative; mechanism not established. Suspected to be related to its potentiation of serotonergic activity in the CNS. Preclinical studies show selective inhibition of neuronal reuptake of serotonin and antagonism at 5-HT-2A/2C serotonin receptors.

PHARMACOKINETICS: Absorption: Well-absorbed; T_{max}=1 hr (fasting), 2 hrs (fed). **Distribution:** Plasma protein binding (89%-95%). **Metabolism:** Liver (extensive); CYP3A4 via oxidative cleavage; m-chlorophenylpiperazine (active metabolite). **Elimination:** Urine (<1% unchanged).

NURSING CONSIDERATIONS

Assessment: Assess for psychiatric history, including family history of suicide, bipolar disorder, and depression, for cardiac disease (eg, recent MI), conditions that may predispose to priapism, penile anatomical deformation, arrhythmias, renal/hepatic impairment, pregnancy/nursing status, and possible drug interactions.

Monitoring: Monitor for signs/symptoms of clinical worsening, suicidality, unusual changes in behavior, serotonin syndrome, QT/QTc interval prolongation, priapism, cardiac arrhythmias, orthostatic hypotension, syncope, bleeding events, hyponatremia, hepatic/renal function, withdrawal symptoms and for other adverse reactions.

Patient Counseling: Inform about the benefits and risks of therapy. Instruct patients and caregivers to notify physician if signs of clinical worsening, changes in behavior, or suicidality occur. Instruct men to immediately d/c use and contact physician if erection lasts >6 hrs, whether painful or not. Inform that withdrawal symptoms (eg, anxiety, agitation, and sleep disturbances) may occur. Caution against performing potentially hazardous tasks (eg, operating machinery/driving). Inform that therapy may enhance response to alcohol, barbiturates, and other CNS depressants. Instruct to notify physician if pregnant, intending to become pregnant, or nursing.

Administration: Oral route. Take shortly after a meal or light snack. Swallow whole or half the tab along the score line. **Storage:** 20-25°C (68-77°F).

TREANDA   RX
bendamustine HCl (Cephalon)

THERAPEUTIC CLASS: Alkylating agent

INDICATIONS: Treatment of chronic lymphocytic leukemia (CLL). Treatment of indolent B-cell non-Hodgkin lymphoma (NHL) that has progressed during or within 6 months of treatment with rituximab or a rituximab-containing regimen.

DOSAGE: *Adults:* CLL: Usual: 100mg/m² IV over 30 min on Days 1 and 2 of a 28-day cycle, up to 6 cycles. Delay administration in the event of Grade 4 hematologic toxicity or clinically significant ≥Grade 2 nonhematologic toxicity. May reinitiate therapy once nonhematologic toxicity has recovered to ≤Grade 1 and/or the blood counts have improved (absolute neutrophil count [ANC] ≥1 x 10⁹/L, platelets ≥75 x 10⁹/L). ≥Grade 3 Hematologic Toxicity: Reduce dose to 50mg/m² on Days 1 and 2 of each cycle; if ≥Grade 3 toxicity recurs, reduce dose to 25mg/m² on Days 1 and 2 of each cycle. ≥Grade 3 Nonhematologic Toxicity: Reduce dose to 50mg/m² on Days 1 and 2 of each cycle. May consider dose re-escalation in subsequent cycles. NHL: Usual: 120mg/m² IV over 60 min on Days 1 and 2 of a 21-day cycle, up to 8 cycles. Delay administration in the event of Grade 4 hematologic toxicity or clinically significant ≥Grade 2 nonhematologic toxicity. May reinitiate therapy once nonhematologic toxicity has recovered to ≤Grade 1 and/or the blood counts have improved (ANC ≥1 x 10⁹/L, platelets ≥75 x 10⁹/L). Grade 4 Hematologic Toxicity: Reduce dose to 90mg/m² on Days 1 and 2 of each cycle; if Grade 4 toxicity recurs, reduce dose to 60mg/m² on Days 1 and 2 of each cycle. ≥Grade 3 Nonhematologic Toxicity: Reduce dose to 90mg/m² on Days 1 and 2 of each cycle; if ≥Grade 3 toxicity recurs, reduce dose to 60mg/m² on Days 1 and 2 of each cycle.

HOW SUPPLIED: Inj: 25mg, 100mg

WARNINGS/PRECAUTIONS: Severe myelosuppression reported; may require dose delays and/or subsequent dose reductions if recovery to the recommended values has not occurred by the 1st day of the next scheduled cycle. Monitor leukocytes, platelets, Hgb, and neutrophils frequently if treatment-related myelosuppression occurs. Infection, including pneumonia, sepsis, septic shock, and death reported. Infusion reactions and severe anaphylactic/anaphylactoid reactions reported; monitor clinically and d/c for severe reactions. Consider measures to prevent severe reactions (eg, antihistamines, antipyretics, corticosteroids) in subsequent cycles in patients who have experienced Grade 1 or 2 infusion reactions. Consider discontinuation for Grade 3 infusion reactions as clinically appropriate; d/c for Grade 4 infusion reactions. Do not rechallenge in patients who experience ≥Grade 3 allergic-type reactions. Tumor lysis syndrome reported; preventive measures include vigorous hydration and close monitoring of blood chemistry, particularly K^+ and uric acid levels. Skin reactions, including rash, toxic skin reactions, and bullous exanthema, reported; monitor closely and withhold or d/c if skin reactions are severe or progressive. Premalignant and malignant diseases (eg, myelodysplastic syndrome, myeloproliferative disorders, acute myeloid leukemia, bronchial carcinoma) reported. Extravasations reported; assure good venous access prior to starting infusion and monitor for infusion-site redness, swelling, pain, infection, and necrosis during and after administration. May cause fetal harm. Caution with mild/moderate renal impairment and with mild hepatic impairment. Do not use with CrCl <40mL/min or with moderate (AST/ALT 2.5-10X ULN and total bilirubin 1.5-3X ULN) or severe (total bilirubin >3X ULN) hepatic impairment.

ADVERSE REACTIONS: Anemia, thrombocytopenia, neutropenia, lymphopenia, leukopenia, N/V, fatigue, diarrhea, pyrexia, constipation, anorexia, cough, headache, decreased weight, stomatitis.

INTERACTIONS: CYP1A2 inhibitors (eg, fluvoxamine, ciprofloxacin) may increase plasma concentrations of bendamustine and may decrease plasma concentrations of active metabolites. CYP1A2 inducers (eg, omeprazole, smoking) may decrease plasma concentrations of bendamustine and may increase plasma concentrations of active metabolites. Use caution or consider alternative treatments if treatment with CYP1A2 inhibitors/inducers is needed. Increased risk of severe skin toxicity with allopurinol.

PREGNANCY: Category D, not for use in nursing.

MECHANISM OF ACTION: Alkylating agent; has not been established. Bifunctional mechlorethamine derivative containing a purine-like benzimidazole ring; forms electrophilic alkyl groups that form covalent bonds with electron-rich nucleophilic moieties, resulting in interstrand DNA crosslinks. Bifunctional covalent linkage can lead to cell death via several pathways. Active against both quiescent and dividing cells.

PHARMACOKINETICS: Distribution: Plasma protein binding (94-96%); V_d=20-25L. **Metabolism:** Extensive via hydrolytic (primary), oxidative, and conjugative pathways; gamma-hydroxy-bendamustine (M3), N-desmethyl-bendamustine (M4) (active minor metabolites) via CYP1A2. **Elimination:** Urine (50%, 3.3% unchanged, <1% as M3 and M4), feces (25%); $T_{1/2}$=40 min, 3 hrs (M3), 30 min (M4).

NURSING CONSIDERATIONS

Assessment: Assess for renal/hepatic impairment, hypersensitivity to drug, pregnancy/nursing status, and possible drug interactions.

Monitoring: Monitor for signs/symptoms of myelosuppression, infections, anaphylaxis/infusion reactions, tumor lysis syndrome, skin reactions, premalignant/malignant diseases, extravasation, infusion-site reactions, laboratory abnormalities, and other adverse reactions. Monitor CBCs and blood chemistry, particularly K^+ and uric acid levels.

Patient Counseling: Inform of the possibility of mild/serious allergic reactions and to immediately report rash, facial swelling, or difficulty breathing during or soon after infusion. Inform that therapy may cause a decrease in WBCs, platelets, and RBCs, and of the need for frequent monitoring of blood counts; instruct to report SOB, significant fatigue, bleeding, fever, or other signs of infection. Advise that therapy may cause tiredness; instruct to avoid driving or operating dangerous tools or machinery if tiredness occurs. Inform that therapy may cause N/V, diarrhea, and mild rash or itching; instruct to report any adverse reactions immediately to physician. Advise women to avoid becoming pregnant and men to use reliable contraception throughout treatment and for 3 months after discontinuation of therapy; instruct to immediately report pregnancy and to avoid nursing while on therapy.

Administration: IV route. Refer to PI for reconstitution/preparation, administration, safe handling, and disposal instructions. **Storage:** Up to 25°C (77°F); excursions permitted up to 30°C (86°F). Protect from light. Final Admixture: Stable for 24 hrs at 2-8°C (36-47°F) or for 3 hrs at 15-30°C (59-86°F) with room light.

TRECATOR   RX
ethionamide (Wyeth)

THERAPEUTIC CLASS: Peptide synthesis inhibitor

INDICATIONS: Treatment of active tuberculosis (TB) in patients with *Mycobacterium tuberculosis* resistant to isoniazid or rifampin, or where there is intolerance to other drugs.

DOSAGE: *Adults:* 15-20mg/kg qd with food. May give in divided doses with poor GI tolerance. Max: 1g/day. Alternate Regimen: Initial: 250mg qd then titrate gradually to optimal doses as tolerated, or 250mg qd for 1-2 days, then 250mg bid for 1-2 days, then 1g/day in 3-4 divided doses. Continue therapy until bacteriological conversion has become permanent and maximal clinical improvement occurs.
Pediatrics: ≥12 Yrs: 10-20mg/kg/day in divided doses given bid or tid with food, or 15mg/kg/day as single dose. Continue therapy until bacteriological conversion has become permanent and maximal clinical improvement occurs.

HOW SUPPLIED: Tab: 250mg

CONTRAINDICATIONS: Severe hepatic impairment.

WARNINGS/PRECAUTIONS: Give with pyridoxine. Rapid development of resistance if used alone; should be used with at least 1 or 2 other drugs. Perform ophthalmologic exams before and periodically during therapy. Measure serum transaminases prior to initiation and monthly thereafter. Risk of hypoglycemia in diabetics; monitor blood glucose prior to initiation then periodically. Hypothyroidism reported; monitor TFTs.

ADVERSE REACTIONS: N/V, diarrhea, abdominal pain, excessive salivation, metallic taste, stomatitis, anorexia, psychotic disturbances, drowsiness, dizziness, hypersensitivity reactions, increase in serum bilirubin, SGOT or SGPT.

INTERACTIONS: D/C all antituberculous medication with elevated serum transaminases until resolved; reintroduce sequentially to determine which drug is responsible. May raise isoniazid levels. May potentiate adverse effects of other antituberculous drugs. Convulsions reported with cycloserine. Risk of psychotic reactions with excessive ethanol ingestion.

PREGNANCY: Category C, not for use in nursing.

MECHANISM OF ACTION: Peptide synthesis inhibitor; may be bacteriostatic or bactericidal in action.

PHARMACOKINETICS: Absorption: Completely absorbed; C_{max}=2.16mcg/mL, T_{max}=1.02 hrs, AUC=7.67mcg•hr/mL. **Distribution:** V_d=93.5L; plasma protein binding (30%); widely distributed into body tissues. **Metabolism:** Liver (extensive). **Elimination:** Urine ≤1%; $T_{1/2}$=1.92 hrs.

NURSING CONSIDERATIONS

Assessment: Assess for severe hepatic impairment, diabetes mellitus, susceptibility test, pregnancy/nursing status, and possible drug interactions.

Monitoring: Monitor for hypersensitivity reactions, and GI and psychotic disturbances. Determination of serum transaminases (SGOT, SGPT), blood glucose, thyroid function, and eye exams should be done periodically.

Patient Counseling: Advise to report vision loss or blurriness, with/without eye pain. Instruct to avoid excessive alcohol ingestion. Instruct to take ud; skipping doses or not completing full course may decrease effectiveness and increase resistance.

Administration: Oral route. **Storage:** 20-25°C (68-77°F). Dispense in tight container.

TRELSTAR   RX
triptorelin pamoate (Watson)

THERAPEUTIC CLASS: Synthetic gonadotropin-releasing hormone analog

INDICATIONS: Palliative treatment of advanced prostate cancer.

DOSAGE: *Adults:* 3.75mg IM every 4 weeks, 11.25mg IM every 12 weeks, or 22.5mg IM every 24 weeks as single dose in either buttock.

HOW SUPPLIED: Inj: 3.75mg, 11.25mg, 22.5mg [vial, Mixject delivery system]

CONTRAINDICATIONS: Women who are or may become pregnant.

WARNINGS/PRECAUTIONS: Administer under the supervision of a physician. Dosage strengths are not additive; select strength based on desired dosing schedule. Anaphylactic shock, hypersensitivity, and angioedema reported; d/c immediately and administer appropriate supportive and symptomatic care if these occur. May cause transient increase in serum testosterone levels; worsening or onset of new symptoms (eg, bone pain, neuropathy, hematuria, urethral/bladder outlet obstruction) may occur during the 1st few weeks of treatment. Spinal cord compression reported; institute standard treatment or consider immediate orchiectomy in extreme cases if spinal cord compression or renal impairment develops. Closely monitor patients with metastatic vertebral lesions and/or with upper or lower urinary tract obstruction during 1st few weeks of therapy. Long-term androgen deprivation therapy prolongs QT interval; consider whether benefits outweigh potential risks in patients with congenital long QT syndrome, electrolyte abnormalities, or congestive heart failure (CHF) and in patients taking Class 1A (eg, quinidine, procainamide) or Class III (eg, amiodarone, sotalol) antiarrhythmics. Hyperglycemia and an increased risk of developing diabetes reported; monitor blood glucose and/or HbA1c periodically. Sudden cardiac death, stroke, and an increased risk of developing myocardial infarction (MI) reported; monitor for signs/symptoms of cardiovascular disease (CVD). Monitor response by measuring serum testosterone levels periodically or as indicated. Chronic or continuous administration in therapeutic doses may suppress pituitary-gonadal axis; diagnostic tests of pituitary-gonadal function conducted during treatment and after cessation of therapy may be misleading.

ADVERSE REACTIONS: Hot flush, HTN, headache, skeletal pain, dysuria, leg edema, erectile dysfunction, testicular atrophy, inj-site pain, leg pain, pain.

INTERACTIONS: Avoid with hyperprolactinemic drugs.

PREGNANCY: Category X, not for use in nursing.

MECHANISM OF ACTION: Synthetic gonadotropin-releasing hormone (GnRH) agonist analog; initially increases circulating levels of luteinizing hormone (LH), follicle-stimulating hormone (FSH), testosterone, and estradiol. Chronic and continuous administration causes a sustained decrease in LH and FSH secretion and marked reduction of testicular steroidogenesis.

PHARMACOKINETICS: Absorption: (IM) C_{max}=28.4ng/mL (3.75mg), 38.5ng/mL (11.25mg), 44.1ng/mL (22.5mg); T_{max}=1-3 hrs. **Distribution:** (0.5mg IV) V_d=30-33L. **Elimination:** (IV) Urine (41.7%, unchanged), $T_{1/2}$=3 hrs.

NURSING CONSIDERATIONS

Assessment: Assess for hypersensitivity to drug/other GnRH agonists/GnRH, metastatic vertebral lesions, urinary tract obstruction, diabetes, congenital long QT syndrome, electrolyte abnormalities, CHF, and possible drug interactions. Obtain baseline serum testosterone levels.

Monitoring: Monitor response to drug and for signs/symptoms of worsening prostate cancer, spinal cord compression, renal impairment, anaphylactic shock, hypersensitivity, angioedema, CVD, QT interval prolongation, and other adverse reactions. Periodically monitor serum testosterone, blood glucose, and/or HbA1c.

Patient Counseling: Inform that patients may experience worsening of symptoms of prostate cancer during the 1st weeks of treatment and that these symptoms should decline 3-4 weeks following administration of therapy. Inform of the increased risk of developing diabetes, MI, sudden cardiac death, and stroke. Advise that allergic reactions could occur and that serious reactions require immediate treatment. Instruct to report any previous hypersensitivity to drug, other GnRH agonists, or GnRH.

Administration: IM route. Administer in either buttock; alternate inj site periodically. Administer immediately upon reconstitution. Refer to PI for reconstitution instructions. **Storage:** 20-25°C (68-77°F). Do not freeze with Mixject.

TREXIMET   RX
naproxen sodium - sumatriptan (GlaxoSmithKline)

> May increase risk of serious cardiovascular (CV) thrombotic events, myocardial infarction (MI), and stroke; increased risk with duration of use and with cardiovascular disease (CVD) or risk factors for CVD. Increased risk of serious GI adverse events (eg, bleeding, ulceration, stomach/intestinal perforation) that can be fatal and occur anytime during use without warning symptoms; elderly patients are at greater risk.

THERAPEUTIC CLASS: 5-HT$_1$-agonist/NSAID

INDICATIONS: Acute treatment of migraine attacks with or without aura in adults.

DOSAGE: *Adults:* Individualize dose. Usual: 1 tab. Max: 2 tabs/24 hrs. Dosing should be at least 2 hrs apart.

HOW SUPPLIED: Tab: (Naproxen-Sumatriptan): 500mg-85mg

CONTRAINDICATIONS: History, symptoms, or signs of ischemic cardiac syndromes (eg, angina pectoris, MI, silent myocardial ischemia), cerebrovascular syndromes (eg, strokes, transient ischemic attacks), or peripheral vascular syndromes (eg, ischemic bowel disease). Other significant CVD, coronary artery bypass graft (CABG) surgery, hepatic impairment, uncontrolled HTN, hemiplegic or basilar migraine, concurrent administration of MAO-A inhibitors or use within 2 weeks of discontinuation of an MAO-A inhibitor, use within 24 hrs of any ergotamine-containing or ergot-type drugs (eg, dihydroergotamine, methysergide) or other 5-HT$_1$ agonists. Patients who have experienced asthma, rhinitis, nasal polyps, or allergic-type reactions after taking aspirin (ASA) or other NSAIDs.

WARNINGS/PRECAUTIONS: May cause coronary artery vasospasm; do not give with unrecognized ischemic/vasospastic coronary artery disease (CAD). Avoid in patients whom unrecognized CAD is predicted by the presence of risk factors (eg, HTN, hypercholesterolemia, smoker, obesity, diabetes, strong CAD family history, menopause, males >40 yrs) unless with a satisfactory CV evaluation; administer 1st dose under medical supervision and consider obtaining an ECG immediately following administration. Signs and symptoms suggestive of decreased arterial flow should be evaluated for atherosclerosis or predisposition to vasospasm. Chest discomfort, jaw or neck tightness, peripheral vascular ischemia, and colonic ischemia reported. Transient and permanent blindness and significant partial vision loss have been reported with the use of sumatriptan. Caution with controlled HTN, fluid retention, and heart failure (HF). Serotonin syndrome may occur. Anaphylactic/anaphylactoid reactions may occur; avoid in patients with ASA-triad. May cause serious skin reactions (eg, exfoliative dermatitis, Stevens-Johnson syndrome, toxic epidermal necrolysis); d/c at 1st appearance of skin rash/hypersensitivity. Avoid in late pregnancy; may cause premature closure of ductus arteriosus. Caution with diseases that may alter absorption/metabolism/excretion, preexisting asthma, history of epilepsy or conditions associated with a lowered seizure threshold. Renal injury reported with long-term use; increased risk with renal/hepatic impairment, HF, and in elderly. Not recommended in patients with CrCl <30mL/min. Exclude potentially serious neurologic conditions before treatment in patients not previously diagnosed with migraine headache or who experience headache that is atypical for them. Anemia may occur; monitor Hgb/Hct if signs/symptoms of anemia develop. May prolong bleeding time; caution with coagulation disorders. D/C if signs and symptoms of liver/renal disease develop, systemic manifestations (eg, eosinophilia) occur, or abnormal LFTs persist or worsen. Use lowest effective dose for the shortest duration possible. Caution with prior history of ulcer disease, GI bleeding, risk factors for GI bleeding, history of inflammatory bowel disease. Overuse may lead to exacerbation of headache.

ADVERSE REACTIONS: CV thrombotic events, MI, stroke, GI events, dizziness, somnolence, nausea, chest discomfort/pain, neck/throat/jaw pain/tightness/pressure.

INTERACTIONS: See Contraindications. Avoid with other naproxen-containing products. Caution with methotrexate; may prolong serum methotrexate levels. Not recommended with ASA. Increased plasma lithium levels; monitor for lithium toxicity. May reduce natriuretic effect of loop (eg, furosemide) or thiazide diuretics; monitor for signs of renal failure and diuretic efficacy. Probenecid may increase levels. May reduce the antihypertensive effect of ACE inhibitors and β-blockers (eg, propranolol). Increased risk of renal toxicity with diuretics and ACE inhibitors. Increased risk of GI bleeding with PO corticosteroids or anticoagulants, warfarin, alcohol use, and smoking. Serotonin syndrome reported, particularly during combined use with SSRIs or SNRIs.

PREGNANCY: Category C, not for use in nursing.

MECHANISM OF ACTION: Naproxen: NSAID; not established. May be related to prostaglandin synthetase inhibition. Sumatriptan: 5-HT$_1$ receptor agonist; mediates vasoconstriction of human basilar artery and vasculature of human dura mater that correlates with the relief of migraine headache.

PHARMACOKINETICS: Absorption: Naproxen: Rapid and complete; bioavailability (95%); T_{max}=5 hrs. Sumatriptan: Bioavailability (15%), T_{max}=1 hr. **Distribution:** Naproxen: V_d=0.16L/kg; plasma protein binding (>99%); found in breast milk. Sumatriptan: V_d=2.4L/kg; plasma protein binding (14-21%); found in breast milk. **Metabolism:** Naproxen: Extensive; 6-0-desmethyl naproxen metabolite. Sumatriptan: Indole acetic acid (metabolite). **Elimination:** Naproxen: Urine (<1% unchanged, <1% 6-0-desmethyl naproxen, 66-92% conjugates), $T_{1/2}$=19 hrs. Sumatriptan: Urine (60%), feces (40%); $T_{1/2}$=2 hrs.

NURSING CONSIDERATIONS

Assessment: Assess for conditions where treatment is contraindicated or cautioned, pregnancy/nursing status, and possible drug interactions. Obtain ECG after 1st administration for those with CAD risk factors.

Monitoring: Monitor for signs/symptoms of cardiac events, colonic ischemia, bloody diarrhea, serotonin syndrome, hypersensitivity reactions, jaw/neck tightness, seizures, headache, signs and symptoms of GI adverse events, and clinical response. For long-term therapy or with CAD risk factors, perform periodic monitoring of CV function. Monitor vital signs, CBC, LFTs, bleeding time, renal function, and ECG periodically.

Patient Counseling: Inform to seek medical advice if symptoms of CV events, GI ulcerations/bleeding, skin/hypersensitivity reactions, unexplained weight gain or edema, hepatotoxicity, anaphylactic/anaphylactoid reactions occur. Instruct to notify physician if pregnant, planning to become pregnant, or nursing. Inform about the risk of serotonin syndrome, particularly during combined use with SSRIs or SNRIs. Advise to use caution with activities that require alertness if they experience drowsiness, dizziness, vertigo, or depression during therapy.

Administration: Oral route. Give 1st dose in physician's office or similar medically staffed and equipped facility unless patient has previously received sumatriptan. Take with or without food. Do not split, crush, or chew tab. **Storage:** 25°C (77°F); excursions permitted to 15-30°C (59-86°F).

T

TRIBENZOR   RX
olmesartan medoxomil - hydrochlorothiazide - amlodipine (Daiichi Sankyo)

D/C when pregnancy is detected. Drugs that act directly on the renin-angiotensin system (RAS) can cause injury/death to the developing fetus.

THERAPEUTIC CLASS: ARB/calcium channel blocker (dihydropyridine)/thiazide diuretic

INDICATIONS: Treatment of HTN.

DOSAGE: *Adults:* Usual: Dose qd. May increase after 2 weeks. Max: 40mg-10mg-25mg qd. Replacement Therapy: May substitute for individually titrated components. Add-On/Switch Therapy: Use if not adequately controlled on any 2 of the following antihypertensive classes: ARBs, calcium channel blockers, and diuretics. With dose-limiting adverse reactions to an individual component while on any dual combination of the components of Tribenzor, may switch to Tribenzor containing a lower dose of that component. Severe Hepatic Impairment/Elderly ≥75 Yrs: Initial: 2.5mg amlodipine.

HOW SUPPLIED: Tab: (Olmesartan-Amlodipine-HCTZ) 20mg-5mg-12.5mg, 40mg-5mg-12.5mg, 40mg-5mg-25mg, 40mg-10mg-12.5mg, 40mg-10mg-25mg

CONTRAINDICATIONS: Anuria, sulfonamide-derived drug hypersensitivity. Coadministration with aliskiren in patients with diabetes.

WARNINGS/PRECAUTIONS: Not for initial therapy of HTN. Avoid use with severe renal impairment (CrCl ≤30mL/min). Renal impairment reported; consider withholding or discontinuing if progressive renal impairment becomes evident. Sprue-like enteropathy with symptoms of severe, chronic diarrhea with substantial weight loss reported; exclude other etiologies if these symptoms develop, and consider discontinuation in cases where no other etiology is identified. Olmesartan: Symptomatic hypotension may occur in patients with an activated RAS (eg, volume-and/or salt-depleted patients receiving high doses of diuretics) after initiation of treatment; initiate treatment under close medical supervision. Oliguria or progressive azotemia and (rarely) acute renal failure and/or death may occur in patients whose renal function may depend on renin-angiotensin-aldosterone system activity (eg, severe congestive heart failure [CHF]). May increase SrCr and BUN levels with renal artery stenosis. Increased blood creatinine levels and hyperkalemia reported. Amlodipine: May develop increased frequency, duration, or severity of angina or acute myocardial infarction (MI), particularly with severe obstructive coronary artery disease (CAD). Rare reports of acute hypotension; caution with severe aortic stenosis. Hepatic enzyme elevations reported. HCTZ: May precipitate azotemia with renal disease, and hepatic coma due to fluid and electrolyte imbalance. Observe for clinical signs of fluid or electrolyte imbalance (eg, hyponatremia, hypochloremic alkalosis, hypokalemia). Hypokalemia may cause cardiac arrhythmia and may sensitize/exaggerate the response of the heart to toxic effects of digitalis. May cause metabolic acidosis, hyperuricemia or precipitation of frank gout, hyperglycemia, manifestation of latent diabetes mellitus (DM), hypomagnesemia, hypersensitivity reactions (with or without a history of allergy or bronchial asthma), exacerbation/activation of systemic lupus erythematosus (SLE), and increased cholesterol and TG levels. Enhanced effects in post-sympathectomy patients. D/C before testing for parathyroid function. May cause idiosyncratic reaction, resulting in acute transient myopia and acute angle-closure glaucoma; d/c as rapidly as possible.

ADVERSE REACTIONS: Dizziness, peripheral edema, headache, fatigue, nasopharyngitis, muscle spasms, nausea.

INTERACTIONS: See Contraindications. Olmesartan: NSAIDs, including selective COX-2 inhibitors, may result in deterioration of renal function, including possible acute renal failure and attenuated antihypertensive effect; monitor renal function periodically. Dual blockade of the RAS is associated with increased risk of hypotension, hyperkalemia, and changes in renal function (including acute renal failure); closely monitor BP, renal function, and electrolytes with concomitant agents that also affect the RAS. Avoid with aliskiren in patients with renal impairment (GFR <60mL/min). Reduced levels with colesevelam; administer at least 4 hrs before colesevelam dose. Amlodipine: May increase simvastatin exposure; limit simvastatin dose to 20mg/day. HCTZ: Increased risk of lithium toxicity; avoid concurrent use. Alcohol, barbiturates, or narcotics may potentiate orthostatic hypotension. Dose adjustment of antidiabetic drugs (eg, oral agents, insulin) may be required. Additive effect or potentiation with other antihypertensives. Anionic exchange resins (eg, cholestyramine, colestipol) may impair absorption. Corticosteroids and adrenocorticotropic hormone may intensify electrolyte depletion, particularly hypokalemia. May decrease response to pressor amines (eg, norepinephrine). May increase response to nondepolarizing skeletal muscle relaxants (eg, tubocurarine). NSAIDs may reduce diuretic, natriuretic, and antihypertensive effects.

PREGNANCY: Category D, not for use in nursing.

MECHANISM OF ACTION: Olmesartan: Angiotensin II receptor antagonist; blocks vasoconstrictor effects of angiotensin II by selectively blocking binding of angiotensin II to AT_1 receptor in vascular smooth muscle. Amlodipine: Calcium channel blocker (dihydropyridine); inhibits trans-membrane influx of Ca^{2+} ions into vascular smooth muscle and cardiac muscle. HCTZ: Thiazide diuretic; has not been established. Affects renal tubular mechanisms of electrolyte reabsorption, directly increasing excretion of Na^+ and Cl^- and indirectly reducing plasma volume.

PHARMACOKINETICS: Absorption: Olmesartan: Rapid; absolute bioavailability (26%); T_{max}=1-2 hrs. Amlodipine: Absolute bioavailability (64-90%); T_{max}=6-12 hrs. HCTZ: T_{max}=1.5-2 hrs. **Distribution:** Olmesartan: V_d=17L; plasma protein binding (99%). Amlodipine: Plasma protein binding (93%). HCTZ: Crosses placenta; found in breast milk. **Metabolism:** Olmesartan: Ester hydrolysis. Amlodipine: Hepatic (extensive). **Elimination:** Olmesartan: Urine (35-50%), feces; $T_{1/2}$=13 hrs. Amlodipine: Urine (60% metabolites, 10% parent), $T_{1/2}$=30-50 hrs. HCTZ: Urine (≥61% unchanged); $T_{1/2}$=5.6-14.8 hrs.

NURSING CONSIDERATIONS

Assessment: Assess for anuria, sulfonamide-derived drug hypersensitivity, history of penicillin allergy, history of allergy or bronchial asthma, renal/hepatic impairment, aortic stenosis, renal artery stenosis, SLE, CHF, volume/salt depletion, electrolyte imbalances, postsympathectomy status, DM, CAD, pregnancy/nursing status, any other conditions where treatment is cautioned, and possible drug interactions.

Monitoring: Monitor for signs/symptoms of hypotension, fluid/electrolyte imbalance, sprue-like enteropathy, exacerbation/activation of SLE, hypersensitivity reactions, idiosyncratic reaction, metabolic disturbances, myopia and angle-closure glaucoma (eg, decreased visual acuity, ocular pain), increased frequency, duration, or severity of angina or acute MI upon starting or at the time of dosage increase, latent DM, and other adverse reactions. Monitor BP, visual acuity, cholesterol levels, TG levels, and renal/hepatic function.

Patient Counseling: Counsel about risks/benefits of therapy and possible adverse effects. Inform of consequences of exposure during pregnancy; instruct to notify physician as soon as possible if pregnant/plan to become pregnant. Caution about lightheadedness, especially during the 1st days of therapy, and advise to report to physician. Instruct to d/c and consult physician if syncope occurs. Caution that inadequate fluid intake, excessive perspiration, diarrhea, or vomiting may lead to an excessive fall in BP, which may result in lightheadedness or syncope.

Administration: Oral route. Take with or without food. **Storage:** 25°C (77°F); excursions permitted to 15-30°C (59-86°F).

TRICOR   RX
fenofibrate (AbbVie)

THERAPEUTIC CLASS: Fibric acid derivative

INDICATIONS: Adjunctive therapy to diet to reduce elevated LDL, total cholesterol, TGs, and apolipoprotein B, and to increase HDL in adults with primary hypercholesterolemia or mixed dyslipidemia. Adjunctive therapy to diet for treatment of adults with severe hypertriglyceridemia.

DOSAGE: *Adults:* Primary Hypercholesterolemia/Mixed Dyslipidemia: Initial/Max: 145mg qd. Severe Hypertriglyceridemia: Initial: 48-145mg/day. Titrate: Adjust dose if necessary following repeat lipid determinations at 4- to 8-week intervals; individualize dose. Max: 145mg qd. Mild to Moderate Renal Impairment: Initial: 48mg/day. Titrate: Increase only after evaluation of effects on renal function and lipid levels. Elderly: Dose based on renal function. Consider reducing the dosage if lipid levels fall significantly below the targeted range. D/C if no adequate response after 2 months of treatment with max dose.

HOW SUPPLIED: Tab: 48mg, 145mg

CONTRAINDICATIONS: Severe renal impairment (including dialysis), active liver disease (including primary biliary cirrhosis and unexplained persistent liver function abnormalities), preexisting gallbladder disease, and nursing mothers.

WARNINGS/PRECAUTIONS: Not shown to reduce coronary heart disease morbidity and mortality in patients with type 2 diabetes mellitus (DM). Increased risk of myopathy and rhabdomyolysis; risk increased with DM, renal insufficiency, hypothyroidism, and in elderly. D/C therapy if marked CPK elevation occurs or myopathy/myositis is suspected or diagnosed. Increases in serum transaminases, hepatocellular, chronic active and cholestatic hepatitis, and cirrhosis (rare) reported; perform baseline and regular periodic monitoring of LFTs, and d/c therapy if enzyme levels persist >3X the normal limit. Elevations in SrCr reported; monitor renal function in patients with renal impairment or at risk for renal insufficiency. May cause cholelithiasis; d/c if gallstones are found. Acute hypersensitivity reactions and pancreatitis reported. Mild to moderate decreases in Hgb, Hct and WBCs, thrombocytopenia, and agranulocytosis reported; periodically monitor RBC and WBC counts during the first 12 months of therapy. May cause venothromboembolic disease. Severe decreases in HDL levels reported; check HDL levels within the 1st few months after initiation of therapy. If a severely depressed HDL level is detected, withdraw therapy, monitor HDL level until it has returned to baseline, and do not reinitiate therapy. Estrogen therapy, thiazide diuretics, and β-blockers may be associated with massive rises in plasma TG; discontinuation of these drugs may obviate the need for specific drug therapy of hypertriglyceridemia.

ADVERSE REACTIONS: Abnormal LFTs, respiratory disorder, abdominal pain, back pain, increased AST/ALT/CPK, headache.

INTERACTIONS: Increased risk of rhabdomyolysis with HMG-CoA reductase inhibitors (statins); avoid combination unless benefit outweighs risk. May potentiate anticoagulant effects of coumarin anticoagulants; use with caution, reduce anticoagulant dosage, and monitor PT/INR frequently. Immunosuppressants (eg, cyclosporine, tacrolimus) may produce nephrotoxicity; consider benefits and risks, use lowest effective dose, and monitor renal function with immunosuppressants and other potentially nephrotoxic agents. Bile acid-binding resins may bind other drugs given concurrently; take at least 1 hr before or 4-6 hrs after the bile acid-binding resin to avoid impeding its absorption. Cases of myopathy, including rhabdomyolysis, reported when coadministered with colchicine; caution when prescribing with colchicine.

PREGNANCY: Category C, not for use in nursing.

MECHANISM OF ACTION: Fibric acid derivative; activates peroxisome proliferator-activated receptor α. Increases lipolysis and elimination of TG-rich particles from plasma by activating lipoprotein lipase and reducing production of apoprotein C-III (lipoprotein lipase activity inhibitor). Also, induces an increase in the synthesis of apolipoproteins A-I, A-II, and HDL.

PHARMACOKINETICS: Absorption: Well-absorbed. T_{max} =6-8 hrs. **Distribution:** Plasma protein binding (99%). **Metabolism:** Rapid by ester hydrolysis to fenofibric acid (active metabolite); conjugation with glucuronic acid. **Elimination:** Urine (60%, fenofibric acid and glucuronate conjugate), feces (25%); $T_{1/2}$=20 hrs.

NURSING CONSIDERATIONS

Assessment: Assess for renal impairment, active liver disease, preexisting gallbladder disease, other medical conditions (eg, DM, hypothyroidism), hypersensitivity to drug, pregnancy/nursing status, and possible drug interactions. Obtain baseline LFTs.

Monitoring: Monitor for signs/symptoms of myositis, myopathy, or rhabdomyolysis; measure CPK levels in patients reporting such symptoms. Monitor for cholelithiasis, pancreatitis, hypersensitivity reactions, pulmonary embolism and deep vein thrombosis. Monitor renal function, LFTs, CBC, and lipid levels. Monitor PT/INR frequently with coumarin anticoagulants.

Patient Counseling: Advise of potential benefits and risks of therapy, and of medications to avoid during treatment. Instruct to follow appropriate lipid-modifying diet during therapy and to take drug qd, at the prescribed dose. Instruct to inform physician of all medications, supplements, and herbal preparations being taken, any changes in medical condition, development of muscle pain, tenderness, or weakness, and onset of abdominal pain or any other new symptoms. Advise to return for routine monitoring.

Administration: Oral route. May be taken without regard to meals. Swallow tab whole. **Storage:** 25°C (77°F); excursions permitted to 15-30°C (59-86°F). Protect from moisture.

TRIGLIDE
fenofibrate (Shionogi)

RX

THERAPEUTIC CLASS: Fibric acid derivative

INDICATIONS: Adjunctive therapy to diet to reduce elevated LDL, total cholesterol, TG, and apolipoprotein B, and to increase HDL in adults with primary hypercholesterolemia or mixed dyslipidemia. Adjunctive therapy to diet for treatment of adults with severe hypertriglyceridemia.

DOSAGE: *Adults:* Primary Hypercholesterolemia/Mixed Dyslipidemia: 160mg qd. Severe Hypertriglyceridemia: Initial: 50-160mg/day. Titrate: Adjust dose if necessary following repeat lipid determinations at 4- to 8-week intervals; individualize dose. Max: 160mg qd. Mild to Moderate Renal Impairment: Initial: 50mg/day. Titrate: Increase only after evaluation of effects on renal function and lipid levels. Elderly: Dose based on renal function. Consider reducing dose if lipid levels fall significantly below the targeted range. D/C if no adequate response after 2 months of treatment with max dose.

HOW SUPPLIED: Tab: 50mg, 160mg

CONTRAINDICATIONS: Severe renal impairment (including dialysis), active liver disease (including primary biliary cirrhosis and unexplained persistent liver function abnormalities), preexisting gallbladder disease, and nursing mothers.

WARNINGS/PRECAUTIONS: Not shown to reduce coronary heart disease morbidity and mortality in patients with type 2 diabetes mellitus (DM). Increased risk of myopathy and rhabdomyolysis; risk increased with DM, renal insufficiency, hypothyroidism, and in elderly. D/C if marked CPK elevation occurs or myopathy/myositis is suspected. Increases in serum transaminases, hepatocellular, chronic active and cholestatic hepatitis, and cirrhosis (rare) reported; perform baseline and regular periodic monitoring of LFTs, and d/c therapy if enzyme levels persist >3X the normal limit. Elevations in SrCr reported. May cause cholelithiasis; d/c if gallstones are found. Acute hypersensitivity reactions and pancreatitis reported. Mild to moderate decreases in Hgb, Hct and WBCs, thrombocytopenia, and agranulocytosis reported; periodically monitor RBC and WBC counts during the first 12 months of therapy. May cause venothromboembolic disease. Severe decreases in HDL levels reported; check HDL levels within the 1st few months after initiation of therapy. If a severely depressed HDL level is detected, withdraw therapy, monitor HDL level until it has returned to baseline, and do not reinitiate therapy. Estrogen therapy, thiazide diuretics, and β-blockers may be associated with massive rises in plasma TG; d/c of these drugs may obviate the need for specific drug therapy of hypertriglyceridemia.

ADVERSE REACTIONS: Abnormal LFTs, respiratory disorder, abdominal pain, back pain, increased AST/ALT/CPK, headache.

INTERACTIONS: Increased risk of rhabdomyolysis with HMG-CoA reductase inhibitors (statins); avoid combination unless benefit outweighs risk. May potentiate anticoagulant effects of coumarin anticoagulants; use with caution, reduce anticoagulant dosage, and monitor PT/INR frequently. Immunosuppressants (eg, cyclosporine, tacrolimus) may produce nephrotoxicity; consider benefits and risks, use lowest effective dose, and monitor renal function with immunosuppressants and other potentially nephrotoxic agents. Bile acid-binding resins may bind other drugs given concurrently; take at least 1 hr before or 4-6 hrs after the bile acid-binding resin to avoid impeding its absorption. Cases of myopathy, including rhabdomyolysis, reported when coadministered with colchicine; caution when prescribing with colchicine. Changes in exposure/levels with atorvastatin, pravastatin, fluvastatin, glimepiride, metformin, and rosiglitazone.

PREGNANCY: Category C, not for use in nursing.

MECHANISM OF ACTION: Fibric acid derivative; activates peroxisome proliferator-activated receptor α. Increases lipolysis and elimination of TG-rich particles from plasma by activating lipoprotein lipase and reducing production of apoprotein C-III (lipoprotein lipase activity inhibitor). Also, induces an increase in the synthesis of apoproteins A-I, A-II, and HDL.

PHARMACOKINETICS: Absorption: Well-absorbed; T_{max}=3 hrs. **Distribution:** Plasma protein binding (99%). **Metabolism:** Rapid by ester hydrolysis to fenofibric acid (active metabolite); conjugation with glucuronic acid. **Elimination:** Urine (60%, fenofibric acid and glucuronate conjugate), feces (25%); $T_{1/2}$=16 hrs.

NURSING CONSIDERATIONS

Assessment: Assess for renal impairment, active liver disease, preexisting gallbladder disease, other medical conditions (eg, DM, hypothyroidism), hypersensitivity to the drug, pregnancy/nursing status, and possible drug interactions. Obtain baseline LFTs.

Monitoring: Monitor for signs/symptoms of myositis, myopathy, or rhabdomyolysis; measure CPK levels in patients reporting such symptoms. Monitor for cholelithiasis, pancreatitis, hypersensitivity reactions, pulmonary embolism, and deep vein thrombosis. Monitor renal function, LFTs, CBC, and lipid levels.

Patient Counseling: Advise of potential benefits and risks of therapy, and medications to be avoided during treatment. Instruct to follow appropriate lipid-modifying diet during therapy, and to take drug ud. Instruct to notify physician of all medications, supplements, and herbal preparations being taken, any changes in medical condition, development of muscle pain, tenderness, or weakness, and onset of abdominal pain, or any other new symptoms. Advise to return for routine monitoring.

Administration: Oral route. May be taken without regard to meals. Swallow tab whole; do not crush, dissolve, or chew. **Storage:** 20-25°C (68-77°F); excursions permitted to 15-30°C (59-86°F). Protect from light and moisture.

TRILEPTAL   RX
oxcarbazepine (Novartis)

THERAPEUTIC CLASS: Dibenzazepine

INDICATIONS: Monotherapy or adjunctive therapy in the treatment of partial seizures in adults. Monotherapy in the treatment of partial seizures in children ≥4 yrs with epilepsy, and adjunctive therapy in children ≥2 yrs with partial seizures.

DOSAGE: *Adults:* Give in a bid regimen. Adjunctive Therapy: Initial: 600mg/day. Titrate: May increase by a max of 600mg/day at weekly intervals. Usual: 1200mg/day. Conversion to Monotherapy: Initial: 600mg/day while reducing dose of other antiepileptic drugs (AEDs). Max dose of therapy should be reached in about 2-4 weeks while other AEDs should be completely withdrawn over 3-6 weeks. Titrate: May increase by a max of 600mg/day at weekly intervals. Usual: 2400mg/day. Initiation of Monotherapy: Initial: 600mg/day. Titrate: Increase by 300mg/day every 3rd day. Usual: 1200mg/day. Renal Impairment (CrCl <30mL/min): Initial: 1/2 of usual starting dose (300mg/day). Titrate: Increase slowly.

Pediatrics: Give in a bid regimen. 4-16 Yrs: Adjunctive Therapy: Initial: 8-10mg/kg/day, not to exceed 600mg/day. Maint: Achieve over 2 weeks. >39kg: 1800mg/day. 29.1-39kg: 1200mg/day. 20-29kg: 900mg/day. Conversion to Monotherapy: Initial: 8-10mg/kg/day while reducing dose of other AEDs. Withdraw other AEDs over 3-6 weeks. Titrate: May increase by a max of 10mg/kg/day at weekly intervals. Usual: Refer to PI for range of maint doses based on weight. Initiation of Monotherapy: Initial: 8-10mg/kg/day. Titrate: Increase by 5mg/kg/day every 3rd day. Usual: Refer to PI for range of maint doses based on weight. 2-<4 Yrs: Adjunctive Therapy: Initial: 8-10mg/kg/day, not to exceed 600mg/day. May consider 16-20mg/kg/day for patients <20kg. Maint: Achieve over 2-4 weeks. Max: 60mg/kg/day. Renal Impairment (CrCl <30mL/min): Initial: 1/2 of usual starting dose (300mg/day). Titrate: Increase slowly.

HOW SUPPLIED: Sus: 300mg/5mL [250mL]; Tab: 150mg*, 300mg*, 600mg* *scored

WARNINGS/PRECAUTIONS: Clinically significant hyponatremia may develop; consider measurement of serum Na⁺ levels during maintenance treatment, particularly if symptoms indicating hyponatremia develop. Anaphylaxis and angioedema involving the larynx, glottis, lips, and eyelids reported; d/c therapy if any of these reactions develop, start alternative treatment, and do not rechallenge. Caution in patients with history of hypersensitivity reactions to carbamazepine; d/c immediately if signs/symptoms of hypersensitivity develop. Serious dermatological reactions (eg, Stevens-Johnson syndrome, toxic epidermal necrolysis) reported; consider discontinuing and prescribing another AED if a skin reaction develops. Increased risk of suicidal thoughts or behavior; monitor for emergence/worsening of depression, suicidal thoughts or behavior, and/or any unusual changes in mood or behavior. Withdraw gradually to minimize the potential of increased seizure frequency. Associated with CNS-related adverse events (cognitive symptoms, somnolence or fatigue, coordination abnormalities). Multiorgan hypersensitivity reactions reported; d/c therapy and start alternative treatment if suspected. Pancytopenia, agranulocytosis, and leukopenia reported; consider discontinuation if any evidence of hematologic events develop. Levels may decrease during pregnancy; monitor patients during pregnancy and through the postpartum period. Associated with decreases in T4, without changes in T3 or TSH. Caution with severe hepatic impairment.

ADVERSE REACTIONS: Dizziness, somnolence, diplopia, fatigue, N/V, ataxia, abnormal vision, tremor, abnormal gait, dyspepsia, abdominal pain, upper respiratory tract infection, headache.

INTERACTIONS: Monitor serum Na⁺ levels during maintenance treatment, particularly with other medications known to decrease serum Na⁺ levels (eg, drugs associated with inappropriate antidiuretic hormone secretion). Verapamil, valproic acid, and strong CYP450 inducers (eg, carbamazepine, phenytoin, phenobarbital) may decrease levels. May decrease levels of dihydropyridine calcium antagonists, oral contraceptives (eg, ethinylestradiol, levonorgestrel), cyclosporine, and felodipine. May induce CYP3A4/5 with potentially important effects on levels of other drugs. May increase levels of phenytoin, phenobarbital, and CYP2C19 substrates; may require dose reduction of phenytoin when using oxcarbazepine doses >1200mg/day. Decreased levels with AEDs that are CYP450 inducers.

PREGNANCY: Category C, not for use in nursing.

MECHANISM OF ACTION: Dibenzazepine; has not been established. Oxcarbazepine and 10-monohydroxy metabolite (MHD) suspected to exert antiseizure effects through blockade of voltage-sensitive Na⁺ channels, resulting in stabilization of hyperexcited neural membranes, inhibition of repetitive neuronal firing, and diminution of propagation of synaptic impulses. Also, increased K⁺ conductance and modulation of high-voltage activated Ca²⁺ channels may contribute to the anticonvulsant effects.

PHARMACOKINETICS: Absorption: (Tab) Complete. T_{max}=4.5 hrs (median). (Sus) T_{max}=6 hrs (median). **Distribution:** Found in breast milk. MHD: V_d=49L; plasma protein binding (40%). **Metabolism:** Liver (extensive); reduction by cytosolic enzymes to MHD (active metabolite). MHD: Conjugation with glucuronic acid. **Elimination:** Urine (>95%, <1% unchanged), feces (<4%); $T_{1/2}$=2 hrs. MHD: $T_{1/2}$=9 hrs.

NURSING CONSIDERATIONS

Assessment: Assess for history of hypersensitivity to drug or to carbamazepine, depression, renal/hepatic function, pregnancy/nursing status, and possible drug interactions.

Monitoring: Monitor for signs/symptoms of hyponatremia, anaphylaxis, angioedema, dermatological reactions, emergence/worsening of depression, suicidal thoughts/behavior, any unusual changes in mood or behavior, cognitive/neuropsychiatric events, multiorgan hypersensitivity reactions, hematologic events, and other adverse reactions. Monitor patients during pregnancy and through the postpartum period.

Patient Counseling: Advise to report symptoms of low Na⁺, and fever to physician. Instruct to d/c and contact physician immediately if signs/symptoms suggesting angioedema develop. Advise to consult physician immediately if experiencing a hypersensitivity reaction, symptoms suggestive of blood disorders, or if a skin reaction occurs. Warn female patients of childbearing age that concurrent use with hormonal contraceptives may render this method of contraception less effective; advise to use additional nonhormonal forms of contraception. Advise of the need to be alert for the emergence/worsening of symptoms of depression, any unusual changes in mood/ behavior, or the emergence of suicidal thoughts, behavior, or thoughts about self-harm; instruct to immediately report behaviors of concern to physician. Instruct to use caution if taking alcohol while on therapy. Advise that drug may cause dizziness and somnolence, and not to drive or operate machinery until effects have been determined. Encourage to enroll in the North American Antiepileptic Drug Pregnancy Registry if patient becomes pregnant.

Administration: Oral route. Take with or without food. Sus and tab may be interchanged at equal doses. (Sus) Shake well before use. Refer to PI for preparation and administration instructions.

Storage: 25°C (77°F); excursions permitted to 15-30°C (59-86°F). (Sus) Use within 7 weeks of 1st opening the bottle.

TRILIPIX RX
fenofibric acid (AbbVie)

THERAPEUTIC CLASS: Fibric acid derivative

INDICATIONS: Adjunct to diet in combination with a statin to reduce TGs and increase HDL in patients with mixed dyslipidemia and coronary heart disease (CHD) or a CHD risk equivalent. Adjunctive therapy to diet to reduce TGs in patients with severe hypertriglyceridemia. Adjunctive therapy to diet to reduce elevated LDL, total cholesterol, TGs, and apolipoprotein B, and to increase HDL in patients with primary hypercholesterolemia or mixed dyslipidemia.

DOSAGE: *Adults:* Severe Hypertriglyceridemia: Initial: 45-135mg qd. Titrate: Adjust dose if necessary following repeat lipid determinations at 4- to 8-week intervals; individualize dose. Max: 135mg qd. Primary Hypercholesterolemia/Mixed Dyslipidemia: 135mg qd. Coadministration Therapy with Statins for Mixed Dyslipidemia: 135mg qd. Avoid max dose of statin unless benefits outweigh the risks. Mild to Moderate Renal Impairment: Initial: 45mg qd. Titrate: Increase only after evaluation of effects on renal function and lipid levels. Elderly: Dose based on renal function.

HOW SUPPLIED: Cap, Delayed-Release: 45mg, 135mg

CONTRAINDICATIONS: Severe renal impairment (including dialysis), active liver disease (including primary biliary cirrhosis and unexplained persistent liver function abnormalities), preexisting gallbladder disease, and nursing mothers.

WARNINGS/PRECAUTIONS: No incremental benefit of fenofibric acid on cardiovascular morbidity and mortality over and above that demonstrated for statin monotherapy has been established. Not shown to reduce CHD morbidity and mortality in patients with type 2 diabetes mellitus (DM). Not indicated for patients who have elevations of chylomicrons and plasma TGs, but have normal VLDL levels. Increased risk of myositis/myopathy and rhabdomyolysis; risk increased with DM, renal failure, hypothyroidism, and in elderly. D/C therapy if markedly elevated CPK levels occur or myopathy/myositis is suspected or diagnosed. Increases in serum transaminases, hepatocellular, chronic active and cholestatic hepatitis, and cirrhosis (rare) reported; perform baseline and regular monitoring of LFTs, and d/c therapy if enzyme levels persist >3X ULN. Reversible elevations in SrCr reported. May cause cholelithiasis; d/c if gallstones are found. Acute hypersensitivity reactions and pancreatitis reported. Mild to moderate decreases in Hgb, Hct and WBCs, thrombocytopenia, and agranulocytosis reported; periodically monitor RBC and WBC counts during the first 12 months of therapy. May cause venothromboembolic disease. Severe decreases in HDL levels reported; check HDL levels within the 1st few months after initiation of therapy. If a severely depressed HDL level is detected, withdraw therapy, monitor HDL level until it has returned to baseline, and do not reinitiate therapy. D/C or change medications known to exacerbate hypertriglyceridemia (eg, β-blockers, thiazides, estrogens) if possible before considering therapy.

ADVERSE REACTIONS: Headache, back pain, nasopharyngitis, nausea, myalgia, diarrhea, upper respiratory tract infection, abnormal LFTs, pain in extremity, arthralgia, dizziness, dyspepsia, sinusitis, constipation, pain.

INTERACTIONS: Increased risk of rhabdomyolysis with HMG-CoA reductase inhibitors (statins). May potentiate anticoagulant effects of coumarin anticoagulants; use with caution, reduce anticoagulant dosage, and monitor PT/INR frequently. Bile acid-binding resins may bind other drugs given concurrently; take at least 1 hr before or 4-6 hrs after the bile acid resin to avoid impeding its absorption. Immunosuppressants (eg, cyclosporine, tacrolimus) may produce nephrotoxicity; consider benefits and risks, and use lowest effective dose with immunosuppressants and other potentially nephrotoxic agents. Cases of myopathy, including rhabdomyolysis, reported when coadministered with colchicine; caution when prescribing with colchicine.

PREGNANCY: Category C, not for use in nursing.

MECHANISM OF ACTION: Fibric acid derivative; activates peroxisome proliferator-activated receptor α. Increases lipolysis and elimination of TG-rich particles from plasma by activating lipoprotein lipase and reducing production of Apo CIII (lipoprotein lipase activity inhibitor). Also induces an increase in the synthesis of HDL and Apo AI and AII.

PHARMACOKINETICS: Absorption: Well-absorbed. Absolute bioavailability (81%); T_{max}=4-5 hrs. **Distribution:** Plasma protein binding (99%). **Metabolism:** Conjugation with glucuronic acid. **Elimination:** Urine; $T_{1/2}$=20 hrs.

NURSING CONSIDERATIONS

Assessment: Assess for renal impairment, active liver disease, preexisting gallbladder disease, other medical conditions (eg, DM, hypothyroidism), hypersensitivity to drug, pregnancy/nursing status, and possible drug interactions. Obtain baseline LFTs.

Monitoring: Monitor for signs/symptoms of myositis, myopathy, or rhabdomyolysis; measure CPK levels in patients reporting such symptoms. Monitor for cholelithiasis, pancreatitis, hypersensitivity reactions, pulmonary embolism, and deep vein thrombosis. Monitor renal function, LFTs, CBC, and lipid levels. Monitor PT/INR frequently with coumarin anticoagulants.

Patient Counseling: Advise of the potential benefits and risks of therapy, and of medications to avoid during treatment. Instruct to follow appropriate lipid-modifying diet during therapy, and to take drug ud. Inform that if drug is coadministered with a statin, they may be taken together. Advise to return for routine monitoring. Instruct to inform physician of all medications, supplements, and herbal preparations being taken, any changes in medical condition, development of muscle pain, tenderness, or weakness, and onset of abdominal pain or any other new symptoms.

Administration: Oral route. May be taken without regard to meals. Swallow cap whole; do not open, crush, dissolve, or chew. **Storage:** 25°C (77°F); excursions permitted to 15-30°C (59-86°F). Protect from moisture.

TRIOSTAT   RX
liothyronine sodium (JHP)

> Drugs with thyroid hormone activity, alone or together with other therapeutic agents, have been used for the treatment of obesity. Doses within the range of daily hormonal requirements are ineffective for weight reduction in euthyroid patients. Larger doses may produce serious or life-threatening manifestations of toxicity, particularly when given in association with sympathomimetic amines, such as those used for their anorectic effects.

THERAPEUTIC CLASS: Thyroid replacement hormone

INDICATIONS: Treatment of myxedema coma/precoma.

DOSAGE: *Adults:* Initial: 25-50mcg IV (emergency treatment) or 10-20mcg IV (with known/suspected cardiovascular disease [CVD]). Initial and subsequent doses should be based on continuous monitoring of clinical status and response to therapy. At least 4 hrs and no more than 12 hrs should elapse between doses. Switching to PO Therapy: Resume as soon as clinical situation has been stabilized and patient is able to take PO medication. D/C therapy, initiate PO therapy at a low dose, and increase gradually according to response. D/C gradually if L-thyroxine rather than liothyronine sodium is used in initiating PO therapy. Elderly: Start at lower end of dosing range.

HOW SUPPLIED: Inj: 10mcg/mL [1mL]

CONTRAINDICATIONS: Uncorrected adrenal cortical insufficiency, untreated thyrotoxicosis, artificial rewarming.

WARNINGS/PRECAUTIONS: Not for IM or SQ route. Use is unjustified for the treatment of male or female infertility unless accompanied by hypothyroidism. Caution with CVD (eg, angina pectoris) or in elderly; monitor cardiac function. Caution in myxedematous patients; start at a low dose level and increase gradually. Supplemental adrenocortical steroids may be necessary in patients with severe and prolonged hypothyroidism. May precipitate a hyperthyroid state or aggravate hyperthyroidism. May aggravate symptoms of diabetes mellitus (DM), diabetes insipidus (DI), or adrenal cortical insufficiency. Monitor and treat infection appropriately in myxedema coma patients. Therapy of myxedema coma requires simultaneous administration of glucocorticoids. Concurrent use with androgens, corticosteroids, estrogens, oral contraceptives containing estrogens, iodine-containing preparations, and salicylates may interfere with thyroid laboratory tests.

ADVERSE REACTIONS: Arrhythmia, tachycardia.

INTERACTIONS: See Boxed Warning. Hypothyroidism decreases and hyperthyroidism increases sensitivity to anticoagulants; monitor PT closely and adjust anticoagulants based on frequent PT determinations. May cause increases in insulin or oral hypoglycemic requirements during thyroid replacement initiation. Estrogens increase thyroxine-binding globulin; increase in thyroid dose may be needed in patients without a functioning thyroid gland. Increased effects of both agents with TCAs (eg, imipramine). May cause HTN and tachycardia with ketamine; use with caution and treat HTN if necessary. May potentiate toxic effects of digitalis. Increased adrenergic effect of catecholamines (eg, epinephrine, norepinephrine). May increase risk of precipitating coronary insufficiency, especially with coronary artery disease (CAD) with vasopressors; use with caution. Caution when administering fluid therapy.

PREGNANCY: Category A, caution in nursing.

MECHANISM OF ACTION: Synthetic thyroid hormone; enhances oxygen consumption by most tissues of the body and increases the basal metabolic rate and metabolism of carbohydrates, lipids, and proteins.

NURSING CONSIDERATIONS

Assessment: Assess thyroid status, CVD (eg, CAD, angina pectoris), DM/DI, adrenal cortical insufficiency, nursing status, and for possible drug interactions.

Monitoring: Monitor for signs/symptoms of precipitation of adrenocortical insufficiency, aggravation of DM/DI, infection, hypersensitivity reactions, and other adverse reactions. Monitor thyroid function periodically. Monitor patient's clinical status and response to therapy. Monitor PT closely in thyroid-treated patients on anticoagulants and adjust anticoagulants based on frequent PT determinations.

Patient Counseling: Inform of the risks/benefits of therapy. Instruct to seek medical attention if symptoms of toxicity, aggravation of DM/DI, or hypersensitivity reactions occur.

Administration: IV route. Refer to PI for further administration instructions. **Storage:** 2-8°C (36-46°F).

TRIZIVIR   RX
abacavir sulfate - zidovudine - lamivudine (ViiV Healthcare)

> Lactic acidosis and severe hepatomegaly with steatosis, including fatal cases, reported with nucleoside analogues. Abacavir: Serious and sometimes fatal hypersensitivity reactions (multiorgan clinical syndrome) reported; d/c as soon as suspected and never restart therapy or any other abacavir-containing product. Patients with HLA-B*5701 allele are at high risk for hypersensitivity; screen for HLA-B*5701 allele prior to therapy. Zidovudine: Associated with hematologic toxicity (eg, neutropenia, severe anemia), particularly with advanced HIV-1 disease. Symptomatic myopathy associated with prolonged use. Lamivudine: Severe acute exacerbations of hepatitis B reported in patients coinfected with hepatitis B virus (HBV) and HIV-1 and have discontinued therapy; closely monitor hepatic function for at least several months. If appropriate, initiation of antihepatitis B therapy may be warranted.

THERAPEUTIC CLASS: Nucleoside reverse transcriptase inhibitor

INDICATIONS: Treatment of HIV-1 infection alone or in combination with other antiretrovirals.

DOSAGE: *Adults:* ≥40kg: CrCl ≥50mL/min: Usual: 1 tab bid.
Pediatrics: Adolescents: ≥40kg: CrCl ≥50mL/min: Usual: 1 tab bid.

HOW SUPPLIED: Tab: (Abacavir Sulfate-Lamivudine-Zidovudine) 300mg-150mg-300mg

CONTRAINDICATIONS: Hepatic impairment.

WARNINGS/PRECAUTIONS: Obesity and prolonged nucleoside exposure may be risk factors for lactic acidosis and severe hepatomegaly with steatosis; suspend therapy if clinical or laboratory findings suggestive of lactic acidosis or pronounced hepatotoxicity develop. Immune reconstitution syndrome reported. Autoimmune disorders (eg, Graves' disease, polymyositis, Guillain-Barre syndrome) reported to occur in the setting of immune reconstitution and can occur many months after initiation of treatment. Redistribution/accumulation of body fat may occur. Cross-resistance potential with nucleoside reverse transcriptase inhibitors reported. Caution with any known risk factors for liver disease and in elderly. Avoid use in adolescents weighing <40kg and in patients requiring dose adjustments (eg, renal impairment [CrCl <50mL/min]). Abacavir: Increased risk of myocardial infarction (MI) reported; consider underlying risk of coronary heart disease (CHD) when prescribing therapy. Lamivudine: Emergence of lamivudine-resistant HBV reported. Zidovudine: Caution with compromised bone marrow evidenced by granulocyte count <1000 cells/mm^3 or Hgb <9.5g/dL; monitor blood counts frequently with advanced HIV-1 disease and periodically in other HIV-1 infected patients. Interrupt therapy if anemia or neutropenia develops.

ADVERSE REACTIONS: Lactic acidosis, severe hepatomegaly with steatosis, hematologic toxicity, myopathy, N/V, headache, malaise, fatigue, hypersensitivity reaction, diarrhea, fever, chills, depressive disorders.

INTERACTIONS: Avoid with other abacavir-, lamivudine-, zidovudine-, and/or emtricitabine-containing products. Hepatic decompensation may occur in HIV-1/hepatitis C virus (HCV) coinfected patients receiving interferon alfa with or without ribavirin; closely monitor for treatment-associated toxicities. Abacavir: Ethanol may decrease elimination, causing an increase in overall exposure. May increase oral methadone clearance. Zidovudine: Avoid with stavudine, doxorubicin, and nucleoside analogues that affect DNA replication (eg, ribavirin). Atovaquone, fluconazole, methadone, probenecid, and valproic acid may increase levels. Clarithromycin, nelfinavir, rifampin, and ritonavir may decrease levels. May increase hematologic toxicity with ganciclovir, interferon alfa, ribavirin, and other bone marrow suppressive or cytotoxic agents. Lamivudine: Nelfinavir and trimethoprim/sulfamethoxazole may increase levels.

PREGNANCY: Category C, not for use in nursing.

MECHANISM OF ACTION: Abacavir: Carbocyclic synthetic nucleoside analogue; inhibits HIV-1 reverse transcriptase (RT) by competing with natural substrate deoxyguanosine-5'-triphosphate and by incorporating into viral DNA. Lamivudine/Zidovudine: Synthetic nucleoside analogue; inhibits RT via DNA chain termination after incorporation of the nucleotide analogue.

PHARMACOKINETICS: Absorption: Rapid. Bioavailability: Abacavir/Lamivudine (86%), zidovudine (64%). **Distribution:** Abacavir: V_d=0.86L/kg; plasma protein binding (50%). Lamivudine: V_d=1.3L/kg; plasma protein binding (low); found in breast milk. Zidovudine: V_d=1.6L/kg; plasma protein binding (low); crosses the placenta; found in breast milk. **Metabolism:** Abacavir: Via alcohol dehydrogenase and glucuronyl transferase; 5'-carboxylic acid, 5'-glucuronide (metabolites). Lamivudine: Trans-sulfoxide (metabolite). Zidovudine: Hepatic via glucuronyl transferase; 3'-azido-3'-deoxy-5'-O-β-D-glucopyranuronosylthymidine (GZDV) (major metabolite). **Elimination:** Abacavir: $T_{1/2}$=1.45 hrs. Lamivudine: (IV) Urine (70%, unchanged); $T_{1/2}$=5-7 hrs. Zidovudine: Urine (14% unchanged, 74% GZDV); $T_{1/2}$=0.5-3 hrs.

NURSING CONSIDERATIONS

Assessment: Assess for history of hypersensitivity reactions, advanced HIV disease, hepatic/renal impairment, risk factors for lactic acidosis, risk factors for liver and CHD, bone marrow compromise, HBV infection, pregnancy/nursing status, and possible drug interactions. Screen for HLA-B*5701 allele prior to initiation of therapy. Assess medical history for prior exposure to any abacavir-containing product.

Monitoring: Monitor for signs/symptoms of hypersensitivity reactions, hematologic toxicity, lactic acidosis, hepatomegaly with steatosis, myopathy, immune reconstitution syndrome (eg, opportunistic infections), autoimmune disorders, fat redistribution/accumulation, MI, and other adverse reactions. Monitor hepatic/renal function and blood counts. Monitor hepatic function closely for at least several months in patients who d/c therapy and are coinfected with HIV-1 and HBV.

Patient Counseling: Inform about hypersensitivity reactions; instruct to contact physician immediately if symptoms develop and not to restart or replace with any drug containing abacavir without medical consultation. Inform about risk for hematologic toxicities and advise on importance of close blood count monitoring while on therapy. Counsel about the possible occurrence of myopathy and myositis with pathological changes during prolonged use and that therapy may cause a rare but serious condition called lactic acidosis with liver enlargement (hepatomegaly). Inform patients coinfected with HBV that deterioration of liver disease has occurred in some cases when treatment was discontinued; instruct to discuss any changes in regimen with physician. Inform that hepatic decompensation has occurred in HIV-1/HCV-coinfected patients receiving combination antiretroviral therapy and interferon alfa with or without ribavirin. Inform that redistribution/accumulation of body fat may occur. Advise that drug is not a cure for HIV-1 infection and that illness associated with HIV-1 may still be experienced. Advise to avoid doing things that can spread HIV-1 infection to others. Inform patients to take all HIV medications exactly as prescribed.

Administration: Oral route. Take with or without food. **Storage:** 25°C (77°F); excursions permitted to 15-30°C (59-86°F).

TROKENDI XR   RX
topiramate (Supernus)

THERAPEUTIC CLASS: Sulfamate-substituted monosaccharide antiepileptic

INDICATIONS: Initial monotherapy in patients ≥10 yrs of age with partial onset or primary generalized tonic-clonic seizures and adjunctive therapy in patients ≥6 yrs of age with partial onset or primary generalized tonic-clonic seizures. Adjunctive therapy in patients ≥6 yrs of age with seizures associated with Lennox-Gastaut syndrome (LGS).

DOSAGE: *Adults:* Monotherapy: Partial Onset/Primary Generalized Tonic-Clonic Seizures: Usual: 400mg qd. Initial: Week 1: 50mg qd. Titrate: Week 2: 100mg qd. Week 3: 150mg qd. Week 4: 200mg qd. Week 5: 300mg qd. Week 6: 400mg qd. ≥17 Yrs: Adjunctive Therapy: Partial Onset/Primary Generalized Tonic-Clonic Seizures/LGS: Initial: 25-50mg qd. Titrate: Increase in increments of 25-50mg every week to achieve effective dose. Partial Onset Seizures/LGS: Usual: 200-400mg qd. Primary Generalized Tonic-Clonic Seizures: Usual: 400mg qd. Hemodialysis: May need supplemental topiramate dose. Elderly (with CrCl <70mL/min): May need to adjust dose. Refer to PI for dose modifications with concomitant phenytoin and/or carbamazepine, and for patients with renal impairment.
Pediatrics: ≥10 Yrs: Monotherapy: Partial Onset/Primary Generalized Tonic-Clonic Seizures: Usual: 400mg qd. Initial: Week 1: 50mg qd. Titrate: Week 2: 100mg qd. Week 3: 150mg qd. Week 4: 200mg qd. Week 5: 300mg qd. Week 6: 400mg qd. 6-16 Yrs: Adjunctive Therapy: Partial Onset/Primary Generalized Tonic-Clonic Seizures/LGS: Usual: 5-9mg/kg qd. Begin titration at 25mg qpm (based on a range of 1mg/kg/day to 3mg/kg/day) for 1st week. Subsequently, increase at 1- or 2-week intervals by increments of 1mg/kg to 3mg/kg. Dose titration should be guided by clinical outcome. Longer intervals between dose adjustments may be used if required. Hemodialysis:

May need supplemental topiramate dose. Refer to PI for dose modifications with concomitant phenytoin and/or carbamazepine, and for patients with renal impairment.

HOW SUPPLIED: Cap, Extended-Release: 25mg, 50mg, 100mg, 200mg

CONTRAINDICATIONS: Patients with recent alcohol use (eg, within 6 hrs prior to and 6 hrs after use), patients with metabolic acidosis taking concomitant metformin.

WARNINGS/PRECAUTIONS: Acute myopia associated with secondary angle-closure glaucoma reported; d/c immediately to reverse symptoms. Oligohydrosis and hyperthermia reported, mostly in pediatric patients; monitor closely for decreased sweating and increased body temperature. Hyperchloremic, non-anion gap, metabolic acidosis reported; conditions or therapies that predispose to acidosis may be additive to the bicarbonate lowering effects. D/C or reduce dose if metabolic acidosis develops/persists. If decision is made to continue therapy, consider alkali treatment. Increased risk of suicidal thoughts/behavior; monitor for the emergence/worsening of depression, suicidal thoughts/behavior, and/or any unusual changes in mood or behavior. Cognitive-related dysfunction, psychiatric/behavioral disturbances, somnolence, or fatigue reported. May cause cleft lip and/or cleft palate in infants if used during pregnancy. D/C gradually to minimize the potential for seizures or increased seizure frequency; appropriate monitoring is recommended when rapid withdrawal is required. Patients with inborn errors of metabolism or reduced hepatic mitochondrial activity may be at an increased risk for hyperammonemia with or without encephalopathy; consider hyperammonemic encephalopathy and measure ammonia levels in patients who develop unexplained lethargy, vomiting, or changes in mental status associated with therapy. Kidney stones formation reported; hydration recommended to reduce new stone formation. Paresthesia may occur. Lab abnormalities may occur.

ADVERSE REACTIONS: Paresthesia, weight decrease, somnolence, anorexia, dizziness, difficulty with memory, upper respiratory tract infection, diarrhea, mood problems, fatigue, nervousness, difficulty with concentration, aggressive reaction, confusion, depression.

INTERACTIONS: See Contraindications. May decrease contraceptive efficacy and increase breakthrough bleeding with combination oral contraceptives. Phenytoin or carbamazepine may decrease levels. Concurrent administration of valproic acid has been associated with hyperammonemia with or without encephalopathy, and hypothermia. Concomitant administration with other CNS depressant drugs or alcohol can result in significant CNS depression. Other carbonic anhydrase inhibitors (eg, zonisamide, acetazolamide, dichlorphenamide) may increase the severity of metabolic acidosis and may also increase the risk of kidney stone formation. Increase in systemic exposure of lithium observed following topiramate doses of ≤600mg/day; monitor lithium levels. Caution with agents that predispose patients to heat-related disorders (eg, carbonic anhydrase inhibitors, anticholinergics).

PREGNANCY: Category D, caution in nursing.

MECHANISM OF ACTION: Sulfamate-substituted monosaccharide antiepileptic; has not been established. Suspected to block voltage-dependent Na$^+$ channels, augment activity of the neurotransmitter gamma-aminobutyrate (GABA) at some subtypes of the GABA-A receptor, antagonize the α-amino-3-hydroxy-5-methyl-4-isoxazolepropionic acid/kainate subtype of the glutamate receptor, and inhibit the carbonic anhydrase enzyme, particularly isoenzymes II and IV.

PHARMACOKINETICS: Absorption: T_{max}=24 hrs (200mg). **Distribution:** Plasma protein binding (15-41%). **Metabolism:** Hydroxylation, hydrolysis, glucuronidation. **Elimination:** Urine (70% unchanged); $T_{1/2}$=31 hrs.

NURSING CONSIDERATIONS

Assessment: Assess for recent alcohol use, metabolic acidosis in patients taking concomitant metformin, predisposing factors for metabolic acidosis, renal dysfunction, inborn errors of metabolism, reduced hepatic mitochondrial activity, pregnancy/nursing status, and possible drug interactions. Obtain baseline serum bicarbonate and blood ammonia levels. Obtain baseline estimated GFR measurement in patients at high risk for renal insufficiency.

Monitoring: Monitor for signs/symptoms of acute myopia, secondary-angle glaucoma, oligohydrosis, hyperthermia, cognitive or neuropsychiatric adverse reactions, kidney stones, renal dysfunction, metabolic acidosis, paresthesias, hyperammonemia, and other adverse reactions. Monitor serum bicarbonate and blood ammonia levels.

Patient Counseling: Instruct to take ud. Advise to completely avoid consumption of alcohol at least 6 hrs prior to and 6 hrs after taking the drug. Instruct to seek immediate medical attention if blurred vision, visual disturbances, periorbital pain, decreased sweating, or increased body temperature occurs. Inform about the potentially significant risk for metabolic acidosis that may be asymptomatic and may be associated with adverse effects on kidneys, bones, and growth in pediatric patients, and on the fetus. Instruct to immediately report to the physician if emergence or worsening of depression, unusual changes in mood/behavior, emergence of suicidal thoughts, or behavior/thoughts about self-harm occurs. Instruct to use caution when engaging in any activities where loss of consciousness may result in serious danger. Inform of pregnancy risks; encourage pregnant women to enroll in the North American Antiepileptic Drug Pregnancy

Registry. Warn about the possible development of hyperammonemia with or without encephalopathy; instruct to contact physician if unexplained lethargy, vomiting, or mental status changes develop. Instruct to maintain an adequate fluid intake to minimize risk of kidney stones. Inform that therapy may cause a reduction in body temperature that can lead to alterations in mental status; if changes are noted, instruct patients to measure their body temperature and to contact physician. Instruct to consult physician if tingling in the arms and legs occurs.

Administration: Oral route. Swallow cap whole and intact; do not sprinkle on food, chew, or crush. **Storage:** 25°C (77°F); excursions permitted to 15-30°C (59-86°F). Protect from moisture and light.

TRUSOPT   RX
dorzolamide HCl (Merck)

THERAPEUTIC CLASS: Carbonic anhydrase inhibitor

INDICATIONS: Treatment of elevated intraocular pressure (IOP) in patients with ocular HTN or open-angle glaucoma.

DOSAGE: *Adults:* 1 drop in the affected eye(s) tid. May be used concomitantly with other topical ophthalmic drug products to lower IOP; administer at least 5 min apart if >1 topical ophthalmic drug is being used.
Pediatrics: 1 drop in the affected eye(s) tid. May be used concomitantly with other topical ophthalmic drug products to lower IOP; administer at least 5 min apart if >1 topical ophthalmic drug is being used.

HOW SUPPLIED: Sol: 2% [10mL]

WARNINGS/PRECAUTIONS: Systemically absorbed. Rare fatalities have occurred due to severe sulfonamide reactions (eg, Stevens-Johnson syndrome, toxic epidermal necrolysis, fulminant hepatic necrosis, agranulocytosis, aplastic anemia, other blood dyscrasias); d/c if signs of hypersensitivity or other serious reactions occur. Sensitization may recur when readministered irrespective of the route of administration. Bacterial keratitis reported with use of multiple-dose containers of topical ophthalmic products that had been inadvertently contaminated by patients with a concurrent corneal disease or a disruption of the ocular epithelial surface. Caution in patients with low endothelial cell counts; increased potential for corneal edema. Local ocular adverse effects (eg, conjunctivitis, lid reactions) reported with chronic use; d/c use and evaluate patient before considering restarting therapy. The management of acute angle-closure glaucoma requires therapeutic interventions in addition to ocular hypotensive agents. Not recommended with severe renal impairment (CrCl <30mL/min). Caution with hepatic impairment.

ADVERSE REACTIONS: Ocular burning/stinging/discomfort, bitter taste, superficial punctate keratitis, ocular allergic reactions, conjunctivitis, lid reactions, blurred vision, eye redness, tearing, dryness, photophobia.

INTERACTIONS: Concomitant administration of oral carbonic anhydrase inhibitor is not recommended due to potential for additive effects. Acid-base and electrolyte disturbances reported with oral carbonic anhydrase inhibitors; drug interactions (eg, toxicity associated with high-dose salicylate therapy) may occur.

PREGNANCY: Category C, not for use in nursing.

MECHANISM OF ACTION: Carbonic anhydrase inhibitor; decreases aqueous humor secretion, presumably by slowing the formation of bicarbonate ions with subsequent reduction in Na^+ and fluid transport, resulting in a reduction in IOP.

PHARMACOKINETICS: Absorption: Systemic. **Distribution:** Plasma protein binding (33%). **Metabolism:** N-desethyl (metabolite). **Elimination:** Urine (unchanged, metabolite); $T_{1/2}$=4 months.

NURSING CONSIDERATIONS

Assessment: Assess for hypersensitivity to drug, acute angle-closure glaucoma, low endothelial cell counts, renal/hepatic impairment, pregnancy/nursing status, and possible drug interactions.

Monitoring: Monitor for sulfonamide hypersensitivity reactions, ocular reactions, bacterial keratitis, and other adverse reactions. Monitor for improvement in IOP.

Patient Counseling: Advise to d/c use if serious or unusual reactions (eg, severe skin reactions, signs of hypersensitivity) occur. Instruct to seek immediate physician's advice concerning the continued use of present multidose container if patients have ocular surgery or develop an intercurrent ocular condition (eg, trauma, infection). Advise to d/c use and seek physician's advice if patient develops any ocular reactions (eg, conjunctivitis, lid reactions). Instruct to avoid allowing tip of dispensing container to contact eye or surrounding structures. Inform that ocular solutions can become contaminated by common bacteria known to cause ocular infections if handled improperly or if the tip of the dispensing container contacts the eye or surrounding structures, and may result in serious damage to the eye and subsequent loss of vision. Instruct to administer at least 5 min apart if >1 topical ophthalmic drug is being used. Instruct to remove contact lenses prior to administration and may be reinserted 15 min after administration.

Administration: Ocular route. **Storage:** 15-30°C (59-86°F). Protect from light.

TRUVADA RX
tenofovir disoproxil fumarate - emtricitabine (Gilead)

Lactic acidosis and severe hepatomegaly with steatosis, including fatal cases, reported with the use of nucleoside analogues in combination with other antiretrovirals. Not approved for treatment of chronic hepatitis B virus (HBV) infection. Severe acute exacerbations of hepatitis B reported in patients coinfected with HBV and HIV-1 and have discontinued therapy; closely monitor hepatic function with both clinical and laboratory follow-up for at least several months. If appropriate, initiation of anti-hepatitis B therapy may be warranted. Drug resistant HIV-1 variants have been identified with use for preexposure prophylaxis (PrEP) indication following undetected acute HIV-1 infection. PrEP use must only be prescribed to individuals confirmed to be HIV-negative immediately prior to initiating and periodically (at least every 3 months) during use; do not initiate if signs or symptoms of acute HIV-1 infection are present unless negative infection status is confirmed.

THERAPEUTIC CLASS: Nucleoside analogue combination

INDICATIONS: Treatment of HIV-1 infection in combination with other antiretroviral agents (eg, non-nucleoside reverse transcriptase inhibitors or protease inhibitors) in adults and pediatric patients ≥12 yrs of age. For PrEP to reduce the risk of sexually acquired HIV-1 in high risk adults, in combination with safer sex practices.

DOSAGE: *Adults:* HIV-1 Infection: ≥35kg: 1 tab qd. CrCl ≥50mL/min: 1 tab q24h. CrCl 30-49mL/min: 1 tab q48h. PrEP: 1 tab qd.
Pediatrics: ≥12 Yrs: HIV-1 Infection: ≥35kg: 1 tab qd.

HOW SUPPLIED: Tab: (Emtricitabine-Tenofovir Disoproxil Fumarate [TDF]) 200mg-300mg

CONTRAINDICATIONS: Individuals with unknown or positive HIV-1 status when used for PrEP. Use in HIV-infected patients without other concomitant antiretroviral agents.

WARNINGS/PRECAUTIONS: Obesity and prolonged nucleoside exposure may be risk factors for lactic acidosis and severe hepatomegaly with steatosis. Caution with known risk factors for liver disease. D/C if findings suggestive of lactic acidosis or pronounced hepatotoxicity develop. Test for the presence of chronic HBV before initiating therapy; offer vaccination to HBV-uninfected individuals. Renal impairment (eg, acute renal failure, Fanconi syndrome) reported; assess CrCl prior to initiating therapy and as clinically appropriate during therapy. In patients at risk of renal dysfunction, including patients who have previously experienced renal events while receiving adefovir dipivoxil, assess CrCl, serum phosphorus (P), urine glucose, and urine protein prior to initiation and periodically during therapy. Do not administer in patients with CrCl <30mL/min or requiring hemodialysis (HIV-1 treatment) or with CrCl <60mL/min (PrEP). Decreased bone mineral density (BMD) and increased biochemical markers of bone metabolism reported; consider assessment of BMD in patients with history of pathologic bone fracture or other risk factors for osteoporosis or bone loss. Osteomalacia associated with proximal renal tubulopathy reported; consider hypophosphatemia and osteomalacia secondary to proximal renal tubulopathy in patients at risk of renal dysfunction who present with persistent or worsening bone or muscle symptoms. Redistribution/accumulation of body fat and immune reconstitution syndrome reported. Autoimmune disorders (eg, Graves' disease, polymyositis, Guillain-Barre syndrome) reported in the setting of immune reconstitution and can occur many months after initiation of treatment. Early virological failure and high rates of resistance substitutions reported with certain regimens that only contain 3 nucleoside reverse transcriptase inhibitors; not recommended to be used as component of triple nucleoside regimen. Use for PrEP only as part of a comprehensive prevention strategy that includes other prevention measures (eg, safer sex practices). Delay starting PrEP therapy for at least 1 month and reconfirm HIV-1 status or use an FDA-approved test to diagnose acute or primary HIV-1 infection if symptoms of acute viral infection are present and recent (<1 month) exposures are suspected. D/C PrEP therapy if symptoms of acute HIV-1 infection develop following potential exposure event until negative status is confirmed using an FDA-approved test. Caution in elderly.

ADVERSE REACTIONS: Lactic acidosis, hepatomegaly with steatosis, diarrhea, nausea, fatigue, headache, dizziness, depression, insomnia, abnormal dreams, rash, abdominal pain, pharyngitis, syphilis.

INTERACTIONS: Avoid with concurrent or recent use of nephrotoxic agents (eg, high-dose or multiple NSAIDs). Do not coadminister with emtricitabine- or TDF-containing products, drugs containing lamivudine, or with adefovir dipivoxil. May increase levels of didanosine; d/c didanosine if didanosine-associated adverse effects develop. TDF decreases atazanavir levels; do not coadminister with atazanavir without ritonavir (RTV). Lopinavir/RTV, atazanavir with RTV, and darunavir with RTV may increase TDF levels; d/c treatment if TDF-associated adverse reactions develop. P-glycoprotein and breast cancer resistance protein transporter inhibitors may increase absorption. Coadministration with drugs eliminated by active tubular secretion (eg, acyclovir, cidofovir, ganciclovir, valacyclovir, aminoglycosides [eg, gentamicin], high-dose or multiple NSAIDs) may increase levels of emtricitabine, TDF, and/or the coadministered drug. Drugs that decrease renal function may increase levels of emtricitabine and/or TDF. Refer to PI for dosing modifications when used with certain concomitant therapies.

PREGNANCY: Category B, not for use in nursing.

MECHANISM OF ACTION: Emtricitabine: Nucleoside analogue of cytidine; inhibits activity of HIV-1 reverse transcriptase (RT) by competing with natural substrate deoxycytidine 5'-triphosphate and by being incorporated into nascent viral DNA, which results in chain termination. TDF: Acyclic nucleoside phosphonate diester analogue of adenosine monophosphate; inhibits activity of HIV-1 RT by competing with the natural substrate deoxyadenosine 5'-triphosphate and, after incorporation into DNA, by DNA chain termination.

PHARMACOKINETICS: Absorption: Emtricitabine: Rapid. (Fasted) Bioavailability (92%) (median); C_{max}=1.8mcg/mL; T_{max}=1-2 hrs; AUC=10mcg•hr/mL. TDF: (Fasted) Bioavailability (25%) (median); C_{max}=0.3mcg/mL; T_{max}=1 hr; AUC=2.29mcg•hr/mL. **Distribution:** Found in breast milk. Emtricitabine: Plasma protein binding (<4%). TDF: Plasma protein binding (<0.7%). **Metabolism:** Emtricitabine: 3'-sulfoxide diastereomers and their glucuronic acid conjugate (metabolites). **Elimination:** Emtricitabine: Urine (86%; 13% metabolites); $T_{1/2}$=10 hrs (median). TDF: Urine (70-80%, unchanged) (IV); $T_{1/2}$=17 hrs (median).

NURSING CONSIDERATIONS

Assessment: Assess for risk factors for lactic acidosis or liver disease, renal dysfunction, HBV infection, pregnancy/nursing status, and possible drug interactions. Confirm a negative HIV-1 test immediately prior to initiating PrEP therapy. In patients at risk of renal dysfunction, assess CrCl, serum P, urine glucose, and urine protein. Assess BMD in patients with history of pathologic bone fracture or other risk factors for osteoporosis or bone loss.

Monitoring: Monitor for signs/symptoms of lactic acidosis, hepatomegaly with steatosis, hepatotoxicity, new onset or worsening renal impairment, bone effects, redistribution/accumulation of body fat, immune reconstitution syndrome (eg, opportunistic infections), autoimmune disorders, and other adverse reactions. Closely monitor hepatic function with both clinical and laboratory follow-up for at least several months in patients coinfected with HBV and HIV-1 and have discontinued therapy. Screen for HIV-1 infection at least once every 3 months when using for PrEP. In patients at risk of renal dysfunction, monitor CrCl, serum P, urine glucose, and urine protein periodically.

Patient Counseling: Inform about the risks and benefits of therapy. Inform that medication is not a cure for HIV-1 and patients may continue to experience illness associated with HIV-1 infection (eg, opportunistic infections). Counsel about the importance of adhering to recommended dosing schedule. Counsel about safe sex practices. Instruct not to breastfeed, share needles or personal items that can have blood or body fluids on them, or d/c without informing physician. For PrEP, inform patients/partners about the importance of knowing their HIV-1 status, obtaining HIV-1 test at least every 3 months, getting tested for other sexually transmitted infections, and immediate reporting to physician if any symptoms of acute HIV-1 infection develop.

Administration: Oral route. Take with or without food. **Storage:** 25°C (77°F); excursions permitted to 15-30°C (59-86°F).

TUDORZA PRESSAIR   RX
aclidinium bromide (Forest)

THERAPEUTIC CLASS: Anticholinergic bronchodilator

INDICATIONS: Long-term maintenance treatment of bronchospasm associated with chronic obstructive pulmonary disease, including chronic bronchitis and emphysema.

DOSAGE: *Adults:* 1 PO inh bid.

HOW SUPPLIED: MDI: 400mcg/actuation [30 doses, 60 doses]

WARNINGS/PRECAUTIONS: Not for initial treatment of acute episodes of bronchospasm (eg, rescue therapy). D/C and consider alternative treatments if immediate hypersensitivity reactions or paradoxical bronchospasm occur. Caution with hypersensitivity to atropine and/or milk proteins. Caution with narrow-angle glaucoma; observe for signs and symptoms of acute narrow-angle glaucoma (eg, eye pain or discomfort, blurred vision, visual halos or colored images in association with red eyes from conjunctival congestion and corneal edema). Caution with urinary retention; observe for signs and symptoms of prostatic hyperplasia or bladder neck obstruction.

ADVERSE REACTIONS: Headache, nasopharyngitis, cough.

INTERACTIONS: Avoid with other anticholinergic-containing drugs; may lead to an increase in anticholinergic effects.

PREGNANCY: Category C, caution in nursing.

MECHANISM OF ACTION: Anticholinergic bronchodilator; inhibits M3-receptors at the smooth muscle in the airways, leading to bronchodilation.

PHARMACOKINETICS: Absorption: Absolute bioavailability (6%), T_{max}=10 min. **Distribution:** (IV) V_d=300L. **Metabolism:** Hydrolysis by esterases. **Elimination:** Urine (0.09%); $T_{1/2}$=5-8 hrs.

NURSING CONSIDERATIONS

Assessment: Assess for hypersensitivity to the drug, milk proteins, and/or atropine, and for narrow-angle glaucoma, urinary retention, pregnancy/nursing status, and possible drug interactions.

Monitoring: Monitor for hypersensitivity reactions, paradoxical bronchospasm, acute narrow-angle glaucoma, prostatic hyperplasia or bladder neck obstruction, and other adverse reactions.

Patient Counseling: Inform on how to correctly use the inhaler. Instruct that if a dose was missed, to take the next dose at the usual time and not to take 2 doses at one time. Inform that the medication is a bid maintenance bronchodilator and should not be used for immediate relief of breathing problems (eg, as a rescue medication). Advise to d/c treatment if paradoxical bronchospasm occurs. Instruct to consult physician immediately if signs/symptoms of acute narrow-angle glaucoma (eg, eye pain, blurred vision, visual halos) occur. Advise that miotic eyedrops alone are not considered to be effective treatment. Inform not to allow the powder to enter into the eyes, as this may cause blurring of vision and pupil dilation. Instruct to consult physician immediately if signs/symptoms of new or worsening prostatic hyperplasia or bladder outlet obstruction (eg, difficulty passing urine, dysuria) occur.

Administration: Oral inhalation route. Refer to PI for further administration instructions. **Storage:** 25°C (77°F); excursions permitted to 15-30°C (59-86°F). Store in a dry place. Store inhaler inside the sealed pouch and only open immediately before use. Discard inhaler 45 days after opening the pouch, after the marking "0" with a red background shows, or when the device locks out, whichever comes 1st.

TUSSICAPS

chlorpheniramine polistirex - hydrocodone polistirex (Mallinckrodt)

CIII

THERAPEUTIC CLASS: Antihistamine/opioid antitussive

INDICATIONS: Relief of cough and upper respiratory symptoms associated with allergy or cold in adults and children ≥6 yrs.

DOSAGE: *Adults:* 1 full-strength cap q12h. Max: 2 caps/24 hrs. Elderly: Start at lower end of dosing range.
Pediatrics: ≥12 Yrs: 1 full-strength cap q12h. Max: 2 caps/24 hrs. 6-11 Yrs: 1 half-strength cap q12h. Max: 2 caps/24 hrs.

HOW SUPPLIED: Cap, Extended-Release: (Chlorpheniramine-Hydrocodone) 8mg-10mg (Full-Strength), 4mg-5mg (Half-Strength)

CONTRAINDICATIONS: Children <6 yrs of age.

WARNINGS/PRECAUTIONS: May produce dose-related respiratory depression and irregular/periodic breathing; may be antagonized by the use of naloxone HCl and other supportive measures when indicated. Caution with postoperative use, pulmonary disease, depressed ventilatory function, narrow-angle glaucoma, asthma, prostatic hypertrophy, severe hepatic/renal impairment, hypothyroidism, Addison's disease, or urethral stricture, and in pediatric patients ≥6 yrs, elderly, or debilitated patients. May have exaggerated respiratory depressant effects and elevation of CSF pressure in patients with head injury, other intracranial lesions, or preexisting increase in intracranial pressure. May obscure clinical course of head injuries and acute abdominal conditions. Chronic use may result in obstructive bowel disease, especially in patients with underlying intestinal motility disorder. Carefully consider benefit to risk ratio, especially in pediatric patients with respiratory embarrassment (eg, croup).

ADVERSE REACTIONS: Sedation, drowsiness, lethargy, anxiety, dysphoria, euphoria, dizziness, rash, pruritus, N/V, ureteral spasm, urinary retention, psychic dependence, mood changes.

INTERACTIONS: Additive CNS depression with narcotics, antihistamines, antipsychotics, antianxiety agents, or other CNS depressants (including alcohol); reduce dose of 1 or both agents when combined therapy is contemplated. Increased effect of either antidepressant or hydrocodone with MAOIs or TCAs. May produce paralytic ileus with other anticholinergics. Increased risk of respiratory depression in pediatric patients treated with concomitant respiratory depressants.

PREGNANCY: Category C, not for use in nursing.

MECHANISM OF ACTION: Hydrocodone: Semisynthetic narcotic antitussive/analgesic; not established. Believed to act directly on cough center. Chlorpheniramine: H_1-receptor antagonist; possesses anticholinergic and sedative activity. Prevents released histamine from dilating capillaries and causing edema of the respiratory mucosa.

T

PHARMACOKINETICS: Absorption: (Extended-Release Sus) Hydrocodone: C_{max}=22.8ng/mL, T_{max}=3.4 hrs. Chlorpheniramine: C_{max}=58.4ng/mL, T_{max}=6.3 hrs. **Elimination:** Hydrocodone: $T_{1/2}$=4 hrs. Chlorpheniramine: $T_{1/2}$=16 hrs.

NURSING CONSIDERATIONS

Assessment: Assess use in postoperative/elderly/debilitated patients, renal/hepatic function, other conditions where treatment is cautioned or contraindicated, drug hypersensitivity, pregnancy/nursing status, and possible drug interactions.

Monitoring: Monitor for signs/symptoms of respiratory depression, hypersensitivity reactions, hepatic/renal function, and development of obstructive bowel disease.

Patient Counseling: Inform that medication may produce marked drowsiness and impair mental and/or physical abilities required for the performance of potentially hazardous tasks. Instruct not to dilute with fluids or mix with other drugs.

Administration: Oral route. **Storage:** 20-25°C (68-77°F).

TWYNSTA   RX
amlodipine - telmisartan (Boehringer Ingelheim)

> D/C when pregnancy is detected. Drugs that act directly on the renin-angiotensin system (RAS) can cause injury/death to the developing fetus.

THERAPEUTIC CLASS: ARB/calcium channel blocker (dihydropyridine)

INDICATIONS: Treatment of HTN alone or with other antihypertensive agents. May also be used as initial therapy in patients likely to need multiple drugs to achieve their BP goals.

DOSAGE: *Adults:* Individualize dose. Initial Therapy: 40mg-5mg qd or, if requiring larger BP reductions, 80mg-5mg qd. Titrate: May be increased after at least 2 weeks. Max: 80mg-10mg qd. Add-On Therapy: May be used if BP not adequately controlled with amlodipine (or another dihydropyridine calcium channel blocker [CCB]) alone or with telmisartan (or another ARB) alone. Patients with dose-limiting adverse reactions to amlodipine 10mg may be switched to telmisartan-amlodipine 40mg-5mg qd. Replacement Therapy: May substitute for individual components; increase dose if BP control is unsatisfactory. Hepatic/Severe Renal Impairment or Patients ≥75 yrs: Titrate slowly.

HOW SUPPLIED: Tab: (Telmisartan-Amlodipine) 40mg-5mg, 40mg-10mg, 80mg-5mg, 80mg-10mg

CONTRAINDICATIONS: Coadministration with aliskiren in patients with diabetes.

WARNINGS/PRECAUTIONS: Symptomatic hypotension may occur in patients with an activated RAS (eg, volume- or salt-depleted patients) and in patients with severe aortic stenosis. Correct volume/salt depletion prior to therapy or start therapy under close medical supervision with a reduced dose. Not recommended for use as initial therapy in patients ≥75 yrs or with hepatic impairment. Amlodipine: Worsening angina and acute myocardial infarction (MI) may develop after starting or increasing the dose, particularly in patients with severe obstructive coronary artery disease (CAD). Closely monitor patients with heart failure (HF). Caution in elderly. Telmisartan: Hyperkalemia may occur, particularly in patients with advanced renal impairment or HF; periodically monitor serum electrolytes. Clearance is reduced in patients with biliary obstructive disorders or hepatic insufficiency. Oliguria and/or progressive azotemia, and (rarely) acute renal failure and/or death, reported in patients whose renal function may depend on RAS (eg, severe congestive HF or renal dysfunction). May increase SrCr/BUN with renal artery stenosis. Dual blockade of the RAS (eg, by adding an ACE inhibitor to an ARB) should include close monitoring of renal function.

ADVERSE REACTIONS: Peripheral edema, dizziness, back pain.

INTERACTIONS: See Contraindications. Amlodipine: Increased exposure to simvastatin reported; limit dose of simvastatin to 20mg daily. Diltiazem may increase systemic exposure. Strong CYP3A4 inhibitors (eg, ketoconazole, itraconazole, ritonavir) may increase concentrations to a greater extent; monitor for symptoms of hypotension and edema when coadministered with CYP3A4 inhibitors. Monitor for adequate clinical effect when coadministered with CYP3A4 inducers. Telmisartan: Avoid with aliskiren in patients with renal impairment (GFR <60mL/min). May increase digoxin concentrations; monitor digoxin levels upon initiation, adjustment, and discontinuation of therapy. Increases in lithium concentrations/toxicity reported; monitor lithium levels during concurrent use. NSAIDs, including selective COX-2 inhibitors, may attenuate antihypertensive effect and may deteriorate renal function. Not recommended with ramipril; ramipril/ramiprilat levels are increased, whereas telmisartan levels are decreased. Increased risk of hyperkalemia with renal replacement therapy, K^+-sparing diuretics, K^+ supplements, K^+-containing salt substitutes, or other drugs that increase K^+ levels. May possibly inhibit metabolism of drugs metabolized by CYP2C19.

PREGNANCY: Category D, not for use in nursing.

MECHANISM OF ACTION: Amlodipine: Dihydropyridine CCB; inhibits transmembrane influx of Ca^{2+} ions into vascular smooth muscle and cardiac muscle. Telmisartan: ARB; blocks vasoconstrictor and aldosterone-secreting effects of angiotensin II by selectively blocking the binding of angiotensin II to the AT_1 receptor in many tissues, such as vascular smooth muscle and adrenal gland.

PHARMACOKINETICS: Absorption: Amlodipine: Absolute bioavailability (64-90%); T_{max}=6-12 hrs. Telmisartan: Absolute bioavailability (42%, 40mg), (58%, 160mg); T_{max}=0.5-1 hr. **Distribution:** Amlodipine: V_d=21L/kg; plasma protein binding (93%). Telmisartan: V_d=500L; plasma protein binding (>99.5%). **Metabolism:** Amlodipine: Liver (extensive). Telmisartan: Conjugation. **Elimination:** Amlodipine: Urine (10% unchanged, 60% metabolites); $T_{1/2}$=30-50 hrs. Telmisartan: Feces (>97%, unchanged), urine (0.49%); $T_{1/2}$=24 hrs.

NURSING CONSIDERATIONS

Assessment: Assess for severe obstructive CAD, severe aortic stenosis, HF, volume/salt depletion, biliary obstructive disorders, renal artery stenosis, diabetes, hepatic/renal dysfunction, hypersensitivity to drug, pregnancy/nursing status, and possible drug interactions.

Monitoring: Monitor for worsening angina, acute MI, and other adverse reactions. Monitor BP, renal function, and serum electrolytes (especially K^+ levels).

Patient Counseling: Inform of consequences if exposure occurs during pregnancy, and of treatment options in women planning to become pregnant. Instruct to report pregnancies to physician as soon as possible.

Administration: Oral route. Take with or without food. **Storage:** 25°C (77°F); excursions permitted to 15-30°C (59-86°F). Do not remove from blisters until immediately before administration. Protect from light and moisture.

TYGACIL   RX
tigecycline (Wyeth)

An increase in all-cause mortality observed in clinical trials; should be reserved for use in situations when alternative treatment are not suitable.

THERAPEUTIC CLASS: Glycylcycline

INDICATIONS: Treatment of complicated skin and skin structure infections (cSSSIs), complicated intra-abdominal infections (cIAIs), and community-acquired bacterial pneumonia (CABP) caused by susceptible strains of indicated pathogens in patients ≥18 yrs of age.

DOSAGE: *Adults:* ≥18 Yrs: Give IV over 30-60 min. Initial: 100mg. Maint: 50mg q12h for 5-14 days (cSSSIs/cIAIs) or for 7-14 days (CABP). Duration of therapy should be guided by severity of infection. Severe Hepatic Impairment (Child-Pugh C): Initial: 100mg. Maint: 25mg q12h.
Pediatrics: Should not be used unless no alternative antibacterial drugs are available. Give IV over 30-60 min. 12-17 Yrs: 50mg q12h. 8-11 Yrs: 1.2mg/kg q12h. Max: 50mg q12h.

HOW SUPPLIED: Inj: 50mg [5mL, 10mL]

WARNINGS/PRECAUTIONS: Not indicated for the treatment of diabetic foot infections and hospital-acquired or ventilator-associated pneumonia. Anaphylaxis/anaphylactoid reactions reported. Caution with known hypersensitivity to tetracycline-class antibiotics. Isolated cases of significant hepatic dysfunction and hepatic failure reported; adverse events may occur after therapy has been discontinued. Acute pancreatitis reported; consider stopping therapy if suspected. May cause fetal harm in pregnant women and permanent tooth discoloration (yellow-gray-brown) when administered during tooth development (last 1/2 of pregnancy to 8 yrs of age). *Clostridium difficile*-associated diarrhea (CDAD) reported; d/c if CDAD is suspected or confirmed. Caution when used for cIAI secondary to clinically apparent intestinal perforation. Structurally similar to tetracyclines; may have similar adverse effects (eg, photosensitivity, pseudotumor cerebri, antianabolic action [may lead to increased BUN, azotemia, acidosis, hyperphosphatemia]). May result in overgrowth of nonsusceptible organisms; take appropriate measures if superinfection develops. Use in the absence of a proven or strongly suspected bacterial infection is unlikely to provide benefit and increases the risk of development of drug-resistant bacteria. Caution in patients with severe hepatic impairment (Child Pugh C) and monitor for treatment response.

ADVERSE REACTIONS: Abdominal pain, asthenia, headache, infection, N/V, phlebitis, diarrhea, anemia, dizziness, rash, abnormal healing, increased alkaline phosphatase/BUN/liver enzymes (SGOT/SGPT), hypoproteinemia.

INTERACTIONS: May render oral contraceptives less effective. Monitor PT or other suitable anticoagulation test with warfarin.

PREGNANCY: Category D, caution in nursing.

T

MECHANISM OF ACTION: Glycylcycline; inhibits protein translation in bacteria by binding to the 30S ribosomal subunit and blocking entry of amino-acyl tRNA molecules into the A site of the ribosome.

PHARMACOKINETICS: Absorption: Single Dose: (100mg) C_{max}=1.45mcg/mL (30 min infusion), 0.90mcg/mL (60 min infusion); AUC=5.19mcg•hr/mL. Multiple Dose: (50mg q12h) C_{max}=0.87mcg/mL (30 min infusion), 0.63mcg/mL (60 min infusion); $AUC_{0-24 hr}$=4.7mcg•hr/mL. **Distribution:** V_d=7-9L/kg; plasma protein binding (71-89%). **Elimination:** Bile (59%), urine (33%, 22% unchanged); $T_{1/2}$=27.1 hrs (single dose), 42.4 hrs (multiple dose).

NURSING CONSIDERATIONS

Assessment: Assess for known hypersensitivity to tetracycline-class antibiotics, hepatic impairment, cIAI secondary to clinically apparent intestinal perforation, culture and susceptibility testing, pregnancy/nursing status, and possible drug interactions.

Monitoring: Monitor for signs/symptoms of hypersensitivity reactions, hepatic impairment, pancreatitis, photosensitivity, superinfection, CDAD and other adverse reactions.

Patient Counseling: Inform that therapy only treats bacterial, not viral, infections. Instruct to take exactly ud even if the patient feels better early in the course of therapy; skipping doses or not completing the full course of therapy may decrease effectiveness and increase risk of bacterial resistance. Advise that diarrhea is a common problem that usually ends when therapy is discontinued; however, if watery and bloody stools (with/without stomach cramps and fever) occur, even as late as 2 or more months after last dose, instruct to contact physician as soon as possible. Advise of risk of fetal harm during pregnancy.

Administration: IV route. Refer to PI for preparation and handling details. **Storage:** Prior to Reconstitution: (Powder) 20-25°C (68-77°F); excursions permitted to 15-30°C (59-86°F). Reconstituted Sol: Room temperature (not to exceed 25°C [77°F]) up to 24 hrs (up to 6 hrs in vial and remaining time in IV bag); use immediately if storage conditions exceed 25°C (77°F). Mixed with 0.9% NaCl Inj or D5 Inj: 2-8°C (36-46°F) for up to 48 hrs following immediate transfer of reconstituted solution into IV bag.

TYKERB RX
lapatinib (GlaxoSmithKline)

Hepatotoxicity may occur; may be severe and deaths have been reported.

THERAPEUTIC CLASS: Kinase inhibitor

INDICATIONS: In combination with capecitabine for the treatment of patients with advanced/metastatic breast cancer whose tumors overexpress human epidermal receptor type 2 (HER2) and who had prior therapy, including an anthracycline, a taxane, and trastuzumab. In combination with letrozole for the treatment of postmenopausal women with hormone receptor-positive metastatic breast cancer that overexpresses the HER2 receptor for whom hormonal therapy is indicated.

DOSAGE: *Adults:* Take at least 1 hr ac or 1 hr pc. HER2-Positive Metastatic Breast Cancer: Usual: 1250mg qd on Days 1-21 continuously with capecitabine 2000mg/m^2/day (2 doses 12 hrs apart) on Days 1-14 in a repeating 21-day cycle. Take capecitabine with food or within 30 min after food. Continue treatment until disease progression or unacceptable toxicity occurs. Hormone Receptor-Positive, HER2-Positive Metastatic Breast Cancer: Usual: 1500mg qd continuously with letrozole 2.5mg qd. Refer to PI for dose modification guidelines.

HOW SUPPLIED: Tab: 250mg

WARNINGS/PRECAUTIONS: Patients should have disease progression on trastuzumab prior to initiation of treatment in combination with capecitabine. Decreased left ventricular ejection fraction (LVEF) reported; confirm normal LVEF prior to therapy and monitor during treatment. Caution with conditions that may impair left ventricular function. Monitor LFTs before treatment, every 4-6 weeks during therapy, and as clinically indicated; d/c if severe liver function changes occur, and do not retreat. Consider reducing dose with severe preexisting hepatic impairment. Diarrhea, including severe cases and deaths, reported; early identification and intervention is critical. Prompt treatment of diarrhea with antidiarrheals (eg, loperamide) after the 1st unformed stool is recommended. Replace electrolytes/fluids, use antibiotics such as fluoroquinolones (especially if diarrhea persists beyond 24 hrs, there is fever, or Grade 3 or 4 neutropenia), and interrupt or d/c therapy if severe diarrhea occurs. Associated with interstitial lung disease and pneumonitis; d/c if pulmonary symptoms indicative of interstitial lung disease/pneumonitis (≥Grade 3) occur. QT prolongation observed; caution in patients who have or may develop prolongation of QTc (eg, taking antiarrhythmics or other drugs that prolong the QT interval, and cumulative high-dose anthracycline therapy). Correct hypokalemia and hypomagnesemia before administration. May cause fetal harm.

ADVERSE REACTIONS: Hepatotoxicity, diarrhea, N/V, stomatitis, dyspepsia, palmar-plantar erythrodysesthesia, rash, dry skin, mucosal inflammation, pain in extremity, back pain, dyspnea, fatigue, headache, alopecia.

INTERACTIONS: Caution with substrates of CYP3A4, CYP2C8, and P-glycoprotein (P-gp); consider dose reduction of the substrate drug. Avoid with strong CYP3A4 inhibitors (eg, keto-conazole, clarithromycin, atazanavir) and inducers (eg, dexamethasone, phenytoin, rifampin); if unavoidable, consider dose modification of lapatinib. Avoid with grapefruit. Increased levels with P-gp inhibitors; use with caution. May increase exposure of paclitaxel and midazolam. May increase levels of digoxin; if digoxin level is >1.2ng/mL, reduce digoxin dose by 1/2.

PREGNANCY: Category D, not for use in nursing.

MECHANISM OF ACTION: Kinase inhibitor; inhibits both epidermal growth factor receptors (EGFR [ErbB1]) and HER2 (ErbB2), resulting in tumor cell growth inhibition.

PHARMACOKINETICS: Absorption: Incomplete and variable. C_{max}=2.43mcg/mL, T_{max}=4 hrs, AUC=36.2mcg•hr/mL. **Distribution:** Plasma protein binding (>99%). **Metabolism:** Liver (extensive); (major) CYP3A4, CYP3A5; (minor) CYP2C19, CYP2C8. **Elimination:** Feces (27% parent, 14% metabolites), urine (<2%); $T_{1/2}$=14.2 hrs (single dose).

NURSING CONSIDERATIONS

Assessment: Assess for severe hepatic impairment, decreased LVEF or conditions that may impair left ventricular function, QT prolongation, hypokalemia, hypomagnesemia, pregnancy/nursing status, drug hypersensitivity, and possible drug interactions. Obtain baseline ECG, LFTs, serum K⁺, and Mg²⁺ levels.

Monitoring: Monitor for hepatotoxicity, diarrhea, bowel changes, pulmonary symptoms indicative of interstitial lung disease or pneumonitis, hypokalemia, hypomagnesemia, decreased LVEF, and QT prolongation. Consider ECG and electrolyte monitoring. Monitor LFTs every 4-6 weeks during therapy and as clinically indicated.

Patient Counseling: Instruct to notify physician if SOB, palpitations, or fatigue occur. Advise that diarrhea is a common side effect and instruct on how it should be managed/prevented; instruct to contact physician immediately if any change in bowel patterns or severe diarrhea occurs. Counsel to report use of any prescription/nonprescription drugs or herbal products. Instruct not to take with grapefruit products. Advise women not to become pregnant while on therapy. Advise against doubling dose the next day for a missed dose.

Administration: Oral route. Take at least 1 hr ac or 1 hr pc. Do not divide the daily dose. **Storage:** 25°C (77°F); excursions permitted to 15-30°C (59-86°F).

Tysabri   RX
natalizumab (Biogen Idec)

> Increases risk of progressive multifocal leukoencephalopathy (PML). Risk factors for development of PML include duration of therapy, prior use of immunosuppressants, and presence of anti-JCV antibodies. Monitor for any new signs/symptoms of PML; withhold therapy at the 1st sign/symptom suggestive of PML. Available only through a special restricted distribution program called the TOUCH Prescribing Program.

THERAPEUTIC CLASS: Monoclonal antibody/VCAM-1 blocker

INDICATIONS: Monotherapy for the treatment of relapsing forms of multiple sclerosis (MS). To induce and maintain clinical response and remission in adults with moderately to severely active Crohn's disease (CD) with evidence of inflammation who have had an inadequate response to, or are unable to tolerate, conventional CD therapies and TNF-α inhibitors.

DOSAGE: *Adults:* 300mg IV infusion over 1 hr every 4 weeks. (CD) In patients starting therapy while on chronic oral corticosteroids, commence steroid tapering as soon as therapeutic benefit has occurred. D/C therapy if no therapeutic benefit by 12 weeks, if patient cannot be tapered off corticosteroids within 6 months of starting therapy, or in patients who require additional steroid use that exceeds 3 months within a calendar yr to control their CD.

HOW SUPPLIED: Inj: 300mg/15mL

CONTRAINDICATIONS: PML or history of PML.

WARNINGS/PRECAUTIONS: Anti-JCV antibody testing should not be used to diagnose PML. Avoid anti-JCV antibody testing for at least 2 weeks following plasma exchange due to the removal of antibodies from the serum. Retest patients with negative anti-JCV antibody test result periodically. PML reported following discontinuation in patient who do not have findings suggestive of PML at the time of discontinuation; monitor for any new signs or symptoms that may be suggestive of PML for at least 6 months following discontinuation. Immune reconstitution inflammatory syndrome (IRIS) reported in patients with PML, who have subsequently discontinued natalizumab; monitor for development of IRIS and treat appropriately. Increases the risk of developing encephalitis and meningitis caused by herpes simplex and varicella zoster viruses; d/c and treat appropriately if herpes encephalitis and meningitis occurs. Liver injury, including acute liver failure requiring transplant, reported; d/c with jaundice or other evidence of significant liver injury (eg, lab evidence). Hypersensitivity reactions, including serious systemic reactions (eg, anaphylaxis) reported; d/c, institute appropriate therapy, and do not retreat. May increase risk for infections. Avoid in patients with systemic medical conditions resulting in significantly compromised immune system function. Induces increases in circulating lymphocytes, monocytes, eosinophils, basophils, and nucleated RBCs or transient decreases in Hgb levels.

ADVERSE REACTIONS: Headache, fatigue, arthralgia, urinary tract infection, depression, lower/upper respiratory tract infection, abdominal discomfort, rash, gastroenteritis, vaginitis, urinary urgency/frequency, diarrhea, abnormal LFTs.

INTERACTIONS: Avoid with immunomodulatory therapy, immunosuppressants (eg, 6-mercaptopurine, azathioprine, cyclosporine, methotrexate) or TNF-α inhibitors. Taper corticosteroids in CD patients when starting natalizumab therapy. Antineoplastic, immunosuppressive, or immunomodulating agents may further increase risk of infections, including PML and other opportunistic infections.

PREGNANCY: Category C, safety not known in nursing.

MECHANISM OF ACTION: Monoclonal antibody/VCAM-1 blocker; recombinant humanized IgG4k monoclonal antibody that binds to α4-subunit of α4β1 and α4β7 integrins expressed on surface of all leukocytes, except neutrophils. Inhibits α4-mediated adhesion of leukocytes to their counter-receptor(s).

PHARMACOKINETICS: Absorption: (MS) C_{max}=110mcg/mL; (CD) C_{max}=101mcg/mL. **Distribution:** Found in breast milk; (MS) V_d=5.7L; (CD) V_d=5.2L. **Elimination:** (MS) $T_{1/2}$=11 days; (CD) $T_{1/2}$=10 days.

NURSING CONSIDERATIONS

Assessment: Assess for risk of PML, history of chronic immunosuppressant or immunomodulatory therapy, immunosuppression, drug hypersensitivity, pregnancy/nursing status, and possible drug interactions. Perform magnetic resonance imaging and CSF analysis. Test for anti-JCV antibody status; retest periodically in patients with negative result.

Monitoring: Monitor for PML, anaphylactic/hypersensitivity reactions, infections, hepatotoxicity, development of IRIS and other adverse reactions. Antibody testing recommended if presence of persistent antibodies is suspected. Evaluate patients 3 and 6 months after the 1st infusion, every 6 months thereafter, and for at least 6 months after discontinuing treatment

Patient Counseling: Inform about TOUCH Prescribing Program. Educate on risks/benefits of therapy. Counsel about the follow-up schedule (3 and 6 months after 1st infusion, every 6 months thereafter, and for at least 6 months after discontinuation). Instruct to seek medical attention if symptoms suggestive of PML develop, including progressive weakness on one side of the body or clumsiness of the limbs, disturbance of vision, and changes in thinking, memory, and orientation leading to confusion and personality changes. Instruct to report symptoms of infections, hypersensitivity reactions, and hepatotoxicity.

Administration: IV route. Do not give as an IV push or bolus. Refer to PI for dilution/administration instructions. **Storage:** 2-8°C (36-46°F). Administer within 8 hrs of preparation. Do not shake or freeze. Protect from light.

TYZEKA   RX
telbivudine (Novartis)

> Lactic acidosis and severe hepatomegaly with steatosis, including fatal cases, reported with nucleoside analogues alone or in combination with other antiretrovirals. Severe acute exacerbations of hepatitis B reported in patients who discontinued therapy; monitor hepatic function closely for at least several months. If appropriate, resumption of anti-hepatitis B therapy may be warranted.

THERAPEUTIC CLASS: Nucleoside reverse transcriptase inhibitor

INDICATIONS: Treatment of chronic hepatitis B in adults with evidence of viral replication and either evidence of persistent elevations in serum aminotransferases (ALT or AST) or histologically active disease.

DOSAGE: *Adults:* ≥16 Yrs: Usual: 600mg tab or 30mL qd. Renal Impairment: CrCl 30-49mL/min: 600mg tab q48h or 20mL qd. CrCl <30mL/min (not requiring dialysis): 600mg tab q72h or 10mL qd. End-Stage Renal Disease: 600mg tab q96h or 6mL qd; administer after hemodialysis when administered on hemodialysis days. Elderly: Adjust dose accordingly.

HOW SUPPLIED: Sol: 100mg/5mL [300mL]; Tab: 600mg

CONTRAINDICATIONS: Combination with pegylated interferon alfa-2a.

WARNINGS/PRECAUTIONS: Initiate only if pretreatment HBV DNA and ALT levels are known. HBV DNA should be <9 $\log_{10}$ copies/mL and ALT should be ≥2X ULN in HBeAg-positive patients prior to therapy. HBV DNA should be <7 $\log_{10}$ copies/mL in HBeAg-negative patients prior to therapy. Institute alternate therapy in patients with incomplete viral suppression (HBV DNA ≥300 copies/mL) after 24 weeks of treatment or if patients test positive for HBV DNA at any time after initial response. Female gender, obesity, and prolonged nucleoside exposure may be risk factors for developing lactic acidosis and hepatomegaly with steatosis; d/c therapy if lactic acidosis or hepatotoxicity develops. Caution with known risk factors for liver disease. Myopathy/myositis and peripheral neuropathy reported; interrupt therapy if suspected and d/c if confirmed. Rhabdomyolysis and uncomplicated myalgia reported. Caution in elderly.

ADVERSE REACTIONS: Fatigue, creatinine kinase increase, headache, cough, diarrhea, abdominal pain, nausea, pharyngolaryngeal pain, arthralgia, pyrexia, rash, lactic acidosis, severe hepatomegaly with steatosis, back pain, dizziness.

INTERACTIONS: See Contraindications. Drugs that alter renal function may alter plasma concentrations. Combination with interferons may be associated with risk of peripheral neuropathy.

PREGNANCY: Category B, not for use in nursing.

MECHANISM OF ACTION: Thymidine nucleoside analogue; inhibits HBV DNA polymerase (reverse transcriptase) by competing with the natural substrate thymidine 5'-triphosphate and causing DNA chain termination after incorporation into viral DNA.

PHARMACOKINETICS: Absorption: (600mg qd) C_{max}=3.69mcg/mL, T_{max}=2 hrs, AUC=26.1mcg•h/mL. Administration with varying degrees of renal function resulted in different pharmacokinetic parameters. **Distribution:** Plasma protein binding (3.3%). **Elimination:** (600mg single dose) Urine (42%), $T_{1/2}$=40-49 hrs.

NURSING CONSIDERATIONS

Assessment: Assess for renal/hepatic impairment, use in women, obesity, nucleoside exposure duration, risk factors for liver disease, pregnancy/nursing status, and possible drug interactions. Obtain HBV DNA and ALT levels prior to therapy.

Monitoring: Monitor hepatic function periodically and for several months after discontinuation. Monitor for exacerbation of HBV after discontinuation, lactic acidosis, hepatomegaly, hepatotoxicity, myopathy, and peripheral neuropathy. Monitor HBV DNA levels at 24 weeks of therapy and every 6 months thereafter. Monitor renal function in elderly patients. Closely monitor for any signs/symptoms of unexplained muscle pain, tenderness, or weakness when initiating with any drug associated with myopathy.

Patient Counseling: Advise patients to remain under care of a physician during therapy and to discuss any new symptoms or concurrent medications. Advise to report promptly unexplained muscle weakness, tenderness or pain, numbness, tingling, and/or burning sensations in the arms and/or legs with or without difficulty walking. Inform that medication is not a cure for hepatitis B and long-term treatment benefits are unknown. Inform that deterioration of liver disease may occur in some cases if treatment is discontinued; advise to discuss any changes in regimen with physician. Inform that therapy has not shown to reduce risk of transmission of HBV to others through sexual contact or blood contamination and counsel on HBV prevention strategies. Advise patients on low-sodium diet that sol contains 47mg sodium/600mg. Advise to dispose of unused/expired drug properly, and to remove all identifying information from the original container prior to disposal.

Administration: Oral route. Take with or without food. Consider oral sol in patients with difficulty swallowing tab. **Storage:** 25°C (77°F); excursions permitted to 15-30°C (59-86°F). (Sol) Use within 2 months after opening. Do not freeze.

ULORIC   RX   U
febuxostat (Takeda)

THERAPEUTIC CLASS: Xanthine oxidase inhibitor

INDICATIONS: Chronic management of hyperuricemia in patients with gout.

DOSAGE: *Adults:* Initial: 40mg qd. Titrate: If serum uric acid (sUA) is not <6mg/dL after 2 weeks, increase dose to 80mg qd.

HOW SUPPLIED: Tab: 40mg, 80mg

CONTRAINDICATIONS: Patients being treated with azathioprine or mercaptopurine.

WARNINGS/PRECAUTIONS: Not recommended for treatment of asymptomatic hyperuricemia. Increase in gout flares observed after initiation; concurrent prophylactic treatment with NSAIDs or colchicine is recommended. Cardiovascular (CV) thromboembolic events (eg, CV deaths, myocardial infarctions [MI], strokes) reported; monitor for signs and symptoms of MI and stroke. Fatal and nonfatal hepatic failure reported; obtain baseline LFTs before initiation. Measure LFTs promptly in patients who report symptoms that may indicate liver injury; d/c if LFTs are abnormal (ALT >3X ULN) and do not restart if no alternative etiology is found. D/C permanently in patients with ALT >3X ULN with serum total bilirubin >2X ULN without alternative etiologies;

use with caution in patients with lesser ALT or bilirubin elevations and with an alternate probable cause. Caution with severe hepatic impairment (Child-Pugh Class C) and severe renal impairment (CrCl <30mL/min). Avoid use in patients whom the rate of urate formation is greatly increased (eg, malignant disease and its treatment, Lesch-Nyhan syndrome).

ADVERSE REACTIONS: Liver function abnormalities, nausea, arthralgia, rash.

INTERACTIONS: See Contraindications. Caution with theophylline.

PREGNANCY: Category C, caution in nursing.

MECHANISM OF ACTION: Xanthine oxidase inhibitor; achieves its therapeutic effect by decreasing sUA.

PHARMACOKINETICS: Absorption: C_{max}=1.6mcg/mL (40mg), 2.6mcg/mL (80mg); T_{max}=1-1.5 hrs. **Distribution:** V_d=50L; plasma protein binding (99.2%). **Metabolism:** Conjugation via uridine diphosphate glucuronosyltransferase enzymes and oxidation via CYP450 enzymes. **Elimination:** Urine (49%, 3% unchanged), feces (45%, 12% unchanged); $T_{1/2}$=5-8 hrs.

NURSING CONSIDERATIONS

Assessment: Assess for asymptomatic hyperuricemia, hepatic/renal impairment, malignant disease, Lesch-Nyhan syndrome, pregnancy/nursing status, and possible drug interactions. Obtain baseline sUA and LFTs.

Monitoring: Monitor sUA levels as early as 2 weeks after initiation of therapy. Monitor for signs/symptoms of liver injury, MI, and stroke.

Patient Counseling: Advise of the potential benefits and risks of therapy. Inform that gout flares, elevated liver enzymes, and adverse CV events may occur. Instruct to notify physician if rash, chest pain, SOB, or neurologic symptoms suggesting a stroke occur. Instruct to inform physician of any other medications, including OTC drugs, currently being taken.

Administration: Oral route. May be taken without regard to food or antacid use. **Storage:** 25°C (77°F); excursions permitted to 15-30°C (59-86°F). Protect from light.

ULTRACET   RX
tramadol HCl - acetaminophen (Janssen)

> Associated with cases of acute liver failure, at times resulting in liver transplant and death. Most cases of liver injury are associated with acetaminophen (APAP) use at doses >4000mg/day and often involve >1 APAP-containing product.

THERAPEUTIC CLASS: Central acting analgesic

INDICATIONS: Short-term (≤5 days) management of acute pain.

DOSAGE: *Adults:* Initial: 2 tabs q4-6h PRN for ≤5 days. Max: 8 tabs/day. CrCl <30mL/min: Max: 2 tabs q12h. Elderly: Dose selection should be cautious.

HOW SUPPLIED: Tab: (Tramadol-APAP) 37.5mg-325mg

CONTRAINDICATIONS: Any situation where opioids are contraindicated, including acute intoxication with alcohol, hypnotics, narcotics, centrally acting analgesics, opioids, or psychotropic drugs.

WARNINGS/PRECAUTIONS: Do not exceed recommended dose. May complicate clinical assessment of acute abdominal conditions. Not recommended in patients with hepatic impairment; increased risk of acute liver failure in patients with underlying liver disease. Not for use in pregnant women prior to or during labor unless benefits outweigh risks. Not recommended for obstetrical preoperative medication or for postdelivery analgesia in nursing mothers. Caution in elderly. Serious and fatal anaphylactic reactions reported; avoid use in patients with a history of anaphylactoid reactions to codeine or other opioids. D/C use if anaphylaxis develops. APAP: Avoid in patients with APAP allergy. May cause serious skin reactions (eg, acute generalized exanthematous pustulosis, Stevens-Johnson syndrome, toxic epidermal necrolysis), which can be fatal; d/c at the 1st appearance of skin rash or any other sign of hypersensitivity. Tramadol: Seizures reported; risk increases in patients with epilepsy, history/risk of seizures, and with naloxone coadministration. Avoid in patients who are suicidal or addiction-prone; caution with emotional disturbances or depression. Reports of tramadol-related deaths with previous history of emotional disturbances, suicidal ideation/attempts, and misuse of tranquilizers/alcohol/CNS-active drugs. Potentially life-threatening serotonin syndrome including mental status changes, autonomic instability, neuromuscular aberrations, and GI symptoms may occur. Caution if at risk for respiratory depression; consider alternative nonopioid analgesic. Caution with CNS depression, head injury, and increased intracranial pressure (ICP). May impair mental/physical abilities. May cause withdrawal symptoms; do not d/c abruptly.

ADVERSE REACTIONS: Acute liver failure, constipation, somnolence, increased sweating, diarrhea, nausea, anorexia, dizziness.

INTERACTIONS: See Contraindications. Do not use concomitantly with alcohol, other APAP- or tramadol-containing products; increased risk of acute liver failure with alcohol ingestion. May alter effects of warfarin; periodically monitor PT with warfarin-like compounds. Tramadol: Increased seizure risk with SSRIs, TCAs, other tricyclic compounds (eg, cyclobenzaprine, promethazine, etc.), MAOIs, other opioids, neuroleptics, and drugs that reduce seizure threshold. Serotonin syndrome may occur when coadministered with SSRIs, SNRIs, TCAs, MAOIs, triptans, α_2-adrenergic blockers, linezolid, lithium, St. John's wort, or drugs that impair tramadol metabolism; observe carefully, especially during initiation and dose increases. Caution and reduce dose with CNS depressants (eg, alcohol, opioids, anesthetics, narcotics, phenothiazines, tranquilizers, sedative hypnotics); increased risk of CNS/respiratory depression. Caution with antidepressants and muscle relaxants; additive CNS depressant effects. CYP2D6 inhibitors (eg, quinidine, fluoxetine, paroxetine, amitriptyline) and/or CYP3A4 inhibitors (eg, ketoconazole, erythromycin) may reduce metabolic clearance; increased risk of serious adverse effects. CYP3A4 inhibitors or inducers (eg, rifampin, St. John's wort) may alter drug exposure. Digoxin toxicity may occur with concomitant use. Carbamazepine may reduce analgesic effect; avoid coadministration.

PREGNANCY: Category C, not for use in nursing.

MECHANISM OF ACTION: Tramadol: Centrally acting synthetic opioid analgesic; has not been established. Suspected to be due to the binding of parent and M1 metabolite to μ-opioid receptors and weak inhibition of reuptake of norepinephrine and serotonin. APAP: Nonopiate, nonsalicylate analgesic, and antipyretic.

PHARMACOKINETICS: Absorption: Tramadol: Absolute bioavailability (75%); T_{max}=2 hrs. APAP: T_{max}=1 hr. **Distribution:** Tramadol: (100mg IV) V_d=2.6L/kg (male), 2.9L/kg (female); plasma protein binding (20%); found in breast milk; crosses the placenta. APAP: V_d=0.9L/kg; plasma protein binding (20%). **Metabolism:** Tramadol: Liver (extensive) via CYP2D6, 3A4; M1 (active metabolite). APAP: Liver via CYP2E1, 1A2, 3A4. **Elimination:** Tramadol: Urine (30% unchanged, 60% metabolites); $T_{1/2}$=5-6 hrs. APAP: Urine (<9% unchanged); $T_{1/2}$=2-3 hrs.

NURSING CONSIDERATIONS

Assessment: Assess for known hypersensitivity to the drug and other opioids, acute intoxication with alcohol, hypnotics, narcotics, centrally acting analgesics, opioids, or psychotropic drugs, epilepsy, seizure and respiratory depression risks, suicidal ideation, emotional disturbance or depression, increased ICP, head injury, drug abuse potential, suicidal or addiction proneness, renal/hepatic impairment, pregnancy/nursing status, and possible drug interactions.

Monitoring: Monitor for acute liver failure, skin hypersensitivity/anaphylactic reactions, respiratory/CNS depression, physical dependence/abuse, misuse, tolerance, seizures, development of serotonin syndrome, withdrawal symptoms with abrupt discontinuation, and other adverse reactions. Periodically monitor PT with warfarin-like compounds.

Patient Counseling: Instruct patient to d/c therapy and notify physician if signs of allergy occur. Advise patients of dose limits. Instruct to seek medical attention immediately upon ingestion of >4000mg/day APAP, even if feeling well. Inform patients not to use with other tramadol or APAP-containing products, including OTC preparations. Advise that seizures and serotonin syndrome may occur when used with serotonergic agents or drugs that reduce the clearance of tramadol. Inform that therapy may impair physical/mental abilities. Instruct to notify physician if pregnant or planning to become pregnant. Inform patients to avoid alcohol-containing beverages while on therapy. Inform about the signs of serious skin reactions and of possible drug interactions.

Administration: Oral route. **Storage:** 25°C (77°F); excursions permitted to 15-30°C (59-86°F).

ULTRAM   RX   U
tramadol HCl (Janssen)

OTHER BRAND NAMES: Ultram ER (Janssen)

THERAPEUTIC CLASS: Central acting analgesic

INDICATIONS: (Tab) Management of moderate to moderately severe pain in adults. (Tab, Extended-Release [ER]) Management of moderate to moderately severe chronic pain in adults who require around-the-clock treatment for an extended period of time.

DOSAGE: *Adults:* Individualize dose. (Tab) ≥17 Yrs: Initial: 25mg/day qam. Titrate: Increase as tolerated by 25mg every 3 days to reach 100mg/day (25mg qid), then increase by 50mg every 3 days to reach 200mg/day (50mg qid). After Titration/Rapid Onset Required: 50-100mg q4-6h PRN. Max: 400mg/day. CrCl <30mL/min: Dose q12h. Max: 200mg/day. Cirrhosis: 50mg q12h. Elderly: Start at lower end of dosing range. >75 Yrs: Max: 300mg/day. (Tab, ER) ≥18 Yrs: Not Currently on Tramadol Immediate-Release (IR): Initial: 100mg qd. Titrate: Increase as necessary by 100mg increments every 5 days. Max: 300mg/day. Currently on Tramadol IR: Initial: Calculate 24-hr tramadol IR dose and initiate total daily dose rounded down to the next lowest 100mg increment. Maint: Individualize. Max: 300mg/day. Elderly: Start at lower end of dosing range.

HOW SUPPLIED: Tab: 50mg*; Tab, ER: 100mg, 200mg, 300mg *scored

CONTRAINDICATIONS: Any situation where opioids are contraindicated, including acute intoxication with alcohol, hypnotics, narcotics, centrally acting analgesics, opioids, or psychotropic drugs.

WARNINGS/PRECAUTIONS: Do not exceed recommended dose. Seizures reported; risk increases in patients with epilepsy, history of seizures, risk of seizures, and with naloxone coadministration. Anaphylactoid reactions and potentially life-threatening serotonin syndrome may occur. Avoid in patients who are suicidal or addiction-prone, and with history of anaphylactoid reactions to codeine and other opioids. Reports of tramadol-related deaths with previous history of emotional disturbances, suicidal ideation/attempts, and misuse of tranquilizers/alcohol/CNS active drugs. Caution if at risk for respiratory depression; consider alternative nonopioid analgesic. Caution with increased intracranial pressure (ICP) or head injury, and in elderly. May impair mental/physical abilities. Do not d/c abruptly; withdrawal symptoms may occur. May complicate clinical assessment of acute abdominal conditions. Not for use in pregnant women prior to or during labor unless benefits outweigh risks. Not recommended for obstetrical preoperative medication or for postdelivery analgesia in nursing mothers. (Tab) Caution with emotional disturbances or depression. (Tab, ER) Avoid with severe renal impairment (CrCl <30mL/min) and severe hepatic impairment (Child-Pugh Class C).

ADVERSE REACTIONS: Dizziness, N/V, constipation, headache, somnolence, sweating, asthenia, dry mouth, diarrhea, pruritus.

INTERACTIONS: See Contraindications. Caution and reduce dose with CNS depressants (eg, alcohol, opioids, anesthetics, narcotics, phenothiazines, tranquilizers, sedative hypnotics, muscle relaxants, antidepressants); increased risk of CNS/respiratory depression. CYP2D6 inhibitors (eg, quinidine, fluoxetine, paroxetine, amitriptyline) and CYP3A4 inhibitors (eg, ketoconazole, erythromycin) may reduce metabolic clearance and increase risk of adverse events. Altered exposure with CYP3A4 inducers (eg, rifampin, St. John's wort). Increased seizure risk with SSRIs, TCAs, other tricyclic compounds (eg, cyclobenzaprine, promethazine), MAOIs, opioids, neuroleptics, and drugs that reduce seizure threshold. Caution with SSRIs, SNRIs, TCAs, MAOIs, α_2-adrenergic blockers, triptans, linezolid, lithium, St. John's wort, and drugs that impair tramadol metabolism, due to potential serotonin syndrome. Not recommended with carbamazepine; decreased analgesic efficacy. Possible digoxin toxicity and altered warfarin effects. (Tab, ER) Use with other tramadol products not recommended.

PREGNANCY: Category C, not for use in nursing.

MECHANISM OF ACTION: Centrally acting synthetic opioid analgesic; has not been established. Suspected to be due to binding of parent and M1 metabolite to μ-opioid receptors and weak inhibition of norepinephrine and serotonin reuptake.

PHARMACOKINETICS: Absorption: Administration of multiple doses resulted in different parameters. **Distribution:** (100mg IV) V_d=2.6L/kg (male), 2.9L/kg (female); plasma protein binding (20%). **Metabolism:** Extensive via CYP2D6, 3A4 and 2B6; N- and O-demethylation and glucuronidation or sulfation (major pathway); M1 (active metabolite). **Elimination:** Urine (30% unchanged, 60% as metabolite); (Tab) $T_{1/2}$=6.3 hrs (drug), 7.4 hrs (M1), (Tab, ER) $T_{1/2}$=7.9 hrs (drug), 8.8 hrs (M1).

NURSING CONSIDERATIONS

Assessment: Assess for known hypersensitivity to the drug and other opioids, acute intoxication with alcohol, hypnotics, narcotics, centrally acting analgesics, opioids, or psychotropic drugs, pain intensity, epilepsy, seizure and respiratory depression risks, suicidal ideation, emotional disturbance or depression, increased ICP, head injury, drug abuse potential, suicidal or addiction proneness, renal/hepatic impairment, pregnancy/nursing status, and possible drug interactions.

Monitoring: Monitor for anaphylactoid reactions, respiratory/CNS depression, physical dependence/abuse, misuse, seizures, development of serotonin syndrome, and withdrawal symptoms with abrupt d/c.

Patient Counseling: Inform that drug may impair physical/mental abilities; use caution when driving or operating machinery. Instruct not to consume alcohol. Inform patients to use caution when taking tranquilizers, hypnotics, or opiate-containing analgesics. Instruct to notify physician if pregnant/nursing or planning to become pregnant. Educate about single-dose and 24-hr dosing limits and time interval between doses; advise not to exceed the recommended dose.

Administration: Oral route. (Tab, ER) Swallow whole; do not chew, crush, or split. **Storage:** 25°C (77°F); excursions permitted to 15-30°C (59-86°F).

UNASYN   RX
ampicillin sodium - sulbactam sodium (Roerig)

THERAPEUTIC CLASS: Beta-lactamase inhibitor/semisynthetic penicillin

INDICATIONS: Treatment of skin and skin structure infections (SSSIs), intra-abdominal infections, and gynecological infections caused by susceptible strains of microorganisms.

DOSAGE: *Adults:* Usual: 1.5-3g (ampicillin + sulbactam) IM/IV q6h. Max: 4g sulbactam/day. Renal Impairment: CrCl ≥30mL/min/1.73m²: 1.5-3g q6-8h. CrCl 15-29mL/min/1.73m²: 1.5-3g q12h. CrCl 5-14mL/min/1.73m²: 1.5-3g q24h.
Pediatrics: ≥1 Yr: SSSI: Usual: 300mg/kg/day (200mg ampicillin + 100mg sulbactam) IV in equally divided doses q6h. ≥40kg: Dose according to adult recommendations. Max: 4g sulbactam/day. Therapy should not routinely exceed 14 days.

HOW SUPPLIED: Inj: (Ampicillin-Sulbactam) 1g-0.5g, 2g-1g. Also available as a Pharmacy Bulk Package. Refer to individual package insert for more information

WARNINGS/PRECAUTIONS: Serious and occasionally fatal hypersensitivity reactions reported; d/c and institute appropriate therapy if allergic reaction occurs. *Clostridium difficile*-associated diarrhea (CDAD) reported and may range in severity from mild diarrhea to fatal colitis; d/c if CDAD is suspected or confirmed. Ampicillin class antibiotics should not be administered to patients with mononucleosis. May result in bacterial resistance in the absence of proven or suspected bacterial infection or a prophylactic indication; d/c and/or take appropriate measures if superinfection develops. Decrease in total conjugated estriol, estriol-glucuronide, conjugated estrone, and estradiol reported in pregnant women. Lab test interactions may occur. Caution with renal impairment.

ADVERSE REACTIONS: Inj-site pain, thrombophlebitis, diarrhea.

INTERACTIONS: Probenecid decreases renal tubular secretion and may increase and prolong blood levels. Increased incidence of rash with allopurinol.

PREGNANCY: Category B, caution in nursing.

MECHANISM OF ACTION: Ampicillin: Semi-synthetic penicillin; acts through inhibition of cell wall mucopeptide biosynthesis. Has a broad spectrum of bactericidal activity against many gram-positive and gram-negative aerobic and anaerobic bacteria. Sulbactam: β-lactamase inhibitor; provides good inhibitory activity against clinically important plasmid mediated β-lactamases most frequently responsible for transferred drug resistance.

PHARMACOKINETICS: Absorption: IV/IM administration of variable doses resulted in different parameters. **Distribution:** Plasma protein binding (28% ampicillin, 38% sulbactam); found in breast milk. **Elimination:** Urine (75-85% unchanged); $T_{1/2}$=1 hr.

NURSING CONSIDERATIONS

Assessment: Assess for history of hypersensitivity to cephalosporins/PCNs or other allergens, mononucleosis, renal impairment, pregnancy/nursing status, and for possible drug interactions. Confirm diagnosis of causative organisms.

Monitoring: Monitor for signs/symptoms of hypersensitivity reactions, CDAD, superinfection, and other adverse reactions. Monitor for changes in estrogen levels in pregnant women.

Patient Counseling: Inform that therapy should only be used to treat bacterial and not viral infections (eg, common cold). Advise to take exactly ud; inform that skipping doses or not completing full course may decrease effectiveness and increase resistance. Inform that diarrhea is a common problem caused by therapy and will usually end upon discontinuation of therapy. Inform that diarrhea may occur as late as ≥2 months after last dose of therapy; instruct to notify physician as soon as possible if watery/bloody stools (with or without stomach cramps and fever) occur.

Administration: IV/IM route. Refer to PI for directions for use. Do not reconstitute with aminoglycosides. (IM) Administer by deep IM inj. (IV) Administer slowly over at least 10-15 min or 15-30 min in greater dilutions. **Storage:** Prior to Reconstitution: ≤30°C (86°F). Reconstituted: Refer to PI for storage requirements.

UNIRETIC   RX
moexipril HCl - hydrochlorothiazide (UCB)

> D/C when pregnancy is detected. Drugs that act directly on the renin-angiotensin system (RAS) can cause death/injury to developing fetus.

THERAPEUTIC CLASS: ACE inhibitor/thiazide diuretic

INDICATIONS: Treatment of HTN.

DOSAGE: *Adults:* Take 1 hr ac. Uncontrolled BP on Moexipril/HCTZ Monotherapy: Initial: 7.5mg-12.5mg, 15mg-12.5mg, or 15mg-25mg qd. Titrate: Based on clinical response. May increase HCTZ dose after 2-3 weeks. Max: 30mg-50mg qd. Controlled BP on 25mg qd HCTZ with Hypokalemia: Switch to 3.75mg-6.25mg (1/2 of 7.5mg-12.5mg tab). Excessive BP Reduction with 7.5mg-12.5mg: Switch to 3.75mg-6.25mg. Replacement Therapy: May substitute for titrated components.

HOW SUPPLIED: Tab: (Moexipril-HCTZ) 7.5mg-12.5mg*, 15mg-12.5mg*, 15mg-25mg* *scored

CONTRAINDICATIONS: History of ACE inhibitor-associated angioedema, anuria, hypersensitivity to sulfonamide-derived drugs. Coadministration with aliskiren in patients with diabetes.

WARNINGS/PRECAUTIONS: Not for initial therapy. Not recommended with severe renal impairment (CrCl ≤40mL/min/1.73m²). Symptomatic hypotension may occur, most likely in patients with salt and/or volume depletion; correct such conditions before therapy. May precipitate hepatic coma with hepatic impairment or progressive liver disease. Caution in elderly. HCTZ: Enhanced antihypertensive effects in postsympathectomy patients. May precipitate azotemia with severe renal disease. May cause idiosyncratic reaction, resulting in acute transient myopia and acute angle-closure glaucoma; d/c as rapidly as possible. May cause exacerbation or activation of systemic lupus erythematosus (SLE), hyperuricemia, precipitation of frank gout or overt diabetes, hypercalcemia, hypophosphatemia, hypomagnesemia, reduced glucose tolerance, and increased cholesterol and TG levels. Observe for signs of fluid and electrolyte imbalance; monitor serum electrolytes periodically. Hypokalemia may sensitize or exaggerate the response of the heart to toxic effects of digitalis. Moexipril: Angioedema of the face, extremities, lips, tongue, glottis, and/or larynx reported; d/c and administer appropriate therapy if symptoms develop. Intestinal angioedema reported; monitor for abdominal pain. More reports of angioedema in blacks than nonblacks. Anaphylactoid reactions reported during desensitization with hymenoptera venom, dialysis with high-flux membranes, and LDL apheresis with dextran sulfate absorption. Excessive hypotension, which may be associated with oliguria or progressive azotemia, and rarely, with acute renal failure and/or death, may occur in congestive heart failure (CHF) patients; monitor closely upon initiation and during first 2 weeks of therapy and whenever dose is increased. May cause changes in renal function. May increase BUN/SrCr in patients with no preexisting renal vascular disease or with renal artery stenosis; monitor renal function during the 1st few weeks of therapy in patients with renal artery stenosis. May cause agranulocytosis and bone marrow depression; monitor WBCs with collagen vascular disease. Rarely, associated with syndrome of cholestatic jaundice, hepatic necrosis, and death; d/c if jaundice or marked hepatic enzyme elevation occurs. Hyperkalemia and persistent nonproductive cough reported. Hypotension may occur with major surgery or during anesthesia.

ADVERSE REACTIONS: Cough, dizziness, angioedema, hypotension, fatigue.

INTERACTIONS: See Contraindications. Dual blockade of the RAS is associated with increased risks of hypotension, hyperkalemia, and changes in renal function (including acute renal failure); closely monitor BP, renal function, and electrolytes with concomitant agents that affect the RAS. Avoid with aliskiren in patients with renal impairment (GFR <60mL/min). NSAIDs, including selective COX-2 inhibitors, may attenuate diuretic, natriuretic, and antihypertensive effects. HCTZ: Potentiation of orthostatic hypotension may occur with alcohol, barbiturates, or narcotics. Dosage adjustment of antidiabetic drugs (oral agents and insulin) may be required. Cholestyramine and colestipol resins may reduce absorption. Corticosteroids and adrenocorticotropic hormone may intensify electrolyte depletion, particularly hypokalemia. May decrease response to pressor amines (eg, norepinephrine). May increase responsiveness to nondepolarizing skeletal muscle relaxants (eg, tubocurarine). Increased absorption with guanabenz or propantheline. May potentiate action of other antihypertensives, especially ganglionic or peripheral adrenergic-blocking drugs. Moexipril: NSAIDs may deteriorate renal function. Increased lithium levels and symptoms of toxicity reported; use with caution and monitor lithium levels. Increased risk of hyperkalemia with K⁺-sparing diuretics (spironolactone, amiloride, triamterene), K⁺ supplements, or K⁺-containing salt substitutes; use with caution and monitor serum K⁺. Nitritoid reactions reported with injectable gold (sodium aurothiomalate).

PREGNANCY: Category D, not for use in nursing.

MECHANISM OF ACTION: Moexipril: ACE inhibitor; decreases angiotensin II formation, leading to decreased vasoconstriction, increased plasma renin activity, and decreased aldosterone secretion. HCTZ: Thiazide diuretic; not established. Affects distal renal tubular mechanisms of electrolyte reabsorption, directly increasing excretion of Na⁺ and Cl⁻ in approximately equivalent amounts.

PHARMACOKINETICS: Absorption: Moexipril: Incomplete. Bioavailability (13%, moexiprilat); T_{max}=0.8 hr, 1.5-1.6 hrs (moexiprilat); C_{max} and AUC reduced by 70% and 40%, respectively, with low-fat breakfast, or 80% and 50%, respectively, with high-fat breakfast. **Distribution:** Moexipril: V_d=2.8L/kg (moexiprilat); plasma protein binding (50%, moexiprilat). HCTZ: V_d=1.5-4.2L/kg; plasma protein binding (21-24%); crosses placenta; found in breast milk. **Metabolism:** Rapid via de-esterification; moexiprilat (active metabolite). **Elimination:** Moexipril: Urine (1% unchanged, 7% moexiprilat, 5% other metabolites), feces (1% unchanged, 52% moexiprilat); $T_{1/2}$=1.3 hrs, 2-9 hrs (moexiprilat). HCTZ: Kidney (>60% unchanged); $T_{1/2}$=5.6-14.8 hrs.

NURSING CONSIDERATIONS

Assessment: Assess for history of ACE inhibitor-associated angioedema, anuria, hypersensitivity to drug or sulfonamide-derived drugs, history of allergy or bronchial asthma, volume/salt depletion, CHF, collagen vascular disease, renal artery stenosis, SLE, risk factors for hyperkalemia, hepatic/renal function, pregnancy/nursing status, and possible drug interactions. Obtain baseline serum electrolytes.

Monitoring: Monitor for signs of angioedema, hypotension, exacerbation/activation of SLE, idiosyncratic reaction, and other adverse reactions. Monitor hepatic/renal function, BP, WBC counts (collagen vascular disease), serum electrolytes, blood glucose, cholesterol, TG, and uric acid.

Patient Counseling: Advise to take therapy 1 hr ac. Instruct to d/c use and report immediately to physician if signs/symptoms of angioedema occur. Inform that lightheadedness may occur, especially during the 1st few days of therapy; instruct to d/c use and consult physician if fainting occurs. Inform that excessive perspiration, dehydration, and other causes of volume depletion may lead to excessive fall in BP; advise to consult physician if these conditions develop. Instruct not to use K⁺ supplements or salt substitutes containing K⁺ without consulting physician, and to report promptly any indication of infection. Inform of the consequences of exposure during pregnancy and discuss treatment options in women planning to become pregnant. Instruct to report pregnancies to physician as soon as possible.

Administration: Oral route. **Storage:** 20-25°C (68-77°F). Protect from excessive moisture.

UNITHROID   RX
levothyroxine sodium (Lannett)

> Do not use for the treatment of obesity or weight loss; doses within range of daily hormonal requirements are ineffective for weight reduction in euthyroid patients. Serious or life-threatening manifestations of toxicity may occur when given in larger doses, particularly when given in association with sympathomimetic amines.

THERAPEUTIC CLASS: Thyroid replacement hormone

INDICATIONS: Replacement or supplemental therapy in congenital or acquired hypothyroidism of any etiology, except transient hypothyroidism during the recovery phase of subacute thyroiditis. Treatment or prevention of various types of euthyroid goiters, including thyroid nodules, subacute or chronic lymphocytic thyroiditis, multinodular goiter, and as an adjunct to surgery and radioiodine therapy for thyrotropin-dependent well-differentiated thyroid cancer.

DOSAGE: *Adults:* Individualize dose. Adjust dose based on periodic assessment of patient's clinical response and laboratory parameters. Take in the am on an empty stomach at least 1/2-1 hr before food. Take at least 4 hrs apart from drugs that are known to interfere with its absorption. Hypothyroidism: Usual: 1.7mcg/kg/day. >200mcg/day seldom required. >50 Yrs/<50 Yrs with Cardiac Disease: Initial: 25-50mcg/day. Titrate: Increase by 12.5-25mcg increments every 6-8 weeks, PRN until euthyroid. Elderly with Cardiac Disease: Initial: 12.5-25mcg/day. Titrate: Increase by 12.5-25mg increments every 4-6 weeks until euthyroid. Severe Hypothyroidism: Initial: 12.5-25mcg/day. Titrate: Increase by 25mcg/day every 2-4 weeks until TSH level normalized. Secondary (Pituitary)/Tertiary (Hypothalamic) Hypothyroidism: Titrate until euthyroid and serum free-T4 level is restored to the upper 1/2 of the normal range. Pregnancy: May increase dose requirements. Subclinical Hypothyroidism: Lower doses may be adequate to normalize the serum TSH level (eg, 1mcg/kg/day). TSH Suppression in Well-Differentiated Thyroid Cancer and Thyroid Nodules: Individualize dose based on the specific disease and the patient being treated. Refer to PI for further details.

Pediatrics: Individualize dose. Adjust dose based on periodic assessment of patient's clinical response and laboratory parameters. Take in the am on an empty stomach at least 1/2-1 hr before food. Take at least 4 hrs apart from drugs that are known to interfere with its absorption. Hypothyroidism: Growth/Puberty Complete: Usual: 1.7mcg/kg/day. >12 Yrs (Growth/Puberty Incomplete): 2-3mcg/kg/day. 6-12 Yrs: 4-5mcg/kg/day. 1-5 Yrs: 5-6mcg/kg/day. 6-12 Months: 6-8mcg/kg/day. 3-6 Months: 8-10mcg/kg/day. 0-3 months: 10-15mcg/kg/day. Infants at Risk for Cardiac Failure: Use lower starting dose (eg, 25mcg/day). Titrate: Increase dose in 4-6 weeks PRN. Infants with Serum T4 <5mcg/dL: Initial: 50mcg/day. Chronic/Severe Hypothyroidism: Children: Initial: 25mcg/day. Titrate: Increase by 25mcg increments every 2-4 weeks until desired effect is achieved. Minimize Hyperactivity in Older Children: Initial: Give 1/4 of full replacement dose. Titrate: Increase on a weekly basis by an amount equal to 1/4 of the full-recommended replacement dose until full recommended replacement dose is reached. May crush tab and mix with 5-10mL of water.

HOW SUPPLIED: Tab: 25mcg*, 50mcg*, 75mcg*, 88mcg*, 100mcg*, 112mcg*, 125mcg*, 137mcg*, 150mcg*, 175mcg*, 200mcg*, 300mcg* *scored

CONTRAINDICATIONS: Untreated subclinical (suppressed serum TSH level with normal T3 and T4 levels) or overt thyrotoxicosis, acute myocardial infarction (MI), uncorrected adrenal insufficiency.

WARNINGS/PRECAUTIONS: Should not be used in the treatment of male or female infertility unless associated with hypothyroidism. Contraindicated in patients with nontoxic diffuse goiter or nodular thyroid disease, particularly in the elderly or with underlying cardiovascular (CV) disease if serum TSH level is already suppressed; use with caution if TSH level is not suppressed and carefully monitor thyroid function. Has narrow therapeutic index; carefully titrate dose to avoid over- or under-treatment. May decrease bone mineral density (BMD) with long-term use; give minimum dose necessary to achieve desired clinical and biochemical response. Caution with

U

CV disorders and the elderly. If cardiac symptoms develop or worsen, reduce or withhold dose for 1 week and then restart at lower dose. Overtreatment may produce CV effects (eg, increase in HR, increase in cardiac wall thickness, increase in cardiac contractility, precipitation of angina or arrhythmias). Monitor patients with coronary artery disease (CAD) closely during surgical procedures; may precipitate cardiac arrhythmias. Caution in patients with diabetes mellitus (DM). Patients with concomitant adrenal insufficiency should be treated with replacement glucocorticoids prior to therapy.

ADVERSE REACTIONS: Fatigue, increased appetite, weight loss, heat intolerance, headache, hyperactivity, irritability, insomnia, palpitations, arrhythmias, dyspnea, hair loss, menstrual irregularities, pseudotumor cerebri (children), slipped capital femoral epiphysis (children).

INTERACTIONS: Concurrent sympathomimetics may increase effects of sympathomimetics or thyroid hormone; may increase risk of coronary insufficiency with CAD. Upward dose adjustments may be needed for insulin and oral hypoglycemic agents. May decrease absorption with soybean flour, cottonseed meal, walnuts, and dietary fiber. May increase oral anticoagulant activity; adjust dose of anticoagulant and monitor PT. May decrease levels and effects of digitalis glycosides. Transient reduction in TSH secretion with dopamine/dopamine agonists, glucocorticoids, octreotide. Decreased thyroid hormone secretion with aminoglutethimide, amiodarone, iodide (including iodine-containing radiographic contrast agents), lithium, methimazole, propylthiouracil (PTU), sulfonamides, and tolbutamide. May increase thyroid hormone secretion with amiodarone and iodide. May decrease T4 absorption with antacids (aluminum and magnesium hydroxides), simethicone, bile acid sequestrants (cholestyramine, colestipol), calcium carbonate, cation exchange resins (kayexalate), ferrous sulfate, orlistat, and sucralfate; administer at least 4 hrs apart. May increase serum thyroxine-binding globulin (TBG) concentrations with clofibrate, estrogen-containing oral contraceptives, oral estrogens, heroin/methadone, 5-fluorouracil, mitotane, and tamoxifen. May decrease serum TBG concentrations with androgens/anabolic steroids, asparaginase, glucocorticoids, and slow-release nicotinic acid. May cause protein-binding site displacement with furosemide (>80mg IV), heparin, hydantoins, NSAIDs (fenamates, phenylbutazone), and salicylates (>2g/day). May alter T4 and T3 metabolism with carbamazepine, hydantoins, phenobarbital, and rifampin. May decrease T4 5'-deiodinase activity with amiodarone, β-adrenergic antagonists (eg, propranolol >160mg/day), glucocorticoids (eg, dexamethasone >4mg/day), and PTU. Concurrent use with tricyclic (eg, amitriptyline) and tetracyclic (eg, maprotiline) antidepressants may increase the therapeutic and toxic effects of both drugs. Coadministration with sertraline in patients stabilized on levothyroxine may result in increased levothyroxine requirements. Interferon-α may cause development of antithyroid microsomal antibodies and transient hypothyroidism, hyperthyroidism, or both. Interleukin-2 has been associated with transient painless thyroiditis. Excessive use with growth hormones (eg, somatropin, somatrem) may accelerate epiphyseal closure. Ketamine may produce marked HTN and tachycardia. May reduce uptake of radiographic agents. Decreased theophylline clearance may occur in hypothyroid patients. Altered levels of thyroid hormone and/or TSH levels with choral hydrate, diazepam, ethionamide, lovastatin, metoclopramide, 6-mercaptopurine, nitroprusside, para-aminosalicylate sodium, perphenazine, resorcinol (excessive topical use), and thiazide diuretics.

PREGNANCY: Category A, caution in nursing.

MECHANISM OF ACTION: Thyroid replacement hormone; mechanism not established. Suspected that principal effects are exerted through control of DNA transcription and protein synthesis.

PHARMACOKINETICS: Administration: Majority absorbed from jejunum and upper ileum. **Distribution:** Plasma protein binding (>99%), found in breast milk. **Metabolism:** Sequential deiodination and conjugation in liver (mainly), kidneys, other tissues. **Elimination:** Urine; feces (20% unchanged); $T_{1/2}$=6-7 days (T4), ≤2 days (T3).

NURSING CONSIDERATIONS

Assessment: Assess for untreated subclinical or overt thyrotoxicosis, acute MI, uncorrected adrenal insufficiency, CAD, CV disorders, nontoxic diffuse goiter, nodular thyroid disease, DM, hypersensitivity, pregnancy/nursing status, and possible drug interactions. In patients with secondary or tertiary hypothyroidism, assess for additional hypothalamic/pituitary hormone deficiencies. Assess TSH levels. In infants with congenital hypothyroidism, assess for other congenital anomalies.

Monitoring: Monitor for CV effects. In patients on long-term therapy, monitor for signs/symptoms of decreased BMD. In patients with nontoxic diffuse goiter or nodular thyroid disease, monitor for precipitation of thyrotoxicosis. In adults with primary hypothyroidism, perform periodic monitoring of serum TSH levels. In pediatric patients with congenital hypothyroidism, perform periodic monitoring of serum TSH levels and total or free T4 levels. In patients with secondary and tertiary hypothyroidism, perform periodic monitoring of serum free-T4 levels. Refer to PI for TSH and T4 monitoring parameters. Closely monitor PT if coadministered with an oral anticoagulant.

Patient Counseling: Instruct to notify physician if allergic to any foods or medicines, pregnant or planning to become pregnant, breastfeeding or taking any other drugs, including prescriptions and OTC preparations. Instruct to notify physician of any other medical conditions, particularly heart disease, diabetes, clotting disorders, and adrenal or pituitary gland problems. Instruct not to stop or change dose unless directed by physician. Instruct to take on empty stomach, at least 1/2 to 1 hr before eating breakfast. Instruct to notify physician if rapid or irregular heartbeat, chest pain, SOB, leg cramps, headache, or any other unusual medical event occurs. Inform that dose may be increased during pregnancy. Instruct to notify physician or dentist prior to surgery about levothyroxine therapy. Advise that partial hair loss may occur during the 1st few months of therapy, but is usually temporary. Inform that drug should not be used as a primary or adjunctive therapy in a weight control program. Inform that drug should not be administered within 4 hrs of agents such as iron/Ca^{2+} supplements and antacids.

Administration: Oral route. **Storage:** 20-25°C (68-77°F); excursions permitted to 15-30°C (59-86°F). Store away from heat, moisture, and light.

UNIVASC   RX
moexipril HCl (UCB)

> D/C when pregnancy is detected. Drugs that act directly on the renin-angiotensin system (RAS) can cause injury/death to the developing fetus.

THERAPEUTIC CLASS: ACE inhibitor

INDICATIONS: Treatment of HTN alone or in combination with thiazide diuretics.

DOSAGE: *Adults:* Take 1 hr ac. Not Receiving Diuretics: Initial: 7.5mg qd. Titrate: Adjust dose according to BP response. If not adequately controlled, may increase or divide dose. Usual: 7.5-30mg/day given in 1 or 2 divided doses. Max: 60mg/day. Receiving Diuretics: D/C diuretic 2-3 days prior to therapy. Resume diuretic if BP is not controlled. If diuretic cannot be discontinued, give initial dose of 3.75mg. CrCl ≤40mL/min/1.73m²: Initial: 3.75mg qd given cautiously. Max: 15mg/day. Elderly: Start at lower end of dosing range.

HOW SUPPLIED: Tab: 7.5mg*, 15mg* *scored

CONTRAINDICATIONS: History of ACE inhibitor-associated angioedema. Coadministration with aliskiren in patients with diabetes.

WARNINGS/PRECAUTIONS: Angioedema of the face, extremities, lips, tongue, glottis, and/or larynx reported; d/c and administer appropriate therapy if symptoms develop. Intestinal angioedema reported; monitor for abdominal pain. More reports of angioedema in blacks than nonblacks. Anaphylactoid reactions reported during desensitization with hymenoptera venom, dialysis with high-flux membranes, and LDL apheresis with dextran sulfate absorption. Symptomatic hypotension may occur, most likely with salt and volume depletion; correct depletion prior to therapy. Excessive hypotension associated with oliguria, azotemia, acute renal failure, or death may occur in congestive heart failure (CHF) patients; monitor closely upon initiation and during first 2 weeks of therapy and whenever dose is increased. May cause agranulocytosis and bone marrow depression; monitor WBCs with collagen vascular disease. Rarely, associated with syndrome of cholestatic jaundice, fulminant hepatic necrosis, and death; d/c if jaundice or marked hepatic enzyme elevation occurs. May cause changes in renal function. Increased BUN and SrCr reported in patients with renal artery stenosis and without preexisting renal vascular disease; reduce dose and/or d/c. Hyperkalemia reported; risk factors include diabetes mellitus (DM) and renal insufficiency. Hypotension may occur with major surgery or during anesthesia. Persistent nonproductive cough reported. Dual blockade of the RAS is associated with increased risks of hypotension, hyperkalemia, and changes in renal function (including acute renal failure); closely monitor BP, renal function, and electrolytes with concomitant agents that also affect the RAS. Caution in elderly.

ADVERSE REACTIONS: Cough increased, dizziness, diarrhea, flu syndrome.

INTERACTIONS: See Contraindications. Avoid with aliskiren in patients with renal impairment (GFR <60mL/min). Hypotension risk and increased BUN and SrCr with diuretics. Increased risk of hyperkalemia with K⁺-sparing diuretics (spironolactone, amiloride, triamterene), K⁺ supplements, or K⁺-containing salt substitutes; use with caution and monitor serum K⁺. Increased lithium levels and lithium toxicity symptoms reported; use with caution and monitor lithium levels. Nitritoid reactions (eg, facial flushing, N/V, hypotension) reported with injectable gold (sodium aurothiomalate). NSAIDs, including selective COX-2 inhibitors, may deteriorate renal function. Antihypertensive effect may be attenuated by NSAIDs.

PREGNANCY: Category D, caution in nursing.

MECHANISM OF ACTION: ACE inhibitor; reduces angiotensin II formation, decreases vasoconstriction and aldosterone secretion, and increases plasma renin.

PHARMACOKINETICS: Absorption: Incomplete. Bioavailability (13%, moexiprilat); T$_{max}$=1.5 hrs (moexiprilat); C$_{max}$ and AUC reduced by 70% and 40%, respectively, with low-fat breakfast, or 80% and 50%, respectively, with high-fat breakfast. **Distribution:** V$_d$=183L (moexiprilat); plasma protein binding (50%, moexiprilat). **Metabolism:** Rapid via deesterification; moexiprilat (active metabolite). **Elimination:** Urine (1% unchanged, 7% moexiprilat, 5% other metabolites), feces (1% unchanged, 52% moexiprilat); $T_{1/2}$=2-9 hrs (moexiprilat).

NURSING CONSIDERATIONS

Assessment: Assess for history of ACE inhibitor-associated angioedema, hypersensitivity to the drug, volume/salt depletion, CHF, collagen vascular disease, renal artery stenosis, DM, cerebrovascular disease, hepatic/renal function, pregnancy/nursing status, and possible drug interactions.

Monitoring: Monitor BP, hepatic/renal function, WBCs (collagen vascular disease), and serum K^+ levels. Monitor for head/neck and intestinal angioedema, anaphylactoid reaction, and hypersensitivity reactions.

Patient Counseling: Instruct to d/c use and report immediately to physician if signs/symptoms of angioedema occur. Inform that lightheadedness may occur, especially during the 1st few days of therapy; instruct to d/c use and consult physician if fainting occurs. Inform that excessive perspiration, dehydration, and other causes of volume depletion may lead to excessive fall in BP; advise to consult physician if these conditions develop. Instruct not to use K^+ supplements or salt substitutes containing K^+ without consulting physician, and to report any signs/symptoms of infection. Inform of the consequences of exposure during pregnancy and instruct to report pregnancies to physician as soon as possible.

Administration: Oral route. **Storage:** 20-25°C (68-77°F). Protect from excessive moisture.

UROXATRAL   RX
alfuzosin HCl (Sanofi-Aventis)

THERAPEUTIC CLASS: Alpha$_1$-antagonist

INDICATIONS: Treatment of signs and symptoms of BPH.

DOSAGE: *Adults:* 10mg qd, with food and with the same meal each day.

HOW SUPPLIED: Tab, Extended-Release: 10mg

CONTRAINDICATIONS: Moderate or severe hepatic impairment (Child-Pugh categories B and C), concomitant use of potent CYP3A4 inhibitors (eg, ketoconazole, itraconazole, ritonavir).

WARNINGS/PRECAUTIONS: Postural hypotension with or without symptoms (eg, dizziness) may develop within few hrs after administration; caution with symptomatic hypotension or in those who had a hypotensive response to other medications. Syncope may occur; caution to avoid situations in which injury could result should syncope occur. Prostate carcinoma and BPH frequently coexist and many of their symptoms are similar; rule out the presence of prostatic cancer prior to therapy. D/C if symptoms of angina pectoris occur or worsen. Caution with severe renal impairment, mild hepatic impairment, and congenital or acquired QT prolongation. Intraoperative floppy iris syndrome (IFIS) observed in some patients during cataract surgery. Priapism rarely reported; this condition can lead to permanent impotence if not properly treated. May impair mental/physical abilities. Not indicated for use in women or children.

ADVERSE REACTIONS: Dizziness, upper respiratory tract infection, headache, fatigue.

INTERACTIONS: See Contraindications. Avoid use with other α-blockers. Cimetidine, atenolol, and moderate CYP3A4 inhibitors (eg, diltiazem) may increase levels. May increase risk of hypotension/postural hypotension and syncope with nitrates and other antihypertensives. Caution with medications that prolong the QT interval. Caution with PDE-5 inhibitors; may potentially cause symptomatic hypotension.

PREGNANCY: Category B, safety not known in nursing.

MECHANISM OF ACTION: α$_1$-antagonist; selectively inhibits α$_1$-adrenergic receptors in lower urinary tract causing smooth muscle in bladder neck and prostate to relax, which results in improved urine flow and decreased symptoms of BPH.

PHARMACOKINETICS: Absorption: Absolute bioavailability (49%), C_{max}=13.6ng/mL, T_{max}=8 hrs, AUC_{0-24}=194ng•hr/mL. **Distribution:** V_d=3.2L/kg (IV); plasma protein binding (82-90%). **Metabolism:** Liver (extensive) via CYP3A4 (oxidation, O-demethylation, N-dealkylation). **Elimination:** Feces (69%), urine (24%, 11% unchanged); $T_{1/2}$=10 hrs.

NURSING CONSIDERATIONS

Assessment: Assess for BPH, prostatic cancer, symptomatic hypotension, history of QT prolongation, hepatic/renal impairment, cataract surgery, hypersensitivity, and possible drug interactions. Rule out the presence of prostatic cancer prior to therapy.

Monitoring: Monitor for postural hypotension, syncope, hypersensitivity reactions, IFIS, QT prolongation, hepatic/renal dysfunction, urine flow, and allergic/hypersensitivity reactions.

Patient Counseling: Inform about possible occurrence of symptoms related to postural hypotension when beginning therapy; caution about driving, operating machinery, or performing hazardous tasks during this period. Advise to inform ophthalmologist about using the product before cataract surgery or other procedures involving the eyes, even if the patient is no longer taking the medication. Advise about the possibility of priapism resulting from treatment and to seek immediate medical attention if it occurs. Instruct to take with food and with the same meal each day. Instruct not to crush or chew tab.

Administration: Oral route. Take with food. Swallow tab whole; do not chew or crush. **Storage:** 25°C (77°F); excursions permitted to 15-30°C (59-86°F). Protect from light and moisture.

VAGIFEM   RX
estradiol (Novo Nordisk)

> Estrogens increase the risk of endometrial cancer. Perform adequate diagnostic measures, including endometrial sampling, to rule out malignancy in postmenopausal women with undiagnosed persistent or recurring abnormal genital bleeding. Should not be used for prevention of cardiovascular disease (CVD) or dementia. Increased risk of myocardial infarction (MI), pulmonary embolism (PE), stroke, invasive breast cancer, and deep vein thrombosis (DVT) in postmenopausal women (50-79 yrs of age) reported. Increased risk of developing probable dementia in postmenopausal women ≥65 yrs reported. Should be prescribed at the lowest effective dose and for the shortest duration consistent with treatment goals and risks.

THERAPEUTIC CLASS: Estrogen

INDICATIONS: Treatment of atrophic vaginitis due to menopause.

DOSAGE: *Adults:* 1 tab intravaginally qd for 2 weeks, followed by 1 tab twice weekly. Reevaluate treatment need periodically.

HOW SUPPLIED: Tab: 10mcg

CONTRAINDICATIONS: Undiagnosed abnormal genital bleeding, known/suspected/history of breast cancer, known/suspected estrogen-dependent neoplasia, active or history of DVT/PE/arterial thromboembolic disease (eg, stroke, MI), known liver impairment/disease, known protein C, protein S, or antithrombin deficiency, or other known thrombophilic disorders, known/suspected pregnancy.

WARNINGS/PRECAUTIONS: Caution in patients with risk factors for arterial vascular disease and/or venous thromboembolism. If feasible, d/c at least 4-6 weeks before surgery of the type associated with increased risk of thromboembolism, or during periods of prolonged immobilization. May increase risk of gallbladder disease requiring surgery, and ovarian cancer. Consider addition of progestin for women with a uterus or with residual endometriosis post-hysterectomy. May lead to severe hypercalcemia in women with breast cancer and bone metastases; d/c and take appropriate measures if hypercalcemia occurs. Retinal vascular thrombosis reported; if visual abnormalities or migraine occurs, d/c pending exam. If exam reveals papilledema or retinal vascular lesions, d/c permanently. May elevate BP, plasma TGs (with preexisting hypertriglyceridemia), and thyroid-binding globulin levels; d/c if pancreatitis occurs. Caution with history of cholestatic jaundice associated with past estrogen use or with pregnancy; d/c in case of recurrence. May cause fluid retention; caution with cardiac/renal dysfunction. Caution with hypoparathyroidism; hypocalcemia may result. May exacerbate symptoms of angioedema in women with hereditary angioedema. May exacerbate endometriosis, asthma, diabetes mellitus (DM), epilepsy, migraine, porphyria, systemic lupus erythematosus (SLE), and hepatic hemangiomas; use with caution. Local abrasion induced by applicator reported, especially in women with severely atrophic vaginal mucosa. May affect certain endocrine and blood components in lab tests.

ADVERSE REACTIONS: Vulvovaginal mycotic infection, vulvovaginal pruritus, back pain, diarrhea.

INTERACTIONS: CYP3A4 inducers (eg, St. John's wort, phenobarbital, carbamazepine, rifampin) may decrease levels, which may decrease therapeutic effects and/or change uterine bleeding profile. CYP3A4 inhibitors (eg, erythromycin, ketoconazole, ritonavir, grapefruit juice) may increase levels, which may result in side effects. Concomitant thyroid hormone replacement therapy may require increased doses of thyroid replacement therapy.

PREGNANCY: Contraindicated in pregnancy, not for use in nursing.

MECHANISM OF ACTION: Estrogen; binds to nuclear receptors in estrogen-responsive tissues. Circulating estrogens modulate the pituitary secretion of the gonadotropins, luteinizing hormone and follicle-stimulating hormone, through a negative feedback mechanism. Reduces elevated levels of these hormones in postmenopausal women.

PHARMACOKINETICS: Absorption: Well-absorbed. Administration of multiple doses resulted in different parameters. **Distribution:** Largely bound to sex hormone-binding globulin and albumin; found in breast milk. **Metabolism:** Liver, to estrone (metabolite) and estriol (major urinary metabolite); enterohepatic circulation via sulfate and glucuronide conjugation in the liver; biliary secretion of conjugates into the intestine; hydrolysis in the gut; reabsorption. **Elimination:** Urine (parent compound and metabolites).

V

NURSING CONSIDERATIONS

Assessment: Assess for abnormal vaginal bleeding, presence/history of breast cancer, estrogen-dependent neoplasia, active or history of DVT/PE/arterial thromboembolic disease, liver impairment/disease, thrombophilic disorders, known anaphylactic reaction or angioedema to the drug, pregnancy/nursing status, other conditions where treatment is cautioned, need for progestin therapy, and possible drug interactions.

Monitoring: Monitor for signs/symptoms of CVD, malignant neoplasms, dementia, gallbladder disease, hypercalcemia, visual abnormalities, BP and plasma TG elevations, pancreatitis, cholestatic jaundice, hypothyroidism, fluid retention, and for other adverse events. Perform annual breast exam; schedule mammography based on age, risk factors, and prior mammogram results. Monitor thyroid function in patients on thyroid hormone replacement therapy. Perform adequate diagnostic measures (eg, endometrial sampling) in patients with undiagnosed persistent or recurring genital bleeding. Perform periodic evaluation to determine treatment need.

Patient Counseling: Inform postmenopausal women of the importance of reporting abnormal vaginal bleeding to physician as soon as possible. Inform of possible adverse reactions. Advise to have yearly breast exams by a physician and perform monthly breast self-exams. Instruct on how to use the applicator.

Administration: Intravaginal route. **Storage:** 25°C (77°F); excursions permitted to 15-30°C (59-86°F). Do not refrigerate.

VALCYTE   RX
valganciclovir HCl (Genentech)

> Clinical toxicity includes granulocytopenia, anemia, and thrombocytopenia. Carcinogenic, teratogenic, and caused aspermatogenesis in animal studies.

THERAPEUTIC CLASS: Synthetic guanine derivative nucleoside analogue

INDICATIONS: (Tab) Treatment of cytomegalovirus (CMV) retinitis in adults with AIDS and prevention of CMV disease in adult kidney, heart, or kidney-pancreas transplant patients at high risk (donor CMV seropositive/recipient CMV seronegative [D+/R-]). (Tab/Sol) Prevention of CMV disease in kidney or heart transplant patients (4 months-16 yrs of age) at high risk.

DOSAGE: *Adults:* Take with food. Treatment of CMV Retinitis: Induction: 900mg bid for 21 days. Maint: 900mg qd following induction treatment or in patients with inactive CMV retinitis. Prevention of CMV Disease: Heart/Kidney-Pancreas Transplant: Usual: 900mg qd starting within 10 days of transplantation until 100 days post-transplantation. Kidney Transplant: Usual: 900mg qd starting within 10 days of transplantation until 200 days post-transplantation. Renal Impairment: CrCl 40-59mL/min: Induction: 450mg bid. Maint/Prevention: 450mg qd. CrCl 25-39mL/min: Induction: 450mg qd. Maint/Prevention: 450mg every 2 days. CrCl 10-24mL/min: Induction: 450mg every 2 days. Maint/Prevention: 450mg 2X weekly. Elderly: Start at lower end of dosing range.
Pediatrics: Take with food. 4 Months-16 Yrs: Prevention of CMV Disease: Recommended qd dose starting within 10 days of transplantation until 100 days post-transplantation is based on BSA and CrCl derived from a modified Schwartz formula. Refer to PI for dose calculations.

HOW SUPPLIED: Sol: 50mg/mL [88mL deliverable volume]; Tab: 450mg

WARNINGS/PRECAUTIONS: Not for use in liver transplant patients. Safety and efficacy have not been established for prevention of CMV disease in solid organ transplants other than those indicated, prevention of CMV disease in pediatric solid organ transplant patients <4 months of age, or for treatment of congenital CMV disease. Severe leukopenia, neutropenia, pancytopenia, bone marrow aplasia, and aplastic anemia reported. Avoid if absolute neutrophil count (ANC) <500 cells/μL, platelet count <25,000/μL, or Hgb <8g/dL. Cytopenia may occur and may worsen with continued dosing; caution with preexisting cytopenias. May cause inhibition of spermatogenesis in men. May cause suppression of fertility in women. Women of childbearing potential should use effective contraception during and for at least 30 days following treatment. Men should practice barrier contraception during and for at least 90 days following treatment. Acute renal failure may occur in elderly and patients without adequate hydration; maintain adequate hydration in all patients. Caution in elderly and patients with renal impairment. Not recommended for adult patients on hemodialysis (CrCl <10mL/min). Do not substitute tab for ganciclovir caps on a one-to-one basis.

ADVERSE REACTIONS: Diarrhea, N/V, pyrexia, neutropenia, anemia, cough, HTN, constipation, upper respiratory tract infection, tremor, graft rejection, thrombocytopenia, granulocytopenia.

INTERACTIONS: May increase levels of mycophenolate mofetil metabolites (with renal impairment), zidovudine, and didanosine (monitor for toxicity). Probenecid (monitor for toxicity) and mycophenolate mofetil (with renal impairment) may increase levels. Zidovudine and didanosine may decrease levels. Caution with nephrotoxic drugs, myelosuppressive drugs, or irradiation.

PREGNANCY: Category C, not for use in nursing.

MECHANISM OF ACTION: Synthetic guanine derivative nucleoside analogue; inhibits viral DNA polymerase synthesis, resulting in inhibition of human CMV replication.

PHARMACOKINETICS: Absorption: (Tab) Ganciclovir: Absolute bioavailability (59.4%); C_{max}=5.61mcg/mL; T_{max}=1-3 hrs; AUC=29.1mcg•h/mL. **Distribution:** Ganciclovir: V_d=0.703L/kg (IV); plasma protein binding (1-2%). **Metabolism:** Intestinal wall, liver; valganciclovir (prodrug) hydrolyzed to ganciclovir. **Elimination:** Ganciclovir: Renal; $T_{1/2}$=4.08 hrs (Tab). Refer to PI for different parameters.

NURSING CONSIDERATIONS

Assessment: Assess for renal impairment, preexisting cytopenia, prior/current irradiation, hydration status, pregnancy/nursing status, and possible drug interactions. Obtain baseline ANC, platelet count, and Hgb.

Monitoring: Monitor for signs/symptoms of hematologic effects (eg, granulocytopenia, anemia, thrombocytopenia, cytopenia), infertility, renal dysfunction, and other adverse reactions. Monitor CBC with differential and platelet counts frequently. Perform ophthalmologic exams at a minimum of every 4-6 weeks during therapy.

Patient Counseling: Advise not to substitute tab for ganciclovir caps on a one-to-one basis. Instruct adults to use tabs, not the oral sol. Inform patients of major toxicities and possible need to adjust dose or d/c. Inform of possible lab abnormalities and the importance of close monitoring of blood counts during therapy. Advise of possible decreased fertility. Instruct women not to use during pregnancy/breastfeeding. Advise women of childbearing potential to use effective contraception during and for at least 30 days following treatment, and men to practice barrier contraception during and for at least 90 days following treatment. Advise that the therapy should be considered a potential carcinogen. Inform that therapy may impair physical/mental ability. Inform that the therapy is not a cure for CMV retinitis and patients may continue to experience progression during or following treatment; advise to have ophthalmologic follow-up exams every 4-6 weeks at minimum while being treated.

Administration: Oral route. Take with food; do not break or crush tabs. Refer to PI for preparation of oral sol. **Storage:** Tab/Dry Powder: 25°C (77°F); excursions permitted to 15-30°C (59-86°F). Constituted Sol: 2-8°C (36-46°F) for no longer than 49 days. Do not freeze.

VALIUM

CIV

diazepam (Roche Labs)

THERAPEUTIC CLASS: Benzodiazepine

INDICATIONS: Management of anxiety disorders or short-term relief of symptoms of anxiety. Symptomatic relief of acute agitation, tremor, impending/acute delirium tremens and hallucinosis in acute alcohol withdrawal. Adjunct therapy for relief of skeletal muscle spasm due to reflex spasm to local pathology (eg, muscle/joint inflammation, secondary to trauma), spasticity caused by upper motor neuron disorders (eg, cerebral palsy, paraplegia), athetosis, and stiff-man syndrome. Adjunct in convulsive disorders.

DOSAGE: *Adults:* Individualize dose. Anxiety Disorders/Anxiety Symptoms: 2-10mg bid-qid depending on severity of symptoms. Acute Alcohol Withdrawal: 10mg tid or qid for first 24 hrs. Titrate: Reduce to 5mg tid or qid PRN. Skeletal Muscle Spasm: 2-10mg tid or qid. Convulsive Disorders: 2-10mg bid-qid. Elderly/Debilitated: Initial: 2-2.5mg qd or bid. Titrate: May increase gradually PRN and as tolerated.
Pediatrics: ≥6 Months: Individualize dose. Initial: 1-2.5mg tid or qid. May increase gradually PRN and as tolerated.

HOW SUPPLIED: Tab: 2mg*, 5mg*, 10mg* *scored

CONTRAINDICATIONS: Acute narrow-angle glaucoma, myasthenia gravis, severe respiratory/hepatic insufficiency, sleep apnea syndrome, and in patients <6 months of age.

WARNINGS/PRECAUTIONS: Not recommended for the treatment of psychotic patients. May increase frequency and/or severity of grand mal seizures and may require an increase in the dose of standard anticonvulsant medication. Abrupt withdrawal may also temporarily increase frequency and/or severity of seizures. May increase risk of congenital malformations and other developmental abnormalities. Neonatal flaccidity, respiratory and feeding difficulties, and hypothermia reported in children born to mothers who have been receiving benzodiazepines late in pregnancy; may also be at some risk of withdrawal symptoms during the postnatal period. Consider use only when clinical situation warrants the risk to the fetus. Caution during labor and delivery; irregularities in fetal HR and hypotonia, poor sucking, hypothermia, and moderate respiratory depression may occur with high single doses. Caution in the severely depressed or with evidence of latent depression or anxiety associated with depression, or suicidal tendencies; protective measures may be necessary. Psychiatric and paradoxical reactions may occur more likely in children and the elderly; d/c if these occur. Lower dose is recommended with chronic respiratory insufficiency. Extreme caution with history of alcohol or drug abuse. In debilitated patients, limit dose to smallest effective amount; ataxia or oversedation may develop. Repeated use for a prolonged time may result in some loss of response. Neutropenia and jaundice reported; periodic CBC and LFTs are advisable during long-term therapy. Abuse and dependence reported. Caution during dose increases to avoid adverse effects.

ADVERSE REACTIONS: Drowsiness, fatigue, muscle weakness, ataxia, confusion, vertigo, constipation, blurred vision, dizziness, hypotension, stimulation, agitation, incontinence, skin reactions, hypersalivation.

INTERACTIONS: Mutually potentiates effects with phenothiazines, antipsychotics, anxiolytics/sedatives, hypnotics, anticonvulsants, narcotic analgesics, anesthetics, sedative antihistamines, narcotics, barbiturates, MAOIs, and other antidepressants. Concomitant use with alcohol is not recommended; enhances sedative effects. Slower rate of absorption with antacids. Concomitant use with compounds which inhibit certain hepatic enzymes (CYP3A and CYP2C19) (eg, cimetidine, ketoconazole, fluvoxamine, fluoxetine, omeprazole) may increase and prolong sedation. Decreased metabolic elimination of phenytoin reported.

PREGNANCY: Category D, not for use in nursing.

MECHANISM OF ACTION: Benzodiazepine; exerts anxiolytic, sedative, muscle-relaxant, anticonvulsant, and amnestic effects. Facilitates GABA, an inhibitory neurotransmitter in the CNS.

PHARMACOKINETICS: Absorption: T_{max}=1-1.5 hrs. **Distribution:** V_d=0.8-1.0L/kg; plasma protein binding (98%); crosses blood-brain/placental barrier, and appears in breast milk. **Metabolism:** Via N-demethylation and hydroxylation by CYP3A4 and CYP2C19 enzymes, glucuronidation; N-desmethyldiazepam, temazepam, oxazepam (active metabolites). **Elimination:** Urine; $T_{1/2}$=48 hrs, 100 hrs (N-desmethyldiazepam).

NURSING CONSIDERATIONS

Assessment: Assess for anxiety disorders/symptoms, acute alcohol withdrawal, skeletal muscle spasm, convulsive disorders, depression, and other conditions where treatment is contraindicated or cautioned. Assess for pregnancy/nursing status and possible drug interactions.

Monitoring: Monitor for hypersensitivity reactions, rebound or withdrawal symptoms, seizures, psychiatric and paradoxical reactions, and respiratory depression.

Patient Counseling: Advise to consult physician before increasing dose or abruptly d/c the drug. Advise against simultaneous ingestion of alcohol and other CNS depressants during therapy. Caution against engaging in hazardous occupations requiring complete mental alertness, such as operating machinery or driving a motor vehicle.

Administration: Oral route. **Storage:** 15-30°C (59-86°F).

VALTREX   RX
valacyclovir HCl (GlaxoSmithKline)

THERAPEUTIC CLASS: Nucleoside analogue

INDICATIONS: Treatment of herpes labialis (cold sores) in patients ≥12 yrs. Treatment of herpes zoster (shingles) in immunocompetent adults. Treatment of initial and recurrent episodes of genital herpes in immunocompetent adults, chronic suppressive therapy of recurrent episodes of genital herpes in immunocompetent and in HIV-1 infected adults, and reduction of transmission of genital herpes in immunocompetent adults. Treatment of chickenpox in immunocompetent patients 2-<18 yrs.

DOSAGE: *Adults:* Herpes Labialis: 2g q12h for 1 day. Start at earliest symptom of cold sore. Genital Herpes: Initial Episode: 1g bid for 10 days. Most effective when given within 48 hrs of the onset of signs/symptoms. Recurrent Episodes: 500mg bid for 3 days. Start at 1st sign/symptom of episode. Suppressive Therapy: Normal Immune Function: 1g qd. History of ≤9 Episodes/Yr: Alternative Dose: 500mg qd. HIV-1 and CD4 ≥100 cells/mm^3: 500mg bid. Reduction of Transmission: History of ≤9 Episodes/Yr: 500mg qd for the source partner. Herpes Zoster: 1g tid for 7 days. Start at the earliest sign/symptom of herpes zoster. Most effective when given within 48 hrs of the onset of rash. Renal Impairment: Refer to PI for dose modifications.
Pediatrics: Herpes Labialis: ≥12 Yrs: 2g q12h for 1 day. Start at earliest symptom of cold sore. Chickenpox: 2-<18 Yrs: 20mg/kg tid for 5 days. Max: 1g tid. Start at earliest sign/symptom.

HOW SUPPLIED: Tab: 500mg, 1g* *scored

WARNINGS/PRECAUTIONS: Thrombotic thrombocytopenic purpura/hemolytic uremic syndrome (TTP/HUS) in immunocompromised patients reported at doses of 8g qd; immediately d/c if signs/symptoms occur. Acute renal failure reported. Maintain adequate hydration. CNS adverse reactions (eg, agitation, hallucinations, confusion, delirium, seizures, encephalopathy) reported in patients with or without reduced renal function and in those with underlying renal disease who received higher than recommended doses for their level of renal function; d/c if these occur. Caution in elderly and with renal impairment.

ADVERSE REACTIONS: Headache, N/V, abdominal pain, dysmenorrhea, arthralgia, nasopharyngitis, fatigue, rash, upper respiratory tract infections, pyrexia, decreased neutrophil counts, diarrhea, elevated ALT/AST.

INTERACTIONS: Caution with potentially nephrotoxic drugs.

PREGNANCY: Category B, caution in nursing.

MECHANISM OF ACTION: Nucleoside analogue DNA polymerase inhibitor; rapidly converted to acyclovir, which stops replication of herpes viral DNA by competitive inhibition of viral DNA polymerase, incorporation into and termination of growing viral DNA chain, and inactivation of viral DNA polymerase.

PHARMACOKINETICS: Absorption: Rapid. Absolute bioavailability (54.5% acyclovir). Oral administration of variable doses resulted in different parameters. **Distribution:** Plasma protein binding (13.5-17.9%, 9-33% acyclovir); found in breast milk. **Metabolism:** Hepatic/Intestinal (1st pass) to acyclovir and L-valine. **Elimination:** Urine (46%), feces (47%); $T_{1/2}$=2.5-3.3 hrs.

NURSING CONSIDERATIONS

Assessment: Assess for hypersensitivity, immunocompromised state, renal impairment, hydration status, pregnancy/nursing status, and possible drug interactions.

Monitoring: Monitor for signs/symptoms of renal toxicity, TTP/HUS, CNS effects, and other adverse reactions.

Patient Counseling: Advise to maintain adequate hydration. Inform that drug is not a cure for cold sores or genital herpes. For patients with cold sores, instruct to initiate treatment at earliest symptom of a cold sore; inform that treatment should not exceed 1 day (2 doses) and that doses should be taken 12 hrs apart. For patients with genital herpes, instruct to avoid contact with lesions or sexual intercourse when lesions and/or symptoms are present to avoid infecting partner(s), and to use safe sex practice in combination with suppressive therapy. For patients with herpes zoster, advise to initiate treatment as soon as possible after diagnosis. For patients with chickenpox, advise to initiate treatment at the earliest sign/symptom.

Administration: Oral route. Use oral sus for pediatrics for whom a solid dosage form is not appropriate. Refer to PI for extemporaneous preparation of oral sus. **Storage:** 15-25°C (59-77°F).

VALTROPIN   RX
somatropin (LG Life)

THERAPEUTIC CLASS: Human growth hormone

INDICATIONS: Treatment of pediatric patients who have growth failure due to inadequate secretion of endogenous growth hormone. Treatment of growth failure associated with Turner syndrome in pediatric patients who have open epiphyses. Long-term replacement therapy in adults with growth hormone deficiency (GHD) of either adult or childhood onset etiology.

DOSAGE: *Adults:* Individualize dose. Initial: 0.33mg/day SQ 6 days a week. Dosage may be increased to individual patient requirement of 0.66mg/day after 4 weeks. Alternative Dosing: 0.2mg/day (Range: 0.15-0.3mg/day). May increase gradually every 1-2 months by 0.1-0.2mg/day based on individual patient requirements.
Pediatrics: Individualize dose. Divide weekly dose into equal amounts given either daily or 6 days a week by SQ injection. GHD: 0.17-0.3mg/kg of body weight/week. Turner Syndrome: Up to 0.375mg/kg of body weight/week.

HOW SUPPLIED: Inj: 5mg

CONTRAINDICATIONS: Pediatric patients with closed epiphyses. Active proliferative and severe non-proliferative diabetic retinopathy. Presence of active malignancy. Acute critical illness due to complications following open heart surgery, abdominal surgery, or multiple accidental trauma, or those with acute respiratory failure. Patients with Prader-Willi syndrome who are severely obese or have severe respiratory impairment.

WARNINGS/PRECAUTIONS: Known sensitivity to supplied diluent (metacresol). Caution in pediatric patients with Prader-Willi syndrome and who have 1 or more risk factors (severe obesity, history of upper airway obstruction or sleep apnea, or unidentified respiratory infection). May decrease insulin sensitivity. Patients with GHD secondary to intracranial lesion should be monitored closely for progression or recurrence of underlying disease process. Intracranial HTN reported. Monitor closely with diabetes mellitus, glucose intolerance, hypopituitarism. Funduscopic exam recommended at initiation and periodically during course of therapy. Monitor carefully for any malignant transformation of skin lesions.

ADVERSE REACTIONS: Headache, pyrexia, cough, respiratory tract infection, diarrhea, vomiting, pharyngitis.

V

INTERACTIONS: Growth-promoting effects may be inhibited by glucocorticoids. May alter clearance of compounds metabolized by CYP450 liver enzymes (eg, corticosteroids, sex steroids, anticonvulsants, cyclosporine); monitor closely. May need insulin adjustment.

PREGNANCY: Category B, caution in nursing.

MECHANISM OF ACTION: Human growth hormone; stimulates linear growth synthesis, metabolizes lipids, reduces body fat stores by increasing cellular protein, and increases plasma fatty acids.

PHARMACOKINETICS: Absorption: C_{max}=43.97ng/mL, T_{max}=4 hrs, AUC=369.9ng•hr/mL. **Metabolism:** Liver, kidneys (protein catabolism). **Elimination:** $T_{1/2}$=3.03 hrs.

NURSING CONSIDERATIONS

Assessment: Assess for hypersensitivity to benzyl alcohol, history of scoliosis, preexisting papilledema, hypothyroidism, diagnostic imaging (pituitary or intracranial tumor), hypopituitarism, possible drug interactions, and any other condition where treatment is contraindicated or cautioned. Obtain baseline funduscopic exam. Prader-Willi syndrome: Evaluate for signs of upper airway obstruction or sleep apnea before initiation. Turner syndrome: Evaluate for otitis media or other ear disorders, and cardiovascular (CV) disorders before initiation.

Monitoring: Monitor fasting blood glucose and thyroid function tests periodically, conduct fundoscopic exam periodically, and monitor weight control (Prader-Willi syndrome), signs/symptoms of malignant transformation of skin lesions, intracranial HTN, slipped capital femoral epiphysis (eg, onset of limp, hip or knee pain), hypersensitivity/allergic reactions, respiratory infections (Prader-Willi syndrome), otitis media or ear disorders, CV disorders, and progression of scoliosis.

Patient Counseling: Instruct thoroughly as to proper usage and disposal. Caution against any reuse of needles and syringes. Instruct to seek medical attention if signs/symptoms of slipped capital femoral epiphysis (eg, onset of limp, hip or knee pain), hypersensitivity/allergic reactions, respiratory infections (Prader-Willi syndrome), otitis media or CV disorders, or progression of scoliosis occur.

Administration: SQ route (thighs). **Storage:** Before reconstitution: 2-8°C (36-46°F). Do not freeze. After reconstitution: 2-8°C (36-46°F) for up to 21 days. Do not freeze.

VANCOCIN ORAL   RX
vancomycin HCl (ViroPharma)

THERAPEUTIC CLASS: Tricyclic glycopeptide antibiotic

INDICATIONS: Treatment of *Clostridium difficile*-associated diarrhea, and enterocolitis caused by *Staphylococcus aureus* (including methicillin-resistant strains).

DOSAGE: *Adults:* Diarrhea: 125mg qid for 10 days. Enterocolitis: 500mg-2g/day in 3 or 4 divided doses for 7-10 days.
Pediatrics: 40mg/kg/day in 3 or 4 divided doses for 7-10 days. Max: 2g/day.

HOW SUPPLIED: Cap: 125mg, 250mg

WARNINGS/PRECAUTIONS: For PO use only; not systemically absorbed. Potential for systemic absorption with multiple PO doses or in some patients with inflammatory disorders of the intestinal mucosa; monitoring of serum concentrations may be appropriate in some instances (eg, renal insufficiency and/or colitis). Nephrotoxicity reported; increased risk in patients >65 yrs. Ototoxicity reported; caution in patients with underlying hearing loss. Consider performing auditory function serial tests during use to minimize ototoxicity risk. May result in bacterial resistance with prolonged use or use in the absence of a proven/suspected bacterial infection or a prophylactic indication; take appropriate measures if superinfection develops. Caution in elderly.

ADVERSE REACTIONS: N/V, abdominal pain, hypokalemia, diarrhea, pyrexia, flatulence, urinary tract infection, headache, peripheral edema, back pain, fatigue, nephrotoxicity.

INTERACTIONS: Monitor serum concentrations with concomitant use of an aminoglycoside antibiotic. Increased risk of ototoxicity when used concurrently with other ototoxic agents (eg, aminoglycosides).

PREGNANCY: Category B, not for use in nursing.

MECHANISM OF ACTION: Tricyclic glycopeptide antibiotic; inhibits cell-wall biosynthesis. Also alters bacterial cell-membrane permeability and RNA synthesis.

PHARMACOKINETICS: Absorption: Poor. **Distribution:** (IV) Found in breast milk. **Elimination:** Urine, feces.

NURSING CONSIDERATIONS

Assessment: Assess for inflammatory disorders of the intestinal mucosa, renal insufficiency, colitis, hearing disturbances, hypersensitivity to the drug, pregnancy/nursing status, and possible drug interactions. Obtain cultures and perform susceptibility tests.

Monitoring: Monitor for signs/symptoms of nephrotoxicity, ototoxicity, superinfection, and other adverse reactions. Monitor serum concentrations when appropriate. Monitor renal function in patients >65 yrs.

Patient Counseling: Inform that drug treats only bacterial, not viral, infections. Instruct to take exactly ud; advise that skipping doses or not completing full course may decrease effectiveness and increase bacterial resistance.

Administration: Oral route. **Storage:** 59-86°F (15-30°C).

VANCOMYCIN HCI   RX
vancomycin HCl (Various)

THERAPEUTIC CLASS: Tricyclic glycopeptide antibiotic

INDICATIONS: Treatment of serious or severe infections caused by susceptible strains of methicillin-resistant (β-lactam-resistant) staphylococci. Indicated for penicillin-allergic patients who cannot receive or have failed to respond to other drugs, and for infections caused by vancomycin-susceptible organisms that are resistant to other antimicrobials. Initial therapy when methicillin-resistant staphylococci are suspected. Effective in the treatment of staphylococcal endocarditis, other infections due to staphylococci, including septicemia, bone infections, lower respiratory tract infections, and skin and skin-structure infections. Effective alone or in combination with an aminoglycoside for endocarditis caused by *Streptococcus viridans* or *S. bovis*. Effective only in combination with an aminoglycoside for endocarditis caused by enterococci (eg, *Enterococcus faecalis*). Effective for treatment of diphtheroid endocarditis. Successfully used in combination with either rifampin, an aminoglycoside, or both in early-onset prosthetic valve endocarditis caused by *Staphylococcus epidermidis* or diphtheroids. Parenteral form may be administered orally for treatment of antibiotic-associated pseudomembranous colitis produced by *Clostridium difficile* and for staphylococcal enterocolitis.

DOSAGE: *Adults:* Usual: 500mg IV q6h or 1g IV q12h. Administer at no more than 10mg/min or over at least 60 min, whichever is longer. Renal Impairment: Initial: Not <15mg/kg. Dosage per day in mg is about 15X the GFR in mL/min (refer to dosage table in PI). Elderly: Require greater dose reductions than expected. Functionally Anephric Patients: Initial: 15mg/kg, then 1.9mg/kg/24 hrs. Marked Renal Impairment: 250-1000mg once every several days. Anuria: 1000mg every 7-10 days. For PO Administration: 500-2000mg/day in 3-4 divided doses for 7-10 days. Max: 2000mg/day. May dilute in 1 oz. of water. May also be administered via NG tube.
Pediatrics: Usual: 10mg/kg IV q6h. Infants/Neonates: Initial: 15mg/kg, then 10mg/kg q12h for neonates in 1st week of life and q8h thereafter until 1 month of age. Administer over at least 60 min. Renal Impairment: Initial: Not <15mg/kg. Dosage per day in mg is about 15X the GFR in mL/min (refer to table in PI). Premature Infants: Require longer dosing intervals. ADD-Vantage vials should not be used in neonates, infants, and children who require doses <500mg. For PO Administration: 40mg/kg/day in 3-4 divided doses for 7-10 days. Max: 2000mg/day. May dilute in 1 oz. of water. May also be administered via NG tube.

HOW SUPPLIED: Inj: 500mg, 1g

WARNINGS/PRECAUTIONS: Oral route not effective for other types of infections. Rapid bolus administration may cause hypotension and cardiac arrest (rare); administer in diluted sol over a period not <60 min. Ototoxicity reported; caution with underlying hearing loss. Caution with renal insufficiency and adjust dose with renal dysfunction. Pseudomembranous colitis reported. May result in bacterial resistance with prolonged use or use in the absence of a proven/suspected bacterial infection or a prophylactic indication; take appropriate measures if superinfection develops. Reversible neutropenia reported; monitor leukocyte count periodically. Administer via IV route. Thrombophlebitis may occur; infuse slowly and rotate inj sites. Safety and efficacy of administration via the intraperitoneal and intrathecal (intralumbar and intraventricular) routes have not been established. Administration via intraperitoneal route during continuous ambulatory peritoneal dialysis has resulted in a syndrome of chemical peritonitis. Caution in elderly.

ADVERSE REACTIONS: Infusion-related events, hypotension, wheezing, pruritus, chest and back muscle spasm or pain, dyspnea, urticaria, nephrotoxicity, pseudomembranous colitis, ototoxicity, neutropenia, phlebitis.

INTERACTIONS: Concomitant use of anesthetic agents associated with erythema, histamine-like flushing, and anaphylactoid reactions. Concurrent and/or sequential systemic or topical use of other potentially neurotoxic and/or nephrotoxic drugs (eg, amphotericin B, aminoglycosides, bacitracin, polymyxin B, colistin, viomycin, cisplatin) requires careful monitoring. Increased risk of ototoxicity with concomitant ototoxic agents (eg, aminoglycoside). Periodic leukocyte count monitoring with drugs that may cause neutropenia. Serial monitoring of renal function and

V

particular care following appropriate dosing to minimize risk of nephrotoxicity with concomitant aminoglycoside.

PREGNANCY: Category C, not for use in nursing.

MECHANISM OF ACTION: Tricyclic glycopeptide antibiotic; inhibits cell-wall biosynthesis, alters bacterial cell membrane permeability and RNA synthesis.

PHARMACOKINETICS: Absorption: (1g at 2 hrs) C_{max}=23mcg/mL; (500mg at 2 hrs) C_{max}=19mcg/mL. **Distribution:** Serum protein binding (55%). **Elimination:** Urine (75%); $T_{1/2}$=4-6 hrs.

NURSING CONSIDERATIONS

Assessment: Assess for renal function, underlying hearing loss, pregnancy/nursing status and possible drug interactions. Perform culture and susceptibility testing.

Monitoring: Monitor for hypersensitivity reactions (eg, Stevens-Johnson syndrome, vasculitis), infusion reactions (eg, hypotension, arrhythmias, "red neck"), thrombophlebitis, ototoxicity, renal function, diarrhea, pseudomembranous colitis, neutropenia, superinfection, and chemical perito-nitis (intraperitoneal route). Monitor leukocyte count periodically.

Patient Counseling: Inform that drug treats bacterial, not viral, infections. Instruct to take ud; skipping doses or not completing full course may decrease effectiveness and increase bacterial resistance. Warn that patient may experience diarrhea; instruct to notify physician if watery/bloody stools, hypersensitivity reactions, or superinfection develops.

Administration: IV, Oral route. Refer to PI for preparation for IV use. Intermittent infusion recom-mended. Physically incompatible with β-lactam antibiotics. Diluted sol may be given via NGT. (PO) Common flavoring syrup may be added to improve taste. **Storage:** 20-25°C (68-77°F). After reconstitution: may refrigerate for 14 days. After further dilution: may refrigerate for 14 days or 96 hrs, depending on diluent used (refer to PI).

Vanos   RX
fluocinonide (Medicis)

THERAPEUTIC CLASS: Corticosteroid

INDICATIONS: Relief of the inflammatory and pruritic manifestations of corticosteroid-respon-sive dermatoses in patients ≥12 yrs of age.

DOSAGE: *Adults:* Limit treatment to 2 consecutive weeks. Psoriasis/Corticosteroid-Responsive Dermatoses: Apply a thin layer to affected skin area(s) qd or bid ud. Atopic Dermatitis: Apply a thin layer to affected skin area(s) qd ud. Max: 60g/week. D/C therapy when control is achieved. Reassess diagnosis if no improvement is seen within 2 weeks.
Pediatrics: ≥12 Yrs: Limit treatment to 2 consecutive weeks. Psoriasis/Corticosteroid-Responsive Dermatoses: Apply a thin layer to affected skin area(s) qd or bid ud. Atopic Dermatitis: Apply a thin layer to affected skin area(s) qd ud. Max: 60g/week. D/C therapy when control is achieved. Reassess diagnosis if no improvement is seen within 2 weeks.

HOW SUPPLIED: Cre: 0.1% [30g, 60g, 120g]

WARNINGS/PRECAUTIONS: For dermatologic use only; not for ophthalmic, oral, or intravagi-nal use. Not for use in rosacea or perioral dermatitis. Do not apply on the face, groin, or axillae. Systemic absorption may produce reversible hypothalamic-pituitary-adrenal (HPA) axis suppres-sion with the potential for glucocorticosteroid insufficiency, Cushing's syndrome, hyperglycemia, and unmasking of latent diabetes mellitus (DM). Periodically evaluate for HPA-axis suppression and if noted, gradually withdraw treatment, reduce frequency of application, or substitute a less potent steroid. Factors predisposing to HPA-axis suppression include use of more potent steroids, use over large surface areas, prolonged use, use under occlusion, use on an altered skin barrier, and use in patients with liver failure. May suppress immune system if used for >2 weeks. Manifestations of adrenal insufficiency may require supplemental systemic corticosteroids. Pediatric patients may be more susceptible to systemic toxicity. Local adverse reactions may be more likely to occur with occlusive use, prolonged use or use of higher potency corticosteroids. Use appropriate antifungal or antibacterial agent if concomitant skin infections are present or develop; if a favorable response does not occur promptly, d/c until infection is controlled. D/C and institute appropriate therapy if irritation develops. Allergic contact dermatitis may occur; confirm by patch testing.

ADVERSE REACTIONS: Headache, application-site burning, nasopharyngitis, nasal congestion.

INTERACTIONS: Use of >1 corticosteroid-containing product at the same time may increase total systemic absorption.

PREGNANCY: Category C, not for use in nursing.

MECHANISM OF ACTION: Corticosteroid; has not been established. Possesses anti-inflammatory and antipruritic actions. Plays a role in cellular signaling, immune function, inflammation, and protein regulation.

PHARMACOKINETICS: Absorption: Percutaneous; extent of absorption is determined by vehicle and integrity of epidermal barrier. **Distribution:** Found in breast milk (systemically administered).

NURSING CONSIDERATIONS

Assessment: Assess for hypersensitivity to the drug, rosacea, perioral dermatitis, skin infections, liver impairment, pregnancy/nursing status, and possible drug interactions.

Monitoring: Monitor for signs/symptoms of HPA-axis suppression, Cushing's syndrome, hyperglycemia, unmasking of latent DM, skin irritation, and other adverse reactions. Monitor for systemic toxicity (eg, adrenal suppression, intracranial HTN) in pediatric patients. Following withdrawal of treatment, monitor for glucocorticosteroid insufficiency. Reassess diagnosis if no improvement is seen within 2 weeks.

Patient Counseling: Instruct to use externally and ud. Advise not to use for any disorder other than for which it was prescribed. Instruct to avoid contact with eyes and not to use on face, groin, and underarms. Instruct not to bandage, cover, or wrap treated skin, unless directed by physician. Counsel to report any signs of local adverse reactions. Advise that other corticosteroid-containing products should not be used without 1st consulting with the physician. Instruct to d/c use when control is achieved and to notify physician if no improvement seen within 2 weeks. Notify physician if contemplating surgery. Counsel to wash hands following application.

Administration: Topical route. **Storage:** 15-30°C (59-86°F).

VANTAS   RX
histrelin acetate (Endo)

THERAPEUTIC CLASS: Synthetic gonadotropin-releasing hormone analog

INDICATIONS: Palliative treatment of advanced prostate cancer.

DOSAGE: *Adults:* 1 implant SQ into the inner aspect of the upper arm for 12 months. Remove after 12 months and may replace with new implant to continue therapy.

HOW SUPPLIED: Implant: 50mg

CONTRAINDICATIONS: Women who are or may become pregnant.

WARNINGS/PRECAUTIONS: Causes a transient increase in serum concentrations of testosterone during the 1st week of treatment; may experience worsening of symptoms or onset of new symptoms (eg, bone pain, neuropathy, hematuria, ureteral or bladder outlet obstruction). Spinal cord compression and ureteral obstruction reported; closely observe patients with metastatic vertebral lesions and/or with urinary tract obstruction during the 1st few weeks of therapy. Difficulty in locating or removing implant may be experienced. Hyperglycemia and an increased risk of developing diabetes reported; monitor blood glucose and/or HbA1c periodically. Increased risk of developing myocardial infarction, sudden cardiac death, and stroke reported. Results of diagnostic tests of pituitary gonadotropic and gonadal functions conducted during and after therapy may be affected.

ADVERSE REACTIONS: Hot flashes, fatigue, implant-site reaction (bruising/pain/soreness/tenderness), testicular atrophy, renal impairment, gynecomastia, constipation, erectile dysfunction.

PREGNANCY: Category X, not for use in nursing.

MECHANISM OF ACTION: Synthetic gonadotropin-releasing hormone analog; acts as a potent inhibitor of gonadotropin secretion when given continuously in therapeutic doses. Desensitizes responsiveness of pituitary gonadotropin, causing reduction in testicular steroidogenesis.

PHARMACOKINETICS: Absorption: C_{max}=1.1ng/mL; T_{max}=12 hrs (median). **Distribution:** V_d=58.4L (SQ bolus). **Metabolism:** C-terminal dealkylation and hydrolysis. **Elimination:** $T_{1/2}$=3.92 hrs (SQ bolus).

NURSING CONSIDERATIONS

Assessment: Assess for hypersensitivity to the drug, metastatic vertebral lesions, urinary tract obstruction, and risk for diabetes and cardiovascular disease (CV).

Monitoring: Monitor for worsening of symptoms, onset of new symptoms, signs/symptoms of CV disease, and other adverse reactions. Monitor response by measuring serum concentrations of testosterone and prostate-specific antigen periodically, especially if the anticipated clinical or biochemical response to treatment has not been achieved. Monitor blood glucose and/or HbA1c periodically.

Patient Counseling: Inform of risks and benefits of therapy. Instruct to refrain from wetting the arm for 24 hrs and from heavy lifting or strenuous exertion of the inserted arm for 7 days after implant insertion. Instruct to contact physician if the implant was expelled from the body or if experiencing unusual bleeding, redness, or pain at insertion site.

Administration: SQ route. Refer to PI for recommended procedure for implant insertion and removal. **Storage:** Implant: 2-8°C (36-46°F); excursions permitted to 25°C (77°F) for 7 days. Keep in the original packaging until the day of insertion. Protect from light. Do not freeze. Implantation Kit: 20-25°C (68-77°F).

VARIVAX   RX
varicella virus vaccine live (Merck)

THERAPEUTIC CLASS: Vaccine

INDICATIONS: Active immunization for the prevention of varicella in individuals ≥12 months of age.

DOSAGE: *Adults:* 2 doses of 0.5mL SQ into the outer aspect of the upper arm (deltoid region) or the anterolateral thigh; administer with a minimum interval of 4 weeks between doses. *Pediatrics:* Inject into the outer aspect of the upper arm (deltoid region) or the anterolateral thigh. ≥13 Yrs: 2 doses of 0.5mL SQ; administer with a minimum interval of 4 weeks between doses. 12 Months-12 Yrs: 0.5mL SQ. If a 2nd dose is administered, there should be a minimum interval of 3 months between doses.

HOW SUPPLIED: Inj: 0.5mL

CONTRAINDICATIONS: History of anaphylactic or severe allergic reaction to neomycin and gelatin, immunosuppressed or immunodeficient individuals (eg, history of primary or acquired immunodeficiency states, leukemia, lymphoma or other malignant neoplasms affecting the bone marrow or lymphatic system, AIDS, or other clinical manifestations of infection with HIV), febrile illness, active untreated tuberculosis (TB), and pregnancy. Concomitant administration with immunosuppressive therapy (including immunosuppressive doses of corticosteroids).

WARNINGS/PRECAUTIONS: Do not administer IV or IM. Adequate treatment provisions, including epinephrine inj (1:1000), should be available for immediate use should anaphylaxis occur. Defer vaccination in patients with family history of congenital/hereditary immunodeficiency until immune status has been evaluated and found to be immunocompetent. The Advisory Committee for Immunization Practices has recommendations on the use of varicella vaccine in HIV-infected individuals. Transmission of vaccine virus may occur; vaccine recipients should attempt to avoid close association with susceptible high-risk individuals for up to 6 weeks following vaccination. May cause temporary depression of tuberculin skin sensitivity, leading to false negative results; perform tuberculin skin testing (with tuberculin purified protein derivative) before vaccination or on the same day, or at least 4 weeks following vaccination. Avoid pregnancy for 3 months following vaccination.

ADVERSE REACTIONS: Fever, inj-site complaints (eg, pain/soreness, swelling, erythema, rash, pruritus, hematoma, induration, stiffness, numbness), varicella-like rash.

INTERACTIONS: See Contraindications. Avoid use of salicylates (aspirin) or salicylate-containing products in patients 12 months-17 yrs of age for 6 weeks after vaccination; Reye's syndrome may occur. Defer vaccination for at least 5 months following blood/plasma transfusions, or administration of immune globulins. Do not give immune globulins for 2 months following vaccination.

PREGNANCY: Contraindicated in pregnancy, caution in nursing.

MECHANISM OF ACTION: Vaccine; induces both cell-mediated and humoral immune responses to varicella zoster virus.

NURSING CONSIDERATIONS

Assessment: Assess for previous hypersensitivity, health/immunity status, immunization history, active untreated TB, pregnancy/nursing status, possible drug interactions, and for any other conditions where treatment is contraindicated or cautioned.

Monitoring: Monitor for anaphylaxis, inj-site reactions, fever, and other adverse reactions.

Patient Counseling: Inform of potential benefits and risks of vaccination. Advise to report any adverse reactions to physician. Inform that the vaccine may not result in protection of all vaccinees. Instruct to avoid pregnancy for 3 months after vaccination. Due to the concern for transmission of vaccine virus, instruct vaccine recipients to attempt to avoid whenever possible close association with susceptible high-risk individuals for up to 6 weeks following vaccination.

Administration: SQ route. Inject into the outer aspect of the upper arm (deltoid region) or anterolateral thigh. Administer immediately after reconstitution; discard if not used within 30 min. Refer to PI for reconstitution instructions. **Storage:** -50°C to -15°C (-58°F to +5°F). Use of dry ice may subject to temperatures colder than -50°C (-58°F). May store at 2-8°C (36-46°F) for up to 72 continuous hrs prior to reconstitution; discard if not used. Protect from light. Diluent: 20-25°C (68-77°F), or in the refrigerator.

VASOTEC
enalapril maleate (Valeant)

> D/C if pregnancy is detected. Drugs that act directly on the renin-angiotensin system (RAS) can cause injury/death to the developing fetus.

THERAPEUTIC CLASS: ACE inhibitor

INDICATIONS: Treatment of HTN, alone or with other antihypertensive agents (eg, thiazide-type diuretics). Treatment of symptomatic congestive heart failure (CHF), usually in combination with diuretics and digitalis. To decrease the rate of development of overt heart failure (HF) and decrease incidence of hospitalization for HF in clinically stable asymptomatic patients with left ventricular dysfunction (ejection fraction ≤35%).

DOSAGE: *Adults:* HTN: If possible, d/c diuretic 2-3 days prior to therapy. Initial: 5mg qd; 2.5mg if with concomitant diuretic with careful monitoring for at least 2 hrs and until BP is stabilized for at least an additional hr. Titrate: Adjust dose according to BP response. Usual: 10-40mg/day given in single dose or 2 divided doses. May add diuretic if BP not controlled. Renal Impairment: Refer to PI for dose adjustment. HF: Initial: 2.5mg qd. Usual: 2.5-20mg bid. Titrate upward, as tolerated, over a few days/weeks. Max: 40mg/day in divided doses. Asymptomatic Left Ventricular Dysfunction: Initial: 2.5mg bid. Titrate: Increase as tolerated to 20mg/day (in divided doses). Hyponatremia or SrCr >1.6mg/dL with HF: Initial: 2.5mg/day. Titrate: May increase to 2.5mg bid, then 5mg bid and higher PRN, usually at intervals of 4 days or more. Max: 40mg/day. *Pediatrics:* 1 Month-16 Yrs: HTN: Initial: 0.08mg/kg (up to 5mg) qd. Titrate: Adjust according to BP response. Max: 0.58mg/kg (or 40mg/day).

HOW SUPPLIED: Tab: 2.5mg*, 5mg*, 10mg*, 20mg* *scored

CONTRAINDICATIONS: History of ACE inhibitor-associated angioedema and in patients with hereditary or idiopathic angioedema. Coadministration with aliskiren in patients with diabetes.

WARNINGS/PRECAUTIONS: Angioedema of the face, extremities, lips, tongue, glottis, and larynx reported; d/c and administer appropriate therapy if any of these occur. Higher incidence of angioedema reported in blacks than nonblacks. Intestinal angioedema reported; monitor for abdominal pain. Patients with history of angioedema unrelated to ACE inhibitor therapy may be at increased risk of angioedema during therapy. Anaphylactoid reactions reported during desensitization with hymenoptera venom, dialysis with high-flux membranes, and LDL apheresis with dextran sulfate absorption. Excessive hypotension sometimes associated with oliguria or azotemia and (rarely) acute renal failure or death may occur; monitor during first 2 weeks of therapy and whenever dose of the drug and/or diuretic is increased. Neutropenia or agranulocytosis and bone marrow depression may occur; monitor WBCs in patients with renal disease and collagen vascular disease. Associated with syndrome that starts with cholestatic jaundice and progresses to fulminant hepatic necrosis, and sometimes death; d/c if jaundice or marked elevations of hepatic enzymes develop. Caution with left ventricular outflow obstruction. May cause changes in renal function. Increases in BUN and SrCr reported with renal artery stenosis; monitor renal function during the 1st few weeks of therapy. Increases in BUN and SrCr reported. Hyperkalemia may occur; caution with diabetes mellitus (DM) and renal insufficiency. Persistent nonproductive cough reported. Hypotension may occur with major surgery or during anesthesia; may be corrected by volume expansion. Avoid in neonates and children with GFR <30mL/min/1.73m².

ADVERSE REACTIONS: Fatigue, headache, dizziness.

INTERACTIONS: See Contraindications. Dual blockade of the RAS is associated with increased risk of hypotension, hyperkalemia, and changes in renal function (including acute renal failure); closely monitor BP, renal function and electrolytes with concomitant agents that also affect the RAS. Avoid with aliskiren in patients with renal impairment (GFR <60mL/min). Hypotension risk and increased BUN and SrCr with diuretics. Coadministration with NSAIDs, including selective COX-2 inhibitors, may decrease antihypertensive effect of ACE inhibitors and may further deteriorate renal function. K⁺-sparing diuretics, K⁺-containing salt substitutes, or K⁺ supplements may increase serum K⁺ levels; use caution and monitor serum K⁺ frequently. Avoid K⁺-sparing agents in patients with HF. Antihypertensives that cause renin release (eg, diuretics) may augment antihypertensive effect. Lithium toxicity reported with lithium; monitor serum lithium levels frequently. Nitritoid reactions reported rarely with injectable gold (eg, sodium aurothiomalate).

PREGNANCY: Category D, not for use in nursing.

MECHANISM OF ACTION: ACE inhibitor; inhibition of ACE results in decreased plasma angiotensin II, which leads to decreased vasopressor activity and decreased aldosterone secretion.

PHARMACOKINETICS: **Absorption:** T_{max}=1 hr, 3-4 hrs (metabolite). **Distribution:** Crosses placenta; found in breast milk. **Metabolism:** Hydrolysis; enalaprilat (metabolite). **Elimination:** Urine and feces (94%); $T_{1/2}$=11 hrs (metabolite).

V

NURSING CONSIDERATIONS

Assessment: Assess for history of angioedema, hypersensitivity, volume/salt depletion, renal dysfunction/disease, collagen vascular disease, renal artery stenosis, ischemic heart disease, cerebrovascular disease, left ventricular outflow obstruction, DM, pregnancy/nursing status, and possible drug interactions.

Monitoring: Monitor for hypotension, anaphylactoid reaction, angioedema, hypersensitivity reactions, and other adverse reactions. Monitor BP, renal function, and serum K+ levels. Monitor WBC periodically in patients with collagen vascular disease and/or renal disease.

Patient Counseling: Inform of pregnancy risks and to notify physician if pregnant/plan to become pregnant as soon as possible; discuss treatment options in women planning to become pregnant. Instruct to d/c therapy and immediately report signs/symptoms of angioedema. Caution about lightheadedness, especially during the 1st few days of therapy and advise to report to physician. Instruct to d/c and consult physician if syncope occurs. Caution that excessive perspiration and dehydration may lead to excessive fall in BP; advise to consult with the physician. Advise not to use K+ supplements or salt substitutes containing K+ without consulting physician. Advise patient to report any indication of infection.

Administration: Oral route. Refer to PI for preparation of sus. **Storage:** 25°C (77°F); excursions permitted to 15-30°C (59-86°F). Protect from moisture.

Vectibix   RX
panitumumab (Amgen)

> Dermatologic toxicities and severe infusion reactions reported. Fatal infusion reactions occurred in postmarketing experience.

THERAPEUTIC CLASS: Monoclonal antibody/EGFR-blocker

INDICATIONS: As a single agent for the treatment of epidermal growth factor receptor (EGFR)-expressing, metastatic colorectal carcinoma (mCRC) with disease progression on or following fluoropyrimidine-, oxaliplatin-, and irinotecan-containing chemotherapy regimens.

DOSAGE: *Adults:* Usual: 6mg/kg IV infusion over 60 min every 14 days. Infuse doses >1000mg over 90 min. Dose Modifications for Infusion Reactions: Reduce infusion rate by 50% with mild or moderate (Grade 1 or 2) infusion reaction for duration of that infusion. Terminate infusion if experiencing severe infusion reactions. Permanently d/c depending on the severity and/or persistence of the reaction. Dose Modification for Dermatologic Toxicity: Withhold for dermatologic toxicities that are ≥Grade 3 or are considered intolerable. Permanently d/c if toxicity does not improve to ≤Grade 2 within 1 month. Resume at 50% of original dose if dermatologic toxicity improves to ≤Grade 2 and symptoms improve after withholding no more than 2 doses. Permanently d/c if toxicities recur. If toxicities do not recur, may increase subsequent doses by increments of 25% of original dose until 6mg/kg is reached.

HOW SUPPLIED: Inj: 20mg/mL [5mL, 10mL, 20mL]

WARNINGS/PRECAUTIONS: Not indicated for treatment with *KRAS* mutation-positive mCRC or for whom *KRAS* mCRC status is unknown. Not indicated in combination with oxaliplatin-based chemotherapy for the treatment of patients with RAS (*KRAS* or *NRAS*) mutation-positive mCRC or for whom RAS status is unknown. Monitor for dermatologic or soft tissue toxicities; withhold or d/c for dermatologic or soft tissue toxicity associated with severe or life-threatening inflammatory or infectious complications. Not indicated for use in combination with chemotherapy; increased incidence of toxicities and mortalities reported when used in combination with chemotherapy. Pulmonary fibrosis and cases of interstitial lung disease (ILD), including fatalities, reported; interrupt therapy for the acute onset or worsening of pulmonary symptoms, and d/c if ILD is confirmed. Hypomagnesemia and hypocalcemia reported; monitor electrolytes periodically during and for 8 weeks after completion of therapy and institute appropriate treatment PRN. Exposure to sunlight may exacerbate dermatologic toxicity. Keratitis and ulcerative keratitis reported; interrupt or d/c therapy if acute or worsening keratitis occurs. Perform EGFR protein expression assessment to identify patients eligible for treatment.

ADVERSE REACTIONS: Skin toxicities (eg, erythema, dermatitis acneiform, pruritus, exfoliation, paronychia, rash), infusion reactions, hypomagnesemia, fatigue, abdominal pain, N/V, diarrhea, constipation, cough.

PREGNANCY: Category C, not for use in nursing.

MECHANISM OF ACTION: IgG2 kappa monoclonal antibody; binds specifically to EGFR on both normal and tumor cells, and competitively inhibits binding of ligands for EGFR.

PHARMACOKINETICS: Absorption: C_{max}=213mcg/mL, AUC_{0-tau}=1306mcg•day/mL. **Elimination:** $T_{1/2}$=7.5 days.

NURSING CONSIDERATIONS

Assessment: Assess for EGFR protein expression, presence or history of interstitial pneumonitis or pulmonary fibrosis, pregnancy/nursing status, and for possible drug interactions. Obtain baseline electrolyte levels.

Monitoring: Monitor for signs/symptoms of dermatologic and soft tissue toxicities, infusion reactions, ILD, pulmonary fibrosis, keratitis, and other adverse reactions. Monitor electrolytes periodically during and for 8 weeks after completion of therapy.

Patient Counseling: Advise to contact physician if signs/symptoms of an infusion reaction, persistent/recurrent coughing, wheezing, dyspnea, new onset facial swelling, diarrhea, dehydration, or skin/ocular changes develop. Instruct to notify physician if pregnant or nursing. Advise of need for adequate contraception in both males and females during and for 6 months after last dose of therapy, and for the need for periodic monitoring of electrolytes. Instruct to limit sun exposure during and for 2 months after the last dose of therapy.

Administration: IV infusion; do not administer as IV push or bolus. Refer to PI for preparation and administration instructions. **Storage:** Vial: 2-8°C (36-46°F). Protect from direct sunlight. Do not freeze. Diluted: Use within 6 hrs if stored at room temperature or within 24 hrs if stored at 2-8°C (36-46°F). Do not freeze.

VECTICAL   RX
calcitriol (Galderma)

THERAPEUTIC CLASS: Vitamin D analog

INDICATIONS: Treatment of mild to moderate plaque psoriasis in adults ≥18 yrs.

DOSAGE: *Adults:* Apply to affected area(s) bid (am and pm). Max: 200g/week.

HOW SUPPLIED: Oint: 3mcg/g [5g, 100g]

WARNINGS/PRECAUTIONS: Not for PO, ophthalmic, or intravaginal use. Hypercalcemia reported; if aberrations in parameters of Ca^{2+} metabolism occur, d/c therapy until these parameters normalize. Increased absorption with occlusive use. Avoid excessive exposure of treated areas to natural or artificial sunlight (eg, tanning booths, sun lamps); avoid or limit phototherapy.

ADVERSE REACTIONS: Laboratory test abnormality, urine abnormality, psoriasis, hypercalciuria, pruritus, hypercalcemia, skin discomfort.

INTERACTIONS: Caution with medications known to increase serum Ca^{2+} level (eg, thiazide diuretics), Ca^{2+} supplements, or high doses of vitamin D.

PREGNANCY: Category C, caution in nursing.

MECHANISM OF ACTION: Vitamin D analog; mechanism of action in the treatment of psoriasis not established.

NURSING CONSIDERATIONS

Assessment: Assess for known/suspected Ca^{2+} metabolism disorder, pregnancy/nursing status, and possible drug interactions.

Monitoring: Monitor for hypercalcemia, aberrations in parameters of Ca^{2+} metabolism, and other adverse reactions.

Patient Counseling: Instruct to use ud. Instruct to apply only to areas of the skin affected by psoriasis; advise not to apply to the eyes, lips, or facial skin. Instruct to rub gently into the skin. Advise to notify their physician if adverse reactions occur. Advise to avoid excessive exposure of treated areas to sunlight, tanning booths, sun lamps, or other artificial sunlight and to inform physician about treatment if undergoing phototherapy.

Administration: Topical route. **Storage:** 25°C (77°F); excursions permitted to 15°-30°C (59°-86°F). Do not freeze or refrigerate.

V

VELTIN   RX
clindamycin phosphate - tretinoin (Stiefel)

THERAPEUTIC CLASS: Lincosamide derivative/retinoid

INDICATIONS: Topical treatment of acne vulgaris in patients ≥12 yrs of age.

DOSAGE: *Adults:* Apply pea-sized amount qpm. Gently rub the medication to lightly cover the entire affected area.
Pediatrics: ≥12 Yrs: Apply pea-sized amount qpm. Gently rub the medication to lightly cover the entire affected area.

HOW SUPPLIED: Gel: (Clindamycin-Tretinoin) 1.2%-0.025% [30g, 60g]

CONTRAINDICATIONS: Regional enteritis, ulcerative colitis, or history of antibiotic-associated colitis.

WARNINGS/PRECAUTIONS: Not for PO, ophthalmic, or intravaginal use. Avoid the eyes, lips, and mucous membranes. Avoid exposure to sunlight, including sunlamps. Avoid use if sunburn is present. Daily use of sunscreen products and protective apparel are recommended. Weather extremes (eg, wind, cold) may be irritating while under treatment. Clindamycin: Systemic absorption has been demonstrated following topical use. Diarrhea, bloody diarrhea, and colitis (including pseudomembranous colitis) reported; d/c if significant diarrhea occurs. Severe colitis reported following PO or parenteral administration with an onset of up to several weeks following cessation of therapy.

ADVERSE REACTIONS: Local-site reactions (eg, dryness, irritation, exfoliation, erythema).

INTERACTIONS: Avoid with erythromycin-containing products due to possible antagonism to clindamycin. May enhance action of neuromuscular-blocking agents; use with caution. Antiperistaltic agents (eg, opiates, diphenoxylate with atropine) may prolong and/or worsen severe colitis.

PREGNANCY: Category C, not for use in nursing.

MECHANISM OF ACTION: Clindamycin: Lincosamide antibiotic; binds to the 50S ribosomal subunit of susceptible bacteria and prevents elongation of peptide chains by interfering with peptidyl transfer, thereby suppressing protein synthesis. Found to have in vitro activity against *Propionibacterium acnes*. Tretinoin: Retinoid; not established; suspected to decrease the cohesiveness of follicular epithelial cells with decreased microcomedone formation. Also, stimulates mitotic activity and increased turnover of follicular epithelial cells causing extrusion of the comedones.

PHARMACOKINETICS: Absorption: Clindamycin: C_{max}=8.73ng/mL; T_{max}=4 hrs. **Distribution:** Clindamycin: Found in breast milk (orally and parenterally administered).

NURSING CONSIDERATIONS

Assessment: Assess for regional enteritis, ulcerative colitis or history of antibiotic-associated colitis, pregnancy/nursing status, and possible drug interactions. Assess use in patients whose occupations require considerable sun exposure.

Monitoring: Monitor for signs/symptoms of diarrhea, bloody diarrhea, colitis, local skin reactions, and other adverse reactions.

Patient Counseling: Instruct to wash face gently with mild soap and water at hs and apply a thin layer over the entire face (excluding the eyes and lips) after patting the skin dry. Advise not to use more than a pea-sized amount and not to apply more than qd (at hs). Advise to avoid exposure to sunlight, sunlamps, UV light, and other medicines that may increase sensitivity to sunlight; instruct to apply sunscreen qam and reapply over the course of the day PRN. Advise that other topical medications with a strong drying effect (eg, abrasive soaps, cleansers) may cause an increase in skin irritation. Inform that medication may cause irritation (eg, erythema, scaling, itching, burning, stinging). Instruct to d/c therapy and contact physician if severe diarrhea or GI discomfort occurs.

Administration: Topical route. **Storage:** 25°C (77°F); excursions permitted to 15-30°C (59-86°F). Protect from light, heat, and freezing.

VENTOLIN HFA   RX
albuterol sulfate (GlaxoSmithKline)

THERAPEUTIC CLASS: Beta$_2$-agonist

INDICATIONS: Treatment or prevention of bronchospasm with reversible obstructive airway disease and prevention of exercise-induced bronchospasm (EIB) in patients ≥4 yrs.

DOSAGE: *Adults:* Treatment/Prevention of Bronchospasm: 2 inh q4-6h or 1 inh q4h. EIB: 2 inh 15-30 min before exercise. Elderly: Start at lower end of dosing range.
Pediatrics: ≥4 Yrs: Treatment/Prevention of Bronchospasm: 2 inh q4-6h or 1 inh q4h. EIB: 2 inh 15-30 min before exercise.

HOW SUPPLIED: MDI: 90mcg/inh [8g, 18g]

WARNINGS/PRECAUTIONS: D/C if paradoxical bronchospasm or cardiovascular (CV) effects occur. More doses than usual may be a marker of destabilization of asthma and may require re-evaluation of the patient and treatment regimen; give special consideration to the possible need for anti-inflammatory treatment (eg, corticosteroids). ECG changes and immediate hypersensitivity reactions may occur. Fatalities reported with excessive use. Caution with CV disorders (eg, coronary insufficiency, arrhythmias, HTN), convulsive disorders, hyperthyroidism, diabetes mellitus (DM), and in patients unusually responsive to sympathomimetic amines. May cause significant hypokalemia. Caution in elderly.

ADVERSE REACTIONS: Throat irritation, viral respiratory infections, upper respiratory inflammation, cough, musculoskeletal pain.

INTERACTIONS: Avoid with other short-acting sympathomimetic aerosol bronchodilators; caution with additional adrenergic drugs administered by any route. Use with β-blockers may block pulmonary effects and produce severe bronchospasm in asthmatic patients; avoid concomitant use. If needed, consider cardioselective β-blockers and use with caution. ECG changes and/or hypokalemia caused by non-K^+-sparing diuretics (eg, loop, thiazide diuretics) may be worsened. May decrease serum digoxin levels. Use extreme caution with MAOIs and TCAs, or within 2 weeks of discontinuation of such agents; consider alternative therapy if taking MAOIs or TCAs.

PREGNANCY: Category C, not for use in nursing.

MECHANISM OF ACTION: $β_2$-agonist; activates $β_2$-adrenergic receptors on airway smooth muscle, leading to the activation of adenylcyclase and to an increase in the intracellular cAMP. Increased cAMP leads to the activation of protein kinase A, which inhibits the phosphorylation of myosin and lowers intracellular ionic Ca^{2+} concentrations, resulting in relaxation of the smooth muscles of all airways, from the trachea to the terminal bronchioles.

PHARMACOKINETICS: Absorption: C_{max}=3ng/mL (higher dose); T_{max}=0.42 hrs. **Elimination:** $T_{1/2}$=4.6 hrs.

NURSING CONSIDERATIONS

Assessment: Assess for history of hypersensitivity to the drug, CV disorders, convulsive disorders, hyperthyroidism, DM, pregnancy/nursing status, and possible drug interactions. Assess use in patients unusually responsive to sympathomimetic amines.

Monitoring: Monitor for paradoxical bronchospasm, deterioration of asthma, CV effects, ECG changes, hypokalemia, immediate hypersensitivity reactions, and other adverse effects. Monitor BP, HR, and blood glucose levels.

Patient Counseling: Counsel not to increase dose/frequency of doses without consulting physician. Advise to seek immediate medical attention if treatment becomes less effective for symptomatic relief, symptoms become worse, and/or there is a need to use the product more frequently than usual. Instruct on how to properly prime, clean, and use inhaler. Instruct to take concurrent inhaled drugs and asthma medications only ud by the physician. Inform of the common adverse effects of treatment. Advise to notify physician if pregnant/nursing. Instruct to avoid spraying in eyes.

Administration: Oral inhalation route. Shake well before each spray. Before using for 1st time, if inhaler has not been used for >2 weeks, or if it has been dropped, prime inhaler by releasing 4 sprays into air, away from face. Refer to PI for further administration instruction. **Storage:** 15-25°C (59-77°F). Store with mouthpiece down. Do not puncture or store near heat or open flame.

VERAMYST RX

fluticasone furoate (GlaxoSmithKline)

THERAPEUTIC CLASS: Corticosteroid

INDICATIONS: Treatment of the symptoms of seasonal and perennial allergic rhinitis in patients ≥2 yrs.

DOSAGE: *Adults:* Initial: 2 sprays/nostril qd. Titrate to minimum effective dose. Maint: 1 spray/nostril qd. Elderly: Start at lower end of dosing range.
Pediatrics: ≥12 Yrs: Initial: 2 sprays/nostril qd. Titrate to minimum effective dose. Maint: 1 spray/nostril qd. 2-11 Yrs: Initial: 1 spray/nostril qd. Titrate: May increase to 2 sprays/nostril qd if inadequate, then return to initial dose when symptoms are controlled.

HOW SUPPLIED: Spray: 27.5mcg/spray [10g]

WARNINGS/PRECAUTIONS: May cause local nasal effects (eg, epistaxis, nasal ulceration, *Candida* infections, nasal septum perforation, impaired wound healing). Avoid with recent nasal ulcers, surgery, or trauma until healing has occurred. Glaucoma and/or cataracts may develop; monitor closely in patients with change in vision, history of increased intraocular pressure (IOP), glaucoma, and/or cataracts. D/C if hypersensitivity reactions occur. May increase susceptibility to infections; caution with active or quiescent tuberculosis (TB), untreated fungal or bacterial infections, systemic viral or parasitic infections, or ocular herpes simplex. Avoid exposure to chickenpox and measles. D/C slowly if hypercorticism and adrenal suppression occur. Risk of adrenal insufficiency and withdrawal symptoms when replacing systemic corticosteroids with topical corticosteroids. May reduce growth velocity in pediatric patients. Caution with severe hepatic impairment and elderly patients.

ADVERSE REACTIONS: Headache, epistaxis, pharyngolaryngeal pain, nasal ulceration, back pain, pyrexia, cough.

INTERACTIONS: Increased exposure with ritonavir; avoid coadmistration. Reduced cortisol levels with ketoconazole; caution with ketoconazole or other potent CYP3A4 inhibitors.

V

PREGNANCY: Category C, caution in nursing.

MECHANISM OF ACTION: Corticosteroid; not established. Shown to have a wide range of actions on multiple cell types (eg, mast cells, eosinophils, neutrophils, macrophages, lymphocytes) and mediators (eg, histamine, eicosanoids, leukotrienes, cytokines) involved in inflammation.

PHARMACOKINETICS: Absorption: Incomplete; (2640mcg/day) absolute bioavailability (0.5%). **Distribution:** (IV) V_d=608L; plasma protein binding (>99%). **Metabolism:** Hepatic via CYP3A4; hydrolysis. **Elimination:** Feces, urine; (IV) $T_{1/2}$=15.1 hrs.

NURSING CONSIDERATIONS

Assessment: Assess for drug hypersensitivity, patients who have not been immunized or exposed to infections (eg, measles, chickenpox), active or quiescent TB, untreated fungal/bacterial infection, systemic viral/parasitic infection, ocular herpes simplex, history of increased IOP, glaucoma or cataracts, recent nasal ulcers/surgery/trauma, hepatic impairment, pregnancy/nursing status, and possible drug interactions.

Monitoring: Monitor for acute adrenal insufficiency and withdrawal symptoms when replacing systemic corticosteroid with topical corticosteroid. Monitor for hypercorticism, chickenpox, measles, epistaxis, nasal ulceration, nasal septal perforation, hypoadrenalism (in infants born to a mother who received corticosteroids during pregnancy), suppression of growth velocity in children, vision changes, glaucoma, cataracts, increased IOP, and hypersensitivity reactions. Examine periodically for evidence of nasal *Candida* infections.

Patient Counseling: Inform of possible local nasal effects, cataracts, glaucoma, immunosuppression, and hypersensitivity reactions. Advise not to use with recent nasal ulcers, surgery, or trauma until healing has occurred. Instruct to d/c if hypersensitivity reaction occurs. Instruct to avoid exposure to chickenpox and measles. Instruct to consult physician if symptoms do not improve, the condition worsens, or change in vision occurs. Inform that growth in children may be slowed; counsel to regularly check patient's growth. Advise to avoid spraying into eyes.

Administration: Intranasal route. Prime pump before 1st time use, if not used >30 days, or cap left off ≥5 days. Shake well before each use. **Storage:** 15-30°C (59-86°F). Store device in upright position with cap in place. Do not freeze or refrigerate. Discard after 120 sprays have been used.

VERDESO   RX
desonide (Aqua)

THERAPEUTIC CLASS: Corticosteroid

INDICATIONS: Treatment of mild to moderate atopic dermatitis in patients ≥3 months of age.

DOSAGE: *Adults:* Apply thin layer to affected area(s) bid. Dispense smallest amount necessary to adequately cover affected area(s). D/C when control is achieved. Max Duration: 4 consecutive weeks. Reassess if no improvement after 4 weeks. Do not use with occlusive dressings. *Pediatrics:* ≥3 Months: Apply thin layer to affected area(s) bid. Dispense smallest amount necessary to adequately cover affected area(s). D/C when control is achieved. Max Duration: 4 consecutive weeks. Reassess if no improvement after 4 weeks. Do not use with occlusive dressings.

HOW SUPPLIED: Foam: 0.05% [100g]

WARNINGS/PRECAUTIONS: May result in systemic absorption and effects, including hypothalamic-pituitary-adrenal (HPA) axis suppression, manifestations of Cushing's syndrome, hyperglycemia, facial swelling, glycosuria, withdrawal syndrome, and growth retardation in children. May suppress immune system if used for >4 weeks. Application over large surface areas, prolonged use, or addition of occlusive dressing may augment systemic absorption. Periodic evaluation of HPA-axis suppression may be required; gradually withdraw, reduce frequency, or substitute a less potent steroid if HPA-axis suppression is noted. Pediatric patients may be more susceptible to systemic toxicity. May cause local skin adverse reactions. D/C and institute appropriate therapy if irritation develops. Institute an appropriate antifungal, antibacterial, or antiviral agent if concomitant skin infections are present or develop; if no prompt favorable response, may need to d/c until infection is controlled. Flammable; avoid fire, flame, and/or smoking during and immediately following application. Cosyntropin (adrenocorticotropic hormone$_{1-24}$) stimulation test may be helpful in evaluating for HPA-axis suppression. Avoid contact with eyes or other mucous membranes. If used during lactation, do not apply on the chest to avoid accidental ingestion by infant. Caution in elderly. Not for oral, ophthalmic, or intravaginal use.

ADVERSE REACTIONS: Upper respiratory tract infection, cough, application-site burning.

INTERACTIONS: Caution with concomitant topical corticosteroids; may produce cumulative effect.

PREGNANCY: Category C, caution in nursing.

MECHANISM OF ACTION: Corticosteroid; has not been established. Plays a role in cellular signaling, immune function, inflammation, and protein regulation.

PHARMACOKINETICS: Absorption: Percutaneous; extent of absorption is determined by product formulation, integrity of the epidermal barrier, and age. **Distribution:** Found in breast milk (systemically administered). **Metabolism:** Liver. **Elimination:** Kidneys, bile.

NURSING CONSIDERATIONS

Assessment: Assess for skin infections, pregnancy/nursing status, and for possible drug interactions.

Monitoring: Monitor for signs/symptoms of HPA-axis suppression, Cushing's syndrome, hyperglycemia, facial swelling, glycosuria, withdrawal syndrome, growth retardation, delayed weight gain, and intracranial HTN in children. Monitor for irritation, concomitant skin infections, and other adverse reactions. Perform periodic monitoring of HPA-axis suppression if medication is used over large BSA, used with occlusive dressing, or with prolonged use of drug. Reassess diagnosis if no improvement is seen within 4 weeks.

Patient Counseling: Instruct to use externally and ud. Advise not to use for any disorder other than that for which it was prescribed. Instruct to avoid contact with eyes or other mucous membranes. Instruct to not bandage, cover, or wrap treated skin area so as to be occlusive unless directed. Counsel to report any signs of local or systemic adverse reactions. Instruct to inform physician about the treatment if surgery is contemplated. Advise to d/c therapy when control is achieved; instruct to contact physician if no improvement seen within 4 weeks. Instruct not to use other corticosteroid-containing products while on medication without consulting the physician. Inform that medication is flammable; avoid fire, flame, or smoking during and immediately after application.

Administration: Topical route. Shake can before use. Dispense foam by inverting the can. In treating areas of the face, dispense foam in hands and gently massage into affected areas until medication disappears; for areas other than the face, foam may be dispensed directly. **Storage:** 20-25°C (68-77°F); excursions permitted between 15-30°C (59-86°F). Do not puncture or incinerate. Do not expose containers to heat, and/or store at temperatures above 49°C (120°F).

VERELAN RX
verapamil HCl (UCB)

THERAPEUTIC CLASS: Calcium channel blocker (nondihydropyridine)

INDICATIONS: Management of essential HTN.

DOSAGE: *Adults:* Individualize dose. Usual: 240mg qam. Elderly/Small People: Initial: 120mg qam. Titrate: If inadequate response with 120mg, increase to 180mg qam, then 240mg qam, then 360mg qam, then 480mg qam based on therapeutic efficacy and safety evaluated approximately 24 hrs after dosing. Switching from Immediate-Release Verapamil: Use same total daily dose. May sprinkle on applesauce. Swallow whole; do not crush or chew.

HOW SUPPLIED: Cap, Sustained-Release: 120mg, 180mg, 240mg, 360mg

CONTRAINDICATIONS: Severe left ventricular dysfunction, hypotension (systolic blood pressure <90mmHg), cardiogenic shock, sick sinus syndrome, 2nd/3rd-degree atrioventricular (AV) block (except in patients with a functioning ventricular pacemaker), atrial fibrillation (A-fib)/atrial flutter (A-flutter), and an accessory bypass tract (eg, Wolff-Parkinson-White, Lown-Ganong-Levine syndromes).

WARNINGS/PRECAUTIONS: May cause congestive heart failure (CHF), pulmonary edema, hypotension, asymptomatic 1st-degree AV block, transient bradycardia, and PR interval prolongation. Marked 1st-degree block or progressive development to 2nd/3rd-degree AV block requires dose reduction, or d/c and institution of appropriate therapy. Elevated transaminases with and without concomitant elevation in alkaline phosphatase and bilirubin reported; monitor LFTs periodically. Hepatocellular injury reported. Ventricular response/fibrillation has occurred in patients with paroxysmal and/or chronic A-fib/flutter and a coexisting accessory AV pathway. Sinus bradycardia, pulmonary edema, severe hypotension, 2nd-degree AV block, and sinus arrest reported in patients with hypertrophic cardiomyopathy. Caution with hepatic/renal impairment; monitor for abnormal PR interval prolongation. May decrease neuromuscular transmission in patients with Duchenne's muscular dystrophy and may cause worsening of myasthenia gravis; decrease dose with attenuated neuromuscular transmission.

ADVERSE REACTIONS: Constipation, dizziness, headache, lethargy.

INTERACTIONS: May increase levels with CYP3A4 inhibitors (eg, erythromycin, ritonavir) and grapefruit juice. May decrease levels with CYP3A4 inducers (eg, rifampin). Hypotension and bradyarrhythmias reported with telithromycin. May cause myopathy/rhabdomyolysis with HMG-CoA reductase inhibitors that are CYP3A4 substrates; limit dose of simvastatin to 10mg/day or lovastatin to 40mg/day, and may need to lower doses of other CYP3A4 substrates (eg, atorvastatin). Additive negative effects on HR, AV conduction, and contractility with β-blockers; avoid with ventricular dysfunction. Asymptomatic bradycardia with atrial pacemaker has been

V

observed with concomitant use of timolol eye drops. Decreased metoprolol clearance reported. Sinus bradycardia resulting in hospitalization and pacemaker insertion has been reported with the use of clonidine; monitor HR. Chronic treatment may increase digoxin levels, which may result in digitalis toxicity. Additive effects with other antihypertensives (eg, vasodilators, ACE inhibitors, diuretics). Excessive reduction in BP with agents that attenuate α-adrenergic function (eg, prazosin). Avoid disopyramide within 48 hrs before or 24 hrs after verapamil. Additive negative inotropic effects and AV conduction prolongation with flecainide. Avoid quinidine with hypertrophic cardiomyopathy. May increase carbamazepine, cyclosporine, and alcohol effects. Increased bleeding time with aspirin. Cimetidine may either reduce or not change clearance. May increase sensitivity to neurotoxic effects of lithium; monitor lithium levels. Rifampin may reduce oral bioavailability. May increase clearance with phenobarbital. Caution with inhalation anesthetics. May potentiate neuromuscular blockers; both agents may need dose reduction.

PREGNANCY: Category C; not for use in nursing.

MECHANISM OF ACTION: Ca^{2+} ion influx inhibitor (nondihydropyridine); inhibits transmembrane influx of ionic Ca^{2+} into arterial smooth muscle as well as in conductile and contractile myocardial cells.

PHARMACOKINETICS: Absorption: Administration of variable doses resulted in different pharmacokinetic parameters. T_{max}=7-9 hrs. (Immediate-release) Absolute bioavailability (20-35%) **Distribution:** Plasma protein binding (90%); crosses placenta; found in breast milk. **Metabolism:** Liver (extensive), norverapamil (metabolite). **Elimination:** Urine (70%, metabolites; 3-4%, unchanged), feces (≥16%, metabolite); $T_{1/2}$=12 hrs.

NURSING CONSIDERATIONS

Assessment: Assess for ventricular dysfunction, cardiac failure symptoms, cardiogenic shock, sick sinus syndrome, hypertrophic cardiomyopathy, Duchenne's muscular dystrophy, attenuated neuromuscular transmission, and/or any conditions where treatment is contraindicated or cautioned. Assess for pregnancy/nursing status and possible drug interactions.

Monitoring: Monitor signs/symptoms of hypotension, CHF, heart block, ventricular fibrillation, renal/hepatic dysfunction, abnormal prolongation of PR interval and hypersensitivity reactions, and other adverse reactions. Periodically monitor LFTs, BP, ECG changes, and HR.

Patient Counseling: Instruct to swallow cap whole; do not crush or chew. Advise that the entire contents of the cap can be sprinkled onto a spoonful of applesauce; instruct to swallow the applesauce immediately without chewing, and follow with a glass of cool water. Caution that the applesauce should not be hot and should be soft enough to be swallowed without chewing. Instruct to consume the mixture immediately and not store for future use; contents should not be subdivided. Advise to seek medical attention if any adverse reactions occur. Counsel not to breastfeed and to report immediately if pregnant.

Administration: Oral route. **Storage:** 20-25°C (68-77°F). Avoid excessive heat. Brief digressions above 25°C, while not detrimental, should be avoided. Protect from moisture.

VERELAN PM   RX
verapamil HCl (UCB)

THERAPEUTIC CLASS: Calcium channel blocker (nondihydropyridine)

INDICATIONS: Management of essential HTN.

DOSAGE: *Adults:* Individualize dose. Usual: 200mg qhs. Renal or Hepatic Dysfunction/Elderly/Low-Weight Patients: Initial: 100mg qhs. If Inadequate Response with 200mg: May titrate upward to 300mg qhs, then 400mg qhs. Upward titration should be based on the therapeutic efficacy and safety evaluated approximately 24 hrs after dosing. May sprinkle on applesauce. Swallow whole; do not crush or chew.

HOW SUPPLIED: Cap, Extended-Release: 100mg, 200mg, 300mg

CONTRAINDICATIONS: Severe left ventricular dysfunction, hypotension (systolic BP <90mmHg), cardiogenic shock, sick sinus syndrome or 2nd/3rd-degree atrioventricular (AV) block (except in patients with a functioning ventricular artificial pacemaker), atrial fibrillation (A-fib)/atrial flutter (A-flutter), and an accessory bypass tract (eg, Wolff-Parkinson-White, Lown-Ganong-Levine syndromes).

WARNINGS/PRECAUTIONS: May cause congestive heart failure (CHF), pulmonary edema, hypotension, asymptomatic 1st-degree AV block, transient bradycardia, and PR interval prolongation. Marked 1st-degree block or progressive development to 2nd/3rd-degree AV block requires dose reduction, or discontinuation and institution of appropriate therapy. Elevated transaminases with and without concomitant elevations in alkaline phosphatase and bilirubin reported; monitor LFTs periodically. Hepatocellular injury reported. Ventricular response/fibrillation has occurred in patients with paroxysmal and/or chronic A-flutter or A-fib and a coexisting accessory AV pathway. Sinus bradycardia, pulmonary edema, severe hypotension, 2nd-degree AV block, and sinus arrest reported in patients with hypertrophic cardiomyopathy. Caution with hepatic/renal impairment; monitor for abnormal PR interval prolongation. May decrease neuromuscular transmission in patients with Duchenne's muscular dystrophy and cause worsening of myasthenia gravis; decrease dose with attenuated neuromuscular transmission.

ADVERSE REACTIONS: Headache, infection, constipation, flu syndrome, peripheral edema, dizziness, pharyngitis, sinusitis.

INTERACTIONS: May increase levels with CYP3A4 inhibitors (eg, erythromycin, ritonavir) and grapefruit juice. May decrease levels with CYP3A4 inducers (eg, rifampin). May cause myopathy/rhabdomyolysis with HMG-CoA reductase inhibitors that are CYP3A4 substrates; limit dose of simvastatin to 10mg/day or lovastatin to 40mg/day, and may need to lower doses of other CYP3A4 substrates (eg, atorvastatin). Additive negative effects on HR, AV conduction, and/or cardiac contractility with β-blockers; avoid with ventricular dysfunction. Asymptomatic bradycardia with a wandering atrial pacemaker has been observed with concomitant use of timolol eye drops. Decreased metoprolol and propranolol clearance and variable effect with atenolol reported. Chronic treatment may increase digoxin levels, which may result in digitalis toxicity. Sinus bradycardia resulting in hospitalization and pacemaker insertion reported with the use of clonidine; monitor HR. Hypotension, bradyarrhythmias, and lactic acidosis may occur with concurrent telithromycin use. Reduced absorption with cyclophosphamide, oncovin, procarbazine, prednisone (COPP) and vindesine, adriamycin, cisplatin (VAC) cytotoxic drug regimens. May decrease clearance of paclitaxel. May increase levels of doxorubicin, carbamazepine, cyclosporine, theophylline, and alcohol effects. May increase bleeding time with aspirin. Additive effects with other antihypertensives (eg, vasodilators, ACE inhibitors, diuretics). Excessive reduction in BP with agents that attenuate α-adrenergic function (eg, prazosin). Avoid quinidine with hypertrophic cardiomyopathy. Avoid disopyramide within 48 hrs before or 24 hrs after administration. Additive negative inotropic effects and AV conduction prolongation with flecainide. May increase sensitivity to neurotoxic effects of lithium with or without an increase in serum lithium levels; monitor carefully. Caution with inhalation anesthetics. May potentiate neuromuscular blockers (eg, curare-like, depolarizing); both agents may need dose reduction. Increased clearance with phenobarbital. Reduced oral bioavailability with rifampin. Reduced or unchanged clearance with cimetidine.

PREGNANCY: Category C, not for use in nursing.

MECHANISM OF ACTION: Calcium channel blocker (nondihydropyridine); inhibits transmembrane influx of ionic Ca^{2+} into arterial smooth muscle as well as in conductile and contractile myocardial cells without altering serum Ca^{2+} concentrations.

PHARMACOKINETICS: Absorption: Administration of variable doses resulted in different pharmacokinetic parameters. T_{max}=11 hrs. (Immediate-release) Bioavailability (33-65% [R-enantiomer], 13-34% [S-enantiomer]). **Distribution:** Plasma protein binding (94% to albumin and 92% to α-1 acid glycoprotein [R-enantiomer], 88% to albumin and 86% to α-1 acid glycoprotein [S-enantiomer]); crosses placenta, found in breast milk. **Metabolism:** Liver (extensive); O-demethylation, N-dealkylation via CYP450; norverapamil (active metabolite). **Elimination:** Urine (70%, metabolites, 3-4%, unchanged), feces (≥16%, metabolites).

NURSING CONSIDERATIONS

Assessment: Assess for ventricular dysfunction, cardiac failure symptoms, cardiogenic shock, sick sinus syndrome, hypertrophic cardiomyopathy, Duchenne's muscular dystrophy, attenuated neuromuscular transmission, and/or any conditions where treatment is contraindicated or cautioned. Assess for pregnancy/nursing status and possible drug interactions.

Monitoring: Monitor signs/symptoms of hypotension, CHF, heart block, ventricular fibrillation, renal/hepatic dysfunction, abnormal prolongation of PR interval, hypersensitivity, and other adverse reactions. Periodically monitor LFTs, BP, ECG changes, and HR.

Patient Counseling: Instruct to swallow tab whole; do not chew, break, or crush. Advise that the entire contents of the capsule can be sprinkled onto a tbsp of applesauce; instruct to swallow the applesauce immediately without chewing, and follow with a glass of cool water. Caution that the applesauce should not be hot and should be soft enough to be swallowed without chewing. Instruct to consume the mixture immediately and not store for future use; contents should not be subdivided. Advise to seek medical attention if any adverse reactions occur. Counsel not to breastfeed and to report immediately if pregnant.

Administration: Oral route. May sprinkle on applesauce. Swallow whole; do not crush or chew.
Storage: 25°C (77°F); excursions permitted to 15-30°C (59-86°F). Protect from moisture.

V

VERSACLOZ RX
clozapine (Jazz)

May cause agranulocytosis which can lead to serious infection and death. Absolute neutrophil count (ANC) must be ≥2000/mm³ and WBC must be ≥3500/mm³ for a patient to begin treatment; regularly monitor ANC and WBC during treatment. D/C and do not rechallenge if ANC is <1000/mm³ or WBC is <2000/mm³. Available only through a restricted program called Versacloz Patient Registry, because of the risk of agranulocytosis. Orthostatic hypotension, bradycardia, syncope, and cardiac arrest may occur and the risk is highest during initial titration period, particularly with rapid dose escalation; caution with cardiovascular/cerebrovascular disease or conditions predisposing to hypotension (eg, dehydration, use of antihypertensive medications). Seizures may occur and risk is dose-related; caution with history of seizures or other predisposing risk factors for seizure (eg, CNS pathology, medications that lower seizure threshold, alcohol abuse). May impair mental/physical abilities. Myocarditis and cardiomyopathy may occur; d/c and obtain cardiac evaluation upon suspicion of these reactions. Do not rechallenge in patients with clozapine-related myocarditis or cardiomyopathy. Elderly patients with dementia-related psychosis treated with antipsychotic drugs are at an increased risk for death. Not approved for the treatment of dementia-related psychosis.

THERAPEUTIC CLASS: Dibenzapine derivative

INDICATIONS: Treatment of severely ill patients with schizophrenia who fail to respond adequately to standard antipsychotic treatment. Reduction of risk of recurrent suicidal behavior in patients with schizophrenia or schizoaffective disorder who are judged to be at chronic risk for reexperiencing suicidal behavior, based on history and recent clinical state.

DOSAGE: *Adults:* Administer in divided doses. Initial: 12.5mg qd or bid. Titrate: May increase total daily dose in increments of 25-50mg/day if well-tolerated. Target Dose: 300-450mg/day by the end of 2 weeks. Subsequent Dosing: May increase in increments of up to 100mg, once or twice weekly. Max: 900mg/day. Maint: Continue on the effective dose beyond the acute episode. Discontinuation: Reduce gradually over 1-2 weeks. Reinitiation (≥2 days since last dose): Reinitiate with 12.5mg qd or bid; if well-tolerated, may increase to previous therapeutic dose more quickly than recommended for initial treatment. Significant Renal or Hepatic Impairment/CYP2D6 Poor Metabolizers: Reduce dose. Concomitant CYP1A2/CYP2D6/CYP3A4 Inhibitors or CYP1A2/CYP3A4 Inducers: Refer to PI.

HOW SUPPLIED: Sus: 50mg/mL [100mL]

CONTRAINDICATIONS: History of clozapine-induced agranulocytosis or severe granulocytopenia.

WARNINGS/PRECAUTIONS: Eosinophilia may occur and may be associated with myocarditis, pancreatitis, hepatitis, colitis, and nephritis. Evaluate promptly for signs/symptoms of systemic reactions if eosinophilia develops and d/c if clozapine-related systemic disease is suspected. QT prolongation, torsades de pointes and other life-threatening ventricular arrhythmias, cardiac arrest, and sudden death reported; caution with risk factors for QT prolongation and serious cardiovascular reactions. D/C if QTc interval exceeds 500msec or symptoms consistent with torsades de pointes or other arrhythmias develop. Caution in patients at risk for significant electrolyte disturbance, particularly hypokalemia; correct electrolyte abnormalities before initiation and monitor levels periodically. Associated with metabolic changes (eg, hyperglycemia sometimes associated with ketoacidosis or hyperosmolar coma, dyslipidemia, weight gain) that may increase cardiovascular and cerebrovascular risk; monitor glucose and lipid levels and weight. Neuroleptic malignant syndrome (NMS) reported; d/c therapy and institute symptomatic treatment. Transient fever may occur and may necessitate discontinuing treatment; rule out agranulocytosis or infection. Pulmonary embolism (PE), deep vein thrombosis (DVT), and tardive dyskinesia (TD) reported; consider discontinuation if TD occurs. Has potent anticholinergic effects; caution with narrow-angle glaucoma, prostatic hypertrophy, and other conditions where anticholinergic effects can lead to significant adverse reactions. Consider dose reduction if hypotension, sedation, or impairment of cognitive/motor performance occurs. Caution in patients with risk factors for cerebrovascular adverse reactions. If abrupt discontinuation is necessary, monitor carefully for the recurrence of psychotic symptoms and adverse reactions related to cholinergic rebound. Caution in elderly. Refer to PI for frequency of WBC count and ANC monitoring during various stages of therapy.

ADVERSE REACTIONS: Agranulocytosis, seizure, myocarditis, cardiomyopathy, sedation, dizziness, tremor, tachycardia, hypotension, syncope, hypersalivation, sweating, visual disturbances, constipation, fever.

INTERACTIONS: See Boxed Warning. Not recommended with strong CYP3A4 inducers (eg, carbamazepine, phenytoin, St. John's wort, and rifampin). Caution with medications that prolong the QT interval (eg, specific antipsychotics [eg, ziprasidone, iloperidone, chlorpromazine, thioridazine, mesoridazine, droperidol, pimozide], specific antibiotics [eg, erythromycin, gatifloxacin, moxifloxacin, sparfloxacin], Class 1A antiarrhythmics [eg, quinidine, procainamide] or Class III antiarrhythmics [eg, amiodarone, sotalol], and others [eg, pentamidine, levomethadyl acetate, methadone, halofantrine, mefloquine, dolasetron mesylate, probucol or tacrolimus]). CYP1A2 inhibitors (eg, fluvoxamine, ciprofloxacin, enoxacin, oral contraceptives, caffeine), CYP2D6 or CYP3A4 inhibitors (eg, cimetidine, escitalopram, erythromycin, paroxetine, bupropion, fluoxetine, quinidine, duloxetine, terbinafine, sertraline) may increase levels. CYP1A2 or CYP3A4 inducers (eg, tobacco) may decrease levels. May increase levels of drugs metabolized by CYP2D6 (eg, certain antidepressants, phenothiazines, carbamazepine, type 1C antiarrhythmics [eg, propafenone, flecainide, encainide]). Caution with anticholinergics. NMS reported with CNS-active medications (eg, lithium).

PREGNANCY: Category B, not for use in nursing.

MECHANISM OF ACTION: Tricyclic dibenzodiazepine derivative; atypical antipsychotic agent. Has not been established. Efficacy may be mediated through antagonism of the dopamine type 2 and the serotonin type 2A receptors. Also acts as an antagonist at the adrenergic, cholinergic, histaminergic, and other dopaminergic and serotonergic receptors.

PHARMACOKINETICS: Absorption: (100mg-800mg qd) C_{max}=275ng/mL, T_{max}=2.2 hrs. **Distribution:** Plasma protein binding (97%); found in breast milk. **Metabolism:** CYP1A2, CYP2D6, CYP3A4; demethylation, hydroxylation, N-oxidation. Norclozapine (active metabolite). **Elimination:** Urine (50%), feces (30%); $T_{1/2}$=8 hrs (75mg single dose), 12 hrs (100mg bid).

NURSING CONSIDERATIONS

Assessment: Assess for history of clozapine-induced agranulocytosis or severe granulocytopenia, previous hypersensitivity to the drug, history of seizures or other predisposing factors for seizure, renal/hepatic impairment, CYP2D6 poor metabolism, pregnancy/nursing status, possible drug interactions, and other conditions where treatment is cautioned or contraindicated. Obtain baseline CBC with differential (WBC, ANC), FPG levels in patients with diabetes mellitus (DM) or at risk for hyperglycemia/DM, lipid evaluations, ECG, and electrolytes (serum K^+ and magnesium levels).

Monitoring: Monitor for clinical response and need to continue treatment. Monitor for agranulocytosis, myocarditis, cardiomyopathy, hypotension, sedation, cognitive/motor impairment, HF, tachycardia, severe respiratory effects, seizures, flu-like symptoms, infection, eosinophilia, fever, DVT, PE, NMS, TD, hyperglycemia, weight gain, dyslipidemias, and other adverse reactions. Monitor for recurrence of psychotic symptoms and adverse reactions related to cholinergic rebound upon abrupt discontinuation. Monitor glucose control in patients with DM and check periodic FPG levels if at risk for hyperglycemia. Monitor electrolytes and ECG periodically. Refer to PI for frequency of WBC count and ANC monitoring during various stages of therapy.

Patient Counseling: Inform that drug is available only through a program designed to ensure the required blood monitoring schedule. Counsel on the significant risks of developing agranulocytosis. Advise to report immediately the appearance of signs or symptoms consistent with agranulocytosis or infection. Inform about the significant risk of seizure during treatment; caution about driving and any other potentially hazardous activity while on treatment. Inform about the risk of orthostatic hypotension and syncope, especially during the period of initial dose titration. Caution about operating hazardous machinery. If dose was missed for >2 days, instruct not to restart medication at same dose but to contact physician for dosing instructions. Advise to notify physician if taking or planning to take any prescription or OTC drugs or alcohol. Instruct to notify physician if patient becomes pregnant or intends to become pregnant during therapy. Advise not to breastfeed if taking the drug.

Administration: Oral route. Take with or without food. Shake bottle for 10 sec prior to each use. Use oral syringes and syringe adaptor provided. Refer to PI for administration instructions. **Storage:** ≤25°C (77°F). Do not refrigerate or freeze. Protect from light. Stable for 100 days after initial bottle opening.

VESICARE   RX
solifenacin succinate (Astellas)

THERAPEUTIC CLASS: Muscarinic antagonist

INDICATIONS: Treatment of overactive bladder with symptoms of urge urinary incontinence, urgency, and urinary frequency.

DOSAGE: *Adults:* Usual: 5mg qd. Titrate: May increase to 10mg qd if 5mg dose is well tolerated. Severe Renal Impairment (CrCl <30mL/min)/Moderate Hepatic Impairment (Child-Pugh B)/With Potent CYP3A4 Inhibitors (eg, ketoconazole): Max: 5mg qd.

HOW SUPPLIED: Tab: 5mg, 10mg

CONTRAINDICATIONS: Urinary/gastric retention and uncontrolled narrow-angle glaucoma.

WARNINGS/PRECAUTIONS: Not recommended with severe hepatic impairment (Child-Pugh C). Angioedema of the face, lips, tongue, and/or larynx, and rare anaphylactic reactions reported; d/c and provide appropriate therapy. Risk of urinary retention. Caution with decreased GI motility, controlled narrow-angle glaucoma, renal/hepatic impairment, and history of QT prolongation. CNS anticholinergic effects (eg, headache, confusion, hallucinations, somnolence) reported; may impair mental/physical abilities. Monitor for signs of anticholinergic CNS effects, particularly after beginning treatment or increasing the dose; consider dose reduction or discontinuation if such effects occur.

ADVERSE REACTIONS: Dry mouth, constipation, nausea, dyspepsia, urinary tract infection, blurred vision.

INTERACTIONS: See Dosage. Ketoconazole, a potent CYP3A4 inhibitor, may increase levels. CYP3A4 inducers may decrease concentrations. Caution with medications known to prolong the QT interval.

PREGNANCY: Category C, not for use in nursing.

MECHANISM OF ACTION: Muscarinic receptor antagonist; inhibits muscarinic receptors, which mediate contractions of urinary bladder smooth muscle and stimulation of salivary secretion.

PHARMACOKINETICS: Absorption: Absolute bioavailability (90%); C_{max}=32.3ng/mL (5mg), 62.9ng/mL (10mg); T_{max}=3-8 hrs. **Distribution:** V_d=600L; plasma protein binding (98%). **Metabolism:** Liver (extensive) via CYP3A4 (N-oxidation, 4R-hydroxylation); 4R-hydroxy solifenacin (active metabolite). **Elimination:** Urine (69.2%, <15% unchanged), feces (22.5%); $T_{1/2}$=45-68 hrs.

NURSING CONSIDERATIONS

Assessment: Assess for hypersensitivity to the drug and for any other conditions where treatment is contraindicated or cautioned. Assess for renal/hepatic impairment, pregnancy/nursing status, and possible drug interactions.

Monitoring: Monitor for angioedema, anaphylactic reactions, signs of anticholinergic CNS effects, and other adverse reactions.

Patient Counseling: Inform that constipation may occur; advise to contact physician if severe abdominal pain or constipation for ≥3 days occurs. Inform that blurred vision or CNS anticholinergic effects may occur; advise to exercise caution in decisions to engage in potentially dangerous activities until effects have been determined. Inform that heat prostration (due to decreased sweating) can occur when used in a hot environment. Inform that angioedema may occur and could result in fatal airway obstruction; advise to promptly d/c therapy and seek immediate attention if edema or difficulty breathing develops.

Administration: Oral route. Take with water and swallow whole, with or without food. **Storage:** 25°C (77°F); excursions permitted from 15-30°C (59-86°F).

VFEND   RX
voriconazole (Pfizer)

THERAPEUTIC CLASS: Azole antifungal

INDICATIONS: Used in patients ≥12 yrs for the treatment of invasive aspergillosis; esophageal candidiasis; candidemia in non-neutropenic patients and the following *Candida* infections: disseminated infections in skin and infections in abdomen, kidney, bladder wall, and wounds; serious fungal infections caused by *Scedosporium apiospermum* and *Fusarium* spp. including *Fusarium solani* in patients intolerant of, or refractory to, other therapy.

DOSAGE: *Adults:* Aspergillosis/Scedosporiosis/Fusariosis: LD: 6mg/kg IV q12h for first 24 hrs. Maint: IV: 4mg/kg q12h; continue for ≥7 days. Switch to PO form when appropriate. PO: ≥40kg: 200mg q12h; increase to 300mg q12h if inadequate response. <40kg: 100mg q12h; increase to 150mg q12h if inadequate response. Candidemia (Non-Neutropenic Patients) and other Deep Tissue *Candida* Infections: LD: 6mg/kg IV q12h for first 24 hrs. Maint: IV: 3-4mg/kg q12h. PO: Follow maint dose for aspergillosis. Treat for ≥14 days after resolution of symptoms or last positive culture, whichever is longer. Esophageal Candidiasis: Maint: PO: Follow maint dose for Aspergillosis. Treat for ≥14 days and for ≥7 days after resolution of symptoms. Intolerant to Dose Increase: IV: Reduce 4mg/kg q12h to 3mg/kg q12h. PO: Reduce by 50mg steps to minimum of 200mg q12h for ≥40kg or 100mg q12h for <40kg. With Phenytoin: Maint: IV: 5mg/kg q12h. PO: ≥40kg: 400mg q12h. <40kg: 200mg q12h. With Efavirenz: Maint: PO: 400mg q12h and decrease efavirenz to 300mg q24h. Mild to Moderate Hepatic Cirrhosis (Child-Pugh Class A and B): Maint: 1/2 of usual maint dose. CrCl <50mL/min: Use PO. Therapy Duration: Consider severity of disease, recovery from immunosuppression, and clinical response.

HOW SUPPLIED: Inj: 200mg; Sus: 40mg/mL; Tab: 50mg, 200mg

CONTRAINDICATIONS: Concomitant terfenadine, astemizole, cisapride, pimozide, quinidine, sirolimus, rifampin, carbamazepine, long-acting barbiturates, high-dose ritonavir (400mg q12h), rifabutin, ergot alkaloids (ergotamine, dihydroergotamine), St. John's wort. Low-dose ritonavir (100mg q12h) should be avoided unless an assessment of benefit/risk justifies the use.

WARNINGS/PRECAUTIONS: Serious hepatic reactions (eg, clinical hepatitis, cholestasis, fulminant hepatic failure) reported (uncommon); monitor LFTs at initiation and during therapy and consider to d/c if liver disease develops. Optic neuritis and papilledema reported with prolonged use; monitor visual function with treatment >28 days. May cause fetal harm. Tabs contain lactose;

V

avoid with hereditary galactose intolerance, Lapp lactase deficiency, or glucose-galactose malabsorption. May prolong QT interval, and arrhythmias may occur; caution with proarrhythmic conditions. Anaphylactoid-type reactions reported with infusion; consider discontinuing infusion if reactions occur. Correct electrolyte imbalance before starting therapy. Associated with elevations in LFTs and liver damage (eg, jaundice); caution with hepatic insufficiency. Acute renal failure may occur. Monitor for pancreatitis in patients with risk factors for acute pancreatitis (eg, recent chemotherapy, hematopoietic stem cell transplantation) during treatment. May cause serious exfoliative cutaneous reactions (eg, Stevens-Johnson syndrome) and photosensitivity skin reaction; d/c if exfoliative cutaneous reaction or skin lesion consistent with squamous cell carcinoma or melanoma develops. Fluorosis and periostitis reported with long-term therapy; d/c if skeletal pain and radiologic findings compatible with fluorosis and periostitis develop.

ADVERSE REACTIONS: Visual disturbances, fever, chills, rash, headache, N/V, increased alkaline phosphatase.

INTERACTIONS: See Contraindications. Avoid with fluconazole. Efavirenz, phenytoin decrease levels. Non-nucleoside reverse transcriptase inhibitors (NNRTIs) may decrease levels. Cimetidine, omeprazole, oral contraceptives (containing ethinyl estradiol and norethindrone), fluconazole increased levels. HIV protease inhibitors (eg, saquinavir, amprenavir, nelfinavir), NNRTIs (eg, delavirdine) may increase levels. Increased levels of efavirenz, oral contraceptives (containing ethinyl estradiol and norethindrone), cyclosporine, fentanyl, alfentanil, oxycodone, NSAIDs (eg, ibuprofen, diclofenac, celecoxib), tacrolimus, phenytoin, prednisolone, omeprazole, methadone. May increase levels of HIV protease inhibitors, NNRTIs, proton pump inhibitors, statins (eg, lovastatin), benzodiazepines (eg, midazolam, triazolam, alprazolam), calcium channel blockers (eg, felodipine), sulfonylureas (eg, tolbutamide, glipizide, glyburide), vinca alkaloids (eg, vincristine, vinblastine). Increased PT with warfarin. May increase levels of oral coumarin anticoagulants and increase PT. Inhibitors or inducers of CYP2C19, CYP2C9, and CYP3A4 may increase or decrease voriconazole systemic exposure, respectively. May increase systemic exposure of other drugs metabolized by CYP2C9, CYP2C19, and CYP3A4.

PREGNANCY: Category D, not for use in nursing.

MECHANISM OF ACTION: Triazole antifungal agent; inhibits fungal CYP450-mediated 14 α-lanosterol demethylation, an essential step in fungal ergosterol biosynthesis. Accumulation of 14 α-methyl-sterols correlates with subsequent loss of ergosterol in fungal cell wall and may be responsible for antifungal activity of voriconazole.

PHARMACOKINETICS: Absorption: Administration of different doses led to varying parameters. T_{max}=1-2 hrs. **Distribution:** V_d=4.6L/kg; plasma protein binding (58%). **Metabolism:** Hepatic via CYP2C19, 2C9, and 3A4; N-oxide (major metabolite). **Elimination:** Urine (80-83%, <2% unchanged).

NURSING CONSIDERATIONS

Assessment: Obtain fungal cultures prior to therapy to properly identify causative organisms. Assess for proarrhythmic conditions, hematological malignancy, known hypersensitivity to drug or excipient, hereditary problems of galactose intolerance, Lapp lactase deficiency or glucose-galactose malabsorption, history of cardiotoxic chemotherapy, cardiomyopathy, hypokalemia, arrhythmias, hepatic/renal insufficiency, electrolyte disturbances, pregnancy/nursing status, and for possible drug interactions. Obtain baseline LFTs.

Monitoring: Monitor visual acuity, visual field, and color perception with therapy >28 days. Monitor for infusion-related reactions, hepatotoxicity, arrhythmias, QT prolongation, acute renal failure, pancreatitis, fluorosis, periostitis, and dermatological reactions (eg, Stevens-Johnson syndrome, exfoliative cutaneous reactions, skin lesions). Monitor for drug toxicity with hepatic insufficiencies. Monitor renal function (SrCr) and hepatic function (LFTs, bilirubin) during therapy.

Patient Counseling: Counsel to take tabs or oral sus at least 1 hr ac or 1 hr pc. Advise to avoid driving at night; drug may affect vision. Avoid hazardous tasks such as driving or operating machinery until it is known how the drug affects the patient and avoid intense or prolonged exposure to direct sunlight. Counsel females to use proper contraception during therapy. Inform of the signs and symptoms of liver problems, allergic reactions, vision changes, and serious skin reactions and advise to call the physician if any of these conditions develop.

Administration: Oral and IV route. Oral Sus/Tab: Take at least 1 hr ac or 1 hr pc. Reconstitute sus by adding 46mL of water to bottle and shake vigorously for about 1 min. Refer to PI for IV preparation instructions. Refer to PI for use with other parenteral drug products. **Storage:** Inj: Unreconstituted: 15-30°C (59-86°F). Reconstituted: 2-8°C (36-46°F) for 24 hrs. Tab: 15-30°C (59-86°F). Oral Sus: Unreconstituted: 2-8°C (36-46°F) for 18 months. Reconstituted: 15-30°C (59-86°F) for 14 days. Do not refrigerate or freeze. Keep container tightly closed.

V

VIAGRA

sildenafil citrate (Pfizer)

RX

THERAPEUTIC CLASS: Phosphodiesterase type 5 inhibitor

INDICATIONS: Treatment of erectile dysfunction (ED).

DOSAGE: *Adults:* Usual: 50mg qd PRN 1 hr (recommended) or anywhere from 30 min to 4 hrs before sexual activity. Titrate: May increase to 100mg qd or decrease to 25mg qd, based on effectiveness and tolerance. Max: 100mg qd. Concomitant α-blocker: Patient should be stable on α-blocker therapy prior to initiating treatment. Initial: 25mg qd. Concomitant Ritonavir: Usual: 25mg prior to sexual activity. Max: 25mg/48hrs. Elderly/Hepatic Impairment (eg, Cirrhosis)/Severe Renal Impairment (CrCl <30mL/min)/Concomitant Strong CYP3A4 Inhibitors (eg, Ketoconazole, Itraconazole, Saquinavir) or Erythromycin: Initial: Consider 25mg qd.

HOW SUPPLIED: Tab: 25mg, 50mg, 100mg

CONTRAINDICATIONS: Concomitant use with nitric oxide donors (eg, organic nitrates/nitrites) in any form, either taken regularly and/or intermittently.

WARNINGS/PRECAUTIONS: Potential for cardiac risk of sexual activity in patients with cardiovascular disease (CVD); do not use in men for whom sexual activity is inadvisable due to underlying cardiovascular status. Has systemic vasodilatory properties that resulted in transient decreases in supine BP. Caution in patients with left ventricular outflow obstruction (eg, aortic stenosis, idiopathic hypertrophic subaortic stenosis); severely impaired autonomic control of BP; history of myocardial infarction (MI), stroke, or life-threatening arrhythmia within the last 6 months; resting hypotension (BP <90/50mmHg) or HTN (BP >170/110mmHg); and cardiac failure or coronary artery disease (CAD) causing unstable angina. Prolonged erection >4 hrs and priapism (painful erections >6 hrs in duration) reported; caution with anatomical penile deformation (eg, angulation, cavernosal fibrosis, Peyronie's disease), or predispositions to priapism (eg, sickle cell anemia, multiple myeloma, leukemia). Nonarteritic anterior ischemic optic neuropathy (NAION) reported; d/c if sudden loss of vision in one or both eyes occurs, which could be a sign of NAION. Caution with underlying NAION risk factors; increased risk in patients with "crowded" optic disc and with previous history of NAION. D/C if sudden decrease or loss of hearing occurs. Bleeding events reported. Does not protect against sexually transmitted diseases (STDs).

ADVERSE REACTIONS: Headache, flushing, dyspepsia, abnormal vision, nasal congestion, back pain, myalgia, nausea, dizziness, rash.

INTERACTIONS: See Contraindications and Dosage. Increased levels with CYP3A4 inhibitors (eg, ritonavir, erythromycin, saquinavir); stronger CYP3A4 inhibitors (eg, ketoconazole, itraconazole) may have greater effects. Potential additive BP-lowering effects with α-blockers and other antihypertensives (eg, amlodipine). Combination with other PDE-5 inhibitors or other erectile dysfunction therapies is not recommended; may further lower BP.

PREGNANCY: Category B, not for use in nursing.

MECHANISM OF ACTION: PDE-5 inhibitor; enhances effect of nitric oxide by inhibiting PDE-5, which then increase the levels of cGMP in the corpus cavernosum, resulting in smooth muscle relaxation and inflow of blood to the corpus cavernosum.

PHARMACOKINETICS: Absorption: Rapid. Absolute bioavailability (41%); T_{max}=60 min (median). **Distribution:** V_d=105L; plasma protein binding (96%). **Metabolism:** Liver, via CYP3A4 (major), CYP2C9 (minor); N-desmethyl sildenafil (major active metabolite). **Elimination:** Feces (80% metabolites), urine (13% metabolites); $T_{1/2}$=4 hrs.

NURSING CONSIDERATIONS

Assessment: Assess for hypersensitivity to drug, renal/hepatic impairment, CVD, left ventricular outflow obstruction, impaired autonomic control of BP, resting hypotension or HTN, cardiac failure, CAD, anatomical penile deformation, predisposition to priapism, risk for NAION, potential underlying causes of ED, possible drug interactions, and history of MI, stroke, or arrhythmia.

Monitoring: Monitor for prolonged erection, priapism, abnormalities in vision, NAION, decrease/loss of hearing, bleeding, and other adverse reactions.

Patient Counseling: Inform of possible drug interactions. Advise patients who experience symptoms (eg, angina pectoris, dizziness, nausea) upon initiation of sexual activity to refrain from further activity and to discuss the episode with their physician. Advise to d/c and seek medical attention if sudden loss of vision in one or both eyes or sudden decrease/loss of hearing occurs. Instruct to seek immediate medical assistance if erection persists >4 hrs. Counsel about protective measures necessary to guard against STDs, including HIV.

Administration: Oral route. May be taken with or without food. **Storage:** 25°C (77°F); excursions permitted to 15-30°C (59-86°F).

V

VIBATIV

RX

telavancin (Theravance, Inc.)

> Increased mortality observed in patients with preexisting moderate/severe renal impairment (CrCl ≤50mL/min) who were treated for hospital-acquired/ventilator-associated bacterial pneumonia (HABP/VABP); consider therapy only when the anticipated benefit outweighs the risk. New onset or worsening renal impairment reported; monitor renal function in all patients. Women of childbearing potential should have a serum pregnancy test prior to administration. Avoid use during pregnancy unless potential benefit to the patient outweighs the potential risk to the fetus. Potential adverse developmental outcomes in humans may occur.

THERAPEUTIC CLASS: Antibacterial agent

INDICATIONS: Treatment of adults with complicated skin and skin structure infections (cSSSI) caused by susceptible Gram-positive microorganisms. Treatment of adults with HABP/VABP caused by susceptible isolates of *Staphylococcus aureus* (including methicillin-susceptible and -resistant isolates).

DOSAGE: *Adults:* cSSSI: 10mg/kg IV over 60 min q24h for 7-14 days. HABP/VABP: 10mg/kg IV over 60 min q24h for 7-21 days. Duration of therapy depends on the severity and site of infection, and patient's clinical progress. Renal Impairment: CrCl 30-50mL/min: 7.5mg/kg q24h. CrCl 10-<30mL/min: 10mg/kg q48h.

HOW SUPPLIED: Inj: 250mg, 750mg

WARNINGS/PRECAUTIONS: Use of telavancin for the treatment of HABP/VABP should be reserved for when alternative treatments are not suitable. Decreased efficacy in patients with cSSSI and preexisting moderate/severe renal impairment (CrCl ≤50mL/min). Renal adverse events were reported more likely to occur in patients with baseline comorbidities known to predispose patients to kidney dysfunction (preexisting renal disease, diabetes mellitus [DM], congestive heart failure [CHF], or HTN). Consider alternative agent if renal toxicity is suspected. Accumulation of the solubilizer hydroxypropyl-β-cyclodextrin may occur in patients with renal dysfunction. Serious and sometimes fatal hypersensitivity reactions, including anaphylactic reactions, may occur after 1st or subsequent doses; d/c at 1st sign of skin rash, or any other signs of hypersensitivity. Caution with known hypersensitivity to vancomycin. Infusion-related reactions (eg, "red man syndrome"-like reactions) may occur with rapid infusion. *Clostridium difficile*-associated diarrhea (CDAD) reported; d/c if CDAD suspected or confirmed. Use in the absence of a proven or strongly suspected bacterial infection is unlikely to provide benefit and increases the risk of development of drug-resistant bacteria. May result in overgrowth of nonsusceptible organisms; take appropriate measures if superinfection develops. QTc interval prolongation reported; avoid in patients with congenital long QT syndrome, known prolongation of the QTc interval, uncompensated heart failure (HF), or severe left ventricular hypertrophy (LVH). May interfere with coagulation tests (eg, PT, INR, PTT, activated clotting time, coagulation-based factor Xa) and other lab tests; collect blood samples for affected coagulation tests as close as possible prior to the next dose. Caution in elderly patients.

ADVERSE REACTIONS: Renal impairment, taste disturbance, N/V, foamy urine, rigors, diarrhea, decreased appetite.

INTERACTIONS: Caution with drugs known to prolong the QT interval. Higher renal adverse event rates reported with concomitant medications known to affect kidney function (eg, NSAIDs, ACE inhibitors, loop diuretics).

PREGNANCY: Category C, caution in nursing.

MECHANISM OF ACTION: Antibacterial agent; a lipoglycopeptide antibiotic that inhibits cell-wall biosynthesis by binding to late-stage peptidoglycan precursors, including lipid II. Binds to the bacterial membrane and disrupts membrane barrier function.

PHARMACOKINETICS: Absorption: (Multiple dose) C_{max}=108mcg/mL, AUC_{0-24}=780mcg•hr/mL. **Distribution:** Plasma protein binding (90%); (Multiple dose) V_d=133mL/kg. **Elimination:** Urine (76%), feces (<1%); (Multiple dose) $T_{1/2}$=8.1 hrs.

NURSING CONSIDERATIONS

Assessment: Assess for hypersensitivity to the drug/vancomycin, renal impairment, renal impairment risk (eg, preexisting renal disease, DM, CHF, HTN), congenital long QT syndrome, known prolongation of the QTc interval, uncompensated HF, severe LVH, pregnancy/nursing status, and possible drug interactions.

Monitoring: Monitor for new onset or worsening renal impairment, hypersensitivity reactions, CDAD, development of drug-resistant bacteria, overgrowth of nonsusceptible organisms, superinfection, infusion-related reactions, QTc prolongation, and other adverse reactions. Monitor renal function (eg, SrCr, CrCl) during treatment (at 48- to 72-hr intervals or more frequently, if clinically indicated), and at the end of therapy.

Patient Counseling: Inform women of childbearing potential about the potential risk of fetal harm if drug is used during pregnancy; instruct to have a pregnancy test prior to therapy, to use

V

effective contraceptive methods to prevent pregnancy during treatment if not pregnant, and to notify physician if pregnancy occurs. Encourage pregnant patients to enroll in pregnancy registry. Inform that diarrhea may occur, even as late as ≥2 months after last dose of therapy; instruct to notify physician as soon as possible if watery/bloody stools (with/without stomach cramps and fever) occur. Inform that antibacterial drugs should only be used to treat bacterial infections and not viral infections. Instruct to take ud; inform that skipping doses or not completing full course may decrease effectiveness and increase resistance. Counsel about common adverse effects; advise to notify physician if any unusual/known symptom persists or worsens.

Administration: IV route. Refer to PI for preparation and administration instructions. **Storage:** 2-8°C (35-46°F); excursions permitted to ambient temperatures (up to 25°C [77°F]). Avoid excessive heat. Diluted/Reconstituted Sol: Use within 4 hrs when stored at room temperature or use within 72 hrs when stored under refrigeration at 2-8°C (36-46°F).

VIBRAMYCIN RX
doxycycline (Pfizer)

OTHER BRAND NAMES: Vibra-Tabs (Pfizer)

THERAPEUTIC CLASS: Tetracycline derivative

INDICATIONS: Treatment of the following infections caused by susceptible microorganisms: Rocky Mountain spotted fever, typhus fever and the typhus group, Q fever, rickettsialpox, tick fevers, respiratory tract infections, lymphogranuloma venereum, psittacosis (ornithosis), trachoma, inclusion conjunctivitis, uncomplicated urethral/endocervical/rectal infections, nongonococcal urethritis, relapsing fever, chancroid, plague, tularemia, cholera, *Campylobacter fetus* infections, brucellosis, bartonellosis, granuloma inguinale, urinary tract infections (UTIs), anthrax. Treatment of infections caused by *Escherichia coli*, *Enterobacter aerogenes*, *Shigella* species, or *Acinetobacter* species. Treatment of uncomplicated gonorrhea, syphilis, yaws, listeriosis, Vincent's infection, actinomycosis, and *Clostridium* species infections when penicillin (PCN) is contraindicated. Adjunct to amebicides in acute intestinal amebiasis. Adjunctive therapy in severe acne. Prophylaxis of malaria due to *Plasmodium falciparum* in short-term travelers (<4 months) to areas with chloroquine and/or pyrimethamine-sulfadoxine resistant strains.

DOSAGE: *Adults:* Usual: 100mg q12h on Day 1. Maint: 100mg/day. Severe Infections (eg, Chronic UTI): 100mg q12h. Streptococcal Infections: Continue for 10 days. Uncomplicated Gonococcal Infections (Except Anorectal in Men): 100mg bid for 7 days or as an alternate single visit dose, 300mg stat followed in 1 hr by a second 300mg dose; may be taken with food, including milk or carbonated beverage, as required. Uncomplicated Urethral/Endocervical/Rectal Infections and Nongonococcal Urethritis: 100mg bid for 7 days. Early Syphilis: 100mg bid for 2 weeks. Syphilis (>1-Yr Duration): 100mg bid for 4 weeks. Acute Epididymo-Orchitis: 100mg bid for ≥10 days. Malaria Prophylaxis: 100mg qd. Begin 1-2 days before travel and continue daily during travel and for 4 weeks after leaving malarious area. Inhalational Anthrax (Postexposure): 100mg bid for 60 days.
Pediatrics: Inhalation Anthrax (Postexposure): ≥100 lbs: 100mg bid for 60 days. <100 lbs: 1mg/lb (2.2mg/kg) bid for 60 days. >8 Yrs: Malaria Prophylaxis: 2mg/kg qd. Max: 100mg/day. Begin 1-2 days before travel and continue daily during travel and for 4 weeks after leaving malarious area. Infections: Usual: >100 lbs: Initial: 100mg q12h on Day 1. Maint: 100mg/day. Severe Infections (eg, Chronic UTI): 100mg q12h. Infections: ≤100 lbs: 1mg/lb bid on Day 1 then 1mg/lb qd or divided into 2 doses, on subsequent days. More Severe Infections: May use up to 2mg/lb. Streptococcal Infections: Continue for 10 days.

HOW SUPPLIED: Cap: (Hyclate) 100mg; Sus: (Monohydrate) 25mg/5mL [60mL]; Syrup: (Calcium) 50mg/5mL [473mL]; (Vibra-Tabs) Tab: (Hyclate) 100mg

WARNINGS/PRECAUTIONS: May cause permanent teeth discoloration (yellow-gray-brown) if used during tooth development (last 1/2 of pregnancy to 8 yrs of age); avoid use in these age groups for indications other than anthrax. Enamel hypoplasia reported. *Clostridium difficile*-associated diarrhea (CDAD) reported; d/c if CDAD suspected or confirmed. Photosensitivity may occur; d/c at 1st evidence of skin erythema. May result in bacterial resistance if used in the absence of a proven/suspected bacterial infection or a prophylactic indication; take appropriate measures if superinfection develops. Associated with intracranial HTN (pseudotumor cerebri); increased risk in women of childbearing age who are overweight or have a history of intracranial HTN. Intracranial pressure can remain elevated for weeks after drug cessation; monitor patients until they stabilize. May decrease fibula growth rate in prematures or cause fetal harm during pregnancy. May increase BUN. When used for malaria prophylaxis, patients may still transmit the infection to mosquitoes outside endemic areas. False elevations of urinary catecholamines may occur due to interference with the fluorescence test. Syrup contains sodium metabisulfite that may cause allergic-type reactions.

ADVERSE REACTIONS: Anorexia, N/V, diarrhea, dysphagia, maculopapular rash, Stevens-Johnson syndrome, toxic epidermal necrolysis, photosensitivity, increased BUN, hypersensitivity reactions, drug rash with eosinophilia and systemic symptoms, hemolytic anemia, thrombocytopenia, neutropenia, eosinophilia.

INTERACTIONS: Avoid concomitant use with isotretinoin; may also cause pseudotumor cerebri. May interfere with bactericidal action of PCN; avoid concurrent use. May depress plasma prothrombin activity; may require downward adjustment of anticoagulant dose. Bismuth subsalicylate, iron-containing preparations, and antacids containing aluminum, Ca^{2+}, or Mg^{2+} may impair absorption. Barbiturates, carbamazepine, and phenytoin may decrease $T_{1/2}$. Fatal renal toxicity reported with methoxyflurane. May render oral contraceptives less effective.

PREGNANCY: Category D, not for use in nursing.

MECHANISM OF ACTION: Tetracycline derivative; has bacteriostatic activity. Inhibits bacterial protein synthesis by binding to the 30S ribosomal subunit.

PHARMACOKINETICS: Absorption: Complete. (200mg dose) C_{max}=2.6mcg/mL, T_{max}=2 hrs. **Distribution:** Plasma protein binding in varying degrees; found in breast milk. **Elimination:** Urine (40%/72 hrs in CrCl 75mL/min, 1-5%/72 hrs in CrCl <10mL/min), feces; $T_{1/2}$=18-22 hrs.

NURSING CONSIDERATIONS

Assessment: Assess for previous hypersensitivity to any tetracyclines, risk of intracranial HTN, pregnancy/nursing status, and possible drug interactions. Document indications for therapy as well as culture and susceptibility testing results. Perform dark-field exam and blood serology when coexistent syphilis is suspected.

Monitoring: Monitor for signs/symptoms of hypersensitivity reactions, photosensitivity, skin erythema, superinfection, CDAD, intracranial HTN, visual disturbance, and other adverse reactions. In venereal disease with coexistent syphilis, conduct blood serology monthly for at least 4 months. Perform periodic lab evaluation of organ systems, including hematopoietic, renal, and hepatic studies in long-term therapy.

Patient Counseling: Apprise pregnant women of the potential hazard to fetus. Inform that the therapy does not guarantee protection against malaria; instruct to use measures that help avoid contact with mosquitoes. Instruct to avoid excessive sunlight/UV light and to d/c therapy if phototoxicity occurs; advise to consider use of sunscreen or sunblock. Inform that drug absorption is reduced when taking bismuth subsalicylate and when taken with food, especially those that contain Ca^{2+}. Instruct to drink fluids liberally. Inform that drug may increase the incidence of vaginal candidiasis. Instruct to take exactly ud; warn that skipping doses or not completing full course may decrease effectiveness and increase resistance. Counsel that therapy should only be used to treat bacterial, not viral, infections. Inform that diarrhea may be experienced and advise to notify physician as soon as possible if watery/bloody stools (with or without stomach cramps and fever) even as late as ≥2 months after last dose occur.

Administration: Oral route. Take caps/tabs with adequate fluids. Take with food or milk if gastric irritation occurs. **Storage:** <30°C (86°F).

VICODIN
hydrocodone bitartrate - acetaminophen (AbbVie)

CIII

> Associated with cases of acute liver failure, at times resulting in liver transplant and death. Most of the cases of liver injury are associated with acetaminophen (APAP) use at doses >4000mg/day, and often involve >1 APAP-containing product.

OTHER BRAND NAMES: Vicodin HP (AbbVie) - Vicodin ES (AbbVie)

THERAPEUTIC CLASS: Opioid analgesic

INDICATIONS: Relief of moderate to moderately severe pain.

DOSAGE: *Adults:* Adjust dose according to severity of pain and response. (Vicodin) Usual: 1 or 2 tabs q4-6h PRN. Max: 8 tabs/day. (Vicodin ES/Vicodin HP) Usual: 1 tab q4-6h PRN. Max: 6 tabs/day. Elderly: Start at lower end of dosing range.

HOW SUPPLIED: Tab: (Hydrocodone-APAP) (Vicodin) 5mg-300mg*; (Vicodin ES) 7.5mg-300mg*; (Vicodin HP) 10mg-300mg* *scored

WARNINGS/PRECAUTIONS: Increased risk of acute liver failure in patients with underlying liver disease. Hypersensitivity and anaphylaxis reported; d/c if signs/symptoms occur. May produce dose-related respiratory depression, and irregular and periodic breathing. Respiratory depressant effects and CSF pressure elevation capacity may be markedly exaggerated in the presence of head injury, other intracranial lesions or a preexisting increased intracranial pressure. May obscure diagnosis or clinical course of head injuries or acute abdominal conditions. Potential for abuse. Caution with hypothyroidism, Addison's disease, prostatic hypertrophy, urethral stricture, severe hepatic/renal impairment, or in elderly/debilitated. Suppresses the cough reflex; caution with pulmonary disease and in postoperative use. Physical dependence and tolerance may develop.

ADVERSE REACTIONS: Acute liver failure, lightheadedness, dizziness, sedation, N/V.

INTERACTIONS: Additive CNS depression with other narcotics, antihistamines, antipsychotics, antianxiety agents, or other CNS depressants (eg, alcohol); reduce dose of one or both agents. Concomitant use with MAOIs or TCAs may increase the effect of either the antidepressant or hydrocodone. Increased risk of acute liver failure with alcohol ingestion.

PREGNANCY: Category C, not for use in nursing.

MECHANISM OF ACTION: Hydrocodone: Opioid analgesic; not established. Suspected to relate to the existence of opiate receptors in the CNS. APAP: Nonopiate, nonsalicylate analgesic and antipyretic; not established. Antipyretic activity is mediated through hypothalamic heat-regulating centers; inhibits prostaglandin synthetase.

PHARMACOKINETICS: Absorption: Hydrocodone: (10mg) C_{max}=23.6ng/mL; T_{max}=1.3 hrs. APAP: Rapid. **Distribution:** APAP: Found in breast milk. **Metabolism:** Hydrocodone: O-demethylation, N-demethylation, and 6-keto reduction. APAP: Liver (conjugation). **Elimination:** Hydrocodone: (10mg) $T_{1/2}$=3.8 hrs. APAP: Urine (85%); $T_{1/2}$=1.25-3 hrs.

NURSING CONSIDERATIONS

Assessment: Assess for level of pain intensity, type of pain, patient's general condition and medical status, or any other conditions where treatment is contraindicated or cautioned. Assess for history of hypersensitivity, renal/hepatic function, pregnancy/nursing status, and possible drug interactions.

Monitoring: Monitor for signs/symptoms of hypersensitivity or anaphylaxis, respiratory depression, elevations in CSF pressure, drug abuse, tolerance, and dependence. In patients with severe hepatic/renal disease, monitor effects with serial hepatic and/or renal function tests.

Patient Counseling: Instruct to look for APAP on package labels and not to use >1 APAP-containing product. Instruct to seek medical attention immediately upon ingestion of >4000mg/day APAP, even if feeling well. Advise to d/c and contact physician if signs of allergy (eg, rash, difficulty breathing) develop. Inform that drug may impair mental/physical abilities, and to use caution if performing potentially hazardous tasks (eg, driving, operating machinery). Instruct to avoid alcohol and other CNS depressants. Inform that drug may be habit-forming; instruct to take only ud.

Administration: Oral route. **Storage:** 20-25°C (68-77°F).

VICOPROFEN
hydrocodone bitartrate - ibuprofen (AbbVie)

OTHER BRAND NAMES: Reprexain (Quinnova)

THERAPEUTIC CLASS: Opioid analgesic

INDICATIONS: Short-term (generally <10 days) management of acute pain.

DOSAGE: *Adults:* Use lowest effective dose or longest dosing interval consistent with individual treatment goals. After observing the response to initial therapy, adjust dose and frequency based on individual patient's need. Usual: 1 tab q4-6h, as necessary. Max: 5 tabs/24 hrs. Elderly: Reduce dose.
Pediatrics: ≥16 Yrs: Use lowest effective dose or longest dosing interval consistent with individual treatment goals. After observing the response to initial therapy, adjust dose and frequency based on individual patient's need. Usual: 1 tab q4-6h, as necessary. Max: 5 tabs/24 hrs.

HOW SUPPLIED: (Hydrocodone-Ibuprofen) Tab: (Vicoprofen) 7.5mg-200mg; (Reprexain) 2.5mg-200mg, 5mg-200mg, 10mg-200mg

CONTRAINDICATIONS: History of asthma, urticaria, or other allergic-type reactions with aspirin (ASA) or other NSAIDs. Perioperative pain in the setting of coronary artery bypass graft (CABG) surgery.

WARNINGS/PRECAUTIONS: Not for treatment of osteoarthritis or rheumatoid arthritis. Not for treatment of corticosteroid insufficiency or substitute for corticosteroids; abrupt discontinuation of corticosteroids may lead to disease exacerbation. May diminish utility of fever and inflammation as diagnostic signs in detecting complications of presumed noninfectious, painful conditions. Not recommended with advanced renal disease; monitor renal function closely during initiation of therapy. Caution in elderly. Ibuprofen: May increase risk of serious cardiovascular (CV) thrombotic events, myocardial infarction (MI), and stroke; increased risk with known CV disease or risk factors for CV disease. May cause serious GI adverse events including inflammation, bleeding, ulceration, and perforation of the stomach and intestine; extreme caution with history of ulcer disease or GI bleeding and caution in debilitated patients. May lead to onset of new HTN or worsening of preexisting HTN; monitor BP closely and caution with HTN. Fluid retention and edema reported; caution in patients with fluid retention or heart failure (HF). Renal papillary necrosis and other renal injury reported after long-term use; caution with impaired renal function, HF, and liver dysfunction. Anaphylactoid reactions may occur; avoid in patients with ASA triad. May cause serious skin adverse events (eg, exfoliative dermatitis, Stevens-Johnson syndrome, and toxic epidermal necrolysis); d/c at 1st appearance of skin rash/hypersensitivity. Avoid in late pregnancy; may cause premature closure of ductus arteriosus. Elevations of LFTs and severe hepatic reactions (eg, jaundice, fatal fulminant hepatitis, liver necrosis, hepatic failure) reported; d/c if liver disease or systemic manifestations (eg, eosinophilia, rash) occur. Anemia reported; monitor Hgb/Hct if signs/symptoms of anemia present with long-term treatment. May inhibit platelet aggregation and prolong bleeding time; monitor with coagulation disorders. Caution with preexisting asthma and avoid with ASA-sensitive asthma. Aseptic meningitis with fever and coma reported. Hydrocodone: May increase risk of misuse, abuse, or diversion. May produce dose-related respiratory depression. Respiratory depressant effects and CSF pressure elevation may be markedly exaggerated in the presence of head injury, intracranial lesions, or preexisting increased intracranial pressure. May obscure diagnosis/clinical course of acute abdominal conditions or head injuries. Caution in debilitated patients, severe renal/hepatic impairment, hypothyroidism, Addison's disease, prostatic hypertrophy, or urethral stricture. Suppresses cough reflex; caution when used postoperatively and with pulmonary disease.

ADVERSE REACTIONS: Headache, somnolence, dizziness, constipation, dyspepsia, N/V, infection, edema, nervousness, anxiety, pruritus, diarrhea, asthenia, abdominal pain, sweating.

INTERACTIONS: ASA may increase adverse effects; concomitant administration is not recommended. Use with other opioid analgesics, antihistamines, antipsychotics, antianxiety agents, or other CNS depressants (eg, alcohol) may exhibit additive CNS depression; reduce dose of one or both agents. Ibuprofen: Increased risk of GI bleeding with oral corticosteroids or anticoagulants, smoking, and alcohol. May increase the risk of renal toxicity with diuretics and ACE inhibitors. Alterations in platelet function may occur with anticoagulants; monitor carefully. May diminish antihypertensive effect of ACE inhibitors. Synergistic effects on GI bleeding with warfarin. May decrease natriuretic effect of furosemide and loop or thiazide diuretics; monitor for renal failure. May increase lithium levels; monitor for lithium toxicity. May enhance methotrexate toxicity; caution with coadministration. Hydrocodone: Use with MAOIs or TCAs may increase the effect of either the antidepressant or hydrocodone. Not recommended for patients taking MAOIs or within 14 days of stopping such treatment. May produce paralytic ileus with anticholinergics. Caution with concurrent agonist/antagonist analgesics (eg, pentazocine, nalbuphine, butorphanol, buprenorphine) use; may reduce analgesic effect of hydrocodone and/or precipitate withdrawal symptoms. May enhance neuromuscular blocking action of skeletal muscle relaxants and increase respiratory depression.

PREGNANCY: Category C, not for use in nursing.

MECHANISM OF ACTION: Hydrocodone: Opioid analgesic and antitussive; has not been established. Suspected to be related to existence of opiate receptors in CNS. Ibuprofen: NSAID; has not been established. May be related to inhibition of cyclooxygenase activity and prostaglandin synthesis. Possesses analgesic and antipyretic activity.

PHARMACOKINETICS: Absorption: Hydrocodone: C_{max}=27ng/mL, T_{max}=1.7 hrs. Ibuprofen: C_{max}=30mcg/mL, T_{max}=1.8 hrs. **Distribution:** Hydrocodone: Plasma protein binding (19-45%). Ibuprofen: Plasma protein binding (99%). **Metabolism:** Hydrocodone: CYP2D6 via O-demethylation to hydromorphone (active metabolite); CYP3A4 via N-demethylation; 6-keto reduction. Ibuprofen: Interconversion from R-isomer to S-isomer; (+)-2-4'-(2hydroxy-2-methyl-propyl) phenyl propionic acid and (+)-2-4'-(2carboxypropyl) phenyl propionic acid (primary metabolites). **Elimination:** Hydrocodone: Urine (primary); $T_{1/2}$=4.5 hrs. Ibuprofen: Urine (50-60% metabolites, 15% unchanged drug and conjugate), $T_{1/2}$=2.2 hrs.

NURSING CONSIDERATIONS

Assessment: Assess for history of asthma, urticaria or allergic-type reactions with ASA or NSAIDS, known hypersensitivity to the drug, perioperative pain in setting of CABG surgery, CV disease and its risk factors, HTN, fluid retention or HF, ulcer disease or GI bleeding, coagulation disorders, renal/hepatic function, pregnancy/nursing status, any other conditions where treatment is contraindicated or cautioned, and for possible drug interactions. Assess for level of pain intensity, type of pain, patient's general condition and medical status.

Monitoring: Monitor for signs/symptoms of CV thrombotic events, MI, stroke, HTN, fluid retention or edema, drug abuse and dependence, tolerance, respiratory depression, elevations in CSF, GI effects, renal/hepatic effects, anaphylactoid reactions, skin reactions, bronchospasm, aseptic meningitis, and other adverse reactions. If signs/symptoms of anemia develop, evaluate Hgb/Hct. Perform periodic monitoring of CBC and chemistry profile with long-term therapy. Monitor for alterations in platelet function with anticoagulants.

Patient Counseling: Caution that drug may impair mental and/or physical abilities required to perform potentially hazardous tasks (eg, operating machinery/driving). Instruct to avoid alcohol and other CNS depressants while on therapy. Warn that drug may be habit-forming; instruct to take only for as long as prescribed, in the amounts prescribed, and no more frequently than prescribed. Instruct to contact physician if CV events (eg, chest pain, SOB, weakness, slurring of speech), GI effects (eg, ulcers, bleeding), unexplained weight gain or edema occurs. Instruct to immediately d/c therapy and contact physician if signs/symptoms of serious skin reactions (eg, rash) or hepatotoxicity (eg, nausea, fatigue, jaundice) develop. Instruct to seek immediate

V

medical attention if signs of anaphylactoid reactions (eg, difficulty breathing, facial/throat swelling) develop. Instruct to report any signs of blurred vision or other eye symptoms. Instruct to avoid use in late pregnancy.

Administration: Oral route. **Storage:** (Vicoprofen) 25°C (77°F); excursions permitted to 15-30°C (59-86°F). (Reprexain) 20-25°C (68-77°F); excursions permitted to 15-30°C (59-86°F).

VICTOZA   RX
liraglutide (rdna origin) (Novo Nordisk)

> Causes dose dependent and treatment duration dependent thyroid C-cell tumors at clinically relevant exposures in animal studies. It is unknown whether drug causes thyroid C-cell tumors (eg, medullary thyroid carcinoma [MTC]) in humans. Contraindicated in patients with a personal or family history of MTC and in patients with multiple endocrine neoplasia syndrome type 2 (MEN 2). It is unknown whether monitoring with serum calcitonin or thyroid ultrasound will mitigate human risk of thyroid C-cell tumors. Counsel patients on the risk and symptoms of thyroid tumors.

THERAPEUTIC CLASS: Glucagon-like peptide-1 receptor agonist

INDICATIONS: Adjunct to diet and exercise to improve glycemic control in adults with type 2 diabetes mellitus (DM).

DOSAGE: *Adults:* Initial: 0.6mg SQ qd for 1 week. Titrate: Increase to 1.2mg qd after 1 week. If acceptable glycemic control is not achieved, increase to 1.8mg qd. Reinitiate at 0.6mg if >3 days have elapsed since the last dose, and titrate ud. With Insulin Secretagogues (eg, Sulfonylureas): Consider reducing the dose of insulin secretagogues. With Insulin: Consider reducing the dose of insulin. Administer as separate inj. May inject in the same body region but the inj should not be adjacent to each other.

HOW SUPPLIED: Inj: 6mg/mL [3mL, prefilled pen]

CONTRAINDICATIONS: MEN 2, personal or family history of MTC.

WARNINGS/PRECAUTIONS: Not recommended as 1st-line therapy with inadequate glycemic control on diet and exercise. Concurrent use with prandial insulin has not been studied. Not a substitute for insulin; do not use in type 1 DM or for the treatment of diabetic ketoacidosis. Refer patients with thyroid nodules and/or elevated calcitonin levels to an endocrinologist for further evaluation. Acute pancreatitis, including fatal and nonfatal hemorrhagic or necrotizing pancreatitis, reported; observe for signs/symptoms of pancreatitis after initiation of therapy, d/c promptly if suspected, and do not restart therapy if confirmed. Consider other antidiabetic therapies in patients with a history of pancreatitis. Acute renal failure and worsening of chronic renal failure reported; caution when initiating/escalating doses in patients with renal impairment. Serious hypersensitivity reactions (eg, anaphylactic reactions, angioedema) reported; d/c if a hypersensitivity reaction occurs. Caution with hepatic impairment. No conclusive evidence of macrovascular risk reduction.

ADVERSE REACTIONS: N/V, diarrhea, constipation, dyspepsia, headache, antibody formation.

INTERACTIONS: Increased risk of hypoglycemia with insulin secretagogues (eg, sulfonylureas) or insulin; consider dose reduction of insulin secretagogues or insulin. May affect the absorption of oral medications; use with caution.

PREGNANCY: Category C, not for use in nursing.

MECHANISM OF ACTION: Human glucagon-like peptide-1 receptor agonist; increases intracellular cyclic AMP, leading to insulin release in the presence of elevated glucose concentrations. Also decreases glucagon secretion in a glucose-dependent manner and delays gastric emptying.

PHARMACOKINETICS: Absorption: Absolute bioavailability (55%), T_{max}=8-12 hrs; (0.6mg) C_{max}=35ng/mL, AUC=960ng•hr/mL. **Distribution:** Plasma protein binding (>98%); (0.6mg) V_d=13L. **Elimination:** Urine (6%), feces (5%); $T_{1/2}$=13 hrs.

NURSING CONSIDERATIONS

Assessment: Assess for previous hypersensitivity reactions, MEN 2, personal or family history of MTC, history of pancreatitis, type of DM, diabetic ketoacidosis, renal/hepatic impairment, pregnancy/nursing status, and possible drug interactions.

Monitoring: Monitor for signs and symptoms of thyroid tumor, pancreatitis, elevated serum calcitonin levels, hypoglycemia, hypersensitivity reactions, and other adverse reactions. Monitor renal function, blood glucose levels, and HbA1c levels.

Patient Counseling: Advise to report symptoms of thyroid tumors to physician. Inform of the potential risk of dehydration due to GI adverse reactions and instruct to take precautions to avoid fluid depletion. Inform of the potential risk for pancreatitis and worsening renal function. Instruct to d/c therapy promptly and contact physician if persistent severe abdominal pain and/or symptoms of hypersensitivity reactions occur. Advise not to share pen with others, even if needle is changed. Counsel on potential risks/benefits of therapy and of alternative modes of therapy, importance of adhering to dietary instructions, regular physical activity, periodic blood glucose monitoring and HbA1c testing, recognition/management of hypoglycemia/hyperglyce-mia, and assessment for diabetes complications. Advise to seek medical advice during periods of stress, if any unusual symptom develops, or if any known symptom persists or worsens. Instruct not to take an extra dose to make up for a missed dose and to resume as prescribed with the next scheduled dose. Advise to reinitiate treatment at 0.6mg if >3 days have elapsed since the last dose and to then titrate the dose as prescribed.

Administration: SQ route. Inject into abdomen, thigh, or upper arm; may be administered qd at any time of the day, independently of meals. Inj site and timing can be changed without dose adjustment. Refer to PI for further administration instructions. **Storage:** Prior to 1st Use: 2-8°C (36-46°F). Do not freeze and do not use if it has been frozen. After Initial Use: 15-30°C (59-86°F) or 2-8°C (36-46°F) for 30 days. Keep the pen cap on when not in use. Always remove and safely discard the needle after each inj; store pen without an inj needle attached. Protect from excessive heat and sunlight.

VICTRELIS   RX
boceprevir (Merck)

THERAPEUTIC CLASS: HCV NS3/4A protease inhibitor

INDICATIONS: Treatment of chronic hepatitis C genotype 1 infection, in combination with peginterferon alfa and ribavirin, in adults with compensated liver disease, including cirrhosis, who are previously untreated or who have failed previous interferon and ribavirin therapy, including prior null responders, partial responders, and relapsers.

DOSAGE: *Adults:* 800mg tid (q7-9h) with food in combination with peginterferon alfa and ribavirin. Give after 4 weeks of treatment with peginterferon alfa and ribavirin regimen. Duration of Therapy: Patients without Cirrhosis Who are Previously Untreated or Who Previously Failed Interferon and Ribavirin Therapy: Based on viral response; refer to PI. Patients with Cirrhosis: Treat with boceprevir in combination with peginterferon alfa and ribavirin for 44 weeks. Refer to PI for dose modification and discontinuation of therapy.

HOW SUPPLIED: Cap: 200mg

CONTRAINDICATIONS: Pregnant women and men whose female partners are pregnant. Coadministration with CYP3A4/5 substrates for which elevated plasma concentrations are associated with serious and/or life-threatening events, or potent CYP3A4/5 inducers where significantly reduced levels may be associated with reduced efficacy (eg, alfuzosin, doxazosin, silodosin, tamsulosin, carbamazepine, phenobarbital, phenytoin, rifampin, dihydroergotamine, ergonovine, ergotamine, methylergonovine, cisapride, St. John's wort, lovastatin, simvastatin, drospirenone, sildenafil or tadalafil when used for treatment of pulmonary arterial HTN, pimozide, triazolam, oral midazolam). Refer to the individual monographs for peginterferon alfa and ribavirin.

WARNINGS/PRECAUTIONS: Women of childbearing potential and men must use at least 2 forms of effective contraception during treatment and for at least 6 months after treatment discontinuation; perform routine monthly pregnancy tests during this time. One of the forms of contraception can be a combined oral contraceptive product containing at least 1mg of norethindrone. Therapy in combination with peginterferon alfa and ribavirin is associated with an additional decrease in Hgb. Thromboembolic events, neutropenia, and serious cases of pancytopenia reported. If peginterferon alfa or ribavirin is permanently discontinued, boceprevir must also be discontinued. Serious acute hypersensitivity reactions (eg, urticaria, angioedema) reported; d/c combination therapy and institute appropriate therapy immediately. Caution in elderly.

ADVERSE REACTIONS: Anemia, neutropenia, N/V, dysgeusia, diarrhea, fatigue, insomnia, chills, decreased appetite, alopecia, irritability, arthralgia, dizziness, dry skin, headache.

INTERACTIONS: See Contraindications. Avoid with colchicine in patients with renal/hepatic impairment; risk of toxicity. Avoid with dexamethasone or use with caution if necessary. Avoid with budesonide, fluticasone, and efavirenz. May decrease levels of atazanavir/ritonavir, darunavir/ritonavir, or lopinavir/ritonavir; coadministration is not recommended. Not recommended with salmeterol or rifabutin. May increase levels of antiarrhythmics, digoxin, trazodone, desipramine, ketoconazole, itraconazole, voriconazole, posaconazole, colchicine, clarithromycin, rifabutin, calcium channel blockers, prednisone (and its active metabolite, prednisolone), budesonide, fluticasone, bosentan, rilpivirine, atorvastatin, pravastatin, cyclosporine, tacrolimus, sirolimus, salmeterol, buprenorphine/naloxone, PDE-5 inhibitors, alprazolam, and IV midazolam. Frequently assess renal function with cyclosporine, tacrolimus, or sirolimus. May decrease levels of etravirine, methadone, ethinyl estradiol, norethindrone, and escitalopram. Individual patients may require additional titration of their methadone dosage when boceprevir is started or stopped. Monitor for signs of estrogen deficiency in patients using estrogens as hormone replacement therapy. Measure serum digoxin concentrations before initiating therapy; continue monitoring digoxin concentrations. May alter levels of warfarin; monitor INR closely. Ketoconazole, itracon-

V

azole, voriconazole, posaconazole, and other CYP3A4/5 inhibitors may increase levels. Ritonavir and CYP3A4/5 inducers (eg, rifabutin, dexamethasone, efavirenz) may decrease levels.

PREGNANCY: Category B, Category X when used with peginterferon alfa and ribavirin, not for use in nursing.

MECHANISM OF ACTION: Hepatitis C virus (HCV) NS3/4A protease inhibitor; covalently, yet reversibly, binds to the NS3 protease active site serine (S139) through an α-ketoamide functional group to inhibit viral replication in HCV-infected host cells.

PHARMACOKINETICS: Absorption: (800mg tid) AUC=5408ng•hr/mL; C_{max}=1723ng/mL. T_{max}=2 hrs (median). **Distribution:** V_d=772L; (800mg single dose) plasma protein binding (75%). **Metabolism:** Aldo-ketoreductase-mediated pathway (primary) and oxidative metabolism via CYP3A4/5. **Elimination:** (800mg single dose) Urine (9%, 3% unchanged), feces (79%, 8% unchanged). $T_{1/2}$=3.4 hrs.

NURSING CONSIDERATIONS

Assessment: Assess for history of hypersensitivity to the drug, men whose female partners are pregnant, pregnancy/nursing status, and possible drug interactions. Obtain baseline CBC (with WBC differential count).

Monitoring: Monitor for hypersensitivity reactions and other adverse reactions. Monitor HCV-RNA levels at treatment Weeks 4, 8, 12, and 24, at the end of treatment, during treatment follow-up, and as clinically indicated. Obtain CBC (with WBC differential count) at treatment Weeks 2, 4, 8, and 12, and as clinically appropriate. Perform routine monthly pregnancy tests. Frequently assess renal function with cyclosporine, tacrolimus, or sirolimus. Monitor INR closely with warfarin.

Patient Counseling: Inform that drug must be used in combination with peginterferon alfa and ribavirin and must not be used alone. Instruct to notify physician immediately in the event of a pregnancy. Advise women of childbearing potential and men to use at least 2 forms of effective contraception during therapy and for at least 6 months after treatment discontinuation. Advise that anemia, neutropenia, and pancytopenia may occur and that laboratory evaluations are required prior to starting therapy and periodically thereafter. Instruct to seek medical advice promptly if symptoms of acute hypersensitivity reactions (eg, itching, hives, swelling of the face/eyes/lips/tongue/throat, trouble breathing or swallowing) occur. Inform of the potential for serious drug interactions, and that some drugs should not be taken concomitantly. Instruct to skip the missed dose if a dose is missed and it is <2 hrs before the next dose, but to take the missed dose and resume the normal dosing schedule if a dose is missed and it is ≥2 hrs before next dose. Inform that the effect of treatment of hepatitis C on transmission is unknown and that appropriate precautions to prevent transmission should be taken.

Administration: Oral route. Take with a meal or light snack. **Storage:** 2-8°C (36-46°F), or at room temperature up to 25°C (77°F) for 3 months. Avoid exposure to excessive heat.

VIDEX EC   RX
didanosine (Bristol-Myers Squibb)

> Fatal and nonfatal pancreatitis reported when used alone or as part of a combination regimen. Suspend therapy in patients with suspected pancreatitis and d/c with confirmed pancreatitis. Lactic acidosis and severe hepatomegaly with steatosis, including fatal cases, reported with the use of nucleoside analogues alone or in combination. Fatal lactic acidosis reported in pregnant women who received the combination of didanosine and stavudine with other antiretroviral agents; use with caution.

OTHER BRAND NAMES: Videx (Bristol-Myers Squibb)

THERAPEUTIC CLASS: Nucleoside reverse transcriptase inhibitor

INDICATIONS: Treatment of HIV-1 infection in combination with other antiretroviral agents.

DOSAGE: *Adults:* Take on an empty stomach. ≥60kg: (Cap) 400mg qd; (Sol) 200mg bid or 400mg qd. <60kg: (Sol) 125mg bid or 250mg qd. 25-<60kg: (Cap) 250mg qd. 20-<25kg: (Cap) 200mg qd. Renal Impairment: CrCl ≥60mL/min: ≥60kg: (Cap) 400mg qd; (Sol) 200mg bid or 400mg qd. <60kg: (Cap) 250mg qd; (Sol) 125mg bid or 250mg qd. CrCl 30-59mL/min: ≥60kg: (Cap) 200mg qd; (Sol) 200mg qd or 100mg bid. <60kg: (Cap) 125mg qd; (Sol) 150mg qd or 75mg bid. CrCl 10-29mL/min: ≥60kg: (Cap) 125mg qd; (Sol) 150mg qd. <60kg: (Cap) 125mg qd; (Sol) 100mg qd. CrCl <10mL/min or Continuous Ambulatory Peritoneal Dialysis/Hemodialysis: ≥60kg: (Cap) 125mg qd; (Sol) 100mg qd. <60kg: (Sol) 75mg qd. Concomitant Tenofovir Disoproxil Fumarate: CrCl ≥60mL/min: ≥60kg: 250mg qd; <60kg: 200mg qd. Refer to PI for more information and for dosing modifications when used with certain concomitant therapies. *Pediatrics:* Take on an empty stomach. (Cap) ≥60kg: 400mg qd. 25-<60kg: 250mg qd. 20-<25kg: 200mg qd. (Sol) >8 Months-18 Yrs: 120mg/m² bid, not to exceed adult dosing recommendation. 2 Weeks-8 Months: 100mg/m² bid. Renal Impairment: Consider dose reduction. Refer to PI for more information and for dosing modifications when used with certain concomitant therapies.

HOW SUPPLIED: Cap, Delayed-Release (EC): 125mg, 200mg, 250mg, 400mg; (Videx) Sol: 2g, 4g

CONTRAINDICATIONS: Coadministration with allopurinol or ribavirin.

WARNINGS/PRECAUTIONS: Increased risk of pancreatitis in patients with advanced HIV-1 infection, especially elderly. Obesity and prolonged nucleoside exposure may be risk factors for lactic acidosis and severe hepatomegaly with steatosis. Caution in patients with known risk factors for liver disease. Suspend treatment in any patient who develops clinical signs/symptoms with/without lab findings consistent with symptomatic hyperlactatemia, lactic acidosis, or pronounced hepatotoxicity. Increased frequency of liver function abnormalities in patients with preexisting liver dysfunction; consider interruption or discontinuation of therapy with evidence of worsening liver disease. Noncirrhotic portal HTN reported, including cases leading to liver transplantation or death; d/c with evidence of noncirrhotic portal HTN. Peripheral neuropathy reported and occurred more frequently in patients with advanced HIV disease or history of neuropathy; consider discontinuation if peripheral neuropathy develops. Retinal changes and optic neuritis reported; consider periodic retinal examinations. Immune reconstitution syndrome reported. Autoimmune disorders (eg, Graves' disease, polymyositis, Guillain-Barre syndrome) reported in the setting of immune reconstitution and can occur many months after initiation of treatment. Body fat redistribution/accumulation reported. Caution in elderly.

ADVERSE REACTIONS: Pancreatitis, lactic acidosis, severe hepatomegaly with steatosis, diarrhea, peripheral neurologic symptoms/neuropathy, headache, N/V, rash, abdominal pain, serum AST/ALT/alkaline phosphatase/amylase/lipase/bilirubin elevation.

INTERACTIONS: See Boxed Warning and Contraindications. Avoid with hydroxyurea with or without stavudine; may be at increased risk for pancreatitis, hepatotoxicity, and peripheral neuropathy. Caution with drugs that may cause pancreatic toxicity or neurotoxicity (eg, stavudine). Administer nelfinavir 1 hr after didanosine. Ganciclovir and tenofovir may increase levels. Methadone may decrease levels. (Sol) Avoid with methadone. Caution with aluminum- or Mg^{2+}-containing antacids. May decrease levels of delavirdine, indinavir, azole antifungals, and quinolone and tetracycline antibiotics.

PREGNANCY: Category B, not for use in nursing.

MECHANISM OF ACTION: Synthetic purine nucleoside analogue; inhibits the activity of HIV-1 reverse transcriptase both by competing with the natural substrate, deoxyadenosine 5'-triphosphate, and by its incorporation into viral DNA causing termination of viral DNA chain elongation.

PHARMACOKINETICS: Absorption: Rapid. Oral bioavailability (42%, adults; 25%, pediatric patients 8 months-19 yrs of age [sol]); T_{max}=0.25-1.5 hrs. **Distribution:** Plasma protein binding (<5%). Refer to PI for other parameters in adult and pediatric patients. **Metabolism:** Cellular enzymes to dideoxyadenosine 5'-triphosphate (active metabolite). **Elimination:** Urine (18%). Refer to PI for $T_{1/2}$.

NURSING CONSIDERATIONS

Assessment: Assess for risk factors for pancreatitis, lactic acidosis, or liver disease, renal/hepatic impairment, history of peripheral neuropathy, pregnancy/nursing status, and possible drug interactions.

Monitoring: Monitor for signs/symptoms of pancreatitis, lactic acidosis, hepatotoxicity, worsening of liver disease, portal HTN, peripheral neuropathy, immune reconstitution syndrome (eg, opportunistic infections), autoimmune disorders, fat redistribution/accumulation, and other adverse reactions. Monitor renal function. Consider appropriate lab testing, including liver enzymes, serum bilirubin, albumin, CBC, INR, and ultrasonography, if portal HTN is suspected. Consider periodic retinal examinations.

Patient Counseling: Inform of risks and benefits of therapy. Caution about the use of medications or other substances, including alcohol, which may exacerbate drug toxicities. Inform that treatment is not a cure for HIV and patients may continue to experience illnesses associated with HIV. Advise to avoid doing things that can spread HIV to others.

Administration: Oral route. (Cap) Take on an empty stomach. Swallow cap intact. (Sol) Refer to PI for reconstitution of the powder. Take on an empty stomach, at least 30 min ac or 2 hrs pc. Shake admixture thoroughly prior to use. **Storage:** (Cap) 25°C (77°F); excursions permitted between 15-30°C (59-86°F). Store in tightly closed containers. (Sol) 15-30°C (59-86°F). Admixture: 2-8°C (36-46°F) for up to 30 days.

VIGAMOX
moxifloxacin HCl (Alcon)

RX

THERAPEUTIC CLASS: Fluoroquinolone

INDICATIONS: Treatment of bacterial conjunctivitis caused by susceptible strains of organisms.

DOSAGE: *Adults:* 1 drop in the affected eye tid for 7 days.
Pediatrics: ≥1 Yr: 1 drop in the affected eye tid for 7 days.

HOW SUPPLIED: Sol: 0.5% [3mL]

WARNINGS/PRECAUTIONS: Not for inj. Do not inject subconjunctivally or introduce directly into the anterior chamber of the eye. Fatal hypersensitivity reactions reported with systemic quinolone therapy. May result in bacterial resistance with prolonged use; take appropriate measures if superinfection develops. Avoid contact lenses when signs and symptoms of bacterial conjunctivitis are present.

ADVERSE REACTIONS: Conjunctivitis, decreased visual acuity, dry eye, keratitis, ocular discomfort/hyperemia, ocular pain/pruritus, subconjunctival hemorrhage, tearing.

PREGNANCY: Category C, caution in nursing.

MECHANISM OF ACTION: Fluoroquinolone antibiotic; inhibits topoisomerase II (DNA gyrase) and topoisomerase IV.

PHARMACOKINETICS: Absorption: C_{max}=2.7ng/mL, AUC=45ng•hr/mL. **Distribution:** Presumed to be excreted in breast milk. **Elimination:** $T_{1/2}$=13 hrs.

NURSING CONSIDERATIONS

Assessment: Assess for proper diagnosis of causative organisms (eg, slit-lamp biomicroscopy, fluorescein staining). Assess for hypersensitivity to other quinolones, and pregnancy/nursing status.

Monitoring: Monitor for signs/symptoms of hypersensitivity or anaphylactic reactions and other adverse reactions. With prolonged therapy, monitor for overgrowth of nonsusceptible organisms (eg, fungi) and for development of superinfection.

Patient Counseling: Instruct not to touch the dropper tip to any surface to avoid contaminating the contents. Instruct to immediately d/c medication and contact physician at the 1st sign of rash or allergic reaction. Instruct not to wear contact lenses if signs and symptoms of bacterial conjunctivitis develop.

Administration: Ocular route. **Storage:** 2-25°C (36-77°F).

VIIBRYD   RX
vilazodone HCl (Forest)

Antidepressants increased the risk of suicidal thoughts and behavior in children, adolescents, and young adults in short-term studies. Monitor closely for clinical worsening and for emergence for suicidal thoughts and behaviors. Not approved for use in pediatrics.

THERAPEUTIC CLASS: Selective serotonin reuptake inhibitor/5-HT$_{1A}$-receptor partial agonist

INDICATIONS: Treatment of major depressive disorder.

DOSAGE: *Adults:* Usual: 40mg qd. Initial: 10mg qd for 7 days. Titrate: Increase to 20mg qd for an additional 7 days, and then an increase to 40mg qd. Reassess periodically to determine the need for maintenance treatment and the appropriate dose for treatment. Concomitant Strong CYP3A4 Inhibitors (eg, Ketoconazole)/Moderate CYP3A4 Inhibitors (eg, Erythromycin) for Patients with Intolerable Events: Reduce to 20mg. Readjust dose to the original level when CYP3A4 inhibitors are discontinued. Concomitant Strong CYP3A4 Inducers (eg, Carbamazepine): Consider increasing vilazodone dose up to 2-fold when concomitantly used for >14 days. Max: 80mg/day. Reduce dose to the original level in 14 days if CYP3A4 inducers are discontinued. Therapy Discontinuation/Switching to/from an MAOI/Use with Other MAOIs (eg, Linezolid, IV Methylene Blue): Refer to PI. Take with food.

HOW SUPPLIED: Tab: 10mg, 20mg, 40mg

CONTRAINDICATIONS: Use of an MAOI for psychiatric disorders either concomitantly or within 14 day of stopping treatment. Treatment within 14 days of stopping an MAOI for psychiatric disorders. Starting treatment in patients being treated with other MAOIs (eg, linezolid, IV methylene blue).

WARNINGS/PRECAUTIONS: Not approved for use in treating bipolar depression. May precipitate mixed/manic episode in patients at risk for bipolar disorder; screen for risk for bipolar disorder prior to initiating treatment. Serotonin syndrome reported; d/c immediately and initiate supportive symptomatic treatment. Caution with seizure disorder. May increase the risk of bleeding events. Activation of mania/hypomania reported; caution with a history or family history of bipolar disorder, mania, or hypomania. Hyponatremia may occur in association with the syndrome of inappropriate antidiuretic hormone secretion; elderly, patients taking diuretics, or who are volume-depleted may be at greater risk. D/C and appropriate medical intervention should be instituted in patients with symptomatic hyponatremia. Avoid abrupt discontinuation.

ADVERSE REACTIONS: Diarrhea, N/V, dizziness, dry mouth, insomnia, abnormal dreams, decreased libido, abnormal orgasm, fatigue, arthralgia, dyspepsia, flatulence, gastroenteritis, somnolence, paresthesia.

INTERACTIONS: See Contraindications and Dosage. Avoid with alcohol. May cause serotonin syndrome with other serotonergic drugs (eg, triptans, TCAs, fentanyl, lithium, tramadol, tryptophan, buspirone, St. John's wort) and with drugs that impair metabolism of serotonin; d/c immediately if this occurs. Caution with other CNS-active drugs. Increased risk of bleeding with aspirin (ASA), NSAIDs, warfarin, and other drugs that affect coagulation/bleeding. Strong CYP3A4 inhibitors (eg, ketoconazole) may increase plasma levels. Strong CYP3A4 inducers may decrease systemic exposure. May increase the biotransformation of mephenytoin. May inhibit the biotransformation of CYP2C8 substrates. Increased free concentrations with other highly protein-bound drugs.

PREGNANCY: Category C, caution in nursing.

MECHANISM OF ACTION: SSRI and 5-HT$_{1A}$ receptor partial agonist; has not been established. Thought to enhance serotonergic activity in the CNS through selective inhibition of serotonin reuptake.

PHARMACOKINETICS: Absorption: Absolute bioavailability (72%, with food); C_{max}=156ng/mL (fed), $AUC_{(0-24\ hrs)}$=1645ng•hr/mL (fed), T_{max}=4-5 hrs (median). **Distribution:** Plasma protein binding (96-99%). **Metabolism:** CYP3A4 (primary), CYP2C19, CYP2D6 (minor), and carboxylesterase. **Elimination:** Urine (1% unchanged), feces (2% unchanged); $T_{1/2}$=25 hrs.

NURSING CONSIDERATIONS

Assessment: Assess for history or family history of bipolar disorder, mania/hypomania, history of seizure disorder, volume depletion, pregnancy/nursing status, and possible drug interactions.

Monitoring: Monitor for clinical worsening, suicidality, unusual changes in behavior, serotonin syndrome, abnormal bleeding, activation of mania/hypomania, hyponatremia, discontinuation symptoms, and other adverse reactions.

Patient Counseling: Counsel about benefits and risks of therapy. Advise to monitor for the emergence of suicidal thoughts/behaviors, especially early during treatment and when the dose is adjusted up or down; advise to notify physician if these occur. Instruct not to take with an MAOI or within 14 days of stopping an MAOI, and to allow 14 days after stopping therapy before starting an MAOI. Caution about the risk of serotonin syndrome. Caution about risk of abnormal bleeding with NSAIDs, ASA, warfarin, or other drugs that affect coagulation. Warn patients about using the medication if they have a history of seizure disorder. Advise to observe for signs of activation of mania/hypomania. Counsel not to d/c therapy without notifying physician. Advise of risk of hyponatremia and to avoid alcohol. Instruct to notify physician if an allergic reaction (eg, rash, swelling, difficulty breathing) occurs, if pregnant/plan to become pregnant, or if breastfeeding/plan to breastfeed. Caution about operating hazardous machinery, including automobiles until reasonably certain that therapy does not adversely affect the ability to engage in such activities.

Administration: Oral route. Take with food. **Storage:** 25°C (77°F); excursions permitted to 15-30°C (59-86°F).

VIMOVO   RX
esomeprazole magnesium - naproxen (Horizon)

> NSAIDs may increase risk of serious cardiovascular (CV) thrombotic events, myocardial infarction (MI), and stroke; increased risk with duration of use and with cardiovascular disease (CVD) or risk factors for CVD. Increased risk of serious GI adverse events (eg, bleeding, ulceration, stomach/intestinal perforation) that can be fatal and occur anytime during use without warning symptoms; elderly patients are at greater risk. Contraindicated for the treatment of perioperative pain in the setting of coronary artery bypass graft (CABG) surgery.

THERAPEUTIC CLASS: NSAID/proton pump inhibitor

INDICATIONS: Relief of signs and symptoms of osteoarthritis, rheumatoid arthritis, and ankylosing spondylitis. Decrease the risk of developing gastric ulcers in patients at risk of developing NSAID-associated gastric ulcers.

DOSAGE: *Adults:* 375mg-20mg or 500mg-20mg bid at least 30 min ac. Elderly: Use the lowest effective dose.

HOW SUPPLIED: Tab, Delayed-Release: (Naproxen-Esomeprazole): 375mg-20mg, 500mg-20mg

CONTRAINDICATIONS: History of asthma, urticaria, or allergic-type reactions with aspirin (ASA) or other NSAIDs. Treatment of perioperative pain in the setting of CABG surgery.

WARNINGS/PRECAUTIONS: Use lowest effective dose for the shortest duration possible. Not recommended for initial treatment of acute pain. GI-symptomatic response does not preclude the presence of gastric malignancy. D/C with active and clinically significant bleeding. Naproxen: May cause HTN or worsen preexisting HTN; monitor BP closely. Fluid retention and edema reported; caution with HTN, fluid retention, or heart failure. Caution with history of ulcer disease, GI bleeding, or risk factors for GI bleeding (eg, prolonged NSAID therapy, older age, poor general health status); monitor for GI ulceration/bleeding and d/c if serious GI event occurs. May exacerbate inflammatory bowel disease (IBD). Renal injury reported with long-term use; increased risk with renal/hepatic impairment, hypovolemia, heart failure, salt depletion, and in elderly. Not recommended with advanced renal disease or moderate to severe renal impairment; closely monitor

V

renal function if therapy is initiated. Anaphylactic reactions may occur; avoid with ASA-triad. May cause serious skin adverse events (eg, exfoliative dermatitis, Stevens-Johnson syndrome, toxic epidermal necrolysis); d/c at 1st appearance of rash or any sign of hypersensitivity. May cause elevated LFTs or severe hepatic reactions; d/c if liver disease or systemic manifestations occur, and if abnormal LFTs persist/worsen. Caution with chronic alcoholic liver disease and other diseases with decreased/abnormal plasma proteins if high doses are administered; dosage adjustment may be required. Avoid with severe hepatic impairment; monitor and consider dose reduction with mild to moderate hepatic impairment. Anemia may occur; monitor Hgb/Hct if anemia develops with long-term use. Periodically monitor Hgb if initial Hgb ≤10g and receiving long-term therapy. May inhibit platelet aggregation and prolong bleeding time; monitor patients with coagulation disorders. Caution with asthma and avoid with ASA-sensitive asthma. Avoid use starting at 30 weeks gestation; may cause premature closure of ductus arteriosus. Not recommended in women who have difficulty conceiving, or who are undergoing investigation of infertility. Not a substitute for corticosteroids nor treatment for corticosteroid insufficiency. May mask signs of inflammation and fever. Caution in elderly and debilitated. Esomeprazole: Atrophic gastritis reported with long-term use. May increase risk of *Clostridium difficile*-associated diarrhea (CDAD), especially in hospitalized patients. May increase risk for osteoporosis-related fractures of the hip, wrist, or spine, especially with high-dose (multiple daily doses) and long-term therapy (≥1 yr). Hypomagnesemia reported rarely; consider monitoring magnesium levels prior to and periodically during therapy with prolonged treatment.

ADVERSE REACTIONS: CV thrombotic events, MI, stroke, GI adverse events, flatulence, diarrhea, nausea, abdominal distension, constipation, dyspepsia, upper respiratory tract infection, upper abdominal pain, dizziness, headache.

INTERACTIONS: May enhance methotrexate (MTX) toxicity; use with caution or consider temporary d/c during high-dose MTX administration. Naproxen: Avoid with other naproxen-containing products and NSAIDs; coadministration with ASA not recommended. Risk of renal toxicity when coadministered with diuretics, ACE inhibitors, or angiotensin II receptor antagonists. Diminished antihypertensive effect of ACE inhibitors and β-blockers (eg, propranolol). Delayed absorption with cholestyramine. Caution with cyclosporine; increased risk of nephrotoxicity. Coadministration may decrease efficacy of thiazides and loop (eg, furosemide) diuretics; monitor for signs of renal failure and diuretic efficacy. May increase lithium levels; monitor for toxicity. Increased risk of GI bleeding with oral corticosteroids, anticoagulants (eg, warfarin, dicumarol, heparin), antiplatelets (including low-dose ASA), smoking, alcohol, and drugs that interfere with serotonin reuptake (eg, SSRIs); monitor carefully. Potential interaction with albumin-bound drugs (eg, sulfonylureas, sulfonamides, hydantoins, other NSAIDs). Increased plasma levels with probenecid. Esomeprazole: Concomitant use results in reduced concentrations of the active metabolite of clopidogrel and a reduction in platelet inhibition; avoid concomitant use. Caution with digoxin or other drugs that may cause hypomagnesemia (eg, diuretics). Increased levels of tacrolimus. Drug-induced decrease in gastric acidity results in enterochromaffin-like cell hyperplasia and increased chromogranin A levels; may interfere with investigations for neuroendocrine tumors. May interfere with absorption of drugs where gastric pH is an important determinant of bioavailability (eg, absorption of ketoconazole, iron salts, and erlotinib may decrease, while absorption of digoxin may increase); monitor for digoxin toxicity. Decreased levels of atazanavir and nelfinavir; coadministration not recommended. Monitor for saquinavir toxicity; consider saquinavir dose reduction. May change levels of other antiretrovirals. Monitor for increases in INR and PT with warfarin. May inhibit metabolism of CYP2C19 substrates; decreased clearance of diazepam. Levels may be increased with combined CYP2C19 and 3A4 inhibitor (eg, voriconazole). Increased concentrations of cilostazol; consider dose reduction of cilostazol. Decreased levels with CYP2C19 or 3A4 inducers; avoid with St. John's wort or rifampin.

PREGNANCY: Category C (<30 weeks gestation) and D (≥30 weeks gestation), caution in nursing.

MECHANISM OF ACTION: Naproxen: NSAID; not established. Analgesic and antipyretic activity may be related to prostaglandin synthetase inhibition. Esomeprazole: Proton pump inhibitor; suppresses gastric acid secretion by specific inhibition of the H^+/K^+ ATPase in the gastric parietal cell.

PHARMACOKINETICS: Absorption: Naproxen: Bioavailability (95%); T_{max}=3 hrs. Esomeprazole: Rapid; T_{max}=0.43-1.2 hrs. **Distribution:** Naproxen: V_d=0.16L/kg; plasma protein binding (>99%); found in breast milk. Esomeprazole: V_d=16L (Healthy); plasma protein binding (97%). **Metabolism:** Naproxen: Liver (extensive) via CYP2C9 and CYP1A2 into 6-0-desmethyl naproxen (metabolite). Esomeprazole: Liver (extensive) via CYP2C19 (major) into hydroxyl and desmethyl metabolites, and via CYP3A4 into sulfone (main metabolite). **Elimination:** Naproxen: Urine (95%, <1% unchanged, <1% 6-0-desmethyl naproxen, 66-92% conjugates), feces (≤3%); $T_{1/2}$=15 hrs. Esomeprazole: Urine (80% metabolites, <1% unchanged), feces; $T_{1/2}$=1.2-1.5 hrs.

NURSING CONSIDERATIONS

Assessment: Assess for history of asthma, urticaria, or allergic-type reactions with ASA or other NSAIDs, ASA-triad, CVD, risk factors for CVD, HTN, fluid retention, heart failure, history of ulcer disease, history of/risk factors for GI bleeding, history of IBD, renal/hepatic impairment, coagulation disorders, preexisting asthma, decreased/abnormal plasma proteins, tobacco/alcohol use, pregnancy/nursing status, possible drug interactions, or any other conditions where treatment is contraindicated or cautioned. Obtain baseline BP, CBC with platelet count, coagulation and chemistry profiles.

Monitoring: Monitor for CV and GI events, active bleeding, anaphylactic/hypersensitivity/skin reactions, anemia, bone fractures, hypomagnesemia, and CDAD. Monitor BP, LFTs, renal function, CBC with platelet count, coagulation and chemistry profiles.

Patient Counseling: Inform to seek medical advice if symptoms of CV events (eg, chest pain, SOB, weakness, slurred speech), GI ulceration/bleeding (eg, epigastric pain, dyspepsia, melena, hematemesis), skin/hypersensitivity reactions (eg, rash, blisters, fever, itching), unexplained weight gain or edema, hepatotoxicity (eg, nausea, fatigue, lethargy, pruritus, jaundice, right upper quadrant tenderness, flu-like symptoms), anaphylactic reactions (eg, face/throat swelling, difficulty breathing), and hypomagnesemia (eg, palpitations, dizziness, seizures, tetany) occur, and for diarrhea that does not improve. Inform that medication should be avoided in late pregnancy. Caution against activities requiring alertness if drowsiness, dizziness, vertigo, or depression occurs. Inform to notify physician of history of asthma or ASA-sensitive asthma.

Administration: Oral route. Swallow whole with liquid. Do not split, chew, crush, or dissolve.
Storage: 25°C (77°F); excursions permitted to 15-30°C (59-86°F). Protect from moisture.

VIMPAT   CV
lacosamide (UCB)

THERAPEUTIC CLASS: Sodium channel inactivator

INDICATIONS: (Tab/Sol) Adjunctive therapy in the treatment of partial-onset seizures in patients ≥17 yrs of age with epilepsy. (Inj) Adjunctive therapy in the treatment of partial-onset seizures in patients ≥17 yrs of age with epilepsy when oral administration is temporarily not feasible.

DOSAGE: *Adults:* Partial-Onset Seizures: Initial: 50mg bid (100mg/day). Titrate: May increase at weekly intervals by 100mg/day given as 2 divided doses based on response and tolerability. Maint: 200-400mg/day given as 2 divided doses. Switching from PO to IV Dosing: Initial total daily IV dosage should be equivalent to total daily dosage and frequency of PO dosing and should be infused over 30-60 min. Switching from IV to PO Dosing: May switch at equivalent daily dosage and frequency of IV administration at the end of IV treatment period. Mild or Moderate Hepatic Impairment/Severe Renal Impairment (CrCl ≤30mL/min)/End-Stage Renal Disease (ESRD): Max: 300mg/day. Consider dosage supplementation of up to 50% following a 4-hr hemodialysis treatment. Concomitant Strong CYP3A4 and CYP2C9 Inhibitors with Renal/Hepatic Impairment: Dose reduction may be necessary. Discontinuation: Gradually withdraw over at least 1 week.
Pediatrics: ≥17 Yrs: Partial-Onset Seizures: Initial: 50mg bid (100mg/day). Titrate: May increase at weekly intervals by 100mg/day given as 2 divided doses based on response and tolerability. Maint: 200-400mg/day given as 2 divided doses. Switching from PO to IV Dosing: Initial total daily IV dosage should be equivalent to total daily dosage and frequency of PO dosing and should be infused over 30-60 min. Switching from IV to PO Dosing: May switch at equivalent daily dosage and frequency of IV administration at the end of IV treatment period. Mild or Moderate Hepatic Impairment/Severe Renal Impairment (CrCl ≤30mL/min)/ESRD: Max: 300mg/day. Consider dosage supplementation of up to 50% following a 4-hr hemodialysis treatment. Concomitant Strong CYP3A4 and CYP2C9 Inhibitors with Renal/Hepatic Impairment: Dose reduction may be necessary. Discontinuation: Gradually withdraw over at least 1 week.

HOW SUPPLIED: Inj: 10mg/mL [20mL]; Sol: 10mg/mL [200mL, 465mL]; Tab: 50mg, 100mg, 150mg, 200mg

WARNINGS/PRECAUTIONS: May increase risk of suicidal thoughts or behavior; monitor for emergence/worsening of depression, suicidal thoughts/behavior, and/or any unusual changes in mood/behavior. May cause dizziness and ataxia; may impair physical/mental abilities. Dose-dependent prolongations in PR interval reported. Further PR prolongation is possible when given with other drugs that prolong PR interval. Caution with known conduction problems (eg, atrioventricular block, sick sinus syndrome without pacemaker, Na$^+$ channelopathies [eg, Brugada syndrome]), concomitant medications that prolong PR interval, or with severe cardiac disease (eg, myocardial ischemia, heart failure, structural heart disease); obtain an ECG before therapy and after therapy is titrated to steady state. May predispose to atrial arrhythmias, especially in patients with diabetic neuropathy and/or cardiovascular disease (CVD). Syncope or loss of consciousness reported in patients with diabetic neuropathy. Withdraw gradually over a minimum of 1 week to minimize potential of increased seizure frequency. Multiorgan hypersensitivity reactions (also known as drug reaction with eosinophilia and systemic symptoms [DRESS]) may occur; d/c and start alternative treatment if suspected. Avoid with severe hepatic impairment. Monitor closely during dose titration with coexisting hepatic/renal impairment and in elderly. (Sol) Contains aspartame, a source of phenylalanine.

V

ADVERSE REACTIONS: Headache, N/V, diplopia, dizziness, fatigue, blurred vision, somnolence, tremor, nystagmus, vertigo, diarrhea, balance disorder, ataxia.

INTERACTIONS: Increased exposure with strong CYP3A4 and CYP2C9 inhibitors in patients with renal or hepatic impairment; dose reduction may be necessary.

PREGNANCY: Category C, not for use in nursing.

MECHANISM OF ACTION: Na^+ channel inactivator; has not been established. Selectively enhances slow inactivation of voltage-gated Na^+ channels, resulting in stabilization of hyperexcitable neuronal membranes and inhibition of repetitive neuronal firing.

PHARMACOKINETICS: Absorption: (Oral) Complete; absolute bioavailability (100%); T_{max}=1-4 hrs. **Distribution:** V_d=0.6L/kg; plasma protein binding (<15%). **Metabolism:** CYP3A4/2C9/2C19; O-desmethyl-lacosamide (major metabolite). **Elimination:** Urine (95%), feces (<0.5%); $T_{1/2}$=13 hrs.

NURSING CONSIDERATIONS

Assessment: Assess for hepatic/renal impairment, history of depression, cardiac conduction problems and/or CVD, diabetic neuropathy, phenylketonuria, pregnancy/nursing status, and possible drug interactions. Obtain baseline ECG in patients with known conduction problems, on concomitant medications that prolong PR interval, or with severe cardiac disease.

Monitoring: Monitor for emergence/worsening of depression, suicidal thoughts or behavior and/or any unusual changes in mood or behavior, dizziness, ataxia, PR interval prolongation, syncope or loss of consciousness, DRESS, and other adverse reactions. Obtain an ECG after titration to steady state in patients with known conduction problems, on concomitant medications that prolong PR interval, or with severe cardiac disease.

Patient Counseling: Inform of the benefits/risks of therapy. Instruct to take ud. Counsel patients/caregivers/families about increased risk of suicidal thoughts and behavior and of the need to be alert for emergence or worsening of symptoms of depression, any unusual changes in behavior/mood, or emergence of suicidal thoughts, behavior, or thoughts about self-harm. Instruct to report any behaviors of concern to physician immediately. Inform that dizziness, double vision, abnormal coordination and balance, and somnolence may occur; advise not to engage in hazardous activities (eg, driving/operating complex machinery) until effects of drug are known. Counsel that therapy is associated with ECG changes that may predispose to irregular heartbeat and syncope; if syncope develops, instruct to lay down with raised legs and to contact physician. Instruct to d/c if a serious hypersensitivity reaction is suspected and to promptly report any symptoms of liver toxicity (eg, fatigue, jaundice, dark urine). Advise to notify physician if patient is pregnant/intends to become pregnant, or is breastfeeding. Encourage patients to enroll in the North American Antiepileptic Drug Pregnancy Registry if they become pregnant.

Administration: Oral/IV route. Take with or without food. (Inj) May be administered without further dilution or may be mixed with diluents. Refer to PI for compatibility and stability information. (Sol) Obtain and use calibrated measuring device. **Storage:** 20-25°C (68-77°F); excursions permitted between 15-30°C (59-86°F). (Inj/Sol) Do not freeze. (Inj) Discard any unused portion. (Sol) Discard any unused portion after 7 weeks of 1st opening bottle.

VIRACEPT   RX
nelfinavir mesylate (Agouron)

THERAPEUTIC CLASS: Protease inhibitor

INDICATIONS: Treatment of HIV-1 infection in combination with other antiretroviral agents.

DOSAGE: *Adults:* 1250mg (five 250mg or two 625mg tabs) bid or 750mg (three 250mg tabs) tid. Max: 2500mg/day. Take with a meal. Refer to PI for dosing modifications when used with certain concomitant therapies.
Pediatrics: ≥13 Yrs: 1250mg (five 250mg or two 625mg tabs) bid or 750mg (three 250mg tabs) tid. Max: 2500mg/day. 2-<13 Yrs: (Powder or 250mg Tab) 45-55mg/kg bid or 25-35mg/kg tid. Take with a meal. Refer to PI for dosing guidelines based on age and body weight and when used with certain concomitant therapies.

HOW SUPPLIED: Powder: 50mg/g [144g]; Tab: 250mg, 625mg

CONTRAINDICATIONS: Concomitant use with drugs that are highly dependent on CYP3A for clearance and for which elevated concentrations are associated with serious and/or life-threatening events (eg, alfuzosin, amiodarone, quinidine, dihydroergotamine, ergotamine, methylergonovine, cisapride, lovastatin, simvastatin, pimozide, sildenafil [for treatment of pulmonary arterial HTN], triazolam, oral midazolam), and drugs that may lead to reduced efficacy of nelfinavir (eg, St. John's wort, rifampin).

WARNINGS/PRECAUTIONS: Do not use in patients with moderate or severe hepatic impairment (Child-Pugh B or C, score ≥7). Powder contains phenylalanine; caution with phenylketonuria. New onset or exacerbation of diabetes mellitus (DM), hyperglycemia, and diabetic ketoacidosis reported; initiation or dose adjustments of insulin or oral hypoglycemic agents may be required.

Increased bleeding, including spontaneous skin hematomas and hemarthrosis, in patients with hemophilia type A and B reported. Redistribution/accumulation of body fat reported. Immune reconstitution syndrome reported. Autoimmune disorders (eg, Graves' disease, polymyositis, and Guillain-Barre syndrome) reported in the setting of immune reconstitution and can occur many months after initiation of treatment.

ADVERSE REACTIONS: Diarrhea, nausea, flatulence, rash, abdominal pain, anorexia, leukopenia, neutropenia.

INTERACTIONS: See Contraindications. Avoid with colchicine in patients with renal/hepatic impairment. Not recommended with salmeterol. May increase levels of dihydropyridine calcium channel blockers, indinavir, saquinavir, trazodone, rifabutin, bosentan, colchicine, HMG-CoA reductase inhibitors (eg, atorvastatin, rosuvastatin), immunosuppressants, fluticasone, azithromycin, PDE-5 inhibitors, and CY3A substrates. May decrease levels of delavirdine, phenytoin, methadone, ethinyl estradiol, and norethindrone. CYP3A or CYP2C19 inhibitors, delavirdine, indinavir, ritonavir, saquinavir, cyclosporine, tacrolimus, and sirolimus may increase levels. CYP3A or CYP2C19 inducers (eg, rifampin), omeprazole, nevirapine, carbamazepine, phenobarbital, phenytoin, and rifabutin may decrease levels. May affect warfarin concentrations; monitor INR. Give didanosine 1 hr before or 2 hrs after administration. Coadministration with proton pump inhibitors may lead to a loss of virologic response and development of resistance.

PREGNANCY: Category B, not for use in nursing.

MECHANISM OF ACTION: HIV-1 protease inhibitor; prevents cleavage of gag and gag-pol polyprotein, resulting in production of immature, noninfectious virus.

PHARMACOKINETICS: Absorption: 28 days: (1250mg bid) C_{max}=4mg/L; AUC=52.8mg•hr/L. (750mg tid) C_{max}=3mg/L; AUC=43.6mg•hr/L. 14 days: (1250mg bid) C_{max}=4.7mg/L; AUC=35.3mg•hr/L. **Distribution:** V_d=2-7L/kg; plasma protein binding (>98%). **Metabolism:** Liver via CYP3A, 2C19 (oxidation). **Elimination:** Feces (78% metabolites, 22% unchanged), urine (1-2%); $T_{1/2}$=3.5-5 hrs.

NURSING CONSIDERATIONS

Assessment: Assess for previous hypersensitivity, hepatic impairment, DM, hemophilia, pregnancy/nursing status, and possible drug interactions. Assess for phenylketonuria if planning to use the powder formulation.

Monitoring: Monitor for hypersensitivity reactions, new onset or exacerbation of DM, hyperglycemia, diabetic ketoacidosis, immune reconstitution syndrome, autoimmune disorders, fat redistribution/accumulation, and other adverse reactions. In patients with hemophilia, monitor for bleeding events.

Patient Counseling: Instruct to take drug ud. Inform that therapy is not a cure for HIV and that illnesses associated with HIV may continue. Advise to avoid doing things that can spread HIV to others. Instruct not to alter the dose or d/c therapy without consulting physician. Inform that if a dose is missed, take the dose as soon as possible and then return to normal schedule. Instruct to not double the next dose if a dose is skipped. Instruct to notify physician if using any other prescription, nonprescription medication, or herbal products, particularly St. John's wort. Advise to use alternative or additional contraceptive measures if taking oral contraceptives. Inform that most frequent adverse event is diarrhea, which can usually be controlled with nonprescription drugs (eg, loperamide). Inform that fat redistribution/accumulation may occur. Alert patients with phenylketonuria that powder formulation contains phenylalanine.

Administration: Oral route. If unable to swallow tabs, may dissolve tabs in a small amount of water. Refer to PI for further administration instructions. **Storage:** 15-30°C (59-86°F). (Powder) If mixture is not consumed immediately, store under refrigeration, but must not exceed 6 hrs.

VIRAMUNE XR   RX   V
nevirapine (Boehringer Ingelheim)

> Severe, life-threatening, and in some cases fatal, hepatotoxicity (particularly in the first 18 weeks) and skin reactions (eg, Stevens-Johnson syndrome [SJS], toxic epidermal necrolysis [TEN], hypersensitivity reactions) reported. Increased risk of hepatotoxicity reported in women and patients with higher CD4+ cell counts, including pregnant women. Hepatic failure reported in patients without HIV taking nevirapine for postexposure prophylaxis (PEP). Use for occupational and non-occupational PEP is contraindicated. D/C therapy and seek medical evaluation immediately if hepatitis, transaminase elevations combined with rash or other systemic symptoms, severe skin rash or hypersensitivity reactions develop; do not restart therapy. The 14-day lead-in period with 200mg daily dosing must be followed; may decrease the incidence of rash. Monitor intensively during the first 18 weeks of therapy, especially the first 6 weeks.

OTHER BRAND NAMES: Viramune (Boehringer Ingelheim)

THERAPEUTIC CLASS: Non-nucleoside reverse transcriptase inhibitor

INDICATIONS: Treatment of HIV-1 infection in combination with other antiretrovirals.

DOSAGE: *Adults:* (IR) Usual: 200mg qd for the first 14 days, followed by 200mg bid. (ER) Not Currently Taking IR Tab: One 200mg IR tab qd for first 14 days, followed by one 400mg ER tab qd. Switching from IR Tab to ER Tab: May switch to 400mg ER tab qd without the 14-day lead-in period of IR tab. Dialysis Patients: Add 200mg IR dose after each dialysis treatment. Refer to PI for further dose adjustments.
Pediatrics: (IR) ≥15 Days: Usual: 150mg/m² qd for the first 14 days, followed by 150mg/m² bid. Max: 400mg/day. Refer to PI for sus volume calculation based on BSA and a dose of 150mg/m². (ER) 6-<18 Yrs: Lead-In Period: 150mg/m² qd (IR tab or sus) up to 200mg/day for the first 14 days. After Lead-In Period with IR: BSA ≥1.17m²: 400mg ER tab qd. BSA 0.84-1.16m²: Three 100mg ER tabs qd. BSA 0.58-0.83m²: Two 100mg ER tabs qd. Max: 400mg/day. Dialysis Patients: Add 200mg IR dose after each dialysis treatment. Refer to PI for further dose adjustments.

HOW SUPPLIED: [Immediate-Release (IR)] Sus: 50mg/5mL [240mL], Tab: 200mg*; Tab, Extended-Release (ER): 100mg, 400mg *scored

CONTRAINDICATIONS: Moderate or severe (Child-Pugh Class B or C) hepatic impairment. Use as part of occupational and non-occupational PEP regimens.

WARNINGS/PRECAUTIONS: Not recommended for adult females with CD4⁺ cell counts >250 cells/mm³ or in adult males with CD4⁺ cell counts >400 cells/mm³. Coinfection with hepatitis B or C and/or increased transaminase elevations at the start of therapy may increase risk of later symptomatic events (≥6 weeks after starting therapy) and asymptomatic increases in AST/ALT. Caution with hepatic fibrosis/cirrhosis; monitor for drug-induced toxicity. Rhabdomyolysis reported in some patients with skin and/or liver reactions. Monitor closely if isolated rash of any severity occurs; delay in stopping treatment after the onset of rash may result in a more serious reaction. Do not use as single agent to treat HIV-1 or add on as a sole agent to a failing regimen; resistant virus emerges rapidly when administered as monotherapy. Consider potential for cross-resistance in the choice of new antiretroviral agents to be used in combination with therapy. Take into account the half-lives of the combination antiretroviral drugs when discontinuing the regimen; nevirapine has a long half-life and resistance may develop if antiretrovirals with shorter half-lives are stopped concurrently. Immune reconstitution syndrome, autoimmune disorders (eg, Graves' disease, polymyositis, Guillain-Barre syndrome) in the setting of immune reconstitution, and redistribution/accumulation of body fat reported. Caution in elderly.

ADVERSE REACTIONS: Hepatotoxicity, skin reactions, diarrhea, nausea, headache, fatigue, abdominal pain.

INTERACTIONS: Avoid with atazanavir, boceprevir, telaprevir, ketoconazole, itraconazole, and rifampin. Not recommended with fosamprenavir (without ritonavir), efavirenz, and St. John's wort or St. John's wort-containing products. May alter levels of other non-nucleoside reverse transcriptase inhibitor (NNRTI) (eg, delavirdine, etravirine, rilpivirine); avoid coadministration. Increased incidence and severity of rash with prednisone during the first 6 weeks of therapy; not recommended to prevent nevirapine-associated rash. May increase levels of 14-OH clarithromycin and rifabutin. May increase levels of antithrombotics (eg, warfarin); monitor anticoagulation levels. May decrease levels of CYP3A/2B6 substrates, clarithromycin, ethinyl estradiol, norethindrone, efavirenz, atazanavir, amprenavir, indinavir, lopinavir, methadone, nelfinavir, boceprevir, telaprevir, antiarrhythmics, anticonvulsants, ketoconazole, itraconazole, calcium channel blockers, cancer chemotherapy, ergot alkaloids, immunosuppressants, motility agents, and opiate agonists. Fluconazole may increase levels and rifampin may decrease levels. Refer to PI for further information when used with certain concomitant therapies.

PREGNANCY: Category B, not for use in nursing.

MECHANISM OF ACTION: NNRTI; binds directly to reverse transcriptase and blocks RNA-dependent and DNA-dependent DNA polymerase activities by causing a disruption of the enzyme's catalytic site.

PHARMACOKINETICS: Absorption: Readily absorbed. IR: Absolute bioavailability (93%, tab), (91%, sus); C_{max}=2mcg/mL; T_{max}=4 hrs. ER (single dose): AUC=161,000ng•hr/mL; C_{max}=2060ng/mL; T_{max}=24 hrs (median). **Distribution:** V_d=1.21L/kg (IV, healthy); plasma protein binding (60%). Crosses placenta; found in breast milk. **Metabolism:** Liver (extensive); glucuronide conjugation, oxidative metabolism via CYP3A and CYP2B6. **Elimination:** $T_{1/2}$=45 hrs (single dose), 25-30 hrs (multiple dosing). IR: Urine (81.3%; <3%, parent drug), feces (10.1%).

NURSING CONSIDERATIONS

Assessment: Assess for hepatic fibrosis/cirrhosis, hepatitis B or C coinfection, pregnancy/nursing status, and possible drug interactions. Obtain baseline LFTs. (ER) Assess the ability to swallow tabs in pediatric patients.

Monitoring: Monitor for hepatotoxicity, skin or hypersensitivity reactions, immune reconstitution syndrome, autoimmune disorders, fat redistribution/accumulation, rhabdomyolysis, and other adverse reactions. Perform intensive clinical and lab monitoring, including LFTs, during the first 18 weeks of therapy and frequently throughout treatment. Measure serum transaminases immediately if signs/symptoms of hepatitis, hypersensitivity reactions, and rash develop. Monitor anticoagulation levels with antithrombotics (eg, warfarin).

Patient Counseling: Inform about the risks and benefits of therapy. Inform that severe liver disease/skin reactions may occur. Counsel about signs/symptoms of hepatotoxicity, skin reactions, and other adverse reactions, and advise to d/c and seek medical evaluation immediately if any occur. Inform to take drug as prescribed. Instruct not to alter the dose without consulting physician. Inform that therapy is not a cure for HIV-1 infection and that illnesses associated with HIV-1 infection, including opportunistic infections, may still occur. Advise to avoid doing things that can spread HIV-1 infection to others (eg, sharing needles or other inj equipment, sharing personal items that can have blood or body fluids on them [toothbrush, razor blades], breastfeeding). Instruct not to have any kind of sex without protection; inform to always practice safe sex by using a latex or polyurethane condom to lower the chance of sexual contact with semen, vaginal secretions, or blood. Advise to notify physician of the use of any other prescription/OTC medication, or herbal products, particularly St. John's wort. Inform women taking therapy that hormonal methods of birth control should not be used as the sole method of contraception. Inform that fat redistribution may occur. Inform not to take IR tabs/sus and ER tabs at the same time. (ER) Advise that soft remnants of the drug may be seen in stool.

Administration: Oral route. Take with or without food. (ER) Swallow whole; do not chew, crush, or divide. (Sus) Shake prior to administration. Use an oral dosing syringe, particularly for volumes of ≤5mL. If dosing cup is used, rinse thoroughly with water and the rinse should also be administered. **Storage:** 25°C (77°F); excursions permitted to 15-30°C (59-86°F).

VIREAD   RX
tenofovir disoproxil fumarate (Gilead)

> Lactic acidosis and severe hepatomegaly with steatosis, including fatal cases, reported with the use of nucleoside analogues in combination with other antiretrovirals. Severe acute exacerbations of hepatitis reported in hepatitis B virus (HBV)-infected patients who have discontinued therapy; closely monitor hepatic function with both clinical and lab follow-up for at least several months. If appropriate, resumption of anti-hepatitis B therapy may be warranted.

THERAPEUTIC CLASS: Nucleotide analogue reverse transcriptase inhibitor

INDICATIONS: Treatment of HIV-1 infection in combination with other antiretroviral agents in adults and pediatric patients ≥2 yrs of age. Treatment of chronic hepatitis B in adults and pediatric patients ≥12 yrs of age.

DOSAGE: *Adults:* Chronic Hepatitis B/HIV-1 Infection: ≥35kg: One 300mg tab qd. If unable to swallow tabs, may use 7.5 scoops of oral powder. CrCl ≥50mL/min: One 300mg tab q24h. CrCl 30-49mL/min: One 300mg tab q48h. CrCl 10-29mL/min: One 300mg tab q72-96h. Hemodialysis: One 300mg tab every 7 days or after a total of approximately 12 hrs of dialysis; administer following completion of dialysis.
Pediatrics: Chronic Hepatitis B/HIV-1 Infection: ≥12 Yrs: ≥35kg: One 300mg tab qd. If unable to swallow tabs, may use 7.5 scoops of oral powder. HIV-1 Infection: 2-<12 Yrs: 8mg/kg qd. Max: 300mg/day. ≥17kg and Able to Swallow Intact Tabs: 1 tab qd based on body weight. Refer to PI for dosing recommendations based on body weight.

HOW SUPPLIED: Powder: 40mg/g [60g]; Tab: 150mg, 200mg, 250mg, 300mg

WARNINGS/PRECAUTIONS: Obesity and prolonged nucleoside exposure may be risk factors for lactic acidosis and severe hepatomegaly with steatosis. Caution with known risk factors for liver disease. D/C if findings suggestive of lactic acidosis or pronounced hepatotoxicity develop. Renal impairment (eg, acute renal failure, Fanconi syndrome) reported; assess CrCl prior to initiating and as clinically appropriate during therapy. In patients at risk of renal dysfunction, including patients who have previously experienced renal events while receiving adefovir dipivoxil, assess CrCl, serum phosphorus (P), urine glucose, and urine protein prior to initiation and periodically during therapy. Use only in HIV-1 and HBV coinfected patients as part of an appropriate antiretroviral combination regimen. Before initiating therapy, offer HIV-1 antibody testing to all HBV-infected patients and test all patients with HIV-1 for presence of chronic hepatitis B. Decreased bone mineral density (BMD) and increased biochemical markers of bone metabolism reported; consider assessment of BMD for patients with history of pathologic bone fracture or other risk factors for osteoporosis or bone loss. Osteomalacia associated with proximal renal tubulopathy reported; consider hypophosphatemia and osteomalacia secondary to proximal renal tubulopathy in patients at risk of renal dysfunction who present with persistent or worsening bone or muscle symptoms. Redistribution/accumulation of body fat and immune reconstitution syndrome reported. Autoimmune disorders (eg, Graves' disease, polymyositis, Guillain-Barre syndrome) reported in the setting of immune reconstitution and can occur many months after initiation of treatment. Early virological failure and high rates of resistance substitutions reported with certain regimens that only contain 3 nucleoside reverse transcriptase inhibitors; use triple nucleoside regimens with caution. Caution in elderly.

V

ADVERSE REACTIONS: Lactic acidosis, hepatomegaly with steatosis, N/V, diarrhea, depression, asthenia, headache, pain, rash, abdominal pain, insomnia, pruritus, dizziness, pyrexia.

INTERACTIONS: Avoid with concurrent or recent use of nephrotoxic agents (eg, high-dose or multiple NSAIDs). Do not coadminister with tenofovir disoproxil fumarate (TDF)-containing products or with adefovir dipivoxil. May increase levels of didanosine; d/c didanosine if didanosine-associated adverse reactions develop. Decreases levels of atazanavir; do not coadminister with atazanavir without ritonavir. Lopinavir/ ritonavir, atazanavir with ritonavir, and darunavir with ritonavir may increase levels; d/c treatment if TDF-associated adverse reactions develop. P-glycoprotein and breast cancer resistance protein transporter inhibitors may increase absorption. Coadministration with drugs that reduce renal function or compete for active tubular secretion (eg, cidofovir, acyclovir, valacyclovir, ganciclovir, valganciclovir, aminoglycosides [eg, gentamicin], high-dose or multiple NSAIDs) may increase levels of tenofovir and/or the levels of other renally eliminated drugs. Refer to PI for dosing modifications when used with certain concomitant therapies.

PREGNANCY: Category B, not for use in nursing.

MECHANISM OF ACTION: Nucleotide analogue reverse transcriptase inhibitor; inhibits activity of HIV-1 reverse transcriptase and HBV reverse transcriptase by competing with natural substrate deoxyadenosine 5'-triphosphate and, after incorporation into DNA, by DNA chain termination.

PHARMACOKINETICS: Absorption: Adults: (Fasted) Bioavailability (25%); (Fasted, 300mg single dose) C_{max}=0.30mcg/mL, T_{max}=1 hr, AUC=2.29mcg•hr/mL. Pediatric Patients: (12-<18 yrs of age, 300mg tab) C_{max}=0.38mcg/mL, AUC=3.39mcg•hr/mL; (2-<12 yrs of age, 8mg/kg oral powder) C_{max}=0.24mcg/mL, AUC=2.59mcg•hr/mL. **Distribution:** Plasma protein binding (<0.7%); V_d=1.3L/kg (1mg/kg IV dose), 1.2L/kg (3mg/kg IV dose); found in breast milk. **Elimination:** (Fed, 300mg qd multiple doses) Urine (32%); (Single dose) $T_{1/2}$=17 hrs.

NURSING CONSIDERATIONS

Assessment: Assess for risk factors for lactic acidosis or liver disease, renal dysfunction, pregnancy/nursing status, and possible drug interactions. In patients at risk of renal dysfunction, assess CrCl, serum P, urine glucose, and urine protein. Test for HIV-1 antibody (in HBV-infected patients) and presence of chronic hepatitis B (in patients with HIV-1). Assess BMD in patients with history of pathologic bone fracture or other risk factors for osteoporosis or bone loss.

Monitoring: Monitor for signs/symptoms of lactic acidosis, hepatomegaly with steatosis, hepatotoxicity, renal impairment, bone effects, redistribution/accumulation of body fat, immune reconstitution syndrome (eg, opportunistic infections), autoimmune disorders, and other adverse reactions. Closely monitor hepatic function with both clinical and lab follow-up for at least several months in HBV-infected patients who have discontinued therapy. In patients at risk of renal dysfunction, monitor CrCl, serum P, urine glucose, and urine protein periodically. Periodically monitor weight in pediatric patients to guide dose adjustment.

Patient Counseling: Inform about risks and benefits of therapy. Inform that therapy is not a cure for HIV-1 and patients may continue to experience illness associated with HIV-1 infection (eg, opportunistic infections). Instruct to avoid doing things that can spread HIV or HBV to others (eg, sharing of needles/inj equipment or personal items that can have blood/body fluids on them). Advise to always practice safer sex by using latex or polyurethane condoms. Instruct not to breastfeed. Instruct not to d/c without 1st informing physician. Counsel about the importance of adhering to regular dosing schedule and to avoid missing doses.

Administration: Oral route. (Powder) Measure only with the supplied dosing scoop. Refer to PI for preparation and administration instructions. (Tab) Take without regard to food. **Storage:** 25°C (77°F); excursions permitted to 15-30°C (59-86°F).

VISTIDE

RX

cidofovir (Gilead)

> Renal impairment is the major toxicity. Cases of acute renal failure resulting in dialysis and/or contributing to death reported with as few as 1 or 2 doses; prehydrate with IV normal saline (NS) and administer probenecid with each dose. Monitor renal function (SrCr and urine protein) within 48 hrs prior to each dose. Modify dose with renal function changes. Contraindicated with nephrotoxic agents. Neutropenia reported; monitor neutrophil counts. Carcinogenic, teratogenic, and hypospermatic in animal studies.

THERAPEUTIC CLASS: Viral DNA synthesis inhibitor

INDICATIONS: Treatment of cytomegalovirus (CMV) retinitis in AIDS patients.

DOSAGE: *Adults:* IV: Induction: 5mg/kg once weekly for 2 weeks. Maint: 5mg/kg once every 2 weeks. SrCr 0.3-0.4mg/dL Above Baseline: Reduce maint from 5mg/kg to 3mg/kg D/C with increase in SrCr ≥0.5mg/dL above baseline or ≥3+ proteinuria. Administer probenecid 2g PO 3 hrs before cidofovir, then 1g at 2 hrs and 8 hrs after completion of the 1 hr cidofovir infusion (for a total of 4g). Administer at least 1L 0.9% NS IV over a 1- to 2-hr period immediately before infusion. If tolerated, give 2nd L over a 1- to 3-hr period at start of or immediately after infusion.

HOW SUPPLIED: Inj: 75mg/mL

CONTRAINDICATIONS: Initiation of therapy in patients with SrCr >1.5mg/dL, CrCl ≤55mL/min, or urine protein ≥100mg/dL (≥2+ proteinuria). Nephrotoxic agents (d/c at least 7 days before therapy), history of clinically severe hypersensitivity to probenecid or other sulfa-containing agents, direct intraocular use.

WARNINGS/PRECAUTIONS: Decreased intraocular pressure (IOP) and visual acuity reported; monitor IOP. Decreased serum bicarbonate associated with proximal tubule injury and renal wasting syndrome (including Fanconi's syndrome) reported. Cases of metabolic acidosis in association with liver dysfunction and pancreatitis resulting in death reported. Do not administer doses greater than recommended or exceed frequency or rate of administration. Uveitis or iritis reported; consider treatment with topical corticosteroids with or without topical cycloplegic agents. Monitor for signs and symptoms of uveitis/iritis.

ADVERSE REACTIONS: Renal toxicity, N/V, neutropenia, proteinuria, decreased IOP, uveitis/iritis, pneumonia, dyspnea, infection, fever, creatinine elevation ≥2mg/dL, decreased serum bicarbonate.

INTERACTIONS: See Contraindications.

PREGNANCY: Category C, not for use in nursing.

MECHANISM OF ACTION: Viral DNA synthesis inhibitor; suppresses CMV replication by selective inhibition of viral DNA synthesis.

PHARMACOKINETICS: Absorption: Administration of variable doses (with or without probenecid) resulted in different parameters. **Distribution:** V_d=537mL/kg (without probenecid), 410mL/kg (with probenecid); plasma protein binding (<6%). **Elimination:** Urine (80-100% unchanged).

NURSING CONSIDERATIONS

Assessment: Assess renal function (SrCr and urine protein) within 48 hrs prior to each dose, history of clinically severe hypersensitivity to probenecid or other sulfa-containing agents, pregnancy/nursing status, and possible drug interactions.

Monitoring: Monitor renal function and adjust dose as required. Give IV hydration to patients with proteinuria and repeat test as necessary. Monitor WBC counts with differential (prior to each dose), and neutrophil count. IOP, visual acuity, and ocular symptoms should be monitored periodically.

Patient Counseling: Inform that drug does not cure CMV retinitis and that patient may continue to experience progression of retinitis during and following treatment. Advise to have regular follow-up ophthalmologic examinations. Advise to temporarily d/c zidovudine administration, or decrease zidovudine dose by 1/2, on days of cidofovir administration only. Inform of the major toxicity of the drug. Counsel on importance of completing a full course of probenecid with each cidofovir dose. Warn of potential adverse events caused by probenecid. Inform that drug may cause tumors in humans. Advise men that testes weight reduction and hypospermia may occur and may cause infertility. Inform of embryotoxicity in animal studies; advise women of childbearing potential to use effective contraception during and for 1 month following therapy and for men to practice barrier contraceptive methods during and for 3 months after therapy.

Administration: IV route. Infuse at constant rate over 1 hr. Refer to PI for method of preparation and administration. **Storage:** Vial: 20-25°C (68-77°F). Admixture: Under refrigeration, 2-8°C (36-46°F), for no more than 24 hrs. If refrigerated, allow admixture to equilibrate to room temperature prior to use.

VITRASERT   RX   V
ganciclovir (Bausch & Lomb)

THERAPEUTIC CLASS: Synthetic guanine derivative nucleoside analogue

INDICATIONS: Treatment of cytomegalovirus (CMV) retinitis in patients with AIDS.

DOSAGE: *Adults:* Each implant releases 4.5mg over 5-8 months. Remove and replace when evidence of retinitis progression is seen.
Pediatrics: ≥9 Yrs: Each implant releases 4.5mg over 5-8 months. Remove and replace when evidence of retinitis progression is seen.

HOW SUPPLIED: Implant: 4.5mg

CONTRAINDICATIONS: Hypersensitivity to acyclovir, patients with any contraindications for intraocular surgery (eg, external infection, severe thrombocytopenia).

WARNINGS/PRECAUTIONS: For intravitreal implantation only. Does not provide treatment for systemic CMV disease; monitor for extraocular CMV disease. Potential complications from surgery include vitreous loss or hemorrhage, cataract formation, retinal detachment, uveitis, endophthalmitis, and decrease in visual acuity. May experience immediate and temporary decrease in visual acuity in the implanted eye which lasts for 2-4 weeks postoperatively. Maintain sterility of the surgical field and implant rigorously. Handle implant by the suture tab only to avoid damaging the polymer coatings. Do not resterilize implant by any method. A high level of surgical skill is required for implantation procedure; a surgeon should have observed or assisted in surgical implantation prior to attempting the procedure.

ADVERSE REACTIONS: Visual acuity loss, vitreous hemorrhage, retinal detachments, cataract formation/lens opacities, macular abnormalities, intraocular pressure spikes, optic disk/nerve changes, uveitis, hyphemas.

PREGNANCY: Category C, not for use in nursing.

MECHANISM OF ACTION: Synthetic guanine derivative nucleoside analogue; inhibits replication of herpes viruses.

NURSING CONSIDERATIONS

Assessment: Assess for proper diagnosis of CMV retinitis, any contraindications for intraocular surgery, hypersensitivity to the drug or acyclovir, and pregnancy/nursing status.

Monitoring: Monitor for extraocular CMV disease, vitreous loss or hemorrhage, cataract formation, retinal detachment, uveitis, endophthalmitis, decrease in visual acuity, and other adverse reactions.

Patient Counseling: Advise that implant is not a cure for CMV retinitis; inform that some immunocompromised patients may continue to experience progression of retinitis. Instruct to have ophthalmologic follow-up examinations of both eyes at appropriate intervals after implantation. Counsel about the potential complications following intraocular surgery. Inform that patient will experience immediate and temporary decrease in visual acuity for 2-4 weeks after surgery. Advise that the implant only treats eyes in which it has been implanted. Instruct women of childbearing potential to avoid pregnancy during therapy. Inform that the medication may cause infertility and may be carcinogenic.

Administration: Intravitreal implantation. Refer to PI for handling and disposal procedure.
Storage: 15-30°C (59-86°F). Protect from freezing, excessive heat, and light.

VIVELLE-DOT   RX
estradiol (Novartis)

Estrogens increase the risk of endometrial cancer. Perform adequate diagnostic measures, including endometrial sampling, to rule out malignancy in postmenopausal women with undiagnosed persistent or recurrent abnormal genital bleeding. Should not be used for the prevention of cardiovascular (CV) disease or dementia. Increased risk of myocardial infarction (MI), pulmonary embolism (PE), stroke, invasive breast cancer, and deep vein thrombosis (DVT) in postmenopausal women (50-79 yrs of age) reported. Increased risk of developing probable dementia in postmenopausal women ≥65 yrs of age reported. Should be prescribed at the lowest effective dose and for the shortest duration consistent with treatment goals and risks.

THERAPEUTIC CLASS: Estrogen

INDICATIONS: Treatment of moderate to severe vasomotor symptoms and/or vulvar/vaginal atrophy due to menopause. Treatment of hypoestrogenism due to hypogonadism, castration, or primary ovarian failure. Prevention of postmenopausal osteoporosis.

DOSAGE: *Adults:* Apply patch 2X/week to clean, dry area of the trunk of the body (including the abdomen or buttocks). Rotate application sites with an interval of at least 1 week allowed between applications to a particular site. Vasomotor Symptoms/Vulvar and Vaginal Atrophy: Initial: 0.0375mg/day 2X/week. Osteoporosis Prevention: Initial: 0.025mg/day 2X/week. Adjust dose as necessary. Not Currently on PO Estrogens or Switching from Another Estradiol Transdermal Therapy: May be initiated at once. Currently taking PO Estrogens: Initiate 1 week after withdrawal of PO hormone therapy, or sooner if menopausal symptoms reappear in <1 week. May give continuously in patients with no intact uterus, or cyclically (eg, 3 weeks on followed by 1 week off drug) with intact uterus. Reevaluate periodically (eg, 3- to 6-month intervals) to determine whether treatment is still necessary.

HOW SUPPLIED: Patch: 0.025mg/day, 0.0375mg/day, 0.05mg/day, 0.075mg/day, 0.1mg/day [8*]

CONTRAINDICATIONS: Undiagnosed abnormal genital bleeding, known/suspected/history of breast cancer, known/suspected estrogen-dependent neoplasia, active/history of DVT/PE, active/history of arterial thromboembolic disease (eg, stroke, MI), liver impairment or disease, known protein C, protein S, antithrombin deficiency or other known thrombophilic disorders, known/suspected pregnancy.

WARNINGS/PRECAUTIONS: D/C immediately if stroke, DVT, PE, or MI occur or are suspected. Caution in patients with risk factors for arterial vascular disease and/or venous

V

thromboembolism. If feasible, d/c at least 4-6 weeks before surgery of the type associated with an increased risk of thromboembolism, or during periods of prolonged immobilization. May increase risk of ovarian cancer and gallbladder disease. May lead to severe hypercalcemia in patients with breast cancer and bone metastases; d/c and take appropriate measures if hypercalcemia occurs. Retinal vascular thrombosis reported; d/c pending exam if sudden partial/ complete loss of vision, sudden onset of proptosis, diplopia, or migraine occurs. D/C therapy permanently if exam reveals papilledema or retinal vascular lesions. Consider addition of progestin for women with a uterus or with residual endometriosis post-hysterectomy. May increase BP and thyroid-binding globulin levels. May elevate plasma TGs, leading to pancreatitis in women with preexisting hypertriglyceridemia; consider discontinuation if pancreatitis occurs. Caution with impaired liver function and history of cholestatic jaundice associated with past estrogen use or with pregnancy; d/c in case of recurrence. May cause fluid retention; caution with cardiac/renal impairment. Caution with hypoparathyroidism as estrogen-induced hypocalcemia may occur. May exacerbate endometriosis, asthma, diabetes mellitus, epilepsy, migraine, porphyria, systemic lupus erythematosus, and hepatic hemangiomas; use with caution. May exacerbate symptoms of angioedema in women with hereditary angioedema. May affect certain endocrine and blood components in lab tests.

ADVERSE REACTIONS: Constipation, dyspepsia, nausea, influenza-like illness, pain, nasopharyngitis, sinusitis, upper respiratory tract infection, arthralgia, headache, depression, insomnia, breast tenderness, intermenstrual bleeding, sinus congestion.

INTERACTIONS: CYP3A4 inducers (eg, St. John's wort preparations, phenobarbital, carbamazepine, rifampin) may decrease levels, which may decrease therapeutic effects and/or change uterine bleeding profile. CYP3A4 inhibitors (eg, erythromycin, clarithromycin, ketoconazole, itraconazole, ritonavir, grapefruit juice) may increase levels, which may result in side effects. Patients concomitantly receiving thyroid hormone replacement therapy and estrogens may require increased doses of thyroid replacement therapy; monitor thyroid function.

PREGNANCY: Contraindicated in pregnancy, not for use in nursing.

MECHANISM OF ACTION: Estrogen; binds to nuclear receptors in estrogen-responsive tissues. Circulating estrogens modulate the pituitary secretion of the gonadotropins, luteinizing hormone and follicle-stimulating hormone, through a (-) feedback mechanism. Reduces elevated levels of these hormones in postmenopausal women.

PHARMACOKINETICS: Absorption: Transdermal administration of variable doses resulted in different parameters. **Distribution:** Largely bound to sex hormone-binding globulin and albumin; found in breast milk. **Metabolism:** Liver to estrone (metabolite), estriol (major urinary metabolite); sulfate and glucuronide conjugation (liver), biliary secretion of conjugates into the intestine, hydrolysis (intestine), reabsorption; CYP3A4 (partial metabolism). **Elimination:** Urine (parent compound and metabolites); $T_{1/2}$=5.9-7.7 hrs.

NURSING CONSIDERATIONS

Assessment: Assess for undiagnosed abnormal genital bleeding, presence or history of breast cancer, estrogen-dependent neoplasia, DVT, PE, arterial thromboembolic disease, liver impairment/disease, drug hypersensitivity, pregnancy/nursing status, any other conditions where treatment is contraindicated or cautioned, need for progestin therapy, and for possible drug interactions.

Monitoring: Monitor for signs/symptoms of CV disease, malignant neoplasms, dementia, gallbladder disease, hypercalcemia, visual abnormalities, BP and plasma TGs elevations, pancreatitis, cholestatic jaundice, fluid retention, exacerbation of endometriosis and other conditions, and other adverse reactions. Perform adequate diagnostic measures (eg, endometrial sampling) in postmenopausal women with undiagnosed persistent or recurring genital bleeding. Perform annual breast exam; schedule mammography based on age, risk factors, and prior mammogram results. Reevaluate periodically (eg, 3- to 6-month intervals) to determine whether treatment is still necessary. Regularly monitor thyroid function if patient on thyroid hormone replacement therapy.

Patient Counseling: Inform that therapy may increase the chance of getting uterine cancer, heart attack, stroke, breast cancer, blood clots, and dementia. Instruct to report to physician any breast lumps, unusual vaginal bleeding, changes in speech, severe headaches, chest pain, SOB, leg pains, changes in vision, or vomiting. Advise to notify physician if pregnant or nursing. Instruct to have yearly breast exams by a physician and perform monthly breast self-exams. Instruct to use patch ud.

Administration: Transdermal route. Apply immediately upon removal from the protective pouch. Refer to PI for further application instructions. **Storage:** 25°C (77°F); do not store unpouched.

V

VIVITROL   RX
naltrexone (Alkermes)

> May cause hepatocellular injury with excessive doses. Contraindicated in acute hepatitis or liver failure; caution with active liver disease. Does not appear to be a heptatotoxin at recommended doses. Warn patient of the risk of hepatic injury and advise to seek medical attention if symptoms of acute hepatitis occur. D/C in the event of symptoms and/or signs of acute hepatitis.

THERAPEUTIC CLASS: Opioid antagonist

INDICATIONS: Treatment of alcohol dependence in patients who are able to abstain from alcohol in an outpatient setting prior to initiation of therapy. Prevention of relapse to opioid dependence, following opioid detoxification.

DOSAGE: *Adults:* 380mg IM gluteal inj every 4 weeks or once a month, alternating buttocks.

HOW SUPPLIED: Inj, Extended-Release: 380mg

CONTRAINDICATIONS: Acute hepatitis or liver failure, concomitant opioid analgesics, physiologic opioid dependence, acute opioid withdrawal, (+) urine screen for opioids or failed naloxone challenge test.

WARNINGS/PRECAUTIONS: Cases of eosinophilic pneumonia and hypersensitivity reactions, including anaphylaxis, reported. May precipitate opioid withdrawal in alcohol-dependent patients using or dependent on opioids. Must be opioid-free for a minimum of 7-10 days prior to initiation of therapy. Perform naloxone challenge test if there is a risk of precipitating withdrawal. May respond to lower doses of opioids than previously used. Opioid overdose with fatal outcomes reported in patients who use opioids at the end of a dosing interval or when missing a dose. Attempts to overcome opioid blockade could lead to fatal overdose. Monitor for development of depression or suicidal thinking. In emergency situations, suggested plan for pain management is regional analgesia or use of nonopioid analgesics. If opioid therapy is required, monitor continuously in an anesthesia care setting. Caution in renal/hepatic impairment. Does not eliminate or diminish alcohol withdrawal symptoms. Inj-site reactions reported; inadvertent SQ injection may increase likelihood of severe inj-site reactions. As with any IM inj, caution with thrombocytopenia or any coagulation disorder (eg, hemophilia, severe hepatic failure). May cross-react with certain immunoassay methods for the detection of drugs of abuse in urine.

ADVERSE REACTIONS: N/V, diarrhea, insomnia, depression, inj-site reactions, somnolence, anorexia, muscle cramps, dizziness, syncope, appetite disorder, hepatic enzyme abnormalities, nasopharyngitis, toothache.

INTERACTIONS: See Contraindications. Antagonizes effects of opioid-containing medicines (eg, cough and cold remedies, antidiarrheals, opioid analgesics).

PREGNANCY: Category C, not for use in nursing.

MECHANISM OF ACTION: Opioid antagonist; blocks the effects of opioids by competitive binding at opioid receptors.

PHARMACOKINETICS: Absorption: T_{max}=2-3 days. **Distribution:** Plasma protein binding (21%); (PO) found in breast milk. **Metabolism:** Extensive, via dihydrodiol dehydrogenase, 6β-naltrexol (primary metabolite). **Elimination:** Urine; $T_{1/2}$=5-10 days.

NURSING CONSIDERATIONS

Assessment: Assess for hepatic failure, hepatitis or active liver disease, opioid use or dependence, thrombocytopenia, coagulation disorder (eg, hemophilia, severe hepatic failure), renal impairment, preexisting subclinical abstinence syndrome, hypersensitivity, pregnancy/nursing status, alcohol intake, and for possible drug interactions. Assess patient's body habitus to assure the needle length is adequate.

Monitoring: Monitor for severe inj-site reactions, signs/symptoms of acute hepatitis, unintended opioid withdrawal, opioid intoxication (respiratory compromise/arrest, circulatory collapse), eosinophilic pneumonia, depression, suicidal thinking, and hypersensitivity reactions. Monitor LFTs and CPK.

Patient Counseling: Alert families and caregivers to monitor for emergence of symptoms of depression and to call a physician immediately if observed. Instruct to carry documentation to alert medical personnel to therapy. Warn that concomitant large doses of opioids may lead to serious injury, coma, or death. Inform that if patient previously used opioids, he/she may be more sensitive to lower doses of opioids after naltrexone is discontinued. Instruct to notify if pregnant/nursing or planning to become pregnant, experience respiratory symptoms (eg, dyspnea, coughing, wheezing), or have any allergic reactions. Inform that inj-site reactions may occur and instruct to seek medical attention for worsening skin reactions. Instruct to avoid opioids for ≥7-10 days before therapy and inform physician of any prior opioid use. Inform that may cause liver injury if liver disease develops from other cause. Instruct to notify physician if signs/symptoms of liver disease and pneumonia develop. Inform that therapy treats alcohol dependence only when used as part of treatment program. Inform that may impair mental/physical abilities. Inform that may cause nausea, which tends to subside. Instruct to receive the next dose as soon as possible if a dose is missed.

Administration: IM route; gluteal region. Must be administrated by a healthcare provider. Not for IV/SQ use. Inspect for particulate matter and discoloration prior to use. Refer to PI for preparation and administration instructions. **Storage:** 2-8°C (36-46°F). Do not freeze. Can be stored at <25°C (77°F) for <7 days prior administration.

VOLTAREN GEL   RX
diclofenac sodium (Novartis Consumer)

NSAIDs may cause an increased risk of serious cardiovascular (CV) thrombotic events, myocardial infarction, stroke and serious GI adverse events including bleeding, ulceration, and perforation of the stomach or intestines, which can be fatal. Patients with cardiovascular disease (CVD) or risk factors for CVD may be at greater risk. Elderly patients are at a greater risk for GI events. Contraindicated for the treatment of perioperative pain in the setting of coronary artery bypass graft (CABG) surgery.

THERAPEUTIC CLASS: NSAID

INDICATIONS: Relief of the pain of osteoarthritis of joints amenable to topical treatment, such as knees and hands.

DOSAGE: *Adults:* Lower Extremities: Apply 4g to affected foot, knee, or ankle qid. Max: 16g/day to any single joint. Upper Extremities: Apply 2g to affected hand, elbow, or wrist qid. Max: 8g/day to any single joint. Total dose should not exceed 32g/day over all affected joints.

HOW SUPPLIED: Gel: 1% [100g]

CONTRAINDICATIONS: Asthma, urticaria, or allergic-type reactions after taking aspirin (ASA) or other NSAID, setting of CABG surgery.

WARNINGS/PRECAUTIONS: Not evaluated for use on spine, hip, or shoulder. Avoid open wounds, eyes, mucous membranes, external heat, natural or artificial sunlight and/or occlusive dressings. May lead to onset of new HTN or worsening of preexisting HTN; monitor BP closely. Fluid retention and edema reported; caution with fluid retention or heart failure (HF). Renal papillary necrosis and other renal injury reported after long-term use. Not recommended for use with advanced renal disease; if therapy must be initiated, monitor renal function. Anaphylactoid reactions may occur. May cause serious skin adverse events (eg, exfoliative dermatitis, Stevens-Johnson syndrome [SJS], and toxic epidermal necrolysis [TEN]). Avoid in late pregnancy; may cause premature closure of ductus arteriosus. Not a substitute for corticosteroids or to treat corticosteroid insufficiency. May cause elevations of LFTs; d/c if liver disease develops or systemic manifestations occur. To minimize the potential for adverse liver-related events, use the lowest effective dose for the shortest duration possible. Caution in elderly. Anemia may occur; with long-term use, monitor Hgb/Hct if signs or symptoms of anemia develop. May inhibit platelet aggregation and prolong bleeding time; monitor with coagulation disorders. Caution with asthma and avoid with ASA-sensitive asthma. Caution in patients with prior history of ulcer or GI bleeding; monitor for signs or symptoms of GI bleeding. May diminish utility of diagnostic signs (eg, inflammation, fever) in detecting infectious complications of presumed noninfectious, painful conditions.

ADVERSE REACTIONS: Application-site reactions, dermatitis, ALT/AST increase, GI effects.

INTERACTIONS: May enhance methotrexate toxicity and cyclosporine nephrotoxicity; caution when coadministering. May diminish antihypertensive effect of ACE-inhibitors and impair response of loop diuretics. May reduce natriuretic effect of furosemide and thiazides; monitor for renal failure. May increase lithium levels; monitor for toxicity. Synergistic effects on GI bleeding with anticoagulants (eg, warfarin) reported. Avoid concomitant use with other topical products, including topical medications, sunscreens, lot, moisturizers, and cosmetics, on the same skin site; may alter tolerability and absorption. Coadministration with oral NSAIDs or ASA may result in increased adverse effects; concomitant administration with ASA not recommended. Caution with concomitant hepatotoxic drugs (eg, antibiotics, antiepileptics). May increase risk of GI bleeding with oral corticosteroids/anticoagulants, tobacco or alcohol use.

PREGNANCY: Category C, not for use in nursing.

MECHANISM OF ACTION: NSAID; inhibits cyclooxygenase, resulting in reduced formation of prostaglandins, thromboxanes, and prostacylin.

PHARMACOKINETICS: Absorption: (4g) C_{max}=15ng/mL; T_{max}=14 hrs; AUC_{0-24}=233ng•h/mL. (12g) C_{max}=53.8ng/mL; T_{max}=10 hrs; AUC_{0-24}=807ng•h/mL.

NURSING CONSIDERATIONS

Assessment: Assess for hypersensitivity to ASA or NSAIDs, history of ulcer or GI bleeding, HTN, fluid retention, congestive HF, asthma, CVD (or risk factors), renal/hepatic impairment, pregnancy/nursing status, and for possible drug interactions. Obtain baseline BP.

Monitoring: Monitor for signs/symptoms of CV events, GI events (eg, ulcerations, bleeding), hepatotoxicity, renal dysfunction, HTN, skin reactions, anemia, blood loss and hypersensitivity reactions. Monitor BP, LFTs, and renal function periodically.

Patient Counseling: Instruct to avoid contact with eyes and mucous membranes; instruct that if contact occurs, to wash with water or saline, and if irritation persists for >1 hr, to call physician. Advise to minimize or avoid exposure of treated areas to natural or artificial sunlight. Inform to avoid late in pregnancy. Advise to seek medical attention for symptoms of CV events (eg, chest pain, SOB, weakness, slurring of speech), GI events (eg, epigastric pain, dyspepsia, melena, hematemesis), hepatotoxicity (eg, nausea, lethargy, flu-like symptoms, right upper quadrant pain, pruritus, fatigue), unexplained weight gain or edema, skin reactions (eg, skin rash, blisters, fever, SJS, TEN, exfoliative dermatitis) or hypersensitivity reactions (eg, difficulty breathing, swelling of face/throat); instruct to d/c at 1st appearance of rash/hypersensitivity reactions. Stress the importance of follow-up. Instruct not to apply to open skin wounds, infections, inflammations, or exfoliative dermatitis. Instruct to avoid concomitant use with other topical products.

Administration: Topical route. Measure onto enclosed dosing card to appropriate 2g or 4g line. Avoid showering or bathing for ≥1 hr after application. Avoid wearing clothing or gloves for ≥10 min after application. **Storage:** 25°C (77°F), excursions permitted to 15-30°C (59-86°F). Keep from freezing.

VOLTAREN OPHTHALMIC

RX

diclofenac sodium (Novartis Ophthalmics)

THERAPEUTIC CLASS: NSAID

INDICATIONS: Treatment of postoperative inflammation in patients who have undergone cataract extraction. Temporary relief of pain and photophobia in patients undergoing corneal refractive surgery.

DOSAGE: *Adults:* Cataract Surgery: 1 drop to the affected eye qid beginning 24 hrs after surgery and continue throughout the first 2 weeks of postoperative period. Corneal Refractive Surgery: 1 or 2 drops to the operative eye within the hr prior to, and within 15 min after surgery. Continue qid for up to 3 days.

HOW SUPPLIED: Sol: 0.1% [5mL]

WARNINGS/PRECAUTIONS: Refractive stability in patients undergoing corneal refractive procedures and treated with diclofenac sodium ophthalmic not established; monitor for 1 yr following use. May cause increased bleeding of ocular tissues (including hyphemas) in conjunction with ocular surgery. Potential for cross-sensitivity to acetylsalicylic acid, phenylacetic acid derivatives, and other NSAIDs. May slow or delay healing. May result in keratitis. Continued use may lead to sight-threatening epithelial breakdown, corneal thinning/erosion/ulceration/perforation; d/c if evidence of corneal epithelial breakdown occurs and monitor for corneal health. Caution in patients experiencing complicated ocular surgeries, corneal denervation, corneal epithelial defects, diabetes mellitus (DM), ocular surface disease (eg, dry eye syndrome), rheumatoid arthritis (RA), repeat ocular surgeries within a short period of time or with known bleeding tendencies. Use >24 hrs prior to surgery or beyond 14 days post-surgery may increase risk for occurrence and severity of corneal adverse events. Avoid in late pregnancy. Use of the same bottles that are used in association with surgery for both eyes is not recommended.

ADVERSE REACTIONS: Transient burning/stinging, elevated intraocular pressure, lacrimation disorder, ocular allergy, abnormal vision, conjunctivitis, eyelid swelling, ocular discharge, iritis, eye itching, corneal deposits/edema/opacity/lesions, eye pain.

INTERACTIONS: Caution with other medications that may prolong bleeding time. May increase the potential for healing problems with topical steroids.

PREGNANCY: Category C, not for use in nursing.

MECHANISM OF ACTION: NSAID; demonstrated anti-inflammatory and analgesic properties. Thought to inhibit the enzyme cyclooxygenase, which is essential for biosynthesis of prostaglandins.

NURSING CONSIDERATIONS

Assessment: Assess for hypersensitivity or cross-sensitivity, history of complicated or repeated ocular surgeries, corneal denervation, corneal epithelial defects, DM, ocular surface diseases (eg, dry eye syndrome), RA, bleeding tendencies, pregnancy/nursing status, and possible drug interactions.

Monitoring: Monitor for corneal thinning, erosion, ulceration, or perforation, healing problems, keratitis, increased bleeding time, bleeding of ocular tissues (hyphemas) in conjunction with ocular surgery and other adverse reactions. Patients who have undergone corneal refractive procedures should be monitored for one year following use.

Patient Counseling: Instruct not to use while currently wearing soft contact lenses except for the use of a bandage hydrogel soft contact lens during the first 3 days following refractive surgery.

Administration: Ocular route. **Storage:** 15-25°C (59-77°F).

VOLTAREN-XR RX
diclofenac sodium (Novartis)

> NSAIDs may cause an increased risk of serious cardiovascular (CV) thrombotic events, myocardial infarction (MI), stroke, and serious GI adverse events including inflammation, bleeding, ulceration, and perforation of the stomach or intestines, which may be fatal. Contraindicated for the treatment of perioperative pain in the setting of coronary artery bypass graft (CABG) surgery.

THERAPEUTIC CLASS: NSAID

INDICATIONS: Relief of signs and symptoms of osteoarthritis (OA), and rheumatoid arthritis (RA).

DOSAGE: *Adults:* OA: Usual: 100mg qd. RA: Usual: 100mg qd-bid.

HOW SUPPLIED: Tab, Extended-Release: 100mg

CONTRAINDICATIONS: Aspirin (ASA) or other NSAID allergy that precipitates asthma, urticaria, or allergic-type reactions. Treatment of perioperative pain in the setting of CABG surgery.

WARNINGS/PRECAUTIONS: Use lowest effective dose for the shortest duration possible. Not a substitute for corticosteroids or to treat corticosteroid insufficiency. May lead to onset of new HTN or worsening of preexisting HTN; monitor BP closely. Fluid retention and edema reported; caution with fluid retention or heart failure (HF). Extreme caution with a prior history of ulcer disease, and/or GI bleeding. Caution when initiating treatment in patients with considerable dehydration. Renal papillary necrosis and other renal injury reported after long-term use. Not recommended for use with advanced renal disease; if therapy must be initiated, monitor renal function. Anaphylactoid reactions may occur; avoid in patients with ASA-triad. May cause serious skin adverse events (eg, exfoliative dermatitis, Stevens-Johnson syndrome [SJS], toxic epidermal necrolysis). Avoid in late pregnancy; may cause premature closure of ductus arteriosus. May cause elevations of LFTs; d/c if liver disease develops or systemic manifestations occur. Caution in elderly and debilitated patients. Anemia may occur; with long-term use, monitor Hgb/Hct if signs or symptoms of anemia develop. May inhibit platelet aggregation and prolong bleeding time; monitor with coagulation disorders. Caution with asthma and avoid with ASA-sensitive asthma.

ADVERSE REACTIONS: Abdominal pain, constipation, diarrhea, dyspepsia, flatulence, gross bleeding/perforation, heartburn, N/V, GI ulcers, renal function abnormalities, anemia, dizziness, edema, elevated liver enzymes.

INTERACTIONS: Increased adverse effects with ASA; avoid use. May enhance methotrexate toxicity and increase nephrotoxicity of cyclosporine; caution with coadministration. May diminish antihypertensive effect of ACE inhibitors. Patients taking thiazides and loop diuretics may have impaired response to these therapies. ACE inhibitors and diuretics may precipitate overt renal decompensation. May reduce natriuretic effect of furosemide and thiazides. May increase lithium levels; monitor for toxicity. Synergistic effects with warfarin on GI bleeding. May increase risk of GI bleeding with oral corticosteroids or anticoagulants, tobacco or alcohol use. Caution with hepatotoxic drugs (eg, antibiotics, antiepileptics). Caution with CYP2C9 inhibitors or inducers (eg, voriconazole, rifampin); dosage adjustment may be warranted.

PREGNANCY: Category C, not for use in nursing.

MECHANISM OF ACTION: NSAID; not known, suspected to inhibit prostaglandin synthetase.

PHARMACOKINETICS: Absorption: Absolute bioavailability (55%); T_{max}=5.3 hrs. **Distribution:** V_d=1.4L/kg; plasma protein binding (>99%). **Metabolism:** Liver (glucuronidation and sulfation). **Elimination:** Urine (65%), bile (35%); $T_{1/2}$=2.3 hrs.

NURSING CONSIDERATIONS

Assessment: Assess for CV disease or risk factors, fluid retention, edema, conditions affected by platelet function alterations, GI events or risk factors, renal/hepatic function, any other conditions where treatment is contraindicated or cautioned, pregnancy/nursing status, and possible drug interactions. Assess baseline BP, CBC, and chemistry profile.

Monitoring: Monitor for signs/symptoms of GI events, CV thrombotic events, congestive HF, HTN, allergic or skin reactions, hematological effects (eg, anemia, prolongation of bleeding time), renal papillary necrosis or other renal injury/toxicity, hepatotoxicity. Monitor BP, CBC, and chemistry profile periodically.

Patient Counseling: Advise to seek medical attention if signs and symptoms of hepatotoxicity, anaphylactic/anaphylactoid reactions, skin reactions, CV events, GI ulceration or bleeding, weight gain, or edema occur. Inform of pregnancy risks and instruct to avoid use during late pregnancy.

Administration: Oral route. **Storage:** Protect from moisture. Do not store above 30°C (86°F).

VOTRIENT

RX

pazopanib (GlaxoSmithKline)

Severe and fatal hepatotoxicity reported; monitor hepatic function and interrupt, reduce, or d/c dosing as recommended.

THERAPEUTIC CLASS: Tyrosine kinase inhibitor

INDICATIONS: Treatment of advanced renal cell carcinoma (RCC). Treatment of advanced soft tissue sarcoma (STS) that has been treated with prior chemotherapy.

DOSAGE: *Adults:* Usual: 800mg qd without food (at least 1 hr ac or 2 hrs pc). Max: 800mg. Dose Modification: RCC: Initial dose reduction should be 400mg, and additional decrease or increase in dose should be in 200mg steps based on tolerability. STS: Decrease or increase should be in 200mg steps based on tolerability. Moderate Hepatic Impairment: Consider alternative therapy or reduce to 200mg/day. Concomitant Strong CYP3A4 Inhibitors (eg, ketoconazole, ritonavir, clarithromycin): Consider an alternate concomitant medication with no or minimal potential to inhibit CYP3A4. If coadministration is warranted, reduce to 400mg. Further dose reductions may be needed if adverse effects occur during therapy. Missed Dose: If a dose is missed, do not take if <12 hrs until the next dose.

HOW SUPPLIED: Tab: 200mg

WARNINGS/PRECAUTIONS: Avoid with preexisting severe hepatic impairment (total bilirubin >3X ULN with any level of ALT). QT prolongation and torsades de pointes reported; caution with history of QT interval prolongation, and relevant preexisting cardiac disease. Cardiac dysfunction (eg, decreased left ventricular ejection fraction [LVEF], congestive heart failure [CHF]) reported; perform baseline and periodic evaluation of LVEF in patients at risk for cardiac dysfunction (eg, previous anthracycline exposure). Monitor BP and manage promptly using a combination of antihypertensives and dose modification of therapy. Hemorrhagic events reported; avoid with history of hemoptysis, cerebral, or clinically significant GI hemorrhage in the past 6 months. Arterial thromboembolic events (eg, myocardial infarction [MI], ischemia, cerebrovascular accident [CVA], transient ischemic attack [TIA]) reported; caution in patients at increased risk for these events or who have had a history of these events and avoid use if an arterial thromboembolic event has occurred within the past 6 months. Venous thromboembolic events (VTE) (eg, venous thrombosis, pulmonary embolus [PE]), and GI perforation/fistula reported. Thrombotic microangiopathy (TMA), including thrombotic thrombocytopenic purpura (TTP) and hemolytic uremic syndrome (HUS) reported; permanently d/c if TMA occurs. Reversible posterior leukoencephalopathy syndrome (RPLS) reported; permanently d/c if RPLS develops. HTN and hypertensive crisis reported; d/c if evidence of hypertensive crisis or if HTN is severe and persistent despite antihypertensive therapy and dose reduction. May impair wound healing; d/c therapy with wound dehiscence and at least 7 days prior to scheduled surgery. Hypothyroidism and proteinuria reported. Interrupt therapy and reduce dose for 24-hr urine protein ≥3g; d/c for repeat episodes despite dose reductions. Serious infections reported; institute appropriate anti-infective therapy promptly and consider interruption or discontinuation if serious infections develop. May cause serious adverse effects on organ development in pediatric patients; not for use in pediatric patients. May cause fetal harm if used during pregnancy.

ADVERSE REACTIONS: Hepatotoxicity, diarrhea, HTN, hair color changes, N/V, anorexia, fatigue, asthenia, headache, weight/appetite decreased, tumor pain, dysgeusia, dyspnea, musculoskeletal pain, skin hypopigmentation.

INTERACTIONS: See dosage. Do not use in combination with other cancer therapy; increased toxicity and mortality reported with pemetrexed and lapatinib. Strong inhibitors of CYP3A4 (eg, ketoconazole, ritonavir, clarithromycin) may increase concentrations; avoid use and consider an alternate concomitant medication with no or minimal potential to inhibit CYP3A4, or reduce dose of pazopanib when it must be coadministered. Avoid grapefruit or grapefruit juice. CYP3A4 inducers (eg, rifampin) may decrease plasma concentrations; consider an alternate concomitant medication with no or minimal enzyme induction potential and avoid pazopanib if chronic use of strong CYP3A4 inducers cannot be avoided. Avoid use with strong inhibitors of P-glycoprotein (P-gp) or breast cancer resistance protein (BCRP), or consider alternative concomitant medicinal products with no or minimal potential to inhibit P-gp or BCRP. Not recommended with agents with narrow therapeutic windows that are metabolized by CYP3A4, CYP2D6, or CYP2C8. Simvastatin may increase incidence of ALT elevations; follow dosing guidelines or consider alternatives to pazopanib or consider to d/c simvastatin. Caution in patients taking antiarrhythmics or other medications that may prolong the QT interval.

PREGNANCY: Category D, not for use in nursing.

MECHANISM OF ACTION: Tyrosine kinase inhibitor; inhibits vascular endothelial growth factor receptor (VEGFR)-1, VEGFR-2, VEGFR-3, platelet-derived growth factor receptor (PDGFR)-α and -β, fibroblast growth factor receptor (FGFR)-1 and -3, cytokine receptor (Kit), interleukin-2 receptor inducible T-cell kinase (Itk), leukocyte-specific protein tyrosine kinase (Lck), and trans-membrane glycoprotein receptor tyrosine kinase (c-Fms).

PHARMACOKINETICS: Absorption: T_{max}=2-4 hrs (median); (800mg dose) AUC=1037mcg•hr/mL, C_{max}=58.1mcg/mL. **Distribution:** Plasma protein binding (>99%). **Metabolism:** CYP3A4 (major), CYP1A2/CYP2C8 (minor). **Elimination:** Feces (primary), urine (<4% administered dose); (800mg dose) $T_{1/2}$=30.9 hrs.

NURSING CONSIDERATIONS

Assessment: Assess for history of QT interval prolongation, cardiac disease, severe hepatic impairment, pregnancy/nursing status, and for possible drug interactions. Assess for history of hemoptysis/cerebral or clinically significant GI hemorrhage, or an arterial thromboembolic event in the past 6 months. Assess if patient is planning to undergo any surgical procedure. Assess thyroid function. Obtain baseline BP, LFTs, ECG, and urinalysis. Obtain baseline LVEF in patients at risk of cardiac dysfunction.

Monitoring: Monitor for signs/symptoms of hepatotoxicity, QT prolongation, torsades de pointes, cardiac dysfunction, hemorrhagic events, arterial thromboembolic events, VTE, TMA, TTP, HUS, PE, RPLS, GI perforation or fistula, HTN/hypertensive crisis, impaired wound healing, proteinuria, infections, and other adverse reactions. Monitor BP early after starting treatment and then frequently to ensure BP control. Perform periodic urinalysis with follow-up measurement of 24-hr urine protein as clinically indicated. Monitor ECG, thyroid function tests, and serum electrolytes. Monitor LFTs at Weeks 3, 5, 7, and 9, at Months 3 and 4, as clinically indicated, and continue periodic monitoring after Month 4. Periodically monitor LVEF in patients at risk of cardiac dysfunction.

Patient Counseling: Advise that lab monitoring will be required prior to and while on therapy. Instruct to report any signs/symptoms of liver dysfunction, HTN, CHF, unusual bleeding, arterial thrombosis, new onset of dyspnea, chest pain, localized limb edema, GI perforation/fistula, infection, and worsening of neurologic function consistent with RPLS (eg, headache, seizure, lethargy, confusion, blindness). Advise to d/c treatment at least 7 days prior to a scheduled surgery. Inform that thyroid function testing and urinalysis will be performed during treatment. Advise on how to manage diarrhea and to notify healthcare provider if moderate to severe diarrhea occurs. Advise women of childbearing potential to avoid becoming pregnant during therapy. Advise to inform healthcare provider of all concomitant medications, vitamins, or dietary and herbal supplements. Advise that depigmentation of the hair or skin may occur during treatment. Instruct that if a dose is missed, do not take if it is <12 hrs until the next dose.

Administration: Oral route. Do not crush tabs. Take without food (at least 1 hr ac or 2 hrs pc). **Storage:** 20-25°C (68-77°F); excursions permitted to 15-30°C (59-86°F).

VYTORIN   RX
ezetimibe - simvastatin (Merck)

THERAPEUTIC CLASS: Cholesterol absorption inhibitor/HMG-CoA reductase inhibitor

INDICATIONS: Adjunct to diet to: Reduce elevated total cholesterol (total-C), LDL, apolipoprotein B, TG, non-HDL, and to increase HDL in patients with primary (heterozygous familial and nonfamilial) hyperlipidemia or mixed hyperlipidemia. Reduce elevated total-C and LDL in patients with homozygous familial hypercholesterolemia (HoFH), as an adjunct to other lipid-lowering treatments (eg, LDL apheresis) or if such treatments are unavailable.

DOSAGE: *Adults:* Initial: 10mg-10mg or 10mg-20mg qpm. Usual: 10mg-10mg to 10mg-40mg qpm. LDL Reduction (>55%): Initial: 10mg-40mg qpm. After initiation or titration, analyze lipid levels after ≥2 weeks and adjust dose, if needed. Restricted Dosing: Use 10mg-80mg dose only in patients who have been taking 10mg-80mg dose chronically (eg, for ≥12 months) without evidence of muscle toxicity. If currently tolerating 10mg-80mg dose and needs to be initiated on drug that is contraindicated or is associated with a dose cap for simvastatin, switch to an alternative statin or statin-based regimen with less potential for drug-drug interaction. Do not titrate to 10mg-80mg, but place on alternative LDL lowering treatment that provides greater LDL lowering, if unable to achieve LDL goal with 10mg-40mg dose. HoFH: Usual: 10mg-40mg qpm. HoFH with Concomitant Lomitapide: Reduce dose by 50% if initiating lomitapide. Max: 10mg-20mg/day (or 10mg-40mg/day for patients who have previously taken simvastatin 80mg/day chronically [eg, for ≥12 months] without evidence of muscle toxicity). Concomitant Verapamil/Diltiazem/Dronedarone: Max: 10mg-10mg qd. Concomitant Amiodarone/Amlodipine/Ranolazine: Max: 10mg-20mg qd. Concomitant Bile Acid Sequestrants: Take either ≥2 hrs before or ≥4 hrs after bile acid sequestrant. Chinese Patients Taking Lipid-Modifying Doses (≥1g/day Niacin) of

V

Niacin-Containing Products: Caution with doses >10mg-20mg qd; do not give 10mg-80mg dose. Chronic Kidney Disease (GFR <60mL/min): 10mg-20mg qpm.

HOW SUPPLIED: Tab: (Ezetimibe-Simvastatin) 10mg-10mg, 10mg-20mg, 10mg-40mg, 10mg-80mg

CONTRAINDICATIONS: Concomitant administration of strong CYP3A4 inhibitors (eg, itraconazole, ketoconazole, posaconazole, voriconazole, HIV protease inhibitors, boceprevir, telaprevir, erythromycin, clarithromycin, telithromycin, nefazodone, cobicistat-containing products), gemfibrozil, cyclosporine, or danazol. Active liver disease or unexplained persistent elevations in hepatic transaminases, women who are or may become pregnant, and nursing mothers.

WARNINGS/PRECAUTIONS: Myopathy (including immune-mediated necrotizing myopathy [IMNM]) and rhabdomyolysis reported; predisposing factors include advanced age (≥65 yrs of age), female gender, uncontrolled hypothyroidism, and renal impairment. Risk of myopathy, including rhabdomyolysis, is dose related and greater with simvastatin 80mg. D/C if markedly elevated CPK levels occur or myopathy is suspected/diagnosed, and temporarily withhold if experiencing an acute or serious condition predisposing to development of renal failure secondary to rhabdomyolysis. Increases in serum transaminases reported; perform LFTs before initiation and as indicated thereafter. Fatal and nonfatal hepatic failure (rare) reported; promptly interrupt therapy if serious liver injury with clinical symptoms and/or hyperbilirubinemia or jaundice occurs and do not restart if no alternate etiology found. Caution with history of liver disease, substantial alcohol consumption, and in elderly. Increases in HbA1c and FPG levels reported. Use doses >10mg-20mg with caution and close monitoring in patients with moderate to severe renal impairment.

ADVERSE REACTIONS: Headache, increased ALT, myalgia, upper respiratory tract infection, diarrhea.

INTERACTIONS: See Contraindications and Dosage. Due to the risk of myopathy/rhabdomyolysis, avoid grapefruit juice and caution with fenofibrates (eg, fenofibrate, fenofibric acid), lipid-modifying doses (≥1g/day) of niacin, colchicine, verapamil, diltiazem, dronedarone, lomitapide, amiodarone, amlodipine, and ranolazine. If coadministered with a fenofibrate, immediately d/c both agents if myopathy is suspected/diagnosed, and perform gallbladder studies/consider alternative lipid-lowering therapy if cholelithiasis is suspected. Simvastatin may slightly elevate plasma digoxin concentrations; monitor patients taking digoxin when therapy is initiated. Reduced ezetimibe levels with cholestyramine; incremental LDL reduction may be reduced. Simvastatin may potentiate effect of coumarin anticoagulants; determine PT before initiation and frequently during therapy. Increased INR reported when ezetimibe was added to warfarin.

PREGNANCY: Category X, not for use in nursing.

MECHANISM OF ACTION: Ezetimibe: Cholesterol absorption inhibitor. Reduces blood cholesterol by inhibiting absorption of cholesterol by the small intestine. Targets the sterol transporter, Niemann-Pick C1-Like 1, which is involved in intestinal uptake of cholesterol and phytosterols. Simvastatin: HMG-CoA reductase inhibitor. Inhibits conversion of HMG-CoA to mevalonate. Also reduces VLDL, TG, and increases HDL.

PHARMACOKINETICS: Absorption: Simvastatin: Bioavailability (<5% as β-hydroxyacid). **Distribution:** Plasma protein binding: Ezetimibe: (>90%). Simvastatin: (95%). **Metabolism:** Ezetimibe: Small intestine, liver via glucuronide conjugation; ezetimibe-glucuronide (active metabolite). Simvastatin: Liver (extensive 1st pass), by hydrolysis via CYP3A4; β-hydroxyacid, 6'-hydroxy, 6'-hydroxymethyl, and 6'-exomethylene (major active metabolites). **Elimination:** Ezetimibe: Feces (78%, 69% ezetimibe), urine (11%, 9% ezetimibe-glucuronide); $T_{1/2}$=22 hrs. Simvastatin: Feces (60%), urine (13%).

NURSING CONSIDERATIONS

Assessment: Assess for history of or active liver disease, unexplained persistent hepatic transaminase elevations, predisposing factors for myopathy, renal impairment, alcohol consumption, drug hypersensitivity, pregnancy/nursing status, possible drug interactions, and any other conditions where treatment is contraindicated or cautioned. Assess lipid profile and LFTs.

Monitoring: Monitor for signs/symptoms of myopathy (including IMNM), rhabdomyolysis, liver dysfunction, increases in HbA1c and FPG levels, and other adverse reactions. Monitor lipid profile, and LFTs. Check PT with coumarin anticoagulants.

Patient Counseling: Inform of benefits/risks of therapy. Advise to adhere to the National Cholesterol Education Program recommended diet, a regular exercise program, and periodic testing of a fasting lipid panel. Inform about substances that should be avoided during therapy, and advise to discuss all medications, both Rx and OTC, with physician. Instruct to report promptly any unexplained muscle pain, tenderness, or weakness, particularly if accompanied by malaise or fever or if these muscle signs or symptoms persist after discontinuation, or any symptoms that may indicate liver injury. Inform patients using the 10mg-80mg dose that the risk of myopathy, including rhabdomyolysis, is increased. Instruct women to use an effective method of birth control to prevent pregnancy while on therapy, to d/c therapy and call physician if pregnant, and not to breastfeed while on therapy.

Administration: Oral route. Take qpm with or without food. **Storage:** 20-25°C (68-77°F).

VYVANSE
lisdexamfetamine dimesylate (Shire)

> CNS stimulants (amphetamines and methylphenidate-containing products) have a high potential for abuse and dependence. Assess the risk of abuse prior to prescribing and monitor for signs of abuse and dependence while on therapy.

THERAPEUTIC CLASS: Sympathomimetic amine

INDICATIONS: Treatment of attention-deficit hyperactivity disorder.

DOSAGE: *Adults:* Initial: 30mg qam. Titrate: May adjust in increments of 10mg or 20mg at weekly intervals. Max: 70mg/day. Elderly: Start at lower end of dosing range.
Pediatrics: ≥6 Yrs: Initial: 30mg qam. Titrate: May adjust in increments of 10mg or 20mg at weekly intervals. Max: 70mg/day.

HOW SUPPLIED: Cap: 20mg, 30mg, 40mg, 50mg, 60mg, 70mg

CONTRAINDICATIONS: Concurrent use with an MAOI or use within 14 days of the last MAOI dose.

WARNINGS/PRECAUTIONS: Sudden death, stroke, and myocardial infarction (MI) reported in adults. Sudden death reported in children and adolescents with structural cardiac abnormalities and other serious heart problems. Avoid use in patients with known structural cardiac abnormalities, cardiomyopathy, serious heart arrhythmia, coronary artery disease, and other serious heart problems. May cause increase in BP and HR; monitor for potential tachycardia and HTN. May exacerbate symptoms of behavior disturbance and thought disorder in patients with a preexisting psychotic disorder. May induce a mixed/manic episode in patients with bipolar disorder; screen for risk factors for developing a manic episode prior to treatment. May cause psychotic or manic symptoms (eg, hallucinations, delusional thinking, mania) in children and adolescents without a prior history of psychotic illness or mania; consider discontinuation if symptoms occur. Associated with weight loss and slowing of growth rate in pediatric patients; closely monitor growth (weight and height). Associated with peripheral vasculopathy, including Raynaud's phenomenon, which generally improves after dose reduction or discontinuation; observe carefully for digital changes during treatment.

ADVERSE REACTIONS: Appetite decreased, insomnia, upper abdominal pain, irritability, N/V, weight decreased, dry mouth, dizziness, affect lability, rash, diarrhea, anxiety, anorexia, jittery feeling, agitation.

INTERACTIONS: See Contraindications. Urinary acidifying agents (eg, ascorbic acid) increase urinary excretion and decrease the $T_{1/2}$ of the amphetamine, while urinary alkalinizing agents (eg, sodium bicarbonate) decrease urinary excretion and extend the $T_{1/2}$ of the amphetamine; adjust dose accordingly.

PREGNANCY: Category C, not for use in nursing.

MECHANISM OF ACTION: Sympathomimetic amine; CNS stimulant. Prodrug of dextroamphetamine. Blocks the reuptake of norepinephrine and dopamine into the presynaptic neuron and increases the releases of these monoamines into the extraneuronal space.

PHARMACOKINETICS: Absorption: Rapid; T_{max}=1 hr (lisdexamfetamine), 3.5 hrs (dextroamphetamine). **Distribution:** Found in breast milk. **Metabolism:** Hydrolysis by RBC; dextroamphetamine (active metabolite). **Elimination:** Urine (96%; 42% amphetamine, 2% unchanged), feces (0.3%); $T_{1/2}$=<1 hr.

NURSING CONSIDERATIONS

Assessment: Assess for presence of cardiac disease (eg, a careful history, family history of sudden death or ventricular arrhythmia, and physical exam), risk of abuse, risk factors for developing a manic episode, psychosis, bipolar disorder, hypersensitivity to the drug or amphetamine products, pregnancy/nursing status, and possible drug interactions.

Monitoring: Monitor for signs of abuse and dependence; periodically reevaluate the need for therapy. Monitor for potential tachycardia, HTN, exacerbation of preexisting psychosis (eg, behavior disturbance, thought disorder), psychotic or manic symptoms (eg, hallucinations, delusional thinking, mania) in children and adolescents, and other adverse reactions. Monitor height and weight in pediatric patients. Further evaluate patients who develop exertional chest pain, unexplained syncope, or arrhythmias. Observe carefully for signs/symptoms of peripheral vasculopathy (eg, digital changes); further clinical evaluation (eg, rheumatology referral) may be appropriate for certain patients.

Patient Counseling: Inform about benefits/risks of treatment, appropriate use, and drug abuse/dependence risk. Advise about serious cardiovascular risks; instruct to contact physician immediately if symptoms of cardiac disease develop. Instruct to monitor for elevations of BP and pulse rate. Inform that treatment-emergent psychotic or manic symptoms may occur. Instruct

V

parents or guardians of pediatric patients that therapy may cause slowing of growth, including weight loss. Advise to notify physician if pregnant or planning to become pregnant and to avoid breastfeeding. Inform that therapy may impair ability of engaging in dangerous activities; instruct patients to assess how the medication affects them before performing dangerous tasks. Inform about the risk of peripheral vasculopathy, including Raynaud's phenomenon; instruct to report to physician any new numbness, pain, skin color change, or sensitivity to temperature in fingers or toes, and to call physician immediately if any signs of unexplained wounds appear on fingers or toes while on therapy.

Administration: Oral route. Take in am with or without food; avoid afternoon doses. May swallow caps whole or empty contents in a glass of water; refer to PI for further instructions. **Storage:** 25°C (77°F); excursions permitted to 15-30°C (59-86°F).

WELCHOL   RX
colesevelam HCl (Daiichi Sankyo)

THERAPEUTIC CLASS: Bile acid sequestrant

INDICATIONS: As monotherapy or in combination with a statin to reduce LDL-C levels in boys and postmenarchal girls 10-17 yrs old with heterozygous familial hypercholesterolemia if after an adequate trial of diet therapy, LDL-C remains ≥190mg/dL or ≥160mg/dL and there is a positive family history of premature cardiovascular disease (CVD), or ≥2 other CVD risk factors are present. (Adults) Adjunct to diet and exercise to reduce elevated LDL-C with primary hyperlipidemia (Fredrickson Type IIa) as monotherapy or with an HMG-CoA reductase inhibitor. Adjunct to diet and exercise to improve glycemic control with type 2 diabetes mellitus (DM).

DOSAGE: *Adults:* Hyperlipidemia/Type 2 DM: (Tab) 3 tabs bid or 6 tabs qd. Take with meal and liquid. (Sus) 3.75g qd or 1.875g bid in 4-8 oz. of water, fruit juice, or diet soft drinks. Stir well and drink. Take with meals. May be dosed at the same time as a statin or the 2 drugs can be dosed apart.
Pediatrics: 10-17 Yrs: Hyperlipidemia: (Sus) 3.75g qd or 1.875g bid in 4-8 oz. of water, fruit juice, or diet soft drinks. Stir well and drink. Take with meals. May be dosed at the same time as a statin or the 2 drugs can be dosed apart.

HOW SUPPLIED: Sus: 1.875g, 3.75g [pkt]; Tab: 625mg

CONTRAINDICATIONS: Serum TG concentrations >500mg/dL, history of hypertriglyceridemia-induced pancreatitis or bowel obstruction.

WARNINGS/PRECAUTIONS: May increase serum TG concentrations; d/c if TG levels >500mg/dL or if hypertriglyceridemia-induced pancreatitis develops. Caution in patients with TG levels >300mg/dL or with susceptibility to deficiencies of vitamin K (eg, malabsorption syndromes, patients on warfarin) or other fat-soluble vitamins. May cause constipation; avoid with gastroparesis, GI motility disorders, those who have had major GI tract surgery, or at risk for bowel obstruction. Has not been studied in type 2 DM as monotherapy or in combination with dipeptidyl peptidase 4 inhibitors or thiazolidinediones, and in Fredrickson Type I, III, IV, or V dyslipidemias. Not for treatment of type 1 DM or diabetic ketoacidosis. (Sus) Contains phenylalanine, caution with phenylketonurics. Always mix with water, fruit juice, or soft drinks to avoid esophageal distress; do not take in its dry form. (Tab) Caution in patients with dysphagia or swallowing disorders.

ADVERSE REACTIONS: Asthenia, cardiovascular events, constipation, dyspepsia, nausea, rhinitis, fatigue, flu syndrome, nasopharyngitis, hypoglycemia, hypertriglyceridemia, headache, influenza, pharyngitis, upper respiratory tract infection.

INTERACTIONS: May increase TG levels with insulin or sulfonylureas. May decrease absorption of vitamins A, D, E, and K. Give drugs known to have reduced GI absorption when given concomitantly and those that have not been tested for interaction, especially those with narrow therapeutic index, at least 4 hours prior to colesevelam. May increase seizure activity or decrease phenytoin levels. May elevate TSH in patients receiving thyroid hormone replacement therapy. May increase levels of metformin extended-release. May decrease levels of cyclosporine, glimepiride, glipizide, glyburide, levothyroxine, olmesartan medoxomil, repaglinide, verapamil sustained-release, and oral contraceptives containing ethinyl estradiol and norethindrone. Concomitant use with warfarin decreases INR; monitor INR.

PREGNANCY: Category B, safety not known in nursing.

MECHANISM OF ACTION: Bile acid sequestrant; non-absorbed, lipid-lowering polymer that binds bile acids in intestine, impeding their reabsorption. Consequently, compensatory effects lead to increased LDL-C clearance from blood, resulting in decreased serum LDL-C levels. Mechanism unknown in the treatment of DM.

PHARMACOKINETICS: Absorption: Not hydrolyzed by digestive enzymes and not absorbed. **Distribution:** Limited to GI tract. **Excretion:** Urine (0.05%).

NURSING CONSIDERATIONS

Assessment: Assess for history/risk of bowel obstruction, gastroparesis or other GI motility disorders, history of major GI tract surgery or hypertriglyceridemia-induced pancreatitis, susceptibility to deficiencies of vitamin K or other fat soluble vitamins, dysphagia or swallowing disorders, pregnancy/nursing status, and possible drug interactions. Obtain baseline lipid parameters (eg, TG, non-HDL-C).

Monitoring: Monitor for hypertriglyceridemia-induced pancreatitis, hypoglycemia, dysphagia, esophageal obstruction, and other adverse events. Periodically monitor lipid profile (eg, TG, non-HDL-C), blood glucose, and coadministered drug levels.

Patient Counseling: Instruct to take with meal and liquid. Inform to take drugs that may interact (eg, cyclosporine, glyburide, levothyroxine, oral contraceptives) at least 4 hrs prior. Advise to consume diet that promotes bowel regularity. Instruct to promptly d/c and seek medical attention if severe abdominal pain/constipation, or symptoms of acute pancreatitis (eg, severe abdominal pain with or without N/V) occur. Counsel to adhere to the recommended diet of the National Cholesterol Education Program, to dietary instructions, regular exercise program, and regular testing of blood glucose. Advise to notify physician if with dysphagia or swallowing disorders. (Sus) Instruct to empty entire contents of 1 pkt into a glass or cup, then add 4-8 oz. of water, fruit juice, or diet-soft drinks before ingesting.

Administration: Oral route. **Storage:** 25°C (77°F); excursions permitted to 15-30°C (59-86°F). Protect from moisture. (Tab) Brief exposure to 40°C (104°F) does not affect the product.

WELLBUTRIN SR   RX
bupropion HCl (GlaxoSmithKline)

> Antidepressants increased the risk of suicidal thoughts and behavior in children, adolescents, and young adults in short-term trials. Monitor closely for worsening, and for emergence of suicidal thoughts and behavior. Advise families and caregivers of the need for close observation and communication with the prescriber. Serious neuropsychiatric reactions reported in patients taking bupropion for smoking cessation; not approved for smoking cessation. (Budeprion SR) Not approved for use in pediatric patients.

OTHER BRAND NAMES: Budeprion SR (Teva)

THERAPEUTIC CLASS: Aminoketone

INDICATIONS: Treatment of major depressive disorder.

DOSAGE: *Adults:* Initial: 150mg/day given as a single daily dose in am. After 3 days, may increase dose to 300mg/day, given as 150mg bid with an interval of at least 8 hrs between successive doses. Usual: 300mg/day, given as 150mg bid. Max: 400mg/day, given as 200mg bid may be considered if no clinical improvement after several weeks of treatment at 300mg/day. Do not exceed 200mg in any single dose. Periodically reassess the appropriate dose and the need for maint treatment. Renal Impairment: Consider reduced frequency and/or dose. Switching to/from an MAOI Antidepressant: Allow at least 14 days between discontinuation of an MAOI antidepressant and initiation of treatment and allow at least 14 days between discontinuation of treatment and initiation of an MAOI antidepressant. Use with Reversible MAOIs (eg, Linezolid, IV Methylene Blue): Refer to PI. (Wellbutrin SR) Moderate-Severe Hepatic Impairment (Child-Pugh Score: 7-15): Max: 100mg/day or 150mg qod. Mild Hepatic Impairment (Child-Pugh Score: 5-6): Consider reduced frequency and/or dose. (Budeprion SR) Severe Hepatic Cirrhosis: Max: 100mg/day or 150mg qod. Mild-Moderate Hepatic Cirrhosis: Consider reduced frequency and/or dose.

HOW SUPPLIED: Tab, Sustained-Release (SR): 100mg, 150mg, 200mg; (Budeprion SR) 100mg, 150mg

CONTRAINDICATIONS: Seizure disorder, current/prior diagnosis of bulimia or anorexia nervosa. Use of MAOIs (intended to treat psychiatric disorders) either concomitantly or within 14 days of discontinuing treatment. Treatment within 14 days of discontinuing treatment with an MAOI. Starting treatment in patients being treated with reversible MAOIs (eg, linezolid, IV methylene blue). (Wellbutrin SR) Undergoing abrupt discontinuation of alcohol, benzodiazepines, barbiturates, and antiepileptic drugs. (Budeprion SR) Treated currently with other bupropion products, undergoing abrupt discontinuation of alcohol or sedatives (including benzodiazepines).

WARNINGS/PRECAUTIONS: Dose-related risk of seizures; titrate dose gradually. D/C and do not restart treatment if a seizure occurs. May precipitate a manic, mixed, or hypomanic manic episode; risk appears to be increased in patients with bipolar disorder or who have risk factors for bipolar disorder. Screen for bipolar disorder; not approved for use in treating bipolar depression. Neuropsychiatric signs and symptoms (eg, delusions, hallucinations, psychosis, concentration disturbance, paranoia, confusion) reported. May result in elevated BP and HTN; assess BP prior to initiating treatment and monitor periodically during treatment. D/C treatment if allergic or anaphylactoid/anaphylactic reactions occur. Arthralgia, myalgia, fever with rash, and other serum-sickness like symptoms suggestive of delayed hypersensitivity reported. Caution with renal/hepatic impairment, and in elderly. False (+) urine immunoassay screening

W

tests for amphetamines reported. (Wellbutrin SR) Caution with conditions that may increase risk of seizure; consider risk before initiating treatment. (Budeprion SR) Extreme caution with history of seizures, cranial trauma, CNS tumor, or other predisposition(s) toward seizure, and severe hepatic cirrhosis. Increased restlessness, agitation, anxiety, and insomnia reported. Altered appetite/weight reported. Caution with recent myocardial infarction and unstable heart disease. (Budeprion SR 100mg) contains tartrazine, which may cause allergic-type reactions (including bronchial asthma) in certain susceptible persons; frequently seen in patients who also have aspirin sensitivity.

ADVERSE REACTIONS: Headache, infection, abdominal pain, dry mouth, N/V, constipation, anorexia, insomnia, dizziness, agitation, anxiety, pharyngitis, sweating, rash, tinnitus.

INTERACTIONS: See Contraindications. Extreme caution with other drugs that lower seizure threshold (eg, other bupropion products, antipsychotics, antidepressants, theophylline, systemic corticosteroids); use low initial doses and increase the dose gradually. Increased risk of seizure with use of illicit drugs (eg, cocaine), abuse or misuse of prescription drugs (eg, CNS stimulants), diabetes mellitus treated with oral hypoglycemic drugs or insulin, use of anorectic drugs, excessive use of alcohol, benzodiazepines, sedative/hypnotics, or opiates. Ritonavir, lopinavir, or efavirenz may decrease exposure; may need to increase bupropion dose but not to exceed max dose. Carbamazepine, phenytoin, and phenobarbital may induce metabolism and decrease exposure. May reduce efficacy of drugs that require metabolic activation by CYP2D6 to be effective (eg, tamoxifen). CNS toxicity reported when coadministered with levodopa or amantadine; use with caution. Minimize or avoid alcohol. Monitor for HTN with nicotine replacement therapy. Altered PT and/or INR, infrequently associated with hemorrhagic or thrombotic complication, reported with warfarin. Potential for drug interactions with CYP2B6 inhibitors/inducers. Increased risk of HTN with MAOIs or other drugs that increase dopaminergic or noradrenergic activity. (Wellbutrin SR) May increase exposure of CYP2D6 substrates (eg, antidepressants [paroxetine, fluoxetine, sertraline], antipsychotics [eg, haloperidol, risperidone, thioridazine], β-blockers [eg, metoprolol], and type 1C antiarrhythmics [eg, propafenone, flecainide]); may need to decrease the dose of CYP2D6 substrates, particularly for drugs with a narrow therapeutic index. CYP2B6 inhibitors (eg, ticlopidine, clopidogrel) may increase bupropion exposure but decrease hydroxybupropion exposure; may need to adjust dose. If used concomitantly with a CYP inducer, it may be necessary to increase the dose of bupropion, but the max recommended dose should not be exceeded. (Budeprion SR) Potential for drug interactions with CYP2B6 substrates. Paroxetine, sertraline, norfluoxetine, nelfinavir, and fluvoxamine may inhibit hydroxylation. Cimetidine may increase levels of some active metabolites. May increase citalopram levels.

PREGNANCY: Category C, (Wellbutrin SR) caution in nursing; (Budeprion SR) not for use in nursing.

MECHANISM OF ACTION: Aminoketone antidepressant; has not been established. Weak inhibitor of the neuronal uptake of norepinephrine and dopamine. Presumed that action is mediated by noradrenergic and/or dopaminergic mechanisms.

PHARMACOKINETICS: Absorption: T_{max}=3 hrs (Wellbutrin SR), 6 hrs (hydroxybupropion). **Distribution:** Plasma protein binding (84%); found in breast milk. **Metabolism:** Extensive. Hydroxylation (CYP2B6), reduction of carbonyl group; hydroxybupropion, threohydrobupropion, and erythrohydrobupropion (active metabolites). **Elimination:** Urine (87%), feces (10%), (0.5% unchanged); $T_{1/2}$=21 hrs, 20 hrs, 33 hrs, 37 hrs (bupropion, hydroxybupropion, erythrohydrobupropion, threohydrobupropion, respectively).

NURSING CONSIDERATIONS

Assessment: Assess for bipolar disorder, hepatic/renal dysfunction, seizure disorders or conditions that may increase risk of seizure, hypersensitivity to the drug, and any other conditions where treatment is contraindicated or cautioned, pregnancy/nursing status, and possible drug interactions.

Monitoring: Monitor for clinical worsening, suicidality, or unusual changes in behaviors, neuropsychiatric symptoms, suicide risk in smoking cessation treatment, seizures, HTN, activation of mania or hypomania, psychosis and other neuropsychiatric reactions, anaphylactoid/anaphylactic reactions, delayed hypersensitivity, and other adverse reactions. Monitor hepatic/renal function, especially in elderly.

Patient Counseling: Inform of benefits/risks of therapy. Advise patients and caregivers of need for close observation for clinical worsening and/or suicidal risks. Educate on the symptoms of hypersensitivity and to d/c if a severe allergic reaction occurs. Instruct to d/c and do not restart if a seizure occurs while on therapy. Inform that therapy may impair mental/physical abilities; advise to use caution while operating hazardous machinery/driving. Inform that excessive use or abrupt discontinuation of alcohol or sedatives may alter the seizure threshold; advise to minimize or avoid alcohol use. Instruct to notify physician if taking/planning to take any prescription or OTC medications. Advise to contact physician if become/intend to be pregnant during therapy.

Administration: Oral route. Take with or without food. Swallow whole; do not crush, divide, or chew. (Budeprion SR) Avoid hs dosing to minimize insomnia. **Storage:** (Wellbutrin SR) 20-25°C

W

(68-77°F); excursions permitted 15-30°C (59-86°F). Protect from light and moisture. (Budeprion SR) 20-25°C (68-77°F). Dispense in tightly closed, light-resistant container.

WELLBUTRIN XL

RX

bupropion HCl (Valeant)

Antidepressants increased the risk of suicidal thinking and behavior (suicidality) in short-term studies in children, adolescents, and young adults with major depressive disorder (MDD) and other psychiatric disorders. Monitor and observe closely for clinical worsening, suicidality, or unusual changes in behavior. Advise families and caregivers of the need for close observation and communication with the prescriber. Not approved for use in pediatric patients. Not approved for smoking cessation; neuropsychiatric reactions reported in patients taking bupropion for smoking cessation.

THERAPEUTIC CLASS: Aminoketone

INDICATIONS: Treatment of MDD. Prevention of seasonal major depressive episodes in patients with seasonal affective disorder (SAD).

DOSAGE: *Adults:* Give in am. MDD: Initial: 150mg qd. Titrate: May increase to 300mg qd on Day 4. Should be an interval of ≥24 hrs between successive doses. Consider an increase to 450mg qd when no clinical improvement noted after several weeks of treatment at 300mg/day. Usual: 300mg qd. Max: 450mg qd. Maint: Reassess periodically to determine need for maintenance treatment and the appropriate dose. SAD: Individualize timing of initiation and duration of treatment based on patient's historical pattern of seasonal major depressive episodes. Should generally initiate treatment in autumn prior to onset of depressive symptoms and continue through winter season. Taper and d/c in early spring. Initial: 150mg qd. Titrate: May increase to 300mg qd after 1 week. If 300mg dose not adequately tolerated, dose can be reduced to 150mg/day. Usual/Max: 300mg qd. If taking 300mg/day during autumn-winter season, taper to 150mg/day for 2 weeks prior to d/c. Mild-Moderate Hepatic Cirrhosis/Renal Impairment: Consider reduced frequency and/or dose. Severe Hepatic Cirrhosis: Max: 150mg qod. Switching from Bupropion Tab/Sustained-Release Tab: Give same total daily dose when possible.

HOW SUPPLIED: Tab, Extended-Release: 150mg, 300mg

CONTRAINDICATIONS: Seizure disorder, treated currently with other bupropion products, current/prior diagnosis of bulimia or anorexia nervosa, undergoing abrupt discontinuation of alcohol or sedatives (including benzodiazepines), and concurrent use of MAOIs or initiation of treatment within 14 days of discontinuation of an MAOI.

WARNINGS/PRECAUTIONS: Should not generally treat prophylactically patients whose seasonal depressive episodes are infrequent or without significant impairment. Dose-related risk of seizures; do not exceed 450mg qd. D/C and do not restart treatment if a seizure occurs. Extreme caution with history of seizures, cranial trauma, CNS tumor, or other predisposition(s) toward seizure, and severe hepatic cirrhosis. May precipitate mixed/manic episodes in patients at risk for bipolar disorder. Screen for bipolar disorder; not approved for use in treating bipolar depression. Neuropsychiatric signs and symptoms (eg, delusions, hallucinations, psychosis, concentration disturbance, paranoia, confusion) reported. Caution with recent myocardial infarction, unstable heart disease, renal/hepatic impairment, and in elderly. D/C treatment if allergic or anaphylactoid/anaphylactic reactions occur. Arthralgia, myalgia, fever with rash, and other symptoms suggestive of delayed hypersensitivity reported. Altered appetite/weight and HTN reported. Increased restlessness, agitation, anxiety, and insomnia reported shortly after initiation of treatment. False-positive urine immunoassay screening tests for amphetamines reported.

ADVERSE REACTIONS: Headache, dry mouth, nausea, insomnia, dizziness, nasopharyngitis, flatulence, tremor, upper respiratory tract infection, myalgia, anxiety, constipation, sinusitis, weight loss, cough.

INTERACTIONS: See Contraindications. Extreme caution with drugs that lower the seizure threshold (eg, other antidepressants, antipsychotics, theophylline, systemic steroids); use low initial doses and gradually titrate. Increased seizure risk with excessive alcohol or sedative use; opiate, cocaine, or stimulant addiction; use of OTC stimulants or anorectics, oral hypoglycemics, or insulin. Minimize or avoid alcohol. Caution with levodopa and amantadine; use low initial doses and gradually titrate. Inhibits CYP2D6; caution with drugs that are metabolized by CYP2D6 (eg, SSRIs, TCAs, antipsychotics, β-blockers, type 1C antiarrhythmics); use low initial dose. May reduce efficacy of drugs that require metabolic activation by CYP2D6 to be effective (eg, tamoxifen). Monitor for HTN with nicotine replacement therapy. Caution with CYP2B6 substrates or inhibitors/inducers (eg, cyclophosphamide, ticlopidine, clopidogrel). Paroxetine, sertraline, norfluoxetine, nelfinavir, fluvoxamine, and efavirenz may inhibit hydroxylation. Carbamazepine, phenytoin, and phenobarbital may induce metabolism. Decreased exposure with ritonavir, or ritonavir/lopinavir, and efavirenz; may need to increase bupropion dose but do not exceed max dose. Cimetidine increased levels of some active metabolites. May increase citalopram levels. Altered PT and/or INR with warfarin.

PREGNANCY: Category C, not for use in nursing.

W

MECHANISM OF ACTION: Aminoketone antidepressant; has not been established. Weak inhibitor of the neuronal uptake of norepinephrine and dopamine. Presumed that action is mediated by noradrenergic and/or dopaminergic mechanisms.

PHARMACOKINETICS: Absorption: T_{max}=5 hrs. **Distribution:** Plasma protein binding (84%); found in breast milk. **Metabolism:** Extensive; via hydroxylation (CYP2B6) and reduction of carbonyl group; hydroxybupropion, threohydrobupropion, and erythrohydrobupropion (active metabolites). **Elimination:** Urine (87%), feces (10%), (0.5% unchanged); $T_{1/2}$=21 hrs, 20 hrs, 33 hrs, 37 hrs (bupropion, hydroxybupropion, erythrohydrobupropion, threohydrobupropion, respectively).

NURSING CONSIDERATIONS

Assessment: Assess for bipolar disorder, hepatic/renal dysfunction, seizure disorders or conditions that may increase risk of seizure, hypersensitivity to the drug, and conditions where treatment is contraindicated or cautioned, pregnancy/nursing status, and possible drug interactions.

Monitoring: Monitor for clinical worsening, suicidality, or unusual changes in behavior, seizures, increased restlessness, agitation, anxiety, insomnia, neuropsychiatric signs/symptoms, changes in weight/appetite, anaphylactoid/anaphylactic reactions, delayed hypersensitivity reactions, HTN, and other adverse effects. Monitor hepatic/renal function, especially in the elderly.

Patient Counseling: Inform of benefits/risks of therapy. Advise patients and caregivers of need for close observation for clinical worsening and/or suicidal risk. Instruct to d/c and do not restart if a seizure occurs while on therapy. Inform that excessive use or abrupt discontinuation of alcohol or sedatives may alter the seizure threshold; advise to minimize or avoid alcohol use. Inform that therapy may impair mental/physical abilities; advise to use caution while operating hazardous machinery/driving. Instruct to notify physician if taking/planning to take any prescription or OTC medications. Advise to contact physician if become/intend to be pregnant during therapy. Inform that it is normal to notice something that looks like a tab in the stool.

Administration: Oral route. Avoid hs dosing. Swallow whole; do not crush, divide, or chew. Take with or without food. **Storage:** 25°C (77°F); excursions permitted to 15-30°C (59-86°F).

XALATAN   RX
latanoprost (Pharmacia & Upjohn)

THERAPEUTIC CLASS: Prostaglandin analog

INDICATIONS: Reduction of elevated intraocular pressure (IOP) in patients with open-angle glaucoma or ocular HTN.

DOSAGE: *Adults:* Usual: 1 drop in affected eye(s) qd in pm. Max: Once-daily dosing. Space dosing with other ophthalmic drugs by at least 5 min.

HOW SUPPLIED: Sol: 0.005% [2.5mL]

WARNINGS/PRECAUTIONS: Changes to pigmented tissues, increased pigmentation of iris (may be permanent), eyelids, and eyelashes (may be reversible); growth of eyelashes reported. Regularly examine patients with noticeably increased iris pigmentation. May cause changes to eyelashes and vellus hair in the treated eye. Macular edema, including cystoid macular edema, reported; mainly occurred in aphakic patients, pseudophakic patients with a torn posterior lens capsule, and patients at risk for macular edema. Caution with history of intraocular inflammation (iritis/uveitis), patients without an intact posterior capsule, and at risk of macular edema. Avoid with active intraocular inflammation. Limited experience in treating angle-closure, inflammatory, or neovascular glaucoma. Bacterial keratitis reported with multidose container. Remove contact lenses prior to instillation; may reinsert 15 min after administration.

ADVERSE REACTIONS: Eyelash changes, eyelid skin darkening, intraocular inflammation, iris pigmentation changes, macular edema, blurred vision, ocular burning/stinging, conjunctival hyperemia, foreign body sensation, ocular itching, punctate epithelial keratopathy, dry eye, excessive tearing, eye pain.

INTERACTIONS: Avoid with other prostaglandins or prostaglandin analogs; may decrease the IOP lowering effect or cause paradoxical IOP elevations.

PREGNANCY: Category C, caution in nursing.

MECHANISM OF ACTION: Prostaglandin analog; selective FP prostanoid receptor agonist believed to reduce IOP by increasing uveoscleral outflow.

PHARMACOKINETICS: Absorption: T_{max}=2 hrs. **Distribution:** V_d=0.16L/kg. **Metabolism:** Cornea, hydrolyzed to active acid; liver, via fatty acid β-oxidation to 1,2-dinor and 1,2,3,4-tetranor (metabolites). **Elimination:** Urine (88% topical, 98% IV); $T_{1/2}$=17 min (IV/Topical).

NURSING CONSIDERATIONS

Assessment: Assess for drug hypersensitivity, history/active intraocular inflammation (iritis/uveitis), risk for macular edema, aphakic or pseudophakic patients with torn posterior lens capsule, angle-closure, inflammatory or neovascular glaucoma, pregnancy/nursing status, and possible drug interactions.

Monitoring: Monitor for increased pigmentation of the iris, periorbital tissue (eyelid), changes in eyelashes and vellus hair, macular edema (eg, cystoid macular edema), and bacterial keratitis.

Patient Counseling: Inform about risk of brown pigmentation of iris (may be permanent) and darkening of eyelid skin (may be reversible after discontinuation). Inform about the possibility of eyelash and vellus hair changes in the treated eye. Advise to avoid touching tip of dispensing container to the eye or surrounding structures to avoid contamination of the sol. Advise to consult physician if having ocular surgery, or an intercurrent ocular condition (eg, trauma, infection) or ocular reaction develops. Instruct to remove contact lenses prior to instillation; reinsert 15 min after administration. Instruct to administer at least 5 min apart if using >1 topical ophthalmic drug.

Administration: Ocular route. Continue with the next dose as normal if one dose is missed.
Storage: Unopened: 2-8°C (36-46°F). Opened: 25°C (77°F) for up to 6 weeks. Protect from light.

XANAX
alprazolam (Pharmacia & Upjohn)

CIV

THERAPEUTIC CLASS: Benzodiazepine

INDICATIONS: Management of anxiety disorders or short-term relief of anxiety symptoms. Treatment of panic disorder, with or without agoraphobia.

DOSAGE: *Adults:* Individualize dose. Anxiety: Initial: 0.25-0.5mg tid. Titrate: May increase at intervals of 3-4 days. Max: 4mg/day in divided doses. Panic Disorder: Initial: 0.5mg tid. Titrate: May increase by ≤1mg/day every 3-4 days; slower titration to doses >4mg/day. Usual: 1-10mg/day. Elderly/Advanced Liver Disease/Debilitated: Initial: 0.25mg bid-tid. Titrate: May increase gradually PRN. Dose Reduction/Discontinuation: May reduce daily dose gradually by ≤0.5mg every 3 days.

HOW SUPPLIED: Tab: 0.25mg*, 0.5mg*, 1mg*, 2mg* *scored

CONTRAINDICATIONS: Acute narrow-angle glaucoma, concomitant ketoconazole or itraconazole.

WARNINGS/PRECAUTIONS: May be used with treated open-angle glaucoma. Increased risk of dependence with doses >4mg/day, treatment for >12 weeks, and in panic disorder patients. Seizures, including status epilepticus, reported with dose reduction or abrupt discontinuation. Early anxiety and emergence of anxiety symptoms between doses reported; give same total daily dose divided as more frequent administrations. Withdrawal reactions may occur; reduce dose or d/c therapy gradually. May impair mental/physical abilities. May cause fetal harm; avoid use during 1st trimester. Hypomania/mania reported in patients with depression. Caution with severe depression, suicidal ideation/plans, impaired renal/hepatic/pulmonary function, elderly, and debilitated patients. Has a weak uricosuric effect. Decreased systemic elimination rate with alcoholic liver disease/obesity.

ADVERSE REACTIONS: Drowsiness, lightheadedness, fatigue/tiredness, irritability, depression, headache, confusion, insomnia, dry mouth, constipation, diarrhea, N/V, tachycardia/palpitations, blurred vision, nasal congestion.

INTERACTIONS: See Contraindications. Not recommended with azole antifungals. Avoid with very potent CYP3A inhibitors. Caution with alcohol, other CNS depressants, diltiazem, isoniazid, macrolides (eg, erythromycin, clarithromycin), grapefruit juice, sertraline, paroxetine, ergotamine, cyclosporine, amiodarone, nicardipine, nifedipine, and other CYP3A inhibitors. Additive CNS depressant effects with psychotropics, anticonvulsants, antihistaminics, ethanol, and other drugs that produce CNS depression. Increased digoxin concentrations reported (especially in patients >65 yrs of age); monitor for signs/symptoms of digoxin toxicity. May increase plasma concentrations of imipramine and desipramine. Fluoxetine, fluvoxamine, nefazodone, cimetidine, and oral contraceptives may increase concentrations. CYP3A inducers (eg, carbamazepine), propoxyphene, and smoking may decrease levels. May require dose adjustment or discontinuation with HIV protease inhibitors (eg, ritonavir).

PREGNANCY: Category D, not for use in nursing.

MECHANISM OF ACTION: Benzodiazepine; has not been established. Presumed to bind at stereo specific receptors at several sites within the CNS.

PHARMACOKINETICS: Absorption: Readily absorbed; T_{max}=1-2 hrs; C_{max}=8-37ng/mL (0.5-3mg). **Distribution:** Plasma protein binding (80%); found in breast milk; crosses the placenta. **Metabolism:** Liver (extensive) via CYP3A4; 4-hydroxyalprazolam and α-hydroxyalprazolam (major metabolites). **Elimination:** Urine; $T_{1/2}$=11.2 hrs.

X

NURSING CONSIDERATIONS

Assessment: Assess for drug hypersensitivity, acute narrow-angle glaucoma, depression, suicidal ideation, renal/hepatic/pulmonary function, debilitation, history of alcohol/substance abuse, history of seizures/epilepsy, pregnancy/nursing status, and possible drug interactions. Assess for risk of dependence among panic disorder patients.

Monitoring: Monitor for dependence, rebound/withdrawal symptoms, early am anxiety and emergence of anxiety symptoms, CNS depression, episodes of hypomania/mania, suicidality, other treatment-emergent symptoms, and adverse reactions. Monitor CBC, urinalysis, and blood chemistry periodically. Periodically reassess usefulness of therapy.

Patient Counseling: Advise to inform physician about any alcohol consumption and medicines taken and if nursing, pregnant, planning to be pregnant, or if pregnancy occurs while on therapy. Advise to avoid alcohol during treatment. Advise not to drive or operate dangerous machinery until becoming familiar with the effects of therapy. Advise not to increase/decrease dose or abruptly d/c therapy without consultation; instruct to follow gradual dosage-tapering schedule. Inform of risks associated with doses >4mg/day.

Administration: Oral route. **Storage:** 20-25°C (68-77°F).

XANAX XR   CIV
alprazolam (Pharmacia & Upjohn)

THERAPEUTIC CLASS: Benzodiazepine

INDICATIONS: Treatment of panic disorder with or without agoraphobia.

DOSAGE: *Adults:* Individualize dose. Initial: 0.5-1mg qd, preferably in the am. Titrate: May increase at intervals of 3-4 days in increments of ≤1mg/day. Maint: 1-10mg/day. Usual: 3-6mg/day. Elderly/Advanced Liver Disease/Debilitated: Initial: 0.5mg qd. Titrate: May increase gradually PRN. Dose Reduction/Discontinuation: May reduce daily dose gradually by ≤0.5mg every 3 days. Switching from Immediate Release (IR) to ER: Refer to PI.

HOW SUPPLIED: Tab, Extended-Release (ER): 0.5mg, 1mg, 2mg, 3mg

CONTRAINDICATIONS: Acute narrow-angle glaucoma, concomitant ketoconazole or itraconazole.

WARNINGS/PRECAUTIONS: May be used with treated open-angle glaucoma. Increased risk of dependence with doses >4mg/day, treatment for >12 weeks, and in panic disorder patients. Seizures, including status epilepticus, reported with dose reduction or abrupt discontinuation. Early am anxiety/emergence of anxiety symptoms between doses reported. Withdrawal reactions may occur; reduce dose or d/c therapy gradually. May impair mental/physical abilities. May cause fetal harm; avoid use during 1st trimester. Caution with severe depression, suicidal ideation/plans, impaired renal/hepatic/pulmonary function, elderly, and debilitated patients. Hypomania/mania reported in patients with depression. Has a weak uricosuric effect. Decreased systemic elimination rate with alcoholic liver disease/obesity.

ADVERSE REACTIONS: Sedation, somnolence, memory impairment, dysarthria, abnormal coordination, fatigue, depression, constipation, mental impairment, ataxia, dry mouth, nausea, decreased libido, increased/decreased appetite/weight.

INTERACTIONS: See Contraindications. Not recommended with azole antifungals. Avoid with very potent CYP3A inhibitors. Caution with alcohol, other CNS depressants, diltiazem, isoniazid, macrolides (eg, erythromycin, clarithromycin), grapefruit juice, sertraline, paroxetine, ergotamine, cyclosporine, amiodarone, nicardipine, nifedipine, and other CYP3A inhibitors. Additive CNS depressant effects with psychotropics, anticonvulsants, antihistaminics, ethanol, and other drugs that produce CNS depression. Increased digoxin concentrations reported (especially in patients >65 yrs of age); monitor for signs/symptoms of digoxin toxicity. May increase plasma concentrations of imipramine and desipramine. Fluoxetine, fluvoxamine, nefazodone, cimetidine, and oral contraceptives may increase concentrations. CYP3A inducers (eg, carbamazepine), propoxyphene, and smoking may decrease levels. May require dose adjustment or discontinuation with HIV protease inhibitors (eg, ritonavir).

PREGNANCY: Category D, not for use in nursing.

MECHANISM OF ACTION: Benzodiazepine; has not been established. Presumed to bind at stereo specific receptors at several sites within the CNS.

PHARMACOKINETICS: Absorption: Readily absorbed (IR); absolute bioavailability (90%); refer to PI for additional parameters. **Distribution:** Plasma protein binding (80%); crosses the placenta; found in breast milk. **Metabolism:** Liver (extensive), via CYP3A4; 4-hydroxyalprazolam and α-hydroxyalprazolam (major metabolites). **Elimination:** Urine; $T_{1/2}$=10.7-15.8 hrs.

NURSING CONSIDERATIONS

Assessment: Assess for drug hypersensitivity, acute narrow-angle glaucoma, depression, suicidal ideation, renal/hepatic/pulmonary function, debilitation, history of alcohol/substance abuse, history of seizures/epilepsy, pregnancy/nursing status, and possible drug interactions. Assess for risk of dependence among panic disorder patients.

Monitoring: Monitor for dependence, relapse, rebound or withdrawal symptoms, early am anxiety and emergence of anxiety symptoms, CNS depression, episodes of hypomania/mania, suicidality, other treatment-emergent symptoms, and other adverse reactions. Monitor CBC, urinalysis, and blood chemistry periodically. Periodically reassess usefulness of therapy.

Patient Counseling: Advise to take in the am and not crush or chew tabs. Advise to inform physician about any alcohol consumption and medicines taken and if nursing, pregnant, planning to be pregnant, or if pregnancy occurs while on therapy. Advise to avoid alcohol during treatment. Advise not to drive or operate dangerous machinery until becoming familiar with the effects of the medication. Advise not to increase/decrease dose or abruptly d/c therapy without consultation; instruct to follow gradual dosage-tapering schedule. Inform of risks associated with doses >4mg/day.

Administration: Oral route. Do not chew, crush, or break tabs. **Storage:** 25°C (77°F); excursions permitted to 15-30°C (59-86°F).

XARELTO   RX
rivaroxaban (Janssen)

> Premature discontinuation increases the risk of thrombotic events. If therapy is discontinued for a reason other than pathological bleeding or completion of a course of therapy, consider coverage with another anticoagulant. Epidural or spinal hematomas have occurred in patients treated with rivaroxaban who are receiving neuraxial anesthesia or undergoing spinal puncture; long-term or permanent paralysis may result. Increased risk of developing epidural or spinal hematomas in patients using indwelling epidural catheters, concomitant use of other drugs that affect hemostasis (eg, NSAIDs, platelet inhibitors, other anticoagulants), history of traumatic or repeated epidural or spinal puncture, history of spinal deformity or spinal surgery, and when optimal timing between the administration of therapy and neuraxial procedure is not known. Monitor frequently for signs/symptoms of neurological impairment; urgent treatment is necessary if neurological compromise occurs. Consider benefits and risks before neuraxial intervention in patients anticoagulated or to be anticoagulated for thromboprophylaxis.

THERAPEUTIC CLASS: Selective factor Xa inhibitor

INDICATIONS: Reduce the risk of stroke and systemic embolism in patients with nonvalvular atrial fibrillation. Treatment of deep vein thrombosis (DVT) and pulmonary embolism (PE). Reduction in the risk of recurrence of DVT and PE following initial 6 months treatment for DVT and/or PE. Prophylaxis of DVT, which may lead to PE in patients undergoing knee or hip replacement surgery.

DOSAGE: *Adults:* Reduction in Risk of Stroke in Nonvalvular Atrial Fibrillation: CrCl >50mL/min: 20mg qd with pm meal. CrCl 15-50mL/min: 15mg qd with pm meal. Treatment of DVT/PE: 15mg bid with food for the first 21 days, then 20mg qd with food, at approximately the same time each day. Reduction in Risk of Recurrence of DVT/PE: 20mg qd with food at approximately the same time each day. Prophylaxis of DVT: 10mg qd. Give initial dose 6-10 hrs after surgery provided that hemostasis has been established. Treatment Duration: Hip Replacement Surgery: 35 days. Knee Replacement Surgery: 12 days. Surgery/Intervention: If anticoagulation must be discontinued with surgery or other procedures, d/c therapy at least 24 hrs before procedure to reduce the risk of bleeding. Weigh risk of bleeding against urgency of intervention to decide whether procedure should be delayed until 24 hrs after last dose. After procedure, restart therapy as soon as adequate hemostasis has been established. Missed Dose: Refer to PI. Switching from or to Warfarin or other Anticoagulants: Refer to PI.

HOW SUPPLIED: Tab: 10mg, 15mg, 20mg

CONTRAINDICATIONS: Active pathological bleeding.

WARNINGS/PRECAUTIONS: May increase risk of bleeding and cause serious or fatal bleeding; risk of thrombotic events should be weighed against risk of bleeding before initiation of treatment. Promptly evaluate any signs/symptoms of blood loss and consider the need for blood replacement; d/c in patients with active pathological hemorrhage. An epidural catheter should not be removed earlier than 18 hrs after last administration of therapy. The next dose should not be administered earlier than 6 hrs after catheter removal. If traumatic puncture occurs, delay administration for 24 hrs. Caution in pregnant women due to the potential for pregnancy-related hemorrhage and/or emergent delivery. Avoid use for prophylaxis of DVT following hip or knee replacement surgery, treatment of DVT/PE, and reduction in risk of recurrence of DVT/PE in patients with CrCl <30mL/min or for nonvalvular atrial fibrillation in patients with CrCl <15mL/min. Avoid with moderate (Child-Pugh B) and severe (Child-Pugh C) hepatic impairment, or with any hepatic disease associated with coagulopathy. Monitor for signs/symptoms of blood loss in patients with CrCl 30-50mL/min in prophylaxis of DVT following hip or knee replacement surgery.

X

D/C therapy if acute renal failure develops. Not recommended in patients with prosthetic heart valves. Initiation of treatment is not recommended acutely as an alternative to unfractionated heparin in patients with PE who present with hemodynamic instability or who may receive thrombolysis or pulmonary embolectomy.

ADVERSE REACTIONS: Bleeding events, back pain.

INTERACTIONS: See Boxed Warning. May result in changes in exposure with inhibitors/inducers of CYP3A4/5, CYP2J2, and P-glycoprotein (P-gp) and ATP-binding cassette G2 transporters. Avoid with combined P-gp and strong CYP3A4 inducers (eg, carbamazepine, phenytoin, rifampin, St. John's wort); may decrease exposure and efficacy. Increased exposure with combined P-gp and CYP3A4 inhibitors (eg, ketoconazole, ritonavir, clarithromycin, erythromycin, fluconazole) may increase bleeding risk; avoid with combined P-gp and strong CYP3A4 inhibitors (eg, ketoconazole, itraconazole, lopinavir/ritonavir, ritonavir, indinavir, conivaptan). Increased exposure and possible increased bleeding risk with combined P-gp and moderate CYP3A4 inhibitors (eg, diltiazem, verapamil, dronedarone, erythromycin) in renally impaired patients; avoid use in patients with CrCl 15-80mL/min who are receiving concomitant combined P-gp and moderate CYP3A4 inhibitors unless potential benefit justifies risk. Concomitant single dose of enoxaparin resulted in an additive effect on anti-factor Xa activity. Concomitant single dose of warfarin resulted in an additive effect on factor Xa inhibition and PT. Concomitant use of other drugs that impair hemostasis (eg, P2Y$_{12}$ platelet inhibitors, other antithrombotic agents, fibrinolytic therapy, NSAIDs/aspirin) increases the risk of bleeding. May increase bleeding time with clopidogrel. Avoid concurrent use with other anticoagulants due to increased bleeding risk unless benefit outweighs risk.

PREGNANCY: Category C, not for use in nursing.

MECHANISM OF ACTION: Selective factor Xa inhibitor; inhibits free factor Xa and prothrombinase activity. Has no direct effect on platelet aggregation, but indirectly inhibits platelet aggregation induced by thrombin. By inhibiting factor Xa, rivaroxaban decreases thrombin generation. Does not require a cofactor for activity.

PHARMACOKINETICS: Absorption: Absolute bioavailability (80-100% [10mg], 66% [20mg, fasted]); T_{max}=2-4 hrs. **Distribution:** V_d=50L (healthy); plasma protein binding (92-95%). **Metabolism:** Oxidative degradation via CYP3A4/5 and CYP2J2; hydrolysis. **Elimination:** Urine (66%, 36% unchanged), feces (28%, 7% unchanged); $T_{1/2}$=5-9 hrs (20-45 yrs of age [healthy]), 11-13 hrs (elderly).

NURSING CONSIDERATIONS

Assessment: Assess for known hypersensitivity, active pathological bleeding, risk factors for developing epidural or spinal hematomas, conditions that may increase risk of bleeding, renal/hepatic impairment, prosthetic heart valves, PE with hemodynamic instability or patients who may receive thrombolysis or pulmonary embolectomy, pregnancy/nursing status, and possible drug interactions.

Monitoring: Monitor for signs/symptoms of bleeding, stroke, thrombotic events, and other adverse reactions. In patients undergoing neuraxial anesthesia or spinal puncture, monitor for epidural or spinal hematomas and neurological impairment. Monitor renal function (eg, CrCl) periodically.

Patient Counseling: Instruct to take only ud. Advise to follow missed dosing instructions. Advise not to d/c without consulting physician. Advise to report any unusual bleeding or bruising. Inform that it may take longer than usual to stop bleeding, and that patients may bruise and/or bleed more easily. Advise patients who had neuraxial anesthesia or spinal puncture to watch for signs and symptoms of spinal/epidural hematoma (eg, back pain, tingling, numbness, muscle weakness, stool/urine incontinence), especially if concomitantly taking NSAIDs or platelet inhibitors; instruct contact physician immediately if symptoms occur. Instruct to inform physician about therapy before any invasive procedure. Instruct to inform physicians and dentists if taking, or plan to take, any prescription, OTC drugs, or herbals. Advise to inform physician immediately if nursing/pregnant or intend to nurse or become pregnant. Advise pregnant women receiving therapy to immediately report to the physician any bleeding or symptoms of blood loss.

Administration: Oral route. 15mg and 20mg should be taken with food, while 10mg can be taken with or without food. Refer to PI for administration options. **Storage:** 25°C (77°F); excursions permitted to 15-30°C (59-86°F).

XELJANZ
tofacitinib (Pfizer)

Increased risk for developing serious infections (eg, active tuberculosis [TB], invasive fungal infections, bacterial/viral infections due to opportunistic pathogens) that may lead to hospitalization or death. Most patients who developed these infections were taking concomitant immunosuppressants (eg, methotrexate [MTX], corticosteroids). If a serious infection develops, interrupt treatment until infection is controlled. Test for latent TB prior to and during therapy; initiate latent TB treatment prior to therapy. Consider risks and benefits prior to initiating therapy in patients with chronic or recurrent infection. Monitor for development of signs and symptoms of infection during and after treatment. Lymphoma and other malignancies reported. Increased rate of Epstein-Barr virus-associated post-transplant lymphoproliferative disorder observed in renal transplant patients with concomitant immunosuppressive medications.

THERAPEUTIC CLASS: Kinase inhibitor

INDICATIONS: Treatment of moderate to severe active rheumatoid arthritis in adults who have had an inadequate response/intolerance to MTX. May be used as monotherapy or in combination with MTX or other nonbiologic disease-modifying antirheumatic drugs (DMARDs).

DOSAGE: *Adults:* 5mg bid. Reduce to 5mg qd in patients with moderate/severe renal insufficiency, moderate hepatic impairment, concomitant potent CYP3A4 inhibitors, or drugs that are both moderate CYP3A4 inhibitors and potent CYP2C19 inhibitors. Refer to PI for dose modifications.

HOW SUPPLIED: Tab: 5mg

WARNINGS/PRECAUTIONS: Avoid with active, serious infection, including localized infections. Caution in patients with chronic/recurrent infections, who have been exposed to TB, with history of a serious/opportunistic infection, who have resided in or traveled to areas of endemic TB/mycoses, or with predisposing factors to infection. Viral reactivation, including herpes virus reactivation (eg, herpes zoster), reported. Consider risks and benefits of treatment in patients with a known malignancy other than a successfully treated non-melanoma skin cancer or when considering continuing treatment in patients who develop a malignancy. GI perforation reported; caution in patients with increased risk for GI perforation (eg, history of diverticulitis). Associated with initial lymphocytosis, neutropenia, increase in lipid parameters, and liver enzyme elevations. Interrupt treatment if drug-induced liver injury is suspected. Use in patients with severe hepatic impairment, absolute lymphocyte count <500 cells/mm^3, absolute neutrophil count (ANC) <1000 cells/mm^3, or Hgb levels <9g/dL is not recommended. D/C if an opportunistic infection or sepsis occurs. Monitor closely and take appropriate measures if new infection develops. Caution in elderly.

ADVERSE REACTIONS: Infections (eg, upper respiratory tract infections, nasopharyngitis), lymphoma, malignancies, diarrhea, headache.

INTERACTIONS: See Boxed Warning. Avoid with live vaccines. Increased immunosuppression with potent immunosuppressive drugs (eg, azathioprine, tacrolimus, cyclosporine); concurrent use with potent immunosuppressants (eg, azathioprine, cyclosporine) or biologic DMARDs is not recommended. Increased exposure with potent CYP3A4 inhibitors (eg, ketoconazole), and drugs that are both moderate CYP3A4 inhibitors and potent CYP2C19 inhibitors (eg, fluconazole). Decreased exposure resulting in loss of or reduced clinical response to treatment with potent CYP3A4 inducers (eg, rifampin); coadministration is not recommended.

PREGNANCY: Category C, not for use in nursing.

MECHANISM OF ACTION: Kinase inhibitor; inhibits Janus kinase, which transmits signals arising from cytokine or growth factor-receptor interactions on the cellular membrane to influence cellular processes of hematopoiesis and immune cell function.

PHARMACOKINETICS: Absorption: Absolute bioavailability (74%); T_{max}=0.5-1 hr. **Distribution:** V_d=87 L; plasma protein binding (~40%). **Metabolism:** Liver via CYP3A4 (primary) and CYP2C19 (minor). **Elimination:** Urine (30% unchanged); $T_{1/2}$=3 hrs.

NURSING CONSIDERATIONS

Assessment: Assess for infections (eg, bacteria, fungi, viruses), including latent TB, predisposing factors to infection, active hepatic disease or impairment, known malignancy, risk of GI perforation, pregnancy/nursing status, and possible drug interactions. Obtain baseline absolute lymphocyte count, ANC, and lipid and Hgb levels.

Monitoring: Monitor for TB (active, reactivation, or latent), invasive fungal infections, or bacterial, viral, and other opportunistic infections during and after therapy. Monitor for viral reactivation, lymphoma, malignancy, lymphoproliferative disorders, and GI perforations. Monitor absolute lymphocyte counts every 3 months. Monitor neutrophil counts and Hgb after 4-8 weeks of treatment and every 3 months thereafter. Routinely monitor LFTs. Monitor lipid parameters approximately 4-8 weeks following initiation.

Patient Counseling: Advise about potential risks/benefits of therapy. Inform that therapy may lower resistance to infection; advise patients not to start taking medication if they have an active infection. Instruct to contact physician immediately if symptoms suggesting an infection appear

X

during treatment to ensure rapid evaluation and appropriate treatment. Inform that medication may increase risk of lymphoma and other cancers; instruct to inform physician of any type of cancer that they have ever had. Inform that certain lab tests may be affected and that blood tests are required before and during treatment. Inform that medication should not be used during pregnancy unless clearly necessary; advise to inform physician right away if pregnant. Advise to enroll in the pregnancy registry for pregnant women who have taken medication during pregnancy.

Administration: Oral route. Take with or without food. **Storage:** 20-25°C (68-77°F).

XELODA   RX
capecitabine (Genentech)

> Altered coagulation parameters and/or bleeding, including death, reported with concomitant coumarin-derivative anticoagulants (eg, warfarin, phenprocoumon). Monitor PT and INR frequently in order to adjust anticoagulant dose accordingly. Postmarketing reports showed clinically significant increases in PT and INR in patients who were stabilized on anticoagulants at start of therapy. Age >60 yrs and a diagnosis of cancer independently predispose to an increased risk of coagulopathy.

THERAPEUTIC CLASS: Fluoropyrimidine carbamate

INDICATIONS: First-line treatment of metastatic colorectal carcinoma and as a single agent for adjuvant treatment in patients with Dukes' C colon cancer who have undergone complete resection of the primary tumor, when treatment with fluoropyrimidine therapy alone is preferred. Treatment of metastatic breast cancer in combination with docetaxel after failure of prior anthracycline-containing chemotherapy. Monotherapy treatment of metastatic breast cancer in patients resistant to both paclitaxel and anthracycline-containing chemotherapy regimen or resistant to paclitaxel and for whom further anthracycline therapy is not indicated.

DOSAGE: *Adults:* Individualize dose. Monotherapy: Metastatic Colorectal Cancer/Metastatic Breast Cancer: Usual: 1250mg/m² bid for 2 weeks followed by a 1-week rest period given as 3-week cycles. Adjuvant Dukes' C Colon Cancer Treatment: 1250mg/m² bid for 2 weeks followed by 1-week rest period, given as 3-week cycles for total of 8 cycles (24 weeks). Combination with Docetaxel: Metastatic Breast Cancer: Usual: 1250mg/m² bid for 2 weeks followed by 1-week rest period, combined with docetaxel 75mg/m² as a 1 hr IV infusion every 3 weeks. Moderate Renal Impairment (CrCl 30-50mL/min): Reduce to 75% of starting dose (from 1250 mg/m² to 950 mg/m² bid). Refer to PI for dose calculation according to BSA, dose modification recommendations, and docetaxel dose reduction schedule. Swallow whole. Take with water within 30 min pc.

HOW SUPPLIED: Tab: 150mg, 500mg

CONTRAINDICATIONS: Known dihydropyrimidine dehydrogenase (DPD) deficiency, severe renal impairment (CrCl <30mL/min), known hypersensitivity to 5-fluorouracil (5-FU).

WARNINGS/PRECAUTIONS: May induce diarrhea; give fluid and electrolyte replacement with severe diarrhea. Cardiotoxicity (eg, myocardial infarction/ischemia, angina, dysrhythmias, cardiac arrest, cardiac failure, sudden death, ECG changes, cardiomyopathy) observed; common in patients with a prior history of coronary artery disease (CAD). Rarely, severe toxicity (eg, stomatitis, diarrhea, neutropenia, neurotoxicity) associated with 5-FU has been attributed to DPD deficiency. Caution with mild and moderate renal impairment. Hand-and-foot syndrome may occur. Hyperbilirubinemia reported; interrupt therapy if drug-related grade 3 or 4 elevations in bilirubin occur until the hyperbilirubinemia decreases to ≤3X ULN. Necrotizing enterocolitis, neutropenia, thrombocytopenia, anemia, and decrease in Hgb reported. Avoid with baseline neutrophil counts of <1.5 x 10⁹/L and/or thrombocyte counts of <100 x 10⁹/L. Caution in elderly; patients ≥80 yrs of age may experience greater incidence of Grade 3/4 adverse events. Caution with mild to moderate hepatic dysfunction due to liver metastases. May cause fetal harm.

ADVERSE REACTIONS: Diarrhea, hand-and-foot syndrome, asthenia, pyrexia, anemia, N/V, fatigue, dermatitis, thrombocytopenia, constipation, taste disturbance, stomatitis, alopecia, abdominal pain, decreased appetite.

INTERACTIONS: See Boxed Warning. May increase the mean area under the curve of S-warfarin. May increase phenytoin levels; reduce phenytoin dose and monitor carefully. Leucovorin may increase levels and toxicity of 5-FU. Caution with CYP2C9 substrates.

PREGNANCY: Category D, not for use in nursing.

MECHANISM OF ACTION: Fluoropyrimidine carbamate; binds to thymidylate synthase to form a covalently bound ternary complex that inhibits the formation of thymidylate from 2'-deoxyuridylate, inhibits DNA synthesis/cell division and interferes with RNA processing and protein synthesis.

PHARMACOKINETICS: Absorption: T_{max}=1.5 hrs. **Distribution:** Plasma protein binding (<60%); primarily bound to human albumin (approximately 35%). **Metabolism:** Extensive enzymatic conversion to 5-FU; hydrogenated to a much less toxic metabolite 5-fluoro-5, 6-dihydro-fluorouracil by DPD; cleavage of the pyrimidine ring to 5-fluoro-ureido-propionic acid; cleavage to α-fluoro-β-alanine (major metabolite). **Elimination:** Urine (95.5%, 3% unchanged, 57% major metabolite), feces (2.6%); $T_{1/2}$=0.75 hr.

NURSING CONSIDERATIONS

Assessment: Assess for hypersensitivity to drug or to 5-FU, DPD deficiency, renal/hepatic dysfunction, history of CAD, pregnancy/nursing status, and possible drug interactions. Obtain baseline neutrophil/thrombocyte counts.

Monitoring: Monitor for severe diarrhea, necrotizing enterocolitis, cardiotoxicity, hand-and-foot syndrome, hyperbilirubinemia, neutropenia, thrombocytopenia, anemia, decreases in Hgb, severe toxicity, and other adverse reactions. Monitor PT and INR frequently with concomitant oral coumarin-derivative anticoagulant therapy.

Patient Counseling: Instruct to d/c therapy immediately if moderate/severe toxicity occurs. Inform of the expected adverse effects of therapy (eg, diarrhea, N/V, hand-and-foot syndrome, stomatitis). Instruct to contact physician if fever (≥100.5°F) or infection occurs. Counsel about pregnancy risks; instruct to avoid pregnancy during therapy.

Administration: Oral route. Swallow tab whole with water within 30 min pc. Do not cut or crush tab. **Storage:** 25°C (77°F); excursions permitted to 15-30°C (59-86°F). Keep tightly closed.

XENICAL RX
orlistat (Genentech)

THERAPEUTIC CLASS: Lipase inhibitor

INDICATIONS: For obesity management including weight loss and weight maintenance when used in conjunction with a reduced-calorie diet. To reduce the risk for weight regain after prior weight loss. For obese patients with an initial BMI ≥30kg/m² or ≥27kg/m² in the presence of other risk factors (eg, HTN, diabetes, dyslipidemia).

DOSAGE: *Adults:* Usual: 120mg tid with each main meal containing fat (during or up to 1 hr pc). Max: 120mg tid. Use with nutritionally balanced, reduced-calorie diet that contains 30% calories from fat; distribute daily intake of fat, carbohydrate, and protein over 3 main meals. Omit dose if a meal is occasionally missed or contains no fat.
Pediatrics: ≥12 Yrs: Usual: 120mg tid with each main meal containing fat (during or up to 1 hr pc). Max: 120mg tid. Use with nutritionally balanced, reduced-calorie diet that contains 30% calories from fat; distribute daily intake of fat, carbohydrate, and protein over 3 main meals. Omit dose if a meal is occasionally missed or contains no fat.

HOW SUPPLIED: Cap: 120mg

CONTRAINDICATIONS: Pregnancy, chronic malabsorption syndrome, cholestasis.

WARNINGS/PRECAUTIONS: Weight loss may affect glycemic control in patients with diabetes mellitus. Severe liver injury with hepatocellular necrosis or acute hepatic failure reported, with some cases resulting in liver transplant or death; d/c therapy and other suspect medications immediately and obtain LFTs. May increase levels of urinary oxalate; caution with a history of hyperoxaluria or calcium oxalate nephrolithiasis. Cases of oxalate nephrolithiasis and oxalate nephropathy with renal failure reported; monitor renal function. May increase risk of cholelithiasis due to substantial weight loss. Exclude organic causes of obesity (eg, hypothyroidism). GI events may increase with a high-fat diet (>30% total daily calories from fat).

ADVERSE REACTIONS: Oily spotting, flatus with discharge, fecal urgency, fatty/oily stool, oily evacuation, increased defecation, fecal incontinence.

INTERACTIONS: Reduced cyclosporine plasma levels reported; take cyclosporine at least 3 hrs before or after administration. Reduced absorption of some fat-soluble vitamins and β-carotene supplement and inhibited absorption of vitamin E acetate supplement reported. Hypothyroidism reported with levothyroxine; administer at least 4 hrs apart and monitor for thyroid function changes. Vitamin K absorption may be decreased; monitor closely for changes in coagulation parameters with chronic stable doses of warfarin. Convulsions reported with concomitant use with antiepileptic drugs; monitor for possible changes in the frequency and/or severity of convulsions. May require reduction in dosage of oral hypoglycemic agents (eg, sulfonylureas) or insulin in diabetics.

PREGNANCY: Category X, caution in nursing.

MECHANISM OF ACTION: Lipase inhibitor; exerts therapeutic activity in the lumen of the stomach and small intestine by forming a covalent bond with the active serine residue site of gastric and pancreatic lipases. The inactivated enzymes are thus unavailable to hydrolyze dietary fats in the form of TGs into absorbable free fatty acids and monoglycerides.

PHARMACOKINETICS: Absorption: Minimal. T_{max}=8 hrs (360mg dose). **Distribution:** Plasma protein binding (>99%). **Metabolism:** M1 and M3 (primary and secondary metabolites). **Elimination:**

(360mg single dose) Feces (97%, 83% unchanged), urine (<2%); $T_{1/2}$=1-2 hrs, 3 hrs (M1), 13.5 hrs (M3).

NURSING CONSIDERATIONS

Assessment: Assess for hypersensitivity to the drug, chronic malabsorption syndrome, cholestasis, history of hyperoxaluria or calcium oxalate nephrolithiasis, organic causes of obesity (eg, hypothyroidism), pregnancy/nursing status, and possible drug interactions. Obtain baseline weight, FPG, and lipid profile.

Monitoring: Monitor for hepatic dysfunction, cholelithiasis, signs/symptoms of hypersensitivity reactions, GI events, and other adverse events. Monitor renal function in patients at risk for renal insufficiency. Monitor closely for changes in coagulation parameters with chronic stable doses of warfarin.

Patient Counseling: Advise to inform physician if taking cyclosporine, β-carotene or vitamin E supplements, levothyroxine, or warfarin, due to potential interactions. Inform of the common adverse events (eg, oily spotting, flatus with discharge, fecal urgency, fatty/oily stool, oily evacuation, increased defecation, fecal incontinence) associated with the use of the drug. Inform of the potential risks that include lowered absorption of fat-soluble vitamins and potential liver injury, increased urinary oxalate, and cholelithiasis. Inform of the potential benefits that therapy may result in, such as weight loss and improvement in obesity-related risk factors. Instruct to report any symptoms of hepatic dysfunction while on therapy. Counsel patient to take drug ud with meals or up to 1 hr pc. Advise to take a multivitamin qd at least 2 hrs before or after administration, or at hs. Advise patients to adhere to dietary guidelines.

Administration: Oral route. **Storage:** 25°C (77°F); excursions permitted to 15-30°C (59-86°F).

XGEVA   RX
denosumab (Amgen)

THERAPEUTIC CLASS: IgG_2 monoclonal antibody

INDICATIONS: Prevention of skeletal-related events in patients with bone metastases from solid tumors. Treatment of adults and skeletally mature adolescents with giant cell tumor of bone that is unresectable or where surgical resection is likely to result in severe morbidity.

DOSAGE: *Adults:* Bone Metastasis from Solid Tumors: 120mg SQ every 4 weeks. Giant Cell Tumor of Bone: 120mg SQ every 4 weeks with additional 120mg doses on Days 8 and 15 of the 1st month of therapy.
Pediatrics: Adolescents: Giant Cell Tumor of Bone: 120mg SQ every 4 weeks with additional 120mg doses on Days 8 and 15 of the 1st month of therapy.

HOW SUPPLIED: Inj: 120mg/1.7mL

WARNINGS/PRECAUTIONS: Not indicated for the prevention of skeletal-related events in patients with multiple myeloma. May cause severe symptomatic hypocalcemia, and fatal cases reported; greater risk in patients with CrCl <30mL/min or receiving dialysis. Correct preexisting hypocalcemia prior to treatment, monitor Ca^{2+} levels and administer Ca^{2+}, Mg^{2+}, and vitamin D as necessary. Osteonecrosis of the jaw (ONJ) may occur; avoid invasive dental procedures during therapy. Perform oral exam and appropriate preventive dentistry prior to initiation of treatment and periodically during treatment. Atypical femoral fracture reported; evaluate patients with thigh/groin pain to rule out an incomplete femur fracture and consider interruption of therapy. May cause fetal harm.

ADVERSE REACTIONS: Fatigue/asthenia, hypophosphatemia, nausea, dyspnea, diarrhea, hypocalcemia, cough, headache, arthralgia, back pain, pain in extremity.

INTERACTIONS: Monitor Ca^{2+} levels more frequently with other drugs that can lower Ca^{2+} levels.

PREGNANCY: Category D, not for use in nursing.

MECHANISM OF ACTION: IgG_2 monoclonal antibody; binds to RANK ligand, a transmembrane or soluble protein essential for the formation, function, and survival of osteoclasts (cells responsible for bone resorption). It prevents RANKL from activating its receptor, RANK, on the surface of osteoclasts, their precursors, and osteoclast-like giant cells.

PHARMACOKINETICS: Absorption: Bioavailability (62%). **Distribution:** Crosses placenta.
Elimination: $T_{1/2}$=28 days.

NURSING CONSIDERATIONS

Assessment: Assess for hypocalcemia, renal impairment, pregnancy/nursing status, and possible drug interactions. Perform oral exam and appropriate preventive dentistry.

Monitoring: Monitor Ca^{2+} levels, for ONJ, and atypical femur fracture. Perform oral exam and appropriate preventive dentistry periodically.

Patient Counseling: Advise to contact a healthcare professional if experiencing symptoms of hypocalcemia (eg, paresthesias or muscle stiffness, twitching, spasms, cramps), symptoms of ONJ (eg, pain, numbness, swelling of or drainage from the jaw, mouth, or teeth), persistent pain or slow healing of the mouth or jaw after dental surgery, or if nursing. Advise of the need for proper oral hygiene and routine dental care, to inform patients' dentist that they are receiving the drug, and to avoid invasive dental procedures during treatment. Advise that denosumab is also marketed as Prolia; instruct to inform healthcare provider if taking Prolia. Advise to report new or unusual thigh, hip, or groin pain. Advise females of reproductive potential to use highly effective contraception during therapy, and for at least 5 months after the last dose of the drug; instruct to contact physician if they become pregnant or a pregnancy is suspected during this time. Advise male patients of potential for fetal exposure to drug when they had unprotected sexual intercourse with a pregnant partner.

Administration: SQ route. Refer to PI for preparation and administration instructions. **Storage:** 2-8°C (36-46°F). Do not freeze. Once removed from the refrigerator, do not expose to >25°C (77°F) or direct light; discard if not used within 14 days. Protect from heat. Avoid vigorous shaking.

XIFAXAN   RX
rifaximin (Salix)

THERAPEUTIC CLASS: Semisynthetic rifampin analog

INDICATIONS: (200mg) Treatment of travelers' diarrhea caused by noninvasive strains of *Escherichia coli* in patients ≥12 yrs of age. (550mg) Reduction in risk of overt hepatic encephalopathy (HE) recurrence in patients ≥18 yrs of age.

DOSAGE: *Adults:* Travelers' Diarrhea: 200mg tid for 3 days. HE: 550mg bid.
Pediatrics: Travelers' Diarrhea: ≥12 Yrs: 200mg tid for 3 days.

HOW SUPPLIED: Tab: 200mg, 550mg

WARNINGS/PRECAUTIONS: Should not be used in patients with diarrhea complicated by fever and/or blood in the stool or diarrhea due to pathogens other than *E. coli*. D/C if diarrhea symptoms worsen or persist >24-48 hrs; consider alternative antibiotic therapy. *Clostridium difficile*-associated diarrhea (CDAD) reported; d/c if CDAD suspected or confirmed. May result in bacterial resistance with prolonged use in the absence of proven or strongly suspected bacterial infection or a prophylactic indication. Caution with severe hepatic impairment (Child-Pugh Class C); may increase systemic exposure.

ADVERSE REACTIONS: Flatulence, headache, abdominal pain, rectal tenesmus, nausea, peripheral edema, dizziness, fatigue, ascites, muscle spasms, pruritus, abdominal distention, anemia, cough, depression.

INTERACTIONS: Caution with P-glycoprotein inhibitors (eg, cyclosporine); may increase systemic exposure.

PREGNANCY: Category C, not for use in nursing.

MECHANISM OF ACTION: Semisynthetic rifampin analog; binds to β-subunit of bacterial DNA-dependent RNA polymerase, resulting in inhibition of bacterial RNA synthesis.

PHARMACOKINETICS: Absorption: Administration with consecutive dosing, fasting/fed conditions, and Child-Pugh Class (A, B, C) resulted in different pharmacokinetic parameters; refer to PI. **Distribution:** (550mg dose) Plasma protein binding (67.5%, healthy), (62%, hepatic impairment). **Elimination:** (400mg, healthy) Feces (96.62% unchanged), urine (0.32% mostly metabolites, 0.03% unchanged).

NURSING CONSIDERATIONS

Assessment: If diarrhea is present, assess for causative organisms and assess if diarrhea is complicated by fever or blood in stool. Assess for hepatic function, pregnancy/nursing status, and possible drug interactions.

Monitoring: Monitor for signs/symptoms of a hypersensitivity reaction, CDAD, development of drug-resistant bacteria, worsening of symptoms, and other adverse reactions.

Patient Counseling: If being treated for travelers' diarrhea, instruct to d/c therapy and contact physician if diarrhea persists for >24-48 hrs or worsens. Advise to seek medical care for fever and/or blood in the stool. Inform that watery and bloody stools (with or without stomach cramps and fever) may occur even as late as ≥2 months after last dose; advise to contact physician as soon as possible. Inform that drug only treats bacterial, not viral (eg, common cold), infections. Inform that skipping doses or not completing full course of therapy may decrease the effectiveness of treatment and increase resistance. Inform that there is an increase systemic exposure to therapy in patients with severe hepatic impairment (Child-Pugh Class C).

Administration: Oral route. Take with or without food. **Storage:** 20-25°C (68-77°F); excursions permitted to 15-30°C (59-86°F).

XOFIGO

RX

radium ra 223 dichloride (Bayer Healthcare)

THERAPEUTIC CLASS: Radiopharmaceutical agent

INDICATIONS: Treatment of castration-resistant prostate cancer, symptomatic bone metastases and no known visceral metastatic disease.

DOSAGE: *Adults:* 50 kBq (1.35 microcurie)/kg given at 4-week intervals for 6 inj. Refer to PI to calculate total volume to be administered. Administer by slow IV inj over 1 min.

HOW SUPPLIED: Inj: 1000 kBq/mL (27 microcurie/mL) [6mL]

CONTRAINDICATIONS: Pregnancy, women of childbearing potential.

WARNINGS/PRECAUTIONS: Bone marrow failure reported. Myelosuppression (eg, thrombocytopenia, neutropenia, pancytopenia, leukopenia) reported; perform hematologic evaluation at baseline and prior to every dose. Before the 1st administration, the absolute neutrophil count (ANC) should be ≥1.5 x 10⁹/L, the platelet count ≥100 x 10⁹/L and Hgb ≥10g/dL. Before subsequent administrations, the ANC should be ≥1 x 10⁹/L and the platelet count ≥50 x 10⁹/L. D/C therapy if there is no recovery to these values within 6-8 weeks after the last administration. Monitor closely and provide supportive care measures in patients with compromised bone marrow reserve; d/c in patients who experience life-threatening complications despite supportive care for bone marrow failure. Caution in elderly.

ADVERSE REACTIONS: N/V, diarrhea, peripheral edema, anemia, lymphocytopenia, leukopenia, thrombocytopenia, neutropenia.

INTERACTIONS: Concomitant use with chemotherapy is not recommended; d/c therapy if chemotherapy, other systemic radioisotopes or hemibody external radiotherapy are administered during treatment period.

PREGNANCY: Category X, not for use in nursing.

MECHANISM OF ACTION: Radiopharmaceutical agent; α particle-emitting isotope radium-223, which mimics Ca^{2+} and forms complexes with the bone mineral hydroxyapatite at areas of increased bone turnover, such as bone metastases. The high linear energy transfer of α emitters leads to a high frequency of double-strand DNA breaks in adjacent cells, resulting in an antitumor effect on bone metastases.

PHARMACOKINETICS: Distribution: Distributed primarily into bone. **Elimination:** Urine (minimal), feces.

NURSING CONSIDERATIONS

Assessment: Asses for compromised bone marrow reserve. Perform hematologic evaluation at baseline.

Monitoring: Monitor for bone marrow failure, myelosuppression, and other adverse reactions. Perform hematologic evaluation prior to every dose.

Patient Counseling: Advise patients to be compliant with blood cell count monitoring appointments, to stay well hydrated, and to monitor oral intake, fluid status, and urine output while on therapy. Explain the importance of routine blood cell counts. Instruct to report signs of bleeding or infections, dehydration, hypovolemia, urinary retention, or renal failure/insufficiency. Inform that there is no restriction regarding contact with other people after receiving therapy. Advise to follow good hygiene practices while on therapy and for at least 1 week after the last inj in order to minimize radiation exposure from bodily fluids to household members and caregivers. Instruct caregivers to use universal precautions for patient care (eg, gloves and barrier gowns when handling bodily fluids). Advise patients who are sexually active to use condoms and their female partners of reproductive potential to use highly effective method of birth control during therapy and for 6 months following completion of treatment.

Administration: IV route. Flush IV access line or cannula with isotonic saline before and after inj. Refer to PI for instructions for use and handling. **Storage:** Room temperature <40°C (104°F) in the original container or equivalent radiation shielding.

XOLEGEL

RX

ketoconazole (Aqua)

THERAPEUTIC CLASS: Azole antifungal

INDICATIONS: Topical treatment of seborrheic dermatitis in immunocompetent adults and children ≥12 yrs of age.

DOSAGE: *Adults:* Apply qd to affected area for 2 weeks.
Pediatrics: ≥12 Yrs: Apply qd to affected area for 2 weeks.

HOW SUPPLIED: Gel: 2% [45g]

WARNINGS/PRECAUTIONS: Not for oral, ophthalmic, or intravaginal use. Flammable; avoid fire, flame, or smoking during and immediately following application. May cause local irritation at application site; d/c if irritation occurs or if disease worsens. If used during lactation and applied to chest, use caution to avoid accidental ingestion by infant. Hepatitis, lowered testosterone and adrenocorticotropic hormone-induced corticosteroid serum levels reported with orally administered ketoconazole.

ADVERSE REACTIONS: Application-site burning.

INTERACTIONS: Coadministration of oral ketoconazole with CYP3A4 metabolized HMG-CoA reductase inhibitors (eg, simvastatin, lovastatin, atorvastatin) may increase risk of skeletal muscle toxicity, including rhabdomyolysis.

PREGNANCY: Category C, caution in nursing.

MECHANISM OF ACTION: Azole antifungal; not established.

PHARMACOKINETICS: Absorption: Day 7: C_{max}=1.35ng/mL; T_{max}=8 hrs (median); AUC_{0-24}=20.8ng•hr/mL. Day 14: C_{max}=0.80ng/mL; T_{max}=7 hrs (median); AUC_{0-24}=15.6ng•hr/mL.

NURSING CONSIDERATIONS

Assessment: Assess pregnancy/nursing status.

Monitoring: Monitor for irritation and worsening of seborrheic dermatitis.

Patient Counseling: Inform that drug is for external use only. Instruct to use ud and to avoid contact with eyes, nostrils, and mouth. Advise to wash hands after application. Instruct not to use for any disorder other than that for which it has been prescribed. Advise to report any signs of adverse reactions to physician.

Administration: Topical route. **Storage:** 25°C (77°F); excursions permitted to 15-30°C (59-86°F).

XOPENEX HFA   RX
levalbuterol tartrate (Sunovion)

THERAPEUTIC CLASS: Beta$_2$-agonist

INDICATIONS: Treatment or prevention of bronchospasm in patients ≥4 yrs of age with reversible obstructive airway disease.

DOSAGE: *Adults:* 2 inh (90mcg) q4-6h; 1 inh (45mcg) q4h may be sufficient in some patients. Elderly: Start at lower end of dosing range.
Pediatrics: ≥4 Yrs: 2 inh (90mcg) q4-6h; 1 inh (45mcg) q4h may be sufficient in some patients.

HOW SUPPLIED: MDI: 45mcg/inh [80, 200 inhalations]

WARNINGS/PRECAUTIONS: If a previously effective dose regimen fails to provide the usual response or if more doses than usual are needed, this may be a marker of destabilization of asthma and may require reevaluation of the patient and treatment regimen; anti-inflammatory treatment (eg, corticosteroids) may be needed. D/C if paradoxical bronchospasm or cardiovascular (CV) effects occur. ECG changes and immediate hypersensitivity reactions may occur. Fatalities reported with excessive use; do not exceed recommended dose. Caution with CV disorders (eg, coronary insufficiency, arrhythmias, HTN), convulsive disorders, hyperthyroidism, or diabetes mellitus (DM), and in patients unusually responsive to sympathomimetic amines. May produce significant hypokalemia. Caution in elderly and when administering high doses in patients with renal impairment.

ADVERSE REACTIONS: Pharyngitis, rhinitis, pain, vomiting, dizziness, asthma, bronchitis.

INTERACTIONS: Avoid with other short-acting sympathomimetic aerosol bronchodilators or epinephrine; caution with additional adrenergic drugs administered by any route. Use with β-blockers may block pulmonary effects and produce severe bronchospasm in asthmatic patients; avoid concomitant use. If needed, consider cardioselective β-blockers and use with caution. ECG changes and/or hypokalemia caused by non-K$^+$-sparing diuretics (eg, loop or thiazide diuretics) may be worsened; use with caution and consider monitoring K$^+$ levels. May decrease digoxin levels; monitor serum digoxin levels. Use extreme caution with MAOIs or TCAs, or within 2 weeks of discontinuation of such agents.

PREGNANCY: Category C, not for use in nursing.

MECHANISM OF ACTION: β_2-agonist; activates β_2-adrenergic receptors on airway smooth muscle, leading to activation of adenylate cyclase and to an increase in cAMP. Increased cAMP leads to the activation of protein kinase A, which inhibits the phosphorylation of myosin and lowers intracellular ionic Ca^{2+} concentrations, resulting in relaxation of the smooth muscles of all airways, from the trachea to the terminal bronchioles.

X

PHARMACOKINETICS: Absorption: Administration of variable doses in different age groups resulted in different pharmacokinetic parameters. **Metabolism:** GI tract via SULT1A3 (sulfotransferase). **Elimination:** Urine (80-100%), feces (<20%).

NURSING CONSIDERATIONS

Assessment: Assess for history of hypersensitivity to drug or racemic albuterol, CV disorders, convulsive disorders, hyperthyroidism, DM, renal impairment, pregnancy/nursing status, and possible drug interactions. Assess use in patients unusually responsive to sympathomimetic amines.

Monitoring: Monitor for paradoxical bronchospasm, deterioration of asthma, CV effects, ECG changes, hypokalemia, immediate hypersensitivity reactions, and other adverse effects. Monitor BP, HR, and ECG changes.

Patient Counseling: Counsel not to increase dose or frequency of doses without consulting physician. Advise to seek immediate medical attention if treatment becomes less effective for symptomatic relief, symptoms become worse, and/or there is a need to use the product more frequently than usual. Inform that drug may cause paradoxical bronchospasm; instruct to d/c if this occurs. Instruct to take concurrent inhaled drugs and other asthma medications only ud. Inform of the common side effects (eg, chest pain, palpitations, rapid HR, tremor, nervousness). Instruct to notify physician if pregnant/nursing.

Administration: Oral inhalation route. Shake well before use. Prime inhaler before use for the 1st time or if not used for >3 days by releasing 4 test sprays into the air, away from face. Avoid spraying in eyes. Refer to PI for further administration information. **Storage:** 20-25°C (68-77°F). Store with mouthpiece down. Protect from freezing and direct sunlight. Contents under pressure; do not puncture or incinerate. Exposure to temperatures >49°C (120°F) may cause bursting.

XTANDI

RX

enzalutamide (Astellas)

THERAPEUTIC CLASS: Nonsteroidal antiandrogen

INDICATIONS: Treatment of patients with metastatic castration-resistant prostate cancer who have previously received docetaxel.

DOSAGE: *Adults:* Usual: 160mg qd. If experience ≥Grade 3 toxicity or intolerable side effect, withhold dosing for 1 week or until symptoms improve to ≤Grade 2, then resume at same or reduced dose (120mg or 80mg), if warranted. Concomitant Strong CYP2C8 Inhibitors: Reduce dose to 80mg qd; if coadministration of strong CYP2C8 inhibitor is discontinued, dose should be returned to dose used prior to initiation of strong CYP2C8 inhibitor.

HOW SUPPLIED: Cap: 40mg

CONTRAINDICATIONS: Women who are or may become pregnant.

WARNINGS/PRECAUTIONS: Seizures reported; caution in engaging in any activity where sudden loss of consciousness could cause serious harm to patient or to others. Caution in elderly.

ADVERSE REACTIONS: Asthenia, back pain, diarrhea, arthralgia, hot flush, peripheral edema, musculoskeletal pain, headache, upper/lower respiratory tract infection, muscular weakness, dizziness, insomnia, spinal cord compression, hematuria.

INTERACTIONS: Avoid with strong CYP2C8 inhibitors (eg, gemfibrozil) if possible. Strong/moderate CYP2C8 inducers (eg, rifampin) may alter plasma exposure; avoid coadministration if possible and selection of concomitant medication with no or minimal CYP2C8 induction potential is recommended. Increased exposure with gemfibrozil and itraconazole (strong CYP3A4 inhibitor). Strong CYP3A4 inducers (eg, carbamazepine, phenobarbital, phenytoin, rifabutin, rifampin, rifapentine) may decrease plasma exposure; avoid coadministration if possible and recommend to select concomitant medication with no or minimal CYP3A4 induction potential. Moderate CYP3A4 inducers (eg, bosentan, efavirenz, etravirine, modafinil, nafcillin) and St. John's wort may reduce plasma exposure; avoid coadministration if possible. May reduce plasma exposure of midazolam (CYP3A4 substrate) and omeprazole (CYP2C19 substrate). May reduce plasma exposure of warfarin; conduct additional INR monitoring if coadministration cannot be avoided. Avoid with narrow therapeutic index drugs that are metabolized by CYP3A4 (eg, alfentanil, cyclosporine, dihydroergotamine, ergotamine, fentanyl, pimozide, quinidine, sirolimus, tacrolimus), CYP2C9 (eg, phenytoin, warfarin), and CYP2C19 (eg, S-mephenytoin).

PREGNANCY: Category X, not for use in nursing.

MECHANISM OF ACTION: Androgen receptor inhibitor; acts on different steps in the androgen receptor signaling pathway. Competitively inhibits androgen binding to androgen receptors and inhibits androgen receptor nuclear translocation and interaction with DNA.

PHARMACOKINETICS: Absorption: C_{max}=16.6mcg/mL, 12.7mcg/mL (major active metabolite); T_{max}=1 hr. **Distribution:** V_d=110L; plasma protein binding (97-98%, 95% active metabolite). **Metabolism:** Hepatic via CYP2C8 and CYP3A4; N-desmethyl enzalutamide (major active metabolite). **Elimination:** Urine (71%), feces (14%, 0.4% unchanged, 1% active metabolite); $T_{1/2}$=5.8 days, 7.8-8.6 days (major active metabolite).

NURSING CONSIDERATIONS

Assessment: Assess for previous hypersensitivity and possible drug interactions.

Monitoring: Monitor for seizures and other adverse events.

Patient Counseling: Instruct to take dose at the same time each day and ud. Inform those receiving a gonadotropin-releasing hormone analog to maintain such treatment during the course of therapy. Inform that therapy has been associated with increased risk of seizure; advise to discuss conditions that may predispose to seizure and medications that may lower seizure threshold. Advise of risk of engaging in any activity where sudden loss of consciousness could cause serious harm to self or others. Inform that dizziness, mental impairment, paresthesia, hypoesthesia, and falls may occur. Instruct not to interrupt, modify dose or d/c therapy without consulting physician. Advise of the common side effects associated with therapy. Instruct to use a condom if having sex with a pregnant woman and to use a condom and another effective birth control method if having sex with a woman of childbearing potential; advise that these measures are required during and for 3 months after treatment.

Administration: Oral route. Take with or without food. Swallow whole; do not chew, dissolve or open cap. **Storage:** 20-25°C (68-77°F); excursions permitted from 15-30°C (59-86°F).

XYREM

CIII

sodium oxybate (Jazz)

> Obtundation and clinically significant respiratory depression occurred at recommended doses; almost all patients in the trials were receiving CNS stimulants. Sodium oxybate is the Na⁺ salt of gamma hydroxybutyrate (GHB); abuse of GHB, alone or in combination with other CNS depressants, is associated with CNS adverse reactions, including seizure, respiratory depression, decreased level of consciousness, coma, and death. Available only through a restricted distribution program (Xyrem Success Program) because of risk of CNS depression, abuse, and misuse; prescribers and patients must enroll in the program.

THERAPEUTIC CLASS: CNS depressant

INDICATIONS: Treatment of cataplexy and excessive daytime sleepiness in narcolepsy.

DOSAGE: *Adults:* Initial: 4.5g/night in 2 equally divided doses (2.25g qhs at least 2 hrs pc, then 2.25g taken 2.5-4 hrs later). Titrate: Increase by 1.5g/night (0.75g/dose) at weekly intervals. Effective Dose Range: 6-9g/night. Max: 9g/night. Hepatic Impairment: Initial: 2.25g/night in 2 equally divided doses (approximately 1.13g qhs at least 2 hrs pc, then 1.13g taken 2.5-4 hrs later). Elderly: Start at lower end of dosing range.

HOW SUPPLIED: Sol: 0.5g/mL [180mL]

CONTRAINDICATIONS: Concomitant use with sedative hypnotic agents and alcohol. Succinic semialdehyde dehydrogenase deficiency.

WARNINGS/PRECAUTIONS: May only be dispensed to patients enrolled in the Xyrem Success Program. May impair physical/mental abilities. Evaluate for history of drug abuse and monitor closely for signs of misuse/abuse. May impair respiratory drive, especially in patients with compromised respiratory function. Increased central apneas, oxygen desaturation events, and sleep-related breathing disorders may occur. Sleep-related breathing disorders tend to be more prevalent in obese patients, postmenopausal women not on hormone replacement therapy, and narcolepsy patients. Caution in patients with history of depressive illness and/or suicide attempt; monitor for emergence of depressive symptoms. Confusion, anxiety, and other neuropsychiatric reactions (eg, hallucinations, paranoia, psychosis, agitation) reported; carefully evaluate emergence of confusion, thought disorders, and/or behavior abnormalities. Parasomnias reported; fully evaluate episodes of sleepwalking. Contains high salt content; consider amount of daily Na⁺ intake in each dose in patients sensitive to salt intake (eg, heart failure [HF], HTN, renal impairment). Caution with hepatic impairment and in elderly.

ADVERSE REACTIONS: Obtundation, respiratory depression, N/V, dizziness, diarrhea, somnolence, enuresis, tremor, attention disturbance, pain, paresthesia, disorientation, irritability, hyperhidrosis.

INTERACTIONS: See Contraindications. Other CNS depressants (eg, opioid analgesics, benzodiazepines, sedating antidepressants or antipsychotics, general anesthetics, muscle relaxants, and/or illicit CNS depressants) may increase risk of respiratory depression, hypotension, profound sedation, syncope, and death; consider dose reduction or discontinuation of ≥1 CNS depressants (including sodium oxybate) if combination therapy is required. Consider interrupting therapy if short-term use of an opioid (eg, post- or perioperative) is required.

PREGNANCY: Category C, caution in nursing.

X

MECHANISM OF ACTION: CNS depressant; has not been established. Hypothesized that therapeutic effects on cataplexy and excessive daytime sleepiness are mediated through $GABA_B$ actions at noradrenergic and dopaminergic neurons, as well as at thalamocortical neurons.

PHARMACOKINETICS: Absorption: Rapid; absolute bioavailability (88%); T_{max} =0.5-1.25 hr. **Distribution:** V_d=190-384mL/kg; plasma protein binding (<1%). **Metabolism:** Krebs cycle, β-oxidation. **Elimination:** Lungs, urine (<5%), feces; $T_{1/2}$=0.5-1 hr.

NURSING CONSIDERATIONS

Assessment: Assess for succinic semialdehyde dehydrogenase deficiency, alcohol intake, history of drug abuse, compromised respiratory function, history of depressive illness and/or suicide attempt, hepatic impairment, sensitivity to salt intake (eg, HF, HTN, renal impairment), pregnancy/ nursing status, and possible drug interactions.

Monitoring: Monitor for obtundation, respiratory depression, CNS depression, signs of abuse/ misuse, sleep-disordered breathing, suicide attempt, confusion, anxiety, other neuropsychiatric reactions, thought disorders, behavior abnormalities, parasomnias, sleepwalking, and other possible adverse reactions.

Patient Counseling: Inform about the Xyrem Success Program. Instruct to see prescriber frequently (every 3 months) to review dose titration, symptom response, and adverse reactions. Instruct to store drug in a secure place, out of reach of children/pets. Inform that patients are likely to fall asleep quickly (within 5-15 min) after taking the drug; instruct to remain in bed after taking 1st dose. Advise not to drink alcohol or take other sedative hypnotics while on therapy. Inform that therapy can be associated with respiratory depression. Instruct to avoid operating hazardous machinery (eg, automobiles, airplanes) until patients are reasonably certain that therapy does not affect them adversely and for at least 6 hrs after the 2nd nightly dose. Advise to contact physician if depressed mood, markedly diminished interest or pleasure in usual activities, significant change in weight and/or appetite, psychomotor agitation or retardation, increased fatigue, feelings of guilt or worthlessness, slowed thinking or impaired concentration, or suicidal ideation develops. Inform that sleepwalking may occur; instruct to notify physician if this occurs. Inform patients who are sensitive to salt intake that drug contains a significant amount of Na^+ and they should limit their Na^+ intake.

Administration: Oral route. Take 1st dose at least 2 hrs pc. Refer to PI for important preparation and administration instructions. **Storage:** 25°C (77°F); excursions permitted to 15-30°C (59-86°F).

XYZAL   RX
levocetirizine dihydrochloride (Sanofi-Aventis/UCB)

THERAPEUTIC CLASS: H_1-antagonist

INDICATIONS: Relief of symptoms associated with seasonal (adults and children ≥2 yrs of age) and perennial (adults and children ≥6 months of age) allergic rhinitis. Treatment of uncomplicated skin manifestations of chronic idiopathic urticaria in adults and children ≥6 months of age.

DOSAGE: *Adults:* Usual: 5mg (1 tab or 2 tsp [10mL]) qpm. Some may be adequately controlled by 2.5mg qpm. Mild Renal Impairment (CrCl 50-80mL/min): 2.5mg qd. Moderate Renal Impairment (CrCl 30-50mL/min): 2.5mg qod. Severe Renal Impairment (CrCl 10-30mL/min): 2.5mg twice weekly (administered once every 3-4 days). Elderly: Start at lower end of dosing range. *Pediatrics:* ≥12 Yrs: Usual: 5mg (1 tab or 2 tsp [10mL]) qpm. Some may be adequately controlled by 2.5mg qpm. Mild Renal Impairment (CrCl 50-80mL/min): 2.5mg qd. Moderate Renal Impairment (CrCl 30-50mL/min): 2.5mg qod. Severe Renal Impairment (CrCl 10-30mL/min): 2.5mg twice weekly (administered once every 3-4 days). 6-11 Yrs: Usual/Max: 2.5mg (1/2 tab or 1 tsp [5mL]) qpm. 6 Months-5 Yrs: Usual/Max: 1.25mg (1/2 tsp [2.5mL]) qpm.

HOW SUPPLIED: Sol: 0.5mg/mL [5 oz.]; Tab: 5mg* *scored

CONTRAINDICATIONS: End-stage renal disease (CrCl <10mL/min) and patients undergoing hemodialysis, children 6 months-11 yrs of age with renal impairment.

WARNINGS/PRECAUTIONS: Somnolence, fatigue, and asthenia reported. May impair mental/ physical abilities. Urinary retention reported; caution with predisposing factors of urinary retention (eg, spinal cord lesion, prostatic hyperplasia). D/C if urinary retention occurs. Caution in elderly.

ADVERSE REACTIONS: Somnolence, nasopharyngitis, fatigue, dry mouth, constipation, diarrhea, cough, pyrexia, pharyngitis, vomiting, otitis media.

INTERACTIONS: Avoid with alcohol or other CNS depressants; additional reductions in alertness and additional CNS performance impairment may occur. Decreased clearance with theophylline. Increased plasma area under the curve with ritonavir.

PREGNANCY: Category B, not for use in nursing.

MECHANISM OF ACTION: H_1-antagonist; antihistamine that selectively inhibits H_1-receptors.

PHARMACOKINETICS: Absorption: Rapid and extensive. Adults: C_{max}=270ng/mL (single dose), 308ng/mL (multiple doses); T_{max}=0.9 hr (tab), 0.5 hr (PO sol). Pediatrics: (Single dose) C_{max}=450ng/mL; T_{max}=1.2 hrs. **Distribution:** V_d=0.4L/kg; plasma protein binding (91-92%); found in breast milk. **Metabolism:** <14% metabolized through aromatic oxidation (via CYP isoforms), N- and O-dealkylation (via CYP3A4), and taurine conjugation pathways. **Elimination:** Urine (85.4%), feces (12.9%); (adults) $T_{1/2}$=8-9 hrs.

NURSING CONSIDERATIONS

Assessment: Assess for renal impairment, hypersensitivity to the drug, predisposing factors of urinary retention, pregnancy/nursing status, and possible drug interactions.

Monitoring: Monitor for somnolence, fatigue, asthenia, urinary retention, and other adverse reactions.

Patient Counseling: Instruct to use caution when engaging in hazardous occupations requiring complete mental alertness and motor coordination (eg, operating machinery, driving). Instruct to avoid alcohol or other CNS depressants, and to not take more than the recommended dose.

Administration: Oral route. Take without regard to food. **Storage:** 20-25°C (68-77°F); excursions permitted to 15-30°C (59-86°F).

YASMIN   RX
drospirenone - ethinyl estradiol (Bayer Healthcare)

> Cigarette smoking increases the risk of serious cardiovascular (CV) side effects from combination oral contraceptive (COC) use. Risk increases with age (>35 yrs of age) and with the number of cigarettes smoked. Should not be used by women who are >35 yrs of age and smoke.

OTHER BRAND NAMES: Ocella (Barr) - Syeda (Sandoz)

THERAPEUTIC CLASS: Estrogen/progestogen combination

INDICATIONS: Prevention of pregnancy.

DOSAGE: *Adults:* 1 tab qd for 28 days, then repeat. Start 1st Sunday after menses begins or on 1st day of menses. Take at the same time each day, preferably pm, pc, or hs.
Pediatrics: Postpubertal: 1 tab qd for 28 days, then repeat. Start 1st Sunday after menses begins or on 1st day of menses. Take at the same time each day, preferably pm, pc, or hs.

HOW SUPPLIED: Tab: (Drospirenone [DRSP]-Ethinyl Estradiol [EE]) 3mg-0.03mg

CONTRAINDICATIONS: Renal impairment, adrenal insufficiency, high risk of arterial/venous thrombotic disease (eg, smoking if >35 yrs of age, presence/history of deep vein thrombosis/ pulmonary embolism, cerebrovascular disease, coronary artery disease, thrombogenic valvular or thrombogenic rhythm diseases of the heart [eg, subacute bacterial endocarditis with valvular disease, or atrial fibrillation], inherited/acquired hypercoagulopathies, uncontrolled HTN, diabetes mellitus [DM] with vascular disease, headache with focal neurological symptoms or migraine with/without aura if >35 yrs of age), undiagnosed abnormal uterine bleeding, presence/history of breast or other estrogen/progestin-sensitive cancer, benign/malignant liver tumors, liver disease, pregnancy.

WARNINGS/PRECAUTIONS: Increased risk of venous thromboembolism (VTE) and arterial thrombosis (eg, stroke, myocardial infarction [MI]). D/C if arterial/venous thrombotic event occurs. D/C at least 4 weeks before and through 2 weeks after major surgery or other surgeries known to have an elevated risk of thromboembolism. Start therapy no earlier than 4 weeks postpartum in women who do not breastfeed. Caution with cardiovascular disease (CVD) risk factors. D/C if there is unexplained loss of vision, proptosis, diplopia, papilledema, or retinal vascular lesions; evaluate for retinal vein thrombosis immediately. May cause hyperkalemia; avoid use in patients predisposed to hyperkalemia. May increase risk of breast and cervical cancer, intraepithelial neoplasia, and gallbladder disease. Hepatic adenoma and increased risk of hepatocellular carcinoma reported; d/c if jaundice or acute/chronic disturbances of liver function occur. Cholestasis may occur with history of pregnancy-related cholestasis. Increased BP reported; d/c if BP rises significantly. May decrease glucose tolerance; monitor prediabetic and diabetic women. Consider alternative contraception with uncontrolled dyslipidemia. May increase risk of pancreatitis with hypertriglyceridemia or family history thereof. May increase frequency/severity of migraine; d/c if new headaches that are recurrent, persistent, or severe develop. Breakthrough bleeding and spotting may occur; rule out pregnancy or malignancy. Caution with history of depression; d/c if depression recurs to a serious degree. May change results of lab tests (eg, coagulation factors, lipids, glucose tolerance, binding proteins). May induce/exacerbate angioedema in women with hereditary angioedema. Chloasma may occur; women with chloasma should avoid sun exposure or UV radiation. Absorption may not be complete in case of severe vomiting or diarrhea; if vomiting occurs within 3-4 hrs after tablet-taking, regard this as a missed tablet.

ADVERSE REACTIONS: Premenstrual syndrome, headache, migraine, breast pain/tenderness/ discomfort, N/V.

Y

INTERACTIONS: Monitor serum K$^+$ concentration during 1st treatment cycle with drugs that may increase serum K$^+$ concentration (eg, ACE inhibitors, angiotensin II receptor antagonists, K$^+$-sparing diuretics, K$^+$ supplementation, heparin, aldosterone antagonists, NSAIDs). Agents that induce certain enzymes, including CYP3A4 (eg, phenytoin, bosentan, rifampicin), may reduce drug effectiveness or increase incidence of breakthrough bleeding. Significant changes (increase/decrease) in plasma estrogen and progestin levels reported with HIV/hepatitis C virus protease inhibitors or non-nucleoside reverse transcriptase inhibitors. Pregnancy reported with antibiotics. Atorvastatin, ascorbic acid, acetaminophen, CYP3A4 inhibitors (eg, itraconazole, ketoconazole) may increase hormone levels. May decrease levels of lamotrigine and reduce seizure control. May need to increase dose of thyroid hormone in patients on thyroid hormone replacement therapy due to increased thyroid-binding globulin.

PREGNANCY: Contraindicated in pregnancy, not for use in nursing.

MECHANISM OF ACTION: Estrogen/progestogen oral contraceptive; acts primarily by suppressing ovulation. Also causes changes in cervical mucus that inhibit sperm penetration and endometrial changes that reduce the likelihood of implantation.

PHARMACOKINETICS: Absorption: DRSP: Absolute bioavailability (76%); (Cycle 13/day 21) C_{max}=78.7ng/mL; T_{max}=1.6 hrs; AUC=968ng•h/mL. EE: Absolute bioavailability (40%); (Cycle 13/day 21) C_{max}=90.5pg/mL; T_{max}=1.6 hrs; AUC=469pg•h/mL. Refer to PI for additional parameters. **Distribution:** Found in breast milk; DRSP: V_d=4L/kg, plasma protein binding (97%). EE: V_d=4-5L/kg; plasma protein binding (98.5%). **Metabolism:** DRSP: Liver via CYP3A4 (minor). EE: Hydroxylation (via CYP3A4), conjugation (glucuronidation and sulfation). **Elimination:** DSRP: Urine, feces; $T_{1/2}$=30 hrs. EE: Urine, feces; $T_{1/2}$=24 hrs.

NURSING CONSIDERATIONS

Assessment: Assess for renal impairment, abnormal uterine bleeding, adrenal insufficiency, and known or suspected pregnancy and other conditions where treatment is cautioned or contraindicated. Assess use in women who are >35 yrs of age and smoke, have CVD and arterial/venous thrombosis risk factors, predisposition to hyperkalemia, pregnancy-related cholestasis, HTN, DM, uncontrolled dyslipidemia, history of hypertriglyceridemia, history of depression, hereditary angioedema, and history of chloasma. Assess for possible drug interactions.

Monitoring: Monitor for bleeding irregularities, venous/arterial thrombotic and thromboembolic events, cervical cancer or intraepithelial neoplasia, retinal vein thrombosis or any other ophthalmic changes, jaundice, acute/chronic disturbances in liver function, new/worsening headaches or migraines, serious depression, cholestasis with history of pregnancy-related cholestasis, and pancreatitis. Monitor K$^+$ levels, thyroid function if receiving thyroid replacement therapy, glucose levels in DM or prediabetes, lipids with dyslipidemia, liver function, and check BP annually.

Patient Counseling: Counsel that cigarette smoking increases the risk of serious CV events from COC use and to avoid COC use in women who are >35 yrs old and smoke. Inform that drug does not protect against HIV infection and other sexually transmitted diseases. Instruct to take at the same time every day, preferably pm pc or hs. Counsel on what to do if pills are missed or if vomiting occurs within 3-4 hrs after tablet-taking. Inform that amenorrhea may occur and pregnancy should be ruled out if amenorrhea occurs in ≥2 consecutive cycles. Advise to inform physician of preexisting medical conditions and/or drugs currently being taken. Counsel to use an additional method of contraception when enzyme inducers are used with COCs. Counsel women who start COCs postpartum and have not yet had a period to use an additional method of contraception until drug is taken for 7 consecutive days. Instruct to d/c if pregnancy occurs during treatment.

Administration: Oral route. **Storage:** (Syeda) 20-25°C (68-77°F). (Yasmin, Ocella) 25°C (77°F); excursions permitted to 15-30°C (59-86°F).

YAZ RX
drospirenone - ethinyl estradiol (Bayer Healthcare)

> Cigarette smoking increases the risk of serious cardiovascular events from combination oral contraceptive (COC) use. Risk increases with age (>35 yrs of age) and with the number of cigarettes smoked. Should not be used by women who are >35 yrs of age and smoke.

OTHER BRAND NAMES: Loryna (Sandoz)

THERAPEUTIC CLASS: Estrogen/progestogen combination

INDICATIONS: Prevention of pregnancy. Treatment of moderate acne vulgaris in women ≥14 yrs of age who have achieved menarche and who desire an oral contraceptive for birth control. (Yaz) Treatment of symptoms of premenstrual dysphoric disorder (PMDD).

DOSAGE: *Adults:* Contraception/Acne/PMDD: 1 tab qd for 28 days, then repeat. Start 1st Sunday after menses begin or 1st day of menses. Take at the same time each day, preferably pm, pc, or hs.
Pediatrics: Postpubertal: Contraception/Acne (≥14 Yrs)/PMDD: 1 tab qd for 28 days, then repeat.

Start 1st Sunday after menses begin or 1st day of menses. Take at the same time each day, preferably pm, pc, or hs.

HOW SUPPLIED: Tab: (Drospirenone [DRSP]-Ethinyl Estradiol [EE]) 3mg-0.02mg

CONTRAINDICATIONS: Renal impairment, adrenal insufficiency, high risk of arterial/venous thrombotic disease (eg, smoking if >35 yrs of age, active or history of deep vein thrombosis/pulmonary embolism, cerebrovascular disease, coronary artery disease, thrombogenic valvular or thrombogenic rhythm diseases of the heart, inherited/acquired hypercoagulopathies, uncontrolled HTN, diabetes mellitus [DM] with vascular disease, headache with focal neurological symptoms or migraine with/without aura if >35 yrs of age), undiagnosed abnormal uterine bleeding, presence/history of breast or other estrogen/progestin-sensitive cancer, benign/malignant liver tumors, liver disease, pregnancy.

WARNINGS/PRECAUTIONS: Increased risk of venous thromboembolism and arterial thromboses (eg, stroke, myocardial infarction). D/C if arterial or deep venous thrombotic events, unexplained loss of vision, proptosis, diplopia, papilledema, or retinal vascular lesions occur; evaluate for retinal vein thrombosis immediately. Caution in women with cardiovascular disease (CVD) risk factors. D/C at least 4 weeks before and through 2 weeks after major surgery or other surgeries known to have an elevated risk of thromboembolism. Avoid use in patients predisposed to hyperkalemia. May increase risk of cervical cancer or intraepithelial neoplasia and gallbladder disease. Hepatic adenoma reported and increased risk of hepatocellular carcinoma reported; d/c if jaundice or acute/chronic disturbances of liver function occur. Cholestasis may occur with history of pregnancy-related cholestasis. Increased BP reported; d/c if BP rises significantly. May decrease glucose intolerance; monitor prediabetic and diabetic women. Consider alternative contraception with uncontrolled dyslipidemias. Increased risk of pancreatitis with hypertriglyceridemia or family history thereof. May increase frequency/severity of migraine; d/c if new headaches that are recurrent, persistent, or severe develop. Unscheduled bleeding and spotting may occur; rule out pregnancies or malignancies. Caution with history of depression; d/c if depression recurs to serious degree. May change results of lab tests. May induce/exacerbate angioedema. Chloasma may occur, especially with history of chloasma gravidarum; avoid sun or UV radiation exposure. Women who do not breastfeed may start therapy no earlier than 4 weeks postpartum.

ADVERSE REACTIONS: Menstrual irregularities, N/V, headache/migraine, breast pain/tenderness, cervical dysplasia.

INTERACTIONS: Risk of hyperkalemia with ACE inhibitors, angiotensin-II receptor antagonists, K^+-sparing diuretics, K^+ supplementation, heparin, aldosterone antagonists, and NSAIDs. Reduced effectiveness or increased breakthrough bleeding with enzyme inducers, including CYP3A4 (eg, phenytoin, bosentan, rifampicin). Significant changes (increase/decrease) in plasma levels with HIV/hepatitis C virus protease inhibitors or non-nucleoside reverse transcriptase inhibitors. Pregnancy reported with use of hormonal contraceptives and antibiotics. Increased levels with atorvastatin, ascorbic acid, acetaminophen, and CYP3A4 inhibitors (eg, itraconazole, ketoconazole). May decrease plasma concentrations of lamotrigine and reduce seizure control; adjust dose of lamotrigine. Increases thyroid-binding globulin; may need to increase dose of thyroid hormone in patients on thyroid hormone replacement therapy.

PREGNANCY: Contraindicated in pregnancy, not for use in nursing.

MECHANISM OF ACTION: Estrogen/progestogen oral contraceptive; acts by primarily suppressing ovulation. Also causes cervical mucus changes that inhibit sperm penetration and endometrial changes that reduce the likelihood of implantation.

PHARMACOKINETICS: Absorption: DRSP: Absolute bioavailability (76%); (Cycle 1/Day 21) C_{max}=70.3ng/mL; T_{max}=1.5 hrs; AUC=763ng•h/mL. EE: Absolute bioavailability (40%); (Cycle 1/Day 21) C_{max}=45.1pg/mL; T_{max}=1.5 hrs; AUC=220pg•h/mL. **Distribution:** Found in breast milk; DRSP: V_d=4L/kg; serum protein binding (97%). EE: V_d=4-5L/kg; serum albumin binding (98.5%). **Metabolism:** DRSP: Liver, via CYP3A4 (minor). EE: Hydroxylation (via CYP3A4), conjugation with glucuronide and sulfate. **Elimination:** DRSP: Urine, feces; $T_{1/2}$=30 hrs. EE: Urine, feces; $T_{1/2}$=24 hrs.

NURSING CONSIDERATIONS

Assessment: Assess for renal impairment, abnormal uterine bleeding, adrenal insufficiency, and known or suspected pregnancy and other conditions where treatment is cautioned or contraindicated. Assess use in women who are >35 yrs of age and smoke, have CVD and arterial/venous thrombosis risk factors, predisposition to hyperkalemia, pregnancy-related cholestasis, HTN, DM, uncontrolled dyslipidemia, history of hypertriglyceridemia, history of depression, hereditary angioedema, and history of chloasma. Assess for possible drug interactions.

Monitoring: Monitor for bleeding irregularities, venous/arterial thrombotic and thromboembolic events, cervical cancer or intraepithelial neoplasia, retinal vein thrombosis or any other ophthalmic changes, jaundice, acute/chronic disturbances in liver function, new/worsening headaches or migraines, serious depression, cholestasis with history of pregnancy-related cholestasis, and pancreatitis. Monitor K^+ levels, thyroid function if receiving thyroid replacement therapy, glucose levels in DM or prediabetes, lipids with dyslipidemia, and check BP annually.

Y

Patient Counseling: Counsel that cigarette smoking increases the risk of serious CV events from COC use and to avoid use of the drug in women who are >35 yrs old and smoke. Inform that drug does not protect against HIV infection and other sexually transmitted diseases. Instruct to take at the same time every day preferably pm pc or hs. Instruct on what to do if pills are missed or vomiting occurs within 3-4 hrs after tablet-taking. Inform that COCs may reduce breast milk production. Inform that amenorrhea may occur and pregnancy should be ruled out if amenorrhea occurs in ≥2 consecutive cycles. Advise to inform physician of preexisting medical conditions and/or drugs currently being taken. Counsel to use additional method of contraception when enzyme inducers are used with COCs. Counsel women who start COCs postpartum and have not yet had a period to use additional method of contraception until drug taken for 7 consecutive days. Instruct to d/c if pregnancy occurs during treatment.

Administration: Oral route. **Storage:** (YAZ) 25°C (77°F); excursions permitted to 15-30°C (59-86°F). (Loryna) 20-25°C (68-77°F).

YERVOY   RX

ipilimumab (Bristol-Myers Squibb)

Can result in severe and fatal immune-mediated adverse reactions due to T-cell activation and proliferation, which may involve any organ system; most common are enterocolitis, hepatitis, dermatitis (eg, toxic epidermal necrolysis [TEN]), neuropathy, endocrinopathy). The majority of these reactions initially manifested during treatment; however, a minority occurred weeks to months after discontinuation of therapy. Permanently d/c therapy and initiate systemic high-dose corticosteroid therapy for severe immune-mediated reactions. Assess for signs/symptoms of enterocolitis, dermatitis, neuropathy, and endocrinopathy and evaluate clinical chemistries (eg, LFTs, thyroid function tests) at baseline and before each dose.

THERAPEUTIC CLASS: Monoclonal antibody/CTLA-4 blocker

INDICATIONS: Treatment of unresectable or metastatic melanoma.

DOSAGE: *Adults:* Usual: 3mg/kg IV over 90 min every 3 weeks for a total of 4 doses. Refer to PI for recommended dose modifications.

HOW SUPPLIED: Inj: 5mg/mL [10mL, 40mL]

WARNINGS/PRECAUTIONS: Withhold scheduled dose for any moderate immune-mediated adverse reactions or for symptomatic endocrinopathy. Permanently d/c therapy for any persistent moderate adverse reactions or inability to reduce corticosteroid dose to 7.5mg prednisone or equivalent/day, failure to complete full treatment course within 16 weeks from administration of 1st dose, and severe or life-threatening adverse reactions (eg, colitis with abdominal pain, fever, ileus, peritoneal signs; increase in stool frequency [≥7 over baseline]; stool incontinence; need for IV hydration >24 hrs; GI hemorrhage/perforation; AST or ALT >5X ULN; total bilirubin >3X ULN; Stevens-Johnson syndrome; TEN; rash complicated by full thickness dermal ulceration or necrotic, bullous, or hemorrhagic manifestations; severe motor or sensory neuropathy; Guillain-Barre syndrome; myasthenia gravis; severe immune-mediated reactions involving any organ system; immune-mediated ocular disease that is unresponsive to topical immunosuppressive therapy).

ADVERSE REACTIONS: Immune-mediated reactions (eg, enterocolitis, hepatitis, dermatitis, neuropathy, endocrinopathy), diarrhea, colitis, pruritus, rash, fatigue.

INTERACTIONS: Increased transaminases with or without concomitant increase in total bilirubin in some patients who received concurrent vemurafenib (960mg bid or 720mg bid).

PREGNANCY: Category C, not for use in nursing.

MECHANISM OF ACTION: IgG1 kappa human monoclonal antibody; binds to and blocks the interaction of cytotoxic T-lymphocyte-associated antigen-4 (CTLA-4) with its ligands, CD80/CD86. Blockade of CTLA-4 has been shown to augment T-cell activation and proliferation. Mechanism of action in patients with melanoma is indirect; possibly through T-cell mediated antitumor immune responses.

PHARMACOKINETICS: Distribution: Crosses placenta. **Elimination:** $T_{1/2}$=15.4 days.

NURSING CONSIDERATIONS

Assessment: Assess for signs/symptoms of enterocolitis, dermatitis, neuropathy, endocrinopathy, and hepatotoxicity. Assess for pregnancy/nursing status and possible drug interactions. Evaluate clinical chemistries, including LFTs and thyroid function tests, at baseline.

Monitoring: Monitor for signs/symptoms of enterocolitis (eg, diarrhea, abdominal pain, mucus or blood in stool), bowel perforation (eg, peritoneal signs, ileus), hepatotoxicity, dermatitis (eg, rash, pruritus), motor or sensory neuropathy (eg, unilateral or bilateral weakness, sensory alterations, paresthesia), hypophysitis, adrenal insufficiency, hyper- or hypothyroidism, and other severe immune-mediated adverse reactions. Monitor clinical chemistries, including LFTs and thyroid function tests, before each dose and as clinically indicated.

Patient Counseling: Inform of the potential risk of immune-mediated adverse reactions. Instruct to read the medication guide before each infusion. Advise women that therapy may cause fetal harm. Advise nursing mothers not to breastfeed while on therapy.

Administration: IV route. Do not shake. Refer to PI for further preparation and administration instructions. **Storage:** 2-8°C (36-46°F). Do not freeze. Protect from light. Diluted Sol: Store for no more than 24 hrs at 2-8°C (36-46°F) or at 20-25°C (68-77°F).

ZALTRAP   RX
ziv-aflibercept (Sanofi-Aventis)

> Severe and sometimes fatal hemorrhage, including GI hemorrhage, reported in combination with 5-fluorouracil, leucovor-
> in, and irinotecan (FOLFIRI). Monitor for signs and symptoms of GI bleeding and other severe bleeding. Do not administer
> in patients with severe hemorrhage. Nonfatal/fatal GI perforation may occur; d/c therapy in patients who experience GI
> perforation. Severe compromised wound healing may occur; d/c in patients with compromised wound healing. Suspend for
> at least 4 weeks prior to elective surgery; do not resume for at least 4 weeks following major surgery and until the surgical
> wound is fully healed.

THERAPEUTIC CLASS: Vascular endothelial growth factor (VEGF) inhibitor

INDICATIONS: In combination with FOLFIRI for the treatment of metastatic colorectal cancer that is resistant to or has progressed following an oxaliplatin-containing regimen.

DOSAGE: *Adults:* 4mg/kg IV infusion over 1 hr every 2 weeks. Administer prior to any component of the FOLFIRI regimen on day of treatment. Continue until disease progression or unacceptable toxicity. With Recurrent or Severe HTN: Temporarily suspend until controlled and permanently reduce dose to 2mg/kg upon resumption. With Proteinuria: Temporarily suspend for proteinuria ≥2g/24 hrs and resume when proteinuria is <2g/24 hrs. If recurrent, suspend until proteinuria is <2g/24 hrs and then permanently reduce dose to 2mg/kg.

HOW SUPPLIED: Inj: 25mg/mL [4mL, 8mL]

WARNINGS/PRECAUTIONS: D/C if severe hemorrhage develops. For minor surgery (eg, central venous access port placement, biopsy, tooth extraction), may initiate/resume therapy once surgical wound is fully healed. Fistula formation involving GI and non-GI sites reported; d/c in patients who develop fistula. Increased risk of Grade 3-4 HTN; treat with appropriate antihypertensives and continue monitoring BP regularly. D/C with hypertensive crisis or hypertensive encephalopathy. Arterial thromboembolic events (ATE), including transient ischemic attack, cerebrovascular accident, and angina pectoris; severe proteinuria; nephrotic syndrome; and thrombotic microangiopathy (TMA) reported. D/C if ATE, nephrotic syndrome, or TMA develops. Higher incidence of neutropenic complications (eg, febrile neutropenia, neutropenic infection) reported; delay therapy until neutrophil count is ≥1.5 x 10⁹/L. Diarrhea and dehydration reported; closely monitor elderly for diarrhea and dehydration. Reversible posterior encephalopathy syndrome (RPLS) reported; confirm diagnosis of RPLS with magnetic resonance imaging and d/c if RPLS develops. Male and female reproductive function and fertility may be compromised during treatment; use highly effective contraception during and up to a minimum of 3 months after the last dose.

ADVERSE REACTIONS: Hemorrhage, GI perforation, compromised wound healing, leukopenia, diarrhea, neutropenia, proteinuria, AST/ALT increased, stomatitis, fatigue, thrombocytopenia, HTN, weight decrease, decreased appetite, epistaxis.

PREGNANCY: Category C, not for use in nursing.

MECHANISM OF ACTION: VEGF inhibitor; binds to VEGF-A, VEGF-B, and P1GF, and thereby inhibits the binding and activation of their cognate receptors. This inhibition can result in decreased neovascularization and decreased vascular permeability.

PHARMACOKINETICS: Elimination: $T_{1/2}$=6 days.

NURSING CONSIDERATIONS

Assessment: Assess for recent surgery, severe hemorrhage, compromised wound healing, HTN, proteinuria, history of ATE, neutropenia, and pregnancy/nursing status. Obtain baseline CBC with differential count.

Monitoring: Monitor for signs/symptoms of bleeding, GI perforation, fistula formation, compromised wound healing, hypertensive crisis/encephalopathy, ATE, nephrotic syndrome, TMA, diarrhea, dehydration, RPLS, and other adverse reactions. Monitor BP every 2 weeks or more frequently as indicated. Monitor proteinuria by urine dipstick analysis and/or urinary protein creatinine ratio (UPCR) for the development or worsening of proteinuria; obtain a 24-hr urine collection in patients with a dipstick of ≥2+ for protein or UPCR >1. Monitor CBC with differential count prior to initiation of each cycle.

Patient Counseling: Advise to contact physician if bleeding/symptoms of bleeding, elevated BP/symptoms from HTN, severe diarrhea, vomiting, severe abdominal pain, or fever or other signs of infection occur. Inform of the increased risk of compromised wound healing and instruct not to undergo surgery or procedures, including tooth extractions, without discussing 1st with the

Z

physician. Inform of an increased risk of ATE. Inform of the potential risks to the fetus or neonate during pregnancy or nursing; instruct to use highly effective contraception in both males and females during and for at least 3 months following last dose of therapy; advise to immediately contact physician or their partner becomes pregnant during treatment.

Administration: IV route. Do not administer as an IV push or bolus. Do not combine with other drugs in the same infusion bag or IV line. Refer to PI for preparation and further administration instructions. **Storage:** 2-8°C (36-46°F). Keep vials in original carton to protect from light. Diluted Sol: 2-8°C (36-46°F) for up to 4 hrs.

ZANAFLEX   RX
tizanidine HCl (Acorda)

THERAPEUTIC CLASS: Alpha$_2$-agonist

INDICATIONS: Management of spasticity.

DOSAGE: *Adults:* Initial: 2mg. May repeat at 6-8 hr intervals, PRN, up to a maximum of 3 doses/24 hr. Titrate: May gradually increase by 2-4mg/dose, with 1-4 days between increases, until a satisfactory reduction in muscle tone is achieved. Max: 36mg/day. Renal Impairment (CrCl <25mL/min)/Hepatic Impairment: Reduce individual doses during titration. If higher doses are required, increase individual doses. Drug Discontinuation: Decrease dose slowly (2-4mg/day), particularly in patients who have been receiving high doses (20-28mg/day) for long periods of time (≥9 weeks) or who may be on concomitant treatment with narcotics. May take with or without food; do not alter regimen once formulation has been selected and the decision to take with or without food has been made.

HOW SUPPLIED: Cap: 2mg, 4mg, 6mg; Tab: 4mg* *scored

CONTRAINDICATIONS: Concomitant use with potent CYP1A2 inhibitors (eg, fluvoxamine, ciprofloxacin).

WARNINGS/PRECAUTIONS: May cause hypotension; may be minimized by dose titration and by focusing attention on signs/symptoms of hypotension prior to dose advancement. May cause hepatocellular liver injury; caution with hepatic impairment. May cause sedation. Associated with hallucinations/psychosis; consider discontinuation if hallucinations develop. May cause anaphylaxis. Caution with renal insufficiency; monitor closely for the onset or increase in severity of the common adverse events (dry mouth, somnolence, asthenia, dizziness). Withdrawal adverse reactions (eg, rebound HTN, tachycardia, hypertonia) may occur. Caution in elderly.

ADVERSE REACTIONS: Dry mouth, somnolence, asthenia, dizziness, urinary tract infection, infection, constipation, LFT abnormality, vomiting, speech disorder, amblyopia (blurred vision), urinary frequency, dyskinesia, nervousness, pharyngitis.

INTERACTIONS: See Contraindications and Dosage. Avoid with other CYP1A2 inhibitors (eg, zileuton, fluoroquinolones other than strong CYP1A2 inhibitors [which are contraindicated], antiarrhythmics [amiodarone, mexiletine, propafenone, verapamil], cimetidine, famotidine, oral contraceptives, acyclovir, ticlopidine]; if use is clinically necessary, initiate therapy with 2mg dose and increase in 2-4mg steps daily based on patient response to therapy. If an adverse reaction such as hypotension, bradycardia, or excessive drowsiness occurs, reduce or d/c therapy. Additive sedative effects with alcohol and other CNS depressants (eg, benzodiazepines, opioids, TCAs); monitor for symptoms of excess sedation. Monitor for hypotension in patients receiving concurrent antihypertensive therapy. Not recommended with other α_2-adrenergic agonists. Withdrawal symptoms are more likely to occur with concomitant use of narcotics.

PREGNANCY: Category C, caution in nursing.

MECHANISM OF ACTION: Centrally acting α_2-agonist: presumably reduces spasticity by increasing presynaptic inhibition of motor neurons.

PHARMACOKINETICS: Absorption: Complete; absolute bioavailability (40%). (Single Dose) T_{max}=1 hr (two 4mg caps/tabs, fasted); T_{max}=85 min (two 4mg tabs, fed); T_{max}=2-3 hrs (two 4mg caps, fed). **Distribution:** (IV, Healthy) V_d=2.4L/kg; plasma protein binding (30%). **Metabolism:** Liver (extensive) via CYP1A2. **Elimination:** Urine (60%), feces (20%); $T_{1/2}$=2.5 hrs, 2 hrs (two 4mg tabs/caps, fasted).

NURSING CONSIDERATIONS

Assessment: Assess for hypersensitivity to drug, hypotension, hepatic/renal impairment, pregnancy/nursing status, and possible drug interactions. Obtain baseline aminotransferase levels.

Monitoring: Monitor for hypotension, hepatocellular liver injury, anaphylaxis, sedation, hallucinations/psychosis, syncope, dry mouth, somnolence, asthenia, dizziness, and other adverse reactions. Monitor aminotransferase levels at 1 month after max dose is achieved or if hepatic injury is suspected. Monitor renal function with renal impairment and in elderly.

Patient Counseling: Advise not to take with fluvoxamine or ciprofloxacin due to increased risk of serious adverse reactions (eg, severe lowering of BP, sedation); instruct to inform physician

Z

if start/stop taking any medication. Instruct to take exactly ud, and not to switch between tab and cap. Advise not to suddenly d/c therapy because rebound HTN and tachycardia may occur. Inform that they may experience hypotension; advise to be careful when changing from lying/sitting to standing position. Inform that medication may cause somnolence or sedation; instruct to be careful when performing activities that require alertness (eg, driving/operating machinery). Inform that sedation may be additive when taken with drugs (baclofen, benzodiazepines) or substances (eg, alcohol) that act as CNS depressants. Inform that medication decreases spasticity; advise to use caution if dependent on spasticity to sustain posture and balance in locomotion, or whenever spasticity is utilized to obtain increased function. Inform of the signs/symptoms of severe allergic reactions; instruct to d/c and seek immediate medical care if these occur.

Administration: Oral route. Take with or without food. **Storage:** 25°C (77°F); excursions permitted to 15-30°C (59-86°F).

ZARAH   RX
drospirenone - ethinyl estradiol (Watson)

> Cigarette smoking increases the risk of serious cardiovascular (CV) side effects from oral contraceptive use. Risk increases with age (>35 yrs of age) and with heavy smoking (≥15 cigarettes/day). Women who use oral contraceptives should be strongly advised not to smoke.

THERAPEUTIC CLASS: Estrogen/progestogen combination

INDICATIONS: Prevention of pregnancy.

DOSAGE: *Adults:* 1 blue tab (active) qd for 21 consecutive days, followed by 1 peach tab (inert) on Days 22-28. Start 1st Sunday after menses begins or 1st day of menses. Should be taken at the same time each day, preferably pm, pc, or qhs. Begin next and all subsequent regimens on the same day of the week on which the 1st regimen began.
Pediatrics: Postpubertal: 1 blue tab (active) qd for 21 consecutive days, followed by 1 peach tab (inert) on Days 22-28. Start 1st Sunday after menses begins or 1st day of menses. Should be taken at the same time each day, preferably pm, pc, or qhs. Begin next and all subsequent regimens on the same day of the week on which 1st regimen began.

HOW SUPPLIED: Tab: (Ethinyl Estradiol [EE]-Drospirenone [DRSP]) 0.03mg-3mg

CONTRAINDICATIONS: Renal or adrenal insufficiency, hepatic dysfunction, thrombophlebitis, thromboembolic disorders, history of deep vein thrombophlebitis or thromboembolic disorders, cerebrovascular or coronary artery disease (CAD), valvular heart disease with thrombogenic complications, severe HTN, diabetes with vascular involvement, headaches with focal neurological symptoms, known or suspected breast carcinoma, endometrial carcinoma or other known or suspected estrogen-dependent neoplasia, undiagnosed abnormal genital bleeding, cholestatic jaundice of pregnancy or jaundice with prior pill use, liver tumor (benign or malignant) or active liver disease, pregnancy, heavy smoking (>15 cigarettes daily) and >35 yrs of age.

WARNINGS/PRECAUTIONS: May cause hyperkalemia in high-risk patients; avoid use in patients predisposed to hyperkalemia (eg, renal insufficiency, hepatic dysfunction, adrenal insufficiency). Monitor K+ levels during 1st treatment cycle with conditions predisposed to hyperkalemia. Increased risk of myocardial infarction (MI), thromboembolism, stroke, gallbladder disease, vascular disease, and hepatic neoplasia. Increased risk of morbidity and mortality in patients with HTN, hyperlipidemia, obesity, and diabetes mellitus (DM). May increase risk of breast cancer and cervical intraepithelial neoplasia. Retinal thrombosis reported; d/c use if unexplained partial or complete loss of vision, onset of proptosis or diplopia, papilledema, or retinal vascular lesions develop. May cause glucose intolerance; monitor prediabetic and diabetic patients. May cause fluid retention. May increase BP; monitor closely with HTN and d/c if significant elevation of BP occurs. D/C with onset or exacerbation of migraine or development of headache with new pattern which is persistent, recurrent, and severe. Breakthrough bleeding and spotting reported; rule out malignancy or pregnancy. Monitor closely with hyperlipidemias. D/C if jaundice develops. Monitor closely with depression and d/c if depression recurs to serious degree. Contact lens wearers who develop visual changes or changes in lens tolerance should be assessed by an ophthalmologist. Should not be used to induce withdrawal bleeding as a test for pregnancy or to treat threatened or habitual abortion during pregnancy. May affect certain endocrine, LFTs, and blood components in lab tests. Does not protect against HIV infection (AIDS) and other STDs.

ADVERSE REACTIONS: N/V, breakthrough bleeding, spotting, amenorrhea, migraine, depression, vaginal candidiasis, edema, weight changes, breast changes, GI symptoms (abdominal cramps and bloating), menstrual flow changes.

INTERACTIONS: Concomitant use with rifampin, anticonvulsants (eg, phenobarbital, phenytoin, carbamazepine), or phenylbutazone may reduce contraceptive effectiveness and increase menstrual irregularities. Pregnancy reported with antimicrobials (eg, ampicillin, tetracycline, griseofulvin). St. John's wort may reduce contraceptive effectiveness and cause breakthrough bleeding. Increased levels with atorvastatin, ascorbic acid, and acetaminophen (APAP). Risk of hyperkalemia with ACE inhibitors, angiotensin-II receptor antagonists, K+-sparing diuretics,

Z

heparin, aldosterone antagonists, and NSAIDs; monitor K⁺ levels during 1st cycle. May increase levels of cyclosporine, prednisolone, and theophylline. May decrease APAP levels and increase clearance of temazepam, salicylic acid, morphine, and clofibric acid.

PREGNANCY: Category X, not for use in nursing.

MECHANISM OF ACTION: Estrogen/progestogen oral contraceptive; suppresses gonadotropins. Inhibits ovulation and produces changes in cervical mucus (increasing difficulty of sperm entry into uterus) and endometrium (reducing likelihood of implantation).

PHARMACOKINETICS: Absorption: DRSP: Absolute bioavailability (76%); (Cycle 13/Day 21) C_{max}=78.7ng/mL; T_{max}=1.6 hrs; AUC=968ng•h/mL. EE: Absolute bioavailability (40%); (Cycle 13/Day 21) C_{max}=90.5pg/mL; T_{max}=1.6 hrs; AUC=469.5pg•h/mL. **Distribution:** Found in breast milk; DRSP: V_d=4L/kg; serum protein binding (97%). EE: V_d=4-5L/kg; serum albumin binding (98.5%). **Metabolism:** DRSP: Liver, via CYP3A4 (minor). EE: Hydroxylation (via CYP3A4), conjugation (glucuronidation and sulfation). **Elimination:** DRSP: Urine, feces; $T_{1/2}$=30 hrs. EE: Urine, feces; $T_{1/2}$=24 hrs.

NURSING CONSIDERATIONS

Assessment: Assess for current or history of thrombophlebitis or thromboembolic disorders, cerebrovascular disorders, or any other conditions where treatment is contraindicated or cautioned. Assess for pregnancy/nursing status and for possible drug interactions. Assess use in patients with contact lenses, HTN, DM, hyperlipidemia, and who are obese.

Monitoring: Monitor for signs/symptoms of MI, thromboembolism, cerebrovascular disease, carcinoma of the breast, cervical intraepithelial neoplasia, hepatic neoplasia, onset or exacerbation of a migraine headache, gallbladder disease, ocular lesions, hypertriglyceridemia, HTN, bleeding irregularities, jaundice, and for fluid retention. Monitor for signs of worsening depression in patients with a history of depression. Monitor lipid levels in patients with a history of hyperlipidemia. Monitor blood glucose levels in patients with DM. Monitor BP in patients with HTN. Perform annual history and physical exam. Monitor K⁺ levels in patients at risk for hyperkalemia. Refer patients with contact lenses to an ophthalmologist if visual changes or changes in contact lens tolerance occur.

Patient Counseling: Inform that drug does not protect against HIV infection (AIDS) and other STDs. Inform of potential risks/benefits of oral contraceptives. Counsel not to smoke while on treatment. Instruct to take medication at the same time daily. Inform that there may be spotting, light bleeding, or nausea during first 1-3 packs; advise not to d/c medication and if symptoms persist, notify physician. Inform that if started later than the 1st day of the menstrual cycle, it should not be considered effective as a contraceptive until after first 7 consecutive days of administration. Instruct what to do in the event pills are missed.

Administration: Oral route. **Storage:** 20-25°C (68-77°F).

ZARONTIN   RX
ethosuximide (Parke-Davis)

THERAPEUTIC CLASS: Succinimide

INDICATIONS: Control of absence (petit mal) epilepsy.

DOSAGE: *Adults:* Initial: 500mg qd. Titrate: Individualize dose according to response. May increase daily dose by 250mg q4-7 days until control is achieved with minimal side effects. Caution with doses >1.5g/day, in divided doses.
Pediatrics: Initial: ≥6 Yrs: 500mg qd. 3-6 yrs: 250mg qd. Titrate: Individualize dose according to response. May increase daily dose by 250mg q4-7 days until control is achieved with minimal side effects. Optimal Dose: 20mg/kg/day. Caution with doses >1.5g/day, in divided doses.

HOW SUPPLIED: Cap: 250mg; Syrup: 250mg/5mL [474mL]

WARNINGS/PRECAUTIONS: Blood dyscrasias and abnormal renal and liver function studies reported; extreme caution with known liver or renal disease. Perform periodic blood counts, urinalysis, and LFTs. Systemic lupus erythematosus (SLE) reported. May increase risk of suicidal thoughts or behavior; monitor for emergence or worsening of depression and any unusual changes in mood or behavior. Serious dermatologic reactions, including Stevens-Johnson syndrome (SJS) reported; d/c at the 1st sign of rash (unless rash is clearly not drug-related) and do not resume and consider alternative therapy if signs/symptoms suggest SJS. Cases of birth defects reported. May increase frequency of grand mal seizures when used alone in mixed types of epilepsy. May precipitate absence (petit mal) status with abrupt withdrawal; adjust dose slowly.

ADVERSE REACTIONS: Anorexia, N/V, abdominal pain, leukopenia, drowsiness, headache, urticaria, SLE, myopia, vaginal bleeding, diarrhea, euphoria, hirsutism, microscopic hematuria.

INTERACTIONS: May interact with other antiepileptic drugs (eg, may increase levels of phenytoin; increased or decreased levels reported with valproic acid); periodically determine serum levels of these drugs.

PREGNANCY: Safety not known in pregnancy, caution in nursing.

MECHANISM OF ACTION: Succinimide; suppresses paroxysmal 3 cycle/sec spike and wave activity associated with lapses of consciousness that is common in absence (petit mal) seizures. Frequency of attacks is reduced by depression of motor cortex and elevation of the CNS threshold to convulsive stimuli.

PHARMACOKINETICS: Distribution: Crosses placenta; found in breast milk.

NURSING CONSIDERATIONS

Assessment: Assess for history of hypersensitivity to succinimides, depression, renal/hepatic impairment, pregnancy/nursing status, and possible drug interactions.

Monitoring: Monitor for blood dyscrasias, signs/symptoms of SLE, dermatologic reactions, renal function, and infection (eg, sore throat, fever). Monitor for occurrence of grand mal seizures in patients with mixed types of epilepsy who are on monotherapy. Monitor CBC, urinalysis, and LFT periodically. Monitor for worsening of depression, suicidal thoughts or behavior and/or any unusual changes in mood or behavior.

Patient Counseling: Inform of the importance of strictly adhering to prescribed dosage regimen. Inform that the therapy may impair mental/physical abilities. Instruct to contact physician if any signs/symptoms of infection (eg, sore throat, fever) develop. Advise to be alert for the emergence or worsening of depression, any unusual changes in mood or behavior, suicidal thoughts/behavior, and to report to physician any behaviors of concern. Instruct to report to physician immediately if rash occurs. If pregnant, encourage to enroll in North American Antiepileptic Drug (NAAED) Pregnancy Registry.

Administration: Oral route. May be coadministered with other anticonvulsants when other forms of epilepsy coexist with absence. **Storage:** (Cap) 25°C (77°F); excursions permitted to 15-30°C (59-86°F). (Syrup) 20-25°C (68-77°F). Preserve in tight containers. Protect from freezing and light.

ZAROXOLYN   RX
metolazone (CellTech)

> Do not interchange rapid and complete bioavailability metolazone formulations for other slow and incomplete bioavailability metolazone formulations; they are not therapeutically equivalent.

THERAPEUTIC CLASS: Quinazoline diuretic

INDICATIONS: Treatment of HTN and of salt and water retention in edema accompanying congestive heart failure or renal disease.

DOSAGE: *Adults:* Edema: 5-20mg qd. HTN: 2.5-5mg qd. Elderly: Start at low end of dosing range.

HOW SUPPLIED: Tab: 2.5mg, 5mg, 10mg

CONTRAINDICATIONS: Anuria, hepatic coma or precoma.

WARNINGS/PRECAUTIONS: Risk of hypokalemia, orthostatic hypotension, hypercalcemia, hyperuricemia, azotemia, and rapid-onset hyponatremia. Cross-allergy with sulfonamide-derived drugs, thiazides, or quinethazone. Sensitivity reactions may occur with 1st dose. Monitor electrolytes. May cause hyperglycemia and glycosuria in diabetics. Caution in elderly or severe renal impairment. May exacerbate or activate systemic lupus erythematosus (SLE).

ADVERSE REACTIONS: Chest pain/discomfort, orthostatic hypotension, syncope, neuropathy, necrotizing angiitis, hepatitis, jaundice, pancreatitis, blood dyscrasias, joint pain.

INTERACTIONS: Furosemide and other loop diuretics prolong fluid and electrolyte loss. Adjust dose of other antihypertensives. Potentiates hypotensive effects of alcohol, barbiturates, and narcotics. Risk of lithium and digitalis toxicity. Corticosteroids and adrenocorticotropic hormone increase salt and water retention and increase risk of hypokalemia. Enhanced neuromuscular blocking effects of curariform drugs. Salicylates and NSAIDs decrease effects. Decreased arterial response to norepinephrine. Decrease in methenamine efficacy. Dose adjustments of anticoagulants and antidiabetic agents may be necessary.

PREGNANCY: Category B, not for use in nursing.

MECHANISM OF ACTION: Quinazoline diuretic; acts primarily to inhibit Na^+ reabsorption at cortical diluting site and, to a lesser extent, in proximal convoluted tubule.

PHARMACOKINETICS: Absorption: T_{max}=8 hrs. **Elimination:** Urine (unchanged).

NURSING CONSIDERATIONS

Assessment: Assess for anuria, SLE, diabetes mellitus, sulfonamide hypersensitivity, history of allergy or bronchial asthma, hepatic/renal impairment, possible drug interactions.

Monitoring: Monitor serum electrolytes periodically. Monitor for signs/symptoms of electrolyte imbalance, exacerbation or activation of SLE, hyperglycemia, hyperuricemia or precipitation of

Z

gout, hypersensitivity reactions (eg, angioedema, bronchospasm, toxic epidermal necrolysis, Stevens-Johnson syndrome), orthostatic hypotension, renal/hepatic dysfunction.

Patient Counseling: Counsel to take medication ud and promptly report adverse reactions. Advise not to interchange formulations. Instruct to seek medical attention if symptoms of electrolyte imbalance (eg, dry mouth, thirst, weakness) or hypersensitivity reactions occur.

Administration: Oral route. **Storage:** 25°C (77°F); excursions permitted to 15-30°C (59-86°F). Protect from light.

ZEBETA   RX
bisoprolol fumarate (Duramed)

THERAPEUTIC CLASS: Selective beta$_1$-blocker

INDICATIONS: Management of HTN alone or in combination with other antihypertensive agents.

DOSAGE: *Adults:* Individualize dose. Initial: 5mg qd. Titrate: May increase to 10mg and then, if necessary, to 20mg qd. Bronchospastic Disease: Initial: 2.5mg qd. Hepatic/Renal Dysfunction (CrCl <40mL/min): Initial: 2.5mg qd; caution with dose titration.

HOW SUPPLIED: Tab: 5mg*, 10mg *scored

CONTRAINDICATIONS: Cardiogenic shock, overt cardiac failure, 2nd- or 3rd-degree atrioventricular (AV) block, marked sinus bradycardia.

WARNINGS/PRECAUTIONS: Avoid abrupt withdrawal; exacerbation of angina pectoris, myocardial infarction (MI) and ventricular arrhythmia in patients with coronary artery disease, and exacerbation of symptoms of hyperthyroidism or precipitation of thyroid storm reported. Reinstitute temporary therapy if withdrawal symptoms occur. May mask manifestations of hypoglycemia or clinical signs of hyperthyroidism (eg, tachycardia). Caution with compensated cardiac failure, diabetes mellitus, bronchospastic disease, and hepatic/renal impairment. May precipitate cardiac failure; d/c at the 1st signs/symptoms of heart failure (HF) or continue therapy while HF is treated with other drugs. Caution with peripheral vascular disease; may precipitate or aggravate symptoms of arterial insufficiency. Caution with history of severe anaphylactic reaction to a variety of allergens; reactivity may increase with repeated challenge.

ADVERSE REACTIONS: Headache, upper respiratory infection, peripheral edema, fatigue, ALT/AST elevation.

INTERACTIONS: Patients with a history of severe anaphylactic reaction to a variety of allergens taking β-blockers may be unresponsive to usual doses of epinephrine. D/C several days before withdrawal of clonidine. Excessive reduction of sympathetic activity with catecholamine-depleting drugs (eg, reserpine, guanethidine); monitor closely. Avoid with other β-blockers. Caution with myocardial depressants or inhibitors of AV conduction, such as calcium antagonists (eg, verapamil, diltiazem) or antiarrhythmics (eg, disopyramide). Increased risk of bradycardia with digitalis glycosides. Increased clearance with rifampin. Caution with insulin or oral hypoglycemic agents. Reversed effects with bronchodilator therapy. Additive BP lowering effects in mild to moderate HTN with HCTZ.

PREGNANCY: Category C, caution in nursing.

MECHANISM OF ACTION: β$_1$-selective adrenoreceptor blocking agent; not established. May decrease cardiac output, inhibit renin release by the kidneys, and diminution of tonic sympathetic outflow from the vasomotor centers in the brain.

PHARMACOKINETICS: Absorption: (10mg) Absolute bioavailability (80%); C$_{max}$=(5mg) 16ng/mL, (20mg) 70ng/mL; (5-20mg) T$_{max}$=2-4 hrs. **Distribution:** Plasma protein binding (30%). **Elimination:** Urine (50%, unchanged), feces (<2%); T$_{1/2}$=9-12 hrs.

NURSING CONSIDERATIONS

Assessment: Assess for conditions where treatment is contraindicated or cautioned, pregnancy/nursing status, and possible drug interactions.

Monitoring: Monitor for hypoglycemia, hyperthyroidism, hepatic/renal function, signs/symptoms of HF, withdrawal and arterial insufficiency. Monitor HR, ECG, CBC with platelet and differential count.

Patient Counseling: Instruct not to interrupt or d/c therapy without consulting physician. Notify physician if difficulty in breathing, signs/symptoms of congestive heart failure or excessive bradycardia develop. Educate about signs/symptoms of drug's potential adverse effects. Advise to exercise caution while driving, operating machinery or engaging in other tasks requiring alertness.

Administration: Oral route. **Storage**: 20-25°C (68-77°F). Protect from moisture.

ZEGERID RX
sodium bicarbonate - omeprazole (Santarus)

THERAPEUTIC CLASS: Proton pump inhibitor/antacid

INDICATIONS: Short-term treatment of erosive esophagitis (EE) diagnosed by endoscopy, active duodenal ulcer, and active benign gastric ulcer. Treatment of heartburn and other symptoms associated with gastroesophageal reflux disease (GERD). Maintenance of healing of EE. (Sus, 40mg-1680mg) Reduction of risk of upper GI bleeding in critically ill patients.

DOSAGE: *Adults:* ≥18 Yrs: Take on an empty stomach at least 1 hr ac. Duodenal Ulcer: 20mg qd for 4-8 weeks. Gastric Ulcer: 40mg qd for 4-8 weeks. Symptomatic GERD (with No Esophageal Erosions): 20mg qd for up to 4 weeks. EE: 20mg qd for 4-8 weeks. May give up to an additional 4 weeks if no response to 8 weeks of therapy. May consider additional 4- to 8-week courses if there is recurrence of EE or GERD symptoms. Maintenance of Healing of EE: 20mg qd. Consider dose reduction with hepatic insufficiency or in Asian population. (Sus, 40mg-1680mg) Risk Reduction of Upper GI Bleeding in Critically Ill Patients: Initial: 40mg, followed by 40mg after 6-8 hrs. Maint: 40mg qd for 14 days.

HOW SUPPLIED: (Omeprazole-Sodium Bicarbonate) Cap: 20mg-1100mg, 40mg-1100mg; Sus: 20mg-1680mg/pkt, 40mg-1680mg/pkt

WARNINGS/PRECAUTIONS: Omeprazole: Symptomatic response does not preclude the presence of gastric malignancy. Atrophic gastritis reported with long-term use. May increase risk of *Clostridium difficile*-associated diarrhea (CDAD), especially in hospitalized patients. May increase risk of osteoporosis-related fractures of the hip, wrist, or spine, especially with high-dose and long-term therapy. Use lowest dose and shortest duration appropriate to the condition being treated. Hypomagnesemia reported; Mg^{2+} replacement and discontinuation of therapy may be required. Drug-induced decrease in gastric acidity results in enterochromaffin-like cell hyperplasia and increased chromogranin A (CgA) levels, which may interfere with investigations for neuroendocrine tumors; temporarily d/c treatment before assessing CgA levels. Sodium Bicarbonate: Consider the Na^+ content when administering to patients on a Na^+-restricted diet. Caution with Bartter's syndrome, hypokalemia, hypocalcemia, and problems with acid-base balance. Chronic use may lead to systemic alkalosis, and increased Na^+ intake may produce edema and weight increase.

ADVERSE REACTIONS: Agitation, anemia, bradycardia, constipation, rash, tachycardia, diarrhea, fever, thrombocytopenia, hypokalemia, hypomagnesemia, hyperglycemia, atrial fibrillation, HTN, hypotension.

INTERACTIONS: Monitor for the need to adjust dose of drugs metabolized via CYP450 (eg, cyclosporine, disulfiram, benzodiazepines). Omeprazole: Reduces pharmacological activity of clopidogrel; avoid concomitant use, and consider alternative antiplatelet therapy. Caution with digoxin or drugs that may cause hypomagnesemia (eg, diuretics). May elevate and prolong methotrexate (MTX) levels, possibly leading to toxicities; consider temporary withdrawal of therapy with high-dose MTX. May interfere with absorption of drugs where gastric pH is an important determinant of bioavailability (eg, ketoconazole, ampicillin esters, iron salts, digoxin). May prolong elimination of drugs metabolized by hepatic oxidation (diazepam, warfarin, phenytoin). Monitor for increases in INR and PT with warfarin. Voriconazole (combined inhibitor of CYP2C19 and CYP3A4) may increase levels. May decrease levels of atazanavir and nelfinavir; coadministration not recommended. May increase levels of saquinavir and tacrolimus; consider dose reduction of saquinavir. CYP2C19 or CYP3A4 inducers may decrease levels; avoid with St. John's wort or rifampin. Sodium Bicarbonate: Long-term use of bicarbonate with Ca^{2+} or milk can cause milk-alkali syndrome.

PREGNANCY: Category C, not for use in nursing.

MECHANISM OF ACTION: Omeprazole: Proton pump inhibitor; suppresses gastric acid secretion by specific inhibition of the (H^+/K^+)-ATPase enzyme system at the secretory surface of the gastric parietal cell. Sodium Bicarbonate: Antacid; raises gastric pH, thus protecting omeprazole from acid degradation.

PHARMACOKINETICS: Absorption: Omeprazole: Rapid; T_{max}=30 min. (Sus) Absolute bioavailability (30-40%); C_{max}=1954ng/mL; $AUC_{(0-inf)}$=1665ng•hr/mL (after Dose 1 of 40mg-1680mg), 3356ng•hr/mL (after Dose 2 of 40mg-1680mg). (Cap) C_{max}=1526ng/mL. **Distribution:** Omeprazole: Plasma protein binding (95%); found in breast milk. **Metabolism:** Omeprazole: Hydroxyomeprazole and corresponding carboxylic acid (metabolites). **Elimination:** Omeprazole: Urine (77% as metabolites), feces; $T_{1/2}$=1 hr (healthy subjects).

NURSING CONSIDERATIONS

Assessment: Assess for risk of osteoporosis, Na^+-restricted diet, Bartter's syndrome, hypokalemia, hypocalcemia, acid-base balance problems, hypersensitivity to the drug, pregnancy/nursing status, and possible drug interactions. Obtain baseline Mg^{2+} levels in patients expected to be on prolonged therapy.

Z

Monitoring: Monitor for signs/symptoms of atrophic gastritis, CDAD, bone fractures, systemic alkalosis, hypersensitivity reactions, and other adverse reactions. Monitor Mg^{2+} levels periodically in patients expected to be on prolonged therapy.

Patient Counseling: Inform that different formulations are not bioequivalent and should not be used as substitute of one for the other. Inform that increased Na^+ intake may cause swelling and weight gain; instruct to contact physician if these occur. Inform that the most frequent adverse reactions associated with therapy include headache, abdominal pain, N/V, diarrhea, and flatulence. Advise that harmful effect of therapy on the fetus cannot be ruled out. Advise to use with caution if regularly taking Ca^{2+} supplements. Advise to immediately report and seek care for diarrhea that does not improve and for any cardiovascular/neurological symptoms (eg, palpitation, dizziness, seizures, tetany).

Administration: Oral route. (Cap) Swallow intact with water; do not use other liquids. Do not open cap and sprinkle contents into food. (Sus) Empty pkt contents into a small cup containing 1-2 tbsp of water; do not use other liquids or foods. Stir well and drink immediately. Refill cup with water and drink. Refer to PI for preparation/administration instructions if to be administered through an NG/orogastric tube. **Storage:** 25°C (77°F); excursions permitted to 15-30°C (59-86°F). Protect from light and moisture.

ZEGERID OTC   OTC
sodium bicarbonate - omeprazole (MSD Consumer)

THERAPEUTIC CLASS: Proton pump inhibitor/antacid

INDICATIONS: Treatment of frequent heartburn (≥2 days a week).

DOSAGE: *Adults:* ≥18 Yrs: 1 cap with a glass of water at least 1 hr before eating qam (q24h) for 14 days. Max: 1 cap/day. May repeat 14-day course every 4 months, if needed.

HOW SUPPLIED: Cap: (Omeprazole-Sodium Bicarbonate) 20mg-1100mg

WARNINGS/PRECAUTIONS: Not for immediate relief of heartburn; may take 1-4 days for full effect. Do not use if patient is vomiting with blood, has trouble or pain swallowing food, or has bloody or black stools. Caution with heartburn >3 months; heartburn with lightheadedness, sweating, or dizziness; chest/shoulder pain with SOB, sweating, pain spreading to arms/neck/shoulders or lightheadedness; frequent chest pain; frequent wheezing with heartburn; unexplained weight loss; N/V; stomach pain; or Na^+-restricted diet. D/C if heartburn continues/worsens, if patient needs to take the product for >14 days, if >1 course of treatment every 4 months is needed, or if diarrhea occurs.

INTERACTIONS: May interact with warfarin, clopidogrel, cilostazol, prescription antifungal/antiyeast medicines or antiretrovirals, diazepam, digoxin, and tacrolimus.

PREGNANCY: Safety not known in pregnancy/nursing.

MECHANISM OF ACTION: Omeprazole: Proton pump inhibitor; acid reducer. Sodium Bicarbonate: Antacid; allows absorption of omeprazole.

NURSING CONSIDERATIONS

Assessment: Assess for allergy to the drug, trouble or pain swallowing food, vomiting with blood, bloody or black stools, other conditions where treatment is cautioned, pregnancy/nursing status, and possible drug interactions.

Monitoring: Monitor for heartburn that continues/worsens, diarrhea, and other adverse reactions.

Patient Counseling: Advise to take ud. Instruct to d/c use and consult physician if heartburn continues/worsens, if patient needs to take the product for >14 days, if >1 course of treatment every 4 months is needed, or if diarrhea occurs. Advise to notify physician of all medication use.

Administration: Oral route. Take with a glass of water at least 1 hr before eating in the am. Do not chew, crush, or open cap and sprinkle on food. **Storage:** 20-25°C (68-77°F). Protect from high heat, humidity, and moisture.

ZELAPAR   RX
selegiline HCl (Valeant)

THERAPEUTIC CLASS: Monoamine oxidase inhibitor (type B)

INDICATIONS: Adjunct in the management of patients with Parkinson's disease being treated with levodopa/carbidopa who exhibit deterioration in the quality of their response to this therapy.

DOSAGE: *Adults:* Initial: 1.25mg qd for at least 6 weeks. Titrate: After 6 weeks, may increase to 2.5mg qd if a desired benefit has not been achieved and the patient is tolerating therapy. Max: 2.5mg/day.

HOW SUPPLIED: Tab, Disintegrating: 1.25mg

CONTRAINDICATIONS: Concomitant use of meperidine and other selegiline products. Initiation of treatment with meperidine or other selegiline products within 14 days of therapy discontinuation. Concomitant use of tramadol, methadone, propoxyphene, and dextromethorphan.

WARNINGS/PRECAUTIONS: Rare cases of hypertensive reactions associated with ingestion of tyramine-containing foods reported. Incidence of orthostatic hypotension and risk of dizziness greater in geriatrics. Monitor for melanomas frequently and on a regular basis. Increased frequency of mild oropharyngeal abnormality (eg, swallowing/mouth pain, discrete areas of focal reddening, multiple foci of reddening, edema, and/or ulceration) reported. May potentiate dopaminergic side effects of levodopa and may cause or exacerbate preexisting dyskinesia; decreasing the dose of levodopa may ameliorate this side effect. Caution with renal/hepatic impairment; consider discontinuation if adverse reactions that seem more frequent or severe than might ordinarily be expected occur. Symptom complex resembling neuroleptic malignant syndrome reported with rapid dose reduction, withdrawal of, or changes in antiparkinsonian therapy. Hallucinations reported. Contains 1.25mg phenylalanine/tab.

ADVERSE REACTIONS: Nausea, dizziness, pain, headache, insomnia, rhinitis, skin disorders, dyskinesia, back pain, dyspepsia, stomatitis, dry mouth, constipation, pharyngitis, rash.

INTERACTIONS: See Contraindications. Severe toxicity reported with TCAs, SSRIs (eg, fluoxetine, fluvoxamine, sertraline, paroxetine) and SNRIs (eg, venlafaxine); avoid concurrent use. Allow at least 5 weeks (longer with chronic/high-dose fluoxetine) between discontinuation of fluoxetine and initiation of therapy. One case of hypertensive crisis reported with ephedrine. Caution with CYP3A4 inducers (eg, phenytoin, carbamazepine, nafcillin, phenobarbital, rifampin).

PREGNANCY: Category C, not for use in nursing.

MECHANISM OF ACTION: MAOI (Type B); has not been established. Increases net amount of dopamine available by blocking catabolism of dopamine.

PHARMACOKINETICS: Absorption: Rapid. C_{max}=3.34ng/mL (1.25mg), 4.47ng/mL (2.5mg), T_{max}=10-15 min. **Distribution:** Plasma protein binding (up to 85%). **Metabolism:** Liver via CYP2B6 and CYP3A4; l-methamphetamine and desmethylselegiline (metabolites). **Elimination:** Urine (mainly as L-methamphetamine metabolite), feces; $T_{1/2}$=1.3 hrs (1.25mg single dose), 10 hrs (steady state).

NURSING CONSIDERATIONS

Assessment: Assess for drug hypersensitivity, dyskinesia, renal/hepatic impairment, pregnancy/nursing status, and possible drug interactions.

Monitoring: Monitor for orthostatic hypotension, dyskinesia, hallucinations, and other adverse reactions. Monitor frequently for melanomas; periodic skin examinations should be performed by qualified individuals (eg, dermatologists).

Patient Counseling: Inform about signs and symptoms of MAOI-induced hypertensive reactions; instruct to immediately report severe headache or other atypical/unusual symptoms not previously experienced. Inform that hallucinations may occur. Advise to notify physician if experiencing new or increased gambling urges, increased sexual urges, or other intense urges.

Administration: Oral route. Take in am before breakfast and without liquid; avoid ingesting food or liquids for 5 min before and after taking the drug. Refer to PI for proper administration. **Storage:** 25°C (77°F); excursions permitted to 15-30°C (59-86°F). Use within 3 months of opening pouch and immediately upon opening individual blister.

ZEMPLAR ORAL   RX
paricalcitol (AbbVie)

THERAPEUTIC CLASS: Vitamin D analog

INDICATIONS: Prevention and treatment of secondary hyperparathyroidism associated with chronic kidney disease (CKD) Stages 3 and 4, or with CKD Stage 5 on hemodialysis or peritoneal dialysis.

DOSAGE: *Adults:* CKD Stages 3 and 4: Initial: Baseline Intact Parathyroid Hormone (iPTH) Level ≤500pg/mL: 1mcg qd or 2mcg 3X/week. Baseline iPTH Level >500pg/mL: 2mcg qd or 4mcg 3X/week. Administer the 3X/week dose not more often than qod. Titrate: Individualize dose and base dose on serum/plasma iPTH levels. Refer to PI for suggested dose titration. CKD Stage 5: Administer 3X/week, not more frequently than qod. Initial: Base dose on a baseline iPTH level (pg/mL)/80. Treat only after baseline serum Ca^{2+} has been adjusted to ≤9.5mg/dL. Titrate: Individualize dose and base dose on iPTH, serum Ca^{2+}, and phosphorus (P) levels. Refer to PI

Z

for suggested dose titration. On a Ca²⁺-Based Phosphate Binder: May decrease or withhold the phosphate-binder dose, or switch to a non-Ca²⁺-based phosphate binder.

HOW SUPPLIED: Cap: 1mcg, 2mcg, 4mcg

CONTRAINDICATIONS: Vitamin D toxicity, hypercalcemia.

WARNINGS/PRECAUTIONS: Excessive administration may cause over suppression of PTH, hypercalcemia, hypercalciuria, hyperphosphatemia, and adynamic bone disease. Overdose may cause progressive hypercalcemia. Acute hypercalcemia may exacerbate tendencies for cardiac arrhythmias and seizures. Chronic hypercalcemia can lead to generalized vascular calcification and other soft-tissue calcification.

ADVERSE REACTIONS: Headache, hypotension, HTN, diarrhea, N/V, constipation, edema, arthritis, dizziness, insomnia, nasopharyngitis, viral infection, hypersensitivity, peritonitis, fluid overload.

INTERACTIONS: May increase risk of hypercalcemia with high doses of Ca²⁺-containing preparations or thiazide diuretics. Concomitant high intake of Ca²⁺ and phosphate may lead to serum abnormalities requiring more frequent patient monitoring and individualized dose titration. Withhold prescription-based doses of vitamin D and its derivatives during treatment to avoid hypercalcemia. Caution with digitalis compounds. Do not coadminister aluminum-containing preparations (eg, antacids, phosphate binders) chronically; increased blood levels of aluminum and aluminum bone toxicity may occur. Increased exposure with strong CYP3A inhibitors (eg, ketoconazole, atazanavir, clarithromycin); may need to adjust paricalcitol dose, and closely monitor iPTH and serum Ca²⁺ concentrations if a patient initiates or discontinues therapy with a strong CYP3A4 inhibitor. Drugs that impair intestinal absorption of fat-soluble vitamins (eg, cholestyramine) may interfere with absorption. Mineral oil or other substances that may affect absorption of fat may influence absorption.

PREGNANCY: Category C, not for use in nursing.

MECHANISM OF ACTION: Vitamin D analog; binds to vitamin D receptor, which results in the selective activation of vitamin D responsive pathways. Shown to reduce PTH levels by inhibiting PTH synthesis and secretion.

PHARMACOKINETICS: Absorption: Absolute bioavailability (72-86%) (healthy and CKD Stage 5). Refer to PI for pharmacokinetic characteristics in CKD patients. **Distribution:** V_d=44-46L (CKD Stages 3 and 4); plasma protein binding (≥99.8%). **Metabolism:** Liver (extensive) via hydroxylation and glucuronidation, by CYP24, CYP3A4, and UGT1A4. **Elimination:** Feces (70%; 2% unchanged), urine (18%); $T_{1/2}$=14-20 hrs (CKD Stages 3, 4, and 5).

NURSING CONSIDERATIONS

Assessment: Assess for vitamin D toxicity, hypercalcemia, pregnancy/nursing status, and possible drug interactions.

Monitoring: Monitor for hypercalcemia, elevated Ca x P, and other adverse reactions. During the initial dosing or following any dose adjustment, monitor serum Ca²⁺, serum P, and serum/plasma iPTH at least every 2 weeks for 3 months, then monthly for 3 months, and every 3 months thereafter.

Patient Counseling: Inform of the most common adverse reactions (eg, diarrhea, HTN, dizziness, vomiting). Advise to adhere to instructions regarding diet and P restriction, and to return for routine monitoring. Instruct to contact physician if symptoms of elevated Ca²⁺ (eg, feeling tired, difficulty thinking clearly, loss of appetite) develop. Advise to inform physician of all medications (eg, prescription and nonprescription drugs, supplements, and herbal preparations) being taken and any change to medical condition.

Administration: Oral route. May be taken without regard to food. **Storage:** 25°C (77°F); excursions permitted between 15-30°C (59-86°F).

ZENPEP   RX
pancrelipase (Aptalis)

THERAPEUTIC CLASS: Pancreatic enzyme supplement

INDICATIONS: Treatment of exocrine pancreatic insufficiency due to cystic fibrosis or other conditions.

DOSAGE: *Adults:* Individualize dose based on clinical symptoms, degree of steatorrhea present, and fat content of diet. Start at the lowest recommended dose and increase gradually. Initial: 500 lipase U/kg/meal. Max: 2500 lipase U/kg/meal (or ≤10,000 lipase U/kg/day) or <4000 lipase U/g fat ingested/day. Half of the dose used for meals should be given with each snack. Refer to PI for dosing limitations.
Pediatrics: Individualize dose based on clinical symptoms, degree of steatorrhea present, and fat content of diet. Start at the lowest recommended dose and increase gradually. ≥4 Yrs: Initial: 500 lipase U/kg/meal. Max: 2500 lipase U/kg/meal (or ≤10,000 lipase U/kg/day) or <4000 lipase U/g

fat ingested/day. Half of the dose used for meals should be given with each snack. >12 Months-<4 Yrs: Initial: 1000 lipase U/kg/meal. Max: 2500 lipase U/kg/meal (or ≤10,000 lipase U/kg/day) or <4000 lipase U/g fat ingested/day. ≤12 Months: 3000 lipase U/120mL of formula or breastfeeding. Administer immediately prior to each feeding. Refer to PI for dosing limitations.

HOW SUPPLIED: Cap, Delayed-Release: (Lipase-Protease-Amylase) 3000 U-10,000 U-16,000 U; 5000 U-17,000 U-27,000 U; 10,000 U-34,000 U-55,000 U; 15,000 U-51,000 U-82,000 U; 20,000 U-68,000 U-109,000 U; 25,000 U-85,000 U-136,000 U

WARNINGS/PRECAUTIONS: Not interchangeable with other pancrelipase products. Fibrosing colonopathy reported; monitor closely for progression to stricture formation. Caution with doses >2500 lipase U/kg/meal (or >10,000 lipase U/kg/day); use only if these doses are documented to be effective by 3-day fecal fat measures indicating significant improvement. Examine patients receiving >6000 lipase U/kg/meal; immediately decrease or titrate dose downward to a lower range. Ensure that no drug is retained in the mouth. Should not be crushed or chewed, or mixed in foods with pH >4.5; may disrupt enteric coating of cap, resulting in early release of enzymes, irritation of oral mucosa, and/or loss of enzyme activity. Caution in patients with gout, renal impairment, or hyperuricemia; may increase blood uric acid levels. Risk for transmission of viral diseases. Caution with known allergy to proteins of porcine origin; severe allergic reactions reported.

ADVERSE REACTIONS: GI disorders (eg, abdominal pain, flatulence, steatorrhea), headache, cough, weight decreased, early satiety, contusion, skin disorders.

PREGNANCY: Category C, caution in nursing.

MECHANISM OF ACTION: Pancreatic enzyme supplement; catalyzes the hydrolysis of fats to monoglycerides, glycerol, and free fatty acids, proteins into peptides and amino acids, and starch into dextrins and short-chain sugars (eg, maltose, maltriose) in the duodenum and proximal small intestine, thereby acting like digestive enzymes physiologically secreted by the pancreas.

NURSING CONSIDERATIONS

Assessment: Assess for gout, renal impairment, hyperuricemia, known allergy to porcine proteins, and pregnancy/nursing status.

Monitoring: Monitor for fibrosing colonopathy, stricture formation, oral mucosa irritation, viral diseases, and allergic reactions. Monitor serum uric acid levels. Monitor glucose levels in patients at risk for abnormal blood glucose.

Patient Counseling: Instruct to take ud and with food. Inform that if a dose is missed, take the next dose with the next meal/snack ud; instruct not to double doses. Inform that cap contents can be mixed with soft acidic foods (eg, applesauce), if necessary. Instruct to notify physician if pregnant/breastfeeding or planning to become pregnant/breastfeed during treatment. Instruct to notify physician before initiating treatment if patient has a history of abnormal glucose levels. Advise to contact physician immediately if allergic reactions develop.

Administration: Oral route. Do not crush/chew cap or cap contents; do not mix directly into formula or breast milk. Refer to PI for proper administration instructions. **Storage:** (Original glass container) 20-25°C (68-77°F); brief excursions permitted to 15-40°C (59-104°F). Avoid excessive heat. Protect from moisture. (Repackaged HDPE container) Store up to 30°C (86°F) for up to 6 months; excursions permitted to 15-40°C (59-104°F) up to 30 days. Avoid excessive heat. Protect from moisture.

ZENTRIP
OTC
meclizine HCl (Sato)

THERAPEUTIC CLASS: Antihistamine

INDICATIONS: Prevention and treatment of N/V, or dizziness associated with motion sickness.

DOSAGE: *Adults:* Dissolve 1-2 strips on tongue qd or ud. Prevention: ≥1 hr prior to travel. *Pediatrics:* ≥12 Yrs: Dissolve 1-2 strips on tongue qd or ud. Prevention: ≥1 hr prior to travel.

HOW SUPPLIED: Strip, Oral: 25mg

WARNINGS/PRECAUTIONS: Avoid use in children <12 yrs of age. Caution with glaucoma, breathing problems (eg, emphysema, chronic bronchitis), and difficulty in urination due to an enlarged prostate gland. D/C use and consult physician if rash, redness, itching, or difficulty in urination occurs, or if symptoms of dry mouth continue or increase. Drowsiness may occur and may impair mental/physical abilities.

ADVERSE REACTIONS: Drowsiness.

INTERACTIONS: Alcohol, sedatives, and tranquilizers may increase drowsiness. Avoid alcohol use.

PREGNANCY: Safety not known in pregnancy and nursing.

MECHANISM OF ACTION: Antihistamine.

NURSING CONSIDERATIONS

Assessment: Assess for breathing problems (eg, emphysema, chronic bronchitis), glaucoma, difficulty in urination due to an enlarged prostate gland, pregnancy/nursing status, and possible drug interactions.

Monitoring: Monitor for drowsiness, rash, redness, itching, difficulty in urination and increased/continued symptoms of dry mouth.

Patient Counseling: Inform that drowsiness may occur; caution when driving a vehicle or operating machinery. Instruct to avoid alcohol use. Instruct to d/c and consult physician if rash, redness, itching, or difficulty in urination occurs, or if symptoms of dry mouth continue or increase. Advise to consult physician before use if taking sedatives or tranquilizers and if pregnant/nursing.

Administration: Oral route. **Storage:** 20-30°C (68-86°F). Protect from light.

ZERIT   RX
stavudine (Bristol-Myers Squibb)

> Lactic acidosis and severe hepatomegaly with steatosis, including fatal cases, reported with nucleoside analogues. Fatal lactic acidosis reported in pregnant women who received the combination of stavudine and didanosine with other antiretroviral agents; use with caution. Fatal and nonfatal pancreatitis reported when used as part of a combination regimen that included didanosine.

THERAPEUTIC CLASS: Nucleoside reverse transcriptase inhibitor

INDICATIONS: Treatment of HIV-1 infection in combination with other antiretroviral agents.

DOSAGE: *Adults:* ≥60kg: 40mg q12h. <60kg: 30mg q12h. Renal Impairment: CrCl 26-50mL/min: ≥60kg: 20mg q12h. <60kg: 15mg q12h. CrCl 10-25mL/min or on Hemodialysis: ≥60kg: 20mg q24h. <60kg: 15mg q24h. Give after the completion of hemodialysis on dialysis days and at the same time of day on non-dialysis days.
Pediatrics: ≥60kg: 40mg q12h. 30-<60kg: 30mg q12h. ≥14 Days Old and <30kg: 1mg/kg q12h. Birth-13 Days Old: 0.5mg/kg q12h.

HOW SUPPLIED: Cap: 15mg, 20mg, 30mg, 40mg; Sol: 1mg/mL [200mL]

WARNINGS/PRECAUTIONS: Female gender, obesity, and prolonged nucleoside exposure may be risk factors for lactic acidosis and severe hepatomegaly with steatosis. Caution in patients with known risk factors for liver disease. Suspend treatment if findings suggestive of symptomatic hyperlactatemia, lactic acidosis, or pronounced hepatotoxicity develop; consider permanent discontinuation with confirmed lactic acidosis. Increased frequency of liver function abnormalities, including severe and potentially fatal hepatic adverse events in patients with preexisting liver dysfunction; monitor accordingly and consider interruption or discontinuation if worsening of liver disease is evident. Motor weakness reported rarely; d/c if this develops. Dose-related peripheral sensory neuropathy reported; occurs more frequently in patients with advanced HIV-1 disease, history of peripheral neuropathy, or receiving other drugs associated with neuropathy (eg, didanosine). Consider permanent discontinuation if peripheral neuropathy develops. Redistribution/accumulation of body fat reported; monitor for signs/symptoms of lipoatrophy or lipodystrophy. Immune reconstitution syndrome reported. Autoimmune disorders (eg, Graves' disease, polymyositis, Guillain-Barre syndrome) reported in the setting of immune reconstitution and can occur many months after initiation of treatment. Caution with renal impairment and in elderly.

ADVERSE REACTIONS: Lactic acidosis, severe hepatomegaly with steatosis, peripheral neurologic symptoms/neuropathy, headache, diarrhea, rash, N/V, increased AST/ALT/amylase.

INTERACTIONS: See Boxed Warning. Suspend combination of stavudine and didanosine and any other agents that are toxic to the pancreas in patients with suspected pancreatitis; caution with reinstitution of stavudine and avoid use in combination with didanosine if pancreatitis is confirmed. Avoid with zidovudine or hydroxyurea with or without didanosine. Hepatic decompensation may occur in combination with interferon and ribavirin in HIV-1/HCV coinfected patients; monitor for clinical toxicities and consider discontinuation if this occurs. Caution with doxorubicin or ribavirin.

PREGNANCY: Category C, not for use in nursing.

MECHANISM OF ACTION: Synthetic thymidine nucleoside analogue; inhibits activity of HIV-1 reverse transcriptase by competing with natural substrate thymidine triphosphate and by causing DNA chain termination following its incorporation into viral DNA. Inhibits cellular DNA polymerases β and gamma and markedly reduces synthesis of mitochondrial DNA.

PHARMACOKINETICS: Absorption: Rapid. Oral bioavailability (86.4%) (adults), (76.9%) (pediatrics); C_{max}=536ng/mL (adults); T_{max}=1 hr; AUC_{0-24}=2568ng•hr/mL (adults). **Distribution:** (IV) V_d=46L (adults), 0.73L/kg (pediatrics). **Metabolism:** Oxidized stavudine, glucuronide conjugates, and N-acetylcysteine conjugate (minor metabolites). **Elimination:** Urine (42%) (IV, adults), (34%) (pediatrics); $T_{1/2}$=1.6 hrs (adults), 0.96 hr (pediatrics).

NURSING CONSIDERATIONS

Assessment: Assess for drug hypersensitivity, risk factors for lactic acidosis or liver disease, renal/hepatic impairment, history of peripheral neuropathy, pregnancy/nursing status, and possible drug interactions.

Monitoring: Monitor for signs/symptoms of lactic acidosis, hepatotoxicity, worsening of liver disease, motor weakness, peripheral neuropathy, pancreatitis, fat redistribution/accumulation, lipoatrophy/lipodystrophy, immune reconstitution syndrome (eg, opportunistic infections), and autoimmune disorders.

Patient Counseling: Inform that therapy is not a cure for HIV and patients may continue to experience illnesses associated with HIV. Advise to avoid doing things that can spread HIV to others (eg, sharing needles, other inj equipment, or personal items that can have blood or body fluids on them; sex without protection; breastfeeding). Advise diabetic patients that oral sol contains 50mg of sucrose/mL. Advise to seek medical attention immediately if symptoms of hyperlactatemia or lactic acidosis syndrome (eg, unexplained weight loss, abdominal discomfort, N/V, fatigue, dyspnea, motor weakness) develop. Instruct to report symptoms of peripheral neuropathy to physician. Advise to avoid alcohol while on therapy. Inform that fat redistribution/accumulation may occur.

Administration: Oral route. Take with or without food. (Sol) Shake vigorously prior to measuring each dose. Refer to PI for method of preparation of oral sol. **Storage:** 25°C (77°F); excursions permitted between 15-30°C (59-86°F). (Sol) Protect from excessive moisture. After Constitution: 2-8°C (36-46°F). Discard any unused portion after 30 days.

ZESTORETIC

RX

hydrochlorothiazide - lisinopril (AstraZeneca)

> D/C when pregnancy is detected. Drugs that act directly on the renin-angiotensin system (RAS) can cause injury/death to the developing fetus.

THERAPEUTIC CLASS: ACE inhibitor/thiazide diuretic

INDICATIONS: Treatment of HTN.

DOSAGE: *Adults:* BP Not Controlled with Lisinopril/HCTZ Monotherapy: Initial: 10mg-12.5mg or 20mg-12.5mg qd depending on current monotherapy dose. Titrate: Base further increases on clinical response. May increase HCTZ dose after 2-3 weeks. May reduce dose of lisinopril after addition of diuretic. Controlled on 25mg HCTZ qd with Hypokalemia: Switch to 10mg-12.5mg qd. Replacement Therapy: May substitute combination for titrated individual components. Elderly: Start at lower end of dosing range.

HOW SUPPLIED: Tab: (Lisinopril-HCTZ) 10mg-12.5mg, 20mg-12.5mg, 20mg-25mg

CONTRAINDICATIONS: History of ACE inhibitor-associated angioedema, hereditary or idiopathic angioedema, anuria, hypersensitivity to other sulfonamide-derived drugs. Coadministration with aliskiren in patients with diabetes.

WARNINGS/PRECAUTIONS: Not for initial therapy of HTN. Not recommended with severe renal impairment (CrCl ≤30mL/min). Caution in elderly. Lisinopril: Head/neck angioedema reported; promptly d/c and administer appropriate therapy. Higher rate of angioedema in blacks than nonblacks. Intestinal angioedema reported; monitor for abdominal pain. Anaphylactoid reactions reported during desensitization with hymenoptera venom, dialysis with high-flux membranes, and LDL apheresis with dextran sulfate absorption. Excessive hypotension may occur in salt/volume-depleted persons (eg, patients treated vigorously with diuretics or on dialysis). Excessive hypotension, which may be associated with oliguria and/or progressive azotemia, and rarely with acute renal failure and/or death, may occur in patients with severe congestive heart failure (CHF); monitor closely during first 2 weeks of therapy and whenever dose is increased. Caution with ischemic heart or cerebrovascular disease in whom an excessive fall in BP could result in a myocardial infarction or cerebrovascular accident. Leukopenia/neutropenia and bone marrow depression may occur. Rarely, associated with a syndrome that starts with cholestatic jaundice or hepatitis and progresses to fulminant hepatic necrosis and (sometimes) death; d/c if jaundice or marked elevations of hepatic enzymes develop. Caution with left ventricular outflow obstruction. May cause changes in renal function. May increase BUN and SrCr in patients with renal artery stenosis or with no preexisting renal vascular disease; monitor renal function during the 1st few weeks of therapy in patients with renal artery stenosis. Hyperkalemia and persistent nonproductive cough reported. Hypotension may occur with major surgery or during anesthesia. HCTZ: May cause idiosyncratic reaction, resulting in acute transient myopia and acute angle-closure glaucoma; d/c as rapidly as possible. May precipitate azotemia in patients with renal disease. Caution with hepatic dysfunction or progressive liver disease; may precipitate hepatic coma. Sensitivity reactions may occur. May cause exacerbation or activation of systemic lupus erythematosus (SLE), hyperuricemia or precipitation of frank gout, manifestation of latent diabetes mellitus (DM), hypomagnesemia, and hypercalcemia. Observe for signs of fluid or electrolyte

Z

imbalance (hyponatremia, hypochloremic alkalosis, hypokalemia). Hypokalemia may sensitize or exaggerate the response of the heart to toxic effects of digitalis. Enhanced effects in postsympathectomy patients. D/C or withhold if progressive renal impairment becomes evident. D/C before testing for parathyroid function. Increased cholesterol and TG levels reported.

ADVERSE REACTIONS: Dizziness, headache, cough, fatigue, orthostatic effects.

INTERACTIONS: See Contraindications. NSAIDs, including selective COX-2 inhibitors, may reduce effects of diuretics and ACE inhibitors, and may deteriorate renal function. Increased risk of lithium toxicity; avoid with lithium. Lisinopril: Dual blockade of the RAS is associated with increased risks of hypotension, hyperkalemia, and changes in renal function (including acute renal failure); closely monitor BP, renal function, and electrolytes with concomitant agents that also affect the RAS. Avoid with aliskiren in patients with renal impairment (GFR <60mL/min). Hypotension risk, and increased BUN and SrCr with diuretics. Increased risk of hyperkalemia with K^+-sparing diuretics (eg, spironolactone, eplerenone, triamterene, amiloride), K^+ supplements, or K^+-containing salt substitutes; use with caution and monitor serum K^+. Nitritoid reactions reported with injectable gold. HCTZ: Potentiation of orthostatic hypotension may occur with alcohol, barbiturates, or narcotics. Dosage adjustment of antidiabetic drugs (oral agents, insulin) may be required. Additive effect or potentiation with other antihypertensives. Anionic exchange resins (cholestyramine, colestipol) may impair absorption. Corticosteroids and adrenocorticotropic hormone may intensify electrolyte depletion, particularly hypokalemia. May decrease response to pressor amines (eg, norepinephrine). May increase responsiveness to nondepolarizing skeletal muscle relaxants (eg, tubocurarine).

PREGNANCY: Category D, not for use in nursing.

MECHANISM OF ACTION: Lisinopril: ACE inhibitor; decreases plasma angiotensin II, which leads to decreased vasopressor activity and decreased aldosterone secretion. HCTZ: Thiazide diuretic; not established. Affects distal renal tubular mechanism of electrolyte reabsorption. Increases excretion of Na^+ and Cl^-.

PHARMACOKINETICS: Absorption: Lisinopril: T_{max}=7 hrs. **Distribution:** Crosses placenta. HCTZ: Found in breast milk. **Elimination:** Lisinopril: Urine (unchanged); $T_{1/2}$=12 hrs. HCTZ: Kidneys (≥61% unchanged); $T_{1/2}$=5.6-14.8 hrs.

NURSING CONSIDERATIONS

Assessment: Assess for hereditary/idiopathic angioedema, anuria, DM, volume/salt depletion, CHF, ischemic heart or cerebrovascular disease, collagen vascular disease, left ventricular outflow obstruction, SLE, history of ACE inhibitor-associated angioedema, hypersensitivity to drug or sulfonamide-derived drugs, renal/hepatic dysfunction, postsympathectomy status, pregnancy/nursing status, and possible drug interactions.

Monitoring: Monitor for signs/symptoms of angioedema, anaphylactoid/idiosyncratic/hypersensitivity reactions, exacerbation/activation of SLE, hyperuricemia or precipitation of gout, latent DM, fluid/electrolyte imbalance, and other adverse reactions. Monitor BP, renal/hepatic function, serum electrolytes, cholesterol, and TG levels. Consider periodic monitoring of WBCs in patients with collagen vascular disease and renal disease.

Patient Counseling: Inform about fetal risks if taken during pregnancy and discuss treatment options in women planning to become pregnant; instruct to report pregnancy to physician as soon as possible. Instruct to d/c therapy and to immediately report signs/symptoms of angioedema. Instruct to report lightheadedness especially during the 1st few days of therapy; advise to d/c therapy and consult with a physician if actual syncope occurs. Inform that excessive perspiration, dehydration, and other causes of volume depletion (eg, diarrhea, vomiting) may lead to fall in BP; advise to consult with physician. Advise not to use salt substitutes containing K^+ without consulting physician. Advise to promptly report any indication of infection (eg, sore throat, fever).

Administration: Oral route. **Storage:** 20-25°C (68-77°F). Protect from excessive light and humidity.

ZESTRIL

RX

lisinopril (AstraZeneca)

> D/C when pregnancy is detected. Drugs that act directly on the renin-angiotensin system (RAS) can cause injury/death to the developing fetus.

THERAPEUTIC CLASS: ACE inhibitor

INDICATIONS: Treatment of HTN alone or with other antihypertensive agents. Adjunctive therapy in management of heart failure (HF) if inadequately responding to diuretics and digitalis. Treatment of hemodynamically stable patients within 24 hrs of acute myocardial infarction (AMI), to improve survival.

DOSAGE: *Adults:* HTN: Not Receiving Diuretics: Initial: 10mg qd. Titrate: Adjust dose according to BP response. Usual: 20-40mg qd. Max: 80mg. May add a low-dose diuretic if BP is not

controlled. Receiving Diuretics: D/C diuretic 2-3 days prior to therapy. Adjust dose according to BP response. If diuretic cannot be discontinued, give initial lisinopril dose of 5mg under medical supervision for at least 2 hrs and until BP has stabilized for at least an additional 1 hr. Renal Impairment: CrCl 10-30mL/min (SrCr ≥3mg/dL): Initial: 5mg qd. CrCl <10mL/min (Usually on Hemodialysis): Initial: 2.5mg/day. Titrate: May increase until BP is controlled. Max: 40mg/day. HF: Initial: 5mg qd. Usual: 5-40mg qd. May increase by increments of no greater than 10mg at intervals of no less than 2 weeks. Adjust dose based on clinical response. Max: 40mg/day. HF with Hyponatremia (serum Na$^+$ <130mEq/L) or CrCl ≤30mL/min or SrCr >3mg/dL): Initial: 2.5mg qd under close medical supervision. AMI: 5mg within 24 hrs of onset of symptoms, followed by 5mg after 24 hrs, 10mg after 48 hrs, and then 10mg qd for 6 weeks. Low Systolic BP (SBP) ≤120mmHg When Treatment is Started or During First 3 Days After the Infarct: 2.5mg. Maint: 5mg qd with temporary reductions to 2.5mg if needed, if SBP ≤100mmHg occurs. D/C if SBP <90mmHg for >1 hr occurs. Elderly: Start at lower end of dosing range.
Pediatrics: ≥6 Yrs: HTN: Initial: 0.07mg/kg qd (up to 5mg total). Titrate: Adjust dose according to BP response. Max: 0.61mg/kg (or 40mg).

HOW SUPPLIED: Tab: 2.5mg, 5mg*, 10mg, 20mg, 30mg, 40mg *scored

CONTRAINDICATIONS: History of ACE inhibitor-associated angioedema, hereditary or idiopathic angioedema. Coadministration with aliskiren in patients with diabetes.

WARNINGS/PRECAUTIONS: Not recommended in pediatrics with GFR <30mL/min. Caution when initiating therapy in AMI patients with renal dysfunction (SrCr >2mg/dL) and in HF patients. Head/neck angioedema reported; d/c and administer appropriate therapy. Intestinal angioedema reported; monitor for abdominal pain. More reports of angioedema in blacks than nonblacks. Anaphylactoid reactions reported during desensitization with hymenoptera venom, dialysis with high-flux membranes, and LDL apheresis with dextran sulfate absorption. Excessive hypotension sometimes associated with oliguria and/or progressive azotemia, and rarely with acute renal failure and/or death; monitor closely. If symptomatic hypotension develops, dose reduction or discontinuation of therapy or concomitant diuretic may be necessary. Rare cases of leukopenia/neutropenia and bone marrow depression reported. Rarely, syndrome that starts with cholestatic jaundice or hepatitis progressing to fulminant hepatic necrosis and (sometimes) death reported; d/c if jaundice or marked hepatic enzyme elevations occur. Caution with left ventricular outflow tract obstruction. May cause changes in renal function. May increase BUN and SrCr in patients with renal artery stenosis or with no preexisting renal vascular disease. Hyperkalemia and persistent nonproductive cough reported. Hypotension may occur with major surgery or during anesthesia. Caution in elderly.

ADVERSE REACTIONS: Chest pain, cough, diarrhea, dizziness, headache, hypotension, hyperkalemia, syncope.

INTERACTIONS: See Contraindications. Hypotension risk and increased BUN and SrCr with diuretics. Increased hypoglycemic risk with insulin or oral hypoglycemics. NSAIDs, including selective COX-2 inhibitors, may cause deterioration of renal function. Antihypertensive effect may be attenuated by NSAIDs. Dual blockade of the RAS is associated with increased risks of hypotension, hyperkalemia, and changes in renal function (including acute renal failure); closely monitor BP, renal function, and electrolytes with concomitant agents that also affect the RAS. Avoid with aliskiren in patients with renal impairment (GFR <60mL/min). Increased risk of hyperkalemia with K$^+$-sparing diuretics, K$^+$-containing salt substitutes, or K$^+$ supplements; use with caution and monitor serum K$^+$ frequently. Concomitant K$^+$-sparing agents should generally not be used with HF. Lithium toxicity reported; monitor serum lithium levels frequently. Nitritoid reactions reported with injectable gold.

PREGNANCY: Category D, not for use in nursing.

MECHANISM OF ACTION: ACE inhibitor; decreases plasma angiotensin II, which leads to decreased vasopressor activity and decreased aldosterone secretion.

PHARMACOKINETICS: Absorption: T_{max}=7 hrs (adults), 6 hrs (pediatrics). **Distribution:** Crosses the placenta. **Elimination:** Urine (unchanged); $T_{1/2}$=12 hrs.

NURSING CONSIDERATIONS

Assessment: Assess for hypersensitivity to the drug, history of ACE inhibitor-associated angioedema, hereditary or idiopathic angioedema, collagen vascular disease, left ventricular outflow tract obstruction, renal artery stenosis, risk factors for hyperkalemia, risk of excessive hypotension, renal impairment, pregnancy/nursing status, and possible drug interactions.

Monitoring: Monitor for angioedema, anaphylactoid reactions, hyperkalemia, hypersensitivity reactions, and other adverse reactions. Monitor WBCs in patients with collagen vascular disease and renal disease. Monitor BP, LFTs, and renal function.

Patient Counseling: Instruct to d/c therapy and to immediately report signs/symptoms of angioedema. Instruct to report lightheadedness, especially during 1st few days of therapy; advise to d/c and consult with a physician if actual syncope occurs. Advise that excessive perspiration, dehydration, diarrhea, or vomiting may lead to fall in BP; instruct to consult with a physician. Advise not to use salt substitutes containing K$^+$ without consulting physician. Advise diabetic patients to closely monitor for hypoglycemia. Instruct to report any indication of infection (eg, sore throat, fever) that may be a sign of leukopenia/neutropenia. Inform about fetal risks if taken during pregnancy and discuss treatment options for women planning to become pregnant; instruct to report pregnancy to physician as soon as possible.

Administration: Oral route. Refer to PI for sus preparation instruction. Shake sus before each use.
Storage: 20-25°C (68-77°F). Protect from moisture, freezing, and excessive heat.

ZETIA   RX
ezetimibe (Merck)

THERAPEUTIC CLASS: Cholesterol absorption inhibitor

INDICATIONS: Adjunct to diet for primary (heterozygous familial and non-familial) hyperlipidemia, alone or in combination with an HMG-CoA reductase inhibitor; mixed hyperlipidemia in combination with fenofibrate; homozygous familial hypercholesterolemia, in combination with atorvastatin or simvastatin; and homozygous sitosterolemia.

DOSAGE: *Adults:* Usual: 10mg qd. May give with a statin (with primary hyperlipidemia) or with fenofibrate (with mixed hyperlipidemia) for incremental effect. Coadministration with Bile Acid Sequestrant: Give either ≥2 hrs before or ≥4 hrs after bile acid sequestrant.

HOW SUPPLIED: Tab: 10mg

CONTRAINDICATIONS: Active liver disease or unexplained persistent elevations in hepatic transaminase levels, women who are or may become pregnant, and nursing mothers when used with statins.

WARNINGS/PRECAUTIONS: Not recommended with moderate to severe hepatic impairment. Should be used in accordance with the product labeling for the concurrently administered drug (eg, specific statin or fenofibrate). Liver enzyme elevations reported with statins. Consider withdrawal of therapy and/or statin if an increase in ALT or AST ≥3X ULN persist. Myopathy and rhabdomyolysis reported; immediately d/c therapy and any concomitant statin or fibrate, if myopathy is diagnosed/suspected. Increased risk for skeletal muscle toxicity with higher doses of statin, advanced age (>65 yrs of age), hypothyroidism, renal impairment, depending on the statin used, and concomitant use of other drugs. Caution and close monitoring when used with simvastatin >20mg in patients with moderate to severe renal impairment.

ADVERSE REACTIONS: Upper respiratory tract infection, diarrhea, arthralgia, sinusitis, pain in extremity.

INTERACTIONS: Caution with cyclosporine; monitor cyclosporine levels. May increase cholesterol excretion into the bile, leading to cholelithiasis with fibrates; avoid with fibrates (except fenofibrate). Consider alternative lipid-lowering therapy if cholelithiasis occurs with fenofibrate. Decreased levels with cholestyramine; incremental LDL-C reduction may be reduced. Monitor INR levels when used with warfarin.

PREGNANCY: Category C, caution in nursing.

MECHANISM OF ACTION: Cholesterol absorption inhibitor; localizes at the brush border of the small intestine and inhibits the absorption of cholesterol, leading to a decrease delivery of intestinal cholesterol to the liver. Targets the sterol transporter, Niemann-Pick C1-like 1, which is involved in intestinal uptake of cholesterol and phytosterols.

PHARMACOKINETICS: Absorption: (Fasted) C_{max}=3.4-5.5ng/mL, 45-71ng/mL (metabolite); T_{max}=4-12 hrs, 1-2 hrs (metabolite). **Distribution:** Plasma protein binding (>90%). **Metabolism:** Small intestine and liver via glucuronide conjugation; ezetimibe-glucuronide (active metabolite). **Elimination:** Feces (78%, 69% unchanged drug), urine (11%, 9% metabolite); $T_{1/2}$=22 hrs.

NURSING CONSIDERATIONS

Assessment: Assess for hepatic impairment, pregnancy/nursing status, and possible drug interactions. Obtain baseline lipid profile (total-C, LDL-C, HDL-C, TG). Assess for conditions where treatment is contraindicated and risk factors for skeletal muscle toxicity. Obtain baseline LFTs (eg, ALT, AST) when used with statin.

Monitoring: Monitor for signs/symptoms of elevated liver enzymes, myopathy, rhabdomyolysis, and other adverse reactions. Perform periodic monitoring of lipid profile. Periodically monitor LFTs during concomitant statin therapy.

Patient Counseling: Advise to adhere to the National Cholesterol Education Program recommended diet, a regular exercise program, and periodic testing of a fasting lipid panel. Counsel about risk of myopathy; instruct to promptly report to the physician if any unexplained muscle pain, tenderness, or weakness occurs. Advise to discuss with physician about all medications, both prescription and OTC, currently being taken. Counsel women of childbearing age to use an effective method of birth control while using added statin therapy and instruct to d/c combination therapy and contact physician if they become pregnant. Instruct breastfeeding women not

Z

to take the medication if concomitantly using statins; advise patients who have lipid disorder and are breastfeeding to discuss the options with their physician.

Administration: Oral route. Take with or without food. **Storage:** 25°C (77°F); excursions permitted to 15-30°C (59-86°F). Protect from moisture.

ZEVALIN

RX

ibritumomab tiuxetan (Spectrum)

> Serious infusion reactions and severe cutaneous/mucocutaneous reactions, some fatal (deaths have occurred within 24 hrs of rituximab infusion), may occur; d/c rituximab and Y-90 ibritumomab if any of these occur. May cause severe and prolonged cytopenias; avoid with ≥25% lymphoma marrow involvement and/or impaired bone marrow reserve. Y-90 ibritumomab dose should not exceed 32mCi (1184MBq).

THERAPEUTIC CLASS: Monoclonal antibody/CD20-blocker

INDICATIONS: Treatment of relapsed or refractory, low-grade or follicular B-cell non-Hodgkin's lymphoma (NHL) and for previously untreated follicular NHL in patients who achieve partial or complete response to 1st-line chemotherapy.

DOSAGE: *Adults:* Premedicate with acetaminophen and diphenhydramine prior to rituximab infusion. Day 1: Administer rituximab 250mg/m² IV initially at 50mg/hr. Escalate in 50mg/hr increments every 30 min to max of 400mg/hr in absence of infusion reactions. Temporarily slow or interrupt rituximab infusion if less severe infusion reactions occur; continue infusion at 1/2 the previous rate if symptoms improve. Day 7, 8, or 9: Administer rituximab 250mg/m² IV initially at 100mg/hr and increase rate by 100mg/hr increments every 30 min to max of 400mg/hr. If infusion reactions occurred on Day 1, administer initially at 50mg/hr, and escalate in 50mg/hr increments every 30 min to max of 400mg/hr. Give Y-90 ibritumomab 0.4mCi/kg if platelets ≥150,000/mm³ or 0.3mCi/kg if platelets 100,000-149,000/mm³ over 10 min IV within 4 hrs after completion of rituximab infusion.

HOW SUPPLIED: Inj: 3.2mg/2mL

WARNINGS/PRECAUTIONS: May alter biodistribution. Myelodysplastic syndrome (MDS) and/or acute myelogenous leukemia (AML) reported. May cause fetal harm. Monitor closely for extravasation; d/c infusion if signs or symptoms occur and restart in another limb. Minimize radiation exposure to patients and medical personnel during and after radiolabeling with Y-90. Contains albumin; carries extremely remote risk for transmission of viral diseases and Creutzfeldt-Jakob disease.

ADVERSE REACTIONS: Infusion reactions, cytopenias, severe cutaneous/mucocutaneous reactions, fatigue, abdominal pain, nausea, nasopharyngitis, asthenia, diarrhea, cough, pyrexia, myalgia, anorexia, night sweats, immunogenicity.

INTERACTIONS: Avoid with live viral vaccines. Avoid with drugs that interfere with platelet function or coagulation; monitor for thrombocytopenia more frequently.

PREGNANCY: Category D, not for use in nursing.

MECHANISM OF ACTION: Human monoclonal IgG1 kappa antibody/CD20 antigen blocker; binds specifically to CD20 antigen, which is expressed on pre-B and mature B lymphocytes, and on B-cell NHL. The β emission from Y-90 induces cellular damage by the formation of free cell radicals in the target and neighboring cells.

PHARMACOKINETICS: Distribution: Crosses placenta; found in breast milk. **Elimination:** Urine (7.2% over 7 days); $T_{1/2}$=30 hrs.

NURSING CONSIDERATIONS

Assessment: Assess for lymphoma marrow involvement, impaired bone marrow reserve, previous infusion reactions to the drug, pregnancy/nursing status, and possible drug interactions.

Monitoring: Monitor for infusion reactions, cutaneous/mucocutaneous reactions, MDS, AML, and extravasation. Monitor CBC and platelet counts following regimen weekly until levels recover or as clinically indicated. Monitor for cytopenias and their complications (eg, febrile neutropenia, hemorrhage) for up to 3 months after regimen.

Patient Counseling: Advise to contact physician if signs/symptoms of infusion reactions, cytopenias, infection (eg, pyrexia), diffuse rash, bullae, or desquamation of skin or oral mucosa occur. Advise to take premedications as prescribed and avoid medications that interfere with platelet function. Counsel patients of childbearing potential to use effective contraceptive methods during treatment and for a minimum of 12 months following therapy, and to d/c nursing during and after treatment. When administered during pregnancy, apprise patient of the potential hazard to fetus. Advise against immunization with live vaccines for 12 months after treatment.

Administration: IV route. Refer to PI for directions for medication preparation, radiochemical purity determination, and radiation dosimetry. **Storage:** 2-8°C (36-46°F). Do not freeze.

ZIAC

RX

bisoprolol fumarate - hydrochlorothiazide (Duramed)

THERAPEUTIC CLASS: Selective beta$_1$-blocker/thiazide diuretic

INDICATIONS: Management of HTN.

DOSAGE: *Adults:* Uncontrolled BP on 2.5-20mg/day Bisoprolol or Controlled BP on 50mg/day HCTZ with Hypokalemia: Initial: 2.5mg-6.25mg qd. Titrate: May increase at 14-day intervals. Max: 20mg-12.5mg (two 10mg-6.25mg tab) qd, as appropriate. Replacement therapy: May substitute for titrated individual components. Renal/Hepatic Impairment: Caution in dosing/titrating. Cessation of therapy: Withdrawal should be achieved gradually over a period of 2 weeks.

HOW SUPPLIED: Tab: (Bisoprolol-HCTZ) 2.5mg-6.25mg, 5mg-6.25mg, 10mg-6.25mg

CONTRAINDICATIONS: Cardiogenic shock, overt cardiac failure, 2nd- or 3rd-degree atrioventricular (AV) block, marked sinus bradycardia, anuria, hypersensitivity to sulfonamide-derived drugs.

WARNINGS/PRECAUTIONS: Caution with impaired hepatic function/progressive liver disease. Bisoprolol: Caution with compensated cardiac failure. May precipitate cardiac failure; consider discontinuation at 1st signs/symptoms of heart failure (HF). Exacerbations of angina pectoris, myocardial infarction, and ventricular arrhythmia with coronary artery disease (CAD) reported upon abrupt discontinuation; caution against interruption or d/c without physician's advice. May precipitate or aggravate symptoms of arterial insufficiency with peripheral vascular disease (PVD); exercise caution. Avoid with bronchospastic disease, but may use with caution if unresponsive/intolerant of other antihypertensives. Chronically administered therapy should not be routinely withdrawn prior to major surgery; however, may augment risks of general anesthesia and surgical procedures. Caution with diabetes mellitus (DM); may mask tachycardia occurring with hypoglycemia. May mask hyperthyroidism and precipitate thyroid storm with abrupt discontinuation. HCTZ: May precipitate azotemia with impaired renal function. D/C if progressive renal impairment becomes apparent. May precipitate hepatic coma with hepatic impairment. May cause idiosyncratic reaction, resulting in acute transient myopia and acute angle-closure glaucoma; d/c as rapidly as possible. Monitor for fluid/electrolyte disturbances (eg, hyponatremia, hypochloremic alkalosis, hypokalemia, hypomagnesemia). Decreased Ca^{2+} excretion and altered parathyroid glands, with hypercalcemia and hypophosphatemia, observed on prolonged therapy. Precipitation of hyperuricemia/gout and sensitivity reactions may occur. Photosensitivity reactions and exacerbation/activation of systemic lupus erythematosus (SLE) reported. Enhanced effects in postsympathectomy patient. D/C prior to parathyroid function test.

ADVERSE REACTIONS: Hyperuricemia, dizziness, fatigue, headache, diarrhea.

INTERACTIONS: May potentiate other antihypertensive agents. Avoid with other β-blockers. Excessive reduction of sympathetic activity with catecholamine-depleting drugs (eg, reserpine, guanethidine); monitor closely. D/C for several days prior to clonidine withdrawal. Caution with myocardial depressants or inhibitors of AV conduction (eg, certain calcium antagonists [particularly phenylalkylamine and benzothiazepine classes], antiarrhythmic agents [eg, disopyramide]). Bisoprolol: Digitalis glycosides may increase risk of bradycardia. Rifampin may increase clearance. May be unresponsive to usual doses of epinephrine. HCTZ: Alcohol, barbiturates, or narcotics may potentiate orthostatic hypotension. Antidiabetic drugs (eg, oral agents, insulin) may require dosage adjustments. Impaired absorption with cholestyramine and colestipol resins. Corticosteroids and adrenocorticotropic hormone may intensify electrolyte depletion, particularly hypokalemia. May decrease response to pressor amines (eg, norepinephrine). May increase response to nondepolarizing skeletal muscle relaxants (eg, tubocurarine). Do not give with lithium; increased risk of lithium toxicity. NSAIDs may reduce diuretic, natriuretic, and antihypertensive effects.

PREGNANCY: Category C, not for use in nursing.

MECHANISM OF ACTION: Bisoprolol: β$_1$-selective adrenoreceptor blocking agent; not established. May decrease cardiac output, inhibit renin release by the kidneys, and decrease tonic sympathetic outflow from vasomotor centers in the brain. HCTZ: Thiazide diuretic; not established. Affects renal tubular mechanisms of electrolyte reabsorption and increases excretion of Na$^+$ and Cl$^-$.

PHARMACOKINETICS: Absorption: Well-absorbed. Bisoprolol: Absolute bioavailability (80%); C_{max}=9ng/mL (2.5mg-6.25mg), 19ng/mL (5mg-6.25mg), 36ng/mL (10mg-6.25mg); T_{max}=3 hrs. HCTZ: C_{max}=30ng/mL; T_{max}=2.5 hrs. **Distribution:** Bisoprolol: Plasma protein binding (30%). HCTZ: Plasma protein binding (40-68%); crosses placenta; found in breast milk. **Elimination:** Bisoprolol: Urine (55% unchanged); feces (<2%); $T_{1/2}$=7-15 hrs. HCTZ: Urine (60% unchanged); $T_{1/2}$=4-10 hrs.

NURSING CONSIDERATIONS

Assessment: Assess for cardiogenic shock, overt/compensated cardiac failure, 2nd- or 3rd-degree AV block, marked sinus bradycardia, anuria, sulfonamide hypersensitivity, CAD, PVD, bronchospastic disease, DM, hyperthyroidism, renal/hepatic impairment, history of sulfonamide/

penicillin allergy, parathyroid disease, SLE, pregnancy/nursing status, and possible drug interactions. Obtain baseline serum electrolytes.

Monitoring: Monitor for signs/symptoms of HF, withdrawal, hypoglycemia, hyperthyroidism, renal/hepatic impairment, idiosyncratic reaction, fluid or electrolyte disturbances, precipitation of hyperuricemia or gout, and hypersensitivity reactions. Perform periodic monitoring of serum electrolytes.

Patient Counseling: Instruct not to d/c therapy without physician's supervision, especially in patients with CAD. Advise to consult physician if any difficulty in breathing occurs, or other signs/symptoms of congestive HF or excessive bradycardia develop. Inform that hypoglycemia may be masked in patients subject to spontaneous hypoglycemia, or diabetic patients receiving insulin or oral hypoglycemic agents; instruct to use with caution. Advise to avoid driving, operating machinery, or engaging in other tasks requiring alertness until reaction to drug is known. Advise that photosensitivity reactions may occur.

Administration: Oral route. **Storage**: 20-25°C (68-77°F).

ZIAGEN RX
abacavir sulfate (ViiV Healthcare)

> Serious and sometimes fatal hypersensitivity reactions (multiorgan clinical syndrome) reported; d/c as soon as suspected and never restart therapy or any other abacavir-containing product. Patients with HLA-B*5701 allele are at high risk for hypersensitivity; screen for HLA-B*5701 allele prior to therapy. Lactic acidosis and severe hepatomegaly with steatosis, including fatal cases, reported with the use of nucleoside analogues alone or in combination.

THERAPEUTIC CLASS: Nucleoside reverse transcriptase inhibitor

INDICATIONS: Treatment of HIV-1 infection in combination with other antiretroviral agents.

DOSAGE: *Adults:* 300mg bid or 600mg qd. Mild Hepatic Impairment (Child-Pugh Score 5-6): 200mg (10mL) bid.
Pediatrics: (Sol) ≥3 Months: 8mg/kg bid. Max: 300mg bid. (Tab) ≥30kg: 300mg (1 tab) bid (am and pm). >21-<30kg: 150mg (1/2 tab) qam, 300mg (1 tab) qpm. 14-21kg: 150mg (1/2 tab) bid (am and pm). Mild Hepatic Impairment (Child-Pugh Score 5-6): 200mg (10mL) bid.

HOW SUPPLIED: Sol: 20mg/mL [240mL]; Tab: 300mg* *scored

CONTRAINDICATIONS: Moderate or severe hepatic impairment.

WARNINGS/PRECAUTIONS: Obesity and prolonged nucleoside exposure may be risk factors for lactic acidosis and severe hepatomegaly with steatosis; caution with known risk factors for liver disease. Suspend therapy if clinical or lab findings suggestive of lactic acidosis or pronounced hepatotoxicity develops. Immune reconstitution syndrome reported. Autoimmune disorders (eg, Graves' disease, polymyositis, Guillain-Barre syndrome) reported to occur in the setting of immune reconstitution and can occur many months after initiation of treatment. Redistribution/accumulation of body fat reported. Increased risk of myocardial infarction (MI) reported; consider the underlying risk of coronary heart disease when prescribing therapy. Caution in elderly.

ADVERSE REACTIONS: Hypersensitivity reaction, lactic acidosis, severe hepatomegaly with steatosis, N/V, headache/migraine, malaise, fatigue, diarrhea, dreams/sleep disorders, fever, chills, skin rashes, depressive disorders.

INTERACTIONS: Ethanol decreases elimination, causing an increase in overall exposure. May increase oral methadone clearance.

PREGNANCY: Category C, not for use in nursing.

MECHANISM OF ACTION: Carbocyclic nucleoside analogue; inhibits HIV-1 reverse transcriptase activity by competing with the natural substrate deoxyguanosine-5'-triphosphate and by its incorporation into viral DNA.

PHARMACOKINETICS: Absorption: Rapid and extensive. Absolute bioavailability (83%) (tab). (300mg bid) C_{max}=3mcg/mL; AUC_{0-12h}=6.02mcg•hr/mL. (600mg qd) C_{max}=4.26mcg/mL; AUC=11.95mcg•hr/mL. **Distribution:** (IV) V_d=0.86L/kg; plasma protein binding (50%). **Metabolism:** Via alcohol dehydrogenase and glucuronyl transferase; carbovir triphosphate (active metabolite). **Elimination:** Urine (1.2% unchanged, 81% metabolites), feces (16%); $T_{1/2}$=1.54 hrs.

NURSING CONSIDERATIONS

Assessment: Assess for previous hypersensitivity to the drug, hepatic impairment, risk factors for lactic acidosis or liver disease, risk of coronary heart disease, pregnancy/nursing status, and possible drug interactions. Screen for HLA-B*5701 allele prior to initiation of therapy. Assess medical history for prior exposure to any abacavir-containing product.

Monitoring: Monitor for hypersensitivity reactions, lactic acidosis, hepatotoxicity, immune reconstitution syndrome (eg, opportunistic infections), autoimmune disorders, fat redistribution/accumulation, MI, and other adverse reactions.

Patient Counseling: Inform about the risk of hypersensitivity reactions; instruct to contact physician immediately if symptoms develop, and not to restart therapy or any other abacavir-containing product without medical consultation. Inform that lactic acidosis (with liver enlargement) and fat redistribution/accumulation may occur. Inform that drug is not a cure for HIV-1 infection and that illnesses associated with HIV-1 may still be experienced. Advise to avoid doing things that can spread HIV-1 to others (eg, sharing needles, other inj equipment, or personal items that can have blood or body fluids on them, having sex without protection, breastfeeding). Instruct to take all HIV medications exactly as prescribed.

Administration: Oral route. May be taken with or without food. **Storage:** 20-25°C (68-77°F). (Sol) Do not freeze. May be refrigerated.

ZIANA   RX
clindamycin phosphate - tretinoin (Medicis)

THERAPEUTIC CLASS: Lincosamide derivative/retinoid

INDICATIONS: Topical treatment of acne vulgaris in patients ≥12 yrs of age.

DOSAGE: *Adults:* Apply at hs, a pea-sized amount onto 1 fingertip, dot onto the chin, cheeks, nose, and forehead, then gently rub over entire face.
Pediatrics: ≥12 Yrs: Apply at hs, a pea-sized amount onto 1 fingertip, dot onto the chin, cheeks, nose, and forehead, then gently rub over entire face.

HOW SUPPLIED: Gel: (Clindamycin-Tretinoin) 1.2%-0.025% [30g, 60g]

CONTRAINDICATIONS: Regional enteritis, ulcerative colitis, or history of antibiotic-associated colitis.

WARNINGS/PRECAUTIONS: Not for oral, ophthalmic, or intravaginal use. Keep away from eyes, mouth, angles of the nose, and mucous membranes. Avoid exposure to sunlight, including sunlamps. Avoid use if sunburn is present. Daily use of sunscreen products and protective apparel are recommended. Weather extremes (eg, wind, cold) may be irritating while under treatment. Clindamycin: Systemic absorption has been demonstrated following topical use. Diarrhea, bloody diarrhea, and colitis (including pseudomembranous colitis) reported; d/c if significant diarrhea occurs. Severe colitis reported following PO or parenteral administration with an onset of up to several weeks following cessation of therapy.

ADVERSE REACTIONS: Nasopharyngitis, local skin reactions (erythema, scaling, itching, burning), GI symptoms.

INTERACTIONS: Caution with topical medications, medicated/abrasive soaps and cleansers, soaps/cosmetics with strong drying effect, products with high concentrations of alcohol, astringents, spices, or lime because skin irritation may be increased. Avoid with erythromycin-containing products. May enhance action of neuromuscular blocking agents; use with caution. Antiperistaltic agents (eg, opiates, diphenoxylate with atropine) may prolong and/or worsen severe colitis.

PREGNANCY: Category C, not for use in nursing.

MECHANISM OF ACTION: Clindamycin: Lincosamide antibiotic; binds to 50S ribosomal subunits of susceptible bacteria and prevents elongation of peptide chains by interfering with peptidyl transfer, thereby suppressing bacterial protein synthesis. Found to have (in vitro) activity against *Propionibacterium acnes*. Tretinoin: Retinoid; not established. Suspected to decrease cohesiveness of follicular epithelial cells with decreased microcomedo formation. Also, stimulates mitotic activity and increased turnover of follicular epithelial cells, causing extrusion of comedones.

PHARMACOKINETICS: Absorption: Tretinoin: Percutaneous (minimal). **Distribution:** Orally and parenterally administered clindamycin found in breast milk. **Metabolism:** Tretinoin: 13-cis-retinoic acid and 4-oxo-13-cis-retinoic acid (metabolites).

NURSING CONSIDERATIONS

Assessment: Assess for regional enteritis, ulcerative colitis, or history of antibiotic-associated colitis, pregnancy/nursing status, and possible drug interactions. Assess use in patients whose occupations require considerable sun exposure.

Monitoring: Monitor for signs/symptoms of diarrhea, bloody diarrhea, colitis, local skin reactions, and other adverse reactions.

Patient Counseling: Instruct to wash face gently with mild soap and warm water at hs and apply a thin layer over the entire face (excluding the eyes and lips) after patting the skin dry. Advise not to use more than recommended amount and not to apply more than qd (at hs). Instruct to apply sunscreen qam and reapply over the course of the day PRN. Advise to avoid exposure to sunlight, sunlamp, UV light, and other medicines that may increase sensitivity to sunlight. Inform that medication may cause irritation (eg, erythema, scaling, itching, burning, stinging). Instruct to d/c therapy and contact physician if severe diarrhea or GI discomfort occurs.

Administration: Topical route. **Storage:** 25°C (77°F); excursions permitted to 15-30°C (59-86°F). Protect from light and freezing. Keep away from heat. Keep tube tightly closed.

ZINACEF   RX
cefuroxime sodium (Covis)

THERAPEUTIC CLASS: Cephalosporin (2nd generation)

INDICATIONS: Treatment of lower respiratory tract (including pneumonia), urinary tract (UTI), skin and skin structure (SSSI), septicemia, meningitis, uncomplicated and disseminated gonorrhea, and bone and joint infections caused by susceptible strains of microorganisms. Preoperative and perioperative prophylaxis in patients undergoing clean-contaminated or potentially contaminated surgical procedures.

DOSAGE: *Adults:* Usual: 750mg-1.5g q8h for 5-10 days. Uncomplicated Pneumonia/UTI/SSSI/ Disseminated Gonococcal Infections: 750mg q8h. Severe/Complicated Infections: 1.5g q8h. Bone and Joint Infections: 1.5g q8h. Life-Threatening Infections/Infections due to Less Susceptible Organisms: 1.5g q6h. Meningitis: Max: 3g q8h. Uncomplicated Gonococcal Infection: 1.5g IM single dose at 2 different sites with 1g PO probenecid. Surgical Prophylaxis: 1.5g IV 0.5-1 hr before initial incision, then 750mg IM/IV q8h with prolonged procedure. Open Heart Surgery (Perioperative): 1.5g IV at induction of anesthesia and q12h thereafter, for total of 6g. Renal Impairment: CrCl >20mL/min: 750mg-1.5g q8h. CrCl 10-20mL/min: 750mg q12h. CrCl <10mL/ min: 750mg q24h. Hemodialysis: Give a further dose at end of dialysis. Continue therapy for a minimum of 48-72 hrs after the patient becomes asymptomatic or after evidence of bacterial eradication has been obtained. *Streptococcus pyogenes* Infections: Treat for ≥10 days. Elderly: Start at the lower end of dosing range.
Pediatrics: ≥3 Months: Usual: 50-100mg/kg/day in divided doses q6-8h. Severe/Serious Infections: 100mg/kg/day (not to exceed max adult dose). Bone and Joint Infections: 150mg/kg/day in divided doses q8h (not to exceed max adult dose). Meningitis: 200-240mg/kg/day IV in divided doses q6-8h. Renal Impairment: Modify dosing frequency consistent with adult recommendations. Continue therapy for a minimum of 48-72 hrs after the patient becomes asymptomatic or after evidence of bacterial eradication has been obtained. *S. pyogenes* Infections: Treat for ≥10 days.

HOW SUPPLIED: Inj: 750mg, 1.5g, 750mg/50mL, 1.5g/50mL

WARNINGS/PRECAUTIONS: Caution in penicillin (PCN)-sensitive patients; determine whether patient has had previous hypersensitivity reactions to cephalosporins, PCN, or other drugs. D/C if an allergic reaction occurs; serious acute hypersensitivity reactions may require treatment with epinephrine and other emergency measures. *Clostridium difficile*-associated diarrhea (CDAD) reported; d/c if CDAD is suspected or confirmed. May result in overgrowth of nonsusceptible organisms with prolonged use; take appropriate measures if superinfection develops. Use in the absence of a proven or strongly suspected bacterial infection or prophylactic indication is unlikely to provide benefit and increases the risk of the development of drug-resistant bacteria. Hearing loss reported in pediatric patients treated for meningitis. Risk of decreased prothrombin activity in patients with renal/hepatic impairment, poor nutritional state, protracted course of therapy, and patients previously stabilized on anticoagulant therapy. Lab test interactions may occur. Caution with impaired renal function, history of GI disease particularly colitis, and in elderly.

ADVERSE REACTIONS: Local reactions, decreased Hgb and Hct, eosinophilia, ALT/AST elevation.

INTERACTIONS: Caution with potent diuretics; may adversely affect the renal function. Nephrotoxicity reported with concomitant aminoglycosides. May decrease prothrombin activity; caution with anticoagulants. May affect the gut flora, leading to lower estrogen reabsorption and reduced efficacy of combined estrogen/progesterone oral contraceptives.

PREGNANCY: Category B, caution in nursing.

MECHANISM OF ACTION: Cephalosporin (2nd generation); bactericidal; inhibits cell-wall synthesis.

PHARMACOKINETICS: Absorption: C_{max}=(750mg) 27mcg/mL (IM), 50mcg/mL (IV). (1.5g) 100mcg/mL (IV); T_{max}(750mg)=45 min (IM), 15 min (IV). **Distribution:** Plasma protein binding (50%); found in breast milk. **Elimination**: Urine (89%); $T_{1/2}$=80 min.

NURSING CONSIDERATIONS

Assessment: Assess for known allergy to cephalosporins, PCN, or other drugs, renal/hepatic impairment, nutritional status, history of GI disease (eg, colitis), pregnancy/nursing status, and possible drug interactions.

Monitoring: Monitor for signs/symptoms of an allergic reaction, CDAD, and development of superinfection. In pediatric patients with meningitis, monitor for hearing loss. Monitor renal function and PT.

Z

Patient Counseling: Inform that drug only treats bacterial, not viral infections. Instruct to take exactly ud; skipping doses or not completing full course of therapy may decrease effectiveness and increase the likelihood of bacterial resistance. Inform that diarrhea may occur and will usually end if therapy is discontinued. Instruct to contact physician as soon as possible if watery/bloody stools (with/without stomach cramps, fever) develop even as late as 2 months after discontinuation, and other adverse reactions occur.

Administration: IV/IM routes. Refer to PI for administration procedures, directions for preparation of sol and sus, use of frozen plastic container, compatibility and stability, and instructions for constitution of TwistVial vials. **Storage:** (Dry State) 15-30°C (59-86°F). Protect from light. Frozen Premixed Sol: Do not store above -20°C.

ZINECARD   RX
dexrazoxane (Pharmacia & Upjohn)

THERAPEUTIC CLASS: EDTA derivative

INDICATIONS: Reduce the incidence and severity of cardiomyopathy associated with doxorubicin administration in women with metastatic breast cancer who received a cumulative doxorubicin dose of 300mg/m² and who will continue doxorubicin therapy to maintain tumor control.

DOSAGE: *Adults:* 10:1 ratio of dexrazoxane: doxorubicin (eg, 500mg/m²: 50mg/m²). Moderate to Severe Renal Dysfunction (CrCl <40mL/min): 5:1 ratio of dexrazoxane: doxorubicin (eg, 250mg/m²: 50mg/m²). Hepatic Impairment: Reduce dose proportionally (maintaining the 10:1 ratio). Administer via rapid IV drip infusion. Give doxorubicin within 30 min of start of dexrazoxane infusion (administer doxorubicin after dexrazoxane infusion completed).

HOW SUPPLIED: Inj: 250mg, 500mg

CONTRAINDICATIONS: Chemotherapy regimens not containing an anthracycline.

WARNINGS/PRECAUTIONS: Not recommended for use with the initiation of doxorubicin therapy. Monitor cardiac function; potential for anthracycline-induced cardiac toxicity still exists. Secondary malignancies, primarily acute myeloid leukemia (AML), reported in patients chronically treated with PO razoxane. May cause fetal harm. Caution in elderly.

ADVERSE REACTIONS: Alopecia, N/V, fatigue, malaise, anorexia, stomatitis, fever, infection, diarrhea, pain on injection, sepsis, neurotoxicity, phlebitis, esophagitis.

INTERACTIONS: Avoid during initiation of FAC (fluorouracil, doxorubicin, cyclophosphamide) therapy; may interfere with the antitumor efficacy of the regimen. Additive myelosuppression with chemotherapeutic agents and cytotoxic drugs. Frequent CBCs are recommended with cytotoxic drugs. Secondary malignancies (eg, AML, myelodysplastic syndrome) reported with anticancer agents known to be carcinogenic.

PREGNANCY: Category D, not for use in nursing.

MECHANISM OF ACTION: EDTA derivative; not established. Suspected to interfere with iron-mediated free radical generation thought to be responsible, in part, for anthracycline induced cardiomyopathy.

PHARMACOKINETICS: Absorption: (500mg/m²) C_{max} =36.5µg/mL. **Distribution:** (500mg/m²) V_d=22.4L/m². (600mg/m²) V_d=22L/m². **Elimination:** (500mg/m²) Urine (42%); $T_{1/2}$=2.5 hrs. (600mg/m²) $T_{1/2}$=2.1 hrs.

NURSING CONSIDERATIONS

Assessment: Assess cardiac/renal/hepatic function, pregnancy/nursing status, and possible drug interactions.

Monitoring: Monitor for myelosuppression, secondary malignancies, and other adverse reactions. Monitor cardiac/renal/hepatic function.

Patient Counseling: Inform about the risk and benefit of therapy. Advise women who have potential to become pregnant that product may cause fetal harm.

Administration: IV route. Do not administer via IV push. Do not mix with other drugs. Refer to PI for handling and disposal instructions, and preparation of reconstituted sol. **Storage:** 25°C (77°F); excursions permitted to 15-30°C (59-86°F). Reconstituted Sol: Stable for 30 min at room temperature or 2-8°C (36-46°F) for up to 3 hrs. Infusion Sol: Stable for 1 hr at room temperature or 2-8°C (36-46°F) for up to 4 hrs.

Z

ZIPSOR

RX

diclofenac potassium (Depomed)

> NSAIDs may cause an increased risk of serious cardiovascular (CV) thrombotic events, myocardial infarction (MI), stroke, and serious GI adverse events including bleeding, ulceration, and perforation of the stomach or intestines. Contraindicated for the treatment of perioperative pain in the setting of coronary artery bypass graft (CABG) surgery.

THERAPEUTIC CLASS: NSAID

INDICATIONS: Relief of mild to moderate acute pain in adults ≥18 yrs of age.

DOSAGE: *Adults:* ≥18 Yrs: 25mg qid. Elderly: Start at low end of dosing range.

HOW SUPPLIED: Cap: 25mg

CONTRAINDICATIONS: Asthma, urticaria, or allergic reactions after taking aspirin (ASA) or other NSAIDs. Hypersensitivity to bovine protein. Treatment of perioperative pain in the setting of CABG surgery.

WARNINGS/PRECAUTIONS: May lead to onset of new HTN or worsening of preexisting HTN; monitor BP closely. Fluid retention and edema reported; caution with fluid retention or heart failure. Caution in patients with considerable dehydration. Renal papillary necrosis and other renal injury reported after long-term use. Not recommended for use with advanced renal disease. If therapy must be initiated, monitor renal function. Anaphylactoid reactions may occur. Contraindicated in ASA triad patients. May cause serious skin adverse events (eg, exfoliative dermatitis, Stevens-Johnson syndrome, toxic epidermal necrolysis). Avoid in late pregnancy; may cause premature closure of ductus arteriosus. May cause elevations of LFTs; d/c if liver disease develops or systemic manifestations occur. Caution in elderly and debilitated. Anemia may occur; with long-term use, monitor Hgb/Hct if signs or symptoms of anemia develop. May inhibit platelet aggregation and prolong bleeding time; monitor with coagulation disorders. Caution with asthma and avoid with ASA-sensitive asthma. May mask symptoms of infection (eg, fever, inflammation). Caution in patients with history of ulcer disease or GI bleeding, or with risk factors for GI bleeding. Not a substitute for corticosteroids or to treat corticosteroid insufficiency.

ADVERSE REACTIONS: Abdominal pain, constipation, diarrhea, dyspepsia, N/V, dizziness, headache, somnolence, pruritus, increased sweating.

INTERACTIONS: Avoid use with other diclofenac products. Increased adverse effects with ASA. May impair therapeutic response to ACE inhibitors, thiazides or loop diuretics; monitor for renal failure. Synergistic effects on GI bleeding with warfarin. May increase lithium levels; monitor for toxicity. May enhance methotrexate toxicity; caution when coadministering. May increase nephrotoxicity of cyclosporine; caution when coadministering. Caution with coadministration of other drugs that are substrates or inhibitors of CYP2C9.

PREGNANCY: Category C <30 weeks gestation, Category D after 30 weeks. Not for use in nursing.

MECHANISM OF ACTION: NSAID (benzeneacetic acid derivative); suspected to inhibit prostaglandin synthetase, exerts anti-inflammatory, analgesic, and antipyretic actions.

PHARMACOKINETICS: Absorption: Mean absolute bioavailability (50%), C_{max}=1087ng/mL, AUC=597ng•h/mL, T_{max}=0.5 hr. **Distribution:** V_s=1.3L/kg; serum protein binding (>99%). **Metabolism:** Metabolites: 4'-hydroxy-, 5-hydroxy-, 3'-hydroxy-, 4',5-dihydroxy- and 3'-hydroxy-4'-methoxy diclofenac. **Elimination:** Urine (65%), bile (35%); $T_{1/2}$= approximately 1 hr.

NURSING CONSIDERATIONS

Assessment: Assess LFTs, renal function, CBC, and coagulation profile. Assess for history of CABG surgery, asthma and allergic reactions to ASA or other NSAIDs, active ulceration, bleeding or chronic inflammation of GI tract, CV disease, pregnancy/nursing status, and possible drug interactions. Note other diseases/conditions and drug therapies.

Monitoring: Monitor for hypersensitivity reactions, cardiac complications, stroke, GI bleeding, asthma, skin side effects. Monitor BP, LFTs, renal function, CBC with differential and platelet count, coagulation profile (especially if on anticoagulation therapy), hyperglycemia.

Patient Counseling: Counsel about potential CV, GI, hepatotoxic and dermatological events, as well as possible weight gain/edema. Take as prescribed. Caution women against using late in pregnancy. Caution patients to avoid taking unprescribed acetaminophen.

Administration: Oral route. **Storage:** 25°C (77°F); excursions permitted to 15-30°C (59-86°F). Protect from moisture. Dispense in tight container.

Z

ZITHROMAX

RX

azithromycin (Pfizer)

THERAPEUTIC CLASS: Macrolide

INDICATIONS: Treatment of the following infections caused by susceptible strains of microorganisms: (Tab [250mg, 500mg]/Sus [100mg/5mL, 200mg/5mL]) Acute bacterial exacerbations of chronic obstructive pulmonary disease (COPD), acute bacterial sinusitis (ABS), community-acquired pneumonia (CAP), pharyngitis/tonsillitis, uncomplicated skin and skin structure infections (SSSIs), urethritis, cervicitis, genital ulcer disease (men), and acute otitis media. (Inj) CAP and pelvic inflammatory disease (PID). (Tab [600mg]/Sus [Single-Dose Pkt]) Treatment of disseminated *Mycobacterium avium* complex (MAC) disease in combination with ethambutol in persons with advanced HIV infection. Prevention of disseminated MAC disease, alone or in combination with rifabutin, in persons with advanced HIV infection. Treatment of nongonococcal urethritis and cervicitis.

DOSAGE: *Adults:* (Inj) Infuse IV over not <60 min. CAP: 500mg IV qd for at least 2 days, then 500mg PO (two 250mg tabs) qd to complete a 7- to 10-day course. PID: 500mg IV qd for 1-2 days, then 250mg PO qd to complete a 7-day course. (PO) CAP (Mild Severity)/Pharyngitis/Tonsillitis (2nd-Line Therapy)/SSSI (Uncomplicated): 500mg single dose on Day 1, then 250mg qd on Days 2-5. Acute Bacterial Exacerbations of COPD (Mild-Moderate): 500mg qd for 3 days or 500mg single dose on Day 1, then 250mg qd on Days 2-5. ABS: 500mg qd for 3 days. Genital Ulcer Disease (Chancroid)/Nongonococcal Urethritis and Cervicitis: 1g single dose. Gonococcal Urethritis and Cervicitis: 2g single dose. Prevention of Disseminated MAC Disease: 1200mg once weekly. May be combined with rifabutin. Treatment of Disseminated MAC Infections: 600mg qd in combination with 15mg/kg/day ethambutol.
Pediatrics: (Inj) ≥16 Yrs: Infuse IV over not <60 min. CAP: 500mg IV qd for at least 2 days, then 500mg PO (two 250mg tabs) qd to complete a 7- to 10-day course. PID: 500mg IV qd for 1-2 days, then 250mg PO qd to complete a 7-day course. (Sus) ≥2 Yrs: Pharyngitis/Tonsillitis: 12mg/kg qd for 5 days. ≥6 Months: Acute Otitis Media: 30mg/kg single dose, or 10mg/kg qd for 3 days, or 10mg/kg single dose on Day 1, then 5mg/kg/day on Days 2-5. CAP: 10mg/kg single dose on Day 1, then 5mg/kg on Days 2-5. ABS: 10mg/kg qd for 3 days. Refer to PI for dosage guidelines based on body weight.

HOW SUPPLIED: Inj: 500mg; Sus: 100mg/5mL [15mL], 200mg/5mL [15mL, 22.5mL, 30mL], 1g [pkt]; Tab: 250mg, 500mg, 600mg

CONTRAINDICATIONS: History of cholestatic jaundice/hepatic dysfunction associated with prior use of azithromycin.

WARNINGS/PRECAUTIONS: Serious allergic reactions (eg, angioedema, anaphylaxis) and dermatologic reactions (eg, Stevens Johnson syndrome, toxic epidermal necrolysis) rarely reported; d/c if an allergic reaction occurs and institute appropriate therapy. Allergic symptoms may recur, after initial successful symptomatic treatment, without further azithromycin exposure. Abnormal liver function, hepatitis, cholestatic jaundice, hepatic necrosis, and hepatic failure reported; d/c immediately if signs/symptoms of hepatitis occur. *Clostridium difficile*-associated diarrhea (CDAD) reported; d/c if CDAD is suspected or confirmed. Prolonged cardiac repolarization and QT interval, with risk of developing cardiac arrhythmia and torsades de pointes reported. Consider risk of QT prolongation that can be fatal for at risk-groups, including patients with known QT interval prolongation, history of torsades de pointes, congenital long QT syndrome, bradyarrhythmias, uncompensated heart failure, ongoing proarrhythmic conditions (eg, uncorrected hypokalemia/hypomagnesemia), and clinically significant bradycardia. Elderly may be more susceptible to drug-associated effects on the QT interval. Caution with hepatic impairment or severe renal impairment (GFR <10mL/min). Exacerbation of myasthenia gravis symptoms and new onset of myasthenic syndrome reported. May result in bacterial resistance if used in the absence of proven or suspected bacterial infection or a prophylactic indication. (Tab [250mg, 500mg]/Sus [100mg/5mL, 200mg/5mL]) Do not use in patients with pneumonia who are judged to be inappropriate for oral therapy due to moderate to severe illness or risk factors. Should not be relied on to treat syphilis. (Sus [Single-Dose Pkt]) Do not use to administer doses other than 1000mg; not for pediatric use. Should not be relied on to treat gonorrhea or syphilis. (Inj) Local IV-site reactions reported.

ADVERSE REACTIONS: Diarrhea/loose stools, N/V, abdominal pain. (Tab [600mg]) Hearing impairment, flatulence, headache, abnormal vision. (Inj) Pain at inj site, local inflammation.

INTERACTIONS: Caution with drugs known to prolong the QT interval, Class IA (quinidine, procainamide), and Class III (dofetilide, amiodarone, sotalol) antiarrhythmic agents. May increase digoxin, terfenadine, cyclosporine, hexobarbital, and phenytoin levels; monitor carefully. May potentiate effects of oral anticoagulants; monitor PT. Increased levels with nelfinavir; closely monitor for known side effects (eg, liver enzyme abnormalities, hearing impairment). May produce modest effect on pharmacokinetics of atorvastatin, carbamazepine, cetirizine, didanosine, efavirenz, fluconazole, indinavir, midazolam, rifabutin, sildenafil, theophylline (PO and IV), triazolam, trimethoprim/sulfamethoxazole, and zidovudine; monitor theophylline levels. Efavirenz or fluconazole may have a modest effect on pharmacokinetics of azithromycin. Acute ergot toxicity may occur with ergotamine or dihydroergotamine. (PO) Aluminum- and Mg^{2+}-containing antacids may reduce levels.

PREGNANCY: Category B, caution in nursing.

Z

MECHANISM OF ACTION: Macrolide; interferes with microbial protein synthesis by binding to the 50S ribosomal subunit of susceptible microorganisms.

PHARMACOKINETICS: Absorption: Administration of variable doses resulted in different parameters. **Distribution:** (PO) V_d=31.1L/kg. **Elimination:** (PO) Biliary (major, unchanged). Urine (11%, IV 1st dose), (14%, IV 5th dose), (6%, PO unchanged). $T_{1/2}$=68 hrs.

NURSING CONSIDERATIONS

Assessment: Assess for hypersensitivity to drug, history of cholestatic jaundice/hepatic dysfunction associated with prior use of azithromycin, risk for QT prolongation, myasthenia gravis, renal/hepatic impairment, pregnancy/nursing status, and possible drug interactions. In patients with sexually transmitted urethritis or cervicitis, perform serologic test for syphilis and appropriate cultures for gonorrhea at the time of diagnosis. Perform appropriate culture and susceptibility testing. (Tab [250mg, 500mg]/Sus [100mg/5mL, 200mg/5mL]) Assess for pneumonia, cystic fibrosis, nosocomial infections, known/suspected bacteremia, debilitation, underlying health problems that may compromise ability to respond to illness (eg, immunodeficiency, functional asplenia), or if requiring hospitalization.

Monitoring: Monitor for signs/symptoms of allergic reactions, hepatotoxicity, CDAD, QT prolongation, new onset of myasthenic syndrome or exacerbation of myasthenia gravis, and other adverse reactions. (Inj) Monitor for local IV-site reactions.

Patient Counseling: Inform to d/c immediately and contact physician if any signs of an allergic reaction occur. Counsel that therapy should only be used to treat bacterial, not viral (eg, common cold), infections. Instruct to take exactly ud. Inform that skipping doses or not completing the full course may decrease effectiveness and increase resistance. Inform that diarrhea is a common problem caused by therapy that usually ends when therapy is discontinued. Instruct to immediately contact physician if watery and bloody stools (with or without stomach cramps and fever) occur, even as late as ≥2 months after the last dose. (PO) Instruct not to take aluminum- or Mg²⁺-containing antacids and azithromycin simultaneously. (Tab) Inform that taking the tabs with food may increase tolerability.

Administration: Oral/IV route. Shake sus well before use. (Sus/Tab) Take with or without food. (Inj) Infusate concentration and rate of infusion should be either 1mg/mL over 3 hrs or 2mg/mL over 1 hr; avoid higher concentrations. Do not give as bolus or as IM inj. Do not add other IV substances, additives, or other medications to inj or infuse simultaneously through same IV line. Refer to PI for reconstitution and dilution instructions. (Sus [Single-Dose Pkt]) Mix entire contents of pkt with 2 oz. of water. Drink immediately; add an additional 2 oz. of water, mix, and drink to assure complete consumption of dosage. **Storage:** (Tab [250mg, 500mg]) 15-30°C (59-86°F). (600mg Tab) ≤30°C (86°F). (Sus [100mg/5mL, 200mg/5mL]) Dry Powder: <30°C (86°F). Constituted Sus: 5-30°C (41-86°F). Use within 10 days. Discard when full dosing is completed. (Sus [Single-Dose Pkt]) 5-30°C (41-86°F). (Inj) Reconstituted Sol: <30°C (86°F) for 24 hrs. Diluted Sol (Final Infusion Sol): ≤30°C (86°F) for 24 hrs or 5°C (41°F) for 7 days.

ZMAX   RX
azithromycin (Pfizer)

THERAPEUTIC CLASS: Macrolide

INDICATIONS: Treatment of mild to moderate community-acquired pneumonia in adults and pediatric patients ≥6 months of age and acute bacterial sinusitis in adults caused by susceptible microorganisms.

DOSAGE: *Adults:* 2g single dose on an empty stomach (at least 1 hr ac or 2 hrs pc). *Pediatrics:* ≥6 Months: ≥34kg: 2g single dose. <34kg: 60mg/kg single dose. Take on an empty stomach (at least 1 hr ac or 2 hrs pc). Refer to PI for pediatric dosage guidelines.

HOW SUPPLIED: Sus, Extended-Release: 2g

CONTRAINDICATIONS: History of cholestatic jaundice/hepatic dysfunction associated with prior use of azithromycin.

WARNINGS/PRECAUTIONS: Serious allergic reactions (eg, angioedema, anaphylaxis, Stevens Johnson syndrome [SJS], toxic epidermal necrolysis [TEN]) reported; institute appropriate therapy if an allergic reaction occurs. Allergic symptoms may recur after initial successful symptomatic treatment without further azithromycin exposure. Abnormal liver function, hepatitis, cholestatic jaundice, hepatic necrosis, and hepatic failure reported, some of which resulted in death; d/c immediately if signs/symptoms of hepatitis occur. *Clostridium difficile*-associated diarrhea (CDAD) reported; d/c if CDAD is confirmed or suspected. Exacerbation of symptoms of myasthenia gravis and new onset of myasthenic syndrome reported. Prolonged cardiac repolarization and QT interval, and torsades de pointes reported; consider the risk of QT prolongation, which can be fatal, when weighing the risks/benefits for at-risk groups (eg, patients with known QT interval prolongation, history of torsades de pointes, congenital long QT syndrome, bradyarrhythmias or uncompensated heart failure [HF], patients with ongoing proarrhythmic

Z

conditions such as uncorrected hypokalemia or hypomagnesemia, clinically significant bradycardia). Caution with GFR <10mL/min; higher incidence of GI adverse events reported. May result in bacterial resistance if used in the absence of a proven/suspected bacterial infection. Consider additional antibiotic if patient vomits within 5 min of administration. Consider alternative therapy if patient vomits between 5 and 60 min after administration. Neither a 2nd dose nor alternative therapy is warranted if patient vomits ≥60 min after administration with normal gastric emptying. Consider alternative therapy in patients with delayed gastric emptying. Caution in elderly.

ADVERSE REACTIONS: Diarrhea/loose stools, N/V, abdominal pain, rash.

INTERACTIONS: Caution with drugs known to prolong QT interval, Class IA (quinidine, procainamide), and Class III (dofetilide, amiodarone, sotalol) antiarrhythmic agents. May potentiate effects of oral anticoagulants (eg, warfarin); monitor PT. Monitor carefully with digoxin, ergotamine or dihydroergotamine, cyclosporine, hexobarbital, and phenytoin.

PREGNANCY: Category B, caution in nursing.

MECHANISM OF ACTION: Macrolide; interferes with microbial protein synthesis by binding to the 50S ribosomal subunit of susceptible microorganisms.

PHARMACOKINETICS: Absorption: Administration in various population resulted in different pharmacokinetic parameters. **Distribution:** V_d=31.1L/kg; plasma protein binding (51% at 0.02μg/mL, 7% at 2μg/mL). **Elimination:** Bile (major route), urine (6%, unchanged); $T_{1/2}$=59 hrs.

NURSING CONSIDERATIONS

Assessment: Assess for previous hypersensitivity to the drug, erythromycin, or any macrolide/ketolide antibiotic, known QT interval prolongation, history of torsades de pointes, congenital long QT syndrome, bradyarrhythmias, uncompensated HF, proarrhythmic conditions, clinically significant bradycardia, myasthenia gravis, delayed gastric emptying, history of cholestatic jaundice/hepatic dysfunction associated with prior use of azithromycin, renal dysfunction, pregnancy/nursing status, and possible drug interactions. Perform appropriate culture and susceptibility tests prior to treatment.

Monitoring: Monitor for signs/symptoms of allergic/skin reactions (eg, angioedema, SJS, TEN), CDAD, GI adverse effects, cardiac repolarization or QT prolongation, torsades de pointes, exacerbation of myasthenia gravis, new onset of myasthenic syndrome, hepatotoxicity, and other adverse reactions.

Patient Counseling: Inform that drug needs time to work and that patient may not feel better right away. Instruct to contact physician if symptoms do not improve in a few days, if any signs of allergic reaction occur, or if watery/bloody stools with or without stomach cramps develop (even as late as ≥2 months after dosing). Instruct to contact physician for further treatment if vomiting occurs within 1st hr of administration. Inform that therapy treats bacterial, not viral (eg, common cold), infections. Instruct to take ud; advise that not taking the complete dose may decrease effectiveness and increase the likelihood of bacterial resistance. Advise to take without regard to antacids containing magnesium hydroxide and/or aluminum hydroxide.

Administration: Oral route. Take on an empty stomach. Constitute with 60mL water. Shake well before using. Use a dosing spoon, medicine syringe, or cup for pediatric patients <34kg. Consume reconstituted sus within 12 hrs. Discard any remaining sus after dosing in pediatric patients. **Storage:** Dry Powder: ≤30°C (86°F). Reconstituted Sus: 25°C (77°F); excursions permitted to 15-30°C (59-86°F). Do not refrigerate or freeze.

ZOCOR RX
simvastatin (Merck)

THERAPEUTIC CLASS: HMG-CoA reductase inhibitor

INDICATIONS: Adjunct to diet to decrease total cholesterol, LDL, apolipoprotein B, and TG levels, and to increase HDL levels in primary hyperlipidemia or mixed dyslipidemia, hypertriglyceridemia, primary dysbetalipoproteinemia, homozygous familial hypercholesterolemia (HoFH), heterozygous familial hypercholesterolemia (HeFH) (boys and girls who are at least 1 yr post-menarche, 10-17 yrs of age), and to reduce risk of coronary heart disease (CHD) mortality and cardiovascular events.

DOSAGE: *Adults:* Initial: 10mg or 20mg qpm. Usual: 5-40mg/day. High Risk for CHD Events: Initial: 40mg/day. Perform lipid determinations after 4 weeks and periodically thereafter. Restricted Dosing: Use 80mg dose only in patients who have been taking simvastatin 80mg chronically (eg, ≥12 months) without evidence of muscle toxicity. If currently tolerating 80mg dose and needs to be initiated on a drug that is contraindicated or is associated with a dose cap for simvastatin, switch to an alternative statin with less potential for drug-drug interaction. Do not titrate to 80mg, but place on alternative LDL-lowering treatment that provides greater LDL lowering, if unable to achieve LDL goal with 40mg dose. HoFH: Usual: 40mg/day qpm. HoFH with Concomitant Lomitapide: Reduce dose by 50% if initiating lomitapide. Max:

Z

20mg/day (or 40mg/day for patients who have previously taken simvastatin 80mg/day chronically [eg, ≥12 months] without evidence of muscle toxicity). Concomitant Verapamil, Diltiazem, or Dronedarone: Max: 10mg/day. Concomitant Amiodarone, Amlodipine, or Ranolazine: Max: 20mg/day. Chinese Patients Taking Lipid-Modifying Doses (≥1g/day Niacin) of Niacin-Containing Products: Caution with doses >20mg/day; do not give 80mg dose. Severe Renal Impairment: Initial: 5mg/day; monitor closely.

Pediatrics: 10-17 Yrs: HeFH: Individualize dose. Initial: 10mg qpm. Titrate: Adjust at ≥4-week intervals. Range: 10-40mg/day. Max: 40mg/day. Concomitant Verapamil, Diltiazem, or Dronedarone: Max: 10mg/day. Concomitant Amiodarone, Amlodipine, or Ranolazine: Max: 20mg/day. Chinese Patients Taking Lipid-Modifying Doses (≥1g/day Niacin) of Niacin-Containing Products: Caution with doses >20mg/day; do not give 80mg dose. Severe Renal Impairment: Initial: 5mg/day; monitor closely.

HOW SUPPLIED: Tab: 5mg, 10mg, 20mg, 40mg, 80mg

CONTRAINDICATIONS: Concomitant administration of strong CYP3A4 inhibitors (eg, itraconazole, ketoconazole, posaconazole, voriconazole, HIV protease inhibitors, boceprevir, telaprevir, erythromycin, clarithromycin, telithromycin, nefazodone, cobicistat-containing products), gemfibrozil, cyclosporine, or danazol. Active liver disease, which may include unexplained persistent elevations in hepatic transaminases, women who are or may become pregnant, and nursing mothers.

WARNINGS/PRECAUTIONS: Myopathy (including immune-mediated necrotizing myopathy [IMNM]) and rhabdomyolysis reported; predisposing factors include advanced age (≥65 yrs of age), female gender, uncontrolled hypothyroidism, and renal impairment. Risk of myopathy, including rhabdomyolysis, is dose related and greater with 80mg doses. D/C if markedly elevated CPK levels occur or myopathy is diagnosed/suspected, and temporarily withhold in any patient experiencing an acute or serious condition predisposing to development of renal failure secondary to rhabdomyolysis. Persistent increases in serum transaminases reported. Fatal and nonfatal hepatic failure (rare) reported; promptly interrupt therapy if serious liver injury with clinical symptoms and/or hyperbilirubinemia or jaundice occurs and do not restart if no alternate etiology found. Increases in HbA1c and FPG levels reported. Caution with severe renal impairment, substantial alcohol consumption, history of liver disease, and in the elderly.

ADVERSE REACTIONS: Abdominal pain, headache, myalgia, constipation, nausea, atrial fibrillation, gastritis, diabetes mellitus, insomnia, vertigo, bronchitis, eczema, upper respiratory infections, urinary tract infections.

INTERACTIONS: See Contraindications and Dosage. Due to the risk of myopathy/rhabdomyolysis, avoid grapefruit juice and caution with fibrates, lipid-modifying doses (≥1g/day) of niacin, colchicine, verapamil, diltiazem, dronedarone, lomitapide, amiodarone, amlodipine, and ranolazine. May slightly elevate digoxin concentrations; monitor patients taking digoxin when therapy is initiated. May potentiate effect of coumarin anticoagulants; determine PT before initiation and frequently during therapy.

PREGNANCY: Category X, not for use in nursing.

MECHANISM OF ACTION: HMG-CoA reductase inhibitor; specific inhibitor of HMG-CoA reductase, the enzyme that catalyzes the conversion of HMG-CoA to mevalonate, an early and rate-limiting step in the biosynthetic pathway for cholesterol. Reduces VLDL and TG and increases HDL.

PHARMACOKINETICS: Absorption: T_{max}=1.3-2.4 hrs. **Distribution:** Plasma protein binding (95%). **Metabolism:** Liver (extensive 1st pass), by hydrolysis via CYP3A4; β-hydroxyacid, 6'-hydroxy, 6'-hydroxymethyl, and 6'-exomethylene derivatives (major active metabolites). **Elimination:** Feces (60%), urine (13%).

NURSING CONSIDERATIONS

Assessment: Assess for history of or active liver disease, unexplained persistent hepatic transaminase elevations, predisposing factors for myopathy, renal impairment, alcohol consumption, drug hypersensitivity, any other conditions where treatment is contraindicated or cautioned, pregnancy/nursing status, and possible drug interactions. Assess lipid profile and LFTs.

Monitoring: Monitor for signs/symptoms of myopathy (including IMNM), rhabdomyolysis, liver dysfunction, increases in HbA1c and FPG levels, and other adverse reactions. Monitor lipid profile, LFTs when clinically indicated, and CPK levels.

Patient Counseling: Inform of benefits/risks of therapy. Advise to adhere to the National Cholesterol Education Program-recommended diet, a regular exercise program, and periodic testing of a fasting lipid panel. Inform about substances that should be avoided during therapy, and advise to discuss all medications, both prescription and OTC, with physician. Instruct to report promptly any unexplained muscle pain, tenderness, or weakness, particularly if accompanied by malaise or fever or if these muscle signs or symptoms persist after discontinuation, or any symptoms that may indicate liver injury. Inform patients using the 80mg dose that the risk of myopathy, including rhabdomyolysis, is increased. Instruct women of childbearing age to use an

Z

effective method of birth control to prevent pregnancy while on therapy, to d/c therapy and call physician if pregnant, and not to breastfeed while on therapy.

Administration: Oral route. **Storage:** 5-30°C (41-86°F).

ZOFRAN
ondansetron (GlaxoSmithKline)

RX

THERAPEUTIC CLASS: 5-HT$_3$ receptor antagonist

INDICATIONS: (Inj) Prevention of postoperative nausea and/or vomiting (PONV) in patients ≥1 month of age. Prevention of N/V associated with initial and repeat courses of emetogenic cancer chemotherapy, including high-dose cisplatin in patients ≥6 months of age. (PO) Prevention of PONV. Prevention of N/V associated with: highly emetogenic cancer chemotherapy, including cisplatin ≥50mg/m²; initial and repeat courses of moderately emetogenic cancer chemotherapy; radiotherapy in patients receiving either total body irradiation, single high-dose fraction to the abdomen, or daily fractions to the abdomen.

DOSAGE: *Adults:* Prevention of N/V Associated with Initial and Repeat Courses of Emetogenic Chemotherapy: (Inj) Three 0.15mg/kg IV doses up to a max 16mg/dose; infuse over 15 min. Give 1st dose 30 min before chemotherapy, then give subsequent doses 4 and 8 hrs after the 1st dose. Prevention of N/V Associated with Highly Emetogenic Chemotherapy: (Tab) 24mg (given as three 8mg tabs) 30 min before start of single-day chemotherapy. Prevention of N/V Associated with Moderately Emetogenic Chemotherapy: (PO) 8mg bid; give 1st dose 30 min before chemo-therapy, then give subsequent dose 8 hrs after 1st dose, then administer 8mg q12h for 1-2 days after completion of chemotherapy. Prevention of PONV: (Inj) 4mg IM/IV undiluted immediately before induction of anesthesia or postoperatively if prophylactic antiemetic was not received and N/V occurs within 2 hrs after surgery. As IV, infuse in not <30 sec, preferably over 2-5 min. (PO) 16mg given 1 hr before induction of anesthesia. (PO) Prevention of N/V Associated with Radiotherapy: Usual: 8mg tid. Total Body Irradiation: 8mg 1-2 hrs before each fraction of radio-therapy administered each day. Single High-Dose Fraction Radiotherapy to the Abdomen: 8mg 1-2 hrs before radiotherapy, then q8h after 1st dose for 1-2 days after completion of radiotherapy. Daily Fractionated Radiotherapy to the Abdomen: 8mg 1-2 hrs before radiotherapy, then q8h af-ter 1st dose for each day radiotherapy is given. (Inj/PO) Severe Hepatic Dysfunction (Child-Pugh ≥10): Max: 8mg/day. (Inj) Give over 15 min beginning 30 min prior to emetogenic chemotherapy. *Pediatrics:* Prevention of N/V Associated with Initial and Repeat Courses of Emetogenic Chemotherapy: (Inj) 6 Months-18 Yrs: Three 0.15mg/kg doses up to a max 16mg/dose; infuse over 15 min. Give 1st dose 30 min before chemotherapy, then give subsequent doses 4 and 8 hrs after the 1st dose. Prevention of N/V Associated with Moderately Emetogenic Cancer Chemotherapy: (PO) ≥12 Yrs: 8mg bid; give 1st dose 30 min before chemotherapy, then give subsequent dose 8 hrs after 1st dose, then administer 8mg q12h for 1-2 days after completion of chemotherapy. 4-11 Yrs: 4mg tid; give 1st dose 30 min before chemotherapy, then give subsequent doses 4 and 8 hrs after 1st dose, then administer 4mg q8h for 1-2 days after completion of chemotherapy. Prevention of PONV: (Inj) 1 Month-12 Yrs: >40kg: 4mg IV single dose. ≤40kg: 0.1mg/kg IV single dose. Infuse in not <30 sec, preferably over 2-5 min immediately before or after induction of anesthesia or postoperatively if prophylactic antiemetic was not received and N/V occurs shortly after surgery. (Inj/PO) Severe Hepatic Dysfunction (Child-Pugh ≥10): Max: 8mg/day. (Inj) Give over 15 min beginning 30 min prior to emetogenic chemotherapy.

HOW SUPPLIED: Inj: (HCl) 2mg/mL [20mL]; Sol: (HCl) 4mg base/5mL [50mL]; Tab (HCl)/Tab, Disintegrating (ODT): 4mg, 8mg

CONTRAINDICATIONS: Concomitant use with apomorphine.

WARNINGS/PRECAUTIONS: Hypersensitivity reactions reported in patients hypersensitive to other selective 5-HT$_3$ receptor antagonists. Dose-dependent QT interval prolongation and torsades de pointes reported. Avoid in patients with congenital QT syndrome. Monitor ECG in patients with electrolyte abnormalities (eg, hypokalemia, hypomagnesemia), congestive heart failure (CHF), bradyarrhythmias, and in patients taking other medications that lead to QT pro-longation. Use in patients following abdominal surgery or with chemotherapy induced N/V may mask a progressive ileus and/or gastric distension. Does not stimulate gastric/intestinal perista-lsis; do not use instead of NG suction. (ODT) Contains phenylalanine; caution in phenylketonuric patients.

ADVERSE REACTIONS: Headache, diarrhea, constipation, dizziness, fever, drowsiness/sedation. (Inj) Inj-site reaction. (PO) Malaise/fatigue.

INTERACTIONS: See Contraindications. Inducers or inhibitors of CYP3A4, CYP2D6, CYP1A2 may change the clearance and T$_{1/2}$. Potent CYP3A4 inducers (eg, phenytoin, carbamazepine, rifampin) may significantly increase clearance and decrease blood concentrations. May reduce analgesic activity of tramadol.

PREGNANCY: Category B, caution in nursing.

Z

MECHANISM OF ACTION: Selective $5\text{-}HT_3$ receptor antagonist; has not been established. Blocks $5\text{-}HT_3$ receptors from serotonin. Released serotonin may stimulate the vagal afferents through $5\text{-}HT_3$ receptors and initiate the vomiting reflex.

PHARMACOKINETICS: Absorption: Various age groups resulted in different parameters. (PO) Well absorbed from GI tract; mean bioavailability (56%). **Distribution:** Plasma protein binding (70-76%). **Metabolism:** Extensive; via CYP3A4, 1A2, 2D6; hydroxylation (primary), glucuronide/sulfate conjugation. **Elimination:** Urine (5% unchanged). Refer to PI for additional pharmacokinetic information.

NURSING CONSIDERATIONS

Assessment: Assess for congenital long QT syndrome, electrolyte abnormalities, CHF, bradyarrhythmias, hepatic impairment, pregnancy/nursing status, previous hypersensitivity to the drug, and possible drug interactions. (ODT) Assess for phenylketonuria.

Monitoring: Monitor for QT interval prolongation, torsades de pointes, hypersensitivity reactions, and other adverse reactions. Monitor ECG in patients with electrolyte abnormalities, CHF, bradyarrhythmias, and in patients taking other medications that lead to QT prolongation. In patients who recently underwent abdominal surgery or in patients with chemotherapy-induced N/V, monitor for masking of signs of a progressive ileus and/or gastric distension.

Patient Counseling: Inform about potential benefits/risks of therapy. Inform that drug may cause serious cardiac arrhythmias (eg, QT prolongation); instruct patients to contact physician if they perceive a change in their HR, if they feel lightheaded, or if they have a syncopal episode. Counsel about risk factors for developing severe cardiac arrhythmias and torsades de pointes. Inform that hypersensitivity reactions may occur; advise to report any signs/symptoms (eg, fever, chills, rash, breathing problems). Advise to report the use of all medications, especially apomorphine to physician. (ODT) Instruct not to remove from the blister until just prior to dosing and not to push through foil. Advise to use dry hands to peel blister backing completely off the blister. Instruct to remove gently and immediately place tab on the tongue to dissolve and swallow with saliva. Inform phenylketonuric patients that ODT contains phenylalanine.

Administration: IM/IV/Oral routes. Refer to PI for preparation instructions. **Storage:** (Inj/Sol/Tab) Protect from light. (Inj/ODT/Tab) 2-30°C (36-86°F). (Sol) 15-30°C (59-86°F); store bottles upright in cartons. (Inj) Diluted Sol: Do not use beyond 24 hrs. Refer to PI for further information on stability and handling.

ZOLADEX 1-MONTH   RX
goserelin acetate (AstraZeneca)

THERAPEUTIC CLASS: Synthetic gonadotropin-releasing hormone analog

INDICATIONS: Palliative treatment of advanced prostatic carcinoma. Palliative treatment of advanced breast cancer in pre- and perimenopausal women. In combination with flutamide for management of locally confined Stage T2b-T4 (Stage B2-C) prostatic carcinoma. Management of endometriosis, including pain relief and reduction of endometriotic lesions for the duration of therapy. Endometrial-thinning agent prior to endometrial ablation for dysfunctional uterine bleeding.

DOSAGE: *Adults:* Administer into anterior abdominal wall below the navel line. Advanced Prostatic Carcinoma/Breast Cancer: One 3.6mg implant SQ every 28 days. Stage B2-C Prostatic Carcinoma: One 3.6mg implant SQ, followed in 28 days by one 10.8mg implant SQ. Start 8 weeks prior to initiating radiotherapy and continue during radiation therapy. Alternatively, 4 SQ injections of 3.6mg implant at 28-day intervals (2 implants preceding and 2 during radiotherapy). Endometriosis: One 3.6mg implant SQ every 28 days for 6 months. Endometrial Thinning: One or two 3.6mg implants SQ (given 4 weeks apart). Perform surgery after 4 weeks (one implant) or within 2-4 weeks after administration of 2nd implant.

HOW SUPPLIED: Implant: 3.6mg

CONTRAINDICATIONS: Pregnancy (unless used for palliative treatment of advanced breast cancer).

WARNINGS/PRECAUTIONS: May cause fetal harm. Exclude pregnancy in women using therapy for benign gynecological conditions prior to therapy. Premenopausal women should use effective nonhormonal contraception during therapy and for 12 weeks following discontinuation of therapy. Initially, may cause transient increase in serum testosterone levels in men and estrogen in women; worsening of symptoms or onset of additional signs/symptoms may occur during the 1st few weeks of treatment. May experience temporary increase in bone pain; manage symptomatically. Ureteral obstruction and spinal cord compression reported with prostate cancer; institute standard treatment if spinal cord compression or renal impairment secondary to ureteral obstruction develops, and in extreme cases in prostate cancer patients, consider an immediate orchiectomy. Hyperglycemia and increased risk of developing diabetes reported in men. Increased risk of developing myocardial infarction (MI), sudden cardiac death and stroke

Z

reported in men. Hypercalcemia reported in patients with bone metastases. Hypersensitivity, antibody formation, and acute anaphylactic reactions reported. May cause an increase in cervical resistance; caution when dilating the cervix for endometrial ablation. Retreatment not recommended for management of endometriosis; consider monitoring bone mineral density (BMD) if further treatment is contemplated. Addition of hormone replacement therapy is effective in reducing bone mineral loss and occurrence of vasomotor symptoms and vaginal dryness associated with hypoestrogenism. Lab test interactions may occur. Intended for long-term administration for the management of advanced prostate/breast cancer unless clinically inappropriate.

ADVERSE REACTIONS: Hot flushes, sexual dysfunction, decreased erections, seborrhea, vasodilatation, breast atrophy, tumor flare, vaginitis, emotional lability, decreased libido, sweating, depression, headache, acne, peripheral edema.

PREGNANCY: Category X (with endometriosis and endometrial thinning) or Category D (with advanced breast cancer), not for use in nursing.

MECHANISM OF ACTION: Synthetic gonadotropin-releasing hormone analog; acts as an inhibitor of pituitary gonadotropin secretion. In males, causes initial increase in serum luteinizing hormone and follicle-stimulating hormone levels, with subsequent increases in serum testosterone levels; chronic administration suppresses pituitary gonadotropins, causing a fall in testosterone levels to post-castration levels. In females, chronic exposure causes decrease in serum estradiol to levels consistent with postmenopausal state, leading to reduction of ovarian size and function, reduction in size of uterus and mammary gland, and regression of sex hormone-responsive tumors.

PHARMACOKINETICS: Absorption: Rapid. (Males) C_{max}=2.84ng/mL, T_{max}=12-15 days, AUC=27.8ng•day/mL; (Females) C_{max}=1.46ng/mL, T_{max}=8-22 days, AUC=18.5ng•day/mL. **Distribution:** (Sol) (250mcg SQ dose) V_d=44.1L (males), 20.3L (females); plasma protein binding (27.3%). **Metabolism:** Hydrolysis of C-terminal amino acids. **Elimination:** Urine (>90%, 20% unchanged); (Sol) $T_{1/2}$=4.2 hrs, 12.1 hrs (with renal impairment [CrCl <20mL/min]).

NURSING CONSIDERATIONS

Assessment: Assess for drug hypersensitivity, cardiovascular risk factors, diabetes, and pregnancy/nursing status. Obtain baseline serum testosterone, estrogen, blood glucose, and/or HbA1c levels.

Monitoring: Monitor for occurrence or worsening of signs/symptoms of prostate/breast cancer, ureteral obstruction, spinal cord compression, renal impairment, hypersensitivity/acute anaphylactic reactions, antibody formation, bone pain, cardiovascular disease, hypercalcemia, and other adverse reactions. Periodically monitor BMD, serum testosterone, estrogen, blood glucose, and/or HbA1c levels.

Patient Counseling: Inform of risks and benefits of therapy. Inform men of the risk of developing ureteral obstruction, spinal cord compression, reduction in BMD, diabetes or loss of glycemic control in patients with preexisting diabetes, MI, sudden cardiac death, and stroke. Advise to contact physician if any adverse events develop. Inform women that menstruation should stop with effective doses; instruct to notify physician if regular menstruation persists. Inform that patient may experience persistent amenorrhea. Inform that drug may cause fetal harm and increase risk for pregnancy loss. Advise against pregnancy and/or breastfeeding except for palliative treatment of advanced breast cancer. Instruct to d/c if pregnancy occurs during treatment for endometriosis/endometrial thinning. Advise premenopausal women to use nonhormonal contraception during and for 12 weeks after treatment ends. Instruct to avoid initiating treatment if the patient has undiagnosed abnormal vaginal bleeding, or is allergic to the drug. Inform of the most frequent side effects associated with hypoestrogenism (eg, hot flushes, headaches, vaginal dryness) and that the addition of hormone replacement therapy may decrease vasomotor symptoms and vaginal dryness associated with hypoestrogenism. Inform that drug may cause a reduction in BMD in women. Advise to avoid use for periods >6 months in treatment of benign gynecological conditions.

Administration: SQ route. Administer using an aseptic technique under the supervision of a physician. Refer to PI for further administration instructions. **Storage:** Room temperature; do not exceed 25°C (77°F).

ZOLADEX 3-MONTH   RX
goserelin acetate (AstraZeneca)

THERAPEUTIC CLASS: Synthetic gonadotropin-releasing hormone analog

INDICATIONS: Palliative treatment of advanced prostatic carcinoma. In combination with flutamide for management of locally confined Stage T2b-T4 (Stage B2-C) prostatic carcinoma.

DOSAGE: *Adults:* Administer into anterior abdominal wall below the navel line. Stage B2-C Prostatic Carcinoma: One 3.6mg implant SQ, followed in 28 days by one 10.8mg implant SQ. Start 8 weeks prior to initiating radiotherapy and continue during radiation therapy. Advanced Prostatic Carcinoma: 10.8mg SQ every 12 weeks.

HOW SUPPLIED: Implant: 10.8mg

CONTRAINDICATIONS: Pregnancy.

WARNINGS/PRECAUTIONS: Initially, may cause transient increase in serum testosterone levels; worsening or onset of new symptoms may occur during the 1st few weeks of treatment. May experience temporary increase in bone pain; manage symptomatically. Ureteral obstruction and spinal cord compression reported; institute standard treatment, and in extreme cases an immediate orchiectomy if spinal cord compression or renal impairment secondary to ureteral obstruction develops. Hypersensitivity, antibody formation, and acute anaphylactic reactions reported. Hyperglycemia and increased risk of developing diabetes reported. Increased risk of developing myocardial infarction (MI), sudden cardiac death and stroke reported. Lab test interactions may occur.

ADVERSE REACTIONS: Hot flashes, sexual dysfunction, decreased erections, pain, asthenia, gynecomastia, pelvic/bone pain.

PREGNANCY: Category X, not for use in nursing.

MECHANISM OF ACTION: Synthetic gonadotropin-releasing hormone analog; inhibits pituitary gonadotropin secretion. Initially increases serum luteinizing hormone and follicle-stimulating hormone levels with subsequent increases in serum levels of testosterone. Chronic administration leads to suppression of pituitary gonadotropins, and a fall in testosterone levels.

PHARMACOKINETICS: Absorption: Rapid. C_{max}=8.85ng/mL; T_{max}=1.8 hrs. **Distribution:** (Sol) V_d=44.1L (250mcg SQ dose). Plasma protein binding (27%). **Metabolism:** Hydrolysis of C-terminal amino acids. **Elimination:** Urine (>90%, 20% unchanged); (SQ, Sol) $T_{1/2}$=4.2 hrs, 12.1 hrs (with renal impairment [CrCl<20mL/min]).

NURSING CONSIDERATIONS

Assessment: Assess for drug hypersensitivity, diabetes, and cardiovascular risk factors. Obtain baseline serum testosterone, blood glucose, and/or HbA1c levels.

Monitoring: Monitor for worsening or occurrence of signs/symptoms of prostate cancer, bone pain, ureteral obstruction, spinal cord compression, renal impairment, hypersensitivity/acute anaphylactic reactions, antibody formation, cardiovascular disease, and other adverse reactions. Periodically monitor serum testosterone, blood glucose and/or HbA1c levels.

Patient Counseling: Inform of risks and benefits of therapy. Inform of the risk of developing ureteral obstruction, spinal cord compression, reduction in bone mineral density, diabetes, loss of glycemic control in patients with preexisting diabetes, MI, sudden cardiac death, and stroke. Advise to contact physician if any adverse events develop.

Administration: SQ route. Administer using an aseptic technique under the supervision of a physician. Refer to PI for further administration instructions. **Storage:** Room temperature; do not exceed 25°C (77°F).

ZOLINZA
vorinostat (Merck)

RX

THERAPEUTIC CLASS: Histone deacetylase inhibitor

INDICATIONS: Treatment of cutaneous manifestations in patients with cutaneous T-cell lymphoma who have progressive, persistent or recurrent disease on or following two systemic therapies.

DOSAGE: *Adults:* Take with food. Usual: 400mg qd. If Intolerant to Therapy: May reduce to 300mg qd; may further reduce to 300mg qd for 5 consecutive days each week, as necessary. Mild to Moderate Hepatic Impairment (Bilirubin 1-3X ULN/AST>ULN): Reduce starting dose to 300mg qd.

HOW SUPPLIED: Cap: 100mg

WARNINGS/PRECAUTIONS: Pulmonary embolism and deep vein thrombosis (DVT) reported; monitor for signs and symptoms of these events, particularly with prior history of thromboembolic events. Dose-related thrombocytopenia and anemia may occur; adjust dosage or d/c treatment as clinically appropriate. GI disturbances (eg, N/V, diarrhea) reported. Adequately control preexisting N/V and diarrhea before beginning therapy. Hyperglycemia observed. Monitor blood cell counts and chemistry tests, including serum electrolytes, Mg^{2+}, Ca^{2+}, glucose, and SrCr every 2 weeks during the first 2 months of therapy and monthly thereafter. Correct hypokalemia and hypomagnesemia prior to therapy. Monitor K^+ and Mg^{2+} more frequently in symptomatic patients (eg, patients with N/V, diarrhea, fluid imbalance, cardiac symptoms). May cause fetal harm. Caution with renal/hepatic impairment and in elderly.

ADVERSE REACTIONS: Diarrhea, fatigue, N/V, thrombocytopenia, anorexia, dysgeusia, decreased weight, muscle spasms, alopecia, dry mouth, increased blood creatinine, chills, constipation, dizziness.

INTERACTIONS: Prolongation of PT and INR observed with coumarin-derivative anticoagulants; monitor PT and INR more frequently. Severe thrombocytopenia and GI bleeding reported with concomitant use with other histone deacetylase inhibitors (eg, valproic acid); monitor platelet counts every 2 weeks for the first 2 months.

PREGNANCY: Category D, not for use in nursing.

MECHANISM OF ACTION: Histone deacetylase inhibitor; catalyzes the removal of acetyl groups from the lysine residues of proteins (including histones and transcription factors), resulting in open chromatin structure and transcriptional activation.

PHARMACOKINETICS: Absorption: (Fasted, single 400mg dose) C_{max}=1.2μM, T_{max}=1.5 hrs, AUC=4.2μM•hr; (Fed, single 400mg dose) C_{max}=1.2μM, T_{max}=4 hrs, AUC=5.5μM•hr. (Fed, multiple 400mg doses) C_{max}=1.2μM, T_{max}=4 hrs, AUC=6.0μM•hr. **Distribution:** Plasma protein binding (71%). **Metabolism:** Liver via glucuronidation, hydrolysis, and β-oxidation. **Elimination:** Urine (<1% unchanged); $T_{1/2}$=2 hrs.

NURSING CONSIDERATIONS

Assessment: Assess for renal/hepatic impairment, history of thromboembolic events, GI disturbances, fluid imbalance, cardiac symptoms, diabetes, hypokalemia, hypomagnesemia, pregnancy/nursing status, and possible drug interactions.

Monitoring: Monitor for signs/symptoms of pulmonary embolism and DVT, thrombocytopenia, anemia, GI disturbances, dehydration, and hyperglycemia. Monitor blood cell counts, chemistry tests, electrolytes, serum glucose, and SrCr every 2 weeks for the first 2 months and monthly thereafter. Monitor K^+ and Mg^{2+} more frequently in symptomatic patients.

Patient Counseling: Inform about risks and benefits of therapy. Instruct to drink at least 2L/day of fluids to prevent dehydration. Advise to promptly report to physician if excessive vomiting or diarrhea, unusual bleeding, signs of DVT, and if other adverse events develop.

Administration: Oral route. Take with food. Do not open or crush caps. Avoid direct contact of powder in cap with skin or mucous membranes; wash thoroughly if such contact occurs. Avoid exposure to crushed and/or broken cap. **Storage:** 20-25°C (68-77°F); excursions permitted between 15-30°C (59-86°F).

ZOLOFT   RX
sertraline HCl (Pfizer)

> Antidepressants increased the risk of suicidal thinking and behavior (suicidality) in children, adolescents, and young adults in short-term studies of major depressive disorder (MDD) and other psychiatric disorders. Monitor and observe closely for clinical worsening, suicidality, or unusual changes in behavior in patients who are started on antidepressant therapy. Not approved for use in pediatric patients except for patients with obsessive compulsive disorder (OCD).

THERAPEUTIC CLASS: Selective serotonin reuptake inhibitor

INDICATIONS: Treatment of MDD, social anxiety disorder (SAD), panic disorder with/without agoraphobia, premenstrual dysphoric disorder (PMDD), and post-traumatic stress disorder (PTSD) in adults. Treatment of OCD in patients ≥6 yrs.

DOSAGE: *Adults:* Administer am or pm. MDD/OCD: 50mg qd. Max: 200mg/day. Panic Disorder/PTSD/SAD: Initial: 25mg qd. Titrate: Increase to 50mg qd after 1 week. Adjust dose at intervals of no less than 1 week. Max: 200mg/day. PMDD: Initial: 50mg qd throughout menstrual cycle or limited to luteal phase of cycle. Titrate: Increase at 50mg increments/cycle up to 150mg/day for throughout menstrual cycle dosing or 100mg/day for luteal phase dosing if needed. If 100mg/day is established for luteal phase dosing, use a 50mg/day titration step for 3 days at the beginning of each luteal phase dosing period. Reassess to determine need for maintenance treatment. Hepatic Impairment: Use lower or less frequent doses. Switching to/from an MAOI for Psychiatric Disorders: Allow at least 14 days between discontinuation of an MAOI and initiation of treatment, and allow at least 14 days between discontinuation of treatment and initiation of an MAOI. Use with Other MAOIs (eg, Linezolid, IV Methylene Blue): Refer to PI.
Pediatrics: Administer am or pm. OCD: Initial: 13-17 Yrs: 50mg qd. 6-12 Yrs: 25mg qd. Titrate: Adjust dose at intervals of no less than 1 week. Max: 200mg/day. Reassess to determine need for maintenance treatment. Hepatic Impairment: Use lower or less frequent doses. Switching to/from an MAOI for Psychiatric Disorders: Allow at least 14 days between discontinuation of an MAOI and initiation of treatment, and allow at least 14 days between discontinuation of treatment and initiation of an MAOI. Use with Other MAOIs (eg, Linezolid, IV Methylene Blue): Refer to PI.

HOW SUPPLIED: Sol: 20mg/mL [60mL]; Tab: 25mg*, 50mg*, 100mg* *scored

CONTRAINDICATIONS: Use of an MAOI for psychiatric disorders either concomitantly or within 14 days of stopping treatment. Treatment within 14 days of stopping an MAOI for psychiatric disorders. Starting treatment in a patient being treated with MAOIs (eg, linezolid or IV methylene blue). Concomitant use with pimozide. (Sol) Concomitant disulfiram.

WARNINGS/PRECAUTIONS: Not approved for treatment of bipolar depression. Serotonin syndrome reported; d/c immediately and initiate supportive symptomatic treatment. Activation of mania/hypomania, altered platelet function and/or abnormal lab results, decreased serum uric acid, and weight loss reported. Adverse events reported upon discontinuation, particularly when abrupt; reduce dose gradually whenever possible. May increase the risk of bleeding events. Seizures reported; caution with seizure disorder. Caution with hepatic impairment and diseases/ conditions that could affect metabolism or hemodynamic responses. Hyponatremia may occur; caution in elderly and volume-depleted patients. Consider discontinuation in patients with symptomatic hyponatremia and institute appropriate medical intervention. May have an effect on pupil size resulting in mydriasis; caution with angle-closure glaucoma or history of glaucoma. Caution in 3rd trimester of pregnancy due to risk of serious neonatal complications. False-positive urine immunoassay screening tests for benzodiazepines reported. (Sol) Dropper dispenser contains dry natural rubber; caution with latex sensitivity.

ADVERSE REACTIONS: Ejaculation failure, dry mouth, increased sweating, somnolence, fatigue, tremor, anorexia, dizziness, headache, diarrhea, dyspepsia, nausea, constipation, agitation, insomnia.

INTERACTIONS: See Contraindications. May cause serotonin syndrome with other serotonergic drugs (eg, triptans, TCAs, fentanyl) and with drugs that impair metabolism of serotonin; d/c immediately if this occurs. Drugs that are tightly bound to protein (eg, warfarin, digitoxin) may cause a shift in plasma concentrations resulting in an adverse effect. Caution with other CNS active drugs. Monitor lithium, phenytoin, and valproate levels with appropriate dose adjustments. May increase levels of drugs metabolized by CYP2D6, especially those with a narrow therapeutic index (eg, TCAs for treatment of MDD, propafenone, flecainide). Rare cases of weakness, hyperreflexia, and incoordination reported with sumatriptan. May induce metabolism of cisapride. Increased risk of bleeding with aspirin (ASA), NSAIDs, warfarin, and other drugs affecting coagulation. Altered anticoagulant effects reported with warfarin. Avoid with alcohol. Increased risk of hyponatremia with diuretics. Cimetidine may increase levels and $T_{1/2}$. May reduce clearance of diazepam and tolbutamide.

PREGNANCY: Category C, caution in nursing.

MECHANISM OF ACTION: SSRI; presumed to be linked to inhibition of CNS neuronal uptake of serotonin.

PHARMACOKINETICS: Absorption: T_{max}=4.5-8.4 hrs. **Distribution:** Plasma protein binding (98%). **Metabolism:** Liver (extensive); N-demethylation, oxidative deamination, reduction, hydroxylation, glucuronide conjugation; N-desmethylsertraline (metabolite). **Elimination:** Urine (40-45%); feces (40-45%, 12-14% unchanged); $T_{1/2}$=26 hrs (sertraline), 62-104 hrs (N-desmethylsertraline).

NURSING CONSIDERATIONS

Assessment: Assess for bipolar depression, conditions where treatment is contraindicated or cautioned, pregnancy/nursing status, and possible drug interactions.

Monitoring: Monitor for worsening of depression, suicidality, or unusual changes in behavior, serotonin syndrome, hyponatremia, abnormal bleeding, mydriasis, activation of mania/hypomania, seizures; and other adverse events. Periodically monitor height and weight of pediatric patients with long-term therapy.

Patient Counseling: Counsel about benefits, risks, and appropriate use of therapy. Advise families and caregivers to be alert for emergence of anxiety, agitation, panic attacks, insomnia, irritability, hostility, aggressiveness, impulsivity, akathisia, hypomania, mania, other unusual changes in behavior, worsening of depression, and suicidal ideation; instruct to report symptoms to physician. Inform about risk of serotonin syndrome with concomitant triptans, tramadol, or other serotonergic agents. Advise to use caution when performing hazardous tasks (eg, operating machinery, driving). Inform that concomitant use with NSAIDs, ASA, warfarin, and other drugs that affect coagulation may increase the risk of bleeding. Counsel to avoid alcohol and to use caution when using OTC products. Advise to notify physician if pregnant, intend to become pregnant, or if breastfeeding.

Administration: Oral route. (Sol) Must be diluted before use. Mix sol with 4 oz. of water, ginger ale, lemon/lime soda, lemonade, or orange juice only; do not mix with any other liquids. Take dose immediately after mixing. **Storage:** 25°C (77°F); excursions permitted to 15-30°C (59-86°F).

ZOLPIMIST

zolpidem tartrate (ECR)

CIV

Z

THERAPEUTIC CLASS: Imidazopyridine hypnotic

INDICATIONS: Short-term treatment of insomnia characterized by difficulties with sleep initiation.

DOSAGE: *Adults:* Use lowest effective dose. Initial: 5mg for women and either 5mg or 10mg for men, taken only once per night immediately before hs with at least 7-8 hrs remaining before the planned time of awakening. Titrate: May increase to 10mg if the 5mg dose is not effective. Max: 10mg qd immediately before hs. Elderly/Debilitated/Hepatic Insufficiency: 5mg qd immediately before hs. Use with CNS Depressants: May need to adjust dose.

HOW SUPPLIED: Spray: 5mg/actuation [60 actuations]

WARNINGS/PRECAUTIONS: Increased risk of next-day psychomotor impairment if taken with less than a full night of sleep remaining (7-8 hrs). May impair mental/physical abilities. Initiate only after careful evaluation; failure of insomnia to remit after 7-10 days of treatment may indicate presence of a primary psychiatric and/or medical illness. Cases of angioedema involving the tongue, glottis, or larynx reported; do not rechallenge if angioedema develops. Abnormal thinking, behavioral changes, and visual/auditory hallucinations reported. Complex behaviors (eg, sleep-driving) reported; consider discontinuation if a sleep-driving episode occurs. Amnesia, anxiety, and other neuropsychiatric symptoms may occur. Worsening of depression, and suicidal thoughts and actions (including completed suicides) reported in primarily depressed patients; prescribe the least amount of drug that is feasible at a time. Caution with compromised respiratory function; prior to prescribing, consider the risks of respiratory depression, in patients with respiratory impairment (eg, sleep apnea, myasthenia gravis). Withdrawal signs and symptoms reported following rapid dose decrease or abrupt discontinuation; monitor for tolerance, abuse, and dependence.

ADVERSE REACTIONS: Drowsiness, headache, dizziness, allergy, sinusitis, lethargy, drugged feeling, pharyngitis, dry mouth, back pain, diarrhea.

INTERACTIONS: See Dosage. Increased risk of CNS depression and complex behaviors with other CNS depressants (eg, benzodiazepines, opioids, TCAs, alcohol). Use with other sedative-hypnotics (eg, other zolpidem products) at hs or the middle of the night is not recommended. Increased risk of next-day psychomotor impairment with other CNS depressants or drugs that increase zolpidem levels. May decrease peak levels of imipramine. Additive effect of decreased alertness with imipramine or chlorpromazine. Additive adverse effect on psychomotor performance with chlorpromazine or alcohol. Sertraline and CYP3A inhibitors may increase exposure. Fluoxetine may increase $T_{1/2}$. Rifampin (a CYP3A4 inducer) may reduce exposure, pharmacodynamic effects, and efficacy. Ketoconazole (a potent CYP3A4 inhibitor) may increase pharmacodynamic effects; consider lower dose of zolpidem.

PREGNANCY: Category C, caution in nursing.

MECHANISM OF ACTION: Imidazopyridine, nonbenzodiazepine hypnotic; interacts with a gamma-aminobutyric acid-BZ receptor complex. Binds the BZ_1 receptor preferentially with a high affinity ratio of the $α_1/α_5$ subunits.

PHARMACOKINETICS: Absorption: Rapid from oral mucosa and GI tract. C_{max}=114ng/mL (5mg), 210ng/mL (10mg); T_{max}=0.9 hrs (5mg, 10mg). **Distribution:** Plasma protein binding (92.5%); found in breast milk. **Elimination:** Renal; $T_{1/2}$=2.7 hrs (5mg), 3 hrs (10mg).

NURSING CONSIDERATIONS

Assessment: Assess for physical and/or psychiatric disorder, depression, compromised respiratory function, sleep apnea, myasthenia gravis, hepatic impairment, history of drug/alcohol addiction or abuse, hypersensitivity to the drug, pregnancy/nursing status, and possible drug interactions.

Monitoring: Monitor for angioedema, emergence of any new behavioral signs/symptoms of concern, respiratory depression, withdrawal signs/symptoms, tolerance, abuse, dependence, and other adverse reactions.

Patient Counseling: Inform about the benefits and risks of treatment. Instruct to take only as prescribed; advise to wait at least 8 hrs after dosing before driving or engaging in other activities requiring full mental alertness. Instruct to contact physician immediately if any adverse reactions (eg, severe anaphylactic/anaphylactoid reactions, sleep-driving, other complex behaviors, suicidal thoughts) develop. Advise not to use the drug if patient drank alcohol that pm or before bed. Instruct patients not to increase the dose and to inform physician if it is believed that the drug does not work.

Administration: Oral route. Take immediately before hs with at least 7-8 hrs remaining before the planned time of awakening. Do not administer with or immediately after a meal. Prime pump before 1st time use (5 sprays) or if not used for at least 14 days (1 spray). Refer to PI for further administration instructions. **Storage:** 25°C (77°F); excursions permitted to 15-30°C (59-86°F). Store upright. Do not freeze. Avoid prolonged exposure to temperatures >30°C (86°F).

Z

ZOMETA   RX
zoledronic acid (Novartis)

THERAPEUTIC CLASS: Bisphosphonate

INDICATIONS: Treatment of hypercalcemia of malignancy. Treatment of multiple myeloma and documented bone metastases from solid tumors, in conjunction with standard antineoplastic therapy. Prostate cancer should have progressed after treatment with at least one hormonal therapy.

DOSAGE: *Adults:* Infuse IV over no less than 15 min. Hypercalcemia of Malignancy: Max: 4mg as a single-dose. May consider retreatment if serum Ca^{2+} does not return to normal or remain normal after initial treatment; wait for a minimum of 7 days before retreatment. Multiple Myeloma/Bone Metastases of Solid Tumors: CrCl >60mL/min: 4mg every 3-4 weeks. CrCl 50-60mL/min: 3.5mg. CrCl 40-49mL/min: 3.3mg. CrCl 30-39mL/min: 3mg. Refer to PI for recommendations regarding withholding treatment with renal deterioration. Administer oral Ca^{2+} supplement of 500mg and multiple vitamins containing 400 IU of vitamin D daily.

HOW SUPPLIED: Inj: 4mg/5mL, 4mg/100mL

WARNINGS/PRECAUTIONS: Monitor renal function; assess SrCr prior to each treatment. Contains same active ingredient as Reclast; do not treat concomitantly with Reclast or other bisphosphonates. Adequately rehydrate patients with hypercalcemia of malignancy prior to administration and throughout the treatment. Monitor standard hypercalcemia-related metabolic parameters (eg, serum Ca^{2+}, phosphate, Mg^{2+}) following initiation of therapy. Caution in patients with hypercalcemia of malignancy with severe renal impairment. Not recommended in patients with bone metastases with severe renal impairment. Osteonecrosis of the jaw (ONJ) reported; perform dental exam with preventive dentistry prior to treatment and if possible, avoid invasive dental procedures while on treatment. Severe and occasionally incapacitating bone, joint, and/or muscle pain reported; d/c if severe symptoms develop. Atypical subtrochanteric and diaphyseal femoral fractures reported; examine contralateral femur in patients who have sustained femoral shaft fracture. Any patient with a history of bisphosphonate exposure who presents with thigh/groin pain in the absence of trauma should be suspected of having an atypical fracture and should be evaluated; consider discontinuation in patients suspected to have an atypical femur fracture. Bronchoconstriction may occur in aspirin (ASA)-sensitive patients. May cause fetal harm. Hypocalcemia, cardiac arrhythmias, and neurologic adverse events reported; correct hypocalcemia before initiating treatment and adequately supplement with Ca^{2+} and vitamin D.

ADVERSE REACTIONS: Bone pain, N/V, insomnia, abnormal SrCr, fatigue, pyrexia, anemia, constipation, dyspnea, diarrhea, weakness, myalgia, cough, arthralgia, edema (lower limb).

INTERACTIONS: Caution with aminoglycosides; may have an additive effect to lower serum Ca^{2+} level for prolonged periods. Loop diuretics may increase risk of hypocalcemia; do not use until the patient is adequately rehydrated and use with caution. Caution with other potentially nephrotoxic drugs.

PREGNANCY: Category D, not for use in nursing.

MECHANISM OF ACTION: Bisphosphonate; not established. Inhibits bone resorption by inhibiting osteoclastic activity and inducing osteoclast apoptosis. Also blocks osteoclastic resorption of mineralized bone and cartilage through its binding to bone.

PHARMACOKINETICS: Elimination: Urine (39%); $T_{1/2}$=146 hrs.

NURSING CONSIDERATIONS

Assessment: Assess for hypocalcemia, risk factors for ONJ, hypersensitivity to drug, ASA sensitivity, pregnancy/nursing status, and possible drug interactions. Assess renal function and hydration status. Perform dental exam with preventive dentistry.

Monitoring: Monitor renal function, standard hypercalcemia-related metabolic parameters, and hydration status. Monitor for ONJ, musculoskeletal pain, atypical femur fracture, bronchoconstriction, hypocalcemia, and other adverse reactions.

Patient Counseling: Instruct to notify physician of kidney problems, if pregnant/planning to become pregnant, breastfeeding, or if ASA-sensitive. Inform of the importance of getting blood tests during the course of therapy. Advise to have dental exam prior to treatment and avoid invasive dental procedures during treatment. Inform of the importance of good dental hygiene and routine dental care. Advise patients with multiple myeloma or bone metastasis of solid tumors to take an oral Ca^{2+} supplement of 500mg and multiple vitamin containing 400 IU of vitamin D daily. Instruct to report any thigh, hip, or groin pain. Inform of the most common side effects that may develop.

Administration: IV route. Infuse over no less than 15 min. Refer to PI for preparation and administration instructions. **Storage:** 25°C (77°F); excursions permitted to 15-30°C (59-86°F). Diluted Sol: If not used immediately, 2-8°C (36-46°F). Equilibrate to room temperature prior to administration. Total time between dilution, storage in the refrigerator, and end of administration must not exceed 24 hrs.

ZOMIG RX
zolmitriptan (Impax)

OTHER BRAND NAMES: Zomig-ZMT (Impax)

THERAPEUTIC CLASS: 5-HT$_{1B/1D}$ agonist

INDICATIONS: Acute treatment of migraine attacks with or without aura in adults.

DOSAGE: *Adults:* (Spray) Individualize dose. Initial: 2.5 mg. Max Single Dose: 5mg. If migraine is not resolved by 2 hrs or returns after a transient improvement, a 2nd dose may be administered at least 2 hrs after the 1st dose. Max Daily Dose: 10mg/24 hrs. Safety of treating an average of >4 headaches in a 30-day period has not been established. With Cimetidine: Limit max single dose to 2.5mg; do not exceed 5mg/24 hrs. (PO) Initial: 1.25mg (tab) or 2.5mg. Max Single Dose: 5mg. If migraine is not resolved by 2 hrs or returns after a transient improvement, a 2nd dose may be administered at least 2 hrs after the 1st dose. Max Daily Dose: 10mg/24 hrs. Safety of treating an average of >3 migraines in a 30-day period has not been established. Moderate to Severe Hepatic Impairment: (Tab) 1.25mg. Limit total daily dose in patients with severe hepatic impairment to no more than 5mg/day. With Cimetidine: Limit max single dose to 2.5mg; do not exceed 5mg/24 hrs. Elderly: Start at lower end of dosing range.

HOW SUPPLIED: Nasal Spray: 2.5mg, 5mg [100 µL]; Tab: 2.5mg*, 5mg; Tab, Disintegrating: (ZMT) 2.5mg, 5mg *scored

CONTRAINDICATIONS: Ischemic coronary artery disease (angina pectoris, history of myocardial infarction [MI], or documented silent ischemia), other significant underlying cardiovascular (CV) disease, or coronary artery vasospasm, including Prinzmetal's angina. Wolff-Parkinson-White syndrome or arrhythmias associated with other cardiac accessory conduction pathway disorders. History of stroke, transient ischemic attack (TIA), or history of hemiplegic or basilar migraine. Peripheral vascular disease. Ischemic bowel disease. Uncontrolled HTN. Recent use of another 5-HT$_1$ agonist, ergotamine-containing medication, or ergot-type medication (eg, dihydroergotamine, methysergide). Concurrent MAOI-A or recent use/discontinuation of MAOI-A (within 2 weeks).

WARNINGS/PRECAUTIONS: If no treatment response for the 1st migraine attack, reconsider diagnosis before treating any subsequent attacks. Not for prevention of migraine attacks. Serious cardiac adverse reactions, including MI, and coronary artery vasospasm (Prinzmetal's angina) reported. Perform CV evaluation in triptan-naive patients who have multiple CV risk factors (eg, increased age, diabetes, HTN, smoking, obesity, strong family history of coronary artery disease [CAD]) prior to therapy; consider administering 1st dose in a medically supervised setting and performing an ECG immediately following administration if CV evaluation is negative. Evaluate CV periodically with long-term intermittent use. Life-threatening cardiac rhythm disturbances, including ventricular tachycardia and ventricular fibrillation, reported; d/c if these disturbances occur. Sensations of tightness, pain, and pressure in the chest, throat, neck, and jaw commonly occur (usually of noncardiac origin). Cerebrovascular events (eg, cerebral/subarachnoid hemorrhage, stroke) reported; exclude other potentially serious neurological conditions before treating headaches in patients not previously diagnosed with migraine, and in migraine patients with atypical migraine symptoms. May cause noncoronary vasospastic reactions (eg, peripheral vascular ischemia, GI vascular ischemia and infarction, Raynaud's syndrome, splenic infarction). Rule out a vasospasm reaction before receiving additional doses if signs/symptoms suggestive of such reactions occur. Transient and permanent blindness and significant partial vision loss reported. Overuse of acute migraine drugs may lead to exacerbation of headache; detoxification may be necessary. Serotonin syndrome may occur; d/c if suspected. HTN reported; monitor BP. Caution in elderly. (Tab, Disintegrating) Caution with phenylketonuria; each 2.5mg and 5mg ODT contains 2.81mg and 5.62mg phenylalanine. (Tab, Disintegrating, Spray) Not recommended in patients with moderate or severe hepatic impairment. (Spray) D/C if cerebrovascular event occurs.

ADVERSE REACTIONS: Neck/throat/jaw pain, paresthesia, asthenia, somnolence, warm/cold sensation, nausea, heaviness sensation, dry mouth. (Tab/Tab, Disintegrating) Unusual taste, hyperesthesia, dizziness.

INTERACTIONS: See Contraindications. Ergot-containing drugs may prolong vasospastic reactions. Increased exposure with MAOI-A. Risk of vasospastic reactions with 5-HT 1B/1D agonists (eg, triptans). Coadministration with SSRIs or SNRIs, TCAs may cause serotonin syndrome. Half-life and blood levels doubled with cimetidine.

PREGNANCY: Category C, not for use in nursing.

MECHANISM OF ACTION: 5-HT$_{1D/1B}$ agonist; binds with high affinity to human recombinant 5-HT$_{1D}$ and 5-HT$_{1B}$ receptors, and moderate affinity for 5-HT$_{1A}$ receptors. Suspected to be due to the agonist effects at the 5-HT$_{1B/1D}$ receptors on intracranial blood vessels (including arteriovenous anastomoses) and sensory nerves of the trigeminal system, which results in cranial vessel constriction and inhibition of pro-inflammatory neuropeptide release.

PHARMACOKINETICS: Absorption: (PO) Well-absorbed, (Spray) rapid; absolute bioavailability (40%); T_{max}=(Tab, Disintegrating/Spray) 3 hrs, (Tab) 1.5 hrs. **Distribution:** V_d=(PO) 7L/kg, (Spray) 8.4L/kg; plasma protein binding (25%). **Metabolism:** N-desmethyl (active metabolite). **Elimination:** (PO) Urine (65%, 8% unchanged), feces (30%); $T_{1/2}$=(Spray) 3 hrs.

NURSING CONSIDERATIONS

Assessment: Confirm diagnosis of migraine before therapy. Assess for ischemic CAD (eg, angina pectoris, history of MI or documented silent ischemia, Prinzmetal's angina, MI or documented silent MI), ECG changes, or any other conditions where treatment is contraindicated or cautioned. Assess for hepatic/renal dysfunction, pregnancy/nursing status, and possible drug interactions. Perform a CV evaluation for patients who have multiple CV risk factors.

Monitoring: Monitor for signs/symptoms of cardiac adverse reactions, cerebrovascular events, vasospastic reactions, tightness/pain/pressure sensations, peripheral vascular ischemia, serotonin syndrome, ophthalmic changes, increased BP, and other adverse reactions. Perform ECG immediately after administration of therapy and monitor CV function in intermittent long-term users. Monitor for medication overuse; exacerbation of headache may occur.

Patient Counseling: Instruct to take ud. Inform that treatment may cause serious CV events (eg, MI, stroke), which may result in hospitalization and even death. Instruct patients to be alert for signs/symptoms of chest pain, SOB, weakness, slurring of speech; notify physician if indicative signs/symptoms are observed. Inform patients that the use of therapy ≥10 days per month may lead to exacerbation of headache; encourage to record headache frequency and drug use. Counsel about the possible drug interactions. Advise to notify physician if pregnant/nursing or planning to become pregnant. (Tab, Disintegrating) Inform patients with phenylketonuria that it contains phenylalanine. (Spray) Counsel on proper administration technique for nasal spray; avoid spraying contents in the eyes.

Administration: Oral/nasal routes. (Spray) Refer to PI for proper administration instructions. (Tab) Manually break the 2.5mg tab in 1/2 to achieve 1.25mg. (Tab, Disintegrating) Do not remove from blister until just prior to dosing. Subsequently, peel blister pack open and place tab on the tongue. Do not break; dissolve on tongue and swallow. **Storage:** 20-25°C (68-77°F)

ZONEGRAN   RX
zonisamide (Eisai)

THERAPEUTIC CLASS: Sulfonamide anticonvulsant

INDICATIONS: Adjunctive therapy in the treatment of partial seizures in adults with epilepsy.

DOSAGE: *Adults:* ≥16 Yrs: Initial: 100mg/day for 2 weeks. Titrate: May increase to 200mg/day for ≥2 weeks. May then increase to 300mg/day, then to 400mg/day in ≥2-week intervals. Renal/Hepatic Disease: May require slower titration. Elderly: Start at low end of dosing range.

HOW SUPPLIED: Cap: 25mg, 100mg

WARNINGS/PRECAUTIONS: Fatal sulfonamide reactions (eg, Stevens-Johnson syndrome, toxic epidermal necrolysis, fulminant hepatic necrosis, blood dyscrasias) rarely reported; d/c immediately if signs of hypersensitivity occurs. Increased risk of oligohidrosis and hyperthermia in pediatric patients; use not approved for pediatrics. May increase risk of suicidal thoughts or behavior; monitor for emergence/worsening of depression, suicidal thoughts or behavior, and/or any unusual changes in mood or behavior. May cause dose-dependent metabolic acidosis; d/c or reduce dose if metabolic acidosis develops/persists. If decision is made to continue therapy in the face of persistent acidosis, consider alkali treatment. Conditions or therapies that predispose to acidosis (eg, renal disease, severe respiratory disorders, status epilepticus, diarrhea, ketogenic diet, specific drugs) may be additive to the bicarbonate lowering effects. Abrupt withdrawal may precipitate increased seizure frequency or status epilepticus; reduce dose or d/c gradually. May cause serious adverse fetal effects. May cause CNS-related adverse events (eg, psychiatric symptoms, psychomotor slowing, somnolence, fatigue). May impair mental/physical abilities. Kidney stone formation, increased SrCr and BUN reported; d/c if acute renal failure or if a clinically significant sustained increase in SrCr/BUN develops. Avoid with renal failure (estimated GFR <50mL/min). Sudden unexplained deaths and status epilepticus reported. May increase serum chloride and alkaline phosphatase and decrease serum bicarbonate, phosphorus, Ca^{2+}, and albumin. Caution with renal/hepatic impairment and in elderly.

ADVERSE REACTIONS: Somnolence, anorexia, dizziness, ataxia, agitation/irritability, difficulty with memory and/or concentration, headache, nausea, fatigue, abdominal pain, confusion, insomnia, diplopia.

INTERACTIONS: Liver enzyme inducers may increase metabolism and clearance and may decrease $T_{1/2}$. CYP3A4 inducers or inhibitors may alter serum concentrations. May cause CNS

Z

depression and other cognitive/neuropsychiatric adverse events; caution with alcohol or other CNS depressants. Other carbonic anhydrase inhibitors (eg, topiramate, acetazolamide, dichlorphenamide) may increase the severity of metabolic acidosis and may also increase the risk of kidney stone formation; monitor for the appearance or worsening of metabolic acidosis. Phenytoin and carbamazepine may increase plasma clearance. Phenytoin, valproate, or phenobarbital and carbamazepine may decrease $T_{1/2}$. Caution with drugs that predispose patients to heat-related disorders (eg, carbonic anhydrase inhibitors, anticholinergics).

PREGNANCY: Category C, not for use in nursing.

MECHANISM OF ACTION: Sulfonamide anticonvulsant; has not been established. Found to block Na^+ channels and reduce voltage-dependent, transient inward currents (T-type Ca^{2+} currents), consequently stabilizing neuronal membranes and suppressing neuronal hypersynchronization. Facilitates both dopaminergic and serotonergic neurotransmission.

PHARMACOKINETICS: Absorption: (200-400mg) C_{max}=2-5mcg/mL, T_{max}=2-6 hrs (fasted), 4-6 hrs (fed). **Distribution:** V_d=1.45L/kg (400mg); plasma protein binding (40%); found in breast milk. **Metabolism:** Liver via reduction by CYP3A4 and acetylation; N-acetyl zonisamide, 2-sulfamoylacetyl phenol (metabolites). **Elimination:** Urine (62%, parent drug and metabolite), feces (3%); $T_{1/2}$=63 hrs.

NURSING CONSIDERATIONS

Assessment: Assess for previous hypersensitivity to sulfonamides or the drug, depression, suicidal thoughts or behavior, conditions or therapies that predispose to acidosis, risk for kidney stones formation, renal/hepatic impairment, pregnancy/nursing status, and possible drug interactions. Obtain baseline serum bicarbonate.

Monitoring: Monitor for signs/symptoms of sulfonamide reactions, hypersensitivity, oligohidrosis, hyperthermia, emergence/worsening of depression, suicidal thoughts or behavior, unusual changes in mood or behavior, metabolic acidosis, seizures (upon withdrawal), CNS-related adverse events, kidney stones, and status epilepticus. Monitor renal function (SrCr, BUN) and serum bicarbonate periodically.

Patient Counseling: Instruct to take only as prescribed. Advise not to drive a car or operate complex machinery until accustomed to effects of medication. Instruct to contact physician if skin rash develops, seizures worsen, signs or symptoms of kidney stone (eg, sudden back pain, abdominal pain, blood in urine) or hematological complications (eg, fever, sore throat, oral ulcers, easy bruising) develop, and if child is not sweating as usual with or without fever. Inform to increase fluid intake to decrease risk of kidney stone formation. Counsel patients, caregivers, and families that therapy may increase risk of suicidal thoughts and behavior. Advise to contact physician if patient develops symptoms of depression, unusual changes in mood or behavior, or suicidal thoughts, behavior, or thoughts about self-harm. Instruct to contact physician if fast breathing, fatigue/tiredness, loss of appetite, irregular heart beat, or palpitations develop. Advise women of childbearing potential to use effective contraception while on therapy. Instruct to notify physician if pregnant, plan to become pregnant, or breastfeeding during therapy. Encourage to enroll in the North American Antiepileptic Drug Pregnancy Registry if patient becomes pregnant.

Administration: Oral route. Swallow caps whole. **Storage:** 25°C (77°F); excursions permitted to 15-30°C (59-86°F), in a dry place. Protect from light.

ZORTRESS   RX
everolimus (Novartis)

> Should only be prescribed by physicians experienced in immunosuppressive therapy and management of organ transplant patients. Immunosuppression may lead to increased susceptibility to infection and possible development of malignancies (eg, lymphoma, skin cancer). Increased risk of kidney arterial and venous thrombosis leading to graft loss reported, mostly within the first 30 days post-transplantation. Increased nephrotoxicity may occur in combination with standard doses of cyclosporine; reduce dose of cyclosporine to reduce renal dysfunction, and monitor cyclosporine and everolimus whole blood trough concentrations. Increased mortality within the first 3 months post-transplantation in heart transplant patients on immunosuppressive regimens with or without induction therapy; not recommended in heart transplantation.

THERAPEUTIC CLASS: Macrolide immunosuppressant

INDICATIONS: Prophylaxis of organ rejection in adults at low-moderate immunologic risk receiving a kidney transplant in combination with basiliximab induction and concurrently with reduced doses of cyclosporine and with corticosteroids. Prophylaxis of allograft rejection in adults receiving a liver transplant administered no earlier than 30 days post-transplant concurrently in combination with reduced doses of tacrolimus and with corticosteroids.

DOSAGE: *Adults:* Initial: Kidney Transplant: 0.75mg bid with reduced dose of cyclosporine. Give as soon as possible after transplantation. Initiate PO prednisone once PO medication is tolerated. Liver Transplant: 1 mg bid with reduced dose of tacrolimus. Start at least 30 days post-transplant. Titrate: May require dose adjustment based on blood concentrations achieved, tolerability, individual response, change in concomitant medications, and clinical situation. Optimally, dose adjustments should be based on trough concentrations obtained 4 or 5 days after a previous dosing change. Steroid doses may be further tapered on an individualized basis, depending on clinical status and function of graft. Recommended Therapeutic Range: 3-8ng/mL (based on LC/MS/MS assay method). Hepatic Impairment: Mild (Child-Pugh Class A): Reduce initial daily dose by 1/3 of normal daily dose. Moderate or Severe (Child-Pugh Class B or C): Reduce initial daily dose to 1/2 of the normal daily dose. Refer to PI for further drug monitoring instructions and for cyclosporine or tacrolimus therapeutic drug monitoring parameters.

HOW SUPPLIED: Tab: 0.25mg, 0.5mg, 0.75mg

WARNINGS/PRECAUTIONS: Limit exposure to sunlight and UV light. Prophylaxis for *Pneumocystis jiroveci (carinii)* pneumonia and cytomegalovirus recommended. Increased risk of hepatic artery thrombosis (HAT), which may lead to graft loss or death; do not give earlier than 30 days after liver transplant. Consider switching to other immunosuppressive therapies if renal function does not improve after dose adjustments or if dysfunction is thought to be drug related. Angioedema, increased risk of delayed wound healing, increased occurrence of wound-related complications, and generalized fluid accumulation reported. Interstitial lung disease (ILD) reported; resolution may occur upon drug interruption with or without glucocorticoid therapy. Consider diagnosis of ILD for symptoms of infectious pneumonia that do not respond to antibiotic therapy and in whom non-drug causes have been ruled out. Increased risk of hyperlipidemia and proteinuria with higher whole blood trough concentrations; use of anti-lipid therapy may not normalize lipid levels. Polyoma virus infections, including polyoma virus-associated nephropathy (PVAN) and progressive multiple leukoencephalopathy (PML), may occur; consider reductions in immunosuppression if evidence of PVAN or PML develops. Concomitant use with cyclosporine may increase risk of thrombotic microangiopathy/thrombotic thrombocytopenic purpura/hemolytic uremic syndrome; monitor hematologic parameters. May increase risk of new-onset diabetes mellitus (DM) after transplant; monitor glucose levels. Azospermia or oligospermia may be observed. Avoid with rare hereditary problems of galactose intolerance (Lapp lactase deficiency, glucose-galactose malabsorption); diarrhea and malabsorption may occur.

ADVERSE REACTIONS: Peripheral edema, constipation, HTN, nausea, anemia, urinary tract infection, hyperlipidemia, diarrhea, pyrexia, increased blood creatinine, hyperkalemia, headache, hypercholesterolemia, insomnia, upper respiratory tract infections.

INTERACTIONS: Caution with drugs known to impair renal function. May increase risk of angioedema with drugs known to cause angioedema (eg, ACE inhibitors). Monitor for development of rhabdomyolysis with HMG-CoA reductase inhibitors and/or fibrates; use of simvastatin and lovastatin are strongly discouraged in patients receiving everolimus and cyclosporine. Coadministration with strong CYP3A4 inhibitors (eg, ketoconazole, clarithromycin, ritonavir) and strong CYP3A4 inducers (eg, rifampin, rifabutin) is not recommended without close monitoring of everolimus whole blood trough concentrations. Avoid with live vaccines, grapefruit, and grapefruit juice. Inhibitors of P-glycoprotein (P-gp) (eg, digoxin, cyclosporine), moderate inhibitors of CYP3A4 and P-gp (eg, fluconazole, macrolide antibiotics, nicardipine), and verapamil may increase levels. Caution with CYP3A4 and CYP2D6 substrates with a narrow therapeutic index. Increased levels with cyclosporine; dose adjustment may be needed if cyclosporine dose is altered. CYP3A4 inducers (eg, St. John's wort, carbamazepine, phenobarbital) may decrease levels. Combination immunosuppressant therapy should be used with caution.

PREGNANCY: Category C, not for use in nursing.

MECHANISM OF ACTION: Macrolide immunosuppressant; inhibits antigenic and interleukin (IL-2 and IL-15) stimulated activation and proliferation of T and B lymphocytes. Binds to a cytoplasmic protein, the FK506 binding protein-12 (FKBP-12), to form an immunosuppressive complex (everolimus: FKBP-12) that binds to and inhibits the mammalian target of rapamycin, a key regulatory kinase in cells.

PHARMACOKINETICS: Absorption: (0.75mg bid) AUC=75ng•h/mL, C_{max}=11.1ng/mL, T_{max}=1-2 hrs. **Distribution:** Plasma protein binding (74%); (0.75mg bid) V_d=110L. **Metabolism:** Via CYP3A4 and P-gp (monohydroxylations and O-dealkylations). **Elimination:** Feces (80%), urine (5%). (0.75mg bid) $T_{1/2}$=30 hrs.

NURSING CONSIDERATIONS

Assessment: Assess for hereditary problems of galactose intolerance, hepatic impairment, hypersensitivity to the drug or to sirolimus, pregnancy/nursing status, and possible drug interactions. Obtain baseline lipid and glucose levels.

Monitoring: Monitor for infections, angioedema, thrombosis, wound-related complications, fluid accumulation, lymphomas and other malignancies, hyperlipidemia, hepatic impairment, proteinuria, PVAN, HAT, ILD, pneumonitis, and other adverse reactions. Monitor everolimus and cyclosporine or tacrolimus whole blood trough concentrations, lipid profile, blood glucose concentrations, renal function, and hematologic parameters.

Patient Counseling: Counsel to avoid grapefruit and grapefruit juice. Inform of risk of developing lymphomas and other malignancies, particularly of the skin; instruct to limit exposure to sunlight

Z

and UV light. Advise that therapy has been associated with an increased risk of kidney arterial and venous thrombosis, resulting in graft loss, usually occurring within the first 30 days post-transplantation. Inform of the risks of impaired kidney function with concomitant cyclosporine as well as the need for routine blood concentration monitoring for both drugs; advise of the importance of SrCr monitoring. Inform of risk of hyperlipidemia and the importance of lipid profile monitoring. Advise women to avoid pregnancy throughout treatment and for 8 weeks after discontinuation. Instruct to notify physician of all medications and herbal/dietary supplements being taken. Inform that therapy has been associated with impaired or delayed wound healing, and fluid accumulation. Inform of increased risk of proteinuria, DM, infections, noninfectious pneumonitis, and angioedema; advise to contact physician if symptoms develop. Instruct to avoid receiving live vaccines.

Administration: Oral route. Do not crush; swallow whole with water. Administer consistently approximately 12 hrs apart with or without food and at the same time as cyclosporine or tacrolimus. **Storage:** 25°C (77°F); excursions permitted to 15-30°C (59-86°F). Protect from light and moisture.

ZORVOLEX   RX
diclofenac (Iroko)

> NSAIDs may increase risk of serious cardiovascular (CV) thrombotic events, myocardial infarction, and stroke; increased risk with duration of use and in patients with cardiovascular disease (CVD) or risk factors for CVD. Contraindicated for the treatment of perioperative pain in the setting of coronary artery bypass graft (CABG) surgery. NSAIDs may increase risk of serious GI adverse events (eg, bleeding, ulceration, perforation of the stomach or intestines) that can be fatal and occur anytime during use without warning symptoms; elderly patients are at greater risk.

THERAPEUTIC CLASS: NSAID

INDICATIONS: Treatment of mild to moderate acute pain in adults.

DOSAGE: *Adults:* 18mg or 35mg tid. Use lowest effective dose for the shortest duration consistent with treatment goals. Hepatic Impairment: Start at the lowest dose. Initial: 18mg tid. D/C use if efficacy is not achieved. Elderly: Start at lower end of dosing range.

HOW SUPPLIED: Cap: 18mg, 35mg

CONTRAINDICATIONS: History of asthma, urticaria, or allergic reactions after taking aspirin (ASA) or other NSAIDs. Treatment of perioperative pain in the setting of CABG surgery.

WARNINGS/PRECAUTIONS: Non-interchangeable with other formulations of diclofenac; do not substitute with similar dosing strengths of other diclofenac products. Caution in patients with history of ulcer disease or GI bleeding. Increased risk for GI bleeding with longer duration of NSAID therapy, older age, and poor general health status. May cause elevations of LFTs; measure transaminases periodically in patients receiving long-term therapy. D/C use if abnormal liver tests persist or worsen, if clinical signs/or symptoms consistent with liver disease develop, or if systemic manifestations occur (eg, eosinophilia, rash, abdominal pain, diarrhea, dark urine) occur. May lead to new onset or worsening of preexisting HTN; caution in patients with HTN. Fluid retention and edema reported; caution with fluid retention or heart failure (HF). Caution in patients with considerable dehydration. Renal papillary necrosis and other renal injury reported after long-term use. Renal toxicity reported in patients in whom renal prostaglandins have a compensatory role in the maintenance of renal perfusion; increased risk with renal/hepatic impairment, HF, and in the elderly. Not recommended for use with advanced renal disease; monitor renal function closely if therapy must be initiated. Anaphylactoid reactions may occur. Contraindicated in ASA triad patients. May cause serious skin adverse events (eg, exfoliative dermatitis, Stevens-Johnson syndrome, toxic epidermal necrolysis); d/c at the 1st appearance of skin rash or any other signs of hypersensitivity. Avoid use starting at 30 weeks gestation; may cause premature closure of the ductus arteriosus. Not a substitute for corticosteroids or to treat corticosteroid insufficiency. May mask inflammation and fever. Anemia may occur; monitor Hgb or Hct if signs/symptoms of anemia or blood loss develop in patients on long-term therapy. May inhibit platelet aggregation and prolong bleeding time; monitor those who may be adversely affected by alterations in platelet function (eg, coagulation disorders). Not indicated for long-term treatment. Caution with asthma and in the elderly.

ADVERSE REACTIONS: Edema, N/V, headache, dizziness, constipation, pruritus, flatulence, pain in extremity.

INTERACTIONS: May increase risk of GI bleeding with oral corticosteroids, anticoagulants, smoking, and alcohol. Carefully monitor patients receiving anticoagulants. Caution with concomitant drugs known to be potentially hepatotoxic (eg, acetaminophen, certain antibiotics, anti-epileptics). Increased GI adverse effects with ASA; avoid concomitant use. Increased risk of renal toxicity with ACE inhibitors and diuretics. May diminish anti-hypertensive effect of ACE inhibitors. May reduce natriuretic effect of furosemide and thiazides; observe closely for signs of renal failure, and to assure diuretic efficacy. May increase plasma lithium levels and reduce renal lithium clearance; monitor for lithium toxicity. May enhance methotrexate toxicity; caution when coadministering. May increase nephrotoxicity of cyclosporine; caution when coadministering. Caution with coadministration of other drugs that are substrates or inhibitors of CYP2C9.

PREGNANCY: Category C prior to 30 weeks gestation, Category D starting at 30 weeks gestation; caution in nursing.

MECHANISM OF ACTION: NSAID; has not been established. May involve inhibition of the COX-1 and COX-2 pathways. May also be related to prostaglandin synthetase inhibition.

PHARMACOKINETICS: Absorption: Absolute bioavailability (50%); T_{max}=1 hr (fasted), 3.32 hrs (fed). **Distribution:** V_d=1.3L/kg (diclofenac potassium); serum protein binding (>99%). **Metabolism:** Via CYP2C9 (major metabolite), glucuronidation/sulfation, CYP3A4 (minor metabolites), acylglucuronidation via UGT2B7 and oxidation via CYP2C8 may also play a role; 4'-hydroxy-diclofenac (major metabolite). **Elimination:** Urine (65%), bile (35%); $T_{1/2}$=2 hrs.

NURSING CONSIDERATIONS

Assessment: Assess that use is not for perioperative pain in the setting of CABG surgery. Assess for previous hypersensitivity to drug, and history of asthma, urticaria, or allergic-type reactions with ASA or other NSAIDs. Assess for CVD or risk factors for CVD, prior history of peptic ulcer disease and/or GI bleeding, fluid retention or HF, any other conditions where therapy is cautioned or contraindicated, pregnancy/nursing status, and for possible drug interactions. Obtain baseline BP, a CBC, and a chemistry profile including liver and renal function tests.

Monitoring: Monitor for anaphylactoid/skin/hypersensitivity reactions, CV thrombotic events, GI events, fluid retention, edema, asthma, and other adverse reactions. Monitor BP, CBC, and chemistry profile including liver and renal function tests.

Patient Counseling: Counsel about signs/symptoms of serious CV events, GI effects, hepatotoxicity, and skin adverse reactions; instruct to contact physician if any signs/symptoms develop. Advise to report to physician signs/symptoms of unexplained weight gain/edema. Inform of the signs of anaphylactic reaction and instruct to seek immediate emergency help if any occur. Caution women against use starting at 30 weeks gestation.

Administration: Oral route. Taking with food may cause a reduction in effectiveness compared to taking on an empty stomach. **Storage:** 25°C (77°F); excursions permitted to 15-30°C (59-86°F). Protect from moisture.

ZOSTAVAX
zoster vaccine live (Merck)

RX

THERAPEUTIC CLASS: Vaccine

INDICATIONS: Prevention of herpes zoster (shingles) in individuals ≥50 yrs of age.

DOSAGE: *Adults:* ≥50 Yrs: Single 0.65mL SQ in the deltoid region of upper arm.

HOW SUPPLIED: Inj: 19,400 PFU/0.65mL

CONTRAINDICATIONS: History of anaphylactic/anaphylactoid reaction to gelatin or neomycin. Immunosuppression or immunodeficiency, including history of primary or acquired immunodeficiency states, leukemia, lymphoma or other malignant neoplasms affecting the bone marrow or lymphatic system, AIDS or other clinical manifestations of infection with HIV, and those on immunosuppressive therapy. Pregnancy.

WARNINGS/PRECAUTIONS: Avoid pregnancy for 3 months following administration. Serious adverse reactions, including anaphylaxis, reported; have adequate treatment provisions (eg, epinephrine inj [1:1000]) available for immediate use. Transmission of vaccine virus may occur between vaccinees and susceptible contacts. Consider deferral in acute illness (eg, fever) or with active untreated tuberculosis (TB). Duration of protection >4 yrs after vaccination is unknown. May not protect all vaccine recipients.

ADVERSE REACTIONS: Inj-site reactions (erythema, pain, tenderness, swelling, pruritus, warmth), headache.

INTERACTIONS: See Contraindications. Reduced immune response to zoster vaccine live with pneumococcal vaccine polyvalent; consider administration of the 2 vaccines separated by at least 4 weeks.

PREGNANCY: Contraindicated in pregnancy, caution in nursing.

MECHANISM OF ACTION: Vaccine; boosts varicella zoster virus-specific immunity and protects against zoster and its complications.

NURSING CONSIDERATIONS

Assessment: Assess for acute illness, active untreated TB, history of anaphylactic/anaphylactoid reaction to gelatin, neomycin, or any other component of the vaccine, immunosuppression/immunodeficiency, pregnancy/nursing status, and possible drug interactions.

Monitoring: Monitor for anaphylactic/anaphylactoid reactions and other adverse reactions.

Z

Patient Counseling: Instruct to inform physician about reactions to previous vaccines. Inform of benefits and risks of vaccine, including potential risk of transmitting vaccine virus to susceptible individuals (eg, immunosuppressed/immunodeficient individuals, pregnant women who have not had chickenpox). Instruct to report any adverse reactions or any symptoms of concern to physician.

Administration: SQ route. Inject in the deltoid region of the upper arm. Do not inject IV or IM. Refer to PI for preparation, reconstitution, and administration instructions. **Storage:** Before Reconstitution: -50°C to -15°C (-58°F to 5°F). Use of dry ice may subject the vaccine to temperatures colder than -50°C (-58°F). May store and/or transport at 2-8°C (36-46°F) for up to 72 continuous hrs prior to reconstitution; discard if not used within 72 hrs of removal from -15°C (5°F). Protect from light. Diluent: 20-25°C (68-77°F) or 2-8°C (36-46°F). After Reconstitution: Administer immediately; discard if not used within 30 min. Do not freeze.

ZOSYN RX
piperacillin - tazobactam (Wyeth)

THERAPEUTIC CLASS: Beta-lactamase inhibitor/broad-spectrum penicillin

INDICATIONS: Treatment of appendicitis (complicated by rupture or abscess), peritonitis, uncomplicated/complicated skin and skin structure infections (eg, cellulitis, cutaneous abscess, ischemic/diabetic foot infections), postpartum endometritis, pelvic inflammatory disease, moderate community-acquired pneumonia, and moderate to severe nosocomial pneumonia caused by susceptible strains of microorganisms.

DOSAGE: *Adults:* Infuse IV over 30 min. Usual: 3.375g q6h for 7-10 days. CrCl 20-40mL/min: 2.25g q6h. CrCl <20mL/min: 2.25g q8h. Hemodialysis/Continuous Ambulatory Peritoneal Dialysis (CAPD): 2.25g q12h. Give one additional dose of 0.75g following each hemodialysis session. Nosocomial Pneumonia: 4.5g q6h for 7-14 days plus an aminoglycoside. CrCl 20-40mL/min: 3.375g q6h. CrCl <20mL/min: 2.25g q6h. Hemodialysis/CAPD: 2.25g q8h. Give one additional dose of 0.75g following each hemodialysis session. Elderly: Start at lower end of dosing range. *Pediatrics:* Infuse IV over 30 min. Appendicitis/Peritonitis: ≤40kg: ≥9 Months: 100mg-12.5mg/kg q8h. 2-9 Months: 80mg-10mg/kg q8h. >40kg: Use adult dose.

HOW SUPPLIED: Inj: (Piperacillin-Tazobactam) 2g-0.25g, 3g-0.375g, 4g-0.5g [vial]; 2g-0.25g/50mL, 3g-0.375g/50mL, 4g-0.5g/100mL [Galaxy]. Also available as a Pharmacy Bulk Package.

CONTRAINDICATIONS: History of allergic reactions to cephalosporins.

WARNINGS/PRECAUTIONS: Serious and occasionally fatal hypersensitivity (anaphylactic/anaphylactoid) reactions, including shock, reported; d/c and institute appropriate therapy if an allergic reaction occurs. Serious skin reactions (eg, Stevens-Johnson syndrome, toxic epidermal necrolysis) reported; monitor closely if skin rash occurs and d/c if lesions progress. *Clostridium difficile*-associated diarrhea (CDAD) reported; d/c if CDAD is suspected or confirmed. Bleeding manifestations, sometimes associated with abnormalities of coagulation tests, reported; d/c and institute appropriate therapy if bleeding manifestations occur. Leukopenia/neutropenia may occur and is most frequently associated with prolonged administration. May cause neuromuscular excitability or convulsions with higher than recommended dose, particularly in the presence of renal failure. Caution with restricted salt intake. Monitor electrolytes periodically with low K⁺ reserves. May result in bacterial resistance with use in the absence of a proven/suspected bacterial infection. Increased incidence of rash and fever in cystic fibrosis patients reported. Lab test interactions may occur. Caution with renal impairment (CrCl ≤40mL/min). Caution in elderly patients.

ADVERSE REACTIONS: Diarrhea, headache, constipation, N/V, insomnia, rash, fever, dyspepsia, pruritus, oral candidiasis.

INTERACTIONS: May inactivate aminoglycosides. May decrease serum concentrations of tobramycin; monitor aminoglycoside serum concentrations in patients with end-stage renal disease. Probenecid prolongs $T_{1/2}$; avoid coadministration unless the benefit outweighs the risk. Test coagulation parameters more frequently with high doses of heparin, oral anticoagulants, or other drugs that may affect blood coagulation system or thrombocyte function. Piperacillin: May prolong neuromuscular blockade of vecuronium or any nondepolarizing muscle relaxants. May increase risk of hypokalemia with cytotoxic therapy or diuretics. May reduce methotrexate clearance; monitor methotrexate concentrations and for toxicity.

PREGNANCY: Category B, caution in nursing.

MECHANISM OF ACTION: Piperacillin: Broad-spectrum penicillin (PCN); exerts bactericidal activity by inhibiting septum formation and cell-wall synthesis of susceptible bacteria. Tazobactam: β-lactamase enzyme inhibitor.

PHARMACOKINETICS: Absorption: IV administration of multiple doses resulted in different parameters. **Distribution:** Plasma protein binding (30%); crosses the placenta. Piperacillin: V_d=0.243L/kg, found in breast milk. **Elimination:** Kidneys. Piperacillin: Urine (68% unchanged).

Tazobactam: Urine (80% unchanged). Refer to PI for information on additional pharmacokinetic parameters.

NURSING CONSIDERATIONS

Assessment: Assess for previous hypersensitivity reaction to PCN, cephalosporins, or other allergens. Assess for history of bleeding disorder, conditions with restricted salt intake, cystic fibrosis, renal impairment, hypokalemia, pregnancy/nursing status, and possible drug interactions.

Monitoring: Monitor hematopoietic function (especially with prolonged therapy [≥21 days]), renal function, and serum electrolytes periodically. Monitor for signs/symptoms of electrolyte imbalance (eg, hypokalemia), hypersensitivity reactions, CDAD, serious skin reactions, leukopenia/neutropenia, bleeding manifestations, and for neuromuscular excitability or convulsions. Monitor for rash and fever in cystic fibrosis patients.

Patient Counseling: Inform about risks/benefits of therapy. Counsel that drug only treats bacterial, not viral (eg, common cold), infections. Instruct to take ud; inform that skipping doses or not completing full course may decrease effectiveness and increase resistance. Advise to d/c and notify physician if watery/bloody diarrhea (with or without stomach cramps and fever) even as late as ≥2 months after the last dose, or an allergic reaction occurs. Instruct to notify physician if pregnant/nursing.

Administration: IV route. Administer by IV infusion over 30 min. Refer to PI for instructions for reconstitution and dilution. **Storage:** Vial: Prior to Reconstitution: 20-25°C (68-77°F). Reconstituted: Use immediately after reconstitution. Discard any unused portion after 24 hours if stored at 20-25°C (68-77°F) or after 48 hours if stored at 2-8°C (36-46°F). Do not freeze vials after reconstitution. Galaxy Container: ≤-20°C (-4°F). Thawed Sol: 2-8°C (36-46°F) for 14 days, or 20-25°C (68-77°F) for 24 hrs. Do not refreeze.

ZOVIRAX ORAL
acyclovir (GlaxoSmithKline)

RX

THERAPEUTIC CLASS: Nucleoside analogue

INDICATIONS: Acute treatment of herpes zoster (shingles). Treatment of initial and recurrent episodes of genital herpes. Treatment of chickenpox (varicella).

DOSAGE: *Adults:* Herpes Zoster: 800mg q4h, 5X/day for 7-10 days. Genital Herpes: Initial Therapy: 200mg q4h, 5X/day for 10 days. Chronic Therapy: 400mg bid or 200mg 3-5X/day up to 12 months, then reevaluate. Intermittent Therapy: 200mg q4h, 5X/day for 5 days; start at 1st sign/symptom of recurrence. Chickenpox: 800mg qid for 5 days; start at earliest sign/symptom. Renal Impairment: Refer to PI for dose modifications.
Pediatrics: ≥2 Yrs: Chickenpox: >40kg: 800mg qid for 5 days. ≤40kg: 20mg/kg qid for 5 days. Start at earliest sign/symptom. Renal Impairment: Refer to PI for dose modifications.

HOW SUPPLIED: Cap: 200mg; Sus: 200mg/5mL [473mL]; Tab: 400mg, 800mg

CONTRAINDICATIONS: Hypersensitivity to valacyclovir.

WARNINGS/PRECAUTIONS: Renal failure sometimes resulting in death reported. Thrombotic thrombocytopenic purpura/hemolytic uremic syndrome (TTP/HUS) in immunocompromised patients reported. Maintain adequate hydration. Caution in elderly.

ADVERSE REACTIONS: N/V, diarrhea, malaise.

INTERACTIONS: Probenecid may increase levels and $T_{1/2}$ of IV formulation. May increase risk of renal impairment and/or CNS symptoms with nephrotoxic agents; use caution.

PREGNANCY: Category B, caution in nursing.

MECHANISM OF ACTION: Synthetic purine nucleoside analogue; stops replication of herpes viral DNA by competitive inhibition of viral DNA polymerase, incorporation into and termination of growing viral DNA chain, and inactivation of viral DNA polymerase.

PHARMACOKINETICS: Absorption: Oral administration of variable doses resulted in different parameters. **Distribution:** Plasma protein binding (9-33%); found in breast milk. **Elimination:** $T_{1/2}$=2.5-3.3 hrs.

NURSING CONSIDERATIONS

Assessment: Assess for immunocompromised state, hypersensitivity to valacyclovir, renal impairment, nursing status, and possible drug interactions.

Monitoring: Monitor for signs/symptoms of TTP/HUS. Monitor BUN and SrCr.

Patient Counseling: Instruct to consult physician if experiencing severe or troublesome adverse reactions, if pregnant/intending to become pregnant, or intending to breastfeed. Advise to maintain adequate hydration. Inform that therapy is not a cure for genital herpes; advise to avoid contact with lesions or intercourse when lesions/symptoms are present.

Administration: Oral route. **Storage:** 15-25°C (59-77°F); protect from moisture.

Z

ZUPLENZ

ondansetron (Praelia)

RX

THERAPEUTIC CLASS: 5-HT$_3$ receptor antagonist

INDICATIONS: Prevention of N/V associated with highly emetogenic cancer chemotherapy, including cisplatin ≥50mg/m². Prevention of N/V associated with initial and repeat courses of moderately emetogenic cancer chemotherapy. Prevention of N/V associated with radiotherapy in patients receiving either total body irradiation, single high-dose fraction to the abdomen, or daily fractions to the abdomen. Prevention of postoperative nausea and/or vomiting (PONV).

DOSAGE: *Adults:* Prevention of N/V Associated with Highly Emetogenic Chemotherapy: 24mg given successively as three 8mg films 30 min before start of single-day chemotherapy. Prevention of N/V Associated with Moderately Emetogenic Chemotherapy: 8mg bid; give 1st dose 30 min before chemotherapy, then give subsequent dose 8 hrs after 1st dose, then administer 8mg q12h for 1-2 days after completion of chemotherapy. Prevention of N/V Associated with Radiotherapy: Usual: 8mg tid. Total Body Irradiation: 8mg 1-2 hrs before each fraction of radiotherapy administered each day. Single High-Dose Fraction Radiotherapy to Abdomen: 8mg 1-2 hrs before radiotherapy, then q8h after 1st dose for 1-2 days after completion of radiotherapy. Daily Fractionated Radiotherapy to Abdomen: 8mg 1-2 hrs before radiotherapy, then q8h after 1st dose for each day radiotherapy is given. Prevention of PONV: 16mg given successively as two 8mg films 1 hr before induction of anesthesia. Severe Hepatic Impairment (Child-Pugh ≥10): Max: 8mg/day.
Pediatrics: ≥12 Yrs: Prevention of N/V Associated with Moderately Emetogenic Chemotherapy: 8mg bid; give 1st dose 30 min before chemotherapy, then give subsequent dose 8 hrs after 1st dose, then administer 8mg q12h for 1-2 days after completion of chemotherapy. 4-11 Yrs: 4mg tid; give 1st dose 30 min before start of chemotherapy, with subsequent doses 4 and 8 hrs after 1st dose, then administer 8mg q8h for 1-2 days after completion of chemotherapy. Severe Hepatic Impairment (Child-Pugh ≥10): Max: 8mg/day.

HOW SUPPLIED: Film, Oral: 4mg, 8mg

CONTRAINDICATIONS: Concomitant use with apomorphine.

WARNINGS/PRECAUTIONS: Hypersensitivity reactions reported in patients hypersensitive to other selective 5-HT$_3$ receptor antagonists; d/c immediately at the 1st sign of hypersensitivity. ECG changes, including QT interval prolongation and torsades de pointes, reported; avoid in patients with congenital long QT syndrome. Monitor ECG in patients with electrolyte abnormalities (eg, hypokalemia, hypomagnesemia), congestive heart failure (CHF), bradyarrhythmias, and in patients taking other medications that lead to QT prolongation. Use in patients following abdominal surgery or with chemotherapy-induced N/V may mask a progressive ileus and/or gastric distension. Does not stimulate gastric/intestinal peristalsis; do not use instead of NG suction.

ADVERSE REACTIONS: Headache, diarrhea, malaise/fatigue, constipation, hypoxia, pyrexia, dizziness, gynecological disorder, anxiety/agitation, urinary retention, pruritus.

INTERACTIONS: See Contraindications. Potent CYP3A4 inducers (eg, phenytoin, carbamazepine, rifampicin) may significantly increase clearance and decrease blood levels. May reduce analgesic activity of tramadol.

PREGNANCY: Category B, caution in nursing.

MECHANISM OF ACTION: Selective 5-HT$_3$ receptor antagonist; not established. Blocks 5-HT$_3$ receptors from serotonin. Released serotonin may stimulate the vagal afferents through 5-HT$_3$ receptors and initiate the vomiting reflex.

PHARMACOKINETICS: Absorption: Well-absorbed from GI tract. (Single 8mg dose, fasted) T$_{max}$=1.3 hrs; AUC=225ng•hr/mL, C$_{max}$=37.28ng/mL. **Distribution:** Plasma protein binding (70-76%). **Metabolism:** Extensive via CYP3A4, 1A2, 2D6; hydroxylation (primary), glucuronide/sulfate conjugation. **Elimination:** Urine (5% parent compound); (Single 8mg dose, fasted, healthy) T$_{1/2}$=4.6 hrs.

NURSING CONSIDERATIONS

Assessment: Assess for previous hypersensitivity to the drug, congenital long QT syndrome, electrolyte abnormalities, CHF, bradyarrhythmias, hepatic impairment, pregnancy/nursing status, and possible drug interactions.

Monitoring: Monitor for QT interval prolongation, torsades de pointes, hypersensitivity reactions, and other adverse reactions. Monitor ECG in patients with electrolyte abnormalities, CHF, bradyarrhythmias, and in patients taking other medications that lead to QT prolongation. In patients who recently underwent abdominal surgery or in patients with chemotherapy-induced N/V, monitor for masking of a progressive ileus and/or gastric distension.

Patient Counseling: Inform about potential benefits/risks of therapy. Inform that drug may cause serious cardiac arrhythmias (eg, QT prolongation); instruct patients to contact physician if they perceive a change in their HR, feel lightheaded, or have a syncopal episode. Inform that chances of developing severe cardiac arrhythmias are higher in patients with a personal/family history of abnormal heart rhythms (eg, congenital long QT syndrome), patients taking medications (eg, diuretics) which may cause electrolyte abnormalities, and in patients with hypokalemia or hypomagnesemia. Inform that drug may cause headache, malaise/fatigue, constipation, and diarrhea; instruct to report the use of all medications, especially apomorphine or any drug of the 5-HT$_3$ antagonist class, to physician. Inform that drug may cause hypersensitivity reactions, some as severe as anaphylaxis and bronchospasm; instruct to report any hypersensitivity reactions to physician. Instruct on how to use drug.

Administration: Oral route. With dry hands, fold pouch along the dotted line to expose the tear notch. While still folded, tear the pouch carefully along the edge and remove the oral soluble film from pouch. Immediately place film on top of the tongue where it dissolves in 4-20 seconds. Once oral soluble film is dissolved, swallow with or without liquid. Allow each film to dissolve completely before administering the next film. Wash hands after taking oral soluble film.
Storage: 20-25°C (68-77°F).

ZYBAN   RX
bupropion HCl (GlaxoSmithKline)

> Serious neuropsychiatric reactions reported in patients taking bupropion for smoking cessation. Weigh risks against benefits of use. Antidepressants increased the risk of suicidal thoughts and behavior in children, adolescents, and young adults in short-term trials. Monitor closely for worsening, and emergence of suicidal thoughts and behavior. Advise families and caregivers of the need for close observation and communication with the prescriber.

THERAPEUTIC CLASS: Aminoketone

INDICATIONS: Aid to smoking cessation treatment.

DOSAGE: *Adults:* Initiate treatment while patient is still smoking. Patients should set a "target quit date" within the first 2 weeks of treatment. Initial: 150mg qd for first 3 days. Titrate: Increase to 300mg/day, given as 150mg bid with an interval of at least 8 hrs between each dose. Usual/Max: 300mg/day given as 150mg bid. Continue treatment for 7-12 weeks. If patient has not quit smoking after 7-12 weeks, d/c and reassess treatment plan. May consider continuing therapy in patients who successfully quit smoking after 12 weeks of treatment but do not feel ready to d/c treatment; base longer treatment on individual patient benefits/risks. May be used with a nicotine transdermal system. Moderate-Severe Hepatic Impairment (Child-Pugh Score: 7-15): Max: 150mg qod. Mild Hepatic Impairment (Child-Pugh Score: 5-6): Consider reducing dose and/or frequency. Renal Impairment (GFR<90mL/min): Consider reducing dose and/or frequency. Switching to/from an MAOI: Allow at least 14 days between discontinuation of an MAOI and initiation of treatment and allow at least 14 days between discontinuation of treatment and initiation of an MAOI. Use with Reversible MAOIs (eg, Linezolid, IV Methylene Blue): Refer to PI.

HOW SUPPLIED: Tab, Sustained-Release: 150mg

CONTRAINDICATIONS: Seizure disorder, current/prior diagnosis of bulimia or anorexia nervosa. Undergoing abrupt discontinuation of alcohol, benzodiazepines, barbiturates, and antiepileptic drugs. Use of MAOIs (intended to treat psychiatric disorders) either concomitantly or within 14 days of discontinuing treatment. Treatment within 14 days of discontinuing treatment with an MAOI. Starting treatment in patients being treated with reversible MAOIs (eg, linezolid, IV methylene blue).

WARNINGS/PRECAUTIONS: Dose-related risk of seizures; do not exceed 300mg/day and titrate gradually. D/C and do not restart treatment if a seizure occurs. May result in elevated BP and HTN. May precipitate a manic, mixed, or hypomanic manic episode; risk appears to be increased in patients with bipolar disorder or who have risk factors for bipolar disorder. Not approved for use in treating bipolar depression. D/C if an allergic or anaphylactoid/anaphylactic reaction occurs. Arthralgia, myalgia, fever with rash, and other serum sickness-like symptoms suggestive of delayed hypersensitivity reported. False (+) urine immunoassay screening tests for amphetamines reported. Caution with renal/hepatic impairment and in the elderly.

ADVERSE REACTIONS: Neuropsychiatric reactions, insomnia, rhinitis, dry mouth, dizziness, nausea, disturbed concentration, constipation, anxiety, dream abnormality, arthralgia, nervousness, diarrhea, rash, myalgia.

INTERACTIONS: See Contraindications. CYP2B6 inhibitors (eg, ticlopidine, clopidogrel) may increase bupropion exposure but decrease hydroxybupropion exposure; may need to adjust bupropion dose. CYP2B6 inducers (eg, ritonavir, lopinavir, efavirenz) may decrease exposure; may need to increase bupropion dose but not to exceed max dose. Carbamazepine, phenytoin, and phenobarbital may induce metabolism and decrease exposure; may be necessary to increase dose of bupropion, but max recommended dose should not be exceeded if used concomitantly with a CYP inducer. May increase exposure of CYP2D6 substrates (eg, venlafaxine, haloperidol, metoprolol); may need to decrease dose of CYP2D6 substrate, particularly for drugs with a narrow therapeutic index. May reduce efficacy of drugs that require metabolic activation by CYP2D6 to be effective (eg, tamoxifen); may require increased doses of the drug. Extreme

Z

caution with other drugs that lower seizure threshold (eg, antipsychotics, theophylline, systemic corticosteroids); use low initial doses and increase the dose gradually. Increased risk of seizure with illicit drugs (eg, cocaine), abuse or misuse of prescription drugs (eg, CNS stimulants), oral hypoglycemic drugs, insulin, anorectic drugs, excessive use of alcohol, benzodiazepines, sedative/hypnotics, and opiates. CNS toxicity reported when coadministered with levodopa or amantadine; use with caution. Minimize or avoid alcohol. Increased risk of HTN with MAOIs or other drugs that increase dopaminergic or noradrenergic activity. Monitor for HTN with nicotine replacement therapy. Altered PT and/or INR, infrequently associated with hemorrhagic or thrombotic complication, reported with warfarin.

PREGNANCY: Category C, caution in nursing.

MECHANISM OF ACTION: Aminoketone; has not been established. Weak inhibitor of the neuronal uptake of norepinephrine and dopamine. Presumed that action is mediated by noradrenergic and/or dopaminergic mechanisms.

PHARMACOKINETICS: Absorption: T_{max}=3 hrs. **Distribution:** Plasma protein binding (84%); found in breast milk. **Metabolism:** Liver (extensive); hydroxylation, hydroxybupropion (active metabolite) (CYP2B6). Reduction of carbonyl group, threohydrobupropion and erythrohydrobupropion (active metabolites). **Elimination:** Urine (87%) and feces (10%), (0.5% unchanged); $T_{1/2}$=21 hrs (bupropion), 20 hrs (hydroxybupropion), 33 hrs (erythrohydrobupropion), 37 hrs (threohydrobupropion).

NURSING CONSIDERATIONS

Assessment: Assess for bipolar disorder, hepatic/renal dysfunction, seizure disorder or conditions that may increase the risk of seizure, hypersensitivity to the drug, any other conditions where treatment is contraindicated or cautioned, pregnancy/nursing status, and possible drug interactions. Assess BP.

Monitoring: Monitor for seizures, suicidality, activation of mania or hypomania, neuropsychiatric reactions, anaphylactoid/anaphylactic reactions, delayed hypersensitivity, and other adverse reactions. Monitor hepatic/renal function. Monitor BP.

Patient Counseling: Inform of benefits/risks of therapy. Inform that quitting smoking may be associated with nicotine withdrawal symptoms or exacerbation of preexisting psychiatric illness. Advise to notify physician immediately if agitation, hostility, depressed mood, changes in thinking or behavior, or suicidal ideation/behavior occurs. Educate on the symptoms of hypersensitivity and to d/c if a severe allergic reaction occurs. Instruct to d/c and not restart if a seizure occurs while on therapy. Inform that excessive use or abrupt discontinuation of alcohol or sedatives may alter the seizure threshold; advise to minimize or avoid alcohol use. Inform that therapy may impair mental/physical abilities; advise to use caution while operating hazardous machinery/driving. Instruct to notify physician if taking/planning to take any prescription or OTC medications. Advise to contact physician if pregnancy occurs or is intended during therapy. Inform that tab may have an odor.

Administration: Oral route. Swallow tab whole; do not crush, divide, or chew. Take with or without food. Avoid hs dosing. **Storage:** 20-25°C (68-77°F); excursions permitted 15-30°C (59-86°F).

ZYFLO CR   RX
zileuton (Cornerstone)

OTHER BRAND NAMES: Zyflo (Cornerstone)

THERAPEUTIC CLASS: 5-lipoxygenase inhibitor

INDICATIONS: Prophylaxis and chronic treatment of asthma in adults and children ≥12 yrs of age.

DOSAGE: *Adults:* (Tab) 600mg qid. May take with meals and at hs. (Tab, ER) 1200mg bid within 1 hr after am and pm meals. Do not chew, cut, or crush.
Pediatrics: ≥12 Yrs: (Tab) 600mg qid. May take with meals and at hs. (Tab, ER) 1200mg bid within 1 hr after am and pm meals. Do not chew, cut, or crush.

HOW SUPPLIED: Tab: 600mg*; Tab, Extended-Release (ER): 600mg *scored

CONTRAINDICATIONS: Active liver disease or transaminase elevations (≥3X ULN).

WARNINGS/PRECAUTIONS: Not for use in reversal of bronchospasm in acute asthma attacks and status asthmaticus. Elevations of serum ALT/bilirubin may occur; increased risk for ALT elevation in females >65 yrs of age and those with preexisting transaminase elevations. Symptomatic hepatitis with jaundice may develop. D/C and follow transaminase levels until normal if signs of liver dysfunction (eg, right upper quadrant [RUQ] pain, nausea, fatigue) or serum transaminase ≥5X ULN occur. Caution in patients who consume substantial quantities of alcohol and/or have a past history of liver disease. Neuropsychiatric events, including sleep disorders and behavior changes, reported; evaluate risks and benefits of continuing treatment.

ADVERSE REACTIONS: Headache, elevation of ALT/bilirubin, nausea, myalgia, upper respiratory tract infection, sinusitis, pharyngolaryngeal pain, diarrhea.

Z

INTERACTIONS: May increase theophylline and propranolol concentrations; monitor levels and reduce dose as necessary. Monitor use with other β-blockers. May increase warfarin levels; monitor PT or other coagulation tests and adjust dose appropriately. (Tab) Not recommended for use with terfenadine. Monitor use with certain drugs metabolized by CYP3A4 (eg, dihydropyridine calcium channel blockers, cyclosporine, cisapride, astemizole). (Tab, ER) Monitor use with CYP3A4 inhibitors such as ketoconazole.

PREGNANCY: Category C, not for use in nursing.

MECHANISM OF ACTION: Leukotriene inhibitor; antiasthmatic agent, inhibits leukotriene (LTB_4, LTC_4, LTD_4, and LTE_4) formation by inhibiting the enzyme 5-lipoxygenase.

PHARMACOKINETICS: Absorption: (Tab) Rapid; T_{max}=1.7 hrs, C_{max}=4.98mcg/mL, AUC=19.2mcg•hr/mL; (Tab, ER) T_{max}=2.1 hrs (fasting), T_{max}=4.3 hrs (fed). **Distribution:** V_d=1.2L/kg; plasma protein binding (93%). **Metabolism:** Liver, via oxidation by CYP1A2, CYP2C9, CYP3A4. **Elimination:** Urine (94.5%; <0.5% unchanged, <0.5% metabolites), feces (2.2%); (Tab) $T_{1/2}$=2.5 hrs; (Tab, ER) $T_{1/2}$=3.2 hrs.

NURSING CONSIDERATIONS

Assessment: Assess for active/history of liver disease, acute asthma attacks, status asthmaticus, preexisting transaminase elevation, neuropsychiatric events, alcohol use, previous hypersensitivity, pregnancy/nursing status, and possible drug interactions.

Monitoring: Monitor serum bilirubin level. Monitor serum ALT prior to therapy, once a month for first 3 months, every 2-3 months for remainder of 1st yr, and periodically thereafter. Monitor for signs/symptoms of hepatitis, jaundice, liver dysfunction (eg, RUQ pain, nausea, fatigue), neuropsychiatric events (eg, sleep disorders, behavior changes). Monitor alcohol consumption and worsening of asthma.

Patient Counseling: Inform that drug is indicated for chronic treatment, not for acute episodes, of asthma. Instruct to take regularly as prescribed. Advise not to reduce dose or d/c other antiasthma medications unless instructed. Instruct to notify healthcare provider if signs/symptoms of liver dysfunction or neuropsychiatric events occur. Advise to consult physician before starting or discontinuing any prescription or OTC medications. Counsel about potential for liver damage and need for liver enzyme monitoring on regular basis. (Tab, ER) Instruct to take within 1 hr after am and pm meals. Do not cut, crush, or chew.

Administration: Oral route. **Storage:** 20-25°C (68-77°F); (Tab, ER) excursions permitted to 15-30°C (59-86°F). Protect from light.

ZYLET   RX
loteprednol etabonate - tobramycin (Bausch & Lomb)

THERAPEUTIC CLASS: Aminoglycoside/corticosteroid

INDICATIONS: Treatment of steroid-responsive inflammatory ocular conditions for which a corticosteroid is indicated and where superficial bacterial ocular infection or a risk of bacterial ocular infection exists.

DOSAGE: *Adults:* 1 or 2 drops q4-6h into the conjunctival sac of the affected eye. May increase dosing frequency to q1-2h during the first 24-48 hrs. Reduce frequency gradually as condition improves. Not more than 20mL should be prescribed initially.

HOW SUPPLIED: Sus: (Loteprednol Etabonate-Tobramycin) 0.5%-0.3% [5mL, 10mL]

CONTRAINDICATIONS: Most viral diseases of the cornea and conjunctiva, including epithelial herpes simplex keratitis (dendritic keratitis), vaccinia, and varicella, and also in mycobacterial infection of the eye and fungal diseases of ocular structures.

WARNINGS/PRECAUTIONS: Prolonged use may result in glaucoma with optic nerve damage, visual acuity and fields of vision defects; caution with glaucoma and monitor intraocular pressure (IOP) if used for ≥10 days. May result in posterior subcapsular cataract formation. May delay healing and increase incidence of bleb formation if used after cataract surgery, or cause perforations in diseases that cause thinning of the cornea or sclera; initial and renewal of prescription should be made only after examination with aid of magnification (eg, slit lamp biomicroscopy, fluorescein staining). Prolonged use may suppress host response and thus increase the hazard of secondary ocular infections. May mask infection or enhance existing infection in acute purulent conditions of the eye. Reevaluate if signs and symptoms fail to improve after 2 days. May prolong the course and exacerbate the severity of many viral infections of the eye (including herpes simplex); caution with history of herpes simplex. Fungal infections of the cornea may develop with long-term application; consider fungal invasion in any persistent corneal ulceration when steroid has been used or is in use. Sensitivity to topically applied aminoglycosides may occur; d/c if hypersensitivity develops and institute appropriate therapy. Do not d/c therapy prematurely.

Z

ADVERSE REACTIONS: Superficial punctuate keratitis, increased IOP, burning/stinging upon instillation, headache, vision disorders, discharge, itching, lacrimation disorder, photophobia, corneal deposits, ocular discomfort, eyelid disorder.

PREGNANCY: Category C, caution in nursing.

MECHANISM OF ACTION: Loteprednol Etabonate: Corticosteroid; has not been established. Suspected to act by induction of phospholipase A_2 inhibitory proteins (lipocortins), which control the biosynthesis of potent inflammatory mediators by inhibiting the release of arachidonic acid. Tobramycin: Aminoglycoside antibiotic; provides action against susceptible organisms.

PHARMACOKINETICS: Distribution: Loteprednol Etabonate: (Systemic) Found in breast milk.

NURSING CONSIDERATIONS

Assessment: Assess for viral diseases of cornea and conjunctiva (eg, dendritic keratitis, vaccinia, varicella), mycobacterial infection of the eye, fungal diseases of ocular structures, glaucoma, diseases that cause thinning of the cornea or sclera, recent cataract surgery, history of herpes simplex, and pregnancy/nursing status.

Monitoring: Monitor for signs/symptoms of hypersensitivity reactions, glaucoma, defects in visual acuity and fields of vision, posterior subcapsular cataract formation, delayed wound healing, incidence of bleb formation, ocular perforations, exacerbation of viral infections of the eye, secondary infection, and fungal infection of the cornea. Monitor IOP if used ≥10 days.

Patient Counseling: Instruct not to allow dropper tip to touch any surface to avoid contamination. Counsel not to wear soft contact lenses during therapy. Advise to consult physician if pain develops, if redness, itching or inflammation become aggravated, or if signs/symptoms fail to improve after 2 days. Instruct to use as directed.

Administration: Ocular route. **Storage:** 15-25°C (59-77°F). Protect from freezing; store upright.

ZYMAR   RX
gatifloxacin (Allergan)

THERAPEUTIC CLASS: Fluoroquinolone

INDICATIONS: Treatment of bacterial conjunctivitis.

DOSAGE: *Adults:* 1 drop q2h while awake, up to 8X/day for 2 days; then 1 drop up to qid while awake for 5 days.
Pediatrics: ≥1 Yr: 1 drop q2h while awake, up to 8X/day for 2 days; then 1 drop up to qid while awake for 5 days.

HOW SUPPLIED: Sol: 0.3% [5mL]

WARNINGS/PRECAUTIONS: Not for injection. Do not inject subconjunctivally or into the anterior chamber of the eye. Superinfection may result with prolonged use. Fatal hypersensitivity reactions reported after 1st dose of systemic quinolone therapy. Avoid contact lenses when symptoms are present.

ADVERSE REACTIONS: Conjunctival irritation, increased lacrimation, keratitis, papillary conjunctivitis, chemosis, conjunctival hemorrhage, dry eye, eye discharge/irritation/pain, red eye, eyelid edema, headache, reduced visual acuity, taste disturbance.

INTERACTIONS: Systemic quinolone therapy may increase theophylline levels, interfere with caffeine metabolism, enhance warfarin effects, and elevate SrCr with cyclosporine.

PREGNANCY: Category C, caution in nursing.

MECHANISM OF ACTION: Fluoroquinolone antibiotic; inhibits topoisomerase II (DNA gyrase) and topoisomerase IV. DNA gyrase is an essential enzyme involved in replication, transcription, and repair of bacterial DNA. Topoisomerase IV is an enzyme known to play a key role in partitioning of chromosomal DNA during bacterial cell division.

NURSING CONSIDERATIONS

Assessment: Assess for proper diagnosis of causative organisms (eg, slit lamp biomicroscopy, fluorescein staining). Assess for hypersensitivity to other quinolones, possible drug interactions, and use in pregnancy/nursing.

Monitoring: Monitor for signs/symptoms of hypersensitivity or anaphylactic reactions (eg, cardiovascular collapse, loss of consciousness, angioedema). Monitor for overgrowth of nonsusceptible organisms (eg, fungi) with prolonged therapy.

Patient Counseling: Advise to avoid contaminating applicator tip with material from eye, fingers, or other sources. Instruct to d/c therapy and contact physician at first sign of rash or allergic reaction. Advise not to wear contact lenses if there are signs/symptoms of bacterial conjunctivitis.

Administration: Ocular route. Do not inject into eye. **Storage:** Store at 15-25°C (59-77°F). Protect from freezing.

ZYMAXID   RX
gatifloxacin (Allergan)

THERAPEUTIC CLASS: Fluoroquinolone

INDICATIONS: Treatment of bacterial conjunctivitis caused by susceptible strains of organisms.

DOSAGE: *Adults:* 1 drop q2h while awake, up to 8X on Day 1, then 1 drop bid-qid while awake on Days 2-7.
Pediatrics: ≥1 Yr: 1 drop q2h while awake, up to 8X on Day 1, then 1 drop bid-qid while awake on Days 2-7.

HOW SUPPLIED: Sol: 0.5% [2.5mL]

WARNINGS/PRECAUTIONS: For ophthalmic use only; should not be introduced directly into the anterior chamber of the eye. Overgrowth of nonsusceptible organisms, including fungi, may result with prolonged use. D/C use and institute alternative therapy if superinfection occurs. Avoid wearing contact lenses if there are signs and symptoms of bacterial conjunctivitis or during the course of therapy.

ADVERSE REACTIONS: Worsening of the conjunctivitis, eye irritation, dysgeusia, eye pain.

PREGNANCY: Category C, caution in nursing.

MECHANISM OF ACTION: Fluoroquinolone antibiotic; inhibition of DNA gyrase and topoisomerase IV. DNA gyrase is an essential enzyme involved in replication, transcription, and repair of bacterial DNA. Topoisomerase IV is an enzyme known to play a key role in partitioning of chromosomal DNA during bacterial cell division.

NURSING CONSIDERATIONS

Assessment: Assess for conjunctivitis, proper diagnosis of causative organisms (eg, slit lamp biomicroscopy, fluorescein staining), and pregnancy/nursing status.

Monitoring: Monitor for adverse events and overgrowth of nonsusceptible organisms (eg, fungi) with prolonged therapy.

Patient Counseling: Inform that sol is for ophthalmic use only and should not be introduced directly into the anterior chamber of the eye. Advise not to wear contact lenses if there are signs and symptoms of bacterial conjunctivitis and during course of therapy. Instruct to avoid contaminating the applicator tip with material from the eyes, fingers, or other sources.

Administration: Ocular route. **Storage:** 15-25°C (59-77°F). Protect from freezing.

ZYPREXA   RX
olanzapine (Lilly)

> Elderly patients with dementia-related psychosis treated with antipsychotic drugs are at an increased risk of death; most deaths appeared to be cardiovascular (eg, heart failure, sudden death) or infectious (eg, pneumonia) in nature. Not approved for the treatment of patients with dementia-related psychosis. When used with fluoxetine, refer to the Boxed Warning section of the PI for Symbyax.

OTHER BRAND NAMES: Zyprexa Zydis (Lilly)

THERAPEUTIC CLASS: Thienobenzodiazepine

INDICATIONS: (PO) Treatment of schizophrenia, acute treatment of manic or mixed episodes associated with bipolar I disorder and maintenance treatment of bipolar I disorder. Adjunct to lithium or valproate for the treatment of manic or mixed episodes associated with bipolar I disorder. In combination with fluoxetine for the treatment of depressive episodes associated with bipolar I disorder. In combination with fluoxetine for the treatment of treatment resistant depression in adults. (IM) Treatment of acute agitation associated with schizophrenia and bipolar I mania in adults.

DOSAGE: *Adults:* (PO) Schizophrenia: Initial: 5-10mg qd. Target Dose: 10mg/day within several days. Adjust dose by increments/decrements of 5mg qd at intervals of not <1 week. Max: 20mg/day. Maint: 10-20mg/day. Periodically reevaluate the long-term usefulness of the drug. Bipolar I Disorder (Manic or Mixed Episodes): Initial: 10mg or 15mg qd. Adjust dose by increments/decrements of 5mg qd at intervals of not <24 hrs. Maint: 5-20mg/day. Periodically reevaluate the long-term usefulness of the drug. Max: 20mg/day. With Lithium or Valproate: Initial: 10mg qd. Max: 20mg/day. Depressive Episodes Associated with Bipolar I Disorder/Resistant Depression in Combination with Fluoxetine: Initial: 5mg with 20mg fluoxetine qpm. Adjust dose based on efficacy and tolerability. Usual: 5-12.5mg with 20-50mg fluoxetine (depressive episodes associated with Bipolar I disorder) or 5-20mg with 20-50mg fluoxetine (resistant depression). Max: 18mg with 75mg fluoxetine. (IM) Agitation: Usual: 10mg. Range: 2.5-10mg. Assess for orthostatic hypotension prior to subsequent dosing. Max: 3 doses of 10mg 2-4 hrs apart. May initiate PO therapy in a range of 5-20mg/day when clinically appropriate. Refer to PI for dosing in special

Z

populations.

Pediatrics: 13-17 Yrs: (PO) Schizophrenia/Bipolar I Disorder (Manic or Mixed Episodes): Initial: 2.5mg or 5mg qd. Target Dose: 10mg/day. Adjust dose by increments/decrements of 2.5mg or 5mg. Max: 20mg/day. Maint: Use lowest dose needed to maintain remission. Periodically reassess the need for maintenance treatment. 10-17 Yrs: Depressive Episodes Associated with Bipolar I Disorder in Combination with Fluoxetine: Initial: 2.5mg with 20mg fluoxetine qpm. Adjust dose based on efficacy and tolerability. Max: 12mg with 50mg fluoxetine.

HOW SUPPLIED: Inj: 10mg; Tab: 2.5mg, 5mg, 7.5mg, 10mg, 15mg, 20mg; Tab, Disintegrating: (Zydis) 5mg, 10mg, 15mg, 20mg

CONTRAINDICATIONS: When used with fluoxetine, refer to the Symbyax monograph. When used with lithium or valproate, refer to the individual monographs.

WARNINGS/PRECAUTIONS: Supervision should accompany therapy in patients at high risk of attempted suicide. Neuroleptic malignant syndrome (NMS) reported; d/c and instill intensive symptomatic treatment and monitoring. Hyperglycemia, in some cases extreme and associated with ketoacidosis or hyperosmolar coma or death, reported; caution in patients with diabetes mellitus or borderline increased blood glucose levels, and regularly monitor for worsening of glucose control. Hyperlipidemia, weight gain, and hyperprolactinemia reported. Tardive dyskinesia (TD) may develop; d/c if signs/symptoms develop unless treatment is required despite the presence of the syndrome. May induce orthostatic hypotension; caution with known cardiovascular disease (CVD), cerebrovascular disease, and conditions that would predispose to hypotension. Leukopenia, neutropenia, and agranulocytosis reported; consider discontinuing at 1st sign of a clinically significant decline in WBC in the absence of other causative factors. D/C if severe neutropenia (absolute neutrophil count <1000/mm³) develops. May cause esophageal dysmotility and aspiration, and disruption of body temperature regulation. Seizures reported; caution with history of seizures or with conditions that potentially lower the seizure threshold. Not approved for treatment of patients with Alzheimer's disease. May impair mental/physical abilities. Caution in patients with clinically significant prostatic hypertrophy, narrow-angle glaucoma, history of paralytic ileus or related conditions, cardiac patients, hepatic impairment, preexisting conditions associated with limited hepatic functional reserve, and in the elderly.

ADVERSE REACTIONS: Postural hypotension, constipation, dry mouth, weight gain, somnolence, dizziness, personality disorder, akathisia, asthenia, dyspepsia, tremor, increased appetite, abdominal pain, headache, insomnia.

INTERACTIONS: May potentiate orthostatic hypotension with diazepam and alcohol. Increased clearance with carbamazepine (CYP1A2 inducer), and omeprazole and rifampin (CYP1A2 inducers or glucuronyl transferase inducers). Decreased clearance with fluoxetine (CYP2D6 inhibitor) and fluvoxamine (CYP1A2 inhibitor); consider lower dose of olanzapine with concomitant fluvoxamine. Caution with other centrally-acting drugs, alcohol, drugs whose effects can induce hypotension, bradycardia, or respiratory/CNS depression, and in patients being treated with potentially hepatotoxic drugs. May enhance effects of certain antihypertensives. May antagonize effects of levodopa and dopamine agonists. Caution with anticholinergic drugs; may contribute to an elevation in core body temperature. (IM) Not recommended with parenteral benzodiazepines. IM lorazepam may potentiate somnolence. (PO) Decreased levels with activated charcoal.

PREGNANCY: Category C, not for use in nursing.

MECHANISM OF ACTION: Thienobenzodiazepine; not established. Proposed that efficacy in schizophrenia is mediated through a combination of dopamine and serotonin type 2 (5HT2) antagonism.

PHARMACOKINETICS: Absorption: (PO) Well-absorbed, T_{max} =6 hrs; (IM) Rapid, T_{max} =15-45 min. **Distribution:** Found in breast milk. (PO) V_d =1000L; plasma protein binding (93%). **Metabolism:** Via direct glucuronidation and CYP450 mediated oxidation; 10-N-glucuronide and 4'-N-desmethyl olanzapine (major metabolites). **Elimination:** (PO) Urine (57%, 7% unchanged), feces (30%); $T_{1/2}$ =21-54 hrs.

NURSING CONSIDERATIONS

Assessment: Assess for CVD, cerebrovascular disease, risk of hypotension, history of seizures or conditions that could lower the seizure threshold, prostatic hypertrophy, narrow-angle glaucoma, history of paralytic ileus, hepatic impairment, history of drug abuse, risk factors for leukopenia/neutropenia, pregnancy/nursing status, and possible drug interactions. Assess for dementia-related psychosis and Alzheimer's disease in the elderly. Obtain baseline lipid profile, CBC, and FPG levels.

Monitoring: Monitor for signs/symptoms of NMS, TD, orthostatic hypotension, seizures, disruption of body temperature regulation, hyperprolactinemia, and other adverse reactions. Periodically monitor FPG, lipid levels, CBC, and weight of patient. In patients with clinically significant neutropenia, monitor for fever or other symptoms/signs of infection. Periodically reassess to determine the need for maintenance treatment.

Patient Counseling: Advise of potential benefits and risks of therapy. Counsel about the signs and symptoms of NMS. Inform of potential risk of hyperglycemia-related adverse events. Inform that medication may cause hyperlipidemia and weight gain. Inform that medication may cause orthostatic hypotension; instruct to contact physician if dizziness, fast or slow heart beat, or fainting occurs. Inform that medication may impair judgment, thinking, or motor skills; instruct to use caution when operating hazardous machinery, including automobiles. Instruct to avoid over-heating and dehydration. Instruct to notify physician if taking, planning to take, or have stopped taking any prescription or OTC products, including herbal supplements. Instruct to avoid alcohol. Inform that orally disintegrating tab contains phenylalanine. Advise to notify physician if pregnant or planning to become pregnant during treatment. Advise to avoid breastfeeding during therapy.

Administration: Oral/IM routes. (Tab, Zydis) Can be taken with or without food. (Inj) Do not administer IV or SQ. Inject slowly, deep into the muscle mass. (Zydis) After opening sachet, peel back foil on blister. Do not push tab through foil. Upon opening the blister, remove tab and place entire tab in the mouth using dry hands. Refer to PI for proper reconstitution procedures and further administration instructions. **Storage:** Tab, Zydis, and Inj (Before Reconstitution): 20-25°C (68-77°F); excursions permitted between 15-30°C (59-86°F). Reconstituted Inj: 20-25°C (68-77°F) for up to 1 hr; excursions permitted between 15-30°C (59-86°F). Tab/Zydis: Protect from light and moisture. Inj: Protect from light. Do not freeze.

ZYPREXA RELPREVV   RX
olanzapine (Lilly)

Adverse events with signs and symptoms consistent with overdose, in particular, sedation (including coma) and/or delirium reported following inj. Must be administered in a registered healthcare facility with ready access to emergency response services. Observe patient for at least 3 hrs after each inj. Available only through a restricted distribution program called Zyprexa Relprevv Patient Care Program and requires prescriber, healthcare facility, patient, and pharmacy enrollment. Elderly patients with dementia-related psychosis treated with antipsychotic drugs are at an increased risk of death; most deaths appeared to be cardiovascular (eg, heart failure, sudden death) or infectious (eg, pneumonia) in nature. Not approved for the treatment of patients with dementia-related psychosis.

THERAPEUTIC CLASS: Thienobenzodiazepine

INDICATIONS: Treatment of schizophrenia.

DOSAGE: *Adults:* ≥18 Yrs: Establish tolerability with PO olanzapine prior to initiating treatment. Usual: 150-300mg IM every 2 weeks or 405mg IM every 4 weeks. Max: 405mg IM every 4 weeks or 300mg IM every 2 weeks. Debilitated/ Predisposition to Hypotension/Slow Metabolizers/ Sensitive to Olanzapine Effects: Initial: 150mg IM every 4 weeks. Titrate: Increase cautiously. Reassess periodically to determine the need for continued treatment. Refer to PI for recommended dosing based on corresponding PO olanzapine doses.

HOW SUPPLIED: Inj, Extended-Release: 210mg, 300mg, 405mg

WARNINGS/PRECAUTIONS: Supervision should accompany therapy in patients at high risk for attempted suicide. Neuroleptic malignant syndrome (NMS) reported; d/c and instill intensive symptomatic treatment and monitoring. Hyperglycemia, in some cases extreme and associated with ketoacidosis or hyperosmolar coma or death, reported; caution in patients with diabetes mellitus (DM) or borderline increased blood glucose levels, and regularly monitor for worsening of glucose control. Hyperlipidemia, weight gain, and hyperprolactinemia reported. Tardive dyskinesia (TD) reported; d/c if signs/symptoms develop unless treatment is required despite the presence of the syndrome. May induce orthostatic hypotension; caution with known cardiovascular disease (CVD), cerebrovascular disease, and conditions that would predispose to hypotension. Leukopenia, neutropenia, and agranulocytosis reported; d/c at 1st sign of clinically significant decline in WBC in the absence of other causative factors or if severe neutropenia (absolute neutrophil count <1000/mm³) develops. May cause esophageal dysmotility and aspiration, and disruption of body temperature regulation. Seizures reported; caution with history of seizures or with conditions that potentially lower the seizure threshold. Not approved for use in patients with Alzheimer's disease. May impair mental/physical abilities. Caution in patients with clinically significant prostatic hypertrophy, cardiac patients, narrow angle glaucoma, history of paralytic ileus or related conditions, hepatic impairment, preexisting conditions associated with limited hepatic functional reserve, and in the elderly.

ADVERSE REACTIONS: Headache, sedation, diarrhea, cough, back pain, N/V, nasal congestion, dry mouth, nasopharyngitis, weight gain, abdominal pain, somnolence, increased appetite.

INTERACTIONS: May potentiate orthostatic hypotension with diazepam and alcohol. Increased clearance with carbamazepine (CYP1A2 inducer), and omeprazole and rifampin (CYP1A2 inducers or glucuronyl transferase inducers). Decreased clearance with fluoxetine (CYP2D6 inhibitor) and fluvoxamine (CYP1A2 inhibitor); consider lower dose of olanzapine with concomitant fluvoxamine. Caution with other centrally acting drugs, alcohol, drugs whose effects can induce hypotension, bradycardia, or respiratory/CNS depression, and in patients being treated with potentially hepatotoxic drugs. May enhance effects of certain antihypertensive agents. May antagonize effects of levodopa and dopamine agonists. Caution with anticholinergic drugs; may contribute

Z

to an elevation in core body temperature. IM lorazepam may potentiate somnolence. Monitor for excessive sedation and cardiorespiratory depression with parenteral benzodiazepines.

PREGNANCY: Category C, not for use in nursing.

MECHANISM OF ACTION: Thienobenzodiazepine; not established. Proposed that efficacy in schizophrenia is mediated through a combination of dopamine and serotonin type 2 ($5HT_2$) antagonism.

PHARMACOKINETICS: Absorption: (IM) Rapid, T_{max}=15-45 min. **Distribution:** V_d=1000L; plasma protein binding (93%); (PO) found in breast milk. **Metabolism:** Via direct glucuronidation and CYP450 mediated oxidation; 10-N-glucuronide, 4'-N-desmethyl olanzapine (major metabolites). **Elimination:** (PO) Urine (57%, 7% unchanged), feces (30%); (IM) $T_{1/2}$=30 days.

NURSING CONSIDERATIONS

Assessment: Assess for tolerability with PO olanzapine, CVD, cerebrovascular disease, risk of hypotension, history of seizures or conditions that could lower the seizure threshold, prostatic hypertrophy, narrow-angle glaucoma, history of paralytic ileus, risk factors for leukopenia/neutropenia, hepatic impairment, pregnancy/nursing status, and possible drug interactions. Assess for dementia-related psychosis and Alzheimer's disease in the elderly. Obtain baseline lipid profile, CBC, and FPG levels.

Monitoring: Monitor for sedation and/or delirium for at least 3 hrs post-inj. Monitor for signs/symptoms of NMS, TD, orthostatic hypotension, seizures, disruption of body temperature regulation, hyperprolactinemia, and other adverse reactions. In patients with clinically significant neutropenia, monitor for fever or other symptoms/signs of infection. In high-risk patients, monitor closely for a suicide attempt. Perform periodic monitoring of FPG, lipid levels, and weight of patient. Perform frequent monitoring of CBC in patients with a history of clinically significant low WBC or drug-induced leukopenia/neutropenia.

Patient Counseling: Advise of potential benefits and risks of therapy. Advise of the risk of post-inj delirium/sedation syndrome following administration; advise not to drive or operate heavy machinery for rest of the day. Counsel about the signs/symptoms of NMS. Inform of potential risk of hyperglycemia-related adverse events. Counsel that medication may cause hyperlipidemia and weight gain. Inform that medication may cause orthostatic hypotension; instruct to contact physician if dizziness, fast or slow heart beat, or fainting occurs. Inform that medication may impair judgment, thinking, or motor skills; instruct to use caution when operating hazardous machinery, including automobiles. Instruct to avoid overheating and dehydration. Instruct to notify physician if taking, planning to take, or have stopped taking any Rx or OTC drugs, including herbal supplements. Instruct to avoid alcohol. Advise to notify physician if pregnant or planning to become pregnant during treatment. Advise to avoid breastfeeding during therapy.

Administration: IM route. Not for IV or SQ use. Refer to PI for reconstitution and administration instructions. **Storage:** Room temperature ≤30°C (86°F). Reconstituted Sol: May store at room temperature for 24 hrs.

ZYTIGA
abiraterone acetate (Janssen)   **RX**

THERAPEUTIC CLASS: Nonsteroidal antiandrogen

INDICATIONS: In combination with prednisone for the treatment of patients with metastatic castration-resistant prostate cancer.

DOSAGE: *Adults:* Usual: 1000mg qd with prednisone 5mg PO bid. Baseline Moderate Hepatic Impairment (Child-Pugh Class B): 250mg qd; use with caution. If elevations in ALT and/or AST >5X ULN or total bilirubin >3X ULN occur in these patients, d/c use and do not retreat. Hepatotoxicity (ALT and/or AST >5X ULN or Total Bilirubin >3X ULN) Development During Treatment: Interrupt treatment. May restart at 750mg qd following return of LFTs to patient's baseline or to AST and ALT ≤2.5X ULN and total bilirubin ≤1.5X ULN. If hepatotoxicity recurs at 750mg qd, may restart retreatment at 500mg qd, following return of LFTs to patient's baseline or to AST and ALT ≤2.5X ULN and total bilirubin ≤1.5X ULN. If hepatotoxicity recurs at 500mg qd, d/c use. Use with Strong CYP3A4 Inducers: If a strong CYP3A4 inducer must be coadministered, increase abiraterone dosing frequency to bid only during the coadministration period (eg, from 1000mg qd to 1000mg bid). Reduce the dose back to the previous dose and frequency, if the concomitant strong CYP3A4 inducer is discontinued. Take with water on an empty stomach.

HOW SUPPLIED: Tab: 250mg

CONTRAINDICATIONS: Women who are or may become pregnant.

WARNINGS/PRECAUTIONS: May cause HTN, hypokalemia, and fluid retention; caution with history of cardiovascular disease (CVD) or with underlying medical conditions that might be compromised by increases in BP, hypokalemia, or fluid retention. Control HTN and correct hypokalemia before and during treatment. Adrenocortical insufficiency reported; use caution and monitor for signs/symptoms, particularly if patients are withdrawn from prednisone, have prednisone dose reductions, or experience unusual stress. Increased dosage of corticosteroids may be indicated before, during, and after stressful situations. Signs/symptoms of adrenocortical insufficiency may be masked by adverse reactions associated with mineralocorticoid excess. ALT/AST increases reported; measure ALT, AST, and bilirubin levels at baseline, every 2 weeks for the first 3 months (or weekly for the 1st month, then every 2 weeks for the following 2 months in patients with baseline moderate hepatic impairment), and monthly thereafter. Promptly measure serum total bilirubin, AST, and ALT if signs/symptoms of hepatotoxicity develop. Avoid with baseline severe hepatic impairment (Child-Pugh Class C).

ADVERSE REACTIONS: Fatigue, joint swelling/discomfort, edema, hot flush, diarrhea, vomiting, cough, HTN, dyspnea, urinary tract infection (UTI), contusion.

INTERACTIONS: See Dosage. Avoid concomitant strong CYP3A4 inducers (eg, phenytoin, carbamazepine, rifampin, rifabutin, rifapentine, phenobarbital) during treatment. Decreased exposure with rifampin (strong CYP3A4 inducer). Increased levels of dextromethorphan (CYP2D6 substrate). Avoid coadministration with CYP2D6 substrates with narrow therapeutic index (eg, thioridazine); if alternative treatments cannot be used, exercise caution and consider dose reduction of the concomitant CYP2D6 substrate. Monitor closely for signs of toxicity related to CYP2C8 substrates if used concomitantly.

PREGNANCY: Category X, not for use in nursing.

MECHANISM OF ACTION: Androgen biosynthesis inhibitor; inhibits 17 α-hydroxylase/C17,20-lyase (CYP17), an enzyme expressed in testicular, adrenal, and prostatic tumor tissues and is required for androgen biosynthesis.

PHARMACOKINETICS: Absorption: T_{max}=2 hrs (median); C_{max}=226ng/mL; AUC=1173ng•hr/mL. **Distribution:** V_d=19,669L; plasma protein binding (>99%). **Metabolism:** Hydrolysis via esterase to abiraterone (active metabolite). **Elimination:** Feces (88%, 55% unchanged), urine (5%); $T_{1/2}$=12 hrs.

NURSING CONSIDERATIONS

Assessment: Assess for history of CVD and underlying medical conditions that might be compromised by increases in BP, hypokalemia, or fluid retention. Assess hepatic function and for possible drug interactions. Obtain baseline AST, ALT, and bilirubin levels. Control HTN and correct hypokalemia before treatment.

Monitoring: Monitor for HTN, hypokalemia, and fluid retention at least monthly, and for signs/symptoms of adrenocortical insufficiency and hepatotoxicity. Monitor ALT, AST, and bilirubin levels every 2 weeks for the first 3 months (or weekly for the 1st month, then every 2 weeks for the following 2 months in patients with baseline moderate hepatic impairment), and monthly thereafter. For patients who resume treatment after development of hepatotoxicity, monitor serum transaminases and bilirubin at a minimum of every 2 weeks for 3 months, and monthly thereafter.

Patient Counseling: Inform that drug is used together with prednisone and instruct to take ud and not to interrupt or stop either of these medications without consulting a physician. Inform those receiving gonadotropin-releasing hormone agonists to maintain such treatment during therapy. Inform that if a daily dose is missed, take the normal dose the following day, but if >1 daily dose is skipped, advise to consult physician. Counsel about the common side effects (eg, peripheral edema, hypokalemia, HTN, elevated LFTs, UTI). Inform that liver function will be monitored using blood tests. Advise that drug may harm a developing fetus and that women who are pregnant or may be pregnant should not handle the drug without protection (eg, gloves). Instruct to use a condom if having sex with a pregnant woman, and to use a condom and another effective method of birth control if having sex with a woman of childbearing potential; advise that these measures are required during and for 1 week after treatment.

Administration: Oral route. No food should be consumed for at least 2 hrs before and 1 hr after the dose is taken. Swallow tab whole with water; do not crush or chew. **Storage:** 20-25°C (68-77°F); excursions permitted from 15-30°C (59-86°F).

Z

Appendix: Reference Tables

ABBREVIATIONS, ACRONYMS, AND SYMBOLS

ABBREVIATIONS	DESCRIPTIONS
- (eg, 6-8)	to (eg, 6 to 8)
/	per
<	less than
>	greater than
≤	less than or equal to
≥	greater than or equal to
α	alpha
β	beta
5-FU	5-fluorouracil
5-HT	5-hydroxytryptamine (serotonin)
aa	of each
ABECB	acute bacterial exacerbation of chronic bronchitis
ac	before meals
ACE inhibitor	angiotensin converting enzyme inhibitor
ACTH	adrenocorticotropic hormone
ad	right ear
ADHD	attention-deficit hyperactivity disorder
A-fib	atrial fibrillation
A-flutter	atrial flutter
AIDS	acquired immunodeficiency syndrome
ALT	alanine transaminase (SGPT)
am or AM	morning
AMI	acute myocardial infarction
ANA	antinuclear antibody
ANC	absolute neutrophil count
APAP	acetaminophen
Apo B	apolipoprotein B
ARB	angiotensin II receptor blocker
as	left ear
ASA	aspirin
AST	aspartate transaminase (SGOT)
au	each ear
AUC	area under the curve
AV	atrioventricular
bid	twice daily
BMI	body mass index
BP	blood pressure

(Continued)

ABBREVIATIONS	DESCRIPTIONS
BPH	benign prostatic hypertrophy
BSA	body surface area
BUN	blood urea nitrogen
Ca^{2+}	calcium
CABG	coronary artery bypass graft
CAD	coronary artery disease
cap	capsule or gelcap
CAP	community-acquired pneumonia
CBC	complete blood count
CCB	calcium channel blocker
CF	cystic fibrosis
CHF	congestive heart failure
CK	creatine kinase
Cl^-	chloride
cm	centimeter
C_{max}	peak plasma concentration
CMV	cytomegalovirus
CNS	central nervous system
COPD	chronic obstructive pulmonary disease
COX-2 inhibitor	cyclooxygenase-2 inhibitor
CPK	creatine phosphokinase
CrCl	creatinine clearance
cre	cream
CRF	chronic renal failure
CSF	cerebrospinal fluid
CTC	common toxicity criteria
CVA	cerebrovascular accident
CVD	cardiovascular disease
CYP450	cytochrome P450
D5	dextrose 5%
D5W	dextrose 5% in water
d/c or D/C	discontinue
DHEA	dehydroepiandrosterone
DM	diabetes mellitus
DVT	deep vein thrombosis
ECG	electrocardiogram
EDTA	edetate disodium
EEG	electroencephalogram
eg	for example
EPS	extrapyramidal symptom

ABBREVIATIONS	DESCRIPTIONS
ER	extended-release
ESRD	end-stage renal disease
fl oz	fluid ounce
FPG	fasting plasma glucose
FSH	follicle-stimulating hormone
g	gram
G6PD	glucose-6-phosphate dehydrogenase
GABA	gamma-aminobutyric acid
GAD	general anxiety disorder
GERD	gastroesophageal reflux disease
GFR	glomerular filtration rate
GGT	gamma-glutamyl transpeptidase
GI	gastrointestinal
GnRH	gonadotropin-releasing hormone
GVHD	graft-versus-host disease
HbA1c	hemoglobin A1c
HCG	human chorionic gonadotropin
Hct	hematocrit
HCTZ	hydrochlorothiazide
HDL	high-density lipoprotein
HF	heart failure
Hgb	hemoglobin
HIV	human immunodeficiency virus
HMG-CoA	3-hydroxy-3-methylglutaryl-coenzyme A
HR	heart rate
hr, hrs	hour, hours
hs	bedtime
HSV	herpes simplex virus
HTN	hypertension
IBD	inflammatory bowel disease
IBS	irritable bowel syndrome
ICH	intracranial hemorrhage
ICP	intracranial pressure
IM	intramuscular/intramuscularly
INH	isoniazid
inh	inhalation
inj	injection
INR	international normalized ratio
IOP	intraocular pressure
IR	immediate-release

(Continued)

ABBREVIATIONS	DESCRIPTIONS
IU*	international unit
IUD	intrauterine device
IV	intravenous/intravenously
K+	potassium
kg	kilogram
KIU	kallikrein inhibitor unit
L	liter
lb, lbs	pound, pounds
LD	loading dose
LDL	low-density lipoprotein
LFT	liver function test
LH	luteinizing hormone
LHRH	luteinizing-hormone releasing hormone
lot	lotion
loz	lozenge
LVH	left ventricular hypertrophy
M	molar
MAC	*Mycobacterium avium* complex
maint	maintenance
MAOI	monoamine oxidase inhibitor
max	maximum
mcg	microgram
mEq	milli-equivalent
mg	milligram
Mg2+	magnesium
MI	myocardial infarction
min	minute (usually as mL/min)
mL	milliliter
mm	millimeter
mM	millimolar
MRI	magnetic resonance imaging
MS*	multiple sclerosis
msec	millisecond
MTX	methotrexate
N/A	not applicable or not available
Na+	sodium
NaCl	sodium chloride
NG	nasogastric
NKA	no known allergies
NMS	neuroleptic malignant syndrome

ABBREVIATIONS	DESCRIPTIONS
NPO	nothing by mouth
NSAID	nonsteroidal anti-inflammatory drug
NV or N/V	nausea and vomiting
NYHA Class	New York Heart Association Class
OA	osteoarthritis
OCD	obsessive-compulsive disorder
od	right eye
oint	ointment
os	left eye
OTC	over-the-counter
ou	each eye
oz	ounce
P	phosphorus
PAT	paroxysmal atrial tachycardia
pc	after meals
PCN	penicillin
PCP	*Pneumocystis carinii* pneumonia
PD	Parkinson's disease
PDE-5 inhibitor	phosphodiesterase-5 inhibitor
PE	pulmonary embolism
P-gp	P-glycoprotein
PID	pelvic inflammatory disease
pkt, pkts	packet, packets
pm or PM	evening
po or PO	orally
PONV	postoperative nausea and vomiting
postop	postoperative/postoperatively
pr	rectally
preop	preoperative/preoperatively
prn or PRN	as needed
PSA	prostate-specific antigen
PSVT	paroxysmal supraventricular tachycardia
PT	prothrombin time
PTSD	post-traumatic stress disorder
PTT	partial thromboplastin time
PTU	propylthiouracil
PUD	peptic ulcer disease
PVD	peripheral vascular disease
q4h, q6h, q8h, etc.	every four hours, every six hours, every eight hours, etc.

(Continued)

ABBREVIATIONS	DESCRIPTIONS
qam	once every morning
qd*	once daily
qh	every hour
qid	four times daily
qod*	every other day
qpm	once every evening
qs	a sufficient quantity
qs ad	a sufficient quantity to make
RA	rheumatoid arthritis
RAAS	renin-angiotensin-aldosterone system
RAS	renin-angiotensin system
RBC	red blood cell
RDS	respiratory distress syndrome
REM	rapid eye movement
Rx	prescription
SAH	subarachnoid hemorrhage
SBP	systolic blood pressure
sec	second
SGOT	serum glutamic-oxaloacetic transaminase (AST)
SGPT	serum glutamic-pyruvic transaminase (ALT)
SIADH	syndrome of inappropriate antidiuretic hormone secretion
SJS	Stevens-Johnson syndrome
SLE	systemic lupus erythematosus
SNRI	serotonin and norepinephrine reuptake inhibitor
SOB	shortness of breath
sol	solution
SQ, SC	subcutaneous/subcutaneously
SrCr	serum creatinine
SSRI	selective serotonin reuptake inhibitor
SSSI	skin and skin structure infection
STD	sexually transmitted disease
sup or supp	suppository
sus	suspension
SVT	supraventricular tachycardia
$T_{1/2}$	half-life
T3	triiodothyronine
T4	thyroxine
tab	tablet or caplet

ABBREVIATIONS	DESCRIPTIONS
tab, SL	sublingual tablet
TB	tuberculosis
TBG	thyroxine-binding globulin
tbl or tbsp	tablespoonful
TCA	tricyclic antidepressant
TD	tardive dyskinesia
TEN	toxic epidermal necrolysis
TFT	thyroid function test
TG	triglyceride
tid	three times daily
T_{max}	time to maximum concentration
TNF	tumor necrosis factor
total-C	total cholesterol
TPN	total parenteral nutrition
TSH	thyroid-stimulating hormone
tsp	teaspoonful
TTP	thrombotic thrombocytopenic purpura
U*	unit
UC	ulcerative colitis
ud	as directed
ULN	upper limit of normal
URTI/URI	upper respiratory tract infection
UTI	urinary tract infection
UV	ultraviolet
V_d	volume of distribution
VLDL	very low density lipoprotein
VTE	venous thromboembolism
WBC	white blood cell
WHO	World Health Organization
X	times (eg, >2X ULN)
yr, yrs	year, years

*The Joint Commission cautions use of these abbreviations on orders and medication-related documentation that is handwritten (including free-text computer entry) or on pre-printed forms. Visit www.jointcommission.org for more information.

CALCULATIONS AND FORMULAS

METRIC MEASURES

1 kilogram (kg)	1000 g
1 gram (g)	1000 mg
1 milligram (mg)	0.001 g
1 microgram (mcg or μg)	0.001 mg; 1×10^{-6} g
1 liter (L)	1000 mL
1 milliliter (mL)	0.001 L; 1 cc (cubic centimeter)

APOTHECARY MEASURES (AP)

1 scruple	20 grains (gr)
1 dram	3 scruples; 27.3 gr
1 ounce (oz)	16 drams; 22 scruples; 437.5 gr
1 pound (lb)	16 oz; 256 drams; 350 scruples; 7000 gr

U.S. FLUID MEASURES

1 fluid dram	60 minims
1 fluid ounce	8 fluid drams; 480 minims
1 pint (pt)	16 fl oz; 7680 minims
1 quart (qt)	2 pt; 32 fl oz
1 gallon (gal)	4 qt; 128 fl oz

AVOIRDUPOIS WEIGHT (AV)

1 ounce	437.5 gr
1 pound	16 oz

CONVERSION FACTORS

1 gram	15.4 gr
1 grain	64.8 mg
1 ounce (Av)	28.35 g; 437.5 gr
1 ounce (Ap)	31.1 g; 480 gr
1 pound (Av)	453.6 g
1 fluid ounce	29.57 mL
1 fluid dram	3.697 mL
1 minim	0.06 mL

COMMON MEASURES

1 teaspoonful	5 mL; ⅙ fl oz
1 tablespoonful	15 mL; ½ fl oz
1 wineglassful	60 mL; 2 fl oz
1 teacupful	120 mL; 4 fl oz
1 gallon	3800 mL; 128 fl oz
1 quart	946 mL; 32 fl oz
1 pint	473 mL; 16 fl oz
8 fluid ounces	240 mL
4 fluid ounces	120 mL
2.2 lb	1 kg

DOSE EQUIVALENTS

WEIGHT (METRIC)	WEIGHT (APOTHECARY)
30 g	1 ounce
15 g	8.5 drams
10 g	5.6 drams
7.5 g	4.2 drams
6 g	92.6 grains
5 g	77.2 grains
4 g	60 grains; 1 dram
3 g	45 grains

(Continued)

| DOSE EQUIVALENTS *(Continued)* ||
WEIGHT (METRIC)	WEIGHT (APOTHECARY)
2 g	30 grains; ½ dram
1.5 g	22 grains
1 g	15 grains
750 mg	12 grains
600 mg	10 grains
500 mg	7½ grains
400 mg	6 grains
300 mg	5 grains
250 mg	4 grains
200 mg	3 grains
150 mg	2½ grains
125 mg	2 grains
100 mg	1½ grains
75 mg	1¼ grains
60 mg	1 grain
50 mg	¾ grain
40 mg	⅔ grain
30 mg	½ grain
25 mg	⅜ grain
20 mg	⅓ grain
15 mg	¼ grain
12 mg	⅕ grain
10 mg	⅙ grain
8 mg	⅛ grain
6 mg	⅟₁₀ grain
5 mg	⅟₁₂ grain
4 mg	⅟₁₅ grain
3 mg	⅟₂₀ grain
2 mg	⅟₃₀ grain
1.5 mg	⅟₄₀ grain
1.2 mg	⅟₅₀ grain
1 mg	⅟₆₀ grain
LIQUID MEASURES (METRIC)	LIQUID MEASURES (APOTHECARY)
1000 mL	1 quart
750 mL	1½ pints
500 mL	1 pint
230 mL	8 fluid ounces
200 mL	7 fluid ounces
100 mL	3½ fluid ounces
50 mL	1¾ fluid ounces
30 mL	1 fluid ounce
15 mL	4 fluid drams
10 mL	2½ fluid drams
8 mL	2 fluid drams
5 mL	1½ fluid drams
4 mL	1 fluid dram
3 mL	45 minims
2 mL	30 minims
1 mL	15 minims
0.75 mL	12 minims
0.6 mL	10 minims
0.5 mL	8 minims
0.3 mL	5 minims
0.25 mL	4 minims
0.2 mL	3 minims

DOSE EQUIVALENTS *(Continued)*	
LIQUID MEASURES (METRIC)	**LIQUID MEASURES (APOTHECARY)**
0.1 mL	1½ minims
0.06 mL	1 minim
0.05 mL	¾ minim
0.03 mL	½ minim

MILLIEQUIVALENT (mEq) AND MILLIMOLE (mmol)

CALCULATIONS

$$\text{moles} = \frac{\text{weight of a substance (grams)}}{\text{molecular weight of that substance (grams)}} \quad \textbf{OR} \quad = \frac{\text{equivalent}}{\text{valence of ion}}$$

$$\text{millimoles} = \frac{\text{weight of a substance (milligrams)}}{\text{molecular weight of that substance (milligrams)}} \quad \textbf{OR} \quad = \frac{\text{milliequivalents}}{\text{valence of ion}} \quad \textbf{OR} \quad = \frac{\text{moles} \times 1000}{\text{valence of ion}}$$

$$\text{equivalents} = \text{moles} \times \text{valence of ion}$$

$$\text{milliequivalents} = \text{millimoles} \times \text{valence of ion} \quad \textbf{OR} \quad = \text{moles} \times 1000 \times \text{valence of ion}$$

CONVERSIONS

mg/100mL to mEq/L	$\text{mEq/L} = \dfrac{(\text{mg/100mL}) \times 10 \times \text{valence}}{\text{atomic weight}}$
mEq/L to mg/100mL	$\text{mg/100mL} = \dfrac{(\text{mEq/L}) \times \text{atomic weight}}{10 \times \text{valence}}$
mEq/L to volume percent of a gas	$\text{volume \%} = \dfrac{(\text{mEq/L}) \times 22.4}{10}$

ACID-BASE ASSESSMENT

DEFINITIONS

PIO_2	Oxygen partial pressure of inspired gas (mmHg); 150 mmHg in room air at sea level
FiO_2	Fractional pressure of oxygen in inspired gas (0.21 in room air)
PAO_2	Alveolar oxygen partial pressure
$PACO_2$	Alveolar carbon dioxide partial pressure
PaO_2	Arterial oxygen partial pressure
$PaCO_2$	Arterial carbon dioxide partial pressure
P_{ATM}	Ambient barometric pressure (eg, 760 mmHg at sea level)
P_{H2O}	Partial pressure of water vapor (eg, usually 47 mmHg)
R	Respiratory quotient (typically 0.8, increases with high-carbohydrate diet, decreases with high-fat diet)

HENDERSON-HASSELBALCH EQUATION

$$pH = 6.1 + \log [HCO_3^- / (0.03) (pCO_2)]$$

ALVEOLAR GAS EQUATION

$$P_{AO2} = [F_{IO2} \times (P_{ATM} - P_{H2O})] - \frac{PaCO_2}{R}$$

$$PaO_2 = PIO_2 - PaCO_2/R$$

ALVEOLAR/ARTERIAL OXYGEN GRADIENT

$$PAO_2 - PaO_2 \quad \textbf{OR} \quad F_{IO2} (P_{ATM} - P_{H2O}) - \frac{PaCO_2}{R}$$

ACID-BASE DISORDERS

DISORDER	pH	HCO₃⁻	PCO₂	COMPENSATION
Metabolic acidosis	<7.35	Primary decrease	Compensatory decrease	1.2 mmHg decrease in PCO_2 for every 1 mmol/L decrease in HCO_3^- **OR** $PCO_2 = (1.5 \times HCO_3^-) + 8 (\pm 2)$ **OR** $PCO_2 = HCO_3^- + 15$ **OR** $PCO_2 =$ last 2 digits of pH × 100 *(Continued)*

ACID-BASE DISORDERS *(Continued)*

DISORDER	pH	HCO$_3^-$	PCO$_2$	COMPENSATION
Metabolic alkalosis	>7.45	Primary increase	Compensatory increase	0.6-0.75 mmHg increase in PCO$_2$ for every 1 mmol/L increase in HCO$_3^-$. PCO$_2$ should not rise above 55 mmHg in compensation.
Respiratory acidosis	<7.35	Compensatory increase	Primary increase	*Acute:* 1-2 mmol/L increase in HCO$_3^-$ for every 10 mmHg increase in PCO$_2$. *Chronic:* 3-4 mmol/L increase in HCO$_3^-$ for every 10 mmHg increase in PCO$_2$.
Respiratory alkalosis	>7.45	Compensatory decrease	Primary decrease	*Acute:* 1-2 mmol/L decrease in HCO$_3^-$ for every 10 mmHg decrease in PCO$_2$. *Chronic:* 4-5 mmol/L decrease in HCO$_3^-$ for every 10 mmHg decrease in PCO$_2$.

ACID-BASE EQUATION

H$^+$ (in mEq/L) = (24 × PaCO$_2$) divided by HCO$_3^-$

OTHER CALCULATIONS

ANION GAP

Anion gap = Na$^+$ - (Cl$^-$ + HCO$_3^-$) = Unmeasured Anions (UA) - Unmeasured Cations (UC)

OSMOLALITY

Definition:
Osmolality is a measure of the total number of particles in a solution.

U.S. units (sodium as mEq/L, BUN [blood urea nitrogen] and glucose as mg/dL)
    Plasma osmolality (mOsm/kg) = 2[Na$^+$] + [(BUN)/2.8] + [(glucose)/18]

SI units (all variables in mmol/L):
    Plasma osmolality (mOsm/kg) = 2[Na$^+$] + [urea] + [glucose]
    Normal range plasma osmolality: 275 - 290 mOsm/kg

Corrected Sodium
Measured Na$^+$ + 0.016 (Serum glucose - 100), **OR**
Measured Na$^+$ + 0.024 (Serum glucose - 100)

Total Serum Calcium Corrected for Albumin Level
[(Normal albumin - patient's albumin) × 0.8] + patient's measured total calcium

Free Water Deficit
0.6 × body weight (kg) $\frac{[(Current\ Na^+)]}{140}$ - 1

Bicarbonate Deficit
[0.4 × weight (kg)] × (HCO$_3^-$ desired - HCO$_3^-$ measured)

CHILD-PUGH SCORE

The Child-Pugh classification is used to assess the prognosis of chronic liver disease, mainly cirrhosis. Child-Pugh is also used to determine the required strength of treatment and the necessity of liver transplantation.

Score:
The score employs five clinical measures of liver disease. Each measure is scored 1-3, with 3 indicating the most severe derangement.

Measure	1 point	2 points	3 points	Units
Bilirubin (total)	<2	2-3	>3	mg/dL
Serum albumin	>3.5	2.8-3.5	<2.8	g/dL
INR[†]	<1.7	1.71-2.3	>2.3	no unit
Ascites	None	Mild (or controlled by diuretics)	Moderate despite diuretic treatment	no unit
Hepatic encephalopathy	None	Grade I-II (or suppressed with medication)	Grade III-IV (or refractory)	no unit

[†]Some older reference works substitute PT prolongation for INR.

Interpretation:
Chronic liver disease is classified into Child-Pugh class A to C, employing the added score from above.

Points	Class	One-year survival	Two-year survival
5-6	A	100%	85%
7-9	B	80%	60%
10-15	C	45%	35%

CREATININE CLEARANCE

Clinically, creatinine clearance is a useful measure for estimating the glomerular filtration rate (GFR) of the kidneys.

Factors	Abbreviations
Creatinine clearance	Cl_{Cr}
Plasma creatinine concentration	P_{Cr}
Serum creatinine concentration	S_{Cr}
Urine creatinine concentration	U_{Cr}
Urine flow rate	V

Calculations:
$$Cl_{Cr} = \frac{U_{Cr} \times V}{P_{Cr}}$$

Example:
Patient with P_{Cr} 1 mg/dL, U_{Cr} 60 mg/dL, and V of 0.5 dL/hr.
$$Cl_{Cr} = \frac{60 \text{ mg/dL} \times 0.5 \text{ dL/hr}}{1 \text{ mg/dL}} = 30 \text{ dL/hr}$$

Cockroft-Gault formula: Estimates creatinine clearance (mL/min).

Male:
$$Cl_{Cr} = \frac{(140 - \text{age}) \times \text{mass (kg)}}{72 \times S_{Cr} \text{ (mg/dL)}}$$

Example:
Male patient, 67 years of age, weight 75 kg, and S_{Cr} 1 mg/dL.
$$Cl_{Cr} = \frac{(140 - 67) \times 75}{72 \times 1} = 76 \text{ mL/min}$$

Female:
$$Cl_{Cr} = \frac{(140 - \text{age}) \times \text{mass (kg)} \times 0.85}{72 \times S_{Cr} \text{ (mg/dL)}}$$

Example:
Female patient, 67 years of age, weight 75 kg, and S_{Cr} 1 mg/dL.
$$Cl_{Cr} = \frac{(140 - 67) \times 75 \times 0.85}{72 \times 1} = 64.6 \text{ mL/min}$$

Note: Using actual body weight (ABW) in obese patients can significantly overestimate creatinine clearance. Adjusted ideal body weight (IBW) can provide a more approximate estimate. Adjusted IBW = IBW + 0.4 (ABW - IBW).

BASAL ENERGY EXPENDITURE (BEE)

Basal energy expenditure: the amount of energy required to maintain the body's normal metabolic activity (eg, respiration, maintenance of body temperature).
W = weight (kg), H = height (cm), A = age (years)
Male:
BEE = 66.67 + 13.75W + 5H - 6.76A
Female:
BEE = 655.1 + 9.56W + 1.85H - 4.68A

BODY MASS INDEX (BMI)

$$BMI = \frac{\text{weight (kg)}}{[\text{height (m)}]^2}$$

BODY SURFACE AREA (BSA)

$$BSA \text{ (m}^2\text{)} = \sqrt{\frac{\text{height (in)} \times \text{weight (lb)}}{3131}}$$
OR
$$BSA \text{ (m}^2\text{)} = \sqrt{\frac{\text{height (cm)} \times \text{weight (kg)}}{3600}}$$

IDEAL BODY WEIGHT (IBW)

Adults (18 years and older; IBW is in kg; height is in inches):
For adults ≥5 feet:
IBW (male) = 50 + [2.3 × (height - 60)]
IBW (female) = 45.5 + [2.3 × (height - 60)]

Children (IBW is in kg; height is in cm):
For children 1-18 years old and with a height <5 feet:
$$IBW (kg) = \frac{(height^2 \times 1.65)}{1000}$$

POUNDS/KILOGRAMS CONVERSION							
1 POUND = 0.45359 KILOGRAM				1 KILOGRAM = 2.2 POUNDS			
lb	kg	lb	kg	lb	kg	lb	kg
1	0.45	105	47.63	210	95.25	315	142.88
5	2.27	110	49.89	215	97.52	320	145.15
10	4.54	115	52.16	220	99.79	325	147.42
15	6.80	120	54.43	225	102.06	330	149.68
20	9.07	125	56.70	230	104.33	335	151.95
25	11.34	130	58.97	235	106.59	340	154.22
30	13.61	135	61.23	240	108.86	345	156.49
35	15.88	140	63.50	245	111.13	350	158.76
40	18.14	145	65.77	250	113.40	355	161.02
45	20.41	150	68.04	255	115.67	360	163.29
50	22.68	155	70.31	260	117.93	365	165.56
55	24.95	160	72.57	265	120.20	370	167.83
60	27.22	165	74.84	270	122.47	375	170.10
65	29.48	170	77.11	275	124.74	380	172.36
70	31.75	175	79.38	280	127.01	385	174.63
75	34.02	180	81.65	285	129.27	390	176.90
80	36.29	185	83.91	290	131.54	395	179.17
85	38.56	190	86.18	295	133.81	400	181.44
90	40.82	195	88.45	300	136.08	405	183.70
95	43.09	200	90.72	305	138.34	410	185.97
100	45.36	205	92.99	310	140.61	415	188.24

TEMPERATURE CONVERSION							
FAHRENHEIT TO CELSIUS = (°F - 32) × ⁵/₉ = °C				CELSIUS TO FAHRENHEIT = (°C × ⁹/₅) + 32 = °F			
°F	°C	°F	°C	°C	°F	°C	°F
0.0	-17.8	50.0	10.0	0.0	32.0	38.0	100.4
5.0	-15.0	55.0	12.8	5.0	41.0	39.0	102.2
10.0	-12.2	60.0	15.6	10.0	50.0	40.0	104.0
15.0	-9.4	65.0	18.3	15.0	59.0	41.0	105.8
20.0	-6.7	70.0	21.1	20.0	68.0	42.0	107.6
25.0	-3.9	75.0	23.9	25.0	77.0	43.0	109.4
30.0	-1.1	80.0	26.7	30.0	86.0	44.0	111.2
35.0	1.7	85.0	29.4	35.0	95.0	45.0	113.0
40.0	4.4	90.0	32.2	36.0	96.8	46.0	114.8
45.0	7.2	91.0	32.8	37.0	98.6	47.0	116.6

TEMPERATURE CONVERSION *(Continued)*

FAHRENHEIT TO CELSIUS = (°F - 32) × $\frac{5}{9}$ = °C				CELSIUS TO FAHRENHEIT = (°C × $\frac{9}{5}$) + 32 = °F			
°F	°C	°F	°C	°C	°F	°C	°F
92.0	33.3	101.0	38.3	48.0	118.4	59.0	138.2
93.0	33.9	102.0	38.9	49.0	120.2	60.0	140.0
94.0	34.4	103.0	39.4	50.0	122.0	65.0	149.0
95.0	35.0	104.0	40.0	51.0	123.8	70.0	158.0
96.0	35.6	105.0	40.6	52.0	125.6	75.0	167.0
97.0	36.1	106.0	41.1	53.0	127.4	80.0	176.0
98.0	36.7	107.0	41.7	54.0	129.2	85.0	185.0
98.6	37.0	108.0	42.2	55.0	131.0	90.0	194.0
99.0	37.2	109.0	42.8	56.0	132.8	95.0	203.0
100.0	37.8	110.0	43.3	57.0	134.6	100.0	212.0
				58.0	136.4	105.0	221.0

PEDIATRIC DOSAGE ESTIMATION FORMULAS

The following formulas can be used to estimate the approximate pediatric dosage of a medication. These formulas are based on the adult dose and either the child's age or weight. These formulas should be used with caution, as the response to any drug is not always directly proportional to the age or weight of the child relative to the usual adult dose. Dosage will also vary based on the formula used. Care should be taken when using any of these methods to calculate the child's dosage. Some products have FDA-approved pediatric indications and dosages; always refer to the full prescribing information first before calculating a pediatric dosage.

BASED ON WEIGHT

Clark's Rule:
[weight (lb)/150] × adult dose = approximate child's dose
Example: If the child's weight is 15 kg (33 lb) and the adult dose is 50 mg then the child's dose is 11 mg.
(33/150) x 50 mg = 11 mg

BASED ON AGE

Dilling's Rule:
[age (years)/20] × adult dose = approximate child's dose
Example: If the child's age is 8 years and the adult dose is 50 mg then the child's dose is 20 mg.
(8/20) x 50 mg = 20 mg

Cowling's Rule:
$\frac{[\text{age at next birthday (years)}]}{24}$ × adult dose = approximate child's dose

Example: If the child is going to turn 8 years old in a few months and the adult dose is 50 mg then the child's dose is 16.7 mg.
(8/24) × 50 mg = 16.7 mg

Young's Rule:
$\frac{[\text{age (years)}]}{\text{age} + 12}$ × adult dose = approximate child's dose

Example: If the child's age is 8 years and the adult dose is 50 mg then the child's dose is 20 mg.
[8/(8 + 12)] x 50 mg = 20 mg

Fried's Rule (younger than 1 year):
$\frac{[\text{age (months)}]}{150}$ × adult dose = approximate infant's dose

Example: If the child's age is 10 months and the adult dose is 50 mg then the child's dose is 3.3 mg.
(10/150) x 50 mg = 3.33 mg

NORMAL LABORATORY VALUES: BLOOD, PLASMA, AND SERUM

TEST	SPECIMEN	CONVENTIONAL UNITS	SI UNITS
Acetoacetate	Plasma	< 1 mg/dL	< 0.1 mmol/L
Acetylcholinesterase (ACE), RBC	Blood	26.7–49.2 U/g Hb	—
Acid phosphatase	Serum	0.5–5.5 U/L	0–0.9 µkat/L
Activated partial thromboplastin time (aPTT)	Plasma	25–35 sec	—
Adrenocorticotropic hormone (ACTH)	Serum	9–52 pg/mL	2–11 pmol/L
Albumin	Serum	3.5–5.5 g/dL	35–55 g/L
Aldosterone:			
Standing	Serum	7–20 ng/dL	194–554 pmol/L
Supine	Serum	2–5 ng/dL	55–138 pmol/L
Alkaline phosphatase (ALP)	Serum	36–92 U/L	0.5–1.5 µkat/L
Alpha$_1$-antitrypsin (AAT)	Serum	83–199 mg/dL	—
Alpha fetoprotein (AFP)	Serum	0–20 ng/dL	0–20 pg/L
δ-Aminolevulinic acid (ALA)	Serum	15–23 µg/L	1.141.75 µmol/L
Aminotransferase, alanine (ALT)	Serum	0–35 U/L	0–0.58 pkat/L
Aminotransferase, aspartate (AST)	Serum	0–35 U/L	0–0.58 pkat/L
Ammonia	Plasma	40–80 µg/dL	23–47 µmol/L
Amylase	Serum	0–130 U/L	0–2.17 µkat/L
Antibodies to extractable nuclear antigen (AENA)	Serum	< 20.0 units	—
Anti–cyclic citrullinated peptide (anti-CCP) antibodies	Serum	≤ 5.0 units	—
Antidiuretic hormone (ADH; arginine vasopressin)	Plasma	< 1.7 pg/mL	< 1.57 pmol/L
Anti–double-stranded DNA (dsDNA) antibodies, IgG	Serum	< 25 IU	—
Antimitochondrial M2 antibodies	Serum	< 0.1 units	—
Antineutrophil cytoplasmic antibodies (cANCA)	Serum	Negative	—
Antinuclear antibodies (ANA)	Serum	≤ 1.0 units	—
Anti–smooth muscle antibodies (ASMA) titer	Serum	≤ 1:80	—
Antistreptolysin O titer	Serum	< 150 units	—
Antithyroid microsomal antibody titer	Serum	< 1:100	—
α_1-Antitrypsin (AAT)	Serum	83–199 mg/dL	15.3–36.6 µmol/L
Apolipoproteins:			
A-I, females	Serum	98–210 mg/dL	0.98–2.1 g/L
A-I, males	Serum	88–180 mg/dL	0.88–1.8 g/L
B-100, females	Serum	44–148 mg/dL	0.44–1.48 g/L
B-100, males	Serum	55–151 mg/dL	0.55–1.51 g/L

(Continued)

TEST	SPECIMEN	CONVENTIONAL UNITS	SI UNITS
Bicarbonate	Serum	23–28 mEq/L	23–28 mmol/L
Bilirubin:			
Direct	Serum	0–0.3 mg/dL	0–5.1 µmol/L
Total	Serum	0.3–1.2 mg/dL	5.1–20.5 µmol/L
Blood volume:			
Plasma, females	Blood	28–43 mL/kg body wt	0.028–0.043 L/kg body wt
Plasma, males	Blood	25–44 mL/kg body wt	0.025–0.044 L/kg body wt
RBCs, females	Blood	20–30 mL/kg body wt	0.02–0.03 L/kg body wt
RBCs, males	Blood	25–35 mL/kg body wt	0.025–0.035 L/kg body wt
Brain (B-type) natriuretic peptide (BNP)	Plasma	< 100 pg/mL	—
Calcitonin, age ≥ 16 yr:			
Females	Serum	< 8 pg/mL	—
Males	Serum	< 16 pg/mL	—
Calcium	Serum	9–10.5 mg/dL	2.2–2.6 mmol/L
Cancer antigen (CA):			
CA 125	Serum	< 35 U/mL	—
CA 15-3	Serum	< 30 U/mL	—
Carbon dioxide (CO_2) content	Serum	23–28 mEq/L	23–28 mmol/L
Carbon dioxide partial pressure (PCO_2)	Blood	35–45 mm Hg	—
Carboxyhemoglobin	Plasma	0.5–5%	—
Carcinoembryonic antigen (CEA)	Serum	< 2 ng/mL	< 2 µg/L
Carotene	Serum	75–300 µg/L	1.4–5.6 µmol/L
CD4:CD8 ratio	Blood	1–4	—
CD4+ T-cell count	Blood	640–1175/µL	$0.64–1.18 \times 10^9$/L
CD8+ T-cell count	Blood	335–875/µL	$0.34–0.88 \times 10^9$/L
Ceruloplasmin	Serum	25–43 mg/dL	250–430 mg/L
Chloride	Serum	98–106 mEq/L	98–106 mmol/L
Cholesterol, desirable level:			
High-density lipoprotein (HDL-C)	Plasma	≥ 40 mg/dL	≥ 1.04 mmol/L
Low-density lipoprotein (LDL-C)	Plasma	≤ 130 mg/dL	≤ 3.36 mmol/L
Total (TC)	Plasma	150–199 mg/dL	3.88–5.15 mmol/L
Coagulation factors:			
Factor I	Plasma	150–300 mg/dL	—
Factor II	Plasma	60–150% of normal	—
Factor IX	Plasma	60–150% of normal	—
Factor V	Plasma	60–150% of normal	—
Factor VII	Plasma	60–150% of normal	—
Factor VIII	Plasma	60–150% of normal	—
Factor X	Plasma	60–150% of normal	—
Factor XI	Plasma	60–150% of normal	—
Factor XII	Plasma	60–150% of normal	—
Complement:			
C3	Serum	55–120 mg/dL	0.55–1.20 g/L
C4	Serum	20–59 mg/dL	0.20–0.59 g/L
Total	Serum	37–55 U/mL	37–55 kU/L
Copper	Serum	70–155 µg/L	11–24.3 µmol/L

TEST	SPECIMEN	CONVENTIONAL UNITS	SI UNITS
Cortisol:			
1 h after cosyntropin	Serum	> 18 μg/dL and usually ≥ 8 μg/dL above baseline	> 498 nmol/L and usually ≥ 221 nmol/L above baseline
At 5 PM	Serum	3–13 μg/dL	83–359 nmol/L
At 8 AM	Serum	8–20 μg/dL	251–552 nmol/L
After overnight suppression test	Serum	< 5 μg/dL	< 138 nmol/L
C-peptide	Serum	0.9–4.3 ng/mL	297–1419 pmol/L
C-reactive protein (CRP)	Serum	< 0.5 mg/dL	< 0.005 g/L
C-reactive protein, highly sensitive (hsCRP)	Serum	< 1.1 mg/L	< 0.0011 g/L
Creatine kinase (CK)	Serum	30–170 U/L	0.5–2.83 μkat/L
Creatinine	Serum	0.7–1.3 mg/dL	61.9–115 μmol/L
D-Dimer	Plasma	≤ 300 ng/mL	≤ 300 μg/L
Dehydroepiandrosterone sulfate (DHEA-S):			
Females	Plasma	0.6–3.3 mg/mL	1.6–8.9 μmol/L
Males	Plasma	1.3–5.5 mg/mL	3.5–14.9 μmol/L
δ-Aminolevulinic acid (ALA)	Serum	15–23 μg/L	1.14–1.75 μmol/L
11-Deoxycortisol (DOC):			
After metyrapone	Plasma	> 7 μg/dL	> 203 nmol/L
Basal	Plasma	< 5 μg/dL	< 145 nmol/L
D-Xylose level 2 h after ingestion of 25 g of D-xylose	Serum	> 20 mg/dL	> 1.3 nmol/L
Epinephrine, supine	Plasma	< 75 ng/L	< 410 pmol/L
Erythrocyte sedimentation rate (ESR):			
Females	Blood	0–20 mm/h	0–20 mm/h
Males	Blood	0–15 mm/h	0–20 mm/h
Erythropoietin	Serum	4.0–18.5 mIU/mL	4.0–18.5 IU/L
Estradiol, females:			
Day 1–10 of menstrual cycle	Serum	14–27 pg/mL	50–100 pmol/L
Day 11–20 of menstrual cycle	Serum	14–54 pg/mL	50–200 pmol/L
Day 21–30 of menstrual cycle	Serum	19–40 pg/mL	70–150 pmol/L
Estradiol, males	Serum	10–30 pg/mL	37–110 pmol/L
Ferritin	Serum	15–200 ng/mL	15–200 μg/L
α-Fetoprotein (AFP)	Serum	0–20 ng/dL	0–20 pg/L
Fibrinogen	Plasma	150–350 mg/dL	1.5–3.5 g/L
Folate (folic acid):			
RBC	Blood	160–855 ng/mL	362–1937 nmol/L
Serum	Serum	2.5–20 ng/mL	5.7–45.3 nmol/L
Follicle-stimulating hormone (FSH), females:			
Follicular or luteal phase	Serum	5–20 mU/mL	5–20 U/L
Midcycle peak	Serum	30–50 mU/mL	30–50 U/L
Postmenopausal	Serum	> 35 mU/mL	> 35 U/L
Follicle-stimulating hormone (FSH), adult males	Serum	5–15 mU/mL	5–15 U/L
Fructosamine	Plasma	200–285 mol/L	—

(Continued)

TEST	SPECIMEN	CONVENTIONAL UNITS	SI UNITS
Gamma-glutamyl transpeptidase (GGT)	Serum	8–78 U/L	—
Gastrin	Serum	0–180 pg/mL	0–180 ng/L
Globulins:	Serum	2.5–3.5 g/dL	25–35 g/L
α_1-Globulins	Serum	0.2–0.4 g/dL	2–4 g/L
α_2-Globulins	Serum	0.5–0.9 g/dL	5–9 g/L
β-Globulins	Serum	0.6–1.1 g/dL	6–11 g/L
γ-Globulins	Serum	0.7–1.7 g/dL	7–17 g/L
β_2-Microglobulin	Serum	0.7–1.8 µg/mL	—
Glucose:			
2-h postprandial	Plasma	< 140 mg/dL	< 7.8 mmol/L
Fasting	Plasma	70–105 mg/dL	3.9–5.8 mmol/L
Glucose-6-phosphate dehydrogenase (G6PD)	Blood	5–15 U/g Hb	0.32–0.97 mU/mol Hb
γ-Glutamyl transpeptidase (GGT)	Serum	8–78 U/L	—
Growth hormone:			
After oral glucose	Plasma	< 2 ng/mL	< 2 µg/L
In response to provocative stimuli	Plasma	> 7 ng/mL	> 7 µg/L
Haptoglobin	Serum	30–200 mg/dL	300–2000 mg/L
Hematocrit:			
Females	Blood	36–47%	—
Males	Blood	41–51%	—
Hemoglobin:			
Females	Blood	12–16 g/dL	120–160 g/L
Males	Blood	14–17 g/dL	140–170 g/L
Hemoglobin A_{1c}	Blood	4.7–8.5%	—
Hemoglobin electrophoresis, adults:			
Hb A_1	Blood	95–98%	—
Hb A_2	Blood	2–3%	—
Hb C	Blood	0%	—
Hb F	Blood	0.8–2.0%	—
Hb S	Blood	0%	—
Hemoglobin electrophoresis, Hb F in children:			
Neonate	Blood	50–80%	—
1–6 mo	Blood	8%	—
> 6 mo	Blood	1–2%	—
Homocysteine:			
Females	Plasma	0.40–1.89 mg/L	3–14 µmol/L
Males	Plasma	0.54–2.16 mg/L	4–16 µmol/L
Human chorionic gonadotropin (hCG), quantitative	Serum	< 5 mIU/mL	—

TEST	SPECIMEN	CONVENTIONAL UNITS	SI UNITS
Immunoglobulins:			
IgA	Serum	70–300 mg/dL	0.7–3.0 g/L
IgD	Serum	< 8 mg/dL	< 80 mg/L
IgE	Serum	0.01–0.04 mg/dL	0.1–0.4 mg/L
IgG	Serum	640–1430 mg/dL	6.4–14.3 g/L
IgG$_1$	Serum	280–1020 mg/dL	2.8–10.2 g/L
IgG$_2$	Serum	60–790 mg/dL	0.6–7.9 g/L
IgG$_3$	Serum	14–240 mg/dL	0.14–2.4 g/L
IgG$_4$	Serum	11–330 mg/dL	0.11–3.3 g/L
IgM	Serum	20–140 mg/dL	0.2–1.4 g/L
Insulin, fasting	Serum	1.4–14 µIU/mL	10–104 pmol/L
International normalized ratio (INR):			
Therapeutic range (standard intensity therapy)	Plasma	2.0–3.0	—
Therapeutic range in patients at higher risk (eg, patients with prosthetic heart valves)	Plasma	2.5–3.5	—
Therapeutic range in patients with lupus anticoagulant	Plasma	3.0–3.5	—
Iron	Serum	60–160 µg/dL	11–29 µmol/L
Iron binding capacity, total (TIBC)	Serum	250–460 µg/dL	45–82 µmol/L
Lactate dehydrogenase (LDH)	Serum	60–160 U/L	1–1.67 µkat/L
Lactic acid, venous	Blood	6–16 mg/dL	0.67–1.8 mmol/L
Lactose tolerance test	Plasma	> 15 mg/dL increase in plasma glucose level	> 0.83 mmol/L increase in plasma glucose level
Lead	Blood	< 40 µg/dL	< 1.9 µmol/L
Leukocyte alkaline phosphatase (LAP) score	Peripheral blood smear	13–130/100/polymorphonuclear (PMN) leukocyte neutrophils and bands	—
Lipase	Serum	< 95 U/L	< 1.58 µkat/L
Lipoprotein (a) [Lp(a)]	Serum	≤ 30 mg/dL	< 1.1 µmol/L
Luteinizing hormone (LH), females:			
Follicular or luteal phase	Serum	5–22 mU/mL	5–22 U/L
Midcycle peak	Serum	30–250 mU/mL	30–250 U/L
Postmenopausal	Serum	> 30 mU/mL	> 30 U/L
Luteinizing hormone, males	Serum	3–15 mU/mL	3–15 U/L
Magnesium	Serum	1.5–2.4 mg/dL	0.62–0.99 mmol/L
Manganese	Serum	0.3–0.9 ng/mL	5.5–16.4 nmol/L
Mean corpuscular hemoglobin (MCH)	Blood	28–32 pg	—
Mean corpuscular hemoglobin concentration (MCHC)	Blood	32–36 g/dL	320–360 g/L
Mean corpuscular volume (MCV)	Blood	80–100 fL	—
Metanephrines, fractionated:			
Metanephrines, free	Plasma	< 0.50 nmol/L	—
Normetanephrines, free	Plasma	< 0.90 nmol/L	—
Methemoglobin	Blood	< 1.0%	—
Methylmalonic acid (MMA)	Serum	150–370 nmol/L	—

(Continued)

TEST	SPECIMEN	CONVENTIONAL UNITS	SI UNITS
Myeloperoxidase (MPO) antibodies	Serum	< 6.0 U/mL	—
Myoglobin:			
Females	Serum	25–58 µg/L	1.4–3.5 nmol/L
Males	Serum	28–72 µg/L	1.6–4.1 nmol/L
Norepinephrine, supine	Plasma	50–440 pg/mL	0.3–2.6 nmol/L
N-Terminal propeptide of BNP (NT-proBNP)	Plasma	< 125 pg/mL	—
5'-Nucleotidase (5'NT)	Serum	4–11.5 U/L	
Osmolality	Plasma	275–295 mOsm/kg H_2O	275–295 mmol/kg H_2O
Osmotic fragility test	Blood	Increased fragility if hemolysis occurs in > 0.5% NaCl	—
		Decreased fragility if hemolysis is incomplete in 0.3% NaCl	
Oxygen partial pressure (PO_2)	Blood	80–100 mm Hg	—
Parathyroid hormone (PTH)	Serum	10–65 pg/mL	10–65 ng/L
Parathyroid hormone–related peptide (PTHrP)	Plasma	< 2.0 pmol/L	—
Partial thromboplastin time, activated (aPTT)	Plasma	25–35 sec	—
pH	Blood	7.38–7.44	—
Phosphorus, inorganic	Serum	3.0–4.5 mg/dL	0.97–1.45 mmol/L
Platelet count	Blood	150–350 x 10^3/µL	150–350 x 10^9/L
Platelet life span, using chromium-51 (^{51}Cr)	—	8–12 days	—
Porphyrins	Plasma	≤ 1.0 µg/dL	—
Potassium	Serum	3.5–5 mEq/L	3.5–5 mmol/L
Prealbumin (transthyretin)	Serum	18–45 mg/dL	—
Progesterone:			
Follicular phase	Serum	< 1 ng/mL	< 0.03 nmol/L
Luteal phase	Serum	3–30 ng/mL	0.1–0.95 nmol/L
Prolactin:			
Females	Serum	< 20 µg/L	< 870 pmol/L
Males	Serum	< 15 µg/L	< 652 pmol/L
Prostate-specific antigen, total (PSA-T)	Serum	0–4 ng/mL	—
Prostate-specific antigen, ratio of free to total (PSA-F:PSA-T)	Serum	> 0.25	—
Protein C activity	Plasma	67–131%	—
Protein C resistance, activated ratio (APC-R)	Plasma	2.2–2.6	—
Protein S activity	Plasma	82–144%	—
Protein, total	Serum	6–7.8 g/dL	60–78 g/L
Prothrombin time (PT)	Plasma	11–13 sec	—
Pyruvate	Blood	0.08–0.16 mmol/L	—
RBC count	Blood	4.2–5.9 x 10^6 cells/µL	4.2–5.9 x 10^{12} cells/L
RBC survival rate, using ^{51}Cr	Blood	$T_{1/2}$ = 28 days	

TEST	SPECIMEN	CONVENTIONAL UNITS	SI UNITS
Renin activity, plasma (PRA), upright, in males and females aged 18-39 yr:			
Sodium-depleted	Plasma	2.9–24 ng/mL/h	—
Sodium-repleted	Plasma	0.6 (or lower)–4.3 ng/mL/h	—
Reticulocyte count:			
Percentage	Blood	0.5–1.5%	—
Absolute	Blood	23–90 x 10^3/μL	23–90 x 10^9/L
Rheumatoid factor (RF)	Serum	< 40 U/mL	< 40 kU/L
Sodium	Serum	136–145 mEq/L	136–145 mmol/L
Testosterone, adults:			
Females	Serum	20–75 ng/dL	0.7–2.6 nmol/L
Males	Serum	300–1200 ng/dL	10–42 nmol/L
Thrombin time	Plasma	18.5–24 sec	—
Thyroid iodine-123 (^{123}I) uptake	—	5–30% of administered dose at 24 h	—
Thyroid-stimulating hormone (TSH)	Serum	0.5–5.0 μIU/mL	0.5–5.0 mIU/L
Thyroxine (T_4):			
Free	Serum	0.9–2.4 ng/dL	12–31 pmol/L
Free index	—	4–11 μg/dL	—
Total	Serum	5–12 μg/dL	64–155 nmol/L
Transferrin	Serum	212–360 mg/dL	2.1–3.6 g/L
Transferrin saturation	Serum	20–50%	—
Triglycerides (desirable level)	Serum	< 250 mg/dL	< 2.82 mmol/L
Triiodothyronine (T_3):			
Uptake	Serum	25–35%	—
Total	Serum	70–195 ng/dL	1.1–3.0 nmol/L
Troponin I	Plasma	< 0.1 ng/mL	< 0.1 μg/L
Troponin T	Serum	≤ 0.03 ng/mL	≤ 0.03 μg/L
Urea nitrogen (BUN)	Serum	8–20 mg/dL	2.9–7.1 mmol/L
Uric acid	Serum	2.5–8 mg/dL	0.15–0.47 mmol/L
Vitamin B_{12}	Serum	200–800 pg/mL	148–590 pmol/L
Vitamin C (ascorbic acid):			
Leukocyte	Blood	< 20 mg/dL	< 1136 μmol/L
Total	Blood	0.4–1.5 mg/dL	23–85 μmol/L
Vitamin D:			
1,25-Dihydroxycholecalciferol (calcitriol)	Serum	25–65 pg/mL	65–169 pmol/L
25-Hydroxycholecalciferol	Serum	15–80 ng/mL	37–200 nmol/L
WBC count	Blood	3.9–10.7 x 10^3 cells/μL	3.9–10.7 x 10^9 cells/L
Zinc	Serum	66–110 μg/dL	10.1–16.8 μmol/L

μkat = microkatal; pkat = picokatal.

From the Merck Manual of Diagnosis and Therapy, edited by Robert Porter. Copyright 2010–2013 by Merck Sharp & Dohme Corp., a subsidiary of Merck & Co., Inc., Whitehouse Station, NJ. Available at: http://www.merckmanuals.com/professional/. Accessed March 2014.

POISON CONTROL CENTERS

The American Association of Poison Control Centers (AAPCC) uses a single, nationwide emergency number to automatically link callers with their regional poison center. This toll-free number, **800-222-1222**, also works for **teletype lines (TTY)** for the hearing-impaired and **telecommunication devices (TDD)** for individuals who are deaf. The ASPCA/Animal Poison Center is not part of the nationwide system, and has its own emergency number. Within each state, centers are listed alphabetically by city, with their corresponding addresses.

ALABAMA

BIRMINGHAM

Regional Poison Control Center
Children's Hospital of Alabama

1600 7th Ave S
Birmingham AL 35233-1711
www.childrensal.org

ALASKA

(PORTLAND, OR)

Oregon Poison Center
Oregon Health & Science University

3181 SW Sam Jackson Park Rd –
Suite CB550
Portland OR 97239
www.ohsu.edu/xd/outreach/
oregon-poison-center

ARIZONA

PHOENIX

Banner Good Samaritan Poison and Drug Information Center
Banner Good Samaritan Medical Center

1111 E McDowell
Phoenix AZ 85006
www.bannerpoisoncontrol.com

TUCSON

Arizona Poison & Drug Information Center
Arizona Health Sciences Center

1295 N Martin, Room B308
Tucson AZ 85721
www.pharmacy.arizona.edu/
poisoncenter

ARKANSAS

LITTLE ROCK

Arkansas Poison and Drug Information Center
College of Pharmacy – UAMS

4301 W Markham St – MS 522-2
Little Rock AR 72205
www.arpoisoncenter.org

ASPCA/Animal Poison Control Center

1717 S Philo Rd – Suite 36
Urbana IL 61802
Business: 217-337-5030
Emergency: 888-426-4435
(not part of nationwide emergency system)
www.aspca.org/apcc

CALIFORNIA

FRESNO/MADERA

California Poison Control System
Fresno/Madera Division
Children's Hospital Central California

9300 Valley Children's Place – MB 15
Madera CA 93638
www.calpoison.org

SACRAMENTO

California Poison Control System
Sacramento Division
UC Davis Medical Center

2315 Stockton Blvd
Sacramento CA 95817
www.calpoison.org

SAN DIEGO

California Poison Control System
San Diego Division
UC San Diego Medical Center

200 W Arbor Dr
San Diego CA 92103-8925
www.calpoison.org

SAN FRANCISCO

California Poison Control System
San Francisco Division

UCSF Box 1369
San Francisco CA 94143
www.calpoison.org

COLORADO

DENVER

Rocky Mountain Poison & Drug Center

777 Bannock St – MC 0180
Denver CO 80204-4028
www.rmpdc.org

CONNECTICUT

FARMINGTON

Connecticut Poison Control Center
University of Connecticut Health Center

263 Farmington Ave
Farmington CT 06030-5365
poisoncontrol.uchc.edu

DELAWARE

(PHILADELPHIA, PA)

The Poison Control Center
The Children's Hospital of Philadelphia

34th & Civic Center Blvd
Philadelphia PA 19104
www.chop.edu/service/
poison-control-center/home.html

DISTRICT OF COLUMBIA

WASHINGTON, DC

National Capital Poison Center

3201 New Mexico Ave NW
Suite 310
Washington DC 20016
www.poison.org

FLORIDA

JACKSONVILLE

Florida/USVI Poison Information Center-Jacksonville

655 W 8th St, Box C23
Jacksonville FL 32209
www.fpicjax.org

(Continued)

MIAMI

Florida Poison Information Center-Miami

Jackson Memorial Hospital/University
of Miami Miller School of Medicine
1611 NW 12th Ave (R-131)
Institute Annex, 3rd Floor
Miami FL 33136
www.miamipoison.org

TAMPA

Florida Poison Information Center-Tampa
Tampa General Hospital

PO Box 1289
Tampa FL 33601
www.poisoncentertampa.org

GEORGIA

ATLANTA

Georgia Poison Center
Hughes Spalding Children's Hospital
Grady Health System

50 Hurt Plaza – Suite 600
PO Box 26066
Atlanta GA 30303
www.georgiapoisoncenter.org

HAWAII

(DENVER, CO)

Rocky Mountain Poison & Drug Center

777 Bannock St – MC 0180
Denver CO 80204-4507
www.rmpdc.org

IDAHO

(OMAHA, NE)

Nebraska Regional Poison Center

8401 W Dodge Rd – Suite 115
Omaha NE 68114
www.nebraskapoison.com

ILLINOIS

CHICAGO

Illinois Poison Center

222 S Riverside Plaza – Suite 1900
Chicago IL 60606
www.illinoispoisoncenter.org

INDIANA

INDIANAPOLIS

Indiana Poison Center
IU Methodist Hospital
Indiana University Health

1701 N Senate Blvd, Room B402
Indianapolis IN 46202
www.indianapoison.org

IOWA

SIOUX CITY

Iowa Statewide Poison Control Center

401 Douglas St – Suite 402
Sioux City IA 51101
www.iowapoison.org

KANSAS

KANSAS CITY

The University of Kansas Hospital Poison Control Center
University of Kansas Medical Center

3901 Rainbow Blvd
Room B-400
Kansas City KS 66160-7231
www.kumed.com/poison

KENTUCKY

LOUISVILLE

Kentucky Regional Poison Center

Medical Towers South
234 E Gray St – Suite 847
Louisville KY 40202
www.kosairchildrenshospital.com/
poisoncontrol

LOUISIANA

SHREVEPORT

Louisiana Poison Center LSUHSC - Shreveport Department of Emergency Medicine - Section of Clinical Toxicology

1455 Wilkinson St
Shreveport LA 71130
www.lapcc.org

MAINE

PORTLAND

Northern New England Poison Center

22 Bramhall St
Portland ME 04101
www.nnepc.org

MARYLAND

BALTIMORE

Maryland Poison Center
University of Maryland School of Pharmacy

220 Arch St, Office Level 1
Baltimore MD 21201
www.mdpoison.com

(WASHINGTON, DC)

National Capital Poison Center

3201 New Mexico Ave NW
Suite 310
Washington DC 20016
www.poison.org

MASSACHUSETTS

BOSTON

Regional Center for Poison Control and Prevention

300 Longwood Ave
IC Smith Building
Boston MA 02115
www.maripoisoncenter.com

MICHIGAN

DETROIT

Children's Hospital of Michigan Regional Poison Control Center

4707 St Antoine – Suite 302
Detroit MI 48201
www.mitoxic.org

MINNESOTA

MINNEAPOLIS

Minnesota Poison Control System
Hennepin County Medical Center

701 Park Ave, Mail Code RL
Minneapolis MN 55415
www.mnpoison.org

MISSISSIPPI

JACKSON

Mississippi Regional Poison Control Center
University of Mississippi Medical Center

2500 N State St
Jackson MS 39216
poisoncontrol.umc.edu

MISSOURI

ST. LOUIS

Missouri Regional Poison Center
Cardinal Glennon Children's Medical Center

7980 Clayton Rd – Suite 200
St. Louis MO 63117
www.cardinalglennon.com/Pages/
missouri-poison-center.aspx

MONTANA

(DENVER, CO)

Rocky Mountain Poison & Drug Center

777 Bannock St – MC 0180
Denver CO 80204-4028
www.rmpdc.org

NEBRASKA

OMAHA

Nebraska Regional Poison Center

8200 W Dodge Rd
Omaha NE 68114
www.nebraskapoison.com

NEVADA

(DENVER, CO)

Rocky Mountain Poison & Drug Center

777 Bannock St – MC 0180
Denver CO 80204-4028
www.rmpdc.org

NEW HAMPSHIRE

(PORTLAND, ME)

Northern New England Poison Center

22 Bramhall St
Portland ME 04102
www.nnepc.org

NEW JERSEY

NEWARK

New Jersey Poison Information and Education System
University of Medicine and Dentistry at New Jersey

140 Bergen St – PO Box 1709
Newark NJ 07107-170
www.njpies.org

NEW MEXICO

ALBUQUERQUE

New Mexico Poison & Drug Information Center

MSC 09 5080
1 University of New Mexico
Albuquerque NM 87131
nmpoisoncenter.unm.edu

NEW YORK

NEW YORK CITY

New York City Poison Control Center
NYC Bureau of Public Health Labs

455 1st Ave – Room 123
Box 81
New York NY 10016
www.nyc.gov/html/doh/html/
environmental/poison-control.shtml

SYRACUSE

Upstate New York Poison Center

750 E Adams St
Syracuse NY 13210
www.upstatepoison.org

NORTH CAROLINA

CHARLOTTE

Carolinas Poison Center
Carolinas Medical Center

PO Box 32861
Charlotte NC 28232
www.ncpoisoncenter.org

NORTH DAKOTA

(MINNEAPOLIS, MN)

Hennepin Regional Poison Center
Hennepin County Medical Center

701 Park Ave, Mail Code RL
Minneapolis MN 55415
www.mnpoison.org

OHIO

CINCINNATI

Cincinnati Drug and Poison Information Center
Regional Poison Control System

3333 Burnett Ave
MLC 9004
Cincinnati OH 45229-9004
www.cincinnatichildrens.org/dpic

CLEVELAND

Northern Ohio Poison Center
University Hospitals

11100 Euclid Ave – B261 MP6007
Cleveland OH 44106-6010
www.uhhospitals.org/rainbow/
services/emergency-medicine/
poison-emergency-and-prevention

COLUMBUS

Central Ohio Poison Center
Nationwide Children's Hospital

700 Children's Dr
Columbus OH 43205
www.bepoisonsmart.com

OKLAHOMA

OKLAHOMA CITY

Oklahoma Poison Control Center
Oklahoma University Health Science Center

940 NE 13th St – Room 3N3510
Oklahoma City OK 73104
www.oklahomapoison.org

OREGON

PORTLAND

Oregon Poison Center
Oregon Health & Science University

3181 SW Sam Jackson Park Rd – CB550
Portland OR 97239
www.oregonpoison.org

PENNSYLVANIA

PHILADELPHIA

The Poison Control Center
Children's Hospital of Philadelphia

34th & Civic Center Blvd
Philadelphia PA 19104
www.chop.edu/service/poison-
control-center

PITTSBURGH

Pittsburgh Poison Center

200 Lothrop St
Pittsburgh PA 15213
www.chp.edu/CHP/poisoncenter

(Continued)

RHODE ISLAND

(BOSTON, MA)

Regional Center for Poison Control and Prevention

300 Longwood Ave
IC Smith Building
Boston MA 02115
www.maripoisoncenter.com

SOUTH CAROLINA

COLUMBIA

Palmetto Poison Center
South Carolina College of Pharmacy

University of South Carolina
Columbia SC 29208
www.poison.sc.edu

SOUTH DAKOTA

(MINNEAPOLIS, MN)

Hennepin Regional Poison Center
Hennepin County Medical Center

701 Park Ave, Mail Code RL
Minneapolis MN 55415
www.mnpoison.org

SIOUX FALLS

Sanford Poison Center
Sanford Health USD Medical Center

1305 W 18th St – PO Box 5039
Sioux Falls SD 57117
www.sdpoison.org

TENNESSEE

NASHVILLE

Tennessee Poison Center

501 Oxford House
1161 21st Ave S
Nashville TN 37232-4632
www.tnpoisoncenter.org

TEXAS

AMARILLO

Texas Panhandle Poison Center
Texas Tech University

HSC School of Pharmacy
1501 S Coulter Dr – Suite 105
Amarillo TX 79106
www.poisoncontrol.org

DALLAS

North Texas Poison Center
Parkland Health & Hospital System

5201 Harry Hines Blvd
Dallas TX 75235
www.poisoncontrol.org

EL PASO

West Texas Regional Poison Center
University Medical Center of El Paso

4815 Alameda Ave
El Paso TX 79905
www.poisoncontrol.org

GALVESTON

Southeast Texas Poison Center
The University of Texas Medical Branch

3.112 Trauma Bldg
Galveston TX 77555-1175
www.poisoncontrol.org

SAN ANTONIO

South Texas Poison Center
The University of Texas Health Science Center-San Antonio

7703 Floyd Curl Dr – MSC 7849
Trauma Bldg
San Antonio TX 78229-3900
www.texaspoison.com

TEMPLE

Central Texas Poison Center
Scott & White Memorial Hospital

2401 S 31st St
Temple TX 76508
www.poisoncontrol.org

UTAH

SALT LAKE CITY

Utah Poison Control Center
University of Utah

30 S 2000 E – Suite 4540
Salt Lake City UT 84112
poisoncontrol.utah.edu

VERMONT

(PORTLAND, ME)

Northern New England Poison Center

2 Bramhall St
Portland ME 04102
www.nnepc.org

VIRGINIA

CHARLOTTESVILLE

Blue Ridge Poison Center

1222 Jefferson Park Ave
PO Box 800774
Charlottesville VA 22908-0774
www.healthsystem.virginia.edu/internet/brpc

RICHMOND

Virginia Poison Center
Medical College of Virginia Hospitals
Virginia Commonwealth University Health System

PO Box 980522
Richmond VA 23298-0522
www.poison.vcu.edu

(WASHINGTON, DC)

National Capital Poison Center

3201 New Mexico Ave NW
Suite 310
Washington DC 20016
www.poison.org

WASHINGTON

SEATTLE

Washington Poison Control Center

155 NE 100th St – Suite 100
Seattle WA 98125-8007
www.wapc.org

WEST VIRGINIA

CHARLESTON

West Virginia Poison Center

3110 MacCorkle Ave SE
Charleston WV 25304
www.wvpoisoncenter.org

WISCONSIN

MILWAUKEE

Wisconsin Poison Center

PO Box 1997, Mail Station C660
Milwaukee WI 53201-1997
www.wisconsinpoison.org

WYOMING

(OMAHA, NE)

Nebraska Regional Poison Center

8401 W Dodge Rd – Suite 115
Omaha NE 68114
www.nebraskapoison.com

CERTIFICATION PROGRAMS FOR NURSES

Organization	Website
American Nurses Credentialing Center (ANCC)	**www.nursecredentialing.org**

American Nurses Credentialing Center (ANCC) — www.nursecredentialing.org
- Acute Care Nurse Practitioner-Board Certified (ACNP-BC)
- Adult Health Clinical Nurse Specialist-Board Certified (ACNS-BC)
- Adult Nurse Practitioner-Board Certified (ANP-BC)
- Adult Psychiatric–Mental Health Clinical Nurse Specialist-Board Certified (PMHCNS-BC)
- Adult Psychiatric–Mental Health Nurse Practitioner-Board Certified (PMHNP-BC)
- Adult-Gerontology Acute Care Nurse Practitioner-Board Certified (AGACNP-BC)
- Adult-Gerontology Clinical Nurse Specialist-Board Certified (AGCNS-BC)
- Adult-Gerontology Primary Care Nurse Practitioner-Board Certified (AGPCNP-BC)
- Advanced Diabetes Management
- Advanced Forensic Nursing-Board Certified (AFN-BC)
- Advanced Public Health Nursing-Board Certified (APHN-BC)
- Ambulatory Care Nursing, Registered Nurse-Board Certified (RN-BC)
- Cardiac Rehabilitation Nursing, Registered Nurse-Board Certified (RN-BC)
- Cardiac-Vascular Nursing, Registered Nurse-Board Certified (RN-BC)
- Certified Vascular Nurse, Registered Nurse-Board Certified (RN-BC)
- Child/Adolescent Psychiatric–Mental Health Clinical Nurse Specialist-Board Certified (PMHCNS-BC)
- Clinical Nurse Specialist-Board Certified (CNS-BC)
- College Health Nursing, Registered Nurse-Board Certified (RN-BC)
- Community Health Nursing, Registered Nurse-Board Certified (RN-BC)
- Emergency Nurse Practitioner-Board Certified (ENP-BC)
- Faith Community Nursing
- Family Nurse Practitioner-Board Certified (FNP-BC)
- Fundamentals of Magnet™ (Certificate Holder in Fundamentals of Magnet)
- General Nursing Practice, Registered Nurse-Board Certified (RN-BC)
- Gerontological Clinical Nurse Specialist-Board Certified (GCNS-BC)
- Gerontological Nurse Practitioner-Board Certified (GNP-BC)
- Gerontological Nursing, Registered Nurse-Board Certified (RN-BC)
- Guided Care Nursing (Certificate Holder in Guided Care Nursing)
- High-Risk Perinatal Nursing, Registered Nurse-Board Certified (RN-BC)
- Home Health Clinical Nurse Specialist-Board Certified (HHCNS-BC)
- Home Health Nursing, Registered Nurse-Board Certified (RN-BC)
- Informatics Nursing, Registered Nurse-Board Certified (RN-BC)
- Medical-Surgical Nursing, Registered Nurse-Board Certified (RN-BC)
- Nurse Executive-Board Certified (NE-BC)
- Nurse Executive, Advanced-Board Certified (NEA-BC)
- Nursing Case Management, Registered Nurse-Board Certified (RN-BC)
- Nursing Professional Development, Registered Nurse-Board Certified (RN-BC)
- Pain Management Nursing, Registered Nurse-Board Certified (RN-BC)
- Pediatric Clinical Nurse Specialist-Board Certified (PCNS-BC)
- Pediatric Nursing, Registered Nurse-Board Certified (RN-BC)
- Pediatric Primary Care Nurse Practitioner-Board Certified (PPCNP-BC)
- Perinatal Nursing, Registered Nurse-Board Certified (RN-BC)
- Psychiatric–Mental Health Nurse Practitioner-Board Certified (PMHNP-BC)
- Psychiatric–Mental Health Nursing, Registered Nurse-Board Certified (RN-BC)
- Public/Community Health Clinical Nurse Specialist-Board Certified (PHCNS-BC)
- School Nurse Practitioner-Board Certified (SNP-BC)
- School Nursing, Registered Nurse-Board Certified (RN-BC)

American Academy of Medical Esthetic Professionals (AAMEP) — www.aamep.org
- Medical Esthetics Practitioner-Certified (MEP-C)

Association for the Advancement of Medical Instrumentation (AAMI) — www.aami.org
- Certified Biomedical Equipment Technician (CBET)
- Certified Laboratory Equipment Specialist (CLES)
- Certified Radiology Equipment Specialist (CRES)

Organization	Website
American Society of Ophthalmic Registered Nurses (ASORN) • Certified Registered Nurse of Ophthalmology (CRNO)	www.asorn.org
American Board of Certification for Gastroenterology Nurses (ABCGN) • Certified Gastroenterology Registered Nurse (CGRN)	www.abcgn.org
National Council of State Boards of Nursing (NCSBN) • Medication Aide Certification Examination (MACE) • National Council Licensure Examination for Practical Nurses (NCLEX-PN) • National Council Licensure Examination for Registered Nurses (NCLEX-RN) • National Nurse Aide Assessment Program (NNAAP) • Nurse Licensure Compact (NLC) • Nurse Practitioner Certification	www.ncsbn.org
National Certification Board for Diabetes Educators (NCBDE) • Certified Diabetes Educator (CDE)	www.ncbde.org
Board of Certification for Emergency Nursing (BCEN) • Certified Emergency Nurse (CEN) • Certified Flight Registered Nurse (CFRN) • Certified Pediatric Emergency Nurse (CPEN) • Certified Transport Registered Nurse (CTRN)	www.bcencertifications.org
HIV/AIDS Nursing Certification Board (HANCB) • HIV/AIDS Nursing	www.hancb.org
Certification Board of Infection Control & Epidemiology (CBIC) • Certification in Infection Control (CIC)	www.cbic.org
Infusion Nurses Society (INS) • Certified Registered Nurse Infusion (CRNI®) Certification	www.ins1.org
National Certification Corporation (NCC) • Electronic Fetal Monitoring (C-EFM) • Inpatient Obstetric Nursing (RNC-OB) • Low Risk Neonatal Nursing (RNC-LRN) • Maternal Newborn Nursing (RNC-MNN) • Neonatal Intensive Care Nursing (RNC-NIC) • Neonatal Nurse Practitioner (NNP-BC) • Neonatal Pediatric Transport (C-NPT) • Women's Health Care Nurse Practitioner (WHNP-BC)	www.nccwebsite.org
Oncology Nursing Certification Corporation (ONCC®) • Advanced Oncology Certified Clinical Nurse Specialist (AOCNS®) • Advanced Oncology Certified Nurse (AOCN®) • Advanced Oncology Certified Nurse Practitioner (AOCNP®) • Blood and Marrow Transplant Certified Nurse (BMTCN™) • Certified Breast Care Nurse (CBCN®) • Certified Pediatric Hematology Oncology Nurse (CPHON®) • Certified Pediatric Oncology Nurse (CPON®) • Oncology Certified Nurse (OCN®)	www.oncc.org
American Academy of Pain Management (AAPM) • Credentialed Pain Practitioner (CPP)	www.aapainmanage.org
Competency & Credentialing Institute (CCI) • Clinical Nurse Specialist Perioperative Certification (CNS-CP) • Perioperative Nursing (CNOR® & CRNFA®)	www.cc-institute.org
American Society of Plastic Surgical Nurses (ASPSN) • Certified Aesthetic Nurse Specialist (CANS) • Certified Plastic Surgical Nurse (CPSN)	www.aspsn.org
American Board of Perianesthesia Nursing Certification (ABPANC) • Certified Ambulatory Perianesthesia Nurse (CAPA®) • Certified Post Anesthesia Nurse (CPAN®)	www.cpancapa.org

Organization	Website
National Board for Certification of School Nurses (NBCSN) • National Certified School Nurse (NCSN)	www.nbcsn.com
Center for Nursing Education and Testing (C-NET®) • Certified Aesthetic Nurse Specialist (CANS) • Certified Board for Urology Nurses & Associates (CBUNA) • Certified Clinical Hemodialysis Technician (CCHT) • Certified Dialysis Nurse (CDN) • Certified Medical-Surgical Registered Nurse (CMSRN®) • Certified Nephrology Nurse (CNN) • Certified Nephrology Nurse-Nurse Practitioner (CNN-NP) • Certified Plastic Surgical Nurse (CPSN) • Certified Radiology Nurse (CRN) • Certified Urology Associate (CUA) • Certified Urology Nurse Practitioner (CUNP) • Certified Urology Registered Nurse (CURN) • Dermatology Certified Nurse Practitioner (DCNP) • Dermatology Nurse Certified (DNC)	www.cnetnurse.com
Prepared Childbirth Educators, Inc. • Certified Breastfeeding Counselor (CBC) • Certified Childbirth Educator (CCE) • Certified Doula (CD) • Certified Infant Massage Instructor/Educator (CIME) • Certified Prenatal/Postnatal Fitness Instructor (CPFI)	www.childbirtheducation.org
American Association of Nurse Anesthetists • Certified Registered Nurse Anesthetist (CRNA)	www.aana.com

PROFESSIONAL ASSOCIATIONS FOR NURSES

COMMUNITY HEALTH

American Academy of Ambulatory Care Nursing
East Holly Ave – Box 56
Pitman NJ 08071-0056
800-262-6877
www.aaacn.org

American Public Health Association
800 I St NW
Washington DC 20001-3710
202-777-APHA (2742)
www.apha.org

CRITICAL CARE

American Association of Critical-Care Nurses
101 Columbia
Aliso Viejo CA 92656-4109
800-899-2226
www.aacn.org

Northeast Pediatric Cardiology Nurses Association
PO Box 261
Brookline MA 02446
www.npcna.org

Society of Critical Care Medicine
500 Midway Dr
Mount Prospect IL 60056
847-827-6869
www.sccm.org

EMERGENCY NURSING

Air & Surface Transport Nurses Association
7995 E Prentice Ave – Suite 100
Greenwood Village CO 80111
800-897-6362
www.astna.org

Emergency Nurses Association
915 Lee St
Des Plaines IL 60016-6569
800-900-9659
www.ena.org

GERIATRICS

The American Geriatrics Society
40 Fulton St, 18th Floor
New York NY 10038
212-308-1414
www.americangeriatrics.org

Gerontological Advanced Practice Nurses Association
East Holly Ave – Box 56
Pitman NJ 08071-0056
866-355-1392
www.gapna.org

The Gerontological Society of America
1220 L St NW – Suite 901
Washington DC 20005
202-842-1275
www.geron.org

MIDWIFERY

American College of Nurse-Midwives
8403 Colesville Rd – Suite 1550
Silver Spring MD 20910
240-485-1800
www.midwife.org

NEONATAL

Association of Women's Health, Obstetric and Neonatal Nurses
2000 L St NW – Suite 740
Washington DC 20036
800-673-8499
www.awhonn.org

National Association of Neonatal Nurses
8735 W. Higgins Rd – Suite 300
Chicago IL 60631
800-451-3795
www.nann.org

NEPHROLOGY

American Nephrology Nurses' Association
East Holly Ave – Box 56
Pitman NJ 08071
888-600-2662
www.annanurse.org

National Kidney Foundation
30 E 33rd St
New York NY 10016
800-622-9010
www.kidney.org

NEUROSCIENCE

American Association of Neuroscience Nurses
8735 W. Higgins Rd – Suite 300
Chicago IL 60631
800-557-2266
www.aann.org

ONCOLOGY

Association of Pediatric Hematology/ Oncology Nurses
8735 W. Higgins Rd – Suite 300
Chicago IL 60631
847-375-4724
www.aphon.org

Oncology Nursing Society
125 Enterprise Dr
Pittsburgh PA 15275
866-257-4ONS (4667)
www.ons.org

PALLIATIVE CARE

Hospice and Palliative Nurses Association
One Penn Center West – Suite 229
Pittsburgh PA 15276
412-787-9301
www.hpna.org

PEDIATRICS

Pediatric Nursing Certification Board
800 S Frederick Ave – Suite 204
Gaithersburg MD 20877-4152
888-641-2767
www.pncb.org

Society of Pediatric Nurses
7044 S. 13th Street
Oak Creek, WI 53154
414-908-4950
www.pedsnurses.org

PREOPERATIVE & PERIOPERATIVE

American Association of Nurse Anesthetists
222 S Prospect Ave
Park Ridge IL 60068-4001
855-526-2262
www.aana.com

American Society of PeriAnesthesia Nurses
90 Frontage Rd
Cherry Hill NJ 08034-1424
877-737-9696
www.aspan.org

American Society of Plastic Surgical Nurses
500 Cummings Center – Suite 4550
Beverly MA 01915
877-337-9315
www.aspsn.org

Association of PeriOperative Registered Nurses (AORN)
2170 S Parker Rd – Suite 400
Denver CO 80231
800-755-2676
www.aorn.org

(Continued)

PSYCHIATRIC

American Psychiatric Nurses Association
3141 Fairview Park Drive – Suite 625
Falls Church VA 22042
855-863-APNA (2762)
www.apna.org

REHABILITATION

Association of Rehabilitation Nurses
8735 W. Higgins Rd – Suite 300
Chicago IL 60631
800-229-7530
www.rehabnurse.org

SCHOOL NURSING

American School Health Association
1760 Old Meadow Rd – Suite 500
McLean VA 22102
703-506-7675
www.ashaweb.org

National Association of School Nurses
1100 Wayne Avenue – Suite 925
Silver Spring MD 20910
240-821-1130
www.nasn.org

STUDENT NURSING

National Student Nurses' Association
45 Main St – Suite 606
Brooklyn NY 11201
718-210-0705
www.nsna.org

WOUND CARE

Wound, Ostomy and Continence Nurses Society
15000 Commerce Pkwy – Suite C
Mount Laurel NJ 08054
888-224-9626
www.wocn.org

PROFESSIONAL ASSOCIATIONS FOR NPs

NATIONAL ASSOCIATIONS

American Association of Nurse Practitioners
PO Box 12846
Austin TX 78711
512-442-4262
www.aanp.org

Gerontological Advanced Practice Nurses Association
East Holly Ave – Box 56
Pitman NJ 08071
866-355-1392
www.gapna.org

National Association of Pediatric Nurse Practitioners
5 Hanover Square – Suite 1401
New York NY 10004
917-746-8300
www.napnap.org

Nurse Practitioners in Women's Health
505 C St NE
Washington DC 20002
202-543-9693
www.npwh.org

STATE ASSOCIATIONS

ALABAMA
Nurse Practitioner Alliance of Alabama
4924 Branch Mill Circle
Mountain Brook AL 35223
npalliancealabama.org

ALASKA
Alaska Nurse Practitioner Association
3701 E Tudor Rd – Suite 208
Anchorage AK 99507
907-222-6847
www.alaskanp.org

ARIZONA
Arizona Nurse Practitioner Council
1850 E Southern Ave – Suite 1
Tempe AZ 85282
480-831-0404
www.arizonanp.com

ARKANSAS
Arkansas Nurses Association
1123 S University – Suite 1015
Little Rock AR 72204
501-244-2363
www.arna.org

CALIFORNIA
California Association for Nurse Practitioners
1415 L St – Suite 1000
Sacramento CA 95814
916-441-1361
www.canpweb.org

COLORADO
Colorado Society of Advance Practice Nurses
PO Box 100158
Denver CO 80250
303-757-7483
http://csapn.enpnetwork.com

CONNECTICUT
Connecticut Advanced Practice Registered Nurse Society
542 Hopmeadow St – PMB 143
Simsbury CT 06070-5405
www.ctaprns.org

DELAWARE
Delaware Nurses Association
4765 Ogletown-Stanton Rd – Suite L10
Newark DE 19713
302-733-5880
www.denurses.org

DISTRICT OF COLUMBIA
Nurse Practitioner Association of DC
PO Box 77424
Washington DC 20013
www.npadc.org

FLORIDA
Florida Nurses Association
PO Box 536985
Orlando FL 32803-6985
407-896-3261
www.floridanurse.org

Florida Nurse Practitioner Network
PO Box 846
Winter Park FL 32790
866-535-3676
www.fnpn.org

GEORGIA
United Advanced Practice Registered Nurses of Georgia
1035 Fielding Park Court
Atlanta GA 30319
843-732-0402
www.uaprn.org

HAWAII
Hawaii Association of Professional Nurses
615 Piikoi St – Suite 511
Honolulu HI 96812
808-255-4442
www.hapnurses.org

IDAHO
Nurse Practitioners of Idaho
967 E Parkcenter Blvd – Suite 225
Boise ID 83706
208-914-0138
www.npidaho.org

ILLINOIS
Illinois Nurses Association
Chicago Office:
105 W Adams St – Suite 1420
Chicago IL 60603
312-419-2900

Springfield Office:
911 S. Second St
Springfield IL 62704
217-523-0783
www.illinoisnurses.com

INDIANA
Coalition of Advanced Practice Nurses of Indiana
PO Box 87925
Canton MI 48187
www.capni.org

IOWA
Iowa Nurse Practitioner Society
www.iowanpsociety.org

KANSAS
Kansas State Nurses Association
1109 SW Topeka Blvd
Topeka KS 66612
785-233-8638
www.ksnurses.com

KENTUCKY
Kentucky Coalition of Nurse Practitioners and Nurse Midwives
1017 Ash St
Louisville KY 40217
502-333-0076
www.kcnpnm.org

LOUISIANA
Louisiana Association of Nurse Practitioners
5713 Superior Dr – Suite A5
Baton Rouge LA 70816
225-293-7950
www.lanp.org

MAINE
Maine Nurse Practitioner Association
11 Columbia St
Augusta ME 04330
207-621-0313
www.mnpa.us

MARYLAND
Nurse Practitioner Association of Maryland
PO Box 540
Ellicott City MD 21041-0540
888-405-NPAM (6726)
www.npamonline.org

MASSACHUSETTS
Massachusetts Coalition of Nurse Practitioners
PO Box 1153
Littleton MA 01460
781-575-1565
www.mcnpweb.org

MICHIGAN
Michigan Council of Nurse
Practitioners
PO Box 87934
Canton MI 48187
734-432-9881
www.micnp.org

MINNESOTA
Minnesota Nurse Practitioners
PO Box 16332
Saint Paul MN 55116
www.mnnp.org

MISSISSIPPI
Mississippi Nurses Association
31 Woodgreen Pl
Madison MS 39110
601-898-0670
www.msnurses.org

MISSOURI
Missouri Nurses Association
1904 Bubba Ln
PO Box 105228
Jefferson City MO 65110
573-636-4623
www.missourinurses.org

MONTANA
Montana Nurses Association
20 Old Montana State Highway
Montana City MT 59634
406-442-6710
www.mtnurses.org

NEBRASKA
Nebraska Nurse Practitioners
www.nebraskanp.com

NEVADA
Nevada Nurses Association
PO Box 34660
Reno NV 89533
757-747-2333
www.nvnurses.org

NEW HAMPSHIRE
New Hampshire Nurse Practitioner
Association
180 Mutton Rd
Webster NH 03303
603-648-2233
www.npweb.org

NEW JERSEY
New Jersey State Nurses Association
1479 Pennington Rd
Trenton NJ 08618
888-UR-NJSNA (876-5762)
www.njsna.org

NEW MEXICO
New Mexico Nurse Practitioner
Council
PO Box 40682
Albuquerque NM 87196-0682
505-366-3763
www.nmnpc.org

NEW YORK
The Nurse Practitioner Association
New York State
12 Corporate Dr
Clifton Park NY 12065
518-348-0719
www.thenpa.org

NORTH CAROLINA
North Carolina Nurses Association
PO Box 12025
Raleigh NC 27605
800-626-2153
www.ncnurses.org

NORTH DAKOTA
North Dakota Nurse Practitioner
Association
www.ndnpa.org

OHIO
Ohio Association of Advanced Practice
Nurses
17 S. High St – Suite 200
Columbus OH 43215
866-668-3839
www.oaapn.org

OKLAHOMA
Association of Oklahoma Nurse
Practitioners
100 Park Ave – Suite 710
Oklahoma City OK 73102
405-445-4874
www.npofoklahoma.com

OREGON
Nurse Practitioners of Oregon
18765 SW Boones Ferry Rd –
Suite 200
Tualatin OR 97062
503-293-0011
www.nursepractitionersoforegon.org

PENNSYLVANIA
Pennsylvania Coalition of Nurse
Practitioners
2400 Ardmore Blvd – Suite 302
Pittsburgh PA 15221
412-243-6149
www.pacnp.org

RHODE ISLAND
Nurse Practitioner Alliance of Rhode
Island
https://npari.enpnetwork.com

SOUTH CAROLINA
South Carolina Nurses Association
1821 Gadsden St
Columbia SC 29201
803-252-4781
www.scnurses.org

SOUTH DAKOTA
Nurse Practitioner Association of
South Dakota
PO Box 2822
Rapid City SD 57709
www.npasd.org

TENNESSEE
Tennessee Nurses Association
545 Mainstream Dr – Suite 405
Nashville TN 37228
615-254-0350
www.tnaonline.org

TEXAS
Texas Nurse Practitioners
4425 S Mopac Expswy – Bldg III –
Suite 405
Austin TX 78735
512-291-6224
www.texasnp.org

UTAH
Utah Nurse Practitioners
PO Box 581084
Salt Lake City UT 84108
http://utahnp.enpnetwork.com

VERMONT
Vermont Nurse Practitioners
Association
PO Box 64773
Burlington VT 05406
www.vtnpa.org

VIRGINIA
Virginia Council of Nurse Practitioners
250 West Main St – Suite 100
Charlottesville VA 22902
434-977-3716
www.vcnp.net

WASHINGTON
ARNPs United of Washington State
10024 SE 240th St – Suite 230
Kent WA 98031
253-480-1035
www.auws.org

WEST VIRGINIA
West Virginia Nurses Association
1007 Bigley Ave – Suite 308
Charleston WV 25302
800-400-1226
304-342-1169
www.wvnurses.org

WISCONSIN
Wisconsin Nurses Association
6117 Monona Dr – Suite 1
Monona WI 53716
608-221-0383
www.wisconsinnurses.org

WYOMING
Wyoming Council of Advanced
Practice Nurses
PO Box 20752
Cheyenne WY 82003
www.wcapn.org

ANTIPYRETIC PRODUCTS

BRAND	INGREDIENT(S)/STRENGTH(S)	DOSAGE
ACETAMINOPHENS		
Children's Tylenol Meltaways Chewable Tablets*†	Acetaminophen 80mg	**Peds 11 yrs (72-95 lbs):** 6 tabs q4h. **Peds 9-10 yrs (60-71 lbs):** 5 tabs q4h. Peds 6-8 yrs (48-59 lbs): 4 tabs q4h. Peds 4-5 yrs (36-47 lbs): 3 tabs q4h. Peds 2-3 yrs (24-35 lbs): 2 tabs q4h. **Max:** 5 doses/24h.
Children's Tylenol Oral Suspension*	Acetaminophen 160mg/5mL	**Peds 11 yrs (72-95 lbs):** 3 tsp (15mL) q4h. **Peds 9-10 yrs (60-71 lbs):** 2.5 tsp (12.5mL) q4h. **Peds 6-8 yrs (48-59 lbs):** 2 tsp (10mL) q4h. **Peds 4-5 yrs (36-47 lbs):** 1.5 tsp (7.5mL) q4h. **Peds 2-3 yrs (24-35 lbs):** 1 tsp (5mL) q4h. **Max:** 5 doses/24h.
FeverAll Children's Suppositories	Acetaminophen 120mg	**Peds 3-6 yrs:** 1 supp q4-6h. **Max:** 5 doses/24h.
FeverAll Infants' Suppositories	Acetaminophen 80mg	**Peds 12-36 months:** 1 supp q4-6h. **Max:** 5 doses/24h. **Peds 6-11 months:** 1 supp q6h. **Max:** 4 doses/24h.
FeverAll Jr. Strength Suppositories	Acetaminophen 325mg	**Adults & Peds ≥12 yrs:** 2 supp q4-6h. **Max:** 6 doses/24h. **Peds 6-12 yrs:** 1 supp q4-6h. **Max:** 5 doses/24h.
Infants' Tylenol Oral Suspension*	Acetaminophen 160mg/5mL	**Peds 2-3 yrs (24-35 lbs):** 1 tsp (5mL) q4h. **Max:** 5 doses/24h.
Jr. Tylenol Meltaways Chewable Tablets*†	Acetaminophen 160mg	**Peds 11 yrs (72-95 lbs):** 3 tabs q4h. **Peds 9-10 yrs (60-71 lbs):** 2.5 tabs q4h. **Peds 6-8 yrs (48-59 lbs):** 2 tabs q4h. **Max:** 5 doses/24h.
PediaCare Children Fever Reducer/ Pain Reliever Acetaminophen Oral Suspension	Acetaminophen 160mg/5mL	**Peds 11 yrs (72-95 lbs):** 3 tsp (15mL) q4h. **Peds 9-10 yrs (60-71 lbs):** 2.5 tsp (12.5mL) q4h. **Peds 6-8 yrs (48-59 lbs):** 2 tsp (10mL) q4h. **Peds 4-5 yrs (36-47 lbs):** 1.5 tsp (7.5mL) q4h. **Peds 2-3 yrs (24-35 lbs):** 1 tsp (5mL) q4h. **Max:** 5 doses/24h.
PediaCare Infants Fever Reducer/ Pain Reliever Acetaminophen Oral Suspension*	Acetaminophen 160mg/5mL	**Peds 2-3 yrs (24-35 lbs):** 1 tsp (5mL) q4h. **Max:** 5 doses/24h.
Triaminic Children's Fever Reducer Pain Reliever Syrup*†	Acetaminophen 160mg/5mL	**Peds 11 yrs (72-95 lbs):** 3 tsp (15mL) q4h. **Peds 9-10 yrs (60-71 lbs):** 2.5 tsp (12.5mL) q4h. **Peds 6-8 yrs (48-59 lbs):** 2 tsp (10mL) q4h. **Peds 4-5 yrs (36-47 lbs):** 1.5 tsp (7.5mL) q4h. **Peds 2-3 yrs (24-35 lbs):** 1 tsp (5mL) q4h. **Max:** 5 doses/24h.
Triaminic Infants' Fever Reducer Pain Reliever Syrup*†	Acetaminophen 160mg/5mL	**Peds 11 yrs (72-95 lbs):** 3 tsp (15mL) q4h. **Peds 9-10 yrs (60-71 lbs):** 2.5 tsp (12.5mL) q4h. **Peds 6-8 yrs (48-59 lbs):** 2 tsp (10mL) q4h. **Peds 4-5 yrs (36-47 lbs):** 1.5 tsp (7.5mL) q4h. **Peds 2-3 yrs (24-35 lbs):** 1 tsp (5mL) q4h. **Max:** 5 doses/24h.
Tylenol 8 HR Caplets†	Acetaminophen 650mg	**Adults & Peds ≥12 yrs:** 2 tabs q8h prn. **Max:** 6 doses/24h.
Tylenol Extra Strength Caplets	Acetaminophen 500mg	**Adults & Peds ≥12 yrs:** 2 tabs q6h prn. **Max:** 6 tabs/24h.

(Continued)

BRAND	INGREDIENT(S)/STRENGTH(S)	DOSAGE
ACETAMINOPHENS *(Continued)*		
Tylenol Regular Strength Tablets	Acetaminophen 325mg	**Adults & Peds ≥12 yrs:** 2 tabs q4-6h. **Max:** 10 tabs/24h. **Peds 6-11 yrs:** 1 tab q4-6h. **Max:** 5 tabs/24h.
NONSTEROIDAL ANTI-INFLAMMATORY DRUGS		
Advil Caplets	Ibuprofen 200mg	**Adults & Peds ≥12 yrs:** 1-2 tabs q4-6h. **Max:** 6 tabs/24h.
Advil Film-Coated Caplets	Ibuprofen 200mg	**Adults & Peds ≥12 yrs:** 1-2 tabs q4-6h. **Max:** 6 tabs/24h.
Advil Film-Coated Tablets	Ibuprofen 200mg	**Adults & Peds ≥12 yrs:** 1-2 tabs q4-6h. **Max:** 6 tabs/24h.
Advil Gel Caplets	Ibuprofen 200mg	**Adults & Peds ≥12 yrs:** 1-2 tabs q4-6h. **Max:** 6 tabs/24h.
Advil Liqui-Gels	Ibuprofen 200mg	**Adults & Peds ≥12 yrs:** 1-2 caps q4-6h. **Max:** 6 caps/24h.
Advil Tablets	Ibuprofen 200mg	**Adults & Peds ≥12 yrs:** 1-2 tabs q4-6h. **Max:** 6 tabs/24h.
Aleve Caplets	Naproxen sodium 220mg	**Adults & Peds ≥12 yrs:** 1 tab q8-12h. May take 1 additional tab within 1h of first dose. **Max:** 2 tabs/8-12h or 3 tabs/24h.
Aleve Gelcaps	Naproxen sodium 220mg	**Adults & Peds ≥12 yrs:** 1 tab q8-12h. May take 1 additional tab within 1h of first dose. **Max:** 2 tabs/8-12h or 3 tabs/24h.
Aleve Liquid Gels	Naproxen sodium 220mg	**Adults & Peds ≥12 yrs:** 1 cap q8-12h. May take 1 additional cap within 1h of first dose. **Max:** 2 caps/8-12h or 3 caps/24h.
Aleve Tablets	Naproxen sodium 220mg	**Adults & Peds ≥12 yrs:** 1 tab q8-12h. May take 1 additional tab within 1h of first dose. **Max:** 2 tabs/8-12h or 3 tabs/24h.
Children's Advil Suspension*	Ibuprofen 100mg/5mL	**Peds 11 yrs (72-95 lbs):** 3 tsp (15mL) q6-8h. **Peds 9-10 yrs (60-71 lbs):** 2.5 tsp (12.5mL) q6-8h. **Peds 6-8 yrs (48-59 lbs):** 2 tsp (10mL) q6-8h. **Peds 4-5 yrs (36-47 lbs):** 1.5 tsp (7.5mL) q6-8h. **Peds 2-3 yrs (24-35 lbs):** 1 tsp (5mL) q6-8h. **Max:** 4 doses/24h.
Children's Motrin Suspension	Ibuprofen 100mg/5mL	**Peds 11 yrs (72-95 lbs):** 3 tsp (15mL) q6-8h. **Peds 9-10 yrs (60-71 lbs):** 2.5 tsp (12.5mL) q6-8h. **Peds 6-8 yrs (48-59 lbs):** 2 tsp (10mL) q6-8h. **Peds 4-5 yrs (36-47 lbs):** 1.5 tsp (7.5mL) q6-8h. **Peds 2-3 yrs (24-35 lbs):** 1 tsp (5mL) q6-8h. **Max:** 4 doses/24h.
Infants' Advil Concentrated Drops	Ibuprofen 50mg/1.25mL	**Peds 12-23 months (18-23 lbs):** 1.875mL q6-8h. **Peds 6-11 months (12-17 lbs):** 1.25mL q6-8h. **Max:** 4 doses/24h.
Infants' Motrin Concentrated Drops	Ibuprofen 50mg/1.25mL	**Peds 12-23 months (18-23 lbs):** 1.875mL q6-8h. **Peds 6-11 months (12-17 lbs):** 1.25mL q6-8h. **Max:** 4 doses/24h.
Junior Strength Advil Chewable Tablets	Ibuprofen 100mg	**Peds 11 yrs (72-95 lbs):** 3 tabs q6-8h. **Peds 9-10 yrs (60-71 lbs):** 2.5 tabs q6-8h. **Peds 6-8 yrs (48-59 lbs):** 2 tabs q6-8h. **Max:** 4 doses/24h.

BRAND	INGREDIENT(S)/STRENGTH(S)	DOSAGE
NONSTEROIDAL ANTI-INFLAMMATORY DRUGS *(Continued)*		
Junior Strength Advil Tablets	Ibuprofen 100mg	**Peds 11 yrs (72-95 lbs):** 3 tabs q6-8h. **Peds 6-10 yrs (48-71 lbs):** 2 tabs q6-8h. **Max:** 4 doses/24h.
Motrin IB Caplets	Ibuprofen 200mg	**Adults & Peds ≥12 yrs:** 1-2 tabs q4-6h. **Max:** 6 tabs/24h.
PediaCare Children Pain Reliever/Fever Reducer IB Ibuprofen Oral Suspension	Ibuprofen 100mg/5mL	**Peds 11 yrs (72-95 lbs):** 3 tsp (15mL) q6-8h. **Peds 9-10 yrs (60-71 lbs):** 2.5 tsp (12.5mL) q6-8h. **Peds 6-8 yrs (48-59 lbs):** 2 tsp (10mL) q6-8h. **Peds 4-5 yrs (36-47 lbs):** 1.5 tsp (7.5mL) q6-8h. **Peds 2-3 yrs (24-35 lbs):** 1 tsp (5mL) q6-8h. **Max:** 4 doses/24h.
PediaCare Infants Pain Reliever/Fever Reducer IB Ibuprofen Concentrated Oral Suspension	Ibuprofen 50mg/1.25mL	**Peds 12-23 months (18-23 lbs):** 1.865mL q6-8h. **Peds 6-11 months (12-17 lbs):** 1.25mL q6-8h. **Max:** 4 doses/24h.
SALICYLATES		
PLEASE REFER TO ASPIRIN PRODUCTS TABLE		

*Multiple flavors available.
†Product currently on recall or temporarily unavailable from manufacturer, but generic forms may be available.

INSOMNIA PRODUCTS

BRAND	INGREDIENT(S)/STRENGTH(S)	DOSAGE
DIPHENHYDRAMINES		
Compoz Maximum Strength Soft Gel Liquid Capsules	Diphenhydramine HCl 50mg	**Adults & Peds ≥12 yrs:** 1 cap hs prn.
Nytol Extra Strength Tablets	Diphenhydramine HCl 25mg	**Adults & Peds ≥12 yrs:** 1 tab 20-30 minutes before hs.
Nytol QuickCaps	Diphenhydramine HCl 25mg	**Adults & Peds ≥12 yrs:** 2 tabs hs.
Simply Sleep Caplets	Diphenhydramine HCl 25mg	**Adults & Peds ≥12 yrs:** 2 tabs hs prn.
Sleepinal Capsules	Diphenhydramine HCl 50mg	**Adults & Peds ≥12 yrs:** 1 cap hs prn.
Sominex Maximum Strength Caplets	Diphenhydramine HCl 50mg	**Adults & Peds ≥12 yrs:** 1 tab hs prn.
Sominex Original Formula Tablets	Diphenhydramine HCl 25mg	**Adults & Peds ≥12 yrs:** 2 tabs hs prn.
Unisom SleepGels	Diphenhydramine HCl 50mg	**Adults & Peds ≥12 yrs:** 1 cap hs prn.
Unisom SleepMelts	Diphenhydramine HCl 25mg	**Adults & Peds ≥12 yrs:** 2 tabs hs prn.
ZzzQuil LiquiCaps	Diphenhydramine HCl 25mg	**Adults & Peds ≥12 yrs:** 2 caps hs prn. **Max:** 1 dose/24 hrs.
ZzzQuil Liquid	Diphenhydramine HCl 50mg/30mL (2 tbsp)	**Adults & Peds ≥12 yrs:** 30mL (2 tbsp) hs prn. **Max:** 1 dose/24 hrs.
DIPHENHYDRAMINE COMBINATIONS		
Advil PM Caplets	Ibuprofen/Diphenhydramine citrate 200mg-38mg	**Adults & Peds ≥12 yrs:** 2 tabs hs. **Max:** 2 tabs/24 hrs.
Advil PM Liqui-Gels	Ibuprofen/Diphenhydramine HCl 200mg-25mg	**Adults & Peds ≥12 yrs:** 2 caps hs. **Max:** 2 caps/24 hrs.
Bayer PM Caplets	Aspirin/Diphenhydramine citrate 500mg-38mg	**Adults & Peds ≥12 yrs:** 2 tabs hs prn.
Excedrin PM Caplets	Acetaminophen/Diphenhydramine citrate 500mg-38mg	**Adults & Peds ≥12 yrs:** 2 tabs hs prn. **Max:** 2 tabs/24 hrs.
Excedrin PM Express Gels	Acetaminophen/Diphenhydramine citrate 500mg-38mg	**Adults & Peds ≥12 yrs:** 2 caps hs prn. **Max:** 2 caps/24 hrs.
Goody's PM Powder	Acetaminophen/Diphenhydramine citrate 500mg-38mg per powder	**Adults & Peds ≥12 yrs:** 2 powders hs prn.
Motrin PM Caplets	Ibuprofen/Diphenhydramine citrate 200mg-38mg	**Adults & Peds ≥12 yrs:** 2 tabs hs. **Max:** 2 tabs/24 hrs.
Tylenol PM Caplets	Acetaminophen/Diphenhydramine HCl 500mg-25mg	**Adults & Peds ≥12 yrs:** 2 tabs hs. **Max:** 2 tabs/24 hrs.
Tylenol PM Geltabs	Acetaminophen/Diphenhydramine HCl 500mg-25mg	**Adults & Peds ≥12 yrs:** 2 tabs hs. **Max:** 2 tabs/24 hrs.
Unisom PM Pain SleepCaps	Acetaminophen/Diphenhydramine HCl 325mg-50mg	**Adults & Peds ≥12 yrs:** 1 tab hs. **Max:** 1 tab/24 hrs.
DOXYLAMINES		
Unisom SleepTabs	Doxylamine succinate 25mg	**Adults & Peds ≥12 yrs:** 1 tab 30 minutes before hs.

SMOKING CESSATION PRODUCTS

BRAND	INGREDIENT(S)/STRENGTH(S)	DOSAGE
Habitrol Nicotine Transdermal System Patch Step 1	Nicotine 21mg	**Adults:** If smoking >10 cigarettes/day: **Weeks 1 to 4:** Apply one 21mg patch/day. **Weeks 5 to 6:** Apply one 14mg patch/day. **Weeks 7 to 8:** Apply one 7mg patch/day. If smoking ≤10 cigarettes/day: **Weeks 1 to 6:** Apply one 14mg patch/day. **Weeks 7 to 8:** Apply one 7mg patch/day.
Habitrol Nicotine Transdermal System Patch Step 2	Nicotine 14mg	Refer to Habitrol Nicotine Transdermal System Patch Step 1 dosing.
Habitrol Nicotine Transdermal System Patch Step 3	Nicotine 7mg	Refer to Habitrol Nicotine Transdermal System Patch Step 1 dosing.
NicoDerm CQ Step 1 Clear Patch	Nicotine 21mg	**Adults:** If smoking >10 cigarettes/day: **Weeks 1 to 6:** Apply one 21mg patch/day. **Weeks 7 to 8:** Apply one 14mg patch/day. **Weeks 9 to 10:** Apply one 7mg patch/day. If smoking ≤10 cigarettes/day: **Weeks 1 to 6:** Apply one 14mg patch/day. **Weeks 7 to 8:** Apply one 7mg patch/day.
NicoDerm CQ Step 2 Clear Patch	Nicotine 14mg	Refer to NicoDerm CQ Step 1 Clear Patch dosing.
NicoDerm CQ Step 3 Clear Patch	Nicotine 7mg	Refer to NicoDerm CQ Step 1 Clear Patch dosing.
Nicorette 2mg Gum	Nicotine polacrilex 2mg	**Adults:** If smoking first cigarette >30 minutes after waking up, use 2mg gum. **Weeks 1 to 6:** 1 piece q1-2h. **Weeks 7 to 9:** 1 piece q2-4h. **Weeks 10 to 12:** 1 piece q4-8h. **Max:** 24 pieces/day.
Nicorette 4mg Gum	Nicotine polacrilex 4mg	**Adults:** If smoking first cigarette ≤30 minutes after waking up, use 4mg gum. **Weeks 1 to 6:** 1 piece q1-2h. **Weeks 7 to 9:** 1 piece q2-4h. **Weeks 10 to 12:** 1 piece q4-8h. **Max:** 24 pieces/day.
Nicorette 2mg Lozenges	Nicotine polacrilex 2mg	**Adults:** If smoking first cigarette >30 minutes after waking up, use 2mg lozenge. **Weeks 1 to 6:** 1 lozenge q1-2h. **Weeks 7 to 9:** 1 lozenge q2-4h. **Weeks 10 to 12:** 1 lozenge q4-8h. **Max:** 5 lozenges/6 hours or 20 lozenges/day.
Nicorette 4mg Lozenges	Nicotine polacrilex 4mg	**Adults:** If smoking first cigarette ≤30 minutes after waking up, use 4mg lozenge. **Weeks 1 to 6:** 1 lozenge q1-2h. **Weeks 7 to 9:** 1 lozenge q2-4h. **Weeks 10 to 12:** 1 lozenge q4-8h. **Max:** 5 lozenges/6 hours or 20 lozenges/day.
Nicorette 2mg mini Lozenges	Nicotine polacrilex 2mg	**Adults:** If smoking first cigarette >30 minutes after waking up, use 2mg lozenge. **Weeks 1 to 6:** 1 lozenge q1-2h. **Weeks 7 to 9:** 1 lozenge q2-4h. **Weeks 10 to 12:** 1 lozenge q4-8h. **Max:** 5 lozenges/6 hours or 20 lozenges/day.
Nicorette 4mg mini Lozenges	Nicotine polacrilex 4mg	**Adults:** If smoking first cigarette ≤30 minutes after waking up, use 4mg lozenge. **Weeks 1 to 6:** 1 lozenge q1-2h. **Weeks 7 to 9:** 1 lozenge q2-4h. **Weeks 10 to 12:** 1 lozenge q4-8h. **Max:** 5 lozenges/6 hours or 20 lozenges/day.

ANTIFUNGAL PRODUCTS

BRAND	INGREDIENT(S)/STRENGTH(S)	DOSAGE
BUTENAFINES		
Lotrimin Ultra Athlete's Foot Cream	Butenafine HCl 1%	**Adults & Peds ≥12 yrs: Athlete's Foot (between/around toes):** Apply bid for 1 week or qd for 4 weeks. **Jock Itch/Ringworm:** Apply qd for 2 weeks.
Lotrimin Ultra Jock Itch Cream	Butenafine HCl 1%	**Adults & Peds ≥12 yrs:** Apply qd for 2 weeks.
CLOTRIMAZOLES		
FungiCure Intensive Liquid	Clotrimazole 1%	**Adults & Peds ≥2 yrs: Athlete's Foot/Ringworm:** Apply bid for 4 weeks. **Jock Itch:** Apply bid for 2 weeks.
FungiCure Maximum Strength Manicure & Pedicure	Clotrimazole 1%	**Adults & Peds ≥2 yrs: Athlete's Foot/Ringworm:** Apply bid for 4 weeks.
Lotrimin AF Athlete's Foot Cream	Clotrimazole 1%	**Adults & Peds ≥2 yrs: Athlete's Foot/Ringworm:** Apply bid for 4 weeks. **Jock Itch:** Apply bid for 2 weeks.
Lotrimin AF Jock Itch Cream	Clotrimazole 1%	**Adults & Peds ≥2 yrs:** Apply bid for 2 weeks.
Lotrimin AF Ringworm Cream	Clotrimazole 1%	**Adults & Peds ≥2 yrs:** Apply bid for 4 weeks.
MICONAZOLES		
Clearly Confident Antifungal Cream	Miconazole nitrate 2%	**Adults & Peds ≥2 yrs:** Apply bid for 4 weeks.
Desenex Liquid Spray	Miconazole nitrate 2%	**Adults & Peds ≥2 yrs:** Apply bid for 4 weeks.
Desenex Powder	Miconazole nitrate 2%	**Adults & Peds ≥2 yrs:** Apply bid for 4 weeks.
Desenex Spray Powder	Miconazole nitrate 2%	**Adults & Peds ≥2 yrs:** Apply bid for 4 weeks.
Lotrimin AF Athlete's Foot Deodorant Powder Spray	Miconazole nitrate 2%	**Adults & Peds ≥2 yrs: Athlete's Foot/Ringworm:** Apply bid for 4 weeks. **Jock Itch:** Apply bid for 2 weeks.
Lotrimin AF Athlete's Foot Liquid Spray	Miconazole nitrate 2%	**Adults & Peds ≥2 yrs: Athlete's Foot/Ringworm:** Apply bid for 4 weeks. **Jock Itch:** Apply bid for 2 weeks.
Lotrimin AF Athlete's Foot Powder	Miconazole nitrate 2%	**Adults & Peds ≥2 yrs: Athlete's Foot/Ringworm:** Apply bid for 4 weeks. **Jock Itch:** Apply bid for 2 weeks.
Lotrimin AF Athlete's Foot Powder Spray	Miconazole nitrate 2%	**Adults & Peds ≥2 yrs: Athlete's Foot/Ringworm:** Apply bid for 4 weeks. **Jock Itch:** Apply bid for 2 weeks.
Lotrimin AF Jock Itch Powder Spray	Miconazole nitrate 2%	**Adults & Peds ≥2 yrs:** Apply bid for 2 weeks.
Micatin Cream	Miconazole nitrate 2%	**Adults & Peds ≥2 yrs: Athlete's Foot/Ringworm:** Apply bid for 4 weeks. **Jock Itch:** Apply bid for 2 weeks.
Tineacide Antifungal Cream	Miconazole nitrate 2%	**Adults & Peds ≥2 yrs: Athlete's Foot (between/around toes):** Apply bid for 4 weeks. **Jock Itch/Ringworm:** Apply bid for 2 weeks.
Ting AF Spray Powder	Miconazole nitrate 2%	**Adults & Peds ≥2 yrs: Athlete's Foot/Ringworm:** Apply bid for 4 weeks. **Jock Itch:** Apply bid for 2 weeks.
Zeasorb Super Absorbent Powder Athlete's Foot	Miconazole nitrate 2%	**Adults & Peds ≥2 yrs:** Apply bid for 4 weeks.
Zeasorb Super Absorbent Powder Jock Itch	Miconazole nitrate 2%	**Adults & Peds ≥2 yrs:** Apply bid for 2 weeks.
TERBINAFINES		
Lamisil AT Cream	Terbinafine HCl 1%	**Adults & Peds ≥12 yrs: Athlete's Foot (between toes):** Apply bid for 1 week. **Athlete's Foot (on side or bottom of foot):** Apply bid for 2 weeks. **Jock Itch/Ringworm:** Apply qd for 1 week.
Lamisil AT Cream for Jock Itch	Terbinafine HCl 1%	**Adults & Peds ≥12 yrs:** Apply qd for 1 week.
Lamisil AT Gel	Terbinafine 1%	**Adults & Peds ≥12 yrs: Athlete's Foot (between toes):** Apply qhs for 1 week. **Jock Itch/Ringworm:** Apply qd for 1 week.

(Continued)

BRAND	INGREDIENT(S)/STRENGTH(S)	DOSAGE
TERBINAFINES (Continued)		
Lamisil AT Spray	Terbinafine HCl 1%	**Adults & Peds ≥12 yrs: Athlete's Foot (between toes):** Apply bid for 1 week. **Jock Itch/Ringworm:** Apply qd for 1 week.
Lamisil AT Spray for Jock Itch	Terbinafine HCl 1%	**Adults & Peds ≥12 yrs:** Apply qd for 1 week.
TOLNAFTATES		
Flexitol Medicated Foot Cream	Tolnaftate 1%	**Adults & Peds ≥2 yrs:** Apply bid for 4 weeks. **Prevention:** Apply qd or bid.
Lamisil AF Defense Spray Powder	Tolnaftate 1%	**Adults & Peds ≥2 yrs:** Apply bid for 4 weeks. **Prevention:** Apply qd or bid.
Nailene Maximum Strength Antifungal Treatment	Tolnaftate 1%	**Adults & Peds ≥2 yrs:** Apply bid for 4 weeks.
Odor-Eaters Foot & Sneaker Spray Powder	Tolnaftate 1%	**Adults & Peds ≥2 yrs: Prevention:** Apply qd or bid.
ProClearz Maximum Strength Fungal Shield	Tolnaftate 1%	**Adults & Peds ≥2 yrs: Athlete's Foot/Ringworm:** Apply bid for 4 weeks.
Tinactin Athlete's Foot Cream	Tolnaftate 1%	**Adults & Peds ≥2 yrs:** Apply bid for 4 weeks. **Prevention:** Apply qd or bid.
Tinactin Athlete's Foot Deodorant Powder Spray	Tolnaftate 1%	**Adults & Peds ≥2 yrs:** Apply bid for 4 weeks. **Prevention:** Apply qd or bid.
Tinactin Athlete's Foot Liquid Spray	Tolnaftate 1%	**Adults & Peds ≥2 yrs:** Apply bid for 4 weeks. **Prevention:** Apply qd or bid.
Tinactin Athlete's Foot Powder Spray	Tolnaftate 1%	**Adults & Peds ≥2 yrs:** Apply bid for 4 weeks. **Prevention:** Apply qd or bid.
Tinactin Athlete's Foot Super Absorbent Powder	Tolnaftate 1%	**Adults & Peds ≥2 yrs:** Apply bid for 4 weeks. **Prevention:** Apply qd or bid.
Tinactin Jock Itch Cream	Tolnaftate 1%	**Adults & Peds ≥2 yrs:** Apply bid for 2 weeks.
Tinactin Jock Itch Powder Spray	Tolnaftate 1%	**Adults & Peds ≥2 yrs:** Apply bid for 2 weeks.
Ting Cream	Tolnaftate 1%	**Adults & Peds ≥2 yrs: Athlete's Foot/Ringworm:** Apply bid for 4 weeks. **Jock Itch:** Apply bid for 2 weeks. **Prevention (Athlete's Foot):** Apply qd or bid.
Ting Spray Liquid	Tolnaftate 1%	**Adults & Peds ≥2 yrs:** Apply bid for 4 weeks.
UNDECYLENIC ACIDS		
DiaDerm Antifungal Cream	Undecylenic acid 10%	**Adults & Peds ≥2 yrs: Athlete's Foot/Ringworm:** Apply bid for 4 weeks. **Jock Itch:** Apply bid for 2 weeks.
Flexitol Anti-Fungal Liquid	Undecylenic acid 25%	**Adults & Peds ≥2 yrs: Athlete's Foot/Ringworm:** Apply bid for 4 weeks.
Fungi Nail Anti-Fungal Solution	Undecylenic acid 25%	**Adults & Peds ≥2 yrs: Athlete's Foot/Ringworm:** Apply bid for 4 weeks.
Fungi Nail Anti-Fungal Solution Pen Brush Applicator	Undecylenic acid 25%	**Adults & Peds ≥2 yrs: Athlete's Foot/Ringworm:** Apply bid for 4 weeks.
Fungi Nail Toe & Foot Ointment	Zinc undecylenate/ Undecylenic acid 20%-5%	**Adults & Peds ≥2 yrs: Athlete's Foot/Ringworm:** Apply bid for 4 weeks. **Toe Fungus:** Apply under nail and around cuticle area bid.
FungiCure Maximum Strength Liquid	Undecylenic acid 25%	**Adults & Peds ≥2 yrs: Athlete's Foot/Ringworm:** Apply bid for 4 weeks.
FungiCure Maximum Strength Liquid Gel	Undecylenic acid 25%	**Adults & Peds ≥2 yrs: Athlete's Foot/Ringworm:** Apply bid for 4 weeks.
Tineacide Foot & Shoe Spray	Undecylenic acid 5%	**Adults:** Apply 2 sprays to foot/shoe biw or tiw.

WOUND CARE PRODUCTS

BRAND	INGREDIENT(S)/STRENGTH(S)	DOSAGE
BACITRACIN, NEOMYCIN, POLYMYXIN B, AND COMBINATIONS		
Bacitracin Ointment	Bacitracin 500 U/gram	**Adults:** Apply a small amount to affected area qd-tid.
Neosporin Original Ointment	Neomycin/Polymyxin B/ Bacitracin 3.5mg-5000 U-400 U/gram	**Adults:** Apply a small amount to affected area qd-tid.
Neosporin Plus Pain Relief Cream	Neomycin/Polymyxin B/Pramoxine HCl 3.5mg-10,000 U-10mg/gram	**Adults & Peds ≥2 yrs:** Apply a small amount to affected area qd-tid.
Neosporin Plus Pain Relief Ointment	Neomycin/Polymyxin B/Bacitracin/ Pramoxine HCl 3.5mg-10,000 U-500 U-10mg/gram	**Adults & Peds ≥2 yrs:** Apply a small amount to affected area qd-tid.
Polysporin First Aid Antibiotic Ointment	Polymyxin B/Bacitracin 10,000 U-500 U/gram	**Adults:** Apply a small amount to affected area qd-tid.
BENZALKONIUM CHLORIDE AND COMBINATIONS		
Bactine Original First Aid Liquid	Benzalkonium chloride/Lidocaine HCl 0.13%-2.5%	**Adults & Peds ≥2 yrs:** Apply a small amount to affected area qd-tid.
Bactine Pain Relieving Cleansing Spray	Benzalkonium chloride/Lidocaine HCl 0.13%-2.5%	**Adults & Peds ≥2 yrs:** Apply a small amount to affected area qd-tid.
Band-Aid Hurt-Free Antiseptic Wash	Benzalkonium chloride/Lidocaine HCl 0.13%-2%	**Adults & Peds ≥2 yrs:** Flush affected area no more than tid.
Neosporin NEO TO GO! Spray	Benzalkonium chloride/Pramoxine HCl 0.13%-1%	**Adults & Peds ≥2 yrs:** Spray a small amount on affected area qd-tid.
Neosporin Wound Cleanser	Benzalkonium chloride 0.13%	**First Aid Antiseptic Use: Adults & Peds ≥2 yrs:** Pump a small amount on affected area qd-tid. **Wound Cleansing: Adults & Peds ≥2 yrs:** Pump a small amount on affected area.
BENZETHONIUM CHLORIDE AND COMBINATIONS		
Lanacane First Aid Spray	Benzethonium chloride/Benzocaine 0.2%-20%	**Adults & Peds ≥2 yrs:** Spray a small amount on affected area not more than qd-tid.
Lanacane Maximum Strength Anti-Itch Cream	Benzethonium chloride/Benzocaine 0.2%-20%	**Adults & Peds ≥2 yrs:** Apply a small amount to affected area not more than qd-tid.
Simply Saline 3-in-1 Wound Wash	Benzethonium chloride 0.13%	**Adults:** Spray a small amount on affected area qd-tid.
Simply Saline Antibacterial Wound Wash	Benzethonium chloride 0.13%	**Adults:** Spray a small amount on affected area qd-tid.
CHLORHEXIDINE GLUCONATES		
Hibiclens	Chlorhexidine gluconate solution 4%	**Adults:** Rinse affected area with water. Apply the minimum amount necessary to cover area, and wash gently. Rinse again.
IODINES		
Betadine Skin Cleanser	Povidone-iodine 7.5%	**Adults:** Wet skin and apply a sufficient amount for lather to cover all surfaces. Wash vigorously for at least 15 sec, rinse and dry thoroughly.
Betadine Solution	Povidone-iodine 10%	**Adults:** Apply a small amount to affected area qd-tid.
MISCELLANEOUS		
Simply Saline Wound Wash	Sterile 0.9% sodium chloride solution	**Adults:** Flush affected area prn.

ANTACID AND HEARTBURN PRODUCTS

BRAND	INGREDIENT(S)/STRENGTH(S)	DOSAGE
ANTACIDS		
Alka-Seltzer Extra Strength Effervescent Tablets	Aspirin/Citric acid/Sodium bicarbonate 500mg-1000mg-1985mg	**Adults ≥60 yrs:** 2 tabs dissolved in 4 oz water q6h. **Max:** 3 tabs/24h. **Adults & Peds ≥12 yrs:** 2 tabs dissolved in 4 oz water q6h. **Max:** 7 tabs/24h.
Alka-Seltzer Fruit Chewable Tablets	Calcium carbonate 750mg	**Adults & Peds ≥12 yrs:** 1-2 tabs q2-4h. **Max:** 10 tabs/24h.
Alka-Seltzer Gold Effervescent Tablets	Citric acid/Potassium bicarbonate/ Sodium bicarbonate 1000mg-344mg-1050mg	**Adults ≥60 yrs:** 2 tabs dissolved in 4 oz water q4h prn. **Max:** 6 tabs/24h. **Adults & Peds ≥12 yrs:** 2 tabs dissolved in 4 oz water q4h prn. **Max:** 8 tabs/24h. **Peds <12 yrs:** 1 tab dissolved in 4 oz water q4h prn. **Max:** 4 tabs/24h.
Alka-Seltzer Heartburn Relief Effervescent Tablets	Citric acid/Sodium bicarbonate 1000mg-1940mg	**Adults ≥60 yrs:** 2 tabs dissolved in 4 oz water q4h prn. **Max:** 4 tabs/24h. **Adults & Peds ≥12 yrs:** 2 tabs dissolved in 4 oz water q4h prn. **Max:** 8 tabs/24h.
Alka-Seltzer Lemon Lime Effervescent Tablets	Aspirin/Citric acid/Sodium bicarbonate 325mg-1000mg-1700mg	**Adults ≥60 yrs:** 2 tabs dissolved in 4 oz water q4h. **Max:** 4 tabs/24h. **Adults & Peds ≥12 yrs:** 2 tabs dissolved in 4 oz water q4h. **Max:** 8 tabs/24h.
Alka-Seltzer Original Effervescent Tablets	Aspirin/Citric acid/Sodium bicarbonate 325mg-1000mg-1916mg	**Adults ≥60 yrs:** 2 tabs dissolved in 4 oz water q4h. **Max:** 4 tabs/24h. **Adults & Peds ≥12 yrs:** 2 tabs dissolved in 4 oz water q4h. **Max:** 8 tabs/24h.
Gaviscon Extra Strength Chewable Tablets	Aluminum hydroxide/Magnesium carbonate 160mg-105mg	**Adults:** 2-4 tabs qid. **Max:** 16 tabs/24h.
Gaviscon Extra Strength Liquid	Aluminum hydroxide/Magnesium carbonate 254mg-237.5mg/5mL	**Adults:** 2-4 tsp (10-20mL) qid. **Max:** 16 tsp (80mL)/24h.
Gaviscon Regular Strength Chewable Tablets	Aluminum hydroxide/Magnesium trisilicate 80mg-14.2mg	**Adults:** 2-4 tabs qid. **Max:** 16 tabs/24h.
Gaviscon Regular Strength Liquid	Aluminum hydroxide/Magnesium carbonate 95mg-358mg/15mL	**Adults:** 1-2 tbl (15-30mL) qid. **Max:** 8 tbl (120mL)/24h.
Maalox Children's Relief Chewable Tablets	Calcium carbonate 400mg	**Peds 6-11 yrs (48-95 lbs):** 2 tabs prn. **Max:** 6 tabs/24h. **Peds 2-5 yrs (24-47 lbs):** 1 tab prn. **Max:** 3 tabs/24h.
Maalox Regular Strength Chewable Tablets	Calcium carbonate 600mg	**Adults:** 1-2 tabs prn. **Max:** 12 tabs/24h.
Mylanta Supreme Liquid	Calcium carbonate/Magnesium hydroxide 400mg-135mg/5mL	**Adults:** 2-4 tsp (10-20mL) between meals & at hs. **Max:** 18 tsp (90mL)/24h.
Mylanta Ultimate Strength Liquid	Aluminum hydroxide/Magnesium hydroxide 500mg-500mg/5mL	**Adults & Peds ≥12 yrs:** 2-4 tsp (10-20mL) between meals & at hs. **Max:** 9 tsp (45mL)/24h.
Pepto-Bismol Children's Pepto Chewable Tablets	Calcium carbonate 400mg	**Peds 6-11 yrs (48-95 lbs):** 2 tabs prn. **Max:** 6 tabs/24h. **Peds 2-5 yrs (24-47 lbs):** 1 tab prn. **Max:** 3 tabs/24h.
Rolaids Extra Strength Chewable Tablets	Calcium carbonate/Magnesium hydroxide 675mg-135mg	**Adults:** 2-4 tabs prn. **Max:** 10 tabs/24h.
Rolaids Extra Strength Softchews	Calcium carbonate 1177mg	**Adults:** 2-3 chews q1h prn. **Max:** 6 chews/24h.
Rolaids Regular Strength Chewable Tablets	Calcium carbonate/Magnesium hydroxide 550mg-110mg	**Adults:** 2-4 tabs prn. **Max:** 12 tabs/24h.
Rolaids Regular Strength Liquid	Calcium carbonate/Magnesium hydroxide 550mg-110mg/5mL	**Adults:** 2-4 tsp (10-20mL) prn. **Max:** 12 tsp (60mL)/24h.
Rolaids Ultra Strength Chewable Tablets	Calcium carbonate/Magnesium hydroxide 1000mg-200mg	**Adults:** 2-3 tabs prn. **Max:** 7 tabs/24h.

(Continued)

BRAND	INGREDIENT(S)/STRENGTH(S)	DOSAGE
ANTACIDS *(Continued)*		
Rolaids Ultra Strength Liquid	Calcium carbonate/Magnesium hydroxide 1000mg-200mg/5mL	**Adults:** 2-3 tsp (10-15mL) prn. **Max:** 7 tsp (35mL)/24h.
Tums Chewy Delights Chewable Tablets	Calcium carbonate 1177mg	**Adults:** 2-3 tabs prn. **Max:** 6 tabs/24h.
Tums Extra Strength 750 Chewable Tablets	Calcium carbonate 750mg	**Adults:** 2-4 tabs prn. **Max:** 9 tabs/24h.
Tums Extra Strength 750 Sugar Free Chewable Tablets	Calcium carbonate 750mg	**Adults:** 2-4 tabs prn. **Max:** 9 tabs/24h.
Tums Freshers Chewable Tablets	Calcium carbonate 500mg	**Adults:** 2-4 tabs prn. **Max:** 15 tabs/24h.
Tums Kids Chewable Tablets	Calcium carbonate 750mg	**Peds >4 yrs (>48 lbs):** 1 tab prn. **Max:** 4 tabs/24h. **Peds 2-4 yrs (24-47 lbs):** ½ tab prn. **Max:** 2 tabs/24h.
Tums Regular Strength Chewable Tablets	Calcium carbonate 500mg	**Adults:** 2-4 tabs prn. **Max:** 15 tabs/24h.
Tums Smoothies Chewable Tablets	Calcium carbonate 750mg	**Adults:** 2-4 tabs prn. **Max:** 10 tabs/24h.
Tums Ultra Strength 1000 Chewable Tablets	Calcium carbonate 1000mg	**Adults:** 2-3 tabs prn. **Max:** 7 tabs/24h.
ANTACIDS/ANTIFLATULENTS		
Gelusil Chewable Tablets	Aluminum hydroxide/Magnesium hydroxide/Simethicone 200mg-200mg-25mg	**Adults:** 2-4 tabs q1h prn. **Max:** 12 tabs/24h.
Gelusil Liquid	Aluminum hydroxide/Magnesium hydroxide/Simethicone 400mg-400mg-40mg/5mL	**Adults & Peds ≥12 yrs:** 2-4 tsp (10-20mL) between meals and at hs. **Max:** 12 tsp (60mL)/24h.
Maalox Advanced Maximum Strength Chewable Tablets	Calcium carbonate/Simethicone 1000mg-60mg	**Adults & Peds ≥12 yrs:** 1-2 tabs prn. **Max:** 8 tabs/24h.
Maalox Advanced Maximum Strength Liquid	Aluminum hydroxide/Magnesium hydroxide/Simethicone 400mg-400mg-40mg/5mL	**Adults & Peds ≥12 yrs:** 2-4 tsp (10-20mL) bid. **Max:** 8 tsp (40mL)/24h.
Maalox Advanced Regular Strength Liquid	Aluminum hydroxide/Magnesium hydroxide/Simethicone 200mg-200mg-20mg/5mL	**Adults & Peds ≥12 yrs:** 2-4 tsp (10-20mL) qid. **Max:** 16 tsp (80mL)/24h.
Mylanta Maximum Strength Liquid	Aluminum hydroxide/Magnesium hydroxide/Simethicone 400mg-400mg-40mg/5mL	**Adults & Peds ≥12 yrs:** 2-4 tsp (10-20mL) between meals and at hs. **Max:** 12 tsp (60mL)/24h.
Mylanta Regular Strength Liquid	Aluminum hydroxide/Magnesium hydroxide/Simethicone 200mg-200mg-20mg/5mL	**Adults & Peds ≥12 yrs:** 2-4 tsp (10-20mL) between meals and at hs. **Max:** 24 tsp (120mL)/24h.
Rolaids Extra Strength Plus Gas Relief Softchews	Calcium carbonate/Simethicone 1177mg-80mg	**Adults:** 2-3 chews q1h prn. **Max:** 6 chews/24h.
Rolaids Multi-Symptom Chewable Tablets	Calcium carbonate/Magnesium hydroxide/Simethicone 675mg-135mg-60mg	**Adults:** 2-4 tabs q1h prn. **Max:** 8 tabs/24h.
BISMUTH SUBSALICYLATES		
Maalox Total Relief Maximum Strength Liquid	Bismuth subsalicylate 525mg/15mL	**Adults & Peds ≥12 yrs:** 2 tbl (30mL) q1h prn. **Max:** 8 tbl (120mL)/24h.
Pepto-Bismol Caplets	Bismuth subsalicylate 262mg	**Adults & Peds ≥12 yrs:** 2 tabs q½-1h prn. **Max:** 8 doses (16 tabs)/24h.
Pepto-Bismol Chewable Tablets	Bismuth subsalicylate 262mg	**Adults & Peds ≥12 yrs:** 2 tabs q½-1h prn. **Max:** 8 doses (16 tabs)/24h.

BRAND	INGREDIENT(S)/STRENGTH(S)	DOSAGE
BISMUTH SUBSALICYLATES *(Continued)*		
Pepto-Bismol InstaCool Chewable Tablets	Bismuth subsalicylate 262mg	**Adults & Peds ≥12 yrs:** 2 tabs q½-1h prn. **Max:** 8 doses (16 tabs)/24h.
Pepto-Bismol Liquid	Bismuth subsalicylate 262mg/15mL	**Adults & Peds ≥12 yrs:** 2 tbl (30mL) q½-1h prn. **Max:** 8 doses (16 tbl or 240mL)/24h.
Pepto-Bismol Max Strength Liquid	Bismuth subsalicylate 525mg/15mL	**Adults & Peds ≥12 yrs:** 2 tbl (30mL) q1h prn. **Max:** 4 doses (8 tbl or 120mL)/24h.
H₂-RECEPTOR ANTAGONISTS		
Pepcid AC Maximum Strength Tablets	Famotidine 20mg	**Adults & Peds ≥12 yrs:** 1 tab prn. **Max:** 2 tabs/24h.
Pepcid AC Original Strength Tablets	Famotidine 10mg	**Adults & Peds ≥12 yrs:** 1 tab prn. **Max:** 2 tabs/24h.
Tagamet HB 200 Tablets	Cimetidine 200mg	**Adults & Peds ≥12 yrs:** 1 tab prn. **Max:** 2 tabs/24h.
Zantac 75 Tablets	Ranitidine 75mg	**Adults & Peds ≥12 yrs:** 1 tab prn. **Max:** 2 tabs/24h.
Zantac 150 Tablets	Ranitidine 150mg	**Adults & Peds ≥12 yrs:** 1 tab prn. **Max:** 2 tabs/24h.
H₂-RECEPTOR ANTAGONISTS/ANTACIDS		
Pepcid Complete Chewable Tablets	Famotidine/Calcium carbonate/ Magnesium hydroxide 10mg-800mg-165mg	**Adults & Peds ≥12 yrs:** 1 tab prn. **Max:** 2 tabs/24h.
Tums Dual Action Chewable Tablets	Famotidine/Calcium carbonate/ Magnesium hydroxide 10mg-800mg-165mg	**Adults & Peds ≥12 yrs:** 1 tab prn. **Max:** 2 tabs/24h.
PROTON PUMP INHIBITORS		
Prevacid 24 HR Capsules	Lansoprazole 15mg	**Adults:** 1 cap qd x 14 days. May repeat 14-day course q4 months.
Prilosec OTC Tablets	Omeprazole 20mg	**Adults:** 1 tab qd x 14 days. May repeat 14-day course q4 months.
Zegerid OTC Capsules	Omeprazole/Sodium bicarbonate 20mg-1100mg	**Adults:** 1 cap qd x 14 days. May repeat 14-day course q4 months.

ANTIDIARRHEAL PRODUCTS

BRAND	INGREDIENT(S)/STRENGTH(S)	DOSAGE*
ABSORBENTS		
Equalactin Chewable Tablets	Calcium Polycarbophil 625mg	**Adults & Peds ≥12 yrs:** 2 tabs qid. **Max:** 8 tabs/24h.† **Peds 6-<12 yrs:** 1 tab qid. **Max:** 4 tabs/24h.† **Peds 3-<6 yrs:** 1 tab qd-bid. **Max:** 2 tabs/24h.†
FiberCon Caplets	Calcium Polycarbophil 625mg	**Adults & Peds ≥12 yrs:** 2 tabs qd. **Max:** Up to qid.‡
Konsyl Fiber Caplets	Calcium Polycarbophil 625mg	**Adults & Peds ≥12 yrs:** 2 tabs qd-qid. **Max:** 8 tabs/24h.‡ **Peds 6-<12 yrs:** 2 tabs qd.‡
ANTIPERISTALTICS		
Imodium A-D Caplets	Loperamide HCl 2mg	**Adults & Peds ≥12 yrs:** 2 tabs after first loose stool; 1 tab after each subsequent loose stool. **Max:** 4 tabs/24h.† **Peds 9-11 yrs (60-95 lbs):** 1 tab after first loose stool; ½ tab after each subsequent loose stool. **Max:** 3 tabs/24h.† **Peds 6-8 yrs (48-59 lbs):** 1 tab after first loose stool; ½ tab after each subsequent loose stool. **Max:** 2 tabs/24h.†
Imodium A-D EZ Chews	Loperamide HCl 2mg	**Adults & Peds ≥12 yrs:** 2 tabs after first loose stool; 1 tab after each subsequent loose stool. **Max:** 4 tabs/24h.† **Peds 9-11 yrs (60-95 lbs):** 1 tab after first loose stool; ½ tab after each subsequent loose stool. **Max:** 3 tabs/24h.† **Peds 6-8 yrs (48-59 lbs):** 1 tab after first loose stool; ½ tab after each subsequent loose stool. **Max:** 2 tabs/24h.†
Imodium A-D Liquid	Loperamide HCl 1mg/7.5mL	**Adults & Peds ≥12 yrs:** 6 tsp (30mL) after first loose stool; 3 tsp (15mL) after each subsequent loose stool. **Max:** 12 tsp (60mL)/24h.† **Peds 9-11 yrs (60-95 lbs):** 3 tsp (15mL) after first loose stool; 1½ tsp (7.5mL) after each subsequent loose stool. **Max:** 9 tsp (45mL)/24h.† **Peds 6-8 yrs (48-59 lbs):** 3 tsp (15mL) after first loose stool; 1½ tsp (7.5mL) after each subsequent loose stool. **Max:** 6 tsp (30mL)/24h.†
Imodium A-D Liquid for Use in Children	Loperamide HCl 1mg/7.5mL	**Adults & Peds ≥12 yrs:** 6 tsp (30mL) after first loose stool; 3 tsp (15mL) after each subsequent loose stool. **Max:** 12 tsp (60mL)/24h.† **Peds 9-11 yrs (60-95 lbs):** 3 tsp (15mL) after first loose stool; 1½ tsp (7.5mL) after each subsequent loose stool. **Max:** 9 tsp (45mL)/24h.† **Peds 6-8 yrs (48-59 lbs):** 3 tsp (15mL) after first loose stool; 1½ tsp (7.5mL) after each subsequent loose stool. **Max:** 6 tsp (30mL)/24h.†
ANTIPERISTALTICS/ANTIFLATULENTS		
Imodium Multi-Symptom Relief Caplets	Loperamide HCl/Simethicone 2mg-125mg	**Adults & Peds ≥12 yrs:** 2 tabs after first loose stool; 1 tab after each subsequent loose stool. **Max:** 4 tabs/24h.† **Peds 9-11 yrs (60-95 lbs):** 1 tab after first loose stool; ½ tab after each subsequent loose stool. **Max:** 3 tabs/24h.† **Peds 6-8 yrs (48-59 lbs):** 1 tab after first loose stool; ½ tab after each subsequent loose stool. **Max:** 2 tabs/24h.†
Imodium Multi-Symptom Relief Chewable Tablets	Loperamide HCl/Simethicone 2mg-125mg	**Adults & Peds ≥12 yrs:** 2 tabs after first loose stool; 1 tab after each subsequent loose stool. **Max:** 4 tabs/24h.† **Peds 9-11 yrs (60-95 lbs):** 1 tab after first loose stool; ½ tab after each subsequent loose stool. **Max:** 3 tabs/24h.† **Peds 6-8 yrs (48-59 lbs):** 1 tab after first loose stool; ½ tab after each subsequent loose stool. **Max:** 2 tabs/24h.†
BISMUTH SUBSALICYLATES		
Kaopectate Extra Strength Liquid (Peppermint Flavor)	Bismuth Subsalicylate 525mg/15mL	**Adults & Peds ≥12 yrs:** 2 tbl (30mL) q1h prn. **Max:** 4 doses (8 tbl)/24h.†
Kaopectate Liquid (Peppermint Flavor)	Bismuth Subsalicylate 262mg/15mL	**Adults & Peds ≥12 yrs:** 2 tbl (30mL) q1h prn. **Max:** 4 doses (8 tbl)/24h.†

(Continued)

BRAND	INGREDIENT(S)/STRENGTH(S)	DOSAGE*
BISMUTH SUBSALICYLATES *(Continued)*		
Kaopectate Liquid (Vanilla Flavor; Cherry Flavor)	Bismuth Subsalicylate 262mg/15mL	**Adults & Peds ≥12 yrs:** 2 tbl (30mL) q½-1h prn. **Max:** 8 doses (16 tbl)/24h.†
Maalox Total Relief Liquid	Bismuth Subsalicylate 525mg/15mL	**Adults & Peds ≥12 yrs:** 2 tbl (30mL) q1h prn. **Max:** 4 doses (8 tbl)/24h.†
Pepto Bismol Caplets	Bismuth Subsalicylate 262mg	**Adults & Peds ≥12 yrs:** 2 tabs q½-1h prn. **Max:** 8 doses (16 tabs)/24h.†
Pepto Bismol Chewable Tablets	Bismuth Subsalicylate 262mg	**Adults & Peds ≥12 yrs:** 2 tabs q½-1h prn. **Max:** 8 doses (16 tabs)/24h.†
Pepto Bismol InstaCool Chewable Tablets	Bismuth Subsalicylate 262mg	**Adults & Peds ≥12 yrs:** 2 tabs q½-1h prn. **Max:** 8 doses (16 tabs)/24h.†
Pepto Bismol Liquid	Bismuth Subsalicylate 525mg/30mL	**Adults & Peds ≥12 yrs:** 2 tbl (30mL) q½-1h prn. **Max:** 8 doses (16 tbl)/24h.†
Pepto Bismol Max Strength Liquid	Bismuth Subsalicylate 1050mg/30mL	**Adults & Peds ≥12 yrs:** 2 tbl (30mL) q1h prn. **Max:** 4 doses (8 tbl)/24h.†

*Some medications must be taken with water. Refer to individual product labeling for additional dosing information.
†Do not use for more than 2 days.
‡Do not use for more than 7 days unless directed by a healthcare provider.

ANTIFLATULENT PRODUCTS

BRAND	INGREDIENT(S)/STRENGTH(S)	DOSAGE
ALPHA-GALACTOSIDASES		
Beano Meltaways Tablets	Alpha-galactosidase 300 GALU	**Adults:** Take 1 tab before meals.
Beano Tablets	Alpha-galactosidase enzyme 300 GALU	**Adults:** Take 2-3 tabs before meals.
ANTACIDS/ANTIFLATULENTS		
PLEASE REFER TO ANTACID AND HEARTBURN PRODUCTS TABLE		
SIMETHICONE/SIMETHICONE COMBINATIONS		
Gas-X Chewable Tablets	Simethicone 80mg	**Adults:** Chew 1 or 2 tabs prn after meals and at hs. **Max:** 6 tabs/24h.
Gas-X Chewable Tablets Extra Strength	Simethicone 125mg	**Adults:** Chew 1 or 2 tabs prn after meals and at hs. **Max:** 4 tabs/24h.
Gas-X Chewable Tablets Extra Strength with Maalox	Simethicone/Calcium carbonate 125mg/500mg	**Adults:** Chew 1-2 tabs prn or ud. **Max:** 4 tabs/24h.
Gas-X Softgels Extra Strength	Simethicone 125mg	**Adults:** Take 1 or 2 caps prn after meals and at hs. **Max:** 4 caps/24h.
Gas-X Softgels Ultra Strength	Simethicone 180mg	**Adults:** Take 1 or 2 caps prn after meals and at hs. **Max:** 2 caps/24h.
Gas-X Thin Strips Extra Strength	Simethicone 62.5mg	**Adults:** Allow 2-4 strips to dissolve prn after meals and at hs. **Max:** 8 strips/24h.
Infants' Mylicon Drops	Simethicone 20mg/0.3mL	**Peds >2 yrs (>24 lbs):** 0.6mL prn after meals and at hs. **Peds <2 yrs (<24 lbs):** 0.3mL prn after meals and at hs. **Max:** 12 doses/24h.
Little Remedies For Tummys Gas Relief Drops	Simethicone 20mg/0.3mL	**Peds ≥2 yrs (≥24 lbs):** 0.6mL prn after meals and at hs. **Peds <2 yrs (<24 lbs):** 0.3mL prn after meals and at hs. **Max:** 12 doses/24h.
Mylanta Gas Maximum Strength Chewable Tablets	Simethicone 125mg	**Adults:** Chew 1-2 tabs prn after meals and at hs. **Max:** 4 tabs/24h.
PediaCare Infants Gas Relief Drops	Simethicone 20mg/0.3mL	**Peds ≥2 yrs (≥24 lbs):** 0.6mL prn after meals and at hs. **Peds <2 yrs (<24 lbs):** 0.3mL prn after meals and at hs. **Max:** 12 doses/24h.

HEMORRHOIDAL PRODUCTS*

BRAND	INGREDIENT(S)/STRENGTH(S)	DOSAGE†
ANESTHETICS/ANESTHETIC COMBINATIONS		
HemAway Cream	Lidocaine/Phenylephrine HCl 5%/0.25%	**Adults & Peds ≥12 yrs:** Apply externally to affected area up to 4 times a day.
Preparation H Maximum Strength Pain Relief Cream	Glycerin/Phenylephrine HCl/Pramoxine HCl/White petrolatum 14.4%/0.25%/1%/15%	**Adults & Peds ≥12 yrs:** Apply externally to affected area up to 4 times a day.
Tronolane Cream	Pramoxine HCl/Zinc oxide 1%/5%	**Adults & Peds ≥12 yrs:** Apply externally to affected area up to 5 times a day.
Tucks Fast Relief Spray	Pramoxine HCl 1%	**Adults & Peds ≥12 yrs:** Apply externally to affected area up to 5 times a day.
Tucks Hemorrhoidal Ointment	Pramoxine HCl/Zinc oxide/Mineral oil 1%/12.5%/46.6%	**Adults & Peds ≥12 yrs:** Apply externally to affected area up to 5 times a day.
HYDROCORTISONES		
Preparation H Anti-Itch Cream	Hydrocortisone 1%	**Adults & Peds ≥12 yrs:** Apply externally to affected area not more than tid-qid.
WITCH HAZELS/WITCH HAZEL COMBINATIONS		
Preparation H Cooling Gel	Phenylephrine HCl/Witch hazel 0.25%/50%	**Adults & Peds ≥12 yrs:** Apply externally to affected area up to 4 times a day.
Preparation H Medicated Wipes	Witch hazel 50%	**Adults & Peds ≥12 yrs:** Use externally on affected area up to 6 times a day.
T.N. Dickinson's Hemorrhoidal Pads	Witch hazel 50%	**Adults & Peds ≥12 yrs:** Use externally on affected area up to 6 times a day.
Tucks Medicated Cooling Pads	Witch hazel 50%	**Adults & Peds ≥12 yrs:** Use externally on affected area up to 6 times a day.
Tucks Take Alongs Medicated Cooling Towelettes	Witch hazel 50%	**Adults & Peds ≥12 yrs:** Use externally on affected area up to 6 times a day.
MISCELLANEOUS		
Calmol 4 Hemorrhoidal Suppositories	Cocoa butter/Zinc oxide 76%/10%	**Adults & Peds ≥12 yrs:** Insert 1 supp up to 6 times a day.
Medicone Hemorrhoidal Ointment	Camphor/Phenol/Tannic acid/Zinc oxide 3%/2.5%/2.2%/6.6%	**Adults & Peds ≥12 yrs:** Apply externally to affected area up to 3 times a day.
Medicone Hemorrhoidal Suppositories	Hard fat/Phenylephrine HCl 88.7%/0.25%	**Adults & Peds ≥12 yrs:** Insert 1 supp up to 4 times a day.
Preparation H Ointment	Mineral oil/Petrolatum/Phenylephrine HCl 14%/74.9%/0.25%	**Adults & Peds ≥12 yrs:** Apply to affected area up to 4 times a day.
Preparation H Suppositories	Cocoa butter/Phenylephrine HCl 88.44%/0.25%	**Adults & Peds ≥12 yrs:** Insert 1 supp up to 4 times a day.
Tronolane Suppositories	Hard fat/Phenylephrine HCl 88.7%/0.25%	**Adults & Peds ≥12 yrs:** Insert 1 supp up to 4 times a day.
Tucks Internal Soothers Suppositories	Topical starch 51%	**Adults & Peds ≥12 yrs:** Insert 1 supp up to 6 times a day.

*Please refer to the *Laxative Products* table for stool softeners or bulk-forming laxatives adjunct therapies.
†Stop use and contact a healthcare provider if condition worsens or does not improve within 7 days.

LAXATIVE PRODUCTS

BRAND	INGREDIENT(S)/STRENGTH(S)	DOSAGE
BULK-FORMING		
Citrucel Caplets	Methylcellulose 500mg	**Adults & Peds ≥12 yrs:** 2 tabs prn up to 6 times/day. **Max:** 12 tabs/day. **Peds 6-11 yrs:** 1 tab prn up to 6 times/day. **Max:** 6 tabs/day.
Citrucel Orange Powder	Methylcellulose 2g/tbl	**Adults & Peds ≥12 yrs:** 1 tbl prn up to tid. **Peds 6-11 yrs:** 2.5 tsp prn up to tid.
Citrucel Orange Sugar Free Powder	Methylcellulose 2g/tbl	**Adults & Peds ≥12 yrs:** 1 tbl prn up to tid. **Peds 6-11 yrs:** 2 tsp prn up to tid.
Equalactin Chewable Tablets	Calcium polycarbophil 625mg	**Adults & Peds ≥12 yrs:** 2 tabs qid. **Max:** 8 tabs/day. **Peds 6-<12 yrs:** 1 tab qid. **Max:** 4 tabs/day. **Peds 3-<6 yrs:** 1 tab qd-bid. **Max:** 2 tabs/day.
FiberCon Caplets	Calcium polycarbophil 625mg	**Adults & Peds ≥12 yrs:** 2 tabs up to qid.
Konsyl Balance Powder	Psyllium/Inulin 2g-2g/tsp	**Adults & Peds ≥12 yrs:** 1 tsp up to tid. **Peds 7-11 yrs:** ½ tsp up to tid.
Konsyl Easy Mix Powder	Psyllium 4.3g/tsp	**Adults & Peds ≥12 yrs:** 1 tsp qd-tid. **Peds 6-<12 yrs:** ½ tsp qd-tid.
Konsyl Fiber Caplets	Calcium polycarbophil 625mg	**Adults & Peds ≥12 yrs:** 2 tabs qd-qid. **Max:** 8 tabs/day. **Peds 6-<12 yrs:** 2 tabs qd.
Konsyl Naturally Sweetened Powder	Psyllium 3.4g/tsp	**Adults & Peds ≥12 yrs:** 1 tsp qd-tid. **Peds 6-<12 yrs:** ½ tsp qd-tid.
Konsyl Orange Powder	Psyllium 3.4g/tbl	**Adults & Peds ≥12 yrs:** 1 tbl qd-tid. **Peds 6-<12 yrs:** ½ tbl qd-tid.
Konsyl Orange Sugar Free Powder	Psyllium 3.5g/tsp	**Adults & Peds ≥12 yrs:** 1 tsp qd-tid. **Peds 6-<12 yrs:** ½ tsp qd-tid.
Konsyl Original Powder	Psyllium 6g/tsp	**Adults & Peds ≥12 yrs:** 1 tsp qd-tid. **Peds 6-<12 yrs:** ½ tsp qd-tid.
Konsyl Psyllium Capsules	Psyllium 520mg	**Adults & Peds ≥12 yrs:** 5 caps qd-tid.
Metamucil Capsules	Psyllium 525mg	**Adults & Peds ≥12 yrs:** 2-6 caps up to tid.
Metamucil Capsules Plus Calcium	Psyllium/Calcium 600mg-60mg	**Adults & Peds ≥12 yrs:** 2-5 caps up to qid.
Metamucil MultiGrain Wafers	Psyllium 3.4g/dose	**Adults & Peds ≥12 yrs:** 2 wafers up to tid.
Metamucil Orange Coarse Powder	Psyllium 3.4g/tbl	**Adults & Peds ≥12 yrs:** 1 tbl up to tid. **Peds 6-11 yrs:** ½ tbl up to tid.
Metamucil Orange Fiber Singles	Psyllium 3.4g/packet	**Adults & Peds ≥12 yrs:** 1 packet up to tid. **Peds 6-11 yrs:** ½ packet up to tid.
Metamucil Orange Smooth Powder	Psyllium 3.4g/tbl	**Adults & Peds ≥12 yrs:** 1 tbl up to tid. **Peds 6-11 yrs:** ½ tbl up to tid.
Metamucil Orange Sugar Free Fiber Singles	Psyllium 3.4g/packet	**Adults & Peds ≥12 yrs:** 1 packet up to tid. **Peds 6-11 yrs:** ½ packet up to tid.
Metamucil Original Coarse Powder	Psyllium 3.4g/tsp	**Adults & Peds ≥12 yrs:** 1 tsp up to tid. **Peds 6-11 yrs:** ½ tsp up to tid.
Metamucil Sugar Free Smooth Powder (Multi-flavor)	Psyllium 3.4g/tsp	**Adults & Peds ≥12 yrs:** 1 tsp up to tid. **Peds 6-11 yrs:** ½ tsp up to tid.
HYPEROSMOTICS		
Fleet Glycerin Suppositories	Glycerin 2g	**Adults & Peds ≥6 yrs:** 1 supp ud.
Fleet Liquid Glycerin Suppositories	Glycerin 5.4g	**Adults & Peds ≥6 yrs:** 1 supp ud.
Fleet Mineral Oil Enema	Mineral oil 100%/118mL	**Adults & Peds ≥12 yrs:** 1 bottle (118mL). **Peds 2-<12 yrs:** ½ bottle (59mL).

(Continued)

BRAND	INGREDIENT(S)/STRENGTH(S)	DOSAGE
HYPEROSMOTICS (Continued)		
Fleet Pedia-Lax Glycerin Suppositories	Glycerin 1g	**Peds 2-<6 yrs:** 1 supp ud.
Fleet Pedia-Lax Liquid Glycerin Suppositories	Glycerin 2.8g	**Peds 2-<6 yrs:** 1 supp ud.
Miralax	Polyethylene glycol 3350, 17g	**Adults & Peds ≥17 yrs:** 1 capful (17g) qd. **Max:** 7 days.
SALINES		
Fleet Enema	Monobasic sodium phosphate/ Dibasic sodium phosphate 19g-7g/118mL	**Adults & Peds ≥12 yrs:** 1 bottle (118mL).
Fleet Enema Extra	Monobasic sodium phosphate/ Dibasic sodium phosphate 19g-7g/197mL	**Adults & Peds ≥12 yrs:** 1 bottle (197mL).
Fleet Pedia-Lax Chewable Tablets	Magnesium hydroxide 400mg	**Peds 6-<12 yrs:** 3-6 tabs qd or in divided doses. **Max:** 6 tabs/day. **Peds 2-<6 yrs:** 1-3 tabs qd or in divided doses. **Max:** 3 tabs/day.
Fleet Pedia-Lax Enema	Monobasic sodium phosphate/ Dibasic sodium phosphate 9.5g-3.5g/59mL	**Peds 5-11 yrs:** 1 bottle (59mL). **Peds 2-<5 yrs:** ½ bottle (29.5mL).
Magnesium Citrate Solution	Magnesium citrate 1.745g/30mL	**Adults & Peds ≥12 yrs:** ½-1 bottle (300mL). **Peds 6-<12 yrs:** ⅓-½ bottle.
Phillips' Caplets	Magnesium 500mg	**Adults & Peds ≥12 yrs:** 2-4 tabs qhs or in divided doses.
Phillips' Chewable Tablets	Magnesium hydroxide 311mg	**Adults & Peds ≥12 yrs:** 8 tabs qhs or in divided doses. **Peds 6-11 yrs:** 4 tabs qhs or in divided doses. **Peds 3-5 yrs:** 2 tabs qhs or in divided doses.
Phillips' Concentrated Milk of Magnesia Liquid	Magnesium hydroxide 2400mg/15mL	**Adults & Peds ≥12 yrs:** 1-2 tbl (15-30mL) qhs or in divided doses.
Phillips' Milk of Magnesia Liquid	Magnesium hydroxide 1200mg/15mL	**Adults & Peds ≥12 yrs:** 2-4 tbl (30-60mL) qhs or in divided doses. **Peds 6-11 yrs:** 1-2 tbl (15-30mL) qhs or in divided doses.
STIMULANTS		
Alophen Tablets	Bisacodyl 5mg	**Adults & Peds ≥12 yrs:** 1-3 tabs qd. **Peds 6-<12 yrs:** 1 tab qd.
Carter's Sodium-Free Tablets	Bisacodyl 5mg	**Adults & Peds ≥12 yrs:** 1-3 tabs (usually 2) qd. **Peds 6-<12 yrs:** 1 tab qd.
Castor Oil	Castor oil	**Adults & Peds ≥12 yrs:** 15-60mL qd. **Peds 2-<12 yrs:** 5-15mL qd.
Dulcolax Pink Tablets	Bisacodyl 5mg	**Adults & Peds ≥12 yrs:** 1-3 tabs qd. **Peds 6-<12 yrs:** 1 tab qd.
Dulcolax Suppositories	Bisacodyl 10mg	**Adults & Peds ≥12 yrs:** 1 supp qd. **Peds 6-<12 yrs:** ½ supp qd.
Dulcolax Tablets	Bisacodyl 5mg	**Adults & Peds ≥12 yrs:** 1-3 tabs qd. **Peds 6-<12 yrs:** 1 tab qd.
Ex-Lax Maximum Strength Pills	Sennosides 25mg	**Adults & Peds ≥12 yrs:** 2 tabs qd-bid. **Peds 6-<12 yrs:** 1 tab qd-bid.
Ex-Lax Regular Strength Chocolate Pieces	Sennosides 15mg	**Adults & Peds ≥12 yrs:** 2 pieces qd-bid. **Peds 6-<12 yrs:** 1 piece qd-bid.
Ex-Lax Regular Strength Pills	Sennosides 15mg	**Adults & Peds ≥12 yrs:** 2 tabs qd-bid. **Peds 6-<12 yrs:** 1 tab qd-bid.
Fleet Bisacodyl Enema	Bisacodyl 10mg/30mL	**Adults & Peds ≥12 yrs:** 1 bottle (30mL).

BRAND	INGREDIENT(S)/STRENGTH(S)	DOSAGE
STIMULANTS *(Continued)*		
Fleet Bisacodyl Tablets	Bisacodyl 5mg	**Adults & Peds ≥12 yrs:** 1-3 tabs qd. **Peds 6-<12 yrs:** 1 tab qd.
Perdiem Overnight Relief Pills	Sennosides 15mg	**Adults & Peds ≥12 yrs:** 2 tabs qd-bid. **Peds 6-<12 yrs:** 1 tab qd-bid.
Senokot Tablets	Sennosides 8.6mg	**Adults & Peds ≥12 yrs:** 2 tabs qd. **Max:** 4 tabs bid. **Peds 6-<12 yrs:** 1 tab qd. **Max:** 2 tabs bid. **Peds 2-<6 yrs:** ½ tab qd. **Max:** 1 tab bid.
SenokotXtra Tablets	Sennosides 17.2mg	**Adults & Peds ≥12 yrs:** 1 tab qd. **Max:** 2 tabs bid. **Peds 6-<12 yrs:** ½ tab qd. **Max:** 1 tab bid.
STIMULANT COMBINATIONS		
Konsyl Senna Prompt Capsules	Psyllium/Sennosides 500mg-9mg	**Adults & Peds ≥12 yrs:** 2-4 caps qd-bid.
Peri-Colace Tablets	Sennosides/Docusate sodium 8.6mg-50mg	**Adults & Peds ≥12 yrs:** 2-4 tabs qd. **Peds 6-<12 yrs:** 1-2 tabs qd. **Peds 2-<6 yrs:** up to 1 tab qd.
Senokot S Tablets	Sennosides/Docusate sodium 8.6mg-50mg	**Adults & Peds ≥12 yrs:** 2 tabs qd. **Max:** 4 tabs bid. **Peds 6-<12 yrs:** 1 tab qd. **Max:** 2 tabs bid. **Peds 2-<6 yrs:** ½ tab qd. **Max:** 1 tab bid.
SURFACTANTS (STOOL SOFTENERS)		
Colace Capsules	Docusate sodium 50mg	**Adults & Peds ≥12 yrs:** 1-6 caps qd. **Peds 2-<12 yrs:** 1-3 caps qd.
Colace Capsules	Docusate sodium 100mg	**Adults & Peds ≥12 yrs:** 1-3 caps qd. **Peds 2-<12 yrs:** 1 cap qd.
DulcoEase Pink Softgels	Docusate sodium 100mg	**Adults & Peds ≥12 yrs:** 1-3 caps qd or in divided doses. **Peds 2-<12 yrs:** 1 cap qd.
Dulcolax Stool Softener Capsules	Docusate sodium 100mg	**Adults & Peds ≥12 yrs:** 1-3 caps qd. **Peds 2-<12 yrs:** 1 cap qd.
Fleet Pedia-Lax Liquid Stool Softener	Docusate sodium 50mg/tbl	**Peds 2-<12 yrs:** 1-3 tbl (15-45mL) qd or in divided doses. **Max:** 3 tbl (45mL)/day.
Fleet Sof-Lax Softgels	Docusate sodium 100mg	**Adults & Peds ≥12 yrs:** 1-3 caps qd. **Peds 2-<12 yrs:** 1 cap qd.
Phillips' Stool Softener Liquid Gels	Docusate sodium 100mg	**Adults & Peds ≥12 yrs:** 1-3 caps qd or in divided doses. **Peds 6-<12 yrs:** 1 cap qd.
Surfak Stool Softener Softgels	Docusate calcium 240mg	**Adults & Peds ≥12 yrs:** 1 cap qd.

NASAL PREPARATIONS

BRAND	INGREDIENT(S)/STRENGTH(S)	DOSAGE
TOPICAL NASAL DECONGESTANTS		
Afrin NoDrip Extra Moisturizing Pump Mist	Oxymetazoline HCl 0.05%	**Adults & Peds ≥6 yrs:** 2-3 sprays per nostril not more than q10-12h. **Max:** 2 doses q24h.*
Afrin NoDrip Original Pump Mist	Oxymetazoline HCl 0.05%	**Adults & Peds ≥6 yrs:** 2-3 sprays per nostril not more than q10-12h. **Max:** 2 doses q24h.*
Afrin NoDrip Severe Congestion Pump Mist	Oxymetazoline HCl 0.05%	**Adults & Peds ≥6 yrs:** 2-3 sprays per nostril not more than q10-12h. **Max:** 2 doses q24h.*
Afrin NoDrip Sinus Pump Mist	Oxymetazoline HCl 0.05%	**Adults & Peds ≥6 yrs:** 2-3 sprays per nostril not more than q10-12h. **Max:** 2 doses q24h.*
Afrin Original Nasal Spray	Oxymetazoline HCl 0.05%	**Adults & Peds ≥6 yrs:** 2-3 sprays per nostril not more than q10-12h. **Max:** 2 doses q24h.*
Afrin Original Pump Mist	Oxymetazoline HCl 0.05%	**Adults & Peds ≥6 yrs:** 2-3 sprays per nostril not more than q10-12h. **Max:** 2 doses q24h.*
Afrin Severe Congestion Nasal Spray	Oxymetazoline HCl 0.05%	**Adults & Peds ≥6 yrs:** 2-3 sprays per nostril not more than q10-12h. **Max:** 2 doses q24h.*
Afrin Sinus Nasal Spray	Oxymetazoline HCl 0.05%	**Adults & Peds ≥6 yrs:** 2-3 sprays per nostril not more than q10-12h. **Max:** 2 doses q24h.*
Benzedrex Inhaler	Propylhexedrine 250mg	**Adults & Peds ≥6 yrs:** 2 inhalations per nostril not more than q2h.*
Dristan 12-Hr Nasal Spray	Oxymetazoline HCl 0.05%	**Adults & Peds ≥12 yrs:** 2-3 sprays per nostril not more than q10-12h. **Max:** 2 doses q24h.*
Little Remedies For Noses Decongestant Nose Drops	Phenylephrine HCl 0.125%	**Peds 2-<6 yrs:** Instill 2-3 drops per nostril not more than q4h.*
Mucinex Sinus-Max Full Force Nasal Spray	Oxymetazoline HCl 0.05%	**Adults & Peds ≥6 yrs:** 2-3 sprays per nostril not more than q10-12h. **Max:** 2 doses q24h.*
Mucinex Sinus-Max Moisture Smart Nasal Spray	Oxymetazoline HCl 0.05%	**Adults & Peds ≥6 yrs:** 2-3 sprays per nostril not more than q10-12h. **Max:** 2 doses q24h.*
Neo-Synephrine Cold & Sinus Extra Strength Nasal Spray	Phenylephrine HCl 1%	**Adults & Peds ≥12 yrs:** 2-3 sprays per nostril not more than q4h.*
Neo-Synephrine Cold & Sinus Mild Strength Nasal Spray	Phenylephrine HCl 0.25%	**Adults & Peds ≥6 yrs:** 2-3 sprays per nostril not more than q4h.*
Neo-Synephrine Cold & Sinus Regular Strength Nasal Spray	Phenylephrine HCl 0.5%	**Adults & Peds ≥12 yrs:** 2-3 sprays per nostril not more than q4h.*
Neo-Synephrine Severe Sinus Congestion Nasal Spray	Oxymetazoline HCl 0.05%	**Adults & Peds ≥6 yrs:** 2-3 sprays per nostril not more than q10-12h. **Max:** 2 doses q24h.*
Nostrilla Original Fast Relief Nasal Spray	Oxymetazoline HCl 0.05%	**Adults & Peds ≥6 yrs:** 2-3 sprays per nostril not more than q10-12h. **Max:** 2 doses q24h.*
Privine Nasal Drops	Naphazoline HCl 0.05%	**Adults & Peds ≥12 yrs:** 1-2 drops per nostril not more than q6h.*
Vicks Sinex 12-Hour Decongestant Nasal Spray	Oxymetazoline HCl 0.05%	**Adults & Peds ≥6 yrs:** 2-3 sprays per nostril not more than q10-12h. **Max:** 2 doses q24h.*
Vicks Sinex 12-Hour Decongestant UltraFine Mist Moisturizing Nasal Spray	Oxymetazoline HCl 0.05%	**Adults & Peds ≥6 yrs:** 2-3 sprays per nostril not more than q10-12h. **Max:** 2 doses q24h.*
Vicks Sinex 12-Hour Decongestant UltraFine Mist Nasal Spray	Oxymetazoline HCl 0.05%	**Adults & Peds ≥6 yrs:** 2-3 sprays per nostril not more than q10-12h. **Max:** 2 doses q24h.*
Vicks VapoInhaler	Levmetamfetamine 50mg	**Adults & Peds ≥12 yrs:** 2 inhalations per nostril not more than q2h.† **Peds 6-<12 yrs:** 1 inhalation per nostril not more than q2h.†

(Continued)

BRAND	INGREDIENT(S)/STRENGTH(S)	DOSAGE
TOPICAL NASAL DECONGESTANTS *(Continued)*		
Zicam Extreme Congestion Relief Nasal Gel	Oxymetazoline HCl 0.05%	**Adults & Peds ≥6 yrs:** 2-3 sprays per nostril not more than q10-12h. **Max:** 2 doses q24h.*
Zicam Intense Sinus Relief Nasal Gel	Oxymetazoline HCl 0.05%	**Adults & Peds ≥6 yrs:** 2-3 sprays per nostril not more than q10-12h. **Max:** 2 doses q24h.*
TOPICAL NASAL MOISTURIZERS		
Ayr Allergy & Sinus Hypertonic Saline Nasal Mist	Sodium chloride 2.65%‡	**Adults & Peds:** 2 sprays per nostril bid-tid prn.
Ayr Saline Nasal Drops	Sodium chloride 0.65%	**Adults & Peds:** 2-6 drops per nostril prn.
Ayr Saline Nasal Gel	Sodium chloride‡	**Adults & Peds:** Apply around nostrils and under nose during the day and hs prn.
Ayr Saline Nasal Gel No-Drip Sinus Spray	Sodium chloride‡	**Adults & Peds:** 1 spray per nostril.
Ayr Saline Nasal Mist	Sodium chloride 0.65%‡	**Adults & Peds:** 1 spray per nostril prn.
Ayr Saline Nasal Neti Rinse Kit	Sodium chloride‡	**Adults & Peds ≥6 yrs:** Use qd-bid or ud.
Ayr Saline Nasal Rinse Kit & Refills	Sodium chloride‡	**Adults & Peds ≥6 yrs:** Use qd-bid or ud.
Baby Ayr Saline Nose Spray/Drops	Sodium chloride 0.65%‡	**Peds:** 2-6 drops/sprays per nostril.
Little Remedies For Noses Saline Spray/Drops	Sodium chloride‡	**Adults & Peds:** 2-6 drops/sprays per nostril prn or ud.
Little Remedies For Noses Sterile Saline Nasal Mist	Sodium chloride	**Adults & Peds:** 1-3 short sprays per nostril.
Ocean Complete Sinus Rinse	Sodium chloride‡	**Adults & Peds:** Use ud.
Ocean Gel Nasal Moisturizer	Purified water, Glycerin, Carbomer 940, Trolamine, Hyaluronan, Methylparaben, Propylparaben	**Adults & Peds:** Apply to affected areas in and around the nose prn.
Ocean for Kids Saline Nasal Spray	Sodium chloride 0.65%‡	**Peds:** Use ud.
Ocean Saline Nasal Spray	Sodium chloride 0.65%‡	**Adults & Peds:** 2 sprays/drops per nostril prn.
Simply Saline Allergy & Sinus Relief	Sodium chloride 3%	**Adults:** Spray into each nostril ud.
Simply Saline Baby Nasal Moisturizer plus Aloe Vera	Sodium chloride‡	**Peds:** Apply around the nose prn.
Simply Saline Baby Nasal Relief	Sodium chloride 0.9%	**Peds:** Spray into each nostril ud.
Simply Saline Baby Swabs	Sodium chloride‡	**Peds:** Apply in nostrils prn.
Simply Saline Extra Strength Nighttime Formula plus Eucalyptus	Sodium chloride 3%‡	**Adults & Peds ≥2 yrs:** Use hs prn or ud.
Simply Saline Nasal Relief	Sodium chloride 0.9%	**Adults & Peds:** Spray into each nostril prn.
Simply Saline Neti Pot Kit	Sodium chloride‡	**Adults & Peds ≥5 yrs:** Use qd-bid or ud.
MISCELLANEOUS		
NasalCrom Nasal Allergy Spray	Cromolyn sodium 5.2mg	**Adults & Peds ≥2 yrs:** 1 spray per nostril q4-6h. **Max:** 6 doses q24h.
Similasan Nasal Allergy Relief Nasal Spray	*Cardiospermum* 6X, *Galphimia glauca* 6X, *Luffa operculata* 6X, *Sabadilla* 6X	**Adults & Peds:** 1-3 sprays per nostril prn.
Similasan Sinus Relief Mist	Kalium bichromicum 6X, *Luffa operculata* 6X, *Sabadilla* 6X	**Adults & Peds:** 1-3 sprays into each nostril prn.
Simply Saline Children's Cold Formula plus Moisturizers	*Luffa operculata* 6X, *Sabadilla* 6X	**Adults & Peds ≥2 yrs:** Use prn.

BRAND	INGREDIENT(S)/STRENGTH(S)	DOSAGE
MISCELLANEOUS *(Continued)*		
Simply Saline Cold Formula plus Menthol	*Luffa operculata* 6X, *Sabadilla* 6X	**Adults & Peds ≥2 yrs:** Use prn.
SinoFresh Nasal & Sinus Care	*Eucalyptus globulus* 20X, Kalium bichromicum 30X	**Adults:** 1-2 sprays per nostril in the morning and evening ud.
Zicam Allergy Relief Nasal Gel	*Luffa operculata* (4X, 12X, 30X), *Galphimia glauca* (12X, 30X), Histaminum hydrochloricum (12X, 30X, 200X), *Sulphur* (12X, 30X, 200X)	**Adults & Peds ≥12 yrs:** 1 pump per nostril q4h ud.

*Do not use for more than 3 days.
†Do not use for more than 7 days.
‡This product contains multiple ingredients. Please check product label for a complete list of ingredients.

IS IT A COLD, THE FLU, OR AN ALLERGY?

	COLD	FLU	AIRBORNE ALLERGY
SYMPTOMS			
Chest discomfort	Mild to moderate	Common; can become severe	Sometimes
Cough	Common (hacking cough)	Common; can become severe	Sometimes
Diarrhea	Never	Usual (more common in children)	Never
Duration	3-14 days	Usually <2 weeks	Weeks (eg, 6 weeks for ragweed or grass pollen seasons)
Exhaustion	Never	Usual; at the beginning of the illness	Never
Fatigue, weakness	Sometimes	Usual; can last up to 2-3 weeks	Sometimes
Fever	Rare	Usual; high (100-102°F; occasionally higher, especially in young children); lasts 3-4 days	Never
General aches, pains	Slight	Usual; often severe	Never
Headache	Rare	Common	Sometimes
Itchy eyes	Rare or never	Rare or never	Common
Runny nose	Common	Common	Common
Sneezing	Usual	Sometimes	Usual
Sore throat	Common	Sometimes	Sometimes
Stuffy nose	Common	Sometimes	Common
Vomiting	Never	Usual (more common in children)	Never
TREATMENT			
	Antihistamines*	Amantadine	Antihistamines*
	Decongestants*	Rimantadine	Nasal steroids*
	Nonsteroidal anti-inflammatories*	Oseltamivir	Decongestants*
		Zanamivir	
PREVENTION			
	Wash your hands often; avoid close contact with anyone with a cold	Annual vaccination Amantadine Rimantadine Oseltamivir Zanamivir	Avoid allergens such as pollen, house dust mites, mold, pet dander, or cockroaches
COMPLICATIONS			
	Sinus infection	Bronchitis	Sinus infections
	Middle ear infection	Pneumonia	Asthma
	Asthma	Can be life-threatening	
		Can worsen chronic conditions	
		Complications more likely in the elderly, those with chronic conditions, young children, and pregnant women	

*Used only for temporary relief of cold symptoms.

Sources:
1. Is It a Cold or the Flu? National Institute of Allergy and Infectious Diseases website. http://www.niaid.nih.gov/topics/Flu/Documents/sick. pdf. Updated November 2008. Accessed on January 23, 2014.
2. Is It a Cold or an Allergy? National Institute of Allergy and Infectious Diseases website. http://www.niaid.nih.gov/topics/allergicDiseases/ Documents/coldallergy.pdf. Updated November 2008. Accessed on January 23, 2014.
3. Understanding Flu Symptoms and Complications. National Institute of Allergy and Infectious Diseases website. http://www.niaid.nih.gov/ topics/Flu/understandingFlu/Pages/sympComp.aspx#. Updated November 14, 2012. Accessed on January 23, 2014.
4. Antiviral Agents for Influenza. Centers for Disease Control and Prevention website. http://www.cdc.gov/flu/professionals/antivirals/ antiviral-agents-flu.htm. Updated October 1, 2013. Accessed on January 23, 2014.

Cough-Cold-Flu-Allergy Products

BRAND NAME	ANALGESIC	ANTIHISTAMINE	DECONGESTANT	COUGH SUPPRESSANT	EXPECTORANT	DOSAGE
ANTIHISTAMINES						
Alavert Orally Disintegrating Tablets*		Loratadine 10mg				**Adults & Peds ≥6 yrs:** 1 tab qd. **Max:** 1 tab/24h.
Benadryl Allergy Dye-Free Liqui-Gels†		Diphenhydramine HCl 25mg				**Adults & Peds ≥12 yrs:** 1-2 caps q4-6h. **Peds 6-<12 yrs:** 1 cap q4-6h. **Max:** 6 doses/24h.
Benadryl Allergy Ultratab Tablets		Diphenhydramine HCl 25mg				**Adults & Peds ≥12 yrs:** 1-2 tabs q4-6h. **Peds 6-<12 yrs:** 1 tab q4-6h. **Max:** 6 doses/24h.
Children's Benadryl Allergy Liquid		Diphenhydramine HCl 12.5mg/5mL				**Peds 6-11 yrs:** 1-2 tsp (5-10mL) q4-6h. **Max:** 6 doses/24h.
Children's Benadryl Dye-Free Allergy Liquid†		Diphenhydramine HCl 12.5mg/5mL				**Peds 6-11 yrs:** 1-2 tsp (5-10mL) q4-6h. **Max:** 6 doses/24h.
Children's Claritin Chewables		Loratadine 5mg				**Adults & Peds ≥6 yrs:** 2 tabs qd. **Max:** 2 tabs/24h. **Peds 2-<6 yrs:** 1 tab qd. **Max:** 1 tab/24h.
Children's Claritin Syrup		Loratadine 5mg/5mL				**Adults & Peds ≥6 yrs:** 2 tsp (10mL) qd. **Max:** 2 tsp (10mL)/24h. **Peds 2-<6 yrs:** 1 tsp (5mL) qd. **Max:** 1 tsp (5mL)/24h.
Children's Zyrtec Allergy Syrup†		Cetirizine HCl 5mg/5mL				**Adults & Peds ≥65 yrs:** 1 tsp (5mL) qd. **Max:** 1 tsp (5mL)/24h. **Adults <65 yrs & Peds ≥6 yrs:** 1-2 tsp (5-10mL) qd. **Max:** 2 tsp (10mL)/24h. **Peds 2-<6 yrs:** ½-1 tsp (2.5-5mL) qd or ½ tsp (2.5mL) q12h. **Max:** 1 tsp (5mL)/24h.
Claritin Liqui-Gels		Loratadine 10mg				**Adults & Peds ≥6 yrs:** 1 cap qd. **Max:** 1 cap/24h.
Claritin RediTabs 12-Hour		Loratadine 5mg				**Adults & Peds ≥6 yrs:** 1 tab q12h. **Max:** 2 tabs/24h.

(Continued)

BRAND NAME	ANALGESIC	ANTIHISTAMINE	DECONGESTANT	COUGH SUPPRESSANT	EXPECTORANT	DOSAGE
ANTIHISTAMINES *(Continued)*						
Claritin RediTabs 24-Hour		Loratadine 10mg				**Adults & Peds ≥6 yrs:** 1 tab qd. **Max:** 1 tab/24h.
Claritin Tablets		Loratadine 10mg				**Adults & Peds ≥6 yrs:** 1 tab qd. **Max:** 1 tab/24h.
PediaCare Children Allergy		Diphenhydramine HCl 12.5mg/5mL				**Peds 6-11 yrs (48-95 lbs):** 1 tsp (5mL) q4h. **Max:** 6 doses/24h.
PediaCare Children's 24 Hour Allergy		Cetirizine HCl 5mg/5mL				**Adults ≥65 yrs:** 1 tsp (5mL) qd. **Max:** 1 tsp (5mL)/24h. **Adults <65 & Peds ≥6 yrs:** 1-2 tsp (5-10mL) qd. **Max:** 2 tsp (10mL)/24h. **Peds 2-<6 yrs:** ½-1 tsp (2.5-5mL) qd or ½ tsp (2.5mL) q12h. **Max:** 1 tsp (5mL)/24h.
Zyrtec Liquid Gels		Cetirizine HCl 10mg				**Adults <65 yrs & Peds ≥6 yrs:** 1 cap qd. **Max:** 1 cap/24h.
Zyrtec Tablets		Cetirizine HCl 10mg				**Adults <65 yrs & Peds ≥6 yrs:** 1 tab qd. **Max:** 1 tab/24h.
ANTIHISTAMINES + DECONGESTANTS						
Alavert D-12 Hour Extended Release Tablets		Loratadine 5mg	Pseudoephedrine sulfate 120mg			**Adults & Peds ≥12 yrs:** 1 tab q12h. **Max:** 2 tabs/24h.
Allerest PE Tablets		Chlorpheniramine maleate 4mg	Phenylephrine HCl 10mg			**Adults & Peds ≥12 yrs:** 1 tab q4h. **Peds 6-<12 yrs:** ½ tab q4h. **Max:** 6 doses/24h.
Children's Benadryl-D Allergy & Sinus Liquid		Diphenhydramine HCl 12.5mg/5mL	Phenylephrine HCl 5mg/5mL			**Adults & Peds ≥12 yrs:** 2 tsp (10mL) q4h. **Peds 6-11 yrs:** 1 tsp (5mL) q4h. **Max:** 6 doses/24h.
Children's Dimetapp Cold & Allergy Chewable Tablets		Brompheniramine maleate 1mg	Phenylephrine HCl 2.5mg			**Adults & Peds ≥12 yrs:** 4 tabs q4h. **Peds 6-<12 yrs:** 2 tabs q4h. **Max:** 6 doses/24h.
Children's Dimetapp Cold & Allergy Syrup		Brompheniramine maleate 1mg/5mL	Phenylephrine HCl 2.5mg/5mL			**Adults & Peds ≥12 yrs:** 4 tsp (20mL) q4h. **Peds 6-<12 yrs:** 2 tsp (10mL) q4h. **Max:** 6 doses/24h.

BRAND NAME	ANALGESIC	ANTIHISTAMINE	DECONGESTANT	COUGH SUPPRESSANT	EXPECTORANT	DOSAGE
ANTIHISTAMINES + DECONGESTANTS *(Continued)*						
Children's Dimetapp Nighttime Cold & Congestion Syrup		Diphenhydramine HCl 6.25mg/5mL	Phenylephrine HCl 2.5mg/5mL			**Adults & Peds ≥12 yrs:** 4 tsp (20mL) q4h. **Peds 6-<12 yrs:** 2 tsp (10mL) q4h. **Max:** 6 doses/24h.
Claritin-D 12 Hour Tablets		Loratadine 5mg	Pseudoephedrine sulfate 120mg			**Adults & Peds ≥12 yrs:** 1 tab q12h. **Max:** 2 tabs/24h.
Claritin-D 24 Hour Tablets		Loratadine 10mg	Pseudoephedrine sulfate 240mg			**Adults & Peds ≥12 yrs:** 1 tab qd. **Max:** 1 tab/24h.
Sudafed PE Sinus+Allergy Tablets†		Chlorpheniramine maleate 4mg	Phenylephrine HCl 10mg			**Adults & Peds ≥12 yrs:** 1 tab q4h. **Max:** 6 tabs/24h.
Triaminic Cold & Allergy Syrup		Chlorpheniramine maleate 1mg/5mL	Phenylephrine HCl 2.5mg/5mL			**Peds 6-<12 yrs:** 2 tsp (10mL) q4h. **Max:** 6 doses/24h.
Triaminic Night Time Cold & Cough Syrup		Diphenhydramine HCl 6.25mg/5mL	Phenylephrine HCl 2.5mg/5mL			**Peds 6-<12 yrs:** 2 tsp (10mL) q4h. **Max:** 6 doses/24h.
Zyrtec-D Tablets		Cetirizine HCl 5mg	Pseudoephedrine HCl 120mg			**Adults <65 & Peds ≥12 yrs:** 1 tab q12h. **Max:** 2 tabs/24h.
ANTIHISTAMINES + DECONGESTANTS + ANALGESICS						
Advil Allergy & Congestion Relief Tablets	Ibuprofen 200mg	Chlorpheniramine maleate 4mg	Phenylephrine HCl 10mg			**Adults & Peds ≥12 yrs:** 1 tab q4h. **Max:** 6 tabs/24h.
Advil Allergy Sinus Caplets	Ibuprofen 200mg	Chlorpheniramine maleate 2mg	Pseudoephedrine HCl 30mg			**Adults & Peds ≥12 yrs:** 1 tab q4-6h. **Max:** 6 tabs/24h.
Alka-Seltzer Plus Cold Formula Effervescent Tablets*	Aspirin 325mg	Chlorpheniramine maleate 2mg	Phenylephrine bitartrate 7.8mg			**Adults & Peds ≥12 yrs:** 2 tabs q4h. **Max:** 8 tabs/24h.
Alka-Seltzer Plus Night Severe Cold, Cough & Flu Powder Packets	Acetaminophen 650mg/packet	Diphenhydramine HCl 25mg/packet	Phenylephrine HCl 10mg/packet			**Adults & Peds ≥12 yrs:** 1 pkt q4h. **Max:** 5 pkts/24h.
Alka-Seltzer Plus Severe Allergy Sinus Congestion & Headache Liquid Gels	Acetaminophen 325mg	Doxylamine succinate 6.25mg	Phenylephrine HCl 5mg			**Adults & Peds ≥12 yrs:** 2 caps q4h. **Max:** 10 caps/24h.
Children's Delsym Cough-Cold Night Time Liquid	Acetaminophen 325mg/10mL	Diphenhydramine HCl 12.5mg/10mL	Phenylephrine HCl 5mg/10mL			**Adults & Peds ≥12 yrs:** 4 tsp (20mL) q4h. **Max:** 6 doses/24h. **Peds 6-<12 yrs:** 2 tsp (10mL) q4h. **Max:** 5 doses/24h.

(Continued)

ANTIHISTAMINES + DECONGESTANTS + ANALGESICS *(Continued)*

BRAND NAME	ANALGESIC	ANTIHISTAMINE	DECONGESTANT	COUGH SUPPRESSANT	EXPECTORANT	DOSAGE
Children's Mucinex Night Time Multi-Symptom Cold Liquid	Acetaminophen 325mg/10mL	Diphenhydramine HCl 12.5mg/10mL	Phenylephrine HCl 5mg/10mL			**Peds 6–<12 yrs:** 2 tsp (10mL) q4h. **Max:** 5 doses/24h.
Contac Cold + Flu Night Caplets	Acetaminophen 500mg	Chlorpheniramine maleate 2mg	Phenylephrine HCl 5mg			**Adults & Peds ≥12 yrs:** 2 tabs q6h prn. **Max:** 8 tabs/24h.
Delsym Cough+Cold Night Time Liquid	Acetaminophen 650mg/20mL	Diphenhydramine HCl 25mg/20mL	Phenylephrine HCl 10mg/20mL			**Adults & Peds ≥12 yrs:** 4 tsp (20mL) q4h. **Max:** 6 doses/24h.
Dristan Cold Multi-Symptom Formula Tablets	Acetaminophen 325mg	Chlorpheniramine maleate 2mg	Phenylephrine HCl 5mg			**Adults & Peds ≥12 yrs:** 2 tabs q4h. **Max:** 12 tabs/24h.
Mucinex Maximum Strength Fast-Max Night Time Cold & Flu Caplets	Acetaminophen 325mg	Diphenhydramine HCl 25mg	Phenylephrine HCl 5mg			**Adults & Peds ≥12 yrs:** 2 tabs q4h. **Max:** 12 tabs/24h.
Mucinex Maximum Strength Fast-Max Night Time Cold & Flu Liquid	Acetaminophen 650mg/20mL	Diphenhydramine HCl 25mg/20mL	Phenylephrine HCl 10mg/20mL			**Adults & Peds ≥12 yrs:** 4 tsp (20mL) q4h. **Max:** 6 doses/24h.
Robitussin Peak Cold Nighttime Nasal Relief Tablets	Acetaminophen 325mg	Chlorpheniramine maleate 2mg	Phenylephrine HCl 5mg			**Adults & Peds ≥12 yrs:** 2 tabs q4h. **Max:** 12 tabs/24h.
Sudafed PE Severe Cold Caplets†	Acetaminophen 325mg	Diphenhydramine HCl 12.5mg	Phenylephrine HCl 5mg			**Adults & Peds ≥12 yrs:** 2 tabs q4h. **Max:** 12 tabs/24h.
Theraflu Cold & Sore Throat Powder Packets	Acetaminophen 325mg/packet	Pheniramine maleate 20mg/packet	Phenylephrine HCl 10mg/packet			**Adults & Peds ≥12 yrs:** 1 pkt q4h. **Max:** 6 pkts/24h.
Theraflu Flu & Sore Throat Powder Packets	Acetaminophen 650mg/packet	Pheniramine maleate 20mg/packet	Phenylephrine HCl 10mg/packet			**Adults & Peds ≥12 yrs:** 1 pkt q4h. **Max:** 6 pkts/24h.
Theraflu Nighttime Severe Cold & Cough Powder Packets	Acetaminophen 650mg/packet	Diphenhydramine HCl 25mg/packet	Phenylephrine HCl 10mg/packet			**Adults & Peds ≥12 yrs:** 1 pkt q4h. **Max:** 6 pkts/24h.
Theraflu Sinus & Cold Powder Packets	Acetaminophen 325mg/packet	Pheniramine maleate 20mg/packet	Phenylephrine HCl 10mg/packet			**Adults & Peds ≥12 yrs:** 1 pkt q4h. **Max:** 6 pkts/24h.
Theraflu Sugar-Free Nighttime Severe Cold & Cough Powder Packets	Acetaminophen 650mg/packet	Diphenhydramine HCl 25mg/packet	Phenylephrine HCl 10mg/packet			**Adults & Peds ≥12 yrs:** 1 pkt q4h. **Max:** 6 pkts/24h.
Theraflu Warming Relief Flu & Sore Throat Syrup	Acetaminophen 325mg/15mL	Diphenhydramine HCl 12.5mg/15mL	Phenylephrine HCl 5mg/15mL			**Adults & Peds ≥12 yrs:** 2 tbl (30mL) q4h. **Max:** 6 doses (12 tbl or 180mL)/24h.